Nephrology

This congress has been executed with the grant of the Commemorative Association for the Japan World Exposition.

Nephrology VOLUME II

PROCEEDINGS OF THE
XITH INTERNATIONAL CONGRESS OF NEPHROLOGY

Editor
Michinobu Hatano

Associate Editors
Nishio Honda · Hyoe Ishikawa · Kenkichi Koiso
Kiyoshi Kurokawa · Tadao Niijima
Nobuhiro Sugino · Susumu Takahashi

With 239 Figures

Springer-Verlag
Tokyo Berlin Heidelberg
New York London Paris
Hong Kong Barcelona

Editor

MICHINOBU HATANO, M.D., Professor of Medicine, Director, Department of Internal Medicine, Nihon University School of Medicine, Tokyo, Japan

Associate Editors

NISHIO HONDA, Tokyo Senbai Hospital, Tokyo
HYOE ISHIKAWA, Nara Medical University, Nara
KENKICHI KOISO, The University of Tsukuba, Ibaraki
KIYOSHI KUROKAWA, University of Tokyo, Tokyo
TADAO NIIJIMA, Tokyo Seamen's Medical College, Tokyo
NOBUHIRO SUGINO, Tokyo Women's Medical College, Tokyo
SUSUMU TAKAHASHI, Nihon University, Tokyo

ISBN 4-413-70074-9 Springer-Verlag Tokyo Berlin Heidelberg New York
ISBN 3-540-70074-9 Springer-Verlag Berlin Heidelberg New York Tokyo
ISBN 0-387-70074-9 Springer-Verlag New York Berlin Heidelberg Tokyo

Library of Congress Cataloging-in-Publication Data
International Congress on Nephrology (11th: 1990: Tokyo, Japan); Nephrology: proceedings of the XIth International Congress of Nephrology / editors, Michinobu Hatano: associate editors, Nishio Honda...[et al.]. p. cm. Congress held in Tokyo, Japan, July 15-20, 1990. Includes bibliographical references. Includes index. ISBN 4-431-70074-9. – ISBN 3-540-70074-9. – ISBN 0-387-70074-9. 1. Kidneys – Diseases – Congresses. 2. Nephrology – Congresses. 3. Kidney Diseases – congresses. 4. Nephrology – congresses. I. Hatano, Michinobu, 1926- . II. Honda, Nishio. III. Title. [DNLM: WJ 300 I59n 1990]. RC902.A2I56 1990. 616.6'1 –dc20. DNLM/DLC. for Library of Congress 91-4651

Typesetting: Publishers Service of Montana, Bozeman, Montana
Printing and binding: Sanbi Printing, Tokyo

Foreword

The proceedings of the XIth International Congress of Nephrology held in Tokyo in 1990, form the most international and complete document of the present state of basic and clinical science in nephrology. In addition, they document the progress made in this field during the 3 years since the London Congress. The result is nothing short of impressive. The material presented by the invited lecturers and the participants of the symposia all show a remarkable pattern; not only the "height" of the science, but also the depth of the specialized knowledge, both prerequisites of excellency in science, which do not necessarily imply narrowness of outlook. On the contrary, this written document of the Tokyo Congress is a witness to the enormous progress made over the last few years in communication between basic scientists and clinical scientists.

The International Society of Nephrology is a fine example of how fruitful and productive this interaction can be, if it is conducted with the desire to understand each other. The members of the Scientific Program Committee of the Tokyo Congress are to be congratulated, not only for a thoughtful and well designed program, but also for carefully selecting those speakers who, besides their own contribution to nephrological science, also have the talent of being able to communicate with a large, international audience. In particular, I would like to express my deep appreciation to the editors of the Proceedings for their commitment and industriousness which made it possible for this publication to appear so soon after the Congress.

Since the first Congress of the International Society of Nephrology in Evian in 1960, nephrologists have witnessed a phenomenal increase in knowledge, a progress which still continues and will do so in the future. The present proceedings are a snapshot of this process. The counterpoint to the intellectual challenge of acquiring deeper understanding is the duty and promise to utilize that understanding for the benefit of our patients.

Klaus Thurau, M.D.
President,
International Society of Nephrology
(1987–1990)

Preface

The XIth International Congress of Nephrology was held in Tokyo, Japan from July 15–20, 1990.

Since the first congress in Evian, France in 1960, this is the first time that this prestigious congress has been held in Asia. Therefore, enthusiastic expectations were held by nephrologists not only in Japan but also throughout the world.

In organizing the congress under the estimable guidance of Prof. Klaus Thurau, President of the International Society of Nephrology, the ISN Executive Committee and the International Advisory Committee, Prof. Michinobu Hatano, Chairman of the local organizing committee as well as the organizing committee made every effort to make the congress a success.

Over three thousand participants from 71 countries attended the congress. These included 1,470 participants from Japan, 472 from the United States, 150 from France, and 128 from Italy. We were particularly pleased to welcome eight representatives from Czechoslavakia as well as an increased participation from other eastern European countries, the Soviet Union, and China. Forty-nine delegates from Taiwan were also in attendance.

The opening ceremony was held at the New Takanawa Prince Hotel in the presence of the Crown Prince, whose address noted that progress in nephrology would contribute greatly to the welfare of patients worldwide.

The scientific program consisted of 15 state-of-the-art lectures, 36 symposia, 11 workshops, 256 oral and 1,778 poster presentations. Following the advice of the ISN Executive Committee, the Scientific Program Committee encouraged the presentation of clinical and research papers at the same time in each session. This ensured that throughout the scientific program, discussions were constructive, and this helped to make the congress both stimulating and fruitful.

A total of 12 ISN satellite symposia, 4 overseas and 8 in Japan, were also held. The specific topics discussed at each symposium, combined with sightseeing tours at each site, contributed greatly to exchanges of both friendship and information.

Finally, we would like to express our sincere thanks and appreciation to the ISN Committee and all the participants of the congress.

KENZO OSHIMA, M.D.
President

YAWARA YOSHITOSHI, M.D.
Vice-President

YASUSHI UEDA, M.D.
Vice-President

HIROSHI ABE, M.D.
Vice-President

XIth International Congress of Nephrology

ORGANIZED BY:	The Organizing Committee of the XIth International Congress of Nephrology
UNDER THE AUSPICES OF:	International Society of Nephrology
SPONSORED BY:	Japanese Society of Nephrology The Kidney Foundation, Japan
IN COOPERATION WITH:	The Japanese Association of Medical Science Japan Medical Association The Japanese Urological Association The Japan Society for Transplantation Japanese Society for Artificial Organs Japanese Society for Dialysis Therapy The Japanese Society of Pediatric Nephrology Japan Incorporated Medical Association for Dialysis
SUPPORTED BY:	Ministry of Education, Science and Culture Ministry of Health and Welfare Science Council of Japan Tokyo Metropolitan Government

The International Society of Nephrology

Management Committee

Council

XIth International Congress Officers

President	Kenzo Oshima
Vice Presidents	Yawara Yoshitoshi Yasushi Ueda Hiroshi Abe

Organizing Committee

Chairman	Michinobu Hatano
Secretary-General	Susumu Takahashi

Members

Yoshio Aso	Tadashi Miyahara
Toshiyuki Furukawa	Toshihiko Nagasawa
Kohei Hara	Mitsuharu Narita
Nishio Honda	Hiromi Nihira
Takeshi Hoshi	Tadao Niijima
Kazunari Iidaka	Teruo Omae
Hyoe Ishikawa	Zensuke Ota
Chuichi Kawai	Fuminori Sakai
Teruo Kitagawa	Takao Sonoda
Kenkichi Koiso	Nobuhiro Sugino
Kiyoshi Kurokawa	Shizuo Tojo
Sunao Maki	

Scientific Program Committee

Chairmen Nobuhiro Sugino
Nishio Honda

Executive Secretary Kiyoshi Kurokawa

Members

Akitoshi Ando
Kikuo Arakawa
Masaaki Arakawa
Hitoshi Endou
Mamoru Fujimoto
Gerhard Giebisch
Takashi Harada
Eiji Higashihara
Kazunari Iidaka
Masashi Imai
Hiroshi Kida
Hikaru Koide
Kenkichi Koiso
Shozo Koshikawa
Akio Koyama
Kenji Maeda
Sunao Maki
Koichi Matsumoto
Toshihiko Nagasawa
Mitsumasa Nagase
Yasushi Nakamoto
Hiroshi Nihei
Michio Odaka
Hiroyuki Ohi
Yoshimasa Orita
Kazuo Ota
Hideto Sakai
Osamu Sakai
Tadasu Sakai
Takao Saruta
Hidekazu Shigematsu
Kenjiro Yamamoto
Nobuyuki Yoshizawa

Fund Raising Committee

Chairmen Tadao Niijima
Hyoe Ishikawa

Members

Keishi Abe
Yoshio Aso
Tohru Azuma
Kohei Hara
Yoshihei Hirasawa
Hiroshi Kida
Joichi Kumazawa
Yuji Nagura
Zensuke Ota
Tsutomu Sanaka
Takao Sonoda
Naohiko Ueda

Finance Committee

Chairman Kenkichi Koiso

Members

Hiroshi Kawamura
Gengo Osawa

Contents of Volume II

Symposia

Cytokines, Mitogens and Their Receptors on Glomerular Cells

Frontiers of Research on Natriuretic Peptides

Polarity of Tubular Epithelia

Masugi Memorial Symposium: Experimental Nephritis and Its Contribution to Nephrology

Nephrolithiasis: New Ideas in Pathophysiology, New Facts in Therapy

Molecular Action of Diuretics

Cystic Diseases of the Kidney

Continuous Ambulatory Peritoneal Dialysis (CAPD)

Autacoids and the Kidney

Ion Channels of the Kidney

Contents of Volume I

State of the Art Lectures

Symposia

Immunological and Cellular Mechanisms of Glomerulonephritis

Role of Potassium in Acid-Base Disturbances

Role of Kidney in the Pathogenesis of Hypertension

Cellular and Integrative Functions of the Juxtaglomerular Apparatus

Systemic Dysfunctions in Renal Failure and Their Management

ATPases of the Kidney

Vitamin D and Uremic Bone Disease

AIDS/AIDS – Nephropathy

Cellular and Integrative Regulation of Renal Circulation

Dietary Factors and Progression of Chronic Renal Failure

Renal Diseases in Asia

Pathobiology of Glomerular and Tubular Basement Membranes

List of Contributors

For contributors' addresses see chapter opening pages

Symposia

Cytokines, Mitogens and Their Receptors on Glomerular Cells

Chair: Gary E. Striker (USA)
Itaru Kihara (Japan)

The Terminal Complement Complex C5b-9: A Possible Mediator of Acute and Chronic Glomerulonephritis

Gertrud Maria Hänsch, Matthias Schönermark, Christof Wagner, Gisela Schieren, and Bernhard Jahn[1]

Summary. Incubation of cultivated glomerular cells with the activated terminal complement components C5b-9 results in binding of C5b-9, but not in the killing of cells. One mechanism of cellular defense is the expression of a surface protein, C8 binding protein (C8bp), which was initially identified on human erythrocytes as an inhibitor of the terminal complement reaction. C8bp was also found on mesangial cells and glomerular epithelial cells. Its expression was enhanced upon complement attack. Even though C5b-9 is not lytic on glomerular cells it nevertheless stimulates the mesangial cells to release prostaglandin E, interleukin 1, tumor necrosis factor, and epithelial cells to synthesize collagen type IV. We propose that by releasing mediators from mesangial cells, C5b-9 contributes to the perpetuation of an acute inflammatory response and, by stimulating collagen synthesis, to the development of sclerosis.

The role of complement in the development of acute inflammation and also in glomerulonephritis is well established. With complement activation, e.g., by antigen-antibody complexes, the chemotactic peptide C5a is generated, which elicits leukocyte infiltration. C5a, as well as C3b, the latter when bound to surfaces, activate leukocytes, e.g., to release proteolytic or collagenolytic enzymes, oxygen radicals or eicosanoids, thus promoting tissue destruction as well as the infiltration of more leukocytes [1–4].

In recent years, another activity of the complement system has also gained increasing interest, namely the action of the terminal complement component C5b-9, known as the lytic entity of the complement cascade. By either classical or alternative pathway activation of complement, a C5b6 complex is generated, which inserts, after binding of C7, C8, and C9, into membrane lipid bilayer to form a transmembrane pore (Fig. 1) (for review see [5,6]). C56 complexes are generated also by complement-independent pathways. Lowering the pH [7], cleavage by proteolytic

[1]Institut für Immunologie der Universität Heidelberg, 6900 Heidelberg 1, Federal Republic of Germany

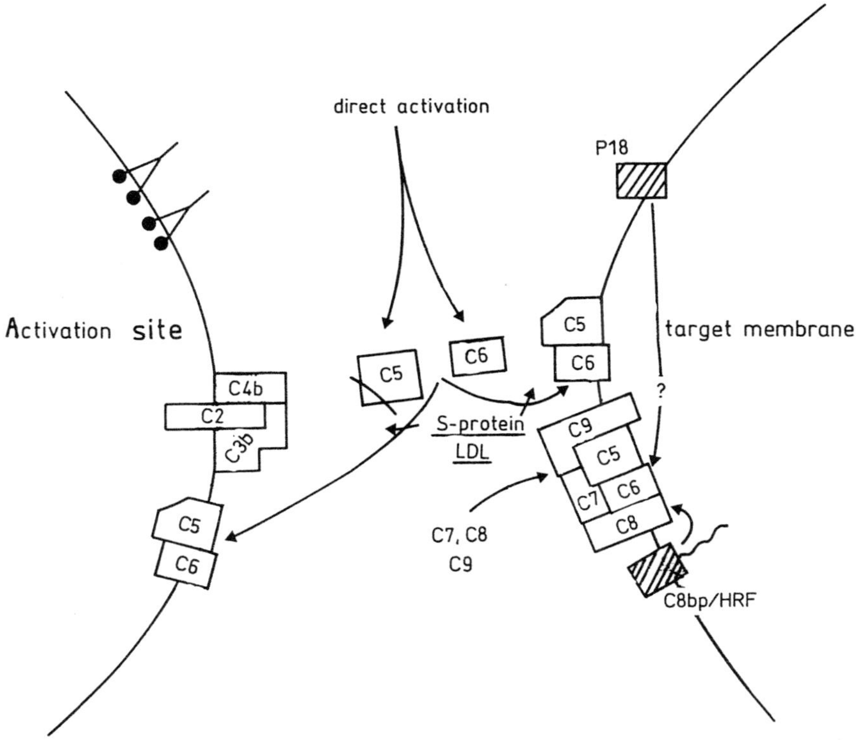

Fig. 1. Control of complement activation: By complement activation, a C5 cleaving enzyme (*C4b2a*) is generated. The cleaved C5, C5b, binds C6 and the ensuing C5b6 complex attaches reversibly to the membrane. Together with C7, C8, and C9 it inserts into the lipid bilayer. Binding of C5b6 can be prevented by fluid phase proteins, e.g., S-protein or low density lipoprotein (*LDL*), and by the efficient formation of C5b-9 by the intrinsic membrane protein C8 binding proteins, C8bp and P18

enzymes [8], or reactive oxygen species [9] are able to directly generate C56 complexes, which, together with C7, C8, and C9, form lytic complexes on membranes.

The C5b6 complex, once generated, does not necessarily bind at the site of activation, but might—for a short period of time—also bind to membranes in the vicinity; the complement reaction up to C9 will then proceed at the "innocent bystander" membrane [10,11].

The activation pathways and the complement attack phase are well regulated (Fig. 1), thus minimizing bystander lysis. S-protein or vitronectin, a serum protein, interferes with the binding of C5b6 and consequently with the formation of membrane-bound C5b-9. Among the inhibitory molecules, cell surface associated proteins, restricting the complement attack in a species-specific manner, are of special interest. With regard to regulation of the terminal complement components, an intrinsic 65kD membrane protein with high affinity for the complement protein C8, and to a minor extent for C9, has been identified, first on human erythrocytes [12],

Table 1. Cell functions elicited by sublytic doses of C5b-9[a]

Release of eicosanoids from
monocytes (human, mouse, rat)
macrophages (rat)
granulocytes (human)
platelets (human)
Kupffer cells (rat)
glomerular mesangial cells (rat, human)
glomerular epithelial cells (rat)
synovial fibroblasts (human)
oligodendrocytes (rat)
Release of interleukin 1 from
glomerular mesangial cells (rat, human)
monocytes (human)
Release of oxygen radicals from
glomerular mesangial cells (rat, human)
granulocytes (human)
Release of collagen type IV from
glomerular epithelial cells (rat, human)
Release of collagenase from
synovial fibroblasts (human)

[a](From [5,6,26])

and later also on other peripheral blood cells [13]. This so-called C8 binding protein, most probably identical to the "homologous restriction factor" [14], interferes with the assembly of the C5b-9 complex by inhibiting the reaction of C8 with C9 [15]. Lack of C8bp, as seen in patients suffering from paroxysmal nocturnal hemoglobinuria, results in an extreme sensitivity of the afflicted erythrocytes to lysis by the terminal complement proteins, which can be fully overcome by incorporating isolated C8bp [16,17]. More recently, a further membrane protein (P18/CD59) with apparent complement-inhibiting activity has been described [18,19]; its mode of action and its relationship to C8bp have, however, not yet been clarified.

In erythrocytes, one single functional channel is enough to cause lysis, due to colloid osmotic swelling. In contrast, nucleated cells survive a limited number of channels [20], most probably due to repair processes, such as shedding or internalization of the complexes [21,22]. When studying these repair mechanisms, we and others found that in response to C5b-9, cells reacted with an enhanced lipid turnover, with liberation of free arachidonic acid, and eventually, with release of prostanoids [23–25]. This observation led to the hypothesis that C5b-9 might not only function

Table 2. Mediator release from cultivated mesangial cells[a]

Eicosanoids
Interleukin 1
Tumor necrosis factor
GM-colony-stimulating factor
Oxygen radicals

[a](From [28,29])

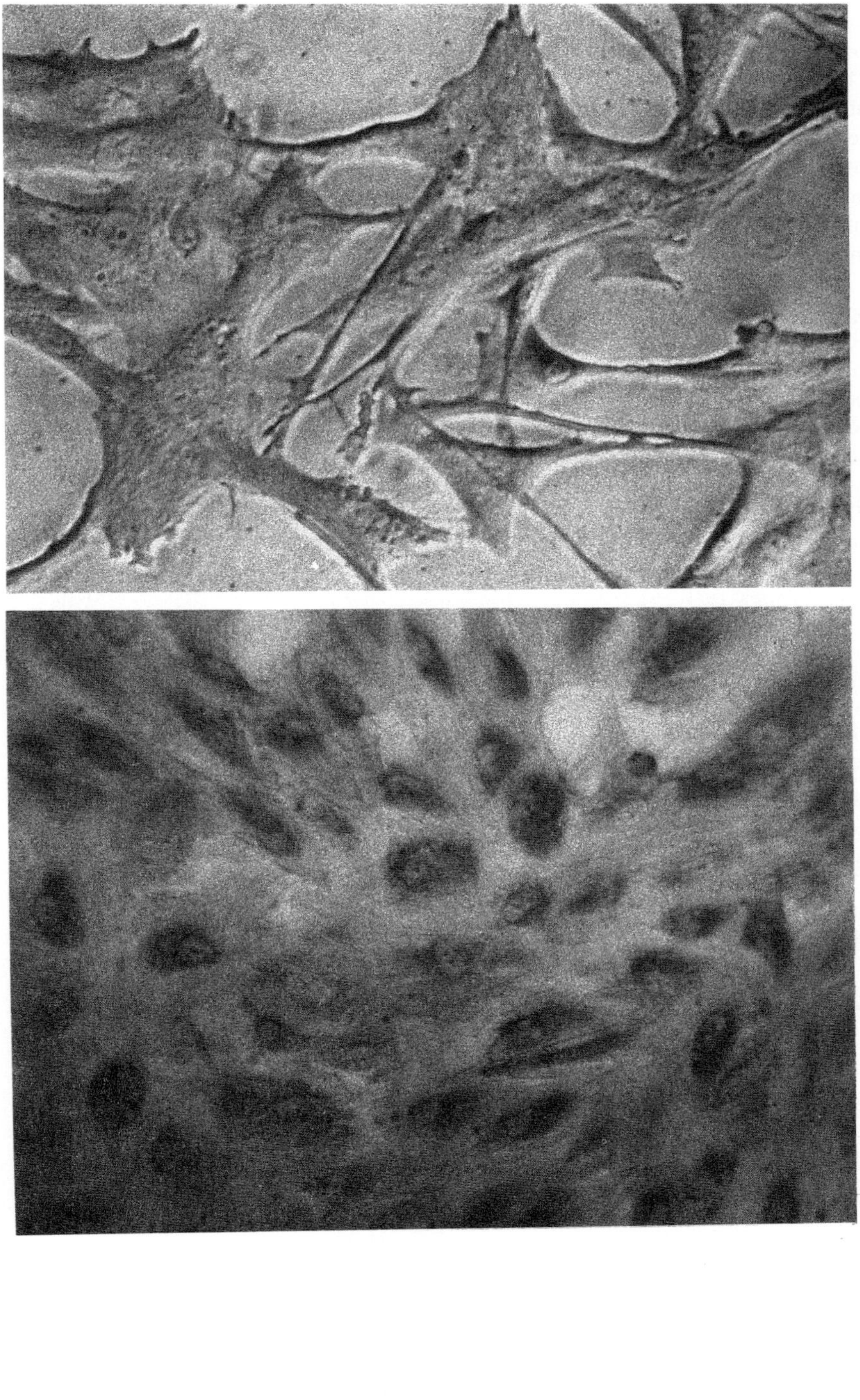

Fig. 2. Presence of C8-binding protein on cultured glomerular epithelial cells (*left*) and mesangial cells (*right*), shown by binding of a specific antibody and a peroxidase-coupled second antibody

as a lytic complex, but might, in sublytic doses, stimulate mediator release. Indeed, stimulation of various cells was found in response to C5b-9, resulting in release of lipid mediators and stimulation of protein synthesis (Table 1). How the C5b-9 stimulated cells is not yet known; increase in intracellular Ca^{2+} has been described, as well as activation of proteinkinase C, and enhanced lipid turnover (for review see [6]).

The question then arose whether the stimulatory function of C5b-9 might be relevant to physiological or pathophysiological events. Looking at glomerulonephritis, several lines of evidence suggested a role of C5b-9. Deposits of C5b-9 complexes are found in various forms of glomerulonephritis and experimental glomerulonephritis. Moreover, evidence for C5b-9 participation has been derived from experimental glomerulonephritis in complement-deficient animals. From these data the conclusion was drawn that proteinuria or the onset of sclerosis was critically dependent on the activity of the terminal complement components. This conclusion was further supported by studies with isolated perfused kidneys (for review see [26,27].

To analyze a possible role of C5b-9 in glomerulonephritis, we studied its interaction with glomerular cells. Since, in recent years, methods of growing cells from isolated glomeruli have been increasingly successful, it has become possible to study the functions of these cells independently of other cells [28,29]. During these studies it became quite obvious that mesangial cells are not only mere bystanders of inflammatory reactions, but that these cells can produce inflammatory mediators (summarized in Table 2). Mesangial cells also release collagenase, which might also contribute to tissue destruction [30]. The release of these proinflammatory mediators can be trig-

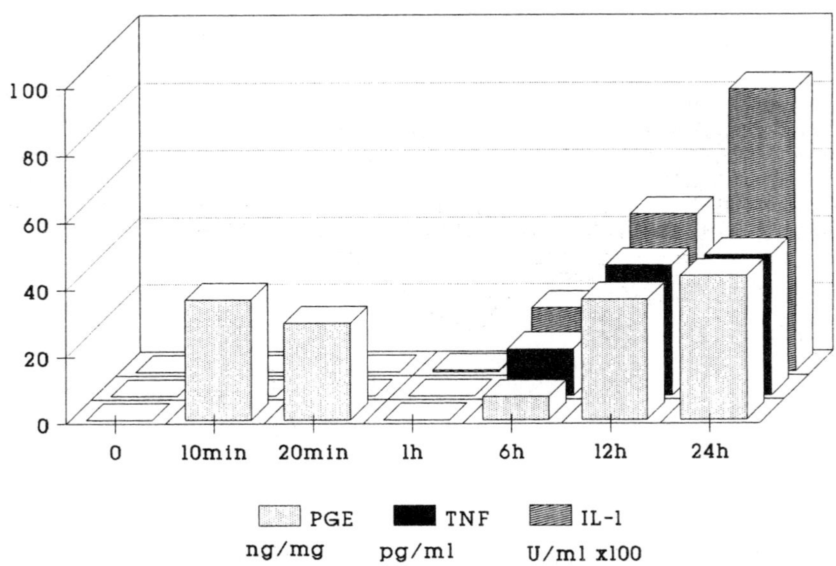

Fig. 3. Mediator release from cultured mesangial cells: The cells were incubated with sublytic doses of preactivated C5b6, C7, C8, and C9. After various times, release of prostaglandin E (*PGE*), interleukin 1 (*IL-1*), and tumor-necrosis factor (*TNF*) was tested by radioimmunoassay

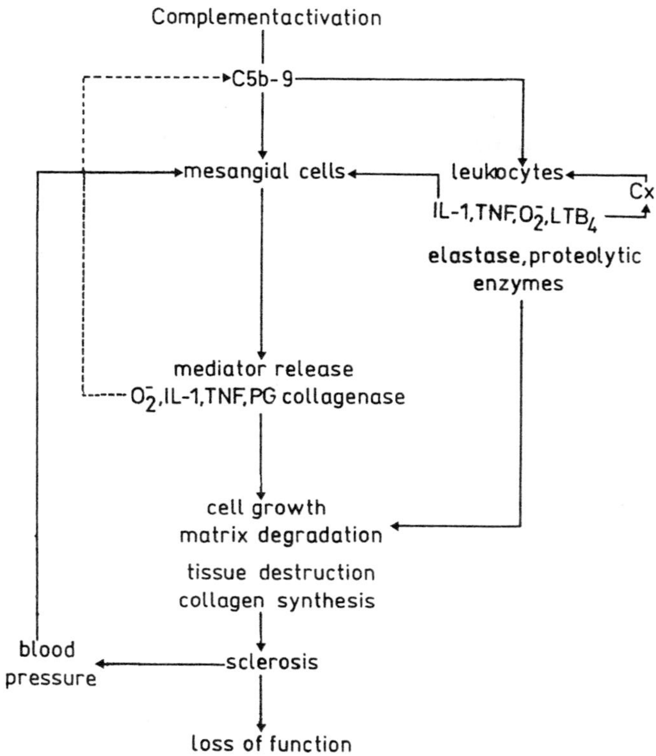

Fig. 4. Role of C5b-9 in acute and chronic inflammation: Activated C5b-9 directly releases inflammatory mediators from mesangial cells, which might promote inflammation. Concomitantly, C5b-9 also activates mediator release from leukocytes. The leukocyte mediators can stimulate other leukocytes, e.g., by causing chemotaxis (*Cx*), but can also affect mesangial cells. Interleukin-I (*IL-1*) might induce proliferation, release of tumor necrosis factor (*TNF*) and of collagenase, leading to tissue destruction. In addition to releasing mediators of acute inflammation, C5b-9 also affects collagen synthesis, thus contributing to the development of sclerosis. PG, prostaglandin; LTB_4, leukotriene B4

gered by other inflammatory mediators, e.g., by interleukin-I (Il-1), but also—and that will presented in more detail here—by the terminal complement components.

When cultured mesangial cells are incubated with purified human C5b6, C7, C8, and C9, rapid binding of C5b-9 is seen. The cells, however, survive the complement attack. On analyzing the molecular basis of complement resistance, we found that after prolonged incubation C5b-9 disappeared gradually from the cell membrane. Concomitantly with the C5b-9 binding, increasing amounts of the complement restricting membrane protein C8bp were expressed on the cell surface. In resident mesangial cells, C8bp is found on the membrane as well as in the cytoplasm (Fig. 2) [31]; by stimulation it is mobilized from the cytoplasmatic reservoirs, thus protecting against the formation of additional lytic complexes.

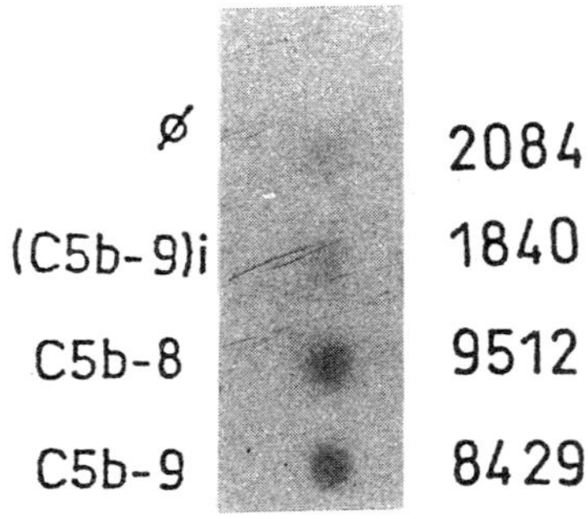

Fig. 5. Induction of collagen type IV synthesis in glomerular epithelial cells: The cells were incubated with sublytic doses of C5b-9, C5b-8, or inactivated C5b-9, respectively. After 2 h collagen type IV mRNA was detected by a cDNA probe (gift of Paul Killen, Ann Arbor, University of Michigan) by dot blot hybridization (*left*). After 24 h the collagen type IV synthesis was also enhanced; this was measured by adsorbing ^{3}H-proline containing protein to an antibody to collagen type IV (* cpm)

Even though mesangial cells are not killed by C5b-9, its interaction with the cell membrane nevertheless results in efficient stimulation of the cells. Rapid release of prostaglandin E is seen, followed by release of interleukin 1 and tumor necrosis factor, followed by a second rise in prostaglandin E (Fig. 3) [31].

By releasing mediators from mesangial cells, C5b-9 might, even in the absence of infiltrating leukocytes, promote an inflammatory reaction. Since C5b-9 also activates leukocytes to release mediators, which then in turn might trigger mesangial cells, other leukocytes, or even platelets, an ongoing inflammatory reaction will be even more enhanced. Considering the fact that complement is readily activated in inflamed tissue, e.g., not only by immune complexes, but also by destroyed cells [32], by exposed basement membrane [33], or by oxygen radicals [9], it is conceivable that even in the absence of the initial triggering event, the acute inflammation turns into a self-perpetuating process (shown schematically in Fig. 4).

One consequence of tissue destruction is tissue repair. By enhanced cell growth, as well as by enhanced matrix production, scar tissue is formed. After extensive destruction, tissue might also be replaced by less differentiated cells, by collagen or mesenchymal matrix, a phenomenon known as sclerosis [34,35].

Sclerosis is a hallmark of chronic glomerulonephritis; many causes for sclerosis have been discussed, especially mechanical stress due to high blood pressure. Alternatively, we tested whether inflammatory mediators might promote sclerosis by directly affecting the synthesis of extracellular matrix proteins.

Collagen type IV is a normal constituent of the basement membrane and it is produced by glomerular epithelial cells. In many forms of chronic glomerulonephritis, however, collagen deposits are also found in the mesangium, most probably due to enhanced synthesis by local cells [36,28].

Glomerular epithelial cells produce some collagen type IV under culture conditions. After incubation with sublytic doses of C5b-9, an increase in collage type IV specific mRNA was seen, 2–4 h after addition of C5b-9 (Fig. 5). After 12–24 h, extracellular collagen type IV was also enhanced; this was measured by biosynthetic labelling with ^{3}H-proline (Fig. 5). With C5b-9, collagen type IV specific mRNA was enhanced about 4–8-fold and protein synthesis was enhanced 5–10-fold, this being in the same range as the enhancement seen after stimulation with interleukin 1 [37].

Mesangial cells also respond to C5b-9 with enhanced collagen synthesis, again, this was tested by enhanced incorporation of radiolabelled proline into collagenase-digestible proteins.

Conclusions

Our data suggest a dual role of C5b-9. Firstly, by triggering the release of proinflammatory mediators such as Il-1 or prostanoids, C5b-9 might enhance the acute inflammatory response. Secondly, by inducing collagen synthesis, C5b-9 might contribute to sclerosis, and thereby to the progression of acute inflammation to chronicity, and finally, to renal failure.

Acknowledgment. This work has been supported by Deutsche Forschungsgemeinschaft Ha 1129/4-2 and Ha 1129/5-1.

References

1. Rother K, Rother U, Hänsch GM (1985) The role of complement in inflammation. Pathol Res Pract 180:117–124
2. Fligiel SEG, Johnson KJ, Ward PA (1988) The role of complement in immune complex induced tissue injury. In: Rother K, Till G (eds) The complement system. Springer, Berlin, pp 487–504
3. Cochrane CG, Unanue ER, Dixon FJ (1965) A role of polymorphonuclear leukocytes and complement in nephrotoxic nephritis. J Exp Med 122:99–116
4. Cochrane CG (1969) Mediation of immunologic glomerular injury. Transplant Proc 1:949–958
5. Hänsch GM (1988) The complement attack phase. In: Rother K, Till G (eds) The complement system. Springer, Berlin, pp 202–230
6. Shin ML, Carney DF (1988) Cytotoxic action and other metabolic consequences of the terminal complement proteins. In: Shin ML (ed) Cytotoxic mediators of inflammation and host defense. Progress in Allergy 40:44–48
7. Rother U, Hänsch GM, Rauterberg EW, Jungfer H, Rother K (1978) Deviated lysis. Lysis of unsensitized cells by complement. V Generation of the activity by low pH and low ionic strength. Z Immun Forsch 155:118–129
8. Wetsel RA, Kolb WP (1982) Complement-independent activation of the fifth component (C5) of human complement. Limited trypsin digestion resulting in the expression of biologic activity. J Immunol 128:2209–2216
9. Vogt W, von Zabern I, Hesse D, Nolte R, Haller Y (1986/87) Generation of an activated form of human C5 (C5b like C5) by oxygen radicals. Immunol Lett 14:209–215
10. Rother U, Hänsch GM, Menzel J, Rother K (1974) Deviated lysis: transfer of complement lytic activity to unsensitized cells. I Generation of the transferable activity on the surface of complement resistant bacteria. Z Immun Forsch 148:172–186
11. Götze O, Müller-Eberhard HJ (1970) Lysis of erythrocytes by complement in the absence of antibody. J Exp Med 132:898–915

12. Schönermark S, Rauterberg EW, Shin ML, Löke S, Roelcke D, Hänsch GM, (1986) Homologous species restriction in lysis of human erythrocytes. A membrane-derived protein with C8-binding capacity functions as an inhibitor. J Immunol 136:1772–1776
13. Blaas P, Berger B, Weber S, Peter HH, Hänsch GM (1988) Paroxysmal nocturnal hemoglobinuria (PNH Type III): enhanced stimulation of platelets by the terminal complement components is related to the lack of C8bp in the membrane. J Immunol 140:4045–4051
14. Zalman LS, Wood LM, Müller-Eberhard HJ (1987) Isolation of a human erythrocyte membrane protein capable of inhibiting expression of homologous complement channels. Proc Natl Acad Sci USA 83:6975–6979
15. Schönermark S, Filsinger S, Berger B, Hänsch GM (1988) A C8 binding protein of the human erythrocyte: interaction with the components of the complement attack phase. Immunology 63:585–590
16. Hänsch GM, Schönermark S, Roelcke D (1987) Paroxysmal nocturnal hemoglobinuria type III: lack of an erythrocytes membrane protein restricting the lysis by C5b-9. J Clin Invest 80:7–12
17. Zalman LS, Wood LM, Frank MM, Müller-Eberhard HJ (1987) Deficiency of the homologous restriction factor in paroxysmal nocturnal hemoglobinuria. J Exp Med 165:572–577
18. Sugita Y, Nakano Y, Tomita M (1988) Isolation of a new membrane protein from human erythrocytes which inhibits the formation of complement transmembrane channels. J Biochem (Tokyo) 104:633–637
19. Davies A, Simmons DL, Lale C, Harrison RA, Tighs H, Lachmann PI, Waldmann H (1989) CD59, an Ly-6-like protein expressed in human lymphoid cells, regulates the action of the complement membrane attack complex on homologous cells. J Exp Med 170: 637–654
20. Koski CL, Ramm LE, Hammer CH, Mayer MM, Shin ML (1983) Cytolysis of nucleated cells by complement: cell death displays multi-hit characteristics. Proc Natl Acad Sci USA 80:3816–3820
21. Carney D, Hammer C, Shin ML (1986) Elimination of the terminal complement intermediates from the plasma membrane of nucleated cells: the rate of disappearance differs for cells carrying C5b-7 or C5b-8 or a mixture of C5b-8 and a limited number of C5b-9. J Immunol 134:1804–1809
22. Morgan PB, Dankert JR, Esser AF (1986) Recovery of human neutrophils from complement attack: removal of the membrane attack complex by endocytosis and exocytosis. J Immunol 138:246–253
23. Imagawa D, Osifchin NE, Paznekas WA, Shin ML, Mayer MM (1983) Consequence of cell membrane attack by complement: release of arachidonate and formation of inflammatory derivatives. Proc Natl Acad Sci USA 80:6647–6651
24. Betz M, Hänsch GM (1984) Release of arachidonic acid: a new function of the late complement components. Immunobiology 166:473–479
25. Hänsch GM, Seitz M, Martinotti G, Betz M, Rauterberg EW, Gemsa D (1984) Macrophages release arachidonic acid, prostaglandin E2 and thromboxane in response to the late complement components. J Immunol 133:2145–2150
26. Couser WG, Baker PJ, Adler S (1985) Complement and the direct mediation of glomerular injury: a new perspective. Kidney Int 2:879–890
27. Rauterberg EW (1987) Demonstration of complement deposits in tissue. In: Rother K, Till G (eds) The complement system. Springer, Berlin, pp 287–326
28. Striker GE, Striker LJ (1985) Biology of disease: glomerular cell culture. Lab Invest 53(2):122–131
29. Lovett DH, Sterzel RB (1986) Cell culture approaches to the analysis of glomerular inflammation. Kidney Int 30:246–254

30. Lovett DH, Sterzel RB, Kashgarian M, Ryan JL (1983) Neutral proteinase activity produced in vitro by cells of the glomerular mesangium. Kidney Int 23:342–348
31. Lovett D, Hänsch, GM, Goppelt M, Resch K (1987) Activation of glomerular mesangial cells by the terminal membrane attack complex of complement. J Immunol 138:2473–2480
32. Baker PJ, Osofsky SG (1980) Activation of human complement by heat-killed human kidney cells grown in culture. J Immunol 124:81–86
33. Williams JD, Czop JK, Abrahamson DR, Davies M, Austin KF (1984) Activation of the alternative complement pathway by isolated human glomerular basement membrane. J Immunol 133:394–399
34. Klahr S, Schreiner G, Ichikawa I (1988) The progression of renal disease. N Engl J Med 318:1657–1666
35. Bruijn JA, Hogendorn PCW, Hoedemaker PJ, Fleuren GL (1988) The extracellular matrix in pathology. J Lab Clin Med 111:140–149
36. Striker LM, Killen PD, Chi E, Striker GE (1984) The composition of glomerulosclerosis and membranoproliferative glomerulonephritis. Lab Invest 51:181–196
37. Torbohm I, Berger B, Schönermark M, von Kempis J, Rother K, Hänsch GM (1989) Modulation of collagen synthesis in human glomerular epithelial cells by interleukin 1. Clin Exp Immunol 75:427–431

The Biosynthesis and Action of Tumor Necrosis Factor α in the Kidney

LAURENT BAUD, BRUNO FOUQUERAY, CAROLE PHILIPPE, and HÉLÈNE AFFRES[1]

SUMMARY. Like other cytokines, tumor necrosis factor alpha (TNF_α) belongs to a network of mediators of cell-to-cell communication. Both monocytes/macrophages and resident glomerular and tubular cells are apparently the cellular source of TNF_α in the kidney. In the glomerulus its cell surface expression and secretion are regulated by the local production of prostaglandins and reactive oxygen species; its secretion is enhanced in experimental models of immune complex glomerulonephritis. Following its synthesis, TNF_α binding to specific cell surface membrane receptors of glomerular mesangial cells and monocytes/macrophages is modulated by the local production of reactive oxygen species. In mesangial cells, this binding is associated with increased prostaglandin synthesis, cyclic AMP accumulation, expression of MHC antigens and of 5′-nucleotidase, and release of procoagulant activity, reactive oxygen species, and proteoglycans. Thus TNF_α appears to promote coagulation, inflammatory response, and sclerosis in the glomerulus.

Cytokines regulate the growth, differentiation, and functions of cells involved in immunity and inflammation. They belong to a network of mediators of cell-to-cell communication, which includes also arachidonic acid metabolites, reactive oxygen species (ROS), and polypeptide hormones. Cytokines were initially named according to their biological effects, and then, after their aminoacid sequence was established, by the term "interleukin" followed by a number [1]. Some of them have retained their original names, such as tumor necrosis factor (TNF) and lymphotoxin (LT), two factors recognized because of their cytotoxic and anti-tumor properties.

TNF was first described by Carswell et al. in the serum of BCG-primed, endotoxin-treated animals. This factor, produced mainly by monocytes/macrophages, has been shown to induce hemorrhagic necrosis of tumors in recipient animals, and to lyse tumor cells in vitro (reviewed in [2]). It was purified to homogeneity and its primary structure was eventually established. This was found to be similar to that of cachectin, a macrophage-derived protein which is able to

[1]INSERM U64, Hôpital Tenon, 4 rue de la Chine, 75020 Paris Cedex 20, France

suppress lipoprotein lipase activity in isolated adipocytes. Lymphocyte-derived LT has been also cloned. Although this factor has cytotoxic properties similar to those of TNF, it exhibits only 30% aminoacid homology. A nomenclature has been adopted that employs the term TNF α for TNF/cachectin, and TNF_β for LT. It is now evident that both TNF_α and TNF_β serve as general mediators of inflammatory processes. The present review will be centered on TNF_α since it has several unique properties which implicate it as an endogenous mediator of renal injury in human and experimental renal diseases.

TNF Gene Expression

The TNF_α gene is located on chromosome 6 in man and is closely linked to the major histocompatibility complex [2,3]. Monocytes/macrophages contain detectable levels of TNF_α messenger RNA (mRNA), prior to induction by bacterial lipopolysaccharide (LPS). Upon exposure to LPS, the transcription of the TNF_α gene is increased approximately threefold; thereafter, its half-life is controlled chiefly by the presence of a highly conserved AU-rich sequence located in the 3′ untranslated region [2]. Such a sequence, which is also found in the mRNA encoding other cytokines, confers instability on messages that contain it. LPS induces a concomitant increase in the production of prostaglandin E_2 (PGE_2) which, in turn, limits the level of transcription of TNF_α mRNA by elevating intracellular cyclic AMP [4]. In addition to LPS, a variety of stimuli are capable of causing TNF_α mRNA expression, including toxic shock syndrome toxin 1, viruses, parasites, cytokines (interferon $_\gamma$: INF_γ; interleukin 2: IL_2), neuropeptides, and immune complexes.

Not only monocytes/macrophages, but also lymphocytes, endothelial and vascular smooth muscle cells, glial cells in the central nervous system, Kupffer cells in the liver, Paneth cells of the intestinal epithelium, and several epithelial tumor cells have been found to exhibit TNF_α mRNA expression upon exposure to these stimuli. Kidney cells express TNF_α mRNA under physiologic conditions, as detected by Northern blotting [5]. After injection of LPS, this expression increases to a greater extent than in other tissues. The precise localization of TNF_α mRNA in the kidney is still unknown, but recent reports suggest that both glomerular mesangial cells [6] and proximal tubular epithelial cells [7] could be responsible for this expression. In LPS-activated rat mesangial cells, TNF_α gene expression is characterized by two hybridizing bands: one strongly hybridizing band and a second weaker band of higher molecular weight which could represent a precursor to the main TNF_α mRNA (6).

Molecular Forms of TNF_α

TNF_α bears a secretory protein signal sequence, and thus, unlike IL_1, is synthesized by the classical secretory pathway through the endoplasmic reticulum and Golgi apparatus. Its synthesis starts with the elaboration of a precursor or prohormone, which is subsequently cleaved during processing to yield the mature protein. The mature human 17 kDa TNF_α consists of 157 aminoacids. The uncleaved precursor of

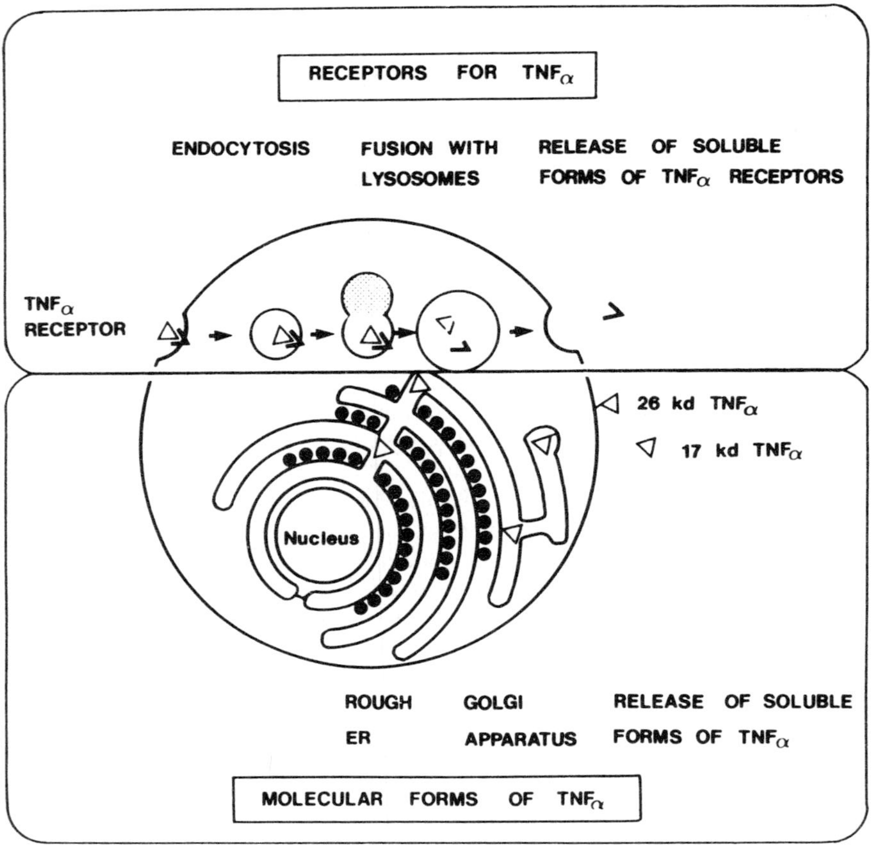

Fig. 1. Schematic view of how TNF_α is synthesized and released and how TNF_α binding to its receptor is followed by rapid internalization and degradation

26 kDa contains 76 supplementary residues, including a long hydrophobic region of 26 aminoacids, allowing it to be expressed as an integral transmembrane protein [8]. How 26 kDa integral transmembrane TNF_α is processed to the 17 kDa secretory component is unknown. But it has been shown that both molecules are active and exhibit possibly different tissue specificities and different biological activities (Fig. 1).

TNF_α molecule is functionally defined as promoting both lysis of the TNF_α-sensitive L929 murine fibroblast cell line, and suppression of lipoprotein lipase activity in adipocytes [6]. In cultured rat mesangial cells [9] as in macrophages [10], cell associated TNF_α activity is demonstrable after less than 1 h exposure to LPS, peaks at 2 h, and decreases progressively thereafter, while TNF_α activity increases in the medium. The progressive rise of TNF_α activity in the medium is followed after 9 h by evident decay. Flow cytometry experiments and immunohistochemical studies reveal that two thirds of LPS-activated macrophages [10] and LPS-activated mesangial cells [9] exhibit TNF_α expression at their surface. The greatest part of these cell-associated TNF_α molecules persists after low pH treatment, indicating that they are integral membrane proteins and not molecules attached to cell surface receptors. Proximal tubular cells, transformed by SV_{40}, which express TNF mRNA upon LPS challenge, do not release TNF_α activity into the medium, whereas they produce membrane-bound TNF_α [11].

The mechanisms whereby cell surface expression and secretion of TNF_α are regulated have been extensively studied, in both macrophages and mesangial cells. Low PGE_2 concentrations enhance, whereas high concentrations (>10 ng/ml) suppress TNF_α release [12]. This complex effect results from the activation of biochemical pathways that have conflicting effects on TNF_α production. Indeed cyclic GMP, which is preferentially increased by low concentrations of PGE_2, stimulates TNF_α release, whereas cyclic AMP, which is increased by high concentrations of PGE_2 [6,12] or by various pharmacologic agents, suppresses it. Because TNF_α is a potent inducer of PGE_2 and cyclic AMP production [13], the inhibition of TNF_α production by PGE_2 is considered as the negative arm of a regulatory circuit which can be blocked by nonsteroidal antiinflammatory drugs. In contrast, the production of TNF_α is positively regulated in macrophages by platelet-activating factor (PAF). Interaction with a specific receptor and subsequent synthesis of 5-lipoxygenase byproducts, including leukotriene B_4 (LTB_4) are required for this effect. The finding that TNF_α induces the release of PAF from macrophages suggests [14], in this case, the existence of a powerful amplification loop.

There is also in vitro evidence of bidirectional interaction between TNF_α and ROS, which are both generated by monocytes/macrophages and mesangial cells. TNF_α is capable of stimulating ROS production by these cells [15], and ROS, in turn, may enhance the release of TNF_α [9,16]. Desferrioxamine (DFX), an iron chelator which prevents the generation of hydroxyl radical via the Haber-Weiss reaction, has been shown to reduce the concentration of TNF_α in culture media of macrophages [16], and mesangial cells [9] through decrease of its release and acceleration of its inactivation [9]. There are at least two different ways in which DFX might decrease the release of TNF_α from LPS-activated mesangial cells. First, DFX could limit TNF_α synthesis at the transcriptional and post-transcriptional levels. Second, DFX could indirectly interfere with the generation of TNF_α when its 26 kDa precursor form is processed to yield a 17 kDa molecule. Because DFX inhibits the release of TNF_α into the medium, but enhances its cell surface expression, it is tempting to speculate that this drug prevents occurrence of the mechanism whereby TNF_α detaches from the membrane. Indeed, hydroxyl radical or its metabolites might induce the cleavage of membrane-associated TNF_α through the activation of latent metalloproteinases and/or the inactivation of proteinase inhibitors [9].

Additionally, different drugs have been shown to affect TNF_α production by monocytes/macrophages and mesangial cells. For instance, corticosteroids and cyclosporine A both reduce TNF_α production by LPS-activated monocytes. Cyclosporine A inhibits the release of TNF_α without modifying its cell-associated form [17]. Antibiotics have similar inhibitory effects. For example, quinolones [18] and aminoglycosides (L. Baud, unpublished observations) decrease extracellular TNF_α production by LPS-activated monocytes in a dose-dependent manner. Collectively, these results may have implications in transplant therapy.

Renal Production of TNF_α in Pathological Processes

Preliminary reports indicate that TNF_α is produced by glomeruli isolated from rats with an accelerated autologous form of nephrotoxic serum nephritis [19]. This is associated with infiltration of the glomeruli by monocytes/macrophages. In support of their contributing role, these cells have been shown to release TNF_α when incubated in vitro with glomerular basement membrane-containing immune complexes [20].

Interestingly, enhanced gene expression for TNF_α has been demonstrated in the renal cortex of two models of spontaneous lupus nephritis, the MRL-1pr [21] and (NZB × NZW)F1 mice [22]. In addition, TNF_α bioactivity has been found in the medium of glomeruli isolated from MRL-1pr mice but not in that from normal congenic MRL++ mice [21]. Again, invading macrophages are the likely source of TNF_α production in the glomerulus. This is in contrast with the observation that peritoneal macrophages from (NZB × NZW)F1 mice express a weak TNF_α bioactivity [23], and with the observation that, in patients with systemic lupus erythematosus, the serum levels of TNF_α are unaltered [24]. The implications of these reports, as well as of other studies on serum TNF_α [25], for the diagnosis and management of renal diseases are still unknown.

Characterization of Receptors for TNF_α and Their Regulation

Studies of the tissue distribution of label after injection of radioiodinated TNF_α demonstrate that 8% of the dose is recovered from the kidneys [26]. This represents a specific binding since reduction of labeling is observed when unlabeled TNF_α is injected together with the tracer. In fact, virtually all somatic tissues, with the exception of erythrocytes, express a receptor for TNF_α. Receptor numbers are highly variable, ranging from 200 to 50,000 sites per cell with a high affinity for TNF_α (Kd of 0.1–3.0 nM). But the biological effects of TNF_α are maximally expressed at receptor occupancies of 5–10%. After binding of TNF_α to its receptor, the TNF_α receptor complex is internalized, without further recycling of the receptor (Fig. 1). Experimental support has accumulated for the upregulation of TNF_α receptors by INF γ and agents that stimulate protein kinase A (PKA) and for their downregulation by corticosteroids, and agents that stimulate protein kinase C (PKC). The mechanisms whereby downregulation by PKC occurs include decreased affinity, reduced density, and increased internalization of TNF_α binding sites. Ding et al. [27] have demonstrated that LPS also promotes the internalization of TNF_α receptors on the surface of macrophages. More recently, we have obtained data indicating that ROS downregulate TNF_α binding, but only slightly increase the degree of internalization of TNF_α receptors [28]. Indeed, exposure of mesangial cells, blood monocytes, or TNF_α-sensitized murine L929 fibroblasts to hydrogen peroxide (H_2O_2) promotes a loss of about 50% in the density of cell membrane TNF_α receptors. This is associated, in L 929 cells, with a decrease in the cytotoxic activity of TNF_α [28]. Conversely, the treatment of blood monocytes with antioxidant drugs such as DFX causes the upregulation of TNF_α receptors through a decrease of their turnover rate (L. Baud, unpublished observations). This further suggests a particular susceptibility of TNF_α receptors to the oxidative damage. It should be noted that the presence of cystein repeats in the extracellular domain of the 55 kDa TNF_α receptor may account for this observation [29].

Soluble forms of the receptors for TNF_α are released from target cells into the plasma and may represent a mechanism by which TNF_α molecules are inactivated [29] (Fig. 1). Such TNF_α binding proteins are found in the urine as well. Uromodulin or Tamm-Horsfall protein, a polypeptide which binds TNF_α with a high affinity via carbohydrate chains, has also been isolated from human urine. However, it does not inhibit the cytotoxic activity of this cytokine. An alternative cause of the inactivation of TNF_α is its degradation by either neutrophil proteolytic enzymes or by hypochlorous acid. In summary, there are several observations in the literature showing that TNF_α efficiency may be modulated at the receptor level. In contrast, to date, there are only few data regarding the intracellular pathways of TNF_α signal transduction and their regulation.

TNF_α Action on Kidney Cells

Only a few of the studies on renal TNF_α action have been performed in vivo. The first to be published described the pattern of lesions induced in suckling mice by daily subcutaneous injections of TNF_α. The kidneys of these mice showed no abnormalities in the glomeruli, but had some cytoplasmic granules in the proximal tubules [30], which probably represented reabsorption of proteins from the lumen. Thereafter, T. Bertani et al. [31] studied glomerular functional and structural changes induced by intravenous infusion of TNF_α to the rabbit. The main finding was the presence of endothelial cell swelling, polymorphonuclear leukocyte accumulation, and fibrin formation in the capillaries. Glomeruli from rats injected with TNF_α also showed a transient influx of neutrophils into capillaries, but no formation of thrombi [32]. Nevertheless, TNF_α administration to rats with antiglomerular basement membrane antibody-mediated nephritis caused a substantial amplification of the glomerular injury, characterized by intra-capillary thrombi and endothelial cell swelling [32]. These structural abnormalities were associated with functional changes, including a dose-dependent increase of proteinuria. Similarly, chronic administration of TNF_α in low doses to mice with spontaneous lupus nephritis increased proteinuria and worsened renal disease and mortality [22], whereas higher doses were protective [23]. This latter event could be the result of changes in cell-mediated immunity more than changes in humoral immunity [33].

There are a number of different ways in which TNF_α might affect the structure and function of both glomerular and tubular cells. They have been identified in in vitro studies.

Prostaglandin Synthesis

TNF_α, either alone or synergistically with IL_1, increases prostaglandin synthesis by glomerular mesangial cells [13, 34–36]. This effect can be measured in vitro as an increased accumulation of PGE_2, $PGF_{2\alpha}$ and 6 keto $PGF_{1\alpha}$, which is the stable breakdown product of PGI_2 [13], in mesangial cell culture medium. This requires a long incubation period, and is inhibited by both actinomycin D and cycloheximide, which is consistent with an increase of transcription and translation. Additionally, TNF_α increases the release of phospholipase A_2 activity [34] together with arachidonic acid [36], and induces cyclooxygenase activity, suggesting possible regulation at two distinct levels.

TNF_α also stimulates cyclic AMP accumulation in the mesangial cell culture medium [13]. Because indomethacin suppresses the effect of TNF_α on prostaglandins but only reduces the effect on cyclic AMP, it is likely that TNF_α stimulates cyclic AMP levels in part independently of its effect on prostaglandin production. Through its effect on prostaglandins and cyclic nucleotides, TNF_α may affect both proliferation and activation of mesangial cells.

Cell Proliferation

There have been reports published both of TNF_α-mediated enhancement and of TNF_α-mediated inhibition of mesangial cell proliferation. Many laboratories have found that TNF_α causes a significant increase of DNA synthesis by rat [37,38] and human [39] mesangial cells, when cultured in serum-free media. This effect has been reported to be not associated with phospholipase C activation and phosphatidic acid production [38]. In contrast, TNF_α does not affect [13] or even inhibits growth of proliferating rat mesangial cells [40]. The origin of this discrepancy is not clear. It is possible that, in serum-enriched media, the endogenous prostaglandin production simultaneously induced by TNF_α antagonizes its growth-promoting effect. Indeed, coincubation of proliferating mesangial cells with TNF_α and indomethacin is associated with an increase of DNA synthesis [37]. Alternatively, because TNF_α-stimulated synthesis of platelet-derived growth factor (PDGF) may be responsible for mesangial cell growth [39], the addition of serum and, hence, of PDGF in excess might mask TNF_α-induced cell proliferation.

Cell Activation

Upon exposure to TNF_α, glomerular and tubular cells may acquire new functions without growth modification. Indeed, in addition to increased production, by glomerular epithelial cells, of a chemotactic factor for polymorphonuclear leukocytes [41], TNF_α may stimulate mesangial cells to express MHC class I and class II antigens [40] and 5′-nucleotidase [42], and to synthesize procoagulant activity [43], ROS [15], and proteoglycans [44]. Thus TNF_α appears to promote coagulation, inflammatory response, and sclerosis in the glomerulus. TNF_α also induces the synthesis of different lipid molecules, including prostaglandins and PAF, which could act as mediators of mesangial cell contraction. It should be noted that this phenomenon might be offset in vivo by the increased synthesis of the potent vasodilatator nitric oxide.

Finally, TNF_α, like IL_1, promotes a marked increase in sodium-dependent uptake of solutes by proximal tubule cells [45]. The TNF_α expression in these cells [11] raises the possibility that, in the absence of inflammatory cells, they may modulate the functions of the proximal nephron.

In conclusion, it is now clear that TNF_α may exert a wide range of action on the kidney. Apparently both monocytes/macrophages and resident kidney cells are sources of this cytokine in pathological and possibly in physiological reaction. Availability of specific TNF_{α} agonists or antagonists should help to extend our knowledge in this field and could open new and interesting methods in therapeutics.

Acknowledgments. Portions of this work were supported by the "Institut National de la Santé et de la Recherche Médicale" and the "Faculté de Médecine Saint-Antoine." The authors thank Mrs Miranda and Mrs Knobloch for secretarial assistance.

References

1. Dinarello CA, Mier JW (1987) Lymphokines. N Engl J Med 317:940–945
2. Beutler B, Cerami A (1986) Cachectin and tumour necrosis factor as two sides of the same biological coin. Nature 320:584–588
3. Beutler B, Cerami A (1988) The common mediator of shock, cachexia, and tumor necrosis. Adv Immunol 42:213–231
4. Kunkel SL, Spengler M, May MA et al. (1988) Prostaglandin E_2 regulates macrophage-derived tumor necrosis factor gene expression. J Biol Chem 263:5380–5384
5. Ulich TR, Guo K, Del Castillo J (1989) Endotoxin-induced cytokine gene expression in vivo. 1. Expression of tumor necrosis factor mRNA in visceral organs under physiologic conditions and during endotoxemia. Am J Pathol 134:11–14
6. Baud L, Oudinet J-P, Bens M et al. (1989) Production of tumor necrosis factor by rat mesangial cells in response to bacterial lipopolysaccharide. Kidney Int 35:1111–1118
7. Wuthrich RP, Glimcher LH, Yui MA et al. (1990) MHC class II, antigen presentation and tumor necrosis factor in renal tubular epithelial cells. Kidney Int 37:783–792
8. Kriegler M, Perez C, de Fay K et al. (1988) A novel form of TNF/cachectin is a cell surface cytotoxic transmembrane protein: Ramifications for the complex physiology of TNF. Cell 53:45–53
9. Affres H, Perez J, Hagege J et al. (to be published) Cell surface expression and release of tumor necrosis factor by lipopolysaccharide-stimulated mesangial cells: effect of desferrioxamine. Kidney Int
10. Chensue SW, Remick DG, Shmyr-Forsch C et al. (1988) Immunohistochemical demonstration of cytoplasmic and membrane-associated tumor necrosis factor in murine macrophages. Am J Pathol 133:564–572
11. Jevnikar AM, Wuthrich RP, Glimcher LH et al. (1990) LPS and $IL\text{-}_{1\alpha}$ stimulated proximal tubular cells produce tumor necrosis factor in vitro (abstract). Kidney Int 37:417
12. Renz H, Gong J-H, Schmidt A et al. (1988) Release of tumor necrosis factor-α from macrophages. Enhancement and suppression are dose-dependently regulated by prostaglandin E_2 and cyclic nucleotides. J Immunol 141:2388–2393
13. Baud L, Perez J, Friedlander G et al. (1988) Tumor necrosis factor stimulates prostaglandin production and cyclic AMP levels in rat cultured mesangial cells. FEBS Lett 239:50–54
14. Camussi G, Bussolino F, Salvidia G et al. (1987) Tumor necrosis factor/cachectin stimulates peritoneal macrophages, polymorphonuclear neutrophils, and vascular endothelial cells to synthesize and release platelet-activating factor. J Exp Med 166:1390–1404
15. Radeke HH, Meier B, Topley N et al. (1990) Interleukin 1-α and tumor necrosis factor-α induce oxygen radical production in mesangial cells. Kidney Int 37:767–775
16. Chaudhri G, Clark IA (1989) Reactive oxygen species facilitate the in vitro and in vivo lipopolysaccharide-induced release of tumor necrosis factor. J Immunol 143:1290–1294
17. Remick DG, Nguyen DT, Eskandari MK et al. (1989) Cyclosporine A inhibits TNF production without decreasing TNF mRNA levels. Biochem Biophys Res Commun 161:551–555

18. Bailly S, Fay M, Gougerot-Pocidalo M-A (1990) Effects of quinolones on TNF production by human monocytes. Pathol Biol Paris 38:267–271
19. Wiggins RC, Eldredge C, Kunkel S (1987) Monokine production by glomeruli at different stages of crescent formation in the rabbit. Proc 4th Int Congress Nephrology, 368 p
20. Vissers MCM, Fantone JC, Wiggins R et al. (1989) Glomerular basement membrane-containing immune complexes stimulate tumor necrosis factor and interleukin-1 production by human monocytes. Am J Pathol 134:1–6
21. Boswell JM, Yui MA, Burt DW et al. (1988) Increased tumor necrosis factor and IL-1_β gene expression in the kidneys of mice with lupus nephritis. J Immunol 141:3050–3054
22. Brennan DC, Yui MA, Wuthrich RP et al. (1989) Tumor necrosis factor and IL-1 in New Zealand black/white mice. Enhanced gene expression and acceleration of renal injury. J Immunol 143:3470–3475
23. Jacob CO, McDevitt HO (1988) Tumour necrosis factor-α in murine autoimmune lupus nephritis. Nature 331:356–358
24. Maury CPJ, Teppo AM (1989) Tumor necrosis factor in the serum of patients with systemic lupus erythematosus. Arthritis Rheum 32:146–151
25. Maury CPJ, Teppo AM (1987) Raised serum levels of cachectin/tumor necrosis factor in renal allograft rejection. J Exp Med 166:1132–1137
26. Beutler BA, Milsark IW, Cerami A (1985) Cachectin/tumor necrosis factor: production, distribution, and metabolic fate in vivo. J Immunol 135:3972–3977
27. Ding AH, Sanchez E, Srimal S et al. (1989) Macrophages rapidly internalize their tumor necrosis factor receptors in response to bacterial lipopolysaccharide. J Biol Chem 264:3924–3929
28. Baud L, Affres H, Perez J et al. (1990) Reduction in tumor necrosis factor binding and cytotoxicity by hydrogen peroxide. J Immunol 145:556–560
29. Schall TJ, Lewis M, Koller KJ et al. (1990) Molecular cloning and expression of a receptor for human tumor necrosis factor. Cell 61:361–370
30. Gresser I, Woodrow D, Moss J et al. (1987) Toxic effects of recombinant tumor necrosis factor in suckling mice. Comparisons with interferon α/β. Am J Pathol 128:13–18
31. Bertani T, Abbate M, Zoja C et al. (1989) Tumor necrosis factor induces glomerular damage in the rabbit. Am J Pathol 134:419–430
32. Tomosugi NI, Cashman SJ, Hay H et al. (1989) Modulation of antibody-mediated glomerular injury in vivo by bacterial lipopolysaccharide, tumor necrosis factor, and Il-1. J Immunol 142:3083–3090
33. Gordon C, Wofsy D (1990) Effect of recombinant murine tumor necrosis factor-α on immune function. J Immunol 144:1753–1758
34. Pfeilschifter J, Pignat W, Vosbeck K et al. (1989) Interleukin 1 and tumor necrosis factor synergistically stimulate prostaglandin synthesis and phospholipase A2 release from rat renal mesangial cells. Biochem Biophys Res Commun 159:385–394
35. Floege J, Topley N, Wessel K et al. (1990) Monokines and platelet-derived growth factor modulate prostanoid production in growth arrested, human mesangial cells. Kidney Int 37:859–869
36. Topley N, Floege J, Wessel K et al. (1989) Prostaglandin E_2 production is synergistically increased in cultured human glomerular mesangial cells by combinations of IL-1 and tumor necrosis factor-α. J Immunol 143:1989–1995
37. Perez J, Baud L, Ardaillou R (1989) Tumor necrosis factor stimulates prostaglandin, cyclic AMP, and DNA synthesis by cultured rat mesangial cells (abstract). Kidney Int 35: 318
38. Nakazato Y, Kester M, Mene P et al. (1989) Tumor necrosis factor stimulates mesangial cell proliferation independent of polyphosphoinositide turnover or phosphatidic acid formation (abstract). Kidney Int 35:179
39. Silver BJ, Jaffer FE, Abboud HE (1989) Platelet-derived growth factor synthesis in mesangial cells: induction by multiple peptide mitogens. Proc Natl Acad Sci USA 86:1056–1060

40. Martin M, Schwinzer R, Schellekens H et al. (1989) Glomerular mesangial cells in local inflammation. Induction of the expression of MHC class II antigens by IFN-γ. J Immunol 142:1887–1894
41. Watanabe K, Nakagawa H (1990) Cytokines enhance the production of a chemotactic factor for polymorphonuclear leukocytes by rat renal glomerular epithelioid cells. Nephron 54:169–175
42. Savic V, Stefanovic V, Ardaillou N et al. (to be published) Induction of ecto-5′-nucleotidase of rat cultured mesangial cells by interleukin-1 and tumour necrosis factor-α. Immunology
43. Wiggins RC, Njoku N, Sedor JR (1990) Tissue factor production by cultured rat mesangial cells. Stimulation by TNF and lipopolysaccharide. Kidney Int 37:1281–1285
44. Davies M, Shewring L, Thomas G et al. (1989) Stimulation of proteoglycan synthesis in rat mesangial cells in response to tumour necrosing factor (abstract) Kidney Int 35:344
45. Schreiner GF, Kohan DE (1990) Regulation of renal transport processes and hemodynamics by macrophages and lymphocytes. Am J Physiol 258:F761–F767

The Renal Biology of Endothelins

Barry M. Brenner[1,2] and Andrew J. King[1,2]

Summary. Endothelin (ET) is distinguished from other endogenous vasoactive peptides by its biphasic pressure response and its sustained duration of action. There is marked regional variability in the sensitivity to either the vasodilatory or the vasoconstrictor effects of ET. The renal vascular bed is exquisitely sensitive and may be an important target organ for ET. The extent to which ET functions as an autocrine, paracrine, or circulating mediator is as yet unclear. Evidence suggests that ET may play a role as a mediator of chronic volume and blood pressure regulation and contribute to sustained renal ischemia in pathophysiological states. Eventual development of effective blockers of ET action will aid in understanding the in vivo effects of ET.

Introduction

It is now well recognized that the endothelium lining the vasculature is capable of transducing hemodynamic and humoral signals into appropriate changes in vascular smooth muscle tone [1]. The effector branch of the endothelial cell response to these mechanical and chemical signals is mediated, at least in part, by auto-production of soluble vasodilating and vasoconstricting factors [2]. Two such vasorelaxants are prostacyclin and endothelium-derived relaxing factor (EDRF). EDRF activity stems in part from nitric oxide (NO), derived from the guanido nitrogen(s) of L-arginine [3], as well as nitrosothiols [4]. Recently, vascular endothelium has also been shown to synthesize endothelin (ET), a 21 amino acid polypeptide with potent vasocon-

[1]Renal Division and Department of Medicine, Brigham and Women's Hospital, Boston, MA 02115, USA

[2]The Harvard Center for the Study of Kidney Diseases, Harvard Medical School, Boston, MA 02115, USA

strictor properties [5]. This review focuses primarily on the role of ET in the modulation of glomerular function.

The original discovery of ET by Yanagisawa et al. [5] stimulated a burst of investigation into the role of this family of peptides in the modulation of regional and systemic hemodynamics. First isolated and purified from porcine aortic endothelial cells, ET-1 is a 21 amino acid peptide encoded by a single gene [5]. Three isoforms have been identified (ET-1,2,3), and are present in all species examined [6]. Isolated vascular rings and muscle strips respond to ET with a sustained contractile response accompanied by a rise in intracellular free calcium and an increase in inositol trisphosphate [5,7]. Intravenous bolus ET leads to a biphasic systemic pressor response, which results from transient systemic vasodilation followed by sustained vasoconstriction [5,6]. The initial vasodilation appears to be due to ET-induced EDRF release in that L-NMMA, an analog of L-arginine (L-Arg) which competitively inhibits the conversion of L-Arg to NO, markedly attenuates the hypotensive effects of ET-1 in anesthetized rats.

Renal Endothelin Receptors

Autoradiographic studies using ^{125}I ET-1 reveal high affinity binding to glomeruli, vasa recta bundles, and the inner medulla, a distribution of binding which is similar to that of atrial natriuretic peptide (ANP) and angiotensin II (AII) [9,10]. High affinity binding sites are also present on cultured glomerular mesangial cells [11–13]. Cross-linking of ^{125}ET-1 to intact rat mesangial cells reveals two binding proteins of 60kDa and 73kDa [12]. Both ET-1 and ET-2 bind to the higher molecular weight receptor, whereas all 3 ET isoforms bind to the smaller protein. An increase in mesangial cytosolic free calcium occurs in response to ET, implying that these binding sites represent true receptors (see below) [7,14,15].

Synthesis of Endothelin

Expression of preproendothelin-1 mRNA in porcine aortic endothelium is increased by a variety of chemical and mechanical stimuli, including the calcium ionophore A23187, thrombin, epinephrine [5], transforming growth factor β (TGF β) [16] and enhanced shear stress [17]. Expression of a 2.3 kb preproendothelin-1 mRNA in cultured bovine glomerular endothelial cells has been shown by Northern analysis using a full length preproendothelin-1 cDNA [18]. This expression is enhanced by co-incubation with agonists known to increase glomerular endothelial cytosolic free calcium, including bradykinin, thrombin, ATP and platelet activating factor [18]. In addition, under basal conditions, glomerular endothelial cells release ET in a time-dependent fashion, a response markedly enhanced by co-incubation with bradykinin [18]. Finally, several renal epithelial cell lines (MDCK, $LLCPK_1$) release ET-1 in a time-dependent fashion [19,20]. Taken together, the evidence for glomerular and renal epithelial cell ET biosynthetic capabilities and the widespread renal ET binding sites strongly suggest a local role for ET in the modulation of renal hemodynamics.

Whole Kidney Responses

When administered intravenously or directly into the renal artery of intact animals, ET induces dose-dependent renal vasoconstriction [11,21,22]. As a renal vasoconstrictor, ET-1 is up to 30 times more potent than AII [21]. As with the systemic response, transient renal vasodilation precedes vasoconstriction.

In anesthetized rats, intravenous boluses of ET-1 result in dose-dependent and sustained reductions of renal plasma flow (RPF) with variable effects on glomerular filtration rate (GFR) [22]. Moderate doses of ET lead to a proportionately greater reduction in RPF than GFR; thus, filtration fraction increases. Higher doses lead to parallel reduction in RPF and GFR [22]. Others have noted parallel reduction of GFR and RPF when ET is infused into the renal artery of rats, or with intravenous infusion in dogs [23]. A similar pattern is seen in isolated perfused kidneys, indicating that the renal response is independent of the systemic effects [21].

Co-infusion of dihydropyridine Ca^{2+} channel blockers with ET into rat renal arteries markedly blunts the vasoconstrictor response, suggesting that renal vasoconstriction is, at least in part, due to the activation of voltage-sensitive Ca^{2+} channels [23]. Co-infusion of pharmacologic doses of ANP, which stimulates particulate guanylate cyclase, also blunts the systemic and renal effects of endothelin [23,24]. Although ET is a potent secretagogue of ANP [25], it is unclear whether ANP exerts a counter-regulatory influence on ET in vivo [23].

Intravenous ET administration, in doses which do not severely compromise filtration, induces a modest natriuresis in rats [22]. When renal perfusion pressure is maintained constant with an aortic snare, the natriuresis is attenuated, suggesting that this effect is, at least in part, pressure-related [22]. In suspensions of rabbit inner medullary collecting duct cells, ET also reduces ouabain-sensitive O_2 consumption, an effect not seen in proximal tubule cells [26]. A reduction of the initial rate of Rb^+ uptake by ET implies decreased Na^+/K^+ ATPase activity. This response is blocked by the cyclooxygenase inhibitor, ibuprofen, suggesting that inhibition of transport is mediated by prostanoids. Indeed, in collecting duct cells, ET stimulates release of PGE_2, a known inhibitor of Na^+/K^+ ATPase in these cells [26]. Autoradiographic labeling of renal parenchyma by ^{125}I ET reveals intense staining of the inner medulla [9,10]. In addition, as noted above, several renal epithelial cell lines synthesize and release ET [19,20] raising the possibility that locally generated ET modulates renal medullary transport functions independent of its renal hemodynamic effects.

Effects of Endothelin on Glomerular Hemodynamics

Afferent and efferent arterioles, the primary resistance vessels of the kidney, are highly sensitive to the vasoconstrictive effects of ET; thus, ET has marked effects on the determinants of glomerular ultrafiltration [14,22,24,27,28]. Studies to date have shown differing sensitivity of the pre- and post-glomerular arterioles, depending primarily on the dose and route of administration. Intravenous infusion of mildly pressor doses of ET (0.63 pmol/min) into anesthetized rats leads to a proportionately greater increase in efferent than in afferent arteriolar resistance, hence an increase in mean glomerular capillary hydraulic pressure ($\bar{P}_{GC}$) [22]. Offsetting this profiltration force is a fall in the glomerular capillary plasma flow rate (Q_A); thus at this low dose, single nephron glomerular filtration rate (SNGFR) remains relatively constant [22]. Higher doses of ET-1 (10 pmol/min) also lead to a proportionately greater increase in efferent than in afferent arteriolar tone [14]. This dose causes more intense renal vasoconstriction, leading to a fall in Q_A. This, in conjunction with a marked reduction in K_f, leads to a fall in SNGFR [14]. In keeping with these findings, studies of isolated perfused glomerular arterioles demonstrate that half-maximal contraction of efferent arterioles ($3.2 \pm 4.0 \times 10^{-12}$M) is achieved with doses 3 orders of magnitude less than for afferent arterioles ($1.4 \pm 2.5 \times 10^{-9}$M) [28]. This vasoconstriction is unaffected by co-infusion of saralasin, an AII receptor antagonist [28]. By contrast, direct infusion of ET (0.16 pmol/min) into a branch of the renal artery leads to predominant afferent arteriolar constriction, a reduction in $\bar{P}_{GC}$, and no significant effect on K_f [29]. A similar pattern of constriction is also noted in isolated perfused hydronephrotic kidneys [27]. Overall, these studies highlight the sensitivity of the glomerular microvasculature to exogenous ET, with nearly all of the determinants of glomerular ultrafiltration being affected.

Effects of Endothelin on Mesangial Cells

Angiotensin II, norepinephrine and arginine vasopressin are each capable of inducing a contractile response in mesangial cells, thereby contributing to the fall in the K_f seen with these agents. Similarly, ET induces dose-dependent contractile effects on cultured mesangial cells [14,30,31]. In these cells ET led to rearrangements of F actin microfilament bundles, consistent with a motile response [31]. As with other vasoconstrictors the contractile effects of ET on mesangial cells may be dampened by concurrent stimulation of prostanoids. Phospholipase A_2 activity is stimulated by ET, leading to increased arachidonate release from mesangial cells as well as release of $PGE_2 > PGI_2 > TXA_2$ [31]. Furthermore, ET-induced PGE_2 production significantly potentiates β agonist-induced cAMP production, which also serves to dampen mesangial contraction [31]. These results suggest that the reduction in K_f by ET is, at least in part, due to mesangial cell contraction.

Mesangial cells respond to low dose (10 pM) ET-1 infusion with a slow rise in cytosolic free calcium, an effect blocked by EGTA but not by nifedipine [15]. Higher doses lead to a brisk increase in intracellular free calcium, followed by a slow return toward baseline. EGTA has no effect on the early rise in Ca^{2+} but abrogates the tonic phase of calcium elevation. These results suggest that, as with the vascular smooth muscle cells, the rapid phase is associated with the release of calcium from intracellular stores, whereas entry of external calcium contributes to the delayed phase. The rise in intracellular Ca^{2+} is paralleled by an increase in inositol phosphate turnover, indicating activation of phospholipase C. Finally, ET is a potent co-mitogen in quiescent mesangial cells, but not in Swiss 3T3 fibroblasts [14,15]. This response may relate to ET-induced activation of Na^+/H^+ exchange. In addition, ET significantly stimulates expression of the proto-oncogenes *c-fos* in mesangial cells and *c-myc/c-fos* in vascular smooth muscle cells, suggesting a possible role for ET in vascular and glomerular hypertrophy [15,32].

Potential Role of Endothelin in Acute Renal Failure

Cyclosporine (CyA) therapy in humans and animals induces marked renal vasoconstriction with a reduction of GFR [33]. Several studies have recently implicated ET in this renal vasoconstrictor response [34,35]. CyA-induced vasoconstriction in isolated perfused rat kidneys is largely overcome by co-infusion of anti-ET antibody, but not by non-immune serum [34]. Studies of intravenous CyA with simultaneous intrarenal artery infusion of anti-ET in rats corroborate these findings in vivo [35]. These studies suggest a role for ET in acute CyA-induced renal vasoconstriction. Whether ET is an important mediator in chronic cyclosporine toxicity awaits further investigation. In addition to augmented ET production, endothelium-dependent vasodilatory responses may also be impaired, since isolated perfused kidneys from CyA-treated rats exhibit shifts of the vasodilatory dose response curves to acetylcholine [36].

Despite an impaired ability of the ischemic kidney to respond to endothelium-dependent vasodilators, there is recent evidence to suggest that ischemia augments ET production. Infusion of anti-ET antibody into a branch of a rat renal artery significantly ameliorates renal vasoconstriction induced by 25 minutes of ischemia [29]. Whether this reflects an increase in local production of ET and/or a change in receptor number or binding is as yet unclear. Of interest, however, ET binding site density of rat cardiac membranes is markedly increased by ischemia [37]. Small changes in affinity occur with ischemia of > 30 minutes duration. Increased binding site density is further enhanced by reperfusion, and is prevented by hypothermic perfusion [37]. Whether similar changes take place in the kidney is not yet known. Taken together, the effects of ischemia on ET receptor density and the stimulation of ET production by CyA may have important implications in the pathogenesis of early renal allograft dysfunction.

Finally, acute infusion of endotoxin in rats is well known to induce renal vasoconstriction [38]. Rats and sheep infused with endotoxin have marked increases in plasma ET concentrations which may contribute to this vasoconstriction [39,40]. Endotoxin also induces NO production from vascular smooth muscle cells [41], which may counterbalance the effects of ET. Plasma levels of ET are elevated in patients with acute renal failure from a variety of causes, and fall with improvement of renal function [42]. Accordingly, future studies are required to determine whether blockade of ET production and/or binding will prove beneficial in the treatment of acute renal failure.

Acknowledgments. Andrew J. King is the recipient of an Individual National Research Service Award of the NIH (1F32DK08003). Studies were supported in part by NIH grant DK35930.

References

1. Brenner BM, Troy JL, Ballermann BJ (1989) Endothelium-dependent vascular responses. Mediators and Mechanisms. J Clin Invest 84:1373–1378
2. Davies PF, Oleson SP, Clapham DE, Morrel EM, Schoen FJ (1988) Endothelial Communication. State of the art lecture. Hypertension 11:563–572

3. Palmer RMJ, Ferrige AG, Moncada S (1987) Nitric oxide release accounts for the biological activity of endothelium-derived relaxing factor. Nature 327:524–526
4. Myers PR, Minor RLJ, Guerra RJ, Bates JN, Harrison DG (1990) Vasorelaxant properties of the endothelium-derived relaxing factor more closely resemble S-nitrocysteine than nitric oxide. Nature 345:161–163
5. Yanagisawa M, Kurihara H, Kimura S, Tomobe Y, Kobayashi M, Mitsui Y, Yazaki Y, Goto K, Masaki T (1988) A novel potent vasoconstrictor peptide produced by vascular endothelial cells. Nature 332:411–415
6. Inoue A, Yanagisawa M, Kimura S, Kasuya Y, Miyauchi T, Goto K, Masaki T (1989) The human endothelin family: three structurally and pharmacologically distinct isopeptides predicted by three separate genes. Proc Natl Acad Sci USA 86:2863–2867
7. Marsden PA, Danthuluri NR, Brenner BM, Ballermann BJ, Brock TA (1989) Endothelin action on vascular smooth muscle involves inositol trisphosphate and calcium mobilization. Biochem Biophys Res Commun 158:86–93
8. Whittle BJR, Lopez-Belmonte J, Rees DD (1989) Modulation of the vasodepressor actions of acetylcholine, bradykinin, substance P and endothelin in the rat by a specific inhibitor of nitric oxide formation. Br J Pharmacol 98:646–652
9. Kohzuki MC, Johnston CI, Chai SY, Casley DJ, Mendelsohn FAO (1989) Localization of endothelin receptors in rat kidney. Eur J Pharmacol 160:193–194
10. Koseki C, Imai M, Hirata Y, Yanagisawa M, Masaki T (1989) Autoradiographic distribution in rat tissues of binding sites for endothelin: a neuropeptide? Am J Physiol 256:R858–R866
11. Badr KF, Munger KA, Sugiura M, Snajdar RM, Schwartzberg M, Inagami T (1989) High and low affinity binding sites for endothelin on cultured rat glomerular mesangial cells. Biochem Biophys Res Commun 161:776–781
12. Martin ER, Brenner BM, Ballermann BJ (to be published) Heterogeneity of cell surface endothelin receptors. J Biol Chem
13. Sugiura M, Snajdar RM, Schwartzberg M, Badr KF, Inagami T (1989) Identification of two types of specific endothelin receptors in rat mesangial cells. Biochem Biophys Res Commun 162:1396–1401
14. Badr KF, Murray JJ, Breyer MD, Takahashi K, Inagami T, Harris RC (1989) Mesangial cell, glomerular and renal vascular responses to endothelin in the rat kidney. J Clin Invest 83:336–342
15. Simonson MS, Wann S, Mene P, Dubyak GR, Kester M, Nakazato Y, Sedor JR, Dunn MJ (1989) Endothelin stimulates phospholipase C, Na/H exchange, c-fos expression, and mitogenesis in rat mesangial cells. J Clin Invest 83:708–712
16. Kurihara H, Yoshizumi M, Takaku M, Yanagisawa M, Masaki T, Hamaoki M, Kato H, Yazaki Y (1989) Transforming growth factor β stimulates the expression of endothelin mRNA by vascular endothelial cells. Biochem Biophys Res Commun 159:1435–1440
17. Yoshizumi M, Kurihara H, Sugiyama T, Takaku F, Yanagisawa M, Masaki T, Yazaki Y (1989) Hemodynamic shear stress stimulates endothelin production by cultured endothelial cells. Biochem Biophys Res Commun 161:859–864
18. Marsden PA, Dorfman DM, Brenner BM, Orkin BJ, Ballermann BJ (1989) Endothelin: gene expression, release and action in cultured cells of the renal glomerulus. Am J Hypertens 2(2):49A
19. Kosaka T, Suzuki N, Matsumoto H, Itoh Y, Yasuhara T, Onda H, Fujino M (1989) Synthesis of the vasoconstrictor peptide endothelin in kidney cells. FEBS Lett 249:42–46
20. Shichiri M, Hirata Y, Emori T, Ohta K, Nakajima T, Sato K, Sato A, Marumo F (1989) Secretion of endothelin and related peptides from renal epithelial cell lines. FEBS Lett 253:203–206
21. Cairns HS, Rogerson ME, Fairbanks LD, Neild GH, Westwick J (1989) Endothelin induces

an increase in renal vascular resistance and a fall in glomerular filtration rate in the rabbit isolated perfused kidney. Br J Pharmacol 98:155–160
22. King AJ, Brenner BM, Anderson S (1989) Endothelin: a potent renal and systemic vasoconstrictor peptide. Am J Physiol 256:F1051–F1058
23. Katoh T, Chang H, Uchida S, Okuda T, Kurakawa K (1990) Direct effects of endothelin in the rat kidney. Am J Physiol 258:F397–F402
24. Hirata Y, Matsuoka H, Kimura K, Fukui K, Hayakawa H, Suzuki E, Sugimoto T, Yanagisawa M, Masaki T (1989) Renal vasoconstriction by the endothelial cell-derived peptide endothelin in spontaneously hypertensive rats. Circ Res 65:1370–1379
25. Mantymaa P, Leppaluoto J, Ruskoaho H (1990) Endothelin stimulates basal stretch-induced atrial natriuretic peptide secretion from the perfused rat heart. Endocrinology 126:587–595
26. Zeidel ML, Brady HR, Kone BC, Gullans SR, Brenner BM (1989) Endothelin, a peptide inhibitor of Na/K ATPase in intact renal tubular epithelial cells. Am J Physiol 257: C1101–C1107
27. Loutzenhiser R, Epstein M, Hayashi K, Horton C (1990) Direct visualization of effects of endothelin on the renal microvasculature. Am J Physiol 258:F61–F68
28. Yuan BH, McMurtry IF, Conger JD (1989) Effect of endothelin on isolated perfused rat afferent and efferent arterioles. Clin Res 37:586A
29. Kon V, Yoshioka T, Fogo A, Ichikawa I (1989) Glomerular actions of endothelin in vivo. J Clin Invest 83:1762–1767
30. Culebras M, Montanes I, Lopez-Farre A, Millas I, Lopez-Novoa JM (1989) Effect of endothelin on renal function and on the contraction of cultured rat mesangial cells. Med Sci Res 17:245–246
31. Sinmonson MS, Dunn MJ (1990) Endothelin-1 stimulates contraction of rat glomerular mesangial cells and potentiates β-adrenergic-mediated cyclic adenosine monophosphate accumulation. J Clin Invest 85:790–797
32. Komuro I, Kurihara H, Sugiyama T, Yoshizumi M, Takaku F, Yazaki Y (1988) Endothelin stimulates c-fos and c-myc expression and proliferation of vascular smooth muscle cells. FEBS Lett. 238:249–252
33. Myers B (1986) Cyclosporine nephrotoxicity. Kidney Int 30:964–974
34. Dedan J, Perico N, Remuzzi G (1990) Role of endothelin in cyclosporine-induced renal vasoconstriction. Kidney Int 37:479A
35. Kon V, Sugiura M, Inagami T, Harvie BR, Ichikawa I, Hoover RL (1990) Role of endothelin in cyclosporin-induced glomerular dysfunction. Kidney Int 37:1487–1491
36. Gerkins JF (1989) Cyclosporine treatment of normal rats produces a rise in blood pressure and decreased renal vascular responses to nerve stimulated, vasoconstrictors and endothelium-dependent dilators. J Pharmacol Exp Ther 250:1105–1112
37. Liu J, Chen R, Casley DJ, Nayler WG. Ischemia and reperfusion increase ^{125}I-labeled endothelin-1 binding in rat cardiac membranes. Am J Physiol 258:H829–H835
38. Badr KF, Kelley VE, Rennke HG, Brenner BM (1986) Roles for thromboxane A and leukotrienes in endotoxin-induced acute renal failure. Kidney Int 30:474–480
39. Morel DR, Lacroix JS, Hemsen A, Steinig A, Pittet JF, Lundberg JM (1989) Increased plasma and pulmonary lymph levels of endothelin during endotoxin shock. Eur J Pharmacol 167:427–428
40. Sugiura M, Inagami T, Kon V (1989) Endotoxin stimulates endothelin-release in vivo and in vitro as determined by radioimmunoassay. Biochem Biophys Res Commun 161:1220–1227
41. Beasley D, Brenner BM, Schwartz JH (1990) Interleukin-1 activates guanylate cyclase in rat vascular smooth muscle cells by inducing nitric oxide. FASEB J 4:685A
42. Tomita K, Ujiie K, Nakanishi T, Tomura S, Matsuda O, Ando K, Shichiri M, Hirata Y, Marumo F (1990) Plasma endothelin levels in patients with acute renal failure (letter). N Engl J Med 321:1127

Effect of Insulin-Like Growth Factor-I on Glomerular Cells in Vitro

Liliane J. Striker[1]

Summary. Since mesangial proliferation is the hallmark of many human glomerular diseases we investigated whether glomerular cells have receptors for insulin-like growth factor-I (IGF-I), a growth peptide. All three glomerular cell types; mesangial, epithelial, and endothelial cells were found to have surface receptors for IGF-I. This peptide was a potent mitogen for mesangial cells in vitro and acted as a progression factor. In addition, IGF-I-like molecules may play an important role in glomerular disease.

Introduction

The insulin-growth factors are a family of peptides that were originally discovered in the late 1950s. The early work was performed by Salmon and Daughaday [1], who established that one of the major effects of growth hormone was mediated through the production of a liver factor which stimulated the incorporation of labeled SO_4 into cartilage, which was therefore called "sulfation-factor." This soluble factor was further characterized and was shown to exert multiple effects on cell mitogenesis and differentiation. The term "Somatomedin," coined in 1972, was further completely replaced by that of Insulin-like growth factor (IGF-I). In 1978, Rinkerknecht and Humbel [2], isolated two peptides, with a molecular weight of 7500, from human plasma. One of these peptides, which contained 70 amino-acids, was basic (pI 8.1–8.5) and had a 48% structural homology with proinsulin. Because of this homology, and because this peptide had some effects comparable to those known for insulin in vivo, these investigators proposed the name of IGF-I for this molecule.

Whereas it was initially assumed that IGF-I was exclusively synthesized in the liver and acted as a hormone on the target organs, it was subsequently shown that this pep-

[1]NIDDK, MDB, National Institute of Health, Building 10, Room 3 N 110, Bethesda, MD 20892, USA

tide was produced locally by multiple tissues [3]. The production of IGF-I was also found to be regulated not only by growth hormone (GH), but also by multiple other factors. In the plasma, IGF-I binds to carrier proteins called IGF-1 binding proteins (IGF-BP) [4,5].

Several lines of evidence support a role for IGF-I in the kidney [6]. The administration of this peptide to intact animals is accompanied by an increase in glomerular filtration rate [7]. In addition, following a unilateral nephrectomy, there is an increase in the level of extractable IGF-I in the remaining kidney, suggesting that this peptide is a growth factor for the kidney [6,8]. We have examined whether glomerular cells had receptors for IGF-I. We found that this peptide was a mitogen for mesangial cells [9,10]. These cells produced IGF-I and IGF-I binding proteins in a coordinate fashion, suggesting that the glomerulus is an important target for this peptide [11]. The present paper reviews the evidence gathered in our laboratory that IGF-I plays a role in the physiology of mouse and human glomerular cells in vitro.

Receptors for IGF-I on Mesangial Cells

Mouse Mesangial Cells

Material and Methods

Mesangial cells were isolated and propagated, according to methods previously published, from a strain of mice which is devoid of glomerular disease [12]. The cells were characterized and subcultured as described [9]. These elongated cells contained long parallel actin filaments, but no cytokeratin or von-Willebrand antigen; these two features characterizing epithelial or endothelial cells, respectively.

All studies were performed on cells between passages 8 and 20. To ensure that these were a representative mesangial population, experiments were repeated on a second cell line, isolated independently from the initial glomerular outgrowth.

All experiments were performed on confluent cells. These were incubated in serum-free medium for 15 hours. The binding studies were performed on monolayers, as reported by Conti et al. [9]. The conditions were optimized for temperature, time, and pH dependency. The specificity of IGF-I binding was determined using unlabeled recombinant IGF-I, porcine insulin, and MSA (rat IGF-II). At the end of the incubation period the monolayers were washed and solubilized in order to measure the cell-associated radioactivity. The radioactivity bound in the presence of an excess of unlabeled IGF-I represented the non-specific binding, which was subtracted from the total to calculate the specific binding.

To assess the mitogenic effect of IGF-I, mesangial cells were plated in medium containing 20% serum. Twenty-four hours later the medium was removed and the cells were repeatedly washed; the medium was then changed to serum-free medium supplemented with 0.1% of bovine serum albumin (BSA). After a period varying from 24 to 72 hours, the cells were incubated in fresh serum-free medium containing IGF-I. Sixteen hours later, ^{3}H thymidine was added for a total of 4 hours. The cell layer was solubilized with NaOH and counted.

Table 1. Analysis according to scatchard

Cell type	Kd	Number of receptors/cell
Human mesangial cells	1.35×10^{-9}	1.04×10^{5}
Mouse mesangial cells	1.27×10^{-9}	0.64×10^{5}
Mouse endothelial cells	2.25×10^{-9}	1.62×10^{5}
Mouse epithelial cells	1.5×10^{-9}	2.45×10^{5}

Results

Radiolabeled IGF-I bound specifically to the mesangial cell surface. The binding was dependent on time and temperature. The pH-dependence of the binding was comparable to that found for other cell types. Non-specific binding accounted for only 10% of total binding. Degradation of the tracer appeared to be minimal. The optimal conditions selected for competition experiments were 150 minutes, 15°C, and a pH of 7.8. A type I receptor was identified in competition studies utilizing unlabeled IGF-I, insulin, and IGF-II. The estimated kd was 1.27×10^{-9}. The number of receptors was calculated to be 64×10^{4} per cell. (Tables 1 and 2). This receptor was further characterized using solubilized cell fractions and wheat-germ agglutinin eluates (WGA). The kd obtained from the receptor preparation and from WGA eluates were, respectively, 2.3×10^{-9} and 3.7×10^{-10}.

The peak of mitogenesis, as detected by thymidine incorporation, occurred 18 hours after the addition of IGF-1. As shown in Table 2, there was a 2.6-fold increase above the levels found for unstimulated cells.

Human Mesangial Cells

Material and Methods

Normal human glomeruli were obtained from the non affected areas of kidneys removed for cancer or from organs not used for transplantation. The initial outgrowth appeared within one week after the initial plating. Patches of elongated cells were selected with cloning rings and were dilute-plated until we obtained homogenous cells which were further identified as mesangial populations. Mesangial cells appeared initially stellate before they reached confluence, after which they formed a multilayer of parallel arrays. The cells contained long filaments of actin, and also contained desmin, myosin, and vimentin intermediate filaments. There was

Table 2. Mitogenesis

Cell type	Dose of IGF-I	Exposure (hours)	Increase over control
Human mesangial cells	10 ng/ml	14	2.1
Mouse mesangial cells	10 ng/ml	18	2.5
Mouse endothelial cells	10 ng/ml	18	1.10
Mouse epithelial cells	10 ng/ml	18	1.47

specific angiotensin-II binding on the surface of the cells, as reported by Doi et al. [10]. All the studies were performed between passages 4 and 9.

The binding experiments were performed using the same method as those described above for mouse mesangial cells. In addition, we examined the effect of various concentrations of a monoclonal antibody directed against the IGF-I receptor (αIR-3) on the IGF-I binding to the receptor. The presence of IGF-I receptors was also examined on the surface of the cells by immunofluorescence microscopy, using the same antibody.

SDS-polyacrylamide gel electrophoresis and autoradiographic studies were performed on immunoprecipitates obtained by incubating αIGF-3 with receptor-enriched preparations obtained by WGA chromatography.

Studies of mitogenesis were completed by an analysis of the labeling index. Briefly, cells were plated on plastic chamber-slides. They were stimulated for optimal periods by the various ligands of interest, in the presence of ^{3}H thymidine. Autoradiography was performed on the slides. The labeling index was expressed as the percentage of nuclei labeled [10].

Results

The binding of radiolabeled IGF-I was measured on cells that had been starved for 0–48 hours. The maximal binding was reached at 12 hours and was 27.2% + 2.6% per 10^6 cells after an incubation period of 150 minutes, with a non-specific binding of 3.8%. Analysis of the data by Scatchard's method indicated that the cells had a single type of receptor with a kd of 1.35×10^{-9}. The estimated number of receptors per cell was 1.04×10^5.

The antibody to the receptor inhibited the IGF-I binding in a dose-dependent manner. By immunofluorescence, this antibody stained a large number of small dots over the cell surface, presumably representing coated pits present on the cell membranes. The identification of the receptor revealed two major bands, of 130 k and 90 k, which are thought to correspond to the α and β subunits of the receptor. A minor band of 150 kd also found in the precipitate was presumed to represent partially reduced α and β fragments.

The mitogenesis was measured by thymidine incorporation after the addition of either IGF-I or insulin. Following the addition of recombinant IGF-I, there was a dose-dependent increase in mitogenesis (Table 1). In contrast, there was only a minor increase in response to high doses of insulin, suggesting that the observed effect was mediated through the IGF-I receptor. The labeling index, which was used to deter-

Table 3. Labeling index

Ligands	Labeling index (% labeled nuclei)
Control	1.06
PDGF	2.01
IGF-I	3.35
PDGF + IGF-I	5.19
PDGF + IGF-I (sequentially)	5.27

mine the number of cells entering S phase, showed that IGF-I was much more efficient if the cells were initially exposed to a competence factor, such as platelet-derived growth factor (PDGF). These data confirm that the effect of IGF-I is that of a progression factor. (Table 3) [10,13,14].

Receptors for IGF-I on Mouse Endothelial and Epithelial Cells

Materials and Methods

Glomerular endothelial and epithelial cells from normal mice were established, maintained, and identified in culture, as previously described [12]. All experiments were performed on cells between passages 14 and 25. Endothelial or epithelial cells were plated in 35mm dishes or 24 well dishes in their respective complete media. Experiments were performed on confluent cells, following a 16 hour preincubation in serum-free medium, as described above for mesangial cells.

To perform IGF-I receptor crosslinking, cells were grown to confluence in 100mm dishes and were incubated with [^{125}I]IGF-I, in the presence or absence of excess cold IGF-I or insulin, under standard binding conditions. The [^{125}I]IGF-I bound to its receptor was cross-linked by the addition of DSS [10]. The cells were solubilized, collected, and concentrated. The sample was then electrophoresed, under reducing conditions, on an SDS-polyacrylamide gel and was exposed for autoradiography.

Results

Specific [^{125}I]IGF-I binding to glomerular endothelial and epithelial cells was time and temperature dependent, and the optimal pH was found to be 7.8. In both cell types non-specific binding accounted for less than 10% of the total binding and it did not increase over time. The kd was 2.25×10^{-9} for endothelial cells and 1.5×10^{-9} for epithelial cells.

A single radioactive band was obtained in both endothelial and epithelial cell extracts. The apparent molecular weight under reducing conditions was 145k and 142k, respectively. This band was no longer detectable when cells were incubated in the presence of unlabeled IGF-I, and its intensity decreased when cells were incubated with insulin [15].

Endothelial and epithelial cells failed to show any mitogenic activity following exposure to IGF-I, using conditions under which this peptide could stimulate mesangial cell mitogenesis (Table 1).

Release of Insulin-Like Growth Factor I by Mesangial Cells in Culture

Materials and Methods

Mesangial cells were grown to approximately 80% confluence, washed with basal medium, and incubated in serum-free medium containing 0.1% BSA. This medium was discarded and the cells were incubated for up to 72 hours in fresh basal medium which was collected for further analysis.

The culture medium was centrifuged and acidified as previously described [11], in order to dissociate free IGF from binding proteins. After concentration, the samples were treated by manual reverse-phase chromatography with Sep-pak c18 cartridges. After extraction, it was found that the recovery of IGF-I was as high as 80%–90%.

IGF-I activity was detected by two methods: a radioimmunoassay, using a polyclonal antibody to human IGF-I (UBK 487) generated by L.E. Underwood, and provided by the NIDDK and the National hormone and pituitary program (University of Maryland, School of Medicine). The antibody was used at a dilution of 1:18 000. Human recombinant IGF-I was used as a standard and [^{125}I]IGF-I was used as the tracer.

In addition, IGF-I was measured by the ability of the cell culture medium to inhibit IGF-I binding to mouse mesangial cell culture in the radioreceptor assay, as described above.

Results

The supernatant of glomerular mesangial cells contained an immunoreactive IGF-I-like molecule. In contrast, supernatants from either endothelial or epithelial cells did not contain immunoreactive IGF-I. These results were confirmed independently, using a radioreceptor assay. The concentration of IGF-I was much higher (tenfold) using this method, as compared to the radioimmunoassay, presumably because the antibody used was directed against human, rather than mouse, IGF-I.

Finally, using reverse-phase chromatography, it was established that samples of supernatants from mesangial cells contained a single peak of IGF-I activity.

In addition, we examined the amount of IGF-I released by mesangial cells and found that it was regulated by cell density. Sparse cells released greater amounts of IGF-I-like molecules than did confluent cells. In parallel, mesangial cells released an IGF-I binding protein.

Discussion

The presence of specific receptors on all three glomerular cell types supports the hypothesis that IGF-I plays a role in glomerular cell physiology. Furthermore, IGF-I acted as a progression factor for mesangial cells when these were made competent after exposure to PDGF. In contrast, endothelial and epithelial cells did not exhibit any mitogenesis after exposure to IGF-I.

Other investigators have reported the presence of receptors for IGF-I in glomerular mesangial cells from other species [16–18]. The significance of these findings in vivo is not yet elucidated. A dysregulation of mesangial cell mitogenesis in vivo may be one of the pathological events leading to glomerular diseases which progress to sclerosis. This would be envisaged in diseases as diverse as diabetes mellitus, IgA disease, light chain systemic disease, and membranoproliferative glomerulonephritis. In this group of disorders, proliferation of resident cells from the mesangial areas constitutes the initial event, which is further followed by increased matrix formation [19,20].

Mesangial cells respond to multiple combinations of growth-related peptides in vitro [21]. Normally, their growth in vivo is tightly regulated and appears minimal, as shown by autoradiographic studies performed in rats and mice [22,23]. These cells are capable not only of responding to IGF-I, but also of releasing an immunoreactive IGF-I molecule.

Furthermore, we found that mesangial cells produced IGF-I binding proteins [24]. In mouse mesangial cells, the release of IGF-BP was coordinately regulated with that of IGF-I molecules. These observations suggest that the IGF-I axis is quite important in the biology of mesangial cells. The normal regulation of IGF-I and IGF-I binding protein release is not yet elucidated. Our preliminary findings suggest, however, that cells which are confluent produce much less IGF-I and IGF-BP than do sparse cells. These observations favor a role for IGF-I in the control of mesangial cell proliferation and suggest that alterations of this regulation could be an important factor in progressive glomerular disease.

The role of IGF-I in vivo is not yet elucidated. In mice transgenic for IGF-I, we have observed an increase in the size of the glomeruli and a mild mesangial proliferation, contrasting with lesions that occur in growth-hormone transgenic mice [25]. Further analysis will be required to establish the role of IGF-I in disease states.

References

1. Salmon WD, Daughaday WH (1957) A hormonally controlled serum factor which stimulates sulfate incorporation by cartilage in vitro. J Lab Clin Med 49:825–836
2. Rinderknecht E, Humbel RE (1978) The amino acid sequence of human insulin-like growth factor-I and its structural homology with proinsulin. J Biol Chem 253:2769–2776
3. D'Ercole AJ, Stiles AD, Underwood LE (1984) Tissue concentrations of somatomedin-C: further evidence for multiple sites of synthesis and paracrine or autocrine mechanisms of action. Proc Natl Acad Sci USA 81:935–939
4. Froesch ER, Schmid C, Schwander J, Zapp J (1985) Actions of insulin-like growth factors. Annu Rev Physiol 47:443–467
5. Rechler MM, Nissley SP (1985) The nature and regulation of the receptors for insulin-like growth factors. Annu Rev Physiol 47:425–442
6. Hammerman MR (1989) The growth hormone-insulin-like growth factor axis in kidney. Am J Physiol 257:F503–F514
7. Hirschberg R, Kopple JD (1989) Evidence that insulin-like growth factor I increases renal plasma flow and glomerular filtration rate in fasted rats. J Clin Invest 83:326–330
8. Fagin JA, Melmed S (1987) Relative increase in insulin-like growth factor I messenger ribonucleic acid levels in compensatory renal hypertrophy. Endocrinology 120:718–724
9. Conti FG, Striker LJ, Lesniak MA, MacKay K, Roth J, Striker GE (1988) Studies on binding and mitogenic effect of insulin and insulin-like growth factor I in glomerular mesangial cells. Endocrinology 122:2788–2795
10. Doi T, Striker LJ, Elliot SJ, Conti FG, Striker GE (1989) Insulin-like growth factor-1 is a progression factor for human mesangial cells. Am J Pathol 134:395–404
11. Conti FG, Striker LJ, Elliot SJ, Andreani D, Striker GE (1988) Synthesis and release of insulin-like growth factor I by mesangial cells in culture. Am J Physiol 255:F1214–F1219
12. MacKay K, Striker LJ, Elliot S, Pinkert CA, Brinster RL, Striker GE (1980) Glomerular epithelial, mesangial, and endothelial cell lines from transgenic mice. Kidney Int 33:677–684
13. Pfeifle B, Boeder H, Ditschuneit H (1987) Interaction of receptors for insulin-like growth factor I, platelet-derived growth factor, and fibroblast growth factor in rat aortic cells. Endocrinology 120:2251–2258

14. Stiles CD, Capone GT, Scher CD, Antoniades HN, Van Wyk JJ, Pledger WJ (1979) Dual control of cell growth by somatomedins and platelet-derived growth factor. Proc Natl Acad Sci USA 76:1279–1283
15. Conti FG, Elliot S, Striker LJ, Striker GE (1989) Binding of insulin-like growth factor-I by glomerular endothelial and epithelial cells: Further evidence for IGF-I action in the renal glomerulus. Biochem Biophys Res Commun 163:952–958
16. Aron DC, Rosenzweig JL, Abboud HE (1989) Synthesis and binding of insulin-like growth factor I by human glomerular mesangial cells. J Clin Endocrinol Metab 68:585–591
17. Arnqvist HJ, Ballerman BJ, King GL (1988) Receptor for and effects of insulin and IGF-1 in rat glomerular mesangial cells. Am J Physiol 23:C411–C416
18. Abrass CK, Raugi GJ, Gabourel LS, Lovett DH (1988) Insulin and insulin-like growth factor I binding to cultured rat glomerular mesangial cells. Endocrinology 13:2432–2439
19. Striker LJ, Doi T, Elliot S, Striker GE (1989) The contribution of mesangial cells to progressive glomerulosclerosis. In: Klahr S (ed) Seminars in nephrology, vol 9. WB Saunders, Philadelphia, pp 318–329
20. Fogo A, Ichikawa I (1989) Evidence for the central role of glomerular growth promoters in the development of sclerosis. In: Klahr S (ed) Seminars in nephrology, vol 9. WB Saunders, Philadelphia, pp 329–343
21. Jaffer F, Saunders C, Shultz P, Throckmorton D, Weinshell E, Abboud HE (1989) Regulation of mesangial cell growth by polypeptide mitogens. Am J Pathol 135:261–269
22. Pabst R, Sterzel RB (1983) Cell renewal of glomerular cell types in normal rats. An autoradiographic analysis. Kidney Int 24:626–631
23. Vancura P, Miller WL, Little JW, Malt RA (1970) Contribution of glomerular and tubular RNA synthesis to compensatory renal growth. Am J Physiol 219:78–88
24. Perfetti R, Conti FG, Elliot S, Striker LJ, Striker GE (1989) Mouse glomerular mesangial cells in culture produce IGF-I binding proteins. 71st annual meeting of Endocrinology, 1989. Seattle, United States
25. Doi T, Striker LJ, Quaife CJ, Conti FG, Palmiter RD, Behringer RR, Brinster RL, Striker GE (1988) Progressive glomerulosclerosis develops in transgenic mice chronically expressing growth hormone and growth hormone releasing factor but not in those expressing insulin-like growth factor-1. Am J Pathol 131:398–403

Frontiers of Research on Natriuretic Peptides

Chair: Thomas Maack (USA)
Fumiaki Marumo (Japan)

Brain Natriuretic Peptide is a Novel Cardiac Hormone Secreted from the Ventricle in Humans

Masashi Mukoyama, Kazuwa Nakao, Yoshihiko Saito, Yoshihiro Ogawa, Kiminori Hosoda, Shin-ichi Suga, Gotaro Shirakami, Hiroo Imura[1], Michihisa Jougasaki, Kenji Obata, and Hirofumi Yasue[2]

Summary. Using a specific radioimmunoassay for human brain natriuretic peptide (hBNP), with a monoclonal antibody against hBNP, we investigated the secretion of this peptide in comparison with that of atrial natriuretic peptide (ANP), in normal and failing human hearts. The plasma BNP-like immunoreactivity (BNP-LI) level in normal subjects was 0.90 ± 0.07 fmol/ml, which was 16% of the ANP-LI level. In contrast, the plasma BNP-LI level increased markedly in patients with congestive heart failure (CHF), with a progressive rise in proportion to the severity of CHF. The plasma BNP-LI level surpassed the ANP-LI level in cases with severe CHF, and the percentage increment of the plasma BNP-LI level in severe cases was one order of magnitude greater than that of the plasma ANP-LI level. There was a significant step-up of the plasma BNP-LI level in the coronary sinus, compared with that in the aortic root, and the difference in plasma BNP-LI levels between the coronary sinus and the aorta, $\Delta_{(CS\text{-}Ao)}$BNP, increased with the severity of CHF. In addition, the difference in BNP-LI levels between the anterior interventricular vein and the aorta ($\Delta_{(AIV\text{-}Ao)}$BNP) was comparable to $\Delta_{(CS\text{-}Ao)}$BNP, indicating that BNP is secreted predominantly from the ventricle. From these results, we conclude that BNP, a novel cardiac hormone, is secreted predominantly from the ventricle in humans, in striking contrast with ANP, which is secreted mainly from the atrium. We further conclude that as the plasma level of hBNP in CHF is more markedly augmented than that of ANP, this suggests a discrete pathophysiological role of BNP in a dual natriuretic peptide system.

[1]Second Division, Department of Medicine, Kyoto University School of Medicine, Kyoto, 606 Japan
[2]Division of Cardiology, Kumamoto University Medical School, Kumamoto, 860 Japan

Introduction

Since the discovery of atrial natriuretic peptide (ANP) in the heart, and subsequently in the brain, ANP has been implicated in body fluid homeostasis and blood pressure control, both as a hormone and as a neuropeptide [1–3]. We and others have demonstrated previously that the synthesis and secretion of ANP in the heart are increased in patients with congestive heart failure (CHF), in a manner related to the severity of CHF [4–8].

More recently, brain natriuretic peptide (BNP) was isolated from the porcine brain [9]; this peptide shows a remarkable sequence homology to ANP and has peripheral and central actions similar to those of ANP [9–12]. We demonstrated that BNP is also synthesized in, and secreted into the circulation from, the porcine heart [13]. Subsequently, we isolated BNP from the rat heart [14]. To date, however, little is known about BNP in humans, since antisera against porcine or rat BNP have failed to detect any BNP-like immunoreactivity (BNP-LI) in human tissues, suggesting a structural diversity of BNP among species.

Recently, we have isolated human BNP (hBNP) from the atrium, and determined its amino acid sequence [15]. Human BNP is composed of 32 amino acid residues, whose sequence is identical to the sequence, [77–108], of the hBNP precursor deduced from the cDNA sequence [16]. In the present study, with a monoclonal antibody against hBNP, we established a specific radioimmunoassay (RIA) for hBNP. Using the RIA, we investigated the secretion of hBNP, in comparison with that of ANP, in normal subjects and in patients with CHF.

Methods

Subjects

Eleven healthy male subjects (aged 25–33 years, mean 29.6 years) and 48 patients with heart disease (33 men and 15 women, aged 16–78 years, mean 55.0 years) were studied. They included 17 patients with coronary artery disease, 13 with valvular heart disease, 7 with dilated cardiomyopathy, 7 with hypertensive heart disease, 2 with congenital heart disease, 1 with hypertrophic obstructive cardiomyopathy, and 1 with myocarditis. According to the functional classification of the New York Heart Association (NYHA) [17], 10 patients, with no limitation of physical activity, were classified as class I, 16 patients were classified as class II, 17 as class III, and 5 as class IV, in the order of increasing cardiovascular disability. None of the patients had evidence of renal failure. Informed consent was obtained from the patients and the study was approved by the ethical committee on human research of Kyoto University (No. 61-9).

Plasma Samples

Blood for peripheral plasma samples was obtained from the antecubital vein while subjects were in a recumbent position. This procedure was performed at 9:00 A.M. after an overnight fast. The blood was transferred to chilled glass tubes containing Na_2EDTA (1 mg/ml) and aprotinin (1000 KIU/ml, Ohkura, Kyoto, Japan); plasma

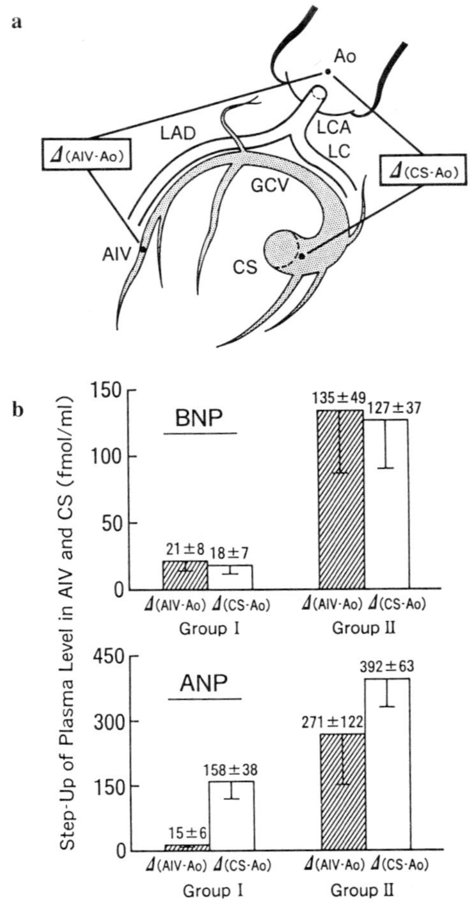

Fig. 1a. Schematic representation of the coronary venous system and three sampling points (*indicated as dots*). AIV, anterior interventricular vein; GCV, great cardiac vein; CS, coronary sinus; Ao, aortic root; LCA, left coronary artery; LAD, left anterior descending artery; LC, left circumflex artery; $\Delta_{(AIV\text{-}Ao)}$, the difference in the plasma level between the AIV and the Ao; $\Delta_{(CS\text{-}Ao)}$, the difference in the plasma level between the CS and the Ao. **b** Step-ups of BNP (*top*) and ANP (*bottom*) levels in the AIV (*hatched columns*) and in the CS (*open columns*). Patients are classified into Group I and Group II according to the level of $\Delta_{(AIV\text{-}Ao)}$ANP, as described in the text

was immediately frozen and stored at −20°C until assay. In 11 patients undergoing diagnostic cardiac catheterization (8 men and 3 women, aged 21–69 years), plasma samples were obtained from various sites, including the coronary sinus (CS), the anterior interventricular vein (AIV), and the aortic root (Ao) (see Fig. 1a). The difference in plasma ANP levels between the AIV and the Ao ($\Delta_{(AIV\text{-}Ao)}$ANP), which reflects the amount of ANP released from the ventricle, was calculated according to methods used in our previous study [8], and the patients were classified into two groups, those with normal (Group I), and those with increased ventricular secretion of ANP (Group II). Among the 6 patients in Group I, 2 were in NYHA class I and 4 were in class II, while of the 5 patients in Group II, 4 were in NYHA class II and 1 was in class III.

RIA for hBNP

Using a monoclonal antibody, we performed an RIA for hBNP, following the RIA method for ANP previously reported [18]. A monoclonal antibody, KY-hBNP-I, raised against hBNP[83–108] conjugated to bovine thyroglobulin, recognized the ring structure of hBNP. The antibody was incubated, either with standard hBNP or with plasma samples (25 μl), in 0.2 ml assay buffer for 24 hours at 4°C, after which 0.05 ml [^{125}I] [Tyr^{82}]-hBNP[83–108] (10000 cpm) was added; the mixture was then further incubated for 24 hours at 4°C. Bound and free ligands were separated by the dextran-coated charcoal method [18]. For the measurement of plasma BNP-LI levels in normal subjects, BNP was extracted from 5–10 ml plasma, using a Sep-Pak C_{18} cartridge (Waters, Milford, Mass.) [13]. The mean recovery of 3–15 fmol/ml standard hBNP added to plasma was 70%. The minimal detectable concentrations of BNP-LI in plasma with and without extraction were 0.4 and 10 fmol/ml, respectively. The intra- and interassay coefficients of variation were 8.4% (n=8) and 6.4% (n=8), respectively. The cross-reactivity with α-hANP in this RIA was less than 0.005% on a molar basis.

RIA for ANP

The RIA for ANP was performed as previously described [18]. The cross-reactivity with hBNP was less than 0.01% on a molar basis.

Statistical Analysis

Data were expressed as means ± SE. Statistical analysis was performed using Student's t-test or Duncan's multiple range test.

Results

Peripheral Plasma BNP-LI Level

Serial dilution curves of plasma samples, with and without extraction, were parallel to the standard curve of hBNP. The plasma BNP-LI level in 11 normal subjects was 0.90 ± 0.07 fmol/ml, which was only 16% ± 2% of their ANP-LI level (6.4 ± 0.9 fmol/ml).

In contrast, the plasma BNP-LI level increased significantly in patients with heart disease (Fig. 2). In patients with mild CHF, the elevation was moderate (NYHA class I, 13 ± 3.1 fmol/ml; class II, 56 ± 24 fmol/ml). However, plasma BNP-LI levels were markedly elevated in patients with severe CHF (NYHA class III, 148 ± 37 fmol/ml; class IV, 267 ± 80 fmol/ml). Thus, a progressive rise in the plasma BNP-LI level, in accordance with the severity of CHF, was observed. The plasma ANP-LI

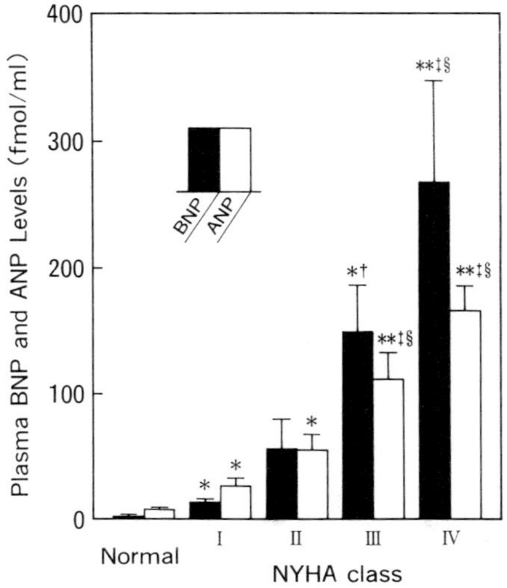

Fig. 2. Plasma BNP (*closed columns*) and ANP (*open columns*) levels in normal subjects and in patients with heart disease. NYHA class, the functional classification of the New York Heart Association. $^*P<0.01$, $^{**}P<0.001$ compared with values in normal group. $^\dagger P<0.05$, $^\ddagger P<0.01$ compared with values in NYHA class I group. $^\S P<0.01$ compared with values in NYHA class II group

level also increased according to the severity of the disease (Fig. 2), but the increase of ANP-LI was less marked than that of BNP-LI. In patients with severe CHF (NYHA classes III and IV), mean plasma BNP-LI levels surpassed mean ANP-LI levels (Fig. 2). When compared with normal levels, the percentage increment of plasma BNP-LI in severe CHF was much more prominent (200–300 times) than that of ANP-LI (20–30 times).

BNP-LI in Plasma Obtained During Cardiac Catheterization

In order to elucidate the source of plasma BNP, BNP-LI levels in plasma taken from various sites during cardiac catheterization were measured in 11 patients (Fig. 1a). Plasma BNP-LI levels in the CS (132 $\pm$ 53 fmol/ml) were 2–3 times higher than those in the Ao near the coronary ostium (66 $\pm$ 33 fmol/ml) in all cases, demonstrating that BNP-LI is secreted from the heart into the circulation through the CS.

In order to further investigate the secretion of hBNP from the heart, we measured the plasma BNP-LI level in the AIV, and analyzed $\Delta_{(AIV\text{-}Ao)}$BNP and $\Delta_{(CS\text{-}Ao)}$BNP (Fig. 1a) in comparison with $\Delta_{(AIV\text{-}Ao)}$ANP and $\Delta_{(CS\text{-}Ao)}$ANP in two groups of patients. Plasma BNP-LI and ANP-LI levels from the peripheral vein in Group I were 22 $\pm$ 10 fmol/ml and 47 $\pm$ 16 fmol/ml, respectively, while those in Group II were 99 $\pm$ 51 fmol/ml and 108 $\pm$ 27 fmol/ml, respectively. The value for $\Delta_{(AIV\text{-}Ao)}$ANP of Group I was less than 50 fmol/ml, indicating that ANP secretion from the ventricle was minimal in these patients. In contrast, $\Delta_{(AIV\text{-}Ao)}$ANP of Group II ranged from 72 to 747 fmol/ml, showing that a significant amount of ANP was secreted from the ventricle in Group II. As shown in Fig. 1b, in Group I patients, $\Delta_{(CS\text{-}Ao)}$ANP was 10 times greater than $\Delta_{(AIV\text{-}Ao)}$ANP. This pattern of ANP secretion in the coronary circulation clearly shows that ANP is secreted predominantly from the atrium. The secretory pattern of hBNP, however, showed a striking contrast with that of ANP. A significant step-up of the BNP-LI level was observed in the AIV, and $\Delta_{(AIV\text{-}Ao)}$BNP was comparable to $\Delta_{(CS\text{-}Ao)}$BNP, indicating that hBNP is secreted predominantly from the ventricle in these patients. In Group II, $\Delta_{(AIV\text{-}Ao)}$BNP, as well as $\Delta_{(CS\text{-}Ao)}$BNP, increased significantly compared with those of Group I, and there was also no difference between $\Delta_{(AIV\text{-}Ao)}$BNP and $\Delta_{(CS\text{-}Ao)}$BNP. Both $\Delta_{(AIV\text{-}Ao)}$ANP and $\Delta_{(CS\text{-}Ao)}$ANP increased in these patients, and an increase of $\Delta_{(AIV\text{-}Ao)}$ANP was evident.

Discussion

The present study demonstrates that hBNP is a novel cardiac hormone, secreted predominantly from the ventricle in humans. The step-up of hBNP concentration in plasma taken at the CS clearly indicates that the major source of circulating hBNP is the heart. Furthermore, a significant step-up in the plasma hBNP level between the Ao and the AIV, which drains the left ventricle but not the atrium [8] (Fig. 1a), clearly demonstrates that hBNP is secreted from the ventricle. Moreover, there was no significant difference between the plasma hBNP levels of the AIV and the CS, suggesting that hBNP secreted from the atrium constitutes a minor portion of hBNP in the CS plasma in these patients. In contrast with hBNP secretion, ANP is secreted predominantly from the atrium, as clearly shown in patients of Group I (Fig. 1b). Although the exact share of the ventricle in hBNP secretion from the whole heart is not clear, it is highly likely that hBNP is secreted predominantly from the ventricle and that the atrial contribution to hBNP secretion is much smaller than its contribution to ANP secretion. These findings in the human heart are consistent with our recent observations of BNP secretion from the rat heart, which showed that approximately 60% of secreted rat BNP was derived from the ventricle [19].

The present study demonstrates that the plasma hBNP level is markedly augmented in patients with CHF, in proportion to the severity of CHF (Fig. 2). The plasma hBNP level reached as high as 500 fmol/ml in the severest cases, although its normal level was 0.90 ± 0.07 fmol/ml. Thus, the percentage increment in the plasma level of hBNP is much greater (one order of magnitude or more) than that of ANP in severe CHF. Furthermore, the present study demonstrates the marked augmentation of $\Delta_{(AIV\text{-}Ao)}$BNP in Group II patients (Fig. 1b), showing augmented secretion of hBNP from the ventricle of the failing heart. In addition to the augmented secretion from the heart, the marked increase in the plasma level of hBNP, out of proportion to that of ANP in CHF, could, at least in part, be due to a decreased clearance of hBNP from the circulation, compared to the clearance of ANP. This decreased clearance could be due to a renal or an extra-renal mechanism. Further studies are needed in order to clarify the regulatory mechanism of hBNP secretion from the heart, the clearance of hBNP from the circulation, and the functional role of the markedly increased plasma hBNP in the setting of CHF.

In conclusion, the present study demonstrates that BNP is a novel cardiac hormone, secreted predominantly from the ventricle in humans, and that, in patients with CHF, the plasma level of hBNP is much more augmented than that of ANP.

Combined with the recent discovery of a biologically active receptor relatively specific for BNP [20], these findings suggest a possible pathophysiological role of BNP, distinct from that of ANP, in cardiovascular control, and, furthermore, the findings suggest the presence of an exquisite dual natriuretic peptide system.

Acknowledgments. We thank Drs. H. Matsuo, N. Minamino (National Cardiovascular Center, Suita, Japan), and K. Kangawa (Miyazaki Medical College, Miyazaki, Japan) for kindly providing synthetic peptides. We also thank Drs. Y. Kambayashi, K. Inouye, and N. Yoshida (Shionogi Research Laboratories, Osaka, Japan) for valuable discussion. The excellent secretarial work of Ms. H. Kato, Ms. A. Kibune, and Ms. Y. Kawabata is also gratefully acknowledged.

References

1. De Bold AJ (1985) Atrial natriuretic factor: a hormone produced by the heart. Science 230:767–770
2. Kangawa K, Matsuo H (1984) Purification and complete amino acid sequence of α-human atrial natriuretic polypeptide. Biochem Biophys Res Commun 118:131–139
3. Nakao K, Morii N, Itoh H, Yamada T, Shiono S, Sugawara A, Saito Y, Mukoyama M, Arai H, Sakamoto M, Imura H (1986) Atrial natriuretic polypeptide in brain—implication of central cardiovascular control—J Hyperten 4(Suppl 6):S492–S496
4. Tikkanen I, Fyhrquist F, Metsarinne K, Leidenius R (1985) Plasma atrial natriuretic peptide in cardiac disease and during infusion in healthy volunteers. Lancet II:66–69
5. Burnett JC Jr, Kao PC, Fu DC, Heser DW, Heublein D, Granger JP, Opgenorth TJ, Reeder GS (1986) Atrial natriuretic peptide elevation in congestive heart failure in the human. Science 231:1145–1147
6. Sugawara A, Nakao K, Morii N, Yamada T, Itoh H, Shiono S, Saito Y, Mukoyama M, Arai H, Nishimura K, Obata K, Yasue H, Ban T, Imura H (1988) Synthesis of atrial natriuretic polypeptide (ANP) in human failing hearts—evidence for altered processing of ANP precursor and augmented synthesis of β-human ANP—. J Clin Invest 81: 1962–1970
7. Saito Y, Nakao K, Arai H, Nishimura K, Okumura K, Obata K, Takemura G, Fujiwara H, Sugawara A, Yamada T, Itoh H, Mukoyama M, Hosoda K, Kawai C, Ban T, Yasue H, Imura H (1989) Augmented expression of atrial natriuretic polypeptide gene in ventricle of human failing heart. J Clin Invest 83:298–305
8. Yasue H, Obata K, Okumura K, Kurose M, Ogawa H, Matsuyama K, Jougasaki M, Saito Y, Nakao K, Imura H (1989) Increased secretion of atrial natriuretic polypeptide (ANP) from the left ventricle in patients with dilated cardiomyopathy. J Clin Invest 83:46–51
9. Sudoh T, Kangawa K, Minamino N, Matsuo H (1988) A new natriuretic peptide in porcine brain. Nature 332:78–81
10. Itoh H, Nakao K, Yamada T, Shirakami G, Kangawa K, Minamino N, Matsuo H, Imura H (1988) Antidipsogenic action of a novel peptide "brain natriuretic peptide" in rats. Eur J Pharmacol 150:193–196
11. Shirakami G, Nakao K, Yamada T, Itoh H, Mori K, Kangawa K, Minamino N, Matsuo H, Imura H (1988) Inhibitory effect of brain natriuretic peptide on central angiotensin II-stimulated pressor response in conscious rats. Neurosci Lett 91:77–83
12. Yamada T, Nakao K, Itoh H, Shirakami G, Kangawa K, Minamino N, Matsuo H, Imura H (1988) Intracerebroventricular injection of brain natriuretic peptide inhibits vasopressin secretion in conscious rats. Neurosci Lett 95:223–228

13. Saito Y, Nakao K, Itoh H, Yamada T, Mukoyama M, Arai H, Hosoda K, Shirakami G, Suga S, Minamino N, Kangawa K, Matsuo H, Imura H (1989) Brain natriuretic peptide is a novel cardiac hormone. Biochem Biophys Res Commun 158:360–368
14. Kambayashi Y, Nakao K, Itoh H, Hosoda K, Saito Y, Yamada T, Mukoyama M, Arai H, Shirakami G, Suga S, Ogawa Y, Jougasaki M, Minamino N, Kangawa K, Matsuo H, Inouye K, Imura H (1989) Isolation and sequence determination of rat cardiac natriuretic peptide. Biochem Biophys Res Commun 163:233–240
15. Kambayashi Y, Nakao K, Mukoyama M, Saito Y, Ogawa Y, Shiono S, Inouye K, Yoshida N, Imura H (1990) Isolation and sequence determination of human brain natriuretic peptide in human atrium. FEBS Lett 259:341–345
16. Sudoh T, Maekawa K, Kojima M, Minamino N, Kangawa K, Matsuo H (1989) Cloning and sequence analysis of cDNA encoding a precursor for human brain natriuretic peptide. Biochem Biophys Res Commun 159:1427–1434
17. The Criteria Committee of the New York Heart Association (1964) Diseases of the heart and blood vessels; nomenclature and criteria for diagnosis, 6th edn. Little, Brown, Boston
18. Nakao K, Sugawara A, Morii N, Sakamoto M, Suda M, Soneda J, Ban T, Kihara M, Yamori Y, Shimokura M, Kiso Y, Imura H (1984) Radioimmunoassay for α-human and rat atrial natriuretic polypeptide. Biochem Biophys Res Commun 124:815–821
19. Ogawa Y, Nakao K, Mukoyama M, Shirakami G, Itoh H, Hosoda K, Saito Y, Arai H, Suga S, Jougasaki M, Yamada T, Kambayashi Y, Inouye K, Imura H (1990) Rat brain natriuretic peptide—tissue distribution and molecular form—. Endocrinology 126:2225–2227
20. Chang MS, Lowe DG, Lewis M, Hellmiss R, Chen E, Goeddel DV (1989) Differential activation by atrial and brain natriuretic peptides of two different receptor guanylate cyclases. Nature 341:68–72

Structural and Functional Relationships of Atrial Peptide Receptor Subtypes

J. Gordon Porter, Forrest H. Fuller, Judith A. Miller, Lisa C. Gregory, and John A. Lewicki[1]

Summary. The atrial natriuretic peptides (ANP) elicit numerous biological effects by interacting with multiple ANP receptors. At least three receptors have been characterized. The ANP A-receptor, and a related receptor, the ANP B-receptor, contain an ANP binding domain and guanylate cyclase catalytic activity in a single polypeptide chain. These receptors promote increases in intracellular cyclic guanosine monophosphate (GMP) which then mediate many of the direct biological actions of the atrial natriuretic peptides. A third receptor, the ANP C-receptor, is not a guanylate cyclase. Rather, this receptor mediates the sequestration and metabolic clearance of ANP from the circulation. A cDNA encoding the human ANP C-receptor was cloned from a human kidney cDNA library. The deduced amino acid sequence is 95% identical to that of the bovine ANP C-receptor. In addition, the extracellular binding domain of the human ANP C-receptor is 33% identical with the human ANP A-receptor. The localization of ANP C-receptor mRNA in human adult and fetal kidney and fetal heart provides further evidence that this receptor is operative in mediating the metabolic clearance of ANP in man.

Introduction

The family of atrial natriuretic peptides elicits a number of biological effects directed at the maintenance of blood pressure and extracellular fluid volume [1]. These effects are mediated by the specific binding of the peptides to cell surface receptors that have been characterized in a variety of target tissues, including vasculature, kidney, adrenal, and brain [2]. Pharmacological and molecular cloning studies have demonstrated heterogeneity of the atrial natriuretic peptide receptors, and at least three forms of atrial natriuretic peptide receptors have been identified [3–6]. The dynamic physiological actions of the atrial peptides are regulated by interactions of the peptides with these multiple receptor subtypes.

[1]California Biotechnology Inc., 2450 Bayshore Parkway, Mountain View, CA 94043, USA

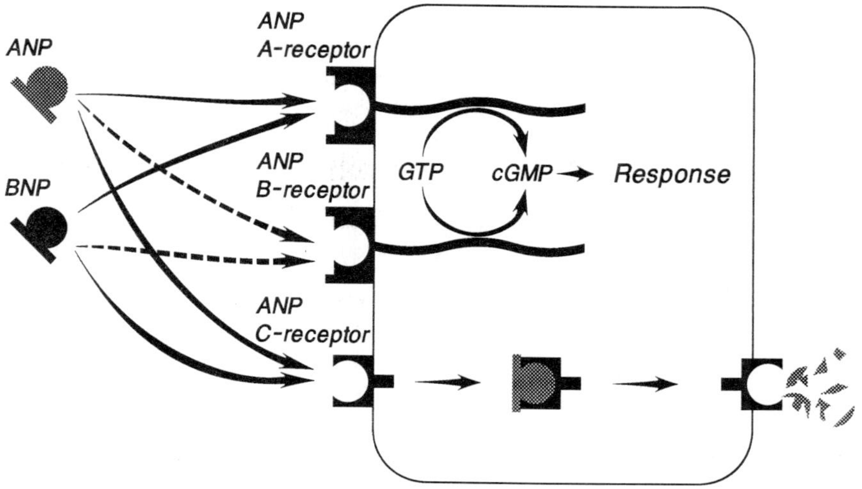

Fig. 1. A model depicting the atrial natriuretic receptor subtypes. GTP, guanosine triphosphate

Our current understanding of the intracellular role and ligand specificity of the ANP receptors is depicted in Fig. 1. The ANP A-receptor has been cloned based on its unique association with particulate guanylate cyclase. The early observations that ANP stimulates particulate guanylate cyclase activity and that ANP binding activity copurifies with particulate guanylate cyclase provided the initial clues for an association between these two molecular entities [7–8]. By screening mammalian cDNA libraries with probes derived from the DNA sequence encoding sea urchin sperm guanylate cyclase, Chinkers et al. were able to identify clones encoding a protein that contains specific ANP binding and guanylate cyclase activity within a single polypeptide chain [5]. This ANP A-receptor is thus characterized by an extracellular ANP binding domain, a single transmembrane region, and an intracellular guanylate cyclase domain. Binding of ANP to this receptor elicits a rise in intracellular levels of cyclic GMP, which presumably then mediates many of the direct biological responses of the peptide. The ANP A-receptor binds both ANP and BNP with high affinity. However, carboxyl terminal truncated ANP analogs interact only weakly with this site.

A related receptor, the ANP B-receptor is similarly comprised of an external ligand binding domain, a single transmembrane domain, and an internal guanylate cyclase region. ANP A- and B- receptors also display several regions of amino acid sequence conservation, particularly in the guanylate cyclase domain. Upon expression in mammalian cells, the ANP B-receptor binds ANP and BNP quite weakly (Kda = 25 μM and 6 μM) and this has led to speculation that an as yet unidentified hormone may be the natural ligand for this site [6].

A third ANP receptor, the ANP C-receptor, mediates the metabolic clearance of ANP [9]. This receptor does not contain a guanylate cyclase domain and is not coupled to the prominent renal, adrenal or hemodynamic actions of these peptides, as specific ANP C-receptor ligands do not have any functional activity in isolated preparations of these tissues. However, this receptor features prominently in the dynamic in vivo actions of the atrial peptides, by regulating the clearance of the hormone, thus affecting circulating ANP levels [10]. This contention is supported by studies in which ANP C-receptor specific ligands are infused into intact animals. By saturating C-receptors, and thus inhibiting clearance of native ANP, these ligands elicit 2–5 fold increases in steady state plasma ANP concentrations, leading to profound natriuresis, diuresis, and suppression of renin and aldosterone [9,11]. The ANP C-receptor is comprised of an external ligand binding domain, a single transmembrane domain, and a short cytoplasmic sequence of 37 amino acids. The C-receptor binds ANP and BNP with high affinity (~1 nM) and also avidly binds small truncated analogs of these peptides, including a linear octapeptide fragment derived from within the 17-membered ring of ANP [12].

The atrial peptide receptors have been cloned from several species. However, the ANP C-receptor has not been well characterized in man. We have now cloned the human ANP C-receptor, and are now able to make a detailed comparison of this protein to the previously described bovine C-receptor and to the human ANP A-receptor.

Materials and Methods

Library Screening

An oligo dT primed human kidney library, propagated in bacteriophage λ gt 11 vector, was plated onto E. coli host strain cf 1600, and transferred in duplicate onto nitrocellulose filters using standard techniques. Approximately 10^6 recombinant phage were screened using nick-translated bovine ANP C-receptor cDNA (ANPRc1/4) (Fuller et al., 1988 [4]) as a hybridization probe, as discussed below. The DNA bound to the nitrocellulose filters was denatured, the filters were baked at 80°C for 2h and prehybridized in a solution containing 50% formamide, 5 × Denhardt's solution, 6X SSC (1X SSC is 0.16 M NaCl, 0.016 M Na Citrate), 50 mM $NaPO_4$, and 10 μg/ml sheared salmon sperm DNA at 42°C. Hybridization was performed in the same solution plus 1.0×10^6 cpm ^{32}P-labelled probe per filter at 42°C. After hybridization, the filters were washed in 6X SSC, 0.1% SDS two times at room temperature, and once each in 6X SSC, 55°C for 15 min and 1X SSC, 55°C for 15 min. Filters were exposed to X-ray film for 1–3 days. Of 11 original hybridizing plaques, 3 were followed through subsequent rounds of purification. DNA inserts from these phage were isolated and subcloned into M13 for sequence determination as described below. One of these clones (clone 1) was used to screen a human placental cDNA library; subsequently a second human kidney library from which clones corresponding to the 5′ half of the cDNA were isolated.

Northern Blot Analysis

Poly(A)$^+$ RNA was isolated from human fetal lung and kidney tissue by the guanidinium isothiocyanate method as described by Chirgwin et al. [13], followed by oligo(dT)-cellulose chromatography. RNA was first denatured in formamide and formaldehyde at 50°C and was then fractionated on a 1.4% agarose gel containing 40 mM morpholinopropanesulfonic acid (pH 7.0), 10 mM sodium acetate, 1 mM

EDTA, and 2.2 M formaldehyde, and was transferred to nitrocellulose. Mobilities of RNA size standards (BRL) were determined by ethidium bromide staining prior to transfer. RNA was attached to nitrocellulose by baking the filters at 80°C for 2 h. The filters were hybridized in 50% formamide, 5X SSC, using, as probe, purified insert DNA from a cDNA clone (clone 1) encoding a portion of the human ANP C-receptor. DNA was radiolabelled with ^{32}P-nucleotide triphosphates by nick-translation. Filters were washed in 6X SSC, 0.1% SDS at room temperature for 20 min, and then in 1X SSC, 0.1% SDS at 65°C for 20 min and were analyzed by autoradiography.

DNA Sequencing

All DNA sequences were determined using the enzymatic method [14] by subcloning into M13 [15] and were confirmed from overlapping DNA strands. Sequences were analyzed using the Gel and Seq programs (Intellicorp, Inc., Mountain View, Calif.).

Results and Discussion

Several partial length cDNA clones encoding the human ANP C-receptor were isolated from human kidney cDNA libraries (see Materials and Methods). An analysis of overlapping sequences and comparison with bovine ANP C-receptor sequences allowed construction of a complete cDNA encompassing the complete coding region. A schematic of the human ANP C-receptor is shown in Fig. 2.

The open reading frame of 1626 nucleotides, deduced by homology with the bovine ANP C-receptor, defines a 541 amino acid sequence containing a signal peptide sequence and a pro-receptor domain. The predicted length of the mature human ANP C-receptor is 496 amino acids. The receptor is highly conserved (95%) and differs from the bovine C-receptor at only 27 of 496 amino acids which are scattered throughout the molecule. The five cysteines within the extracellular domain are conserved in both species and are likely to be important for receptor conformation. Four consensus sequences for N-linked glycosylation sites are completely conserved, although glycosylation of the human C-receptor has not yet been demonstrated.

A schematic of the human A-receptor, derived from the sequence of Lowe et al. [16], is also shown in Fig. 2. The extracellular domains of these two proteins are 33% homologous, but the protein sequence diverges completely in the cytoplasmic region. The ANP C-receptor contains only 37 cytoplasmic amino acids, while the ANP A-receptor is comprised of 568 amino acids within the cell. It is noteworthy that if the ANP C-receptor has a function in addition to clearance, the signalling mechanism would have to be contained in this abbreviated intracellular region. An analysis of the two proteins reveals that the cysteine residues of the C-receptor are conserved in the A-receptor. However, the extracellular domain of the A-receptor contains two additional cysteines. Thus, the tertiary structure of the two proteins may differ. This would not be surprising in view of the differential ligand specificity of the two receptors.

With respect to potential ligand binding domains, it is interesting to note that a 28 amino stretch of the ANP A-receptor and the ANP C-receptor (amino acid residues 132–159) is more than 75% conserved between these receptors [16]. It seems quite significant that this 28 amino acid region is completely identical in the human and bovine

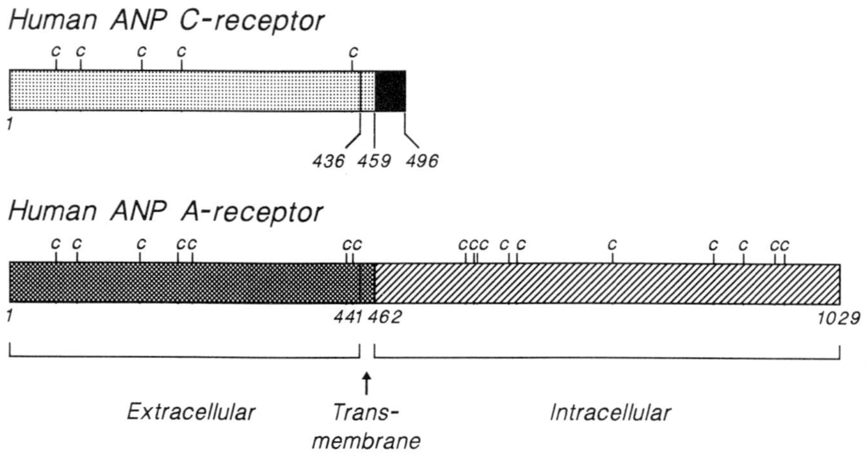

Fig. 2. Schematic representations of the human ANP A-receptor and human ANP C-receptor. *C* denotes cysteine residues. The *numbers below* each receptor represent amino acid positions beginning with the first Met of the predicted open reading frame

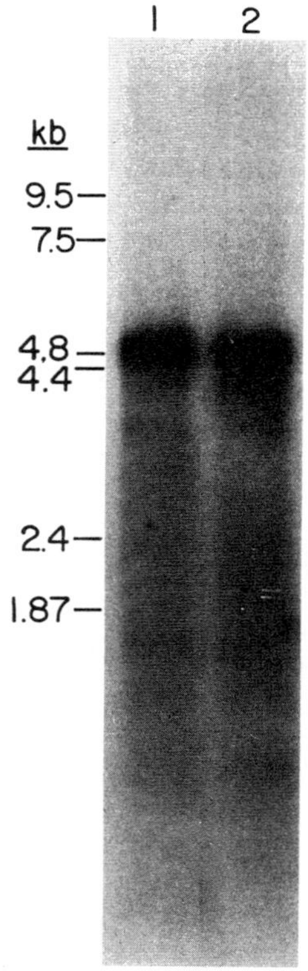

Fig. 3. Northern blots of human ANP C-receptor mRNA from human fetal lung (*lane 1*) or fetal heart (*lane 2*). Northern blots were performed as described in Materials and Methods

ANP C-receptors. Competition binding experiments with 125_{I-ANP} following transient expression of the human and bovine ANP C-receptors in mammalian cells demonstrated comparable high affinity for ANP (6×10^{-9}M), suggesting that this conserved extracellular region may be important in ligand recognition. Further studies are necessary to define the potential significance of this region of the molecule.

The functional significance of the ANP C-receptor in man is supported by its presence in several human tissues. Northern blots of poly A^+ mRNA from human fetal heart and kidney are shown in Fig. 3. Unlike the mRNA for the bovine C-receptor, which exhibits size heterogeneity in a number of tissues and cell lines [4], the human receptor is encoded by a single 5.4 kb mRNA in these tissues. Similar hybridization intensity is observed in both tissues, suggesting a comparable abundance of ANP C-receptor mRNA in each tissue. While the clearance function of the C-receptor has been well characterized in kidney, its possible role in the heart is unclear. While it has been suggested recently that the C-receptor may also be coupled to signal transduction [13], further data is needed to validate this proposal. Nevertheless, it is interesting to speculate on a possible role for the ANP C-receptor in regulating cardiac function, or perhaps in the release of ANP in man.

In summary, molecular cloning studies have afforded a detailed understanding of the structural relationships between the ANP receptor subtypes. It is anticipated that similar studies may uncover additional atrial peptide receptors in the upcoming months. When coupled with our current understanding of the functional role of these receptors, this information provides an appreciation of the complex and dynamic manner in which the natriuretic peptides regulate cardiovascular and renal homeostasis.

References

1. Baxter JD, Lewicki JA, Gardner DG (1988) Atrial natriuretic peptide. Bio/Technology 6:529–546
2. Leitman DC, Andresen JW, Kuno T, Kamisaki Y, Chang JK, Murad F (1986) Identification of multiple binding sites for atrial natriuretic factor by affinity cross-linking in cultured endothelial cells. J Biol Chem 261:11650–11655
3. Scarborough RM, Schenk DB, McEnroe G, Arfsten A, Kang L-L, Schwartz K, Lewicki JA (1986) Truncated atrial natriuretic peptide (ANP) analogs: comparison between receptor binding affinity and cyclic GMP stimulation in cultured aortic smooth muscle cells. J Biol Chem 261:12960–12964
4. Fuller F, Porter G, Arfsten A, Miller J, Schilling J, Scarborough RM, Lewicki JA, Schenk D (1988) Atrial natriuretic peptide clearance receptor: complete sequence and functional expression of cDNA clones. J Biol Chem 263:9395–9401
5. Chinkers M, Garbers DD, Chang M-S, Lowe DG, Chin H, Goeddel DV, Schulz S (1989) A membrane form of guanylate cyclase is an atrial natriuretic peptide receptor. Nature 338:78–83
6. Chang M-S, Lowe DG, Lewis M, Hellmin R, Chen E, Goeddel DV (1989) Differential activation by atrial and brain natriuretic peptides of two different receptor guanylate cyclases. Nature 341:68–71
7. Waldman S, Rapoport RM, Murad F (1984) Atrial natriuretic factor selectively activates particulate guanylate cyclase and elevates cyclic GMP in rat tissues. J Biol Chem 259:14322–14344

8. Kuno T, Andresen JW, Kamisaki Y, Waldman SA, Chang LY, Saheki S, Leitman DC, Nakane M, Murad F (1986) Co-purification of an atrial natriuretic factor receptor and particulate guanylate cyclase from rat lung. J Biol Chem 261:5817–5823
9. Maack T, Suzuki M, Almeida FA, Nussenzveig D, Scarborough RM, McEnroe GA, Lewicki JA (1987) Physiological role of silent receptors of atrial natriuretic factor. Science 238:675–678
10. Almeida FA, Suzuki M, Scarborough RM, Lewicki JA, Maack T (1989) Clearance function of type C receptors of atrial natriuretic factor in rats. Am J Physiol 256:R469–R475
11. Gregory LC, Scarborough RM, Metzler CH, McEnroe GA, Maack T, Lewicki JA (1988) Effects of acute infusion of a C-ANP receptor specific compound in conscious dog. J Cell Biochem [Suppl] 12A:23
12. Scarborough RM, Arfsten A, Kang L-L, Schwartz K, McEnroe GA, Porter JG, Suzuki M, Maack T, Lewicki JA (1988) Linear fragments of ANPs bind to C-ANP receptors with high affinity. J Cell Biochem [Suppl] 12A:20
13. Chirgwin JM, Pryzbyla AE, MacDonald RJ, Rutter NJ (1979) Isolation of biologically active ribonucleic acid from sources enriched in ribonuclease. Biochemistry 18:5294–5299
14. Sanger F, Nicklen S, Coulsen AR (1977) DNA sequencing with chain-terminating inhibitors. Proc Natl Acad Sci USA 74:5463–69
15. Messing J (1983) New M13 vectors for cloning. In: Grossman L, Moldave K (eds) Methods enzymology 101. Academic, New York, pp 20–78
16. Lowe DG, Chang M-S, Hellmin R, Chen E, Singh S, Garbers DL, Goeddel DV (1989) Human atrial natriuretic peptide receptor defines a new paradigm for second messenger signal transduction. EMBO J 8:1377–1384
17. Anand-Srivastava MB, Sairam MR, Cantin M (1990) Ring-deleted analogs of atrial natriuretic factor inhibit adenylate cyclase/cAMP system. J Biol Chem 265:8566–8572

Functional Properties and Cell Biology of Renal and Vascular Receptors of Atrial Natriuretic Factor

DANIEL R. NUSSENZVEIG, BEATRIZ M.A. FONTOURA, JURAJ OKOLICANY, AKIRA OWADA, and THOMAS MAACK[1]

Introduction

Atrial natriuretic factor (ANF) is secreted mainly by the heart atria in response to volume expansion and increases in atrial pressure or stretch. The hormone has important effects in several tissues, resulting in modulation of plasma volume, extracellular fluid volume, and blood pressure (for review, see [1,2]). There are two general classes of ANF receptors in peripheral tissues. Biological receptors proper (B-ANF receptors) mediate the ANF-induced increase in cGMP and many, if not all, of the physiological effects of the hormone [3]. These receptors were shown to contain guanylate cyclase in the cytoplasmic domain of their molecules [4]. This is a first example of a biological receptor which directly catalyzes the formation of a small second messenger upon hormone binding [4]. The other class of ANF receptors is widely distributed, at orders of magnitude larger in density than B-ANF receptors, in several tissues and cells, including kidney cortex, endothelial and vascular smooth muscle cells, and fibroblasts. The functional and biochemical nature of this receptor (named C-ANF receptor) has been fully characterized [5,6]. C-ANF receptors do not mediate any of the known effects of the hormone, but have an important role in the removal of ANF from the circulation [5]. This is a first example of a separate class of clearance receptors for a circulating polypeptide hormone. The extracellular domains of B-ANF receptors and C-ANF receptors have considerable homology [4], explaining the finding that both receptors have a similar very high affinity for native ANF_{1-28} [3,7].

In this overview, we will briefly consider some of the work done by our laboratory on the distribution and function of renal and vascular receptors of ANF.

[1]Department of Physiology and Cardiovascular Center, Cornell University Medical College, New York, NY 10021, USA

Renal Receptors of ANF

Renal Effects of ANF

ANF has complex renal vascular, hemodynamic, and tubular effects [1,2,8–20]. ANF increases glomerular filtration without necessarily increasing renal blood flow [8–14]. This is due to an efferent vasoconstrictive effect of ANF that may or may not be accompanied by an afferent dilation [8,10,11,13,14]. As a result, glomerular capillary hydrostatic pressure rises, increasing glomerular filtration rate (GFR) [10,13]. In addition, ANF is a potent antagonist of renal vasoconstriction induced by hormonal or nonhormonal agents [8,11]. ANF may also increase the glomerular ultrafiltration coefficient, which further contributes to the increase in GFR [13]. Consistent with these effects are the autoradiographic findings showing that ANF receptors are distributed in glomerular and vascular structures of the kidney cortex [21,22].

More controversial is whether or not ANF has direct or even indirect proximal tubular actions. Attempts to detect such effects by micropuncture or isolated perfused tubule techniques were, in general, negative [14]. Nevertheless, the increase in fractional lithium clearance and the increase in phosphate excretion have been interpreted to suggest a proximal tubular action of the hormone [12]. However, up to the present, investigators have been unable to detect ANF receptors or ANF-induced increase in cGMP in proximal tubule preparations [23]. Recently, however, it has been shown that ANF is able to antagonize angiotensin II-induced increase in proximal tubule sodium and water reabsorption [19].

ANF has marked effects on the renal papilla, decreasing the hypertonicity of its interstitium [1,2,9] and directly or indirectly impairing load-reabsorption balance of sodium in papillary collecting ducts [15]. In view of the close apposition of vascular, interstitial, and epithelial structures in the renal papilla, autoradiographic studies on the localization of ANF receptors in this kidney region are inconclusive [21,22]. ANF specific binding and generation of cGMP was detected in isolated papillary collecting duct, but not in outer medullary segments of collecting ducts, and only to a very small extent in thick ascending limb of Henle's loop and cortical collecting ducts [24]. Accordingly, specific binding, generation of cGMP, and inhibition of sodium uptake occur in purified suspensions of cells from papillary collecting duct but not in those from medullary collecting duct or Henle's loop [16,17]. Patch clamp experiments in cultured inner papillary collecting duct cells indicate that ANF is able to block an amiloride-sensitive cation channel in these cells [25]. Furthermore, ANF directly inhibits NaCl cotransport in isolated perfused cortical collecting ducts of the rat [22]. Finally, we recently detected major specific binding of ANF and generation of cGMP in cultured renomedullary interstitial cells from the rat (see below).

ANF Receptors in the Rat Kidney

Studies in the isolated perfused rat kidney show that the kidney cortex contains more than 95% of the total renal population of ANF receptors. Cortical receptors of ANF have a very high density (Bmax = 7 pmoles/g tissue) and affinity (Kd = 50 pM). On the other hand, the renal papilla contains fewer than 2% of the renal binding sites of ANF, but the density of these sites is fairly high (Bmax = 3 pmoles/g tissue) [26].

In the isolated rat kidney there is an almost perfect identity between the binding curves of ANF_{1-28} in the kidney cortex and the dose-response curves of renal vascular (relaxation of pre-constricted renal vasculature), hemodynamic (increase in GFR and filtration fraction (FF)) and excretory (increase in excretion of fluid and electrolytes) effects of ANF [26]. Specific binding and renal effects of ANF are detectable at ANF perfusate concentrations of 10–100 pM, which are near normal plasma levels of ANF in the rat. Furthermore, the ED_{50} of ANF effects is very close to its Kd of binding (50–100 pM), and maximal effects are observed at ANF concentrations that lead to saturation of its specific binding sites (1–10 nM). The very high affinity of cortical binding sites, together with the low ED_{50} of ANF effects, is further evidence that this hormone is an important endogenous modulator of renal vascular resistance, glomerular filtration rate, and fluid and electrolyte excretion.

Clearance Receptors of ANF in the Kidney

The overwhelming majority of renal receptors of ANF is constituted by C-ANF receptors that, in contrast to B-ANF receptors, do not mediate any of the known renal effects of the hormone. Binding and effects of ring-C terminal deleted analogues of ANF such as Des[Gln^{18}, Ser^{19}, Gly^{20}, Leu^{21}, Gly^{22}]rANF4-23-NH_2 (henceforth referred to as C-ANF$)_{4-23}$ were tested in the isolated perfused rat kidney preparation [5]. C-ANF_{4-23}, similarly to ANF_{1-28}, displaced more than 95% of [^{125}I]-ANF_{1-28} from its binding sites in whole kidney and kidney cortex at a perfusate concentration of 100 nM. On the other hand, in the renal papilla C-ANF_{4-23} displaced only 50% of [^{125}I]-ANF_{1-28} from its binding sites. Competition binding studies further demonstrated that the apparent affinity of C-ANF_{4-23} for ANF receptors was very high, only 5–10 times lower than that of native ANF_{1-28}. These experiments demonstrated that C-ANF_{4-23} binds with high affinity to the overwhelming majority of ANF receptors in whole kidney and kidney cortex.

Excess prefusate concentration of C-ANF_{4-23} (1 μM) had no effects on its own in any of the measured renal function parameters in the isolated perfused rat kidney, including GFR, FF, renal vascular resistance, and fluid and electrolyte excretion. Furthermore, this excess concentration also did not alter the dose-response curves of ANF_{1-28} on the above mentioned parameters. Thus, C-ANF_{4-23} had no agonist or antagonist action, in spite of occupying more than 95% of the total ANF receptor population in the isolated rat kidney [5]. On the basis of these results, we concluded that the overwhelming majority of renal receptors of ANF is biologically silent, in the sense that they did not mediate any of the known renal effects of the hormone. We further postulated that these receptors, which we named C-ANF receptors, may serve as peripheral storage/clearance binding sites for ANF and that in this manner they play an important role in the removal of ANF from the circulation and in the plasma homeostasis of the hormone [5]. Conclusive evidence that this is indeed the case is summarized below.

The Clearance Role of C-ANF Receptors in the Rat

C-ANF_{4-23} was administered to intact conscious and/or anesthetized rats to determine whether blockage of C-ANF receptors increased plasma levels of endogenous immunoreactive (ir)ANF, induced renal and systemic effects, and altered the metabolism of ANF.

Constant infusion of C-ANF_{4-23} practically doubled plasma levels of endogenous irANF [5,7]. The increase in plasma irANF induced by blockage of C-ANF receptors in anesthetized rats was accompanied by expected renal and systemic effects [5,7]. Mean blood pressure decreased slightly, but significantly, by approximately 10 mmHg and GFR, urine volume, and sodium excretion were significantly increased. The quantitative effects of the infusion of 1 μg/kg per min of C-ANF_{4-23} corresponded to those obtained by an infusion of native ANF_{1-28} (0.02–0.03 μg/min per Kg body wt) that increased plasma irANF to the same extent as that obtained by the infusion of C-ANF_{4-23}. The results of these studies indicate that blockage of C-ANF receptors increases plasma levels of endogenous ANF, which in turn leads to natriuretic and blood pressure lowering effects. The results of these experiments also show that relatively modest increases in plasma ANF are biologically effective, which further attests to the significance of this hormone as a modulator of plasma volume and blood pressure.

Administration of C-ANF_{4-23} (1 μg/min per Kg body wt) markedly altered the pharmacokinetics of a single bolus injection of [^{125}I]-ANF_{1-28} in intact anesthetized rats [27]. Thus, C-ANF_{4-23} reduced the apparent volume of distribution at steady state (Vss) and metabolic clearance rate (MCR) to half of the control value, consistent with the doubling of the plasma levels of endogenous irANF by this dose of the C-ANF receptor ligand. Saturating doses of C-ANF_{4-23} (10 μg/min per Kg body wt) led to further reduction of Vss to one-third, and of MCR to one-quarter of control values. With the higher dose there was a significant increase in plasma half-life of administered [^{125}I]-ANF_{1-28}. These results demonstrate that binding to C-ANF receptors is responsible for the very large apparent volume of distribution of ANF and that these receptors are importantly involved in the removal of the hormone from the circulation. Correspondingly, blockage of C-ANF receptors also led to a marked delay in the appearance of [^{125}I]-ANF_{1-28} hydrolytic products in plasma. This further demonstrates that a major fraction of ANF metabolism in the rat is due to C-ANF receptor-mediated hydrolysis of the peptide.

In our laboratory we have recently shown that small linear peptide analogues of ANF, containing 5 amino acids of the ring structure of native ANF_{1-28}, bind to C-ANF but not to B-ANF receptors. The effects of these small linear peptide analogues on plasma levels, volume of distribution, and metabolic clearance rate of ANF were similar to those described above for C-ANF_{4-23} [28]. These findings raise hopes for the future development and use of orally active ligands of C-ANF receptors.

ANF Receptor Subtypes in Isolated Glomeruli

Glomeruli are a major site for ANF action and also receive a large fraction of the cardiac output. Accordingly, isolated glomeruli were shown to contain a high density of ANF receptors and to generate cGMP in a dose-dependent manner when incubated with biologically active atrial peptides [29]. Studies in our laboratory have demonstrated that the majority (approximately 80%) of the total ANF receptor population in isolated glomeruli is constituted by C-ANF receptors [30].

ANF Receptor Subtypes in Cultured Glomerular Mesangial Cells

Saturation binding studies using [^{125}I]-ANF$_{1-28}$ showed that the density of total ANF receptors in cultured mesangial cells was 28 fmoles/million cells with a Kd of 77 pM [30,31]. Saturation binding studies with [^{125}I]-(Y^3)-C-ANF$_{3-23}$, a specific ligand of C-ANF receptors, show a similar affinity (Kd = 83 pM) but a lower density of binding sites (Bmax = 9.6 fmoles/million cells) than that obtained for the total ANF receptor population [32]. Saturation binding studies with [^{125}I]-ANF$_{1-28}$ in the presence of 0.1 μM C-ANF$_{4-23}$, a concentration that occupies all C-ANF receptors available, showed a receptor density of 20.0 fmoles/million cells with a Kd of 241 pM. Thus, C-ANF receptors constitute approximately 30% of the total ANF receptor population in mesangial cells. This value is much lower than the proportion of C-ANF receptors in whole isolated glomeruli (80%). Different passages of cultured glomerular mesangial cells express the proportion of surface ANF receptors variably. Thus in later passages (after the 20th passage) of cloned cultured glomerular mesangial cells we found that surface C-ANF receptor became undetectable, whereas there was no change or even an increase in density of surface B-ANF receptors compared to the earlier passages.

ANF$_{1-28}$ generates a dose-related increase in cGMP in cultured mesangial cells, with a maximal generation of 106 ± 9 pmoles of cGMP/2 min per million cells and an ED$_{50}$ of 5 nM. C-ANF$_{4-23}$ (1 μM) did not generate cGMP and did not potentiate or antagonize the cGMP generating effect of ANF$_{1-28}$ [31]. Thus, cultured glomerular mesangial cells have functionally distinct B-ANF and C-ANF receptors with a similar very high affinity for native ANF$_{1-28}$. Furthermore, it is apparent that B-ANF and C-ANF receptors do not interact as far as generation of the second messenger (cGMP) is concerned.

ANF Receptor Subtypes in Cultured Renomedullary Interstitial Cells (RMIC)

Binding studies in the isolated perfused rat kidney preparation have revealed that the renal papilla contains B-ANF and C-ANF receptors at fairly high densities and in almost identical proportions [26]. Freshly prepared suspensions of inner medullary collecting duct cells were shown to contain guanylate cyclase-coupled B-ANF receptors [16,17], but their receptor density is too low to account for the whole receptor density that we observed in the papilla. Since renomedullary interstitial cells are a prevalent cell type of the renal medulla, we developed a culture of renomedullary interstitial cells (RMIC) from the rat to determine ANF receptor subpopulations in these cells [32]. Electron microscopy of the cultured cells showed the typical features of RMIC in vivo, including prominent lipid droplets. Equilibrium saturation and competition binding studies showed a very high density of high affinity binding sites for the native form of the hormone, ANF$_{1-28}$ (Bmax = 23,000 sites/cell; Kd = 50 pM). There was only minimal binding of C-ANF$_{4-23}$, a specific ligand of C-ANF receptors. ANF$_{1-28}$ markedly increased cGMP from 1.3 ± 0.3 to 106 ± 22 pmoles cGMP/2 min per million cells, with an ED$_{50}$ of 1.2 nM. The effect of ANF$_{1-28}$ on cGMP was nearly additive to that of sodium nitroprusside and was not potentiated or antagonized by C-ANF$_{4-23}$. The results demonstrate that in contrast to the whole kidney tissue, the overwhelming majority of ANF receptors in RMIC are guanylate cyclase coupled B-ANF receptors. The density of B-ANF receptors in RMIC is the highest reported to date in the literature for any cell type. The maximal ANF-induced generation of cGMP is equivalent to that found in glomerular mesangial cells in our laboratory and is also one of the highest reported to date in other cells. The results indicate that RMIC are an important target cell for ANF in the renal papilla. This suggests that RMIC may mediate some of the known effects of ANF in this kidney region and/or may influence the secretion of an anti-hypertensive substance(s) by these cells. Further work is needed to clarify the exact role of the effects of ANF in renomedullary interstitial cells.

Cellular Mechanisms of C-ANF Receptor-Mediated Hydrolysis of ANF

Specific receptor-mediated endocytosis and lysosomal hydrolysis is a common mechanism by which peptide hormones, as well as non-hormonal proteins, are disposed of by cells [33]. Lysosomotropic weak bases, such as NH_4Cl or chloroquine, by virtue of increasing the normally low pH of lysosomes, are universal and specific inhibitors of lysosomal hydrolysis of peptidic substances. Therefore, in order to test whether lysosomal hydrolysis is implicated in the metabolism of ANF mediated by C-ANF receptors we first determined the effects of NH_4Cl on the hydrolysis of ANF in the isolated perfused rat kidney [34]. In this preparation, NH_4Cl as well as chloroquine practically abolished the renal hydrolysis of $[^{125}I]I\text{-}ANF_{1\text{-}28}$, demonstrating that lysosomal hydrolysis is the major mode of renal metabolism of ANF. Since binding to C-ANF receptors accounts for $> 95\%$ of the total accumulation of ANF in the kidney, these results are consistent with the interpretation that renal metabolism of ANF is due to C-ANF receptor-mediated endocytosis with subsequent delivery of ANF to lysosomes where it undergoes complete hydrolysis to amino acids. To gain further insights into this process we used cultured cells with an absolute predominance and high density of C-ANF receptors. Results of these studies are briefly summarized below.

Metabolism of ANF Mediated by C-ANF Receptors in 3T3 Swiss Albino Mouse Fibroblasts

Binding studies in cultured 3T3 Swiss albino mouse fibroblasts have shown that these cells have high affinity C-ANF receptors with a density of approximately 20000 receptors/cell, but no detectable B-ANF receptors [35]. Experiments of cell internalization and metabolism of $[^{125}I]\text{-}ANF_{1\text{-}28}$ have shown that radioiodinated $ANF_{1\text{-}28}$ is internalized in a temperature-dependent manner: there is no receptor internalization at 4°C, receptors are internalized at an initial rate of 4% of occupied C-ANF receptors/min at 22°C and 12% of occupied C-ANF receptors/min at 37°C. Of the internalized peptide, 51% and 74% is released as $[^{125}I]$-monoiodotyrosine to the medium by 15 min of incubation at 22°C and 37°C, respectively. NH_4Cl had no effect on the rate of internalization of $[^{125}I]\text{-}ANF_{1\text{-}28}$, but markedly reduced the appearance of $[^{125}I]$-monoiodotyrosine in the medium to 4% and 40% of the internalized peptide by 15 min of incubation at 22°C and 37°C, respectively. Blockage of C-ANF receptors by $C\text{-}ANF_{4\text{-}23}$ or $ANF_{1\text{-}28}$ practically abolished the internalization and hydrolysis of [^{125}I]ANF$_{1-28}$ [35]. These results demonstrate that C-ANF receptor-mediated endocytosis and delivery of the ligand to lysosomes is the basic mechanism of ANF removal from the circulation.

C-ANF Receptor-Mediated Internalization of ^{125}I-ANF$_{1-28}$ and Receptor Recycling in Cultured Aorta Smooth Muscle Cells

To further study the cell physiology of C-ANF receptor-mediated clearance of ANF, we determined internalization and recycling, as well as retroendocytosis and lysosomal hydrolysis, of atrial peptides in cultured bovine vascular smooth muscle cells [36,38]. These cells have the highest density of C-ANF receptors (200000–500000 sites/cell) reported to date in the literature [30]. At 37°C, C-ANF receptors internalized at a rate of 4.7% of occupied receptors/min. After 30 min incubation, 50% of [^{125}I]-ANF$_{1-28}$ initially bound to C-ANF receptors was hydrolysed and the product of hydrolysis ([^{125}I]-monoiodotyrosine) was released to the medium. Hydrolysis of [^{125}I]-ANF$_{1-28}$ was practically abolished when cells were incubated in the presence of NH_4Cl (10 mM) or excess (0.1 μM) C-ANF$_{4-23}$ or ANF$_{1-28}$. Retroendocytosis of intact [^{125}I]-ANF$_{1-28}$ was also detected when intracellular accumulation of the intact labeled peptide was maximized by previous incubation with NH_4Cl. Experiments designed to study the fate of internalized C-ANF receptors revealed that these receptors recycle back to the cell surface after dissociation from their ligand in endosomes. In this manner, surface C-ANF receptor density decreased to 56% and then returned to 93% of its initial value by incubation with saturating concentrations of [^{125}I]-ANF$_{1-28}$, for 15 and 60 min, respectively. At 60 min, the amount of labeled peptide which was hydrolyzed corresponded to one complete cycle of the total population of surface C-ANF receptors [36,38]. Similar results were obtained with [^{125}I](Y^3)-C-ANF$_{3-23}$, a labeled specific ligand of C-ANF receptors [37]. Cycloheximide, a potent protein synthesis inhibitor, does not interfere with cell surface C-ANF receptor replenishment. Detergent solubilization and cell surface receptor trypsinization have shown that the intracellular C-ANF receptor pool is small and cannot account for the cell surface C-ANF receptor replenishment. Consequently, these results demonstrate that cell surface C-ANF receptor replenishment is due to receptor reutilization [38]. Furthermore, experiments showed that C-ANF receptor internalization and recycling did not depend on the presence of the ligand.

In summary, the results of this study demonstrate that ANF molecules bound to C-ANF receptors are rapidly internalized. After dissociation from their receptors in endosomes, ANF molecules are delivered to lysosomes, where they undergo complete hydrolysis. There is some retroendocytosis of receptor-ligand complexes, but the actual degree and physiological role of this process remain to be elucidated. Internalized C-ANF receptors are rapidly recycled to the cell membrane, thus becoming available to mediate another cycle of internalization and lysosomal hydrolysis of ANF. This process is independent of the presence of the ligand. From the data it can be calculated that in cultured vascular smooth muscle cells, the entire population of C-ANF receptors is internalized and recycled every hour. Finally, due to rapid and complete recycling, there is no short-term down regulation of C-ANF receptors by ANF.

The effectiveness of C-ANF receptors in the exercise of their clearance function is due to the combination of a very high affinity for ANF, wide distribution in strategic organs and tissues, rapid internalization, and constant availability due to rapid recycling.

Conclusions

In this brief review of recent studies in our laboratory we have summarized the evidence showing that there are two functionally distinct classes of ANF receptors. B-ANF receptors mediate the ANF-induced increase in cGMP and the known renal and systemic effects of the hormone; these receptors are found in many tissues and cells including adrenal, vascular smooth muscle, and endothelial cells. They are also prevalent kidney structures, particularly in glomerular mesangial cells and renomedullary interstitial cells. C-ANF receptors do not mediate increases in cCMP or any of the known renal or systemic effects of ANF, but have a major role in the removal of ANF from the circulation. However, it cannot be ruled out at present that C-ANF receptors may also mediate some unknown effect of ANF. C-ANF receptors constitute the overwhelming majority of the total ANF receptor population in several tissues, including the kidney cortex. They are strategically located for their clearance function, with prevalent localization in vascular smooth muscle cells, glomeruli, endothelial cells, and fibroblasts. The cellular mechanisms of the clearance function of C-ANF receptors were recently elucidated in our laboratory. ANF binds with high affinity to these receptors and the receptor-ligand complex is rapidly internalized. The internalized hormone is delivered to lysosomes, where it undergoes complete hydrolysis to amino acids, whereas the internalized C-ANF receptors are rapidly recycled to the cell surface. In this manner, the location, high density, high affinity, and rapid recycling of C-ANF receptors make them ideally suited to remove ANF from the circulation.

The results of our studies provide the first evidence of a separate class of clearance receptors for a polypeptide hormone. The full physiological implications of this finding remain to be elucidated, but it is likely that C-ANF receptors contribute importantly to the plasma homeostasis of ANF by acting as a hormonal buffer system. In addition, specific ligands of C-ANF receptors may be therapeutically useful since, by blocking the clearance function of this receptor, they increase the plasma levels of endogenous ANF and, consequently, increase desirable natriuretic and blood pressure lowering effects.

Acknowledgment. Research was supported by NIH Grant DK 14241.

References

1. Maack T (1986) Atrial natriuretic factor: a physiological link between the heart and the kidney. In: Bromm B, Luggers DW (eds) Physiologie Aktuell, vol 2. Gustav Fisher, Stuttgart, pp 59–85
2. Atlas SA, Maack T (1987) Effects of atrial natriuretic factor on the kidney and the renin-angiotensin-aldosterone system. Endocrinol Metab Clin North Am 16:107–143
3. Leitman DC, Murad F (1987) Atrial natriuretic factor receptor heterogeneity and stimulation of particulate guanylate cyclase and cyclic GMP accumulation. Endocrinol Metab Clin North Am 16:79–105

4. Chinkers M, Garbers DL, Chang MS, Lowe DG, Chin HM, Goeddel DV, Schulz S (1989) A membrane form of guanylate cyclase is an atrial natriuretic peptide receptor. Nature 338:78–83
5. Maack T, Suzuki M, Almeida FA, Nussenzveig D, Scarborough RM, McEnroe GA, Lewicki JA (1987) Physiological role of silent receptors of atrial natriuretic factor. Science 238:675–678
6. Fuller F, Porter JG, Arfsten AE, Miller J, Schilling JW, Scarborough RM, Lewicki JA, Schenk DB (1988) Atrial natriuretic peptide clearance receptor. Complete sequence and functional expression of cDNA clones. J Biol Chem 263:9395–9401
7. Maack T, Suzuki M, Nussenzveig DR, Owada A, Scarborough RM, Lewicki JA, Almeida FA (1988) Clearance receptors of atrial natriuretic factor. In: Needleman P (ed) UCLA symposia on molecular and cellular biology new series. Alan R. Liss, New York, pp 57–76 (Biological and molecular aspects of atrial factors, vol 81)
8. Camargo MJ, Kleinert HD, Atlas SA, Sealey JE, Laragh JH, Maack T (1984) Ca-dependent hemodynamic and natriuretic effects of atrial extract in isolated rat kidney. Am J Physiol 246: 2)-P F447–F455
9. Maack T, Marion DN, Camargo MJ, Kleinert HD, Laragh JH, Vaughan ED Jr, Atlas SA (1984) Effects of auriculin (atrial natriuretic factor) on blood pressure, renal function, and the renin-aldosterone system in dogs. Am J Med 77:1069–1075
10. Dunn BR, Ichikawa I, Pfeffer JM, Troy JL, Brenner BM (1986) Renal and systemic hemodynamic effects of synthetic atrial natriuretic peptide in the anesthetized rat. Circ Res 59:237–246
11. Maack T, Camargo MJ, Kleinert HD, Laragh JH, Atlas SA (1985) Atrial natriuretic factor: structure and functional properties. Kidney Int. 27:607–615
12. Burnett JC Jr, Granger JP, Opgenorth TJ (1984) Effects of synthetic atrial natriuretic factor on renal function and renin release. Am J Physiol 247: 2)-P F863–F866
13. Fried TA, McCoy RN, Osgood RW, Stein JH (1986) Effect of atriopeptin II on determinants of glomerular filtration rate in the in vitro perfused dog glomerulus. Am J Physiol 250: 2)-P F1119–F1122
14. Huang CL, Lewicki J, Johnson LK, Cogan MG (1985) Renal mechanism of action of rat atrial natriuretic factor. J Clin Invest 75:769–773
15. Sonenberg H, Honrath U, Chong CK, Wilson DR (1986) Atrial natriuretic factor inhibits sodium transport in medullary collecting duct. Am J Physiol 250: 2)-P F963–F966
16. Zeidel ML, Silva P, Brenner BM, Seifter JL (1987) cGMP mediates effects of atrial peptides on medullary collecting duct cells. Am J Physiol 252: 2)-P F551–F559
17. Zeidel ML (1988) In: Davidson AM (ed) Nephrology: V1. Balliere Tindall, London, pp 145–154
18. Maack T (1988) In: Davidson AM (ed) Nephrology: V1. Balliere Tindall, London, pp 123–136
19. Harris PJ, Thomas D, Morgan TO (1987) Atrial natriuretic peptide inhibits angiotensin-stimulated proximal tubular sodium and water reabsorption. Nature 326:697–698
20. Nonoguchi H, Sands JM, Knepper MA (1989) ANF inhibits NaCl and fluid absorption in cortical collecting duct of rat kidney. Am J Physiol 256: 2)-P F179–F188
21. Bianchi C, Gutkowska J, Thibault G, Garcia R, Genest J, Cantin M (1985 Radioautographic localization of 125I-atrial natriuretic factor (ANF) in rat tissues. Histochemistry 82: 441–452
22. Koseki C, Hayashi Y, Torikai S, Furuya M, Ohnuma N, Imai M (1986) Localization of binding sites for alpha-rat atrial natriuretic polypeptide in rat kidney. Am J Physiol 250: 2)-P F210–F216
23. Stokes TJ Jr, McConkey CL Jr, Martin KJ (1986) Atriopeptin III increases cGMP in glomeruli but not in proximal tubules of dog kidney. Am J Physiol 250: 2)-P F27–F31

24. Nonoguchi H, Knepper MA, Manganiello VC (1987) Effects of atrial natriuretic factor on cyclic guanosine monophosphate and cyclic adenosine monophosphate accumulation in microdissected nephron segments from rats. J Clin Invest 79:500–507
25. Light DB, Schweibert EM, Karlson KH, Stanton BA (1989) Atrial natriuretic peptide inhibits a cation channel in renal inner medullary collecting duct cells. Science 243: 383–385
26. Suzuki M, Almeida FA, Nussenzveig DR, Sawyer D, Maack T (1987) Binding and functional effects of atrial natriuretic factor in isolated rat kidney. Am J Physiol 253: 2)-P F917–F922
27. Almeida FA, Suzuki M, Scarborough RM, Lewicki JA, Maack T (1989) Clearance function of type C receptors of atrial natriuretic factor in rats. Am J Physiol 256: 2)-P R469–R477
28. Okolicany J, Scarborough B, McEnroe G, Kang L-L, Lewicki J, Maack T (1990) Specific blockage of C-ANF receptors by small linear peptide analogues causes natriuresis in the rat (abstract). Kidney Int 37:342
29. Ballermann BJ, Hoover RL, Karnovsky MJ, Brenner BM (1985) Physiologic regulation of atrial natriuretic peptide receptors in rat renal glomeruli. J Clin Invest 76:2049–2056
30. Nussenzveig DR, Scarborough R, Lewicki J, Maack T (1988) Clearance receptors of atrial natriuretic factor (C-ANF receptors) in isolated glomeruli and mesangial cells in culture (abstract). Kidney Int 33:279
31. Nussenzveig DR, Owada A, Scarborough R, Arfsten A, Maack T (1988) Biological (B) and clearance (C) receptors of ANF in cultured mesangial cells and fibroblasts (abstract). Am J Hypertens 1:121A
32. Fontoura BMA, Nussenzveig DR, Pelgon KA, Maack T (1990) Atrial natriuretic factor receptors in cultured renomedullary interstitial cells. Am J Physiol 258:C692–C699
33. Wall DA, Maack T (1985) Endocytic uptake, transport, and catabolism of proteins by epithelial cells. Am J Physiol. 248:C12–C20
34. Owada A, Nussenzveig DR, Maack T (1988) Receptor-mediated hydrolysis of atrial natriuretic factor (ANF) in isolated perfused rat kidney (IK) (abstract). Am J Hypertens 1:121A
35. Nussenzveig DR, Fontoura BMA, Scarborough R, Lewicki J, Maack T (1989) Clearance (C) receptors mediate internalization and lysosomal hydrolysis of ANF in fibroblasts (abstract). Kidney Int 35:285
36. Nussenzveig DR, Lewicki JA, Maack T (1989) Internalization, recycling and function of clearance receptors of atrial natriuretic factor (ANF) in vascular smooth muscle cells (abstract). In: Proceedings of the 71st annual meeting of the endocrine society. Seattle, United States. p 1113
37. Nussenzveig DR, Lewicki JA, Maack T (1990) Cellular mechanisms of the clearance function of C-ANF receptors (abstract). Kidney Int 37:341
38. Nussenzveig DR, Lewicki JA, Maack T (1990) Cellular mechanisms of the clearance function of type C receptors of atrial natriuretic factor. J Biol Chem 265:(in press)

Polarity of Tubular Epithelia

Chair: Eberhard Frömter (FRG)
Gerhard Malnic (Brazil)

Comparison Between Apical and Basolateral Transporters in Tubular Epithelia: A Dual Location of Na^+/H^+-Exchange with Different Properties

VALERIA CASAVOLA, CORINNA HELMLE-KOLB, and HEINI MURER[1]

SUMMARY. Na^+/H^+-exchange located in the plasma membrane of epithelial cells may fulfill a dual role: i) epithelial transport functions, such as in bicarbonate reabsorption and ii) cell homeostatic functions ("housekeeping"). A dual location of the Na^+/H^+-exchange has been documented for renal tubular epithelia, such as rabbit proximal tubule S_3 segment [1,2]. By microspectrofluorometry, we have analyzed for the polarized expression of the Na^+/H^+-exchange in an established renal cell line LLC-PK_1/PKE_{20}. In agreement with previous data on tracer flux measurements [3,4], we observed Na^+/H^+-exchange activities on both cell surfaces; we found that apical Na^+/H^+-exchange is less sensitive to ethylisopropyl-amiloride inhibition than basolateral activity. Forskolin and 8 Br-cAMP (i.e., activation of kinase A) lead to inhibition of apical and basolateral Na^+/H^+-exchange; phorbolester (i.e., activation of kinase C) leads to inhibition of apical and stimulation of basolateral Na^+/H^+-exchange activities. Vasopressin and calcitonin lead to inhibition of apical Na^+/H^+-exchange and stimulation of basolateral Na^+/H^+-exchange activity. Thus, renal epithelial cells may contain two different Na^+/H^+-exchange activities which show different pharmacological and regulatory properties and may serve different functions.

Introduction

Vectorial epithelial transport of solutes requires different transport properties of plasma membrane domains facing the apical and serosal (basolateral) compartments, respectively. For example, in absorptive secondary active transport functions, e.g., Na^+-coupled glucose absorption, Na^+-solute cotransport systems can mediate uphill influx at the apical cell side and Na^+-independent efflux at the basolateral cell pole will complete transcellular solute movement [5]. It should be noted, however, that

[1]Department of Physiology, University of Zürich, CH - 8057 Zürich, Switzerland

epithelial polarity with respect to transport functions can also be based on more subtile differences in transport properties. For amino acid reabsorption in the proximal tubule, Na^+-dependent transport pathways can be found on both cell surfaces; vectorial flux will then be determined by differences either in their capacities and/or kinetics or in their mode of energetization (e.g., Na^+/solute coupling coefficients, [5]).

For bicarbonate absorbing epithelia, the proton-secretory mechanism is usually on the apical cell surface; in renal proximal tubule this is a Na^+/H^+-exchange mechanism [6]. Besides this "epithelial" apical Na^+/H^+-exchange activity, basolateral Na^+/H^+-exchange activity may coexist in epithelial cells. This has been shown for small intestinal epithelial cells [7] as well as for rabbit S_3 proximal tubular epithelia [1,2].

LLC-PK_1/PKE_{20}, a renal epithelial cell line, was selected on the basis of its amiloride-resistance in a selection protocol and was found to have high Na^+/H^+-exchange activities in the apical as well as in the basolateral cell surface [3,4]. We have used this tissue culture model system to ask questions related to differences in the basic properties, as well as differences in regulatory characteristics, between apical and basolateral Na^+/H^+-exchange activities. Interestingly, we have observed that apical and basolateral Na^+/H^+-exchange activities are not only different with respect to their sensitivity to amiloride inhibition, but also with respect to hormonal regulatory phenomena [8,9,10].

Methods

For the studies to be summarized in this report we have used LLC-PK_1/PKE_{20}-cells grown on collagen coated teflon filters to confluent monolayers [8,9,10]; PKE_{20}-cells were obtained from Dr. C.W. Slayman (New Haven, Conn., USA, [3,4]). After mounting confluent monolayers on permeant support in a specially constructed "sandwich" chamber [11] and separate perfusion of the apical and basolateral compartment, intracellular pH (pH_i) was recorded by using the intracellular pH-indicator BCECF (Molecular Probes) [11,12,13]. Na^+/H^+-exchange was defined as Na^+-dependent recovery from a NH_4Cl-preload induced intracellular acidification; this Na^+-dependent recovery mechanism was competitively inhibited by ethylisopropylamiloride [8,9,10,14].

Results and Discussion

In agreement with trace flux studies [3,4], we have found Na^+/H^+-exchange activities on the apical as well as on the basolateral cell surface of LLC-PK_1/PKE_{20}-cell monolayers; the capacity of the apical Na^+/H^+-exchange activity was 20%–30% higher than basolateral activity [9,10]. Na^+-saturation kinetics revealed an apparent K_m-value of 25 mM and no difference between apical and basolateral activity [8,9,10]. Similar experiments performed previously in our laboratory with the same technique showed only apical Na^+/H^+-exchange activity in an established renal cell line derived from opossum kidney (OK-cells) [12,13] and only basolateral activity in wild type LLC-PK_1-cells [11] as well as in LLC-PK_1/$Clone_4$-cells, the parent cell line of LLC-PK_1/PKE_{20} [8,9,10]. These initial experiments clearly document a dual location of Na^+/H^+ exchange in the cultured renal epithelial cell line LLC-PK_1/PKE_{20}.

Inhibition of Apical and Basolateral Na^+/H^+-Exchange in LLC-PK_1/PKE_{20} Monolayers by Ethylisopropylamiloride (EIPA)

The amiloride analogue EIPA is known to be a competitive inhibitor of Na^+/H^+-exchange activities [14]. Na^+-dependent pH_i-recovery from an acid load due to superfusion with 20 mM Na was inhibited by 94% $\pm$ 2% at the basolateral cell surface but only by 31% $\pm$ 4% at the apical cell surface; in the presence of 140 mM Na^+ in the perfusate, inhibition at the basolateral cell surface was 66% $\pm$ 15% and at the apical surface was 16% $\pm$ 9%. These results [8,9,10] are clear evidence for a relative resistance to inhibition by EIPA of apical Na^+/H^+-exchange in LLC-PK_1/PKE_{20} as compared to Na^+/H^+-exchange at the basolateral cell surface of the same cell and evidence for a competitive interaction between Na^+ and EIPA. Thus, two Na^+/H^+-exchange activities with different inhibitory properties seem to be expressed at the two different cell surfaces of LLC-PK_1/PKE_{20}-cells.

Effect of Pharmacological Activation of Proteinkinase A and Proteinkinase C on Apical and Basolateral Na^+/H^+-Exchange Activities in LLC-PK_1/PKE_{20}

Plasma membrane Na^+/H^+-exchange is usually inhibited by cAMP/kinase A mediated pathways and stimulated by diacylglycerol/kinase C mediated pathways [13,14]. In a recent study on OK-cells we found parathyroid hormone-dependent inhibition of apical Na^+/H^+-exchange; this hormone-dependent inhibition of Na^+/H^+-exchange could be mimicked by 8 Br-cAMP and by forskolin—both leading to activation of proteinkinase A—as well as by phorbolester leading to activation of kinase C [17,18]. The LLC-PK_1/PKE_{20}-cell system offers the possibility of looking for regulation of two differently located Na^+/H^+-exchange activities within the same cell (single cell microspectrofluorometry). Apical Na^+/H^+-exchange activity in LLC-PK_1/PKE_{20}-cells was inhibited within minutes by 8 Br-cAMP (2.5×10^{-4} M; 42% $\pm$ 8%), forskolin (10 μM; 65% $\pm$ 7%), phorbolester (TPA, 0.1 μM; 56% $\pm$ 5%) and phorbolester plus forskolin (above concentrations; 40% $\pm$ 1%). Basolateral Na^+/H^+-exchange activity was inhibited by 8 Br-cAMP (2.5×10^{-4} M; 42% $\pm$ 8%) and forskolin (10 μM; 48% $\pm$ 5%); it was stimulated by phorbolester (TPA, 0.1 μM; 37% $\pm$ 3%) and by phorbolester plus forskolin (above concentrations (40% $\pm$ 8%). These data document separate regulatory control of apically and basolaterally located Na^+/H^+-exchange activities and, further, suggest the coexistence of two separately controlled Na^+/H^+-exchange activities in LLC-PK_1/PKE_{20}-cells [8,9,10].

Effect of Vasopressin and Calcitonin on Apical and Basolateral Na^+/H^+-Exchange Activities in LLC-PK_1/PKE_{20}

LLC-PK_1-cells are known to express V_1-receptors (coupled to phospholipase C) as well as V_2-receptors coupled to adenylatecyclase [19]; receptors for calcitonin have also been described [19]. Thus, it was of interest to analyze for the relative importance of proteinkinase A and proteinkinase C mediation in vasopressin or in calcitonin mediated control of apical or basolateral Na^+/H^+-exchange in LLC-PK_1/PKE_{20}-cells. Vasopressin leads, within minutes, to inhibition of apical Na^+/H^+-exchange (2×10^{-6} M; 26% ± 1%); basolateral Na^+/H^+-exchange activity was stimulated by the same vasopressin treatment (17% ± 2%) [8,9,10].

This result suggests that either the kinase A and the kinase C regulatory pathways are activated together or that only the kinase C regulatory pathway is activated by vasopressin. Additional experiments indicated that the same treatment leads to a cellular accumulation of cAMP [10]. Thus, vasopressin exerts a dual effect on the two differently located Na^+/H^+-exchangers; this is best explained by vasopressin's actions via V_1 (cAMP-independent)- and via V_2 (cAMP-dependent)-receptor events.

Similar effects are observed for calcitonin. Calcitonin treatment leads, within minutes, to inhibition of apical Na^+/H^+-exchange (3×10^{-7} M; 25% ± 2%) and to stimulation of basolateral Na^+/H^+-exchange activities (27% ± 8%). These data, together with a measured increase in cAMP, again suggest that calcitonin effects must be mediated by two pathways, cAMP-dependent and cAMP-independent regulatory cascades.

Conclusions

Epithelial cells may contain two Na^+/H^+-exchange activities which are under different hormonal control and which can also be distinguished by their sensitivity to amiloride inhibition. Figure 1 summarizes the main observations obtained in our study on LLC-PK_1/PKE_{20}-monolayers, a tissue culture model for (proximal) tubular epithelia [3,4,8,9,10,19]. It should be noted that a similar dual location of Na^+/H^+-exchange activity might also be present in native proximal tubular epithelia [1,2], although regulatory hormones in the proximal tubule would not include vasopressin and calcintonin, but could be related to other agonists. In LLC-PK_1/PKE_{20}-cell monlayers, apical Na^+/H^+-exchange, as compared to basolateral activity, is resistant to EIPA inhibition. Proteinkinase A activation (by cAMP) leads to inhibition of apically and basolaterally located Na^+/H^+-exchange activities; proteinkinase C activation by diacylglycerol (DAG) leads to inhibition of apical, but

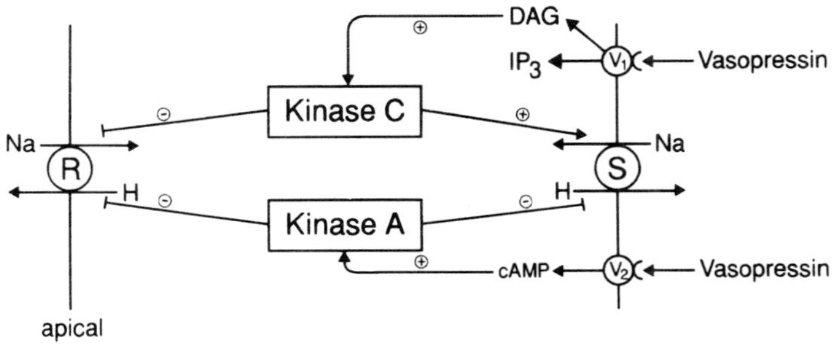

Fig. 1. Dual location of Na^+/H^+-exchange in LLC-PK_1/PKE_{20} monolayers and vasopressin-induced regulatory control. R, amiloride-resistant; S, amiloride-sensitive; DAG, diacylglycerol; IP_3, inositoltrisphosphate

stimulation of basolateral Na^+/H^+-exchange activity. As illustrated in Fig. 1 vasopressin exerts contrasting effects on apical and basolateral Na^+/H^+-exchange activities: apical activity is inhibited and this can be mediated by both kinase A and kinase C; basolateral activity is stimulated, and inhibition can be mediated only by activation of kinase C.

Acknowledgments. The financial support of the Swiss National Science Foundation (Grant Nr. 3.851.088), the "Stiftung für wissenschaftliche Forschung an der Universität Zürich," the "Hartman Müller Stiftung," the "Geigy-Jubiläumsstiftung," and the "Sandoz Stiftung" are gratefully acknowledged. We are grateful to Dr. C.F. Slayman for giving us access to LLC-PK_1/PKE_{20}- and LLC-PK_1/$Clone_4$-cells.

References

1. Kurtz I (1989) Basolateral membrane Na^+/H^+ antiport, Na^+/base cotransport, and Na^+-independent Cl^-/base exchange in the rabbit S_3 proximal tubule. J Clin Invest 83:616– 622
2. Kurtz I (1987) Apical Na^+/H^+ antiporter and glycolysis-dependent H^+-ATPase regulate intracellular pH in the rabbit S_3 proximal tubule. J Clin Invest 80:928–935
3. Haggerty JG, Agarwal N, Reilly RF, Adelberg EA, Slayman CW (1988) Pharmacologically different Na^+/H^+-antiporters on the apical and basolateral surfaces of cultured kidney cells (LLC-PK_1). Proc Natl Acad Sci USA 85:6797–6801
4. Haggerty JG, Agarwal N, Cragoe EJ, Adelberg EA, Slayman CW (1988) LLC-PK_1 mutant with increased Na^+/H^+-exchange and decreased sensitivity to amiloride. Am J Physiol 255:C495–C501
5. Kinne R (1986) Epithelial transport: The interplay between ionic gradients and cell polarity. In: Alvarado F, van Os C (eds) Ion gradient-coupled transport (INSERM symposium 26). Elsevier, Amsterdam, pp 255–273
6. Alpern RJ (1990) Cell mechanisms of proximal tubule acidificiation. Physiol Rev 70:79–114
7. Barros F, Dominguez P, Velasco G, Lazo PS (1986) Na^+/H^+-exchange is present in basolateral membranes from rabbit small intestine. Biochem Biophys Res Commun 134:827–834
8. Casavola V, Helmle-Kolb C, Murer H (1989) Separate regulatory control of apical and basolateral Na^+/H^+-exchange in renal epithelial cells. Biochem Biophys Res Commun 165:833–837
9. Casavola V, Helmle-Kolb C, Montrose MH, Murer H (1990) Polarized expression of Na^+/H^+-exchange activities in clonal LLC-PK_1 cells ($Clone_4$ and PKE_{20}): 1. Basic characterization (in preparation)
10. Casavola V, Helmle-Kolb C, Montrose MH, Murer H (1990) Polarized expression of Na^+/H^+-exchange activities in clonal LLC-PK_1 cells ($Clone_4$ and PKE_{20}):2. Hormonal regulation (in preparation)
11. Montrose MH, Friedrich T, Murer H (1987) Measurements of intracellular pH in single LLC-PK_1 cells: Recovery from acid load via basolateral Na^+/H^+-exchange. J Membr Biol 97:63–78
12. Montrose MH, Murer H (to be published) Regulation of intracellular pH by cultured opossum kidney (OK) cells. Am J Physiol
13. Montrose MH, Murer H (to be published) Polarity and kinetics of Na^+/H^+-exchange in cultured opossum kidney (OK) cells. Am J Physiol
14. Vigne P, Frelin C, Cragoe EJ, Lazdunski M (1983) Ethylisopropylamiloride: a new and highly potent derivative of amiloride for the inhibition of the Na^+/H^+-exchange system in various cell types. Biochem Biophys Res Commun 116:86–90

15. Grinstein S, Rothstein A (1986) Mechanisms of regulation of the Na^+/H^+-exchanger. J Membr Biol 90:1–12
16. Frelin C, Vigne P, Ladoux A, Lazdunski M (1988) The regulation of the intracellular pH in cells from vertebrates. Eur J Biochem 174:3–14
17. Helmle-Kolb C, Montrose MH, Stange G, Murer H (1990) Regulation of Na^+/H^+-exchange in opossum kidney cells by parathyroid hormone, cyclic AMP and phorbol esters. Pflugers Arch 415:461–470
18. Helmle-Kolb C, Montrose MH, Murer H (to be published) PTH-Regulation of Na^+/H^+-exchange in opossum kidney cells: Polarity and mechanisms. Pflugers Arch
19. Gstraunthaler GJA (1988) Epithelial cells in tissue culture. Renal Physiol Biochem 11:1–42

Electrophysiological Localization of Transporters in the Distal Nephron Segments

Koji Yoshitomi, Masashi Imai[1], Toshikatsu Shimizu[2], Junichi Taniguchi[3], and Fumiaki Yamasaki[4]

Summary. The distal convoluted tubule (DCT) and the connecting tubule (CNT) from the rabbit kidney were investigated by electrophysiological techniques, isotopic flux measurement, and microfluorometry, in order to characterize the ion transport properties of cell membranes. When the DCT and the CNT were perfused in vitro, the transepithelial voltage (V_T) displayed lumen negative, and the transepithelial resistances (R_T) were relatively low, as in the category of leaky epithelia. Random cellular impalement revealed that the basolateral membrane voltage (V_B) of the DCT showed Gaussian distribution, whereas the CNT consisted of two cell populations, having different V_B and different fractional resistance of the apical membrane (fR_A). The CNT cell had a high V_B and lower fR_A and the intercalated (IC) cell in the CNT had a low V_B and higher fR_A. Using ion substitution and channel inhibitors, the conductive properties of DCT cells and CNT cells revealed that the luminal membrane had both Na^+ and K^+ conductances and that the basolateral membrane had both K^+ and Cl^- conductances. Intercalated cells of CNT had only a Cl^- conductance in the basolateral membrane. Besides Na^+ conductance in the luminal membrane of CNT cells, two other modes of Na^+ entry process were observed. One pathway was the Na/Cl cotransporter, revealed by isotopic ion flux studies, which was inhibitable with thiazide diuretics, and the other was a nonselective cation conductance, which was not sensitive to amiloride and was opened by parathyroid hormone (PTH). From intracellular calcium measurement and calcium flux studies, it was found that the latter mode serves as a route for calcium entry pathway in CNT cells.

[1]Department of Pharmacology, Jichi Medical School, Minamikawachi 3311-1, Tochigi, 329-04 Japan

[2]Shionogi Research Laboratories, Shionogi and Co., Ltd., Fukushima, Osaka, 553 Japan

[3]Research Institute, National Cardiovascular Center, Suita, Osaka, 565 Japan

[4]Fuji Central Research Lab., Mochida Pharmaceutical Co. Ltd., Gotenba, Shizuoka, 412 Japan

Introduction

It has generally been accepted that the function of the distal convoluted tubule (DCT) is reabsorption of NaCl and Ca^{2+} and secretion of K^+. This knowledge is based mainly on micropuncture studies on rat in vivo. However, the transitions from DCT to connecting tubule (CNT), or from CNT to cortical collecting duct (CCD), are gradual and several cell types are mixed within the transitional portion. In vitro microperfusion of DCT (and CNT) isolated from rabbit kidney has an advantage over the in vivo micropuncture studies of rat distal nephron, since the transition from DCT to CNT is clear. The DCT is characterized by its special location and shape, together with its calcitonin sensitivity in the distal nephron segments. For years, the exact mechanism of ion transport has been unknown, because of the difficulty of isolating the tubule. However, we have succeeded in identifying several membrane characteristics by elecctrophysiological means [1–5]. In the first step we found the exact location and appearance of DCT from collagenase-treated kidney, since microdissection from the collagenase-treated kidney was very easy. Eventually we used intact tubules for macroconductance measurements, together with patch clamp studies in collagenase-treated tubules. Thus far we have found that the DCT plays a significant role in the reabsorption of NaCl and Ca^{2+} and the secretion of potassium. We also found that DCT had an ability to increase the reabsorption rate of NaCl when dietary intake of NaCl was increased [3].

The connecting tubule (CNT) is a nephron segment located between the distal convoluted tubule (DCT) and the cortical collecting duct (CCD). The functional significance of this segment had been neglected for a long time, until Morel and his associates [6] reported that the CNT was a unique segment with respect to adenylate cyclase response to hormones. Subsequently, Imai [7] confirmed this view by observing that the changes in transmural voltage ($_t$) in response to hormones are distinct from those observed in the DCT and in the CCD. Limited numbers of studies [2,8–10] suggest that the CNT plays a significant role in the renal tubular transport of Na^+, K^+, Cl^-, HCO_3^- and Ca^{2+}. According to these studies, the CNT is assumed to be one of the target sites of isoproterenol, parathyroid hormone (PTH), and thiazide diuretics.

Material and Methods

In Vitro Microperfusion of Isolated DCT and CNT

Isolated nephron segments were perfused in vitro according to the method of Burg et al. [11]. With slight modification [2,12]. Male Japanese white rabbits weighing 2.0–2.5 kg were maintained on standard rabbit chow and tap water ad libitum. The animals were anesthetized with pentobarbital (35 mg/kg,i.v.). The kidneys were removed and coronal slices were placed in ice-cold intracellular-fluid-like solution of the following composition (mM): 14 KCl, 44 K_2HPO_4, 14 KH_2PO_4, 9 $NaHCO_3$, and 160 sucrose. The connecting tubule was isolated by free hand dissection under a stereo microscope, according to the criteria reported previously [7,10]. A tubular segment was transferred to a bath chamber mounted on an inverted microscope (Olympus, IMT-2) and was perfused with in vitro microperfusion equipment developed by Narishige (Tokyo, Japan). The bathing fluid was supplied through a heating water jacket and was allowed to flow at a rate of 6–9 ml/min. The temperature of the bathing solution was maintained at 37°C. The tubular lumen was perfused under gravity at a rate of 10–20 nl/min.

Electrical Measurement

The transepithelial voltage (V_T) and voltage deflection (dV_o) were measured through the lumen of the perfusion pipette, which was connected to one channel of a dual electrometer (Duo 773, WP Instruments, New Haven, Conn., USA) with 1 mol/l agar bridge and calomel half cell. A flowing boundary 1 mol/l KCl electrode or 1 mol/l KCl agar bridge, which was connected to a calomel half cell, was placed at the outflow of the bath and served as a system ground. In the case of cable analysis, the tubules were cannulated with double barrelled perfusion pipettes (theta borosilicate glass, no.1402401, Hilgenberg, Malsfeld, FRG) as reported previously [2,12]. Through one barrel of the perfusion pipette, current (I_o) was passed into the tubular lumen via an Ag-AgCl wire, then the transepithelial resistance (R_T) and the fractional resistance of the apical membrane (fR_A) were measured. The current was passed from a stimulator (SEN-7103, Nihon Kohden, Tokyo, Japan) with a stimulus isolator (S-1540, Nihon Kohden, Tokyo, Japan), which served as a constant current source. The voltage deflection at the distal end of the tubule (dV_L) was measured by a 1 mol/l KCl agar bridge cannulated into the collecting pipette, which was connected to the other channel of the dual electrometer. The cable parameters were determined using cable equations was reported previously [2,12], assuming that both ends of the cable were closed.

The basolateral membrane voltage (V_B) was measured with conventional microelectrodes, which were pulled from borosilicate glass tubing of 1.5 mm OD and 0.87 mmID (Hilgenberg, no.14033521, Malsfeld, FRG) on a vertical puller (PE-2, Narishige, Tokyo, Japan). They were filled with 1 mol/l KCl solution and had a resistance of 150–200 megaohm and negligible tip potentials (<5 mV). They were fixed to a microelectrode holder containing a Ag-AgCl pellet and were connected to an electrometer (8100, Single electrode system, Dagan, Minneapolis, USA). To impale a tubular cell, a microelectrode was positioned against the basolateral membrane with a hydraulic micromanipulator (MO-102N, Narishige, Tokyo, Japan) which was mounted in another micromanipulator (MN-1, Narishige, Tokyo, Japan) fixed to the stage of a microscope (IMT-2, Olympus, Tokyo, Japan). The microelectrode advanced into the cell by using current oscillations ("Buzz").

All the voltages were monitored by a digital storage oscilloscope (VC-6050, HITACHI, Tokyo, Japan) and stored on an FM-tape recorder (XR-30, TEAC, Tokyo, Japan).

Solutions

The artificial solution used in this study contained in mmol/l; NaCl 110, KCl 5, Na_2HPO_4 0.8, $CaCl_2$ 1.5, $MgCl_2$ 1.0, D-glucose 8.3. L-alanine 5, L-glutamate 3.5, and $NHCO_3$ 25. The solution was gassed with 5% CO_2/95% O_2. In the experiment with Na^+ removal from the control solution, NaCl and $NaHCO_3$ were replaced by equimolar choline Cl and choline HCO_3. In the case of increasing K^+ concentration, 45 mmol/l NaCl was replaced by KCl (50 mmol/l K^+ solution). In the experiment with Cl^- reduction, NaCl was replaced by Na gluconate, and $CaCl_2$ was increased around 6.0 mmol/l, in order to keep ionic Ca^{2+} activity constant (19 mmol/l Cl^- solution). Amiloride HCl was purchased from Sigma Chemicals (St. Louis, Mo., USA).

Statistical Analysis

All the values were expressed as the means ± SEM. Comparison between two groups was made using either a paired or non-paired Student *t*-test when appropriate. *P* values less than 0.05 were considered to be significant.

Results

Mechanism of Ion Transport in DCT

Basic Electrical Properties

When the DCT was perfused with symmetrical solution, the transepithelial voltage displayed lumen negative, indicating the presence of Na^+ channel [1–5]. The transepithelial resistance was 21.8 ohm·cm², indicating that DCT is in the category of leaky epithelia [2]. It is of interest that the magnitude of V_T is dependent on the luminal flow rate, as described by Imai [1,7] and Shimizu et al. [10]. As the flow rate becomes higher, V_T shows lower lumen negativity. Whether this phenomenon is explained by flow rate or by luminal pressure is presently unknown. The distribution of the basolateral membrane voltage (V_B) is nearly Gaussian, with an average V_B of −77.8 mV. The fractional resistance of the luminal membrane was 0.78, indicating the ionic conductive pathway(s) in the luminal membrane [2].

The Luminal Membrane

Amiloride decreased the V_T and the luminal membrane was hyperpolarized by 5 mV. Na^+ removal from the lumen also hyperpolarized the luminal membrane by 8 mV. Addition of Ba^{2+}, or luminal perfusion with high K^+ solution, depolarized the luminal membrane, by 42.6 mV and 37.5 mV, respectively, indicating the presence of K^+ channel [2]. Decrease in luminal Cl^- concentration did not change the luminal membrane voltage, suggesting the absence of Cl^- conductance.

The Basolateral Membrane

When the K^+ concentration in the bathing fluid was increased, or when Ba^{2+} was added to the bath, the basolateral membrane was depolarized by 45.8 mV and 18.3 mV, respectively [2]. Using the patch clamp technique, Taniguchi et al. [4] were able to observe two kinds of K^+ channel in the basolateral membrane. One type was a Ba^{2+} sensitive K^+ channel of 50–60 pS single channel conductance, and the other was a flickering and Ba^{2+} insensitive K^+ channel of 77 pS. Reduction of Cl^- concentration in the bath caused only by a small positive deflection of V_B; however, 14 mV depolarization was observed in the presence of Ba^{2+} with the same maneuver. These data indicate that a small Cl^- conductance exists in the basolateral membrane.

Effect of Calcitonin on Ca^{2+} Transport

Net Ca^{2+} flux was measured by using Fura-2 in the perfusate [5]. This revealed that significant Ca^{2+} reabsorption, which is stimulated by calcitonin and cyclic AMP, takes place in DCT. Furthermore, Ca^{2+} reabsorption was decreased in the presence of ouabain, or when Na^+ was removed from the bath, indicating the existence of secondary active Ca^{2+} transport which is coupled to Na^+, namely the Na/Ca exchanger. In order to transport Ca^{2+} from lumen to bath, there must be an entry step in the luminal membrane. However, with respect to the entry pathway for Ca^{2+} in the luminal membrane, we have no data at present.

Mechanism of Ion Transport in the Connecting Tubule

Electrical Properties of CNT

When the tubule was perfused with symmetrical solutions, the transepithelial voltage (V_T) displayed -3.0 ± 0.4 mV ($n=49$), lumen being negative. This observation was consistent with the finding which was reported previously from our laboratory [5,7–10,13]. Cable analysis of the CNT revealed that the transepithelial resistance (R_T) was 28.9 ± 2.5 ohm·cm² ($n=19$), indicating that the CNT is also in the category of leaky epithelia.

Evidence for Two Cell Populations; CNT and IC Cells

Although morphological studies have disclosed that the CNT has a cellular heterogeneity, namely CNT cells and IC cells, no report is available at present with respect to the conductive nature of the CNT cell. Therefore we impaled the cells of the CNT with conventional microelectrodes in order to investigate the electrical properties of the cell membranes [13]. Random impalement of the CNT revealed that there were two groups of cells having different basolateral membrane voltage. One group had a V_B of -73.1 ± 1.1 mV ($n=77$) and the other group had a V_B of (-28.1 ± 1.8 mV) ($n=39$). The low V_B cell, by analogy with the cortical collecting duct or the medullary collecting duct, is assumed to be an intercalated cell. In 19 cases of cable analysis with cellular impalement of electrodes, the fractional resistance of the luminal membrane (fR_A) was also divided into two groups. In all cases, the low fR_A group (0.50 ± 0.05, $n=22$) corresponded to high V_B cells and the converse held for the high fR_A group (0.96 ± 0.01, $n=9$). Thus, the low V_B and high fR_A cells in the CNT are analogous to the IC cells in the collecting duct. By exclusion, the other type of cell must be the CNT cell.

The Luminal Membrane of the CNT Cell

Since the transepithelial voltage always displayed lumen negative, suggesting the existence of Na^+ channel in the luminal membrane, we applied amiloride to the tubular lumen. When the tubular lumen was perfused with 10^{-5} mol/l amiloride, the transepithelial voltage was decreased from -14.3 ± 2.1 to -0.1 ± 0.2 mV ($n=4$, $P<0.01$) and the basolateral membrane in the CNT cell was hyperpolarized slightly, by 2.8 ± 1.4 mV ($n=4$, NS). No change of V_B was observed in the IC cell (0.3 ± 0.3 mV, $n=4$, NS) upon amiloride application. In order to confirm that the changes of V_T and V_B in response to amiloride were driven by the changes in luminal membrane conductance of the CNT cell, the fractional resistance of the apical membrane (fR_A) was monitored by current injection. Indeed this was true, since the transepithelial resistance (R_T) was increased from 36.1 ± 6.4 to 42.8 ± 7.6 ohm·cm^2 ($n=4$, $P<0.05$) and the fR_A of the CNT cell was increased from 0.49 ± 0.06 to 0.66 ± 0.05 ($n=4$, $P<0.001$). The fR_A of the IC cell did not change at all (0.97 ± 0.01 vs. 0.97 ± 0.01, $n=4$). These results indicate that the luminal membrane of the CNT cell has a Na^+ conductance which is inhibitable with amiloride.

When the luminal concentration of K^+ was changed from 5 to 50 mmol/l, V_T increased from -2.4 ± 0.5 to -7.9 ± 1.7 mV ($n=14$, $P<0.05$) and the basolateral membrane of the CNT cell was depolarized by 35.6 ± 1.1 mV ($n=14$, $P<0.001$). To further confirm this result, the lumen was perfused with Ba^{2+} (2 mmol/l). The transepithelial voltage increased from -6.3 ± 1.3 to -11.1 ± 1.1 mV ($n=4$, $P<0.05$) and the basolateral membrane was depolarized by 18.8 ± 3.1 mV ($n=4$, $P<0.01$). These results indicate that K^+ conductance is also present in the luminal membrane of the CNT cells.

The Basolateral Membrane of the CNT Cell

In order to examine the conductive properties of the basolateral membranes in the CNT cells, concentration changes of K^+ or Cl^- in the bathing solution were applied. In the CNT cells, an increase in K^+ concentration from 5 to 50 mmol/l in the bathing solution depolarized the basolateral membrane from -78.3 to -34.8 mV. Further, a reduction in Cl− concentration from 120 to 19 mM in the bath depolarized the basolateral membrane by 13.7 mV.

To examine the barium sensitivity of K^+ conductance, 2 mmol/l of $BaCl_2$ was added to the bathing solution. The basolateral membrane of the CNT cell was depolarized by 35.3 ± 2.1 mV ($n=9$), on average. When a sudden reduction in Cl^- concentration was applied in the presence of Ba^{2+} in the bath, CNT cells displayed a sharp depolarization of the basolateral membrane (24.3 ± 2.6 mV, $n=8$) which was larger than in the absence of Ba^{2+}.

Effect of PTH on Ca^{2+} Transport and V_T

When PTH was applied to CNT from the bath, net Ca^{2+} flux was markedly increased and the transepithelial voltage (V_T) displayed a biphasic response: initial increase in lumen negativity, followed by gradual and sustained decrease in V_T [14]. This phenomenon was mimicked by cyclic AMP. In the presence of amiloride in the lumen, we could observe only the initial phase, indicating that the second phase could be attributed to the inhibition of Na^+ conductance. The same disappearance of second phase was observed when the lumen was made Ca^{2+} free, suggesting that the increase in cell Ca^{2+} in response to PTH might be related to the inhibition of the Na^+ channel. The first phase of increase in V_T was abolished only when the lumen was perfused with Na^+ free solution, indicating that PTH has a role in opening the amiloride-insensitive cation conductance, which can carry Ca^{2+} together with Na^+. This was confirmed by cell Ca^{2+} measurement using Fura-2 [15]. PTH caused a sustained increase in cell Ca^{2+}, and gradual decrease, under the baseline level of cell Ca^{2+}, was observed after PTH withdrawal, indicating the dual effects of PTH: stimulating both the entry process and the extrusion mechanism.

In the basolateral membrane, there must be a Ca^{2+} extrusion mechanism. PTH-stimulated increase in Ca^{2+} flux was abolished in the presence of ouabain or in the absence of Na^+ ion in the bath. These results indicated the existence of a secondary active Ca^{2+} transport which is coupled to Na^+, namely the Na/Ca exchanger. Cell Ca^{2+} measurement confirmed the view that Na^+ removal from the bath caused an exaggerated increase in cell Ca^{2+} in CNT cells.

Discussion

General Transport Properties of DCT and CNT

Morphological study shows that the distal convoluted tubule (DCT) consists of a homogeneous cell type (the DCT cell), whereas the connecting tubule (CNT) consists of heterogeneous cell types (CNT cells and intercalated cells). Morel et al. [6] were the first to report that, among distal nephron segments, the DCT and CNT were unique with regard to response of adenylate cyclase activity to various hormones, such as calcitonin, isoproterenol, vasopressin, and PTH. Subsequently, Imai [7] confirmed this view by observing that the voltage responses to these hormones in the DCT, CNT, and CCD were distinct. He also reported that the water permeabilities of the DCT and CNT were very low, compared with that of the cortical collecting duct. Recently, we have examined other aspects of these segments, using electrophysiological studies and ion flux measurement of Ca^{2+}, Na^+, K^+, and cell Ca^{2+} movement in response to the above mentioned hormones and in response to changes in dietary intake of NaCl.

Distribution of Transporters in DCT and CNT

Almeida and Burg [8] reported that the transepithelial resistance of the CNT was low (31 ohm·cm^2). In the present study, we also confirmed this value (28.9 ohm·cm^2). It is of interest to note that all distal tubules, including the distal straight tubule (DST), distal convoluted tubule (DCT), and CNT, are leaky segments. The transepithelial resistances found so far are very low in all these segments. However, there is a tendency for the resistance to increase along the axis of the nephron. In contrast, the transepithelial resistance of the collecting duct is very high.

In the present study, we confirmed previous observations [1–5,7–10,13] that both DCT and CNT generate lumen negative voltage. Shimizu et al. [3,10] reported that addition of 10^{-5} M amiloride to the lumen abolished the lumen negative V_T, suggesting that Na^+ conductance in the luminal membrane is critical for negative V_T. This notion has become definite since the finding that amiloride in the lumen increased transepithelial resistance and fractional apical resistance, together with hyperpolarizing the luminal membrane [2]. The luminal membrane in the DCT and CNT also has K^+ channels which are inhibitable with Ba^{2+}. Therefore, the conductive properties of the luminal membrane are very similar to those of the collecting duct cell. However, particularly in the CNT cell, we observed other modes of Na^+ transport in the luminal membrane: namely the Na/Cl cotransporter, which is inhibitable with thiazide [10], and a non-selective cation conductance, which is able to carry Na^+ and Ca^{2+} [14]. The significance of the latter transport will be discussed later.

Both DCT and CNT cells were characterized by high V_B and fR_A, of 0.50 – 0.78. An fR_A lower than unity may be accounted for by the existence of both Na^+ and K^+ conductances in the luminal membranes of both cells, conductances which were inhibitable with amiloride and Ba^{2+}, respectively. The basolateral membrane of the CNT had a large K^+ conductance and a small Cl^- conductance. The apparent transference numbers for K^+ and Cl^- were calculated to be 0.75 and 0.16 in DCT cells, and 0.71 and 0.28 in CNT cells, respectively. Thus, almost 90%–99% of the ionic conductance in the basolateral membrane is accounted for by K^+ and Cl^- conductances, with K^+ conductance being preferential.

Physiological Significance of DCT and CNT

The major task of the DCT and the CNT is considered to be the reabsorption of NaCl. Secretion of K^+ [16] and absorption of Ca^{2+} [1,9] would be considered as phenomena secondary to active Na^+ transport, since K^+ secretion takes place as a backleak from the cell, via luminal K^+ conductance, and Ca^{2+} reabsorption has recently been shown to be related to the Na^+/Ca^{2+} exchanger in the basolateral membrane [5,14,15,17]. Ca^{2+} transport is specifically stimulated by calcitonin and PTH in the DCT and the CNT, respectively.

The DCT cell has a special ability to reabsorb NaCl, in that the rate of NaCl reabsorption and K^+ secretion changes depending on the volume of dietary NaCl intake. When animals were given an increased NaCl intake, DCT cells became large and both net Na^+ reabsorption and net K^+ secretion were increased. It was demonstrated that the sizes of the Na^+ and K^+ conductances were increased together with increased Na-K-ATPase activity [3].

Among the distal nephron segments, the net Na^+ reabsorption in CNT is the highest [8,10]. This corresponds to the activity of Na-K-ATPase. Na-K-ATPase activity is 6 times greater in the CNT than in the CCD. The net Na^+ flux across the CNT has been reported to be 20.3 $pmol{\cdot}cm^{-1}{\cdot}s^{-1}$ [8], whereas the net Na^+ fluxes of the DCT and the CCD were 13.7 [16] and 2.7 – 5.7 $pmol{\cdot}cm^{-1}{\cdot}s^{-1}$, respectively. In CNT, trichlormethiazide, one of the potent thiazide diuretics, was shown to inhibit lumen-to-bath Na^+ flux by 32.3% and net Cl^- flux by 30.6%, by inhibiting the Na^+/Cl^- cotransporter in the luminal membrane [10]. In the present study, when amiloride (10^{-5} mol/l) was applied to the lumen, the magnitude of decrease in the equivalent short circuit current (V_T/R_T) was calculated to be 395 $\mu A/cm^2$, corresponding to 30.8 $pmol{\cdot}cm^{-1}{\cdot}s^{-1}$. This value is consistent with the magnitude of the decrease in lumen-to-bath Na^+ flux, 32.5 $pmol{\cdot}cm^{-1}{\cdot}s^{-1}$ (46.1%), found in our previous study [10]. Thus, in the CNT the sum of Na^+/Cl^- cotransport and amiloride-sensitive Na^+ conductance yields around 78% of the total transepithelial Na^+ flux. The remaining 22% could be mediated by the Na^+/H^+-Cl^-/HCO_3^- exchanger and by an amiloride-insensitive cationic conductance. It has recently been suggested, by Shimmizu et al. [14], that the latter mechanism is the entry pathway for Ca^{2+} at the luminal membrane.

References

1. Imai M, Nakamura R (1982) Function of distal convoluted and connecting tubules studied by isolated nephron fragments. Kidney Int 22:465–472
2. Yoshitomi K, Shimizu T, Taniguchi J, Imai M (1989) Electrophysiological characterization of rabbit distal convoluted tubule. Pflugers Arch 414L457–463
3. Shimizu T, Yoshitomi K, Taniguchi J, Imai M (1989) Effect of high NaCl intake on Na and K transport in rabbit distal convoluted tubule. Pflugers Arch 414:500–508
4. Taniguchi J, Yoshitomi K, Imai M (1989) K^+ channel currents in basolateral membrane of distal convoluted tubule of rabbit kidney. Am J Physiol 256:F246–F254
5. Shimizu, T, Yoshitomi K, Nakamura M, Imai M (1990) Effects of PTH, calcitonin, and cAMP on calcium transport in rabbit distal nephron segments. Am J Physiol 259:F408–F414
6. Morel F, Chabardes D, Imbert M (1976) Functional segmentation of the rabbit distal tubule by microdetermination of hormone-dependent adenylate cyclase activity. Kidney Int 9:264–277
7. Imai M (1979) The connecting tubule: A functional subdivision of the rabbit distal nephron segments. Kidney Int 15:346–356
8. Almeida AJ, Burg MB (1982) Sodium transport in the rabbit connecting tubule. Am J Physiol 243:F330–F334
9. Imai M (1981) Effect of parathyroid hormone and N′,O′-dibutyryl cyclic AMP on Ca transport across the rabbit distal nephron segments perfused in vitro. Pflugers Arch 390: 145–151
10. Shimizu T, Yoshitomi K, Nakamura M, Imai M (1988) Site and mechanism of action of trichlormethiazide in rabbit distal nephron segments perfused in vitro. J Clin Invest 82:721–730
11. Burg MB, Grantham J, Abramow M, Orloff J (1966) Preparation and study of fragments of single rabbit nephrons. Am J Physiol 210:1293–1298
12. Yoshitomi K, Koseki C, Taniguchi J, Imai M (1987) Functional heterogeneity in the hamster medullary thick ascending limb of Henle's loop. Pflugers Arch 408:600–608
13. Yoshitomi K, Shimizu T, Imai M (1988) Functional cellular heterogeneity in the rabbit connecting tubule. Kidney Int 33:430
14. Shimizu T, Yoshitomi K, Nakamura M, Imai M (1990) Effect of parathyroid hormone on the connecting tubule from the rabbit kidney; biphasic response of transmural voltage. Pflugers Arch 416:254–261
15. Shimizu T, Yamasaki F, Imai M, Yoshitomi K (1990) Regulation of calcium transport in the distal nephron segments. Kidney Int 37:461
16. Shareghi GR, Stoner LC (1978) Calcium transport across segments of the rabbit distal nephron in vitro. Am J Physiol 235:F367–F375
17. Bourdeau JE, Lau K (1989) Effects of parathyroid hormone on cytosolic free calcium concentration in individual rabbit connecting tubules. J Clin Invest 83:373–379

Vesicle Trafficking and Membrane Polarity in Epithelial Cells: Relationship to Intercalated Cell Function in Kidney Collecting Ducts

Dennis Brown[1]

Summary. Many plasma membrane components are delivered to their appropriate membrane domain in membrane-bounded vesicles, and the control of vesicle targeting and fusion are, therefore, critical elements in epithelial cell function. This review discusses some current concepts of how the specificity of this targeting process may be determined, including protein structure, microtubule pathways, and GTP-binding proteins as fusion factors. These concepts of epithelial cell polarity generation and maintenance are of tremendous functional importance to the kidney, because epithelial cells lining the kidney collecting duct have developed highly-specialized, yet independent systems for the rapid modulation of the composition of their plasma membranes in response to different stimuli. In particular, the ability of subpopulations of collecting duct intercalated cells to insert a proton pumping ATPase into opposite plasma membrane domains is a remarkable cell biological feat that provides a unique opportunity for investigating mechanisms of protein targeting in epithelia.

Introduction

The plasma membrane composition of virtually all eucaryotic cells is established, maintained, and modified by the process of membrane recycling. Specific plasma membrane components are inserted by exocytosis of transport vesicles, and are removed by endocytosis of segments of the membrane in which particular proteins are concentrated. It is particularly important for kidney function that epithelial cells lining the urinary tubule can respond rapidly to changes in the composition of their environment; epithelial cells lining the kidney collecting duct have developed highly-specialized, yet independent systems for the rapid modulation of the composition of their plasma membranes in response to different stimuli [1]. Vasopressin induces the

[1]Renal Unit, Massachusetts General Hospital and Department of Pathology, Harvard Medical School, Boston, MA 02114, USA

cycling of vesicles that are thought to carry water channels to and from the apical plasma membrane of principal cells, thus rapidly modulating the water permeability of this membrane. In the intercalated cells of the collecting duct, hydrogen ion secretion is controlled by the recycling of vesicles carrying proton pumps to and from the plasma membrane. In both cell types, "coated" carrier vesicles are involved, but whereas clathrin-coated vesicles participate in water channel recycling, the vesicles in intercalated cells are coated with the cytoplasmic domains of proton pumps. In addition to these rapidly recycling membrane components, kidney epithelial cells are highly polarized with respect to many other membrane proteins that play an integral role in tubular function in all regions of the urinary tubule. These molecules have been localized using a variety of techniques from physiological measurements of tubular function to immunocytochemical detection at the light and/or electron microscopical level. This review will first examine some of the potential mechanisms by which integral membrane proteins may find their way to specific plasma membrane domains, and will then summarize studies related to the polarized distribution of a proton pumping ATPase in kidney epithelial cells.

Generation of Polarity in Epithelial Cells

Because epithelia function as selective barriers separating two different types of extracellular milieux, it is necessary for them to generate and maintain the polarity of a wide variety of plasma membrane proteins and lipids. Many plasma membrane components are delivered to the appropriate membrane domain in membrane-bounded vesicles, and so the control of vesicle targeting and fusion are critical elements in epithelial cell function. A considerable amount of work is now aimed at understanding the molecular mechanisms that determine the selectivity of vesicle movement and fusion, and some of the key areas of current investigation are:

The Role Played by Targeting Sequences that Form Part of the Structure of Individual Proteins

Some amino acid sequences allow proteins to be inserted into mitochondrial membranes [2], while others are required for clustering of proteins into clathrin-coated pits on the cell surface [3]. Other covalent modifications of proteins, such as the addition of mannose-6-phosphate groups to carbohydrate side chains, are required to direct lysosomal hydrolases to lysosomes [4]. Yet other amino acid sequences cause proteins to be retained in the rough endoplasmic reticulum, and prevent their transfer to the Golgi apparatus [5]. Recently, it has been proposed that a phosphatidylinositol-glycan anchor that links a special class of proteins to the lipid bilayer may be a signal for incorporation of these proteins into the apical plasma membrane of epithelial cells [6]. Based on these studies, and others examining the role of cytoplasmic domains of viral glycoproteins in the targeting process [7], it is generally believed that the amino acid sequence of a given protein will play a large part in determining its final destination in a cell. For this reason, our finding that subpopulations of intercalated cells in the kidney collecting duct can insert a proton pumping ATPase into the apical or basolateral plasma membrane domain is intriguing [8], since most plasma membrane proteins appear to be restricted to one pole of the cell or the other.

The Role of Cytoskeletal Elements in Directing Vesicular Traffic in Cells

Considerable data have accumulated showing that microtubule disruption by agents such as colchicine can interfere severely with intracellular membrane traffic, secretory processes, lysosomal distribution, and the processing and packaging of proteins at the level of the Golgi apparatus [9–14]. In an earlier study, we showed that colchicine interferes with the processing, packaging, and stimulated secretion of newly-synthesized amylase from the rat parotid gland, but that it does not affect secretion of pre-formed amylase that had already been packed into secretory granules [12]. In the same study, we also showed that colchicine severely disrupts the structure of the Golgi apparatus, causing the ordered cisternae to be replaced by swarms of small vesicles. Recently, it has been shown that following Golgi disruption by nocodazole, the reclustering of scattered Golgi elements occurs along microtubules [15].

Despite these dramatic effects on the secretory apparatus, whether microtubules are involved in the generation and maintenance of epithelial cell polarity is still an unresolved issue. Conflicting results [16,17] have been obtained in virally-infected cells concerning the importance of microtubules for the polarized insertion of membrane proteins (in this case, viral proteins). Much less work has been performed using endogenous proteins, but recent data indicate that nocodazole inhibits the normal insertion of an endogenous apical membrane protein in cultured cells [18], and microtubule disruption has a dramatic effect on cell polarity in intestinal epithelial cells, resulting in the formation of patches of brush-border microvilli and the appearance of normally apical proteins such as alkaline phosphatase on the basolateral plasma membrane [9,13,19]. How microtubules may influence the intracellular movement of organelles and transporting vesicles is emerging as a result of the discovery of so-called microtubule motors (kinesin and cytoplasmic dyneins); these proteins, isolated from cytosolic fractions of cells, have the capacity to induce ATP-dependent organelle movement along isolated microtubules in either an anterograde or retrograde direction [20]. Recent observations on the pH dependence of lysosomal distribution in fibroblasts have been suggested to result from the selective switching on or off of different microtubule motors at different cytoplasmic pH values [10]. The possibility that microtubules are involved in the movement of transporting vesicles to the apical pole of epithelial cells, and that this movement may be pH-dependent, is of clear relevance to the physiological response of collecting duct intercalated cells to different acid-base conditions. Indeed, in turtle bladder, acidification in response to CO_2 is inhibited by colchicine [21].

The actin-based microfilamentous system is also of importance to intracellular vesicle trafficking, although the effects of cytochalasins, which disrupt the structure and function of actin filaments, are less consistent than those of microtubule disrupting agents. For example, in some endocrine cells, cytochalasin B causes an increase in the initial secretory response [22], whereas in the toad urinary bladder it causes a decrease in the vasopressin-stimulated increase in transepithelial water permeability, a process which also involves exocytotic events [14,23]. It is apparent from our examination of 3-dimensional electron micrographs of freeze-dried, rotary shadowed epithelial cells, that cytoplasmic organelles and vesicles have a complex interaction

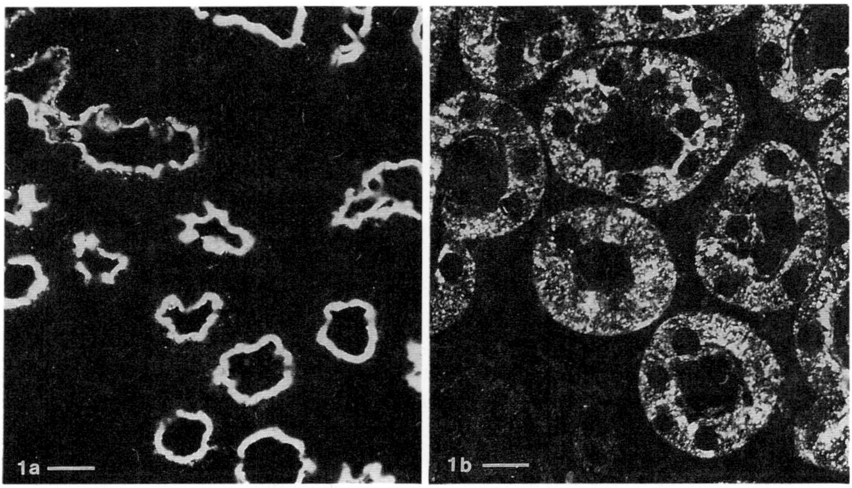

Fig. 1a,b. Frozen sections of control (**a**) and colchicine-treated (**b**) rat cortex stained with antibodies against gp330. In control kidney, gp330 is concentrated at the apical pole of proximal tubule cells, whereas after colchicine-induced disruption of microtubules, it is present on vesicles scattered throughout the cytoplasm (see [29]). Bar = 20 μm

with microfilaments, and in many cases appear to be almost entirely "cocooned" in the dense subapical network of actin filaments (Hartwig and Brown, unpublished results). Furthermore, there are reports in the literature that the charged surface of artificial liposomes can act as a surface that induces actin polymerization in vitro [24]. In addition, there is accumulating evidence that many transmembrane proteins are linked either directly or indirectly to the cytoskeleton [25,26]. Of particular interest to the mechanism of proton and bicarbonate transport in the kidney is the well-known interaction of band 3 with spectrin in the erythrocyte [25], and with non-erythrocyte spectrin (fodrin) in intercalated cells [27]; the sodium-potassium ATPase has also been found to be linked to cytoskeletal elements in MDCK cells [28]. These transmembrane linkages certainly play an important role in the maintenance of polarized membrane domains. Clearly, the potential interaction between microtubules, microfilaments and intracellular vesicles requires that the contributions of all three elements be considered in any scheme of vesicle trafficking and the generation and maintenance of cell polarity.

GTP-Binding Proteins and Vesicle Targeting

Once vesicles containing a specific cargo of protein and lipid have been formed and transported to the vicinity of their site of fusion in the cell cytoplasm, how is the final process of fusion with their target membrane controlled? Our recent studies using an apical membrane glycoprotein of the proximal tubule brush border, gp330, have shown that colchicine treatment of rats results in a dramatic redistribution of this glycoprotein in the cell (Fig. 1a,b). Instead of its usual exclusively apical localization, it is found on many vesicles scattered throughout the cytoplasm after drug treatment

[29]. However, despite the fact that many of these vesicles are found close to the basolateral plasma membrane, no evidence for a significant incorporation of gp330 into the basolateral membrane was found. This suggests that the mere proximity of a vesicle to a membrane is not sufficient to ensure fusion, and that most probably a second level of control is exerted that requires some specific recognition signal between the vesicle and the target membrane domain. The microtubules would, then, be required to direct vesicles to the apical pole of the cell, and thereby to increase the local concentration of fusion-competent vesicles beneath the apical plasma membrane. As discussed above, however, colchicine-treatment of intestinal epithelial cells *does* result in the appearance of apical markers on the basolateral membrane. One potential explanation for this is that these proteins are packaged into the "wrong" transporting vesicles after microtubule disruption. Thus, the targeting error in these cells is made at the level of sorting in the Golgi apparatus, not at the level of vesicle-plasma membrane interaction. In the proximal tubule, the vesicles containing gp330 that redistribute throughout the cell may be derived mainly from the apical plasma membrane, owing to the high rate of apical membrane recycling in this cell type. For this reason, they may not be able to fuse with the basolateral membrane. The contribution of newly-synthesized gp330 to the total, redistributed intracellular pool is unknown.

In view of the undoubted specificity of intracellular fusion events which is necessary to maintain the characteristic protein/lipid fingerprint of individual membranes, it is likely that some type of "ligand-receptor" interaction between donor and acceptor membranes is required, and one developing area of research concerns the role of guanine-nucleotide binding proteins (G-proteins) in this process. The G-proteins that are linked to signal transduction events at the cell surface, and also control the gating of a number of ion channels on the cell membrane, are heterotrimeric structures consisting of alpha, beta and gamma subunits [30]. These G-protein subunits combine with a receptor protein and an effector such as adenylyl cyclase to form a functional unit, and all these elements are associated in the same membrane microdomain to provide selectivity and amplification in the signalling pathway. The intrinsic GTPase activity of the alpha subunit that hydrolyses GTP to GDP to stop the transduction of the signal is an important "timer" element in the signal transduction cascade.

However, recent work has shown that GTP-binding proteins are also associated with some intracellular compartments, and that a distinct class of ras-like small molecular weight G-proteins (SMGs) [31, 32] may play a role in vesicle trafficking and fusion events [33]. These small molecular weight G-proteins appear to be widely distributed in both membranes and cytosol, and some are also substrates for ADP-ribosylation induced by bacterial toxins, particularly those from *Clostridium botulinum* [32], *Clostridium perfringens* [34], and cholera toxin [35].

While the analogy with heterotrimeric G-proteins has led to the assumption that each of these proteins participates in a signal transduction pathway, this assumption remains unproven. In particular, all of the SMGs studied to date lack one or more of the essential elements required for signal transduction. For example, while all, by definition, bind GTP, some have little (ras) [36] or no (ARF) [37] GTPase activity. However, this "timer" function can be served by a distinct cytosolic protein, GAP (GTPase activating protein), which enhances the GTPase activity of two of the SMGs, ras and rho [38]. In addition, another SMG, ARF [37], is able to stimulate the cholera-toxin induced ADP ribosylation of the alpha subunit of Gs, indicating that some degree of crosstalk may exist between SMGs and the heterotrimeric G-proteins.

This discussion leads to the idea that these SMGs are ideal candidates to be involved in vesicle targeting, because the sequential and selective interactions between these proteins and the other proteins necessary for them to function in "signal transduction" would ensure that only when a vesicle carrying a particular SMG met with a membrane carrying another necessary component to reconstitute function, would vesicle fusion ensue. According to a hypothesis proposed by Bourne [33], an integral membrane protein present on an intracellular vesicle would form a membrane-associated complex with a specific G-protein. A docking protein on a recipient (target) membrane would then recognize this G-protein complex on the vesicle, and thereby induce GTP hydrolysis, resulting in vesicle fusion. This hydrolysis of GTP to GDP should be blocked by non-hydrolyzable GTP analogues and should inhibit vesicle fusion; this is precisely what has been demonstrated in isolated vesicle fractions from the Golgi region [39]. Furthermore, secretory processes in mast cells and neutrophils have also been linked to G-proteins [40], and G-proteins have been localized on the membranes of secretory granules in yeast and chromaffin cells [41, 42]. Most recently, a soluble NEM-sensitive factor that resembles the SEC18 gene product of yeast [43], and a second soluble fusion factor found in cytosol have been proposed to interact with an integral membrane protein to control vesicle fusion at the level of the Golgi apparatus [44]; the same NEM-sensitive factor is also required for vesicle mediated transport between the RER and the Golgi [45], a known function of SEC18 in yeast [46]. Most recently, three integral membrane proteins that are necessary for vesicle fusion to occur have been isolated from Golgi membranes [47]. These data support the idea outlined above that multiple protein interactions may be required to reconstitute a functional complex that catalyses membrane fusion events.

Polarized Function in Kidney Intercalated Cells

Proton Pump Localization and Recycling in Intercalated Cells

The concepts of epithelial cell polarity outlined above are of tremendous functional importance to the kidney. Distinctive morphological alterations occur in intercalated cells during an increase in H^+ secretion by collecting ducts [48, 49]. Following induced acidosis in rats, an increase in the apical surface area of intercalated cells is accompanied by a decrease in the number of specialized cytoplasmic vesicles, known as tubulovesicles [48], presumably as a result of their exocytotic fusion with the apical plasma membrane. Previous studies in turtle bladder and the collecting duct had shown that vesicles containing proton pumps are inserted into the apical membrane of these carbonic anhydrase rich cells during acidosis [49, 50]. Tracer studies with horseradish peroxidase demonstrated that these specialized coated vesicles were also involved in endocytotic events [51]. Specific antibodies against different subunits of the proton pumping ATPase from bovine kidney medulla were used to show that the vesicle coating material contained defined subunits of the proton pump [8, 52]. The "coat" seen on the cytoplasmic side of the plasma membrane of some intercalated cells also contained the same pump subunits and the structure of the membrane coat was elucidated, using the rapid-freeze, deep-etch technique, in which high resolution

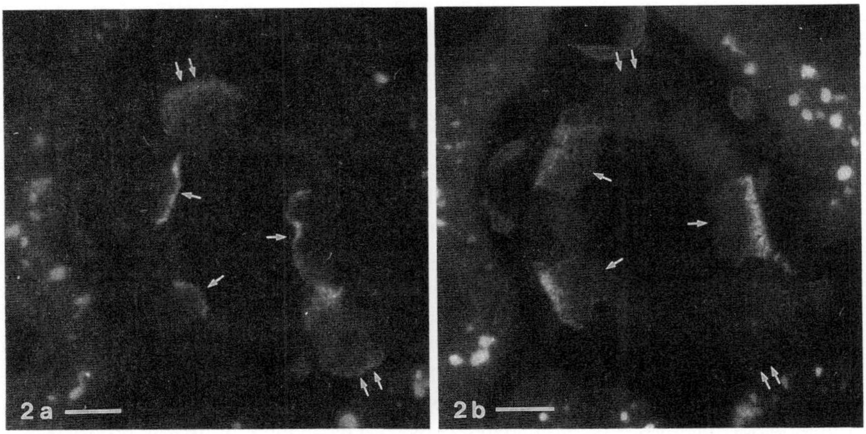

Fig. 2a,b. Consecutive semithin 1 μm sections showing a cortical collecting duct stained with antibodies against a proton pumping ATPase (**a**) and a band 3-like anion exchanger (**b**). A-type intercalated cells show basolateral staining for band 3 and apical staining for the proton pump (*single arrows*). In contrast, B-type intercalated cells with basolateral or diffuse/bipolar proton pump staining (*double arrows*) are not labeled with anti band 3 antibodies. (See [57]). The brightly fluorescent spots in proximal tubules are autofluorescent lysosomes. Bar = 10 μm

microscopic images of proteins can be obtained. It was shown that the membrane-coating material had a structure that was identical to that of immunoaffinity-purified proton pumps, incorporated into phospholipid liposomes [52], thus confirming its identity as part of the proton pumping ATPase responsible for distal urinary acidification.

Opposite Polarity of Proton Pumps in A and B Intercalated Cells

This and other work suggested that tubulovesicles fuse with the apical plasma membrane during acidosis and incorporate their membrane into this plasma membrane domain. However, in the cortical collecting duct [48] and in the turtle urinary bladder [53], two morphological variants of "carbonic anhydrase-rich" cell have been described, which are believed to be proton-secreting (A-cells) or bicarbonate-secreting (B-cells). Both types co-exist in kidney cortical collecting ducts, in accord with the ability of this tubule segment to secrete either net acid or net base under different physiological conditions of acidosis or alkalosis. Using anti-proton pump antibodies, we demonstrated that while all medullary intercalated cells have proton pumps associated with their apical plasma membrane, cortical intercalated cells had three patterns of labeling (Fig. 2a): apical, basolateral, and diffuse cytoplasmic or bipolar [8]. This finding provided direct support for the idea that different intercalated cells in the cortex are responsible for either proton (apical pumps) or bicarbonate (basolateral pumps) secretion into the tubule lumen. It is possible that the cells with a diffuse staining might be an intermediate or transitional cell type. There was an inverse relationship between the number of cells stained diffusely or basolaterally, while the number of apically-stained cells was relatively constant among different animals.

Cellular Remodelling in Intercalated Cells

Provocative data by Schwartz et al. [54] suggested that A and B cells may be interconvertible, and may change their functional polarity by inserting proton pumps into either apical or basolateral plasma membranes, depending on prevailing acid-base conditions of the animal. However, more recent work reported that A and B cells do not interconvert during alterations in acid-base status [55]. While this question has not yet been clearly resolved, several observations are pertinent. The A cells have a basolateral band 3-like chloride-bicarbonate exchanger [27, 56], whereas no chloride-bicarbonate exchanger has yet been located by immunocytochemistry in type B cells, either in the apical or the basolateral plasma membrane. Double staining studies show that all B-type intercalated cells with basolateral or diffuse proton pump staining lack detectable band 3, while the vast majority of cells with apical proton pumps show strong basolateral band 3 staining (Fig. 2). However, we consistently found a small (1%) population of cortical intercalated cells with apical proton pumps but no basolateral band 3 [57]. Whether this cell type is a distinct population or a transitional type of intercalated cell is unknown. The absence of band 3-like antigenicity on the apical surface of all intercalated cells demonstrates that if a simple exchange of transporting molecules from apical to basolateral plasma membrane and vice-versa occurs in these cells during adaptation to acid-base loads, then the apical anion exchanger must be modified in some way that renders it undetectable by a range of anti-band 3 antibodies [27, 56, 57]. In acidotic animals, functionally-detectable apical anion exchangers appear to be internalized by B-intercalated cells [58], but whether or not proton pumps are subsequently inserted into the apical membrane of the same cells is still unclear. By immunofluorescence microscopy, a decrease in the number of basolaterally stained intercalated cells is found in the cortex of rats with metabolic acidosis; the number of cells with "apical" proton pumps increases both after acute (6h) gavage with NH_4Cl (D. Brown, I. Sabolic, and S. Gluck, unpublished), as well as after chronic 14 day NH_4Cl treatment [59]. Whether these "apical" pumps are associated with the plasma membrane or are present in subapical vesicles remains to be determined.

Role of Microtubules in Vesicle Trafficking in Intercalated Cells

Whether or not the same intercalated cell is able to transfer membrane transporters from one pole of the cell to the other, the observation that intercalated cell subpopulations can maintain an opposite polarity with respect to proton pumps remains a finding of great cell biological interest. One possibility that might explain differential targeting of proton pumps is that the apical and basolateral versions of the proton ATPase may not be identical in subunit composition; this difference could confer domain specificity on the targeting process. Another possibility is that the microtubular network is somehow different in cells with apical or basolateral proton pumps, and that vesicles containing the pumps move selectively to only one pole of the cell. As discussed above, it has been proposed that microtubule tracks are important for the delivery of apical proteins, but that basolateral proteins are routed to the

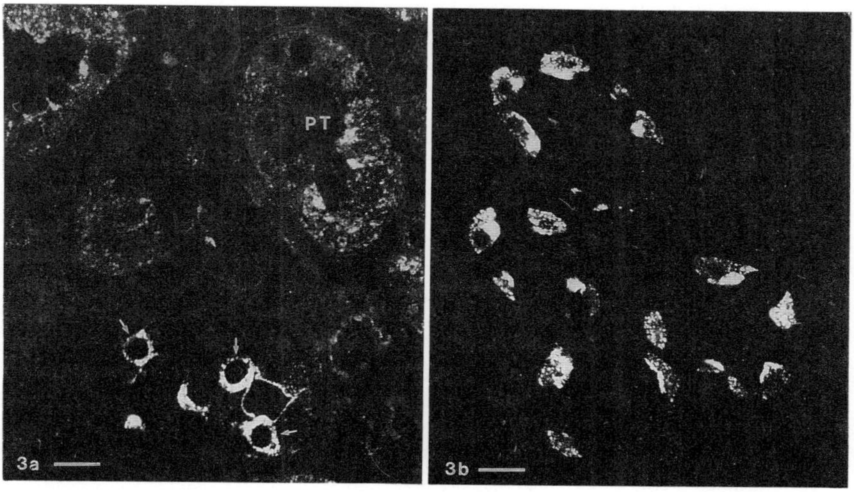

Fig. 3a,b. Part of the cortex (**a**) and inner stripe (**b**) of colchicine-treated rat kidney stained with antibodies against a proton pumping ATPase. In the cortex, proton pumps are distributed on vesicles scattered throughout the cytoplasm of both proximal tubule epithelial cells, and intercalated cells (*arrows*). In the inner stripe of the outer medulla, vesicles containing proton pumps are also distributed throughout the cytoplasm of heavily-labeled intercalated cells. This study was performed in collaboration with Dr. Ivan Sabolic (MGH, Boston) and Dr. Stephen Gluck (Washington University Jewish Hospital, St. Louis, Mo). Bar = 20 μm

base of the cell by a default pathway. In this way, microtubule depolymerization might be expected to result in basolateral, rather than apical insertion of proton pumps. This prediction assumes that vesicles carrying proton pumps are competent to fuse with either apical or basolateral plasma membranes, and that the specificity of the process lies exclusively in the delivery of the vesicles to the appropriate membrane domain. However, this is clearly not the case with another apical membrane protein, gp330, which is present in vesicles that do not fuse with the wrong (i.e., the basolateral) plasma membrane (see above).

This prediction was tested in animals treated for up to 24h with colchicine to induce microtubule depolymerization. In these animals, proton pumps were no longer polarized to one pole of the cell, but they were concentrated in numerous vesicles scattered throughout the cytoplasm (D. Brown, I. Sabolic and S. Gluck, submitted for publication). A similar scattered distribution was seen in A and B intercalated cells, as well as in epithelial cells of the proximal tubule (Fig. 3a). Of particular note is that A-type cells in the inner stripe of the outer medullar did not concentrate proton pumps in their basolateral plasma membranes (Fig. 3b). These results indicate that microtubule depolymerization alone is not sufficient to account for the final differences in the membrane distribution of proton pumps seen in A and B intercalated cells. As is also the case for gp330-containing vesicles in the proximal tubule, an additional level of control must govern the final fusion process between these re-routed vesicles and their target membrane region. The nature of this control process is unknown, but any of the factors discussed in the initial part of this review could be involved.

References

1. Brown D (1989) Membrane recycling and epithelial cell function. Am J Physiol 256: F1–F12
2. Verner K, Schatz G (1988) Protein translocation across membranes. Science 241:1307–1313
3. Davis CG, Lehrman MA, Russell DW, Anderson RGW, Brown MS, Goldstein JL (1986) The J. D. mutation in familial hypercholesterolemia: amino acid substitution in cytoplasmic domain impedes internalization of LDL receptors. Cell 45:15–24
4. Sly WS, Fisher HD (1982) The phosphomannosyl recognition system for intracellular and intercellular transport of lysosomal enzymes. J Cell Biochem 18:319–347
5. Rose JK, Doms RW (1988) Regulation of protein export from the endoplasmic reticulum. Ann Rev Cell Biol 4:257–288
6. Lisanti MP, Caras IW, Dovitz MA, Rodriguez-Boulan E (1989) A glycophospholipid membrane anchor serves as an apical targeting signal in polarized epithelial cells. J Cell Biol 109:2145–2156
7. Garoff H (1985) Using recombinant DNA techniques to study protein targeting in the eucaryotic cell. Ann Rev Cell Biol 1:403–445
8. Brown D, Hirsch S, Gluck S (1988) An H^+ ATPase is present in opposite plasma membrane domains in subpopulations of kidney epithelial cells. Nature 331:622–624
9. Achler C, Filmer D, Merte C, Drenckhahn D (1989) Role of microtubules in polarized delivery of apical membrane proteins to the brush border of the intestinal epithelium. J Cell Biol 109:179–189
10. Heuser J (1989) Changes in lysosome shape and distribution correlated with changes in cytoplasmic pH. J Cell Biol 108:855–864
11. Matteoni R, Kreis TE (1987) Translocation and clustering of endosomes and lysosomes depends on microtubules. J Cell Biol 105:1253–1265
12. Patzelt C, Brown D, Jeanrenaud B (1977) Inhibitory effect of colchicine on amylase secretion by rat parotid glands. Possible localization in the Golgi area. J Cell Biol 73:578–593
13. Pavelka M, Ellinger A, Gangl A (1983) Effect of colchicine on rat small intestinal adsorptive cells I. Formation of basolateral microvillus borders. J Ultrastruct Res 85:249–259
14. Taylor A (1977) Role of microtubules and microfilaments in the action of vasopressin. In: Andreoli TE, Grantham JJ, Rector FC (eds) Disturbances in Body Fluid Osmolality. Am Physiol Soc, Bethesda, pp 97–124
15. Kreis T (1989) Reclustering of scattered Golgi elements occurs along microtubules. Eur J Cell Biol 48:250–263
16. Salas P, Misek D, Vega-Salas D, Gundersen D, Cereijido M, Rodriguez-Boulan E (1986) Microtubules are not critically involved in the biogenesis of epithelial cell surface polarity. J Cell Biol 102:1853–1867
17. Rindler MJ, Ivanov IE, Sabatini DD (1987) Microtubule-acting drugs lead to the nonpolarized delivery of the influenza hemagglutinin to the cell surface of polarized Madin-Darby canine kidney cells. J Cell Biol 104:231–241
18. Eilers U, Klumperman J, Hauri HP (1989) Nocodazole, a microtubule-active drug, interferes with apical protein delivery in cultured intestinal epithelial cells. J Cell Biol 108: 13–22
19. Hasegawa H, Watanabe K, Nakamura T, Nagura H (1987) Immunocytochemical localization of alkaline phosphatase in absorptive cells of rat small intestine after colchicine treatment. Cell Tiss Res 250:521–529
20. Vale RD (1987) Intracellular transport using microtubule-based motors. Ann Rev Cell Biol 3:347–378
21. Stetson DL, Steinmetz PR (1983) Role of membrane fusion in CO_2 stimulation of proton secretion by turtle bladder. Am J Physiol 245:C113–C120

22. Orci L, Gabbay KH, Malaisse WJ (1972) Pancreatic beta-cell web: its possible role in insulin secretion. Science 175:1128–1130
23. Muller J, Kachadorian WA, DiScala VA (1980) Evidence that ADH-stimulated intramembrane particle aggregates are transferred from cytoplasmic to luminal membranes in toad bladder epithelial cells. J Cell Biol 85:83–95
24. Laliberte A, Gicquad C (1988) Polymerization of actin by positively-charged liposomes. J Cell Biol 106:1221–1227
25. Bennett V (1985) The membrane skeleton of human erythrocytes and its implications for more complex cells. Annu Rev Biochem 54:273–304
26. Nelson WJ, Veshnock PJ (1986) Dynamics of membrane-skeleton (fodrin) organization during development of polarity in Madin-Darby kidney epithelial cells. J Cell Biol 103: 1751–1765
27. Drenkhahn D, Schluter K, Allen DP, Bennett V (1985) Co-localization of Band 3 with ankyrin and spectrin at the basal membrane of intercalated cells in the rat kidney. Science 230:1287–1289
28. Nelson WJ, Hammerton RW (1989) A membrane-cytoskeletal complex containing Na^+, K^+-ATPase, ankyrin, and fodrin in Madin-Darby canine kidney (MDCK) cells: implications for the biogenesis of epithelial cell polarity. J Cell Biol 108:893–902
29. Gutmann EJ, Niles JL, McCluskey RT, Brown D (1989) Colchicine-induced redistribution of an endogenous apical membrane glycoprotein (gp 330) in kidney proximal tubule epithelium. Am J Physiol 257:C397–C407
30. Gilman AG (1987) G-proteins: transducers of receptor-generated signals. Annu Rev Biochem 56:615–649
31. McGrath JP, Capon DJ, Goeddel DV, Levinson AD (1984) Comparative biochemical properties of normal and activated human ras p21 protein. Nature 310:644–649
32. Bokoch GM, Mumby SM (1988) Purification and characterization of the 22,000-Dalton GTP-binding protein substrate for ADP-ribosylation by botulinum toxin, G_{22K*}. J Biol Chem 263:16744–16749
33. Bourne HR (1988) Do GTPases direct membrane traffic in secretion? Cell 53:669–671
34. Aktories K, Weller U, Chhatwal GS (1987) Clostridium botulinum type C produced a novel ADP-ribosyltransferase distinct from botulinum C2 toxin. FEBS Lett 212:109–113
35. Heyworth CM, Whetton AD, Wong S, Martin RB, Houslay MD (1985) Insulin inhibits the cholera-toxin-catalysed ribosylation of a Mr-25,000 protein in rat liver plasma membranes. Biochem J 228:593–603
36. Barbacid MA (1987) Ras genes. Annu Rev Biochem 56:779–827
37. Kahn RA, Gilman AG (1986) The protein cofactor necessary for ADP-ribosylation of Gs by cholera toxin is itself a GTP binding protein. J Biol Chem 261:7906–7911
38. Trahey M, McCormick F (1987) A cytoplasmic protein stimulates normal N-ras p21 GTPase, but does not affect oncogenic mutants. Science 238:542–545
39. Melancon P, Glick BS, Malhotra V, Weidman PJ, Serafini T, Gleason ML, Orci L, Rothman JE (1987) Involvement of GTP-binding "G" proteins in transport through the Golgi stack. Cell 51:1053–1062
40. Nuβe O, Lindau M (1988) The dynamics of exocytosis in human neutrophils. J Cell Biol 107:2117–2123
41. Toutant M, Aunis D, Bockaert J, Homburger V, Rouot B (1987) Presence of three pertussis toxin substrates and Go alpha immunoreactivity in both plasma and granule membranes of chromaffin cells. FEBS Lett 215:339–344
42. Goud B, Salminen A, Walworth NC, Novick PJ (1988) A GTP-binding protein required for secretion rapidly associates with secretory vesicles and the plasma membrane in yeast. Cell 53:753–768
43. Wilson DW, Wilcox CA, Flynn GC, Chen E, Huang WK, Henzel WJ, Block MR, Ullrich A, Rothman JE (1989) A fusion protein required for vesicle-mediated transport in both mammalian cells and yeast. Nature 339:355–359

44. Weidman PJ, Melancon P, Block MR, Rothman JE (1989) Binding of and N-ethylmaleimide-sensitive fusion protein to Golgi membranes requires both a soluble protein and an integral membrane receptor. J Cell Biol 108:1589–1596
45. Beckers CJM, Block MR, Glick BS, Rothman JE, Balch WE (1989) Vesicular transport between the endoplasmic reticulum and the Golgi stack requires the NEM-sensitive fusion protein. Nature 339:397–398
46. Novick P, Ferro S, Schekman R (1981) Order of events in the yeast secretory pathway. Cell 25:461–469
47. Clary D, Rothman JE (1990) Purification of three related peripheral membrane proteins needed for vesicular transport. J Biol Chem 265:10109–10117
48. Madsen KM, Tisher CC (1986) Structure-function relationships along the distal nephron. Am J Physiol 250:F1–F15
49. Schwartz GJ, Al-Awqati Q (1985) Carbon dioxide causes exocytosis of vesicles containing H^+ pumps in isolated perfused proximal and collecting tubules. J Clin Invest 75:1638–1644
50. Gluck S, Cannon C, Al-Awqati Q (1982) Exocytosis regulates urinary acidification in turtle bladder by rapid insertion of H^+ pumps into the luminal membrane. Proc Natl Acad Sci USA 79:4327–4331
51. Brown D, Weyer P, Orci L (1987) Non-clathrin coated vesicles are involved in endocytosis in kidney collecting duct intercalated cells. Anat Rec 218:237–242
52. Brown D, Gluck S, Hartwig J (1987) Structure of the novel membrane-coating material in proton-secreting epithelial cells and identification as an H^+ ATPase. J Cell Biol 105:1637–1648
53. Stetson DA, Steinmetz PR (1985) A and B types of carbonic anhydrase-rich cells in turtle bladder. Am J Physiol 249:F553–F565
54. Schwartz GJ, Barasch J, Al-Awqati Q (1985) Plasticity of functional epithelial polarity. Nature 318:368–371
55. Verlander JW, Madsen KM, Tisher CC (1988) Effect of acute respiratory acidosis on two populations of intercalated cells in rat cortical collecting duct. Am J Physiol 253:F1142–F1156
56. Schuster VL, Bonsib SM, Jennings ML (1986) Two types of collecting duct mitochondria-rich (intercalated) cells: lectin and band 3 cytochemistry. Am J Physiol 251:C347–C355
57. Alper SL, Natale J, Gluck S, Lodish HF, Brown D (1989) Subtypes of intercalated cells in rat kidney collecting duct defined by antibodies against erythroid band 3 and renal vacuolar H^+-ATPase. Proc Natl Acad Sci USA 86
58. Satlin LM, Schwartz GJ (1989) Cellular remodelling of HCO_3^- secreting cells in rabbit renal collecting duct in response to an acidic environment. J Cell Biol 109:1279–1288
59. Bastani B, Purcell H, Hemken P, Gluck S (1990) Adaptational changes in rat kidney H^+ ATPase after chronic acid (AC) or alkali (AL) loading. Kidney Int 37:532a

Sorting of Surface Proteins and Lipids in Epithelial Cells

Kai Simons[1]

Summary. The sorting of newly synthesized apical and basolateral proteins in epithelial cells seems to follow three different scenarios. In Madin-Darby canine kidney (MDCK) cells, apical and basolateral proteins are sorted primarily on the exocytic route in the trans Golgi network. In hepatocytes they are sorted on the endocytic-transcytotic route. In intestinal Caco-2 cells both pathways are used. We have proposed that all the data can be accommodated by a model in which sorting to the apical domain is signal-mediated, while delivery to the basolateral domain represents a default pathway [1].

Introduction

Epithelial cells are polarized to carry out their vectorial functions in secretion, absorption, and ion transport. The plasma membrane of each epithelial cell is divided into two domains with distinct protein and lipid compositions [2,3]. An apical domain confronts the organism's exterior and a basolateral domain, attached to an underlying extracellular matrix, faces the interior. The proteins in the apical domain seem to vary according to epithelial cell type and function, whereas the basolateral domain is more like the plasma membrane of non-polarized cells and contains proteins responsible for nutrient uptake, for regulation of intracellular ionic environment, and for growth control, in addition to epithelial-specific junctional and adhesion proteins. The two plasma membrane domains are separated by circumferential tight junctions which form an occluding barrier between neighboring cells and simultaneously prevent intermixing of apical and basolateral components [4,5].

One central problem in the field of epithelial cell biology is how the polarized distribution of newly synthesized surface proteins and lipids is achieved. Three different

[1]European Molecular Biology Laboratory, Meyerhofstr. 1, Postfach 10.2209, D-6900 Heidelberg, Federal Republic of Germany

scenarios are now known. The first one is the best studied and derives from analysis of biosynthetic membrane traffic in filter-grown kidney MDCK cells. When epithelial cells are cultured on permeable supports, they form a tightly polarized cell layer that mimics the epithelial organization observed in vivo [2]. Both exogenous viral glycoproteins and endogenous surface proteins are sorted before they reach the plasma membrane, most likely in the trans-Golgi network (TGN) of the Golgi complex [2,3,1,6]. In the TGN of MDCK cells, apical and basolateral proteins are packaged into separate apical and basolateral carrier vesicles which transport the proteins to their surface destinations [7]. In addition to resident apical and basolateral proteins that carry out their functions in the apical or the basolateral membranes respectively, there is another class of epithelial surface proteins that function in transporting ligands from one surface domain to the other across the cell [8]. These transcytosing receptors include the polymeric immunoglobulin receptor (plgR) which transports IgA and IgM from the basolateral to the apical side in a variety of epithelia [9]. This receptor is not present in MDCK cells, but when the cDNA encoding the rabbit plgR is expressed in these cells, the newly synthesized receptor is routed from the Golgi complex to the basolateral side, and after endocytosis from the basolateral membrane, plgR undergoes transcytosis to the apical side [10]. Such transcytosing proteins can therefore be present on both the basolateral and the apical membranes. Recent studies have confirmed that endogenous proteins present on both sides of MDCK cells are involved in transcytosis in both directions [11].

MDCK cells also secrete newly synthesized proteins into the apical and the basolateral media. Secretion is polarized, e.g., laminin and heparan proteoglycan are secreted in the basolateral direction, while glycoprotein (GP) 80 is predominantly secreted into the apical medium [12,13]. The mechanism responsible for the polarity of secretion is not yet known, but, most likely, secretory proteins bind to sorting receptors in the Golgi complex; the complexes are then sorted into apical and basolateral carrier vesicles in a way which is analogous to the mechanism by which mannose 6-phosphate containing enzymes are bound to mannose 6-phosphate receptors; these carrier vesicles are in turn sorted into clathrin-coated vesicles for delivery to the endocytic pathway [14]. If exogenous secretory proteins such as lysozyme are expressed in MDCK cells, they become secreted in an unpolarized fashion [15,16]. Since the cells presumably lack the appropriate sorting receptors for these exogenous proteins, they distribute passively into the luminal contents of both the apical and the basolateral carrier vesicles. In this way, they are delivered indiscriminately to both sides of the epithelium.

Not only are the proteins of the apical and basolateral plasma membrane domains different, but their lipid compositions also differ [17]. The lipid constituents of the apical membrane are unusual because of their high content of sphingolipids. This layer of glycolipids facing the exterior protects the cells from outside injuries. The basolateral membrane, on the other hand, has a lipid composition similar to that of the plasma membrane of non-polarized cells. Differences in lipid compositions of the epithelial membrane domains also seem to be generated during biosynthetic membrane traffic. Sphingolipid sorting has been studied in filter-grown MDCK cells [18]. The data suggest that glycosphingolipid sorting, like protein sorting, takes place in the TGN and that the sphingolipids are included in the same exocytic carrier vesicles as the membrane proteins.

The second scenario for sorting proteins to the epithelial cell surface is provided by studies with hepatocytes. Each hepatocyte has several apical poles, which line the bile canaliculi and are separated from the intervening basolateral membranes by tight junctions. Hubbard et al. have shown that both apical and basolateral membrane proteins are delivered from the Golgi complex to the basolateral membrane before sorting occurs [19]. The apical proteins are sorted after endocytosis to basolateral early endosomes and are then delivered by transcytosis to the apical side. The apical proteins that have been studied seem to follow the route taken by the transcytosing pIgR. They probably have no other alternative because the apical route from the TGN appears to be missing in hepatocytes. The massive amounts of albumin and other secretory proteins produced by hepatocytes are secreted constitutively from the basolateral (sinusoidal) membrane. Proteins found in the bile seem to be derived from the blood, either by transcytosis across the liver cell or by passage between the cells. The reason for the lack of a direct secretory route from the TGN to the apical side may be the need to avoid the loss of newly synthesized plasma proteins into the bile. If membrane traffic from the TGN to the hepatocyte cell surface were possible only by transport along the basolateral route, then sorting receptors would not be required for exocytosis. Constitutive secretion could occur simply by default.

The third scenario for epithelial protein sorting is derived from recent studies with intestinal CaCo-2 cells [20]. These cells seem to use features from both the MDCK and the hepatocyte sorting mechanisms. Some apical proteins (such as sucrase-isomaltase) are routed directly from the TGN, while other apical proteins (amino peptidase N and dipeptidyl peptidase IV) use both the direct route to the apical membrane and the transcytotic pathway via the basolateral membrane. Secretion of proteins in CaCo-2 cells occurs mainly in the basolateral direction [21,22]. Expression of exogenous immunoglobulin kappa light chains leads to secretion of 90% of the protein into the basolateral medium, while only 10% is secreted apically. The available data thus suggest that the apical route from the TGN exists but it may not have as high a capacity in CaCo-2 cells as in MDCK cells.

The simplest model for explaining these results is to postulate that only one of the two epithelial pathways for delivery of surface proteins operates by signal-recognition (Fig. 1). We have suggested that apical sorting from the TGN is the pathway that requires specific sorting signals, whereas the basolateral pathway from the TGN operates by default, as proposed for membrane traffic to the cell surface from the TGN in non-polarized cells [1,6,17]. The differences in routing from the TGN would be reduced to either the non-existence of an apical route from the TGN in hepatocytes, or to differences in the affinities of apical proteins for the sorting machinery in the TGN of CaCo-2 cells. Apical proteins not sorted into apical carrier vesicles would be included in the basolateral default vesicles for delivery to the basolateral side. The sorting of the apical proteins from the basolateral side requires an additional sorting step that probably takes place immediately after endocytosis from the basolateral plasma membrane into early endosomes from which the transcytotic carrier vesicles form [1,6] (Fig. 2).

This model for epithelial sorting specifies that apical membrane protein should have specific sorting signals whereas basolateral membrane proteins require none. Is this model compatible with what is known of epithelial sorting signals? Unfortunately, an affirmative answer is not possible from available data [12,23]. Despite numerous attempts, identification of the sorting signals for transmembrane proteins

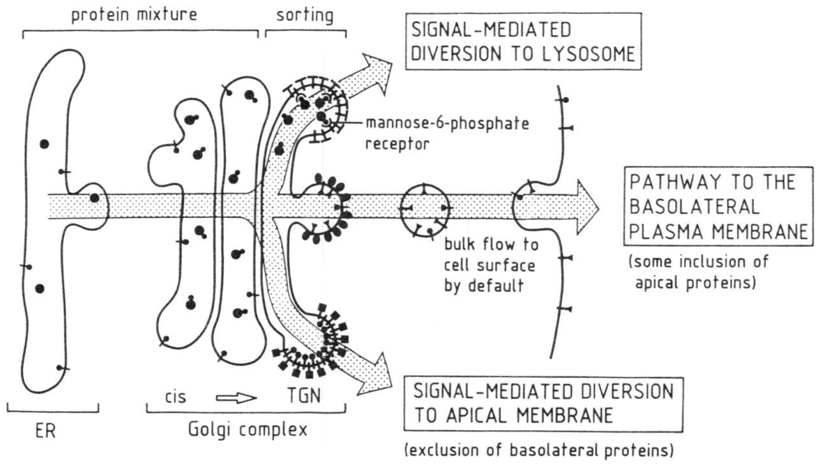

Fig. 1. Working model for sorting from the trans-Golgi network (*TGN*) in MDCK cells. Three possible exit routes from the trans-Golgi network are indicated; two of which lead to the plasma membrane and one which leads to lysosomes [14]. Inclusion in the apical transport vesicles requires specific signals and unrecognized proteins are specifically excluded. The basolateral transport vesicles represent the bulk flow route and carry those proteins to the surface which have not been segregated by selective sorting processes. Constitutive secretory proteins are not indicated, but their vectorial delivery is assumed to be dependent on binding to membrane-bound receptors. In the absence of recognition, soluble proteins would be free to be carried with the fluid phase to both membrane domains. (Model from [6])

has not been successful. Most studies would agree that the sorting information is in the extracytoplasmic domain of both apical and basolateral proteins. Expression of chimeric proteins are usually routed to the apical cell surface if they contain the extracytoplasmic part of an apical protein. However, several notable exceptions are known [24–26]. The observed results can, however, be accommodated by apical-specific sorting and delivery to basolateral membranes by default. Sorting into apical vesicles would have to depend on both signal-mediated inclusion and specific exclusion of both basolateral proteins and proteins which contain apical sorting signals, but have cytoplasmic domains with structures that are incompatible with the formation of the specific protein-protein interactions which are necessary for the assembly of the apical carrier vesicle [1]. It is possible that post-translational modifications, e.g., phosphorylation, can regulate whether exclusion occurs or not [24]. Another possibility is that the binding of an accessory protein to the cytosolic domain leads to exclusion.

The open question is whether glycolipid sorting operates in all epithelial cells [17] and whether or not transcytosis involves glycolipid sorting. Does basolateral to apical transcytosis involve the same machinery as that which is used for making apical carrier vesicles in the TGN? Or is it a different machinery with its own sorting specificity? Since the magnitude of transcytotic traffic is considerable [27], it is difficult to envisage transcytosis without both protein and lipid sorting. Otherwise, the two plasma membrane domains would slowly intermix. The sorting of sphingolipids in

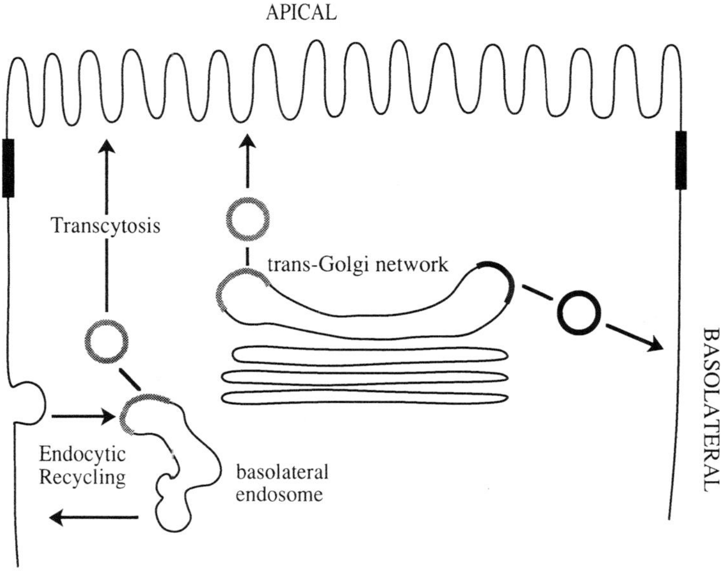

Fig. 2. Sorting pathways for newly synthesized apical and basolateral proteins in epithelial cells. Apical proteins that are not sorted in the apical direction in the trans-Golgi network (*TGN*) leave the Golgi by the postulated default pathway to the basolateral side. Here the apical proteins become internalized by endocytosis in the early endosomes (see [29] and [30]). The proteins can be recycled back to the basolateral domain or sorted into transcytosic vesicles that carry the proteins to the apical surface domain. One important difference between sorting from the trans-Golgi network and from the basolateral early endosomes is the time spent in the sorting compartment. Newly synthesized apical proteins reside only a short time in the Golgi complex before exiting, while apical proteins at the basolateral cell surface can recycle back and forth between the plasma membrane and the early endosome before being included into a transcytotic carrier vesicle. Proteins with a low affinity to the postulated sorting protein in the trans-Golgi network might leave the trans-Golgi network by the basolateral route before being sorted. These apical proteins can be slowly sorted to the apical side from the basolateral endosome by transcytosis [1]. ER, endoplasmic reticulum

the TGN of MDCK cells has been postulated to be coupled to protein sorting [17]. Apical proteins have been proposed to interact with sorting receptors, which in turn interact with glycosphingolipid clusters to form a subdomain in the TGN membrane which is induced to bud with putative accessory proteins into a carrier vesicle. Basolateral proteins and lipids would be excluded because they cannot participate in the cooperative bonding process. An interesting group of proteins are those with glycophospholipid anchors. In several epithelial cell types, these are predominantly localized to the apical membrane [28]. Recent studies have shown that the glycophospholipid anchors themselves contain the apical sorting signals. It is, therefore, possible that these proteins are sorted into the apical carrier vesicles in the same way as glycolipids are.

Concluding Remarks

The challenge in the field of epithelial protein and lipid sorting is the identification of the proteins which are responsible for apical and basolateral sorting and specific targeting to the correct membrane domain. The first steps in this direction have been taken by the isolation of apical and basolateral carrier vesicles, derived from the trans-Golgi network of MDCK cells [7]. It is now possible to study the individual proteins of these vesicles and to study their function in sorting and vesicle targeting.

References

1. Simons K, Wandinger-Ness A (1990) Polarized sorting in epithelia. Cell 62:207–210
2. Simons K, Fuller SD (1985) Cell surface polarity in epithelia. Annu Rev Cell Biol 1:243–288
3. Rodriguez-Boulan E, Nelson J (1989) Morphogenesis of the polarized epithelial cell phenotype. Science 245:718–725
4. Gumbiner B, Simons K (1987) The role of uvomorulin in the formation of epithelial occluding junctions. John Wiley and Sons, New York, pp 168–180
5. Simons K (1990) The epithelial tight junction: occluding barrier and fence. In: Edelman GM, Cunningham BA, Thiery J-P (eds) Morphoregulatory molecules, vol 2. John Wiley and Sons, New York 341–356
6. Wandinger-Ness A, Simons K (1991) The polarized transport of surface proteins and lipids in epithelial cells. In: Hanover J, Steer C (eds) Intracellular Trafficking of Proteins. Cambridge University Press, Cambridge 575–612
7. Wandinger-Ness A, Bennett MK, Antony C, Simons (1990) Distinct transport vesicles mediate the delivery of plasma membrane proteins to the apical and basolateral domains of MDCK Cells. J Cell Biol 111:987–1000
8. Van Deurs B, Petersen OW, Olsnes S, Sandvig K (1989) The ways of endocytosis. Int Rev Cytol 117:31–178
9. Mostov KE, Simister NE (1985) Transcytosis. Cell 43:389–390
10. Mostov KE, Deitcher DL (1986) Polymeric immunoglobulin receptor expressed in MDCK cells transcytoses IgA. Cell 46:613–621
11. Brändli AW, Parton RG, Simons K (1990) Transcytosis in MDCK cells: identification of glycoproteins transported bidirectionally between both plasma membrane domains. J Cell Biol, in press
12. Caplan M, Matlin KS (1989) Sorting of membrane and secretory proteins in polarized epithelial cells. Mod Cell Biol 8:71–127
13. Urban J, Parczyk K, Leutz A, Kayne M, Kondor-Koch C (1987) Constitutive apical secretion of an 80-kDa sulfated glycoprotein complex in the polarized epithelial Madin-Darby canine kidney cell line. J Cell Biol 105:2735–2743
14. Kornfeld S, Mellman I (1989) The biogenesis of lysosomes. Annu Rev Cell Biol 5:483–525
15. Gottlieb TA, Beaudry G, Rizzolo L, Colman M, Rindler M, Adesnik M, Sabatini DD (1986) Secretion of endogenous and exogenous proteins from polarized MDCK cell monolayers. Proc Natl Acad Sci USA 83:2100–2104
16. Kondor-Koch CB, Bravo R, Fuller SD, Cutler D, Garoff H (1985) Exocytic pathways exist to both the apical and the basolateral cell surface of the polarized epithelial cell MDCK. Cell 43:297–306
17. Simons K, van Meer G (1988) Lipid sorting in epithelial cells. Biochemistry 27:6197–6202

18. van Meer G, Stelzer EHK, Wijnaendts-van-Resandt R, Simons K (1987) Sorting of sphingolipids in epithelial (Madin-Darby canine kidney) cells. J Cell Biol 105:1623–1635
19. Hubbard AL, Stieger B, Bartles JR (1989) Biogenesis of endogenous plasma membrane proteins in epithelial cells. Annu Rev Physiol 51:735–770
20. Matter K, Brauchbar M, Bucher K, Hauri H-P (1990) Sorting of endogenous plasma membrane proteins occurs from two sites in cultured human intestinal epithelial cells. Cell 60:429–437
21. Traber MG, Kayden HJ, Rindler MJ (1987) Polarized secretion of newly synthesized lipoproteins by the Caco-2 human intestinal cell line. J Lipid Res 28:1350–1363
22. Hughson EJ, Cutler DF, Hopkins CR (1989) Basolateral secretion of kappa light chain in the polarized epithelial cell line, Caco-2. J Cell Sci 94:327–332
23. Roth MG (1989) Molecular Biological Approaches to Protein Sorting. Annu Rev Physiol 51:797–810
24. Casanova JE, Breitfeld PP, Ross SA, Mostov KE (1990) Phosphorylation of the polymeric immunoglobulin receptor required for its efficient transcytosis. Science 248:742–745
25. Roth MG, Ktistakis N, Shia S-P, Zwart D, Thomas D, Brewer C (1990) Recombinant glycoproteins as probes for sorting events occurring during intracellular transport (abstract). FASEB J 4:A2180
26. Hunziker W, Mellman I (1989) Expression of macrophage-lymphocyte receptors in MDCK cells: polarity and transcytosis differ for isoforms with or without coated pit localization domains. J Cell Biol 109:3291–3302
27. von Bonsdorff C-H, Fuller SD, Simons K (1985) Apical and basolateral endocytosis in MDCK cells grown on nitrocellulose filters. EMBO J 4:2781–2792
28. Lisanti MP, Rodriguez-Boulan E (1990) Glycophospholipid membrane anchoring provides clues to the mechanism of protein sorting in polarized epithelial cells. TIBS 15:113–118
29. Bomsel M, Prydz K, Parton RG, Gruenberg J, Simons K (1989) Endocytosis in filter-grown Madin-Darby canine kidney cells. J Cell Biol 109:3243–3258
30. Parton RG, Prydz K, Bomsel M, Simons K, Griffiths G (1989) Meeting of the apical and basolateral endocytic pathways of the Madin-Darby canine kidney cell in late endosomes. J Cell Biol 109:3259–3272

Masugi Memorial Symposium: Experimental Nephritis and Its Contribution to Nephrology

Chair: Hidekazu Shigematsu (Japan)
Curtis B. Wilson (USA)

Matazo Masugi and Nephrotoxic Nephritis

Yozo Masugi[1]

Matazo Masugi, the author's father and the discoverer of nephrotoxic serum nephritis, was born in Japan almost 100 years ago – in 1896 in Ohtsu, a city near Kyoto. The house where he was born still stands, and he lived there with his parents until 1917, at which time, having graduated from Senior high school in Kyoto, he went to Tokyo to enter the Medical School of Tokyo Imperial University.

In 1921, upon graduation, he entered the Department of Pathology of this university. After undergoing fundamental training in pathological anatomy for several years, in 1925 he was given an opportunity to further his studies in basic medical science in Europe.

At that time, the main overseas destination for medical scholars funded by the Japanese government was Germany. Possibly for this reason, he first went to the Institute of Pathology, known as Aschoff House, at Freiburg University. There, under the guidance of Professor Aschoff, he continued studies into the relationship between monocytes and histiocytes [1] that had been initiated by the late Professor Kiyono of Kyoto University.

In the following year, on completion of this work, he transferred to the Pathology Institute of Basel University in Switzerland. There, under Professor Rössle, he engaged in the study of specific anti-serum action on monocellular organisms such as paramecium, in order to develop prototypes of cytotoxic cellular damage. As a consequence of these studies, he concluded that the action of cytotoxin on paramecia caused an initial paralysis in the organisms that ultimately led to death [2]. Because of his involvement in this research, it can be assumed that his general interest in the actions of cytotoxin was thus developed.

In October 1927, he returned to Japan via the United States, and soon after, at the age of 32, he was appointed the Professor of Pathology at Chiba Medical School. During this period, maintaining his original interest in cytotoxic cells and tissue damage, he began to study kidney and liver changes in rats after respective adminis-

[1]Department of Pathology, Nippon Medical School, Tokyo, 113, Japan

trations of nephrotoxin or hepatotoxin. Each cytotoxin prepared for this purpose was made from immunized rabbits.

Two years later, in 1929, at a convention of the Japanese Pathological Society [3], he reported the first results of his investigations into cytotoxic organ changes, wherein he concluded that cytotoxin could produce damage in targeted parenchymal cells, such as the damage to urinary tubuli of the kidney produced by nephrotoxin, or the damage produced in hepatic cells by hepatotoxin administration. At the same time, however, he noted a generalized anaphylactic shock that occurred in some animals. Therefore, he also presented the associated evidence of a functional derangement of the vascular system that occurred through reversed anaphylaxis, due to antibody conjugation to the vascular tissues.

In retrospect, this observation appears to be the first step toward his later discovery of nephrotoxic serum nephritis. Still, he apparently did not focus much attention on glomerular changes in these experiments.

In any event he was not greatly satisfied with the results that he obtained regarding cytotoxic organ changes in these provisional experiments. Thus, during the next few years, he continued to experiment on rats, administering nephrotoxin or hepatotoxin, concentrating his search on the primary effect of cytotoxin on the targeted organ.

Finally, after many experiments, he came to realize that the primary target of the cytotoxin must be the vascular system of the target organ, such as the glomerular capillaries of the kidney in the case of nephrotoxin administration. Therefore, damage to the parenchymal cells, such as to the tubular epithelia, which hitherto had been generally thought to be the target, was secondary to the glomerular change. Using this same reasoning, the effect of the hepatotoxin on the liver was also interpreted as being due to vascular change, in this case, change in the periportal areas. In conclusion, he speculated that the changes produced by nephrotoxin in the kidney of rat were similar to the changes of human glomerulonephritis, and that the changes produced by hepatotoxin in the liver corresponded to the changes of human eclampsia.

In later years, he recalled how difficult it was to upset the previously unchallenged concept of the cytotoxin target, especially that of nephrotoxin. In any event, he reported these findings to the annual review of the Japanese Pathological Society in 1931 [4], and later he contributed an article to Ziegler's Beitrage zur path. Anatomie in 1933 [5], although this latter article had no accompanying microscopic pictures of the target organs.

Confident of his findings, he decided to use larger animals, such as rabbits, for successive experiments. For preparing the anti-rabbit kidney serum he used duck, the animal that was then usually used for the production of antisera to blood group-specific substances. Further, in pursuing his experiments, he not only studied each rabbit kidney histologically, but also followed the clinical and the laboratory data of each experimental animal given nephrotoxin.

In this manner, he concluded that the nephrotoxic serum nephritis of his experimental rabbits was similar, both pathologically and clinically, to human glomerulonephritis. Further, he was able to create many kinds of diffuse glomerulonephritis in his experimental animals. According to the anti-kidney antibody titer of the antiserum he used and by varying the amount of the administered volume, he was able to induce acute, subacute, or chronic, diffuse glomerulonephritis, as well as an acute variety that terminated in a diffuse, glomerular fibrin thrombus formation.

Based on this capability, he came to decide that this specific antigen-antibody reaction, i.e., the allergic reaction occurring at the glomerular capillaries, was the pathogenetic factor responsible for diffuse glomerulonephritis.

In 1932, he contributed this evidence to the annual review of the Japanese Pathological Society [6]. Two years later, he submitted his findings to Ziegler's Beitrage zur path. Anatomie, along with a series of histological pictures of his experimental animals and their pertinent clinical charts [7]. This latter article had a considerable impact on the medical world, and the existence of nephrotoxic serum nephritis gradually came to be accepted internationally, and was later verified through many other experimental reports.

Among the many studies of cytotoxic organ changes that he pursued, only nephrotoxic serum nephritis became accepted as having a pathogenetic significance. As I have mentioned previously, he also thought that the periportal vascular change that occurred in the liver of rats after hepatotoxin administration was similar to human eclamptic liver change, although this observation did not gain acceptance.

He also pursued studies of heart changes produced in rats after administration of an anti-heart serum, i.e., a cardiotoxin prepared from rabbits. However, he was unable to induce a rheumatoid heart, although he did report the finding of sporadic vascular changes in the interstitium of the heart that he felt were general manifestations of cytotoxic organ change [8]. Additionally, in 1938, in the field of human pathology, he is thought to have been the first person to describe the vascular changes of diffuse schlerodermia in the skin [9].

He would have continued to expand his research, but he began to suffer from persistent anemia of unknown origin, and in March 1939 he had to be hospitalized, thus making it impossible for him to pursue his studies independently.

His lecture on allergy and its pathologic significance [10], which he had been asked to give at the convention of the Japanese Pathological Society in April 1939, had to be read by someone else. This lecture covered not only nephrotoxic serum nephritis, but also multiple allergic disorders in experimental animals and in human diseases that he had studied.

In April 1942, his days as a professor officially ended, and in March 1944, he retired from Chiba Medical School due to illness. Shortly after, in August 1945, World War II in Asia ended. The following year, though his health was very poor, he took on professorial work in pathology at some private medical schools in Tokyo.

His post-war days, however, were numbered, and in September 1947, after being confined to bed for two weeks, he died at the age of 51. An autopsy disclosed a massive bilateral hemothorax and diffuse pericardial adhesions of an undetermined nature.

This briefly covers my father's career and the work that he accomplished. It is said that the administration of nephrotoxin in experimental animals was originated as a procedure by Lindemann in 1900 [11]. The achievement of Matazo Masugi, however, was that he altered a prevailing idea, proving that the target of nephrotoxin was not the tubular epithelia, but the glomeruli in the kidney. Moreover, he clarified the significance of the allergic reaction that occurs at the glomerular capillaries in the pathogenesis of diffuse glomerulonephritis.

Permit a final observation. Matazo Masugi speculated that the apparent period of latency in rabbit nephrotoxic nephritis, brought about by the administration of duck antiserum, was due to the necessary lag time for the nephrotoxin and the glomeruli to combine.

Retrospectively, I regret that he may not have read Kay's two phase theory, concerning the occurrence of nephrotoxic nephritis, that was published in November 1940 [12]. The world was at war, so that he may not have been able to read this paper, and thus we are deprived of his learned opinion.

References

1. Masugi M (1927) Über die Beziehungen zwischen Monozyten und Histiocyten. Beitr Path Anat 76:396–443
2. Masugi M (1927) Über die Wirkung des Normal- sowie des spezifischen Immunserums auf die Paramäzien. Über die Immunität derselben gegen die beiden Serumwirkungen. Krhtforschg 5:375–402
3. Masugi M (1929) Über die spezifisch zytotoxische Wirkung des Antinieren- und -leberserums sowie über die sog. umgekehrte Anaphylaxie. Trans Jpn Path Soc 19:132–137
4. Masugi M, Tomizuka Y (1931) Über die spezifisch zototoxischen Veränderungen der Niere und der Leber durch das spezifische Antiserum (Nephrotoxin und Hepatotoxin). Zugleich ein Beitrag zur Pathogenese der Glomerulonephritis. Trans Jpn Path Soc 21:329–341
5. Masugi M (1933) Über das Wesen der spezifischen Veränderungen der Niere und der Leber durch das Nephrotoxin bzw. das Hepatotoxin. Zugleich ein Beitrag zur Pathogenese der Glomerulonephritis und der eklamptischen Lebererkrankung. Beitr Path Anat 91:82–112
6. Masugi M, Sato Y, Murasawa S, Tomizuka Y (1932) Über die experimentelle Glomerulonephritis durch das spezifische Antinierenserum. Trans Jpn Path Soc 22:614–628
7. Masugi M (1934) Über die experimentelle Glomerulonephritis durch das spezifische Antinierenserum. Ein Beitrag zur Pathogenese der diffusen Glomerulonephritis. Beitr Path Anat 92:429–466
8. Masugi M, Sato Y, Todo S (1935) Über die Veränderungen des Herzens durch das spezifische Antiherzserum. Experimentelle Untersuchungen über die allergischen Gewebsschäden des Herzens. Trans Jpn Path Soc 25:211–216
9. Masugi M, Yä S (1938) Die difuse Sklerodermie und ihre Gefässveränderung. Virchows Arch [A] 302:39–62
10. Masugi M (1939) Die Allergie und ihre pathologische Bedeutung. Trans Jpn Path Soc 29:603–631
11. Lindemann W (1900) Sur le mode d'action de certains poisons renaux. Ann Inst Pasteur 13:49–59
12. Kay CF (1940) The mechanism by which experimental nephritis is produced injected with nephrotoxic duck serum. J Exp Med 72:559–572

In Situ Immune Complex Nephritis

ARNOLD VOGT[1]

Introduction

Until the beginning of the nineteen eighties it was generally believed that glomerulonephritis was a "soluble complex disease" [1–3], the exception being that induced by anti-GBM antibody. Glomerular injury was considered to be the result of antigen-antibody deposits, with inflammation-inducing properties, which had previously been formed within the circulation [4]. This way of looking at things—for a long time it almost had the status of a dogma—was eventually challenged by Couser and Salant [5], who pointed at observations in passive Heymann nephritis, where the disease is not the result of circulating immune complexes but arises from combinations of the anti Fx1A antibody with particular surface structures of the glomerular epithelial cells [6,7]. The main target molecule has been identified as a glycoprotein of 330 kD, known as gp 330 [8].

The target molecule in passive Heymann nephritis is an intrinsic structure of the glomerulus, as in Masugi nephritis. In human immune complex nephritis the putative nephritogenic antigens are more likely to be non-glomerular components, of exogenous—in the case of postinfectious glomerulonephritis (GN)—or autologous—in the case of an autoimmune associated GN like Lupus nephritis—origin.

Antigens Possessing Affinity for the Glomerular Basement Membrane (GBM)

Postulating that there is an in situ mechanism of immune complex formation with an exogenous antigen in most forms of human immune complex glomerulonephritis (ICGN), one readily hits on the idea that the nephritogenic antigen should possess a

[1]Institute of Medical Microbiology, D-78 Freiburg, Federal Republic of Germany

particular quality which is responsible for its binding to distinct structures in the glomerulus. Izui, prompted by in vitro findings, was the first to propose such an affinity for DNA in systemic lupus erythematosus (SLE) associated nephritis [9]. Though it turns out that DNA alone does not possess an affinity for the GBM in vivo [10], the idea of a "planted antigen" stimulated a body of interesting experimental work. In 1979 Golbus and Wilson showed that Concanavalin A can be planted in the GBM and can act as a target for subsequently injected antibody [11]. A number of lectins can bind to various structures in the kidney [12], but it is questionable whether lectins are included among nephritogenic antigens. In the beginning of the 1980s, three groups independently drew attention to cationic antigens and their potential role as planted antigens. Border's groups [13,14], working with the experimental model of chronic serum sickness, found cationized antigen to be far more effective in inducing nephritis than the native anionic molecule.

Gallo and co-workers, studying the fate of passively administered preformed immune complexes, observed a predominantly capillary localization when complexes were prepared from cationized antigen, in contrast to the mesangial deposition of complexes prepared from unmodified (anionic) antigen [15–17]. Our group studied the influence of the charge and size of protein molecules on their capability of acting as planted antigens for circulating antibodies [18–22]. All authors unanimously emphasized the ability of both cationic antigens and cationic immune complexes to form subepithelial deposits. Complexes prepared from unmodified (anionic) antigen localize predominantly within the mesangium or in the subendothelial space [23,24]. Only when complexes were prepared in high antigen excess, or when small complexes were obtained with low avidity antibody, have subepithelial deposits been noted [25].

Influence of Charge and Size on the Affinity of Proteins for the GBM

Polycations not only have more easy access to the glomerular filtration barrier, they also interact with the anionic structures of the GBM [21]. In contrast to unmodified proteins, circulating molecules will accumulate along the glomerular capillary wall when highly cationized, and they may persist in the GBM for a while. To interact with and persist in the GBM, the cationic molecule must fulfill certain requirements. In addition to having a high positive overall charge (pI greater than 8.5) the size is critical (>40 kD). Accumulation of cationic molecules in the GBM increases with increasing size. Small molecules like monomeric lysozyme (MW 14400, pI 11.3) are not retarded within the GBM even though they are highly positively charged. Intravenously injected ovalbumin (40 kD) only becomes detectable along the GBM when heavily cationized (pI > 10.0). Ferritin, on the other hand, will already fix to the GBM when its pI is about 9.0 [21]. The persistence of cationized proteins in the GBM is clearly governed by charge and size. While highly cationized ferritin can be detected in the glomeruli of rats up to 16h after intravenous injection of 5 to 10 mg per animal, highly cationized ovalbumin is demonstrable for less than 2 hours.

In Situ Immune Complex Formation

From the foregoing it is clear that for an injected antibody to reach a planted antigen the antibody has to be administered within a relatively short interval after antigen administration. With highly cationized HuIgG and ferritin, an interval of 15 minutes–2 hours between antigen and antibody administration will result in massive subepithelial immune deposits. From electronmicroscopic studies with ferritin we learned that the immune complexes were formed primarily on the endothelial site, and were transferred, with time, to the subepithelial region, where they persisted for weeks [21].

Though massive subepithelial immune complex formation occurs after intravenous injection of both antigen and antibody, nephritis can be induced only when the cationized antigen is perfused intrarenally, followed by intravenous injection of the specific antibody. This puzzling aspect of the experimental model of in situ immune complex nephritis is also seen in the active model, where the cationized antigen has to be injected intrarenally into the immunized animal [22]. The reason for this is not known. It may be connected with the influence of cationized proteins on the clotting and complement systems or it may be due to the fact that antibody binds less well to cationized antigens [26]. The latter reason, however, is less likely to be true because very small amounts, i.e., a few micrograms of cationized antigen and antibody, are sufficient to induce a fullblown, unilateral nephritis [20].

Polycations can Mediate the Glomerular Deposition of Polyanions

The glomerular deposition of highly anionic molecules can be mediated by polycations. Native ferritin (ESR 61 Å), which, due to its size (500 kD) and negative charge (pI 4.5–4.8), is not able to enter the GBM, accumulates massively within the lamina rara of an animal which has been previously injected with the polycation polethyleneimine [27,28]. We have explored this idea with polydisperse DNA fragments and the naturally occurring polycation histone. In contrast to the general assumption that DNA and anti-DNA-antibodies are essentially involved in the pathogenesis of SLE associated GN, we propose that binding of histones to the GBM is the initiating event in the development of Lupus nephritis. DNA alone does not possess any affinity for the GBM. After intravenous injection no significant deposition of DNA in the isolated glomeruli can be detected [10]; however, when histone, which like (PEI), possesses a high affinity for the GBM, has been injected previously then massive deposits of DNA fragments can be found along the glomerular capillary wall [29].

Our hypothesis that histones are one of the nephritogenic antigens involved in the pathogenesis of Lupus nephritis is supported by the finding that histones can frequently be detected by indirect immunofluorescence staining in glomerular deposits of Lupus nephritis. This holds true for kidneys of diseased NZB/NZW F_1 mice [30], graft versus host mice, and for kidney biopsies obtained from patients with Lupus nephritis (unpublished work). In this connection it is of interest that antibodies to histones can be found regularly in the sera of patients with Lupus nephritis [31].

Cationic Antigens Involved in the Pathogenesis of Postinfectious GN

Our efforts to identify nephritogenic cationic proteins from bacteria associated with postinfectious GN were at first less successful than the studies reported above. The expectation in 1982 that we had, for the first time, identified a nephritogenic antigen from an infectious agent, proved to be premature. The streptococcal antigen found in the glomerular deposits [32] was identified as a cationic streptococcal protease, which had been described and characterized earlier by Liu and Elliot [33] and which possessed, as we had to learn, no affinity for the GBM in its monomeric form. In fact, none of the three streptococcal antigens so far accused of being involved in the pathogenesis of acute post-streptococcal glomerulonephritis (APSGN)—the nephritis strain associated protein (NSAP) of Zabriskies' group [34], the endostreptosin of Lange's group [35] or our cationic streptococcal protease—fulfill the most important of Koch's postulates, that is, they are not capable of inducing nephritis in experimental models.

Outlook

The search for nephritogenic antigens in postinfectious GN has to continue. I believe that the model of in situ immune complex nephritis, as experience with Lupus nephritis has taught us, can lead us to a successful strategy for finding or identifying nephritogenic candidates from infectious agents.

The most important message from the experimental model is that nephritogenic antigens, most likely, will have an affinity for the GBM. Thus the logical first step is to screen for bacterial or viral proteins which reveal affinity for the GBM. Highly cationic proteins with a critical size do possess an affinity for the GBM. Our proposed strategy at the moment is to isolate fractions of cationic proteins from infectious agents which are known to cause postinfectious ICGN. After intravenous injection of the ^{125}I labelled fraction the glomeruli are isolated and the proteins bound to the glomeruli are separated on SDS-PAGE and detected by autoradiography. Comparison of the bands found in the isolated glomeruli with the injected fractions after SDS-PAGE-autoradiography enables one to identify and (hopefully) to isolate and to evaluate the nephritogenicity of the protein which possesses affinity for the GBM.

Using this procedure we were able to identify cationic proteins, both with strong affinity for the GBM, from two bacteria: *Yersinia enterocolitica* (pI $>$ 10.0) [36] and *Staphylococcus aureus* (pI $>$ 10.0) [37]. The Yersinia protein is composed of a 19 kD polypeptide, but occurs in dimeric and aggregated form with a size exceeding 65 kD (as judged from gel filtration). The staphylococcal protein migrates in SDS-PAGE as a 31 kD band. With the latter antigen we were able to induce proteinuria and kidney damage after a single intravenous injection into immunized rats. The nephritogenic potency of the Yersinia antigen is under study.

Thus, the model of in situ ICGN may lead us to a successful method for identifying cationic nephritogenic antigens involved in naturally occurring ICGN.

References

1. Cameron JS (1983) The pathogenesis of glomerulonephritis. In: Bertani T, Remuzzi G (eds) Glomerular injury. 300 years after Morgagni. Wichtig Edition, Milan, pp 11–30
2. Dixon FJ (1968) The pathogenesis of glomerulonephritis. Am J Med 44:493–498
3. Wilson CB, Dixon FJ (1981) The renal response to immunological injury. In: Brenner BM, Rector FC (eds) The kidney. WB Saunders, Philadelphia, p 1237
4. Cochrane CG, Koffler D (1973) Immune complex disease in experimental animals and in man. Adv Immunol 16:185–264
5. Couser WG, Salant DJ (1980) In situ immune complex formation and glomerular injury (editorial review). Kidney Int 17:1–13
6. Van Damme BJC, Fleuren GJ, Bakker WW, Vernier RL, Hoedemaeker PJ (1978) Experimental glomerulonephritis in the rat induced by antibodies directed against tubular antigens. IV. Fixed glomerular antigens in the pathogenesis of heterologous immune complex glomerulonephritis. Lab Invest 38:502–510
7. Couser WG, Steinmuller DR, Stilmant MM, Salant DJ, Lowenstein LM (1978) Experimental glomerulonephritis in the isolated perfused rat kidney. J Clin Invest 62:1275–1287
8. Kerjaschki D, Farquhar MG (1983) Immunocytochemical localization of the Heymann nephritis antigen (GP 330) in glomerular epithelial cells of normal Lewis rats. J Exp Med 157:667–685
9. Izui S, Schur PH, Kunkel HG (1967) Immunologic studies concerning the nephritis of systemic lupus erythematosus. J Exp Med 126:607–623
10. Stoeckl F, Schmiedeke T, Sugisaki Y, Mertz A, Batsford S, Vogt A (1990) DNA has no affinity for the GBM in vivo: binding is mediated by histone (abstract). Kidney Int 37:434
11. Golbus SM, Wilson CB (1979) Experimental glomerulonephritis induced by in situ formation of immune complexes in the glomerular capillary wall. Kidney Int 16:148–157
12. Holthofer H (1983) Lectin binding sites in kidney: A comparative study of 14 animal species. J Histochem Cytochem 31:431–537
13. Ward HJ, Cohen AH, Border WA (1984) In situ formation of subepithelial immune complexes in the rabbit glomerulus: requirement of a cationic antigen. Nephron 36:257–264
14. Border WA, Ward HJ, Kamil ES, Cohen AH (1982) Induction of membranous nephropathy in rabbits by administration of an exogenous cationic antigen: Demonstration of a pathogenic role for electrical charge. J Clin Invest 69:451–461
15. Gallo GR, Caulin-Glaser T, Lamm ME (1981) Charge of circulating immune complexes as a factor in glomerular basement membrane localization in mice. J Clin Invest 67:1305–1313
16. Caulin-Glaser T, Gallo GR, Lamm EM (1983) Nondissociating cationic immune complexes can deposit in glomerular basement membrane. J Exp Med 158:1561–1572
17. Gallo GR, Caulin-Glaser T, Emancipator SN, Lamm ME (1983) Nephritogenicity and differential distribution of glomerular immune complexes related to immunogen charge. Lab Invest 48:353–362
18. Batsford SR, Takamiya H, Vogt A (1980) A model of in situ immune complex glomerulonephritis in the rat induced by planted, cationized antigen. Clin Nephrol 14:211–216
19. Batsford SR, Oite T, Takamiya H, Vogt A (1980) Anionic binding sites in the glomerular basement membrane: possible role in the pathogenesis of immune complex glomerulonephritis. Renal Physiol 3:336–340
20. Oite T, Batsford SR, Mihatsch MJ, Takamiya H, Vogt A (1982) Quantitative studies of in situ immune complex glomerulonephritis in the rat induced by planted, cationized antigen. J Exp Med 155:460–474

21. Vogt A, Rohrbach R, Shimizu F, Takamiya H, Batsford S (1982) Interaction of cationized antigen with rat glomerular basement membrane: In situ immune complex formation. Kidney Int 22:27–35
22. Oite T, Shimizu F, Suzuki Y, Vogt A (1985) Ultramicroscopic localization of cationized antigen in the glomerular basement membrane in the course of active, in situ complex glomerulonephritis. Virchows Arch [Cell Pathol] 48:107–118
23. Koyama A, Niwa Y, Shigematsu H, Taniguchi M, Tada T (1978) Studies on passive serum sickness. II. Factors determining the localization of antigen-antibody complexes in murine renal glomerulus. Lab Invest 38:253–262
24. Germuth FG Jr, Rodriguez E (1973) Immunopathology of the renal glomerulus. Immune complex deposit and anti-basement membrane disease. Little, Brown, Boston
25. Germuth FG Jr, Rodriguez E, Lorelle CA, Trump ER, Milano LL, Wise O (1979) Passive immune complex glomerulonephritis in mice: Models for various lesions found in human disease: II. Low avidity complexes and diffuse proliferative glomerulonephritis with subepithelial deposits. Lab Invest 41:366–371
26. Koyama A, Inage H, Kobayashi M, Ohta Y, Narita M, Tojo S, Cameron JS (1986) Role of antigenic charge and antibody avidity on the glomerular immune complex localization in serum sickness of mice. Clin Exp Immunol 64:606–614
27. Barnes JL, Radnik RA, Gilchrist EP, Venkatachalam MA (1984) Size and charge selective permeability defects induced in glomerular basement membrane by a polycation. Kidney Int 25:11–19
28. Barnes JL, Ventakachalam MA (1984) Enhancement of glomerular immune complex deposition by a circulating polycation. J Exp Med 160:286–293
29. Schmiedeke TMJ, Stöckl FW, Weber R, Sugisaki Y, Batsford S, Vogt A (1989) Histones have high affinity for the glomerular basement membrane: relevance for immune complex formation in Lupus nephritis. J Exp Med 169:1879–1894
30. Schmiedeke T, Stoeckl F, Muller S, Mertz A, Vogt A (1990) Detection of histone H3 and H2A in glomerular deposits of Lupus mice (abstract). Kidney Int 37:430
31. Gioud M, Ait Kaci M, Montier JC (1982) Histone antibodies in systemic Lupus erythematosus. Arthritis Rheum 25:407–413
32. Vogt A, Batsford S, Rodriguez-Iturbe B, Garcia R (1983) Cationic antigens in poststreptococcal glomerulonephritis. Clin Nephrol 20:271–279
33. Liu TY, Elliot SD (1971) Streptococcal proteinase. In: Buyer (ed) The enzymes, vol 3, 3rd edn. Academic, pp 609–647
34. Johnston KH, Zabriskie JB (1986) Purification and partial characterization of the nephritis strain-associated protein from streptococcus pyogenes, group A. J Exp Med 163:697–712
35. Lange K, Seligson G, Cronin W (1983) Evidence for the in situ origin of poststreptococcal glomerulonephritis: glomerular localization of endostreptosin and the clinical significance of the subsequent antibody response. Clin Nephrol 19:3–16
36. Mertz A, Batsford S, Stoeckl F, Vogt A (1990) *Yersinia enterocolitica* induced acute GN: Possible role of nucleic acid-binding proteins in immune complex formation (abstract). Kidney Int 37:423
37. Yousif Y, Mertz A, Batsford S, Vogt A (to be published) Cationic staphylococcal antigens have affinity for renal basement membrane: possible pathogenetic role in glomerulonephritis. Proceedings of the VIth international symposium on staphylococci and staphylococcal infections, September 4–8 1989 Warsaw, Poland. Jeljaszewicz J (ed) Gustav Fischer, Stuttgart

Pathogenesis of IgA Immune Complex-Mediated Glomerulonephritis

ABDALLA RIFAI[1]

SUMMARY. In a period of less than ten years, complementary experimental and clinical observations have contributed greatly to our understanding of various aspects of IgA immune complexes and their pathogenetic potential in IgA nephropathy. The primary mechanism of glomerular IgA deposition has been discussed in the light of experimental data. These findings indicate that the molecular form of IgA is critical for the formation of large- and intermediate-sized complexes that result in glomerular deposition. Glomerular IgA deposits, however, appear to develop in a continuum of preformed polymeric IgA complexes and in situ formed monomeric IgA complexes. Removal of IgA immune complexes from the circulation is mediated by the liver, with no evidence of any removal dysfunction in IgA nephropathy patients. IgA macromolecules are unable to activate the complement pathway in vitro or as a glomerular deposit. Complement activation, however, is shown to be an antigen-mediated process. Participation of the complement system in induction of glomerular injury associated with IgA nephropathy needs further investigation. Experimental evidence supports the hypothesis that in IgA immune complex-mediated nephropathy, the repertoire of IgA immune complexes that induce mesangial proliferation and glomerular sclerosis consists of IgA-bound nephritogenic antigens which determine the extent and outcome of glomerular injury.

Introduction

Glomerular IgA deposits represent the diagnostic hallmark of primary IgA nephropathy. This feature is also a consistent finding in and characteristic of Schonlein-Henoch purpura-associated glomerulonephritis. A secondary form of IgA nephro-

[1]Departments of Pathology, Rhode Island Hospital and Brown University, Providence, RI 02903, USA

pathy with identical glomerular immunohistochemical features is occasionally associated with alcoholic liver disease, portal systemic shunt, celiac disease, dermatitis herpetiformis, ankylosing spondylitis, and a number of other diverse diseases [1–3].

Several abnormalities are implicated in the pathogenesis of primary and secondary IgA nephropathy. Some of these abnormalities include: bacterial infections, viral infections, decreased T cell suppressor function, increased T cell helper function, increased polyclonal B cell activation, increased polymeric IgA synthesis, enhanced alpha chain switch region expression, IgM autoantibodies, IgG antibodies, IgA rheumatoid factors, collagen binding IgA, fibronectin-binding IgA, IgA anti-galactosyl reactivity, genetic predisposition, familial association, complement dysfunction, phagocytic dysfunction, anti-endothelial antibodies, anti-bovine serum albumin, anti-gluten, and anti-idiotypic antibodies. If at least 20 such abnormalities are to be accommodated in an experimental model, then the simple factorial rule (n!) would yield 2.4×10^{18} combinatorial models. Undoubtedly, no single experimental model aimed at elucidating the pathogenesis of IgA nephropathy can be developed to include all these abnormalities. IgA immune complexes, however, remain the most commonly reported and implicated immunopathologic abnormality. Accordingly, we have focused our studies on the mechanisms that lead to glomerular IgA immune deposit formation and, in particular, the potential role of the IgA, complement, and antigen in the development of glomerular injury.

IgA Immune Complexes

The first described experimental model for IgA nephropathy examined the ability of IgA immune complexes (IgA-IC) to induce glomerular injury [4]. This model took advantage of two important technical approaches. First, a well characterized monoclonal IgA (MOPC 315) anti-dinitrophenol was used as a source of purified antibody. Second, the hapten dinitrophenol (DNP) could be conjugated to a variety of carrier molecules, such as bovine serum albumin (DNP-BSA), or a chemically modified polysaccharide (DNP-Ficoll) to serve as an antigen. Thus, well characterized IgA-IC could be prepared in vitro and used for passive administration. Complexes of IgA-DNP-BSA prepared over a wide range of antigen/antibody ratio resulted in glomerular IgA immune deposits with the characteristic granular immunofluorescent patterns of IgA and complement component C3. The immunofluorescent pattern of bovine serum albumin in the deposits was identical with the IgA and confirmed the immune complex nature of the mesangial IgA.

Using two different experimental protocols, glomerular IgA immune deposits were also induced in vivo. In the first protocol, DNP-BSA administered to normal mice was followed by the injection of IgA. In the second protocol, DNP-BSA was administered to mice bearing the MOPC 315 myeloma, with predetermined levels of circulating IgA anti-DNP. Both protocols resulted in histopathological changes, representing primarily glomerular PAS positive material, that correlated well with the level of circulating IgA and administered antigen. Of importance in these findings were the mesangial IgA immune deposits which developed over a wide concentration range of IgA (antibody excess) and antigen (antigen excess) in the complexes.

There are seminal clinical observations that support the causal role of IgA-IC. First, the granular immunofluorescent pattern of the IgA and C3 deposits is usually indicative of an immune deposit. Second, electron dense deposits, a common feature of IgA nephropathy, were identified immunohistochemically to be IgA [5]. Third, extrarenal systemic vascular IgA deposits have also been reported in patients with IgA nephropathy. Fourth, a vast number of studies have reported the presence of circulating IgA-IC in primary and secondary forms of IgA nephropathy [6–9]. Most importantly, a correlation between serum level of circulating macromolecular IgA (IgA immune complexes) and hematuria has also been documented [10].

Mechanisms of Glomerular IgA Deposits Formation

The primary pathogenetic mechanism of immune complex-mediated glomerulonephritis is the formation or glomerular deposition of the IC. In IgA nephropathy, the role that the IgA molecular form (monomeric or polymeric) plays in the development of glomerular immune deposits is based largely on experimental observations. Large amounts of purified monomeric IgA anti-DNP mixed with DNP-BSA at different antigen-antibody ratios did not induce glomerular deposits. In contrast, smaller amounts of polymeric IgA were potent in inducing glomerular immune deposits [4]. In a comparative analytical study, in vitro preformed monomeric IgA and polymeric IgA immune complexes prepared with the same antigen (DNP-Ficoll) showed, by gradient polyacrylamide gel electrophoresis, that monomeric IgA formed only small-sized complexes. In contrast, polymeric IgA formed large- and intermediate-sized complexes. These results suggest that the size of the IgA immune complex plays a critical role in glomerular deposition [11].

To determine the relationship between immune complex formation, size, and glomerular deposition, analytical and kinetic double radioisotope studies were performed in vivo. In those studies, ^{131}I-antigen (DNP-Ficoll) was injected intravenously and ^{125}I-labelled monomeric or polymeric IgA anti-DNP were administered intraperitoneally [12]. At timed intervals, plasma samples were obtained and analyzed by gradient gel electrophoresis. Two important findings were revealed by these studies. First, large- and intermediate-sized IgA-IC composed only of polymeric IgA emerged in the circulation prior to glomerular deposition. Thus, glomerular IgA deposits were detectable only in mice that received polymeric IgA and DNP-Ficoll. A second important finding was that although monomeric IgA failed to bind or complex with polymeric IgA-IC in the circulation it did bind to the polymeric IgA immune deposits in the glomerulus. These findings indicate that glomerular IgA immune deposits evolve through a continuum process, initiated by the localization of preformed circulating polymeric IgA complexes and perpetuated by an in situ monomeric IgA-mediated complex formation.

Several clinical studies, utilizing immunohistochemical techniques, demonstrated that polymeric IgA is present in the glomerular immune deposits in patients with IgA nephropathy. The presence of J chain, the binding of secretory component to IgA immune deposits, and size analysis of renal eluates all confirmed the presence or predominance of polymeric IgA [13,14]. The participation or contribution of monomeric IgA to immune deposit formation, however, awaits further clinical investigation.

Removal of IgA Immune Complexes from Circulation

The presence of circulating and glomerular deposits of IgA-IC in IgA nephropathy patients propelled a series of experimental investigations to determine the kinetics, tissue distribution, and fate of IgA immune complexes. Because the antigen usually affects the clearance of immune complexes [15], we used model IgA immune complexes, prepared by covalent cross-linking of purified IgA anti-DNP with a specific affinity labeling antigen (Bis-dinitrophenyl pimelic acid ester). Removal of model IgA-IC from circulation was according to size. Large-sized IgA macromolecules were removed rapidly ($t_{1/2} < 2$ min), whereas small-sized polymers persisted in the circulation. Through the use of these covalently cross-linked IgA oligomers, we were able to determine the minimal composition of four dimeric IgA which was required for rapid elimination [16]. Tissue distribution results showed the liver as the major organ for removal of macromolecular IgA. Immunofluorescence microscopy and electron microscopy autoradiography showed macromolecular IgA to be associated with Kupffer cells [17]. With increasing doses of injected macromolecular IgA the clearance velocity approached a maximum, thus prolonging the circulation of macromolecular IgA. Further kinetic, morphologic, and binding specificity studies demonstrated in vivo the presence of specific receptors on Kupffer cells that bind and remove macromolecular IgA from circulation.

An impairment in the reticulophagocytic function of patients with IgA nephropathy has been postulated as the potential cause for the persistence of IgA immune complexes in the circulation that consequently lead to their glomerular deposition [18,19]. Since the fate and removal mechanisms of circulating macromolecular IgA are unknown in humans, equipped by our experience from animal studies, we examined the blood clearance and organ uptake of purified human IgA macromolecules and polymers in patients with IgA nephropathy and in normal controls [20]. The IgA macromolecules, serving as a probe of IgA-IC, were prepared by covalent cross-linking of purified human polymeric IgA with a heterobifunctional reagent, N-Succinimidyl 3-(2-pyridyldithio) proprianate. After intravenous injection, large-sized IgA macromolecules were removed from the circulation of patients ($t_{1/2} = 3.8 \pm 1.0$ min) and normal controls ($t_{1/2} = 4.9 \pm 1.5$ min). Dynamic gamma camera scintigraphy revealed the liver as the major organ that mediates the removal of the macromolecular IgA, with no significant difference in the rate of hepatic uptake for patients ($t_{1/2} = 3.4 \pm 0.6$ min) and controls ($t_{1/2} = 3.3 \pm 0.9$ min). No significant amount of radioactivity could be detected in the lungs, kidneys, and spleen. These findings have general significance in showing the liver as a major organ for removal of macromolecular IgA. In addition, the results have specific importance in showing that patients with IgA nephropathy do not suffer from an IgA-removal dysfunction. Collectively, the similarity of these clinical and experimental results emphasizes the value of the experimental model.

IgA Immune Complexes and Complement

Although the central component (C3) of the classical and alternative pathways is found in mesangial deposits in many cases of IgA nephropathy, clinical studies have failed to detect systemic activation of the complement system [21]. Detection of other components of the alternative pathway and the membrane attack complex [22] have focused attention on the potential role of the complement system as mediator of glomerular injury.

The ability of aggregated human IgA to activate the complement system has been a subject of several conflicting reports. To address this issue in a manner relevant to IgA nephropathy, we examined in vitro the interaction of covalently cross-linked IgA macromolecules or naturally occurring IgA immune complexes with fresh normal human serum [23]. We demonstrated the lack of activation of C3 or factor B. Similar studies by Waldo and Cochrane [24] confirmed our findings. Administration of human IgA immune complexes or IgA macromolecules to mice resulted in glomerular deposition. Despite the presence of intense glomerular IgA deposits no C3 was detected. Collectively, these findings suggest that neither soluble nor renal localized human IgA deposits activate the complement system.

Although the above studies demonstrate the inability of human IgA to activate the complement system, the cause of the presence of complement in the glomerular deposits remains unknown. We entertained the possibility that the antigen might cause complement activation. A series of experiments were performed in order to determine how IgA immune complex activates complement and generates the mesangial complement deposits [25]. The first experiment was designed to determine whether the presence of an antigen within a glomerular IgA deposit is required for complement activation. In these experiments, covalently cross-linked model IgA macromolecules of anti-DNP with free antigen-binding sites were administered into two groups of mice. Following disappearance of the majority of macromolecules from circulation, either DNP-conjugated antigen or buffer was injected. After six hours both groups were killed. As expected, both groups showed glomerular IgA deposits. Yet only the group that received the DNP-conjugate, a known activator of the alternative pathway, showed C3 deposits. In the second series, a paired comparison of IgA immune complexes prepared with the same monoclonal IgA anti-phosphorylcholine and antigen-carrier, but differing only in a single antigenic feature (DNP), also demonstrated that glomerular C3 deposits developed with a DNP-conjugated antigen. The third series of experiments also showed, using immunoassay analysis, negligible or no conversion of normal serum C3 to inactive C3b (iC3b) upon treatment with soluble or insoluble large-sized IgA aggregates. In contrast, the antigen alone was able to induce maximal conversion of C3 to iC3b. Collectively, these findings indicate that the nature of the antigen in a glomerular IgA immune deposit is the major mediator of complement activation.

Although complement activation can be induced by the antigen in glomerular IgA deposits it is unknown whether such activation causes glomerular injury. Experimentally, we could not detect any histologic features that differentiated between glomeruli with or without C3 deposits within the same renal biopsy. Also, comparative experiments of induced glomerular IgA immune complexes in C3-depleted mice and normal mice showed no histopathologic difference. A number of studies have reported intense C3 deposits with no or minimal glomerular changes in IgA nephropathy. Although there is an agreement between clinical and preliminary experimental observations that the complement system does not appear to mediate glomerular injury, complement activation may be of importance in induction of hematuria, as shown experimentally by Emancipator et al. [26].

Influence of Antigen on Glomerular Injury

One of the most poorly defined areas relative to the role of immune complexes in IgA nephropathy is precise identification of the antigen involved. The close temporal relationship between upper respiratory tract or gastrointestinal infection and episodes of gross hematuria has been described as a frequent feature of IgA nephropathy [27]. The fact that this has also been associated with circulating IgA immune complexes [28] strongly implicates infectious agents as the source of antigen.

In most passive and active experimental models of immune complex-mediated glomerulonephritis, the antigen used is usually a heterologous serum protein consigned to aggregating the antibody without itself being detrimental. In IgG immune complex-mediated glomerulonephritis, the effector function of IgG, as in complement activation, is considered to be the main cause of glomerular injury. As described above, however, IgA has very little or lacks the ability to activate the complement system. As also emphasized, despite intense C3 deposits there is little or no evidence of glomerular injury in several cases of IgA nephropathy. The antigen may then be the major variable that may account for the spectrum of histopathologic patterns observed in IgA nephropathy.

In order to test the pathogenetic potential of the antigen in IgA-IC-mediated glomerulonephritis, we compared the effect of immune complexes formed in vivo with the same IgA anti-phosphorylcholine, and two different antigens, pneumococcal C-polysaccharide and phosphorylcholine-conjugated Ficoll (PC-Ficoll) that share phosphorylcholine (PC) as a common antigenic determinant [29]. Only the C-polysaccharide-containing IgA immune complexes resulted in renal injury. Recently we developed an animal model whereby glomerular IgA immune deposits, composed exclusively of IgA or IgA/IgA-IC, can capture circulating antigens in situ [30]. In this model, glomerular IgA deposits (IgA/IgA-IC) were induced by administration of a constant amount of IgA anti-DNP (antibody) and DNP-conjugated IgA anti-PC as antigen. The latter also served as antibody to capture, in situ, circulating PC-containing antigens. Mice that received only IgA/IgA-IC developed glomerular IgA and C3 deposits and a focal increase in mesangial cells and matrix, but no evidence of renal damage. Diffuse increase in mesangial cells and matrix developed in mice treated with IgA/IgA-IC and either PC-Ficoll or PC-conjugated bovine serum albumin. No significant alterations were noted in these groups. In contrast, mice that received IgA/IgA-IC and pneumococcal C-polysaccharide developed severe diffuse mesangial hypercellularity with segmental necrosis and thrombosis. These mice also developed proteinuria and hematuria. These studies demonstrate that the antigen plays a critical role in the development of glomerulonephritis associated with IgA immune complexes.

Conclusion

The experimental model of IgA immune complex-mediated glomerulonephritis has come of age. Conceptual and technical approaches have begun to provide accurate information regarding the factors and mediators that are involved in pathogenesis. In composing this review I have focused on an experimental system with emphasis on its relevance to human IgA nephropathy. I realize that this course is accompanied by obvious risks of misinterpretation. I hope that the benefits of intellectual challenge outweigh the pitfalls of misconception, and trust my composition provides adequate distinction between fact and fantasy. Finally, I predict that many of the observations made in this model, that appear now to be intriguing, will serve as a lead in the investigation of the pathogenesis of IgA nephropathy, once they are demystified by acquisition of thorough, substantiated information.

Acknowledgments. The presented experimental work was supported by NIH grant 32379. I am indebted to my collaborators whose contributions made this work possible. To the many investigators who have not been cited due to publisher restrictions, but who have contributed to the development of the knowledge presented in this review, my apologies and thanks. The secretarial assistance of Laura Gantt is highly appreciated.

References

1. Clarkson AR, Woodroffe AJ, Aarons I, Hiki Y, Hale G (1987) IgA nephropathy. Annu Rev Med 38:157–68
2. D'Amico G (1987) The commonest glomerulonephritis in the world: IgA nephropathy. Q J Med 245:709–27
3. Emancipator SN, Lamm ME (1989) IgA nephropathy: pathogenesis of the most common form of glomerulonephritis. Lab Invest 60:168–83
4. Rifai A, Small PA, Teague PO, Ayoub EM (1979) Experimental IgA nephropathy. J Exp Med 150:1161–73
5. Kanatsu K, Doi T, Sekita K, Yoshida H, Nagai H, Hamashima Y (1983) A comparative immunologic study of IgA nephropathy. Am J Kidney Dis 2:618–25
6. Woodroffe AJ, Gormly AA, McKenzie PE, Wootton AM, Thompson AJ, Seymour AE, Clarkson AR (1980) Immunologic studies in IgA nephropathy. Kidney Int 18:366–74
7. Hall RP, Stachura I, Cason J, Whiteside TL, Lawely TJ (1983) IgA-containing circulating immune complexes in patients with IgA nephropathy. Am J Med 74:56–63
8. Coppo R, Basolo B, Piccoli G, Mazzucco G, Roccatello D (1984) IgA1 and IgA2 immune complexes in primary IgA nephropathy and Henoch-Schonlein nephritis. Clin Exp Immunol 57:583–90
9. Egido J Sancho J, Rivera F, Hernando L (1984) The role of IgA and IgG immune complexes in IgA nephropathy. Nephron 36:52–9
10. Valentijn RM, Kauffmann RH, de la Riviere GB, Daha MR, van Es LA (1983) Presence of circulating macromolecular IgA in patients with hematuria due to primary IgA nephropathy. Am J Med 74:375–81
11. Rifai A, Millard K (1985) Glomerular deposition of immune complexes prepared with monomeric or polymeric IgA. Clin Exp Immunol 60:363–68
12. Chen A, Wong SS, Rifai A (1988) Glomerular immune deposits in experimental IgA nephropathy: A continuum of circulating and in situ formed immune complexes. Am J Pathol 130:216–22
13. Bene MC, Faure G, Duheille J (1982) IgA nephropathy: characterization of the polymeric nature of mesangial deposits by in vitro binding of secretory component. Clin Exp Immunol 47:527–34
14. Monteiro RC, Halbwachs-Mecarelli L, Roque-Barreira, Noel LH, Berger J, Lesavre P (1985) Charge and size of mesangial IgA in IgA nephropathy. Kidney Int 28:666–71

15. Finbloom DS, Magilavy DB, Harford JB, Rifai A, Plotz PH (1981) The influence of antigen on immune complex behavior in mice. J Clin Invest 68:214–24
16. Rifai A, Mannik M (1983) Clearance kinetics and fate of mouse IgA immune complexes prepared with monomeric or dimeric IgA. J Immunol 130:1826–32
17. Rifai A, Mannik M (1984) Clearance of circulating IgA immune complexes is mediated by a specific receptor on Kupffer cells in mice. J Exp Med 160:125–37
18. Lawrence S, Pussel BA. Charlesworth JA (1983) Mesangial IgA nephropathy: Detection of defective reticulophagocytic function in vivo. Clin Nephrol 16:280–83
19. Nicholls K, Kincaid-Smith P (1984) Defective in vivo Fc- and C3b-receptor function in IgA nephropathy. AM J Kidney Dis 4:128–34
20. Rifai A, Schena FP, Montinaro V, Mele M, D'Addabbo A, Nitti L, Pezzullo JC (1989) Clearance kinetics and fate of macromolecular IgA in patients with IgA nephropathy. Lab Invest 61:381–388
21. Miyazaka R, Kuroda M, Akiyama T, Tofuku Y, Takeda R (1984) Glomerular deposition and serum levels of complement control proteins in patients with IgA nephropathy. Clin Nephrol 21:335–40
22. Rauterberg EW, Lieberknecht HM, Wingen AM, Ritz E (1987) Complement membrane attack (MAC) in idiopathic IgA-glomerulonephritis. Kidney Int 31:820–29
23. Imai H, Chen A, Wyatt RJ, Rifai A (1988) Lack of complement activation by human IgA immune complexes. Clin Exp Immunol 73:479–83
24. Waldo FB, Cochran AM (1989) Mixed IgA-IgG aggregates as a model of immune complexes in IgA nephropathy. J Immunol 142:3841–3846
25. Rifai A, Chen A, Imai H (1987) Complement activation in experimental IgA nephropathy: an antigen-mediated process. Kidney Int 32:838–44
26. Emancipator SN, Ovary Z, Lamm ME (1987) The role of mesangial complement in the hematuria of experimental IgA nephropathy. Lab Invest 57:269–76
27. Indraprasit S, Boonpucknavig V, Boonpucknavig S (1985) IgA nephropathy associated with enteric fever. Nephron 40:219–22
28. Davin JC, Malaise M, Foidart J, Mahieu P (1987) Anti-alpha-galactosyl antibodies and immune complexes in children with Henoch-Schonlein purpura or IgA nephropathy. Kidney Int 31:1132–9
29. Imai H, Chen A, Endoh M, Rifai A (1987) Influence of the antigen on experimental IgA nephropathy. Semin Nephrol 7:283–285
30. Montinaro et al. (to be published)

Anti-Thymocyte Antibody Induced Mesangiolytic Nephritis

Nobuaki Yamanaka and Masamichi Ishizaki[1]

Summary. Recently, an experimental model of mesangiolytic nephritis, induced by the anti-thy 1 antibody, was established. The thy 1 antigen is known as the cell surface antigen of the mouse thymocyte and is found to be expressed also on the rat mesangial cell membrane, as thy 1.1 antigen. A single intravenous administration of anti-thymocyte serum (ATS) immediately induces complement-mediated mesangiolytic destruction of the glomerulus, followed by proliferative changes of mesangial cells. Reconstruction of the glomerular structure results from the mesangial proliferation associated with revascularization. Between day 30 and day 45 after administration of ATS, most of the glomeruli had reverted to almost their original structure, with occasional focal and segmental defective changes. This model is characterized by acute mesangial proliferation and the rapid repair process of a drastically deformed glomerular structure, demonstrating the self-repair function of the glomerulus.

Overloading some conditions on this model, such as repeated injection of ATS or renal lymphatic ligation after ATS administration, for example, modifies the natural course of this self-limited proliferative change and is useful for analyzing the glomerular lesions.

This experimental model will make a contribution as a good tool for use in elucidating not only the mechanisms of proliferative glomerulonephritis, but also for elucidating the various functions of mesangial cells.

Introduction

Following the significant influence contributions made toward elucidating glomerular injuries by studies based on Masugi's experimental animal models of nephrotoxic nephritis, there have been recent similar attempts to adapt normal glomerular com-

[1]Department of Pathology, Nippon Medical School, 1-1-5, Sendagi, Bunkyo-ku, Tokyo, 113 Japan

ponents other than glomerular basement membrane (GBM), as antigen sources in aiming toward the establishment of a new experimental model. Such components as the epithelial cell [1], endothelial cell [2], mesangial cell, [3] and mesangial matrix, have been selected [4,5]. Selective injuries of mesangial cells induced by the immune mechanism will contribute to the analysis of many aspects of proliferative changes in the glomerulus. However, the appropriate experimental model whose target antigen is in the mesangium has not been successful, although some trials have been reported [3–5]. Recently, an experimental model of mesangiolytic nephritis which is induced by the anti-thymocyte antibody in the rat has been in the spotlight, because the antibody reacts with the mesangial cell itself with a high incidence of successive proliferative changes.

Thy 1 Antigen and Mesangial Cells

In 1980, Ishizaki found that the thy 1 antigen, which is known as the cell surface marker antigen of the mouse thymocyte, is also expressed on the cell surface of the rat mesangial cell [6]. In the same year, Morris et al., based on their immunofluorescent study of thy 1 cell surface differentiation antigen in connective tissue, briefly described the fact that this antigen is expressed in the rat mesangial cell [7]. Following this description, the studies of Harada et al. [8], Paul et al. [9], Bagchus et al. [10], and Yamamoto et al. [11], established the fact that this antigen is present on the cell surface of the rat mesangial cell.

The presence of thy 1 antigen is recognized in other tissue cells in mouse as well as in rat thymocytes [12]. It is known that there are two sorts of thy 1 antigen, thy 1.1 and thy 1.2 antigens [13]. Only thy 1.1 antigen was found on the surface of the rat mesangial cell. In our laboratory, it was found that the thy 1.1 antigen is also expressed on the surface of mesangial cells of the Mongolian gerbil [14]. This animal, which lives in the desert, is commonly called the sand rat. So far, no other species have been found to express thy 1 antigen in mesangial cells. Interestingly, neither thy 1.1 nor thy 1.2 antigen are present in the mouse mesangial cell.

Immunofluorescent microscopy, using mouse monoclonal antibody against thy 1.1 antigen, shows that the antigen has limited distribution, exclusively in the mesangial area, and in some regions it appears to exist circumferentially. Immunoelectron microscopy, using mouse monoclonal antibody, reveals that thy 1.1 antigen localizes on the surface of mesangial cells of the rat.

Anti-Thymocyte Antibody Induced Mesangial Lesions

In 1980, in his paper (in Japanese), Ishizaki briefly described this phenomenon: an intravenous administration of anti-rat thymocyte rabbit serum in the rat induced destruction of the mesangium, which was followed by segmental proliferation of mesangial cells [15]. We have continued to study the details of this phenomenon, and we have published our analysis of the results, in English this time [16]. In the same year Bagchus et al., using mouse monoclonal antibody against the rat thymocytes, had almost the same results [17,18]. Yamamoto et al., using polyclonal antithymocyte serum, also demonstrated an extensive analysis of similar glomerular lesions [11,19,20]. The methods and results of these three different groups are somewhat different in details; however, the main evolution of the disease is basically the same. That is to say, the heterologous antibody binds to the mesangial cell in the short term, subsequent autologous complement activation is induced, and as a result, cytolysis of the mesangial cell occurs, followed by mesangial proliferation.

According to our data [16], in immunofluorescent microscopy, rabbit IgG localizes in the region of the rat mesangium from at least 5 minutes after the intravenous administration of anti-thymocyte serum (ATS) and completely fixes within 15 minutes. The localization of rat C3 in the rat glomerulus is observed within 30 minutes of the administration of ATS. It demonstrates almost the same positive pattern as the distribution of rabbit IgG.

The electron micrograph reveals that 30 minutes after the administration of ATS, the mesangial cell severely degenerates, with shrinkage and dark appearance of the cytoplasm, suggesting an ongoing necrotic process. Two hours after the administration of ATS, a majority of mesangial cells lyse and disappear from the mesangial area, while GBM is always well preserved. Endothelial cells are also preserved in spite of the significant destruction of the mesangium. In the lysed mesangial areas, there is an accumulation of blood components, including blood plasma and blood cells. Yamamoto et al. [19] and Bagchus et al. [18] demonstrated that the C5b–C9 complement components are also positive in almost the same pattern as mesangial C3 deposition, thus establishing the involvement of the membrane attack complex in this cytolytic process. Yamamoto et al. performed studies on the depletion of complement activation by using cobra venom and proved the complement-dependency of the lytic phenomenon in the mesangium in this model [19]. Bagchus et al. demonstrated that IgG 1, which is a subclass of IgG and is unable to activate rat complement, is able to bind to the antigen on the mesangial cell, but is not able to induce subsequent cytolytic changes. On the other hand, IgG 2, which is able to activate rat complement, can cause cytolysis [17].

Aneurysmal cystic lesion of the glomerular capillary is observed 24 hours after administration of ATS, with margination of leukocytes and an accumulation of platelets and fibrin. The lesion highly resembles the glomerular lesion induced by snake venom and is regarded as an extremely severe state of mesangiolysis [21]. The GBM is usually preserved and the evidence of rupture is rare.

Figure 1 shows chronological glomerular changes followed by mesangiolysis demonstrated by methenamine silver staining. At 24 hours after ATS administration, the glomerulus exhibits a cystic mesangiolytic lesion containing accumulated cells with neutrophils (Fig. 1a). The glomerulus shows leukocytic infiltration with a predominance of monocytes, and the initiation of mesangial cell proliferation from day 2 to day 4 after ATS administration (Fig. 1b). The matrix component is rarely present in this region. The glomerulus in Fig. 1c exhibits the changes on day 8. It shows the significant proliferation of mesangial cells in a segmental fashion, with a decreased number of leukocytes, which is equivalent to the state of proliferative glomerulonephritis. The silver-positive matrix components among the proliferated mesangial cells are recognized, as well as the regression of the diseased segment, together with irregular increase of capillary lumens. On day 18, there is a decrease of cell proliferation, with evident reconstruction of capillary structure, decrease of matrix components, and disappearance of leukocytes in the segmental lesion (Fig. 1d). These findings appear to be the expression of rapid repair of the drastic cystic lesion of

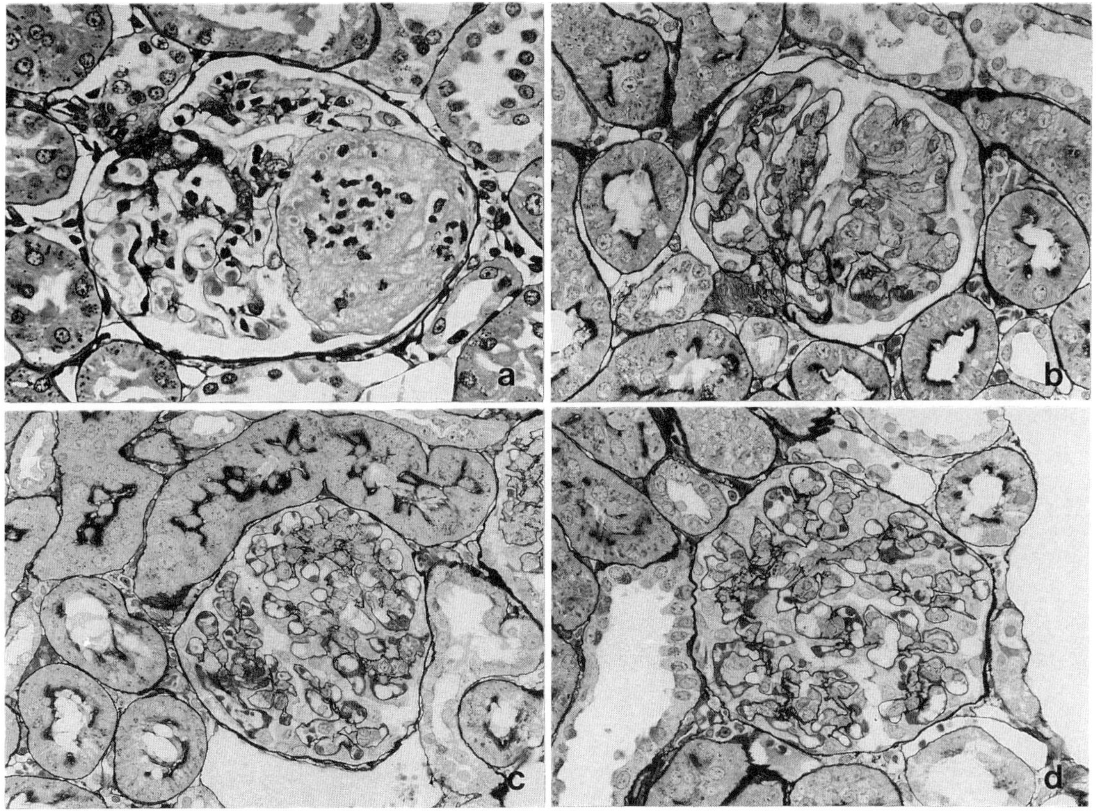

Fig. 1a-d. Chronological glomerular changes after administration of ATS (PAM stain). **a** 24 hours: cystic mesangiolytic lesion with accumulated neutrophils, **b** 2–4 days: initiation of mesangial proliferation with monocyte infiltration, **c** 8 days: proliferation of mesangial cells with a decreased number of leukocytes and increased matrix components, **d** 18 days: decrease of cell proliferation and matrix components with reconstruction of capillary structure

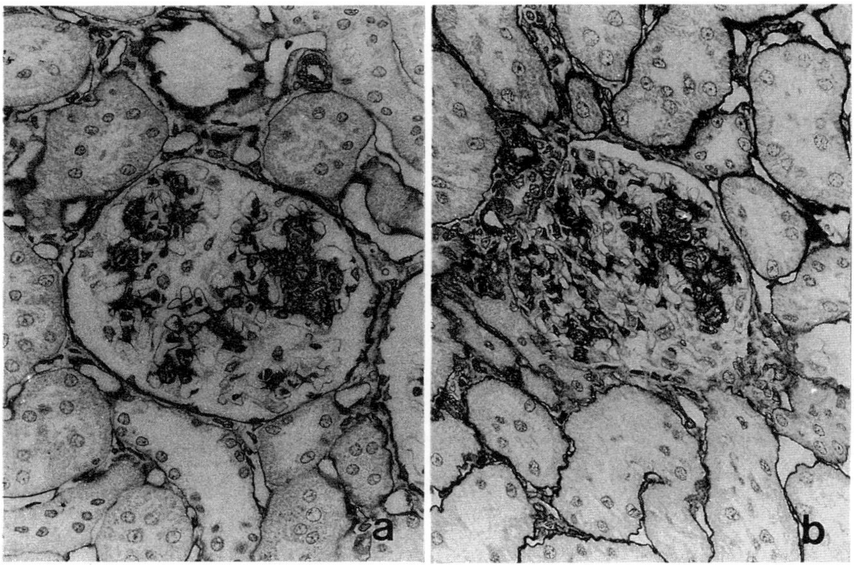

Fig. 2a,b. Immunostaining of increased matrix components in the injured glomerulus 12 days after ATS administration, demonstrated by immunoperoxidase (*PAP*) method. **a** type IV collagen, **b** laminin

mesangiolysis. The electron micrograph from around day 6 exhibits prominent mesangial proliferation with evident increase of the matrix, which occupies the site of the preforming cystic mesangiolytic change. Proliferation of endothelial cells and reconstruction of the glomerular vasculature are also demonstrated.

The process of protein excretion shows massive transient proteinuria with the peak around day 4 and gradual decrease to a normal level until around day 21. This movement of proteinuria is well correlated with the morphological changes of rapid reconstruction of the glomerular structure.

From day 30 to day 45 after the administration of ATS, most of the glomeruli had virtually reverted to their original structure, with focal and segmental sclerosis, partial appearance of collagen fibers or focal remnants of proliferative change, and occasional deformation. No proteinuria was detected at this stage. This model shows the characteristics of the rapid repair process of a drastically deformed glomerulus with mesangiolysis in the case of a one-shot charge of antibody. This model indicates that the glomerulus has a self-repair function which can reconstruct the breaking of its structure, and the proliferation of the mesangial cells in such situations may be the expression of the repair reaction of the living body.

Another characteristic of the model is that, in the rat, there is only heterologous reaction and no autologous antibody formation. It is probable that this defect of the autologous phase is the cause of the rapid recovery of the glomerular lesions.

Detection of changes in the matrix components in these diseased processes by the immunohistological method, reveal an overt increase of type IV collagen associated with mesangial cell proliferation. The distribution of laminin shows almost the same

Table 1. Evolution of anti-thymocyte antibody-induced glomerular injury

Antigen-antibody binding followed by activation of complement
Complement-mediated cytolysis of mesangial cell
Various degrees of mesangiolysis
Mesangial hypercellularity with leukocytic infiltration
1 Polymormphonuclear neutrophils (PMN) → monocyte-macrophage, aggregation of platelets
2 monocyte-macrophage + mesangial cell proliferation
Mesangial cell proliferation and increase of matrix components
Mesangial cell proliferation with revascularization
Remodelling of the glomerular structure
Defect healing with occasional focal segmental sclerosis

pattern as that of type IV collagen (Fig. 2). Proliferated mesangial cells and increased matrix components are reorganized in the stalk regions in accordance with the reconstitution of the glomerulus due to revascularization; gradually these components distribute in an almost normal fashion. These processes resemble mesangial development during glomerular embryogenesis [22].

The process of glomerular injury caused by anti-thymocyte antibody will progress in the manner proposed in Table I. The characteristics of this experimental model are as follows: 100% of the glomerular lesions will be induced by the administration of heterologous antibody; these lesions will be followed by complement-dependent drastic mesangiolysis. In the initial stage, there are inflammatory changes characterized by leukocyte infiltration and aggregation of platelets, followed by a prominent proliferation of mesangial cells. The increase of matrix components occurs among the proliferated mesangial cells, as does revascularization, which will contribute to the reconstruction of glomerular structure. In the case of a one-shot charge of antibody, most of the glomeruli repair morphologically within a short period of from 30 to 45 days.

Our studies on this model reveal that the degree of mesangiolysis induced by ATS administration is varied, and that mild mesangiolysis is a more common finding than aneurysmal cystic lesions. The proliferative response to mild mesangiolysis is rapid and mild mesangial cell proliferation tends to occur in the early period. Judging from these processes, the mesangial proliferation in this model may be the expression of the mesangial repair mechanism.

Bagchus et al. demonstrated these mesangiolytic glomerular changes by using only a small amount of monoclonal antibody [17,18]. Their results are very important because they show that these continuous histological changes of glomerular proliferation can be induced by administration of monoclonal antibody.

Thy 1 Antigen in Newborn Rat Kidney

Using mouse monoclonal antibody, the distribution of thy 1.1 antigen in the newborn rat kidney is found to reveal positive immunofluorescence in the cleft of the S-shaped body, which is the most immature glomerulus. Positive findings increase in accordance with the maturity of the primitive glomeruli. The most mature glomerulus in the newborn rat shows overt positive fluorescence encircling each mesangial cell in

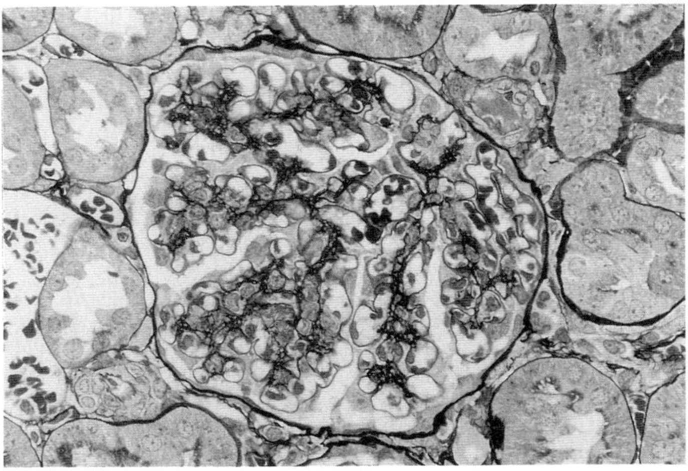

Fig. 3. Prolonged mesangial cell proliferation with increased matrix components due to repeated charges of ATS (PAM stain)

the simplified glomerular structure. These findings suggest the possibility of the induction of a mesangial lesion even in such primitive glomeruli.

Repeated Charges of ATS

According to our ongoing studies with repeated charges of polyclonal anti-thymocyte serum in the rat, the repair process of the damaged glomerulus is markedly retarded, demonstrating significant widening of the mesangial area due to diffuse increase of the cellular components and matrix (Fig. 3). These findings resemble the histological findings of chronic proliferative glomerulonephritis in human material. Appropriate applications of this experimental model will contribute to the analysis of the mechanism of human glomerulonephritis.

Influences of Lymphatic Ligation

In our laboratory, we have observed retardation of mesangial pathway flow by carrying out complete ligation of the renal lymph vessels at the renal hilus in the rat. In the ligated groups, the mesangiolytic changes of the glomerulus are mild, compared to those in the non-ligated groups, and no cystic lesions of mesangiolysis were observed (Fig. 4). These observations are interpreted as hindrance of antigen-antibody binding on the mesangial cell surface caused by retardation of flow through the mesangial pathway. In our observation of the glomerular changes which occurred after one-shot administration of ATS, the repair process progressed through a relatively short period in the nonligated group; however, this repair process was markedly hindered in the lymphatic ligated group during the mesangiolytic stage,

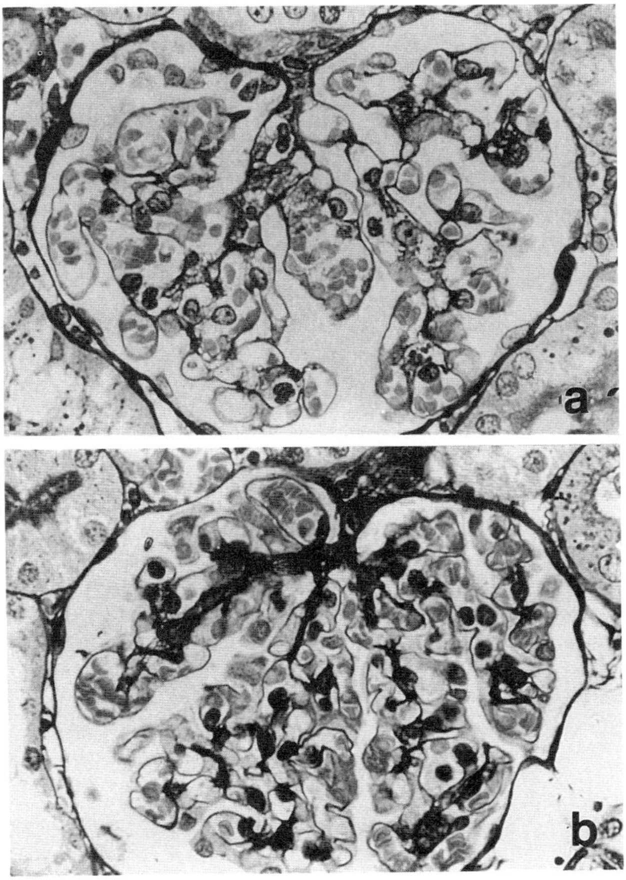

Fig. 4a,b. Influence of lymphatic ligation at renal hilus before ATS administration (PAM stain). **a** overt mesangiolytic change with no lymphatic ligation, **b** mild mesangiolytic change with lymphatic ligation

due to retardation of the mesangial pathway flow. As shown in these examples, by overloading some conditions on this self-limited proliferative model, the creation of an experimental setting for continuous mesangial change will be possible.

Conclusions

We will be able to analyze various factors in mesangial proliferation by using this model. Johnson et al., for example, reported on platelet mediation in glomerular cell proliferation by using this anti-thymocyte antibody model [23]. Sophisticated utilization of this experimental condition will contribute not only to analyzing the mechanism of glomerulonephritis, but also to elucidating the various functions of the mesangial cell. We now have great expectations for the use of this simple and clear model as a good tool in the elucidation of various problems in nephrology, other than the problem of mesangial proliferation.

References

1. Kerjaschki D, Farquhar MG (1983) Immunocytochemical localization of the Heymann nephritis antigen (gp330) in glomerular epithelial cells of normal Lewis rats. J Exp Med 157:667–686
2. Matsuo S, Fukatsu A, Taub ML, Caldwell PRB, Brentjens JR, Andres G (1987) Glomerulonephritis induced in the rabbit by antiendothelial antibodies. J Clin Invest 79:1798–1811
3. Seelig HP, Seelig R, Roth E (1975) Antibodies reacting with the glomerular mesangium; isolation and immunopathology. Virchows Arch [A] 336:313–330
4. Mendrick DL, Rennke HG (1986) Immune deposits formed in situ by a monoclonal antibody recognizing a new intrinsic rat mesangial matrix antigen. J Immunol 137:1517–1526
5. Batsford SR, Rohrback R, Takamiya H, Kluthr R, Vogt A (1979) Autoantibody specific for the glomerular mesangium and Bowman's capsule in man. Clin Nephrol 12:163–167
6. Ishizaki M, Sato S, Sano J, Fukuda Y, Sugisaki Y, Masugi Y (1980) The presence of Thy-1.1 antigen in rat glomerular mesangial cells. Biomed Res 1:438–442
7. Morris RJ, Ritter MA (1980) Association of Thy-1 cell surface differentiation antigen with certain connective tissues in vivo. Cell Tissue Res 206:459–475
8. Harada K, Yamamoto T, Hara M, Kihara I (1982) Antigenic association between kidney and thymocyte. Acta Pathol Jpn 32:483–489
9. Paul LC, Rennke HG, Milford EL, Carpenter CB (1984) Thy-1.1 in glomeruli of rat kidneys. Kidney Int 25:771–777
10. Bagchus WM, Donga J, Ronzing J, Hoedemaeker PhJ, Bakker WW (1984) The specificity of nephritogenic antibodies. IV. Binding of monoclonal anti-thymocyte antibodies to rat kidney. Transplantation 41:739–745
11. Yamamoto T, Yamamoto K, Kawasaki K, Yaoita E, Shimizu F, Kihara I (1986) Immunoelectron microscopic demonstration of Thy-1 antigen on the surface of mesangial cells in the rat glomerulus. Nephron 43:293–298
12. Douglas TC (1972) Occurrence of a theta-like antigen in rats. J Exp Med 136:1054–1062
13. Reif AE, Allen JM (1966) Mouse thymic iso-antigens. Nature 209:521–523
14. Ishizaki M, Shimizu M, Shichinoe K, Masuda Y, Sugisaki Y, Yamanaka N, Masugi Y (1989) The presence of Thy-1.1 antigen in Mongolian gerbils. Biomed Res 10:413–416
15. Ishizaki M (1980) The presence of Thy 1.1 antigen in rat glomerular mesangial cells (in Japanese, with abstract in English). Allergy 29:816–826
16. Ishizaki M, Masuda Y, Fukuda Y, Sugisaki Y, Yamanaka N, Masugi Y (1986) Experimental mesangioproliferative glomerulonephritis in rats induced by intravenous administration of anti-thymocyte serum. Acta Pathol Jpn 36:1191–1203
17. Bagchus WM, Hoedemaeker PJ, Rozing J, Bakker WW (1986) Acute glomerulonephritis after intravenous injection of monoclonal antithymocyte antibodies in the rat. Immunol Lett 12:109–113
18. Bagchus WM, Hoedemaeker PJ, Rozing J, Bakker WW (1986) Glomerulonephritis induced by monoclonal anti-Thy 1.1 antibodies. A sequential histological and ultrastructural study in the rat. Lab Invest 55:680–687

19. Yamamoto T, Wilson CB (1987) Complement dependence of antibody induced mesangial injury in the rat. J Immunol 138:3758–3765
20. Yamamoto T, Wilson CB (1987) Quantitative and qualitative studies of antibody-induced mesangial cell damage in the rat. Kidney Int 32:514–525
21. Morita T, Churg J (1983) Mesangiolysis. Kidney Int 24:1–9
22. Yamanaka N (1988) Development of the glomerular mesangium. Pediatr Nephrol 2:85–91
23. Johnson R, Garcia RI, Pitzl P, Alpers CE (1990) Platelets mediate glomerular cell proliferation in immune complex nephritis induced by anti-mesangial cell antibodies in the rat. Am J Pathol 136:369–374

Experimental Nephritis—Other Models and Future Directions

CURTIS B. WILSON[1]

SUMMARY. Almost all of the advances in understanding the nephritogenic process responsible for human immune, glomerular, and tubulointerstitial renal injury have their basis in animal models. A large number of model systems are now available, with recent interest focused on producing selective glomerular cell injury. Anti-mesangial cell and anti-epithelial cell surface antigens participate in these processes. An almost parallel set of models are available for understanding the immune processes responsible for tubulointerstitial nephritis. These processes, which include immune deposit formation through antibody reactions with structural and cellular antigens, immune complex formation, and cellular immune reactions, are reviewed. Possible future directions for model use are described. A search for models of disease produced by antigens present only in activated or stimulated cells is suggested and should lead to a better understanding of the immunopathogenesis of vasculitis. Extensions of current model systems to better define the contribution of cytokine and growth factor cascades responsible for glomerular and renal cell contributions to injury are discussed, including the use of the isolated perfused kidney. A number of other possible extensions are mentioned, including selective immunotherapies using antibodies to the T cell receptor Vbeta gene, utilization of SCID mice for development of models of human autoimmunity, the possible role of transgenic mice, and, finally, the utilization of models of selective renal cell injury to further the understanding of renal pathophysiology.

Studies of model systems have produced great strides in understanding the immunologic basis of glomerular disease since the early work of Lindemann, Masugi, Kay, and von Pirquet (Table 1). These studies have been the subject of review [1,2]. The classical Masugi nephritis employs heterogenous anti-glomerular basement membrane (GBM) antibodies (Abs), reactive with a variety of GBM components, to cause acute glomerular capillary wall damage and glomerulonephritis

[1]Department of Immunology, Research Institute of Scripps Clinic, La Jolla, CA 92037, USA

Table 1. Immune models of glomerular injury

Ab reactions with glomerular Ags to form immune deposits
Basement membrane and extracellular matrix Ags
Trapped or planted Ags
Immune complex formation/dynamic interchange
Glomerular cell surface Ags
?? Ab reactions without immune deposits
Cellular immune mechanisms
?? Activation of immune mediator pathways

(GN) in a dose-dependent fashion, largely through the recruitment of systemic mediator systems. This model, combined with the models inducing autoimmune anti-GBM reactions in sheep introduced by Stebley and co-workers, laid the groundwork for recognition of the role of anti-GBM Ab-related injury in humans. The heterologous anti-GBM Ab bound to the GBM in the Masugi model, in turn, served as a trapped antigen (Ag) during the autologous phase of injury, when the host's own Ab response to it caused a second wave of inflammation. The trapped Ag concept now encompasses a wide variety of Ags capable of binding to the glomerular capillary for a number of physicochemical reasons, including lectin binding and charge interactions.

The concept of selective glomerular localization or trapping of a potentially nephritogenic Ag in the glomerular capillary wall for subsequent Ab reaction, and the concept of Ag/Ab reactions in the circulation which form immune complexes (ICs) that can subsequently accumulate in the glomerular capillary, provide a complicated interface between planted Ag mechanisms and IC-based immunopathogenic processes. Except for instances in which Ag can be trapped before the appearance of Ab, as in the Masugi nephritis model, Ag and Ab are typically present together, making quantitative separate or trapping with in situ Ab reaction from IC formation and accumulation difficult. No matter what the major factor is in initiating the glomerular and vascular accumulation of IC, the subsequent dynamic interaction of Ag and Ab in the deposit causes considerable reshaping of the deposit relative to the concentrations of Ag and Ab in the immediate environment; the interchange is modified by physicochemical factors that retain Ag or Ab at the site. Secondary immune reactions, such as anti-idiotypic Abs or rheumatoid factor production, also alter this interchange, depending on the degree of cross-linking produced.

The concept of Ab reactions with the glomerular capillary wall of the Masugi nephritis model has recently been expanded by the recognition of specific reactions with glomerular cell surface Ags, leading to selective injury or modulation of individual glomerular cell types. The mesangial cell lesions, associated with an Ab reactive with a Thy-1-like Ag on the mesangial cell surface, caused complement-mediated cell death and subsequent proliferation of residual mesangial cells, which resolved with focal mesangial matrix increase [3,4]. As with the Masugi nephritis model, quantitative features of anti-Thy-1 Ab binding can be related to the extent of cell injury, degree of proliferation, or to re-injury by additional Ab. The ability to selectively damage one glomerular cell type allows the study of the cell's function and pathophysiology.

Necrotizing and crescentic GN, associated with vasculitis, can occur in patients without evidence of immune deposits, suggesting that other mechanisms of immune injury remain to be defined (see ahead). Cellular immune mechanisms are not pre-

Table 2. Ab reactions with glomerular cell Ags leading to immune deposit formation and/or cell injury

Fx1A-associated Ags (gp330, dipeptidyl peptidase IV, etc), Thy-1, ACE, other Ags recognized by monoclonal Abs, ? infectious agents, phagocytosed materials, ?MHC Ags, ? trapped Ags, ? expressed Ags

ACE, angiotensin converting enzyme

dominant in most instances of GN; however, interesting models in chickens and a recent example in rats indicate the need for additional study [5,6]. Activation of immune mediator systems may also participate, as in Type II membranoproliferative GN.

A topic which originally was planned to be the subject of a separate discussion during the symposium was that of the Ab reactions with a glomerular cell in the long-studied Heymann's nephritis model. Initially, this model was considered to be an example of an autologous IC mechanism involving a proximal tubular brush border Ag. More recently, evidence has accumulated that a selective reaction of Ab with Ags, in particular gp330, shared between the glomerular epithelial cell podocytes and the brush border of the proximal renal tubule, is responsible [7,8]. The molecule has cysteine-rich 40-amino acid repeats, which are also a feature of the human low-density lipoprotein (LDL) receptor; similarity with some regions of epidermal growth factor precursor is also present [9]. A 76 kDa serum protein is reported that may be a ligand for gp330; the 76 kDa material also binds with nephritogenic autoAb eluted from glomerular deposits [10]. Additional Ags may be involved in the full blown Heymann's nephritis lesion. The membrane attack complex of complement (MAC) pays a major role in mediation of this non-inflammatory glomerular lesion [11,12].

In Heymann's nephritis, the mechanism of injury is related to Ab-induced cross-linking of the epithelial cell surface Ag, with shedding of the complex as an immune deposit at the subepithelial aspect of the GBM, where the podocytes abut the GBM [13,14]. Other epithelial Ags, including dipeptidyl peptidase IV, lead to more transient Ab binding [15–17] (see Table 2). It remains difficult to completely exclude ICs, due to the complexity of different crude Ags used for induction and the possibility of anti-idiotypic contributions. The relationship of the Heymann's nephritis model to human membranous glomerulopathy remains unclear, although there are occasional reports of possible anti-gp330 reactions and reports that some anti-glomerular epithelial cell antibodies can react with human or monkey glomeruli with redistribution of surface Ag [18,19]. A spontaneous GN, with subepithelial deposits in rabbits, may represent a similar type of immune mechanism with a glomerular Ag that is also prominent in human glomeruli [20].

We have learned a lot from these models regarding the effects of antibody binding; in terms of quantity and tempo, the site of binding, the accessibility of the reactive antigen which governs these parameters, and the ever increasing complexity of the mediator systems, both systemic and intrinsic, within the glomerular cells themselves, that can produce the injury signaled by the specific interaction of antibody molecules.

It is now apparent that virtually all the immune mechanisms defined in the study of glomerular injury models have counterparts in tubulointerstitial nephritis (TIN) as well (Table 3) (reviewed in [21]). In some of these models, cellular immune mechanisms play major roles. The tubular basement membranes (TBMs) are prominent Ags

Table 3. Immune tubulointerstitial nephritis (TIN)

Ab reactions with tubular Ags to form immune deposits
Basement membrane and extracellular matrix Ags
TBM, TBM/GBM, ? TBM/Drug conjugates
?? Trapped or planted Ags
Drugs, microbial Ags, DNA, etc.
Immune complex formation/dynamic interchange
Serum proteins, drugs, products of infectious agents, tissue components, idiotypic Ags, etc.
Tubular cell surface Ags
Brush border Ags, Tamm Horsfall protein
Cellular immune mechanisms
Ags associated with delayed type hypersensitivity
Aggregated proteins, cell surface Ags, TBM Ags, ? drugs
Ags in cellular forms of TIN
Isologous kidney, homologous renal basement membrane, heterologous TBM, tubular Ag/TBM Ag in kdkd mice, ?non-native materials (drugs, infectious agents, etc.)
?? Activation of immune mediator pathways

which, when used as immunogens in adjuvants, can elicit predominantly humoral (guinea pigs, rats) or cellular (mice) immune mononuclear leukocyte-dominated reactions, surrounding the tubules with linear Ig deposits in the TBM. The circulating and eluted anti-TBM Abs react with Ags confined to the proximal TBM; the Ags are genetically variable in rats and in humans [22]. The allotypic differences can induce anti-TBM Ab in association with renal transplantation. TBM/drug conjugates have been suggested to induce anti-TBM antibody reactions in humans [23]. Sodium aurothiomalate and mercuric chloride can also induce Ab reactive with TBM [24,25]. A different set of immune reactions in rats is directed toward Ags shared with GBM/TBM, as seen in human anti-GBM Ab disease and Goodpasture's syndrome.

The anti-TBM Ab disease of the guinea pig or rat is transferable with immune serum. In the rat, the kinetics of binding have been studied, and reveal a gradual increase in fixation over 5–6 days, suggesting that the Ag is relatively sequestered [26]. The molecule carrying the reactive Ag may vary somewhat in size depending on extraction methods. It has been termed 3M-1 and is about 30 kDa in mice, 42–45 or 48 kDa in rats, and 48 kDa in rabbits and humans (reviewed in [27]). cDNA defines the 3M-1 as a complex, novel structure containing five distinct amino acid termini, all sharing a common framework domain [28]. Comparisons of the anti-TBM Ab binding sequence suggest a 37% non-repetitive structural similarity with some intermediate filament-associated proteins (E.G. Neilson personal communication). A peptide fragment synthesized from the sequence encoding this common framework domain was able to bind to a monoclonal 3M-1 reactive anti-TBM Ab and stimulate the growth of 3M-1-reactive helper T cells, as well as induce nephritogenic effector T cells capable of producing TIN (E.G. Neilson personal communication). These findings indicate that a small and unique, immunodominant region of the 3M-1 Ag, evolutionarily related to the family of intermediate filament-associated proteins, provides a sufficient recognition structure for the model of TIN.

Reactions with renal tubular cell Ags also occur in models that parallel, to some extent, those reactive with glomerular cell Ags. Active or passive immunization to Fx1A type Ags leads to immune deposits in and around the proximal tubular cell;

striking damage to the brush border is found when the Ab gains access to the tubular urine [29]. The reaction is thought to represent another example of Ab-induced cross-linking of Ag [30]. Numerous Ags would be candidates for this type of reaction and anti-tubular brush border Abs are sometimes identified in humans with tubular damage (reviewed in [27]). Another tubular protein that has been studied in a similar type of reaction is the Tamm-Horsfall protein [31] and angiotensin converting enzyme which may react with the basolateral compartment of the proximal tubular cell [32]. A wide variety of monoclonal Abs reactive with tubular cell Ags have a similar potential. The concept of molecular mimicry, in which short segments of amino acid homology are shared between molecules, can also lead to cross-reactions with renal tubular Ags. For example, we have found that a number of monoclonal anti-viral Abs also react with renal tubular (or glomerular) structures.

As they do in immune glomerular injury, ICs can accumulate in the tubulointerstitial tissues in serum sickness, and in murine and human examples of systemic lupus erythematosus (SLE) or presumed IC disease. Regarding circulating versus in situ formed ICs, the same factors as those in the glomeruli must be taken into consideration, as well as the dynamic interchange of Ag and Ab (see above). The possibility of trapping of Ag within the tubulointerstitial tissue for subsequent Ab reaction is another possibility, although good models are lacking as yet.

In TIN, cellular immune reactions play a more striking role than in GN, and a variety of models of delayed type hypersensitivity reactions are described (reviewed in [27]). The TIN of SJL mice induced by immunization with heterologous TBM, as noted above, is largely cellular in nature, with the development of a MHC class I restricted, Lyt-2$^+$ effector cell which can adaptively transfer the disease [33–36]. The proximal tubular epithelial cell line producing the 3M-1 Ag expresses MHC class II Ags and can support the proliferation of MHC class II restricted helper T cell lines in culture [37]. Anti-3M-1 Abs down regulate MHC class II expression of the 3M-1 synthesizing cells in vitro [38]. Proximal tubular enhancement of MHC class II expression is also found in the MRL/1pr lupus mice [39]. The SJL model is being used very successfully to explore therapeutic approaches, including the evaluation of suppressor cell networks capable of inhibiting the disease, via injection of spleen cells coupled with TBM Ag [40]. At least two suppressor subsets are defined and soluble factors from spleen cells of mice treated to induce suppressor cells are able to inhibit development of interstitial lesions in an Ag-specific, genetically restricted manner [41,42]. These models hold considerable promise for better understanding of treatment (see ahead).

Lewis rats (lacking reactive TBM Ag), when immunized with Brown Norway rat TBM, develop a severe nodular granulomatous form of TIN [43]. The lesion is easily transferred with immune cells and there is little evidence for an Ab role in the model. The kdkd mouse, a congenic subline of the CBA/Ca strain, also appears to have a cell-mediated form of TIN [44]. As considered in glomerular disease, immune mediation activation, particularly that of complement, may occur in the tubulointerstitial tissue, associated with ammonia increases during compromised renal function.

The models of GN and TIN are responsible for our current understanding of the immunopathogenesis of renal disease. The growth of knowledge in the past few years, based on molecular biologic techniques and glomerular cell culture, has been outstanding, but much of it is yet to be transferred to the intact kidney models or the human counterparts. The models can be expected to play a more prominent role as the basic information is translated in vivo. The request by the program organizers to look into the next century is difficult and it is a bit presumptuous to predict how the current or new models will be used; however, some suggestions will be made.

A new mechanism of injury, such as that recently defined by the glomerular cell surface reactions, may emerge in the broad field of Ag accessibility and induced Ag expression. In the former case, evidence is accumulating that alveolar basement membrane Ags are not readily available for anti-GBM Ab reaction unless the integrity of the alveolar wall is first altered, as determined in model studies [45]. If this is also true for human anti-GBM Abs, it could explain episodes of pulmonary hemorrhage in Goodpasture's syndrome. In the case of Ag expression, the renal syndromes associated with vasculitis serve as a starting point. In these conditions, glomerular disease may be severe, without the usual evidence of immune deposits. This suggests a new immunopathogenic mechanism. In Kawasaki's syndrome, for example, the Abs present are capable of lysis of activated, but not normal, cultured human endothelial cells [46,47]. In one type, IgG and IgM Abs lyse interleukin-1 (IL-1) and tumor necrosis factor (TNF)-treated endothelial cells. In the other type, IgM Abs lyse INF gamma treated endothelial cells via different Ags. Complement-fixing IgG and IgM Abs are reported in acute hemolytic uremic syndrome, which can lyse umbilical vein endothelial cells, but not after INF treatment [48]. A number of less well defined anti-endothelial cell Abs have been reported in Wegener's granulomatosis, other vasculitis, and IgA nephropathy. The cytokine effects on endothelium have been reviewed [49] and, in addition to modulating a number of coagulation related proteins, including tissue factor, thrombomodulin, and PAI, they also increase surface adhesion of leukocytes. The latter is via expression of endothelial leukocyte adhesion molecule (ELAM-1) and intracellular adhesion molecule (ICAM-1, CD54)J. ICAM-1 is a ligand for LFA-1 (CD11a/CD18) of the leukocyte adhesion CD11/18 complex, which also includes Mac-1 and p150,95, all having common beta chains and unique alpha chains (reviewed in [50]).

In addition to changes in the endothelium with the expression of Ags, one must also consider a similar observation in the neutrophil, the target of anti-neutrophil (and macrophage) cytoplasmic Ab (ANCA), subsets of which are seen in various forms of vasculitis and in idiopathic necrotizing and crescentic GN [51,52]. Of great interest is the recent observation that neutrophils may need to be "activated" with cytokines to be able to express the reactive Ag on their surface [53]. These Ag expression observations should serve as a base for a new use of model systems in advancing understanding of the immunopathogenesis of the poorly understood class of vasculitis-associated renal injury that occurs without the usual immune deposit formation.

The models of glomerular injury have been widely used to study systemic mediator pathways of immune GN, and, to a lesser extent, TIN, injury (Table 4). Almost all that we know was derived first from observation of possible reactants and subsequent mediator depletion in models. These studies have been coupled, in many instances, with identification of similar factors in humans. It is to be expected that the models will continue to be used for these purposes. In addition, there has been an explosion of information derived from glomerular cell culture and application of molecular biologic techniques. This incorporation points to the potential large contribution of factors from the glomerular cells themselves to the inflammatory process and to the sclerosis that often follows (Table 5). It is in this area that the models, particularly the models in which selective glomerular cell damage can be produced, will have a great deal of play

Table 4. Models and isolated kidney for the study of systemic mediators of inflammation

Ab effects and the MAC
? Integrins, glomerular cell products
Neutrophils and macrophages
Oxidants, proteinases, cationic proteins, eicosanoids, cytokines, growth factors, coagulation factors
Platelets
Neutrophil interaction, PAF, platelet factor 4, eicosanoids
Lymphocytes

MAC, membrane attack complex; PAF, platelet activating factor

in the next few years. The determination of cytokine/growth factor cascades in glomerular inflammation will employ molecular biology techniques, bioassays, and cytochemical staining in models employing selective systemic mediator depletion. It is also expected that the isolated perfused kidney will find great usefulness in the study of immune injury in the absence of systemic mediators. The perfused kidney can also be used to study the direct glomerular effects of initial factors in the cascades, to confirm their roles. It is anticipated that the isolated perfused kidney will be used to manipulate pivotal factors, using Ab, peptide, or molecular techniques, so that the most suitable approaches for therapy in the intact models and, subsequently, in human glomerular disease can be determined. Interference with receptor binding, with peptide blocking such as the RGD (arg-gly-asp) sequence [54], or with gene expression, through the administration of anti-sense RNA, [55] has potential usefulness that can be tested in the isolated perfused kidney and in the models.

The T cell-mediated models will be used to advantage to study the effects of immunologically specific therapy, such as that utilizing T cell receptor Vbeta-specific antibodies, as in experimental allergic encephalomyelitis [56,57]. In experimental allergic encephalomyelitis, only two T cell receptor Vbeta gene segments, Vbeta8.2 and Vbeta13, and two distinct Valpha gene segments, Valpha2.3 and Valpha4.3, are identified in the myelin basic protein-specific T helper cells. This limited use of the T cell receptor V region genes, in response to myelin basic protein, allowed the specific treatment of the disease, including reversal of paralysis, with a combination of monoclonal Vbeta8.2 and Vbeta13 specific antibodies [58].

The recent identification of the SCID mice, which have sufficient immunodeficiency to allow implantation and growth of human immune cells, allows the construction of models of laboratory animal based human disease. In mice given peripheral blood leukocytes from patients with systemic lupus erythematosus, antinuclear antibodies develop and glomerular immune deposits resembling lupus nephritis are found [59]. The model expands the potential for directly evaluating the

Table 5. Potential contribution of glomerular cells to inflammation

Interleukin −1(IL-1alpha, beta), Tumor necrosis factor (TNF), interleukin-6 (IL-6), insulin-like growth factor (IFG-I), tissue plasminogen activator (t-PA), plasminogen activator inhibitor (PAI), platelet activating factor (PAF), platelet derived growth factor (PDGF), tissue factor (TF), oxidative products, neutral proteinase and its inhibitor, thrombospondin, renin, eicosanoids, endothelial cell adhesion molecules
Growth factors; epidermal growth factor (EGF), receptors for transforming growth factor beta (TGFbeta), beta1-integrin, fibronectin production

influence of cellular and humoral functions in the progression of the disease and expands the potential for evaluating various possible therapies in several mice from the same donor. We have been successful in establishing anti-GBM Ab production in SCID mice, with transfer of peripheral blood leukocytes from patients with active disease, so that the study of numerous autoimmune diseases with renal features appears to be possible.

The development of mesangial proliferative GN has been noted in IL-6 transgenic mice [60], and mesangial proliferation and progressive glomerulosclerosis has been observed in mice expressing growth hormone and growth hormone releasing factor [61,62]. The heavy metal-inducible promoter of the mouse metallothione in I gene, among others, can be used to express genes in the kidneys of transgenic mice. It is much easier, currently, to express a gene than to delete the function of one. As currently employed, the technique of homologous recombination used for the latter is demanding [63]. It is to be expected that systems will be available, however, which will use transgenic animals to alter gene expression for a variety of purposes in the study of immune renal injury. Extensions of the studies evaluating the role of cytokines and growth factors should be possible, as noted above. Alteration in Ag expression and manipulation of Ab production or T cell receptor functions should also be of interest.

Another use of the models, either of those now available or of those that could be developed, would be in the examination of the pathophysiologic effects of selective glomerular or tubular cell injury. We have used the anti-mesangial cell injury model to look at the effect of acute mesangial cell lysis at 24 hours after antibody administration; we found a reduction in glomerular ultrafiltration coefficient as plasma was shunted into the lytic mesangial space away from the filtering surface [64]. During the proliferative phase of injury, 3–5 days later, the ultrafiltration coefficient remained low during the increase in mesangial volume and decreased capillary luminal volume and surface area.

Acknowledgments. This work was supported in part by USPHS Grants Nos. AI-07007, DK20043, DK32353, DK40251, AG04342, and Biomedical Research Support Grant RR0-5514.

References

1. Wilson CB (to be published) The renal response to immunological injury. In: Brenner BM, Rector FC Jr (eds) The kidney, 4th edn. Saunders, Philadelphia
2. Wilson CB (1988) Antibody reactions with native or planted glomerular antigens producing nephritogenic immune deposits or selective glomerular cell injury. IN: Wilson CB (guest ed) Contemporary issues in nephrology, vol 18. Churchill-Livingstone, New York, pp 1–34
3. Yamamoto T, Wilson CB (1987) Complement dependence of antibody-induced mesangial cell injury in the rat. J Immunol 138:3758–3765
4. Yamamoto T, Wilson CB (187) Quantitative and qualitative studies of antibody-induced mesangial cell damage in the rat. Kidney Int 32:514–525
5. Bolton WK, Tucker FL, Sturgill BC (1984) New avian model of experimental glomerulonephritis consistent with mediation by cellular immunity. Nonhumorally mediated glomerulonephritis in chickens. J Clin Invest 73:1263–1276

6. Rennke HG, Klein PS, Mendrick DL (1990) Cell-mediated immunity (CMI) in hapten-induced interstitial nephritis and glomerular crescent formation in the rat (abstract). Kidney Int 37:428
7. Kerjaschki D, Farquhar MG (1982) Identification of membrane glycoprotein from kidney brush border as the pathogenic antigen of Heymann's nephritis. Proc Natl Acad Sci USA 79:5557–5561
8. Ronco P, Neale TJ, Wilson CB, Galceran M, Verroust P (1986) An immunopathologic study of a 330-kD protein defined by monoclonal antibodies and reactive with anti-RTE-alpha-5 antibodies and kidney eluates from active Heymann nephritis. J Immunol 136:125–130
9. Raychowdhury R, Niles JL, McCluskey RT, Smith JA (1989) Autoimmune target in Heymann nephritis is a glycoprotein with homology to the LDL receptor. Science 244:1163–1165
10. Kanalas JJ, Makker SP (1988) A possible ligand of serum origin for the kidney autoantigen of Heymann nephritis. J Immunol 141:4152–4157
11. Salant DJ, Belok S, Madaio MP, Couser WG (1980) A new role for complement in experimental membranous nephropathy in rats. J Clin Invest 66:1339–1350
12. Cybulsky AV, Rennke HG, Feintzeig ID, Salant DJ (1986) Complement-induced glomerular epithelial cell injury. Role of the membrane attack complex in rat membranous nephropathy. J Clin Invest 77:1096–1107
13. Andres G, Brentjens JR, Caldwell PRB, Camussi G, Matsuo S (1986) Formation of immune deposits and disease. Lab Invest 55:510–520
14. Kerjaschki D, Miettnen A, Farquhar MG (1987) Initial events in the formation of immune deposits in passive Heymann nephritis. J Exp Med 166:109–128
15. Mendrick DL, Rennke HG (1988) Epitope specific induction of proteinuria by monoclonal antibodies. Kidney Int 33:831–842
16. Quigg RJ, Abrahamson DR, Cybulsky AV, Badalamenti J, Minto AWM, Salant DJ (1989) Studies with antibodies to cultured rat glomerular epithelial cells. Subepithelial immune deposit formation after in vivo injection. Am J Pathol 134:1125–1133
17. Verroust PF (1989) Kinetics of immune deposits in membranous nephropathy. Kidney Int 35:1418–1428
18. Fukatsu A, Yuzawa Y, Olson L, Miller J, Milgrom M, Zamlauski-Tucker, Van Liew JB, Campagnari A, Niesen N, Patel J, Doi T, Striker L, Striker G, Milgrom F, Brentjens J, Andres G (1989) Interaction of antibodies with human glomerular epithelial cells. Lab Invest 61:389–403
19. Makker SP, Kanalas JJ (1989) Autoantibodies to human gp330 in sera of patients with idiopathic membranous nephropathy. Kidney Int 35:211
20. Neale TJ, Woodroffe AJ, Wilson CB (1984) Spontaneous glomerulonephritis in rabbits: Role of a glomerular capillary antigen. Kidney Int 26:701–711
21. Wilson CB (1989) Study of the immunopathogenesis of tubulointerstitial nephritis using model systems. Kidney Int 35:938–953
22. Wilson CB, Lehman DH, McCoy RC, Gunnells JC Jr, Stickel DL (1974) Antitubular basement membrane antibodies after renal transplantation. Transplantation 18:447–452
23. Border WA, Lehman DH, Egan JD, Sass HJ, Glode JE, Wilson CB (1974) Antitubular basement-membrane antibodies in methicillin-associated interstitial nephritis. N Engl J Med 291:381–384
24. Ueda S, Wakashin M, Wakashin Y, Yoshida H, Iesato K, Mori T, Mori Y, Akikusa B, Okuda K (1986) Experimental gold nephropathy in guinea pigs: Detection of autoantibodies to renal tubular antigens. Kidney Int 29:539–548
25. Guery C-J, Hedrich HJ, Mercier P, Reetz IC, Mandet C, Mahieu P, Neilson EG, Druet P (1989) Mapping of a gene for the M_r 48000 tubular basement membrane antigen in the rat. Immunogenetics 29:350–354

26. Bannister KM, Wilson, CB (1985) Transfer of tubulointerstitial nephritis in the Brown Norway rat with anti-tubular basement membrane antibody: Quantitation and kinetics of binding and effect of decomplementation. J Immunol 135:3911–3917
27. Wilson CB (to be published) Nephritogenic tubulointerstitial antigens. Kidney Int
28. Neilson EG, Sun MJ, Emergy J, Kelly CJ, Haverty T, Clayman M, Cooke NE (1989) Molecular cloning of the 3M-1 nephritogenic antigen (abstract). Kidney Int 35:358
29. Noble B, Mendrick DL, Brentjens Jr, Andres GA (1981) Antibody-mediated injury to proximal tubules in the rat kidney induced by passive transfer of homologous anti-brush border serum. Clin Immunol Immunopathol 19:289–301
30. Brodkin M, Noble B (1988) Antibody-mediated proliferation of proximal tubule cells requires cross-linking of antigenic determinants. Clin Exp Immunol 72:315–320
31. Ishidate T, Hoyer JR, Seiler MW (1983) Influence of altered glomerular permeability on renal tubular immune complex formation and clearance. Lab Invest 49:582–588
32. Fukatsu A, Yuzawa Y, Niesen N, Matsuo S, Caldwell PRB, Brentjens JR, Andres G (1988) Local formation of immune deposits in rabbit renal proximal tubules. Kidney Int 34:611–619
33. Neilson EG, Phillips SM (1982) Murine interstitial nephritis. I. Analysis of disease susceptibility and its relationship to pleiomorphic gene products defining both immune-response genes and a restrictive requirement for cytotoxic T cells at H-2K. J Exp Med 155: 1075–1085
34. Zakheim B, McCafferty E, Phillips SM, Clayman M, Neilson EG (1984) Murine interstitial nephritis II. The adoptive transfer of disease with immune T lymphocytes produces a phenotypically complex interstitial lesion. J Immunol 133:234–239
35. Mann R, Kelly CJ, Hines WH, Clayman MD, Blanchard N, Sun MJ, Neilson EG (1987) Effector T cell differentiation in experimental interstitial nephritis. I. The development and modulation of effector lymphocyte maturation by I-J$^+$ regulatory T cells. J Immunol 138:4200–4208
36. Kelly CJ, MoK H, Neilson EG (1988) The selection of effector T cell phenotype by contrasuppression modulates susceptibility to autoimmune injury. J Immunol 141:3022–3028
37. Haverty TP, Kelly CJ, Hines WH, Amenta PS, Wattanabe M, Harper RA, Kefalides NA, Neilson, EG (1988) Characterization of a renal tubular epithelial cell line which secretes the autologous target antigen of autoimmune experimental interstitial nephritis. J Cell Biol 107:1359–1368
38. Haverty TP, Wattanabe M, Neilson EG, Kelly CJ (1989) Protective modulation of class II MHC gene expression in tubular epithelium by target antigen-specific antibodies. Cell-surface directed down-regulation of transcription can influence susceptibility to murine tubulointerstitial nephritis. J Immunol 143:1133–1141
39. Wuthrich RP, Yui MA, Mazoujian G, Nabavi N, Glimcher LH, Kelley VE (1989) Enhanced MHC class II expression in renal proximal tubules precedes loss of renal function in MRL/1pr mice with lupus nephritis. Am J Pathol 134:45–51
40. Neilson EG, McCafferty E, Mann R, Michaud L, Clayman M (1985) Tubular antigen-derivatized cells induce a disease-protective, antigen-specific, and idiotype-specific suppressor T cell network restricted by I-J and Igh-V in mice with experimental interstitial nephritis. J Exp Med 162:215–230
41. Mann R, Neilson EG (1986) Murine interstitial nephritis. V. The auto-induction of antigen-specific Lyt2$^+$ suppressor T cells diminishes the expression of interstitial nephritis in mice with antitubular basement membrane disease. J Immunol 136:908–912
42. Neilson EG, Kelly CJ, Clayman MD, Hines WH, Haverty T, Sun MJ, Blanchard N (1987) Murine interstitial nephritis. VII. Suppression of renal injury after treatment with soluble suppressor factor TsF^1_1. J Immunol 139:1518–1524
43. Bannister KM, Ulich TR, Wilson CB (1987) Induction, characterization, and cell transfer of autoimmune tubulointerstitial nephritis in the Lewis rat. Kidney Int 32:642–651

44. Kelly CJ, Neilson EG (1987) Contrasuppression in autoimmunity. Abnormal contrasuppression facilitates expression of nephritogenic effector T cells and interstitial nephritis in kdkd mice. J Exp Med 165:107–123
45. Queluz TH, Pawlowski I, Brunda MJ, Brentjens JR, Vladutiu AO, Andres G (1990) Pathogenesis of an experimental model of Goodpasture's hemorrhagic pneumonitis. J Clin Invest 85:1507–1515
46. Leung DYM, Geha RS, Newburger JW, et al. (1986) Two monokines, interleukin 1 and tumor necrosis factor, render cultured vascular endothelial cells susceptible to lysis by antibodies circulating during Kawasaki syndrome. J Exp Med 164:1958–1972
47. Leung Dym, Collins T, Lapierre LA, et al. (1986) Immunoglobulin M antibodies present in the acute phase of Kawasaki syndrome lyse cultured vascular endothelial cells stimulated by gamma interferon. J Clin Invest 77:1428–1435
48. Leung DYM, Moake JL, Havens PL, et al. (1988) Lytic anti-endothelial cell antibodies in haemolytic-uraemic syndrome. Lancet II:183–186
49. Cotran RS, Pober JS (1989) Effects of cytokines on vascular endothelium: Their role in vascular and immune injury. Kidney Int 35:969–975
50. Arnaout MA (1990) Structure and function of the leukocyte adhesion molecules CD11/CD18. Blood 75:1037–1050
51. Falk RJ, Jennette JC (1988) Anti-neutrophil cytoplasmic autoantibodies with specificity for myeloperoxidase in patients with systemic vasculitis and idiopathic necrotizing and crescentic glomerulonephritis. N Engl J Med 318:1651–1657
52. Cohen Tervaert JW, Goldschmeding R, Elema JD, et al. (1990) Autoantibodies against myeloid lysosomal enzymes in crescentic glomerulonephritis. Kidney Int 37:799–806
53. Falk RJ, Terrell RS, Charles LA, Jennette JC (1990) Anti-neutrophil cytoplasmic autoantibodies induce neutrophils to degranulate and produce oxygen radicals in vitro. Proc Natl Acad Sci USA 87:4115–4119
54. Hynes RO (1986) Fibronectins. Sci Am 254:42–51
55. Stein CA, Cohen JS (1988) Oligodeoxynucleotides as inhibitors of gene expression: a review. Cancer Res 48:2659–2668
56. Urban JL, Kumar VK, Kono DH, Gomez C, Horvath SJ, Clayton J, Ando DG, Sercarz EE, Hood L (1988) Restricted use of T cell receptor V genes in murine autoimmune encephalomyelitis raises possibility of antibody therapy. Cell 54:577–592
57. Acha-Orbea H, Mitchell DJ, Timmermann L, Wraith DC, Tausch GS, Waldor MK, Zamvil SS, McDevitt HO, Steinman L (1988) Limited heterogeneity of T cell receptors from lymphocytes mediating autoimmune encephalomyelitis allows specific immune intervention. Cell 54:263–273
58. Zaller DM, Osman G, Kanagawa O, Hood L (1990) Prevention and treatment of murine experimental allergic encephalomyelitis with T cell receptor Vbeta-specific antibodies. J Exp Med 1943–1955
59. Duchosal MA, McConahey PJ, Robinson CA, Dixon RJ (to be published) Transfer of human systemic lupus erythematosus in SCID mice. J Exp Med
60. Suematsu S, Matsuda T, Aozasa K, Akira S, Nakano N, Ohno S, Miyazaki J, Yamamura K, Hirano T, Kishimoto T (1989) IgG1 plasmacytosis in interleukin 6 transgenic mice. Proc Natl Acad Sci USA 86:7547–7551
61. Doi T, Striker LJ, Quaife C, Conti FG, Palmiter R, Behringer R, Brinster R, Striker GE (1988) Progressive glomerulosclerosis develops in transgenic mice chronically expressing growth hormone and growth hormone releasing factor but not in those expressing insulin-like growth factor-1. Am J Pathol 131:398–403
62. Quaife CJ, Mathews LS, Pinkert CA, Hammer RE, Brinster RL, Palmiter RD (1989) Histopathology associated with elevated levels of growth hormone and insulin-like growth factor I in transgenic mice. Endocrinology 124:40–48

63. Zijlstra M, Li E, Sajjadi F, Subramani S, Jaenisch R (1989) Germ-line transmission of a disrupted beta$_2$-microglobulin gene produced by homologous recombination in embryonic stem cells. Nature 342:435–438
64. Yamamoto T, Mundy C, Wilson CB, Blantz RC (1988) Antibody induced mesangial cell (MC) lysis and proliferation: Glomerular hemodynamic consequences (abstract). Kidney Int 33:327

Nephrolithiasis: New Ideas in Pathophysiology, New Facts in Therapy

Chair: Philippe Jaeger (Switzerland)
Kenkichi Koiso (Japan)

Idiopathic Hypercalciuria: Proposal for a New Cascade

Pierre Bataille, Albert Fournier, Bernard Boudailliez, Pierre François Westeel, Najeh El Esper, Jean Michel Achard[1], Catherine Bergot[2], and Roger Bouillon[3]

SUMMARY. Idiopathic hypercalciuria (IH) is defined by a 24 hour urinary excretion of calcium greater than 4 mg or 0.1 mmol/kg of body weight on a calcium diet of 1 g and greater than 3 mg or 0.07 mmol/kg on a Ca diet of 400 mg, while there is no excess of sodium (120–180 mmol) nor of protein (1–1.3 g/kg per day). IH with fasting hypercalciuria but without secondary hyperparathyroidism represents in our experiece the most prevalent subtype of IH. Since bone mineral density has been shown to be decreased in this undetermined subtype (Pak's classification), as in patients with absorptive hypercalciuria type I or with renal hypercalciuria, the clinical relevance of this classification is questioned. A primary bone hyperresorption seems to be the main explanation of IH, since in this group as a whole, fasting hypercalciuria is correlated positively with fasting hydroxyprolinuria which is higher than in controls. This bone resorption may be favored by protein intake of non-dairy origin due to a higher meat intake and hypersensitivity of bone resorption to meat intake, as evidenced by a higher daily urinary excretion of urea on a diet without dairy products and a steeper slope of the regression of fasting calciuria versus 24 hour urea excretion. Furthermore, calcitriol synthesis is increased, probably because of a hypersensitivity of 25 OH vitamin D 1α hydroxylase to phosphate, as evidenced by the fact that plasma calcitriol correlates negatively with plasma phosphate which, however, remains in the normal range. High plasma calcitriol is not responsible for the bone hyperresorption, since it correlates negatively with fasting hypercalciuria and positively with bone density and postprandial calciuria (an index of calcium absorption).

Since Pacifici has recently shown that Ca stone formers with fasting hypercalciuria have an increased synthesis of interleukin I by their peripheral monocytes, and that interleukin I may stimulate prostaglandin E2, which can be responsible for both bone resorption and increased activity of the 25 OH vitamin D 1α hydroxylase, a new cascade of pathophysiological events originating from a monocyte disease has been

[1]Hôpital Sud, Service de Néphrologie du CHRU d'Amiens, 80054 Amiens Cédex, France
[2]Service de Radiologie de l'Hôpital St. Louis, Paris, France
[3]Laboratoire d'Endocrinologie, Université de Leuven, Leuven, Belgium

presented. The therapeutic consequences of these new pathophysiological insights are: 1/ dietary restriction in protein of non dairy origin, so that the calcium intake remains around 1000 mg to prevent worsening of bone loss; 2/ thiazide therapy which decreases calciuria not only by a direct tubular effect, but also by a decrease of prostaglandin E2 synthesis.

Introduction

Hypercalciuria is found in about one-half of patients with idiopathic calcium lithiasis, i.e., Ca lithiasis not explained by a well individualized disease which is responsible either for secondary hypercalciuria, such as primary hyperparathyroidism, sarcoidosis, distal tubular acidosis, neoplasia, hyperthyroidism, Cushing's syndrome, vitamin D intoxication and milk alkali syndrome, or for frank hyperoxaluria (primary or enteric hyperoxaluria). Hypercalciuria is therefore the most frequent risk factor of idiopathic Ca lithiasis. Despite recent advances in the knowledge of its pathogenesis, hypercalciuria is still a controversial subject for many reasons: 1/ the statistical difficulty of assigning an upper limit of calcium excretion in a normal population; 2/ the role of dietary factors other than calcium intake; and 3/ the interrelation of many metabolic abnormalities.

In this paper, we shall consider successively the definition of hypercalciuria, the dietary factors influencing calcium excretion, the classical types and subtypes of idiopathic hypercalciuria as proposed by Pak, the evidence for disordered calcitriol synthesis, the evidence for bone involvement, and data suggesting a primary monocyte disorder which could be an overall explanation for the spectrum of this so called idiopathic hypercalciuria.

Definition of Hypercalciuria and its Relation with Dietary Factors Influencing Calcium Excretion

Because of an upward skew of calciuria values in a normal population on a free diet, it is preferable to take as the upper limit of normal not the sum of the mean plus 2 standard deviations, but the limit below which is found the calciuria of 90% of the population [1]. There is a considerable overlap between calciuria histograms of controls and stone-formers, the latter being shifted upwards by 75 mg/day [2,3].

Calciuria is an extremely variable parameter, which depends on a constitutional parameter such as weight and dietary parameters: intakes not only of calcium, but also of protein, phosphate, sodium, and carbohydrate.

The expression of calciuria adjusted to the creatinine excretion or, as is more usually done, to the body weight, makes unnecessary the use of the term "*constitutional hypercalciuria*" proposed by Broadus [4] to describe high values of calciuria in relation only to larger patient size, and not to specific metabolic abnormalities.

Increasing calcium intake from 400 mg/day to 1000 mg/day induces an increase of calciuria both in normal controls and in Ca stone formers, but this increase is much greater in the latter (120 mg/24h) than in the normals (40 mg/24h) [5]. In evaluating calciuria, it is thus necessary to have data for calciuria measured in controls who are on the same known dietary intake of calcium as the Ca stone formers.

Dietary protein intake is likewise an important determinant of urinary calcium. In a normal subject, calcium excretion doubles as daily protein intake increases from 0.5 g/kg of body weight to 2g/kg. As a matter of fact, daily urea excretion, which is an index of protein intake, is positively correlated with calciuria [6]. The mechanism of the dependency of calcium excretion upon protein intake is not clear. Initially it was thought to be linked to an increased fixed acid production producing mild metabolic acidosis, which would increase calcium excretion by inhibition of tubular calcium reabsorption and by stimulation of bone resorption related to skeletal buffering of retained acids [5]. Actually the decreased tubular calcium reabsorption seems rather to be linked to the increase of urinary sulfate concentration observed after protein loads rich in methionine. Sulfate is a poorly reabsorbed anion which is available for complexing urinary calcium; this thus limits its tubular reabsorption [7]. Indeed, this explains the fact that prevention of metabolic acidosis does not correct the protein-induced hypercalciuria [7]. Whatever the actual mechanism of protein-induced hypercalciuria, high dietary protein intake induces a negative calcium balance which favors bone loss [8,9].

Dietary phosphate intake variation in the usual range, from 600 to 1500 mg/day, does not significantly influence calciuria. However, extreme phosphate restriction (<300 mg of phosphate/day) is accompanied by hypercalciuria which is responsible for a negative calcium balance, in spite of a fall in parathyroid hormone (PTH) secretion [7].

Infusion of sodium chloride or increasing dietary sodium intake increases urinary calcium. In controls, urinary calcium increases by about 25 mg per 100 mEq of additional dietary sodium chloride and a strong relationship is observed between daily urinary sodium and urinary calcium excretions [10,11]. The sodium load depresses both proximal and distal tubular calcium reabsorption. After 28 days, sodium-induced hypercalciuria is, however, no longer observed in normal subjects [12]. In calcium stone formers the dependence of calcium excretion upon sodium intake exists on a short term basis (1 week) [13] and persists after 2 months [14]. The influence of sodium intake on calciuria is so strong in Ca stone formers that it influences even fasting calciuria, so that high Na intake may be responsible for factitious renal hypercalciuria (see Pak's classification) [13].

Refined carbohydrates increase calcium excretion by inducing hyperinsulinism, which enhances tubular sodium reabsorption and decreases tubular calcium reabsorption [15,16]. Alcohol also seems to favor hypercalciuria probably by way of an identical mechanism. The clinical importance of alcohol and carbohydrate excess remains unclear for the moment.

The importance of dietary factors is all the more great in that *the hypercalciuric effect of protein and sodium is more pronounced in Ca stone-formers than in normal subjects.* The slopes of the relationship between calcium and sodium or urea excretion are, respectively, 3 times [13] and 5 times [6,17] greater in stone-formers.

Thus, in order to appropriately evaluate calcium excretion, results must be weight or creatinine adjusted and interpreted in relation to calcium, sodium, protein, and, possibly, carbohydrate intakes. According to our own data [17] and those in the literature, *we propose the following values as upper limits of normal for calciuria according to diet:*

1) 4 mg or 0.1 mmol/kg per day on a diet providing 1 g calcium, 130 mmol of sodium, and 1–1.3 g/kg of protein daily;

2) 3 mg or 0.07 mmol/kg per day after 4 days of low calcium intake (excluding all dairy products ≈ 400 mg calcium daily) and 115 mmol of sodium and 1–1.3 g/kg of protein daily.

In clinical practice it is, however, important to first evaluate the patient, as an outpatient, on his or her usual diet, i.e., the diet followed spontaneously before any dietary advice, for at least 2 days (because of the variability of calciuria). Then, to properly classify the calciuria, it is important to measure it again, in 24 hour urine, for at least 4 days while the patient is on a known calcium intake. We recommend evaluating the patients on both 1000 mg and 400 mg calcium diets. As a matter of fact, a 1000 mg calcium diet is now the diet recommended for calcium stone formers in order to prevent bone loss (see below) and marginal hyperoxaluria induced by calcium restriction [17]; a 400 mg calcium diet is the diet recommended so that fasting calciuria according to Pak [18] can be appropriately evaluated.

Calciuria exceeding the upper limit of normal on 400 and 1000 mg Ca diets while sodium, protein, and carbohydrate intakes are concomitantly controlled defines true idiopathic hypercalciuria, once well defined diseases responsible for secondary hypercalciuria have been eliminated (see introduction). It must be pointed out that in most previous reports in the literature, authors have classified patients as having idiopathic hypercalciuria, without taking into account sodium, protein, and carbohydrate intakes. Thus, dietary hypercalciuria, an expression which was formerly used to designate only hypercalciuria related to gluttony for calcium-rich food, may now also be applied to hypercalciuria related to gluttony for salt-, protein-, and carbohydrate-rich food, although these types of hypercalciuria were formerly classified as idiopathic hypercalciuria.

Classification of Idiopathic Hypercalciuria (IH) According to Pak

Some years ago, Pak proposed to classify IH into two main types, namely absorptive hypercalciuria (AH), and renal hypercalciuria (RH) [18].

In AH, he further distinguished 3 subtypes (Table I): *type II*, actually a dietary hypercalciuria related to an excess calcium intake; *type I*, due to a primary selective jejunal hyperabsorption of calcium, since the calcitriol levels are normal or low [19]; and *type III*, in which the hyperabsorption of calcium is linked to an increased synthesis of calcitriol, secondary to a hypophosphoremia induced by a primary tubular leak of phosphate. This phosphate leak hypothesis is supported by several pieces of evidence: (*1*) the high prevalence of hypophosphatemia and decreased Tm P/GFR in patients with IH [2,4,7]; (*2*) the increased levels of circulating calcitriol in response to hypophosphatemia observed in normal subjects [20] and the partial reversal of the syndrome in patients after treatment with oral phosphate [21,22]; (*3*) the inverse relationship between plasma calcitriol level and phosphate concentration [23,24]; and (*4*) the recently described syndrome of IH with renal phosphate leak and increased plasma calcitriol occurring in a Bedouin tribe, some of whose members presented with hereditary hypophosphatemic rickets along with hypercalciuria [25].

Renal hypercalciuria (RH) is differentiated from AH mainly on the basis of fasting hypercalciuria (fasting UCa/UCr > 0.12 mg/mg or > 0.33 mmol/mmol) and of secondary hyperparathyroidism. As a matter of fact it is thought to be due to a primary renal leak of calcium which would promote negative calcium balance which would

Table 1. Possible primary mechanisms of hypercalciuria and their pathophysiological consequences

	Primary mechanism		Excessive dietary intake of				Primary	Hypersecretion of calcitriol			Primary	
		Primary	Ca	Na	Protein	Sugar alcohol	intestinal Ca hyperabsorption	Renal PO4 leak	Renal Ca leak	Primary	bone resorption	Monocyte disease[e]
	Pak's classification[a]	hyperparathyroidism	AH II	–	–	–	AH I	AH III	RH	–	–	–
Pathophysiological consequences	24 hour calciuria on fixed Ca intake[b]	↗	N	↗	↗	↗	↗	↗	↗	↗	↗	↗
	Fasting calciuria[c]	↗	N	↗	↗	N	N	N	↗	?	↗	↗
	Δ UCa after 1 g of oral Ca[d]	↗	N	?	?	?	↗	↗	↗	↗	N	↗
	Fractional intestinal absorption of Ca	↗	N	?	?	?	↗	↗	↗	↗	N	↗
	Plasma calcium	↗	N	N	N	N	N	N	N	N	N	N
	Plasma phosphate	↘·N	N	N	N	N	N	↘	N	N	N	N
	PTH or nephrogenic cAMP											
	fasting	↗	N·↘	?	?	?	N·↘	N·↘	↗	N·↘	N·↘	N·↘
	after Ca load	↗	↘	?	?	?	N·↘	N·↘	N	N·↘	N·↘	N·↘
	Fasting plasma calcitriol	↗	↘·N	?	?	?	N	↗	↗	↗	N·↘	↗
	Hydroxyprolinuria	↗	N	?	↗	?	N	?	↗	?	↗	↗
	Bone density	↘	N	?	↘	?	N·↘·?	?	↘	?	↘	↘

[a]According to Pak: AHI - II - III, absorptive hypercalciuria type I - II - III; RH, renal calciuria
[b]Upper limit of normal per kg BW/day is 4 mg or 0.1 mmol on 1000 mg of Ca, and 3 mg or 0.07 mmol on 400 mg of Ca
[c]Upper limit of normal of fasting hypercalciuria is <0.12 mg/mg creatinine or 0.33 mmol/mmol creatinine
[d]The upper limit of normal increase of calciuria after 1 g of oral calcium is <0.17 mg/mg creatinine or 0.50 mmol/mmol
[e]Monocyte disease responsible for hypersecretion of interleukin I, hypersecretion of calcitriol and bone resorption
N, normal; ↗, increased; ↘, decreased, ?, uncertain or unknown; PTH, parathyroid hormone

therefore stimulate, primarily PTH secretion and secondarily, calcitriol synthesis and increase intestinal absorption of calcium. This secondary hyperparathyroidism is, however, suppressed by an oral calcium load [24], as shown by the normalization of plasma PTH or nephrogenic cAMP in the urine.

However, this clear-cut classification has been challenged for various reasons:

1) the classification does not take into account the dependence of IH on dietary factors other than calcium intake [6];
2) the overprevalence of AH I in Pak's experience (60%) is in blatant contradiction with the calcium balance data which show a negative balance in two-thirds of patients [2,26] (the average calcium balance for the hypercalciuric stone former is -1.0 ± 2.7 mmol/day, whereas it is $+0.7\pm2.4$ mmol/day in healthy controls [2]);
3) primary disorders of intestinal calcium absorption and tubular reabsorption of calcium or phosphate appear to be variously associated in the same patients, making their classification within distinct pathogenetic subtypes not always possible [4,26,27];
4) Pak's classification is not able to classify all patients, namely those with fasting hypercalciuria not related to a high sodium diet: most of these patients, in fact, do not have high plasma concentrations of PTH, but on the contrary, have normal or low PTH levels, excluding the hypothesis of renal hypercalciuria [24,28]. In patients with fasting hypercalciuria not associated with secondary hyperparathyroidism a subtle renal leak of calcium may, however, be suspected. In patients with fasting hypercalciuria, a proximal tubular defect has been demonstrated by successive acute administration of diuretics [27]. These subtle renal disorders could explain the hypersensitivity to sodium, acidosis, or high protein diet in IH patients, discussed previously (Fig. 1).

Increased Calcitriol Production

Plasma calcitriol concentration is extremely sensitive to variations in calcium intake in normal controls as well as in patients with IH. Most of the studies which have taken calcium diet into account have shown increased levels of plasma calcitriol in calcium stone-formers with IH and normal PTH levels [7]. Direct evidence for a disordered control of calcitriol production has been clearly demonstrated by Broadus in patients with AH. In these patients, when a high normal calcium diet is continued for several weeks, calcitriol plasma levels initially decrease, but after 2 weeks an escape phenomenon with a rebound increase in circulating calcitriol level and a pronounced fall in T mP/GFR [29] is observed.

The mechanism accounting for this increased calcitriol synthesis remains controversial. As discussed above, several pieces of evidence favor a tubular phosphate leak. However, the frequency of hypophosphatemia in IH is controversial, probably because of a lack of data regarding diurnal variations in serum phosphate; this impedes detection of subtle hypophosphatemia. For instance, in normal man, a decrease of dietary phosphorus which induces a 35% decrease of afternoon serum phosphate, induces a 58% increase in fasting serum levels of calcitriol, while no change is observed in the morning fasting levels of phosphorus [30]. In patients with IH, we observed a negative correlation between plasma calcitriol and plasma phos-

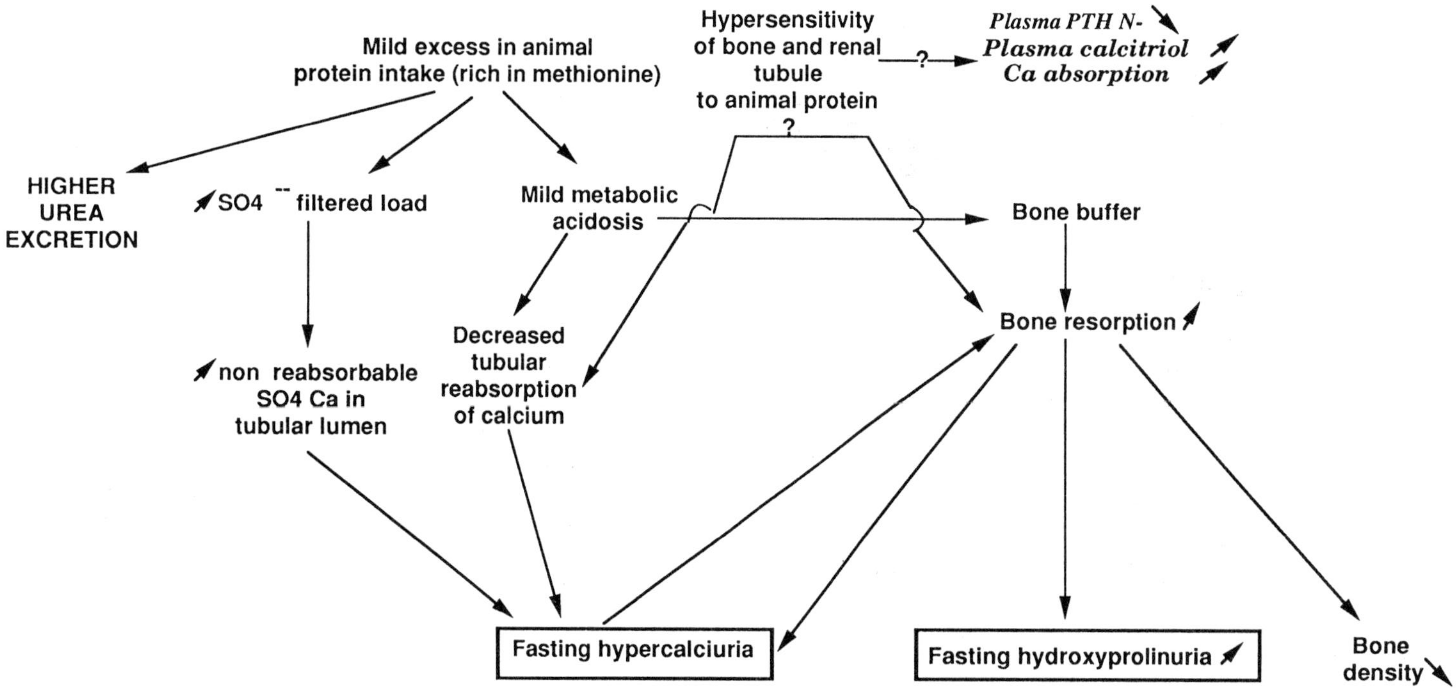

Fig. 1. This figure is an attempt to put into perspective the pathophysiological events derived from the exaggerated protein-induced hypercalciuria observed in calcium stone formers with idiopathic hypercalciuria (*IH*). Mild excess in meat intake and hypersensitivity of the renal tubule and skeleton to mild acidosis secondary to the protein-induced production of acids (especially H_2SO_4 derived from methionine) may explain the fasting hypercalciuria. The fasting hyperhydroxyprolinuria is an index of increased bone resorption, which may be secondary to the primary renal calcium leak because of sulfate overproduction and mild acidosis and the consumption of bone buffer because of the mild acidosis. This scheme does not account for the fact that in IH, parathyroid hormone (*PTH*) levels are normal or low while plasma calcitriol levels and intestinal absorption of calcium are increased. ☐ Parameter correlating positively with 24 hour UREA EXCRETION on Ca restricted diet

phate which, however, remained in the normal range [17]. On the basis of this negative correlation, we suggest that the increased synthesis of calcitriol in IH may be due to a hypersensitivity of 25 OH vitamin D 1α hydroxylase to phosphate.

An alternative hypothesis which would explain this disordered control of calcitriol and the tendency to hypophosphatemia would be hypersensitivity of 25 OH vitamin D 1α hydroxylase to PTH. This possibility remains dubious because no correlation exists between PTH and calcitriol and because PTH levels are normal or low in most patients with fasting hypercalciuria.

Finally, as will be discussed below, another explanation for increased calcitriol synthesis could be a monocyte disease.

Bone Involvement in Idiopathic Hypercalciuria

While overt bone disease with pain and fractures is extremely rare in hypercalciuric patients, the frequently observed mild negative calcium balance suggests that bone may be the primary source of the extra calcium appearing in the urine. This possibility is supported by the positive relationships observed between fasting calcium and hydroxyprolinuria [17,31,32] or fasting calciuria and alkaline phosphatases [31], and by radiocalcium kinetic data showing increased bone turnover [33].

Indeed, loss of bone mass has been detected by various techniques in calcium stone formers with hypercalciuria: photonabsorptiometry of the distal radius [34] or the lumbar spine [35], radiological density of the proximal radial shaft [36], in vivo neutron activation of the trunk and upper thighs [37], and single energy computerized tomography (CT) densitometry of the vertebrae [17,38].

In most of these studies the type of hypercalciuria was not clearly defined. In Lawoyin's study [39] this was done and decreased bone mineral content of the radius was observed only in renal hypercalciuria patients, but not in absorptive hypercalciuria patients. In the study of Pacifici et al. [38] vertebral mineral density was decreased in all calcium stone formers, whether with normocalciuria, absorptive hypercalciuria, or fasting hypercalciuria with normal PTH, but the decrease was greater in the last-mentioned group. In our experience [17] vertebral mineral density was decreased comparably in fasting hypercalciuria with normal PTH, in one case of renal hypercalciuria, and in absorptive calciuria type I, but not in absorptive calciuria type II.

Moreover, scarce histomorphometric evaluations have shown bone abnormalities, such as increased bone resorption with normal bone formation [40] and normal bone resorption with decreased bone formation and mineralization rate [41]. The recent study of 33 patients with recurrent stone formation and idiopathic hypercalciuria with hypophosphatemia and normal PTH carried out by Steiniche et al. [42] confirms the existence of a moderate mineralization defect (reduced adjusted appositional rate, prolonged mineralization lag time), with increased eroded surfaces but without decrease of the trabecular bone volume.

What is the origin of this increased bone loss? In most of these patients mild hyperparathyroidism is excluded by normal or low values of plasma PTH. A bone resorbing effect of calcitriol has been suspected according to the following observations: (1) in normal subjects put on a low calcium diet fasting calciuria is increased by oral calcitriol elevating serum 1,25 (OH)2 D3 concentration [43]; (2) in organ cultures of bone, 1,25 (OH)2 D3 has a bone resorbing effect [44]. Therefore, in IH patients put on a low calcium diet, a high level of calcitriol could lead to bone loss in spite of a normal PTH level. However, this is probably not the case, at least in our experience: after 4 days of low calcium diet, plasma calcitriol was, on the contrary, negatively correlated with fasting calciuria and was positively correlated with vertebral mineral density and with calcium absorption (as assessed by calciuria increase after oral calcium load). These data suggest that a high level of calcitriol has a protective effect which is mediated by increased intestinal calcium absorption [17].

Nutritional factors also have to be considered. A dietary restriction of calcium, as treatment for hypercalciuric patients, may worsen the bone problem. Sequential measurements of bone density have shown that patients chronically submitted to a low calcium diet increase their bone loss [36,45].

A high protein intake has also been shown to favor osteoporosis [46]. Urea excretion on a low calcium diet was significantly higher in our IH patients than in the controls, suggesting that their protein intake of non dairy origin (i.e., meat) was greater than that of the controls. Furthermore, plasma bicarbonates were lower than in controls and the correlation between fasting calciuria and 24 hour urea excretion of the previous day was much steeper in this group of patients than in controls. The urea excretion of the IH patients was also correlated with fasting hydroxyprolinuria [17]. These data support the hypothesis that in our patients with IH, higher protein intake could favor bone loss by inducing mild acidosis (Fig. 1). In Ca stone formers, Fellström [47] has demonstrated that a short term animal protein intake simultaneously increases calciuria and hydroxyprolinuria.

Thus, such nutritional factors as low calcium diet and high meat intake may favor bone loss in IH. However, they do not account for all the observed metabolic abnormalities, especially the high plasma calcitriol levels along with normal-low PTH levels and increased calcium absorption. This leads to a search for a broader disorder which could encompass all these various data. Such a disorder could be an immunological disorder involving the monocyte. This could be proposed as a global explanation depending on a new cascade of mechanisms which we now wish to discuss.

Idiopathic Hypercalciuria as a Monocyte Disease

Some recent data favor an immunological involvement in bone resorption. Pacifici et al. [38] have recently described an increased production of interleukin I. The interleukin I is produced by peripheral blood monocytes in association with increased hydroxyproline excretion and decreased vertebral mineral density. Interleukin I activity was related positively to hydroxyprolinuria and negatively to vertebral mineral density, suggesting that interleukin I may induce bone resorption. This bone resorbing effect might either be direct or be mediated by prostaglandins, well known bone resorbing agents, which have been shown to be stimulated by interleukin I [48]. In patients with fasting hypercalciuria, the administration of a powerful prostaglandin synthesis inhibitor, with (diclofenac) or without (sulindac) effect on the renal cyclooxygenase system, decreases calcium excretion with a rise in PTH levels [48]. These results suggest that in fasting IH, the hypercalciuria is secondary to a prostaglandin mediated bone resorption which suppresses PTH secretion. This interpretation of the results excludes the alternative explanation for the association of increased interleukin I production by monocyte and increased bone resorption,

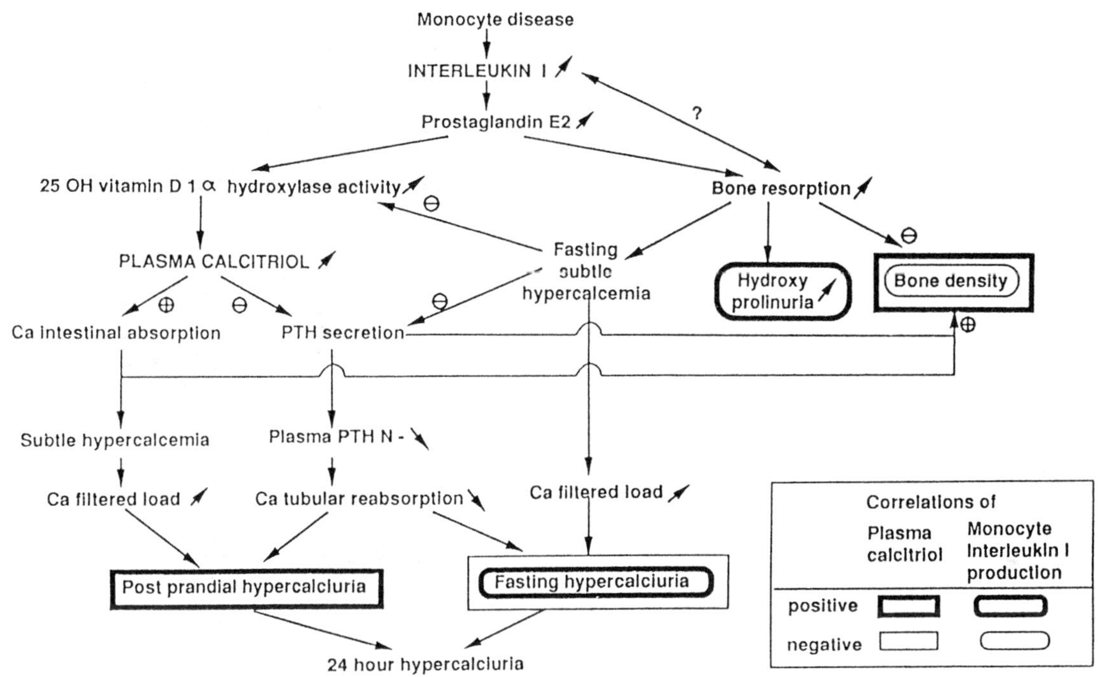

Fig. 2. A monocyte disease leading to increased production of interleukin I favors bone resorption directly or by stimulating prostaglandin E2 synthesis. Increased bone resorption explains fasting calciuria, fasting hyperhydroxyprolinuria, and decreased bone density. Therefore there are positive correlations of interleukin I production with fasting calciuria and hydroxyprolinuria, and a negative correlation between interleukin I production and bone density. The activity of 25 OH vitamin D 1α hydroxylase is increased because of increased production of prostaglandin E2. Resulting high plasma calcitriol levels explain calcium intestinal hyperabsorption and parathyroid hormone (*PTH*) suppression (together with the calcium coming from bone): these factors favor post prandial hypercalciuria (hence the positive correlation between plasma calcitriol and post prandial hypercalciuria).

The effect of calcitriol on calcium absorption and PTH secretion has a beneficial effect on bone density, thus explaining the positive correlation of plasma calcitriol and bone density

namely, that products such as TGFβ, coming from resorbing bones, stimulate the production of Interleukin I.

The disordered control of calcitriol synthesis found in IH may also be explained by the same immunological cascade (Fig. 2). In idiopathic hypercalciuria with normal vitamin D nutritional status, the disordered control of calcitriol synthesis is characterized by its dependence upon plasma 25 OH D, as is the case in vitamin D depleted patients [49]. In IH, an increase of plasma calcitriol induced by ultraviolet radiation is associated with increased plasma levels of calcitriol [50], whereas such a phenomenon is not observed in normal men [51] and plasma calcitriol is positively correlated to plasma calcidiol [17]. The nature and the site of this disturbed metabolism is unknown. A disordered monocyte, mimicking, for instance, what is observed in granulomatous disease such as sarcoidosis would be a possible explanation. As a matter of fact, a very high and positive correlation between plasma calcidiol and plasma calcitriol is observed in patients with hypercalcemic-sarcoidosis [52]. An abnormal monocyte,, producing interleukin I in excess, could induce increased calcitriol synthesis mediated by prostaglandins [53]. In IH, urinary prostaglandins have been shown to be increased [54,55].

Therefore an abnormality of the monocyte in calcium stone-formers provides a seductive explanation for an apparent primary bone disease and a disturbed 1,25 dihydroxyvitamin D metabolism. The cascade of events (Table I and Fig. 2) could be: increased interleukin I production by abnormal monocyte stimulates the synthesis of prostaglandins E2, which have been proven to stimulate the synthesis of prostaglandins E2, which have been proven to stimulate both bone resorption and calcitriol synthesis. Thus, the two apparently contradictory phenomena that we have found in our patients with IH, namely, increased bone resorption leading to reduction of bone density and the protective effect of high plasma calcitriol levels [17], could be explained by a monocyte disease recently discovered by Pacifici et al.

Therapeutic Implications

The observation of decreased bone mineral content in patients with idiopathic hypercalciuria and the two new cascades that we propose for explaining hypercalciuria, namely the protein cascade, and the monocyte cascade, suggest the following therapeutic conclusions:

1) Protein intake of non-dairy origin should be restricted, so that the total daily intake is of the order of 1 g/kg per day.
2) Dairy products should, however, not be restricted so that calcium intake will be 800–1000 mg/day in order to prevent bone loss worsening and to prevent the marginal hyperoxaluria of the Ca stone former. This hyperoxaluria increases when dietary calcium is decreased, leading to a lack of improvement in the probability index of stone formation in idiopathic hypercalciuria [56].
3) Thiazides appear to be an appropriate therapy for all types of idiopathic hypercalciuria, since we have found decreased vertebral mineral density in all subtypes [17]. As a matter of fact, thiazides have a hypocalciuric effect explained not only by a direct tubular effect, but also by the inhibition of prostaglandin E synthesis, this latter accounting for a decrease of 25 OH vitamin D 1α hydroxylase activity [57] and a decrease of prostaglandin mediated bone resorption [58].

Because thiazides have already been proven both to decrease the recurrence of Ca stones [2] and to decrease the risk of femoral neck fracture [59], they should be considered as the treatment of reference. Pending the results of ongoing trials, prostaglandin synthetase inhibitors which can reduce hypercalciuria and bone resorption cannot presently be recommended, especially considering their possible long term hazards on renal function.

References

1. Hodgkinson A, Pyrah LN (1958) The urinary excretion of calcium and inorganic phosphate in 344 patients with calcium stone of renal origin. Br J Surg 46:10–11
2. Lemann J (1980) Idiopathic hypercalciuria. In: Coe FL, Brenner BM, Stein IH (eds) Nephrolithiasis. Churchill Livingstone, New York, pp 86–115
3. Robertson WG, Peacock M, Marshall BW, et al. (1978) Risk factors in calcium stone disease of the urinary tract. Br J Urol 50:449–454
4. Broadus AE, Burdis WJ, Oren DA (1987) Concerning the pathogenesis of idiopathic hypercalciuria. In: Linari F, Marangella M (eds) The pathogenesis and treatment of nephrolithiasis. Contrib Nephrol 36:127–136
5. Lemann J, Adams NC, Gray BW (1979) Urinary calcium excretion in human beings. N Engl J Med 301:535–541
6. Goldfard S (1988) Dietary factors in the pathogenesis and prophylaxis of nephrolithiasis. Kidney Int 34:544–555
7. Lemann J, Worcester ER (1989) Nephrolithiasis. In: Massry S, Glassock R (eds) Textbook of nephrology. Williams and Wilkins, Baltimore, pp 920–941
8. Walker RM, Linkswiler HM (1972) Calcium retention in the adult human male as affected by protein intake. J Nutr 102:1297–1302
9. Aller LH, Oddoye EA, Margen S (1979) Protein induced hypercalciuria a longer term study. Am J Clin Nutr 32:741–749
10. Kleeman CR, Bohannan J, Bernstein D, Living S, Maxwell MH (1964) Effect of variations in sodium intake on calcium excretion in normal humans. Soc Exp Biol Med 115:29–32
11. McCarron DA, Rankin LI, Bennet WM (1981) Urinary calcium excretion at extremes of sodium intake in normal man. Am J Nephrol 1:84–90
12. Kirkendall WM, Connar WE, Abbou DF, Rastogi SP, Anderson TA, Fry M (1976) The effect of dietary sodium chloride on blood pressure, body fluids, electrolytes, renal function of normotensive man. J Lab Clin Med 87:418–434
13. Muldowney FP, Freaney B, Moloney MF (1982) Importance of dietary sodium in the hypercalciuric syndrome. Kidney Int 22:292–296
14. Bataille P, Fournier A, Locquet P, Idrissi A, Renaud H, Finet M, Leflon P, Rogez JC, Plaquet R (1987) Hydrochlorothiazide-amiloride association in calcium stone formers: increase of oxalate tolerance and critical role of calcium and sodium intake on their hypocalciuric effect. In: Puschett JB, Greenberg A (eds) Diuretic II: chemistry, pharmacology and clinical applications. Elsevier Science, pp 438–444
15. Lemann J (1985) Urinary calcium excretion and net acid excretion: effects of dietary protein, carbohydrate and calories. In: Schwille PO, Smith LH, Robertson WG, Finlayson B (eds) Urolithiasis and Related Clinical Research. Plenum, New York, pp 53–60
16. Ulmann A, Aubert J, Bourdeau A (1982) Effects of weight and glucose ingestion on urinary calcium and phosphate excretion: implications for urolithiasis. J Clin Endocrinol Metab 54:1063–1068
17. Bataille P, Fournier A, Bouillon R (to be published) Vertebral mineral density in hypercalciuric Ca stone formers. Its relation to calcium and protein intake and vitamin D

metabolism. Evidence for primary bone resorption in dietary calcium independent hypercalciuria favored by high protein intake of non dairy origin and suppressed by high plasma concentration of calcitriol. Kidney Int (submitted)
18. Pak CYC, Galosy RA (1979) Fasting urinary calcium and cyclic adenosine 3′, 5′ monophosphate: a discriminant analysis for the identification of renal absorptive hypercalciuria. J Clin Endocrinol Metab 48:260–265
19. Pak CYC, Britton F, Petterson R (1980) Ambulatory evaluation of nephrolithiasis. Am J Med 69:19–30
20. Gray BW, Wilz DR, Caldas AE (1977) The importance of phosphate in regulating plasma 1,25 (OH)2 vitamin D levels in humans: studies in healthy subjects, in calcium stoneformers and in patients with primary hyperparathyroidism. J Clin Endocrinol Metab 45:299–306
21. Van Den Berg CY, Kumar B, Wilson DM, Heath H, Smith LH (1980) Orthophosphate therapy decreases urinary calcium excretion and serum 1,25 dihydroxyvitamin D concentrations in idiopathic hypercalciuria. J Clin Endocrinol Metab 51:998–1001
22. Barilla DE, Zerwekh JE, Pak CYC (1979) A critical evaluation of the role of phosphate in the pathogenesis of absorptive hypercalciuria. Min Electrol Metab 2:301–309
23. Shen FH, Baylink DJ, Nielsen RL (1977) Increased serum 1,25 (OH)2 D3 in patients with idiopathic hypercalciuria. J Lab Clin Med 90:955–961
24. Bataille P, Bouillon R, Fournier A (1986) Increased plasma concentrations of total and free 1,25 (OH)2 D3 in calcium stone formers with idiopathic hypercalciuria. In: Linari F, Marengella M (eds) Pathogenesis and treatment of nephrolithiasis. Contrib Nephrol 58: 50–53
25. Tieder M, Modai D, Samuel B (1987) "Idiopathic" hypercalciuria and hereditary hypophosphatemic rickets. N Engl J Med 316:125–129
26. Coe FL, Bushinsky DA (1984) Pathophysiology of hypercalciuria. Am J Physiol 247: F1–F13
27. Sutton R, Walker V (1980) Responses to hydrochlorothiazide and acetazolamide in patients with calcium stones. Evidence suggesting a defect in renal tubular function. N Engl J Med 302:709–715
28. Burckhardt P, Jaeger P (1981) Secondary hyperparathyroidism in idiopathic renal hypercalciuria: fact or theory? J Clin Endocrinol Metab 53:550–551
29. Broadus AE, Insogna KL, Lang R (1984) Evidence for disordered control of 1,25 (OH)2 D production in absorptive hypercalciuria. N Engl J Med 311:73–80
30. Portale A, Halloran BP, Morris C (1989) Physiologic regulation of the serum concentration of 1,25 dihydroxyvitamin D by phosphorus in normal men. J Clin Invest 83:1494–1499
31. Messa P, Mioni G, Montanaro D (1987) About primitive osseous origin of the so-called idiopathic hypercalciuria. In: Linari F, Marangella M (eds) Pathogenesis and treatment of nephrolithiasis. Contrib Nephrol 58:106–110
32. Sutton R, Walker V (1986) Bone resorption and hypercalciuria in calcium stone formers. Metabolism 6:485–486
33. Liberman V, Sperling O, Atsman A (1969) Metabolic and calcium kinetic studies in idiopathic hypercalciuria. J Clin Invest 47:2580–2590
34. Alhava EM, Juuti M, Karjalainen P (1976) Bone mineral density in patients with urolithiasis. Scand J Urol Nephrol 10:154–156
35. Malvasi L, Sartori L, Giannini S, Al Awady M, Musaio F, Varotto S, D'Angelo A (1988) Mineral metabolism and bone mineral content in calcium nephrolithiasis with and without hyperparathyroidism. Urological Res 16:190
36. Velentzas C, Oreopoulos DG, Meema S, Meema HE, Nutsuga T, Alison E, Katirtzoglou A, Crassweller P (1981) Dietary calcium restriction may be good for patients' stones but not for their bones. In: Smith LH, Robertson WG, Finlayson B (eds) Urolithiasis clinical and basic research. Plenum, New York, pp 847–854

37. Barkin J, Wilson DR, Manuel MA, Bayley A, Murray T, Harrison J (1985) Bone mineral content in idiopathic calcium nephrolithiasis. Min Electrol Metab 11:19–24
38. Pacifici R, Rothstein M, Rifas L, Lau KHW, Baylink DG, Avioli LV, Hruska K (1990) Increased monocyte interleukin-I activity and decreased vertebral bone density in patients with fasting hypercalciuria. J Clin Endocrinol Metab
39. Lawoyin S, Sismilich S, Browne B, Pak CYC (1979) Bone mineral content in patients with calcium orolithiasis. Metabolism 28:1250–1254
40. Bordier P, Ryckwaert A, Gueris J (1977) On the pathogenesis of the so-called idiopathic hypercalciuria. Am J Med 63:398–402
41. Malluche HH, Tschoepe W, Ritz E (1980) Abnormal bone histology in idiopathic hypercalciuria. J Clin Endocrinol Metab 50:654–658
42. Steiniche T, Mosekilde L, Christensen MS, Melsen F (1989) A histomorphometric determination of iliac bone remodeling in patients with recurrent renal stone formation and idiopathic hypercalciuria. A.P.M.I.S. 4:309–316
43. Maierhofer W, Lemann JJ, Gray R (1984) Dietary calcium and serum 1,25 (OH)2 D concentrations as determinants of calcium balance in healthy men. Kidney Int 26:752–759
44. Raisz DG, Trummel CL, Holick MF, De Luca MF (1972) 1,25 dihydroxycholecalciferol: a potent stimulator of bone resorption in tissue culture. Science 175:768–769
45. Fuss M, Pepersack T, Van Geel J, Corvilain J, Vandewall JC, Bergman P, Simon P (1990) Involvement of low-calcium diet in the reduced bone mineral content of idiopathic renal stone formers. Calcif Tissue Int 46:9–13
46. Wachman A, Bernstein DS (1968) Diet Osteoporosis. Lancet I:958–959
47. Fellström B, Danielson BG, Karlström B (1986) Effect of high intake of dietary animal protein on mineral metabolism and urinary supersaturation of calcium oxalate in renal stone formers. Brit J Urol 56:263–269
48. Filipponi P, Mannarelli C, Pacifici R, Grossi E, Moretti I, Tini S, Carloni C, Blass A, Morucci P, Hruska KA, Avioli LV (1988) Evidence for a prostaglandin-mediated bone resorptive mechanism in subjects with fasting hypercalciuria. Calcif Tissue Int 43:61–66
49. Bouillon R, Auwery JH, Lissens WD, Pelemans W (1987) Vitamin D status in the elderly: seasonal substrate deficiency causes 1,25 dihydroxycholecalciferol deficiency. Am J Clin Nutr 45:755–763
50. Varghese M, Godman JS, William CG (1989) The effect of ultraviolet B radiation treatment on calcium excretion and vitamin D metabolites in kidney stone formers. Clin Nephrol 31:225–231
51. Bell NH, Greene V, Sharry J, Shaw J (1986) Evidence that 25-hydroxyvitamin D has a role in the regulation of calcium metabolism in man (abstract). J Bone Mineral Res 1:380
52. Sandler LM, Winearls CG, Fraher LJ, Clemens TL, Smith R, O'Riordan JLH (1984) Studies on the hypercalcemia of sarcoidosis: effect of steroids and exogenous vitamin D3 on the circulating concentrations of 1,25 dihydroxyvitamin D3. Q J Med New Series 53:165–180
53. Yamade M, Matrumoto T, Takahashi N, Suda T, Ogada E (1983) Stimulatory effect of prostaglandin E2 on 1α 25 dihydroxyvitamin D3 synthesis in rats. Biochem J 216:237–240
54. Roche CH, Rodriguez-Iturbe B, Henera J, Parra G (1988) Increased urinary excretion of prostaglandin E in patients with idiopathic hypercalciuria. Clin Sci 75:581–587
55. Houser M, Zimmerman B, Davidson M, Smith C, Smaiko A, Fish A (1984) Idiopathic hypercalciuria associated with hyperreninemia and high urinary prostaglandin E. Kidney Int 26:176–182
56. Bataille P, Charransol G, Grégoire I, Daigre JC, Fournier A (1983) Effect of calcium restriction on renal excretion of oxalate and the probability of stones in the various pathophysiological groups with calcium stones. J Urol 130:218–223
57. Calo L, Cantaro S, Marchini F, Giannini S, Castrignano B, Gambaro G, Antonello A, Baggio B, D'Angelo A, Williams H, Borsatti A (1990) Is hydrochlorothiazide-induced hypocalciuria due to inhibition of prostaglandin E2 synthesis? Clin Sci 78:321–325

58. Lemann J, Gray RW, Maïerhofer WJ, Cheung HS (1985) Hydrochlorothiazide inhibits bone resorptions in men despite experimentally elevated serum 1,25 dihydroxy vitamin D concentrations. Kidney Int 28:951–958
59. Lacroix AZ, Wienpahl J, White LR, Wallace RB, Scherr PA, George LK, Cornoni-Huntley J, Ustfeld AM (1990) Thiazide diuretic agents and the incidence of hip fracture. N Engl J Med 322:286–290

Extracorporeal Shock Wave Lithotripsy (ESWL): Past, Present, and Future

CHRISTIAN G. CHAUSSY[1] and GERHARD J. FUCHS[2]

SUMMARY. Extracorporeal shock wave lithotripsy (ESWL) has now been in clinical use for 10 years and has replaced other treatment techniques for the majority of surgical calculi located in the upper urinary tract. For the first time it provides a completely noninvasive method for the treatment of renal and ureteral stones. The current range of its indications includes approximately 70% of nonselected urinary stone patients. An additional 25% of patients with more complex stones in the upper urinary tract can receive treatment with the lithotripter (E.S.W.L. (R)) when combining the method with endourological procedures (see Table 1).

Introduction

The first experimental efforts at using extracorporeally induced shock waves to disintegrate human kidney stones were made in Munich (West Germany) in 1972. After extensive in vitro testing had proven the disintegration of stones of various chemical composition by focussed shock wave energy to be feasible, an animal stone model was finally used to demonstrate that shock waves generated outside the body could noninvasively disintegrate kidney stones to a size allowing their spontaneous passage [1–5].

In February 1980, extracorporeal shock wave lithotripsy (ESWL) was introduced clinically at the Department of Urology, University of Munich, as the first noninvasive method to treat patients suffering from upper urinary tract stones [3,4]. It only took a short time to prove the efficacy, safety, and reliability of the method, dramatically changing the management of upper urinary stones.

[1]Department of Urology, Staedtisches Krankenhaus, München-Harlaching, Federal Republic of Germany

[2]UCLA Stone Center, Division of Urology, Los Angeles, CA 90024, USA

Table 1. Historical development of ESWL

1972–1980	Development of extracorporeal shock wave lithotripsy (ESWL)	
ä	Ludwig Maximillian Universität, Departments of Surgical Research and Urology, München,	
ü	Germany Dornier Medical Systems, Friedrichshafen, Germany	
2/80–5/82	Human model no 1 (HM-1)	Indications
ü	-First clinical application of ESWL (München, Germany) 200 patients	renal pelvic stones + caliceal stones <1 cm. (approx. 20%)*
5/82–10/83	Human model no 2 (HM-2)	
ü	(München, Germany) 800 patients	+ selected ureteral stones + infected stones + stones up to 2.5 cm. + partial staghorn stones (approx. 60–70%)*
10/83	Human model no 3 (HM-3)	
	-Beginning of series production and distribution of the lithotripter	+ staghorn stones + combination with percutaneous surgery (approx. 95%)
12/1984	Food and Drug Administration (U.S.A.) -PMA Approval for Dornier HM-3 lithotripter	
1984-Present	-More than 2.000.000 treatments Distribution to 700 centers in 32 countries worldwide Clinical trials with new second generation lithotripters (Table 2)	

*percentage of unselected stone patients eligible for ESWL(R)

Physical Principles

The underlying physical principles of shock wave treatment of calculi in the human urinary tract are 1) generation of shock waves outside the body, 2) focusing of the shock wave onto an area distant from the generation area, 3) coupling of the shock wave into the body and, 4) localization and positioning of the respective treatment target into the treatment focus. The selective utilization of the destructive potential of shock waves for the disintegration of brittle stone material without damage to surrounding tissues constitutes a major breakthrough of modern medical technology [1–5].

Lithotripter Hardware Features

In the recent past, clinical trials involving new lithotripters have been performed at a number of centers in Europe, Japan, and the United States. The basic features of these devices are described in Table 2 [6,7]. Preliminary clinical data and product information furnished by the various manufacturers indicate that changes of the

Table 2. Comparison of technology of various shock wave lithotripters

Lithotripter	Energy source	Focusing device	Coupling medium	Localization	Anesthesia
Dornier HM-3	Spark gap	Ellipsoid	Bath	X-ray	regional, SDA
modified Dornier HM-4	Spark gap	Ellipsoid	Membrane	X-ray	SDA
Dornier MPL 9000	Spark gap	Ellipsoid	Membrane	Ultrasound	No, SDA
Dornier MFL 5000	Spark gap	Ellipsoid	Membrane	X-ray	No, SDA
Technomed	Modified spark gap	Ellipsoid	Limited bath	Ultrasound, X-ray	No, SDA
Yashiyoda	Microexplosive	Ellipsoid	Bath	X-ray	SDA
Siemens	Electromagnetic	Lens	Membrane	X-ray	SDA
Wolf	Piezoelectric	Bowl	Limited bath	Ultrasound	No
EDAP	Piezoelectric	Bowl	Membrane	Ultrasound	No, (SDA)
Medstone	Spark gap	Ellipsoid	Membrane	X-ray	SDA
Direx	Spark gap	Ellipsoid	Membrane	X-ray	SDA
Nitech	Spark gap	Ellipsoid	Membrane	Ultrasound	SDA

SDA, Sedoanalgesia

major lithotripter components (energy source, focusing device, coupling medium, stone localization system) result in distinctly different treatment parameters.

Preliminary results with the new lithotripters indicate that the various energy sources are all effective in fragmenting kidney stones [7]. Compared to the original device, however, a lower percentage of stone fragmentation is noted for most of the new devices, resulting in a higher number of repeat treatments [7].

In particular, the non spark gap devices, the PESE and EMSE energy sources currently used, fall short in this regard. Focusing of the shock wave onto a distant focal area utilizes different principles, as depicted in Table 2.

Depending on the characteristic features of the focusing devices (ellipsoid, acoustical lens, self-focusing), areas of high energy density ranging from 0.3 cm times 0.6 cm to 4.5 cm times 6.0 cm are measured. Energy density at the skin level and the maximum energy applied determines the need for anesthesia. Since the introduction of ESWL several anesthesia techniques have been employed.

Most groups working with the original device utilize regional anesthesia (epidural catheter anesthesia); only about 25% of users routinely employ general anesthesia. Several centers use local infiltration anesthesia of the skin entry area in an effort to reduce the amount of anesthetic required. Some of the newer devices require much less anesthesia (IV sedation and IM analgesics) due to changed physical parameters of shock wave generator energy and focusing devices [7]. Other devices even offer the prospect of anesthesia free shock wave treatment, owing to the different characteristics of the shock wave at the skin entry site and lower overall energy density [6,7]. This mainly applies to the piezoelectric devices, to machines using larger ellipsoids in conjunction with lower generator energy levels, and to the EMSE system. Clinical trials have shown this concept to be applicable at the expense of a significantly higher number of repeat treatments.

Ultrasound as a means of stone localization is utilized with several of the newer devices (Table 2). With the use of sophisticated ultrasound equipment this may offer reduced X-ray exposure and cost savings. Preliminary results of groups using ultrasound localizing devices, who have extensive experience with conventional shock wave lithotripsy, are encouraging. The problem areas are the technical limitations of

Table 3. Exclusion criteria for ESWL

Medical	-uncorrected bleeding disorder -uncorrected hypertension -pregnancy (stone treatment rarely necessary, placement of internal stent or percutaneous nephrostomy) -aortic or renal artery aneurysm (calcifications of aorta and renal artery are relative contraindications) -pacemakers (standby–cardiologist recommended)
Technical	-depending on type of lithotripter -general problems: stone location relative to energy source and patient positioning system (determinants: patient size, patient obesity, skeletal anomalies and ectopic kidneys, radio-opacity of stone)
Urological	-severe anatomical or functional alterations precluding proper elimination of debris -stenosis distal to the stone (calyceal neck, ureteropelvic junction, ureter, hypertrophy of prostate requiring surgical correction, urethral stricture) -stone bearing calyx grossly distended (especially dependent calyces) -functional impairment of ureteral mobility (neurogenic, immobile patient)

current ultrasound equipment, the unfamiliarity of many lithotripter operators with proper ultrasound interpretation, and the time needed for proper ultrasound localization [7]. Owing to the difficulty of detecting ureteral stones with ultrasound, the range of indications for these stones is limited.

Current State of the Clinical Use of Extracorporeally Induced Shock Waves

Contraindications

Less than 5% of all stone patients are excluded from ESWL routine treatment as they present with one of the still existing contraindications (Table 3). High risk patients, i.e., patients with bleeding disorders, hypertension or a heart condition have been treated with extracorporeal shock wave lithotripsy (ESWL) [5,7–9].

Indications

The range of indications, initially established in Munich, was soon confirmed by other centers [6, 8–10]. Owing to the high success rate of extracorporeal shock wave lithotripsy, the low rate of periprocedural complications, and the absence of long term adverse effects, the range of indications has been expanded over the years to include most of the urinary stones (Tables 4 and 5). Approximately 70% of non-selected stone patients are eligible for extracorporeal shock wave lithotripsy monotherapy [5–7,9,11–14]. This group includes single and multiple stones of an added stone mass of up to 2.5 cm in the kidney, selected ureteral stones above the iliac crest and below the pelvic brim (pelvic window), and staghorn stones which fill a non-dilated collecting system (in the absence of intrarenal stenosis or dilatation). The aforementioned stones are found in approximately 70%–80% of patients that are referred to a urinary stone center, depending on certain referral biases. The

Table 4. Selection criteria for extracorporeal shockwave lithotripsy of renal stones

Variables determining treatment approach
-stone burden (period of stone passage and rate of auxiliary procedures increase proportionally with stone size)
-intrarenal stone distribution (pelvis vs. calyces)
-presence of intrarenal stenosis
-isolated dilatation of calyces
-stone composition (calcium-oxalate monohydrate and cystine stones respond poorly to ESWL)
-patient compliance (prolonged period of time before treatment is completed, depending on stone size)

remainder of patients present with more complex stone disease, or with stones which need auxiliary procedures to maximize the advantage of extracorporeal shock wave lithotripsy. Into the latter group fall radiolucent and small semiopaque stones which need to be made visible by use of contrast medium, as they cannot be primarily identified on the X-ray screen (with the exception of ultrasound based localization lithotripters).

Controversy still exists over the treatment of staghorn stones and ureteral stones. For these two subgroups, different treatment strategies have evolved (monotherapy with extracorporeal shock wave lithotripsy vs the combined treatment of endourological procedures and subsequent extracorporeal shock wave lithotripsy) [5–11,15]. Success with extracorporeal shock wave lithotripsy of kidney stones is dependent upon (1) the overall stone burden in the kidney, (2) the shape of the renal collecting system, (3) the architecture of the dependent calyces, and (4) stone composition [5,6,8–11,13,15,16]. Based on these criteria the following guidelines for the treatment of staghorn stones have been established at our institution. In partial and complete staghorn stones, monotherapy with extracorporeal shock wave lithotripsy (in conjunction with the use of indwelling ureteral catheters) is preferable to other treatment modalities only in cases where the stone fills a nondilated collecting system [5–7,9]. A planned staged extracorporeal shock wave lithotripsy procedure is usually performed in staghorn stones which fill a slightly dilated collecting system [7,9]. It has to be pointed out, however, that with increasing stone burden the rates for second sessions and follow up complications are considerably higher than those encountered with smaller stones.

Also, the period of stone passage is significantly prolonged compared to percutaneous stone surgery or the combination therapy. The liberal use of indwelling ureteral catheters has not had any proven effect on these parameters; however, it reduces perioperative morbidity and the need for auxiliary procedures to relieve ureteral obstruction. Auxiliary procedures, namely percutaneous nephrostomy tube placement and

Table 5. Selection criteria for extracorporeal shock wave lithotripsy of ureteral stones

Variables determining treatment approach
-approach individualized according to expansion space and stone location
-no standard treatment protocol for all ureteral stones available
-depending on lithotripter used (X-ray or ultrasound stone localization)
-depending on endourological experience

ureteroscopic ureteral manipulations are required in approximately 60% of patients after ESWL treatment of large branched stones [5–7,9,13].

Thus, in staghorn stones with (1) a large stone mass, filling a dilated renal collecting system, and (2) with intrarenal anatomical alterations, a percutaneous procedure is performed first for debulking the stone. In a second session, extracorporeal shock wave lithotripsy is employed for the disintegration of the remaining caliceal stone parts and under the same anesthesia the patient undergoes a second percutaneous procedure for removal of the stone gravel [5–7,9]. Although inherently more invasive than monotherapy with extracorporeal shock wave lithotripsy, this approach is of great benefit for the patient with regard to stone free rates, hospitalizations, and time lost from work.

Although 80% of all stones which become symptomatic are ureteral stones, only 10%–15% of those stones require interventional treatment; the remainder pass spontaneously. Ureteral stones have been primarily amenable to extracorporeal shock wave lithotripsy only if located above the bony pelvis in the mid or upper third of the ureter [5,7,9,10,12,14–16]. Only recently, stones in the terminal ureter below the pelvic brim have been treated successfully with ESWL through the pelvic window [7,14,17]. The prone position has been advocated for stones overlying the bony pelvis.

When ultrasound stone localization systems are used, treatment of ureteral stones becomes more difficult, especially for stones below the level of the lower pole of the kidney [7]. Experience has shown that even with a stone in a favorable position, the success rate of stone disintegration is dependent on particle expansion, which is low or nonexistent in the ureter surrounding an impacted stone [5–7,9,14]. To obviate this unfavorable condition, two modalities are available—namely, repositioning the stone(s) into the renal pelvis, and/or passing a ureteral catheter about the calculus. With both procedures the expansion chamber is increased, thereby resulting in a high rate of stone disintegration (>97%) [5–7,9,14]. Ureteral stones overlying the bony pelvis below the iliac crest and above the pelvic brim become amenable to extracorporeal shock wave lithotripsy only when repositioned into the upper ureter or ideally into the renal pelvis in a retrograde or antegrade fashion. Otherwise the shock wave energy would be absorbed by the bony structures and would therefore not suffice to fragment the stone. Prone positioning is a time-consuming alternative with less than optimal success rates. Stones which cannot be manipulated, or ESWL treatment failures are best managed ureteroscopically [5–7,9,14].

Although nephrolithiasis is a relatively rare incident in the pediatric age group, the advent of a noninvasive treatment modality for children was especially appreciated. Treatment by ESWL is particularly advantageous in this patient population, as it can be repeated without adverse effect.

Concerns have been raised with regard to the effect of high energy shock waves on immature bony tissue, growing renal tissue, long-term renal function, or the induction of hypertension [7,18]. The available clinical results indicate that extracorporeal shock wave lithotripsy does not lead to deterioration of long-term renal function or affect renal development; no juvenile hypertension has been noted after extracorporeal shock wave lithotripsy. Recently conducted research on the effects of high energy shock waves on immature bony tissue and renal growth confirms the safety of this treatment modality. Cautious use of the energy, however, is advocated [7].

Table 6. Results with extracorporeal shock wave lithotripsy (München, Dornier HM-1,2,3)

Extracorporeal shock wave lithotripsy	
Results of the Munich group	
(1980–1983)	
Stone free	90%
Spontaneously passable	9.3%
Surgery	0.7%
Renal function unchanged	
(n = 50, 1980–1984)	

Results with Extracorporeal Shock Wave Lithotripsy

The initial results of the Munich group for the first three years, when extracorporeal shock wave lithotripsy was used in Munich alone, revealed a success rate of 99%. Ninety percent of patients became completely stone free within a three month period. Only small and spontaneously passable fragments remained in 9.3% of patients. In 0.7% of cases an open surgical or endourological procedure was indicated to relieve a persisting ureteral obstruction (Table 6) [4,15,16].

Evaluation of pre and post-lithotripsy renal function showed no evidence of any adverse effects of extracorporeal shock wave lithotripsy on renal function. Over a four year period, it was found that the renal function of those patients treated with extracorporeal shock wave lithotripsy actually improved with time, which is attributable to those cases where obstructing stones had been successfully treated (Table 6). Comparison of these results with the results from other institutions using the same lithotripter, and with those results achieved with different machines is difficult, since there is no commonly accepted nomenclature or stratification system. It would therefore seem reasonable to agree on a nomenclature encompassing stone size, location, anatomy of the urinary tract, and stone composition. The reported annual stone recurrent rates of 4%–8% are reassuringly low and compare favorably to those of other treatment modalities. Approximately 25% of residual stones increase in size over a 2 year followup period. Long-term observation of the clinical fate of these patients is necessary to decide whether or not the regrowth rate and the associated need for auxiliary procedures are acceptable.

Complications of Extracorporeal Shock Wave Lithotripsy

Transient macroscopic hematuria is reported to occur in most patients, regardless of the energy source used. However, clinically significant bleeding with the development of perirenal hematoma is a rare exception (0.1%–0.66%) [7,9,18]. Recent discussion has focused on the relevance of short-term shockwave induced alterations on renal morphology, long-term function, and the possibility of so far unappreciated long-term adverse effects. With the advent of more sensitive imaging technology immediate changes in renal morphology, such as subcapsular bleeding, perirenal fluid collections and loss of corticomedullary differentiation, have been described in as many a 63% of patients following shockwave treatment for renal stones. Animal studies have revealed renal injury secondary to shock wave energy, including disruption of renal vessels, damage to tubular epithelium, and eventual formation of focal and segmental interstitial fibrosis when higher than clinically recommended levels of energy were employed. These studies identified the amount of energy used as a common denominator of damage. Unless exceedingly high levels of energy were used, however, the shock wave induced morphological changes were found to be transient. Clinically, no long-term adverse effects have been reported until recently, when various retrospective studies suggested an incidence of new onset hypertension of up to 8% within a 2 year period following extracorporeal lithotripsy treatment [7,18].

These figures, however, were obtained from retrospective observations and have not been reproduced so far in prospective studies, reflecting the difficulties of reliable assessment of small changes in blood pressure within a relatively short period. Urological post-lithotripsy complications are secondary to either insufficient stone disintegration or to ureteral obstruction with stone debris. Discomfort or pain is found in between 5% and 25% of all cases. Auxiliary procedures after extracorporeal shock wave lithotripsy are indicated when obstructive pyelonephritis (2%–6%) has to be relieved to prevent urosepsis. In our service we use percutaneous nephrostomy tube drainage liberally. This, together with appropriate antibiotic treatment, quickly relieves the acute symptoms (pain and/or infection). When ureteral Steinstrasse (accumulation of disintegrated stone debris in the ureter) is present without signs of infection, obstruction persistent for 4 weeks prompts us to use percutaneous nephrostomy drainage. In many cases fragments are then spontaneously discharged within a reasonable period, thus reducing the necessity for more invasive auxiliary procedures.

Conclusion

Undoubtedly, extracorporeal shock wave lithotripsy has become a most valuable asset to the urologist and greatly benefits urological stone patients. During the short time since the advent of extracorporeal shock wave lithotripsy the management of urinary stone disease has completely changed. Extracorporeal shock wave lithotripsy has almost completely supplanted open surgical and, to a lesser extent, endourological approaches.

Experience has shown that approximately 70% of patients can benefit from extracorporeal shock wave lithotripsy as monotherapy. More complex stones require auxiliary procedures, namely endourological procedures or, at times, open surgery. Those 25%–30% of cases which require combined endourological or open surgical techniques are technically demanding and should be reserved for the stone centers, where extensive experience with all alternative techniques of urinary stone treatment exists.

We certainly have not yet reached the endpoint of the development of this method and its clinical applications in urology and other medical fields. At this point it is certain that the progress of ESWL represents a dramatic change in the management of urinary stones, by which invasive approaches have been superseded by a noninvasive procedure. We, the urologists, and of course over and above all, the patient himself who gets rid of his stones, avoiding open surgery, have learned to appreciate the outstanding achievements of the recent past. From now on all other methods employed for the treatment of urinary stones will have to be judged against the results of this new methodology.

References

1. Chaussy C, Eisenberger F, Wanner K, Forssmann B, Hepp W (1976) The use of shock waves for the destruction of renal calculi without direct contact. Urol Res 4:175
2. Chaussy C, Schmiedt E, Forssmann B, Brendel W (1979) Contact free renal stone destruction by means of shock waves. Eur Surg Res 11:36
3. Chaussy C, Brendel W, Schmiedt E (1980) Extracorporeally induced destruction of kidney stones by shock waves. Lancet 12.3:1265
4. Chaussy C, Schmiedt E, Jocham D, Brendel W, Forssmann B, Walther W (1981) First clinical experience with extracorporeally induced destruction of kidney stones by shock waves. J Urol 125:417–420
5. Chaussy C, Schmiedt E, Jocham D, Fuchs G, Brendel W (1986) Extracorporeal shock wave lithotripsy, 2nd ed. In: Chaussy CG (ed) Karger, Munich
6. Fuchs G, Chaussy C (1987) Worldwide experience with, and future concepts of ESWL, In: Riehle R, Newman D (eds) Principles of extracorporeal shock wave lithotripsy. Livingstone, New York
7. Chaussy C, Fuchs G (1989) Current state and future development of noninvasive treatment of human stones with extracorporeal shockwave lithotripsy. J Urol 141:790
8. Drach G, Dretler S, Fair W, Finlayson B, Gillenwater J, Griffith D, Lingeman J, Newman D (1986) Report of the United States cooperative study of extracorporeal shock wave lithotripsy. J Urol 135:1127
9. Chaussy C, Fuchs G (1986) Extracorporeal shock wave lithotripsy (ESWL) for the treatment of urinary stones. In: Gillenwater J (ed) Textbook on adult and pediatric urology. Year Book Publishers, Chicago
10. Fuchs G, Miller K, Rassweiler J, Eisenberger F (1985) Extracorporeal shock wave lithotripsy: One-year experience with the Dornier Lithotripter. Eur Urol 11:145
11. Eisenberger, F, Fuchs G, Miller K, Rassweiler J (1985) Extracorporeal shock wave lithotripsy and endourology—an ideal combination for the treatment of kidney stones. World J Urol 3:41–47
12. Miller K, Fuchs G, Rassweiler J, Eisenberger F (1985) Treatment of ureteral stone disease: the role of ESWL and endourology. World J Urol 3:445
13. Winfield H, Clayman R, Chaussy C, Weyman P, Fuchs G, Lupu A (1988) Monotherapy of staghorn calculi: Comparative study between percutaneous nephrolithotomy and extracorporeal shock wave lithotripsy. J Urol 139:895
14. Fuchs G, Chaussy C, Riehle R (1987) The Use of ESWL for ureteral stones. In: Riehle R, Newman D (eds) Principles of extracorporeal shock wave lithotripsy. Livingstone, New York
15. Schmiedt E, Chaussy C (1984) Extracorporeal shock wave lithotripsy of kidney and ureteric stones. Urol Int 39:193–198
16. Chaussy C, Schmiedt E (1983) Shock wave treatment for stones in the upper urinary tract. N Amer Clin Urol vol 10, No 4:743–750
17. Chaussy C, Fuchs G (1987) Extracorporeal shock wave lithotripsy of distal ureteral calculi: Is it worthwhile? J Endourol 1:1
18. Lingeman J, Evan A (1987) Bioeffects of ESWL. J Endourol 1:89
19. Jocham D, Liedl B, Chaussy C, Schmiedt E (1987) Preliminary clinical experience with the HM-4 bath-free Dornier lithotriptor. World J Urol 5:4, 208

Extracorporeal Shock Wave Lithotripsy (ESWL): Late Consequences

JOHN C. PETERSON[1]

SUMMARY. Since its introduction, ESWL has had a great impact on the treatment of renal stone disease. This treatment is 90% successful for upper urinary tract stones less than 2 centimeters in diameter. The initial reports created tremendous enthisiasm and related few complications. Subsequent studies have raised concerns about stone recurrence rates and renal dysfunction, as well as hypertension, following lithotripsy. Studies on stone recurrence rates have yielded reassuringly low rates; however, the duration of follow-up in these studies is only 2 years and certainly more data concerning the 10%–30% of patients with remnant stone fragments are needed. Initial reports of tissue damage, consisting of subcapsular hematomas immediately following treatment and localized areas of interstitial fibrosis in more chronic animal models, provide a possible explanation for the reports of decreased renal blood flow correlated with hypertension in human subjects studied up to 4 years after lithotripsy. These studies contain small numbers of patients and corroborative studies are needed to document the risks of such complications.

Introduction

Renal stone disease accounts for approximately 1% of all hospital admissions in the United States and has an annual incidence of 7–21 cases per 10000 persons. Its peak incidence is between ages 20 and 30 years, thus it affects individuals during the height of career development [1]. Realizing the economic impact of this disease and the extraordinary technologic developments in its treatment over the past decade, the Office of Medical Applications of Research of the National Institute of Health (NIH) convened a Consensus Development Conference on the Prevention and Treatment of

[1]Division of Nephrology, Hypertension and Transplantation, University of Florida College of Medicine, Gainesville, FL 32610-0224, USA

Kidney stones in March of 1988. One of the topics discussed was the role of lithotripsy in treatment of renal stone disease. Their summary statement included the following comment: "Since ESWL is relatively new, the long-term effects of this therapy are unknown. Concerns relative to the effects of kidney function,. . . increased new stone growth, and subsequent diseases, such as hypertension will require long term evaluation [1]."

Extracorporeal shock wave lithotripsy (ESWL) was first used by Chaussy in 1980 [2], was introduced to the United States in 1984 and, almost immediately, became the treatment of choice for the majority of cases of symptomatic upper urinary tract nephrolithiasis [3–5]. Initial reports suggested that ESWL had very few deleterious effects [6–7]. Early in our experience (late 1984) with ESWL, one patient developed flank pain and abrupt onset of hypertension within hours of treatment, and was found to have a markedly reduced effective renal plasma flow (by radionuclide renography) with a perirenal hematoma (by magnetic resonance imaging). This experience prompted a prospective study showing acute effects of ESWL on morphology and renal function [8], and a retrospective review of our first 79 patients suggested an increase in diastolic blood pressure several months following ESWL [9]. Subsequently, other reports have corroborated these findings [10–12] and reports concerning tissue effects—both acute and chronic—have suggested that ESWL does have a measurable effect on renal and on other tissues [13–16].

This paper will review the reported experience of long-term consequences of ESWL as enumerated by the NIH-convened consensus report, i.e., increased stone growth, effects on kidney function, and hypertension [1].

Increased or Recurrent Stone Growth

There is no debate concerning the efficacy of ESWL in removing stones which previously would have required surgery. Several large series have reported success rates of approximately 90% when pre-treatment stone diameter is less than 2 centimeters [17,18]. These success rates generally include 10%–30% of patients who are left with small (0.3–0.4 centimeters) stone fragments at the time of discharge, which subsequently pass, leaving the patient "stone-free" or with a remarkably reduced stone burden at 3 months as evaluated by plain film radiography. Whether these remnant stone fragments serve as a nidus for further stone formation was not addressed by these initial studies. Since the natural history of nephrolithiasis suggests that 40% of patients will have a recurrent stone (15% will recur in the first year) within five years after the first episode [19], the presence of stone fragments in 10%–30% of patients after 3 months is bothersome. Two recent reports show reassuringly low rates of new stone formation, approximating 6% [20,21]; however, these evaluations were at 19–26 months after ESWL and thus the long-term effects on stone recurrence must await further studies at longer time periods after ESWL. Additionally, the issue of regrowth of residual fragments will also require further study, since the values in different reports are not consistent. Since the clinical effectiveness of ESWL seems to be greater than its stone-removal (or stone-free) efficacy, future reports will need to include clinical correlation and to contain follow-up for periods longer than the current two-year studies.

Kidney Function and Hypertension

The second and third concerns enumerated by the NIH Consensus Report involve kidney function and hypertension, as well as the tissue effects of ESWL [1]. I shall attempt a collated discussion of these subjects, since it seems rational to suppose that long-term decrements in renal function are attributable to tissue damage incurred during ESWL, and recent evidence indicates a significant correlation between decrement in estimated renal plasma flow (ERPF) and increment in systolic and diastolic blood pressure [22].

As related above, our initial experience with hypertension, reduced renal plasma flow, and a perirenal hematoma in a single patient led us to do a retrospective study in which we found an increased diastolic blood pressure in 4% (3 out of 79) of patients up to several months after ESWL. Because all 3 cases had perirenal or subcapsular hematomas which subsequently resolved while the blood pressure remained elevated, we suggested the pathophysiology might involve a phenomenon known as the Page kidney [9]. In the same symposium, Kaude and co-workers, using magnetic resonance imaging, documented loss of corticomedullary demarcation and subcapsular hemorrhage in 24% of patients [23]. Studies in dog kidneys demonstrated pathologic changes in the kidney, which were dose-dependent on the number of shocks delivered [24], and demonstrated that fibrosis was a predictable event in the resolution of intraparenchymal hemorrhage following ESWL [14,15].

In the interim, in 1987 Lingeman and Kulb [10] reported a retrospective evaluation of 900 patients treated with ESWL; of follow-up patients examined, 8.2% (24 out of 295) had become hypertensive. Bomanji and co-workers then reported a significant decrement in glomerular filtration rate immediately after ESWL [25].

In 1988, Williams and co-workers reported an overall prevalence of hypertension, at 18 months after treatment, of 8% (7 out of 91). In a subgroup of 21 patients with decreased blood flow, 5 were hypertensive [12]. Sixteen of these patients were restudied 4 years after treatment and showed a further decline in blood flow to the treated kidney, with hypertension severe enough to require treatment present in 4 of 16 patients (25%). Interestingly, the decreased blood flow to the treated kidney correlated significantly with the increments in both systolic and diastolic blood pressure [22]. Lingeman and co-workers have recently reported results of follow-up blood pressure measurements in 731 patients at least 1 year after ESWL. They found no difference in annualized incidence of diastolic hypertension compared to a control group of patients who received urethroscopy or passed stones spontaneously (171 patients); however, the group as a whole had a significant rise in diastolic blood pressure after ESWL. Unfortunately their definition of hypertension included only diastolic values and no systolic values were reported [11]. A recent report from the same center documented findings in 8 patients with solitary kidneys who received ESWL five years ago. They showed a significant rise in serum creatinine, new onset of hypertension in 2 of 8 patients, and a decrement in renal blood flow that did not reach statistical significance (pre-327 ml/min and post-294 ml/min) [26].

In summary, although the numbers of patients studied are small and uncontrolled, the data to date suggest that hypertension and reduced renal function occur after ESWL and are maintained for at least 4 years. Even if further studies corroborate these findings, ESWL will continue to have a massive impact on the treatment of kidney stones. The stage has been set for the development of a multi-center, prospective evaluation of the long-term consequences of ESWL. This is currently underway and the results will be eagerly awaited.

References

1. Consensus development summaries (1988) Prevention and treatment of kidney stones. National Institutes of Health. Conn Med 52(7):415–420
2. Chaussy CG, Brendel W, Schmiedt E (1980) Extracorporeally induced destruction of kidney stones by shock waves. Lancet II:1265–1268
3. Fuchs G, Miller K, Rassweiler J, Eisenberger F (1985) Extracorporeal shock wave lithotripsy. Eur Urol 11:145–149
4. Lingeman JE, Newman DM, Mertz JHO, Mosbaugh PG, Steele RE, Kahnoski RJ, Coury TA, Woods JR (1986) Extracorporeal shock wave lithotripsy. J Urol 135:1134–1137
5. Drach G, Dretler SP, Fair W, Finlayson B, Gillenwater J, Griffith D, Lingeman J, Newman D (1986) Report of the United States cooperative study of extracorporeal shock wave lithotripsy. J Urol 135:1127–1133
6. Chaussy CG, Schmiedt E, Jocham D, Brendel W, Forssman B, Walther V (1982) First clinical experience with extracorporeally induced destruction of kidney stones by shock waves. J Urol 127:417–420
7. Chaussy CG, Schmiedt E (1983) Shock wave treatment for stones in the upper urinary tract. Urol Clin North Am 10:743–750
8. Kaude JV, Williams MC, Millner MR, Scott KN, Finlayson B (1985) Renal morphology and function immediately after extracorporeal shock wave lithotripsy. AJR 145:305–313
9. Peterson JC, Finlayson B (1986) Effects of ESWL on blood pressure. In: Gravenstein JS, Peter K (eds) Extracorporeal shock wave lithotripsy for renal stone disease. Butterworth, Stoneham, pp 145–150
10. Lingeman JE, Kulb TB (1987) Hypertension following extracorporeal shock wave lithotripsy. J Urol 137:142A
11. Lingeman JE, Woods JR, Toth PD (1990) Blood pressure changes following extracorporeal shock wave lithotripsy and other forms of treatment of nephrolithiasis. JAMA 263(13):1789–1794
12. Williams CM, Kaude JV, Newman RC, Peterson JC, Thomas WC (1988) ESWL: Long-term complications. AJR 150:311–315
13. Lingeman JE, McAteer JA, Kempson SA, Evan AP (1988) Bioeffects of extracorporeal shock wave lithotripsy. Urol Clin North Am 15:507–514
14. Newman R, Hackett R, Senior D, Feldman J, Sosnowski J, Finlayson B (1987) ESWL: pathologic effects on canine renal tissues. Urology 29:194–200
15. Jaeger P, Redha G, Uhlschmid G, Hauri D (1988) Morphological changes in canine kidneys following extracorporeal shock wave treatment. Urol Res 16:161–166
16. Haupt G, Haupt A, Donovan JM, Drach GW, Chaussy C (1989) Short-term changes of laboratory values after extracorporeal shock wave lithotripsy. J Urol 142:259–262
17. Roth RA, Beckmann CF (1988) Complications of extracorporeal shock wave lithotripsy and percutaneous nephrolithotomy. Urol Clin North Am 15(2):155–166
18. Schmiedt E, Chaussy C (1984) Extracorporeal shock wave lithotripsy of kidney and ureteric stones. Urol Int 39:193–198
19. Williams RE (1969) The natural history of renal lithiasis. In: Hodgkinson A, Nordin BEC (eds) Renal stone research symposium, Leeds (1968). Churchill, London, pp 65–70
20. Miles SG, Kaude JV, Newman RC, Thomas WC, Williams CM (1988) Extracorporeal shock wave lithotripsy: prevalence of renal stones 3 to 21 months after treatment. AJR 150:307–309

21. Graff J, Diederichs W, Schulze H (1987) Long-term follow-up in 1003 extracorporeal shock wave lithotripsy patients. J Urol 140:479–483
22. Williams CM, Thomas WC (1989) Permanently decreased renal blood flow and hypertension after lithotripsy. N Engl J Med 321:1269–1270
23. Kaude JV, Williams CM, Millner M, Finlayson B (1986) Magnetic resonance imaging of the kidney after ESWL. In: Extracorporeal shock wave lithotripsy for renal stone disease: technical and clinical aspects. Butterworth, Stoneham, pp 125–129
24. Delius M, Enders G, Xuan Z, Liebisch HG, Brendel W (1988) Biological effects of shock waves. Ultrasound Med Biol 14:117–122
25. Bomanji J, Boddy SAM, Britton KE, Nimmon CC, Whitfield HN (1987) Radionuclide evaluation pre- and post-extracorporeal shock wave lithotripsy for renal calculi. J Nucl Med 28:1284–1289
26. Brito CG, Lingeman JE, Newman DM, Kight JL, Heck LL (1990) Long term follow-up of renal function in ESWL-treated patients with solitary kidney. J Urol 143(4):299A

Nephrolithiasis – Extracorporeal Shock Wave Lithotripsy (ESWL): Current Status in Japan

Hiroshi Tazaki[1]

Introduction of ESWL to Japan

In December 1983, a survey team was sent to Munich and Stuttgart, Federal Republic of Germany, to study new lithotripters. Drs. Tazaki and Higashihara were there; they reported that the machine was effective for disintegrating kidney stones and that the side effects were minor. In 1984, four machines were installed in four institutions in Japan and treatments were initiated. The spark gap system ESWL was found to be so useful that the number of machines had increased to ten by the end of 1986. Membrane type and piezo type ESWL were introduced in 1987 and 1988. In November, 1989 at the seventh world congress of endourology and ESWL in Kyoto, all kinds of lithotripters were displayed at the exhibit and discussed. Multipurpose types of ESWL became more popular; since 1989 the Piezo type ESWL with ultrasound focusing has tended to be the preferred type.

As of the end of June, 1990, 244 ESWL machines are being operated in this country; the regional distribution and types of ESWL are shown in Figs. 1 and 2. Regional populations and patient ratio to machine are shown in Table 1. Wide differences in each region become more apparent when comparisons are made between prefectures. More ESWL machines are found on the Pacific coast; there are no machines in two prefectures along the sea of Japan; however, the incidence of stone disease is apparently higher on the Pacific side of Japan.

Clinical Investigation of ESWL

Results of clinical studies on urinary stone disintegration, using various types of ESWL, have been published. The results are almost the same as the reports from

[1]Department of Urology, School of Medicine, Keio University, 35, Shinanomachi, Shinjuku-ku, Tokyo, 160 Japan

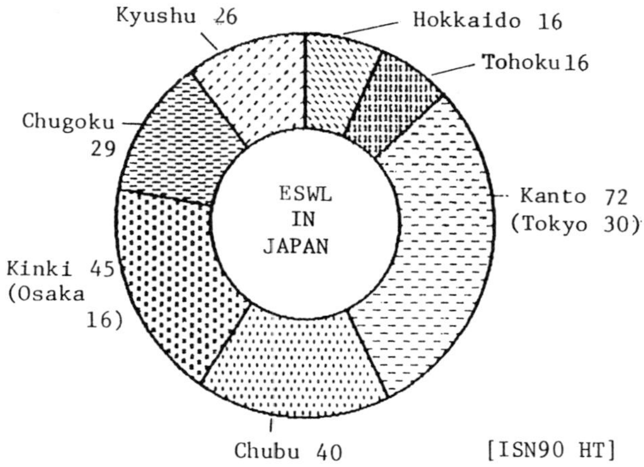

Fig. 1. Regional distribution of ESWL (June 1990)

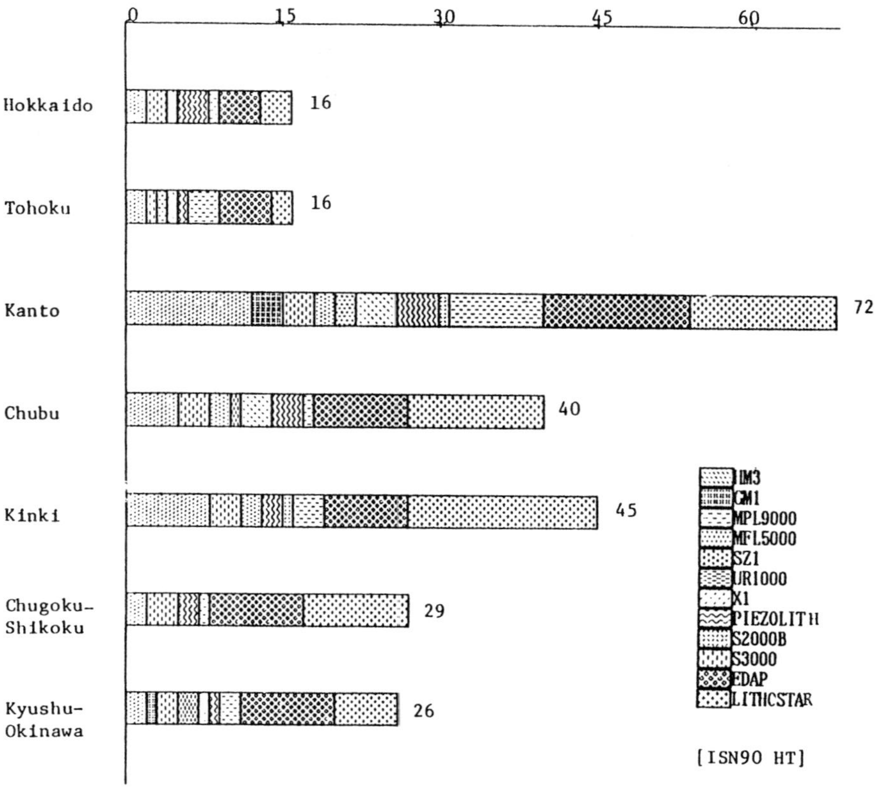

Fig. 2. Regional distribution of ESWL in Japan (June 1990)

Table 1. ESWL distribution and regional population

	Number of ESWL	Population (million)	Ratio (1: $\times 10^3$)
Hokkaido	16	5.6	350
Tohoku	16	9.8	610
Kanto	72	35.6	490
(Tokyo)	(30)	(11.5)	(380)
Chubu	40	20.3	510
Kinki	45	21.4	480
(Osaka)	(16)	(8.4)	(520)
Chugoku-Shikoku	29	12.0	410
Kyushu-Okinawa	26	14.3	550
	244	120.0	350–610

other countries, and so far on simple single stones in the renal pelvis the success rate has been shown to be nearly 90%. Some of these reports are summarized as follows:

HM3

The most significant report on the results of clinical investigation using HM3 was published by Higashihara et al. in the *Journal of Endourology and ESWL* in 1988 [1]. The study summarized 3702 cases treated with HM3 at 11 hospitals in Japan. Of these, 93% were treated by ESWL monotherapy; 7% of the cases required additional therapies such as percutaneous nephrolithotripsy (PNL), percutaneous nephrostomy (PCN), and transurethral ureterolithotripsy (TUL); the incidence of these therapies was 50%, 21% and 29%, respectively (Fig. 3). At 6 month follow-up in the same study residual fragments of 4mm or less were seen in 17% of cases; fragments over 4mm in size were seen in 4% of cases; however, 79% of cases were free of residual

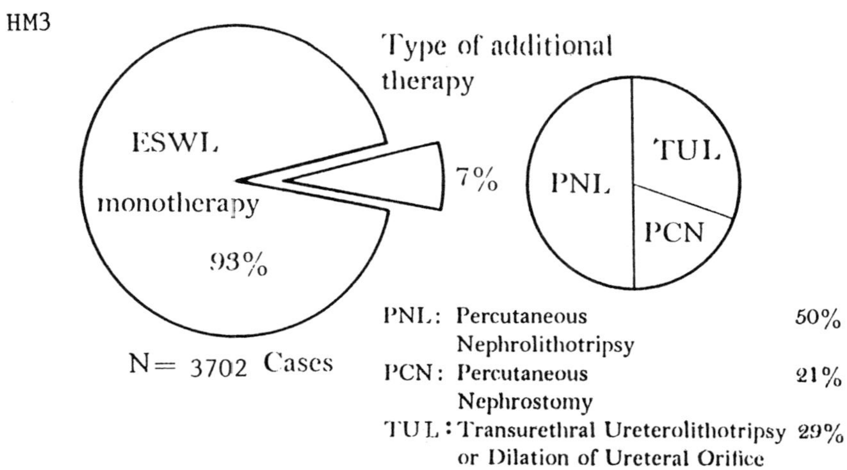

Fig. 3. Type of additional therapy. (From [1])

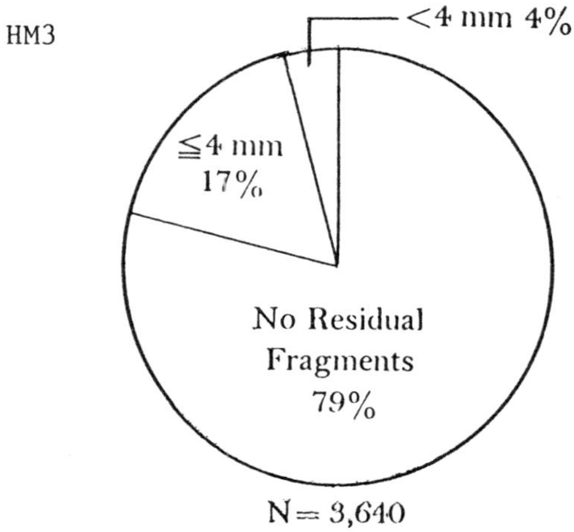

Fig. 4. Residual fragments at 6-month follow-up. (From [1])

fragments (Fig. 4). More reports on staghorn stones and complicated cases have been seen in 1989–1990, which have fairly good results using combinations of various endourological techniques.

Lithostar

Konishi et al. [2] reported their experience of 323 cases treated with the electromagnetic lithotripter, Lithostar, in 1988 and 1989. The study included 123 cases (35.1%) of upper ureteral stones (Table 2); good results were achieved. Many other reports have described the advantages to be gained with this ESWL machine.

Piezolith

Our experience with 183 cases, [3] using the piezoelectric type lithotripter, Piezolith 2200, at Keio University Hospital are shown in Tables 3 and 4. A great advantage of using this ESWL machine that it is anesthesia free; none of these 183 patients

Table 2. Lithostar

Number of cases	323 cases
Male:female	227:96
Age	13 ~ 89 (mean 49.6)
Stone location	
Kidney	111 (31.6%)
Upper ureter	123 (35.1%)
Middle ureter	39 (11.1%)
Lower ureter	70 (19.9%)
Bladder	8 (2.3%)

(From [2])

Table 3. Keio University Hospital, Tokyo Piezolith 117 cases in 1989

Location	No. of stones evaluated	Largest diameter (mm)
Pelvis and calyx	39	15.5±6.5
Calyx	103	8.4±5.4
UPJ	11	11.2±4.1
Upper ureter	7	9.0±3.2
Ureter:Pelvis (flush up)	23	7.8±2.3
Total	183	9.3±5.8

(From [3])

required even pretreatment sedation. Ultrasonographic imaging for focusing is good, but in cases with small stones focusing is difficult, especially in the ureter.

Other Studies and Complications

Experience with EDAP LT01, Sonolith 2000B, and other machines has been reported. Yachiyoda SZ1 is a Japanese made ESWL, using microexplosives for its energy source of shock waves; its characteristics are shown in Table 5. The results of the study described by Honda et al. in 1988 [4] indicate that, because of its lower residual stone rates, this ESWL machine has greater power to disintegrate stones with microexplosives.

Complications have been reported. Subcapsular hematomas, endotoxin shock and possibilities of hypertension have been reported following the therapy. From our experience with Piezolith, temporary elevation of plasma renin activity has been described by Baba et al. [3]; however, this may not indicate persistent hypertension so much as late complications; also, it is not specific to the piezoelectric system.

Socioeconomic Background of ESWL

In the early stages of the introduction of ESWL to Japan nobody could have predicted that this new therapeutic modality would take over from traditional treatments within 5 years. Apparently the government was so interested in new trends that reconsidera-

Table 4. Keio University Hospital, Tokyo Piezolith 117 cases in 1989

	Stone Size 3 Months after Tx.		
Stone free	<3mm	3~5mm	>5mm
66.7%	11.1%	7.4%	14.8%
67.0%	13.9%	2.6%	5.2%
81.8%	9.1%	9.1%	0%
85.7%	0%	14.3%	0%
95.7%	4.3%	0%	0%
73.8%	12.8%	3.7%	7.5%

(From [3])

Table 5. Characteristics of microexplosive ESWL

	Characteristics
• Energy source	Microexplosion (10 mg silver azide)
• Focus	X-rays
• Target	Moving the chair by computer control
• Coupling	Water bath
• Patient's position	Sitting
• Anesthesia	Not required
• Clinical results	Satisfactory (almost equivalent to conventional ESWL)
• Complications	Not severe (almost comparable with conventional ESWL)
• Cost of construction	Not expensive

(From [4])

tion of the socialized medical care system resulted in the formation of a new system called "High Technology Medicare" in 1985. However, ESWL and endourology were excluded from the system and the government set the treatment cost at the lowest level of 20000 points per treatment. This resulted in the installation of low running cost machines becoming preferable.

On the other hand, private insurance for stone disease can cover most expenses. As the aged population increases, those patients are not covered for a 100% increase and they must go to a local doctor for conventional therapy. The distribution of ESWL machines is greater in large cities and is still inadequate. Endourology is established in this country, but people wish to have totally non-invasive therapy, as they do in other countries. Other problems occurring coincidentally such as gall bladder stones can be treated. Most surgeons still like open surgery, but patients like less invasiveness. Organization in society is needed to promote ESWL and exclude endourology in the near future. As the machines become more sophisticated the cost per treatment becomes higher; new types of ESWL will replace old models.

Conclusion and the Remarks on the Future

Introducing ESWL to Japan was a culture shock. The shock continued for the next 5 years. At present the status of this therapy is in an early stage of recovery. The recovery must be complete with no scar remaining. The coming era will see the replacement of the 1st and 2nd generation machines by Japanese-made machines. It will be done serenely and peacefully.

References

1. Higashihara E (1988) Jpn J Endourol ESWL 1:24–25
2. Konishi T et al. (1989) Jpn J Endourol ESWL 2:105–109
3. Baba S et al. (1989) Jpn J Endourol ESWL 2:114–120
4. Honda M et al. (1988) Jpn J Endourol ESWL 1:28–29

New Drugs to Prevent Recurrence of Renal Stone Disease

Bo G. Danielson, B. Fellström, M. Lindsjö, S. Ljunghall, and B. Wikström[1]

SUMMARY. Many patients who are stone formers have recurrent stone formation, for which detailed clinical and biochemical work-up is necessary. Even if conventional treatments with thiazides, orthophosphate, or magnesium or potassium citrate are effective in many stone formers, their use may be limited by their way of acting or by their side effects. This is particularly the case in patients with increased urinary oxalate excretion.

Therefore, during recent years, two new approaches have been tried. Since it is known that glycosaminoglycans are potent inhibitors of calcium oxalate crystal growth, aggregation, and possibly also crystal adherence to the walls of the urinary tract, a pentosan polysulfate (PPS), has been tried as a prophylactic treatment in stone formers. Of the patients on PPS treatment 75% were free of recurrences, despite severe stone disease with previous frequent recurrences. Another 10% of the patients experienced considerable reduction in the frequency of the stone episodes.

In patients with enteric hyperoxaluria and severe stone disease, treatment with an organic marine hydrocolloid (OMH)—trade name Ox—absorb—was used to reduce gastrointestinal oxalate absorption. The OMH was shown to bind oxalate in vitro, and to reduce urinary oxalate by oxalate binding in the gut. It was very well tolerated, improved bowel function, showed promising effects on stone episode rate, and had very few side effects.

Introduction

During recent years less interest has been focused on basic mechanisms of stone formation and prophylactic treatment than on extracorporeal shock wave lithotripsy (ESWL) treatment and its consequences.

---

[1]Department of Internal Medicine, University Hospital, S-751 85 Uppsala, Sweden

However, there are many patients with severe stone disease, with frequent recurrences where repeated shock-wave treatment is less suitable and where prophylactic medical treatment is more advisable. Even if ESWL may be the easiest way to treat the stone former when he or she presents with a stone, the strategy for long-term treatment has to be considered. Therefore a clinical and metabolic work up of the recurrent stone former is essential.

Renal stone formation is basically a consequence of an imbalance between supersaturation of the urine and the inhibition of crystal formation, growth and aggregation [1]. Urine contains many substances which are claimed to modify the rate of crystallization of calcium oxalate and calcium phosphate.

Increased renal excretion of calcium, oxalate, and phosphate contributes to an increased risk of stone formation. The risk can be influenced by the presence of various promoters of nucleation, growth, and aggregation which could contribute to matrix formation and also to epitaxial growth.

However, the urine also contains many substances which inhibit crystal formation through one or two possible mechanisms. Firstly, they may act by complexing either calcium or oxalate ions, thereby reducing the level of calcium oxalate and calcium phosphate supersaturation in the crystallizing solution. Of the urinary inhibitors, citrate and magnesium fall into this group. The other group of inhibitors acts at relatively low concentrations by adsorbing to the surface of the crystals, thereby retarding the rate of crystal growth and agglomeration. Among this group could be mentioned pyrophosphate, heparinoids or glycosaminoglycans (GAGs) like chondroitin sulfate, heparin, heparan sulfate, dermatane sulfate, nephrocalcin, and Tamm-Horsefall mucopolysaccharide. Glycosaminoglycans including chondroitin sulfate, heparin sulfate, keratan sulfate and dermatane sulfate are naturally occurring in human urine. Heparin, however, is not excreted in human urine. It has been shown previously in experimental work that the inhibitor potential of GAGs is dependent on the degree of sulfation and that the inhibitor effect takes place because of reversible binding of the GAGs to the crystal surface, whereby further crystal growth and aggregation become blocked. Experimental studies have also included a pentosan polysulfate (PPS), which has been used for clinical trials in the treatment of urolithiasis.

In Vitro Study of PPS

The inhibition of calcium oxalate crystal growth was investigated by seeded crystal procedure, whereby seeded crystals of calcium oxalate were added to metastable calcium oxalate solution together with the inhibitor to be studied. The inhibition of calcium oxalate crystal growth by polyanionic GAGs, Tamm-Horsefall glycoprotein, and pyrophosphate was compared [2]. Using the same system, PPS was also added in order to compare the inhibitory effect. On a concentration basis pyrophosphate was found to be the most inefficient inhibitor tested. Among the polyanions, heparin was the most effective inhibitor, whereas chondroitin sulfate exerted about 40% of the inhibitory activity of heparin. The inhibitory effect of PPS was about 80% of the inhibitory activity found for heparin. The inhibition was directly proportional to the logarithm of the concentration of the polyanions.

In order to investigate the mechanism of inhibition, experiments were performed with radioactive-labeled heparin, chondroitin sulfate, and pentosan polysulfate, binding to calcium oxalate crystals; subsequent displacements were induced by increasing the amounts of non-radioactive ligands or by increasing ionic strength. It was then found that ligands with a high charge density bound more readily and with a seemingly higher affinity than ligands with a low charge density, but the former were also more suspectible to displacement when the ionic strength was increased [3]. It could be concluded that the higher affinity of the crystals may be the reason why highly charged glycosaminoglycans are more efficient inhibitors of calcium oxalate crystal growth.

Pharmacokinetic Studies of PPS

Following intravenous injection of PPS the plasma curve could be described by an exponential decline, indicating a two-compartment distribution [4]. The distribution half-life was 25 min for the first compartment and the plasma half-life, i.e., elimination phase, was 24 h. Renal clearance was about 4 ml/min and the renal excretion of unchanged PPS was 8%–10%.

When tritium-labeled PPS was given orally to healthy volunteers, about 3% of the given dose appeared unchanged in the urine, which is significantly more than the amount found using unlabeled PPS.

The distribution of PPS has also been studied using autoradiographic techniques, where it was found that PPS could be observed in the urinary tract, urinary bladder, the pelvis of the kidney, and in the urethra.

Clinical Results with PPS as Prophylactic Treatment

With these experimental and pharmacokinetic data as background, a clinical trial was started where PPS was evaluated as a prophylactic agent in renal calcium stone disease [5]. One hundred patients with recurrent renal calcium stones were the subjects; PPS treatment was given at a dose of 400 mg/day. The drug was given in the form of capsules two hours after meals. When the results were evaluated, patients who had been on the treatment for more than 12 months were included. The average follow-up time was nearly 3 years (12–56 months). The patients were 66 males and 34 females with a mean age of 47 years. The duration of the stone disease was 15 ± 10 years with the range between 1 and 43 years. Six patients had experienced more than 50 stones each and, when these were excluded, the average number of total stone episodes was 11 ± 9 stones, or 1.3 stones/year. About half of the patients had had surgical intervention because of stones. Each of the patients had had an average of 1.8 operations.

Of the 100 patients, 76 patients were free of recurrences. Of the 96 patients who were evaluated, 20 formed new stones during the main treatment time of 22 months. Four of these 20 patients had enteric disorders, one patient had celiac disease, and three had regional enteritis. One patient acquired a urinary tract infection caused by *Proteus*. Eight of the other 15 patients had fewer and smaller stones than before treatment.

Of the 100 patients initially included in the study, 16 patients were withdrawn because of side effects or other concomitant events. Nine of the patients had nausea, diarrhea, and other related gastrointestinal problems, their susceptibility perhaps related in part to a history of previous ulcers or gastritis found in many of them. Two patients were withdrawn because of pregnancy, one had a myocardial infarction, one died of intercurrent disease, one had eczema (probably not related to PPS), and two patients with regional enteritis and severe stone disease which continued were withdrawn.

The excretion of urinary electrolytes such as calcium, oxalate, magnesium, urate and citrate was not altered in response to treatment.

It could be concluded that the experimental and clinical results favoured the concept of PPS as a potent inhibitor of calcium oxalate crystal growth. The clinical results showed that about 75% of the patients who had been on treatment for more than 12 months had been free of recurrences of stone production and another 10% of the patients were improved.

However, gastrointestinal side effects may occur, particularly in patients with a history of enteric disease. Special attention has therefore to be focussed on how the drug is administered, in order to reduce the gastrointestinal side effects. A lower effective dose and administration of the drug together with meals could help to reduce adverse reactions. However, in patients with inflammatory or intestinal bowel disease the risk that the uptake of the drug may be reduced has to be considered. From the clinical results it seems that pentosan polysulfate inhibits calcium oxalate growth and may also inhibit stone formation by preventing microcrystal adherence to the wall of the urinary tract.

Treatment of Patients with Enteric Hyperoxaluria and Renal Stones

Calcium oxalate is the main constituent of most renal stones. Urinary oxalate is of great significance for stone formation, since even a small increase of urinary oxalate concentration exerts a great influence on the degree of urinary saturation. A group with often severe kidney stone disease are those patients with enteric hyperoxaluria due to gastrointestinal disorders, i.e., inflammatory bowel disease. (For a review, see [6]).

Oxalate is basically a non-essential metabolic end product in man. Under normal circumstances about 90% of urinary oxalate is derived from endogenous oxalate and only 10% from exogenous oxalate in the diet. Ascorbate and glyoxalate are the main precursors of oxalate, each contributing 30%–50% to urinary oxalate. The gastrointestinal absorption of oxalate is mainly a passive diffusion process, which takes place in the entire intestine. More than half of the dietary oxalate in man is decomposed by bacteria in the large intestine.

The intestinal absorption of oxalate in healthy subjects is in the range of 5%–14%, dependent on the amounts given and whether the subjects were fasting or not. A substantial decrease in urinary oxalate excretion occurs during a low oxalate diet, not only in patients with enteric hyperoxaluria, but also in healthy individuals. The uptake of oxalate is also known to be influenced by various dietary components, such as calcium, but magnesium, iron, trace metals, fatty acids, bile salts, and perhaps fibers can also influence the absorption. Binding of oxalate to calcium in the gut lowers the concentration of free oxalate and reduces the oxalate uptake. Conversely oxalate absorption increases when calcium is restricted. Intraluminal fatty acids bind calcium, which will reduce the amount of calcium available for binding of oxalate. Bile salts may increase the absorption of oxalate in the colon by altering mucosa permeability. It has also been suggested that fibers and fatty acids might affect oxalate absorption, mainly by binding to calcium, leaving more oxalate available for absorption.

In contrast to healthy subjects, where the fractional gastrointestinal oxalate absorption is in the range of 5%–10%, idiopathic stone formers may have moderately increased oxalate absorption of up to 15%, but patients with enteric hyperoxaluria caused by, e.g., regional enteritis, celiac disease, or intestinal bypass operations could have significantly increased absorption of oxalate—up to 60% of the ingested oxalate.

Urinary oxalate intake in the ordinary western diet is less than 500 μmol/24 h. In various groups of idiopathic stone formers a moderately increased urinary oxalate excretion could be found, up in the range of 400–600 μmol/24 h.

A diagnosis called mild metabolic hyperoxaluria has been suggested, where typical findings for oxalate excretion are in the range of 500–800 μmol/24 h, in combination with renal calcium stone formation and a raised urinary glycolate concentration, indicating a metabolic and not absorptive cause of hyperoxaluria. Some of these patients have been reported to have responded to pyridoxine treatment.

In patients with enteric hyperoxaluria increased urinary oxalate, in the range of 600–1200 μmol/24 h, is found. This disease is often complicated with severe renal stone disease and is due to gastrointestinal disorders, i.e., inflammatory bowel disease, celiac disease, and pancreatic insufficiency. In some patients the increased oxalate excretion is due to previous surgical intervention, e.g., small bowel resection or jejunoileal bypass operations, done for example, because of obesity. The origin of the increased urinary oxalate in patients with enteric hyperoxaluria is the diet.

This group of patients also has fat malabsorption; a strong correlation between urinary oxalate and degree of steatorrhea has been found. Non-absorbed fatty acids form soaps with interluminal calcium, which leaves unbound oxalate available for absorption. In addition, non-absorbed fatty acids and bile acids in the colon are supposed to increase colonic permeability to oxalate. In healthy subjects oxalate absorption takes place along the entire gastrointestinal tract, but in patients with enteric hyperoxaluria, increased oxalate absorption is due to increased absorption in the colon. In patients with ileostomy no hyperoxaluria has been observed.

A particular group of patients are those who have undergone jejunoileal bypass operations because of obesity. They have an increased risk of renal stone formation and also an increased risk of interstitial nephritis with renal failure, probably due to renal tubular dysfunction and renal tubular acidosis. They often have low excretion of citrate and magnesium, but high oxalate excretion.

Treatment of Hyperoxaluria

The contribution of the diet to hyperoxaluria may be reduced by dietary measures. A logical approach to treatment of enteric hyperoxaluria is to avoid oxalate-rich foodstuffs. A low fat diet has been shown to further reduce urinary oxalate. Binding of the oxalate in the gut seems logical; aluminum or cholestyramin have been used for this purpose, but have not always been successful. Cholestyramin may also bind bile salts and fatty acids and could then reduce the effect of the increased colonic permeability for calcium.

Calcium supplementation has been reported to reduce urinary oxalate by binding oxalate in the gut. However, there is a risk of increased calcium absorption and increase of urinary calcium, which may counteract the binding of the oxalate in the gut. Magnesium therapy can result in an increase of both urinary magnesium and citrate, which may be beneficial, but it may cause further deterioration of bowel function. Potassium citrate, by complexing calcium, has also been reported to have favourable clinical effects on patients with low citrate excretion, but may be of disadvantage in patients with hyperoxaluria. Orthophosphate has also been used in stone patients with primary hyperoxaluria and has been shown to have a beneficial effect on the stone recurrence rate in patients with primary and mild metabolic hyperoxaluria. Pyridoxine deficiency may occasionally be a cause of hyperoxaluria; pyridoxine treatment could be of value in patients with primary hyperoxaluria, but is probably not of any value in patients with enteric hyperoxaluria.

Reduction of Gastrointestinal Oxalate Absorption with OMH

In patients with enteric hyperoxaluria a markedly increased gastrointestinal absorption of oxalate leads to high urinary oxalate excretion. One approach to therapy might therefore be to reduce the gastrointestinal uptake of oxalate by binding dietary oxalate in the gut. In the present study an organic marine hydrocolloid (OMH) used in the treatment of enteric hyperoxaluria was investigated [7]. This group of substances consist of polymers of high molecular weight, derived from alginates and carrageenans extracted from plants and seaweeds. The OMH (Ox-Absorb, Vitaline, Ashland, Oregon, USA) used for this purpose was specially processed and charged with calcium and zinc. It can be formulated as tablets or capsules. In this case each 1 g tablet contained 100 mg calcium and 1.2 mg of zinc. The OxAbsorb was given 3 tabl t.i.d. with meals. This group of substances have no toxic properties and are also licensed as food additives. They also have the capacity to increase water binding, which might be of beneficial effect to soften and enlarge patients' stools. This hydrocolloid was investigated with respect to its capacity to bind oxalate, its effect on oxalate excretion, and also its effect on crystal inhibition in recurrent stone formers with hyperoxaluria.

In Vitro Binding Experiments with OMH

Binding of oxalate to OMH was studied in vitro by incubation of the substance with sodium oxalate at different pH. For measurements of the oxalate binding ^{14}C-oxalate was used. The results showed that a maximum binding of 3.4 mmol of oxalate/g OMH was achieved.

Patient Studies with OMH

Patients with recurrent renal stone formation and hyperoxaluria due to jejunoileal bypass or MbCrohn with ileal resection were included in two studies, namely a *short-*

term (two-week pilot study where 5 females and 4 males, mean age 46 years, as well as one patient with ulcerative colitis and ileostomy with normal urinary oxalate excretion were included) and a *long-term study* (six months, where 18 females and 2 males, mean age 41 years, range 22–63 years, were included). The main purpose of these two studies was to measure the urinary oxalate excretion during short- and long-term treatment, respectively. In the two-week pilot study there was a significant reduction of the 24-hour urinary oxalate excretion with a mean reduction of 133 ± 92 μmol/24 h. There was no difference in the excretion of electrolytes such as calcium, magnesium, phosphate, or urate. During the long-term study urinary oxalate excretion was also significantly reduced.

A simple estimate of the ionic product for calcium oxalate (AP_{CaOx}) was calculated on each 24 h collection of the patients who participated in the long-term study. The activity product index decreased significantly despite a moderate increase of urinary calcium excreted on treatment. The activity product index decreased in 8 of the 10 patients included in the study. Even if the studies were too short to evaluate the stone episode rate, it was found, in addition to biochemical effects, that 7 of the 10 patients with diarrhea reported considerable improvement in bowel function. Although OMH is capable of binding water and swelling, the marked clinical improvement may also have been due to the binding of free fatty acids in the bowel. The patient studies referred to here do not permit any evaluation with respect to the effects of treatment on the long-term risk of stone formation. However, in a few patients who have been on treatment for up to 5 years, there has been a prompt reduction of stone formation, which encourages further clinical trials with this group of substances.

Conclusions

It can therefore be concluded that patients with enteric hyperoxaluria often have severe kidney stone disease. It has been shown that OMH (Ox-Absorb) binds oxalate in vitro. Treatment with this marine hydrocolloid, in patients with enteric hyperoxaluria, resulted in reduced gastrointestinal absorption and urinary excretion of oxalate, often with drastic improvement of diarrheas. In the few patients treated so far on a long-term basis, substantial reduction in stone formation was achieved.

References

1. Robertson WG, Hughes H, Barkworth SA, Walker VR (1988) Competition between the known inhibitors and promoters of calcium oxalate crystallization in urine. In: Martelli A, Buli P, Marchesini B (eds) Inhibitors of Crystallization in Renal Lithiasis and their Clinical Application. Acta Medica, Bologna, pp 193–195
2. Fellström B, Danielson BG, Ljunghall S, Wikström B (1986) Crystal inhibition: the effects of polyanions on calcium oxalate crystal growth. Clin Chim Acta 158:229–235
3. Fellström B, Lindsjö M, Danielson BG, Karlsson FA, Ljunghall S (1989) Binding of glycosaminoglycan inhibitors to calcium oxalate crystals in relation to ionic strength. Clin Chim Acta 3:213–220
4. Fellström B, Björklund U, Danielson BG, Eriksson H, Odlind B, Tengblad A (1986) Pentosan polysulphate (Elmiron): pharmacokinetics and effects on the urinary inhibition of crystal growth. Fortschr Urol Nephrol 25:340–344

5. Danielson BG, Fellström B, Wikström B (1989) Glycosamino-glycans as inhibitors of renal stone formation. In: Walker VR, Sutton RAL, Cameron ECB, Pak CYC, Robertson WG (eds) Urolithiasis. Plenum, New York, pp 101–104
6. Lindsjö M (1989) Oxalate metabolism in renal stone disease. Scand J Urol Nephrol [Suppl] 119:1–54
7. Lindsjö M, Fellström B, Ljunghall S, Wikström B, Danielson BG (1989) Treatment of enteric hyperoxaluria with a calcium containing organic marine hydrocolloid. Lancet II:701–704

Molecular Action of Diuretics

Chair: Neil A. Kurtzman (USA)
Yoshimasa Orita (Japan)

The Mode of Action of Diuretics

E. LOHRMANN[1], R.B. NITSCHKE[1], R. NITSCHKE[1], I. BURHOFF[1], B. MASEREEL[2], B. PIROTTE[2], E. SCHLATTER[1], J. DELARGE[2], H.J. LANG[3], H.C. ENGLERT[3], M. SALOMONSSON[4], A.E.G. PERSSON[4], O. EIDELMAN[5], Z.I. CABANTCHIK[5], and R. GREGER[1]

SUMMARY. This review will address several recent findings regarding the interaction of so called loop diuretics of the furosemide type with the $Na^+2Cl^-K^+$ cotransporter in the thick ascending limb of the loop of Henle (TAL): (i) The organ selectivity of these transport inhibitors is caused by their secretion by the proximal tubule leading to an increase in their luminal concentration. We have examined whether probenecid, a selective inhibitor of proximal organic anion secretion, reduces the diuretic effect of known loop diuretics. We show that all compounds tested: furosemide (FUR), piretanide (PIR), bumetanide (BUM), and azosemide (AZO) lose part of their diuretic effect when administered in the presence of probenecid. (ii) Previously, we have shown that all loop diuretics of the furosemide type require an acidic group for binding to the $Na^+2Cl^-K^+$ cotransporter. This is a carboxylate group in the case of FUR, PIR, and BUM; a tetrazolic acid group in the case of AZO; and a sulfonylurea group in the case of torasemide (TOR). Now we show that TOR-derivates with an even less acidic sulfonylurea group ($pK_a > 8$) are still very potent inhibitors of the $Na^+2Cl^-K^+$ cotransporter. Experiments at various pH values indicate that, even for these substances, it is only the anionic form which inhibits the $Na^+2Cl^-K^+$ cotransporter. (iii) Most of the loop diuretics, with the exception of TOR, are rather hydrophilic (FUR, PIR, BUM, AZO). Now we have examined whether one can design compounds which sustain their inhibitory effect on the $Na^+2Cl^-K^+$ cotransporter, although they are highly lipophilic. We found that cyclo-alkyl substitutions at the tolyl- and sulfonylurea-moieties of TOR led to highly lipophilic compounds with very high affinity for the $Na^+2Cl^-K^+$ cotransporter. (iv) Previous data suggested that loop diuretics bind to the $Na^+2Cl^-K^+$ cotransporter at the extracellular side of the

[1]Albert-Ludwigs-Universität, Freiburg, Federal Republic of Germany
[2]Institut de Pharmacie, Université de Liège, Belgium
[3]Hoechst Pharma, Frankfurt/Main, Federal Republic of Germany
[4]Department of Physiology and Biophysics, University of Lund, Sweden
[5]Department of Biological Chemistry, Hebrew University, Jerusalem, Israel

luminal membrane. Now we have designed impermeable macromolecular derivatives of PIR and we show that these macromolecular probes inhibit the $Na^+2Cl^-K^+$ cotransporter as well as PIR. (v) Previous data indicated that loop diuretics interrupt the macula densa feedback mechanism, and circumstantial evidence suggested that the uptake of Cl^- and/or Na^+ by macula densa cells may occur via the $Na^+2Cl^-K^+$ cotransporter. Now we show that macula densa cells sense the luminal NaCl concentration via FUR sensitive $Na^+2Cl^-K^+$ cotransport.

The Mode of Action of Loop Diuretics

Loop diuretics bind to the $Na^+2Cl^-K^+$ cotransporter of the thick ascending limb (TAL) of the loop of Henle [1,2] and inhibit the coupled uptake of all participating ions. This effect is instantaneous and easily reversible. The inhibition of Na^+ influx reduces the requirement to remove Na^+ from the cell via $(Na^+ + K^+)$-ATPase, and thus reduces the ATP [3,4] and O_2 consumption of TAL cells [5]. Hence this nephron segment is protected against hypoxic or ischemic damage [6]. From studies with a large number of derivatives [7–10] we have some understanding of the molecular requirements for interaction of a compound with the $Na^+2Cl^-K^+$ cotransporter. Figure 1 shows several loop diuretics: furosemide (FUR), piretanide (PIR), bumetanide (BUM), azosemide (AZO), and torasemide (TOR), and gives the concentrations for the half maximal inhibition (IC_{50}) of active NaCl reabsorption in the rabbit cortical thick ascending limb of the loop of Henle (cTAL). It is important to note that all these molecules have several properties in common: (1) All substances are more or less acidic. The pK_a-values of the -COOH group (FUR, PIR, BUM) are around 4, the value for the tetrazolic group (AZO) is around 5, and that for the sulfonylurea (TOR) is around 7. (2) All substances except TOR possess a sulfonamide group. In the case of TOR, the nitrogen of the pyrimidine ring, probably serves the same function [11]. (3) All substances possess a secondary or tertiary amine, and (4) all have apolar residue. Still, most of these substances, except for TOR, are rather hydrophilic.

In the following paper we will address, on the basis of recent findings from our laboratories, a few loosely related questions regarding (1) the secretion of loop diuretics by the proximal tubule and the inhibition of this secretion by probenecid, (2) the relevance of the acidic moiety of loop diuretics, (3) the lipophilicity of loop diuretics, (4) the site of interaction of loop diuretics with the TAL, and (5) the effect of FUR on macula densa cells.

Secretion by the Proximal Tubule, a Prerequisite for the Inhibitory Effect of Loop Diuretics

It has recently been shown [12] that loop diuretics are secreted by the proximal tubule via basolateral uptake through the so-called PAH-system. This prompted us to ask whether the secretion of all used loop diuretics is equally sensitive towards an inhibitor of basolateral anion uptake, namely, probenecid [13]. This question could be clinically relevant because it cannot be anticipated that proximal secretion of all loop diuretics would be equally affected by other organic acids such as probenecid.

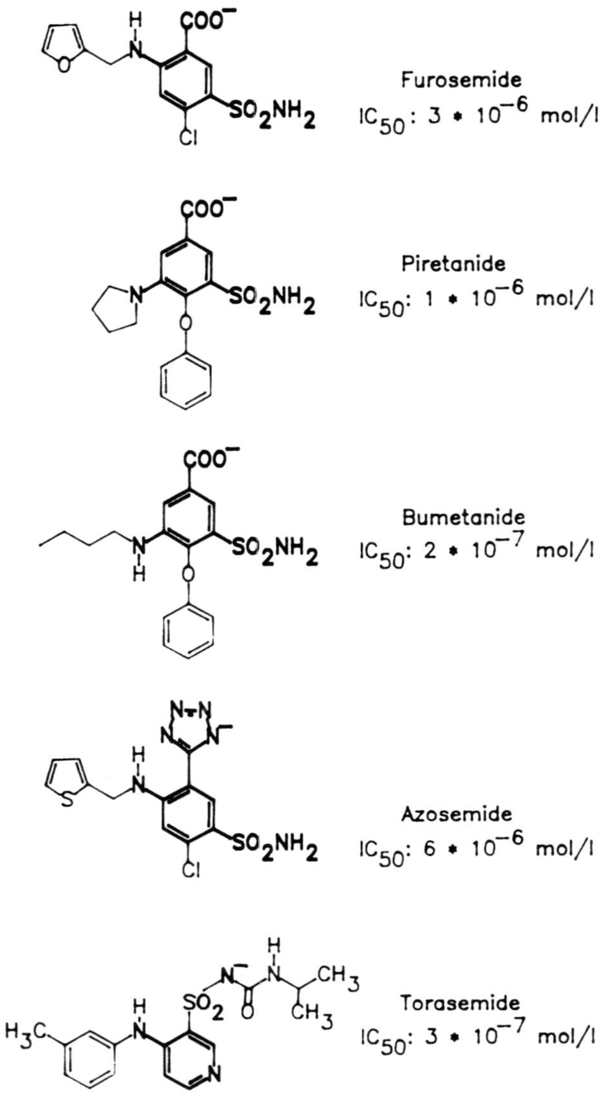

Fig. 1. Chemical structures of diuretics and the concentrations required for half maximal inhibition of equivalent short circuit current (IC_{50} values) in isolated in vitro perfused rabbit thick ascending limbs of Henle's loop

Figure 2 summarizes the results from rat clearance experiments for PIR, BUM, FUR, and AZO. It is evident that comparable diuretic responses to any of these diuretics were almost equally attenuated by increasing doses of probenecid. These findings indicate: (1) The secretion of all these loop diuretics is highly relevant for their effect in the TAL segment. The increase in luminal concentration by secretion

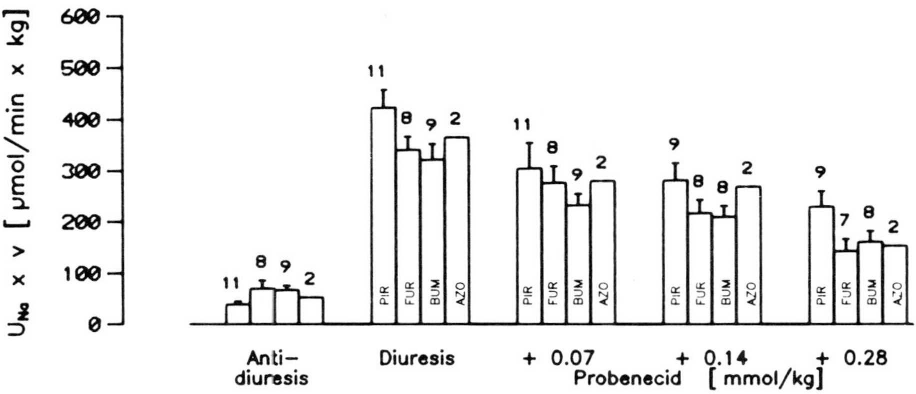

Fig. 2. Rat clearance experiments. Urinary Na^+ (U_{Na}) excretion is given for the control period, after the respective diuretic, and after additional application of probenecid. Note that probenecid attenuates the natriuretic response equally well for all diuretics used. Attenuation of the diuretic response to FUR, furosemide, 90 μmol/kg prime and same dose over one hour; PIR, piretanide, 17 μmol/kg and same dose over one hour; BUM, bumetanide, 27 μmol/kg and same dose over one hour; and AZO, azosemide, 90 μmol/kg and same dose over one hour, by increasing doses of probenecid (0.07–0.28 mmol/kg)

and by water reabsorption is the only cause for the organ selectivity of these drugs. In fact, the $Na^+2Cl^-K^+$ cotransporter is present in many cells of the body, and its sensitivity towards loop diuretics appears to be similar in all these cells [2,14]. (2) None of the diuretics tested has any detectable advantage over the others, i.e., a comparable diuretic effect is attenuated in a comparable way by probenecid, irrespective of the diuretic used. This finding is surprising, since the doses of the diuretics used were quite different: 17 μmol/kg of PIR, 27 μmol/kg of BUM, 90 μmol/kg of FUR and AZO. The finding may be explained by the presence of affinity sequences for the basolateral membrane organic anion transporter comparable to those on the $Na^+2Cl^-K^+$ cotransporter.

All Loop Diuretics Inhibit in Their Anionic Form

Previous data has suggested that all loop diuretics act in their anionic form [7]. For example, the pK_a of 3.6 for FUR predicts that some 99.9% of the total luminal concentration of FUR will be in the anionic form. On the other hand, we have found that TOR and its derivatives are also strong inhibitors of the $Na^+2Cl^-K^+$ cotransporter [8,15], but the pK_a values of these compounds are much less acidic. Recently, we examined even less acidic derivatives [16] with pK_a values as high as 9.0, and found that these substances were still strong inhibitors of the $Na^+2Cl^-K^+$ cotransporter in the rabbit cTAL segment. In the case of the compound BM 10 (cf Fig. 4), pK_a value 9.0, only 2.5% would be anionic at pH 7.4, at which pH we carried out the experiments. Rabbit cTAL segments were perfused with solutions containing 0.5 μmol/l

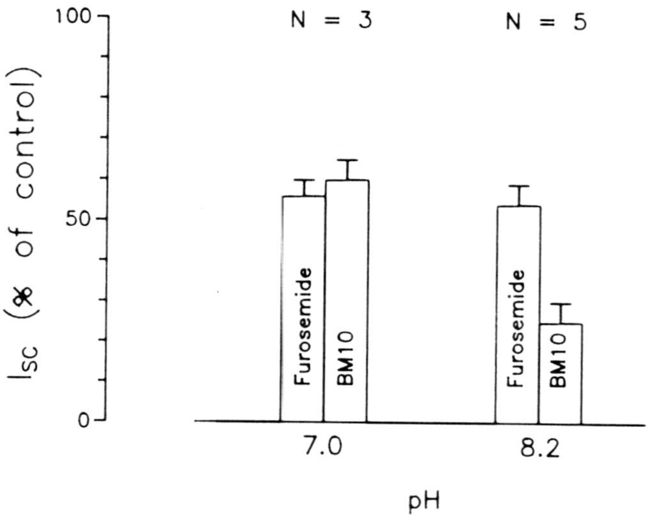

Fig. 3. pH dependence of the inhibitory effect of a sulfonylurea diuretic (BM 10, structural formula c.f. Fig. 4) in isolated perfused rabbit cTAL segments. The remaining equivalent short circuit current (I_{SC}) (in percent of control) is shown for different luminal pH values. The total concentration of BM 10 was 0.5 μmol/l at both pH values. The anionic form was 0.005 and the protonated form 0.495 μmol/l at pH 7.0, and 0.07 and 0.43 μmol/l, respectively, at pH 8.2. Note that the anionic form determines the inhibitory effect

BM 10 at various pH-values. The results are shown in Fig. 3. It is evident that the inhibitory effect is enhanced with alkaline pH. This indicates that only the anionic moiety of this compound interacts with the $Na^+2Cl^-K^+$ cotransporter. By extension, this finding implies that the IC_{50}-value for this compound, which was determined at pH 7.4, would be almost two decades lower if expressed as the concentration of the anionic moiety of this compound (IC_{50} = 12 nmol/l instead of 0.5 μmol/l).

Inhibitors of the $Na^+2Cl^-K^+$ Cotransporter can be Designed as Highly Lipophilic Compounds

Most loop diuretics are rather hydrophilic (FUR, PIR, BUM, AZO). Only TOR shows an octanol/water partition of around 3. It was tempting to examine whether one could design even more lipophilic compounds related to TOR, which would still be inhibitors of the $Na^+2Cl^-K^+$ cotransporter [16]. This effort was triggered by the hypothesis that such compounds would dissolve into a larger volume of distribution and, hence, would be excreted more slowly. Furthermore, such compounds might be able to cross the blood brain barrier more easily and have direct effects on the volume of glial cells (BM and JD unpublished work). Figure 4 shows several derivates of TOR and summarizes the pK_a values, the octanol/water partition (as log P = [octanol]/[water]), and the IC_{50} value in rabbit cTAL segments. It is evident that the

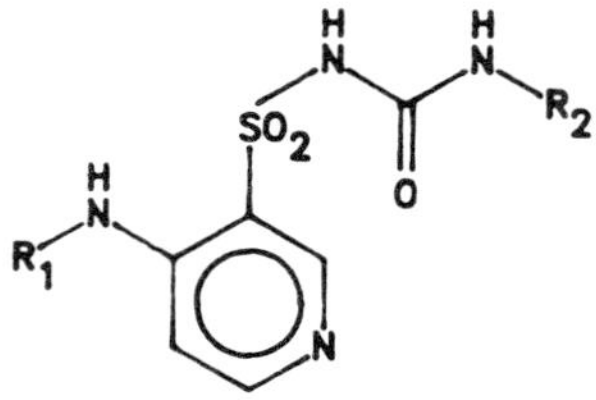

	R_1	R_2	pKa	log P	IC_{50} (umol/l)	IC_{50}^{cor}
TOR	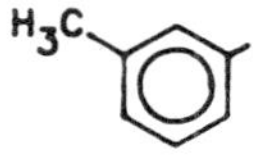	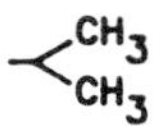	6·82	0·449	0·30	0·24
BM2	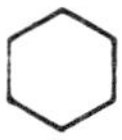	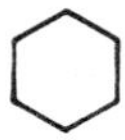	9·03	1·331	19	0·43
BM8	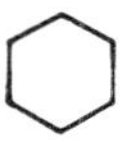	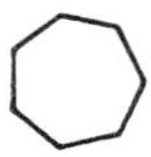	9·39	1·717	9·6	0·097
BM4	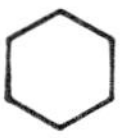	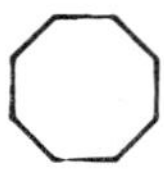	9·15	2·074	14	0·24
BM3	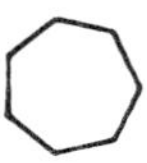	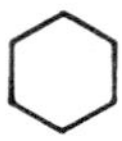	9·30	1·665	3·5	0·043
BM27	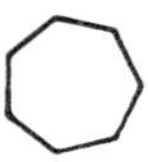	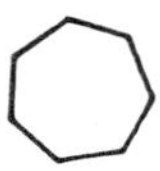	n·t·	2·062	2·8	n·t·
BM10	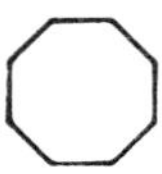	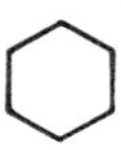	8·98	2·063	0·47	0·012
BM6	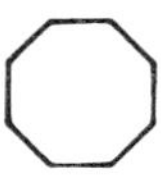	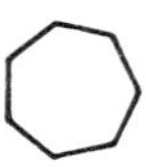	9·13	2·449	2·0	0·036
BM9	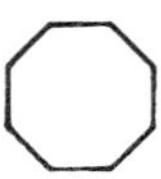	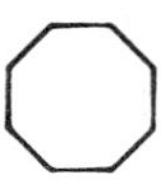	7·70	2·704	0·56	0·18

Fig. 4. Lipophilic sulfonylurea diuretic compounds. The chemical structure, the pK_a value, the log of the octanol/water partition (log P), the total luminal concentration for half maximal inhibition of equivalent short circuit current in isolated perfused rabbit cTAL segments (IC_{50} in μmol/l), and the concentration of the anionic form (IC_{50}^{cor}) are given for the individual compounds. Note that the highly lipophilic compound BM 10 has a very strong inhibitory effect R_1, radical 1; R_2, radical 2

tolyl and isopropyl residues of TOR can be replaced by cyclo-alkyls. This leads to an increase in the octanol/water partition, an increase in pK_a value, and a reduction in the IC_{50} value, indicating that these compounds have a very high affinity for the $Na^+2Cl^-K^+$ cotransporter. An optimal structure is, e.g., the compound BM 10, with apparent IC_{50} values of 0.5 μmol/l. The IC_{50} values would be even smaller if one took into account the finding above that the inhibition was caused only by the anionic moiety (IC_{50}^{cor} values in Fig. 4). We conclude that it is possible to design highly lipophilic loop diuretics which may offer some therapeutical advantages.

The Interaction with the $Na^+2Cl^-K^+$ Cotransporter in the Luminal Membrane of the cTAL Segment Occurs at an Extracellular Binding Site

Several findings have suggested that drugs like FUR need not be incorporated into the cTAL cell to exert their effect. (i) We have noted that the effect of FUR [1] and of PIR [4] was instantaneous and rapidly reversible. Inhibition occurred as rapidly as we were able to change the lumen perfusate ($\ll 1$ s), and recovery after removal of the drugs was complete within a few seconds. These findings would not be expected for a compound entering the cell. (ii) We measured the cytosolic Cl^--activity with ion selective microelectrodes in cTAL cells [17]. The used ion exchanger was several hundreds of times more sensitive for FUR when compared to Cl^-. Still, we were able to show that the apparent cytosolic Cl^--activity signal fell rapidly after the addition of furosemide. Both arguments, even though strongly suggestive, do not prove that FUR interacts at the extracellular side. Therefore, we designed macromolecular probes of piretanide, with a molecular mass of 5300 daltons, and examined their effects in rabbit cTAL segments [18]. We found that dextran as well as polyethyleneglycol macromolecules inhibited the $Na^+2Cl^-K^+$ cotransporter with IC_{50} values very similar to those for PIR. Hence, we conclude that the binding site for loop diuretics of the $Na^+2Cl^-K^+$ cotransporter is easily accessible at the extracellular side of the luminal membrane. These and other macromolecular probes of PIR are currently used to design antibodies against the $Na^+2Cl^-K^+$ carrier. When given systematically these macromolecular PIR derivatives show only a very moderate diuresis. This indicates that these substances cannot be secreted by the proximal tubule (c.f. above).

Macula Densa Cells Sense Luminal NaCl Concentration via Furosemide Sensitive $Na^+2Cl^-K^+$ Cotransport

It has been known for some time that loop diuretics inhibit the so called feedback response between macula densa cells and single nephron filtration rate [19]. Furthermore, it has been shown that the feedback response is produced by luminal Na^+ [20] or Cl^- concentration [21]. This has prompted us to examine directly whether macula densa cells possess the $Na^+2Cl^-K^+$ cotransporter. We used an electrophysiological approach to examine this question. Rabbit cTAL segments with the glomerulus and

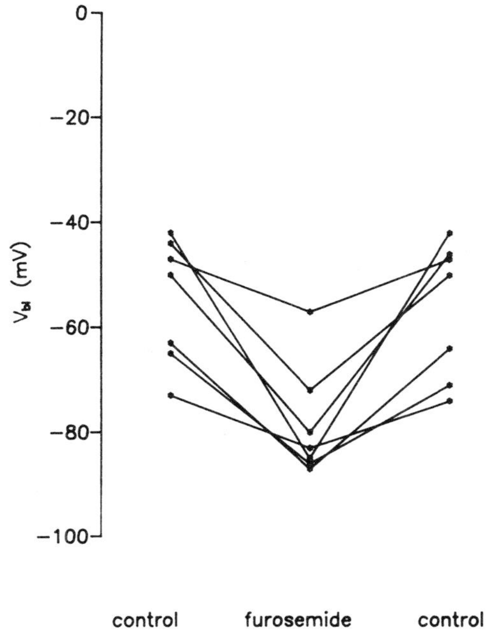

Fig. 5. Basolateral membrane voltage (V_{bl}) of macula densa cells of isolated in vitro perfused rabbit cTAL segments containing the macula densa region. Note that V_{bl} is hyperpolarized by luminal furosemide (10 μmol/l)

the macula densa segment attached were perfused in vitro and the transepithelial voltages, as well as the membrane voltage across the basolateral membrane, of macula densa cells was examined [22]. The key finding is shown in Fig. 5. The basolateral membrane voltage (V_{bl}) of macula densa cells hyperpolarized by some 14 mV when FUR was added to the luminal perfusate. Similarly, a hyperpolarization of V_{bl} was observed when the NaCl concentration in the lumen was reduced from 150 to 30 mmol/l. Examination of the conductance properties of these cells revealed that the luminal membrane was K^+-, and the basolateral membrane was Cl^--conductive [22]. All these findings are compatible with the view that the luminal membrane of macula densa cells is equipped with the $Na^+2Cl^-K^+$ cotransporter, and that the general cell model of the macula densa cells is identical to that described for the TAL segment [2,23]. It should be noted, however, that the transport rates across macula densa cells are much lower than those across the TAL segment [22]. Thus, it is likely that the $Na^+2Cl^-K^+$ carrier-mediated uptake in macula densa cells serves to sense the concentrations in the tubule lumen and to trigger a, thus far unknown, transducing mechanism which translates the cytosolic signal in macula densa cells into the response of renin producing cells.

Acknowledgments. Supported by Deutsche Forschungsgemeinschaft Gr 480/10 and by German Israeli Foundation GIF I-86-100.1/88.

References

1. Greger R, Schlatter E (1983) Cellular mechanism of the action of loop diuretics on the thick ascending limb of Henle's loop. Klin Wochenschr 61:1019–1027
2. Greger R (1985) Ion transport mechanisms in thick ascending limb of Henle's loop of mammalian nephron. Physiol Rev 65:760–797
3. Greger R (1985) Wirkung von Scheifendiuretika auf zellulärer Ebene. Nieren-Hochdruckkrankheiten 14(6):217–220
4. Greger R, Wangemann PH (1987) Loop diuretics. Renal Physiol 10:174–183
5. Eveloff J, Bayerdörffer E, Silva P, Kinne R (1981) Sodium-chloride transport in the thick ascending limb of Henle's loop. Oxygen consumption studies in isolated cells. Pflugers Arch 389:263–270
6. Brezis M, Rosen S, Silva P, Epstein FH (1984) Renal ischaemia: A new perspective. Kidney Int 26:375–383
7. Schlatter E, Greger R, Weidtke C (1983) Effect of "high ceiling" diuretics on active salt transport in the cortical thick ascending limb of Henle's loop of rabbit kidney. Correlation of chemical structure and inhibitory potency. Pflugers Arch 396:210–217
8. Wittner M, Di Stefano A, Wangemann P, Delarge J, Ligeois JF, Greger R (1987) Analogues of torasemide-structure function relationships. Experiments in the thick ascending limb of the loop of Henle of rabbit nephron. Pflugers Arch 408:54–62
9. Greger R, Lang HJ, Englert HC, Wangemann P (1987) Blockers of the $Na^+2Cl^-K^+$ carrier and of chloride channels in the thick ascending limb of the loop of Henle. In: Puschett JB (ed) Diuretics II. Elsevier, Amsterdam, pp 33–38
10. Greger R, Wangemann P, Wittner M, Di Stefano A, Lang HJ, Englert HC (1987) Blockers of active transport in the thick ascending limb of the loop of Henle. In: Andreucci VE, Dal Canton A (eds) Diuretics: Basic, pharmacological, and clinical aspects. Martinus Nijhoff, Boston, pp 33–38
11. Wangemann P, Wittner M, Di Stefano A, Englert HC, Lang HJ, Schlatter E, Greger R (1987) Cl^--channel blockers in the thick ascending limb of the loop of Henle. Structure activity relationship. Pflugers Arch 407(Suppl 2):S128–S141
12. Ullrich KJ, Rumrich G, Klöss S (1989) Contraluminal organic anion and cation transport in the proximal renal tubule: V. Interaction with sulfamoyl- and phenoxy diuretics, and with β-lactam antibiotics. Kidney Int 36:78–88
13. Braitsch R, Lohrmann E, Greger R (1990) Effect of probenecid on loop diuretic induced saluresis and diuresis. In: Puschett J (ed) Diuretics III, chemistry, pharmacology, and clinical applications. Elsevier, New York, pp 137–139
14. Greger R (1986) Chlorid-transportierende Epithelien. In: Bromm B (ed) Physiologie Aktuell, Band 2. Gustav Fischer, Stuttgart, pp 47–58
15. Wittner M, Di Stefano A, Schlatter E, Delarge J, Greger R (1986) Torasemide inhibits NaCl reabsorption in the thick ascending limb of the loop of Henle. Pflugers Arch 407:611–614
16. Lohrmann E, Masereel B, Nitschke R, Pirotte B, Delarge J, Greger R (1990) Action of diuretics at the cellular level. In: Reyes AJ (ed) Diuretics. Gustav Fischer, Stuttgart, in press
17. Greger R, Oberleithner H, Schlatter E, Cassola AC, Weidtke C (1983) Chloride activity in cells of isolated perfused cortical thick ascending limbs of rabbit kidney. Pflugers Arch 399:29–34
18. Nitschke R, Schlatter E, Eidelman O, Lang HJ, Englert HC, Cabantchik ZI, Greger R (1989) Piretanide-dextran and piretanide-polyethylene glycol interact with high affinity with the $Na^+ 2Cl^- K^+$ cotransporter in the thick ascending limb of the loop of Henle. Pflugers Arch 413:559–561

19. Wright FS, Schnermann J (1974) Interference with feedback control of glomerular filtration rate by furosemide, triflocin and cyanide. J Clin Invest 53:1695–1708
20. Thurau K, Schnermann J (1965) Die Natriumkonzentration an den Macula Densa Zellen als regulierender Faktor für das Glomerulumfiltrat (Mikropunktionsversuche). Klin Wochenschr 43:410–413
21. Schnermann J, Ploth DW, Hermle M (1976) Activation of tubuloglomerular feedback of chloride transport. Pflugers Arch 362:229–240
22. Schlatter E, Salomonsson M, Persson AEG, Greger R (1989) Macula densa cells sense luminal NaCl concentration via the furosemide sensitive Na-2Cl-K cotransporter. Pflugers Arch 414:286–290
23. Greger R, Schlatter E (1981) Presence of luminal K^+, a prerequisite for active NaCl transport in the thick ascending limb of Henle's loop of rabbit kidney. Pflugers Arch 392:92–94

Biochemical Action of Loop Diuretics

Yoshimasa Orita[1], Masaru Yamazaki[2], and Yoshifumi Fukuhara[3]

Summary. We have investigated the quantum-chemical and physico-chemical properties of hydrochlorothiazide and its related molecules. Negative charge of the 7th carbon in the benzothiadiazine ring, hydrophobicity, and van der Walls volume, play important roles in contacting the sodium chloride channel of the renal tubule. Binding of hydrochlorothiazide to erythrocytes of human and rabbit was analyzed. Three different binding sites were demonstrated. This property could contribute to the high bioavailability and long duration of mild diuretic activity of hydrochlorothiazide. Ethacrynic acid acts as both an uncoupler and an inhibitor of the electron transport system of mitochondria. These biochemical properties of ethacrynic acid might be one of the causes of its inhibition of sodium chloride transport in the thick ascending limb of Henle's loop.

Introduction

The site of action of diuretics in the nephron has been extensively studied [1,2]. The physiological basis of the mode of action of diuretics also has been explored [3,4]. But few studies on the biochemical properties of diuretics have been reported. Since physiological function is supported by biochemical reaction or process, attention should be paid to the biochemical properties of diuretics. Recently, the molecular structure of transporter and channel was clarified by molecular biological techniques [5]. The interaction of these molecules and diuretics under physico-chemical forces might be expected. The physico-chemical properties of diuretics should be explored.

---

[1]College of Biomedical Technology Osaka University, 1-1, Machikaneyama-cho, Toyonaka, 560 Japan

[2]Faculty of Pharmaceutical Science Osaka University, 1-6, Yamadaoka, Suita, 565 Japan

[3]Department of Medicine, Osaka University Medical School, 1-1-50, Fukushima, Fukushima-ku, Osaka, 553 Japan

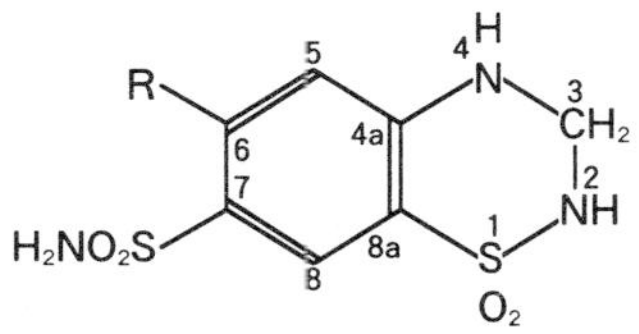

R	diuretic activity
Cl	++++
NO_2	+++
OCH_3	++
CH_3	+
F	+
NH_2	−
H	−

Fig. 1. Diuretic activity of hydrochlorothiazide and its related molecules (deStevens)

Quantum-Chemical and Physico-Chemical Properties of Hydrochlorothiazide

The chemical structure of hydrochlorothiazide and its related molecules are shown in Fig. 1 [6]. The molecular geometry of hydrochlorothiazide is cited from an X-ray crystallographic study [7]. To examine the electronic effect of the sulfamoyl group on the benzothiadiazine ring, the electronic state of imaginary molecules with substituents in the 7th carbon of the benzothiadiazine ring were also calculated. The substituents were chloride, methyl, amino, fluorine, methoxy, hydrogen, and amino [8]. Molecular orbital calculation with CNDO/2 (complete neglect of differential overlap, all valenced electron approximation with 3dπ) was carried out.

The van der Waals volume of the substituents of the 7th carbon was calculated by Bondi's method. The hydrophobic parameter of Hansch was used. It was found that the negative charge of the 7th carbon in the benzothiadiazine ring seems to be essential to diuretic activity. Diuretic activity, van der Waals volume, and the hydrophobic parameter of the substituent of the 6th carbon in hydrochlorothiazide and its related molecules are shown in Table 1. The highest index of correlation was obtained by the regression equation

Table 1. Diuretic activity, van der Waals volume, and the hydrophobic parameter of hydrochlorothiazide and its related molecules

Substituent of the 6th position	Diuretic activity[a]	van der Waals volume[b]	Hydrophobic parameter[c]
Cl	4+	0.178	0.71
CH_3	1+	0.167	0.56
OCH_3	2+	0.248	−0.02
NO_2	3+	0.200	−0.28
H	−	0.013	0.00
NH_2	−	0.112	−1.23

[a]By deStevens in the dog
[b]By Bondi's method
[c]By C. Hansch

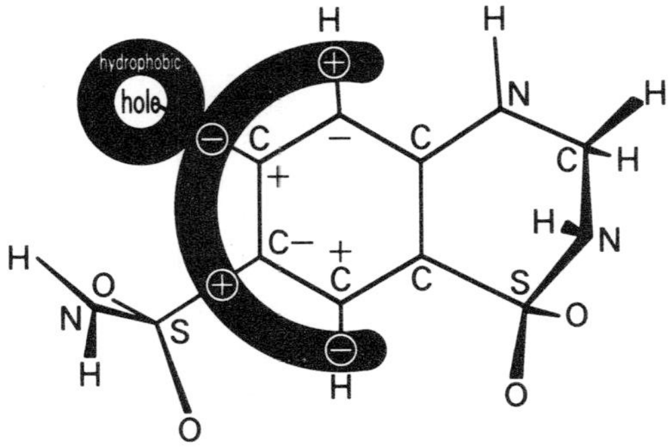

Fig. 2. A proposed model of the interaction site for thiazide diuretics in the apical membrane of the distal convoluted tubule. (From [8] with permission)

$$\ln y = 0.2695 \times 10^{-3}\, \pi + 7.62535\ \text{V.W.} + 15.7681\ Fc_7 + 0.98501$$

where $r = 0.980$ ($P < 0.01$)

π, hydrophobic parameter of the substituent of the 6th carbon;
V.W., van der Waals volume of the substituent of the 6th carbon;
Fc_7, the formal charge of the 7th carbon.

We proposed a model of the action site of hydrochlorothiazide in the tubular membrane, particularly the apical side of the distal convoluted tubule (Fig. 2). This site consisted of a rather larger hydrophobic (lipophilic) hole and an electrostatic reaction with a positive charge to the negative charge of the 7th carbon of the benzothiadiazine ring of hydrochlorothiazide. The result shown in Table 1 suggests that the van der Waals volume has a close relation to diuretic activity. The significance of the van der Waals volume in the biological membrane has been pointed out [9,10]. Considering the lipid rich biological membrane and an electrostatic interaction between diuretics and the sodium chloride channel consisting of polypeptide, the proposed site of action of hydrochlorothiazide in the sodium chloride channel in the distal convoluted tubule seems to be reasonable. Hydrochlorothiazide has been reported to be excreted in the urine in unchanged form [11,12]. Hydrochlorothiazide could act on the channel of the distal convoluted tubule before being excreted in the urine.

Binding of Hydrochlorothiazide to Erythrocyte

We have already reported that concentrations of hydrochlorothiazide in the erythrocytes of humans and animals were always about ten times higher than those in plasma [11]. We have attempted to clarify the kinetics of hydrochlorothiazide binding to erythrocyte [13]. Fresh blood was drawn from rabbits and immediately centrifuged to separate erythrocytes. The erythrocytes were suspended in phosphate buffered saline (PBS) containing varying amounts of hydrochlorothiazide (1, 10, 100 μg/ml). These samples were incubated at 37°C for up to 4 hours; after incubation, the samples were centrifuged and hemolyzed. Hydrochlorothiazide concentration in erythrocytes was determined using column chromatography on Sephadex G-75 [14].

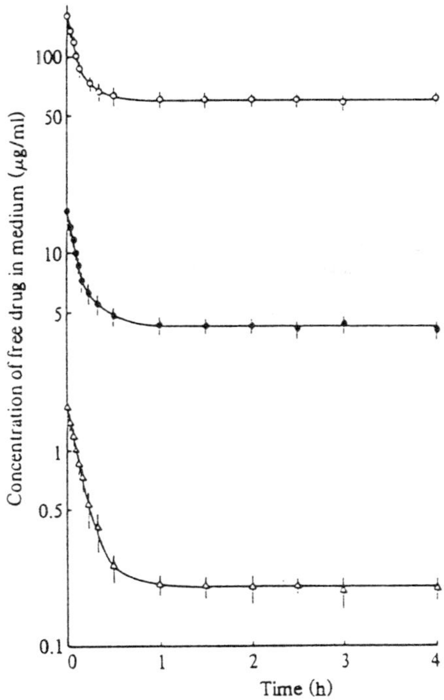

Fig. 3. Decrease of hydrochlorothiazide in the incubation medium by uptake by erythrocytes. Each point represents the mean ± S.D. of four data. Initial concentration in erythrocyte suspension: 100 μg/ml (○), 10 μg/ml (●), 1 μg/ml (△). (From [13] with permission)

Using a similar experimental method, the effect of $HgCl_2$ or acetazolamide on hydrochlorothiazide binding to erythrocytes was studied.

The disappearance kinetics of hydrochlorothiazide in PBS for up to 4 hours are shown in Fig. 3. The kinetics showed similar monoexponential curves. Percentage binding by erythrocytes was 65%, 75%, and 88% at 100, 10, and 1 μg/ml of the initial hydrochlorothiazide concentration respectively. Preincubation of erythrocytes with $HgCl_2$ had no affect on the uptake amount of hydrochlorothiazide (Table 2). On

Table 2. Effect of $HgCl_2$ and acetazolamide on the binding of hydrochlorothiazide to erythrocyte

Inhibitor	Concentration (μM)	Amount of hydrochlorothiazide in erythrocyte (%)
$HgCl_2$	0	100.0 ± 1.2
	5.00	102.2 ± 2.8
	10.00	97.6 ± 3.5
Acetazolamide	1.67	98.6 ± 2.9
	16.7	87.4 ± 2.3
	167.00	73.2 ± 5.3

Each value represents the mean ± S.D. of 5 experiments. The concentration of hydrochlorothiazide in suspension is 16.7 μM. (From [13] with permission)

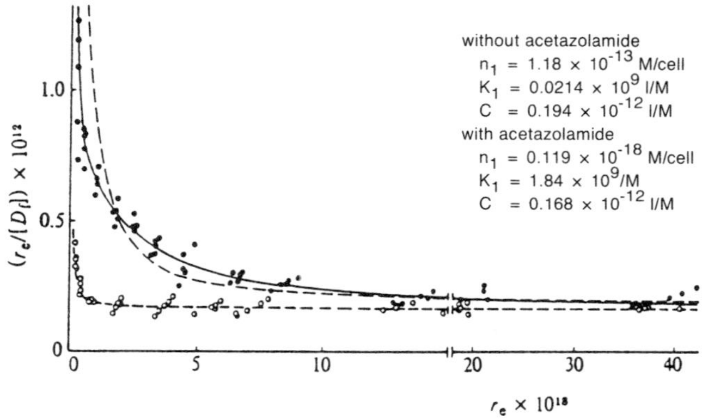

Fig. 4. Scatchard plot of the binding of hydrochlorothiazide with (○) and without (●) acetazolamide. The *broken lines* are the least-square regression line obtained from Eq. 3 as 3-parameter model. The *solid line* is obtained from Eq. 4 as 5-parameter model. (See text for equations). (From [13] with permission)

the other hand, acetazolamide, an inhibitor of carbonic anhydrase, dose-dependently significantly decreased the uptake of hydrochlorothiazide (Table 2). These data were converted to a Scatchard plot (Fig. 4); r_e is the number of moles of hydrochlorothiazide bound per erythrocyte and $[D_f]$ is the concentration of free hydrochlorothiazide. The curve for hydrochlorothiazide binding without acetazolamide has a curvature with nearly horizontal asymptote at higher r_e. The addition of acetazolamide discharged the majority of the first phase observed at lower r_e, but the phase characterized by extremely high affinity and low capacity still remained. Blanchard et al. [15] reported a model with three parameters to describe binding data involving multiple binding sites (equation 3).

$$r/[D_f] = n_1K_1/(1 + K_1[D_f]) + C$$

$$r = [D_b]/[M_t]$$

where r is the number of moles of preservative bound per mole of macromolecule;
$[D_f]$ and $[D_b]$ are the concentrations of free and bound drug, respectively;
$[M_t]$ is the concentration of macromolecule;
K_1 is the association constant;
n_1 is the number of binding sites per macromolecule;
$C = n_2K_2$

The parameters were calculated by the non-linear least-squares computer program MULTI [16]. The theoretical lines obtained are illustrated as broken lines in Fig. 4.

By analysis of the curve of hydrochlorothiazide binding with acetazolamide, the presence of binding sites showing an extremely high binding affinity was observed. The model with five parameters was used and the plots for hydrochlorothiazide binding without acetazolamide were fitted for the equation (equation 4) which is written as:

$$\frac{r_e}{[D_f]} = \frac{n_1K_1}{1 + K_1[D_f]} + \frac{n_2K_2}{1 + K_2[D_f]} + C$$

The parameters obtained were as follows: K_1, 1.84 × 10^9 l/M; K_2, 0.158 × 10^6l/M; n_1, 0.119 × 10^{-18} M/cell; n_2, 3.21 × 10^{-18} M/cell; C, 0.170 × 10^{-12} l/M

r_c: the number of moles of drug preservatively bound per mole of macromolecule

K_1,K_2: the association constant of the first binding site and the second binding site, respectively;

n_1,n_2: the number of the first binding sites per macromolecule and the second binding sites per maculomolecule respectively

The theoretical line obtained by this equation is shown as the solid line in Fig. 4. This line fitted well to the plots of hydrochlorothiazide binding without acetazolamide.

The presence of a high capacity binding site in erythrocytes implies a high bioavailability of hydrochlorothiazide [17,18]. In a therapeutic range, the second sites (inhibited by acetazolamide) seem to play an important role, because serum hydrochlorothiazide concentration is about 1–10 μM. Long acting diuretic activity is explained by this binding ability of hydrochlorothiazide to erythrocytes.

Effect of Ethacrynic Acid on Mitochondrial Electron Transport System and Oxidative Phosphorylation

The physiological basis of the site of action of ethacrynic acid has been well defined [19,20]. However, some questions remain concerning the biochemical properties of ethacrynic acid. One perplexing problem is whether or not ethacrynic acid acts as an uncoupler [21–23]. We have attempted to determine whether ethacrynic acid is an uncoupler or not and whether it is an inhibitor of the electron transport system in mitochondria. The mitochondrial enzymes which are sensitive to ethacrynic acid

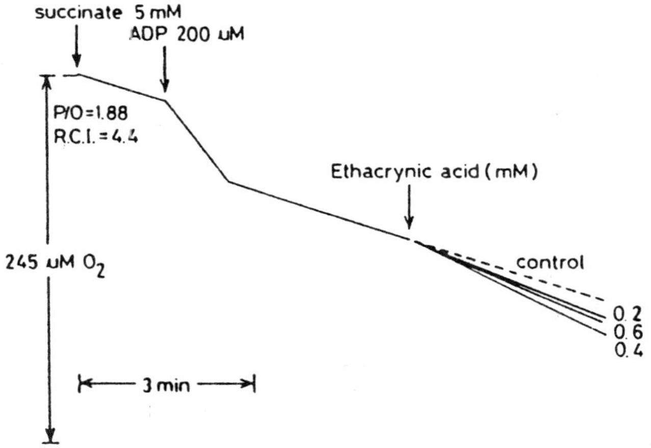

Fig. 5. The effect of ethacrynic acid on succinate oxidation in intact rat liver mitochondria (state 4). The final mitochondrial concentration was about 0.5 mg protein/ml. The cell volume of the oxygen electrode apparatus was 2.7 ml. (From [24] with permission)

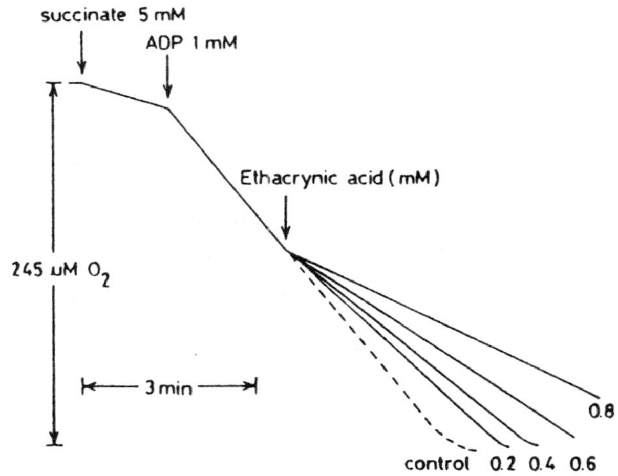

Fig. 6. The effect of ethacrynic acid on succinate oxidation in intact rat liver mitochondria (state 3). The final mitochondrial concentration was about 0.5 mg protein/ml. (From [24] with permission)

have not been identified. Another aim of this study was to identify the enzymes affected by ethacrynic acid.

Mitochondria were obtained from the liver, the renal cortex, and the renal medulla of the rat [24]. Further, mitochondria were obtained from the heart of freshly slaughtered cows [25].

Measurement of oxygen consumption was made with a galvanic electrode in each incubation medium [24]. Oxygen consumption of the mitochondria of rat liver, renal

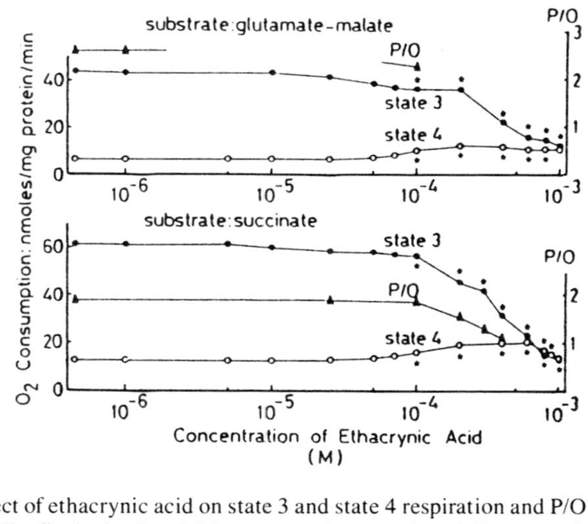

Fig. 7. The effect of ethacrynic acid on state 3 and state 4 respiration and P/O ratio of rat liver mitochondria. The final mitochondrial concentration was about 0.5 mg protein/ml. The results are the means of from two to eight experiments. $*P<0.05$. (From [24] with permission)

cortex, and renal medulla was measured. Oxygen consumption of rat liver mitochondria treated with oligomycin was also measured. The P/O ratio was calculated by the method of Chance [26]. Using frozen bovine heart mitochondria, the enzyme activities of NADH (reduced form of nicotinamide adenine dinucleotide)-DCIP (2,6-dichloroindophenol) reductase, NADH-cytochrome c reductase, succinate dehydrogenase, and succinate-cytochrome c reductase were assayed [27].

As shown in Fig. 5, state 4 respiration of rat liver mitochondria in succinate oxidation was stimulated by ethacrynic acid.

Figure 6 shows that ethacrynic acid dose-dependently inhibited the respiration of phosphorylating mitochondria (state 3) in succinate oxidation. Ethacrynic acid stimulated state 4 respiration (substrate; glutamate-malate). On the other hand, ethacrynic acid inhibited state 3 respiration (substrate; glutamate-malate). Figure 7 shows the relationship between the concentration of ethacrynic acid and the respiration of mitochondria in rat liver. A slight, but significant, stimulation was observed at the concentration of 10^{-4}M/l. A significant inhibition of state 3 respiration was observed dose-dependently from the concentration of 10^{-4} M/l. The same effects of ethacrynic acid on mitochondria were observed in the mitochondria of renal cortex (Fig. 8). Ethacrynic acid at concentrations of 10^{-4}M/l, 5×10^{-4}M/l, and 10^{-3}M/l

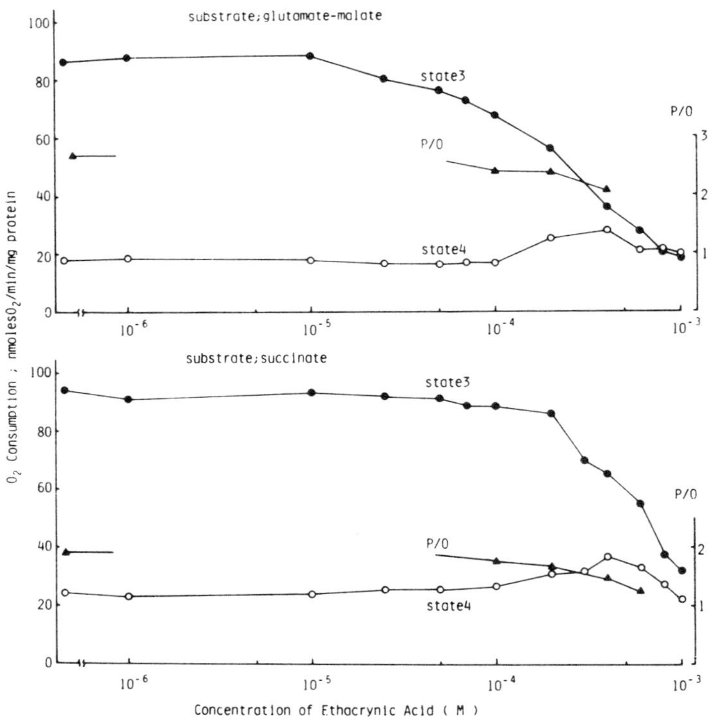

Fig. 8. The effect of ethacrynic acid on state 3 and state 4 respiration and P/O ratio in rat renal cortex mitochondria. Final mitochondrial concentrations used were about 0.5 mg protein/ml. The results are means of two to eight experiments. (From [24] with permission)

Table 3. The effects of ethacrynic acid on respiration inhibited by oligomycin

	Substrate: glutamate-malate	*n*	Substrate: succinate	*n*
Control (ADP 500 μmol/l + oligomycin 1 μmol/l)	14.9 ± 0.6	4	15.1 ± 0.7	4
Ethacrynic acid (mmol/l)				
0.1	16.3 ± 0.3*	4	16.8 ± 0.4*	4
0.5	21.4 ± 0.6***	4	20.0 ± 0.8**	
1.0	17.9 ± 0.7*	4	14.1 ± 0.3	4
10.0	11.8 ± 0.6**	4	11.1 ± 0.4**	4

Rate of oxygen consumption expressed as nmol/mg protein per min
$^*P < 0.01$, $^{**}P < 0.005$, $^{***}P < 0.001$
(From [24] with permission)

Table 4. The effects of ethacrynic acid (*EA*) on enzyme activities of bovine heart mitochondria

Enzyme	Control	*n*	EA 1 mmol/l	*n*	% inhibition
NADH-DCIP reductase[a]	150.0 ± 2.1	4	128.8 ± 2.5	4	14.2 $P < 0.001$
NADH-cytochrome c reductase[b]	440.7 ± 34.3	5	277.7 ± 12.3	5	37.0 $P < 0.005$
Succinate dehydrogenase[a]	106.7 ± 5.1	4	79.6 ± 2.2	4	25.4 $P < 0.005$
Succinate-cytochrome c reductase[b]	335.9 ± 7.7	4	255.9 ± 8.1	4	23.8 $P < 0.001$

[a]Expressed as nmol DCIP reduced/mg protein per min
[b]Expressed as nmol cytochrome c reduced/mg protein per min
(From [24] with permission)

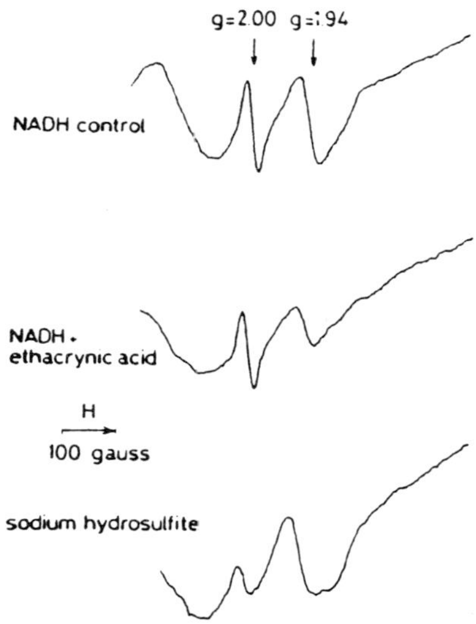

Fig. 9. The effect of ethacrynic acid on EPR absorption spectrum of bovine heart mitochondria. The EPR absorption spectrum is shown in the region between g = 3.0 and g = 1.0. Mitochondria were suspended at a concentration of about 30 mg protein/ml in 0.1 mol/l potassium phosphate buffer at pH 8.0 and 20°C and were frozen in liquid nitrogen after 1 min incubation with 0.2 mmol/l NADH at 20°C. All spectra were recorded at a sample temperature 100°K. The EPR absorption spectrum of fully reduced mitochondria by the addition of hydrosulfite is shown in the *bottom* panel. EPR, electron paramagnetic resonance. (From [24] with permission)

stimulated the respiration of rat liver mitochondria inhibited by oligomycin, but a much higher concentration of ethacrynic acid (10^{-2}M/l) significantly inhibited this respiration when the substrate was glutamate-malate. When the substrate was succinate, ethacrynic acid at 10^{-4}M/l and 5×10^{-4}M/l stimulated the respiration of rat liver mitochondria inhibited by oligomycin. But a much higher concentration of ethacrynic acid (10^{-2}M/l) significantly inhibited this respiration (Table 3).

Ethacrynic acid at the concentration of 10^{-3}M/l significantly inhibited the activity of NADH-DCIP reductase and the activity of NADH-cytochrome c reductase in mitochondria of the frozen-thawed bovine heart (Table 4). The activity of succinate dehydrogenase and that of succinate-cytochrome c reductase were significantly inhibited by 10^{-3}M/l of ethacrynic acid.

Ethacrynic acid at the concentration of 10^{-3}M/l remarkably reduced the signal height in electron paramagnetic resonance (EPR) at electron value $g = 1.94$ of mitochondria of frozen-thawed bovine heart after 1 min incubation with 0.2 mM/l NADH (Fig 9). In contrast, when the substrate was succinate, reduction of signal height, $g = 1.94$ was not observed (Fig. 10).

The results obtained are summarized in Fig. 11. In general, uncouplers, such as dinitrophenol and pentachlorophenol, stimulate state 4 respiration at lower concentration and inhibit electron transport at higher concentration [28]. However, ethacrynic acid stimulates state 4 respiration and inhibits the electron transport system at the same concentration. To identify the site of electron transport inhibition,

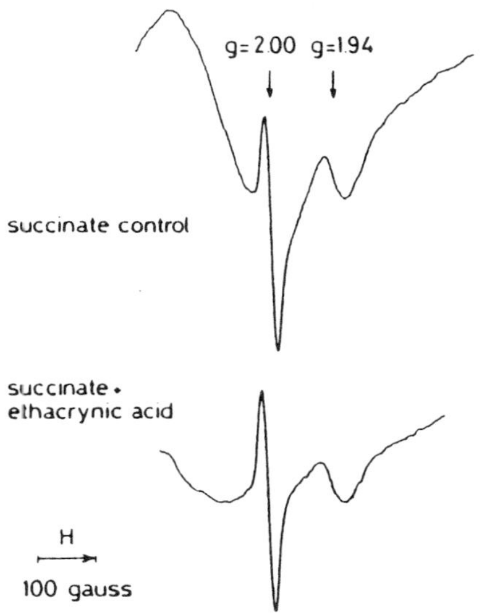

Fig. 10. The effect of ethacrynic acid on EPR absorption spectrum of bovine heart mitochondria. The EPR absorption spectrum is shown in the region between $g = 3.0$ and $g = 1.0$. Mitochondria were suspended at a concentration of about 30 mg protein/ml in 0.1 mol/l potassium phosphate buffer at pH 7.4 and 20°C and were frozen in liquid nitrogen after 1 min incubation with 10 mmol/l succinate at 20°C. All spectra were recorded at a sample temperature 100°K. EPR, electron paramagnetic resonance. (From [24] with permission)

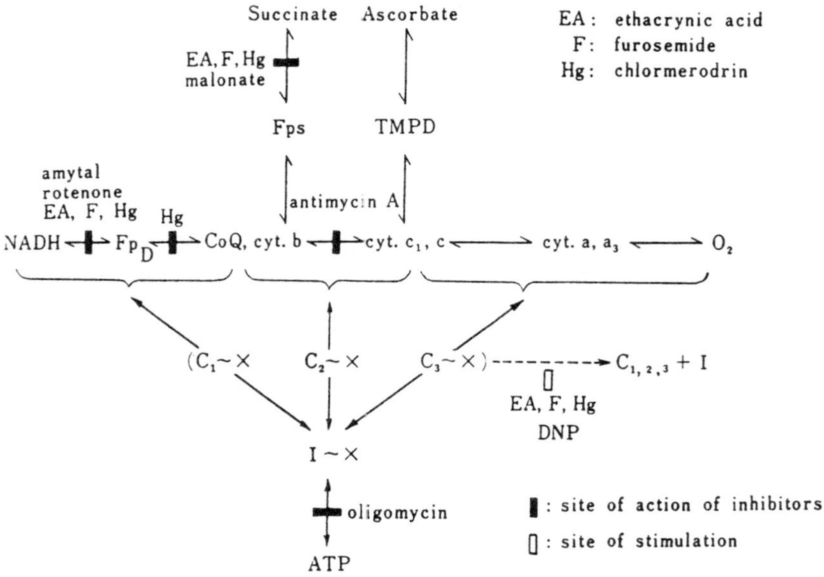

Fig. 11. A possible inhibitory site by some diuretics in the mitochondrial electron transport system. EA, ethacrynic acid; F, furosemide; Hg, chlormerodrin; TMPD, tetramethyl-*p*-phenyline-diamine; Fps, flavoproteins; DNP, 2,4-dinitrophenol

the effects of ethacrynic acid on the enzyme activities of the electron transport system were studied. The method of Hatefi [27] was used to purify the enzymes from bovine heart mitochondria. No differences have been observed between animal species and tissue types in the properties of electron transfer systems [29]. Our experimental results suggest that ethacrynic acid inhibits mitochondrial NADH dehydrogenase, since ethacrynic acid inhibited NADH-cytochrome c reductase more strongly than it inhibited NADH-DCIP reductase. Further, the results suggest that ethacrynic acid inhibits succinate dehydrogenase, but does not inhibit the electron transport system between succinate dehydrogenase and cytochrome c. In order to clarify the site of electron transport inhibition between NADH dehydrogenase and cytochrome c, the effects on ethacrynic acid of the reduction of nonhem iron were studied. The reduced form of nonhem iron has an EPR absorption at low temperature with a characteristic electron g value [29]. We have determined the reduction of nonhem iron by the signal height of the EPR spectrum at $g = 1.94$. Our results suggest that ethacrynic acid inhibits the electron transport system from flavin of NADH dehydrogenase to nonhem iron. Therefore, ethacrynic acid could inhibit the activity of NADH-cytochrome c reductase more strongly than it inhibits the activity of NADH-DCIP reductase, and could inhibit the activities of succinate dehydrogenase and succinate-cytochrome c reductase to a similar extent. We submit that ethacrynic acid inhibits the mitochondrial electron transport system at several sites: NADH dehydrogenase, succinate dehydrogenase, and the reduction of nonhem iron. Ethacrynic acid is considered to be one of the phenol derivatives [31]. The electron accepting nature of phenol derivatives was reported to be important for their uncoupling activity [32]. We have previously reported the electron accepting nature of ethacrynic acid [33]. These biochemical actions of ethacrynic acid were noted at concentrations above 10^{-4}M/l. This concentration is more than ten times that required to inhibit sodium transport of the isolated, perfused renal tubule [19]. However, in kidney slices ethacrynic acid was reported to accumulate in a concentration almost ten times that of the incubation medium [34]. This raises the possibility that ethacrynic acid inhibits sodium reabsorption by interfering with energy generation in the renal tubule.

References

1. Greger R, Frömter E (1980) Time course of oubain and furosemide effects on transepithelial potential difference in cortical thick ascending limbs of rabbit nephron. In: Kidney and body fluids. Pergamon, Budapest, p 375
2. Burg MB, Stoner L, Cardina J, Green N (1973) Furosemide effect on isolated perfused tubules. Am J Physiol 225:119–124
3. Malnic G, Klose RM, Giebisch G (1966) Micropuncture study of distal tubular potassium and sodium transport in rat nephron. Am J Physiol 211:529–547
4. Grantham JJ, Burg MB, Orloff J (1970) The nature of transtubular Na and K transport in isolated rabbit renal collecting duct. J Clin Invest 49:1815–1826
5. Hediger MA, Coady MJ, Ikeda TS, Wright EM (1987) Expression, cloning and cDNA sequencing of Na+/glucose co-transporter. Nature 330:379–381
6. deStevens G (1963) Diuretics, chemistry and pharmacology. Academic, New York, p 99
7. Dupont L, Diedeberg O (1972) Structure cristalline et l'Hydrochlorothiazide. Acta Cryst B 28:2340–2347
8. Orita Y, Ando A, Yamabe S, Nakanishi T, Arakawa Y, Abe H (1983) Quantum-chemical and physico-chemical properties of hydrochlorothiazide. Arzneimittelforsch 33:688–691
9. Hansch C, Rockwell SD, Jow PY, Leo A, Stellar EE (1972) Substituent constants of correlation analysis. J Med Chem 20:304–308
10. Moriguchi I, Kanada Y (1977) Use of van der Waals volume in structure-activity studies. Chem Pharm Bull (Tokyo) 25:926–935
11. Orita Y, Nakanishi T, Nakahama H, Fukuhara Y, Ando A, Abe H, Yamazaki M, Itoh S, Itoh Y (1984) Diuretics I, Chemistry, Pharmacology, Clinical Applications. Elsevier, New York, pp 546–548
12. Patel RB, Patel UR, Rogge MC, Shah VP, Prasad VK, Selen A, Welling PG (1984) Bioavailability of hydrochlorothiazide from tablets and suspensions. J Pharm Sci 73:359–361
13. Yamazaki M, Itoh S, Okuda T, Tanabe K, Nakahama H, Fukuhara Y, Orita Y (1989) Binding of hydrochlorothiazide to erythrocytes. J Pharmacobiodyn 12:423–428
14. Dieterle W, Wangere J, Faigle J (1976) Binding of chlorthalidone to blood components in man. Eur J Clin Pharmacol 10:37–42
15. Blanchard J, Fink W, Duffy J (1977) Effect of sorbitol on interaction of phenolic preservatives with polysorbate. J Pharm Sci 66:1470–1473
16. Yamaoka K, Tanigawara Y, Nakagawa T, Uno T (1981) A pharmacokinetic analysis program (MULTI) for microcomputer. J Pharmacobiodyn 4:879–885
17. Yamazaki M, Itoh T, Yaginuma H, Itoh S, Kamada A, Orita Y, Nakama H, Nakanishi T, Ando A (1984) High-performance liquid chromatographic method of determination of hydrochlorothiazide in plasma, urine, blood cells and bile. Chem Pharm Bull (Tokyo) 32:2387–2394

18. Welling PG (1986) Pharmacokinetics of the thiazide diuretics. Biopharm Drug Dispos 7:501–535
19. Burg MB, Green N (1973) Effect of ethacrynic acid on the thick ascending limb of Henle's loop. Kidney Int 4:301–308
20. Greger R (1985) Ion transport mechanisms in thick ascending limb of Henle's loop of mammalian nephron. Physiol Rev 65:760–797
21. Sawa H, Weinman EJ, Hyde SE, Ekynoyan G (1976) Renal and hepatic mitochondrial effect of diuretics in the rat. Biochem Pharmacol 25:2649–2655
22. Mannuel MA, Weiner MW (1976) Effects of ethacrynic acid and furosemide on isolated rat kidney mitochondria. J Pharmacol Exp Ther 198:209–221
23. Landon EJ, Fritzpartick DF (1972) Ethacrynic acid and kidney cell metabolism. Biochem Pharmacol 21:1561–1568
24. Yanase M, Orita Y, Fukuhara Y, Okada N, Ando A, Abe H (1983) Effect of ethacrynic acid on mitochondrial electron transport system and oxidative phosphorylation. Arzneimittelforsch 33:120–124
25. Azzone GF, Colonna R, Zieche B (1979) Preparation of bovine heart mitochondria in high yield. Methods Enzymol 55:46–50
26. Chance B, Williams GR (1956) The respiratory chain and oxidative phosphorylations. Adv Enzymol 17:65–134
27. Hatefi Y, Haavik AG, Jurtshuk P (1961) Studies on the electron transport system, DPNH-cytochrome reductase. Biochim Biophys Acta 52:106–118
28. Heytler PG (1979) Uncouplers of oxidative phosphorylation. Methods Enzymol 55:462–472
29. Singer TP (1979) Mitochondrial electron-transport inhibitors. Methods Enzymol 55:454–462
30. Lehninger AL (1975) Biochemistry. Worth, New York, pp 477–508
31. Schultz EM, Cragoe EJ Jr, Bricking JB, Bolhofer WA, Sprague JM (1962) α, β-unsaturated ketone derivatives of aryloxyacetic acid acids, A new class of diuretics. J Med Pharmacol Chem 5:660–662
32. Kean EA (1968) An ihibitor of mitochondrial oxidations. Arch Biochem Biophys 127:528–533
33. Orita Y, Ando A, Takamitsu Y, Shirai D, Urakabe S, Furukawa T, Abe H (1968) A quantum biological analysis of thiazide diuretics and ethacrynic acid. Jpn Circ J 32:547–554
34. Charnock JS, Almeida AF (1972) Ethacrynic acid accumulation by renal tissue. Biochem Pharmacol 21:647–655

Molecular Properties of the Na-K-Cl-Cotransporter

ROLF K.H. KINNE[1]

SUMMARY. Since 1980, when the transporter was first characterized in Ehrlich Ascites tumor cells [1], the Na-K-Cl cotransport system has been found to play a major role in volume regulation in cells in general, and in transepithelial active chloride transport in epithelia in particular [2]. This contribution first summarizes our still very limited knowledge on the molecular properties, in the strictest sense, of the transport system and then deals with some peculiarities of the transporter which set it apart from other "simple" sodium cotransport systems: i.e., the polyfunctionality and variability of the transport activity. Finally the question of the intrarenal distribution of the transporter is addressed.

Molecular Properties

During recent years various laboratories have aimed to define the molecular weight of the cotransport system and to isolate it in an active form. A summary of these attempts is given in Table 1 [3–7]. In most instances the protein was identified by, or purified via, its interaction with loop diuretics. This interaction is dependent on the presence of sodium and potassium and requires in addition a small amount of chloride, higher chloride concentrations being inhibitory. These results indicate that the loop diuretics interact with the Na-K-Cl cotransport system at one of its anion binding sites [8]. Thus far the molecular weights proposed for the transporter vary, however, quite substantially. This might be due to a lack of specificity of labeling or might reflect an oligomeric structure of the protein – similar to that of the sodium-D-glucose cotransport system [9,10].

With regard to the specificity and affinity of the transporter for anions and cations the transport system has been relatively well characterized, as summarized in Table 2 [11–15]. The points worth mentioning are the very high affinity of the sodium and

[1]Max-Planck-Institut für Systemphysiologie, Rheinlanddamm 201, 4600 Dortmund, Federal Republic of Germany

Table 1. Tentative molecular mass of the Na-K-Cl cotransporter

Author	Method of identification	Material	Molecular mass	Comments
Haas & Forbush [4]	Photolabeling with [^{3}H]-BSTBA, high affinity, potassium, sodium, and chloride dependence	Dog kidney membranes	~150 kDa	Nonreducing SDS-PAGE
Haas & Forbush [5]	Photolabeling with [^{3}H]-bumetanide, high affinity	Dog kidney membranes	~150 kDa	Nonreducing SDS-PAGE
Feit et al. [6]	Affinity chromatography on bumetanide column	Ehrlich ascites cell plasma membranes	~135 kDa	Cholate gel
Kinne et al. (unpublished work)	Radiation inactivation	Rabbit kidney outer medulla microsomes	~76 kDa ~83 kDa	Reducing SDS-PAGE
Deutscher et al. (unpublished work)	Photolabeling with [^{3}H]-bumetanide, chloride dependence	Shark rectal gland plasma membranes	~42 kDa	Reducing SDS-PAGE
	Affinity chromatography on piretanide column, chloride-dependent labeling of isolated protein with [^{3}H]-bumetanide	Shark rectal gland plasma membranes	~42 kDa	Reducing SDS-PAGE
Haas & Forbush [4]	Photolabeling with [^{3}H]-BSTBA, low affinity, sodium dependence of labeling	Dog kidney membranes	~50 kDa	Nonreducing SDS-PAGE
Jørgensen et al. [7]	Photolabeling with [^{3}H]-bumetanide, competition with cold bumetanide	Rabbit kidney membranes	~34 kDa	Reducing SDS-PAGE

BSTBA, 4-benzoyl-5-sulfamoyl-3-(3-phenyloxy) benzoic acid; SDS-PAGE, sodium dodecylsulfate polycarylamide gel electrophoresis

Table 2. Properties of the Na-K-Cl cotransporter in various renal cells

	Rabbit TALH [2,11–13]	$LLC-PK_1$ [14]	MDCK Cells [15]
Sodium binding site			
Affinity	1.8-3.5 mM	0.5 mM	9 mM
Specificity	$Na > Li >> NH_4$	ND	$Na > Li$
Potassium binding site			
Affinity	0.3 mM	ND	9 mM
Specificity	$K = Rb > NH_4 > Cs$	ND	$K = Rb > NH_4 > Cs$
Chloride binding site 1			
Affinity	~1.0 mM	~5.1 mM	ND
Specificity	$Br = Cl >> J = NO_3 = SCN$	ND	$Br = Cl$
Chloride binding site 2			
Affinity	~15 mM	~55.2 mM	~48 mM
Specificity	$Br > Cl > J = NO_3 = SCN$	ND	ND
Interaction with loop diuretics			
Affinity (bumetanide)	~10^{-6} M	~10^{-6} M	ND
Specificity	bumetanide > piretanide > furosemide		

TALH, thick ascending limb of Henle's loop; ND, not done

the potassium site of the transporter and the presence of two different anion binding sites. One site has a high affinity and selectivity for chloride (and bromide) and a second which, when the first binding site is occupied by chloride, shows a broad substrate specificity and is probably one site of interaction of the loop diuretics with the carrier. As depicted in Fig. 1 one diuretic with a very high affinity for the transporter is a molecule which carries a SO_3 at C_1 (Hoe 758) instead of a COO^- as does furosemide. The SO_3 group probably interacts with the second anion binding site of the transporter as demonstrated recently by Shetlar et al. in Xenopus oocytes (R. Shetlar et al., unpublished work). However, substitutions at other positions of the diuretic also change the apparent affinity of the diuretic to the transporter. This holds, as demonstrated in Fig. 2, for positions at the aromatic ring, as well as for the deletion of the sulfamoyl group [16,17]. These results suggest a very complex and very flexible (cooperative) interaction of the transporter with its substrates as well as with its inhibitors.

With regard to the amino acid residues essential for these interactions, the study of George and Turner [18] is worth mentioning. In isolated basal-lateral plasma membrane vesicles of salivary glands it was demonstrated that N-ethylmaleimide—which interacts mainly with SH-groups—inhibits KCl-dependent ^{22}Na uptake. Substrate protection studies suggest that this SH-group is closely associated with the anion binding site to which loop diuretics also bind.

Further studies are needed to unravel the molecular basis of the Na-K-Cl cotransporter—a challenge endowed with a higher probability of success after the cloning of the Na-glucose cotransporter has been achieved [19].

Polyfunctionality of the Transporter

As is evident from the data presented in Table 2 on the substrate specificity of the Na-K-Cl cotransporter, NH_4 can very effectively and with a high affinity replace potassium at its binding site [20]. It can also substitute for potassium as a cotransported

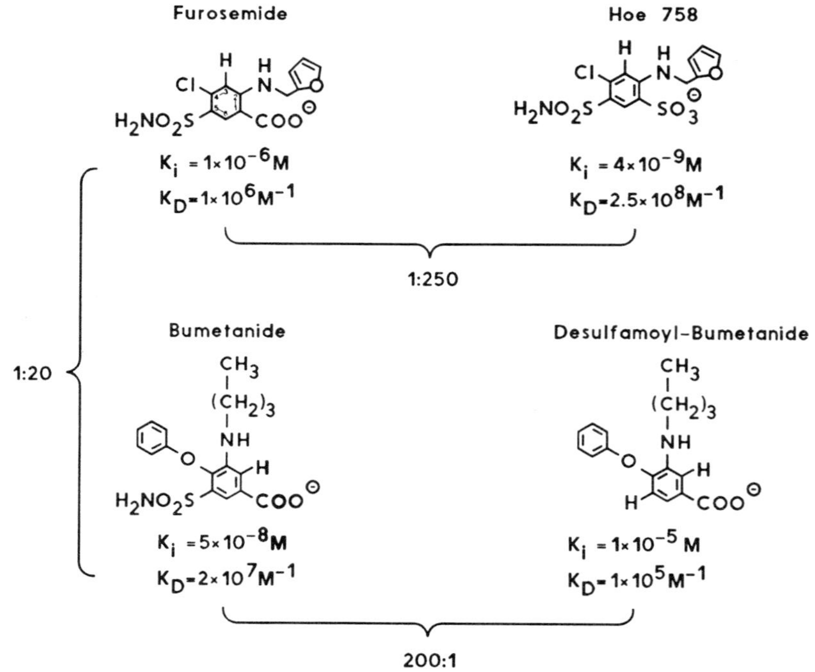

Fig. 1. Effect of side group modifications on the affinity of loop diuretics. K_i = concentration of the diuretic which led to 50% inhibition of transport activity in chloride-containing modified Ringer's solution. The numbers given in the figure compare relative affinities based on the ratios of the dissociation constants K_D. K_D values represent the reciprocals of the K_i values. (Data from [16] and [17])

ion. This results in a Na-NH_4-Cl cotransport which, together with a rather low permeability of the luminal thick ascending limb of Henle (TALH) membrane for NH_3, forms the basis for active ammonium reabsorption in this segment [21]. Thus, application of loop diuretics also interferes with the way in which ammonium is handled by the kidney. The same holds for anions other than chloride; as physiologically relevant iodide, which is also accepted by the anion binding site of the cotransporter, might be mentioned [13].

Variability of Cotransport Activity

Due to its high stoichiometry for chloride translocation and the coupling of sodium and chloride movement to an uptake of potassium into the cell, this transport system is exquisitely sensitive to alterations in transmembrane driving forces. Such an example is shown in Table 3, where the driving forces for the transporter at the beginning and at the end of the TALH have been estimated [22]. Assuming that the intracellular ion composition is identical, the decrease in intratubular sodium and chloride

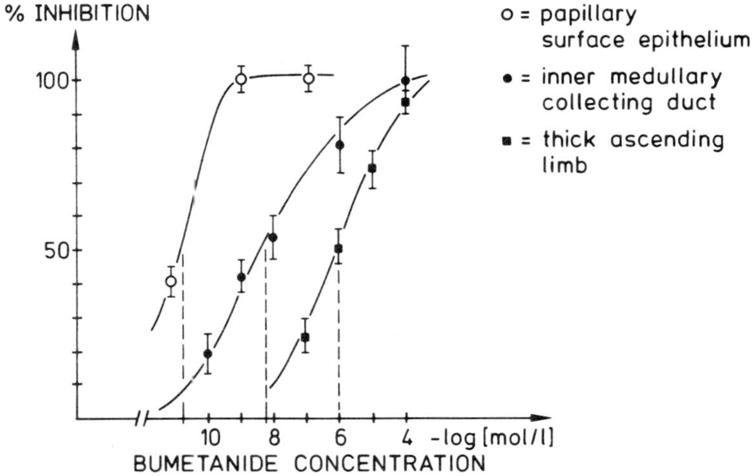

Fig. 2. Effect of bumetanide on Na-K-Cl cotransport in various renal epithelia. Data for the papillary surface epithelia are from [23]; data for the inner medullary collecting duct are from [24]. (After [3] with permission)

suffices to reduce the driving forces, and thereby active chloride transport, to zero. The same can be achieved by lowering the extracellular potassium content. Experiments in low potassium medium suggest that in such instances the transporter acts as a major potassium leak for the cell [15]. Similarly, changes in intracellular ion composition markedly affect the rate of Na-K-Cl cotransport. Thus, a decrease in intracellular chloride by stimulation of an independent chloride channel increases the rate of transport, as does an activation of the Na-K-ATPase [11]. Therefore, sometimes the responsiveness of the transporter to inhibitors such as the loop diuretics, as well as to endogenous regulators such as cAMP, cGMP, and antidiuretic hormone (ADH) might vary, depending on the experimental conditions employed. This different *set-point* of the transporter can explain the sometimes contradictory results [23].

Table 3. Driving forces for the Na-K-Cl cotransporter

	Luminal sodium	Luminal chloride	Luminal potassium	Driving force
Initial TALH	137 mM E_{Na} = 66 mV	150 mM E_{Cl} = 96 mV	2.5 mM E_K = −100 mV	+62 mV
End of TALH	25–40 mM E_{Na} = 23–34 mV	25–40 mM E_{Cl} = 6.4–30 mV	6.0 mM E_K = −79 mV	−49 / −15 mV
Intracellular ions	Na 10 mM K 140 mM Cl 22 mM			

Intrarenal Distribution of the Na-K-Cl Cotransport System

The renal Na-K-Cl cotransport system was first demonstrated in the thick ascending limb of Henle's loop (TALH) of mammals and in the diluting segment of amphibia and was considered to represent a transport system specific for this renal segment [11]. Accordingly, it was assumed that loop diuretics acted exclusively on this part of the nephron. In recent years, however, Na-K-Cl cotransport activity has been detected in the papillary surface epithelium of the rabbit [24], covering the surface of the renal papilla, and in isolated inner medullary collecting duct cells of rat kidney [25]. The sensitivity of these three renal Na-K-Cl cotransporters to inhibition by bumetanide is compared in Fig. 2. It is evident that within the rabbit kidney the transport system in the papillary surface epithelium is much more sensitive to the loop diuretic than the transport system in the TALH. The consequences of this additional action of loop diuretics have not been investigated thus far. It is interesting to note that the papillary surface epithelium has been postulated to participate in the exchange of water and solutes between pelvic urine and medullary tissue [26] and to facilitate the function of pelvic refluxes in aiding the diluting processes of the urine.

The transport activity found in rat inner medulla also seems to have a high sensitivity to loop diuretics. This transport system, as in other cells [27], is activated by cell shrinkage and mediates regulatory volume increase [28]; an inhibition of this system by diuretics might impair the capability of the collecting duct cells to regulate volume.

Conclusion

The renal Na-K-Cl cotransport system is thus far only poorly characterized with regard to its biochemical molecular properties; the biophysical events which ultimately lead to the translocation of the four ions are essentially unknown. Similarly, the detailed interactions of diuretics with the transporter remain to be elucidated. Phenomenologically and thermodynamically, the transporter is well characterized and some peculiarities such as high cooperativity, polyfunctionality, and variability of transport activity can be explained based on these phenomenological parameters. In considering the renal site of action of loop diuretics, recent evidence suggests that the transport system is not only present in the thick ascending limb of Henle's loop, but is also present distally in the inner medullary collecting duct and in the papillary surface epithelium. The extent to which the latter locations contribute to the action of diuretics or the extent to which they may lead to unexpected side effects remains to be determined.

Acknowledgment. The travel support by Hoechst Japan and Hoechst Germany is gratefully acknowledged. The skillful secretarial work of Mrs. D. Mägdefessel is also greatly appreciated.

References

1. Geck P, Heinz E (1986) The Na-K-2Cl cotransport system. J Membr Biol 91:97–105
2. Kinne R, Hannafin JA, König B (1985) Role of NaCl-KCl cotransport system in active chloride absorption and secretion. Ann NY Acad Sci 456:198–206

3. Kinne RKH (1989) The Na-K-Cl cotransporter in the kidney. Ann NY Acad Sci 574:63–74
4. Haas M, Forbush III B (1987) Photolabeling of a 150-kDa (Na + K + Cl) cotransport protein from dog kidney with a bumetanide analogue. Am J Physiol 253:C243–C250
5. Haas M, Forbush III B (1987) Na,K,Cl-cotransport system: characterization by bumetanide binding and photolabelling. Kidney Int 32:S134–S140
6. Feit PW, Hoffmann EK, Schiødt M, Kristensen P, Jessen F, Dunham PB (1988) Purification of proteins of the Na/Cl cotransporter from membranes of Ehrlich ascites cells using a bumetanide-sepharose affinity column. J Membr Biol 103:135–147
7. Jørgensen PL, Petersen J, Rees WD (1984) Identification of a Na^+, K^+, Cl^--cotransporter protein of M_r 34000 from kidney by photolabeling with [^{3}H]bumetanide. The protein is associated with cytoskeleton components. Biochim Biophys Acta 775:105–110
8. Haas M, McManus TJ (1983) Bumetanide inhibits (Na + K + Cl) cotransport at a chloride site. Am J Physiol 245:C235–C240
9. Lin J-T, Szwarc K, Kinne R, Jung CY (1984) Structural state of the Na^+/D-glucose cotransporter in calf kidney brush-border membranes. Target size analysis of Na^+-dependent phlorizin binding and Na^+-dependent D-glucose transport. Biochim Biophys Acta 777:201–208
10. Jung CY (1987) Radiation target size measurement of glucose transport function in animal cells. In: Venter JC, Jung CY (eds) Target-Size Analysis of Membrane Proteins. Alan R. Liss, New York, pp 137–151
11. Greger R (1985) Ion transport mechanisms in thick ascending limb of Henle's loop of mammalian nephron. Physiol Rev 65:760–797
12. Kinne RKH (1988) Sodium cotransport systems in epithelial secretion. Comp Biochem Physiol [A] 90:721–726
13. Kinne R, Kinne-Saffran E, Schölermann B, Schütz H (1986) The anion specificity of the sodium-potassium-chloride cotransporter in rabbit kidney outer medulla: Studies on medullary plasma membranes. Pflügers Arch 407:S168–C173
14. Brown CDA, Murer H (1985) Characterization of a Na:K:2Cl cotransport system in the apical membrane of a renal epithelial cell line (LLC-PK_1). J Membr Biol 87:131–139
15. Saier Jr MH, Boyden DA (1984) Mechanism, regulation and physiological significance of the loop diuretic-sensitive NaCl/KCl symport system in animal cells. Mol Cell Biochem 59:11–32
16. Schlatter E, Greger R, Weidtke C (1983) Effect of "high ceiling" diuretics on active salt transport in the cortical thick ascending limb of Henle's loop of rabbit kidney. Correlation of chemical structure and inhibitory potency. Pflügers Arch 396:210–217
17. Amsler K, Kinne R (1986) Specific irreversible inhibition of Na^+-K^+-Cl^- cotransport activity by exposure to bumetanide and near UV light. In: Alvarado F, van Os CH (eds) Ion-Gradient-Coupled Transport. INSERM Symposium No. 26. Elsevier, Amsterdam, pp 295–298
18. George JN, Turner RJ (1989) Inactivation of the rabbit parotid Na/K/Cl cotransporter by N-ethylmaleimide. J Membr Biol 112:51–58
19. Hediger MA, Turk E, Pajor AM, Wright EM (1989) Molecular genetics of the human Na^+/glucose cotransporter. Klin Wochenschr 67:843–846
20. Kinne R, Kinne-Saffran E, Schütz H, Schölermann B (1986) Ammonium transport in medullary thick ascending limb of rabbit kidney. Involvement of the Na^+,K^+,Cl^--cotransporter. J Membr Biol 94:279–284
21. Garvin JL, Burg MB, Knepper MA (1988) Active NH_4^+ absorption by the thick ascending limb. Am J Physiol 255:F57–F65
22. Kinne R (to be published) Selectivity and direction: Plasma membranes in renal transport. Am J Physiol
23. Haas M (1989) Properties and diversity of (Na-K-Cl) cotransporters. Annu Rev Physiol 51:443–457

24. Sands JM, Knepper MA, Spring KR (1986) Na-K-Cl cotransport in apical membrane of rabbit renal papillary surface epithelium. Am J Physiol 251:F475–F484
25. Grupp C, Pavenstädt-Grupp I, Grunewald RW, Stokes III JB, Kinne RKH (1989) A Na-K-Cl cotransporter in isolated rat papillary collecting duct cells. Kidney Int 36:201–209
26. Schmidt-Nielsen B (1990) Function of the pelvis. Comp Physiol 2:103–140
27. Geck P (1990) Volume regulation in Ehrlich Cells. Comp Physiol 4:26–58
28. Grunewald JM, Grunewald RW, Kinne RKH (1990) Osmoregulation in isolated rat renal inner medullary collecting duct (IMCD) cells. FASEB J 4:A563

The Cellular Receptor for Thiazide-Type Diuretics

DARRELL D. FANESTIL, ZUOFANG CHEN, JOHAN M. TRAN, DUKE A. VAUGHN, and KEVIN BEAUMONT[1]

SUMMARY. ^{3}H-metolazone has been developed by our laboratory as a marker for the density of the thiazide diuretic receptor. The identity of the high affinity binding site for ^{3}H-metolazone with the receptor for thiazide-type diuretics is supported by three lines of investigation: (i) pharmacological specificity, (ii) autoradiographic localization in distal nephron, and (iii) the influence of the presumed transported ions, sodium and chloride, on the affinity. This development is beginning to impact upon our understanding of the renal regulation of excretion of sodium and chloride. Heretofore, there has been a lack of attention to the potential role of physiological and pathophysiological regulation of the thiazide-sensitive segment of the nephron in the homeostatic control of sodium, chloride, calcium, and acid-base homeostasis. The published and unpublished studies reviewed in this paper point out that the thiazide-sensitive transporter can be rapidly (within minutes) regulated, is influenced by both sex and adrenal steroid hormones, and is altered in two types of pathophysiological condition – experimental genetic hypertension and experimental genetic hypercalciuria. We predict with confidence that future work will provide additional appreciation for the role of the thiazide-sensitive Na-Cl transporter in renal physiology and pathophysiology.

Introduction

Thiazide diuretics (benzothiadiazides) have been utilized since the 1950s for the treatment of edema and hypertension [1]. Relatively little is known about the molecular and cellular mechanisms of action of thiazides, despite this long history of clinical utility in edema and hypertension. Moreover, the mode of their antihypertensive action is not firmly established [2]. However, thiazide-type diuretics are known to

[1]Division of Nephrology, Department of Medicine, University of California San Diego, La Jolla, CA 92093-0623, USA

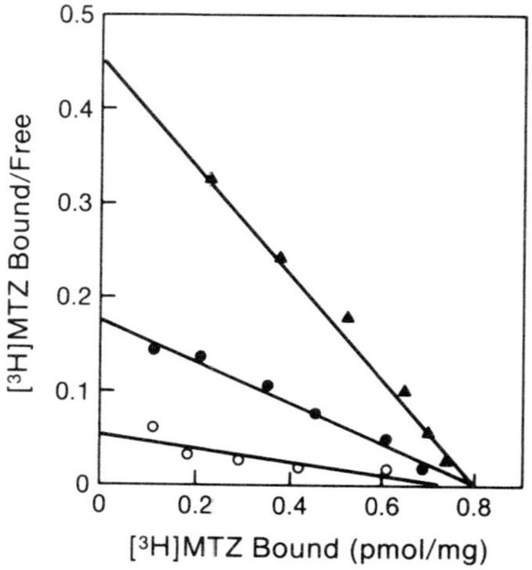

Fig. 1. Effect of sodium and of chloride on the binding of ^{3}H-metolazone by rat kidney membranes. Membranes were incubated with various concentrations of ^{3}H-metolazone in the presence of no added salt (*solid circles*), 25 mM Na_2SO_4 (*triangles*), or 50 mM NaCl (*open circles*). Results are plotted according to Scatchard, in which the intercept with the abscissa defines the maximal binding capacity and the slope of the line reflects the affinity. The maximal binding of ^{3}H-metolazone was not affected by the ions. In contrast, the apparent affinity of the binding of ^{3}H-metolazone, expressed as the equilibrium dissociation constant, was 3.56 nM in the absence of salt (n=10), 1.32 nM in the presence of 50 mM sodium (n=5), and 9.27 nM (n=10) in the presence of 50 mM sodium chloride. (From [9] with permission of The American Physiological Society)

inhibit reabsorption of NaCl and increase reabsorption of calcium from the renal tubule [3,4], probably by inhibition of a Na-Cl electroneutral symporter in the distal nephron [5,6,7].

Identification and Model of the Thiazide Receptor

The deficit in knowledge about the cellular and molecular mechanism of action of this important class of diuretics is undergoing rapid rectification. Our laboratory has recently developed and utilized ^{3}H-metolazone to identify the putative pharmacological receptor for thiazide-type diuretics by ligand-binding technology [8,9]. Two classes of binding sites for ^{3}H-metolazone, distinguished by differing affinities, were identified. The binding of ^{3}H-metolazone to the class of sites with lower affinity could be inhibited by a variety of drugs with calcium channel-blocking activity (at micromolar concentration). In contrast, the high affinity binding site for ^{3}H-metolazone exhibited characteristics expected of the pharmacological receptor for thiazide diuretics. Indeed, the identity of the high-affinity specific binding site for ^{3}H-metolazone with the thiazide receptor is indicated by three major sets of data. *First*, the pharmacological specificy of the binding of ^{3}H-metolazone to rat kidney membranes is as expected for the receptor for thiazide-type diuretics [8]. The biological potency of 12 thiazide-type diuretics correlated (r=0.75, P<0.01) with their

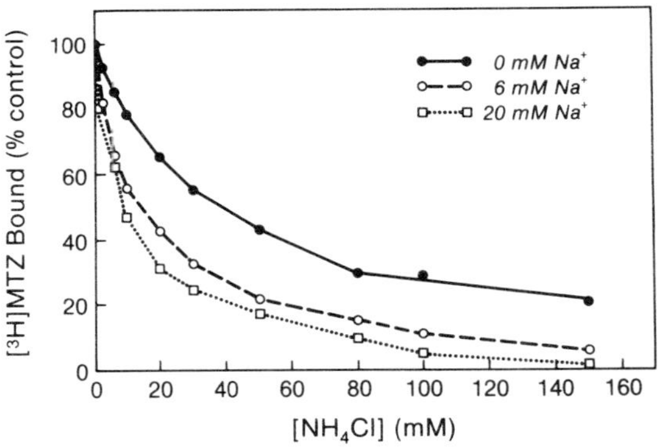

Fig. 2. Effect of Sodium on the ability of chloride to inhibit binding of ^{3}H-metolazone. Renal membranes were incubated with 1 nM ^{3}H-metolazone in the absence or presence of the indicated concentrations of sodium (as the SO_4 salt) and in the presence of the indicated concentrations of chloride (as the ammonium salt). (From [9] with permission of The American Physiological Society)

affinity for the putative receptor [8]. *Second*, the high affinity site for ^{3}H-metolazone has been localized by autoradiography to short and sparsely distributed segments of renal cortical tubules [10], a pattern consistent with a localization to the distal convoluted tubule (DCT). *Third*, the affinity of the binding of ^{3}H-metolazone is altered by the presumed transported ions [9]. The affinity of the thiazide receptor for ^{3}H-metolazone is increased by sodium ions and is decreased by chloride ions, as shown in Fig. 1. Moreover, the ability of chloride to inhibit binding of ^{3}H-metolazone to the thiazide receptor is modulated by the presence of cations. The concentration of chloride needed to produce 50% inhibition of binding (IC_{50}) of ^{3}H-metolazone in the presence of no added cation was 47 ± 3 mM. However, the IC_{50} decreased in the presence of 6 and 20 mM Na^+ to 19 ± 3 and 10 ± 2 mM chloride, respectively (Fig. 2). An additional important observation was that the Hill slopes characterizing the stimulation of binding by sodium and the inhibition of binding by chloride were not significantly different from unity. Therefore, there is no need to implicate more than one class of binding sites for either cation or anion. These findings enabled Tran et al. [9] to propose a conservative model for the transport of sodium/chloride by the transporter (see Fig. 3). The model predicts (a) that the transporter contains two binding sites, one for sodium and one that recognizes chloride and metolazone in a mutually exclusive/competitive fashion and (b) that occupancy of the sodium site increases the affinity of the second site for chloride/metolazone. Normally, the carrier is loaded with sodium from the tubular fluid (Step II, Fig. 3), resulting in an increase in the affinity for chloride, which is loaded in turn (Step III). The lower concentration of sodium in the tubular cell (from the action of Na-K-ATPase) provides a tubular fluid to intracellular concentration gradient for sodium that enables a favorable conformational change in the loaded Na-Cl carrier, such that sodium dissociates into the cell. This decreases the affinity of the carrier for the Cl and, consequently, results in the dissociation of Cl from the carrier into the cell (Step IV). Metolazone and other thiazide-type diuretics exert their action by binding to the transporter from the

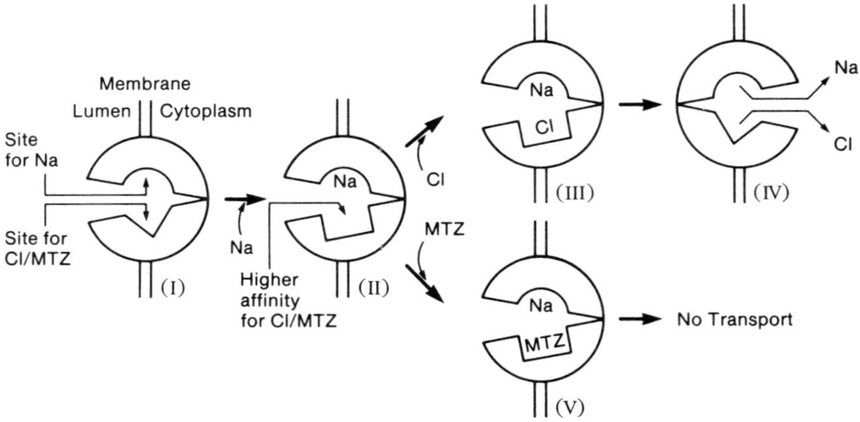

Fig. 3. Model for the mechanism of NaCl cotransport by the thiazide receptor. (From [9] with permission of The American Physiological Society)

tubular side, where their binding affinity is increased as a result of the loading of the carrier with sodium. However, the Na-thiazide carrier complex prevents the loading of chloride, and hence its transport, by the carrier (Step V).

Role of Thiazide-Sensitive Transport in Sodium Homeostasis

Regulation of the reabsorption of sodium by the renal tubule has been under long-term and extensive investigation by numerous laboratories. These studies have led to the following (admittedly overly simplified) appreciation of the complexity of the renal regulation of excretion of sodium. (i) In the proximal tubule, current evidence indicates that sodium transport regulators include angiotensin, the sympathetic nervous system, and dopamine. (ii) In the thick ascending limb of Henle, sodium transport regulators include antidiuretic hormone (in some species), PGE_2, and parathyroid hormone. (iii) In the collecting tubule and ducts, sodium transport regulators include aldosterone, antidiuretic hormone, atrial natriuretic peptide and others. In contrast, there is a paucity of information about regulation of transport of sodium by the DCT.

The lack of information about regulation of the handling of sodium and chloride by the DCT is now in the process of change. Kaissling and Stanton [11,12] and Ellison et al. [13] have recently shown that the DCT responds to increased sodium delivery by changing morphology, including an increase in the basolateral surface area of DCT cells, and an increase in the rate at which sodium is reabsorbed by the DCT.

Our development of ^{3}H-metolazone as a new method for quantitating specific binding sites for thiazide-type diuretics provides the opportunity to determine for the first time if the density of the thiazide receptor is regulated by physiological or pathophysiological conditions. We have learned the following about the regulation of the density of the thiazide receptor in vivo.

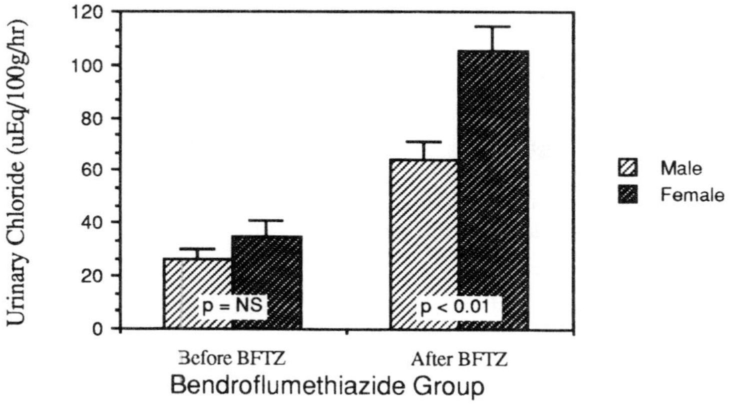

Fig. 4. Effect of treatment with bendroflumethiazide (BFTZ) on urinary excretion of chloride in males and females. The figure shows the hourly rate of excretion of chloride during six hours after treatment with vehicle (before BFTZ) or drug (after BFTZ) in 12 animals of each gender. (Data from [14])

The Thiazide Receptor is Regulated by Gender/Sex Hormone Status

Chen and co-workers [14] have found the following regarding the thiazide receptor in Sprague-Dawley rats: (a) a greater density in 12-week-old female (0.770 ± 0.048 pmol/mg protein) than in age-matched male animals (0.433 ± 0.040 pmol/mg protein); (b) a decrease in density after ovariectomy (0.529 ± 0.051 pmol/mg protein); and (c) an increase in density after orchiectomy (0.793 ± 0.076 pmol/mg protein). Importantly, in unpublished studies, the gender-related difference in binding of ^{3}H-metolazone was accompanied by a demonstrable difference in the renal response to administration of bendroflumethiazide (BFTZ). (Bendroflumethiazide was selected because of its low carbonic anhydrase inhibitory activity.) Urinary excretion of sodium, potassium, and chloride was quantitated during six hours after intraperitoneal administration of diluent or BFTZ. Bendroflumethiazide increased the excretion of sodium in both sexes and the magnitude of the increase was not different between the sexes. In contrast, the excretion of chloride after BFTZ rose to a greater extent in females than in males (Fig. 4). The rate of excretion of chloride was not significantly different between the sexes before BFTZ, but was greater ($P < 0.01$) in females than in males after BFTZ. Since urine pH was less than 6.0 in all animals after BFTZ, the drug did not appreciably inhibit carbonic anhydrase. This greater chloriuresis in females than in males is a finding consistent with the greater density of the thiazide receptor in females than in males.

The Thiazide Receptor is Altered by Adrenocortical Status

Our preliminary studies indicate that the thiazide receptor: (a) decreased in density 5 days post adrenalectomy ($0.248 \pm .027$ pmol/mg protein) vs that in sham operated, age matched control males (0.597 ± 0.048); (b) in another experiment, increased in density after 7 days from 0.117 ± 0.012 pmol/mg in adrenalectomized animals receiving diluent via minipump to 0.383±0.010 pmol/mg in adrenalectomized animals receiving aldosterone (5 μg/100 g per day for 7 days by osmotic minipump), and to 0.445±0.24 pmol/mg in adrenalectomized animals receiving dexamethasone (30 μg/100 g per day for 7 days). This level of replacement of aldosterone was chosen in order to produce a plasma level of aldosterone that was intermediate between that found in animals on a normal vs a low salt diet [15]. This level of administration of dexamethasone was selected in order to produce a maximal glucocorticoid effect, as judged by the ability to decrease the weight of the thymus [16].

The Thiazide Receptor is Increased by Adrenomedullectomy

In unpublished studies (M. Ziegler), adrenal medullectomy resulted in a 50% increase in density from 0.431±.036 pmol/mg in control animals to 0.652±0.025 pmol/mg 4 days post adrenomedullectomy. The adequacy of the medullectomy was confirmed by measurement of adrenal epinephrine content.

The Thiazide Receptor is Altered by Prior Administration of Chloriuretic Diuretics [17]

The density of the binding of ^{3}H-metolazone was increased 47% by acute (60 min) administration of hydrochlorothiazide and 39% by acute administration of furosemide (Fig. 5). In contrast, acute acetazolamide produced no change in binding (Fig. 5), though eliciting a dramatic diuresis, natriuresis, and kaliuresis. Acetazolamide did not produce chloriuresis. Chronic hydrochlorothiazide (5 days) and chronic furosemide (7 days) increased binding of ^{3}H-metolazone by 46% and 101%, respectively. In contrast, variation in dietary sodium intake over a range that allowed normal growth of the animal and that produced urinary excretion of sodium varying from 0.28–2.62 mEq/100gm per day failed to alter the density of the binding of ^{3}H-metolazone. These results do not support the postulate that the receptor is "upregulated" by increased sodium at the lumen of the distal convoluted tubule, since the acetazolamide-treated animals undoubtedly had increased delivery of sodium to the distal convoluted tubule [18,19]. However, we cannot eliminate either of two other postulates regarding the potential signal or mechanism whereby these changes in the density of the thiazide receptor are elicited: The increase in density of the thiazide receptor might be regulated (i) by increased delivery or concentration of chloride in distal convoluted tubular fluid or (ii) by occupancy of the thiazide receptor by either chloride or diuretic.

The Thiazide Receptor is Decreased by Anoxia/Ischemia

Ten minutes of in situ ischemia (produced by cross-clamping the renal pedicle) decreased the density of binding by 90%. Subsequent reperfusion (produced by releasing the cross-clamp) for 10 minutes restored binding ⅔ of the way to normal [20]. In pursuing the in vivo effects of ischemia in vitro, we determined that small segments of rat kidney incubated in physiological salt solution also responded to anoxia or to inhibitors of oxidative phosphorylation with a decrease in density of the thiazide receptor. The in vitro effect of anoxia was reversible upon restoration of oxy-

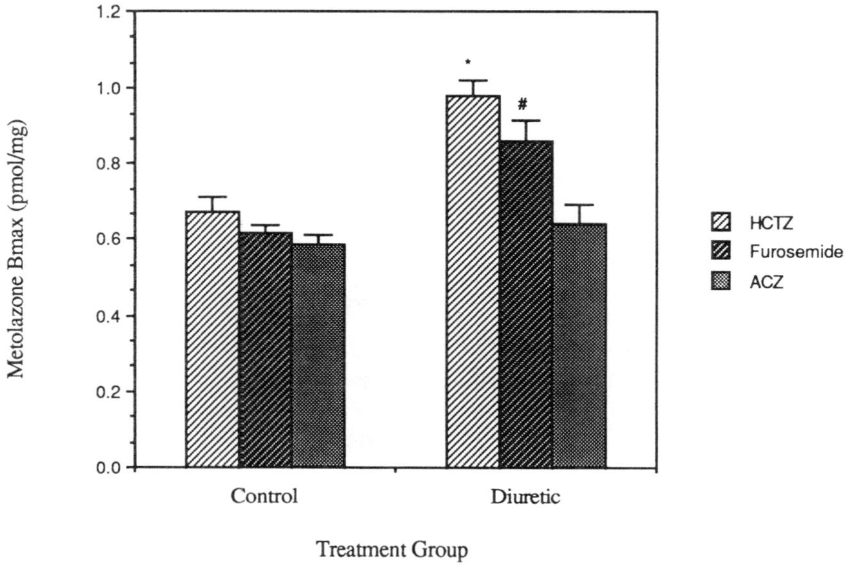

Fig. 5. Acute effect of diuretics on binding of ^{3}H-metolazone. Animals were treated with hydrochlorothiazide (*HCTZ*), furosemide or acetazolamide (*ACZ*) 60 min prior to removal of the kidneys for determination of the density of the thiazide receptor. * and # indicate significantly different from the respective, simultaneously analyzed control groups at $P \leq 0.01$. (Data from [17])

gen (just as in vivo ischemia had been), even after 30 minutes of incubation under a 100% nitrogen environment [20].

The Thiazide Receptor is Increased in Genetic Hypercalciuria

Dr. David Bushinsky has selectively bred rats for hypercalciuria [21]. He presented convincing evidence that the primary defect is gastrointestinal hyperabsorption of calcium, since the animals are in positive calcium balance. We have collaborated in a preliminary study on the thiazide receptor in these animals. The rationale was: if the thiazide-sensitive transporter were so intimately related to control of urinary excretion of calcium as is suggested by the pharmacological actions of thiazide-type diuretics on the DCT, an appropriate homeostatic response to hyperabsorption of calcium would be secondary hyperactivity of the thiazide-sensitive system, in order to facilitate excretion of the increased body burden of calcium. Dr. Bushinsky harvested and rapidly froze kidneys from hypercalciuric animals and their normocalciuric controls. The daily rate of excretion of calcium by the hypercalciuric animals was increased about 5-fold above the control. The kidney weights from the two groups of animals did not differ. However, the density of the thiazide receptor, measured by saturation binding studies with ^{3}H-metolazone, was increased from $0.872 \pm .045$ pmol/mg to $1.102 \pm .057$, $P = .005$.

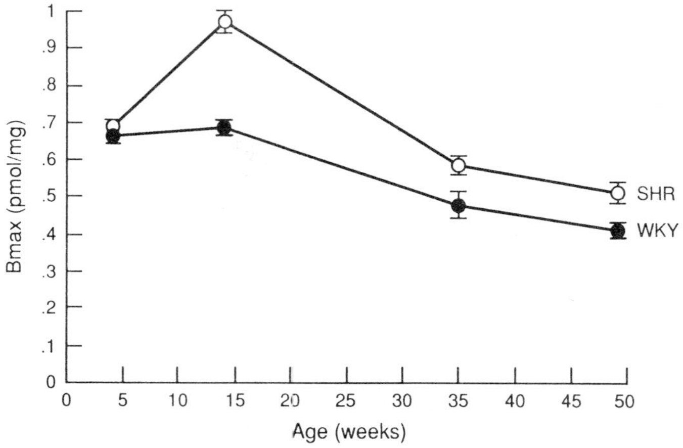

Fig. 6. Alteration of the density of the thiazide diuretic receptor in kidneys from female spontaneously hypertensive (*SHR*) and Wistar Kyoto control (*WKY*) rats. Values are means ± sem for 6–9 animals in each group. SHR and WKY differ significantly at all except 4 weeks of age. (From [22] by courtesy of Marcel Dekker, Inc.)

The Thiazide Receptor is Increased in the Spontaneously Hypertensive Rat (SHR)

Fig. 6 shows a comparison of the density of the receptor in SHR females at several ages, compared with the normotensive Wistar-Kyoto control (WKY) [22]. There was increased receptor density at 14, 35, and 49 weeks of age in female animals and at 35 weeks of age in male animals (the only age tested in males – data not shown). The density was not different in SHR females at 4 weeks of age. Since GFR is low in 5-week-old SHR but normal in older SHR [23,24,25], the density of the thiazide receptor per unit of GFR is likely greater in SHR than in WKY at all ages tested. Thus, the thiazide receptor could mediate increased reabsorption of sodium/chloride per unit GFR in SHR at all ages! An intuitive interpretation of these findings would be that the increase in thiazide receptor in SHR would lead to retention of sodium/chloride and cause or contribute to the generation of hypertension. It is important to note that the increase in thiazide receptor density in hypertensive SHR was not a non-specific effect of elevated renal perfusion pressure, since the receptor density was not different in the clipped vs. unclipped kidney in 2 Kidney-1 Clip animals whose systemic systolic blood pressure was at a level similar to that of the SHR [22]. The relationship between the genes that cause hypertension in SHR and the development of the increased density of the thiazide receptor are fruitful areas for future investigation. Moreover, this finding raises the possibility that the alteration in calcium homeostasis known to occur in SHR [26,27] might be secondary, in SHR, to alteration in calcium reabsorption in the thiazide-sensitive segment of the renal tubule.

The Thiazide Receptor is Dependent Upon Age

The density of the receptor decreases in spontaneously hypertensive (SHR) and Wistar Kyoto control (WKY) females after 15 weeks of age (Fig. 6). This observation has been confirmed in Sprague-Dawley animals in our laboratory (unpublished data).

Conclusions

Development of ^{3}H-metolazone as a marker for the density of the thiazide diuretic receptor is beginning to impact upon our understanding of the renal regulation of excretion of sodium and chloride. Heretofore, there has been a lack of attention to the potential role of physiological and pathophysiological regulation of the thiazide-sensitive segment of the nephron in the homeostatic control of sodium, chloride, calcium, and acid-base homeostasis. The published and unpublished studies reviewed in this paper point out that the thiazide-sensitive transporter can be rapidly (within minutes) regulated, is influenced by both sex and adrenal steroid hormones, and is altered in two types of pathophysiological conditions – experimental genetic hypertension and experimental genetic hypercalciuria. We predict with confidence that future work will provide additional appreciation for the role of the thiazide-sensitive Na-Cl transporter in renal physiology and pathophysiology.

References

1. Wilkins RW, Hollander W, Chobanian AV (1959) Chlorothiazide in hypertension: studies on its mode of action. Ann NY Acad Sci 71:465–472
2. O'Connor DT, Preston RA, Mitas JA, Frigon RP, Stone RA (1981) Urinary kallikrein activity and renal vascular resistance in the antihypertensive response to thiazide diuretics. Hypertension 3:139–147
3. Costanzo LS, Windhager EE (1978) Calcium and sodium transport by the distal convoluted tubule of the rat. Am J Physiol 246:F492–F506
4. Costanzo LS (1985) Localization of diuretic action in microperfused rat distal tubules: Ca and Na transport. Am J Physiol 248:F527–F535
5. Velazquez H, Good DW, Wright FS (1984) Mutual dependence of sodium and chloride absorption by renal distal tubule. Am J Physiol 247:F904–F911
6. Ellison DH, Velazquez H, Wright FS (1987) Thiazide-sensitive sodium chloride cotransport in the early distal tubule. Am J Physiol 253:F546–F554
7. Kunau RT, Weller DR, Webb HL (1975) Clarification of the site of action of chlorothiazide in the rat nephron. J Clin Invest 56:401–407
8. Beaumont K, Vaughn DA, Fanestil DD (1988) Thiazide diuretic receptors in rat kidney: identification with [3-H]metolazone. Proc Natl Acad Sci USA 85:2311–2314
9. Tran JM, Farrell MA, Fanestil DD (1990) Effect of ions on the binding of the thiazide-type diuretic metolazone to kidney membranes. Am J Physiol 258:F908–F915
10. Beaumont K, Vaughn DA, Healy DP (1989) Thiazide diuretic receptors: Autoradiographic localization in rat kidney with [3H]-metolazone. J Pharmacol Exp Ther 250:414–419
11. Kaissling B, Stanton BA (1988) Adaptation of distal tubule and collecting duct to increased sodium delivery. I. Ultrastructure. Am J Physiol 255:F1256–F1268

12. Stanton BA, Kaissling B (1988) Adaptation of distal tubule and collecting duct to increased Na delivery. II. Na^+ and K^+ transport. Am J Physiol 255:F1269–F1275
13. Ellison DH, Velazquez H, Wright FS (1989) Adaptation of the distal convoluted tubule of the rat. Structural and functional effects of dietary salt intake and chronic diuretic infusion. J Clin Invest 83:113–126
14. Chen Z, Vaughn DA, Cochoit J, Fanestil DD (to be published) Influence of gender, sex hormone status and pregnancy on binding of 3H-metolazone in kidney.
15. Martin RS, Jones WJ, Hayslett JP (1983) Animal model to study the effect of adrenal hormones on epithelial function. Kidney Int 24:386–391
16. Khalid BAK, Lim AT, Funder JW (1982) Steroid effects on protein synthesis: Mineralocorticoids and glucocorticoids, thymus and pituitary. Excerpta Medica 598:289–294
17. Chen Z, Vaughn DA, Beaumont K, Fanestil DD (1990) Effects of diuretic treatment and of dietary sodium on renal binding of 3H-metolazone. J Am Soc Nephrology 1:91–98
18. Cogan MG, Maddox DA, Warnock DG, Lin ET, Rector JFC (1979) Effect of acetazolamide on bicarbonate reabsorption in the proximal tubule of the rat. Am J Physiol 237:F447–F454
19. Kunau RT (1972) The influence of the carbonic anhydrase inhibitor benzolamide (Al-11,366) on the reabsorption of chloride, sodium and bicarbonate in the proximal tubule of the rat. J Clin Invest 51:294–306
20. Beaumont K, Vaughn DA, Maciejewski AR, Fanestil DD (1989) Reversible downregulation of thiazide diuretic receptors by acute renal ischemia. Am J Physiol 256:F329–F334
21. Bushinsky DA, Favus MJ (1988) Mechanism of hypercalciuria in genetic hypercalciuric rats. J Clin Invest 82:1585–1591
22. Beaumont K, Vaughn DA, Casto RL, Printz MP, Fanestil DD (1990) Thiazide diuretic receptors in spontaneously hypertensive rats and 2-kidney 1-clip hypertensive rats. Clin Exp Hypertens [A]12:215–226
23. Arendshorst WJ, Beierwaltes WH (1979) Renal tubular reabsorption in spontaneously hypertensive rats. Am J Physiol 237:F38–F47
24. Arendshorst WJ, Beierwaltes WH (1979) Renal and nephron hemodynamics in spontaneously hypertensive rats. Am J Physiol 237:F246–F251
25. Beierwaltes WH, Arendshorst WJ, Klemmer PJ (1982) Electrolyte and water balance in young spontaneously hypertensive rats. Hypertension 4:908–915
26. Hsu CH, Chen P-S, Smith DE, Yang C-S (1986) Pathogenesis of hypercalciuria in spontaneously hypertensive rats. Min Electrol Metab 12:130–141
27. McCarron DA (1989) Calcium metabolism and hypertension. Kidney Int 35:717–736

Application of the Amiloride Series in the Study of Ion Transport

Thomas R. Kleyman[1]

Summary. Amiloride and amiloride analogs have been extensively used as inhibitors of Na^+-selective transport proteins. The interaction of amiloride analogs with the epithelial Na^+ channel, Na^+/H^+ exchanger, and Na^+/Ca^{2+} exchanger is summarized. The potential use of amiloride analogs as biochemical probes for amiloride-sensitive transport proteins, and as immunologic tools for development of antibodies directed against these proteins is discussed, as are some of the limitations and problems encountered using amiloride analogs as "specific" inhibitors of defined transport proteins.

Introduction

The search for diuretics with antikaliuretic properties lead to the generation of the amiloride series [1,2]. Both the natriuresis and antikaliuresis following oral administration of amiloride occur as a result of inhibition of the epithelial Na^+ channel present in the distal nephron [3]. The concentration of amiloride required to inhibit the epithelial Na^+ channel by 50% (IC_{50}) is less than 1 μM. Higher concentrations inhibit other transport proteins (see Table 1) including Na^+/H^+ exchanger, Na^+/Ca^{2+} exchanger, Na^+,K^+-ATPase, Na^+-d-glucose cotransporter, Na^+-1-alanine cotransporter, Na^+-PO_4^{3-} cotransporter, voltage-gated Na^+ channel, voltage-gated Ca^{2+} channel, delayed rectifier K^+ channel, and the nicotinic acetylcholine receptor (for review, see [4]).

Amiloride inhibits most Na^+-selective transport proteins, and kinetic studies of amiloride's interaction with the Na^+/H^+ exchanger [5], Na^+/Ca^{2+} exchanger [6], and Na^+-hexose cotransporter [7] suggest that amiloride binds to a Na^+ recognition or binding site on these transporters. Studies of the interaction of amiloride with the epithelial Na^+ channel in several model systems have also suggested that amiloride

[1]Renal and Electrolyte Section—700 CRB, University of Pennsylvania, Philadelphia, PA 19104-6144, USA

Table 1. Amiloride-sensitive transport proteins

Epithelial Na^+ channel
Na^+/H^+ exchanger
Na^+/Ca^{2+} exchanger
Na^+,K^+-ATPase
Na^+-d-glucose cotransporter
Na^+-l-alanine cotransporter
Na^+-PO_4^{3-} cotransporter
Voltage-gated Na^+ channel
Voltage-gated Ca^{2+} channel
Delayed rectifier K^+ channel
Nicotinic acetylcholine receptor

and Na^+ share a common binding or recognition site, which is presumably in or near the pore of the channel [8,9,10]. However, examination of the site of interaction of amiloride with the Na^+ channel is complicated by the voltage-dependent interaction of amiloride (a monovalent cation) with the channel [11,12], as the varied Na^+ concentrations used in these studies could change the electric potential across the plasma membrane and, as a secondary effect, alter the binding of amiloride.

Inhibition of Transport Proteins

Amiloride is a substituted pyrazinoylguanidine. Its structure is illustrated in Fig. 1. In addition, two major classes of amiloride analogs have been used as ion transport inhibitors. These include analogs with hydrophobic groups on the terminal nitrogen of the guanidino moiety of amiloride, such as benzamil (Fig. 1), and analogs with hydrophobic groups on the 5-amino moiety of the pyrazine ring, such as EIPA

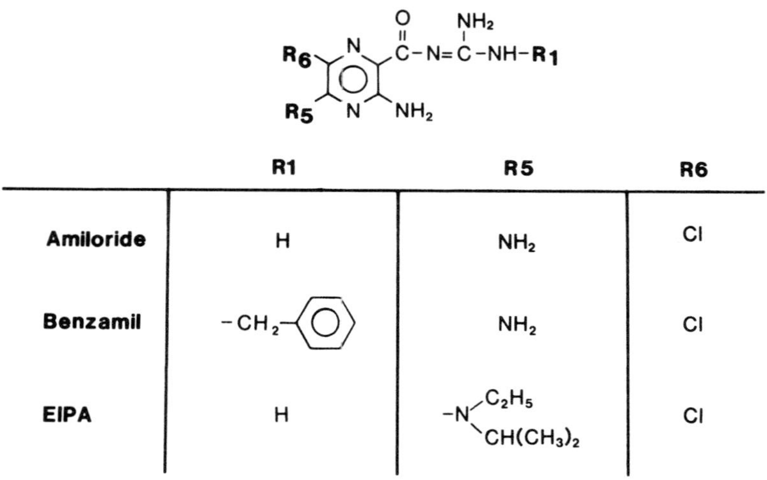

Fig. 1. Structures of amiloride and the amiloride analogs benzamil and EPIA

Table 2. IC_{50} (μM) of amiloride or amiloride analogs

	Na^+ channel	Na^+/H^+ exchange	Na^+/Ca^{2+} exchange
Amiloride	0.35	84	1,100
Benzamil	0.04	>1,000	100
EIPA	>10	0.38	140

The concentrations of amiloride, benzamil, and EIPA required to achieve half maximal inhibition (IC_{50}) of the A6 cell epithelial Na^+ [4] channel, neutrophil Na^+/H^+ exchanger [15], and GH_3 cell Na^+/Ca^{2+} [6] exchanger are listed

(Fig. 1). Amiloride is a reversible inhibitor of ion transport and it is the protonated form of amiloride which is required to block transport [6,13,14]. The interaction of amiloride or amiloride analogs with ion transporters has been most extensively characterized in three systems: the epithelial Na^+ channel, Na^+/H^+ exchange, and Na^+/Ca^{2+} exchange. A summary of the IC_{50}s of amiloride, benzamil, and EIPA for the apical epithelial Na^+ channel [4], Na^+/H^+ exchanger (in neutrophils) [15], and Na^+/Ca^{2+} exchanger [6] is listed in Table 2.

Epithelial Na^+ Channel

The epithelial Na^+ channel is expressed on the apical plasma membrane of high-resistance, Na^+-transporting epithelia, such as renal collecting tubule, distal colon, urinary bladder, and trachea (for review, see [16]). Amiloride inhibits the Na^+ channel at a site which is accessible from extracellular fluid. The IC_{50} for amiloride is in the range of 0.1–0.5 μM, when measured in the presence of a physiologic concentration of Na^+ [4]. Lowering the extracellular Na^+ concentration will decrease the IC_{50} by up to ~10 fold [4,17]. As discussed above, the kinetics of amiloride binding to the Na^+ channel in the presence of a varying apical plasma membrane potential suggest that amiloride senses between 10%–45% of the membrane electric field [11,12]. This observation, together with studies in voltage-clamped cells demonstrating that amiloride binding kinetics are altered by Na^+ or Li^+ loading cells in order to generate an outward current through the channel [18,19], support the notion that the amiloride-binding site is likely within the pore of the channel, possibly at a Na^+ binding or recognition site.

Amiloride analogs with hydrophobic groups on the guanidino moiety tend to lower the IC_{50} and increase the specificity for the Na^+ channel [4,20]. Analogs with hydrophobic groups on the 5-amino moiety of the pyrazine ring both raise the IC_{50} and decrease the specificity for the channel [4,20].

Na^+ channels with a low affinity for amiloride (IC_{50}s in the range of 1–20 μM) have recently been described [21,22]. The interaction of these channels with amiloride analogs differs from that observed with the high affinity Na^+ channels described above, in that the IC_{50}s for amiloride analogs with hydrophobic groups on the guanidino moiety or on the 5-amino moiety of the pyrazine ring are similar to the IC_{50} for amiloride. These channels were described in membrane vesicles isolated from urinary bladder and colon. A Na^+ conductive pathway, with an IC_{50} for amiloride of 13 μM, was recently observed in the basolateral plasma membrane of toad urinary bladder [23], suggesting that these channels are expressed on the basolateral plasma membrane of high-resistance, Na^+-transporting epithelia.

Na^+/H^+ Exchange

The Na^+/H^+ exchanger is a 110 kDa glycoprotein [24] which is constitutively expressed in most mammalian cells and participates in regulation of intracellular pH [25]. This transporter is also expressed at the apical plasma membrane of low-resistance epithelia and facilitates vectorial transport of Na^+ and HCO_3^- (or H^+) [25]. Amiloride inhibits the Na^+/H^+ exchanger with an IC_{50} in the range of 3–30 μM, when measured in the presence of a low Na^+ concentration [5,14,26,27]. The IC_{50} is dependent on the extracellular Na^+ concentration, in that lowering the extracellular Na^+ concentration will decrease the IC_{50}. Certain amiloride analogs with hydrophobic groups on the 5-amino moiety of the pyrazine ring have a lower IC_{50}, relative to amiloride, for the exchanger and at low concentrations are specific inhibitors of the exchanger [4,14,15,26,27]. In contrast, analogs with hydrophobic groups on the guanidino moiety inhibit the Na^+/H^+ exchanger with IC_{50}s greater than amiloride.

In epithelia, basolateral and apical transporters differ in their apparent affinity for amiloride. The apical transporter has a higher IC_{50} for both amiloride and the analog EIPA, relative to the basolateral transporter. The IC_{50} of EIPA for the basolateral transporter is ~300-fold lower than that for the apical transporter [28].

Na^+/Ca^{2+} Exchange

The Na^+/Ca^{2+} exchanger is expressed at the plasma membrane of a variety of cell types and participates in intracellular Ca^{2+} regulation. Amiloride's IC_{50} is ~ 1 mM [6]. The IC_{50} for amiloride is dependent on the extracellular Na^+ concentration, in that lowering the extracellular Na^+ concentration will decrease the IC_{50}. Analogs with hydrophobic groups on either the 5-amino moiety of the pyrazine ring and/or on the guanidino moiety lower the IC_{50} for the exchanger [4,6]. Certain amiloride analogs which inhibit Na^+/Ca^{2+} exchange may inhibit Ca^{2+} channels with equal or lower IC_{50}s [29].

Amiloride Analogs as Probes for Na^+-Selective Transport Proteins

Aside from the use of amiloride analogs as inhibitors of ion transporters, amiloride analogs have been successfully used as probes for biochemical characterization of transport proteins. Radioactive amiloride derivatives have been used to examine binding of amiloride analogs to the Na^+ channel and Na^+/H^+ exchanger [30–33]. Two groups have recently used the binding of a radiolabeled amiloride analog as a marker to purify the epithelial Na^+ channel [32,34].

Photoactive amiloride analogs have also been used to identify the amiloride-binding subunit of the epithelial Na^+ channel. Two classes of photoactive amiloride

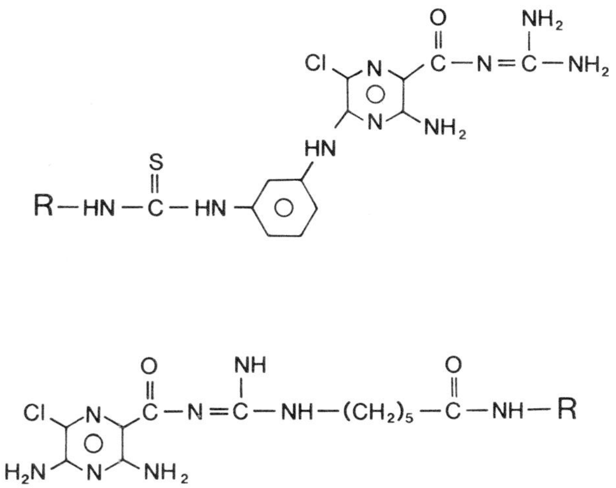

Fig. 2. Structures of amiloride analogs coupled to carrier protein (*R*). Amiloride was coupled to albumin either through the 5-amino group on the pyrazine ring or through the guanidino group

analogs with different reactive groups were used to affinity label the amiloride-binding subunit of the Na^+ channel [30,34,35]. The first class of compounds, which include bromobenzamil and bromomethylamiloride, utilize the halide (bromo) on the 6-position of the pyrazine ring on the amiloride molecule as the photoreactive moiety. A second class of photoactive amiloride analogs was developed with an aromatic ether attached to amiloride through its guanidino moiety. One member of this group, 2-methoxy-5-nitrobenzylamiloride, was used to label the amiloride-binding subunit of the Na^+ channel [35]. The 2-methoxy-5-nitrobenzyl group undergoes photoactivation and incorporates into proteins through a mechanism of aromatic nucleophilic photosubstitution [36]. This type of photochemical reaction has several major advantages. First, it is a high efficiency reaction, as labeling of more than 30% of amiloride-binding sites was noted [35]. Second, only one reactive intermediate is formed, with a half-life of less than 10^{-7} s [36], which markedly reduces nonspecific photolabeling. The Na^+ channel is an oligomeric protein [34]. The amiloride-binding subunit of the channel identified in photoaffinity labeling studies is a polypeptide subunit with an apparent molecular weight in the range of 130–180 kDa [30,34,35].

Amiloride analogs with spacer arms have been synthesized with terminal carboxyl or amino groups to allow for coupling to immobilized resins or to carrier protein (see Fig. 2) [37,38]. Since amiloride analogs with hydrophobic groups on the guanidino moiety of amiloride are specific high affinity inhibitors of the Na^+ channel, amiloride coupled through its guanidino group to albumin was used as an immunogen to raise anti-amiloride antibodies. These antibodies bind amiloride analogs in a manner similar to that of the Na^+ channel [39]. In contrast, antibodies raised against amiloride conjugated to albumin through its 5-amino group bound amiloride analogs in a manner similar to that of the Na^+/H^+ exchanger [39]. These antibodies raised against the different amiloride-albumin conjugates recognize distinct epitopes on amiloride.

The anti-amiloride antibodies have proven to be useful in detecting a photoactive amiloride analog covalently bound to the Na^+ channel [35], and as tools for raising anti-idiotypic antibodies which recognize the Na^+ channel. This approach for raising anti-Na^+ channel antibodies is based on the apparent structural mimicry of the amiloride-binding domain on the anti-amiloride antibody and on the Na^+ channel. The anti-idiotypic antibody can mimic the effect of amiloride by inhibiting Na^+ transport across a Na^+-transporting epithelium (A6 cells) (Kleyman TR, Kraehenbuhl JP, and Ernst SA, J. Biol. Chem. in press).

Problems Encountered Using Amiloride Analogs as Ion Transport Probes

Amiloride analogs are often added to extracellular fluid in order to inhibit ion transport proteins expressed on the plasma membrane. Unfortunately, amiloride analogs do not remain in the extracellular space and will accumulate within cells. The cellular uptake of amiloride occurs by simple diffusion [40,41], although transport across the plasma membrane has been observed in hepatocytes [42]. The intracellular concentration may reach levels greater than the extracellular concentration, assuming that measured "cellular" amiloride was free in solution and not bound to lipid, nor compartmentalized. In neutrophils 75% of the intracellular amiloride was considered to be in the lysozomal compartment [40]. In other cell types, the extent to which intracellular amiloride is compartmentalized is uncertain. Amiloride diffuses across red blood cell and neutrophil plasma membranes with a permeability coefficient of approximately 10^{-7} cm•sec^{-1} [40,41]. As amiloride is a permeable weak base, cellular accumulation of amiloride could alter intracellular pH.

Amiloride and amiloride analogs have gained widespread use as inhibitors of ion transport proteins. However, the specificity of these drugs may be limited by inhibition of cellular processes other than ion transport. Amiloride binds to or inhibits a number of enzymes, which are listed in Table 3 (for review, see [4]). The inhibition of protein kinase activity is competitive with respect to ATP, suggesting that amiloride interacts with, or binds to an ATP binding site on protein kinases [43]. As inhibition of a particular enzyme might have a direct (or indirect) influence on a specific

Table 3. Amiloride-sensitive enzymes

Acetylcholinesterase
Adenylate cyclase
DNA Topoisomerase II
Monoamine oxidase
Na^+,K^+-ATPase
Renal kallikrein
Urokinase type plasminogen activator
Type I cAMP dependent protein kinase
Type II cAMP dependent protein kinase
Epidermal growth factor receptor protein kinase
Platelet derived growth factor receptor protein kinase
Insulin receptor protein kinase
Protein kinase C

ion transporter protein, it is of value to be cognizant of the effects of amiloride analogs on these enzymes when using amiloride analogs as "selective" inhibitors of ion transport.

Amiloride analogs have been observed to effect other cellular processes as well. These include inhibition of oxidative phosphorylation and depletion of cellular ATP levels, and inhibition of DNA, RNA, and protein synthesis [14,26,42,44] (for review, see [4]). The extent of inhibition may vary with the cell type studied. These effects may be both direct, as well as indirect, as a result of inhibition of ion transport [14].

Amiloride is a fluorescent aromatic compound with excitation maxima at 286 and 360 nm and emission maxima at 410–414 nm [4,43]. The major absorption peaks of amiloride are at 360–370 nm, 265–290 nm, and 215–235 nm [4]. The fluorescence and absorption properties of amiloride may interfere with techniques which utilize fluorescent probes to measure intracellular pH and intracellular Ca^{2+}.

Protonation of the guanidino group is required for amiloride to inhibit ion transport. The pK_a of the guanidino group is 8.8, and at a pH of 7.4, more than 95% of amiloride will be protonated [4]. However, the pK_a is significantly lowered in certain amiloride analogs with substituents on the guanidino group, which can considerably alter the concentration of the amiloride analog which is in its active, or protonated form.

Review

The amiloride series was initially developed with the goal of identifying new diuretics with antikaliuretic properties. These compounds subsequently found widespread use as inhibitors of Na^+-selective transport proteins. Amiloride or amiloride analogs are often used as specific inhibitors of ion transporters; however, the use of these compounds as selective inhibitors should be tempered by knowledge of their effects on enzymes and other cellular processes which could indirectly alter ion transport. Despite these limitations, amiloride analogs have provided valuable probes for the isolation and biochemical characterization of the epithelial Na^+ channel, and for the generation of antibodies directed against this channel. As amiloride and its analogs bind to a Na^+ recognition or binding site on several of the Na^+-selective transport proteins, these compounds may provide useful tools to define structural features on these proteins which participate in Na^+ binding.

Acknowledgments. This work was supported by grants from the Cystic Fibrosis Foundation and the Department of Veterans Affairs.

References

1. Cragoe EJ Jr, Woltersdorf OW Jr, Bicking JB, Kwong SF, Jones JH (1967) Pyrazine diuretics. II. N-amidino-3-amino-5-substituted 6-halopyrazine-carboxamides. J Med Chem 10:66–75
2. Cragoe EJ Jr (1983) Pyrazine diuretics. In: Cragoe EJ Jr (ed) Diuretics: chemistry, pharmacology, and medicine. John Wiley and Sons, New York, pp 303–343

3. Kleyman TR, Cragoe EJ Jr (1988) Mechanism of action of amiloride. Semin Nephrol 8:242–248
4. Kleyman TR, Cragoe EJ Jr (1988) Amiloride and its analogs as tools in the study of ion transport. J Membr Biol 105:1–21
5. Kinsella JL, Aronson PS (1981) Amiloride inhibition of the Na^+/H^+ exchanger in renal microvillus membrane vesicles. Am J Physiol 241:F374–F379
6. Kaczorowski GJ, Barros F, Dethmers JK, Trumble MJ (1985) Inhibition of Na^+/Ca^{2+} exchange in pituitary plasma membrane vesicles by analogues of amiloride. Biochemistry 24:1394–1403
7. Cook JS, Shaffer C, Cragoe EJ Jr (1987) Inhibition by amiloride analogues of Na^+-dependent hexose uptake in LLC-PK_1/CL_4 cells. Am J Physiol 253:C199–C204
8. Li JH-Y, Lindemann B (1983) Competitive blocking of epithelial sodium channels by organic cations: the relationship between macroscopic and microscopic inhibition constants. J Membr Biol 76:235–251
9. Cuthbert A (1981) Sodium entry step in transporting epithelia – results of ligand-binding studies, In: Schultz S (ed) Ion transport by epithelia. Raven, New York, pp 181–196
10. Gottlieb GP, Turnheim K, Frizzell RA, Schultz SG (1978) p-Chloromercuribenzene sulfonate blocks and reverses the effect of amiloride on sodium transport across rabbit colon in vitro. Biophys J 22:125–129
11. Palmer LG (1984) Voltage-dependent block by amiloride and other monovalent cations of apical sodium channels in the toad urinary bladder. J Membr Biol 80:153–165
12. Hamilton K, Eaton D (1985) Single-channel recordings from amiloride-sensitive epithelial sodium channel. Am J Physiol 249:C200–C207
13. Benos DJ, Simon SA, Mandel LJ, Cala PM (1976) Effect of amiloride and some of its analogues on cation transport in isolated frog skin and thin lipid membranes. J Gen Physiol 68:43–63
14. L'Allemain G, Franchi A, Cragoe EJ Jr, Pouyssegur J (1984) Blockade of the Na^+/H^+ antiport abolishes growth factor-induced DNA synthesis in fibroblasts. Structure-activity relationships in the amiloride series. J Biol Chem 259:4313–4319
15. Simchowitz L, Cragoe EJ Jr (1986) Inhibition of chemotactic-factor activated Na^+/H^+ exchange in human neutrophils by analogues of amiloride: structure-activity relationships in the amiloride series. Mol Pharmacol 30:112–120
16. Sariban-Sohraby S, Benos DJ (1986) The amiloride-sensitive sodium channel. Am J Physiol 250:C175–C190
17. Cuthbert AW, Shum WK (1974) Amiloride and the sodium channel. Naunyn Schmiedebergs Arch Pharmacol 281:261–269
18. Li JH-Y, Lindemann B (1982) Movement of Na and Li across the apical membrane of frog skin. In: Emrich HM, Aldenhoff JB, Lux DH (eds) Basic mechanisms in the action of lithium. Excerpta Medica, Amsterdam, pp 28–35
19. Van Driessche W, Erlij P (1983) Noise analysis of inward and outward Na^+ currents across the apical border of ouabain-treated frog skin. Pflugers Arch 398:179–188
20. Cuthbert AW, Fanelli GM (1978) Effects of some pyrazinecarboxamides on sodium transport in frog skin. Br J Pharmacol 63:139–149
21. Asher C, Cragoe EJ Jr, Garty H (1987) Effects of amiloride analogues on Na^+ transport in toad bladder membrane vesicles. J Biol Chem 262:8566–8573
22. Bridges RJ, Cragoe EJ Jr, Frizzell RA, Benos DJ (1989) Inhibition of colonic Na^+ transport by amiloride analogues. Am J Physiol 256:C67–C74
23. Garty H, Warncke J, Lindemann B (1987) An amiloride-sensitive Na^+ conductance in the basolateral membrane of toad urinary bladder. J Membr Biol 95:91–103
24. Sardet C, Counillon L, Franchi A, Pouyssegur J (1990) Growth factors induce phosphorylation of the Na/H antiporter, a glycoprotein of 110 kD. Science 247:723–726

25. Seifter JL, Aronson PS (1986) Properties and physiologic roles of the plasma membrane sodium-hydrogen exchanger. J Clin Invest 78:859–864
26. Zhuang Y, Cragoe EJ Jr, Shaikewitz T, Glaser L, Cassel D (1984) Characterization of potent Na/H exchange inhibitors from the amiloride series in A431 cells. Biochemistry 23:4481–4488
27. Vigne P, Frelin C, Cragoe EJ Jr, Lazdunski M (1984) Structure-activity relationships of amiloride and certain of its analogues in relation to the blockade of the Na^+/H^+ exchange system. Mol Pharmacol 25:131–136
28. Haggerty JG, Agarwal N, Reilly RF, Adelberg EA, Slayman CW (1988) Pharmacologically different Na/H antiporters on the apical and basolateral surfaces of cultured porcine kidney cells (LLC-PK_1). Proc Natl Acad Sci USA 85:6797–6801
29. Garcia ML, King VF, Shevell JL, Slaughter RS, Suarez-Kurtz G, Winquist RJ, Kaczorowski GJ (1990) Amiloride analogs inhibit L-type calcium channels and display calcium entry blocker activity. J Biol Chem 265:3763–3771
30. Kleyman TR, Yulo T, Ashbaugh C, Landry D, Cragoe EJ Jr., Karlin A, Al-Awqati Q (1986) Photoaffinity labeling of the epithelial sodium channel. J Biol Chem 261:2839–2943
31. Sariban-Sohraby S, Benos DJ (1986) Detergent solubilization, functional reconstitution, and partial purification of epithelial amiloride binding protein. Biochemistry 25:4639–4646
32. Barbry P, Chassande C, Vigne P, Frelin C, Ellory C, Cragoe EJ Jr, and Lazdunski M (1987) Purification and subunit structure of the [^{3}H]phenamil receptor associated with the renal apical Na^+ channel Proc Natl Acad Sci USA 84:4836–4840
33. Vigne P, Frelin C, Aucinot M, Borsotto M, Cragoe EJ Jr, Lazdunski M (1984) [^{3}H]ethylpropylamiloride, a radio-labelled diuretic for the analysis of the Na^+/H^+ exchange system. EMBO J 3:2647–2651
34. Benos DJ, Saccomani G, Sariban-Sohraby S (1987) The epithelial sodium channel. Subunit number and localization of the amiloride binding site. J Biol Chem 262:10613–10618
35. Kleyman TR, Cragoe EJ Jr, Kraehenbuhl JP (1989) The cellular pool of Na^+ channels in the amphibian cell line A6 is not altered by mineralocorticoids. Analysis using a new photoactive amiloride analog in combination with anti-amiloride antibodies. J Biol Chem 264:11995–12000
36. Cornelisse J, Havinga E (1975) Photosubstitution reactions of aromatic compounds. Chem Rev 75:353–388
37. Kleyman TR, Rajagopalan R, Cragoe EJ Jr, Erlanger BF, Al-Awqati Q (1986) New amiloride analogue as hapten to raise anti-amiloride antibodies. Am J Physiol 250:C165–C170
38. Cassel D, Rotman M, Cragoe EJ Jr, Igarashi P (1988) Preparation of 6-^{125}I-labeled amiloride derivatives. Anal Biochem 170:63–67
39. Kleyman TR, Kraehenbuhl JP, Rossier BC, Cragoe EJ Jr, Warnock DG (1989) Distinct epitopes on amiloride. Am J Physiol 257:C1135–C1141
40. Simchowitz L, Woltersdorf OW Jr, Cragoe EJ Jr (1987) Intracellular accumulation of potent amiloride analogues by human neutrophils. J Biol Chem 262:15875–15975
41. Benos DJ, Reyes J, Shoemaker DG (1983) Amiloride fluxes across erythrocyte membranes. Biochim Biophys Acta 734:99–104
42. Leffert HL, Koch KS, Fehlmann M, Heiser W, Lad PJ, Skelly H (1982) Amiloride blocks cell-free protein synthesis at levels attained inside cultured rat hepatocytes. Biochem Biophys Res Commun 108:738–745
43. Davis RJ, Czech MP (1985) Amiloride directly inhibits growth factor receptor tyrosine kinase activity. J Biol Chem 260:2543–2551
44. Koch KS, Leffert HL (1979) Increased sodium ion influx is necessary to initiate rat hepatocyte proliferation. Cell 18:153–163

Target Cell Metabolism of Corticosteroids Mediating Antisteroid Effects

KLAUS HIERHOLZER, HELMUT BÜHLER, and FRANK H. PERSCHEL[1]

Introduction

Anticorticosteroid hormones have attracted attention, since they not only provide useful tools for evaluating mechanisms of corticosteroid (CS) action but also since they constitute powerful therapeutic agents. Thus, antimineralocorticosteroids are applied in treating hypertension, antiglucocorticosteroids are useful in counteracting glucocorticosteroid (GCS) excess syndromes, and antiprogestins are widely used in interrupting the luteal phase, in counteracting early pregnancy, and may be useful in inhibiting mammary tumor growth.

In Principle, Antisteroid Effects Can Be Induced

1) By interfering with CS production either at the level of the adrenals or by reducing the availability of releasing and/or trophic hormones,
2) by interfering with CS effects in target cells, i.e., by anti-CS action in the classical sense which (competitively) binds to target cell receptors and inhibits the function of endogenous agonists; or
3) by interfering with steps subsequent to hormone-receptor interaction at the transcriptional level, or even further downstream.

Recent developments in the field have been covered in several excellent publications [1–22].

[1]Institut für Klinische Physiologie, Klinikum Steglitz, Freie Universität Berlin, Hindenburgdamm 30, 1000 Berlin 45, Federal Republic of Germany

A fourth principle of modulating physiological CS effects is inhibition (or stimulation) of CS-metabolizing enzymes. This aspect has recently attracted attention. It can be documented that many target organs are equipped with CS transforming enzymes that share the potency to convert CS to metabolites with biological properties which may differ quantitatively, as well as qualitatively, from the respective mother hormones. It is this fourth aspect which shall be addressed in the present paper. This is pertinent for the present discussion, since the 11-hydroxysteroid dehydrogenase (11-HSD) system constitutes a diuretic principle and, in turn, inhibition of 11-HSD results in Na^+ and fluid retention.

Materials and Methods

Experiments were performed with male Sprague Dawley rats (250–400 g). Renal tissue slices, microsomes and solubilized 11-HSD were incubated in vitro with ^3H-labelled corticosterone (B) or 11-dehydro B. Metabolites were identified by reversed phase high pressure liquid chromatography (RP-HPLC). The techniques used are described in detail elsewhere [23–26].

Sources of steroids and chemicals were: 1] ^3H-B from New England Nuclear, Dreieich, FRG, 2] ^3H-11 dehydro B prepared in our laboratory from 1, 3] β-glycyrrhetinic acid from Sigma, Deisenhofen, FRG, 4] detergents: CHAPS series from Calbiochem, Frankfurt/Main, FRG, Triton X-100 from Boehringer Mannheim, FRG, 5] bile acids from Calbiochem and Sigma, and 6] ginseng root extract and ginsenosides from Tsumura Co., Japan.

CS Metabolism in Peripheral Target Organs

Figure 1 indicates the sites of the steroid skeleton where metabolic transformations occur, as shown, in different tissues such as kidney, liver, intestinal tract, salivary glands, gonads, placenta, toad bladder, and fish gills (for references see [24,25]).

In our studies we initially concentrated on the rat kidney. Isolated perfused organs, tissue slices, and subcellular fractions such as microsomes, nuclei, mitochondria and cytoplasm were incubated with the respective endogenous ^3H-CS; the metabolites formed were identified by HPLC and mass spectrometry [23,27]. It can be shown that mammalian renal tissue converts aldosterone into reduced di- and tetrahydro metabolites. B is converted at C_{11} and C_{20} and is subsequently reduced to pregnane. From a quantitative point of view the enzyme 11-HSD seems to be most important. Thus, we concentrated on this enzyme (system).

Some of the relevant properties of the enzyme are listed in Table 1. Of particular interest seem to be results obtained in microbiochemical studies with microdissected single tubules, which demonstrated highest activities of 11-HSD in the proximal pars recta [28]. Furthermore, a peculiar distribution pattern of immunoreactive enzyme in cortex and papilla was obtained in immunohistochemical studies using a specific mouse anti-11-HSD monoclonal antibody. The latter studies identified intra-epithelial localization of 11-HSD in cortex and interstitial cell staining in renal

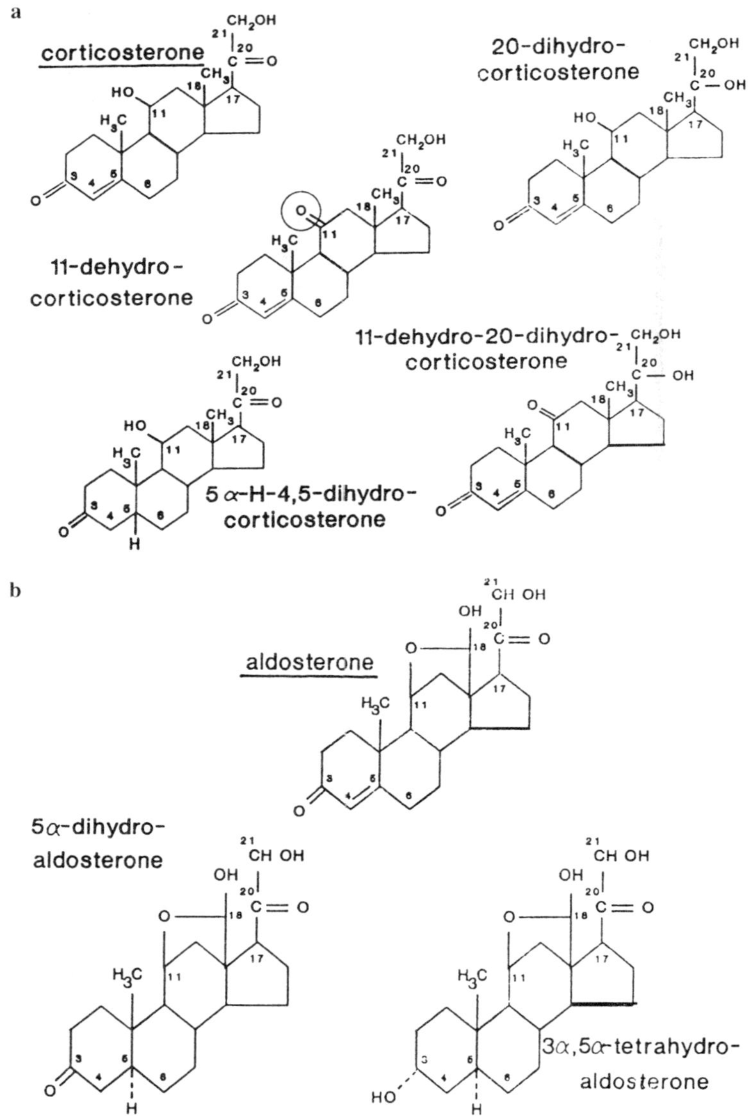

Fig. 1a,b. Structure of corticosterone with possible sites of renal metabolism **a**, corticosterone **b**, aldosterone

Table 1. 11-Hydroxysteroid-dehydrogenase (rat kidney)

(E.C. 1.1.1.146)
- Membrane bound (micros., nuclear)
- Identified in a) liver, gonads b) transporting epithelia (kidney, GIT, lung, placenta, toad bladder)
- Bidirectional? (oxidoreductase?) 11–OH–CS ⟷ 11=O–CS
- Properties:
  a) molecular weight 34 kDa
  b) $K_m \sim 10^{-7}$ M
  c) $P_I \sim 5.9$ (ox. and red)
  d) pH $opt_{ox} \sim 9$, pH $opt_{red} \sim 6$–7
- Biological significance:
  CGS (in)activation
  Control of apparent MCS specificity

medulla [29]. The potential biological relevance of this differing distribution pattern has recently been discussed [30,31].

Inhibitors of 11-HSD (and other CS Transforming Enzymes)

The evaluation of the potential biological significance of the 11-HSD enzyme system has recently benefitted from experiments with specific enzyme inhibitors [30–36].

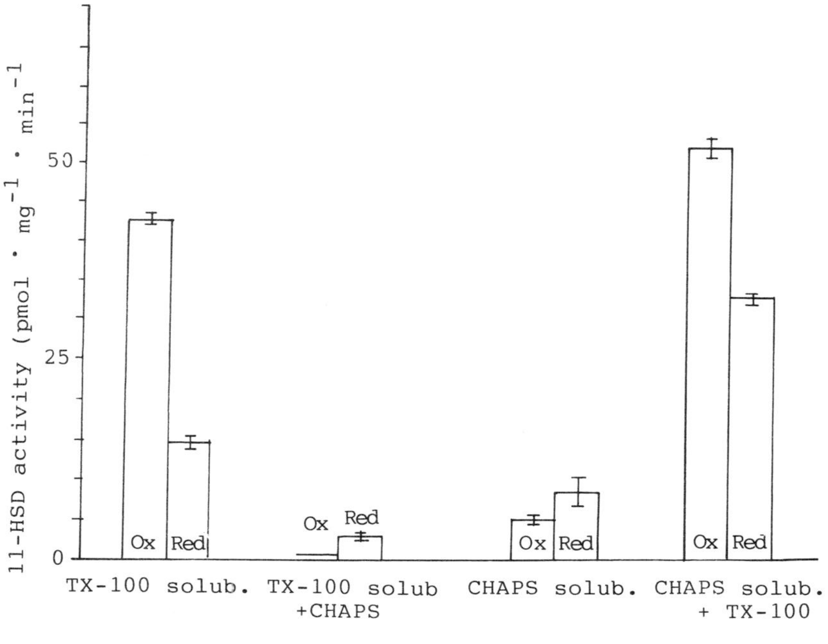

Fig. 2. Interference of different detergents with 11-HSD. Triton X (*TX*)-100 solubilized 11-HSD was incubated with 0.1% CHAPS; CHAPS solubilized 11-HSD was incubated with 0.1% Triton X-100. Ox, Oxidase; Red, Reductase. (X±SEM) (From [25])

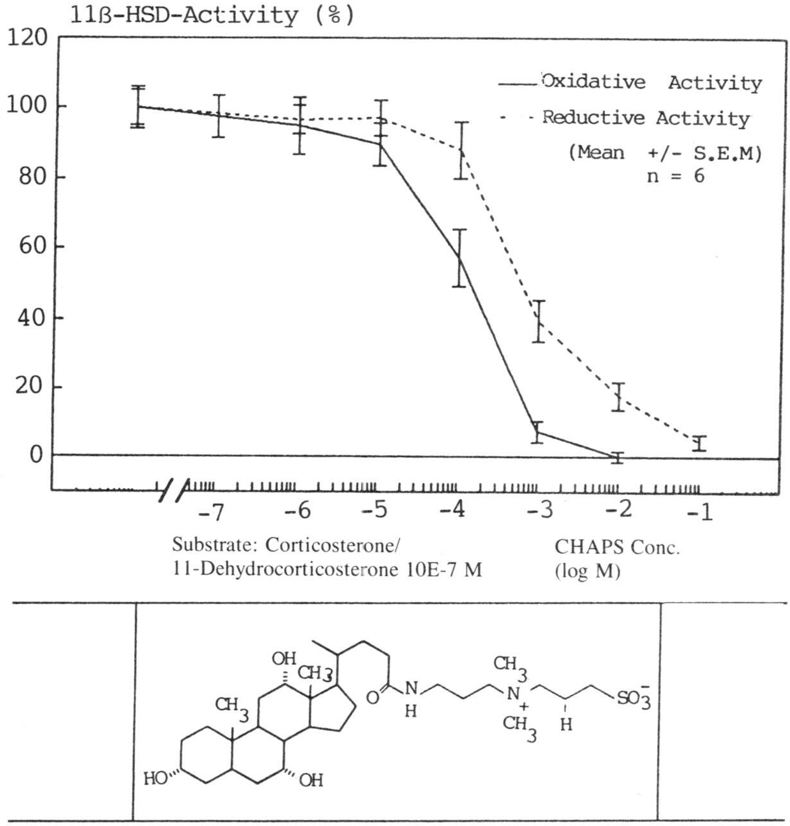

Fig. 3. Inhibition of 11-HSD by CHAPS. Aliquots of rat renal microsomes (adjusted to 20 μg protein/ml HEPES buffer) were incubated (pH 8, 37°C, 30 min). Corticosterone (*B*) + ^{3}H-B or 11-dehydro B + ^{3}H-11-dehydro B (10^{-7} M) and cosubstrates ($NADP^+$ or NADPH, 10^{-3} M) were added; metabolites were measured using RP-HPLC. (Adapted from [31])

Exogenous Inhibitors of 11-HSD

A first group of inhibitors was detected when we tried to solubilize 11-HSD from rat renal microsomes with different detergents, such as TX-100, Zwittergent, N-octylglucoside, and the CHAPS series. In contrast to all mentioned nonsteroidal detergents, CHAPS seemed to be rather ineffective in solubilizing oxidative activity [25]. Since the oxidative activity of the solubilized fraction could be reconstituted in vitro simply by dilution of the CHAPS concentration to less than 0.01% (Fig. 2) [25] we tested whether or not CHAPS, a steroidal detergent, might inhibit 11-HSD. The results shown in Fig. 3 document that both oxidative, and to a lesser degree, reductive activities are inhibited by concentrations ranging from 10^{-5} to 10^{-1} M. Comparable results were obtained with Big CHAP and Deoxy Big CHAP, which differ from CHAPS only in the hydrophilic head segment.

Table 2. Effects of licorice (L.) and/or glycyrrhetinic acid (Gl.Ac.)

– L. exerts DOC-like activity	Moluysen et al.	(1950), [37]
– L. causes hypertension, hypokalemia, ↓ plasma renin-activity (PRA), ↑ aldosterone	Epstein et al.	(1977), [38]
– Gl.Ac. binds to CS-receptors	Ulmann et al.	(1975), [39]
– Addision patients and adx. rats do not respond to L.	Borse et al.	(1953), [40]
	Card et al.,	(1953), [44]
– L. causes high urinary cortisol (at normal plasma cortisol)	Epstein et al.	(1978), [41]
– L. effect inhibited by spironolactone	Salassa et al.	(1982), [42]
– L. effect inhibited by dexamethasone	Hoefnagels et al.	(1983), [43]
– Gl.Ac. inhibits 11-HSD	Stewart et al.	(1987), [32]

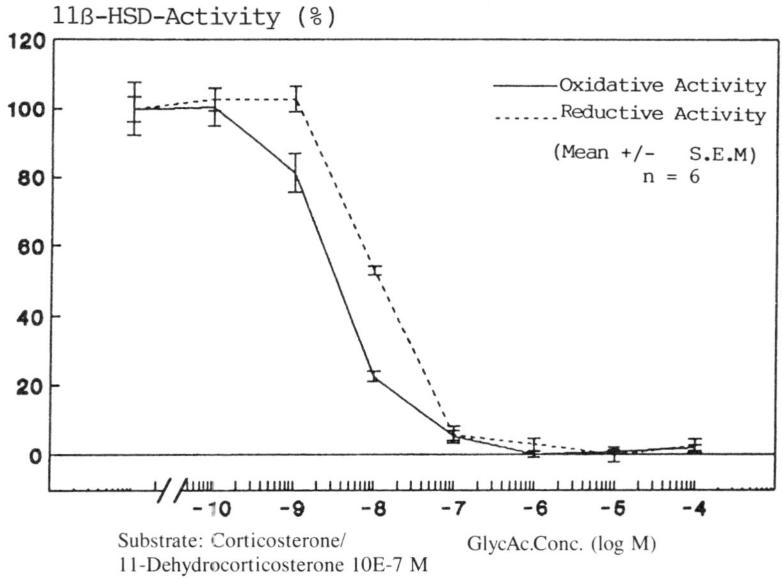

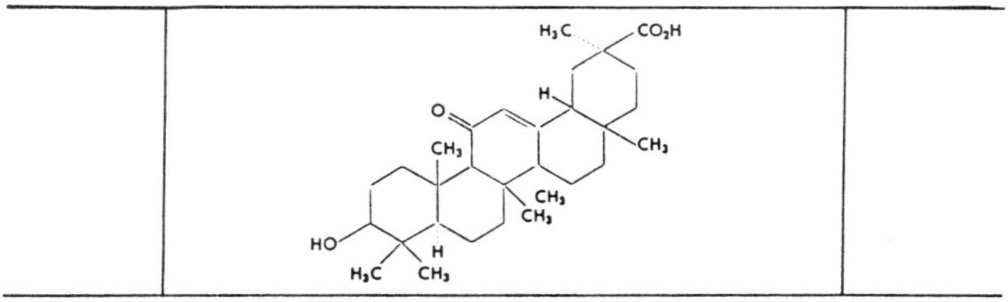

Fig. 4. Inhibition of 11-HSD by β-glyc. acid; experiments and presentation as in Fig. 3 glyc., glycyrrhetinic acid (Adapted from [31])

A second group of inhibitors of 11-HSD consists of licorice and its active principles, glycyrrhitic acid, glycyrrhetinic acid, and the succinate ester carbenoxolone [30–36]. As shown in Table 2 this group gained attention when clinical studies pointed to a desoxycorticosterone (DOC)-like effect of licorice which could not be explained on the basis of the weak binding properties of the active principle to mineralocorticosteroid (MCS)-receptors, but could apparently be explained by its effect on cortisol metabolism [32,37–44].

Stewart et al. [32] were the first who demonstrated that glycyrrhetinic (glyc.) acid was a potent inhibitor of 11β-HSD; they proposed the concept that the inhibitor plays an important role in controlling the access of GCS such as B and cortisol (F) to the MCS-receptor. Relevant data from our laboratory are shown in Fig. 4. It was demonstrated that glyc. acid inhibited 11-HSD in vitro in a dose-dependent manner; effective concentrations ranged from 10^{-9} to 10^{-6} M.

Similar results have been obtained with a mixture of glycyrrhitic acid, cysteine, and glycine (REMEFA S kindly provided by Dr. Falk, Pharma GmbH, Freiburg, Federal Republic of Germany, distributed in Japan as "Stronger Neo-Minophagen C").

The biologic function of glyc. acid as an 11-HSD inhibitor has been tested in invitro preparations. Thus, Dr. Fromm in our laboratory was able to show that addition of the inhibitor (10^{-6} M) to totally stripped rat rectal colon unmasked an apparent MCS effect of B (10^{-8} M) on amiloride inhibitable short circuit current. The apparent MCS effect was indistinguishable from the maximal aldosterone effect [31]. Comparable effects have been observed in isolated toad bladders by Gaeggeler et al. [45] and by Brem et al. [46].

A third class of inhibitors stems from Japanese traditional medicine. We have come across the fact that ginseng root contains steroid-like compounds which might exhibit

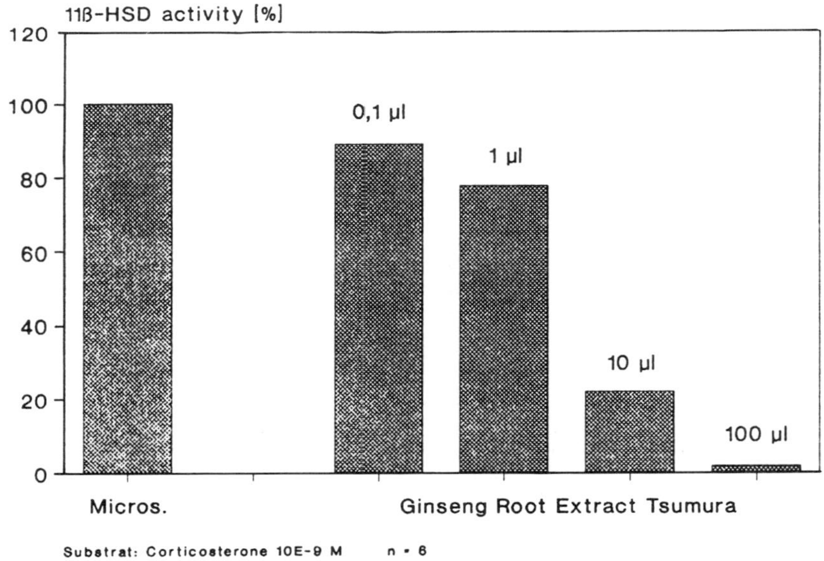

Fig. 5. Effect of ginseng root extract on activity of 11-HSD

Table 3. Inhibition of rat renal 11β-HSD

Compound	Mol. conc. at 50% inhibition	
	Oxidase	Reductase
CHAPS	1.4×10^{-4}	6.1×10^{-4}
Big CHAP	2.8×10^{-6}	6.0×10^{-6}
Deoxy Big CHAP	7.1×10^{-5}	–[a]
Glycyrrhetinic acid	3.4×10^{-9}	1.2×10^{-8}
Remefa[b]	7.1×10^{-7}	1.2×10^{-6}

Substrate: corticosterone/11-dehydrocorticosterone 10^{-7} M $n = 6$–12
[a]No inhibition within range of solubility. When solubilized 11-HSD was used instead of microsomes deoxyBigCHAP inhibited 50% of reductase at 4.0×10^{-4} M
[b]Conc. of active principle: glycyrrhizin (From [53])

affinity to the active center of 11-HSD. Therefore, extracts of ginseng root and subsequently isolated and purified ginsenosides (kindly provided by Tsumura Co., Tokyo, Japan) were tested in vitro using, again, rat renal microsomal 11-HSD. Figure 5 shows the results of pilot experiments which demonstrate that total extract inhibits the enzyme. This is of particular interest, since the extract contains several steroidal compounds of comparable structure and thus may provide a means of testing the structural details which have a bearing upon inhibitor affinity to the enzyme. So far, only one member of the group seems to exert inhibitory effects. Obviously, the results of further experiments, which are under way, will have to be waited for. Table 3 summarizes results hitherto established in our laboratory. It is pertinent to note that glyc. acid is the most effective exogenous inhibitor so far.

Endogenous Inhibitors of 11-HSD

The observations presented above tempted us to search for the possible existence of endogenous inhibitors of 11-HSD. Bile acids were likely candidates, since they resemble CHAPS, as far as the hydrophobic tail segment is concerned, and differ only in the hydrophilic head. So far we have tested cholic acid and chenodeoxycholic acid, deoxycholic acid and lithocholic acid, as well as ursodeoxycholic acid as primary, secondary, and tertiary bile acids, respectively. Studies with conjugated bile acids are under way.

Figure 6 shows an inhibitory curve of both oxidative and reductive activity of 11-HSD, obtained with cholic acid. The experiments were carried out with renal cortical microsomes. As demonstrated, enzymatic oxidative and reductive activities are inhibited in a dose dependent manner. Table 4 lists molar bile acid concentrations which are required in order to induce a 50% inhibition under experimental conditions in vitro.

From these studies we conclude that, in principle, bile acids can act as modulators of 11-HSD and possibly of other CS-degrading enzyme systems. This is important in view of older reports which have pointed to an abnormal cortisol metabolism in liver cirrhosis, in extrahepatic biliary obstruction, and after ingestion of bile acids [47–49].

Figure 7 summarizes the sites of steroidal compounds which may be of strategic importance in controlling the fitting of an inhibitor to 11-HSD. An oxygen function

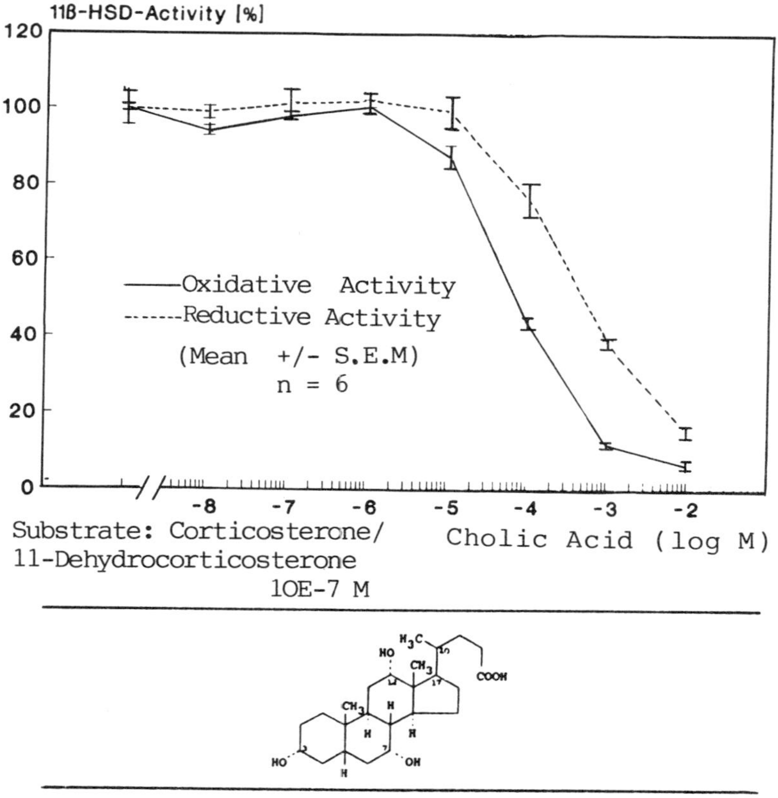

Fig. 6. Inhibition of 11-HSD by cholic acid; experiments and presentation as in Fig. 3. (Adapted from [54])

at C_3, either in the α- or β-position, is present in all inhibitors so far tested. The C_7 can carry a hydroxyl- or a keto group, or can be deoxidized as in deoxycholate; the same holds for C_{11}. The C_{12} can be hydroxylated, as in cholic acid. The hemiacetal configuration (C_{11}–C_{18}) does not prevent fitting (data not shown), but prevents metabolism of aldosterone. Glycyrrhetinic acid, the strongest inhibitor presently

Table 4. Inhibition of rat renal 11β-HSD by different bile acids

			50% Inhibition	
Class of bile acid	Compound	*n*	Ox.	Red.
Primary bile acids	Cholic acid	6	$7.1*10^{-5}$	$5.0*10^{-4}$
	Chenodeoxycholic acid	6	$2.1*10^{-6}$	$8.0*10^{-6}$
Secondary bile acids	Deoxycholic acid	8	$8.0*10^{-5}$	$3.1*10^{-3}$
	Lithocholic acid	6	$2.3*10^{-6}$	$3.1*10^{-5}$
Tertiary bile acid	Ursodeoxycholic acid	6	$2.3*10^{-5}$	$3.1*10^{-3}$

(From [54])

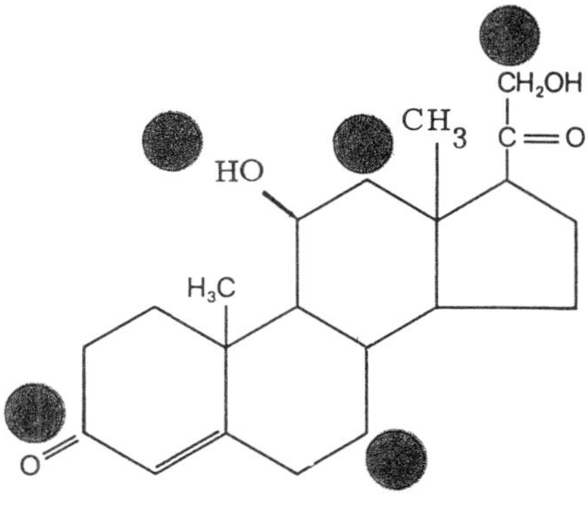

Fig. 7. Properties of inhibitors of 11-HSD

available, is characterized by a 5-ring configuration. Interestingly, large hydrophilic side chains can be tolerated, as demonstrated by the results obtained with the CHAPS-series. We realize that this is only a first overview, which needs further evaluation on the basis of three-dimensional data.

Conclusions

These experiments have demonstrated that the 11-HSD system serves several important functions. First, it effectively inactivates GCS such as F and B by oxidative degradation at C_{11}. The primary importance of the system may lie in GCS-signal inactivation; however, since 11-HSD in essence is an oxido-reductase system, it is conceivable that under certain metabolic conditions the intracellular concentrations of active GCS can be raised by conversion of cortisone to cortisol and/or 11-dehydro B to B. This would in essence constitute signal activation. Intracellular stores of inactivated GCS might, therefore, serve as a pool for active GCS and permit adjustment of local activation and inactivation of GCS, e.g., in cells like those of the proximal pars recta, which is a site of nicotinamide-adenine-dinucleotide phosphate $(NADP)^+/H$ dependent enzymatic reactions [50].

More relevant for the present discussion is the notion that GCS transformation via 11-HSD may control access of CS signals to MCS receptors, as suggested by Steward et al. [32]. The situation, which is in accord with experimental data, is depicted in Fig. 8. In essence, 11-HSD constitutes a diuretic principle in preventing access of large concentrations of GCS to receptors of limited MCS- versus GCS-specificity.

Inhibition of the system, whether genetically determined, as in "apparent MCS excess syndrome" [51], or whether caused by exogenous inhibitors such as medically used glyc. acid preparations or possibly caused by endogenous inhibitors of the bile acid type, thus exerts MCS agonist effects. This is not only of theoretical value, but also of great practical importance in view of the widespread use of, e.g., glyc. acid in chronic hepatitis and AIDS or as an additive.

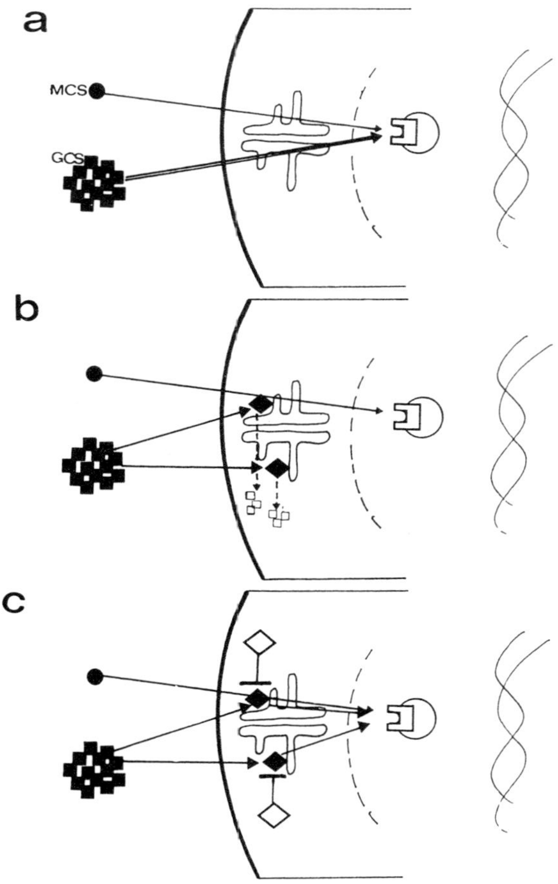

Fig. 8. Schematic presentation of different models of CS interaction with target cells: **a** due to the lack of 11-HSD, both MCS and GCS gain access to CS receptors **b** 11-HSD prevents access of 11-hydroxylated GCS by oxidative inactivation at C_{11}, **c** inhibition of 11-HSD as caused by glyc. acid, CHAPS, or bile acids converts the target cells essentially into the type shown in **a**. MCS, mineralocorticosteroids; GCS, glucocorticosteroids

Most relevant to this discussion of diuretics are recent reports that at least one inhibitor, glyc. acid, not only affects 11-HSD but induces accumulation of DH- and TH-aldosterone [35,52] and, thus, may also interfere with other CS-degrading enzymes.

Acknowledgments. KH was supported by the Deutsche Forschungsgemeinschaft Hi 97/16 1-4. Expert technical assistance of Ingrid Lichtenstein and Harald Siebe, and expert secretarial assistance of Helga Gräbener is acknowledged.

References

1. Corvol P, Claire M, Oblin ME, Geering K, Rossier B (1981) Mechanism of the antimineralocorticoid effects of spirolactones. Kidney Int 20:1–6
2. Agarwal MK (1984) An original multifaceted antihormone in vivo. Adrenal steroid antagonism. In: Proceedings of Workshop 7th International Congress Endocrinology Canada. W. De Gruyter, Berlin
3. Clark CR (1985) Intracellular localization of steroid receptors. In: Sluyser M, Horward E (eds) Interaction of steroid hormone receptors with DNA. Ellis Horwood, Chichester, pp 7–56
4. Henderson D (1987) Antiprogestational and antiglucocorticoid activities of some novel 11β-aryl substituted steroids. In: Furr BJA, Wakeling AE (eds) Pharmacology and clinical uses of inhibitors of hormone secretion and action. Bailliere Tindall, London, 184–211
5. Munck A, Holbrook NJ (1988) Cyclic, nonequilibrium models of glucocorticoid antagonism: role of activation, nuclear binding and receptor recycling. J Steroid Biochem 31 (4B):599–606
6. Kloosterboer HJ, Deckers GHJ, van der Heuvel MJ, Loozen HJJ (1988) Screening of antiprogestagens by receptor studies and bioassays. J Steroid Biochem 31 (4B):567–571
7. Teutsch G, Ojasoo T, Raynaud JP (1988) 11β-substituted steroids, an original pathway to antihormones. J Steroid Biochem 31 (4B):549–565
8. Chrousos GP, Laue L, Nieman LK, Kawai S, Udelsman RU, Brandon DD, Loriaux DL (1988) Glucocorticoids and glucocorticoid antagonists: lesson from RU 486. Kid Int 34 (Suppl 26):18–23
9. Baulieu EE (1988) Molecular mechanism of antisteroid hormones at the receptor level. Kid Int 34 (Suppl 26):2–7
10. Waeber B, Nüssberger J, Brunner HR (1988) Clinical applications of antimineralocorticoids. J Steroid Biochem 31 (4B):739–744
11. Duax WL, Griffin JF, Weeks CM, Wawrzak Z (1988) The mechanism of action of steroid antagonists: insights from crystallographic studies. J Steroid Biochem 31 (4B):481–492
12. Schmidt TJ (1989) Comparison of in vivo activation of triamcinolone acetonide- and RU 38486-receptor complexes in the CEM-C7 and IM-9 Human leukemic cell lines.[1] Cancer Res 49:4390–4395
13. Raaka BM, Finnerty M, Samuels HH (1989) The glucocorticoid antagonist 17α-methyltestosterone binds to the 10 S glucocorticoid receptor and blocks agonist-mediated dissociation of the 10 S oligomer to the 4 S deoxyribonucleic acid-binding subunit. Molecular Endocrinol 3 (2):332–341
14. Beier HM, Mootz U, Hegele-Hartung CH (1989) Studies on the establishment of mammalian pregnancy: synchronization of the maternal and the embryonic systems. Reprod Biol Med 210–223
15. Baulieu EE (1989) RU-486 as an antiprogesterone steroid. From receptor to contragestin and beyond. JAMA 262 (13):1808–1814
16. Michna H, Schneider MR, Nishino Y, El Etreby MF (1989) Antitumor activity of the antiprogestins ZK 98.299 and RU 38.486 in hormone dependent rat and mouse mammary tumors: mechanistic studies. Breast Cancer Res Treat 14:275–288
17. Schneider MR, Michna H, Nishino Y, El Etreby MF (1989) Antitumor activity of the progesterone antagonists ZK 98.299 and RU 38.486 in the hormone-dependent MXT mammary tumor model of the mouse and the DMBA- and the MNU-induced mammary tumor models of the rat. Eur J Cancer Clin Oncol 25 (4):691–701
18. Agarwal MK, Kalimi M (1989) Analysis of the mineralocorticoid receptor in rat heart with the aid of two new spirolactone derivatives. Biochem Med Metabol Biol 41:36–45
19. Brooks VL (1989) Vasporessin and ANG II in the control of ACTH secretion and arterial and atrial pressures. Am J Physiol 256:R339–R347

20. Zhu Q, Bateman A, Singh A, Solomon (1989) Isolation and biological activity of corticostatic peptides (anti-ACTH). Endocr Res Commun 15 (1,2):129–149
21. Lamberts SWJ, Bruining HA, Marzouk H, Zuiderwijk J, Uitterlinden P, Blijd JJ, Hackeng WHL, De Jong FH (1989) The new aromatase inhibitor CGS-16949A suppresses aldosterone and cortisol production by human adrenal cells in vitro. J Clin Enocrinol Metab 69 (4):896–901
22. van der Schoot P, Uilenbroek JThJ, Slappendel EJ (1990) Effect of the progesterone antagonist mifepristone on the hypothalamo-hypophysial-ovarian axis in rats. J Endocrinol 124:425–432
23. Hierholzer K, Schöneshöfer M, Siebe H, Tsiakiras D, Weskamp P (1984) Corticosteroid metabolism in isolated rat kidney in vitro I. Formation of lipid soluble metabolites from corticosterone (B) in renal tissue from male rats. Pflügers Arch 400:363–371
24. Kobayashi N, Schulz W, Hierholzer K (1987) Corticosteroid metabolism in rat kidney in vitro IV. Subcellular sites of 11β-hydroxysteroid dehydrogenase activity. Pflügers Arch 408:46–53
25. Schulz W, Lichtenstein I, Siebe H, Hierholzer K (1989) Isoelectric focusing analysis of detergent extracted renal 11β-hydroxysteroid dehydrogenase. J Steroid Biochem 32:581–590
26. l'Allemand D, Siebe H, Tsiakiras D, Hoyer GA, Vecsei P, Hierholzer K (1988) Aldosterone metabolism in rat renal tissue in vitro. Formation of lipid soluble metabolites. Pflügers Arch 411:529–539
27. Hoyer GA, Tsiakiras D, Siebe H, Hierholzer K (1984) Corticosteroid metabolism in isolated rat kidney in vitro III. Structure analysis of lipid soluble metabolites of corticosterone. Pflügers Arch 400:377–380
28. Spieth A, Hierholzer K (1987) Longitudinal heterogeneity of renal corticosterone metabolism in mouse nephron. Pflügers Arch 408:R42
29. Castello R, Schwarting R, Müller C, Hierholzer K, Lichtenstein I (1989) Immunohistochemical localization of 11-hydroxysteroid dehydrogenase in rat kidney with a monoclonal antibody. Renal Physiol Biochem 12:320–327
30. Hierholzer K, Castello R, Kobayashi N, Fromm M (1989) Sites and significance of renal corticosteroid metabolism. In: Berliner RW, Honda N, Ullrich KJ (eds) The frontiers of nephrology, Elsevier, Amsterdam, pp 67–76
31. Hierholzer K, Siebe H, Fromm M (1990) Inhibition of 11β-hydroxysteroid dehydrogenase and its effect on epithelial sodium transport. Kidney Int 38:673–678
32. Stewart PM, Valentino R, Wallace AM, Burt D, Shackleton CHL, Edwards CRW (1987) Mineralocorticoid activity of liquorice: 11β-hydroxysteroid dehydrogenase deficiency comes of age. Lancet II:821–24
33. Edwards CRW, Stewart PM, Burt D, Brett L, McIntyre MA, Sutanto WS, De Kloet ER, Monder C (1988) Localisation of 11β-Hydroxysteroid dehydrogenase-tissue specific protector of the mineralocorticoid receptor. Lancet 29:986–989
34. Edwards CRW, Burt D, Stewart PM (1989) The specificity of the human mineralocorticoid receptor: Clinical clues to a biological conundrum. J Steroid Biochem 32 (1B):213–216
35. Morris DJ, Souness GW (1990) The 11β-OHSD inhibitor, carbenoxolone, enhances Na retention by aldosterone and 11-deoxycorticosterone. Am J Physiol 258:F756–F759
36. Funder JW, Pearce PT, Smith R, Smith AI (1988) Mineralocorticoid action: Target tissue specificity is enzyme, not receptor, mediated. Science 242:583–585
37. Molhuysen JA, Gerbrandy J, De Vries IA (1950) A liquorice extract with "deoxycortone-like" action. Lancet II:381–386
38. Epstein MT, Espiner EA, Donald RA, Hughes H (1977) Liquorice toxicity and the renin-angiotensin-aldosterone axis in man. Br Med J [Clin Res] 1:209–210
39. Ulmann A, Menard J, Corvol P (1975) Binding of glycyrrhetinic acid to kidney mineralocorticoid and glucocorticoid receptors. Endocrinology 97:46–51

40. Borst JGG, Tenholt SP, De Vries LA, Molhuysen JA (1953) Synergistic action of liquorice and cortisone in Addison's and Simmonds's disease. Lancet II:657–663
41. Epstein MT, Espiner EA, Donald RA, Hughes H, Cowles RJ, Lun S (1978) Licorice raises urinary cortisol in man. J Clin Endocrinol Metab 47:397–400
42. Salassa RM, Mattox VR, Rosevear JW (1982) Inhibition of the "mineralocorticoid" activity of licorice by spironolactone. J Clin Endocrinol Metab 22:1156–1159
43. Hoefnagels WHL, Kloppenburg PWC (1983) Antimineralocorticoid effects of dexamethasone in subjects treated with glycyrrhetinic acid. J Hypertens 1 (Suppl 2):313–315
44. Card WI, Mitchell W, Strong JA, Taylor NRW, Tompsett SL, Wilson JMG, (1953) Effects of liquorice and its derivatives on salt and water metabolism. Lancet II:663–667
45. Gaeggeler HP, Edwards CRW, Rossier BC (1989) Steroid metabolism determines mineralocorticoid specificity in the toad bladder. Am J Physiol 257:F690–F695
46. Brem AS, Matheson KL, Conca T, Morris DJ (1989) Effect of corbenoxolone on glucocorticoid metabolism and Na transport in toad bladder. Am J Physiol 257:F700–F704
47. Zumoff B, Bradlow HL, Gallagher TF, Hellamn L (1967) Cortisol metabolism in cirrhosis. J Clin Invest 46:1735–1742
48. Zumoff B, Bradlow HL, Gallagher TF (1971) Cortisol metabolism in total extrahepatic biliary obstruction. J Clin Endocrinol Metab 32:36–41
49. Gerdes H, Riemenschneider H, Littmann KP (1971) Effect of bile acids and some biliary excreted drugs on the metabolism of cortisol. Acta Endocrinol (Copenh) 173:10
50. Guder WG, Ross BD (1984) Enzyme distribution along the nephron. Kidney Int 26:101–111
51. Ulick S, Levine LS, Gunczler P, Zanconato G, Ramirez LC, Rauh W, Rösler A, Bradlow HL, New MI (1979) A syndrome of apparent mineralocorticoid excess associated with defects in the peripheral metabolism of cortisol. Endocrinol Soc 49:757–764
52. Latif SA, Conca TJ, Morris DJ (1990) The effects of the licorice derivative, glycyrrhetinic acid, on hepatic 3α- and 3β-hydroxysteroid dehydrogenases and 5α- and 5β-reductase pathways of metabolism of aldosterone in male rats. Steroids 55:52–58
53. Bühler H, Kobayashi N, Lichtenstein I, Perschel FH, Siebe H, Hierholzer K (1990) Reversible inhibition of renal 11-hydroxysteroid dehydrogenase (11-HSD) by steroids, structure-function-relationship. Nieren + Hochdruckkrankheiten 19:374
54. Perschel FH, Bühler H, Siebe H, Lichtenstein I, Hierholzer K (1990) Bile acids as endogenous inhibitors of 11β-hydroxysteroid dehydrogenase (11-HSD). Nieren + Hochdruckkrankheiten 19:406

Glomerular Cells and Extracellular Matrix

Chair: R. Bernd Sterzel (FRG)
Fujio Shimizu (Japan)

Ultrastructure of the Mesangial Matrix

WILHELM KRIZ and MARLIES ELGER[1]

Introduction

The glomerular mesangium and the glomerular capillaries are enclosed in a single compartment bounded by a common basement membrane. The capillary-mesangium interface consists only of a fenestrated endothelium. There is no basement membrane at this interface. Thus, a discrete hydraulic barrier is not established. Therefore, the range of hydraulic pressure in the mesangium, i.e., in the mesangial matrix, can be expected to be of the same magnitude as the range of glomerular capillary pressure. Tracer studies [1,2], which show the rapid entry of macromolecular compounds into the mesangium from the blood, support this postulate. As a result, the transmural hydraulic pressure difference across the perimesangial glomerular basement membrane (GBM) should also be of about the same magnitude as that across the capillary wall. These hydraulic pressure differences have to be counteracted to prevent capillary and mesangial expansion [3,4].

As shown by recent studies, counteraction is established by the connection of the GBM to the contractile apparatus of mesangial cells [3–5]. By these connections the GBM is pulled centrally to the axial region of the mesangium. These connections are most prominent at mesangial angles, but are found along the entire perimesangial GBM. In addition to direct attachments of mesangial cells to the GBM, the mesangial matrix has been suggested to be the connecting element [6]. In our view, the ultrastructural equivalent underlying this mechanical function is represented by a *microfibrillar network*. This review summarizes the findings on this subject.

Ultrastructure and Composition of the Mesangial Matrix

The mesangial matrix may be regarded as a specific interstitial space, filled with a matrix of relatively high electron density. Ultrastructurally, the mesangial matrix has

[1]Institut für Anatomie und Zellbiologie, Universität Heidelberg, D-6900 Heidelberg, Federal Republic of Germany

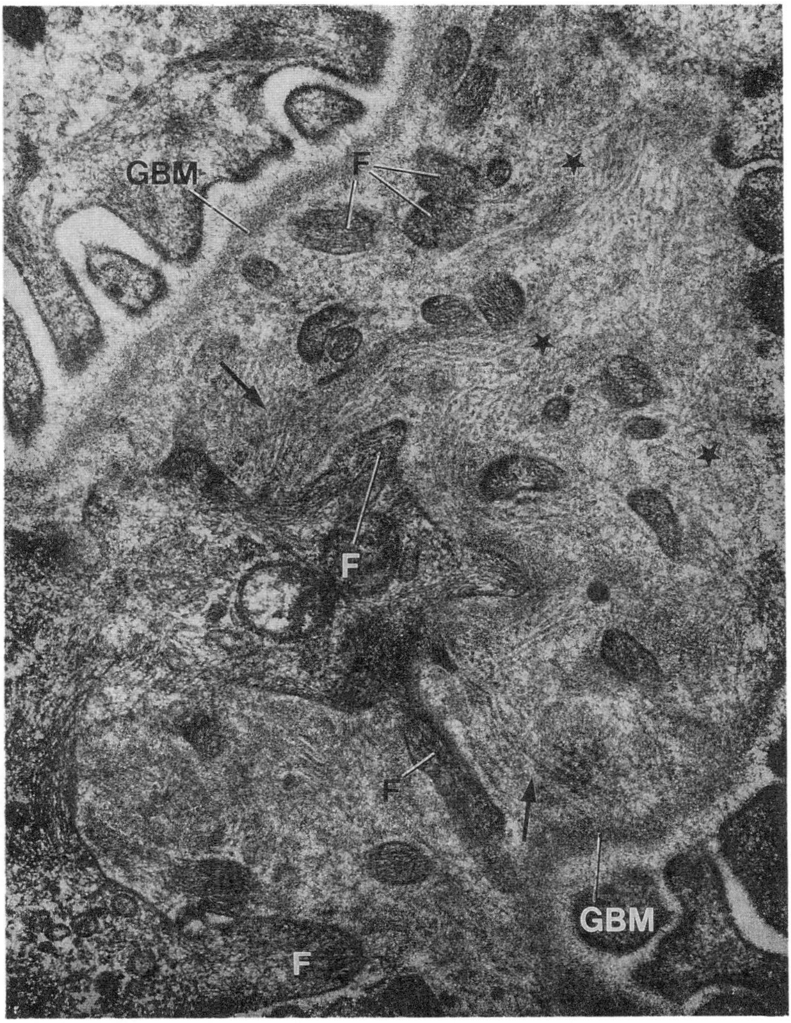

Fig. 1. Rat glomerulus; section through the mesangium, which is bounded by the glomerular basement membrane (*GBM*). The numerous processes of the mesangial cells contain microfilament bundles (*F*). In the mesangial matrix abundant microfibrils are seen, which form a network (*asterisks*) or are arranged in bundles (*arrows*). Transmission electron micrograph (*TEM*), × 37000

been described as similar to but clearly different "from the basement membrane proper by its looser texture and by the presence of small bundles of fine fibers (D = 100 Å) embedded in its feltwork of finer fibrils" [7]. Microfibrils can be identified clearly in cross section by their tubular structure. Several authors, using this criterion, have described microfibrils as a component of the mesangial matrix [8,9]. By

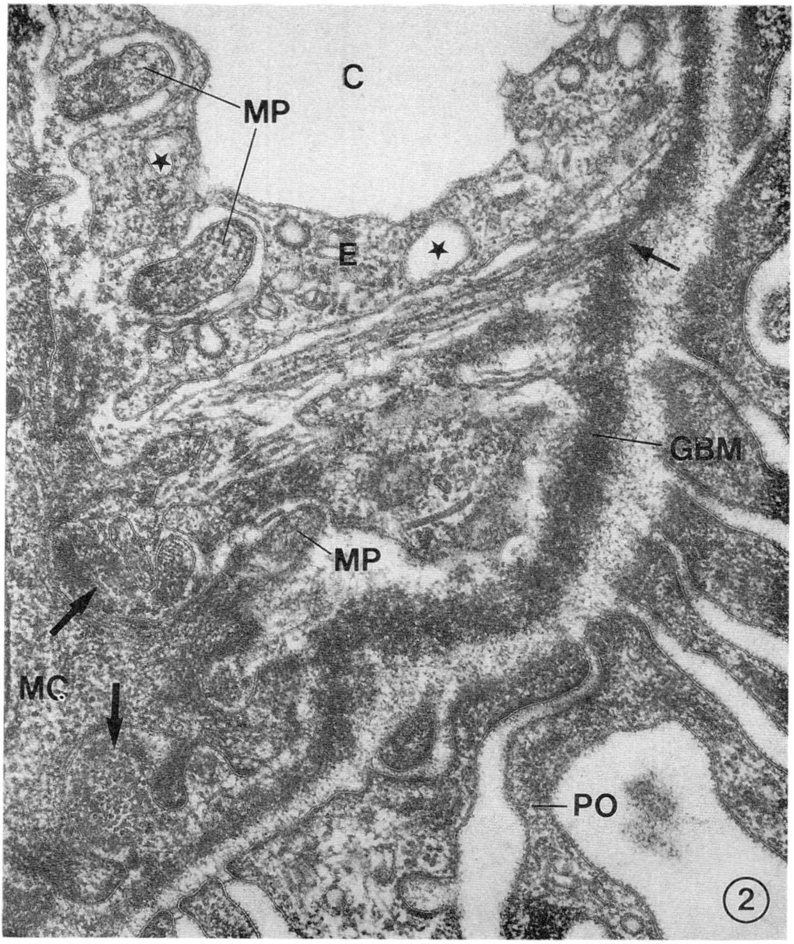

Fig. 2. Rat glomerulus; tangential section through the capillary-mesangial interface. Beneath the endothelium (*E*) a bundle of microfibrils is seen attaching to the GBM at a mesangial angle (*thin arrow*). Mesangial cell processes (*MP*) and part of a mesangial cell body (*MC*) are seen. Thick bundles of microfibrils are entrapped within invaginations of the cell body (*thick arrows*). Note that there is no basement membrane between the endothelium and the mesangium; the endothelium is fenestrated (*asterisks*). C, capillary lumen; PO, foot processes of podocytes. TEM, × 40000

combining tannic acid staining with a dehydration technique in the cold, we found that the mesangial matrix basically consists of a dense network of microfibrils [5,10] (Fig. 1).

Microfibrils represent a specific extracellular entity, characterized structurally by their typical appearance as hollow, nonbranching fibrils of undefined length. In the mesangial matrix we measured a very uniform thickness of almost exactly 15 nm

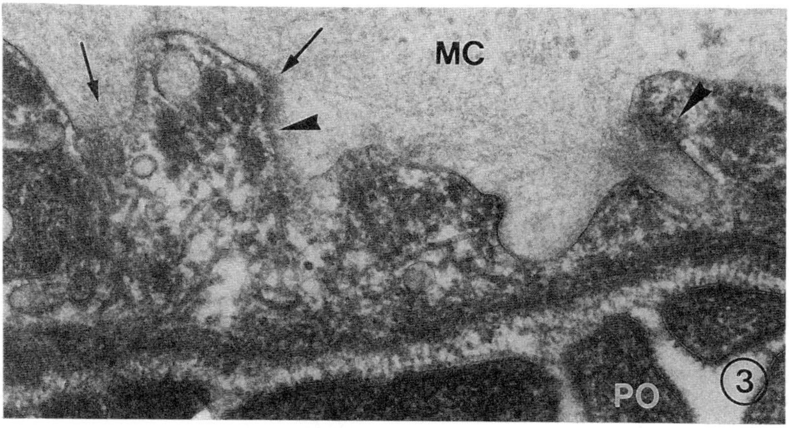

Fig. 3. Part of a mesangial cell (*MC*) with small processes running towards the GBM. The faint staining of the cell (the tissue has not been treated by OsO_4 and was stained with tannic acid, see [10]) allows identification of the narrow association of extracellular microfibrils (*dark stained*) and intracellular microfilaments (*faintly stained*) along the cell membrane (*arrows*). At favorable sites microfibrils are found in close relation to periodically spaced substructures on the outside of the cell membrane (*arrowheads*). PO, foot processes of podocytes. TEM, × 60000

[10]. This thickness is in good agreement with microfibril diameters measured at other sites and in other species [9,11–14].

Various elaborations of the mesangial microfibrillar network have to be considered. First, discrete microfibrillar connections are found between processes of mesangial cells and the GBM. They are most prominent at mesangial angles [3–5] (Fig. 2). In these connections, microfibrils appear to be attached to sites in the mesangial cell membrane that serve for the anchorage of intracellular actin filaments (Fig. 3). At opposite sites these bundles of microfibrils are closely associated with the GBM: at favorable sites microfibrils can clearly be recognized to penetrate into the lamina densa of the GBM (Fig. 2).

Second, in between these distinct connections, a network of interwoven microfibrils is found (Fig. 1), which attaches to the inner surface of the GBM and to the surface of mesangial cells at countless sites and is also associated with the discrete mesangial cell/GBM-connections described above.

Third, cross sections of microfibrillar bundles are regularly recognized running within bay-like cytoplasmic invaginations of mesangial cells (Fig. 2). They seem to run fairly parallel to the cell surface. They are more frequently found associated with cell bodies and larger processes than with peripheral parts of mesangial cells. Their course, their beginning, and their termination are unclear.

By means of immunocytochemistry, collagen type IV, V, and VI [15,16], fibronectin [17–19], laminin [19], and entactin [20] have been detected as components of the mesangial matrix. Among them fibronectin is the most abundant. This is in agreement with the ultrastructural observation that the mesangial matrix basically consists of a microfibrillar network, since microfibrils have been shown to be consistently associated with fibronectin [18,21]. The abundant mesangial fibronectin has been interpreted as serving for the linkage of mesangial cell surfaces to extracellular structures [2,18]. In addition, one may suggest that fibronectin interconnects the interwoven microfibrils at their crossing points, thus stabilizing the matrix net. Very recently, a 340 kDa protein, representing a major component of elastic microfibrils, has also been detected in the glomerular mesangium in the rat [22].

Functional Relevance

A function of the mesangial matrix as a connecting structure between mesangial cells and the GBM has been proposed previously, in studies in which the supposed failure of such a connection may have produced microaneurysms [23–25]. The microfibrillar network establishes a solid base of contact between mesangial cells and the GBM. In addition to direct attachments of mesangial cell processes to the GBM, microfibrils represent the connecting element between the contractile apparatus of mesangial cells and the GBM. Probably, the fundamental relevance of this system is that it counteracts the distending forces which are exerted on the GBM by high intracapillary and intramesangial pressures. The microfibrillar network of the mesangial matrix appears to be capable of balancing distending forces which act essentially in all directions.

Acknowledgments. We thank Ms Hiltraud Hosser for skillful technical assistance and Ms Ingrid Ertel for photographic work. Secretarial help was provided by Ms Helene Dehoust. Supported by Deutsche Forschungs-gemeinschaft, Kr 546/5–3, Forschergruppe "Niere," Heidelberg.

References

1. Michael AF, Keane WF, Raij L, Vernier RL, Mauer SM (1980) The glomerular mesangium. Kidney Int 17:141–154
2. Latta H, Fligiel S (1985) Mesangial fenestrations, sieving, filtration, and flow. Lab Invest 52:591–598
3. Kriz W, Elger M, Lemley K, Sakai T (1990) The structure of the glomerular mesangium: a biomechanical interpretation. Kidney Int 38 (suppl 30):52–59
4. Kriz W, Elger M, Lemley KV, Sakai T (1990) Mesangial cell-glomerular basement membrane connections counteract glomerular capillary and mesangium expansion. Am J Nephrol 10 (suppl 1):4–13
5. Sakai T, Kriz W (1987) The structural relationship between mesangial cells and basement membrane of the renal glomerulus. Anat Embryol (Berl) 176:373–386
6. Latta H, Maunsbach AB, Madden SC (1960) The centrolobular region of the renal glomerulus studied by electron microscopy. J Ultrastruct Res 4:455–472
7. Farquhar MG, Palade GE (1962) Functional evidence for the existence of a third cell type in the renal glomerulus. Phagocytosis of filtration residues by a distinctive "third" cell. J Cell Biol 13:55–87
8. Farquhar MG (1964) Glomerular permeability investigated by electron microscopy. In: Siperstein MD, Colwell AR, Meyer K (eds) Proceedings of the conference on small blood

vessel involvement in Diabetes Mellitus, 1963. Warrenton, USA. Am Inst Biol Sci, Washington, pp 31–80
9. Reale E, Luciano L, Kühn KW, Stolte H, Brod J (1981) Glomerular basement membrane and mesangial matrix. A comparative study in different vertebrates. In: Thomas S, Berlyne GM (eds) Renal physiology. Karger, Basel, pp 85–89
10. Mundel P, Elger M, Sakai T, Kriz W (1988) Microfibrils are a major component of the mesangial matrix in the glomerulus of the rat kidney. Cell Tissue Res 254:183–187
11. Ross R, Bornstein P (1969) The elastic fiber: I. The separation and partial characterization of its macromolecular components. J Cell Biol 40:366–381
12. Hsu H-C, Churg J (1979) Glomerular microfibrils in renal disease: A comparative electron microscopic study. Kidney Int 16:497–504
13. Cleary EG, Gibson MA (1983) Elastin-associated microfibrils and microfibrillar proteins. Int Rev Connect Tissue Res 10:97–209
14. Inoué S, Leblond CP (1986) The microfibrils of connective tissue: I. Ultrastructure. Am J Anat 176:121–138
15. Roll JF, Madri JA, Albert J, Futhmayr H (1980) Codistribution of collagen types IV and AB2 in basement membranes and mesangium of the kidney: an immunoferritin study of ultrathin frozen sections. J Cell Biol 85:597–616
16. Karkavelas G, Kefalides NA (1988) Comparative ultrastructural localization of collagen types III, IV, VI and laminin in rat uterus and kidney. J Ultrastruct Mol Struct Res 100:137–155
17. Oberley TD, Mosher DF, Mills MD (1979) Localization of fibronectin within the renal glomerulus and its production by cultured glomerular cells. Am J Physiol 96:651–658
18. Courtoy PJ, Kanwar YS, Hynes RO, Farquhar MG (1980) Fibronectin localization in the rat glomerulus. J Cell Biol 87:691–696
19. Madri JA, Roll FJ, Furthmayr H, Foidart J-M (1980) Ultrastructural localization of fibronectin and laminin in the basement membranes of the murine kidney. J Cell Biol 86:682–687
20. Bender BL, Jaffe R, Carlin B, Chung AE (1981) Immunolocalization of entactin, a sulfated basement membrane component in rodent tissues, and comparison with GP-2(laminin). Am J Pathol 103:419–426
21. Schwartz E, Goldfischer S, Coltoff-Schiller B, Blumenfeld OO (1985) Extracellular matrix microfibrils are composed of core proteins coated with fibronectin. J Histochem Cytochem 33:268–274
22. Gibson MA, Kumaratilake JS, Cleary EG (1989) The protein components of the 12-nanometer microfibrils of elastic and nonelastic tissues. J Biol Chem 264:4590–4598
23. Bloodworth JMB (1978) A re-evaluation of diabetic glomerulosclerosis 50 years after the discovery of insulin. Hum Pathol 9:439–453
24. Morita T, Churg J (1983) Mesangiolysis. Kidney Int 24:1–9
25. Saito Y, Kida H, Takeda S-I, Yoshimura M, Yokoyama H, Koshino Y, Hattori N (1988) Mesangiolysis in diabetic glomeruli: Its role in the formation of nodular lesions. Kidney Int 34:389–396

The Proteoglycans of Glomerular Mesangial Cells

MALCOLM DAVIES, GARETH J. THOMAS, LORNA SHEWRING[1], and ROGER M. MASON[2]

Introduction

Proteoglycans are located on cell membranes, in basement membranes and extracellular matrices, and are widely distributed in tissues [1]. They have many important biological roles, including cell adhesion, migration, and proliferation [2]. In the kidney they are of particular interest, because proteoglycans in the glomerular basement membrane (GBM) form the main charge and steric exclusion barriers to transcapillary passage of plasma proteins [3]. Loss of anionic sites is associated with proteinuria and has been noted in several nephropathies, including diabetic nephropathy, congenital nephrotic syndrome, and autologous immune complex disease. The anionic sites in the glomerular filter are mainly due to the presence of heparan sulfate proteoglycan (HSPG) [4]. Other proteoglycans, however, have been localised in the glomerulus, including chondroitin sulfate proteoglycan (CSPG) [5–7]. This proteoglycan is not present in the GBM in any significant amount, but does appear to be localised in the mesangium. In this chapter, investigations on the localization, biosynthesis, and metabolic turnover of mesangial proteoglycans from our own and other laboratories are reviewed. A short section which speculates on the possible role of CSPG in mesangial cell function is also included.

Chondroitin Sulphate Proteoglycans

Proteoglycans are a heterogenous and complex family of macromolecules composed of a core protein to which a number of charged linear polysaccharides called glycosaminoglycans (GAG) are covalently linked [1]. The GAG chains are made up

[1]Institute of Nephrology, University of Wales College of Medicine, Cardiff CF2 1SZ, Wales, UK
[2]Department of Biochemistry, Charing Cross and Westminster Hospital Medical School, London, UK

of repeating disaccharide units of a hexuronic acid and an N-acetylhexosamine to which a sulfate group may be coupled via ester or amide linkage. At present, proteoglycans are classified according to their glycosaminoglycan chain but as more information becomes available on core proteins these components may provide a better means of classification. Five main classes have been identified: hyaluronan, keratan sulfate, heparan sulfate (including heparin), chondroitin sulfate (CS) and dermatan sulfate (DS). Of these, the latter two are the subject of this chapter. In CS-GAG the disaccharide repeat unit consists of D-glucuronic acid linked β (1–3) to N-acetyl galactosamine. The hexosamine residue carries ester-linked sulfated groups either at the C-4 position (CS-4-SO_4) or at C-6 (CS-6-SO_4). Dermatan sulfate is an epimer of chondroitin sulfate and the uronic acid residue in the repeat disaccharides is iduronic acid, i.e., L-iduronic acid linked α(1–3) to N-acetylgalactosamine. Chondroitin sulfate-GAG and DS-GAG can best be distinguished from each other by their susceptibility to fragmentation by chondroitin ABC lyase and chondroitin AC-II lyase. Chondroitin sulfate-GAG is degraded by both glycosidases to disaccharides whereas DS-GAG is degraded by chondroitin ABC lyase but is insensitive to chondroitin AC-II lyase. Since CS-GAG and DS-GAG are both resistant to deamination with nitrous acid not only is it possible to distinguish these glycosaminoglycans from each other but it is also possible to distinguish them from heparan sulfate (HS-GAG).

Localization of Proteoglycans in the Glomerular Mesangium

The proteoglycans that have been localised in the mesangium of the glomerulus are summarized in Table 1. The first evidence that the mesangium is enriched in CS-GAG was obtained by Kanwar et al. [5]. These authors used radiolabelled cationized ferritin as a probe for in situ labeling of the glomerular anionic sites. The localization of CS-GAG chains was demonstrated by a combination of enzymatic digestion with chondroitin ABC lyase and quantitative electron microscopy. Prior perfusion of the kidney with the enzyme revealed a decrease in binding of the radiolabelled probe to the anionic sits of the mesangial matrix but not in glomerular basement membrane. The presence of CS-GAG on the mesangium was confirmed by immuno-

Table 1. Mesangial proteoglycans detected by immunostaining and other procedures

Location	Method	Proteoglycan	Reference
Mesangial matrix	EM-Autoradiography	Chondroitin-dermatan	Kanwar et al. [5]
	IMS	Heparan sulfate	Miettinen et al. [8] Mynderse et al. [9] Isemura et al. [10]
	IMS	Chondroitin-4-sulfate	Couchman et al. [6]
	IMS	Basement membrane chondroitin sulfate	McCarthy et al. [7]
	Tissue culture/IMS	Basement membrane chondroitin sulfate	Shewring et al. [11]
	Tissue culture/IMS	Dermatan sulfate (PGII)	Shewring et al. [11]
Mesangial cell surface	IMS	Heparan sulfate	Farquhar et al. [3]

IMS, immunostaining

histochemical staining with monoclonal antibody against CS-4-SO_4 and CS-6-SO_4 [6]. Both these antibodies stained the mesangial matrix but not the GBM. Recently the same author [7] showed that four monoclonals with anti-CSPG specificity immunostained different rat basement membranes but not the GBM. All these macromolecules did, however, stain the kidney mesangium. The CSPG used in the preparation of these monoclonals was extracted from Reichert's membrane and characterized as a large macromolecule (Mr ~500 kD) with a protein core of approximately Mr 150 kD and GAG chains of Mr 15–18 kD. Identical elution profiles after treatment of the glycosaminoglycan chains with both chondroitin ABC and AC-II lyase indicated the absence of iduronic acid rich regions in the chains and identified the molecules as CS and not as DS proteoglycan. This proteoglycan has been termed a basement membrane-CSPG. A similar proteoglycan was extracted and partially purified from rat kidney [7].

Thus, immunostaining data suggest that different sub-classes of CSPG are located in the mesangial matrix.

Biosynthesis and Characterization of Mesangial Cell Proteoglycans

Investigations on the biosynthesis of glomerular proteoglycans have utilized techniques of radiolabelling in vivo, organ perfusion with medium containing ^{35}S-sulphate, or incubation of isolated glomeruli with ^{35}S-sulphate, or ^{3}H-glucosamine in vitro [12]. Based on the information included in Table 1 it has been widely accepted that newly synthesized radiolabelled CS/DS proteoglycans extracted from the glomeruli in these experiments are all derived from the biosynthetic activity of mesangial cells. However, this assumption is open to criticism. For example, the proportion of ^{35}S-proteoglycans that were accounted for as CS/DS-like molecules varied between the in vivo and in vitro studies. Kidneys perfused in situ or in vivo synthesized a comparatively low proportion of CS/DS GAG chains (~15% of the total ^{35}S-GAGs) whereas in vitro these molecules represented 65% of the total ^{35}S-proteoglycans. One possible explanation is that the pattern of synthesis in vitro is due to the preferential survival or activation of the mesangial cells. Another is that glomeruli in culture change their proteoglycan phenotype. These and other explanations, together with the advantages and disadvantages of the different experimental protocols, have been reviewed by us [12].

The labelled ^{35}S-proteoglycans synthesized by isolated glomeruli in vitro have been extensively characterized by Klein et al. [13]. Two major ^{35}S-DSPG were described. One (DS-tll) was extracted from the tissue eluted from DEAE-Sephacel with 0.56 M NaCl (i.e. high charge density) and by dissociative Sepharose CL-4B chromatography was estimated to have a Mr 500 kD. It was not displaced from the tissue with heparin. The second (DS-MII) was present in the medium only and was considerably smaller (Mr 200 kD) than DS-tII. In addition, a small dermatan sulfate (DS-tIA) was extracted from the glomeruli. It was a minor component and accounted for 5% of the total ^{35}S-proteoglycans compared to DS-tII and DS-IIM, which represented 29% and 32% respectively. This proteoglycan was released from the glomeruli

Table 2. ^{35}S-Proteoglycans synthesized by glomeruli[a] and mesangial cells[b] in culture

Species	Proteoglycan	Location	Mr (kD)	Core protein (kD)	Comment	Reference
Rat[a]	DSPG	Tissue extract	150	na	Displaced by heparin	Klein et al. [13]
		Tissue extract	500	na	–	
		Tissue extract	200	na	–	
Rat[b]	DSPG	Medium	220	45	Biglycan (PGI)	Border et al. [15]
		Medium	120	45	Decorin (PGII)	
Rat[b]	CSPG	Layer	230	na	Biglycan ?	Yaoita et al. [16]
		Layer	150	na	Decorin ?	
		Medium	135	na	Decorin ?	
Rat[b]	Basement membrane/ CSPG	Medium	–	na	Identified with Mab 2D6	Shewring et al. [11]
	DSPG	Medium/layer	220	na	Cell layer PG hydrophobic	
	DSPG	Medium/layer	110	na	Cell layer PG hydrophobic	
Human[b]	CS/DS-PG	Medium	na	na	–	Striker et al. [17]
Human	CSPG	Layer/ medium	>1000	400	Cell layer hydrophobic	Davies et al. [18]
	DSPG	Layer/ medium	450	40		
		Medium	200	40		

by incubation with heparin. These findings, taken together with pulse-chase experiments, suggested that DS-tIA, once synthesized, was intercalated into cell membranes and then rapidly released into the medium. Since DS-tII required extraction with dissociative buffer it was suggested that this molecule is associated with matrix GAG binding sites. Radiolabelled DSPG similar to DS-tIA and DS-MII were separated from cultures of glomeruli labelled in vitro by Beavan et al. [14]. In addition, a large CSPG (Kav 0.3 on Sepharose CL4B) of high charge density was extracted from a GBM fraction and may be a product of mesangial cells.

Recent studies have used well established renal cell cultures to investigate proteoglycans synthesized by different glomerular cells. These studies have allowed information to determine whether particular proteoglycans are intercalated into cell membranes or are destined for export and integration with receptors for GAGs in the extracellular matrix. Proteoglycans synthesized by rat [15,16] and human [17,18] mesangial cell lines have been characterized and in general appear similar to those isolated from the in vitro experiments described above (Table 2). Moreover, these tissue culture studies indicate that the predominant GAG synthesized by mesangial cells are chondroitin and dermatan sulfate.

In human mesangial cells the majority of the proteoglycans synthesized are small DSPG which are released extracellularly. These were resolved into two sub-classes, namely DSPGI and DSPGII, in a ratio of 4:1. Both these DSPG have similar size protein cores (Mr ~40 kD) and identical size GAG chains (Mr 25 kD). The difference in their overall molecular size (DSPGI ~400000; DSPGII ~200000) is most likely due to the number of GAG chains covalently linked to the protein core. Thus DSPGI and DSPGII have physical properties similar to, but not identical to, biglycan (also known as PGI) [19] and decorin (also known as PGII) [20], respectively. Furthermore DSPGII was recognized in a dot, blot assay by an antiserum raised against human fibroblast PGII (i.e., decorin).

In the cell extract DSPGI and DSPGII are also present, but as minor components. Indeed, pulse-chase experiments indicated that the majority of these proteoglycans, once synthesized, were rapidly released into the culture medium.

The prominent species in the cell extract of human mesangial cells is a high molecular weight CSPG (CSPGI Mr > 1000 kD). The GAG chains of this CSPG were totally sensitive to chondroitin ABC lyase and ACII lyase digestion. Thus CSPGI does not contain iduronic acid residues and can be classified as a chondroitin sulphate. The CSPGI in the cell layer was accessible to mild trypsin treatment, bound to octyl-Sepharose, and could be inserted into liposomes, indicating that this proteoglycan originated from cell surfaces where it is intercalated via its core protein into the cell membrane.

Two large HSPG (Mr ~1000 and 450 kD) are synthesized by human mesangial cells in vitro [18]. They comprise about 20% of the total ^{35}S-proteoglycans. Both these proteoglycans are considerably larger than the HSPG extracted from human glomerular epithelial cells [21,22].

Chondroitin sulfate/DS proteoglycans synthesized by cultures of rat mesangial cells have also been recently characterized and found to be similar to those found in the human cultures above (Table 2). Border et al. [15] separated two DSPG from the culture medium using gradient SDS-polyacrylamide gel electrophoresis. These, on the basis of their Mr, were identified as biglycan and decorin.

In their studies Yaoita et al. [16], using cesium chloride density gradient centrifugation and column chromatography, also identified several sub-classes of small DS proteoglycans. Two of these (Mr 230 and 150 kD) may be associated with the plasma membrane, while a third (Mr 135 kD) was only present in the culture medium. Data on their core proteins were not given, but it is likely that these DS proteoglycans are related to biglycan and decorin.

We can confirm that rat mesangial cells synthesize mainly small DSPG. In addition we have used an affinity column prepared by coupling monoclonal 2D6 (which recognizes the basement membrane-CSPG from Reichert's membrane [7]) to investigate the ^{35}S-proteoglycans synthesized by rat mesangial cells [11]. Approximately 6% of the total ^{35}S-proteoglycans extracted from the medium bound to this column. The radiolabelled GAG released by alkaline-borohydride treatment of the bound material were completely susceptible to digestion with chondroitin ABC and ACII lyase. The hydrodynamic size of the intact proteoglycan was similar to the CSPG isolated from Reichert's membrane. The same monoclonal used for the affinity column also immunostained rat mesangial cells, as did the other three monoclonal antibodies described by McCarthy et al. [7]

Thus, at least four populations of CS/DS proteoglycans that differ in respect to hydrodynamic size and glycosaminoglycan composition as well as location, have been identified in mesangial cells. These proteoglycans show striking similarities to those found in aortic medial smooth muscle cells [23].

Turnover of Mesangial Cell Proteoglycans

Recently we have reported an in vivo model designed to follow the metabolism of proteoglycans in the rat glomerulus [24]. An important feature of the experimental design was that, after labelling experiments in which rats were given repeated intraperitoneal injections of ^{35}S-sulphate, the newly synthesized ^{35}S-proteoglycans were fixed in the tissue by perfusing the kidney in situ with 0.1% cetyl pyridinium chloride [14]. This approach ensured complete recovery of labelled molecules. The ^{35}S-GAGs accounted for 80% of the labelled macromolecules, the remainder being due to ^{35}S-glycoproteins. Of the ^{35}S-GAGs synthesized, 85% were HS-GAG and the remainder were CS-GAG [24]. A pulse-chase experiment was undertaken to determine the metabolic half-life of the ^{35}S-proteoglycans in the rat glomeruli. At defined times after the pulse with ^{35}S-sulphate, glomeruli were isolated and analyzed for ^{35}S-labelled macromolecules by autoradiographic and immunochemical methods, and by biochemical analysis. Together, these methods allowed the measurement of turnover times for the different proteoglycans in the glomerulus. Overall, the results showed a complex turnover pattern of ^{35}S-labelled macromolecules consisting of a rapid phase followed by a slower phase. The total population of ^{35}S-HSPG had a metabolic half-life ($t_{1/2}$) of 20 h and 60 h in the first and second phases, respectively. The turnover of basement membrane ^{35}S-HSPG was even faster and revealed $t_{1/2}$ of 5 h and 20 h, respectively. In contrast, the turnover of ^{35}S-CSPG differed from that of HSPG. Whilst it decreased initially with a $t_{1/2}$ of 20 h, the ^{35}S-CSPG pool showed little or no turnover during the second phase. One possible inference from this finding is that the turnover of mesangial cell proteoglycans is different from that of other cells of the glomerulus (endothelial and epithelial). This finding and the above discussion on the glomerular localization of CSPG suggest that mesangial cell proteoglycans may have a relatively slow turnover. Interestingly, the metabolism of ^{35}S-proteoglycans by cultured human glomerular mesangial cells is considerably slower than in human glomerular epithelial cells (Fig. 1). Thus, with mesangial cells after an 8 h chase, 70% of the initial proteoglycans remain associated with the cell layer. More detailed analysis of individual proteoglycans shows that a relatively small amount of DSPG enters the degradative pathway and that loss of proteoglycan from the cell layer is largely accounted for by release of DSPG into the medium.

Growth Factor and Mesangial Cell Proteoglycans

Studies on cultured glomerular cells indicate that enhancement of mesangial matrix synthesis is subject to modulation by cytokines. Tumor necrosis factor (TNFα) [25] and transforming growth factor (TGF-β) [15] have both been shown to be stimulators of mesangial cell proteoglycan production. The effects of the stimulatory cytokines were dose and time-dependent and were not the result of alteration in cell number. These cytokines did not alter the distribution of proteoglycans between the cell layer and culture medium, neither did they appear to have any significant effects on the quality of proteoglycans produced. These observations suggest a role for soluble DSPG in mesangial cell functions, possibly in the control of growth and proliferation. It is possible that the secreted DSPG interact with extracellular matrix com-

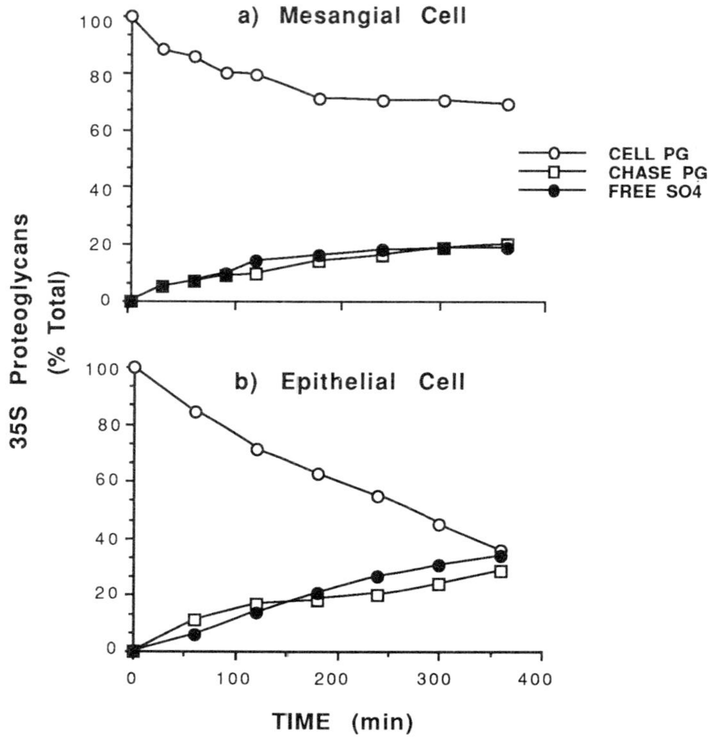

Fig. 1a,b. Pulse chase experiments with (**a**) human mesangial cells and (**b**) human glomerular epithelial cells. Cells were cultured with ^{35}S-sulfate for 24 h, the medium decanted and the cells chased for up to 6 h in fresh medium. At each time point the amount of ^{35}S-proteoglycans remaining in the cell layer (○) and released into the medium (□) was determined after chromatography on Sepharose CL-4B as well as free SO_4 (●). PG, proteoglycan

ponents such as fibronectin, with integrins, or with cytokines themselves to effect the regulation of mesangial cell growth. Such interactions have been reported in other cells [2].

Conclusions

At present it is only possible to speculate on the function of CS/DS proteoglycans in the mesangium. Table 3 contains a list of possible functions. It is possible that the basement membrane CSPG interacts, either through its protein core or GAG component, with other mesangial matrix components such as fibronectin or laminin. In this way it may serve to stabilize the architecture of the matrix. Mesangial basement membrane-CSPG co-exist with HSPG and the combined polyanionic nature of these molecules must contribute to the negative charge of the mesangium. It has been argued that proteoglycans, due to their charge, trap certain types of circulating immune complexes within the mesangium [5]. Cell surface proteoglycans possess binding sites for one or more extracellular proteins and therefore potentially link cells to matrix. Thus the large mesangial cell membrane CSPG could interact with GAG binding sites in the mesangial matrix and form part of a transmembrane cytoskeletal-matrix linkage. Such an interaction would favour cell adhesion. On the other hand, the soluble large CSPG may destabilize adhesion by "substratum conditioning," which then renders the matrix unsuitable for adhesion [26]. The small DSPG could also interact with GAG binding sites or fibronectin and interfere with cell attachment due to steric exclusion or charge repulsion [2]. Such an interaction would favour migration of cells. It is interesting to note that migration of mesangial cells into the pericapillary space between endothelium and GBM is a prominent feature in mesangio-capillary forms of glomerulonephritis [27].

Extensive research should be undertaken to shed more light on the functional and structural relationships between mesangial cell CS/DS and the other components of the mesangial matrix. In view of the known interactions of proteoglycans and fibronectin [2] and the abundance of fibronectin in the mesangial matrix, interactions between CS/DS proteoglycan may provide new insights into the function of the mesangial cell in the normal physiology of the kidney and possibly in the pathophysiology of glomerular disease. Furthermore, the observations that small DSPG are involved in cell-cell interactions and are themselves regulated by cytokines is of direct relevance to the architecture of the mesangial matrix.

Acknowledgments. Part of this work was supported by a MRC Partnership Award to MD and RMM. LS is the recipient of a Kidney Research Unit Foundation for Wales postgraduate award. The authors gratefully acknowledge Dr. John Couchman, University of Alabama at Birmingham, USA for making available Mab 2D6, 2B5, 5A3 and 4D5.

References

1. Poole AR (1986) Proteoglycans in health and disease: structure and functions. Biochem J 236:1–14
2. Ruoslahti E (1989) Proteoglycans in cell regulation. J Biol Chem 264:13369–13372
3. Farquhar MG, Lemkin MC, Stow JL (1984) Role of proteoglycans in glomerular function and pathology. In: Robinson RR (Ed) Nephrology. Springer, New York Berlin Heidelberg Tokyo, pp 580–600
4. Farquhar MG (1986) Characterisation and immunolocalization of glomerular basement membrane proteoglycans. In: Evered D, Whelan J (eds) Functions of the proteoglycans, Ciba Foundation symposium. John Wiley, Chichester, pp 223–240
5. Kanwar YS, Jakubowski ML, Rosenweig LJ (1983) Distribution of sulfated glycosaminoglycans in the glomerular basement membrane and mesangial matrix. Eur J Cell Biol 31:290–295
6. Couchman JR, Caterson B. Christner JE, Baker JR (1984) Mapping by monoclonal antibody detection of glycosaminoglycans in connective tissues. Nature 307:650–652
7. McCarthy KJ, Accavitti MA, Couchman JR (1989) Immunological characterization of a basement membrane–specific chondroitin sulfate proteoglycan. J Cell Biol 109:3187–3198

8. Miettinen A, Stow JL, Mentone S, Farquhar MG (1986) Antibodies to basement membrane heparan sulfate proteoglycans bind to the laminae rarae of the glomerular basement membrane (GBM) and induce subepithelial GBM thickening. J Exp Med 163:1064–1084
9. Mynderse LA, Hassell JR, Kleinman HK, Martin GR, Martinez-Hernandez A (1983) Loss of heparan sulfate proteoglycan from glomerular basement membrane of nephrotic rats. Lab Invest 48:292–302
10. Oomura A, Nakamura T, Arakawa M, Ooshima A, Isemura M (1989) Alterations in the extracellular matrix components in human glomerular diseases. Virchows Arch [A] 415:151–159
11. Shewring L, McCarthy K, Couchman J, Davies M (1990) Rat mesangial cells synthesize mainly chondroitin/dermatan sulphate proteoglycans. XIIth meeting of European Connective Tissue Societies, Poland.
12. Mason RM, Beavan LA, Davies M (1988) The biosynthesis and metabolic turnover of glomerular proteoglycans. In: Gubler M-C, Sternberg M (eds) Progress in basement membrane research; renal and related aspects. J Libbey, London, pp 77–89
13. Klein DJ, Brown DM, Oegema TR (1986) Partial characterization of heparan and dermatan sulfate proteoglycans synthesized by normal rat glomeruli. J Biol Chem 261:16636–16652
14. Beavan LA, Davies M, Mason RM (1988) Renal glomerular proteoglycans: An in vivo investigation of their synthesis using an in situ fixation technique. Biochem J 251:411–418
15. Border WA, Okuda S, Languino LR, Ruoslahti E (1990) Transforming growth factor-β regulates production of proteoglycans by mesangial cells. Kidney Int 37:689–695
16. Yaoita E, Oguri K, Okayama E, Kawasaki K, Koyayashi S, Kihara I, Okayama M (1990) Isolation and characterization of proteoglycans synthesized by cultured mesangial cells. J Biol Chem 265:522–531
17. Striker GE, Killen PD, Farin FM (1980) Human glomerular cells in vitro: Isolation and characterization. Transplant Proc 12:88–99
18. Davies M, Thomas GJ, Jenner L, Mason RM (1988) Human glomerular epithelial and mesangial cells produce different populations of proteoglycans. In: Gubler MC, Sternberg M (eds) Progress in basement membrane research; renal and related aspects. J Libbey, London, pp 35–42
19. Krusius T, Ruoslahti E (1986) Primary structure of an extracellular matrix proteoglycan core protein deduced from cloned cDNA. Proc Natl Acad Sci USA 83:7683–7687
20. Fisher LW, Termine JD, Young MF (1989) Deduced-protein sequence of bone small proteoglycan I (biglycan) shows homology with proteoglycan II (decorin) and several non-connective tissues in a variety of species. J Biol Chem 264:4571–4576
21. Thomas GJ, Jenner L, Mason RM, Davies M (1990) Human glomerular epithelial cell proteoglycans. Arch Biochem Biophys 278:11–20
22. Klein DJ, Oegema TR, Fredeen TS, van der Woude F, Kim Y, Brown DM (1990) Partial characterization of proteoglycans synthesized by human glomerular epithelial cells in culture. Arch Biochem Biophys 277:389–401
23. Wight TN, Lark WL, Kinsella MG (1987) Blood vessel proteoglycans. In: Wight TN, Meacham RP (eds) Biology of extracellular matrix: Biology of proteoglycans. Academic Press, Orlando, pp 267–300
24. Beavan LA, Davies M, Couchman JR, Williams MA, Mason RM (1988) In vivo turnover of the basement and cell-associated heparan sulphate proteoglycans of rat glomerulus. Arch Biochem Biophys 269:576–585
25. Shewring L, Thomas GJ, Davies M (1989) Proteoglycan synthesis is stimulated by TNF in rat mesangial cells in vitro. Clin Sci 76:S20
26. Funderburg FM, Markwald RR (1986) Conditioning of native substrates by chondroitin sulphate proteoglycan during cardiac mesenchymal cell migration. J Cell Biol 103:2475–2487
27. Sterzel RB, Lovett DH, Stein HD, Kashgarian M (1982) The mesangium and glomerulonephritis. Klin Wochenschr 60:1077–1094

Cell and Matrix in Monoclonal Antibody-Induced Mesangiolysis

FUJIO SHIMIZU[1]

SUMMARY. In order to investigate the mutual relationship between mesangial cells and matrix, we used a monoclonal antibody (mAb) to develop an experimental model in rats, in which the rats have transient but massive proteinuria and mesangiolysis, followed by an increase in cell number and an increase of matrix size in the mesangial area.

Proteinuria was induced immediately after a single intravenous injection of mAb (IgG3), which binds, in vitro, to the limited mesangial cell surface facing endothelial cells; proteinuria peaked on day 5, with average values of over 150mg/day. Deposition of mouse IgG and rat C3 in the mesangial area, as well as infiltration of polymorphonuclear cells and degenerative signs of mesangial cells, was observed 30 minutes after mAb injection. Mesangiolytic change occurred 24 or 48 hours after mAb injection, followed by an increase in cell number (4 or 6 days after injection) and an increase in matrix size (2 or 4 weeks after injection) in the mesangial area.

Preliminary study using this model revealed some alterations in cell and mesangial matrix composition (e.g., abnormal production of type I collagen) during the course of this experiment.

We regard this model as a valuable tool for investigating, in vivo, the interrelationship between mesangial cells and matrix.

Introduction

There is increasing evidence that cell structure and function are deeply influenced by the extracellular matrix [1,2].

[1]Department of Immunology, Institute of Nephrology, Niigata University School of Medicine, Asahimachi-dori, Niigata, 951 Japan

A growing interest has been taken in the interrelationship between mesangial cells and matrix in order to better understand the mechanism of proliferation of mesangial cells and matrix leading to progressive glomerular sclerosis.

The information accumulated on this mutual relationship has been obtained mainly from in vitro studies [3].

However, it is well known that cultured mesangial cells are structurally and functionally different from those in vivo. For example, mesangial cells in vitro synthesize mainly type I collagen [4], which cannot be immunohistochemically demonstrated in the normal glomerular mesangium.

The remarkable effects of matrix on the morphology, growth rate, and proteoglycan synthesis of mesangial cells were reported by Yaoita [5]. He demonstrated that mesangial cells, cultured in E gel (prepared from EHS tumor), showed characteristics of morphology and growth rate similar to those in vivo. These findings suggested the possibility that we could partly mimic in vivo surroundings. However, even in his system, mesangial cells cultured in E gel synthesized mainly chondroitin sulphate proteoglycan. Thus, such an imitation has its limits.

In vivo models, used to examine the mutual relationship between mesangial cells and matrix, have been developed by Ishizaki et al. [6] and Yamamoto et al. [7]. According to their reports, mesangiolysis, followed by cellular and matrix increase in the mesangial area, was induced in rats with intravenous injection of anti-rat thymocyte serum. However, lesions are not so uniformly induced by polyclonal anti-thymocyte serum, especially those lesions which relate to the degree of proteinuria. If we could use an antibody which is always identical and monospecific against a limited epitope, it would be ideal for minimizing individual differences and also for further analysis of this model. A monoclonal antibody is the best tool for such purposes.

We have produced a monoclonal antibody (mAb) which also induces mesangiolysis in rats with a single intravenous injection [8]. In this paper, we describe the details of this model and the preliminary results on the alteration of cell and matrix components which were obtained during the course of this experiment.

Monoclonal Antibody-Induced Mesangial Lesions

As reported by Kawachi et al. [8], an intravenous injection of mAb 1–22–3 (IgG3) in rats can induce a massive but transient proteinuria with mesangiolysis, followed by an increase in cell number and an increase in matrix size, in the mesangial area.

This mAb reacts with the limited mesangial cell surface facing endothelial cells. Reactivity of this mAb to thymus, brain, and intestine could also be observed.

Urinary protein excretion started immediately following 500ug mAb injection and peaked on day 5, with average values of over 150mg/day; this was followed by a gradual decline and virtual normalization by day 18. Deposition of mouse IgG and rat C3 in the mesangial area and the infiltration of neutrophils and lymphocytes were observed in rats 30 minutes after mAb injection. Twenty four hours after injection, the staining intensity of IgG or rat C3 decreased.

Mesangiolytic change occurred 24 or 48 hours after mAb injection, followed by an increase in cell number (4 or 6 days after injection) and an increase in matrix size (2 or 4 weeks after injection) in the mesangial area [8].

Mesangial Area Cells in This Model

Preliminary examination with monoclonal antibodies (anti-thy-1, anti-macrophage) revealed that the cells which accumulated after mesangiolysis in this model have more characteristics of intrinsic mesangial cells.

Mesangial Matrix in This Model

Preliminary examination with polyclonal anti-laminin, anti-fibronectin and monoclonal anti-type I, type IV collagen antibodies demonstrated positive fluorescence for laminin and fibronectin in the increased matrix.

Positive staining for type I collagen was observed 2 or 4 weeks after injection.

Type I collagen, not detectable in normal rat glomeruli, may be produced by the cells which are no longer regulated by the matrix, which has disappeared or become disorganized.

We are planning to develop an ideal model for chronic progressive sclerotic lesions, varying the dose and intervals of mAb administration. Applying many advanced techniques in basic cell biology and genetics, the kinetics of cells and matrix in this model will be further examined, with special reference to the influence of cytokines.

Acknowledgments. This work was supported, in part, by a research grant from the Ministry of Education, Science, and Culture (01480163) and from the Ministry of Health and Welfare, Japan (1989).

References

1. Kashgarian M (1985) Mesangium and glomerular disease. Lab Invest 52:569–571
2. Border WA, Okuda S, Nakamura T (1989) Extracellular matrix and glomerular disease. Semin Nephrol 9:307–317
3. Lovett PH, Sterzel RB (1986) Cell culture approaches to the analysis of glomerular inflammation. Kidney Int 30:246–252
4. Haralson MA, Jacobson HR, Hoover RL (1987) Collagen polymorphism in cultured rat kidney mesangial cells. Lab Invest 57:513–519
5. Yaoita E (1989) Behavior of rat mesangial cells cultured within extracellular matrix. Lab Invest 61:410–418
6. Ishizaki M, Masuda Y, Fukuda Y, Sugisaki Y, Yamanaka N, Masugi Y (1986) Experimental mesangioproliferative glomerulonephritis in rats induced by intravenous administration of anti-thymocyte serum. Acta Pathol Jpn 36:1191–1203
7. Yamamoto T, Wilson CB (1987) Complement dependence of antibody-induced mesangial cell injury in the rat. J Immunol 138:3758–3765
8. Kawachi H, Orikasa M, Matsui K, Morioka T, Oite T, Shimizu F (1990) Induction of proteinuria and morphological change in the rat by a monoclonal antibody against mesangial cell surface (abstract). Kidney Int 37:418

Regulation of Collagen IV Expression

Paul D. Killen, Cynthia A. DeMeester, Robert A. Long, Erin O'Brien, and Joseph P. Grande[1]

Summary. Recent advances in the molecular biology of basement membrane components have resulted in new tools for the study of basement membrane metabolism during normal renal development and growth. Collagen IV, the major structural protein of basement membranes, is assembled from at least 5 distinct gene products. mRNA encoding the α1(IV) and α2(IV) chains vary in a precise temporal and spatial fashion during nephronogenesis. Inflammation, such as that observed in anti-glomerular basement membrane (GBM) nephritis or in the metabolic or hemodynamic disturbances exemplified by diabetes mellitus, leads to increased steady-state levels of mRNA for these basement membrane components. Increased transcription of these genes may, in part, account for the increase. These two genes are separated by a 130 bp bidirectional promoter which is regulated by sequences contained within the genes. We have directly measured transcription of each gene by the nuclear run-on method and have correlated this with the steady-state mRNA level for each chain. The data suggest that transcriptional attenuation may play an important role in determining the ratio of α1(IV)/α2(IV) mRNA as well as the relative abundance of these mRNA in different tissues. These methods should provide new insights into the mechanism of collagen IV gene expression during renal development and in experimental disease models.

Introduction

Basement membranes play an important role during tissue morphogenesis [1]. By providing a substratum for adhesion, the basement membrane orients cells for the maintenance of cell polarity and a differentiated phenotype [2] and it acts as a template for the restoration of normal tissue architecture following injury [3]. Further,

[1]Department of Pathology, School of Medicine, University of Michigan, Ann Arbor, MI 48109-0602, USA

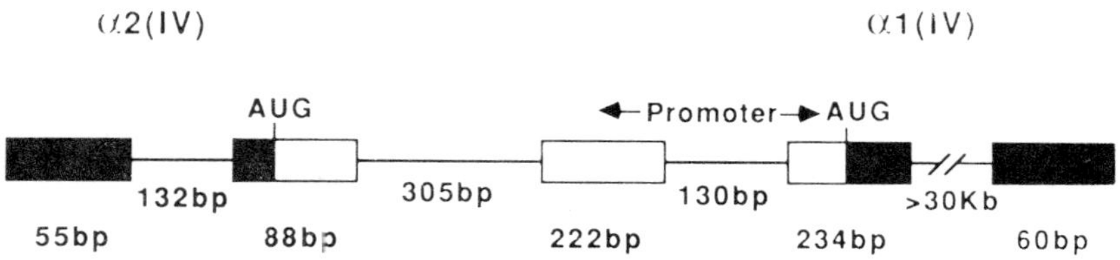

Fig. 1. Bidirectional transcription of collagen IV genes

it constitutes an important permeability barrier for the filtration of plasma to form urine [4]. Changes in the abundance or morphological appearance of glomerular matrices characterize the glomerular response to inflammatory, hemodynamic, or metabolic disorders. The deposition of this extracellular matrix is currently viewed as irreversible and inexorable, leading to diminished function or organ failure. The mechanisms regulating the synthesis of these matrix components during renal development or in response to injury are unknown.

Collagen IV occurs uniquely in basement membranes where it provides tensile strength. Each triple helical molecule is assembled from an assortment of 5 genetically distinct α chains. All basement membranes contain α1(IV) and α2(IV) collagen chains, whereas α3-5(IV) have a restricted anatomic distribution [5–7]. The abundance of the α1(IV) and α2(IV) mRNA vary widely between [8] and within tissues [9]. The molecular mechanisms regulating the steady-state levels of these MRNA are not known. The α1(IV) and α2(IV) genes are clustered with the 5′ ends of the genes, separated by a 130 bp (in the mouse) bidirectional promoter [10,11] (Fig. 1). Differential transcription of these genes could cause the observed differences in the abundance of these MRNA. In order to directly assess the transcription of these genes, we have studied transcription of the α1(IV) and α2(IV) genes by expressing and non-expressing cell types in vitro. Our results suggest that differences in transcription elongation may, in part, regulate the abundance of these mRNA.

Methods

Cell Culture

NIH-3T3 cells were obtained from the American Type Culture Collection. PF-HR9 cells were the generous gift of R. Kramer, UCSF. Cells were maintained in Dulbecco's modified Eagle's medium (DMEM) supplemented with 1 mM L-glutamine, penicillin/streptomycin (100U/1μg per ml) and 10% calf serum. In some experiments, calf serum was incubated, with stirring, with activated charcoal for 60 minutes.

Quantitation of Collagen IV mRNA

Total cellular RNA was purified from confluent cultures of NIH-3T3 cells or PF-HR9 cells as previously described [11]. Then 10 μg of denatured RNA were electrophoresed in a 2.2 M formaldehyde 1% agarose gel and the RNA was transferred to nylon

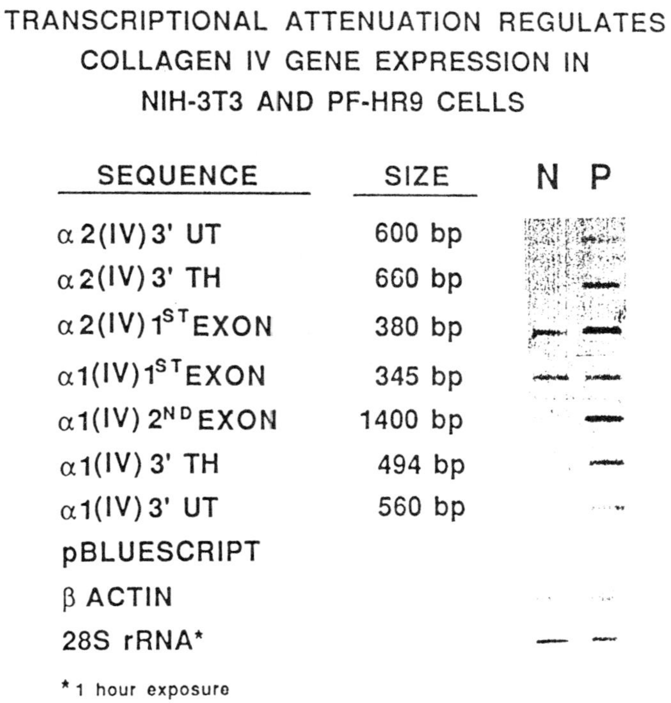

Fig. 2. Transcriptional attenuation regulates collagen IV gene expression in NIH-3T3 and PF-HR9 cells

filters by capillary blotting. Serial dilutions of RNA were directly applied to the filters with the aid of a vacuum manifold. RNA was fixed to the filters by baking in vacuo at 80°C for 2 hours. Purified fragments of the murine α1(IV), α2(IV), or β-actin cDNA [12] were labeled with $\alpha^{32}P$ dCTP to a specific activity of 10^9 dpm/μg [13]. Filters were hybridized and washed as previously described [8]. X-OMAT AR film (Kodak) was preflashed, and exposed to the filters at −80°C with intensifying screens. The Northern blot was intentionally overexposed. The relative abundance of the α1(IV) or α2(IV) mRNA in these cells was determined with a laser densitometer.

Nuclear Run-on Transcription

Direct assessment of α1(IV) gene transcription was determined by the nuclear run-on method. In brief, nuclei were isolated following cell lysis in NP-40 and incubated for 30 minutes at 30°C in 45 mM TRIS, pH 8.3, 6 mM $MgCl_2$, 150 mM KCl, 250 μM ATP, CTP, GTP and 0.33 μM $\alpha^{32}P$ UTP (3000 Ci/mM) essentially as described by McKnight and Palmiter [14]. The labeled RNA transcripts were precipitated, and separated from unincorporated nucleotides on mini-spin columns of G-100. The RNA was partially hydrolyzed with alkali, precipitated, and redissolved at a final concentration of 5×10^6 dpm/ml in hybridization buffer. Five μg of denatured DNA was applied to nitrocellulose with a slot blot manifold. Fragments from the 5′ end of the murine α1(IV) or α2(IV) gene and from cDNAs encoding the 3′ end of the triple helical domain or from the 3′ untranslated region served as test sequences. Special attention was given to the potential of cross hybridization of the collagen IV transcripts. In particular, it was observed in preliminary studies that hybridization to a NCl domain encoding sequence was approximately twice the expected radiodensity for its length. Presumably, both α1 and α2 transcripts were hybridizing to this sequence due to the high homology between the NCl domain encoding sequences of the two genes. Positive and negative controls included β-actin [12], the 28S rRNA gene [15], and pBluescript KSM13^{+} (Stratagene, La Jolla). Filters were hybridized for 72 hours at 65°C in equal volumes of 10 mM TES, pH 7.4, 0.3 M NaCl, 10 mM EDTA, 0.2% SDS containing 1X Denhardt's solution, and 0.25 mg/ml E. Coli RNA. Filters were washed three times at 65°C in 2X SSC, 0.1% SDS, and twice in 0.1X SSC, 0.1% SDS. Autoradiograms were prepared as described above.

Results

Northern blots of total cellular RNA isolated from PF-HR9 and 3T3 cells hybridized with cDNA probes specific for the α1(IV) or α2(IV) chain demonstrated strong signals of the expected size in RNA from the PF-HR9 cells. In contrast, NIH 3T3 cells displayed a weak signal which required several days exposure to adequately visualize. No differences in the steady-state level of β-actin mRNA were observed between the two cell types. Since the cDNA probes hybridized specifically, the relative abundance of these mRNA could be determined by serial dilutions of RNA on "dot blots." Laser densitometry demonstrated that the collagen IV mRNA were more than 50-fold more abundant in the PF-HR9 cells than in the NIH 3T3 cells.

In order to directly measure the transcription of each gene, we subcloned in pBluescript, segments of the α1(IV) and α2(IV) gene which lacked repetitive sequence as assessed by hybridization with ^{32}P labeled murine genomic DNA in plasmids. In addition, fragments of cDNAs were also subcloned. Fragments of the α1(IV) gene included a 345 bp fragment containing the first exon, a 1.4 kb fragment containing the second exon, a 494 bp cDNA fragment encoding the 3′ portion of the triple-helical (3′TH) domain, and a 560 bp segment of the 3′ untranslated sequence (3′UT) proximal to the first polyadenylation site. Fragments of the murine α2(IV) gene included a 380 bp fragment containing the first exon, a 660 bp cDNA fragment encoding the 3′TH domain, and a 600 bp segment of the 3′UT sequence downstream from the B2 repeat but upstream from the polyadenylation site [16]. No significant hybridization was observed with the negative control, pBluescript. Hybridization to the 28S rRNA gene sequences were similar in the two cell types, indicating that the specific activity of the labeled transcripts was similar for the two filters. Furthermore, the hybridization to the β-actin cDNA was similar in the two cell types. When transcription of the two collagen IV genes was compared in the PF-HR9 cells, transcript initiation, as detected by the sequences containing the first exon, was nearly equally efficient in the α2(IV) or α1(IV) directions. However, there was a modest decrease in transcriptional efficiency along the length of the gene. Hybridization to the 3′UT sequences was significantly weaker than the first exon, and the predicted signal (assuming 100% completion of transcripts) should be greater than the first exon due to the greater length of the 3′UT sequences.

If differences in the abundance of the α1(IV) and α2(IV) mRNA were exclusively due to differences in transcription, then hybridization of these transcripts to the collagen IV gene transcripts should be more than 50-fold less than that observed with the PF-HR9 cells. Surprisingly, transcription initiation, as reflected by hybridization of transcripts to the first exon, was nearly identical in the two cell types. However, hybridization to the 3′UT sequences was virtually undetectable in NIH 3T3 cells. Thus, somewhere within the gene, there is significant attenuation of transcription. Indeed, in the case of the α1(IV) gene transcript elongation must be blocked in the first intron.

Discussion

The expression of collagen IV genes is highly regulated in both space and time. The α1(IV) and α2(IV) mRNA appear early in nephronogenesis and reach a maximal level at birth or shortly thereafter [17]. Subsequently, the abundance of these mRNA rapidly falls to a low level, which in the adult kidney, is less than 10% of maximal. In situ hybridization demonstrates these transcripts in a characteristic pattern that changes with renal development and growth [18]. Renal injury alters the abundance of these mRNA in adult animals. For instance, within 4 days of administration of anti-GBM antibody, α1(IV) mRNA are increased some 9-fold in rabbit kidney cortex [19]. Increases in collagen IV mRNA have also been noted in diabetic and spontaneously hypertensive rat kidneys (unpublished work). Whether these changes are due to changes in the transcription of the collagen IV genes or due to changes in mRNA stability is unknown.

In order to develop methods for the analysis of collagen IV gene transcription in vivo, we have studied the expression of collagen IV genes in cell lines in vitro. We compared PF-HR9 cells, which constitutively synthesize collagen IV chains, to NIH 3T3 cells, which do not synthesize these proteins. Our results indicate that differences in transcription, in part, underlie the differences in collagen IV gene expression. However, this may not be due to differences in transcript initiation by the collagen IV promoter, but rather may be due to differences in the efficiency of transcript elongation, as has been observed with other genes [20–22]. This observation may explain why the collagen IV promoter resembles promoters of "housekeeping" genes [23]. Initiation of transcripts may occur in all cells, but elongation of transcripts may occur in a cell- or tissue-specific fashion. The transcriptional block occurs in the first intron of the α1(IV) gene, as has been observed for the proto-oncogenes c-myb and c-myc [21,22]. In studies reported at this meeting [24], we have found that sequences within the first intron of the α1(IV) gene are capable of decreasing transcription of heterologous promoters in NIH 3T3 cells. These sequences bind specifically to proteins in nuclear extracts from NIH 3T3. Future studies will determine whether differences in transcription initiation and elongation regulate expression of collagen IV genes during renal development or in pathological contexts.

Acknowledgments. We gratefully acknowledge the many helpful discussions with Craig Thompson during the course of these studies and the assistance of Kimberly

Drake in the preparation of this manuscript. This work was supported in part by NIH grant, HL-31963. JPG is supported by NIH training grant, HL-07517.

References

1. Ekblom P, Vestweber D. Kemler R (1986) Cell-matrix interactions and cell adhesion during development. Annu Rev Cell Biol 2:27–47
2. Sugrue SP, Hay ED (1986) The identification of extracellular matrix (ECM) binding sites on the basal surface of embryonic corneal epithelium and the effect of ECM binding on epithelial collagen production. J Cell Biol 102:1907–1916
3. Vracko, R (1974) Basal lamina scaffold-anatomy and significance for maintenance of orderly tissue structure. Am J Pathol 77:314–346
4. Maddox DA, Brenner BM (1977) Glomerular filtration of fluid and macromolecules: the renal response to injury. Annu Rev Med 28:91–102
5. Saus J, Wieslander J, Langveld JP, Quinones S, Hudson BG (1988) Identification of the Goodpasture antigen as the α3(IV) chain of collagen IV. J Biol Chem 263:13374–13380
6. Kleppel MM, Santi PA, Cameron JD, Wieslander J, Michael AF (1989) Human tissue distribution of novel basement membrane collagen. Am J Pathol 134:813–825
7. Hostikka S, Eddy RL, Byers MG, Hoyhtya M, Shows TB, Tryggvason K (1990) Identification of a distinct type IV collagen alpha chain with restricted kidney distribution and assignment of its gene to the locus of X chromosome-linked Alport syndrome. Proc Natl Acad Sci USA 87:1606–1610
8. Kleinman HK, Ebihara I, Killen PD, Sasaki M, Cannon FB, Yamada Y, Martin GR (1987) Genes for basement membrane proteins are coordinately expressed in differentiating F9 cells but not in normal adult murine tissues. Dev Biol 122:373–378
9. Boot-Hanford RP, Kurkinen M, Prockop DJ (1987) Steady-state levels of mRNAs for the type IV collagen and laminin polypeptide chains of basement membranes exhibit marked tissue-specific stoichiometric variations in the rat. J Biol Chem 262:12475–12478
10. Burbelo PD, Yamada Y, Martin GR (1988) Alpha 1(IV) and alpha2(IV) collagen genes are regulated by a bidirectional promoter and a shared enhancer. Proc Natl Acad Sci USA 85:9679–9682
11. Poschl E, Pollner R, Kuhn K (1988) The genes for the alpha 1 (IV) and alpha 2(IV) chains of human basement membrane collagen IV are arranged head-to-head and separated by a bidirectional promoter of unique structure. EMBO J 7:2687–2695
12. Cleveland DW, Lopata MA, McDonald RJ, Cowan NJ, Rutter WJ (1980) Number and evolutionary conservation of α- and β-tubulin and cytoplasmic β- and γ-actin genes using specific cloned cDNA probes. Cell 20:95–105
13. Feinberg A, Vogelstein B (1982) A technique for radiolabeling DNA restriction endonuclease fragments to high specific activity. Anal Biochem 132:6–13
14. McKnight GS, Palmiter RD (1979) Transcriptional regulation of the ovalbumin and conalbumin genes by steroid hormones in chick oviduct. J Biol Chem 254:9050–9058
15. Chan YL, Olvera J, Wool IG (1983) Structure of rat 28S ribosomal ribonucleic acid inferred from the sequence of nucleotides in a gene. Nucleic Acids Res 11:7819–7831
16. Oberbaumer I, Magdolen U (1988) The 3′ untranslated region of the murine mRNA for the alpha 2 chain of type IV collagen contains a B1-like element. Nucleic Acids Res 16:7181
17. Ebihara I, Killen PD, Laurie GW, Huang T, Yamada Y, Martin GR, Brown KS (1988) Altered mRNA expression of basement membrane components in a murine model of polycystic kidney disease. Lab Invest 58:262–269
18. Laurie GW, Horikoshi S, Killen PD, Segui-Real B, Yamada Y (1989) In situ hybridization reveals temporal and spatial changes in cellular expression of mRNA for a laminin recep-

tor, laminin, and basement membrane (type IV) collagen in the developing kidney. J Cell Biol 109:1351–1362
19. Merrit S, Killen PD, Wiggins R (to be published) Analysis of α1(I) procollagen, α1(IV) collagen β and β-actin mRNA in glomeruli and cortex of rabbits with experimental anti-GBM disease. Evidence of early extraglomerular collagen biosynthesis. Lab Invest
20. Bender TP, Thompson CB, Kuehl WM (1987) Differential expression of c-*myb* mRNA in murine B lymphomas by a block to transcription elongation. Science 237:1473–1476
21. Lindstein T, June CH, Thompson CB (1988) Multiple mechanisms regulate c-*myc* expression during normal T cell activation. EMBO J 7:2787–2794
22. Lindsten T, June CH, Thompson CB, Leiden JM (1988) Regulation of 4F2 heavy-chain gene expression during normal human T-cell activation can be mediated by multiple distinct molecular mechanisms. Mol Cell Biol 8:3820–3826
23. Killen PD, Burbelo PD, Martin GR, Yamada Y (1988) Characterization of the promoter of the α1(IV) collagen gene. J Biol Chem 263:12310–12314
24. Killen PD, DeMeester CA, Long R, O'Brien E (1991) Identification of sequences which enhance or repress collagen IV gene transcription. Proceedings of the XIth International Congress of Nephrology, July 15–20 1990. Tokyo, Japan

Renal Tubular Acidosis

Chair: Robert J. Alpern (USA)
Teruo Kitagawa (Japan)

Proximal Renal Tubular Acidosis (RTA): Normal Proximal Tubule Function and Evidence of Cellular Defects

SEI SASAKI[1]

SUMMARY. During the last ten years, the mechanisms and regulation of HCO_3^-/H^+ transport across the cell membranes of proximal tubule cells, have been extensively studied. The generally accepted view is that tubular acidification is performed by H^+ secretion into the lumen. This secretion is mostly due to a luminal Na/H exchange; a small portion is mediated by an ATP-dependent H^+ pump. Most basolateral HCO_3^- exit is through a Na-$(HCO_3)_3$ cotransport; a small fraction (15%) is mediated by Na^+ coupled Cl^-/HCO_3^- exchange. The amount of passive HCO_3^- leak from the peritubular to the tubular lumen is relatively small compared to the active H^+ secretion. Based on this concept, I will discuss possible mechanisms of proximal RTA; (1) decreased luminal H^+ secretion, (2) decreased basolateral HCO_3^- exit, (3) inhibition of Na-K-ATPase pump, (4) decreased generation of ATP, and (5) increased passive permeability of HCO_3^-.

Introduction

Proximal renal tubular acidosis (RTA) is a clinical syndrome characterized by hyperchloremic metabolic acidosis, which is caused by a defect in proximal tubular acidification. Proximal tubule reabsorbs most of the filtered water and solutes. As shown in Fig. 1, the data in rat free flow micropuncture studies have shown that proximal tubule reabsorbs 85% of filtered HCO_3^-, 98% of glucose, 90% of amino acids, 50% of phosphate, and about 60% of the organic anions, such as acetate, citrate, and uric acid [1]. One important characteristic of the reabsorption of these solutes is a coupling with Na^+. For example, HCO_3^- is reabsorbed by proton secretion, mediated by luminal Na^+/H^+ exchange, into the lumen. The driving force of this exchange is an electrochemical gradient of Na^+ across the luminal membrane. Cell Na^+ is maintained at a low level by the basolateral Na-K-ATPase pump, and intracellular potential is highly negative. Following this large electrochemical gradient of Na^+ across the cell mem-

[1]Second Department of Internal Medicine, Tokyo Medical and Dental University, 1-5-45 Yushima, Bunkyo-ku, Tokyo, 113 Japan

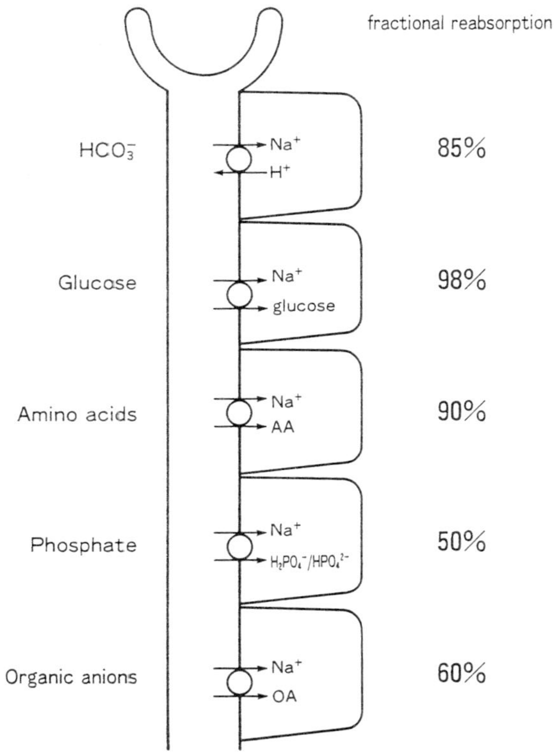

Fig. 1. Solute reabsorption in the proximal tubules. Most glomerular filtered solutes are reabsorbed in the proximal tubules. Generalized defects of proximal reabsorption will cause inhibition of the reabsorption of these solutes. One important character of these transports is a coupling with Na. AA, amino acids; OA, organic anions

brane, Na^+ goes inside the cell and proton is extruded from the cell. Reabsorption of other solutes also uses this Na^+ electrochemical gradient. Thus, reabsorption of solutes in the proximal tubule is, in general, mediated by secondary active processes.

Proximal RTA can be divided into two forms. One form, "the Fanconi syndrome," is a proximal acidification defect which is accompanied by a generalized proximal reabsorption defect. The other form, which is rare, is a selective defect of proximal acidification. A simple expectation from Fig. 1 is that if this electrochemical gradient of Na^+ is not maintained, this lack of maintenance will cause a generalized defect of proximal solute reabsorption, i.e., the Fanconi syndrome.

Normal Proximal Acidification

During the last 10 years, mechanisms of proximal acidification have been clarified by advances in experimental techniques, such as ion selective microelectrodes, fluorescent measurements, and vesicle studies. Figure 2 shows a currently accepted

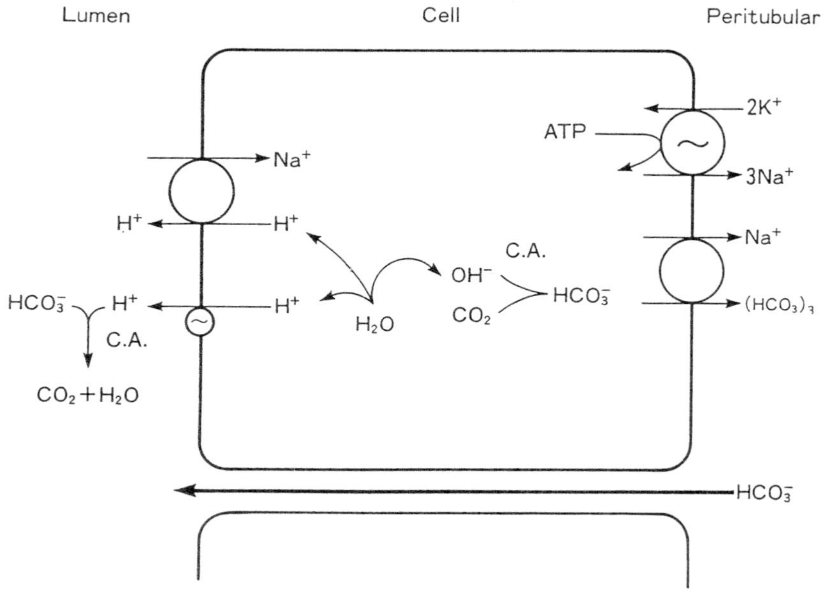

Fig. 2. Mechanisms of proximal acidification. Luminal proton secretion is mediated by Na/H exchange and ATP dependent pump. Basolateral HCO_3 exit is mainly mediated by Na-HCO_3 cotransporter. A small portion of reabsorbed HCO_3 leaks back to the lumen through a paracellular shunt pathway. C.A., carbonic anhydrase

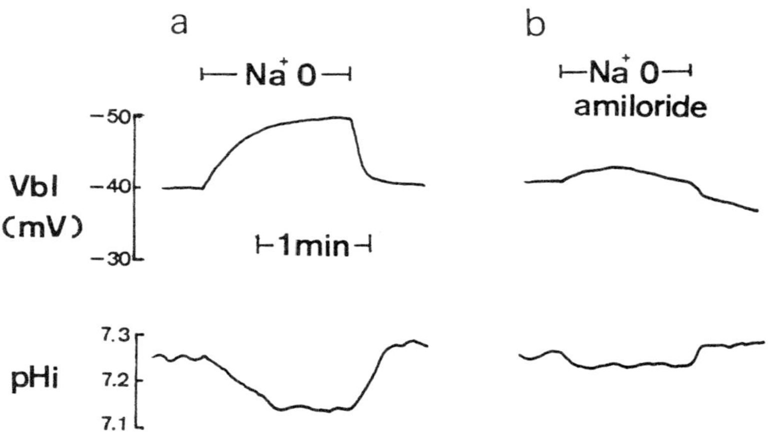

Fig. 3a,b. Luminal Na/H exchange examined by pH-selective microelectrode. In response to luminal Na removal, cell pH (*pHi*) was acidified (**a**) and this effect was inhibited by amiloride (**b**). Vbl, basolateral membrane potential. (From [4] with permission)

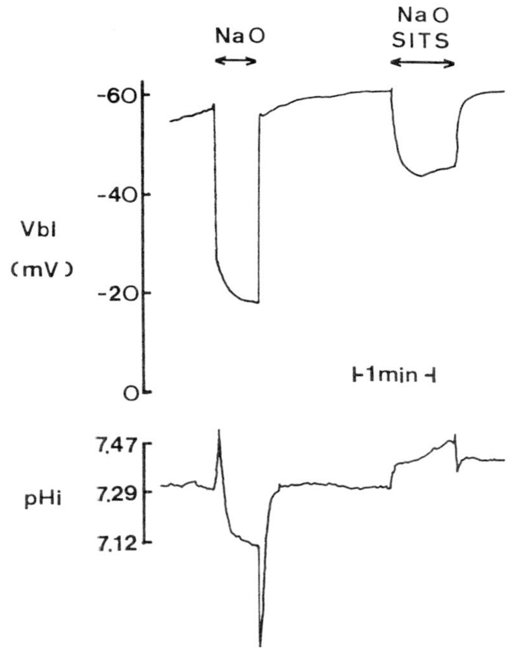

Fig. 4. Basolateral Na-HCO_3 cotransporter examined by pH electrode. Bath Na removal decreased cell pH. This cell acidification was accompanied by a large depolarization of basolateral membrane potential (*Vbl*). These effects were inhibited by the anion transport inhibitor, SITS. (Data from [4] with permission)

model of proximal acidification, in which an important step is proton secretion across the luminal membrane. Most of the proton secretion is performed by the luminal Na^+/H^+ antiporter. In addition to the antiporter, a small amount of proton is secreted by a luminal ATP-dependent H^+ pump [2]. Secreted H^+ titrates luminal HCO_3^-, making CO_2 and water in the presence of luminal carbonic anhydrase (CA). Inside the cell, OH^- is left, and this OH^- reacts with CO_2 to make HCO_3^-.

This process is also CA-dependent. Most of the generated HCO_3^- exits the basolateral membrane through the Na-$(HCO_3)_3$ cotransporter. Stoichiometry of this cotransport has been shown as 1 Na^+: 3 HCO_3^-. As already described, luminal Na^+/H^+ exchange is driven by a Na^+ electrochemical gradient, and the basolateral NaK-ATPase pump maintains this Na^+ electrochemical gradient.

Figure 3 shows our data, obtained by pH sensitive microelectrode which examined the luminal Na^+/H^+ exchange in rabbit proximal straight tubules [4]. Removal of luminal Na^+ caused a significant cell pH decrease. This cell pH decrease was partly inhibited by a high dose of amiloride, an inhibitor of Na^+/H^+ exchange, thus demonstrating the presence of a Na^+/H^+ exchange. An example of an experiment which examined the basolateral Na^+-HCO_3^- cotransport is shown in Fig. 4 [4,5]. Na^+ removal from basolateral fluid rapidly decreased cell pH. This cell acidification was accompanied by a large cell membrane depolarization, indicating the electrogenic nature of this transport. This Na^+ coupled HCO_3^- transport was inhibited by SITS, an anion transport inhibitor, indicating the presence of Na^+-HCO_3^- cotransport across the basolateral membrane. Further studies have shown that a small fraction (15%) of basolateral HCO_3^- transport is mediated by Na^+-dependent Cl^-/HCO_3^- exchange [6].

Defects of Proximal Acidification: Increased Passive Leak vs Inhibited Active Proton Secretion

Defects of proximal acidification can be caused by either of two mechanisms; increased passive leak of reabsorbed solutes and/or inhibited active reabsorption. Because proximal tubule epithelium is leaky, and because a large concentration gradient is generated between tubular lumen and peritubular cells, reabsorbed solutes can diffuse back to the tubular lumen along their chemical gradient. Therefore, increased passive permeability (presumably through the paracellular shunt), can, theoretically, cause a generalized defect in proximal solute reabsorption.

Figure 5 shows a summary of active and passive fluxes of HCO_3^- and glucose, based on kinetic analysis of rat proximal convoluted tubule. Active HCO_3^- reabsorption is 800 peq/min per single proximal convoluted tubule in normal condition. On the other hand, passive leak flux is 100, which is 13% of the value for active flux [7]. Thus, a large change in passive flux may not affect total HCO_3^- flux very much. Indeed, Alpern et al. showed that a 50% increase in passive HCO_3^- permeability did not appreciably change net HCO_3^- reabsorption [8]. In the case of glucose reabsorption, the difference between active and passive fluxes is more striking. Passive flux is only 6% of active reabsorptive flux [9]. Thus, these calculations indicate that the

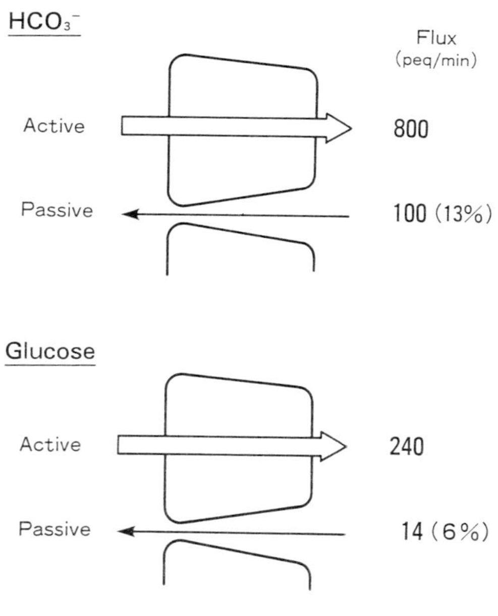

Fig. 5. Active reabsorption and passive leak in proximal solute reabsorption. Data are taken from rat micropuncture studies. In HCO_3 reabsorption, active reabsorption is 800 peq/min per single proximal convoluted tubule, whereas the value for passive leak is only 100, demonstrating the small contribution made by passive leak flux

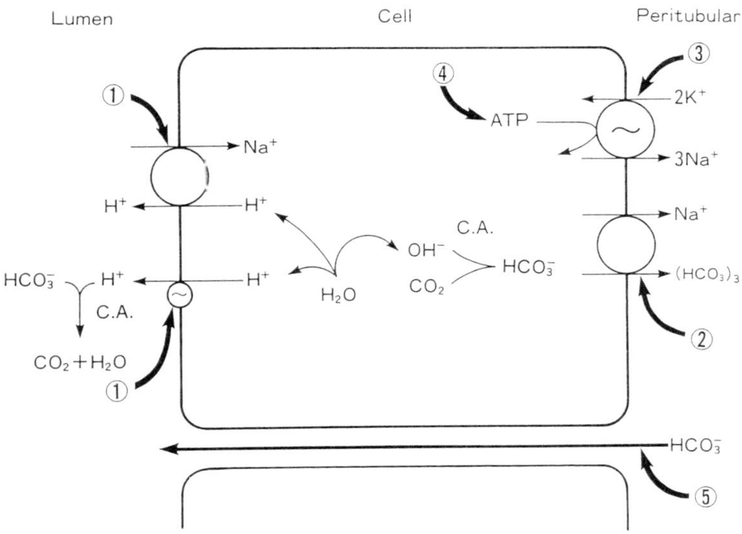

Fig. 6. Possible mechanisms of proximal RTA. See text (under heading "Pathogenesis of RTA") for details. C.A., carbonic anhydrase

contribution of increased passive fluxes of solutes to the genesis of RTA may be small. Furthermore, the existence of selective defects of passive leak may be unlikely. Defects in passive leak would accompany more generalized cell function defects, and generalized cell function defects would affect active reabsorption, which has a dominant role in net solute reabsorption.

Pathogenesis of Proximal RTA

In theory, proximal RTA can be introduced through defects in any of the H^+/HCO_3^- transporters shown in Fig. 2. Defects in the transporters are caused by many mechanisms, for example, chemical modification of transporters, such as phosphorylation; decreased numbers of transporting proteins, decreased energy supply for transporters; and decreased driving force for secondary active transporters. Figure 6 shows possible mechanisms of proximal acidification defects. 1) Decreased luminal H^+ extrusion through the Na^+/H^+ exchange and proton pump causes an acidification defect. This defect may be caused by chemical modification of these transport proteins and the decreased number of these transporters. We have recently shown that parathyroid hormone (PTH) causes an inhibition of proximal acidification, which is mediated by decreased Na^+/H^+ antiporter activity, which in turn is due to phosphorylation by cAMP dependent A-kinase. Also, lack of luminal carbonic anhydrase inhibits luminal H^+ excretion by increasing luminal H^+ concentration. An inherited syndrome which accompanies RTA has been reported to be due to a deficiency of carbonic anhydrase II [10].

2) Proximal acidification defects can be caused by inhibition of basolateral HCO_3^- exit. This may be due to inhibition of either Na^+-HCO_3^- cotransport or inhibition of Na^+-dependent Cl^-/HCO_3^- exchange. An example of this type defect is obtained by administration of carbonic anhydrase inhibitors. We have shown that acetazolamide, a carbonic anhydrase inhibitor, inhibits basolateral HCO_3^- exit by reducing intracellular HCO_3^- availability [11].

3) Inhibition of the Na-K-ATPase pump can cause a proximal acidification defect by reducing electrochemical driving force for Na^+ across the luminal membrane. It is interesting that activation of protein kinase C has been reported to inhibit NaK-ATPase in rat proximal tubules [12]. This result may indicate the possibility that stimulation of protein kinase C decreases luminal acidification. A recent study in rabbit proximal tubules supports this expectation [13].

4) Decreased supply of ATP to the pumps, NaK-ATPase and the luminal H^+ pump, decreases proximal acidification. A decreased level of ATP in renal cortical homogenate has been reported in an experimental model of Fanconi's syndrome produced by maleic acid infusion [14]. This type of defect can easily affect generalized proximal solute reabsorption. In hereditary fructose intolerance, which causes proximal RTA, intracellular accumulation of fructose-1-phosphate occurs, inducing intracellular phosphate depletion, which in turn causes a decreased generation of ATP [15].

5) Increased passive leak of reabsorbed solutes can cause Fanconi syndrome. However, as described above, the contribution of this mechanism may be small. Recent experimental data, in which the passive permeability of HCO_3^- was measured, denied the contribution of this mechanism [16,17].

References

1. Rector FC (1983) Sodium, bicarbonate, and chloride absorption by the proximal tubule. Am J Physiol 244:F461–F471
2. Preisig PA, Ives HE, Cragoe EJ, Alpern RJ, Rector FC (1987) Role of the Na/H antiporter in rat proximal tubule bicarbonate absorption. J Clin Invest 80:970–978
3. Yoshitomi K, Burckhardt B-Ch, Fromter E (1985) Rheogenic sodium-bicarbonate cotransport in the peritubular cell membrane of rat renal proximal tubule. Pflugers Arch 405:360–366
4. Sasaki S, Shiigai T, Takeuchi J (1985) Intracellular pH in the isolated perfused rabbit proximal straight tubule. Am J Physiol 249:F417–F423
5. Sasaki S, Shiigai T, Yoshiyama N, Takeuchi J (1987) Mechanism of bicarbonate exit across basolateral membrane of rabbit proximal straight tubule. Am J Physiol 252:F11–F18
6. Sasaki S, Yoshiyama N (1988) Interaction of chloride and bicarbonate transport across the basolateral membrane of rabbit proximal straight tubule. Evidence for sodium coupled chloride/bicarbonate exchange. J Clin Invest 81:1004–1011
7. Alpern RJ, Rector FC (1985) A model of proximal tubular bicarbonate absorption. Am J Physiol 248:F272–F281
8. Alpern RJ, Cogan MG, Rector FC (1983) Effects of extracellular fluid volume and plasma bicarbonate concentration on proximal acidification. J Clin Invest 71:736–746

9. Barfuss DW, Schafer JA (1981) Differences in active and passive glucose transport along the proximal nephron. Am J Physiol 241:F322–F332
10. Sly WS, Whyte MP, Sundaram V, Tashian RE, Hewett-Emmett D, Guibaud P, Vainsel M, Baluarte HJ, Gruskin A, Al-Mosawi M, Sakati N, Ohlsson A (1985) Carbonic anhydrase II deficiency in 12 families with the autosomal recessive syndrome of osteopetrosis with renal tubular acidosis and cerebral calcification. N Engl J Med 313:139–145
11. Sasaki S, Marumo F (1989) Effect of carbonic anhydrase inhibitors on basolateral base transport of rabbit proximal straight tubule. Am J Physiol 247:F947–F952
12. Bertorello A, Aperia A (1989) Na-K-ATPase is an effector protein for protein kinase C in renal proximal tubule cells. Am J Physiol 256:F370–F373
13. Baum M, Hays SR (1988) Phorbol myristate acetate and dioctanoylglycerol inhibit transport in rabbit proximal convoluted tubule. Am J Physiol 254:F9–F14
14. Kramer HJ, Gonick HC (1970) Experimental Fanconi syndrome. I. Effect of maleic acid on renal cortical Na-K-ATPase activity and ATP levels. J Lab Clin Med 76:799–808
15. Burch HB, Choi S, Dence CN, Alvey TR, Cole BR, Lowry OH (1980) Metabolic effects of large fructose loads in different parts of the rat nephron. J Biol Chem 255:8239–8244
16. Bank N, Aynedjian HS, Mutz BF (1986) Microperfusion study of proximal tubule bicarbonate transport in maleic acid-induced renal tubular acidosis. Am J Physiol 250:F476–F482
17. Salmon RJ, Baum M (1990) Intracellular cystine loading inhibits transport in the rabbit proximal convoluted tubule. J Clin Invest 85:340–344

Cellular Mechanisms of Type 2 Renal Tubular Acidosis/Fanconi Syndrome

R. CURTIS MORRIS[1]

Introduction

As depicted in Fig. 1, impaired proximal bicarbonate reabsorption might result from a selective disorder of the acidification process affecting: 1) the Na^+/H^+ antiporter required for hydrogen ion secretion (labeled 1); 2) the Na^+/HCO_3^- symporter responsible for bicarbonate exit from the proximal tubule cell (labeled 2); 3) the carbonic anhydrases (labeled 3 and 4) or possibly luminal H^+ ATPase. An abnormality in the mechanism by which intracellular sodium concentration is maintained at a normally low level would dictate a diminished reabsorption of all solutes that depend on a Na^+-coupled transport, including not only most of bicarbonate but also glucose, amino acids, phosphate and uric acid, and hence the expression of renal tubule acidosis Type 2 (RTA-2) combined with the Fanconi syndrome (RTA2/FS) [1]. Such a global abnormality might result from several mechanisms: a large increase in cell sodium permeability (labeled 5); diminished activity of the Na^+/K^+-ATPase pump itself (labeled 6); diminished availability of phosphate/impaired metabolic generation of ATP needed to energize the pump (labeled 7); impaired membrane recycling, vacuolar transport or trafficking (labeled 8) and loss of epithelial mass.

Acute RTA2/FS

Hereditary Fructose Intolerance (HFI)

The renal tubular disorder reversibly induced within minutes by intravenous administration of fructose in patients with HFI [2] can be both a dramatic clinical cause of RTA-2/FS and, uniquely, an acute experimental model of RTA-2/FS in humans. The

[1]General Clinical Research Center, School of Medicine, Moffitt Hospital, San Francisco, CA 94143-0126, USA

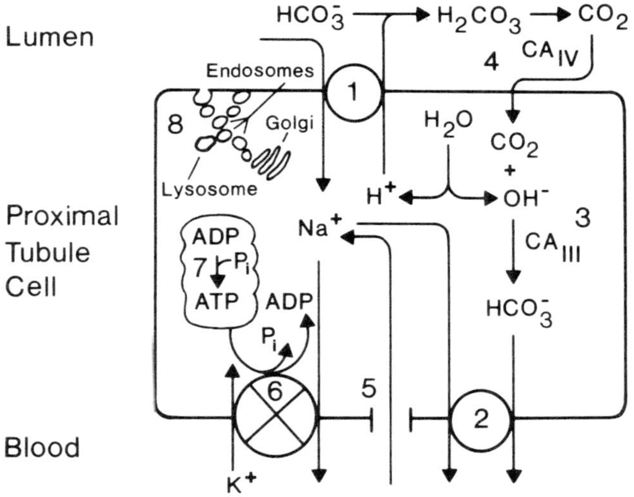

Fig. 1. Potential cellular mechanisms of proximal (Type II) RTA. Possible causes of impaired proximal acidification include defects in the luminal Na^+-H^+ antiport (*1*); the basolateral Na^+-HCO_3^- symport (*2*); the intracellular (*3*) or luminal (*4*) carbonic anhydrases (*CA*); sodium permeability (*5*); The Na-K ATPase (*6*); the intracellular generation of ATP (*7*); or membrane recycling, metabolism, or trafficking (*8*)

pathogenesis of this acute form of RTA2/FS is presumed to depend on an induced incapacity of the proximal tubule to generate the energy necessary to drive its Na^+-coupled resorptive transport processes. Aldolase B, the genetically defective enzyme in HFI, is a cytoplasmic enzyme which catalyzes the cleavage of fructose-1-phosphate. The enzyme normally occurs only in the liver, small bowel, and proximal renal tubule. When patients with HFI are acutely exposed to fructose, their enzymatic defect dictates in the cells of these tissues the near immediate occurrence of a rapid sequence of biochemical events: accumulation of F-1-P → depletion of P_i → depletion of ATP. In these tissues, the acute P_i depletion 1) triggers a massive degradation of preformed total adenine nucleotides (ATP, ADP, and AMP) by activating cytoplasmic AMP deaminase, and 2) restricts the rate at which mitochondria can regenerate ATP. In the fructose-loaded rat, prior phosphate loading largely prevents the otherwise striking reduction of ATP and total adenine nucleotides in the renal cortex despite doubling its concentration of F-1-P.

In patients with HFI given fructose experimentally, phosphate loading initiated beforehand attenuates the severity of the RTA-2/FS, as well as that of the attendant hyperuricemia and hyperinosinuria, phenomena entrained by the P_i depletion-dependent breakdown of preformed adenine nucleotides. In a woman with HFI in whom fructose was administered intravenously over two 1-hour periods, which were interrupted by a period of 100 min, phosphate loading initiated before the second period prevented the occurrence of RTA2/FS. Accordingly, and since fructose-induced depletion of hepatic adenine nucleotides in humans persists for at least 2 hours, it seems likely that phosphate loading attenuated the renal tubular dysfunc-

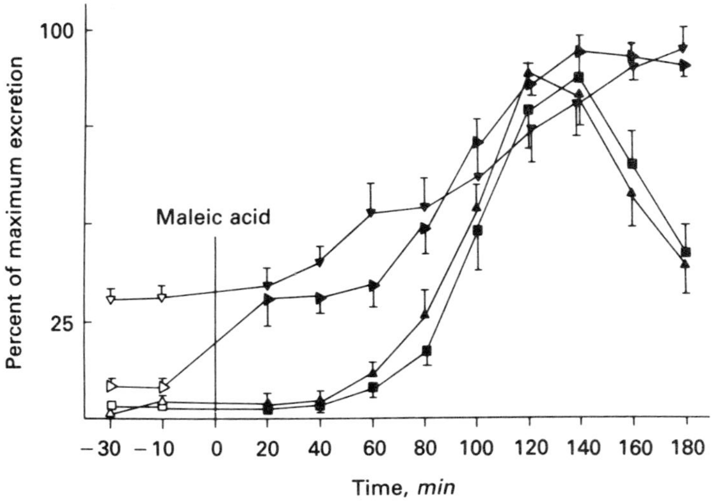

Fig. 2. Time course of the maleic acid-induced increases in urinary excretion of N-acetyl-β-glucosaminidase (NAG) (■), lysozyme (▲, alpha-amino nitrogen (▼), and sodium (►). Values are expressed as percent of the maximal excretion rates attained after administration of maleic acid

tion despite continued, severely reduced concentrations of ATP and total adenine nucleotide in the proximal renal tubule, possibly by enhancing this tissue's mitochondrial respiration and rate of regeneration of ATP.

The Experimental Model Induced by Maleic Acid (MA)

The experimental model of RTA-2/FS acutely induced by fructose in patients with HFI has striking parallels with the experimental model of RTA-2/FS acutely induced within minutes of initiating parenterally administered MA in the dog and rat [1] (Fig. 2). From clearance studies in the dog studied during water diureses, Al-Bander et al. concluded that MA induced the proximal tubule to reject greatly increased amounts of HCO_3^- (and sodium and chloride) that accounted for the maleate-induced bicarbonaturia of RTA2 [3]. On the basis of microperfusion studies of the proximal tubule in rats given maleate, Bank et al. and Reboucas et al. [4] concluded that the maleate-induced, acute reduction of net reabsorption of HCO_3^- in the proximal tubule did not result from back-flux of HCO_3^- through an abnormally leaky membrane, but rather from impaired active reabsorption of HCO_3^-, i.e., impaired H^+ secretion. In microperfusion studies of MA-induced aminoaciduria, Gunther and his coworkers concluded that MA inhibits the saturable reabsorption of amino acids along the proximal tubule; they showed that MA does not induce a greater efflux of amino acid into the lumen at distal sites of the nephron [5].

Although not occurring in nature, maleic acid is the cis isomer of fumaric acid, and like that naturally occurring metabolite of the Krebs oxidative cycle, readily metabolized by renal cortical mitochondria. At doses that induce RTA-2/FS, maleic acid induces in the proximal renal tubule striking structural abnormalities in the mitochondria, an impairment in their oxidative metabolism, and a reduced renal cortical concentration of ATP and activity of Na^+/K^+ ATPase [6]. Presumably, in part by impairing mitochondrial oxidation, maleic acid also induces in the renal cortex greatly increased rates of glucose uptake and glycolysis and increased concentrations of phosphorylated glycolytic intermediates [7]. That the increase in glycolysis induced by maleic acid might participate in the pathogenesis of its nephrotoxicity is suggested by one of Berliner's original observations [1]. Whereas maleic acid administered alone induced only transient renal dysfunction, it induced persisting renal failure when administered in combination with previously initiated glucose loading [1]. The metabolic pathogenesis of RTA 2/FS acutely induced by maleic acid could then involve a positive feedback loop in cells of the proximal renal tubule: impaired mitochondrial oxidation → increased glucose uptake → increased formation and concentration of phosphorylated glycolytic intermediates → limitation on the availability of cellular P_i → more severely impaired mitochondrial oxidative metabolism and possibly increased production of lactic acid [8]. In support of this hypothesis, Al-Bander et al. observed in the dog given maleic acid that prior phosphate loading attenuated RTA2/FS, whereas glucose loading exacerbated it, even when initiated after the dysfunction had already occurred [8]. Consistent with this hypothesis and its possible relevance to the pathogenetic mechanism of chronic clinical RTA2/FS is the recent observation by Jonas et al. that urinary excretion of lactic acid and d-glyceraldehyde is greatly increased in patients with chronic RTA2/FS in whom the plasma concentrations of lactate and d-glyceraldehyde are not increased [9]. The phenomenon was observed in a group of 16 patients affected with RTA2/FS, most of whom had cystinosis; others had cytochrome *c* oxidase deficiency, tyrosinosis, glycogenosis, and Lowe's syndrome, respectively, and in one the disorder was judged to be idiopathic. Hyperlacticaciduria without hyperlacticacidemia in combination with "tubular" proteinuria, which included B_2 microglobin, has also been reported as the earliest finding in young children affected with an autosomal dominant renal disorder that is expressed in early childhood as RTA2/FS and sometime later as severe renal insufficiency as well. In those described with this disorder, the severity of aminoaciduria and hyperlacticaciduria has increased with age.

Lysozymuria, Lysosomal Enzymuria – Pathogenetic Implications

Whether occurring as part of either an acute experimental disorder or as a chronic clinical disorder, RTA2/FS is attended by a reduction in renal tubular reabsorption of lysozyme and other low molecular weight proteins (LMWP) readily filtered by the normal glomerulus. Normally these LMWP are almost completely reabsorbed in the proximal renal tubule by a vacuolar transport system of some selectivity [10]. Given the extensive system of clathrin coated pits located at the base of the microvilli in the proximal tubule [11], and the active participation of clathrin in the process of receptor-mediated endocytosis, it seems likely that at least some of the selective reabsorption of LMWP represents a form of receptor-mediated endocytosis [10]. The reabsorbed LMWP, which also include B_2 microglobulin, insulin, immunoglobulin L Chain, and ribonuclease, first attach to the luminal membrane, presumably in coated pits, when they are internalized in apical endocytic vesicles and subsequently conveyed through endosomes [10] to a prelysosomal compartment, and finally to lysosomes, where they are enzymatically degraded [10]. In the experimental model of FS/RTA2 induced acutely in the rat given maleic acid, Christensen and Maunsbach reported the direct histochemical demonstration of impaired renal tubular uptake and vacuolar transport of lysozyme to lysosomes, an impairment which occurred restrictively in the proximal tubule and within 20 minutes of administering maleic acid [12].

Also observed whenever sought in either experimental or clinical FS/RTA2 is the phenomenon of increased urinary excretion of lysosomal enzymes such as N-acetyl-β-Glucosaminidase (NAG) [13]. Although too large to be filtered by the normal glomerulus, these proteins normally occur in the renal tubule, predominantly segregated in lysosomes of the proximal tubule in whose cells they are synthesized in the endoplasmic reticulum. An increased urinary excretion of NAG and other lysosomal enzymes is generally inferred to reflect "damage" or "injury" to the proximal tubule, and simple leakage of lysosomal enzymes from its damaged lysosomes.

But hyperexcretion of lysosomal enzymes could reflect much more complex mechanisms. Since the process of endocytosis is dynamically coupled to that of exocytosis [14], the combined hyperexcretion of lysozyme and lysosomal enzymes in FS/RTA2 could reflect a complex proximal tubular disorder of vacuolar transport affecting both endocytosis and exocytosis. In accordance with this hypothesis, Al-Bander et al. [15] observed in the dog that minutes after the onset of maleate-induced RTA2/FS, the urinary excretion of lysosomal enzymes, N-Acetyl-β-Glucosaminidase, β-Glucuronidase and β-Galactosidase increased simultaneously with the anticipated increase in renal clearance of lysozyme (Figs. 2–3). The severities of all these enzymurias increased rapidly and in parallel, all reaching a peak some 80–100 minutes after onset, then decreasing rapidly and in parallel. Sodium phosphate loading strikingly attenuates, and glucose loading exacerbates, the severities of both the RTA2/FS and hyperexcretion of lysozyme and lysosomal enzymes [15] (Fig. 4). These observations suggest that in the RTA2/FS induced by maleic acid in the dog, a P_i-dependent disorder of carbohydrate metabolism in the cells of the proximal renal tubule underlies both its dysfunction of transepithelial solute transport and derangement of protein handling [15]. In the RTA-2/FS acutely induced by intravenously administering fructose to patients with HFI, an acute, rapidly reversible hyperexcretion of lysozyme and lysosomal enzymes also occurs.

The process of endocytosis and exocytosis are coupled such that they constitute opposing limbs of cyclic continua in which membrane fragments of endocytotic vacuoles are recycled to exocytotic vacuoles through endosomes and to the plasma membrane, the recycling occurring within minutes. The process is energy dependent, as is that of orderly clathrin assembly/disassembly. In the proximal renal tubule cells of the rat, just minutes after its receipt of maleate, large endocytic apical vacuoles accumulate, most of the apical tubules disappear [11,12], coated pits lose their clathrin coat [11], and the corresponding coated pits membrane, which normally remains restricted to the base of the microvilli during endocytosis, becomes internalized to the newly formed, large apical vacuoles [11]. The membrane incorporated into these vacuoles appears not to derive from either microvillar membranes or lysosomal membranes [11]. If, as seems likely, apical tubules function to return membrane material from the endocytic vacuoles to the luminal plasma membrane [12], the maleate-induced disappearance of these tubules would indicate altered recycling of membrane to the luminal membrane [12].

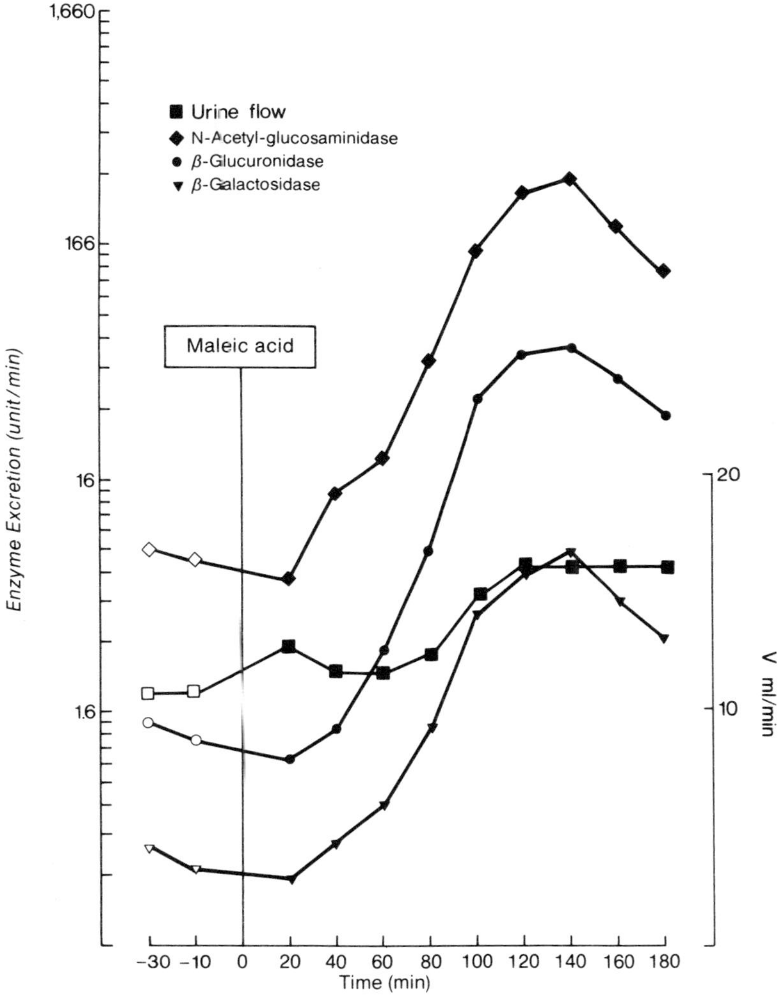

Fig. 3. Urine flow (■) and urinary excretion of N-acetyl-β-glucosaminidase (♦), β-glucuronidase (●), and β-galactosidase (▼) before (*open symbols*) and after (*closed symbols*) administration of maleic acid in 8 dogs. Values are the mean. Data are plotted on a semilog basis. Parallel lines indicate relatively constant enzyme excretion ratios

Since a variety of cells can be induced to secrete newly synthesized lysosomal enzymes with enzymatic activity, the lysosomal enzymes hyperexcreted in RTA2/FS may not be the mature, smaller enzymes normally segregated in renal lysosomes. In both acquired and genetically transmitted human disease, increased amounts of newly synthesized, larger lysosomal enzymes exit affected cells and occur in "pathological" urine [16,17]. In fact, both newly synthesized and mature lysosomal enzymes occur in the urine of normal humans, the first apparently being secreted by a non-lysosomal pathway, the second by a lysosomal pathway [16].

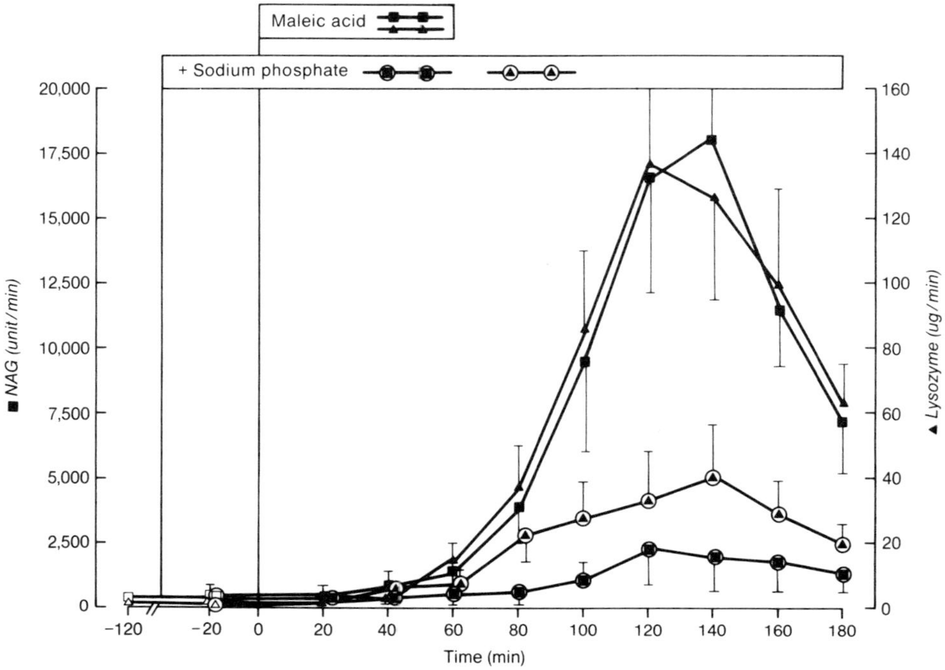

Fig. 4. Urinary excretion of lysozyme (▲ μg/min, *right scale*) and N-acetyl-β-glucosaminidase (*NAG*, ■ U/min, *left scale*) before (*open symbols*) and after (*circled symbols*) intravenous administration of maleic acid alone (8 studies) or after sodium phosphate loading (8 studies, circled symbols). Values are the mean ± SEM

After their synthesis in rough endoplasmic reticulum, enzymes destined for segregation in lysosomes traverse the Golgi complex. There, most of these proteins gain phosphomannosyl residues which bind them to mannose-6-phosphate receptors and thereby "address" them to lysosomes [18]. The ligand-receptor complexes exit the trans-Golgi network, the last station along the Golgi pathway, in clathrin-coated vesicles and proceed to a "late" endosome "prelysosomal compartment." The more acidic interior of this compartment effects the disassociation of the ligand-receptor complex, thus allowing the released enzymes to be segregated in lysosomes and the unoccupied receptors to be recycled to the Golgi apparatus and plasma membrane. In normal rat kidney cells, the prelysosomal compartments appears to be stationed on the "main endocytic route" from the plasma membrane to the lysosomes [19]. In consequence, both lysosomal enzymes bound to mannose-6-phosphate receptors in the Golgi network and proteins endocytosed by receptor mediation accumulate attached to their receptors in the prelysosomal compartment, immediately before either dissociates from its receptor and is transferred to lysosomes [19].

By rendering the "late" endosome prelysosomal compartment less acidic and thus retarding the dissociation of ligand-receptor complexes, certain weak bases like chloroquine and NH_4Cl, or genetically decreased activity of endosomal H^+ATPase, can restrict the recycling of unoccupied mannose-6-phosphate receptors to the Golgi apparatus. Accordingly, these bases and this enzymatic disorder can effect the constitutive secretion of immature, mannose-6-phosphate-bearing lysosomal enzymes and impair receptor-mediated endocytosis. Caplan and his colleagues recently reported that treatment of canine renal tubule cells (Mardin-Darby canine kidney cell line) with NH_4Cl induced secretion of newly synthesized cathepsin "D," a lysosomal enzyme, into both apical and basolateral media [20]. In preliminary studies chloroquine has been reported to inhibit endocytic reabsorption of protein in the isolated perfused rabbit proximal renal tubule [21]. While it remains to be demonstrated that the lysosomal enzymes hyperexcreted in RTA2/FS contain mannose-6-phosphate, Tager and his colleagues have demonstrated the occurrence in urine of normal subjects a mannose-6-phosphate-bearing immature lysosomal enzyme, α glucosidase, as well as a smaller, mature form of this enzyme that contained no mannose-6-phosphate residues [22]. In acute RTA2/FS, rapidly reversible, coordinate hyperexcretion of lysozyme and mannose-6-phosphate-bearing immature lysosomal enzymes could then result from a rapidly reversible loss of normal acidity in the late endosome prelysosomal compartment in cells of the proximal renal tubule. This loss could be caused by a reversible reduction in function of endosomal H^+-ATPase consequent to impaired metabolic generation of ATP.

Whatever the details of its character and mechanism, the fact of the coordinate, rapidly reversible lysozymuria/lysosomal enzymuria characteristic of acute RTA2/FS, in conjunction with the loss of apical tubules in cells of the proximal tubule, and the accumulation there of large apical vacuoles containing membrane normally restricted to the base of microvilli, almost certainly reflects a severe disordering of endocytosis/exocytosis and membrane recycling in the proximal tubule. This disordering could impair exocytotic replenishment of transport components of its luminal membrane and thereby entrain varied and complex disturbances of its physiological functions [1,4], somewhat as proposed by Bergeron et al. [23]. Such a disordering could impair exocytotic insertion into the luminal membrane of not only electrogenic H^+ ATPase, but possibly also the endosomal electroneutral H^+/Na^+ antiporter recently described in the proximal tubule. Impaired mitochondrial generation of ATP induced in the proximal tubule by maleic acid in animals, or by fructose in patients with HFI, might then be pathogenetically linked to RTA2/FS through diminished activity of both basolateral Na^+-K^+ ATPase and apical H^+ ATPase and consequent impairment of not only electroneutral H^+/Na^+ exchange and electrogenic H^+ secretion, but possibly also impairment of net luminal plasma membrane transport of such normally reabsorbed solutes as glucose and phosphate.

The Junk Mail Message Hypothesis

If patients with RTA-2/FS, or FS alone, hyperexcrete immature enzymes bearing mannose-6-phosphate (because these enzymes are constitutively secreted by metabolically disordered proximal tubules), the consequent occurrence of increased concentrations of these glycoproteins in the tubular lumen fluid and peritubular blood (basolateral secretion) [20] could have important pathogenetic implications. The mannose-6-phosphate receptor (cation independent) that normally ferries immature lysosomal enzymes from the Golgi (and the plasma membrane) to the prelysosomal compartment [19], is also the insulin-like growth factor (IGF)-II receptor [24]. Specifically, a single protein binds and transports mannose-6-phosphate-liganded lysosomal enzymes and IGF-II. Mannose-6-phosphate and IGF-II can modulate each others binding to this dual ligand receptor. The receptor occurs both on the brush border and basolateral membrane of the mammalian proximal renal tubule and in the glomeruli. Hammerman and his colleagues [25] have recently demonstrated that mannose-6-phosphate amplifies the biological effect of IGF-II at the basolateral membrane of the proximal renal tubule of the rat: At this site, mannose-6-phosphate amplifies the capacity of IGF-II to stimulate phospholipase C, as measured by increased production of inositol triphosphate, a reaction product of phosphoinositide hydrolysis. While the physiological consequences of this phenomenon are by no means clear, it is clear that IGF-II can evoke a number of biological phenomena, and stimulation of phospholipase C and the consequent production of inositol triphosphate (and diacylglycerol) are critical to signal transmission of a variety of hormones and growth factors. It is also clear that mannose-6-phosphate-bearing lysosomal enzymes can modulate the binding of IGF-II to the IGF-II/mannose-6-phosphate receptor [26]. Thus, in patients with RTA-2/FS the IGF-II/mannose-6-phosphate receptor might be pathologically modulated at multiple sites of the renal tubule by increased concentrations of mannose-6-phosphate-bearing lysosomal enzymes.

Chronic RTA2/FS – Cystinosis

In patients with cystinosis, the most common cause of RTA2/FS in children, "storage" of cystine in lysosomes may be a primary pathogenetic event in many tissues affected [27,28], and the occurrence of this phenomenon in the proximal renal tubule might underlie RTA2/FS. In so-called nephropathic or "infantile" cystinosis, lysosomal accumulation of cystine occurs prenatally, RTA/FS is expressed within the first 12 months of life, progressive reduction in glomerular filtration rate leads to uremia by midchildhood, and the free-cystine content of leukocytes is 80 times normal.

Cystine is the only aminoacid stored in cystinotic lysosomes. A defect in carrier mediated transport of cystine across lysosomal membrane accounts for its massive accumulation in the lysosomes of those homozygous for infantile cystinosis [28]. Lysosomal accumulation of cystine occurs throughout the kidney, particularly in the interstitium and glomerulus, and apparently also in the cells of the proximal tubule. The phenomenon of cystine "storage" would seem to be important to the pathogenesis of the glomerulopathy and progressive renal failure characteristic of cystinosis in childhood. Cysteamine depletes intracellular cystine stores. In cystinotic children, early treatment with cysteamine, which greatly reduces lysosomal cystine concentration in leukocytes, can attenuate and perhaps prevent the otherwise predictable occurrence of both the progressive reduction of GFR and the severe stunting of somatic growth characteristic of this disease. Yet, with one apparent exception, institution of cysteamine, even in the first weeks of life, has failed to either prevent the occurrence of RTA2/FS or to attenuate established RTA2/FS. This failure might reflect restricted access of cysteamine to cystine-laden lysosomes in the proximal renal tubule. It is not clear, however, that lysosomal accumulation of cystine, per se, in the proximal tubule, or whatever "destruction" such accumulation might entrain there, accounts for either the RTA2/FS of cystinosis or the massive urinary excretion of lysosomal enzymes characteristic of this disease. Portale and his associates have recently studied a young girl with RTA-2/FS, massively increased urinary excretion of N-acetylglucosaminidase, and the classic clinical characteristics of cystinosis, including photophobia and retarded growth. Yet excessive cystine was demonstrably not present in leucocytes or fibroblasts. Renal biopsy revealed no evidence of cystinosis.

It might be noted that neither RTA2/FS nor any of the other clinical features of cystinosis have been described in I cell disease, a disorder in which cystine also accumulates in lysosomes because of its impaired transport, and in which urinary excretion of newly synthesized lysosomal enzymes is also increased. In I cell disease newly synthesized lysosomal enzymes, and perhaps also component proteins of lysosomal membrane transport systems, fail to acquire the mannose-6-phosphate residues that "address" them to lysosomes and are thus diverted from their normal lysosomal destination and secreted. Lacking mannose-6-phosphate, these proteins would not be expected to modulate binding of IGF II to its receptor on the plasma membrane of the renal tubule (see above).

Recent observations with cystine dimethylester may provide a clue to the mechanism through which cystine might evoke RTA-2/FS in patients with cystinosis. Foreman, Segal, and their coworkers [29] demonstrated that parenteral administration of this substance for four days led to an increased urinary volume and excretion of phosphate, glucose and α-amino nitrogen and various amino acids. Cystine dimethylester treatment did not affect the creatinine clearance. In studies of isolated renal tubules, preincubation with cystine dimethylester greatly inhibited the uptake of lysine, glycine and α-methylglucoside. In the isolated perfused rabbit proximal renal tubule, Salmon and Baum [30] demonstrated that cystine dimethylester added to the bath induced, within 10 minutes, large reductions in J_V, bicarbonate transport (J_{TCO_2}) and glucose transport. The methylesters of leucine and tryptophan had no effect on these transport systems. Cystine dimethylester had no effect on mannitol or bicarbonate permeability. Thus, the inhibition of transport observed was due to inhibition of active transport.

Incubation of renal tubules with cystine dimethylester led to an increased tissue concentration of cystine, comparable to that measured in kidney tissue of cystinotics who had nephrectomies before renal transplantation. Additionally, there was a five-fold increase in cysteine. Intraperitoneal administration of cystine which induced features of the FS resulted in increased renal concentration of cysteine, but neither cystine nor cystine dimethylester was detected. In the isolated perfused proximal convoluted tubule, addition of cysteine methylester to the bath induced a transport impairment like that induced by cystine dimethylester, but only with four times higher concentrations. Preliminary observations by Baum and Salmon would indicate that cystine dimethylester induces an immediate 50% reduction in ATP and O_2 consumption of renal tubules. Thus, the mechanism through which cystinosis gives rise to RTA-2/FS may involve impaired mitochondrial oxidative metabolism in the proximal renal tubule. Such a mechanism has obvious parallels with that inferred in both the RTA-2/FS induced by fructose in patients with hereditary fructose intolerance and that induced by maleate in experimental animals.

References

1. Berliner RW, Kennedy TJ, Hilton JG (1950) Effect of maleic acid on renal function. Proc Soc Exp Biol Med 75:791–794

2. Morris RC Jr, Sebastian A (1983) Renal Tubular Acidosis and Fanconi Syndrome. In: Stanbury JB, Wyngaarden JB, Fredrickson DS, Goldstein JL, Brown MS (eds) The metabolic basis of inherited disease. McGraw-Hill, New York, pp 1808–1866
3. Al-Bander HA, Weiss RA, Humphreys MH, Morris RC Jr (1982) Dysfunction of the proximal tubule underlies maleic acid-induced type II renal tubular acidosis. Am J Physiol 243:F604–F611
4. Bank N, Aynedjian HS, Mutz BF (1986) Microperfusion study of proximal tubule bicarbonate transport in maleic acid-induced renal tubular acidosis. Am J Physiol 250:F476–F482
5. Gunther R, Silbernagl S, Deetjen P (1979) Maleic acid induced aminoaciduria studied by free flow micropuncture and continuous microperfusion. Pflugers Arch 382:109–114
6. Kramer HJ, Gonick HC (1970) Experimental Fanconi syndrome. I. Effect of maleic acid on renal cortical Na-K-ATPase activity and ATP levels. J Lab Clin Med 76:799–808
7. Rogulski J, Strzelecki T, Pacanis A, Kaminska E, Angielski S (1975) Effects of maleate on renal carbohydrate metabolism in vivo and in vitro. In: Angielski S, Dubach UC (eds) Biochemical aspects of renal function. Huber, Bern, pp 106–110
8. Al-Bander H, Etheredge SB, Paukert T, Humphreys MH, Morris RC Jr (1985) Phosphate loading attenuates renal tubular dysfunction induced by maleic acid in the dog. Am J Physiol 248:F513–F521
9. Jonas AJ, Lin S-N, Conley SB, Schneider JA, Williams JC, Caprioli RC (1989) Urine glyceraldehyde excretion is elevated in the renal Fanconi syndrome. Kidney Int 35:99–104
10. Wall DA, Maack T (1985) Endocytic uptake, transport, and catabolism of proteins by epithelial cells. Am J Physiol 248:C12–C20
11. Rodman JS, Seidman L, Farquhar MG (1986) The membrane composition of coated pits, microvilli, endosomes, and lysosomes is distinctive in the rat kidney proximal tubule cell. J Cell Biol 102:77–87
12. Christensen EI, Maunsbach AB (1980) Proteinuria induced by sodium maleate in rats: Effects on ultrastructure and protein handling in renal proximal tubule. Kidney Int 17:771–787
13. Kunin CM, Chesney RW, Craig WA, England AD, DeAngelis C (1978) Enzymuria as a marker of renal injury and disease: Studies of N-acetyl-beta-glucosaminidase in the general population and in patients with renal disease. Pediatrics 620:751–760
14. Steinman RM, Mellman IS, Muller WA, Cohn ZA (1983) Endocytosis and the recycling of plasma membrane. J Cell Biol 96:1–27
15. Al-Bander HA, Mock DM, Etheredge SB, Paukert TT, Humphreys MH, Morris RC Jr (1986) Coordinately increased lysozymuria and lysosomal enzymuria induced by maleic acid. Kidney Int 30:804–812
16. Kress BC, Hirani S, Freeze HH, Little L, Miller AL (1982) Mucolipidosis III B-N-acetyl-D-hexosaminidase; A purification and properties. Biochem J 207:421–428
17. Zuhlsdorf M, Imort M, Hasilik A, von Figura K (1983) Molecular forms of B-hexosaminidase and cathepsin D in serum and urine of healthy subjects and patients with elevated activity of lysosomal enzymes. Biochem J 213:733–740
18. Dahms NM, Lobel P, Kornfeld S (1989) Mannose 6-phosphate receptors and lysosomal enzyme targeting. J Biol Chem 264:12115–12118
19. Griffiths G, Hoflack B, Simons K, Mellman I, Kornfeld S (1988) The mannose 6-phosphate receptor and the biogenesis of lysosomes. Cell 52:329–341
20. Caplan MJ, Stow JL, Newman AP, Madri J, Anderson HC, Farquhar MG, Palade GE, Jamieson JD (1987) Dependence on pH of polarized sorting of secreted proteins. Nature 329:632–635
21. Park CH, Clapp WL, Madsen KM, Tisher CC (1987) Structure and function of endosomal-lysosomal (EL) system in the proximal tubule (PT) (abstract). Xth International Congress of Nephrology 589

22. Oude Elferink RPJ, Brouwer-Kelder EM, Surya I, Strijland A, Kroos M, Reuser AJJ, Tager JM (1984) Isolation and characterization of a precursor form of lysosomal alpha-glucosidase from human urine. Eur J Biochem 139:489–495
23. Bergeron M, Dubord L, Hausser C (1976) Membrane permeability as a cause of transport defects in experimental Fanconi syndrome: A new hypothesis. J Clin Invest 57:1181–1189
24. Morgan DO, Edman JC, Standring DN, Fried VA, Smith MC, Roth RA, Rutter WJ (1987) Insulin-like growth factor II receptor as a multifunctional binding protein. Nature 329:301–307
25. Hammerman MR (1989) The growth hormone-insulin-like growth factor axis in kidney. Am J Physiol 257:F503–F514
26. Kiess W, Blickenstaff GD, Sklar MM, Thomas CL, Nissley SP, Sahagian GG (1988) Biochemical evidence that the type II insulin-like growth factor receptor is identical to the cation-independent mannose 6-phosphate receptor. J Biol Chem 263:9339–9344
27. Schneider JA, Schulman JD (1983) Cystinosis. In: Stanbury JB, Wyngaarden JB, Fredrickson DS, Goldstein JL, Brown MS (eds) The metabolic basis of inherited disease. McGraw-Hill, New York, pp 1844–1866
28. Gahl WA, Renlund M, Thoene JG (1989) Lysosomal transport disorders: Cystinosis and Sialic Acid Storage. In: Scriver CR, Beaudet AL, Sly WS, Valle D (eds) The metabolic basis of inherited disease. McGraw-Hill, New York, pp 2619–2648
29. Foreman JW, Bowring MA, Lee J, States B, Segal S (1987) Effect of cystine dimethylester on renal solute handling and isolated renal tubule transport in the rat: a new model of the Fanconi syndrome. Metabolism 36:1185–1191
30. Salmon RF, Baum M (1990) Intracellular cystine loading inhibits transport in the rabbit proximal convoluted tubule. J Clin Invest 85:340–344

Mechanism of Distal Acidification: Relevance to Distal RTA

ROBERT J. ALPERN[1]

SUMMARY. Acid secretion in the distal nephron is mediated by a cell with an apical membrane ATP-coupled H pump and a basolateral membrane Cl/HCO_3 exchanger. Considering H secretion as a function of luminal pH, defects in distal acidification can be divided into three broad groups: an abnormal *leak* where net H secretion is normal in the absence of a pH gradient but becomes abnormal as luminal pH decreases; a *rate* defect where minimal urinary pH is normal but the rate of acidification is decreased at higher luminal pH; and a *voltage* defect where the rate of H secretion at all luminal pH is decreased and the minimal urinary pH is increased. The U-$BPCO_2$ has been used to assess the rate of H secretion in the presence of a minimal gradient for back diffusion. The presence of hyperkalemia indicates that the disease process involves the cortical collecting tubule where H and K are both secreted, or indicates an abnormality in aldosterone which stimulates H and K secretion. Lastly, the response of urinary pH and urinary K to an increase in distal Na delivery can be used to examine cortical collecting tubule function.

Normal Physiology

In considering the pathophysiologic basis of distal RTA, it is best to view this in the context of normal mechanisms of H secretion in the collecting duct. We will therefore start by defining the mechanisms of H transport in the H secreting cell of the collecting duct. This cell type has been best studied in the in vitro perfused inner stripe of the rabbit outer medullary collecting duct [1–4]. In this segment, a number of transporters have been defined, as shown in Fig. 1. The apical membrane contains an H ATPase which is most likely of the vacuolar type [3,5]. This transporter utilizes the chemical energy of ATP to transport H ions energetically uphill. In addition, data has

[1]Division of Nephrology, Department of Internal Medicine, University of Texas Southwestern Medical Center, 5323 Harry Hines Blvd., Dallas, TX 75235-8856, USA

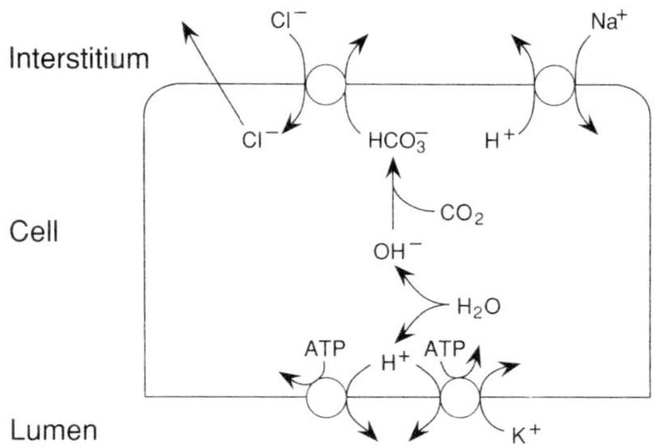

Fig. 1. Model of H secreting cell in collecting duct

been presented suggesting that during K deficiency an HK ATPase, similar to that present in gastric mucosa, is inserted into the apical membrane of these cells [4]. Hays and Alpern could not find evidence for this transporter in outer medullary collecting tubules harvested from normal animals [3]. Base, which is generated within the cell by the H pumps, then exits across the basolateral membrane on a Cl/HCO_3 exchanger. This Cl/HCO_3 exchanger appears to be similar to, but not identical to, the red cell band 3 Cl/HCO_3 exchanger. The difference resides in alternate splicing of the mRNA leading to truncation of the amino terminal portion of the exchanger in the kidney form [6,7]. Lastly, a basolateral membrane Na/H antiporter has been identified in this cell [1,2]. This transporter would not be expected to contribute to transepithelial H secretion, and in fact would decrease the rate. Most likely, this transporter serves certain housekeeping functions such as cell pH defense and cell volume defense during changes in medullary tonicity.

Also of relevance to the understanding of distal RTA is an understanding of axial heterogeneity in the distal nephron. The cortical collecting tubule possesses three cell types: a principal cell which absorbs Na and secretes K, a type A intercalated cell which secretes H, and a type B intercalated cell which secretes HCO_3. This allows the cortical collecting tubule to secrete either acid or base, in response to changes in dietary acid. In addition, this allows H secretion from the cortical collecting tubule to be regulated by changes in transepithelial voltage secondary to changes in Na transport. The medullary collecting tubule, on the other hand, appears to secrete only H ions. There is no capacity for HCO_3 secretion and there is no net Na transport. In states of chronic K deficiency, this segment is capable of absorbing K, most likely using the apical membrane HK ATPase described above [4].

Relevance to Distal RTA

The turtle urinary bladder has been used as a model to examine the regulation of H secretion by the collecting duct. Using this model, Steinmetz, Al-Awqati, and coworkers have demonstrated that the rate of H secretion is a linear function of luminal

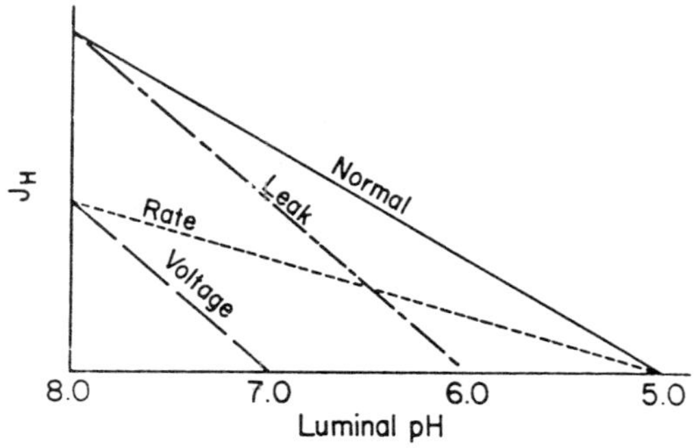

Fig. 2. Potential mechanisms for defects in distal H secretion. (From [9] with permission of McGraw Hill Inc.)

pH [8]. This is shown as the line labelled normal in Fig. 2. In addition, these investigators demonstrated that changes in luminal pH and in transepithelial voltage had similar effects on H secretion when considered as the electrochemical gradient. Thus, a tenfold pH gradient was found to be similar to a 60 mV change in voltage. Using this approach, one can consider different forms of defects in H secretion and how they would be expressed as a function of luminal pH. This then allows one to predict whether patients will be able to acidify their urine maximally in the presence of these defects.

The first defect is that of an increased leak. During normal urinary acidification, the lumen of the collecting tubule becomes markedly acidified compared to the pH of the interstitium. This sets up driving forces for leak of H, H_2CO_3 or HCO_3. As can be seen in Fig. 2, if luminal pH is similar to that of the interstitium, there is no driving force for leaks and therefore no effect on the rate of H secretion. However, as luminal fluid becomes more acid, there is increased leak and thus a greater defect in net acidification. This type of lesion has been referred to as a gradient lesion, because it is anticipated that patients would be unable to acidify their urine maximally. The best example of this lesion is the amphotericin-induced lesion.

A second category of defect is a rate defect. Here the H secreting cell is able to establish a normally acid luminal fluid, but the rate of H secretion at any luminal pH is slower than in control. Thus, if luminal flow rate is sufficiently slow, or if luminal buffer content is sufficiently low, a normally acid urine can be achieved. However, in the presence of normal rates of buffer delivery and normal tubular fluid flow rates, the slow rates of H secretion will lead to an inappropriately alkaline urine. The best example of this defect is that of aldosterone deficiency [8]. When ammoniagenesis is suppressed in these patients by hyperkalemia, they can acidify their urine normally. When hyperkalemia is corrected, ammonia synthesis is normal, and the urine is inappropriately alkaline due to the rate defect.

The last possible defect is a voltage defect. Here, the apparatus for secreting H is intact, but due to abnormalities in NaCl transport, the normal lumen-negativity of the cortical collecting tubule is not present. Because changes in voltage are additive to changes in luminal pH (see above), the line drawn in Fig. 2 is parallel to, but beneath the normal line. Thus, these patients should be unable to achieve maximally acidified urines. The best example of this phenomenon is seen in amiloride administration to experimental animals. While in theory aldosterone deficiency would also inhibit Na transport and decrease transepithelial voltage, this effect appears to be minor compared to the rate defect, as patients can normally acidify their urine in the presence of low buffer delivery.

Based on the schema presented in Fig. 2, the ability to acidify the urine normally can be extremely useful in classifying patients with distal RTA. It is also useful to measure the rate of H secretion in the distal nephron in the absence of a pH gradient. This can be done with the U-B PCO_2 (urine minus blood PCO_2). This will be described in further detail by the subsequent speakers. In general, in the presence of a HCO_3 diuresis, accumulation of carbonic acid in the lumen will lead to a high PCO_2 in the urine. As the major cause of high luminal carbonic acid concentration is H secretion, this parameter has been considered to be useful in assessing the ability of the collecting tubule to secrete H. Thus, a low U-B PCO_2 in the presence of marked bicarbonaturia can be due to decreased H secretion, back diffusion of secreted H, or back diffusion of H_2CO_3. It has been argued that back diffusion of H and H_2CO_3 would be unlikely to occur in this setting, because of the high concentration of HCO_3 in the lumen and thus an anticipated high luminal pH. However, because carbonic anhydrase is absent in the lumen of most of the collecting tubule, luminal pH is not in equilibrium with HCO_3 and is actually lower than would be predicted from the HCO_3 concentration. Thus, it remains possible that a driving force would persist for back diffusion of H and H_2CO_3.

The presence of hyperkalemia in patients with distal RTA suggests the coexistence of defects in K secretion and H secretion. This occurs in a number of clinical settings. The most common cause is aldosterone deficiency. Because aldosterone stimulates the rate of K and H secretion in the collecting tubule, aldosterone deficiency is accompanied by defects in both K and H secretion. Pseudohyperaldosteronism type I is a condition where aldosterone levels are normal, but aldosterone is unable to regulate transport in the collecting tubule (? receptor defect). Any defect in voltage in the cortical collecting tubule would also be expected to decrease H and K secretion. Lastly, any disease process which damaged the cortical collecting tubule would be expected to interfere with K and H secretion.

Some investigators have argued that the response to increased distal Na delivery is also useful in defining the mechanism of distal RTA. This will be further discussed below. In general, distal Na delivery can be increased by administration of furosemide, sodium sulfate, or sodium phosphate. If this maneuver leads to a decrease in urinary pH and an increase in urinary K, the cortical collecting tubule should be relatively intact. If increasing distal Na delivery has no effect on urine pH but increases urine K normally, there is a defect in H secretion in the cortical collecting tubule. Lastly, if increasing distal Na delivery has no effect on urine pH or on urine K, there is either a combined H and K secretory defect in the cortical collecting tubule, or there is an inability of this maneuver to alter voltage (voltage defect).

Thus, by measuring urine pH, U-B PCO_2, serum K, and the response to increased distal Na delivery, one can define the mechanisms responsible for a defect in distal acidification. In general, the urine pH and serum K are the most useful clinically. The next two chapters will further discuss the mechanisms responsible for distal RTA and the approach to the patient with distal RTA.

References

1. Hays SR, Alpern RJ (1990) Basolateral membrane Na^+-independent Cl^-/HCO^-_3 exchange in the inner stripe of the rabbit outer medullary collecting tubule. J Gen Physiol 95:347–367
2. Breyer MD, Jacobson HR (1989) Regulation of rabbit medullary collecting duct cell pH by basolateral Na^+/H^+ and Cl^-/base exchange. J Clin Invest 84:996–1004
3. Hays SR, Alpern RJ (1990) Apical and basolateral membrane H^+ extrusion mechanisms in the inner stripe of the rabbit outer medullary collecting tubule. Am J Physiol 259 (Renal Fluid Electrolyte Physiol 28):F628–F635
4. Wingo CS (1989) Active proton secretion and potassium absorption in the rabbit outer medullary collecting duct. J Clin Invest 84:361–365
5. Stone DK, Xie X-S (1988) Proton translocating ATPases: Issues in structure and function. Kidney Int 33:767–774
6. Kudrycki KE, Shull GE (1989) Primary structure of the rat kidney band 3 anion exchange protein deduced from a cDNA. J Biol Chem 264:8185–8192
7. Brosius FC III, Alper SL, Garcia AM, Lodish HF (1989) The major kidney band 3 gene transcript predicts an amino-terminal truncated band 3 polypeptide. J Biol Chem 264: 7784–7787
8. Al-Awqati Q (1978) H^+ transport in urinary epithelia. Am J Physiol 235 (Renal Fluid Electrolyte Physiol 4):F77-F88
9. DuBose TD, Alpern RJ In: Metabolic basis of inherited disease, 6th edn. McGraw Hill

Pathophysiological Basis of Distal Renal Tubular Acidosis: Lessons from Animal Models

Thomas D. DuBose Jr[1]

Summary. A number of potential defects may impair acidification either directly or indirectly in segments of the distal nephron. Papillary micropuncture studies have validated the urine minus blood PCO_2 (U-B PCO_2) obtained during a bicarbonate diuresis as a reliable qualitative index of distal nephron proton pump integrity. Microelectrode determination of both PCO_2 and disequilibrium pH in the papillary collecting duct in a number of experimental models of distal renal tubular acidosis (DRTA) have demonstrated at least four types of defects: 1) The permeability or "gradient" defect is best exemplified by the amphotericin B lesion, where reduction in net acid excretion is the result of backleak of bicarbonate during excretion of an acid urine. During bicarbonate loading, the U-B PCO_2 is normal, however, demonstrating that the pump is not defective; 2) Voltage-dependent rate defects are induced by amiloride or lithium. As a result of the decrease in voltage in the cortical collecting tubule (CCT) both H^+ and K^+ secretion are reduced; 3) Nonvoltage mediated pump defects occur in the postobstructed kidney and, when corrected for voltage, are present in aldosterone deficiency; 4) Impaired buffer delivery or production compromises net acid excretion. Ammonium production is decreased in chronic hyperkalemia and with reduction of GFR. Ammonium excretion is impaired in hyperkalemia because a decrease in ammonium transport by the TALH reduces ammonium accumulation in the inner medulla and, thus, impedes transfer of ammonia into the inner medullary collecting duct. Mixed defects also exist, e.g., in aldosterone deficiency hyperkalemia impairs ammonium excretion while aldosterone deficiency compromises the capacity of the proton pump.

Introduction

The pathophysiological basis of the various types of distal renal tubular acidosis (DRTA) have not yet been described fully. Progress has been made recently, however,

[1]Division of Nephrology, Departments of Internal Medicine, Physiology, and Biophysics, University of Texas Medical Branch, Galveston, TX 77550, USA

especially with respect to the understanding of disorders involving abnormalities in "distal" nephron acidification. This presentation will review, in detail, findings from sstudies employing experimental models of DRTA which have been investigated by a number of techniques in vivo and in vitro.

Mechanism of Distal Acidification

Since most of the filtered bicarbonate is reabsorbed by the proximal tubule (90%), the distal nephron (distal convoluted tubule (DCT); cortical collecting tubule (CCT); and medullary collecting duct (MCD)) serves to reabsorb the remainder of this load, and, in addition, to secrete an additional quantity of protons which approximates the quantity of the acid load generated by metabolism [1]. Net acid excretion is facilitated, and the approach to limiting transepithelial pH gradients mitigated, by the availability of urinary buffers and by the excretion of ammonium (NH_4^+). Proton secretion mediates transepithelial bicarbonate reabsorption in the distal convoluted tubule, the cortical collecting duct, and the medullary collecting tubule, and titrates the urinary buffers as well. The cellular mechanism for this process, apical membrane secretion of hydrogen ions, appears to be similar in each of these "distal nephron" segments. Micropuncture studies which have measured the disequilibrium pH in the superficial distal tubule and inner medullary collecting duct have supported this view unequivocally [2,3]. Numerous studies have demonstrated that active proton secretion at the apical membrane is mediated by a proton-translocating, electrogenic, ATP-dependent pump [4–8].

Since the rates of net proton secretion are relatively low in these distal segments, in vitro analysis usually requires the quantitation of bicarbonate reabsorption during in vitro perfusion with bicarbonate concentrations exceeding the load delivered in vitro. A different approach has been taken to assess acidification in these terminal segments in whole kidney studies by measurement of urinary PCO_2 [9]. Micropuncture studies which have measured both acid disequilibrium pH and an elevated urinary CO_2 tension during high bicarbonate delivery to the distal tubule and medullary collecting tubule (MCT), have consistently demonstrated that the magnitude of the elevation in urinary PCO_2 (referred to as the urine-minus-blood PCO_2, or U-B PCO_2, or Δ PCO_2) is quantitatively related to distal nephron proton secretion [2]. The degree of bicarbonaturia achieved in such protocols allows the examination of distal nephron hydrogen ion secretion in the absence of blood-to-lumen bicarbonate gradients. The generation of high inner medullary and urinary CO_2 tension occurs during a bicarbonate diuresis because of the absence of luminal (or membrane-bound) carbonic anhydrase in segments of the distal nephron, and is the result of secretion of protons into bicarbonate-containing tubule fluid, with subsequent slow dehydration of carbonic acid [3].

Classification of Subtypes of DRTA

Permeability ("Leak") Defects

The best experimental model representative of a permeability defect is that induced by amphotericin-B. This antibiotic forms aqueous channels when inserted into lipid

Table 1. Pathophysiological classification of distal renal tubule acidification defects

I. Permeability or "gradient" defect
A. Amphotericin-B
B. Classical DRTA-(normal U-B PCO_2)
II. Rate-dependent defect
A. Voltage-dependent
1. Amiloride (primary impairment of Na^+ reabsorption)
2. Lithium (secondary impairment of Na^+ reabsorption)
*3. Postobstructed kidney
4. Pseudohypoaldosteronism Type II (enhanced chloride shunt)
*5. Selective aldosterone deficiency
B. Nonvoltage-mediated pump defects
*1. Selective aldosterone deficiency
*2. Postobstructed kidney
3. Carbonic anhydrase II deficiency
4. Classical DRTA (low U-B PCO_2)
III. Reduction in ammonium excretion
1. Chronic hyperkalemia
*2. Selective aldosterone deficiency
3. Tubulointerstitial disease
*4. Nephrocalcinosis

*Denotes mixed disorders

membranes [10]. Steinmetz and associates [11] reported that amphotericin-B was associated with a reduction in net hydrogen secretion only as the pH gradient across the turtle bladder was increased, and not in the absence of a pH gradient between mucosa and serosa. Such findings are compatible with a "gradient" lesion, and indicate that an acidification defect, under such a circumstance, would be most apparent when the filtered load of bicarbonate was low and the requirement to excrete a maximally acid urine was necessary. Animals treated chronically with amphotericin-B are unable to acidify the urine maximally under control conditions, or after an acid challenge. With combined acidosis and Na_2SO_4 infusion, a maximally acid urine pH can be achieved, however [12]. In contrast, during bicarbonate-loading, the U-B PCO_2 is normal [12–14]. Microelectrode studies by our laboratory have demonstrated a normal acid disequilibrium pH during this condition in the inner medullary collecting duct (IMCD) in vivo (indicative of a normal rate of H^+ secretion) [14]. In addition, papillary PCO_2 was elevated to levels similar to that observed in controls. Thus, the features of this defect are consistent with a gradient lesion, i.e., the rate of hydrogen secretion is normal during bicarbonate loading, and the reduction in net acid excretion is most likely the result of backleak of bicarbonate, not H^+-ions, H_2CO_3, or non-bicarbonate buffers. Backleak of these latter moieties would be expected to reduce the U-B PCO_2.

Voltage-Dependent Rate Defects

Lithium administration in the rat is consistently associated with a mild metabolic acidosis and an inappropriately alkaline urine pH which does not decrease further following an acid challenge, but responds (falls below pH 5.5) after infusion of sodium sulfate [15,16]. Studies done by our laboratory in the rat receiving lithium have demonstrated, in contrast to the amphotericin-B defect, that hydrogen secretion (failure to generate an acid disequilibrium pH), was clearly impaired. Moreover, urinary and inner medullary collecting duct PCO_2 was also reduced significantly [14]. In turtle urinary bladder under open-circuited conditions, lithium impairs proton secretion by virtue of a detrimental effect on the electrical gradient, favoring H^+ secretion [17]. Since sodium sulfate infusion reduces urine pH appropriately (below pH 5.5) in lithium-induced DRTA [14–17], it is possible that lithium treatment results in a mild voltage dependent impairment by competing with sodium entry across the apical membrane. Nevertheless, potassium secretion is not impaired, since animals treated chronically do not develop hyperkalemia [14]. Since urine flow rate is an important determinant of K^+ secretion by the distal nephron, the accompanying defect in urinary concentration may maintain K^+ secretion, thus avoiding hyperkalemia.

In contrast to the findings observed during lithium treatment, the chronic administration of amiloride to rats is associated with metabolic acidosis, hyperkalemia, and an inappropriately alkaline urine pH unresponsive to infusion of sodium sulfate [18]. Moreover, net proton secretion is markedly impaired and papillary pCO_2 is reduced [14]. The amiloride model differs from the lithium-induced defect in several respects. Amiloride has no effect on H^+ secretion in turtle bladder [19] or in the CCT [20], independent of voltage. As a result of the decreased voltage, both K^+ and H^+ secretion are reduced [20]. Amiloride does not affect bicarbonate transport or voltage in the outer medullary collecting tubule [21], but reduces volume flux in the inner medullary collecting tubule [22]. Therefore, amiloride inhibits acidification predominantly through a voltage-mediated defect in the CCT. The possibility of an additional effect on proton secretion in the inner MCT is suggested, however, by the observation of obliteration, by amiloride, of the disequilibrium pH in this segment.

Non-Voltage Dependent Rate Defects

Postobstructed Kidney (POK)

Experimental studies evaluating the acidification defect occurring after 18–24 hours of unilateral ureteral obstruction have reported findings similar to those observed in the amiloride model. Similarly, we have demonstrated impaired proton secretion and an inability to generate normal papillary CO_2 tensions after bicarbonate administration in the POK [14]. Bicarbonate reabsorption and transepithelial voltage in cortical collecting tubules harvested from rabbits have also been shown to be reduced [23]. In contrast, however, a more recent in vitro study has shown by paired analysis that the medullary, not the cortical collecting tubule, exhibited a marked decrease in bicarbonate reabsorption after 2 days or more of obstruction. Transepithelial voltage in the CCT was unaffected [24]. Finally, recent preliminary studies from the same laboratory have examined (Na^- + K^+) ATPase and N-ethylmaleimide (NEM)-sensitive ATPase activities in microdissected cortical and medullary collecting tubule fragments. NEM-sensitive ATPase (H^+-ATPase activity) was most markedly reduced in the medullary collecting tubule (75%), not in the CCT (25% reduction) [25]. (Na^+ + K^+) ATPase activity decreased 80% in both collecting duct segments.

Thus, the POK model may represent a combination of voltage-mediated and direct proton pump impaired defects. In this respect the POK resembles the type of defect associated with aldosterone deficiency.

Selective Aldosterone Deficiency

The CCT is responsible for reabsorption of a portion of the filtered load of sodium by an aldosterone-dependent process which increases transepithelial voltage, favoring secretion of both K^+ and H^+. Therefore, aldosterone deficiency may cause hyperkalemia and metabolic acidosis. The outer medullary collecting duct also serves as a target organ for aldosterone by increasing net proton secretory capacity independent of sodium transport [21]. Recent studies in our laboratory have demonstrated that selective aldosterone deficiency is associated with imnpaired H^+ secretion in the inner medullary collecting duct [26]. In this same study ammonia transfer into inner medullary collecting ducts was markedly impaired, so that ammonium excretion was reduced dramatically. Moreover, as a result of impaired ammonia production, ammonium delivery to the loop of Henle was also reduced. Thus, a decrease in inner medullary ammonium accumulation accounted for a portion of the reduction in ammonia transfer and inner medullary addition. Since papillary PCO_2 was reduced during bicarbonate loading [26], the rate of proton secretion also was clearly compromised. In these and other studies, when one corrects for voltage changes, it appears that the "rate" defect is quantitatively more important than the "voltage" defect in hypoaldosteronism, and thus the direct effect of aldosterone on H^+-secretion (H^+-ATPase) surpasses the indirect effects mediated through voltage changes.

Impaired Buffer Production and/or Excretion

Recent studies in our laboratory in a rat model of chronic hyperkalemia have affirmed that whole kidney ammonium excretion is reduced significantly in hyperkalemia [27]. This decrease in excretion was a result of a marked reduction in whole kidney ammonium production, which occurred even in the face of coexistent chronic metabolic acidosis. Nevertheless, chronic hyperkalemia had no effect on net transport of ammonium by the superficial proximal tubule [28]. Rather, it was demonstrated that a major nephron site of regulation of ammonium transport in response to hyperkalemia was the medullary thick ascending limb of Henle's loop [27]. Chronic hyperkalemia, by inhibition of active NH_4^+ absorption by this segment, impairs accumulation of total ammonia in the inner medulla and compromises significantly the transfer of ammonia into the inner medullary collecting duct [29].

Other disorders accompanied by chronic hyperkalemia would be expected to exhibit similar adverse effects on ammonium production and transport. Selective aldosterone deficiency could represent, therefore, a mixed model of defective acidification in which hyperkalemia impairs ammonium production and excretion, while hypoaldosteronism impairs acid secretion by the ATP-dependent proton pump. By extension of this view, it seems logical to assume that medullary interstitial disease might be associated with a defect in ammonium accumulation and transfer into the inner medulla, but it would be expected that the superficial proximal tubule would maintain intact ammonium production. Impaired ammonium production might be present in advanced renal insufficiency with metabolic acidosis (reduced functional renal mass), or in circumstances in which glutamine availability or metabolism could be compromised.

Acknowledgments. The participation in these studies by Carlton R. Caflisch and David W. Good was invaluable. I also wish to acknowledge the excellent secretarial assistance of Suzanne Rambin. Studies in the author's laboratory were supported in part by research grant DK30603 awarded by the National Institutes of Health.

References

1. Alpern RJ, Warnock DG, Rector FC Jr (1986) Renal acidification Mechanisms. In Brenner BM, Rector FC Jr (eds) The Kidney, 3rd edn. Saunders, Philadelphia, pp 206–249
2. DuBose TD Jr (1982) Hydrogen ion secretion by the collecting duct as a determinate of the urine to blood PCO_2 gradient in alkaline urine. J Clin Invest 69:145–156
3. DuBose TD Jr (1983) Application of the disequilibrium pH method to investigate the mechanism of urinary acificiation. Am J Physiol 245 (Renal Fluid Electrolyte Physiol 14):F443–F449
4. Gluck S, Al-Awqati Q (1984) An electrogenic proton-translocating adenosine triphosphatase from bovine kidney medulla. J Clin Invest 73:1704–1710
5. Stone DK, Xie XS, Racker E (1984) Comparison of the proton ATPase and chloride transporter from bovine clathrin-coated vesicles and renal medullary vesicles. Kidney Int 25:283 (A)
6. Diaz-Diaz FD, Labelle EF, Eaton DC, et al. (1986) ATP-dependent proton transport in human renal medulla. Am J Physiol 20:F297–F302
7. Kaunitz JD, Gunther RD, Sachs G (1985) Characterization of an electrogenic ATP and chloride-dependent proton translocating pump from rat renal medulla. J Biol Chem 260:11567–11571
8. Gluck S, Hirsch S, Brown D (1987) Immunocytohistochemical localization of H^+-ATPase in rat kidney. Kidney Int 31:167 (A)
9. Halperin ML, Goldstein MB, Haig A, et al. (1974) Studies on the pathogenesis of type I (distal) renal tubular acidosis as revealed by the urinary PCO_2 tension. J Clin Invest 53:669–677
10. Capasso G, Schultz H, Vickermann B, et al. (1986) Amphotericin B and amphotericin B methylester: Effect on brush border membrane permeability. Kidney Int 30:311–317
11. Steinmetz PR, Lawson LR (1970) Defect in acidification induced in vitro by amphotericin B. J Clin Invest 49:596–601
12. Garg LC (1979) Lack of effect of amphotericin-B on urine-blood $PCVO_2$ gradient in spite of urinary acidification defect. Pflugers Arch 381:137–142
13. Julka N, Arruda JAL, Kurtzman NA (1979) The mechanism of amphotericin-induced distal acidification defect in rats. Clin Sci 56:555–562
14. DuBose TD Jr, Caflisch CR (1985) Validation of the difference in urine and blood CO_2 tension during bicarbonate loading as an index of distal nephron acificiation in experimental models of distal renal tubular acidosis. J Clin Invest 75:1116–1123
15. Batlle DC, Sehy JT, Roseman MK, et al. (1981) Clinical and pathophysiologic spectrum of acquired distal renal tubular acidosis. Kidney Int 20:389–396
16. Batlle DC, Gavira M, Grupp M (1982) Distal nephron function in patients receiving chronic lithium therapy. Kidney Int 21:477–485
17. Arruda JAL, Dytko G, Mola R, et al. (1980) On the mechanism of lithium-induced distal renal tubular acidosis: Studies in the turtle bladder. Kidney Int 17:196–204
18. Arruda JAL, Subbarayudu K, Dytko G, et al. (1980) Voltage dependent distal acidification defect induced by amiloride. J Lab Clin Med 95:407–416
19. Husted RF, Steinmetz PR (1979) The effects of amiloride and ouabain on urinary acidification by turtle bladder. J Pharmacol Exp Ther 210:264–268
20. Allen GG, Barrat LJ (1979) An in vivo study of voltage-dependent renal tubular acidosis induced by amiloride. Kidney Int 35:1107–1110

21. Stone DS, Seldin DW, Kokko JP, et al. (1983) Mineralocorticoid modulation of rabbit medullary collecting duct acidification. A sodium-independent acidification. J Clin Invest 72:77–83
22. Ullrich KJ, Papavassiliou F (1979) Sodium reabsorption in the papillary collecting duct of rats. Pflugers Arch 379:49–52
23. Hanley MJ, Davidson K (1982) Isolated nephron segments from rabbit models of obstructive uropathy. J Clin Invest 69:165–174
24. Laski ME, Sabo C, Morgan VE, et al. (to be published) Site of the distal acidification defect in obstructive uropathy. Min Elect Metab
25. Sabatini S (1989) Pathophysiologic mechanisms of abnormal collecting duct function. Sem in Nephr 9:179–202
26. DuBose TD Jr, Caflisch CR (1988) Effect of selective aldosterone deficiency on acidification in nephron segments of the rat inner medulla. J Clin Invest 82:1624–1632
27. DuBose TD Jr, Caflisch CR, Good DW (1990) Effects of chronic hyperkalemia on ammonium transport in inner medulla of the rat. Kidney Int 37:535 (A)
28. DuBose TD Jr, Caflisch CR, Good DW (1989) Effects of chronic hyperkalemia on renal ammonium transport. Kidney Int 35:452 (A)
29. Good, DW (1987) Effect of potassium on ammonium transport by medullary thick ascending limb of the rat. J Clin Invest 80:1358–1365

Classification and Characterization of Types of Distal Acidification Defects in Humans

DANIEL C. BATTLE[1] and TAHA KEILANI

Introduction

The distal renal tubular acidosis (RTA) syndromes are usually characterized by the presence of a hyperchloremic type of metabolic acidosis often associated to either hypokalemia (classic RTA) or hyperkalemia (hyperkalemic types of RTA). Some patients, however, have subtle defects in urinary acidification not manifested by hyperchloremic metabolic acidosis. The identification and classification of the various types of RTA are best approached from a mechanistic point of view and should take into consideration the site of the nephron responsible for the defect in acidification.

In this article we will present a classification of distal RTA based on the deranged cellular mechanism of urinary acidification (Table 1). As discussed recently, some of the proposed mechanisms are represented by relatively well defined clinical entities whereas others are still theoretical [1].

Permeability Defects

A remarkable property of the collecting tubule is that H^+ secretion can occur against a transepithelial H^+ gradient until the H^+ concentration in the mucosal fluid is approximately 1,000 times greater than in the serosal fluid. When this large H^+ gradient is attained (collecting tubule pH $\approx$ 4.4), H^+ secretion ceases. Backleak of H^+ from mucosal fluid into the serosal site is virtually negligible. The existence of a defect in membrane permeability, however, could impair net acidification by causing either H^+ backleak or an increased HCO_3 influx into the lumen [2]. Studies in the turtle urinary bladder and in mammalian collecting tubules have shown that ampho-

[1]Northwestern University Medical School, Morton 3-615, 303 East Chicago, Chicago, IL 60611, USA

Table 1. Classification of Distal RTA subtypes

Type	Example
I. *Permeability/defects*	
a. H^+ backleak	Amphotericin B
b. Enhanced HCO_3 secretion	Unknown
II. *Secretory/defects*	
a. Diffuse collecting tubule H^+ pump defect	Chronic Kidney transplant rejection
b. Medullary collecting tubule H^+ pump defect	Nephrocalcinosis (some cases)
c. Diffuse proton pump failure K^+ secretory defect	Obstructive nephropathy
d. Medullary H^+/K^+ ATPase defect (?)	Endemic hypokalemic distal RTA (?)
III. *Rate-dependent/defects*	
a. Voltage-dependent defect	Amiloride
b. Enhanced chloride transport	Gordon's syndrome
c. Aldosterone deficiency	Selective Aldosterone deficiency
d. Aldosterone resistance	Pseudohypoaldosteronism
e. Reduced urinary buffer	Hyperkalemia
f. Reduced intracellular H^+ anhydrase deficiency	Cytosolic carbonic
g. Reduced H^+ conductance	Toluene

tericin B, applied to the mucosal site, results in H^+ backdiffusion (lumen to blood). The drug also increases potassium permeability (which may explain the occurrence of hypokalemia) but does not affect HCO_3 permeability. On the basis of these experimental findings, it has been inferred that H^+ backleak is the mechanism causing hypokalemic distal RTA in patients receiving amphotericin B [1–5].

As in most types of distal RTA, urine pH in patients treated with amphotericin B is higher than 5.5, despite acidemia. The inability to lower urine pH despite unimpaired H^+ secretion is attributable to H^+ backleak, which is more evident when the tubular urine is acidic [1–5]. Theoretically, it is conceivable that the creation of a large transtubular electrical gradient (lumen-negative) by the administration of sodium sulfate or furosemide could attenuate H^+ backleak and permit lowering of urine pH to normally low values. H^+ backleak should be minimized when the urine is made highly alkaline. That this is the case is suggested by the finding of a normal rise in urine PCO_2 when sodium bicarbonate is infused to amphotericin B-treated rats [6]. As a point of fact, this is the only known experimental model of distal RTA in which urine PCO_2 in a highly alkaline urine is normal (i.e., more than 70 mm Hg) [1]. Further, this is the only type of experimental distal RTA in which an acid disequilibrium pH in the collecting tubule has been documented during the infusion of sodium bicarbonate [6]. This finding strongly suggests that amphotericin B causes DRTA by a mechanism other than impaired collecting tubule H^+ secretion.

It must be emphasized that so far there are no patients described who displayed all of the features outlined in the amphotericin B model of experimental H^+ backleak distal RTA. At present, it seems highly unlikely that any form of hereditary or acquired distal RTA, other than that associated with amphotericin B, is caused by a H^+ backleak mechanism. Some forms of drug-induced hypokalemic distal RTA, such as that caused by toluene sniffing, originally thought to originate from H^+ backleak do not appear to cause it. This can be inferred from the finding of failure to increase urine PCO_2 after bicarbonate infusions in individuals with hypokalemic distal RTA associated with toluene sniffing [7]. Further, in turtle urinary bladders exposed to high concentrations of toluene, the rate of H^+ secretion is reduced, but unlike in amphotericin B-treated bladders, there is no discernible H^+ backleak [7].

Conceivably, a defect in collecting tubule permeability causing an increase in HCO_3 secretion could also result in a decrease in net collecting tubule acidification, thereby leading to distal RTA (Table 1). There is no experimental or clinical evidence, however, for such a defect.

Secretory Defects

Under this terminology will be considered any alteration causing an impairment of collecting tubule acidification by primarily interfering with active H^+ secretion. The collecting tubule contains a proton pump at its luminal surface. This pump, a proton translocating ATPase, secretes H^+ in an electrogenic manner (i.e., is capable of translocating a net positive charge into the lumen) and can operate independently of sodium transport and despite an unfavorable transtubular electrical gradient. The rate of sodium transport and the electrical voltage, however, importantly influence the rate of H^+ secretion. Alterations in transepithelial voltage caused by either inhibition of sodium transport or enhancement of chloride transport can reduce the rate of H^+ secretion and thereby cause distal RTA. These alterations are considered under the heading of rate-dependent defects (see below). A primary H^+ secretory defect, by definition, is limited to the proton pump.

The existence of a secretory type of distal RTA has been reasonably well characterized in patients with different diseases causing acquired distal RTA [8–10]. Derangements of collecting tubule function determined genetically (e.g., hereditary distal RTA), associated with structural abnormalities (e.g., medullary sponge kidney), immunologically mediated (e.g., chronic renal transplant rejection), or caused by impaired metabolic cell function, could all interfere with the proton pump secretory apparatus. One can envision a spectrum of secretory defects ranging from reduction in the number of proton pumps to severe proton pump dysfunction, as well as defects in the active transport pathway due to altered metabolic energy production or use. Given the variety of disease states causing distal RTA and the numerous basic mechanisms on which they could have an impact, there is no reason to believe that they all have to alter the proton secretory apparatus in the same way. There is also no a priori reason to believe that proton pump dysfunction has to involve the entire collecting tubule [10]. It is conceivable that the lesion causing proton pump dysfunction may be confined to a portion of the collecting tubule. For instance, one could anticipate from the anatomic distribution of some disease states causing distal RTA that their defect in acidification would be confined to the medullary collecting tubule [10]. The possible ways to evaluate clinically the site of abnormal H^+ secretion within the collecting tubule are discussed below.

The general features characteristic of a secretory type of distal RTA are as follows. Urine pH during spontaneous acidosis or after acid loading cannot be lowered below 5.5, and the rate of acid excretion is decreased. Ammonium excretion is reduced, a finding that can be inferred at bedside from the finding of a positive urine anion gap [11]. The urine PCO_2 measured after bicarbonate loading does not increase normally, reflecting that the rate of collecting tubule H^+ secretion is reduced [12]. This feature is useful in distinguishing a secretory from a permeability defect [7]. It is not useful, however, in differentiating a secretory from a voltage-dependent defect, which also decreases the rate of H^+ secretion (albeit indirectly). The value of measuring urine PCO_2 in a highly alkaline urine stems from its exquisite sensitivity in portraying the rate of H^+ secretion. For instance, environmental factors that reduce collecting tubule H^+ secretion, such as an alkaline diet or exposure to hypocapnia, are associated with a subnormal rise in urine PCO_2 during bicarbonate loading. Any perturbation leading to a decrease in the rate of collecting tubule H^+ secretion should thus impair the generation of a high urine PCO_2 in a highly alkaline urine. Administration of neutral sodium phosphate also stimulates distal H^+ secretion and should retard acid backleak. The rise in urinary PCO_2 normally seen after the administration of neutral sodium phosphate does not occur when H^+ secretion in the collecting tubule is impaired [8,9].

Rate-Dependent Defects

One can classify under the heading of rate-dependent defects a variety of alterations that have in common that the rate of H^+secretion in the collecting tubule is reduced, not because of primary proton pump failure, but rather as a consequence of reduced availability of intracellular H^+ or reduced urinary buffer content or other defects (Table 1). Failure to sustain an adequate transtubular electrical gradient (voltage-dependent defects), aldosterone deficiency, and aldosterone resistance could all be viewed as rate-dependent defects (Table 1). The latter three entities will be considered separately because their clinical features are quite distinctive (see below).

A mechanism that could result in a decrease in the rate of collecting tubule H^+ secretion is reduced availability of intracellular H^+. Since an intracellular OH^- is generated for each H^+ secreted by the H^+ pump into the tubular lumen, the ability to remove OH^- is required for continued H^+ secretion. The removal of OH^- is facilitated by cytosolic carbonic anhydrase, an enzyme that catalyzes the reaction of OH^- with CO_2. Deficiency of cytosolic carbonic anhydrase in the renal intercalated cells of the collecting tubule (carbonic anhydrase type II) could, therefore, slow down the rate of H^+ secretion by interfering with intracellular OH^- disposal. Likewise, a defect in the exit step for HCO_3 (or OH^-) could reduce the rate of collecting tubule H^+. In patients with hereditary carbonic anhydrase deficiency, urine pH is higher than 5.5 during acidosis. The defect in H^+ should also impair urine PCO_2 formation after bicarbonate loading, but data on this parameter are not available.

The rate of H^+ secretion may be decreased owing to a lack of buffer in the tubular fluid. The rate of H^+ secretion by the collecting tubules is higher when the tubular fluid is alkaline (HCO_3 accepts secreted H^+) than when it is acid. In the absence of H^+ acceptors, tubular fluid is acidified rapidly, and the H^+ pump inhibits its own transport rate by the pH gradient it generates [2]. In quantitative terms, ammonia is the most important H^+ acceptor. Disease states causing decreased ammonia production, such as advanced renal insufficiency, hyperkalemia, and aldosterone deficiency – usually acting in combination – result in impaired ammonium excretion [13–15]. Delivery of ammonia to the medullary collecting tubule may be decreased, thereby limiting H^+ secretion. This situation occurs whenever the kidneys are underperfused. Phosphate depletion not only results in decreased titratable acidity from hypophosphaturia but also interferes with ammonium excretion.

In a restricted sense, the term "rate dependent" distal RTA was first introduced to designate patients with a pattern of urinary acidification characterized by failure to increase urine PCO_2 in a highly alkaline urine, but otherwise intact ability to lower urine pH during ammonium chloride-induced acidosis [16]. Since urinary pH could be lowered in the presence of mild acidosis we felt that a proton secretory defect, per se, was unlikely. Many of the patients were not acidotic but had clinical evidence of tubulointerstitial renal disease, which prompted us to initiate investigation of urinary acidification [16]. In this regard, it represents a variant of incomplete distal RTA. This pattern is also common among patients on well-controlled chronic lithium therapy [17]. The concentration of lithium in the urine of these patients ranges from 10–40 mmoles/liter, a concentration sufficient to inhibit voltage-dependent H^+ secretion in the turtle urinary bladder and in rabbit cortical collecting tubules perfused in vitro [18]. The reduced rate of collecting tubule H^+ secretion, disclosed in vivo by the failure to increase urine PCO_2 in a highly alkaline urine, has been inferred to result from failure to generate a normal transtubular voltage (lumen-negative) when lithium is present in the lumen of the cortical collecting tubule. This cation appears to compete for sodium reabsorption. The impairment in sodium reabsorption, in turn, may lessen the voltage (lumen-negative) required for optimal H^+ and K^+ secretion [18]. Hyperkalemia, however, is not a feature of lithium-treated patients, possibly because of the high urine flow (due to impaired concentrating capacity) which increases K^+ secretion.

Voltage-Dependent Renal Tubular Acidosis

Examples of voltage-dependent defects in collecting tubule acidification due to an isolated impairment of sodium transport are so far confined to lithium and to drugs that primarily block apical sodium transport, such as amiloride and triamterene. There are patients with hyperkalemic RTA in whom furosemide or sodium sulfate administration does not result in lowering of urine pH below 5.5 [10,19]. The kaliuretic response to these agents also is blunted. These findings suggest that voltage-dependent (i.e., sodium-dependent) H^+ and K^+ secretion in the cortical collecting tubule is impaired [10]. In addition to hyperkalemic hyperchloremic metabolic acidosis, one would anticipate a salt-wasting tendency, reflecting impairment of sodium transport, in such patients. Although systematic studies of sodium balance have not been performed, clinical observations of defective sodium conservation have been made on occasional patients [14]. Some of them may display sodium wastage on a normal salt diet, whereas others may manifest sodium wastage only when they are salt restricted. A consequence of salt wastage is the functional deterioration of GFR, which is reversible on fluid replacement.

Although inhibition of sodium transport in the cortical collecting tubule results in a decrease in the rate of H^+ secretion, this could be compensated by enhanced H^+ in the medullary collecting tubule, a segment with a greater capacity for urinary acidification. Unlike individuals treated with amiloride or lithium, these patients develop marked metabolic acidosis, a finding that suggests a more diffuse impairment of collecting tubule acidification. Patients with this form of hyperkalemic distal RTA probably have a proton pump secretory defect that involves the entire collecting tubule [1].

Selective Aldosterone Deficiency

Hyperkalemic metabolic acidosis associated with selective aldosterone deficiency (SAD) is the most common type of RTA in adults [13,14]. It also is the commonest cause of hyperkalemia among patients with mild to moderate insufficiency. Most of these patients have evidence of tubulointerstitial renal disease and reduced GFR. The rate of collecting tubule H^+ secretion is stimulated by aldosterone and reduced in its absence. The urine of these patients is acidic (pH 5.0–5.5) during mild metabolic acidosis. Relative to their reduced rate of ammonium excretion, however, urine pH is slightly higher than that of normal subjects made acidotic by ammonium chloride [11]. This finding reflects that the rate of collecting tubule H^+ secretion is reduced. The PCO_2 in a highly alkaline urine should be reduced, but data from patients are not available regarding this parameter. In addition to the direct stimulatory effect of aldosterone on the rate of collecting tubule H^+ secretion and its indirect effect mediated by changes in distal sodium transport, aldosterone increases ammonia production. Aldosterone deficiency is thus expected to be associated with decreased ammonia production. Further, the development of hyperkalemia causes a marked suppression of ammonium excretion.

Indeed, the main factor responsible for the acidosis of patients with SAD is a decrease in ammonium excretion. In this regard, this type of RTA could be mechanistically classified under the category of reduced concentration of urinary buffers (ammonia) (Table 1). Correction of hyperkalemia, no matter how accomplished, results in amelioration of metabolic acidosis by enhancement of ammonium excretion. Some of the patients with aldosterone deficiency also display end-organ resistance to the action of the hormone, as evidenced by the persistence of hyperkalemia despite chronic administration of large amounts of mineralocorticoid. The typical patient, however, responds reasonably well to mineralocorticoid administration. It is important to recognize that some patients have a combination of both SAD and hyperkalemic distal RTA [19]. Such patients have low ammonium excretion and low aldosterone levels and, in addition, cannot lower urinary pH below 5.5 regardless of the degree of acidosis. The clinical implication of this observation is that a patient with hyperkalemic acidosis with an inappropriately high urine pH (i.e., 5.5) has, by definition, hyperkalemic distal RTA, regardless of whether plasma aldosterone is low, normal, or high [19]. If the patient has low aldosterone and cannot lower urinary pH below 5.5 in the face of acidosis, he or she suffers from both hyperkalemic distal RTA and SAD.

Types of Renal Tubular Acidosis Associated with Aldosterone Resistance and Normal Glomerular Filtration Rate

The term "aldosterone resistance" (or pseudohypoaldosteronism) is used to designate those patients with hyperkalemic hyperchloremic metabolic acidosis in whom aldosterone deficiency clearly is not present and in whom there is no evidence of diffuse tubulointerstitial nephropathy. Two clinical pictures fit this definition: (1) the syndrome of classic pseudohypoaldosteronism of infancy, characterized by salt-wastage and hypotension and (2) a rare syndrome of aldosterone-resistant acidosis and hyperkalemia usually characterized by salt retention and hypertension (chloride shunt type of disorder).

The clinical picture of classic pseudohypoaldosteronism is characterized by dehydration and hyponatremia due to renal salt wastage, hyperkalemia, and hyperchloremic metabolic acidosis. It occurs in infants as a congenital disorder. The severity of salt wastage and potassium retention diminishes with time, but hyponatremia and hyperkalemia may recur if dietary salt is restricted. This condition appears to be a pure form of tubular aldosterone resistance not associated with discernible tubulointerstitial damage at kidney biopsy. It has been proposed that the syndrome results from a deficiency of Na^+, K^+-ATPase, because absence of this enzyme from proximal and distal nephron segments was documented in kidney biopsy material obtained from one patient with classic pseudohypoaldosteronism.

As in any state of end-organ responsiveness, the circulating levels of the hormone are greatly elevated in patients with pseudohypoaldosteronism. The features characteristic of the acidification defect associated with aldosterone resistance should be identical to those seen in states of aldosterone deficiency. Data on urinary acidification from patients with pseudohypoaldosteronism of infancy, however, are sparse. Like patients with aldosterone deficiency, those with aldosterone resistance should have a low urine pH during acidosis, but reduced rates of ammonium excretion. Whether the rate of collecting tubule H^+ secretion, assessed by the rise in urine PCO_2 in a highly alkaline urine, is diminished or not remains to be investigated.

Another aldosterone-resistant type of disorder associated with normal GFR and hyperchloremic hyperkalemic metabolic acidosis has been characterized and is referred to as type II pseudohypoaldosteronism [20]. This disorder corresponds to a similar clinical picture known as Gordon's syndrome. Evidence for aldosterone resistance in such patients is inferred from the persistence of hyperkalemia despite the administration of exogenous mineralocorticoid. In contrast, potassium excretion increases markedly after the administration of sodium sulfate or sodium bicarbonate. Hyperkalemia and metabolic acidosis can be corrected by restriction of dietary sodium or by the administration of thiazide diuretics. The primary abnormality is believed to be a tubular defect characterized by increased chloride reabsorption in the distal nephron. This results in increased NaCl reabsorption, thereby resulting in volume expansion and low-renin hypertension. Plasma aldosterone also may be suppressed and remains low relative to the prevailing hyperkalemia. Enhanced chloride transport limits the sodium-dependent and mineralocorticoid-dependent voltage driving force for potassium and hydrogen ion secretion. This defect could be classified as a voltage-dependent type of distal RTA due to enhanced chloride transport. Unlike the voltage-dependent defect caused by amiloride, the one caused by a chloride shunt type of defect does not appear to interfere with lowering of urine pH during acidosis.

Plasma Potassium and Distal RTA

Abnormalities in plasma potassium are a major feature of the various subtypes of distal RTA. The classic form of RTA is usually accompanied by hypokalemia which has been ascribed to renal K wastage [21–23]. The precise cause of hypokalemia, in our opinion, has not been completely clarified. A permeability defect, causing passive K secretion, would readily explain it but, as stated above, a permeability defect has only been shown to occur with Amphotericin B administration. It is generally held that potassium wastage occurs in the absence of abnormal collecting tubule permeability for potassium, simply because of accelerated potassium secretion in the face of impaired H^+ secretion. The enhancement in K secretion is said to be driven by secondary hyperaldosteronism which may be a feature of distal RTA [23,24]. Aldosterone oversecretion could be expected as a result of sodium wastage which has been documented in some patients with distal RTA [24]. While this may be a reasonable explanation, it is nevertheless intriguing that some patients present with striking hypokalemia whereas others do not. Further, it is unlikely that aldosterone levels would be elevated in the face of protracted potassium depletion and, indeed, few studies have reported aldosterone data from patients with hypokalemic distal RTA. It is, thus, possible that factors other than secondary hyperaldosteronism are responsible for the development of severe hypokalemia, at least in some cases of distal RTA.

A particularly attractive mechanism that could account for hypokalemia is the existence of a defect in the renal K^+/H^+ ATPase pump. Renal K excretion is determined not only by active K secretion localized largely to the distal tubule and cortical collecting tubule, but also by active K absorption localized, at least in part, to the outer medullary collecting tubule [25]. Under conditions of dietary K deprivation or extrarenal K wastage, profound K depletion would ensue unless there were a compensatory increase in K absorptive flux in more terminal nephron segments. Activation of a K conservation mechanism in the outer medullary collecting tubule could prevent further K wastage, while producing enhanced proton secretion. If the K^+/H^+ ATPase pump recently found in the medullary collecting tubule of the rabbit [25–27] were defective, one would expect the development of both hypokalemia and metabolic acidosis. Thus, the capital features of classic RTA could be readily explained by such a defective mechanism.

While the presence of a renal defect in potassium conservation does not need to be a universal defect of hypokalemic distal RTA it is a reasonable possibility, at least for those cases associated with severe hypokalemia. In some patients with distal RTA, gastric hypoactivity has been documented [28]. This suggests the existence of a defect in the H^+/K ATPase of both gastric parietal cells and renal collecting tubule cells. A partial defect in this pump could explain well the development of both hypokalemia and metabolic acidosis, especially under conditions of dietary K deprivation or enhanced extrarenal losses. In this regard, it is intriguing that the occurrence of severe hypokalemic RTA in an endemic area in the Northeastern part of Thailand peaks in the summer months [28]. Heat exposure in the summer could initiate potassium depletion, which would be aggravated by defective renal conservation owing to a K^+/H^+ ATPase defect. In this theoretical scenario we would predict that

Table 2. Theoretical distinction between collecting tubule H^+ pump defects

	H^+ ATPase defect	H^+/K^+ ATPase defect
Acidosis	+++	++
Hypokalemia	+	+++
Urine pH	>5.3	>5.3
Urine K	↑	↑↑
Correction K deficit	No effect or worsening acidosis*	Improvement of acidosis

*by removing a potent stimulus for NH_3 formation

K supplementation alone should ameliorate the metabolic acidosis by enhancing the operation of a defective K^+/H^+ pump. In contrast, a defect in the H^+ pump should not be corrected by K supplementation. In fact, the acidosis should worsen owing to correction of the hypokalemia, a potent stimulus for ammonia production. A purely theoretical list of distinctive features for the two types of defects is offered in Table 2.

Clinical Localization of Segmental Defects in Collecting Tubule H^+ Secretion

Although patients with distal RTA usually display an abnormally high urine pH during acidemia, they may or may not lower urine pH normally in response to the administration of sodium sulfate or loop diuretics. The response to the latter two maneuvers has been proposed as a way of localizing the site of the H^+ secretory defect within the collecting tubule [10]. The collecting tubule, a major site of urinary acidification within the distal nephron, displays axial heterogeneity both anatomically and functionally. In the cortical collecting tubule (CCT) active sodium reabsorption generates an electrical potential (lumen-negative) that favors the secretion of H^+ and potassium. In contrast, in outer medullary collecting tubules, H^+ secretion does not appear to be under the influence of sodium transport and is accompanied by chloride secretion. In this segment, the potential difference is oriented lumen-positive, presumably as a result of electrogenic H^+ secretion. This is in contrast with the lumen-negative electrical potential usually prevailing in the cortical segment, that is thought to be generated by active sodium reabsorption (Fig. 1). Although the relative contribution of each of these two nephron segments to net acidification in vivo has not been delineated, there is remarkable agreement from various studies, using rabbit isolated tubules perfused in vitro, showing that the rate of acidification is considerably greater in the medullary than in the cortical segment of the collecting tubule.

The clinical evaluation of the function of the collecting tubule is, to some extent, possible using maneuvers that either stimulate or inhibit proton secretion in this nephron site. A segmental approach would require a maneuver that acts selectively in each portion of the collecting tubule. The acidemic stimulus, usually provided by the administration of ammonium chloride, is not selective, because acidemia enhances acidification throughout the entire distal nephron. Because H^+ secretion in the medullary collecting tubule is sodium-dependent, one can assume that maneuvers that produce a sodium-dependent increase or decrease in H^+ secretion do not have an impact on this nephron segment. Amiloride, at low doses that inhibit apical sodium conductance but not Na^+/H^+ exchange, inhibits sodium-dependent acidification and potassium secretion in the cortical collecting tubule [10]. Loop diuretics, by blocking NaCl reabsorption in the thick ascending loop of Henle, increase Na delivery to the collecting tubule. Part of the sodium delivered to the cortical collecting tubule is reabsorbed, whereas chloride is not, resulting in the creation of a favorable transtubular voltage (lumen-negative) for H^+ and K^+ secretion. That the increase in distal Na reabsorption secondary to furosemide administration results in enhancement of voltage-dependent acidification in the cortical collecting tubule, can be inferred from the finding that the fall in urine pH and the increase in net acid excre-

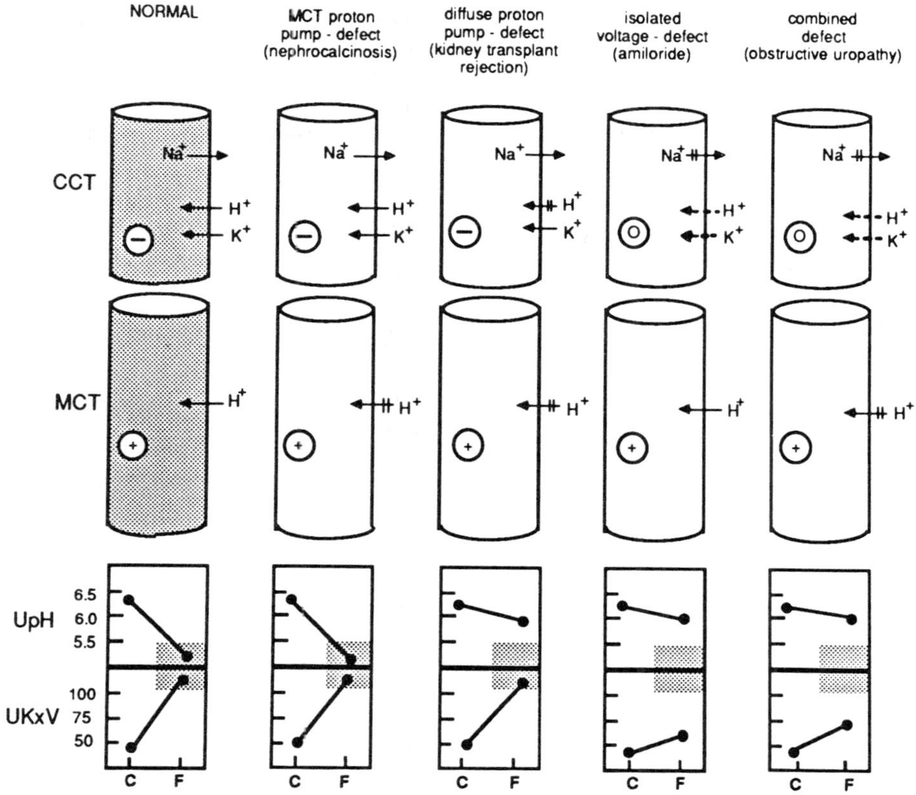

Fig. 1.

tion elicited by furosemide are obliterated by amiloride [10]. Amiloride also lessens the kaliuretic effect of furosemide, indicating that the increase in K^+ secretion observed when furosemide is given alone is due, in part, to an increase in transepithelial voltage. An additional effect of furosemide on renal K^+ excretion, independent of its indirect effect on transepithelial voltage, is apparent from the finding that K^+ excretion increases linearly as a function of urine flow. The difference in K^+ excretion observed at comparable urine flow rates when furosemide is given alone and when it is given with amiloride reflects the contribution of the amiloride-sensitive (that is, sodium-dependent) component of distal nephron H^+ secretion [10].

Sodium-dependent acidification also can be stimulated by the infusion of sodium sulfate. The infusion of sodium sulfate provides a poorly reabsorbable anion as well as Na load that, when reabsorbed by the cortical collecting tubule, results in an increase in transepithelial voltage. An increase in the cortical collecting tubule transepithelial voltage in response to furosemide would occur only if Na were to be reabsorbed well in excess of Cl. Both furosemide and sodium sulfate administration result in enhanced tubular reabsorption of Na, but differ in that Cl reabsorption relative to

Na is depressed after furosemide administration, because in this circumstance Cl behaves as a poorly reabsorbable anion [10].

A scheme for the interpretation of the distinctive responses to furosemide and sodium sulfate found in patients with distal RTA is presented in Fig. 1. This scheme assumes that with administration of these agents, tubular fluid pH falls below 5.3 at the level of the cortical collecting tubule as a consequence of enhanced Na-dependent H^+secretion. This nephron segment could be deranged in that either the number (or function) of proton pumps is reduced, or in that the ability to transport sodium and thereby generate a transepithelial voltage (lumen-negative) is impaired. The latter alteration is seen when amiloride is given to normal subjects [10]. Under these conditions, urine pH cannot be lowered below 5.3, and the kaliuretic effect of furosemide is blunted (Fig. 1). If the proton pump only were impaired, the administration of either furosemide or sodium sulfate should increase transepithelial voltage in the cortical collecting tubule. In this situation, K^+ excretion would increase normally, but urine pH could not be lowered maximally, owing to failure of the proton pump. According to this scheme, patients who exhibit a normal increase in K^+ excretion but are unable to lower urine pH below 5.3 after furosemide or sodium sulfate administration can be classified as having a proton pump defect involving the cortical collecting tubule.

In some patients with distal RTA, K^+ secretion increases and urine pH falls below 5.3 after either furosemide or sodium sulfate administration [19]. The fall in urine pH suggests that the cortical collecting tubule has sufficient intact proton pumps to secrete H^+ when a favorable transepithelial voltage is imposed by these maneuvers. By exclusion, their defect in distal acidification, uncovered by the failure to lower urine pH despite acidemia, must be located in the medullary collecting tubule and confined to this nephron segment (Fig. 1). This notion has the support of experimental work showing that acidemia causes a fall in luminal pH in the medullary collecting tubule. One could argue that normal lowering of urine pH after furosemide or sodium sulfate in some patients with distal RTA simply denoted the existence of a mild proton pump defect. Inasmuch as the response to these agents in some patients with distal RTA is similar to that observed in normal individuals, however, it seems reasonable to conclude that sodium-dependent H^+ secretion in the cortical collecting tubule of such patients is normal.

In some patients with hyperkalemic distal RTA, the response to sodium sulfate and furosemide is characterized by both inability to lower urine pH and a subnormal K excretion [10,19]. In patients with hyperkalemic metabolic acidosis associated with selective aldosterone deficiency, furosemide and sodium sulfate administration result in lowering of urine pH below 5.3 [13]. The pattern found in the former patients could be explained solely on the basis of an isolated voltage-dependent defect in the cortical collecting tubule, such as is seen in normal subjects given amiloride (Fig. 1). In addition to a voltage-dependent defect in the cortical collecting tubule, patients with hyperkalemic distal RTA likely have a proton pump defect affecting the entire collecting tubule (Fig. 1). Thus, these patients are best classified as having a diffuse proton pump secretory defect in the collecting tubule that is associated with impaired sodium and potassium transport in the cortical collecting tubule. This kind of structural involvement could also be anticipated from the type of renal disease (e.g., obstructive uropathy) usually associated with this form of hyperkalemic distal RTA [19].

References

1. Batlle DC (1989) Renal tubular acidosis. In: Seldin DW, Giebisch G (eds) The regulation of acid-base balance. Raven, New York, pp 353–390
2. Steinmetz PR, Lawson WJ (1970) Defect in urinary acidification induced in vitro by amphotericin B. J Clin Invest 49:596–601
3. Arruda JAL, Kurtzman NA (1980) Mechanism and classification of deranged distal urinary acidification. Am J Physiol 8:F515–523
4. Batlle DC, Kurtzman NA (1982) Distal renal tubular acidosis: Pathogenesis and classification. Am J Kidney Dis 1:128–144
5. DuBose TD Jr, Alpern RJ (1989) In: The metabolic basis of inherited disease. McGraw Hill pp 2539–2568
6. DuBose TD Jr, Calflisch CR (1985) Validation of the difference in urine and blood carbon dioxide transport during bicarbonate loading as an index of distal nephron acidification in experimental models of distal renal tubular acidosis. J Clin Invest 75:1116–1123
7. Batlle DC, Sabatini S, Kurtzman NA (1988) On the mechanism of toluene-induced renal tubular acidosis. Nephron 49:210–218
8. Batlle DC, Sehy JT, Roseman MK, Arruda JAL, Kurtzman NA (1981) Clinical and pathophysiologic spectrum of acquired distal renal tubular acidosis. Kidney Int 20:389–396
9. Batlle DC, Moses MF, Manaligod J, Arruda JAL, Kurtzman NA (1981) The pathogenesis of hyperchloremic metabolic acidosis associated with renal transplantation. Am J Med 70:786–796
10. Batlle DC (1986) Segmental characterization of defects in collecting tubule acidification. Kidney Int 30:546–553
11. Batlle DC, Hizon M, Cohen E, Gutterman C, Gupta R (1988) The use of the urinary anion gap in the diagnosis of hyperchloremic metabolic acidosis. N. Engl J Med 318:594–599
12. Halperin ML, Goldstein MB, Haig A, et al. (1974) Studies on the pathogenesis of type 1 (distal) renal tubular acidosis as revealed by the urinary pCO_2 tensions. J Clin Invest 53:669–677
13. Batlle DC (1986) Sodium-dependent urinary acidification in patients with aldosterone deficiency and adrenalectomized rats. Metabolism 35:852–860
14. Batlle DC (1981) Hyperkalemic hyperchloremic metabolic acidosis associated with selective aldosterone deficiency and distal renal tubular acidosis. Semin Nephrol 1:260–274
15. Sebastian A, Schambelan M, Lindenfeld S, et al. (1977) Amelioration of metabolic acidosis with fluorocortisone therapy in hyporeninemic hypoaldosteronism. N Engl J Med 297:576–589
16. Batlle DC, Grupp M, Gaviria M, Kurtzman NA (1982) Distal renal tubular acidosis with intact ability to lower urine pH. Am J Med 72:751–7510
17. Batlle DC, Gaviria M, Grupp M, Arruda JAL, Wynn J, Kurtzman NA (1982) Distal nephron function in patients receiving chronic lithium therapy. Kidney Int 21:477–485
18. Laski ME, Kurtzman NA (1983) Characterization of acidification in the cortical and medullary collecting tubule of the rabbit. J Clin Invest 72:2050–2059
19. Batlle DC, Arruda JAL, Kurtzman NA (1981) Hyperkalemic distal renal tubular acidosis associated with obstructive uropathy. N Engl J Med 304:373–380
20. Schambelan M, Sebastian A, Rector FC Jr (1981) Mineralocorticoid-resistant renal hyperkalemia without salt wasting (type II pseudohypoaldosteronism): Role of increased renal chloride reabsorption. Kidney Int 19:716
21. Rodriguez-Soriano J, Boichis H, Edelmann CM Jr (1967) Bicarbonate reabsorption and hydrogen ion excretion in children with renal tubular acidosis. J Pediatr 71:802–813
22. Caruana RJ, Buckalew VM Jr (1988) The syndrome of distal (Type I) renal tubular acidosis. Medicine, (Baltimore) 67:84

23. Sebastian A, McSherry E, Morris RC Jr (1971) Renal potassium wasting in renal tubular acidosis (RTA). J Clin Invest 50:667
24. Sebastian A, McSherry E, Morris RC Jr (1976) Impaired renal conservation of sodium and chloride during sustained correction of systemic acidosis in patients with Type I, classic renal tubular acidosis. J Clin Invest 58:454–469
25. Wingo CS, Straub SC (1989) Active Proton Secretion and Potassium Absorption in the Rabbit Outer Medullary Collecting Duct. J Clin Invest 84:361–365
26. Doucet A, Marsy S (1987) Characterization of K-ATPase activity in distal nephron: stimulation by potassium depletion. Am J Physiol 253 (Renal Fluid Electrolyte Physiol 22):F418–F423
27. Garg LC, Narang N (1988) Ouabain-insensitive K-adenosine triphosphatase in distal nephron segments of the rabbit. J Clin Invest 81:1204–1208
28. Nilwarangkur S, Nimmannit S, Chaovakul V, Susaengrat W, Ong-aj-yooth S, Vasuvattakul S, Pidetcha P, Malasit P (1989) Endemic Primary Distal Renal Tubular Acidosis in Thailand. Q J Med 74:275,289–301

Endothelin and the Kidney

Chair: Tomoh Masaki (Japan)
Michael J. Dunn (USA)

Endothelin in Renal Diseases

VALENTINA KON[1]

SUMMARY. Injurious stimuli can activate endothelin production and elevate circulating levels of endothelin. However, continuous elevation of endothelin is not necessary for its profound effects. Instead, local endothelin activity, which encompasses local concentration of endothelin or receptor and post-receptor mechanisms, may be of primary importance in mediating the abnormal vascular function following renal injury.

Introduction

It is well recognized that, following any of the numerous insults which lead to acute renal failure, the vascular function of the kidney is profoundly disturbed. The reduced rate of glomerular filtration, central in these disorders, is typically accompanied by decreased renal blood flow, and reflects increased vascular resistance. Even when the rate of blood flow to the kidneys normalizes or is experimentally reestablished to the normal range, the vascular responsiveness of the kidney remains aberrant, including impairment in autoregulation and paradoxical vasoconstriction [1,2]. Although some humoral and neural factors have been implicated in the persistent vasoconstriction, the mechanisms for abnormal vascular function have remained largely unresolved. It has recently been appreciated that endothelial cells are important active regulators in the complete expression of vascular dilation and constriction. Therefore, it appears likely that processes which affect endothelial cell integrity may adversely influence renal vascular function by promoting the elaboration of endothelin (also by impairing the release of other endothelium-derived substances, such as endothelium-derived relaxing factor and/or prostaglandins).

A number of pathophysiologic factors enhance endothelin production. Specifically, hypoxia, anoxia, epinephrine, thrombin, transforming growth factor (TGF)-β,

[1]Pediatric Nephrology, Vanderbilt University School of Medicine, Nashville, TN 37232-2584, USA

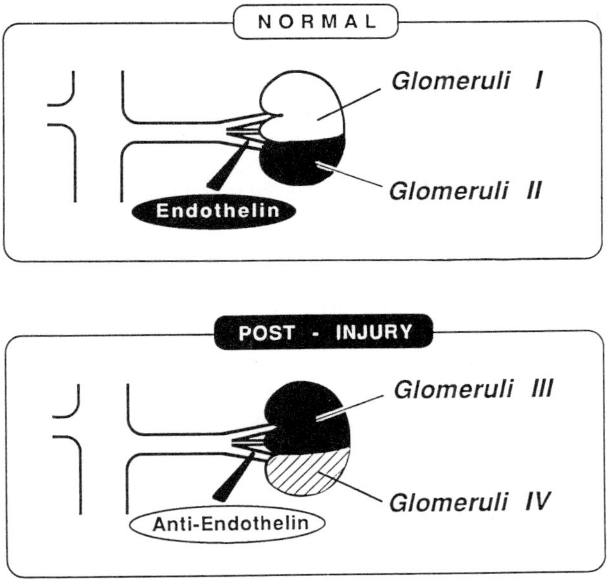

Fig. 1. Schematic illustration of infusing a branch of the main renal artery. This permits specific treatments of different populations of glomeruli within the same kidney. (*Top*) A normal kidney undergoing infusion of endothelin. Glomeruli I represent nephrons not exposed to endothelin; Glomeruli II are nephrons infused with endothelin. (*Bottom*) Kidney which has previously sustained a generalized injury to all the glomeruli. Glomeruli III reflect nephron function following the generalized injury, e.g., renal artery occlusion or intravenous infusion of cyclosporine, while Glomeruli IV represent nephron function from the same damaged kidney subsequently also exposed to anti-endothelin serum. (Reprinted from *Kidney International* with permission [18])

neuropeptide Y, interleukin-1, endotoxin, cyclosporine, and shear stress are factors known to precipitate or contribute to renal injury which can increase endothelin gene expression and/or its synthesis in vitro [3–12]. It has also been shown that the circulating level of endothelin is increased in several experimental settings and in clinical disorders, including acute renal failure, congestive heart failure, cardiogenic shock, hypertension, cyclosporine toxicity, and endotoxemia [5,13–20]. In many of these conditions, systemic hypertension and/or increased vascular resistance, which are features typically observed with exogenous infusion of endothelin, have been documented. Thus, infusion of endotoxin or cyclosporine is followed by an increased level of circulating endothelin, which is associated with systemic hypertension and vasoconstriction of renal, pulmonary, and splenic vascular beds [18,21]. While there is little doubt that injurious stimuli can enhance endothelin production in vitro and that endothelin is a circulating substance whose levels are increased in vivo in conditions where vasoconstriction prevails, it is not yet clear whether the converse is true, namely, that persistently elevated levels of circulating endothelin are necessary to maintain powerful and prolonged vasoconstriction. As will be discussed below, this appears not to be the case.

Endothelin appears to affect all vessels, although its actions on different vascular beds are not uniform. The renal circulation is particularly susceptible to endothelin's vasoconstrictory effects. Ultrasonic inter-organ assessment of blood flow in the pig reveals that the renal vasculature is ten-fold more sensitive to endothelin than the other vascular beds, including coronary, bronchial, and femoral vessels [21]. Similar results have been obtained in the squirrel monkey [22], whose vasoconstrictor response was also found to be most pronounced in the renal vessels, such that a dose of endothelin (3 μg/kg) which reduced blood flow in the heart by 46%, caused virtual cessation of blood flow in the kidney [22]. The reasons for renal susceptibility to this peptide have not been well delineated, but may be related to differences in endothelin production capability and/or differences in the binding capacity for endothelin among various tissues.

Given that the potential targets for endothelin actions include renal and nonrenal vasculature, a method was devised for administration of endothelin that achieved high concentrations but did not cause the striking systemic hemodynamic changes typical of intravenous administration of endothelin [3,22]. For this purpose, a micropipette was inserted into a first-order branch of the main renal artery of Munich-Wistar rats (Fig. 1). Through this micropipette, endothelin was infused (0.4 ng/min). In the absence of changes in systemic blood pressure or arterial hematocrit, the glomerular hemodynamics were profoundly different in glomeruli exposed *versus* those not exposed to the endothelin within the same kidney [23]. Thus, single nephron glomerular filtration rate (SNGFR) was some 35% lower in glomeruli exposed to endothelin compared with glomeruli not infused with endothelin, or with SNGFR values prior to any infusion. Similarly, the glomerular plasma flow rate was some 38% lower in the endothelin-exposed glomeruli. This hypoperfusion and hypofiltration reflected an increase in the resistances in afferent and efferent arterioles. There was no difference in the glomerular capillary ultrafiltration coefficient in these two populations of glomeruli.

Postischemic Renal Failure

In view of the previous observations that vasoconstricting substances are elaborated by the vascular endothelium in response to anoxia and hypoxia [11,24], the possibility that the vasoconstriction which characteristically follows renal ischemia depends upon endogenous endothelin was assessed in functional studies. Forty-eight hours after 25 minutes of renal artery clamping, kidneys were micropunctured while rabbit anti-porcine endothelin serum was being infused into one of the branches of the main renal artery, using the branch infusion technique shown in Fig. 1 [23]. When compared with glomeruli not exposed to the antiserum, glomeruli which were infused with the antiserum showed a remarkable amelioration in post-ischemic renal vasoconstriction, with an almost 60% increase in the SNGFR and a doubling in the glomerular plasma flow rate. Compared with non-infused glomeruli, there was also an increase in the glomerular capillary pressure and a fall in both afferent and efferent arteriolar resistances in previously ischemic glomeruli exposed to anti-endothelin serum. In this regard, Shibuota recently observed that the endothelin concentration in kidney tissues increased 20 hours following 45 minutes of bilateral renal artery occlusion [25]. Of interest, the circulating level of endothelin in these experimental animals was not different from normal controls. Treatment with a monoclonal antibody to endothelin (5 minutes before and 5 minutes, 1 and 2 hours after release of renal occlusion) lessened the accumulation of blood urea nitrogen (BUN) and creatinine, protected cells from development of renal edema and histological damage, and suppressed accumulation of calcium in necrotic tissue [25]. Taken together, ischemia appears to stimulate endothelin release which contributes to renal vascular constriction after ischemic injury.

In addition, it appears that tissue ischemia potentiates endothelin's vasoconstricting and toxic effects. Rats made hypoxemic (by lowering the ventilation volume) showed a doubling of the vasoconstrictor potency of exogenous endothelin and an increase in its myocardial toxicity [26]. It was postulated that this enhanced effect might be related to changes in the receptor characteristics or in the efficiency of coupling to effector mechanisms. In this regard, ischemia has been shown to increase endothelin-1 binding density in rat cardiac membranes [27]. In particular, 60 minutes of cardiac ischemia increased the crude plasma membrane binding density, suggesting upregulation of surface receptors, while the light membrane fraction, presumably representing the intracellular component, fell [27]. These results were taken to show that ischemia increases endothelin binding by externalizing cardiac binding sites for endothelin.

It should be noted that hypoperfusion, and therefore the potential for tissue hypoxia, is a regular feature of injuries which lead to renal dysfunction. Thus, any disorder which has *hypoperfusion* as a feature may activate and/or potentiate a pathophysiologic role for endothelin.

Endotoxemia

Endotoxin-mediated endothelial cell damage has been implicated as central in the pathogenic mechanism of endotoxic injury. Thus, in cultured endothelial cells of bovine transformed thoracic aorta, the addition of E. coli endotoxin to the culture medium increased the release of endothelin in a dose-dependent manner (Fig. 2). Intravenous injection of the endotoxin into rats was associated with a prompt (occurring in 10–15 minutes) increase in circulating endothelin: ~120 pg/ml compared with <2 pg/ml in control rats [5]. In comparison studies, it was shown that while intravenous infusion of endotoxin was followed by a marked reduction in glomerular filtration rate (GFR) in both kidneys, endothelin antiserum infused into the left main renal artery ameliorated renal hypofiltration in that kidney, but not in the contralateral kidney, of the same endotoxemic animals [28].

Cyclosporine Toxicity

Cyclosporine A is an immunosuppressant which has dramatically improved graft survival of a variety of organ transplants during the last decade. Among its recognized adverse side effects, which include hepatotoxicity, hypertension, and central nervous system toxicity, nephrotoxicity is the most important and may be the inevitable consequence of cyclosporine treatment [29,30]. Early renal involvement appears to reflect intense, reversible renal vasoconstriction and has been linked to the renin-

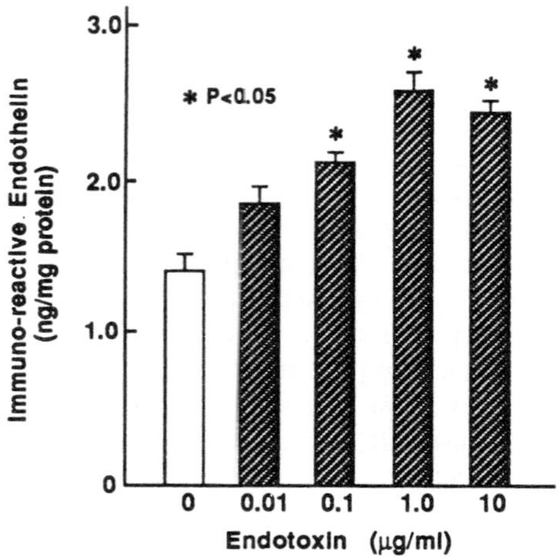

Fig. 2. Dose-dependent stimulating effect of endotoxin on endothelin secretion. Each *bar* represents the mean value in cultured endothelial cells of triplicate experiments. (Adapted from [5])

angiotensin and adrenergic systems and to vasoconstricting thromboxane (A_2). It is likely that cyclosporine-induced vasospasm, at least in part, also reflects altered vascular reactivity due to endothelial cell damage.

Cyclosporine added directly to cultured human vascular cells increases the level of endothelin in the culture medium [6]. An in vivo experimental study showed that intravenous administration of cyclosporine (20 mg/kg) caused an increase in the circulating endothelin level (43 pg/ml, as compared with <2 pg/ml of endothelin found

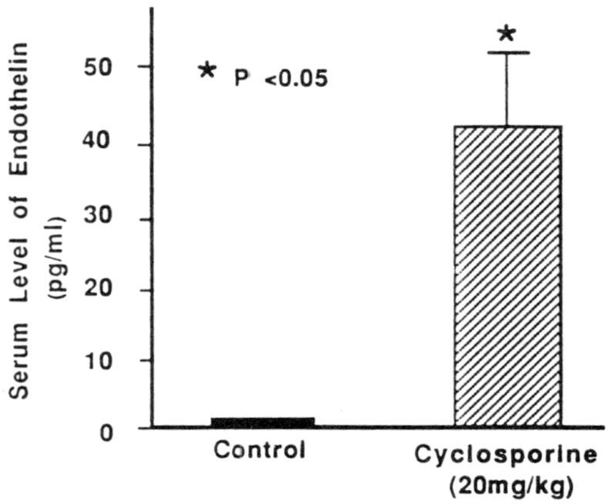

Fig. 3. Circulating levels of endothelin in cyclosporine and vehicle treated rats. (Reprinted from *Kidney International* with permission [18])

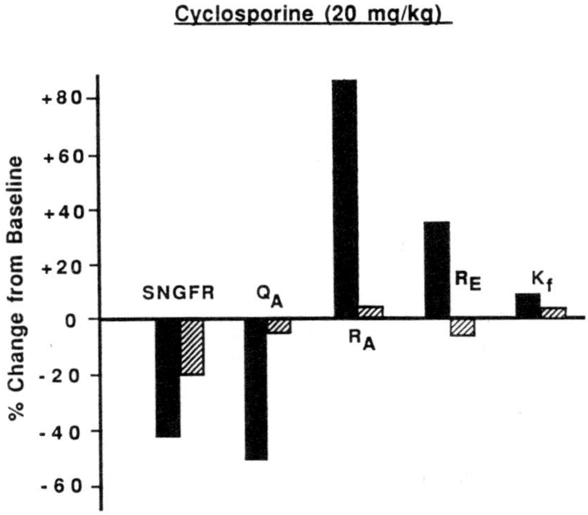

Fig. 4. Change from baseline values in microcirculatory parameters in cyclosporine treated kidneys comparing glomeruli which were not exposed (*black bars:* Glomeruli III in Fig. 1) with those which were exposed to anti-endothelin serum (*stippled bars:* Glomeruli IV in Fig. 1). (Reprinted from *Kidney International* with permission [18])

in identically instrumented rats not given cyclosporine) (Fig. 3) [18]. The elevation in endogenous circulating endothelin occurred in association with an increase in the systemic blood pressure (115 mmHg at baseline versus 133 mmHg at the time of blood collection), an observation in agreement with the well recognized pressor effect of exogenous endothelin.

In a different group of rats, the functional consequences of cyclosporine treatment on glomerular hemodynamics were examined. One hour following cyclosporine administration, rabbit anti-porcine endothelin serum was infused continuously into a first order branch of the main renal artery, whereupon the glomeruli not infused with endothelin antiserum as well as those infused with endothelin antiserum were simultaneously assessed by micropuncture (Fig. 1). A dramatically different hemodynamic pattern was seen in these two groups of nephrons (Fig. 4). The SNGFR fell by more than 40% in glomeruli after cyclosporine administration, while SNGFR in glomeruli of the same injured kidneys which were exposed to endothelin antiserum was only 20% lower than the baseline value. Amelioration of hypoperfusion in association with lower afferent and efferent arteriolar resistances was also apparent in cyclosporine-injured glomeruli infused with endothelin antiserum, when compared with glomeruli not infused with endothelin antiserum. Perico et al. also found that endothelin antiserum ameliorated renal hypoperfusion and hypofiltration following intravenous administration of cyclosporine in rats [31].

It is clear that injurious stimuli, including cyclosporine, can promptly stimulate endogenous endothelin production; however, as noted above, *persistent elevation in the circulating endothelin* level is not necessary to effect its compelling actions. That is, by sixty minutes after cyclosporine administration, at a time when glomerular hypoperfusion and hypofiltration prevail, the circulating level of endothelin is near normal. These findings correlate with the observations that, despite its short estimated half-life (< 1 minute), the biological actions of endothelin are long-lasting [3]. These findings imply persistent activation of vascular smooth muscles at the receptor or post receptor level. In this regard, the endothelin binding characteristics are strikingly different in cyclosporine-treated versus normal rats. In preliminary studies, Awazu et al. found increased endothelin binding in glomeruli of cyclosporine-treated animals [32]. This increased binding appeared specific for endothelin, since cyclosporine treatment did not alter the receptor binding characteristics for another vasoconstrictor, namely, angiotensin [32]. There was also no difference in endothelin binding in hepatic tissue between cyclosporine and control rats. Nambi et al. also showed that cyclosporine treatment (50 mg/kg intraperitoneally) for four days resulted in decreased GFR and a 60% increase in endothelin receptor density in renal tissue [33]. It appears, therefore, that cyclosporine-induced glomerular dysfunction involves upregulation of glomerular endothelin receptors and that this alteration in endothelin receptors is specific to the kidney. These findings concur with the enhanced susceptibility of renal tissue to the effects of both cyclosporine and endothelin.

References

1. Conger JD, Robinette JB, Schrier RW (1988) Smooth muscle calcium and endothelium-derived relaxing factor in the abnormal vascular responses of acute renal failure. J Clin Invest 82(2):532–537
2. Williams RH, Thomas CE, Navar LG, Evan AP (1981) Hemodynamic and single nephron function during the maintenance phase of ischemic acute renal failure in the dog. Kidney Int 19:503–515
3. Yanagisawa M, Kurihara H, Kimura S, Tomobe Y, Kobayashi M, Mitsui Y, Yazaki Y, Goto Y, Masaki T (1988) A novel potent vasoconstrictor peptide produced by vascular endothelial cells. Nature 332:411–415
4. Yoshizumi M, Kurihara H, Morita T, Yamashita T, Oh-hashi Y, Sugiyama T, Takaku F, Yanagisawa M, Masaki T, Yazaki Y (1990) Interleukin-1 increases the production of endothelin-1 by cultured endothelial cells. Biochem Biophys Res Commun 166(1):324–329
5. Sugiura M, Inagami T, Kon V (1989) Endotoxin stimulates endothelin-release in vivo and in vitro as determined by radioimmunoassay. Biochem Biophys Res Commun 161(3): 1220–1227
6. Bunchman TE, Brookshire CA (1990) Cyclosporine stimulated synthesis of endothelin by human endothelial cells in tissue culture. Kidney Int 37(1):A365
7. Xuan Y-T, Whorton AR, Shearer-Poor E, Boyd J, Watkins WD (1989) Determination of immunoreactive endothelin in medium from cultured endothelial cells and human plasma. Biochem Biophys Res Commun 164(1):326–332
8. Emori T, Hirata Y, Ohta K, Shichiri M, Marumo F (1989) Secretory mechanisms of immunoreactive endothelin in cultured bovine endothelial cells. Biochem Biophys Res Commun 160(1):93–100
9. Boarder MR, Marriott DB (1989) Characterization of endothelin-1 stimulation of catecholamine release from adrenal chromaffin cells. J Cardiovasc Pharmacol 13(Suppl 5):S223–S224
10. Kohno M, Murakawa K, Yokokawa K, Yasunari K, Horio T, Kurihara N, Takeda T (1989) Production of endothelin by cultured porcine endothelial cells: modulation by adrenaline. J Hypertens 7(Suppl 6):S130–S131

11. Rubanyi GM, Vanhoutte PM (1985) Hypoxia releases a vasoconstrictor substance from the canine vascular endothelium. J Physiol 364:45–56
12. Sato M, Ohshima N (1990) Effect of wall shear rate on thrombogenesis in microvessels of the rat mesentery. Circ Res 66(4):941–949
13. Totsune K, Mouri T, Takahashi K, Ohneda M, Sone M, Saito T, Yoshinaga K (1989) Detection of immunoreactive endothelin in plasma of hemodialysis patients. FEBS Lett 249(2): 239–242
14. Koyama H, Nishzawa Y, Morii H, Tabata T, Inoue T, Yamaji T (1989) Plasma endothelin levels in patients with uraemia. Lancet I:991–992
15. Saito Y, Nakao K, Mukoyama M, Imura H (1989) Increased plasma endothelin level in patients with essential hypertension. N Engl J Med 322(3):205
16. Saliminen K, Tikkanen I, Saijonmaa O, Nieminen M, Fyhrquist F, Frick MH (1989) Modulation of coronary tone in acute myocardial infarction by endothelin. Lancet II:747
17. Nomura A, Uchida Y, Kameyama M, Saotome M, Oki K, Hasegawa S (1989) Endothelin and bronchial asthma. Lancet II:747–748
18. Kon V, Sugiura M, Inagami T, Harvie BR, Ichikawa I, Hoover RL (1990) Role of endothelin in cyclosporine-induced glomerular dysfunction. Kidney Int 37(6):1487–1491
19. Robertson RM, Susawa T, Sugiura M, Haile V, Inagami T (1990) Circulating endothelin levels: modulation by heart failure in man. Clin Res 38(2):414A
20. Tomita K, Ujiie K, Nakanishi T, Tomura S, Matsuda O, Ando K, Shichiri M, Hirata Y, Marumo F (1989) Plasma endothelin levels in patients with acute renal failure. N Engl J Med 321(16):1127
21. Pernow J, Hemsen A, Lundberg JM (1989) Increased plasma levels of endothelin-like immunoreactivity during endotoxin administration in the pig. Acta Physiol Scand 137(2):317–318
22. Clozel M, Clozel J-P (1989) Effects of endothelin on regional blood flows in squirrel monkeys. J Pharmacol Exp Ther 250(3):1125–1131
23. Kon V, Yoshioka T, Fogo A, Ichikawa I (1989) Glomerular actions of endothelin in vivo. J Clin Invest 83:1762–1767
24. DeMay JG, Vanhoutte PM (1983) Anoxia and endothelium-dependent reactivity of the canine femoral artery. J Physiol (London) 335:65–74
25. Shibouta Y, Suzuki N, Shino A, Matsumoto H, Terashita Z-I, Kondo K, Nishikawa K (1990) Pathophysiological role of endothelin in acute renal failure. Life Sci 46(22): 1611–1618
26. MacLean MR, Randall MD, Hiley CR (1989) Effects of moderate hypoxia, hypercapnia and acidosis on haemodynamic changes induced by endothelin-1 in the pithed rat. Br J Pharmacol 98:1055–1065
27. Liu J, Casley DJ, Nayler WG (1989) Ischaemia causes externalization of endothelin-1 binding sites in rat cardiac membranes. Biochem Biophys Res Commun 164(3):1220–1225
28. Kon V, Badr KF (to be published) Biologic actions and pathyphysiologic significance of endothelin in the kidney. Kidney Int
29. Myers BD (1986) Cyclosporine nephrotoxicity. Kidney Int 30(6):964–974
30. Kahan BD (1989) Medical intelligence: Cyclosporine. N Engl J Med 321(25):1725–1738
31. Perico N, Dadan J, Remuzzi G (1990) Endothlin mediates the renal vasoconstriction induced by cyclosporine in the rat. JASN 1(1):76–8332
32. Awazu M, Sugiura M, Inagami T, Kon V (1990) Cyclosporine-induced renal dysfunction involves upregulation of glomerular receptors for endothelin. Clin Res 38(2):464A
33. Nambi P, Pullen M, Contino LC, Brooks DP (1990) Upregulation of renal endothelin receptors in rats with cyclosporine A-induced nephrotoxicity. FASEB J 4(3):458A

The Cell Biology of Endothelin Peptides: Insights From Studies of Glomerular Mesangial Cells

Michael S. Simonson[1], Tomohiro Osanai[2], and Michael J. Dunn[3]

Summary. Endothelins are regulatory peptides synthesized by selected endothelial and epithelial cells, and within cells of the nervous system. This ever-expanding family of peptides mediates such diverse biological processes as vasoconstriction, mitogenesis, and neurotransmission. Research efforts aimed at understanding the pathways of transmembrane signaling evoked by endothelin (ET) peptides might provide a framework for elucidating the physiological and pathophysiological roles for these peptides. Here we review recent progress towards this goal using cultured glomerular mesangial cells as a model system. Endothelin peptides evoke a phosphoinositide-based Ca^{2+} signaling system with a well-documented role mediating cell contraction. Endothelin peptides also activate alternative signaling pathways such as Na^+/H^+ exchange, prostaglandin synthesis, and *c-fos* expression, which might contribute to ET's action as a growth factor.

Introduction

Endothelins (ETs) are a family of acidic, 21-amino acid peptide hormones [1–3]. The ETs exist in at least four distinct isoforms, namely ET-1, ET-2, ET-3, and vasoactive intestinal contractor, or VIC [4–6]. Both in structure and in function ETs are closely related to sarafotoxin peptides isolated from venom of *Atractaspis engaddensis*, and it seems likely that the two peptide familes share a common evolutionary origin [7]. As shown in Fig. 1, all ET peptides and sarafotoxins share a common design including (*i*) two disulfide bonds that form a hairpin loop containing polar charged side chains and (*ii*) a hydrophobic C-terminus (residues 16–21) containing the aromatic indole side chain at Trp^{21}.

Departments of Medicine[1], Physiology[2], and Biophysics[3], School of Medicine, Case Western Reserve University, Division of Nephrology, University Hospital of Cleveland, Cleveland, OH 44106, USA

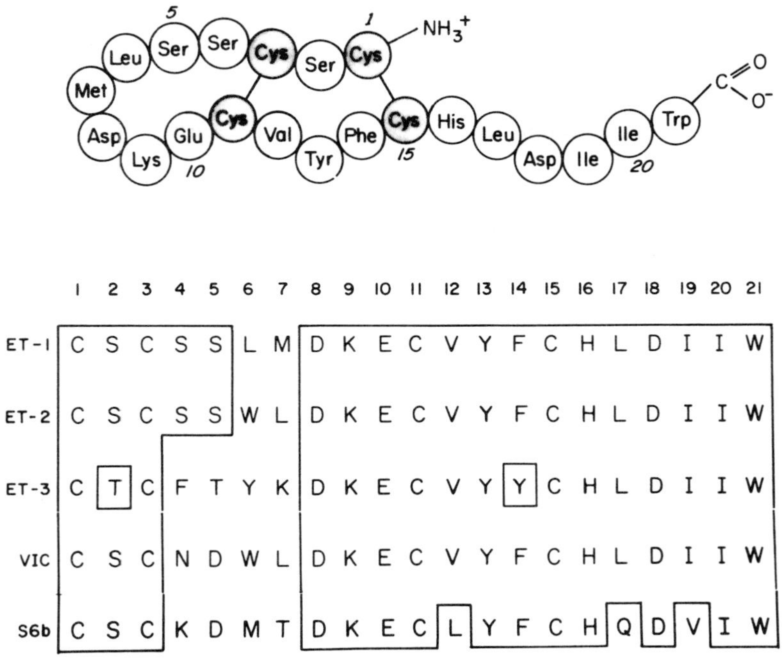

Fig. 1. The structure and sequence homologies of ET isopeptides and S6b. Homologous regions between peptide isoforms are enclosed

In a manner analogous to other peptide hormones, ETs arise via proteolytic processing of isopeptide-specific prohormones. PreproETs are large peptides ($\approx$200 amino acids) that demonstrate species- and isopeptide-specific differences in amino acid sequence [1,5]. Conversion of proET to ET involves a protease with chymotrypsin-like activity and is essential for bioactivity. Although ET was first thought to be synthesized exclusively in the vascular endothelium, it is now clear that numerous extra-vascular tissues synthesize ETs. These extra-vascular sites include epithelial layers in the lung and kidney [8–10], neural tissues in the brain and spinal cord [8,11,12], and cells in the hypothalamus and posterior pituitary [13]. Release of ET requires induction of preproET gene expression. Some stimuli of ET gene expression include Ca^{2+} ionophores, phorbol esters, transforming growth factor β, and fluid-mechanical shear stress [2,14–16].

ETs are regulatory peptides with a surprisingly diverse range of biological activities. Depending on the target cell, ET can act as a vasoactive agent, growth factor, or even as a neuropeptide [2,3]. In this respect ETs are similar to other hormones, including arginine vasopressin, angiotensin II, bombesin, bradykinin, and serontonin [17]. In order to understand how ETs evoke such diverse biological actions it is necessary to define the pathways of transmembrane signaling following activation of ET receptors. Cultured mesangial cells provide a useful in vitro model for understanding the biology of ET peptides in cells of the connective tissue family [18]. Here we review our recent work analyzing the biological actions and signaling pathways of ETs in glomerular mesangial cells.

ET Peptides Have Potent Contractile and Promitogenic Actions

Contractile Activity of ET-1

At 0.1 μM ET-1 causes contraction of mesangial cells cultured on hydrated, three-dimensional collagen gels [19]. Contraction occurs along the long axis of the cell, but in many cells the cell body is also reduced. Cross-sectional area in contractile cells falls by an average of 42%, but in some cells reductions of 60–70% are common. Also induced by ET-1 are complex rearrangements of actin microfilament bundles in mesangial cells [19]; these rearrangements are consistent with an agonist-induced transition from stationary cells expressing stress fibers to motile cells elaborating a diffuse meshwork organization. The contractile state of mesangial cells in vivo is thought to be one factor regulating the glomerular ultrafiltration coefficient, and it seems possible that ET-stimulated contraction of mesangial cells might contribute to regulation of glomerular ultrafiltration. Alternatively, contraction of fibroblasts on collagen gels is thought to mimic a wound healing response, and ET might stimulate similar actions in mesangial cells and thereby contribute to the glomerular response to injury.

Promitogenic Actions of ET-1

One of the interesting biological actions of ETs is the ability to act as a mesangial growth factor [20,21]. As shown in Fig. 2, when ET-1 is added to quiescent cells they reenter G_1 and proceed to S phase 12–18 h later. The mitogenic action of ET-1 is similar to that of 2.5% fetal bovine serum. [^{3}H]Thymidine uptake in response to ET-1 is dose-dependent with a threshold at 0.1 nM, EC_{50} at 0.9 nM, and maximal stimulation at 10 nM. By itself, ET-1 is unable to stimulate mitogenesis and requires either low concentrations of fetal bovine serum (i.e., 0.5%) or a competence factor such as insulin [20]. Thus ET-1 acts as a growth factor for mesangial cells, and the promitogenic action of ET-1 has since been demonstrated in fibroblasts [22,23], vascular smooth muscle cells [24,25], and glial cells [12].

ET Peptides Evoke the Phosphoinositide Cascade

Activation of phospholipase C appears to be the initial transmembrane event following activation of ET receptors in mesangial cells [20,21]. As illustrated in Fig. 3, ET-1 causes a dose-dependent increase in phosphatidylinositol (PtdIns) turnover measured at 15 min in the presence of LiCl. Endothelin-1 stimulates greater PtdIns turnover than 0.1 μM arginine vasopression, a potent phospholipase C-linked agonist in mesangial cells [20]. Analysis of the InsP isomers reveal that both Ins(1,4,5)P_3 and Ins(1,3,4,5)P_4 are elevated by ET-1 (see Fig. 3). Ins(1,4)P_2 and Ins(1,3,4)P_3 probably result from 5-phosphomonoesterase-catalyzed dephosphorylation of Ins(1,4,5)P_3 and Ins(1,3,4,5)P_4, respectively. Activation of phospholipase C

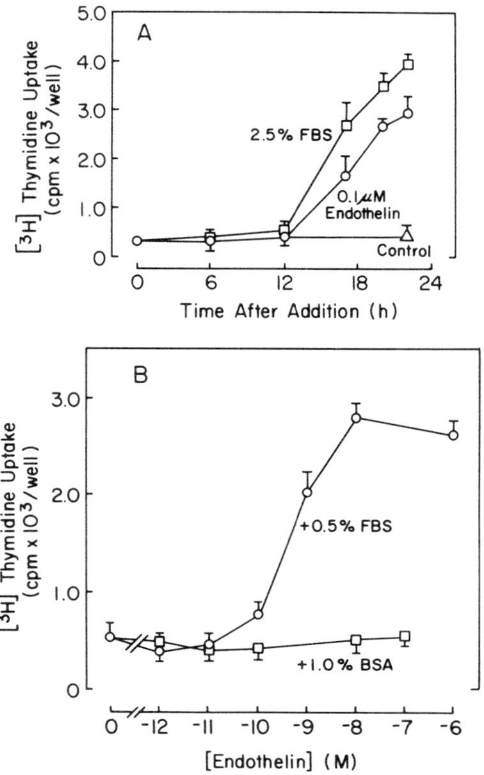

Fig. 2A,B. ET-1 stimulates mitogenesis in quiescent mesangial cells. **A** Time course of [^{3}H]thymidine uptake in response to serum and ET-1 added to DME/F12 medium (plus 0.5% FBS) at zero time **B** Dose-response and cofactor requirements for ET-1-stimulated [^{3}H]thymidine uptake. (From [20] with permission)

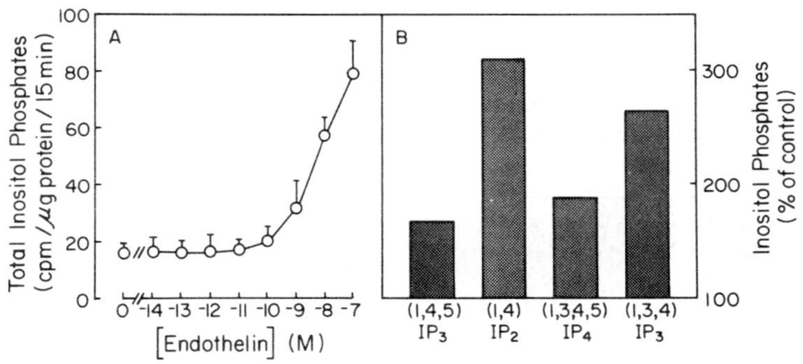

Fig. 3A,B. ET-1 activates phospholipase C to produce inositol phosphate (*InsP*) isomers. **A** Dose-dependence of total InsP turnover following addition of 0.1 μM ET-1 **B** Distribution of InsP isomers 30 sec after addition of ET-1. InsP isomers were analyzed by high pressure liquid chromatography as described in [20]. (From [18] with permission)

produces at least two second messengers: (*i*) the neutral diacylglycerol, which remains within the plane of the plasma membrane and activates protein kinase C, and (*ii*) the water-soluble Ins(1,4,5)P_3, which diffuses and binds to a receptor-gated Ca^{2+} channel to release Ca^{2+} from specialized stores within the endoplasmic reticulum, or calciosome [26]. Induction of the phosphoinositide cascade undoubtedly mediates many of the biological actions of ETs, and the next section discusses the complex patterns of Ca^{2+} signaling by ET peptides.

Ca^{2+} Signaling by ET Peptides

ETs and Sarafotoxin S6b Increase $[Ca^{2+}]_i$ by Two Distinct Mechanisms

We investigated Ca^{2+} signaling by ET peptides in mesangial cells loaded with the fluorescent Ca^{2+} indicator, fura-2 [20,27,28]. As shown in Fig. 4, ET isopeptides cause a biphasic increase in $[Ca^{2+}]_i$ consisting of a rapid (2–5s) spike increase followed by a lesser but sustained phase. Similar results are observed with all ET peptides and Sb6 [27]. The duration of the sustained phase was especially pronounced with ET-1 and ET-2; in some coverslips $[Ca^{2+}]_i$ returned to basal levels only after 20 min (Fig. 4). ET-1-induced Ca^{2+} signaling required conversion of proET-1 to ET-1 [27]. The peak $\Delta[Ca^{2+}]_i$ was dose-dependent with ET-2 $\approx$ ET-1 > S6b > ET-3, demonstrating that ET isopeptides and S6b evoke similar elevations of $[Ca^{2+}]_i$ in mesangial cells but with dissimilar potencies and kinetics.

Two distinct but interdependent mechanisms contribute to ET-induced increments in $[Ca^{2+}]_i$. First, ET stimulates release of Ca^{2+} from intracellular stores, presumably via the action of Ins(1,4,5)P_3 to gate an intracellular Ca^{2+} channel in calciosomes. Second, ET increases influx of extracellular Ca^{2+} into the cytosol. ET-activated Ca^{2+} influx appears to occur through plasma membrane Ca^{2+} ion channels, which might also allow influx of other ions (see below). It is important to note, however, that these two mechanisms work in concert to produce an integrated Ca^{2+} signal. For example, the spike increase in $[Ca^{2+}]_i$ results from both intracellular release of Ca^{2+} *and* extracellular influx of Ca^{2+}, whereas the sustained phase of $[Ca^{2+}]_i$ depends on extracellular influx [27].

Mechanisms of ET-Induced Ca^{2+} Entry

Influx of Ca^{2+} from the extracellular space can occur through voltage-operated channels or through receptor-operated, voltage-independent channels [28]. Our experiments in cultured rat and human mesangial cells demonstrate that ET promotes Ca^{2+} entry via receptor-operated Ca^{2+} channels [27,28]. By using Mn^{2+} as a probe of Ca^{2+}-permeable channels [27,29], we documented rapid (<5 s) increases in Ca^{2+} influx following activation of ET receptors. Endothelin-mediated Ca^{2+} influx occurs independent of dihydropyridine- and voltage-sensitive Ca^{2+} chennels and did not require prior release of intracellular Ca^{2+}. Although the biochemical mechanisms and functions of receptor-mediated Ca^{2+} entry are incompletely understood [26,28], it seems likely that receptor-mediated Ca^{2+} entry by ET contributes to rapid or localized Ca^{2+} signaling or to maintenance of the sustained elevation of $[Ca^{2+}]_i$. It is important to note that in vascular smooth muscle cells ET not only activates receptor-mediated

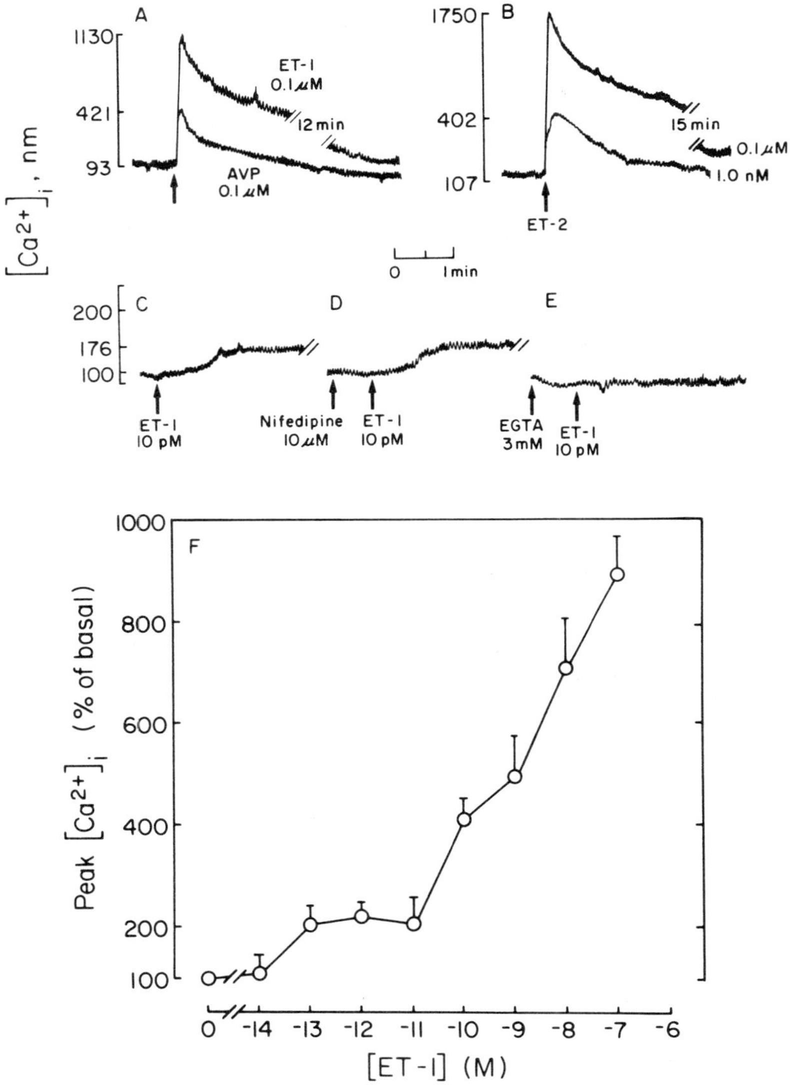

Fig. 4A-F. ET peptide evokes Ca^{2+} signaling in glomerular mesangial cells. Changes in cytosolic free $[Ca^{2+}]_i$ were measured in mesangial cells loaded with the fluorescent probe, fura-2. **A,B** Biphasic increases in $[Ca^{2+}]_i$ by ET-1 and ET-2 **C-E** Slow but sustained increases in $[Ca^{2+}]_i$ in response to low concentrations of ET-1 **F** Dose-dependence of peak $[Ca^{2+}]_i$ in response to ET-1. (From [18] with permission)

Ca^{2+} entry but also indirectly modulates the activity of L-type voltage-operated Ca^{2+} channels [30,31]. Thus, ET evokes multiple, cell-specific pathways of Ca^{2+} influx to produce diverse Ca^{2+} signals.

ET Causes Oscillations of $[Ca^{2+}]_i$ in Human Mesangial Cell Monolayers

In human mesangial cells high concentrations of ET-1 and ET-2 (0.1 μM) stimulate periodic oscillations of $[Ca^{2+}]_i$ following the spike increase [29]. These oscillations can be initiated but not sustained in the absence of extracellular Ca^{2+}. Oscillations induced by ET are especially interesting in that they occur in monolayers and represent synchronized Ca^{2+} signaling in a population of cells, as opposed to the commonly observed oscillations at a single cell level [26]. Similar results with different hormones have been observed in monolayers of ciliated tracheal epithelium [32] and cardiac trabeculae [33], and it seems likely that in human mesangial cells the ET-stimulated increment in $[Ca^{2+}]_i$ passes through gap junctions to trigger a wave of Ca^{2+} in neighboring cells. In this way ET peptides might recruit local populations of mesangial cells to function as a synctium.

ET Stimulates Contraction via Pharmacomechanical Coupling

What biological actions are triggered by ET-induced Ca^{2+} increments? Collectively, the observations that ET stimulates phospholipase C and elevates $[Ca^{2+}]_i$ suggest that ET causes contraction in mesangial cells via pharmacomechanical coupling [19]. This hypothesis is supported by the observation that contraction in response to ET occurs only at concentrations that stimulate phospholipase C. Elevation of $[Ca^{2+}]_i$ with ionomycin, to similar concentrations of $[Ca^{2+}]_i$ observed with ET, also stimulates contraction. Most important, however, ET-induced contraction is unaffected by dihydropyridine Ca^{2+} channel blockers and occurs under conditions where mesangial cells demonstrate little or no voltage-operated Ca^{2+} channel activity [19,27]. While a role for Ca^{2+} in the vasoactive properties of ET seems clear, a link between the phosphoinositide cascade and mitogenesis is less certain. Further work is necessary to evaluate alternative pathways of signal transduction in the mitogenic response to ET.

Down-Regulation of ET-Induced Ca^{2+} Signaling

The previous section discussed the mechanisms by which ET elevates $[Ca^{2+}]_i$, but, like most transduction systems, ET-mediated Ca^{2+} signaling is tightly regulated. At least three major mechanisms function as negative-feedback signals to regulate Ca^{2+} signaling by ET peptides.

Protein Kinase C (PKC)-Dependent Attenuation of Ca^{2+} Signaling

Protein Kinase C is a Ca^{2+}- and phospholipid-dependent protein kinase that modulates Ca^{2+} channel activity and Ca^{2+} signaling [26]. Phorbol esters and diacyglycerol analogs, which activate protein kinase C, fail to increase $[Ca^{2+}]_i$ in mesangial cells loaded with fura-2, suggesting that PKC does not independently increase $[Ca^{2+}]_i$ [27]. However, a 1 min preincubation with phorbol esters or diacyglycerol analogs markedly attenuates both the spike and sustained phases of Ca^{2+} signaling by ET peptides. The number and affinity of ET binding sites are unaffected by preincubation with phorbol esters (Baldi and Dunn, unpublished work). Thus, these data suggest a role for PKC in down-regulating ET-induced increments in $[Ca^{2+}]_i$. Further support for this hypothesis comes from studies in cells depleted of PKC to test the *requirement* of PKC activity in ET-activated Ca^{2+} signaling. In cells depleted of PKC, ET-1 stimulates greater increases of $[Ca^{2+}]_i$ than in concurrent controls. Because Mn^{2+} influx was similar in control and PKC-depleted cells, we conclude that activation of PKC by ET acts as a negative feedback signal to attenuate release of Ca^{2+} from intracellular stores [27]. The exact mechanism by which PKC down-regulates Ca^{2+} signaling remains unclear, but it might relate to heterologous effects on phosphoinositide metabolism [26] or it might act by inhibiting refilling of intracellular Ca^{2+} stores.

PKC-Independent Desensitization by ET Ligands

Desensitization (i.e., tachyphalyxis) induced by ligands is a common adaptive response to many hormones and neurotransmitters, including ET [27,29]. Endothelin isopeptides and S6b desensitize the increase in $[Ca^{2+}]_i$ caused by subsequent additions of the same ET agonist. In fact, preincubation with any ET isopeptide or S6b (0.1 μM) diminishes the $[Ca^{2+}]_i$ increase stimulated by the subsequent, eqimolar addition of any other isopeptide. Even low concentrations of ET-3 (10 nM), which produce only a modest increase in $[Ca^{2+}]_i$, markedly reduce the Ca^{2+} signal produced by 0.1 μM ET-2. Ligand-mediated desensitization persists in cells depleted of PKC, suggesting that this adaptive response is independent of PKC [27]. Many investigators report complex, partially irreversible binding of ET to its receptor [2,3]. Thus, continued receptor occupancy might account for some of the desensitization observed in our studies. Further experiments are necessary to define the exact mechanisms involved.

ET-Dependent Ca^{2+} Efflux Pathway(s)

In preliminary experiments we have used an inhibitor of the endoplasmic reticular Ca^{2+}-ATPase – 2,5-Di-(tert-buty)-1,4-benzohydroquinone (tBuBHQ) – to identify a Ca^{2+} efflux pathway stimulated by ET [27]. In diverse cell types tBuBHQ causes a sustained increase in $[Ca^{2+}]_i$ by preventing reuptake into the intracellular stores [34]. When ET is added to mesangial cells during the tBuBHQ-stimulated increase in $[Ca^{2+}]_i$ it causes a steady decline in $[Ca^{2+}]_i$ to basal levels [27]. That ET-stimulated Ca^{2+} influx is unaffected by tBuBHQ is confirmed by measurements of Mn^{2+} influx. Taken together, these data demonstrate that ET-stimulated Ca^{2+} signaling is attenuated by a ligand-mediated Ca^{2+} efflux pathway independent of Ca^{2+} reuptake into the microsomal pool. This pathway might constitute a mechanism whereby ET terminates its own Ca^{2+} signal. Similar results have been observed by Kass et al. [34] for other Ca^{2+}-mobilizing hormones.

Other Pathways of Signal Transducation

Studies in mesangial cells show that an increase in $[Ca^{2+}]_i$ following activation of ET receptors is only one of several possible pathways of transmembrane signaling for ET peptides. Although the increase in $[Ca^{2+}]_i$ undoubtedly mediates some short-term actions of ET peptides such as secretion and contraction [2,3,19,35], other potential pathways have been described. In mesangial [19] and other cells [2,3] ET fails to stimulate adenylate cyclase. However, ET-1 can potentiate β-adrenergic-stimulated cAMP accumulation via a mechanism involving PGE_2 [19]. Endothelin-1 is also a potent stimulus for phospholipase A_2 [19], which increases the free concentration of arachidonate to provide substrate for the cyclooxygenase and lipoxygenase pathways. Endothelin also stimulates phospholipase D activity to increase the intracellular concentration of phosphatidic acid (Kester et al., unpublished work). The increase in phosphatidic acid might contribute to the sustained increase in $[Ca^{2+}]_i$ following addition of ET peptides. Given the mitogenic action of ET in some target cells, it is interesting to note that ET stimulates electroneutral Na^+/H^+ exchange in mesangial cells [20]. In addition, the finding that ET is a mitogen for mesangial cells [20] demonstrates that ET differentially regulates gene expression to produce long-lasting response as well. In this vein it is worth noting that ET induces the gene for *c-fos* [20]. *c-Fos* is the prototype for a group of inducible genes (i.e., "immediate-early" genes) that convert short-term transmembrane signals into long-term responses requiring transcriptional regulation of target genes (See [36]). Thus activation of the "immediate-early" genes by ET peptides could play an important role in altering cell plasticity and in regulating long-term adaptive responses.

Conclusions

Cultured mesangial cells provide a useful model for investigating the cell biology of ET peptides. Although our knowledge of many components is incomplete, the outline of ET-activated pathways of signal transduction is clear and bears striking resemblance to phosphoinositide-linked signaling systems activated by other regulatory peptides. It is well-documented that ET peptides evoke complex patterns of Ca^{2+} signaling, mediating contractile and/or motile responses, but evidence regarding the role of other transduction systems remains meager. Further research into the mechanisms of cellular signaling employed by ET peptides should reveal how these peptides elicit such diverse biological events in target cells.

Acknowledgments. We gratefully acknowledge the advice and collaboration of our colleagues Drs. George Dubyak, Antonio Scarpa, Elizabetta Baldi, Mark Kester, Paolo Mene', John Sedor, and Shianq Wann. The original work, from the authors' laboratory, presented in this review was supported by National Institutes of Health Grants HL-22563 and HL-37117 to M.J.D.

References

1. Yanagisawa M, Kurihara H, Kimura S, Tombe Y, Kobayashi M, Mitsui Y, Yazaki Y, Goto K, Masaki T (1988) A novel potent vasoconstrictor peptide produced by vascular endothelial cells. Nature 332:411–415

2. Yanagisawa M, Masaki T (1989) Endothelin, a novel endothelium-derived peptide. Biochem Pharmacol 38:1877–1883
3. Simonson MS, Dunn MJ (1990) Cellular signaling by peptides of the endothelin gene family. FASEB J 4:2989–3000
4. Yanagisawa M. Akihiro I, Ishikawa T, Kasuya Y, Kimura S, Kumagaye SH, Nakajima K, Watanabe T, Sakakibara S, Goto K, Masaki T (1988) Primary structure, synthesis and biological activity of rat endothelin, and endothelium-derived vasoconstrictor peptide. Proc Natl Acad Sci USA 85:6964–6967
5. Inoue A, Yanagisawa M, Kimura S, Kasuya Y, Miyauchi T, Goto K, Masaki T (1989) The human endothelin family: Three structurally and pharmacologically distinct isopeptides predicted by three separate genes. Proc Natl Acad Sci USA 86:2863–2867
6. Saida K, Mitsui Y, Ishida N (1989) A novel peptide, vasoactive intestinal constrictor, of a new (endothelin) peptide family. J Biol Chem 264:14613–14616
7. Kloog Y, Sokolovsky M (1989) Similarities in mode and sites of action of sarafotoxins and endothelins. Trends Pharmacol Sci 10:212–214
8. MacCumber MW, Ross CA, Glaser BM, Synder SH (1989) Endothelin: Visualization of mRNAs by in situ hybridization provides evidence for local action. Proc Natl Acad Sci USA 86:7285–7289
9. Kosaka T, Suzuki N, Matasumoto H, Itoh Y, Yasuhara T, Onda H, Fujino M (1989) Synthesis of the vascoconstrictor peptide endothelin in kidney cells. FEBS Lett 249:42–46
10. Shichiri M, Hirata Y, Emori T, Ohta K, Nakajima T, Sato K, Sato A, Marumo F (1989) Secretion of endothelin and related peptides from renal epithelial cell lines. FEBS Lett 253:203–206
11. Giaid A, Gibson SJ, Ibrahim N, Legon S, Bloom SR, Yanagisawa M, Masaki T, Varndell IM, Polak JM (1989) Endothelin 1, an endothelium-derived peptide, is expressed in neurons of the human spinal cord and dorsal root ganglia. Proc Natl Acad Sci USA 86:7634–7638
12. MacCumber MW, Ross CA, Snyder SH (1990) Endothelin in brain: Receptors, mitogenesis, and biosynthesis in glial cells. Proc Natl Acad Sci USA 87:2359–2363
13. Yoshizawa T, Shinmi O, Giaid A, Yanagisawa M, Gibson SJ, Kimura S, Uchiyama Y, Polak JM, Masaki T, Kanazawa I (1990) Endothelin: A novel peptide in the posterior pituitary system. Science 247:462–464
14. Kurihara H, Yoshizumi M, Sugiyama T, Takaku F, Yanagisawa M, Masaki T, Hamaoki M, Kato H, Yazaki Y (1989) Transforming growth factor-b stimulates the expression of endothelin mRNA by vascular endothelial cells. Biochem Biophys Res Commun 159:1435–1440
15. Yoshizuma M, Kurihara H, Sugiyama T, Takaku F, Yanagisawa M, Masaki T, Yazaki Y (1989) Hemodynamic shear stress stimulates endothelin production by cultured endothelial cells. Biochem Biophys Res Commun 161:859–864
16. Schini VB, Hendrickson H, Heublein DM, Burnett JC, Vanhoutte PM (1989) Thrombin enhances the release of endothelin from cultured porcine aortic endothelial cells. Eur J Pharmacol 165:2–3
17. Seuwen K, Pouyssegur J (1990) Serotonin as a growth factor. Biochem Pharmacol 39:985–990
18. Simonson MS, Dunn MJ (1990) Endothelin: Pathways of transmembrane signaling. Hypertension 15(Suppl 1):I5–I12
19. Simonson MS, Dunn MJ (1990) Endothelin-1 stimulates contraction of rat glomerular mesangial cells and potentiates b-adrenergic-mediated cyclic adenosine monophosphate accumulation. J Clin Invest 85:790–797
20. Simonson MS, Wann S, Mene P, Dubyak G, Kester M, Nakazato Y, Sedor JR, Dunn MJ (1989) Endothelin stimulates phospholipase C, Na^+/H^+ exchange, c-fos expression, and mitogenesis in rat mesangial cells. J Clin Invest 83:708–712

21. Badr KF, Murray JJ, Breyer MD, Takahashi K, Inagami T, Harris RC (1989) Mesangial cell, glomerular, and renal vascular responses to endothelin in the kidney. J Clin Invest 83:336–342
22. Takuwa N, Takuwa Y, Yanagisawa M, Yamashita K, Masaki T (1989) A novel vasoactive peptide endothelin stimulates mitogenesis through inositol lipid turnover in Swiss 3T3 fibroblasts. J Biol Chem 264:7856–7861
23. Brown KD, Littlewood CJ (1989) Endothelin stimulates DNA synthesis in Swiss 3T3 cells. Synergy with polypeptide growth factors. Biochem J 263:977–980
24. Komuro I, Kurihara H, Sugiyama T, Takaku F, Yazaki Y (1988) Endothelin stimulates c-fos and c-myc expression and proliferation of vascular smooth muscle cells. FEBS Lett 238:249–252
25. Dubin D, Pratt RE, Cooke JP, Dzau VJ (1989) Endothelin, a potent vasoconstrictor, is a vascular smooth muscle mitogen. J Vasc Med Biol 1:150–154
26. Berridge MJ, Irvine RF (1990) Inositol phosphates and cell signaling. Nature 341:197–205
27. Simonson MS, Dunn MJ (to be published) Ca^{2+} signaling by distinct endothelin peptides in glomerular mesangial cells. Exp Cell Res
28. Hallam TJ, Rink TJ (1989) Receptor-mediated Ca^{2+} entry: diversity of function and mechanism. Trends Pharmacol Sci 10:8–10
29. Simonson MS, Osnai T, Dunn MJ (to be published) Endothelin isopeptides evoke Ca^{2+} signaling and oscillations of cytosolic free $[Ca^{2+}]$ in human mesangial cells. Biochim Biophys Acta
30. Silberberg SD, Poder TC, Lacerda AE (1989) Endothelin increases single-channel calcium currents in coronary arterial smooth muscle cells. FEBS Lett 247:68–72
31. Inoue Y, Oike M, Nakao K, Kitamura K, Kuriyama H (1990) Endothelin augments unitary calcium channel currents on the smooth muscle cell membrane of guinea-pig portal vein. J Physiol (Lond) 423:171–191
32. Sanderson MJ, Chow I, Dirksen ER (1988) Intercellular communication between ciliated cells in culture. Am J Physiol 254:C63–C74
33. Mulder BJM, deTombe PP, terKeurs HE (1989) Spontaneous and propagated contractions in rat cardiac trabeculae. J Gen Physiol 93:943–961
34. Kass GEN, Duddy SK, Moore GA, Orrenius S (1989) 2,5-Di-(tert-butyl)-1,4-benzohydroquinone rapidly elevates cytosolic Ca^{2+} concentration by mobilizing the inositol 1,4,5-trisphosphate-sensitive Ca^{2+} pool. J Biol Chem 264:15192–15198
35. Stojilkovic SS, Merelli F, Iida T, Krsmanovic LZ, Catt KJ (1990) Endothelin stimulation of cytosolic calcium and gonadotropin secretion in anterior pituitary cells. Science 248:1663–1666
36. Sassone-Corsi P, Lamph WW, Verma IM (1988) Regulation of proto-oncogene fos: A paradigm for early response genes. Cold Spring Harbor Symp Quant Biol 53:749–760

Endothelin Action and Production in Renal Tubular Cells

Shunya Uchida, Masahiro Naruse, Shinya Kaname, Mitsuko Horie, Etsuro Ogata[1], Kiyoshi Kurokawa[2], Masashi Yanagisawa, and Tomoh Masaki[3]

SUMMARY. Recent studies suggest that the renal tubule is not only a target of endothelin-1 (ET-1) but is also a possible source of endothelin. Thus, we attempted to detect specific preproET-1 messenger RNA (mRNA) as well as immunoreactive ET-1 secretion in renal epithelial cell lines. Madin-Darby canine kidney (MDCK) cells expressed a single 2.3 kb preproET-1 mRNA. In medium conditioned by MDCK for 24 hours there was a significant amount of immunoreactive ET-1 detected by sandwich type immunoassay. Both mRNA expression and mature ET-1 secretion were stimulated by an addition of transforming growth factor (TGF)-β to the basolateral side in a time-dependent manner, but the increase in peptide secretion lagged behind ET-1 mRNA expression by several hours. The basal secretion of ET-1 was polarized, with 2.3-fold greater secretion into the basolateral side over the apical side, while the difference was augmented to 7.5-fold by TGF-β. In contrast, LLC-PK_1 (pig kidney) cells secreted little ET-1 associated with a lower level of ET-1 mRNA expression. Regarding the effect of ET-1, it elicited $[Ca^{2+}]_i$ transients in LLC-PK_1, but not in MDCK. These data clearly show that renal tubules can express preproET-1 mRNA, synthesize mature ET-1, and secrete it preferentially to the basolateral side of the tubule cells, all of which are enhanced by TGF-β. The data suggest that ET-1 produced by the renal tubule may function as a paracrine hormone in regulating tubular functions.

Introduction

Direct renal tubular action of endothelin has been documented recently and it has been found that endothelin may play possible important roles in the renal tubules.

---

[1]Fourth and [2]First Departments of Internal Medicine, University of Tokyo School of Medicine, 3-28-6 Mejirodai, Bunkyo-ku, Tokyo, 112 Japan

[3]Department of Pharmacology, Institute of Basic Medical Sciences, University of Tsukuba, Ibaraki, 112 Japan

Endothelin tubular action was first speculated by others and ourselves, based on hemodynamic data, using in vivo perfusion studies [1–3]. Thus it has been shown that despite falls in glomerular filtration rate (GFR) and renal plasma flow (RPF), (FE_{Na}) did not decline. This finding implied possible inhibition by endothelin of Na reabsorption in the terminal segment of the tubule. Also, a binding study of endothelin in the whole kidney revealed intensive binding to inner medulla in addition to glomeruli. The direct action of endothelin was demonstrated by Zeidel and his colleagues [4]. They found that ET may inhibit ouabain-sensitive Na^+-K^+-ATPase in inner medullary collecting duct (IMCD) cells, since it inhibited oxygen consumption. More recently Tomita et al., using rat intact tubules, found that ET inhibits vasopressin-stimulated cAMP production in the same nephron segments [5]. These data indicate that ET acts directly on renal tubules, especially in the collecting ducts.

Since ET was originally identified in endothelial cells by Yanagisawa and his colleagues [6], many cell types were found to be capable of producing it. Regarding ET production in the kidney, ET-like immunoreactivity was first extracted, by high-performance liquid chromatography (HPLC), from the inner medulla of pig and rat kidney [7]. This finding, however, suggests two possibilities; production and/or strong binding of ET in inner medulla. Using cultured cells, Kosaka, Suzuki, and their colleagues demonstrated that several epithelial cell lines, including renal tubular epithelial cell line MDCK, could produce ET-1 [8,9]. Similar results were reported by Shichiri et al. using another renal epithelial line, LLC-PK_1 [10]. Thus, it is possible that renal tubules, probably collecting duct cells, are not only a target of ET-1, but also a possible site of ET-1 production.

Therefore, we first examined the direct action of ET-1 on the tubules by monitoring cell calcium in response to ET-1, because the 2nd messenger of ET signal transduction in many cell types is now widely accepted to be an increase in cell calcium.

Furthermore, we examined ET-1 gene expression in MDCK cells as a renal tubular cell model. We used a cultured cell line because it is impossible to obtain a sufficient amount of mRNA for Northern hybridization from microdissected nephron segments.

Methods

Isolation of Individual Nephron Segments

Kidney slices from 4–6 week old male mice were incubated at 37°C for 10min in HHM (Hanks buffer containing Eagle's minimum essential medium (MEM), amino acids and vitamins, 10mM HEPES, 0.1% bovine serum albumin (BSA) and 0.1% collagenase. Dissection and identification of individual nephron segments were performed under a stereomicroscope in ice-cold HHM-BSA buffer within 40 min of sacrifice of the animal. A few pieces of 0.5–1.0mm long tubules were transferred onto thin glass slips and were kept on ice until use.

Cell Culture

MDCK (ATCC CCL34) and LLC-PK_1 cell lines (ATCC CL101) were cultivated in standard Dulbecco's modified Eagle's medium supplemented with 10% fetal calf serum (FCS) (regular DMEM) under humidified 5%CO_2/95%air.

Measurements of Intracellular Free Calcium Concentration

Isolated tubules or cultured cells, both attached on glass slips, were incubated with 10mM fura-2/AM (Dojin Biochemical, Kumamoto, Japan) at 37°C for 30–60min. The glass slip was then superfused on the microscope stage at 37°C with a solution containing 137 NaCl, 6 KCl, 1.2 $CaCl_2$, 1.0 $MgCl_2$, 5.5 glucose, and 20 HEPES (in mM) at pH 7.4. Cells were excited at 340 and 380 nm and emission was monitored at 500nm using a photon detector–CAM-220 (Nippon Bunko, Tokyo). $[Ca^{2+}]_i$ was calculated using the formula described by Grynkiewicz et al. [11].

Isolation of Total RNA and Purification of Poly(A)⁺ RNA from MDCK and Cultured Mesangial Cells

At the end of the experimental incubation, cells were harvested for total RNA extraction by means of guanidine thiocyanate/CsCl cushion centrifuge at 25000 rpm for 18h at 20°C. Poly$(A)^+$ RNA was purified using oligo-dT column chromatography.

Northern Blots

Five μg of poly$(A)^+$ RNA was size fractionated on a 1% agarose, 2.2M formaldehyde denaturing gel, and transferred by capillary blotting to Biodyne Transfer Membrane. For detecting preproET-1 mRNA, we used 1.8kb EcoR1 fragments of a full length cDNA for preproET-1 cloned from porcine aorta endothelial cells [6]. In order to normalize the preproET-1 signals for loaded amounts and transfer efficiencies, β-actin mRNA levels were used [12]. PreproET-1 and β-actin cDNA probes were nick-translated using a kit (Amersham, Buckinghamshire, U.K.) and $[\alpha\text{-}^{32}P]$dCTP (10mCi/ml, New England Nuclear, Wilmington, Del).

Prehybridization was carried out at 42°C for 3–4 hours, and hybridization was carried out at 42°C overnight (usually $>$12h). Washes were conducted with 1x SSC, 0.1% SDS, five times at room temperature; and with 0.1x SSC, 0.1% SDS, at 42°C for 30min. Autoradiography exposures were carried out for several days with two intensifying screens at −80°C.

Assay for Immunoreactive Endothelin-1 and Big-Endothelin-1

After 24 hours of incubation the medium was collected for assay. Cell proteins lysed in 0.5ml 1N NaOH were measured using a kit (Bio-Rad, Richmond, Calif.) with γ-globulin as standard. Enzyme-linked immunoassays (EIA) for ET-1 and big-ET-1 were essentially the same as reported elsewhere [9,13]. Cross reactivities of ET-1 EIA for ET-3, big-ET-1, and so-called ET-related peptides, and those of big-ET-1 EIA for ET-1, ET-3, and ET-related peptides were all less than 0.5% [9].

Polarity of Endothelin Secretion

To examine from which side of the cells ET-1 might be secreted, MDCK cells were grown to confluence on collagen (rat tail, type I, Collaborative Research, Boston, Mass.) coated Millicell-CM (Millipore Products Division, Bedford, Mass.). Each bath contained 2ml culture medium to equal the levels of both media. Permeability of the monolayers was ascertained by lack of leakiness of creatinine, where 0.4mM creatinine was placed only in the basolateral bath. In some experiments, 200pM TGF-β (TGF-β1; human platelets, R & D Systems, Minneapolis, Minn.) was added to either the apical or the basolateral bath.

Analysis of Data and Statistics

Each experiment consisted of at least three separate experiments. Data are presented as mean ± SD, and were analyzed using paired or unpaired *t*-tests as appropriate. *P* values less than 0.05 were considered significant.

Results

ET-1 Evoked Ca^{2+} Transients in Mouse Collecting Ducts

Using isolated tubules we found that ET-1 elicited Ca^{2+} transients in cortical, outer medullary, and inner medullary collecting ducts microdissected from mouse kidneys. Other tubule segments failed to increase cell Ca^{2+}. Cell Ca^{2+} increase was biphasic, with an initial peak and second sustained phase, and the response was dose-dependent between 10^{-9}M and 10^{-6}M ET-1. By removing extracellular Ca^{2+} in concert with addition of 0.5mM EDTA to the superfusate, cell Ca^{2+} increase was markedly abolished.

We previously demonstrated that arginine vasopressin (AVP) elicited Ca^{2+} transients in the cortical collecting ducts through both V_1 and V_2 receptors [14]. The effect of ET-1 on a rise in cell Ca^{2+} was independent of that of AVP. There was no additive activity regarding the effects of ET-1 and AVP. Moreover the second challenge of ET-1 failed to evoke Ca^{2+} increase, data consistent with the notion that ET does not easily dissociate from the receptors once it is bound. Thus, we speculate that these two peptide hormones increase cell Ca^{2+} by distinct mechanisms. Since ET-1 inhibits AVP-stimulated cAMP production in collecting ducts, these two peptides may act on the same cell type, probably on principal cells.

PreproET-1 mRNA Expression and ET-1 Secretion

A single 2.3kb preproET-1 mRNA was clearly expressed at the basal state in MDCK cells. This size was compatible with the one expressed in endothelial cells. TGF-β (200pM), one of the known stimulators for preproET-1 mRNA in endothelial cells, markedly upregulated this mRNA level by several-fold in 6 hours.

An increased mRNA level following 100pM TGF-β was observed as early as 30min, the earliest time point tested. TGF-β increased preproET-1 mRNA dose-dependently in 6 hours, the maximal effect appearing at 20pM and a half maximal effect at 10pM. This is regarded as a physiological concentration.

In fact, MDCK secreted mature ET-1 into the medium. TGF-β increased this secretion 2–3 times at 24 hours. It is of interest that TGF-β had no effect within 6 hours, despite dramatic upregulation of ET-1 mRNA. Thus, there seems to be a time lag of some several hours between the mRNA level and mature ET-1 secretion.

The rate of ET-1 secretion was also examined. Secretion rate was virtually unchanged until 6–12 hours after TGF-β addition, when it began to rise steeply; the rate remained several-fold greater than the basal level for up to 4 days, unless TGF-β was removed. The peak response occurred at around 2 days.

The mechanism whereby TGF-β increases mRNA level is generally thought to be a transcriptional regulation. However, since the half life of preproET-1 mRNA is quite short, actually 15 min, degradation of the transcripts may also be regulated. We investigated the change in half life of preproET-1 mRNA after TGF-β treatment.

PreproET-1 mRNA declined after addition of 10μg/ml actinomycin D to MDCK cells with or without TGF-β. However, preproET-1 mRNA was less degraded in TGF-β treated cells than in control cells. Apparent half lives were 15 min in the basal condition and longer than 30 min in the TGF-β treated condition. Similar mechanisms have been shown in other cell types for procollagen mRNA upregulation by TGF-β.

Effects of TPA on PreproET-1 mRNA and Peptides

Phorbol esters, stimulators of protein kinase C, upregulate preproET-1 mRNA rapidly and dramatically in endothelial cells [15]. Therefore, we examined the effect of TPA, one of the phorbol esters, on the mRNA levels in MDCK.

At as early as 15–30min, 0.5μM TPA increased the preproET-1 mRNA level, which reached a maximum at 45min, and then decreased below control level. No messages were found between 2 and 6 hours. These results are consistent with results reported previously using endothelial cells [15]. We next examined whether this rapid and short increase in preproET-1 mRNA was associated with actual secretion of mature peptides. ET-1 and big-ET-1 secretion from MDCK treated with TPA increased by as early as 1 hour and then by 6 hours it reached the maximum. Although peptide secretion lagged behind mRNA expression, the time courses of ET-1 and big-ET-1 secretion agree well with the profile of the mRNA time course obtained in phorbol ester experiments. The transient increases in mRNA and mature peptide secretion induced by TPA are probably due to a depletion of protein kinase C substrates.

ET-1 Secretion Was Polarized in MDCK Monolayers

One of the characteristics of epithelial cells is that they form cell polarity. Thus, we were interested in seeing to which side of the cells ET-1 secreted. To this end we utilized permeable filter chambers, which allow the separate collection of two compartments, apical baths and basolateral baths. At basal state ET-1 was released to the basolateral side twice as much as to the apical bath. Then 200pM TGF-β was added either to the apical or to the basolateral bath and cells were incubated for 24 hours; media were collected after the last 6 hours. When TGF-β was added to the apical bath, no changes were observed. However, when it was added to the basolateral bath, the amount of ET-1 secreted to the basolateral side of the monolayers increased 3–4-fold, whereas the amount in the apical bath did not increase. Thus, a stimulus like TGF-β may increase ET-1 secretion exclusively to the basolateral or to the capillary side of epithelial cells. The data also suggest that MDCK cells may have TGF-β receptors at the basolateral membranes.

ET-1 Evoked Ca^{2+} Transients in LLC-PK_1 Cells

The pattern of Ca^{2+} rise was quite similar to the patterns seen in intact collecting ducts. Again, ET-elicited Ca^{2+} transient was independent of AVP-evoked Ca^{2+} increase. Furthermore there was no additive activity of these two agonists. In contrast, MDCK cells, which produce substantial amounts of ET-1, failed to respond to ET-1. However, despite a lack of response to ET-1, MDCK cells dramatically increased cell Ca^{2+} when bradykinin was used as a positive control.

Discussion

The results of the present study clearly indicate that MDCK cells, a cell line of canine renal tubular origin, clearly express ET-1 mRNA and are capable of producing and secreting mature ET-1. The mRNA we detected was ~2.3 kb, a size compatible with preproET-1 mRNA [6]. Recent studies have shown that the kidney may express mRNAs for both ET-1 and ET-3 and that the sizes of these mRNAs were ~2.3 kb and ~3.7 kb, respectively ([16], M. Yanagisawa, unpublished work). The cDNA probe used in the present study is specific to ET-1 mRNA, and does not hybridize 3.7 kb transcripts of ET-3. Therefore, the present results do not exclude the possibility of ET-3 mRNA expression in MDCK.

The results achieved by using a specific enzyme-immunoassay for ET-1 clearly demonstrate that MDCK cells secrete mature ET-1, data consistent with an earlier report by Kosaka et al. [8]. Our present EIA system is specific to ET-1 and ET-2, and does not detect ET-3. Taken together with the mRNA data, our present findings show specific production of ET-1 by MDCK cells, but do not exclude a possible production of ET-3 by these cells.

The mRNA expression of ET-1 and secretion of ET-1 by MDCK cells increased in response to TGF-β in a time-dependent manner. Recent observations of ET-1 production and secretion have shown that ET-1 is released in response to stimuli such as thrombin, catecholamine, and TGF-β, and is not stored in the intracellular organelles such as secretory granules. Rather, ET-1 secretion occurs constitutively, so that mRNA level is a predominant determinant of ET-1 production and secretion. Our present findings in MDCK cells are consistent with this current notion of ET-1 production and secretion.

Using a specific device which allows examination of the polarized function of epithelial cells, we found that MDCK cells secrete ET-1 predominantly to the basolateral side of the cells under the basal, unstimulated condition, as well as in response to stimulation by TGF-β. At the basal state, the ratio of ET-1 secreted into the basolateral side of the cells to that secreted into the apical side was 2:3. In response to TGF-β, ET-1 mRNA level increased several-fold in 6 hours and polarized ET-1 secretion into the basolateral bath was 7.5-fold that into the apical bath between 18 and 24 hours. These data demonstrate that increased ET-1 mRNA expression with TGF-β is associated with almost exclusive increase in ET-1 secretion to the basolateral side of the epithelia with little increase in its secretion to the apical side. These data thus suggest that, in addition to the constitutive secretory process present both in the apical and in the basolateral membranes, there must exist a specific mechanism which, following certain stimuli, augments ET-1 secretion

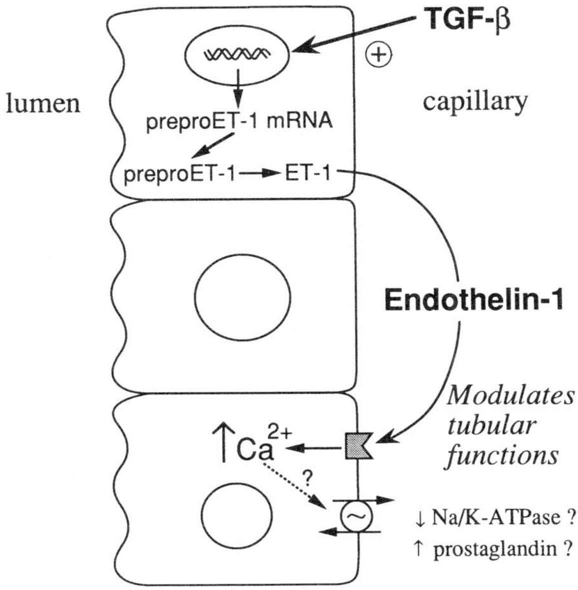

Fig. 1. Schematic model of ET-1 synthesis and secretion, and its paracrine function in the renal tubules. ET-1 can be synthesized in a tubular cell type at the basal state. TGF-β is capable of stimulating preproET-1 mRNA level, both at transcriptional steps and by inhibiting preproET-1 mRNA degradation. Mature ET-1 processed from preproET-1 is secreted by a constitutive pathway, with two-fold greater secretion through basolateral membranes, while the enhanced secretion of ET-1 by TGF-β is more polarized, leading newly produced ET-1 to enter the blood stream. Downstream, ET-1 may act on another tubule cell type, via increase in $[Ca^{2+}]_i$, as a paracrine hormone which modulates water and electrolyte transport, cell metabolism, and cell function, possibly including proliferation

preferentially into the basolateral side of the tubular cells. A mechanism which renders de novo ET that enters capillary blood flow seems physiologically tenable, in view of the fact that ET-1 secreted from apical membranes has no chance of exerting its biological effects, since ET-1 appears to act only from the basolateral side of intact renal tubules (M. Naruse, unpublished work).

Stimulation by TGF-β of ET-1 mRNA levels and ET-1 secretion in MDCK cells is similar to the stimulation reported in endothelial cells [17]. Moreover, the effects of TGF-β could be shown only when this growth factor was added to the basolateral side of MDCK cells, indicating the presence of putative TGF-β receptors on this side of the tubular cells.

TGF-β is a unique growth factor, in that this peptide inhibits the cell growth of certain cell types, including renal tubules [18] and mesangial cells [19]. Most recently we found that cultured rat mesangial cells expressed TGF-β mRNA and that this level was stimulated by fetal calf serum and phorbol ester, suggesting its protein kinase C-dependent activation mechanism [20]. Thus, mesangial cells may be one of the intrarenal sources of TGF-β, which may have access to the collecting duct system via the intrarenal circulation. The physiological implications of the axis of TGF-β-ET-1-

collecting duct system await further investigation. However, it is speculated that this system may play some role in tubular growth and fibrosis.

Regarding the action of ET-1, it evoked a transient rise in $[Ca^{2+}]_i$ in LLC-PK_1 cells, but not in MDCK cells, data indicating that LLC-PK_1 cells are a target of ET-1. Moreover, an absence of any effect of additive activity between ET-1 and AVP clearly indicates that these two peptides evoke rises in $[Ca^{2+}]_i$ through different mechanisms. Recent studies have demonstrated massive ET-1 binding in inner medulla as well as in glomeruli [21,22] and have shown direct action of ET-1 on the renal tubules. Indeed, ET-1 has been shown to inhibit Na^+,K^+-ATPase, and thus Na^+ transport, of the inner medullary collecting ducts, through mechanisms dependent on prostaglandin production [4]. The present findings of ET-1-elicited $[Ca^{2+}]_i$ increase in LLC-PK_1 cells support the presence of a direct tubular action of ET-1. More studies are required in order to elucidate the mechanisms of ET-1 action and the effects of ET-1 on specific segments of the nephron.

Our demonstration of the production and preferential, polarized secretion of ET-1, as well as its action on distinct renal tubular cell lines, clearly suggests the possibility that ET-1 produced by the renal tubules may be secreted into the basolateral side of the tubules, thence reaching another tubular segment downstream of the local blood flow, and modulating the function thereof (Fig. 1). Such a scheme suggests possible roles of ET-1 as an intrarenal paracrine hormone regulating renal tubular functions.

References

1. King AJ, Brenner BM, Anderson S (1989) Endothelin: a potent renal and systemic vasoconstrictor peptide. Am J Physiol 256:F1051–F1058
2. Kon V, Yoshioka T, Fogo A, Ichikawa I (1989) Glomerular actions of endothelin in vivo. J Clin Invest 83:1762–1767
3. Katoh T, Chang H, Uchida S, Okuda T, Kurokawa K (1990) Direct effects of endothelin in the rat kidney. Am J Physiol 258:F397–F402
4. Zeidel ML, Brady HR, Kone BC, Gullans SR, Brenner BM (1989) Endothelin, a peptide inhibitor of Na^+-K^+-ATPase in intact renal tubular epithelial cells. Am J Physiol 257:C1101–C1107
5. Tomita K, Nonoguchi H, Marumo F (1990) Effects of endothelin on peptide-dependent cyclic adenosine monophosphate accumulation along the nephron segments of the rat. J Clin Invest 85:2014–2018
6. Yanagisawa M, Kurihara H, Kimura S, Tomobe Y, Kobayashi M, Mitsui Y, Yazaki Y, Goto K, Masaki T (1988) A novel potent vasoconstrictor peptide produced by vascular endothelial cells. Nature 332:411–415
7. Kitamura K, Tanaka T, Kato J, Eto T, Tanaka K (1989) Regional distribution of immunoreactive endothelin in porcine tissue: abundance in inner medulla of kidney. Biochem Biophys Res Commun 161:348–352
8. Kosaka T, Suzuki N, Matsumoto H, Itoh Y, Yasuhara T, Onda H, Fujino M (1989) Synthesis of the vasoconstrictor peptide endothelin in kidney cells. FEBS Lett 249:42–46
9. Suzuki N, Matsumoto H, Kitada C, Kimura S, Fujino M (1989) Production of endothelin-1 and big-endothelin-1 by tumor cells with epithelial-like morphology. J Biochem (Tokyo) 106:736–741
10. Shichiri M, Hirata Y, Emori T, Ohta K, Nakajima T, Sato K, Sato A, Marumo F (1989) Secretion of endothelin and related peptides from renal epithelial cell lines. FEBS Lett 253:203–206

11. Grynkiewicz G, Poenie M, Tsien RY (1985) A new generation of Ca^{2+} indicators with greatly improved fluorescence properties. J Biol Chem 260:3440–3450
12. Nakajima-Iijima S, Hamada H, Reddy P, Kakunaga T (1985) Molecular structure of the human cytoplasmic b-actin gene: Interspecies homology of sequences in the introns. Proc Natl Acad Sci USA 82:6133–6137
13. Suzuki N, Matsumoto H, Kitada C, Masaki T, Fujino (1989) A sensitive sandwich-enzyme immunoassay for human endothelin. J Immunol Methods 118:245–250
14. Naruse M, Uchida S, Ogata E, Kurokawa K (1990) Vasopressin increases intracellular free Ca by stimulating Ca entry via V_2 receptor in cAMP independent manner in mouse cortical, outer and inner medullary collecting tubule cells. Kidney Int 37:362
15. Yanagisawa M, Inoue A, Takuwa Y, Mitsui Y, Kobayashi M, Masaki T (1989) The human preproendothelin-1 gene: possible regulation by endothelial phosphoinositide turnover signaling. J Cardiovasc Pharmacol 13:S13–S17
16. MacCumber MW, Ross CA, Glaser BM, Snyder SH (1989) Endothelin: Visualization of mRNAs by in situ hybridization provides evidence for local action. Proc Natl Acad Sci USA 86:7285–7289
17. Kurihara H, Yoshizumi M, Sugiyama T, Takaku F, Yanagisawa M, Masaki T, Hamaoki M, Kato H, Yazaki Y (1989) Transforming growth factor-β stimulates the expression of endothelin mRNA by vascular endothelial cells. Biochem Biophys Res Commun 159:1435–1440
18. Fine LG, Holley RW, Nasri H, Badie-Dezfooly B (1985) BSC-1 growth inhibitor transforms a mitogenic stimulus into a hypertrophic stimulus for renal proximal tubular cells: Relationship to Na^+/H^+ antiport activity Proc Natl Acad Sci USA 82:6163–6166
19. MacKay K, Striker LJ, Stauffer JW, Doi T, Agodoa LY, Striker GE (1989) Transforming growth factor-β. J Clin Invest 83:1160–1167
20. Kaname S, Uchida S, Ogata E, Kurokawa K (1990) Transforming growth factor-beta (TGF-β) gene expression in cultured rat mesangial cells. Kidney Int 37:197
21. Koseki C, Imai M, Hirata Y, Yanagisawa M, Masaki T (1989) Autoradiographic distribution in rat tissues of binding sites for endothelin: A neuropeptide? Am J Physiol 256:R858–R866
22. Kohzuki M, Johnson CI, Chai SY, Casley DJ, Mendelsohn FAO (1989) Localization of endothelin receptors in rat kidney. Eur J Pharmacol 160:193–194

Transplantation

Chair: Kazuo Ota (Japan)
Henri Kreis (France)

A Novel Immunosuppressive Agent, Deoxyspergualin

Kota Takahashi and Kazuo Ota

Summary. A new immunosuppressive agent, deoxyspergualin (DSG), has been reported elsewhere to prolong survival of xenografts in animal models and was effective in the treatment of hyperacute rejection in our previous report of ABO-incompatible kidney transplantation, which was thought to be similar to xenograft transplantation.

A new administration modality of DSG, its prophylactic use for the prevention of acute rejection in patients with kidney transplantation from ABO-incompatible or preformed antibody-positive donors, was tried, and satisfactory clinical results were obtained.

The evidence showed that DSG was very effective in the prevention of acute rejection in patients with kidney transplantation from ABO-incompatible or preformed antibody-positive living related donors, and that DSG was also very effective in the treatment of rejection in kidney transplantation.

Introduction

Although immunosuppressive agents are indispensable in organ transplantations, at present fewer than ten agents are in clinical use. The need for new agents for clinical use is therefore very high.

Following mizoribine, deoxyspergualin (DSG) is the second immunosuppressive agent to be developed and clinically applied in Japan. It has become the focus of much attention as efforts are being made to confirm its effectiveness.

This paper summarizes our findings concerning the effectiveness of DSG in the prevention and treatment of acute rejection in kidney transplantation.

[1]Department of Urology, Tokyo Women's Medical College, 8-1, Kawada-cho, Shinjuku-ku, Tokyo, 162 Japan

$$\overset{(\pm)}{}$$

$$H_2N\underset{\underset{NH}{\|}}{C}NH(CH_2)_6CONH\underset{\underset{OH}{|}}{C}HCONH(CH_2)_4NH(CH_2)_3NH_2 . 3HCl$$

M.W. 497

Fig. 1. Structural formula of DSG

Description of Deoxyspergualin

In 1981, Takeuchi et al. isolated a new antibiotic, which was given the name spergualin from its chemical structure, from the culture filtrate of a bacillus. This antibiotic demonstrated an anti-tumor and immunosuppressive effect, and led to the synthesis of a number of derivatives, of which deoxyspergualin, or DSG, was singled out for further development.

Deoxyspergualin has a molecular weight of 497 and is characterized by the removal of a hydroxide group from spergualin, at the 15-position, as shown in Fig. 1. It comes in the form of lumpy white powder and is highly hygroscopic and deliquescent. It is easily dissolved in water, methanol, and formic acid.

At present, DSG is supplied for intravenous injection only, and is, unfortunately, not yet available in oral form, due to absorption problems. The development of an oral form is, however, expected in the near future.

Immunosuppressive Effects

Figure 2 shows the most probable mechanism for the immunosuppressive effects of DSG, based on our current knowledge of DSG characteristics described in the previous section. Possibly, DSG suppresses clonal amplification of cytotoxic T lymphocytes (CTL) through direct action on these cells, by which the functions of the suppressor T-lymphocytes are relatively enhanced. Subsequent direct action on B-lymphocytes causes the suppression of antibody production through suppression of the amplification of B-lymphocytes and plasma cells.

As described above, one of the characteristic of DSG is the suppression of antibody production by direct action on the B-cell system.

DSG was used in the induction phase to prevent kidney transplant rejections, those due to ABO-incompatibility closely related with humoral antibodies, and rejections due to preformed antibodies. The results of these efforts, as well as the use of DSG in the post-transplant treatment of rejections, are described in the following sections.

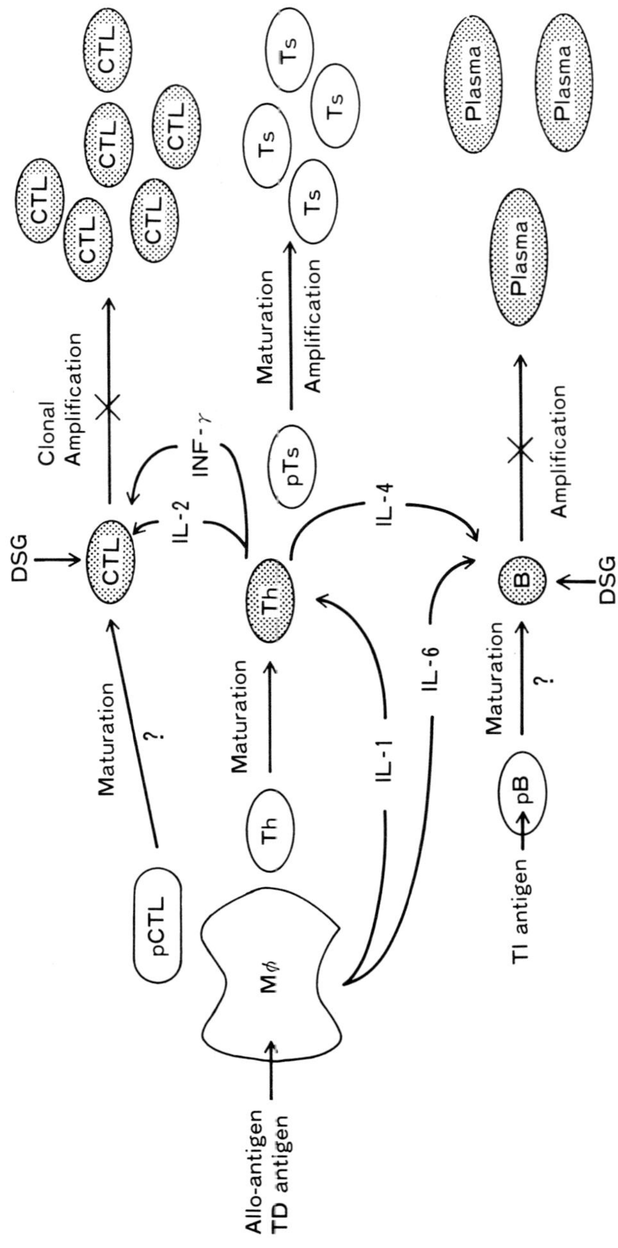

Fig. 2. Immunosuppressive mechanism of DSG

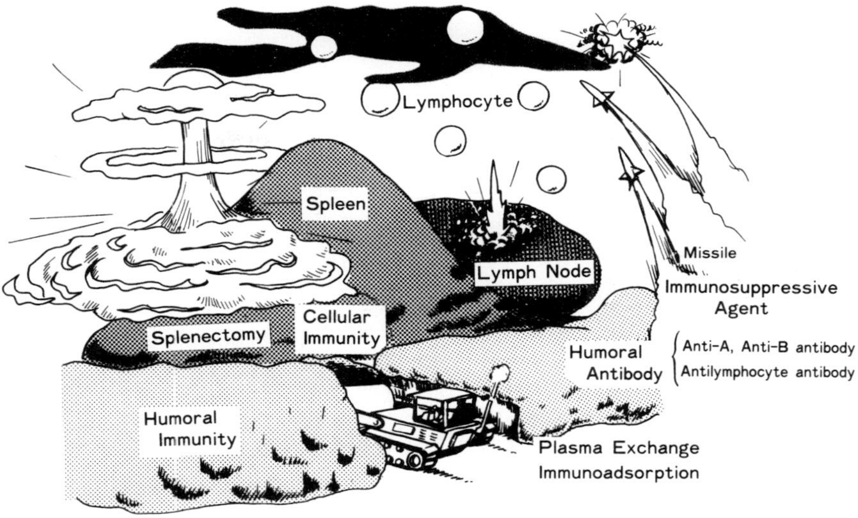

Fig. 3. ABO-incompatible and preformed antibody-positive kidney transplantation

Prophylactic Use of DSG in Kidney Transplantation from ABO-Incompatible and Preformed Antibody-Positive Donors (Fig. 3)

Patients

The patients studied were immunological high responders, consisting of 13 ABO-incompatible kidney transplant recipients and 3 preformed antibody-positive kidney transplant recipients (Table 1). In order to suppress antibody production, DSG was administered to all of these patients.

Methods

ABO-Incompatible Kidney Transplantation

Prior to surgery, anti-A or anti-B antibodies were removed from the recipients by means of double filtration plasmapheresis and immunoadsorption (using a Biosysorb column), thus lowering their anti-A and anti-B antibody titers to 1:8 or less.

In Case 1, an immunosuppressive regimen, consisting of methylprednisolone (MP), cyclosporin (CYA), azathioprine (AZ), and antilymphocyte globulin (ALG), resulted in decreased urinary output three hours after the transplantation. Due to a diagnosis of hyperacute rejection, the patient was given DSG, which resulted in increased urinary output that indicated a recovery of renal function. Based on our observation of Case 1, DSG and the same four-drug regimen were administered in cases 2–13.

Administration of MP started on the day of the transplantation, at a dose of 500 mg/day, which was reduced to a maintenance dose of 8 mg/day in the 4th month.

Table 1. ABO-incompatible kidney transplantation

Case	Sex	Age	Orginal disease	ABO blood type Donor→Recipient	HLA-A, B, DR mismatch No.	MLC fway S.I.	Rejection AAR	Rejection AR	Serum Cr. mg/dℓ 1day	1W	2W	1M	2M	3M	6M	1Y	Anti A, Anti B antibody	1W	1M	2M	3M	6M	9M	1Y	Complication
1 M.N.	M	27	Chronic nephritis	B→O	3	75.0	HAR 2	(−)	6.8	2.4	1.4	1.6	4.4	2.1	2.2	Death	IgM	2	2	4	8	8	8		CMV infection Malignant B cell lymphoma
																	IgG	4	16	4	8	8	8		
2 T.S.	M	28	Chronic nephritis	B→O	3	68.5	(−)	1	4.3	1.3	1.3	1.7	1.7	1.5	1.5	1.5	IgM	1	32	16	8	8	4	4	CMV infection
																	IgG	1	4	8	2	2	2	2	
3 Y.Y.	M	42	Chronic nephritis	B→A_1	0	1.0	(−)	(−)	4.7	1.3	1.3	1.4	1.4	1.4	1.5		IgM	0	2	2	2	2	2		(−)
																	IgG	1	2	2	4	4	4		
4 T.F.	M	13	Chronic nephritis	A_1B→A_1	3	1.7	(−)	1	2.0	0.8	0.8	1.1	1.0	1.0	0.7		IgM	0	1	1	1	1			UTT
																	IgG	0	0	1	1	1			
5 T.S.	M	27	Chronic nephritis	A_1→O	1	15.2	(−)	4	5.9	2.2	4.0	3.5	3.2	2.8	3.0		IgM	4	8	8	8	8			(−)
																	IgG	2	8	8	8	8			
6 N.I.	F	17	Chronic nephritis	A_1B→B	1	12.2	(−)	(−)	2.4	0.9	1.0	1.3	1.2	1.1	1.1		IgM	16	32	8	8	8			CMV infection
																	IgG	8	4	4	8	8			
7 E.S.	M	27	Chronic nephritis	B→O	2	16.4	(−)	(−)	2.9	1.1	1.2	1.3	1.2	1.2	1.2		IgM	1	1	4	4	4			(−)
																	IgG	1	1	2	2	2			
8 E.H.	F	32	Chronic nephritis	B→O	2	3.6	(−)	4	2.9	1.0	0.9	1.2	7.8	2.3	2.2		IgM	2	4	16	16	16			(−)
																	IgG	2	8	16	16	16			
9 T.K.	M	31	Chronic nephritis	A_1→O	1	35.6	(−)	(−)	4.9	1.1	1.1	1.4	1.4	1.4			IgM	2	8	16					Adenovirus Hemorrhagic cystitis
																	IgG	4	16	32					
10 H.T.	M	23	Chronic nephritis	A_1→O	4	11.2	(−)	1	7.1	1.7	1.6	1.8	1.6	1.6			IgM	2	8	16					(−)
																	IgG	4	4	16					
11 S.S.	M	55	Chronic nephritis	A_1→O	3	25.7	(−)	1	1.1	1.1	1.2	AR	Graftloss	Death			IgM	1	128	32					Cerebral haemorrhage
																	IgG	1	128	32					
12 S.K.	F	58	Chronic nephritis	A_1→O	5	16.4	(−)	(−)	1.4	1.3	1.3	1.3	1.3	1.3			Ig	4	4						(−)
																	IgG	4	4						
13 Y.S.	M	53	Polycystic kidney	A_1B→O	5	4.1	(−)	(−)	5.5	2.2	2.0	2.0					A IgM	4	4	4	4				(−)
																	A IgG	4	4	4	4				
																	B IgM	4	4	4	4				
																	B IgG	4	4	4	4				

Oral administration of CYA, at a dose of 8–10 mg/kg per day, started 2 days before the transplantation; drip infusion of CYA, at a dose of 3 mg/kg per day, was administered on the day of the transplantation. Administration of CYA was then adjusted to maintain a CYA through-level in whole blood of between 150 and 200 mg/ml for a duration of 1 or 2 months after the transplantation and a CYA through-level of between 80 and 150 ng/ml thereafter.

Administration of AZ, at a dose of 2 mg/kg per day, was started 2 days before the transplantation and was continued for a period of 1 week, after which the dose was reduced to 1 mg/kg per day and adjusted according to the patient's peripheral white blood cell count.

Administration of ALG, at a dose of 30 mg/kg per day, was begun 2 days before the transplantation and, basically, continued for 14 days. Administration of ALG was discontinued when the platelet count decreased to 50,000/cmm or less. Then DSG was administered, at a dose of 5 mg/kg per day, for 5 days, starting from the day of the transplantation; local X-ray irradiation was performed, at a dose of 150 rad, on the 1st, 3rd, and 5th day after the transplantation. Kidney transplantation surgery was performed according to Murray's method, and, in all cases, a splenectomy was performed at the time of transplantation.

In the treatment of acute rejection episodes, a basic dose of 500 mg of MP was administered for 2 days. When no remission occurred, muromonab CD3 (OKT3), at a dose of 5mg/kg per day, was administered for 10 days, or DSG, at a dose of 5 mg/kg per day, was administered for 5 days. Before the administration of DSG, which remains an experimental drug, prior written consent was obtained from the patients.

Preformed Antibody-Positive Kidney Transplantation

From among the preformed antibody-positive kidney transplant patients, we selected three whose T-cell antibody counts had not become negative 6 months or more after the pre-transplant cross match tests had been carried out. In these cases, double filtration plasmapheresis was conducted a total of two to four times and transplantation was performed following the disappearance of the T-cell antibodies.

In those cases in which T-cell antibodies did not disappear after 6 months, an immunosuppressive regimen, consisting of CYA, at a dose of 2 mg/kg per day, MP, at a dose of 8 mg/day, and MZ, at a dose of 1 mg/kg per day, was administered three times per week following hemodialysis, until the time of the transplantation. After the transplantation, the same immunosuppressive regimen as that employed in ABO-incompatible cases was used. None of the three cases, however, underwent splenectomy.

Table 2 shows the maximum values of the results of cross match tests conducted prior to transplantation.

Results

ABO-Incompatible Kidney Transplantation

Of the ABO-incompatible kidney transplant cases, rejection did not occur in 4 cases, hyperacute rejection occurred once in 1 case, accelerated acute rejection occurred 2 times in 2 cases, and acute rejection occurred 12 times in 6 cases (i.e., four times

Table 2. Preformed antibody-positive kidney transplantation (Tx)

Patient	Age	Sex	Blood type	Original disease	HLA, A, B. DR mismatch No.	Cause of Senitization	Crossmatch test		
							T	BW	BC%
1 F. S.	32	F	O/O	Purpura nephritis	12.5	Pregnancy ? Blood transfusion	30	100	0
2 S. T.	40	M	O/B	Chronic nephritis	12.7	Blood transfusion	20	90	90
3 K. O.	44	F	A/A	Chronic nephritis	12.8	DST	100	100	100

Patient	Treatment before Tx		Immunosuppression		Serum Cr. value	Rejection				Complication
	Immunosupp.	Plasma exchange	Induction phase	Maintenance		HR	AAR	AR	CR	
1 F. S.	CYA, MP MZ	DFPP 2	CYA, MP AZ, DSG, ALG	MP CYA, AZ	1.1 mg/dℓ 1Y1M	(−)	(−)	(−)	(−)	(−)
2 S. T.	CYA, MP MZ	DFPP 3	CYA, MP AZ, DSG, ALG	MP CYA, AZ	1.5 mg/dℓ 1Y	(−)	(−)	(−)	(−)	(−)
3 K. O.	CYA, MP MZ	DFPP 6	CYA, MP AZ, DSG, ALG	MP CYA, AZ	1.6 mg/dℓ 3M	(−)	1	(−)	(−)	(−)

in 2 cases and once in 4 cases). Graft loss caused by rejection occurred in only 1 of the 13 cases.

Regarding anti-A or anti-B titers after transplantation, both IgM and IgG levels were maintained at 1:32 in all cases except patient 11, whose anti-A antibody titers rose to 1:128. In this case, immunoadsorption was performed four times, combined with DSG administration. Although the titer level decreased to 1:32, the rejection led to graft loss.

Complications included three cases of cytomegalovirus (CMV) infection and one case each of urinary tract infection and hemorrhagic cystitis caused by adenovirus type 11.

CMV infection was treated with ganciclovir and CMV high-titer gamma-globulin, while hemorrhagic cystitis was treated with glycyrrhizin.

There were two deaths. One patient died of malignant B cell lymphoma in the 8th month, with the causal relationship between the fatal disease and Epstein-Barr virus infection remaining unclear. The other patient died of cerebral hemorrhage in the 2nd month after transplantation.

Clinical Course

This section describes a typical post-operative course.

Case 2 consisted of a 28-year-old male with type O blood and an original diagnosis of chronic nephritis. The patient received a kidney from his living elder brother, whose blood type was B.

To lower the patient's serum antibody titers, one session of double filtration plasmapheresis (DFPP) and four sessions of immunoadsorption were performed before the transplantation, reducing his serum anti-B IgM and IgG levels to 1:4, or less, immediately before the operation. The kidney transplantation was preceded by splenectomy and the immunosuppressive regimen was carried out according to the method described above (Fig. 4).

After the transplantation, anti-B IgM and IgG titers of up to 1:32 and 1:8, respectively, were maintained. The patient suffered one acute reaction (AR), but recovered fully through MP pulse therapy. At present, 1 year after the transplantation, the patient shows a serum creatinine level of 1.6 mg/dl, which indicates satisfactory functioning of the transplanted kidney.

Preformed Antibody-Positive Kidney Transplantation

The survival rate for patients and grafts ranged from two months to a year after the transplantation, with all cases showing satisfactory functioning of the transplanted kidney and a serum creatinine level of 1.1–1.6 mg/dl.

One patient experienced an AR episode, but recovered through MP pulse therapy.

Clinical Course

The clinical course of a recent case follows:

Case 3 was a 44-year-old female with type A blood and an original diagnosis of chronic nephritis. The patient showed poor histocompatibility with her 64-year-old

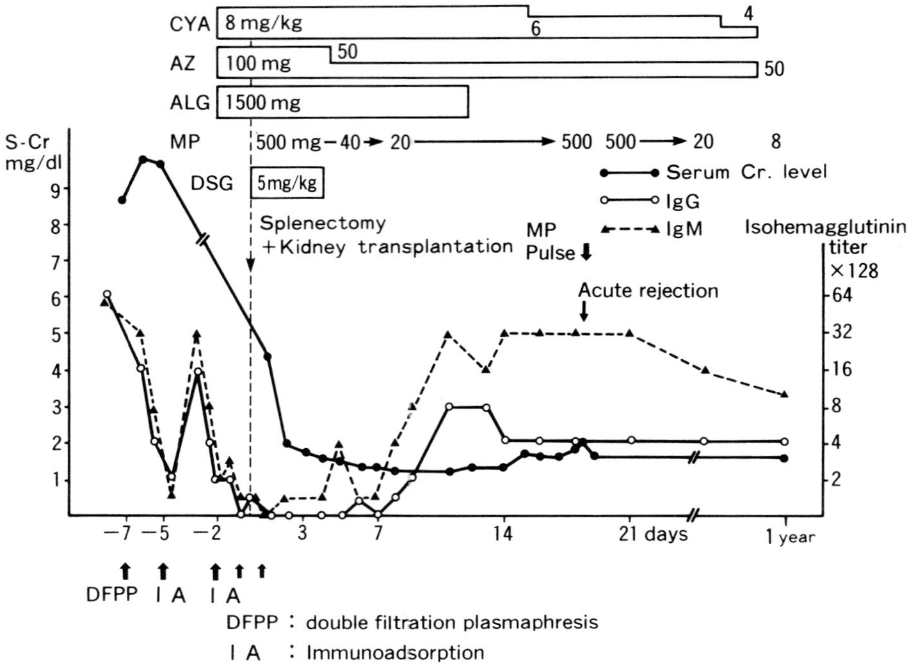

Fig. 4. ABO-incompatible kidney transplantation No. 2. T.S. 28-year-old male ($B^+ \rightarrow O^+$)

mother (i.e., HLA-A, B, DR 3 mismatches and an MLC 1 way S.I. 23). Prior to the transplantation, the patient received a 200-ml donor-specific blood transfusion (DST).

In a crossmatch test performed five months after the DST, the patient showed a 100% T-cell level and was B-cell antibody positive. The patient remained 100% antibody positive in later crossmatch tests over the 6-month clinical course observation which followed. Doses of CYA, at 2 mg/kg per day, were therefore administered three times a week after hemodialysis. Six months later, T-cell antibodies had decreased to 20% and warm and cold B-cell antibodies had decreased to 80%. The patient was then admitted to the hospital and underwent double filtration plasmapheresis four times over a period of 10 days. As a result, T-cell and B-cell antibodies became negative, and the transplantation was then performed. On the 6th day after the transplantation, the patient developed accelerated acute rejection, but recovered through MP pulse therapy. At present, 2 months after the transplantation, the patient shows a serum creatinine level of 1.3 mg/dl, which indicates satisfactory functioning of the transplanted kidney.

The efficacy of DSG against rejection after transplantations, previously detailed at the IVth Congress of the European Society for Organ Transplantation in 1989, is briefly described.

Efficacy of DSG in Treating Rejection Reactions After Kidney Transplantation

We used DSG in 52 rejection episodes which occurred in 44 kidney transplant cases. The 52 rejection episodes consisted of nine accelerated acute rejections (AAR), 24 acute rejections (AR), 11 late acute rejections (LAR), and 8 acute on chronic rejections (AOCR).

DSG was administered by drip infusion, in doses of 3, 5, or 7 mg/kg per day, and the efficacy of DSG against rejection reactions was evaluated on the basis of decreases in the serum creatinine level.

DSG was effective in 38 (73%) of the 52 rejection episodes. In terms of rejection type, DSG was effective in 6/9 (67%) of the cases of AAR, in 20/24 (83%) of the cases of AR, in 10/11 (91%) of the cases of LAR, and in 2/8 (25%) of the cases of AOCR (Table 3).

In cases in which remission was achieved, the serum creatinine level showed a gradual decrease, which, in most cases, started after DSG administration had been completed.

Side effects included leukopenia, which developed 14 times (or in 27% of the rejections) and thrombocytopenia, which developed 4 times (or in 8% of the rejections). There were also two cases of abdominal distension and one case each of lip numbness and facial suffusion. The severity of all side effects was slight, and no complications were observed.

Conclusions

Based on the results of our study, we arrived at the following conclusions:

1) DSG is effective in prophylactic use and in the treatment of rejection in kidney transplantation.
2) Compared to OKT3, DSG has a weaker effect on severe rejection reactions.
3) Compared to steroid pulse therapy, the effect of DSG is slowly manifested; i.e., DSG lowers serum creatinine levels gradually over a period of 3–5 days.
4) DSG has a stronger effect on late acute rejection than does OKT3 or methylprednisolone.
5) DSG suppresses the B-cell system, and therefore antibody production, and is thus effective in ABO-incompatible kidney transplantation involving humoral immunity, and in preformed antibody-positive kidney transplantation.
6) Regarding side effects, DSG slightly suppresses bone marrow function, thus leading to leukopenia and thrombocytopenia. However, granulocyte colony stimulating factor (CSF) proved to be effective in the treatment of leukopenia.
7) DSG causes fewer complications than OKT3 and steroid agents, especially in regard to infectious diseases.

References

1. Amemiya H, Suzuki S, Ota K, Takahashi K, Sonoda T, Ishibashi M, Omoto R, Koyama I, Dohi K, Fukuda Y, Fukao K (1990) A novel rescue drug, 15-deoxyspergualin. Transplantation 19:337–343

2. Takahashi K, Ota K, Tanabe K, Oba S, Teraoka S, Toma H, Agishi T, Kawaguchi H, Ito K (1990) Effect of a novel immunosuppressive agent, deoxyspergualin, on rejection in kidney transplant recipients. Transplant Proc 22:1606–1612

Therapeutic Use of Monoclonal Antibodies in Renal Transplantation

H. KREIS, C. LEGENDRE, and L. CHATENOUD[1]

Introduction

A wide variety of antilymphocyte monoclonal antibodies (MoAb) is now available for therapeutic use (Table 1). The majority of them, produced in mice and in rats, are directed against lymphocyte membrane antigens and/or receptors which are categorized in cluster of differentiation (CD). Each lymphocyte subset can be recognized according to the various CD expressed on their surface

One of the major advantages of MoAb is their homogeneous specificity and properties [1]. Monoclonal-induced immunosuppression has, therefore, greater selectivity, as each MoAb recognizes only one epitope of its target molecule. Therefore, the therapeutic use of MoAb allows: (1) more selective immunosuppression leading to decreased infectious risks, (2) a reduced rate of serum sickness because of the small amount of immunoglobulin needed, (3) blocking of the immune response at a selected level according to the role of the target molecule.

Combination of various MoAb, either simultaneously or consecutively, will probably allow better immunosuppression with risks lower than those of polyclonal antibodies and/or nonspecific chemical immunosuppressive agents.

A wide range of MoAb is already available for human use. They can be classified into three groups according to the function of the target antigen.

MoAb Directed Against the TCR/CD3 Complex

The TCR/CD3 complex allows T lymphocytes to recognize alloantigens in association with either MHC Class I or Class II molecules, and to be further activated [2]. The TCR/CD3 complex has two major parts (Fig. 1). One, devoted to antigen recognition, is made of two chains, an α chain and a β chain and represents the TCR. The

[1]Service de Transplantation and INSERSM U25 Hôpital Necker, Paris 75015, France

Table 1. Major monoclonal antibodies for therapeutic use

Anti CD_2	T11-2	(IgG_1)	E Rosette receptor
	T11-3	(IgG_2 a)	
Anti CD_3	OKT_3	(IgG_2 a)	T_3 (TCR)
	BMA	(IgG_2 b)	TCR αβ
Anti CD_4	OKT_4	(IgG_2 b)	T_4
	OKT_4 a	(IgG_2 a)	
Anti CD_7	RFT_2	(IgG_2 a)	T-Lymphoblasts
	CHH 380	(H-IgG_1 + M-IgG_2 a)	
Anti CD_8	OKT_8	(IgG_1)	T_8
Anti CD_{25}	33B3.1	(IgG_2 a)	
	Anti TAC		RIL-2 (a)
	CAMPATH-6		

other, the CD3 molecule allows the transduction of the activation signal produced by the recognition of the alloantigen. It is made of three chains, γ, δ, and ε. The specificity for an antigen is determined by the variable and constant parts of TCR. Blocking either the TCR or the CD3 will prevent lymphocyte activation and further proliferation and differentiation toward cytotoxic lymphocytes.

Anti-CD3 Monoclonal Antibodies

Anti-CD3 antibodies were the first to be used in the treatment of allograft rejection by Cosimi et al. [3,4]. Based on the very encouraging results reported in a small

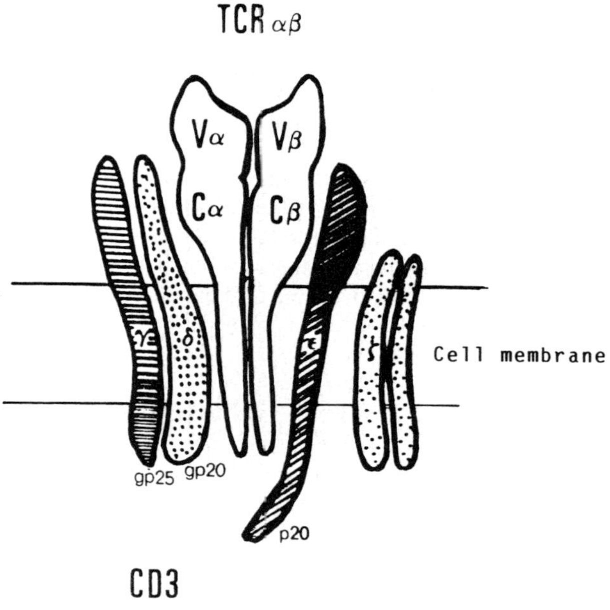

Fig. 1. The TCR/CD3 complex

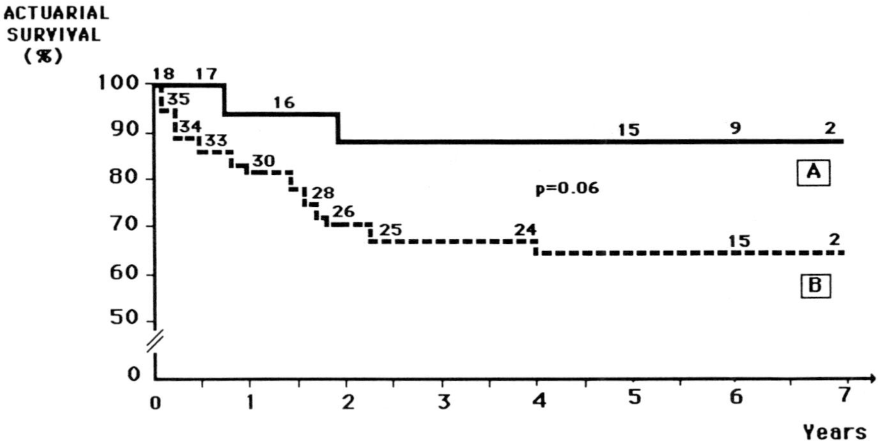

Fig. 2. Actuarial graft survival of OKT3-treated patients versus conventionally treated patients. All patients had at least 5 years of follow-up as of January 1, 1990

series of patients, a multicenter trial was performed in the United States, which demonstrated the efficacy of OKT3 used in first-line treatment of the first acute rejection episode occurring in renal transplantations, as compared with conventional high-dose steroids [5].

It was shown thereafter that OKT3 was also effective in the rescue treatment of patients undergoing rejection, who were resistant to conventional high-dose steroids and/or antithymocyte globulins [6,7]. Our group was the first to prove the efficacy (Fig. 2) of OKT3 when used as a prophylactic agent in association with conventional immunosuppressive agents which were useful in decreasing anti-OKT3 response [8–10]. Using a slightly different protocol, a multicenter trial in the United States confirmed that prophylactic OKT3 gave better results than cyclosporine A (personal communication). We have recently reported [11] that using OKT3 prophylactically was probably more effective than using it to treat ongoing acute rejection episodes (Fig. 3). OKT3 is now generally recognized as major immunosuppressive agent. However, it must not be used without knowledge of the following points.

Treatment Protocols

When used to treat acute rejection episodes, 5 mg i.v. OKT3 is usually given during a 7–10 day period without increasing or adding other immunosuppressive agents. A similar protocol is used to rescue steroid- and ATG-resistant rejection episodes [7]. However, it has recently been shown by our group that inflammatory cells infiltrating rejecting grafts were not completely cleared after 10 days of OKT3 treatment [12]. It is probable, but not yet demonstrated, that a combination treatment of OKT3 and steroids would be more effective than OKT3 used alone.

Used prophylactically, OKT3 has been administered according to two different protocols.

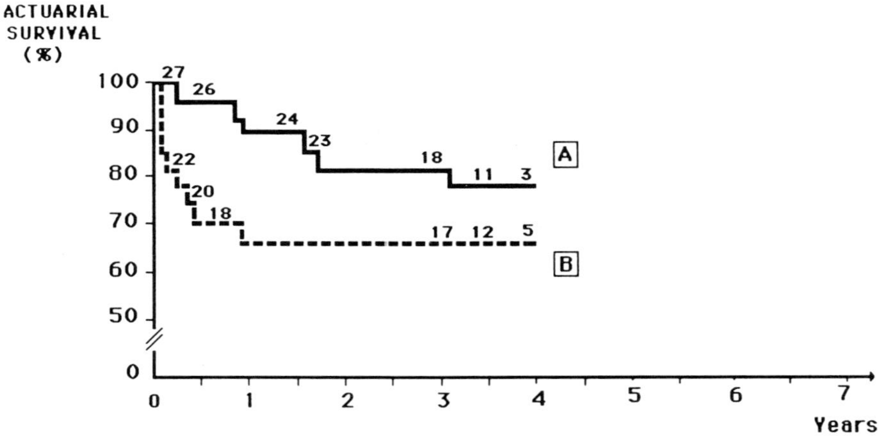

Fig. 3. Actuarial graft survival of patients receiving prophylactic treatment with OKT3 versus patients receiving OKT3 for the treatment of acute rejection episodes only

In our group [9], OKT3 is given during a maximum 30-day-period, in combination with 2–3 mg/kg per day Azathioprine and low doses of steroids. At the end of the one-month treatment period, OKT3 is withdrawn without adding any new immunosuppressive agents. It is thus possible to obtain results similar to those reported with cyclosporine A but without using that drug.

In other prophylactic protocols, OKT3 is used with either simultaneous or sequential cyclosporine A. In the latter case, cyclosporine A is started a few days before discontinuing OKT3, in order to get effective cyclosporine blood levels after MoAb withdrawal (personal communication).

Whatever the protocol, the daily dose in adults is always 5 mg per day. Attempts to decrease this dosage have always led to a higher degree of anti-OKT3 immunization and therefore to a lower activity of the MoAb (unpublished data). In contrast, increasing the daily dose to 10 or 15 mg in patients developing anti-OKT3 immunization allows the maintenance of effective OKT3 blood levels in about 50% of patients, without significantly increasing the so-called "first dose" syndrome [11].

In fact, no real attempts were made in adult patients to use drug dosage per body weight as is frequently done in children. This would probably be more appropriate than the use of reduced drugs.

Monitoring MoAb Treatment

As early as 1 hour after the first injection OKT3 MoAb induces a dramatic and concomitant decrease in T3+, T4+ and T8+ cells [4,10]. However, the impact of the MoAb on lymphocytes within the reticuloendothelial system is not well known. In mice, with similar dosages of an anti-CD3 antibody, partial T3+ cell depletion was observed in spleen and lymph nodes [13].

It is well known that after 3–5 days a significant proportion of T3−, T4+ and T3−, T8+ cells reappears in the circulation, indicating the presence of T3 modulating lymphocytes [14].

Similarly, noncirculating T lymphocytes can also demonstrate modulation of the CD3 molecule. CD3 modulating T lymphocytes were thus observed on sequential transplant biopsies performed in OKT3-treated patients [12]. It is highly probable, but not yet clearly demonstrated, that increasing the treatment dose will lead to a higher percentage of CD3 modulating cells within the lymphoreticularendothelial system, and will thus induce a more profound immunosuppression with an increased risk of infectious or mitogenic complications.

As the CD3 molecule is closely associated with the TCR, OKT3-induced antigenic modulation leads, in fact, to the modulation of the whole TCR/CD3 complex. Therefore, these cells are immunoincompetent. However, a few hours after OKT3 discontinuation, OKT3 blood levels drop below the level of efficacy and a rapidly growing number of T lymphocytes exhibiting the TCR/CD3 complex reappear. This can be observed not only in the blood, but also in the graft, where CD3 modulating lymphocytes, which have not all been cleared, reexpress the TCR/CD3 complex, making them immunocompetent again.

Therefore, monitoring the number of circulating CD3+ cells at least 3 times a week in OKT3-treated patients is mandatory. As soon as more than 10% of circulating CD3 lymphocytes are present, OKT3 must be either discontinued or increased [11]. Monitoring OKT3 blood levels and/or appearance of anti-OKT3 IgG has no clinical use. However, it will help to understand any unusual situation.

Anti-CD3 Side Effects

Among the various side effects that can be induced by OKT3 MoAb, the first-dose syndrome [8,9], induced by a transient T cell activation [15], is directly related to the drug itself. Another side effect, anti-MoAb immunization [10,16–18] appears as a consequence of a xenoprotein and is observed with all xenogeneic MoAb. The last side effect, the risk induced by overimmunosuppression, that is, infectious and mitogenic complications, is shared by all potent immunosuppressive agents, and more especially by all combinations of potent immunosuppressive agents.

The First-Dose Syndrome

Immediately following the first OKT3 injection, a clinical syndrome composed of high fever, chills, headache, diarrhea, and vomiting can be observed [8]. Fever at least is always present, attesting to the efficacy of the MoAb. Dyspnea, tachycardia, hypotension, skin rash, arthralgia, and psychiatric behavior are seldom observed. Respiratory distress with pulmonary edema does not usually occur when the patient has no fluid overload before the first OKT3 injection [4,5,9,19]. Most of these symptoms generally disappear after 2–3 days. Nevertheless, they can last throughout the treatment period in transplant recipients of HLA identical kidneys (unpublished data). This first-dose syndrome is not observed, at least with similar intensity, with other anti-T cell MoAbs. It has been shown by our group [15,20], as well as by others [21], that due to OKT3-induced monocyte activation a number of cytokines are released in the blood immediately after the first OKT3 injection. Among them are tumor necrosis factor (TNF), interferon γ (IFNγ), interleukin-2 (IL-2), IL-3, and IL-6. Cytokine levels were back to normal after 24 hours despite persistent OKT3 treatment.

Although other anti-T lymphocyte MoAb can induce T cell opsonization and depletion, only OKT3 has been held responsible for the cytokine release syndrome [22–24]. In our group [25], it has been possible to reproduce in mice a similar first-dose syndrome using an anti-CD3 MoAb. In this study, pathological studies demonstrated that organs such as liver and lung exhibited major changes. These observations could, at least partially, explain the increased incidence of transient renal failure sometimes observed after the first OKT3 injection. High doses of MoAb were correlated with significant mortality.

It is now well established that high-dose steroids, administered at least 1 hour before OKT3 injection, can drastically reduce the release of cytokines that follows the first injection of OKT3 [26–28,30] (L. Chatenoud et al., unpublished data). Clinical symptoms that follow OKT3 injection are significantly less severe in mice when steroids are administered 30–60 minutes before the MoAb [25]. In man, however, the first-dose syndrome does not seem to have decreased intensity, whether steroids are given 1 hour before, or simultaneously with OKT3 injection (L. Chatenoud et al., unpublished data).

The severity of the first-dose syndrome in kidney graft recipients is probably related to: (1) the number of activated T lymphocytes already present at the time of the first OKT3 injection and (2) the lack of steroid therapy before and during OKT3 treatment. Thus, more severe reactions were observed in recipients of an HLA-identical kidney who were treated by Azathioprine and prophylactic OKT3 without steroids, than in treatment of acute rejection episodes or in the prophylactic treatment of cadaveric kidney recipients.

Corticosteroids are not only anti-inflammatory agents, but also exhibit an inhibitory effect on cytokine production.

Anti-MoAb Immunization

Monoclonal antibodies available today are produced in animals (mice or rats). Therefore, xenogeneic immunization is one of the major side effects which can limit all MoAb utilization. When OKT3 is used as the sole immunosuppressive regimen, almost all patients develop anti-OKT3 antibodies within a short time (usually before the end of a 10-day period) [8,10,16,17,18]. We have shown [9,17] that combining OKT3 with conventional immunosuppression (Azathioprine 2–3 mg/kg per day and low doses of steroids) or cyclosporine A can drastically reduce both the frequency and the intensity of anti-OKT3 immunization and can delay its occurrence. A very small number of patients will develop anti-OKT3 immunization in a 10- to 14-day treatment course, and we observed [11] IgG anti-OKT3 antibodies in only 50% of kidney graft recipients treated prophylactically for 30 days. In fact, 32% of the patients thus treated developed anti-MoAb IgG during the treatment period, whereas in the other 18% they appeared after OKT3 discontinuation. However, there is no close correlation between the occurrence of IgG and blood repopulation by T3+ cells, as in some patients having a low antibody response, OKT3 can still be in excess although at non-effective levels as compared to the amount of IgG. This explains why monitoring cells exhibiting CD3 is more important than monitoring IgG levels.

Anti-OKT3 response is usually composed of IgM and IgG, but only the latter are neutralizing for OKT3 [10,17]. It has been shown by Baudrihaye et al. [16] and Chatenoud et al. [31] that anti-OKT3 antibodies have a very restricted specificity, as only anti-isotypic IgG2a and anti-idiotypic (F(ab), F(ab′) 2) were demonstrated. Anti-idiotypic antibodies neutralize OKT3 immunosuppressive activity by preventing its linkage with T lymphocytes.

We also observed [11] that about half of our patients exhibited an early and strong anti-OKT3 immune response, whereas in the other half the response occurred later with a much lower intensity. In this latter group of patients, increasing the daily dose of OKT3 to 10–15 mg allowed restoration of the percentage of T3+ cells to 0, whereas in the early responders this percentage was not influenced by increasing the OKT3 dose to 15 mg.

It has recently been shown (personal communication) that previous anti-OKT3 immunization did not preclude the re-use of OKT3 for the treatment of a second rejection episode (or a first one, when immunization occurred during a prophylactic course), even though mild levels of anti-OKT3 were still present at the time of retreatment. This is a very strong argument in favor of using OKT3, either as prophylactic treatment or as first-line for the treatment of acute rejection.

Anti-TCR Monoclonal Antibodies

The only MoAb directed against the constant part of TCR which is so far available for human use is BMA 031, a mouse IgG2b [32,33]. Its mode of action differs from that of OKT3 in many ways: (1) There is only partial T cell depletion after BMA injection, ranging from 5 to 50 mg/day; (2) If modulation of the TCR/CD3 complex is also observed with BMA, not all T cells are modulating, and BMA coated cells are always present [32], which, in particular, is never observed with OKT3.

In addition, anti-BMA immunization always occurred rapidly and with a high intensity. This high immunogenicity is probably related to a lower immunosuppressive capacity, as compated with OKT3.

As a matter of fact, the prophylactic use of BMA in our hands (unpublished data), either at 5 or 20 mg/day has never been associated with good graft results. Almost all patients developed relatively severe graft dysfunction after only a few days, either due to rejection because of neutralization of BMA by anti-BMA antibodies or because of serum sickness related to high production of BMA anti-BMA complexes (Table 2).

However, it has been suggested by the Munich group [34] that short prophylactic treatment consisting of two boluses of 50 mg BMA each at days 0 and 2 could significantly improve the results of kidney grafts. This is in the process of being confirmed by a multicenter trial. On the other hand, it must be said that the tolerance of BMA is far better than that of OKT3 and with BMA the first-dose syndrome is either not observed or is seen on a very mild basis which consists of low fever after the first BMA injection [34]. After the first injection, only TNF were increased, without any

Table 2. Rejection episodes in cadaveric kidney recipients treated by a prophylactic course of either 20 mg/day (*I*) or 5 mg/day (*II*) of BI 51 013 (*BMA*) monoclonal antibody

Protocol	No. of patients	Rejection episodes	Reversible rejection	Mean time of onset
I	5	4	3	11 ± 2 d
II	3	3	2	9 ± 3 d

increase in IFNγ or in IL-2 [32,35]. This is in agreement with the low in vitro mitogenic capacity of BMA.

Monoclonal Antibodies Directed Against Cytokine Receptors

A wide variety of cytokines appear as important mediators during the immune response process [36,37]. Cytokines usually act through a specific receptor which is present on the surface membrane of target cells. So far the only MoAb anti cytokine receptors which are available for human use are directed against the IL-2 receptor. This receptor is present only on activated T cells [38], which explains the interest in MoAb able either to destroy this specific T cell subset or to block its function without modifying T cell subsets which are not involved in an immune process. High affinity RIL-2 is composed of two chains, an α chain and a β chain, each chain representing a low affinity receptor. So far the only anti-RIL-2 MoAbs which are available for human use are directed against the α chain of the receptor, which has a molecular weight of 55 kDa (p55) and expresses the Tac or CD25 antigen.

Kirkman et al. [39] were the first to demonstrate better survival of cardiac allografts in mice receiving an anti-CD25 MoAb. Only MoAb able to block IL-2 linkage with the IL-2 receptor have an immunosuppressive effect.

In human renal transplantation, Soulillou in Nantes [24], using the 33B3.1 MoAb directed against the α chain of RIL-2 and Strom in Boston [40], using the anti-Tac MoAb were able to prevent the occurrence of acute rejection episodes. In their hands, these two MoAbs gave results similar to those obtained with polyclonal antilymphocyte globulins, but with a lower incidence of side effects. Cyclosporine A seems to be a necessary adjunct for the anti-Tac MoAb but not for the 33B3.1.

The first attempts made with these MoAb in the treatment of acute rejection episodes were disappointing, although a large number of activated T cells expressing the IL-2 receptor were present. The fact that these MoAb are directed only against the low affinity receptor may explain these poor results.

A multicenter study using the 33B3.1 MoAb, which is in progress, will be necessary to confirm the good results already obtained in single center trials.

Monoclonal Antibodies Directed Against Cell Adhesion Molecules

Various molecules present on T cell membranes allow better adhesion between T lymphocytes and antigen-presenting cells. Among them are LFA1 (Fig. 4), CD2, CD4, and CD8 molecules and their ligand, ICAM-1 and LFA3 molecules and MHC Class II and I, respectively. Monoclonal antibodies directed against these molecules can prevent, or at least decrease, the adhesion capacity of T cells during the process of alloantigen recognition, and can therefore minimize its consequences.

Today, only anti-LFA1 MoAb have been studied in man and have allowed good survival rates of nonrelated bone marrow grafts. It is still too early to know whether anti-LFA1 MoAb will also be helpful in organ transplantation, in combination with

Fig. 4. Adhesion molecules involved in the process of alloantigen recognition by T lymphocytes

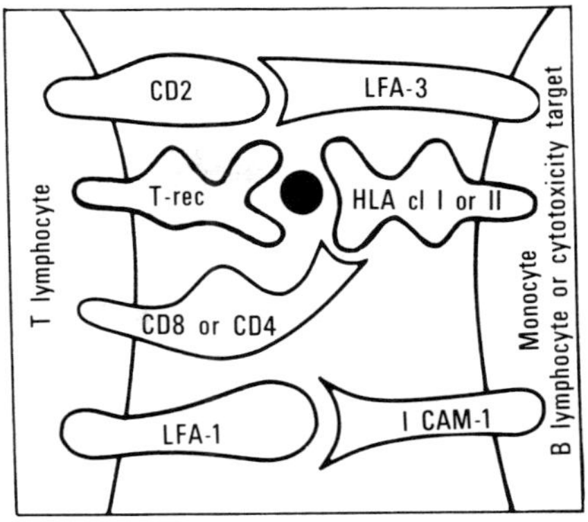

conventional immunosuppression, or in combination with other MoAb such as those directed against the TCR/CD3 complex.

CD4-bearing lymphocytes recognize MHC Class II restricted alloantigens [41]. Therefore, it can be postulated that anti-CD4 MoAb could prevent the recognition of alloantigens by CD4+ T lymphocytes and thus block the immune response process.

This immunosuppressive capacity of anti-CD4 MoAb has been shown in a number of animal experiments concerning either the prevention or the treatment of various autoimmune diseases [42–45]. Interestingly, it seems that anti-CD4 MoAb are able to induce immune tolerance for various antigens. Such tolerance can be observed without CD4 lymphocyte depletion and can be maintained indefinitely, provided antigen injection is periodically repeated [46–48]. The latter effect appears especially interesting in organ transplantation.

As human anti-CD4 MoAb also recognize primate T cells, the first experiments with anti-CD4 MoAb were performed in monkeys. These experiments were performed both by Cosimi [49] and by Jonker [50,51]. Using isolated OKT4A, or a combination of OKT4 and OKT4A, they were able to significantly prolong kidney allografts in Rhesus or Cynomolgus monkeys. Human studies using anti-CD4 MoAb are only starting. According to Chatenoud et al. [35], it seems that another anti-CD4 MoAb, BL4, led to only partial and transient CD4+ cell depletion, but that all CD4+ T cells were coated with the MoAb without any observed antigenic modulation of the CD4 molecule. In addition, none of the patients thus treated had increased cytokine levels and none presented any side effects other than xenoimmunization. A protocol using OKT4A prophylactic treatment of renal grafts in man is now in progress in Boston. MoAb directed against other cell adhesion molecules have not yet been used in organ transplantation.

However, in the years to come, a wide variety of monoclonal antibodies will be available in man, allowing, by their selectivity, and by their combined administration, either consecutively or simultaneously as "poly-monoclonal" sera, a more specific type of immunosuppression. Antixenogeneic immunization will probably be avoided by humanized constructs of MoAb, such as the anti-CD7 (SDZ CHH 380), which is in the process of being studied in man. We are still only at the dawn of immunosuppression in organ transplantation, but monoclonal antibodies are certain to constitute a fundamental new step toward specific tolerance.

References

1. Kohler G, Milstein C (1975) Continuous cultures of fused cells secreting antibody of predefined specificity. Nature 256:495–497
2. Kronenberg M, Siu G, Hood LE, Shastri N (1986) The molecular genetics of the T-cell antigen recognition. Annu Rev Immunol 4:529–591
3. Cosimi AB, Colvin RB, Burton RC, Rubin RH, Godstein G, Kung PC, Hansen WP, Delmonico FL, Russel PS (1981) Use of monoclonal antibodies to T-cell subsets for immunologic monitoring and treatment in recipients of renal allograft. N Engl J Med 305:308–314
4. Cosimi AB, Burton RC, Colvin B, Goldstein G, Delmonico FL, Laquaglia MP, Tolkoff-Rubin N, Rubin RH, Herrin JT, Russel PS (1981) Treatment of acute renal allograft rejection with OKT3 monoclonal antibody. Transplantation 32:535–539
5. Ortho multicenter transplant study group (1985) A randomized clinical trial of OKT3 monoclonal antibody for acute rejection of cadaveric renal transplant. N Engl J Med 313:337–342
6. Goldstein G, Norman DJ, Shield CF. Kreis H, Burdick J, Flye MW, Rivolta E, Starzl T, Monaco A (1986) OKT3 monoclonal antibody reversal of acute renal allograft rejection unresponsive to conventional immunosuppressive treatments. In: Meryman HT (ed) Transplantation approaches to graft rejection. Alan R. Liss, New York, pp 239–249
7. Norman DJ, Barry JM, Bennett WM, Leone M, Henell K, Funnell B, Hubert B (1988) The use of OKT3 in cadaveric renal transplantation for rejection that is unresponsive to conventional anti rejection therapy. Am J Kidney Dis 11:90–93
8. Vigeral P, Chkoff N, Chatenoud L, Campos H, Lacombe M, Droz D, Goldstein G, Bach JF, Kreis H (1986) Prophylactic use of OKT3 monoclonal antibody in cadaver kidney recipients. Utilization of OKT3 as the sole immunosuppressive agent. Transplantation 41:730–733
9. Debure A, Chkoff N, Chatenoud L, Lacombe M, Campos H, Noël LH, Goldstein G, Bach JF, Kreis H (1988) One-month prophylactic use of OKT3 in cadaver kidney transplant recipients. Transplantation 45:546–553
10. Chatenoud L, Baudrihaye MF, Chkoff N, Kreis H, Bach JF (1983) Immunologic follow up of renal allograft recipients treated prophylactically by OKT3 alone. Transplant Proc 15:643–645
11. Kreis H, Chkoff N, Chatenoud L, Debure A, Lacombe M, Chrétien Y, Legendre C, Caillat S, Bach JF (1989) A randomized trial comparing the efficacy of OKT3 used to prevent or to treat rejection. Transplant Proc 21:3–6
12. Caillat-Zucman S, Blumenfeld N, Legendre C, Noël LH, Bach JF, Kreis H, Chatenoud L (to be published) Human in vivo antigenic modulation induced by the anti-T cell OKT3 monoclonal antibody. Transplantation
13. Hirsch R, Eckhaus M, Auchincloss H, Sachs DH, Bluestone JA (1988) Effects of in vivo administration of anti-T3 monoclonal antibody on T cell function in mice: immunosuppression of transplantation response. J Immunol 140:3766–3772
14. Chatenoud L, Baudrihaye MF, Schindler J, Kreis H, Goldstein G, Bach JF (1982) Human in vivo antigenic modulation induced by the anti-T cell OKT3 monoclonal antibody. Eur J Immunol 12:979–982
15. Chatenoud L, Ferran C, Legendre C, Thouard I, Reuter A, Gevaert Y, Kreis H, Franchimont P, Bach JF (to be published) In vivo cell activation following OKT3 administration: systemic cytokine release and modulation by corticosteroids. Transplantation
16. Baudrihaye MF, Chatenoud L, Kreis H, Goldstein G, Bach JF (1984) Unusually restricted anti-isotype human immune response to OKT3 monoclonal antibody. Eur J Immunol 14:686–691
17. Chatenoud L (1986) The immune response against therapeutic monoclonal antibodies. Immunol Today 7:367–368

18. Chatenoud L, Jonker M, Villemain F, Goldstein G, Bach JF (1986) The human immune response to the OKT3 monoclonal antibody is oligoclonal. Science 232:1406–1408
19. Thistlethwaite JR, Gaber AO, Haag BW, Aronson AJ, Broelsh CE, Suart JK, Stuart FP (1987) OKT3 treatment of steroid-resistant renal allograft rejection. Transplantation 43:176–184
20. Chatenoud L, Ferran C, Reuter A, Legendre C, Gevaert Y, Kreis H, Franchimont P, Bach JF (1989) Systemic reaction to the anti-T-cell monoclonal antibody OKT3 in relation to serum levels of tumor necrosis factor and interferon γ. New Engl J Med 320: 1420–1421
21. Abramowicz D, Schandenne L, Goldman M, Crusiaux A, Vereerstraeten O, De Pauw L, Wybran J, Kinneart P, Dupont E, Toussaint C (1989) Release of tumor necrosis factor, interleukin 2 and gamma-interferon in serum after injection of OKT3 monoclonal antibody in kidney transplant recipients. Transplantation 47:606–608
22. Kirkman RL, Araujo JL, Brush GF, Carpenter CB, Milford EL, Reinherz EL, Schlossman SF, Strom TB, Tilney NL (1983) Treatment of acute renal allograft rejection with monoclonal anti-T12 antibody. Transplantation 36:620–626
23. Jonker M, Goldstein G, Balner H (1983) Effects of in vivo administration of monoclonal antibodies specific for human T cell subpopulations on the immune system in a Rhesus monkey model. Transplantation 35:521–529
24. Soulillou JP, Peyronnel P, Le Mauff B, Hourmant M, Olive D, Mawas C, Delaage M, Hirn M, Jacques Y (1987) Prevention of rejection of kidney transplants by monoclonal antibody directed against interleukin-2 receptor. Lancet I:1339–1342
25. Ferran C, Sheehan K, Dy M, Schreiber R, Landais P, Noël LH, Grau G, Bluestone J, Bach JF, Chatenoud L (to be published) Cytokine related syndrome following injection of anti-CD3 monoclonal antibody: further evidence for transient in vivo T cell activation. Eur J Immunol
26. Gyure PM, Girard MT, Morganelli PM, Manganiello PD (1988) Glucocorticoid effects on the production and actions of immune cytokines. J Steroid Biochem 30:89–93
27. Kern JA, Lamb RJ, Reed JC, Daniele RP, Nowell PC (1988) Dexamethasone inhibition of interleukin 1 beta production by human monocytes. Posttranscriptional Mechanisms. J Clin Invest 81:237–244
28. Reed JC, Abidi AH, Alpers JD, Hoover RG, Robb RJ, Nowell PC (1986) Effect of cyclosporin A and dexamethasone on interleukin 2 receptor gene expression. J Immunol 137: 150–154
29. Sariban E, Imamura K, Luebbers R, Kufe D (1988) Transcriptional and posttranscriptional regulation of tumor necrosis factor gene expression in human monocytes. J Clin Invest 81:1506–1510
30. Waage A, Bakke O (1987) Glucocorticoids suppress the production of tumour necrosis factor by lipopolysaccharide-stimulated human monocytes. Immunology 63:299–302
31. Chatenoud L, Baudrihaye MF, Chkoff N, Kreis H, Goldstein G, Bach JF (1986) Restriction of the human in vivo immune response against the mouse monoclonal antibody OKT3. J Imunol 137:830–838
32. Chatenoud L, Ferran C, Legendre C, Kurrle R, Kreis H, Bach JF (to be published) Immunological follow-up of renal allograft recipients treated with the BMA 031 (anti-TCR) monoclonal antibody. Transplant Proc
33. Nashan B, Wonigeit K, Schwinzer R, Schlitt HJ, Kurrle R, Pichlmayr R (1987) Fine specificity of a panel of antibodies against the TCR/CD3 complex. Transplant Proc 19:4270–4272
34. Hillebrand G, Rothang E, Hammer C, Illner WD, Schleibner S, Racenberg J, Gurland HJ, Land W (1989) Experience with a new monoclonal antibody in clinical kidney. Transplantation 21:1776–1777

35. Chatenoud L, Ferran C, Bach JF (1990) Utilisation clinique des anticorps anti-lymphocytes T. In: Flammarion (ed) Actualitées Néphrologiques, Hôpital Necker, Paris, pp 183–203
36. Balkwill F (1988) Cytokinea-soluble factors in immune responses. Curr Opin Immunol 1:241–249
37. Balkwill FR, Burke F (1989) The cytokine network. Immunol Today 10:299–301
38. Waldmann TA (1988) The multichain interleukin-2 receptor: A target for immunotherapy of patients with adult T cell leukemia, autoimmune disorders and individuals receiving allografts. J Autoimmunity 1:641–653
39. Kirkman RL, Barett LV, Gaulton GN, Kelley VE, Ythier A, Strom TB (1985) Administration of anti-interleukin 2 receptor monoclonal antibody prolongs cardiac allograft survival in mice. J Exp Med 162:358–362
40. Shapiro MD, Kirkman RL, Carpenter CB, Milford EL, Tilney NL, Waldmann TA, Zimmerman CE, Ramos EL, Strom TB (1988) Initial trials of the anti-human IL-2 receptor monoclonal antibody anti-Tac in clinical renal transplantation. Transplant Proc 21:1766–1768
41. Swain SL (1983) T cell subsets and the recognition of MHC class. Immunol Rev 74:129–142
42. Wofsy D, Ledbetter JA, Hendler PL, Seaman WE (1985) Treatment of murine lupus with monoclonal anti T-cell antibody. J Immunol 134:852–857
43. Shizuru MA, Tayloedwards C, Bank BA, Gregory AK, Fathman CG (1985) Immunotherapy of the non-obese diabetic mouse: treatment with an antibody to T helper lymphocytes. Science 240:659–661
44. Waldor MK, Sriram S, Hardy R, Herzenberg LA, Lamer L, Lim M, Steinman L (1985) Reversal of experimental allergic encephalomyelitis with monoclonal antibody to a T-cell subset marker. Science 227:415–417
45. Ranges GE, Sriram S, Copper SM (1985) Prevention of type II collagen-induced arthritis by in vivo treatment with anti-L3T4. J Exp Med 162:1105–1110
46. Benjamin RJ, Waldmann H (1986) Induction of tolerance of monoclonal antibody therapy. Nature 320:449–451
47. Benjamin RJ, Qin S, Wise MP (1988) Monoclonal antibodies for tolerance induction: a possible role for the CD4 (L3T4) and CD11a (LFA-1) molecules in self-nonself discrimination. Eur J Immunol 18:1079–1088
48. Gutstein NL, Seaman WE, Scott JH. Wofsy D (1986) Induction of immune tolerance by administration of monoclonal antibody to L3T4. J Immunol 137:1127–1132
49. Cosimi AB, Burton RC, Kung RC, Colvin R, Goldstein G, Lifter H, Rhodes W, Russel PS (1981) Evaluation in primate renal allograft recipients of monoclonal antibody to human T-cell subclasses. Transplant Proc 13:499–503
50. Jonker M, Neuhaus P, Zurcher C, Fucello A, Goldstein G (1985) OKT4 and OKT4A antibody treatment as immunosuppression for kidney transplantation in rhesus monkeys. Transplantation 39:247–253
51. Jonker M, Nooij FJM, Chatenoud L (1986) Immunosuppression by monoclonal anti-T cell antibodies. Transplant Proc 18:1287–1290

Long-Term Follow-Up of Renal Transplantation—Chronic Rejection and Recurrence of Nephritis

RICHARD N. FINE[1]

SUMMARY. Graft loss in long-term (> 10 years) surviving recipients occurs at a rate of 3%–5% annually. The most frequent cause of graft loss is chronic rejection. Unfortunately, no current therapeutic intervention is uniformly successful in forestalling the inevitable decline in graft function. The proposal that hyperfiltration is a significant factor contributing to nephron loss in long-term surviving grafts is interesting; however, controlled clinical trials of protein restricted diets, with concomitant accurate serial measurements of graft function are required before such an approach can be recommended.

Acute rejection and non-compliance with the immunosuppressive medications should be considered with abrupt declines in graft function in long-term recipients. Since such reduction in graft function is often asymptomatic, it is important that surveillance be continued in long-term recipients.

Recurrence of the original disease in the graft contributes minimally to graft loss in long-term surviving grafts. However, the incidence of recurrence causing graft failure during the second decade of function is <5%. Recurrence of diabetic nephropathy may take >20 years to become clinically manifest. The simultaneous transplantation of both the pancreas and kidney may ultimately arrest the recurrence of diabetic nephropathy.

Introduction

In the 21 reports [1] between 1974 and 1988 detailing long-term (> 10 years) patient and graft survival following renal transplantation the mortality rate was 3–5% per annum after 10 years. For patients alive after 10 years, 72–85% survived an additional 5 years. Graft loss after 10 years paralleled patient mortality, with 71–90% of the grafts still functioning at 15 years. Therefore, deterioration of graft function in

[1]Department of Pediatrics, School of Medicine, State University of New York at Stony Brook, Stony Brook, NY 11794-8111, USA

long-term (>10 years) surviving renal allograft recipients is not an unusual occurrence. The potential causes of declining graft function are: (1) chronic rejection, (2) non-immunological phenomenon, (3) acute rejection, (4) recurrence of the primary disease in the graft, (5) non-compliance with immunosuppressive drugs, (6) de novo glomerulonephritis, (7) nephrotoxic drugs, (8) renal artery stenosis, (9) hypertension, (10) concomitant infection, and (11) volume depletion. Although all of the above phenomena require consideration anytime there are perturbations of renal function in a long-term surviving renal allograft recipient, I will discuss only the first five entities in any detail in this manuscript.

Results and Discussion

Chronic Rejection

The *clinical manifestations* of chronic rejection are: (1) a progressive deterioration of graft function which ultimately results in graft loss, (2) proteinuria which frequently is associated with the nephrotic syndrome, and (3) hypertension [2]. The *histological manifestations* of chronic rejection are: (1) *Transplant glomerulopathy* with splitting and reduplication of the glomerular basement membrane without evidence of immune complex deposition by either immunofluorescence or electron microscopy; and (2) *Vascular rejection* manifested by nephron loss with interstitial fibrosis and tubular atrophy [3].

The incidence of graft loss from chronic rejection in grafts surviving >10 years has been variable; however, it is the most common cause of graft loss in long-term functioning grafts [1]. In 6 series from centers in the United States, Europe, and Australia which were reported between 1982 and 1989 the incidence has varied from 8%–24% (Table 1) with 5 of the 6 centers indicating an incidence between 8% and 11% [4–9].

Once chronic rejection is present no treatment has been uniformly successful in changing the clinical course of inevitable decline in graft function with ultimate graft loss. Feehally et al. [10] state that "no immune-modulating maneuver is consistently successful once chronic rejection is established with histopathological evidence of nephron loss and mesangial sclerosis." These authors further state that "no treatment has yet been shown to change the rate of decline in renal function in recipients with chronic rejection." Consequently, once the diagnosis of chronic rejection is established, treatment should be directed toward optimizing the conservative management of chronic renal failure. The admonition against the use of additional corticosteroid

Table 1. Incidence of chronic rejection in grafts surviving >10 years

Report	Center	Year	% Chronic rejection
Mahoney et al. [4]	Sydney	1982	8
Gueco et al. [5]	Cambridge	1985	24
Grapin et al. [6]	Paris/Tenon	1987	9
Lee et al. [7]	Richmond	1987	8
LeFrançois et al. [8]	Lyon	1987	11
Rao et al. [9]	Minneapolis	1989	9

treatment in a setting of chronic rejection is emphasized by Kirkman et al. [11] who note that "increased dosages of corticosteroids may have contributed to the deaths of 2 of 22 patients" with chronic rejection who were treated with increased dosages on one or more occasions.

Non-Immunologic Phenomenon

Feehally et al. [10] hypothesized that chronic renal transplant failure was primarily related to non-immune mechanisms. These authors postulated that hyperfiltration of the remnant nephrons of the graft was the dominant factor leading to the unrelenting decline of graft function. In order to test this hypothesis the authors presecribed a low protein (0.6 gm/kg per day) diet to 5 recipients with chronic renal transplant failure. Following initiation of the diet there was a significant decrease in the slope of the 1/serum creatinine curve for a period of 2–12 months. This hypothesis was further supported by Schmidt [12] who discontinued azathioprine in 5 recipients with chronic rejection and noted that the rate of loss of graft function, as indicated by the slope of 1/serum creatinine, did not change. From these data he concluded "that immunologic mechanisms do not play a major role in the predictable loss of graft function" from chronic rejection. Although this hypothesis is interesting, it is obvious that more detailed studies, on a larger number of recipients, are required before the concept receives additional support. Controlled clinical trials utilizing precise measurements of glomerular filtration rate may be indicated in the future.

Acute Rejection

Acute rejection in the early post-transplant period is well described; however, there is a paucity of information detailing acute rejection episodes in recipients surviving a second decade with a functioning graft. Rao et al. [9] analyzed the incidence, clinical and histological data, and outcome of 69 recipients who survived >10 years with a functioning graft. During the second decade of graft function, 15 recipients developed 20 acute rejection episodes. *Clinical manifestations*—proteinuria (0.7–6.3 gm), hypertension, fluid retention, and congestive heart failure—were present in only 8 of the 20 (40%) episodes of acute rejection, whereas in 12 of the 20 (60%) episodes the recipients were asymptomatic. *Histologic manifestations* were interstitial edema and interstitial mononuclear cell infiltrate without involvement of the glomeruli and blood vessels. These histologic changes were at times superimposed upon evidence of chronic rejection. Thirteen of the acute rejection episodes in 8 recipients were treated with intravenous corticosteroids. The response to treatment was as follows: complete response, 6 out of 13 (46%); partial response, 4 out of 13 (31%); and no response, 3 out of 13 (23%). Of the 8 recipients 2 died of septic complications within one month of treatment and 2 recipients resumed dialysis at 6 and 12 months following corticosteroid treatment. These authors concluded that: (1) long-term surveillance of recipients with long-term surviving renal allografts is required, because the majority of recipients who manifested acute rejection during the second decade of graft function were asymptomatic, (2) the potential response of a late occurring acute rejection episode to intravenous corticosteroids is excellent, and (3) a precise diagnosis is imperative in order to avoid unnecessary corticosteroid treatment of chronic rejection without any potential salutary effect.

Non-Compliance

In a recent report by Schweizer et al. [13] the *incidence* of non-compliance with immunosuppressive therapy following renal transplantation was determined, both prospectively and retrospectively. Between 1971 and 1984 the incidence of non-compliance was determined retrospectively and was found to be 18% (47 out of 269), whereas in the prospective analysis from 1984–1987 the incidence was 15% (30 out of 196). Didlake et al. [14] noted an incidence of non-compliance of 4.7% (25 out of 531) between 1980 and 1986, and stated that all graft losses after 36 months occurred in patients with documented non-compliance. The latter data are from patients transplanted in the cyclosporine era, and therefore the contribution of non-compliance to long-term (>10 years) graft dysfunction could not be determined. Potter et al. [15] described the course of 29 pediatric recipients who had a functioning graft for >10 years and a serum creatinine level of <2.0 mg/dl. During the second post-transplant decade 2 recipients, of whom one was non-compliant, each lost their graft and 5 recipients, 2 of whom were non-compliant, had an increase in the serum creatinine level of >1.0 mg/dl. Therefore, non-compliance can contribute to both *early* and *late graft dysfunction*. In the report of Schweizer et al. [13] rejection and/or death occurred in 91% of the non-compliant recipients in the retrospective analysis and in 37% of the recipients in the prospective study. Early identification of the non-compliant recipient, with subsequent treatment of the acute rejection episode, followed by reinstitution of the maintenance immunosuppressive regimen may be effective in sustaining long-term graft function in the non-compliant recipient.

Recurrence of Primary Disease

Recurrence of either a metabolic or a glomerular primary disease accounts for <2% of all graft failures, whereas the overall incidence of recurrence is probably 5–10 times more common [16]. Most recurrence occurs in the early post-transplant period; only rarely does recurrence from such primary renal diseases as membranoproliferative glomerulonephritis types I and II, IgA nephropathy, and focal glomerulosclerosis contribute to late graft failure [16].

Starzl et al. [17] in 1974, reporting on a decade of follow-up in early cases of renal transplantation, noted "transmission glomerulonephritis" in 8 of 35 graft biopsies obtained at 2 years post-transplant. Seven of the 8 grafts failed at 27–77 months following transplantation. The precise definition of "transmission glomerulonephritis" was not provided. In 1982, Kirkman et al. [11] reported that biopsy proven recurrent glomerulonephritis was evident at 10–11 years post-transplant in 3 out of 32 (9%) grafts which were lost >5 years post-transplant. Of the 21 reports [1] detailing the outcome of long-term (>10 years) surviving renal allografts, only 4 [6,8,18,19] mention recurrent disease as a cause of late graft failure. In these 4 reports the incidence of graft failure from recurrence was <5% and no specific data was provided regarding the type of primary disease (Table 2).

The incidence of recurrent disease in diabetic recipients is currently underestimated because, from recurrence of the diabetic lesion, a mean time of about 20 years for graft failure to occur seems likely [16]. However, there is the possibility that combined pancreas and kidney transplantation may protect the kidney from recurrence of the diabetic lesion. Bohman et al. [20] noted that the glomerular basement

Table 2. Recurrence in long-term (> 10 years) functioning renal allografts

Report	Year	No. of patients	No. of recurrences	
			< 10 Years	> 10 Years
Vanrenterghem et al. [18]	1987	93	2	1
Grapin et al. [6]	1987	90		1
LeFrançois et al. [8]	1987	64		3
McGeown et al. [19]	1988	62	4	

membrane thickening and mesangial expansion typical of diabetic nephropathy in all kidneys >2 years post-transplant were not seen in diabetic recipients who received simultaneous pancreas and kidney transplants.

References

1. Mahony JF (1989) Long term results and complications of transplantation: The kidney. Transplant Proc 21:1433–1434
2. Kreis H (1981) Transplanted kidney: Natural history. In: Hamburger J, Crosnier J, Bach J, Kreis H (eds) Renal transplantation theory and practice. Williams and Wilkins, London, pp 177–231
3. Zhang P, Rao RV, Anderson WR (1988) An ultra-structural study of the memranoproliferative variant of transplant glomerulopathy. Ultrastruct Pathol 12:185
4. Mahony JF, Savdie E, Caterson RJ, Furlong T, Storey BG, Stewart JH, Sheil AGR (1986) The natural history of cadaveric renal allografts beyond ten years. Transplant Proc 18:135–137
5. Gueco IP, Evans DB, Calne RY (1985) Prolonged survival after renal transplantation: A study of 54 patients who lived ten or more years after operation with functioning allografts. Transplant Proc 17:108–109
6. Grapin C, Michel F, Charpentier B, Frantz F, Fries D, Kuss R, Legrain M, Luciani H, Mohamedi D, Poisson J, Thibault P, Sraer JD (1987) Long-term prognosis of renal transplantation: A retrospective study of 90 patients living more than 10 years with a functioning allograft. Transplant Proc 19:3765–3766
7. Lee HM, Mendez-Picon G, Goldman MH, Mohanakumar T, Posner MP (1985) The course of long-term survival in kidney transplantation: One center's experience. Transplant Proc 17:106–107
8. LeFrançois N, Elmghabbar N, Chossegros P, Betuel H, Faure JL, Revillard JP, Traeger J, Dubernard JM, Touraine JL (1987) Long-term results in kidney transplantation: Patient and graft survival, causes of graft failure and mortality, renal function and complications after 10 years. Transplant Proc 19:3767–3768
9. Rao KV, Kasiske BL, Bloom PM (1989) Acute graft rejection in the late survivors of renal transplantation: Clinical and histological observations in the second decade. Transplantation 47:290–292
10. Feehally J, Harris KPG, Bennett SE, Walls J (1986) Is chronic renal transplant rejection a non-immunological phenomenon? Lancet II:486–488
11. Kirkman RL, Strom TB, Weir MR, Tilney NL (1982) Late mortality and morbidity in recipients of long-term renal allografts. Transplantation 34:347–351
12. Schmidt P (1986) Is chronic renal transplant rejection a non-immunological phenomenon? Lancet II:693
13. Schweizer RT, Rovelli M, Palmeri D, Vossler E, Hull D, Bartus S (1990) Noncompliance in organ transplant recipients. Transplantation 49:374–377

14. Didlake RH, Dreyfus K, Kerman RH, Van Buren CTm, Kahan BD (1988) Patient noncompliance: A major cause of late graft failure in cyclosporine-treated renal transplants. Transplant Proc 20:63–69
15. Potter D, Feduska N, Melzer J, Garovoy M, Hopper S, Duca R, Salvatierra O (1986) Twenty years of renal transplantation in children. Pediatrics 77:465–470
16. Mathew TH (1988) Recurrence of disease following renal transplantation. Am J Kidney Dis 12:85–96
17. Starzl TE, Porter KA, Halgrimson CG, Husberg BS, Penn I, Putnam CW (1974) A decade follow-up in early cases of renal homotransplantation. Ann Surg 180:606–617
18. Vanrenterghem Y, Roels L, Lerut T, Waer M, Gruwez J, Michielsen P (1987) Long-term prognosis after cadaveric kidney transplantation. Transplant Proc 19:3762–3764
19. McGeown MG, Douglas JF, Donaldson RA, Hill CM, Kennedy JA, Loughridge WGG, Middleton D (1988) Ten-year results of renal transplantation with azathioprine and prednisone as only immunosuppression. Lancet I:983–985
20. Bohman SO, Wilczek H, Tyden G, et al. (1987) Recurrent diabetic nephropathy in renal allografts placed in diabetic patients and protective effect of simultaneous pancreatic transplantation. Transplant Proc 19:2290–2293

Advances in Managements of Vasculitis and Lupus Nephritis

Chair: D. Keith Peters (UK)
Pao-Hsii Feng (Singapore)

The Specificity of the Autoimmune Response in Vasculitis

L.A. van Es, M.R. Daha, C. Halma, F.J. van der Woude[1], J.W. Cohen Tervaert, C.G.M. Kallenberg[2], A.E.G.Kr van dem Borne, and R. Goldschmeding[3]

Introduction

Systemic vasculitis is one of the most elusive subjects of human pathology. The vasculitides differ in pathology, and in the caliber and localization of the affected blood vessels. The definition and classification of vasculitides is still a matter of debate. The most acceptable classification distinguishes the so-called leukocytoclastic vasculitides, or small vessel vasculitides, the polyarteritis group (polyarteritis nodosa, overlap syndromes, microscopic polyarteritis, and Kawasaki's disease), and the group of granulomatous vasculitides (Wegener's granulomatosis, relapsing polychondritis, Churg-Strauss syndrome, lymphatoid granulomatosis, giant cell arteritis, and Takayasu's disease). To the group of leukocytoclastic vasculitides belong allergic vasculitis, anaphylactoid purpura (Henoch-Schoenlein purpura), hypocomplementemic urticarial vasculitis, postinfectious vasculitis, rheumatoid vasculitis, and vasculitis in systemic lupus erythematosus (SLE) and in Sjögren's syndrome, and in mixed cryoglobulinemia.

As a result of the diversity of clinical presentation of systemic vasculitides, a wide variety of clinical specialists are involved in the management of this relatively rare group of patients. Only few clinical centers have the opportunity to study sufficiently large groups of patients in each category of vasculitis. Therefore, for further progress, national and international collaboration is essential. Most of the data presented

[1]Department of Nephrology, Academish Ziekenhuis Leiden, University Hospital Postbus 9600, 2300 Leiden, The Netherlands

[2]Department of Clinical Immunology, University Hospital, Groningen, The Netherlands

[3]Department of Immunohaematology, Central Laboratory of Bloodtransfusion Service, Amsterdam, The Netherlands

in this review are the result of collaboration between three groups of investigators in the Netherlands.

The Pathogenetic Significance of Autoimmune Antibodies in Vasculitis

Since the detection of antinuclear antibodies in patients with SLE, autoimmune phenomena have received great attention. It is now clear that antinuclear antibodies (ANA) are not specific for SLE. They occur in many other disorders, including infectious diseases. The most useful application of the ANA-test is to exclude the possibility that a patient has SLE. The level of ANA does not correlate with the severity of the disease. A correlation between the level of anti-double stranded DNA (dsDNA) and the severity of lupus nephritis has been claimed by some, but has not been confirmed by others.

Several criteria can be used to demonstrate the pathogenetic significance of autoimmune antibodies. These antibodies should recognize autoantigens in those tissues that are affected by the disease process (the so called target organ). Secondly, disease activity should fluctuate with antibody levels. Artificial removal of antibodies by plasma exchange should result in improvement. On the other hand, transplacental passive transfer of the antibodies to a newborn child should induce the disease manifestations, as has been demonstrated for several autoimmune diseases. Finally, the pathogenetic effect of the antibodies should be reproducible in experimental animals. Except for anti-glomerular basement membrane (GBM) disease, which fulfils most of these criteria, no other auto-antibodies associated with systemic vasculitis meet these criteria. Most of these autoantibodies are considered to be autoimmune phenomena without a causal relationship to the disease process. An important exception to this rule could be made for the so called anti-neutrophil cytoplasmic antibodies (ANCA). These antibodies were first described by Davies in 1982, in patients with crescentic glomerulonephritis possibly caused by arbovirus [1]. In 1984 Hall et al. described these antibodies in patients with vasculitis and glomerulonephritis [2]. In 1985 we described the diagnostic significance of ANCA in patients with Wegener's granulomatosis [3]. The level of these antibodies also correlated with the activity of the disease. In 1988 Falk and Jenette described two types of ANCA: the cytoplasmic type, or c-ANCA, and the perinuclear type, or p-ANCA [4]. The latter frequently, but not always, represent autoantibodies directed against myeloperoxidase (MPO).

The Specificity of c-ANCA

ANCA was discovered by applying patients's serum onto the fixed granulocytes of healthy donors. Fixation by formaldehyde or absolute alcohol influences the immunofluorescence pattern of p-ANCA [4]. Using the indirect immunofluorescence technique it could be demonstrated that ANC detects an antigen present in the polymorphonuclear (PMN) leukocytes and monocytes of humans and chimpanzees but not in lower animals (Goldschmeding, unpublished work). The antigen can first be detected at the stage of differentiation of promyelocyte and promonocyte. Interestingly, it can also bind an antigen in the HL60 cell line that does not contain specific granules or alkaline phosphatase [5]. The antigen cannot be demonstrated in lymphocytes, erythrocytes, or platelets.

Several groups of investigators have attempted to isolate the antigen recognized by c-ANCA in order to develop radioimmunoassays or enzyme-linked immunosorbent assays (ELISA) for objective detection and accurate quantification of ANCA. Lockwood et al. have used an acid extract of sonicated neutrophil cytoplasmic components [6]. After purification by gel filtration and high performance liquid chromatography (HPLC), Wegener's granulomatosis (WG) sera bound to 100, 6.2, and 1.8 kDa components. The 100 kDa component shared epitopes with alkaline phosphatase. Daha et al. [7] isolated, by ion exchange chromatography and gel filtration, a protein that migrated on SDS-PAGE analysis as a 91 kDa protein and on HPLC gel filtration had a molecular weight of 68 kDa. A monoclonal antibody was raised against this antigen. The antigen was found to react with the cytoplasmic area of PMN leukocytes and it recognized, on immunoblots, the 29 kDa triplet isolated by Goldschmeding et al. [8]. Goldschmeding and colleagues used nitrogen bomb cavitation and subcellular fractionation of PMN leukocytes by Percoll density gradient centrifugation. With the use of marker proteins they could demonstrate, by Western blot analysis, that sera from patients with Wegener's granulomatosis (WG) bound to a 29 kDa protein in the α-fraction, representing azurophilic or primary granules [8]. By extraction in a buffer containing 3.5 M urea and 1 M KCl, followed by radioiodination and immunoprecipitation, it could be shown that the ANCA antigen migrates as a triplet of bands with M_r 29000, 30500, and 32000. All 12 c-ANCA-positive WG sera, but not the 23 ANCA-negative control sera, specifically precipitated the 29 kDa antigen. Sera with high ANCA titers precipitated two additional bands at M_r 30500 and 32000. The c-ANCA antigen was found to be a saline-soluble triplet present in azurophilic granules of normal neutrophils [8]. Using ^{3}H-labeled diisopropylfluorophosphate (DFP), it could be shown that ^{3}H-DFP was coprecipitated by WG serum together with the radioionated c-ANCA antigen. The binding of DFP indicates that the ANCA antigen is a serine protease. Using polyclonal antibodies to elastase and cathepsin G, it could be demonstrated by sequential immunoprecipitation that the c-ANCA antigen is not identical to elastase or to cathepsin [8]. Recently, a third serine protease (protease 3) has been described in azurophilic granules [9]. Lüdeman et al. [10] have purified the ANCA-antigen from the supernatant of stimulted PMN by immunoaffinity chromatography, using purified IgG from an ANCA-positive serum. The characteristics of this antigen are very similar to the described properties of protease 3 [9]. Lüdeman et al. have determined the [17] NH_2-terminal amino acid sequence of the c-ANCA antigen [10].

They found it to be:

I–V–G–G–H–E–A–Q–P–H–I–R–P–I–Y–M–A.

A similar study by Niles et al. [11] revealed a similar, but not identical, amino acid sequence:

I–V–G–G–H–E–A–Q–P–H–S–X–P–Y–M–A–S–L–Q–M

These N-terminal sequences show a striking homology with other serine proteases [11].

Table 1. Stimulation of peripheral blood lymphocytes from five healthy donors (*HD*) and four patients with Wegener's granulomatosis (*WG*)

	Proliferative response (pm $\times 10^{-3}$)			
Donor	Medium	91 kDa	29 kDa	PWM
HD-1	1.3	1.0	1.2	17.5
HD-2	1.4	0.9	1.3	18.2
HD-3	1.0	1.2	1.1	31.5
HD-4	1.6	1.3	1.5	18.6
HD-5	1.2	0.5	1.4	24.3
WG-1	1.2	13.3	12.1	18.7
WG-2	1.5	14.7	13.8	19.3
WG-3	1.3	16.9	16.9	20.9
WH-4	1.4	2.3	4.1	23.7

PWM, pokeweed mitogen

Specificity of the Cellular Response in WG

In preliminary experiments, we exposed peripheral blood lymphocytes from five healthy donors and four WG patients to the 91 kDa sputum antigen isolated by Daha and to the 29 kDa antigen isolated by Goldschmeding (Table 1). The proliferative responses of the normal controls in the presence of these two specific antigens did not differ from the proliferation in medium alone (Daha, unpublished work). Peripheral blood lymphocytes from the four WG patients showed a significantly higher proliferative response in the presence of either the 91 kDa or the 29 kDa antigen. The two groups did not differ in their response to pokeweed mitogen. These data indicate that patients with WG not only develop a humoral autoimmune response against 91 kDa and 29 kDa, but also a cellular autoimmune response against these neutrophil antigens.

Specificity of p-ANCA

The specificity of p-ANCA is less clear than the specificity of c-ANCA. First of all, alcohol fixation may not only lead to perinuclear staining, but also to nuclear staining. This artefact is caused by solubilization of nucleophilic constituents of the azurophilic granules which diffuse and bind to the nuclei [12].

In a prospective study, it was found that not only patients with WG, but also patients with microscopic polyarteritis (MPA) have ANCA [13]. MPA has been defined as a primary systemic vasculitis with segmental necrotizing glomerulonephritis [14]. In practice, this definition also includes patients with leukocytoclastic vasculitis (i.e., venulitis). The majority of these patients have crescent formation in their glomeruli. Later ANCA was also detected in sera of patients with primary or idiopathic crescentic glomerulonephritis [4]. In contrast to WG sera, these sera frequently show a p-ANCA. Most, but not all, of these p-ANCA could be explained by a specificity for myeloperoxidase (MPO), another constituent of the azurophilic granules of PMN leukocytes [4].

At Groningen University Hospital, of 42 biopsies taken from patients with crescentic glomerulonephritis, 35 showed no or scanty immune deposits in the glomeruli [15]. All patients with biopsy proven WG ($n=9$) had c-ANCA. Of patients who were suspected to have WG, two-thirds ($n=10$) had c-ANCA and one third ($n=5$) had p-ANCA [15]. Of 8 patients with idiopathic crescentic glomerulonephritis (GN), only 2 had c-ANCA and the remaining 6 patients had p-ANCA. All patients with p-ANCA also had autoimmune antibodies to MPO, as first described by Falk and Jenette [4].

In a few cases, p-ANCA can be based on autoimmune antibodies directed against elastase. However, the p-ANCA observed in SLE patients usually do not have a specificity for MPO or for elastase. The perinuclear and nuclear staining pattern of p-ANCA is indistinguishable from a staining pattern described earlier by Wiik [16] for granulocyte-specific antinuclear antibodies (GS-ANA). These antibodies were originally described in a patient with Felty's syndrome. They are found in 75% of patients with active rheumatoid arthritis, especially in cases having autoimmune neutropenia [17].

References

1. Davies DJ, Moran JE, Nial JF, Ryan GB (1982) Segmental necrotising glomerulonephritis with antineutrophil antibody: possible arbovirus aetiology? Br Med J [Clin Res] 285:606
2. Hall JB, Waldham BMcN, Wood CJ, Ashton V, Adam WR (1984) Vasculitis and glomerulonephritis: a subgroup with an antineutrophil cytoplasmic antibody. Aust NZ J Med 14:277–278
3. Van der Woude FJ, Rasmussen N, Lobatto S, Wiik A, Permin H, Van Es LA, Van der Giessen M, Van der Hem GK, The TH (1985) Autoantibodies against neutrophils and monocytes: tool for diagnosis and marker of disease activity in Wegener's granulomatosis. Lancet I:425–429
4. Falk RJ, Jenette JC (1988) Anti-neutrophil cytoplasmic autoantibodies with specificity for myeloperoxidase in patients with systemic vasculitis and idiopathic necrotizing and crescentic glomerulonephritis. N Engl J Med 318:1651–1657
5. Charles LA, Falk RJ, Jenette JG (1989) Reactivity of anti-neutrophil cytoplasmic autoantibodies with HL-60 cells. Clin Immunol Immunopathol 53:243–253
6. Lockwood CM, Bakes D, Jones S, Whitaker KB, Moss DW, Savage COS (1987) Association of alkaline phosphatase with an autoantigen recognized by circulating anti-neutrophil antibodies in systemic vasculitis. Lancet I:716–720
7. Daha MR, Leusen J, Kramps JA, Schrama E, Van Es LA, Van der Woude FJ (1990) Isolation from purulent sputum of an antigen reactive with antibodies in serum of patients with Wegener's granulomatosis. Neth J Med 36:117–120
8. Goldschmeding R, Van der Schoot CE, Ten Bokkel Huinink D, Hack CE, Van den Ende ME, Kallenberg CGM, Von dem Borne AEGKr (1989) Wegener's granulomatosis antibodies identify a novel diisopropylfluorophosphate-binding protein in the lysosomes of normal human neutrophils. J Clin Invest 84:1577–1587
9. Kao RC, Wehner NG, Skubitz KM, Gray BH, Hoidal JR (1988) Proteinase 3. A distinct human polymorphonuclear leukocyte proteinase that produces emphysema in hamsters. J Clin Invest 82:1963–1973
10. Lüdeman J, Utecht B, Gross WL (1990) Anti-neutrophil cytoplasm antibodies in Wegener's granulomatosis recognize an elastinolytic enzyme. J Exp Med 171:357–362

11. Niles JL, McCluskey RT, Ahmad MF, Arnaout MA (1989) Wegener's granulomatosis autoantigen is a novel neutrophil serine protease. Blood 74:1888–1893
12. Falk RJ, Hogan S, Wilkman AS, Terrell RS, Lautizen S, Charles LA, Jenette JC (1990) Myeloperoxidase specific anti-neutrophil cytoplasmic autoantibodies (MPO-ANCA). Neth J Med 36:121–125
13. Savage LOS, Winearls CG, Jones S, Marshall PD, Lockwood CM (1987) Prospective study of radioimmunoassay for antibodies against neutrophil cytoplasm in diagnosis of systemic vasculitis. Lancet I:1389–1393
14. Savage LOS, Winearls CG, Evans DJ, Rees AJ, Lockwood M (1985) Microscopic polyarteritis: presentation, pathology and prognosis. Q J Med 56:467–483
15. Cohen Tevaert JW, Goldschmeding R, Elema JD, Van der Giessen M, Huitema MG, Van der Hem GK, The TH, Von dem Borne AEGKr, Kallenberg CGM (1990) Autoantibodies against myeloid lysosomal enzymes in crescentic glomerulonephritis. Kidney Int 37:799–806
16. Wiik A (1987) The value of specific ANA determination in rheumatology. Allergy 42: 241–261
17. Wiik A (1980) Granulocyte-specific antinuclear antibodies? Possible significance for the pathogenesis, clinical features and diagnosis of rheumatoid arthritis. Allergy 35:362–389

New Perspectives on Systemic Vasculitis: Implications for Diagnosis and Treatment

C. MARTIN LOCKWOOD[1]

Introduction

There is now growing evidence that autoimmune mechanisms play an important role in the systemic vasculitides: their demonstration forms the basis of the first diagnostic laboratory test for this group of diseases and their manipulation constitutes the first advance towards specific immunotherapy for their treatment [1,2]. The systemic vasculitides form a loosely associated group which have as their pathological basis a chronic necrotizing inflammation which affects vessels of varying sizes at varying sites throughout the body. There are primary and secondary forms, primary, which involve blood vessels exclusively and which are the subject of this article, and secondary, which arise in association with disease elsewhere, for example, vasculitis secondary to Crohn's disease. Some primary forms are associated with granulomata, for example, Takayasu's disease and Wegener's granulomatosis. Because so little is known of their pathogenesis, a morphological approach has been adopted toward their classification, see Table 1. Because of the same uncertainty, the evolution of a treatment strategy has been mainly empirical, driven by the high morbidity and mortality rates if no therapy was given. Thus, until recently, the best evidence that autoimmune processes played an important role in the systemic vasculitides came from evidence that powerful immunosuppressive agents were beneficial, [3] and that these might be humoral mechanisms was supported by the finding that additional plasma exchange was useful in the management of severe forms of these diseases, particularly rapidly progressive nephritis [4].

In 1982, Davies et al. reported that patients with polyarteritis and renal vasculitis had circulating autoantibodies which reacted with the cytoplasm of normal granulocytes [5]. A similar report in 1985 by Van der Woude et al. documented the same phenomenon occurring in patients with Wegener's granulomatosis [6]. These auto-

[1]Department of Medicine, University of Cambridge School of Clinical Medicine, Addenbrooke's Hospital, Cambridge, CB2 2QQ, UK

Table 1. Morphological classification of systemic vasculitides

	Granulomata	
Vessel size	Present	Absent
Large	Takayasu's[a]	Giant cell arteritis
Medium	Churg-Strauss[a]	Polyarteritis nodosa
Small	Wegener's granulomatosis[a]	Microscopic polyarteritis[a] Kawasaki disease[a] Henoch-Schönlein purpura[a]

[a]Denote vasculitides in which anti-neutrophil cytoplasm antibodies have been reported

antibodies were detected by indirect immunofluorescence techniques which were subjective and relatively insensitive. The development of solid phase immunoradiometric assays obviated both problems and showed that detection of autoantibodies to neutrophil cytoplasm antigens (ANCA) by these techniques provided both sensitive and specific means for diagnosis of the common primary vasculitides [7]. That these autoimmune mechanisms operate in systemic vasculitis has provided new perspectives on these diseases, with consequent implications for diagnosis and treatment.

ANCA and Disease Activity

The close association of ANCA with the development of certain vasculitides indicated that serial measurements might reflect disease activity, which could be useful not only in managing treatment, but also in predicting disease relapse. Van der Woude showed that by indirect immunofluorescence assays ANCA levels correlated with disease activity [6] and we also used this test in a retrospective study of patients' progress after discharge from hospital. We monitored 18 patients over a period of three years. Eight had become ANCA negative during their initial inpatient treatment but 10 still had detectable ANCA at the beginning of the study. No relapses occurred in the ANCA negative group, but eight relapses occurred in the ANCA positive group. In six of the eight who relapsed, relapses seemed to occur in relation to reductions in immunosuppressive therapy. This underlined the connection between ANCA and active disease. However, there were some patients who remained ANCA positive without symptomatology. In such patients further studies showed the importance of other factors in promoting disease expression, for example, ANCA isotype (see below).

This early experience led us to adopt a treatment strategy aimed at inducing both clinical and serological remission. We then tested the assay's predictive performance in a prospective fashion by assessing patients' progress at regular intervals both clinically and serologically. We have now studied 20 patients who were in clinical and serological remission at the beginning of the study, for a mean of 48 patient weeks. The patients were assessed clinically at monthly intervals. ANCA seroconversion was taken to indicate serological relapse and the Creative protein (CRP) level was used as a nonspecific indicator either of this or other inflammatory events (such as intercurrent infection). We observed 11 relapses in 9 patients. A rise in ANCA preceded relapse in eight and occurred at the same time in two; no seroconversion could be detected in one relapse. On two occasions ANCA tests became positive, but disease did not follow.

Only on one occasion did a rise in CRP precede relapse. Thus, although a rise in CRP was not a good predictive test, ANCA seroconversion was useful. Furthermore, since the mean time to relapse after seroconversion was one month, this raised the prospect that monthly patient follow-up might be carried out remote from specialist centers, with recall if ANCA titers rose.

Class and Subclass of ANCA

In Wegener's disease and microscopic polyarteritis, ANCA are usually of IgG isotype. Rarely, patients with a polyarteritis pulmonary-renal syndrome have been identified where ANCA are restricted to IgM isotype [8]. These patients have severe disease, readily responsive to plasma exchange, an appropriate treatment since IgM is predominantly confined to the intravascular compartment. With treatment a late isotype switch (to IgG) has been documented in three patients as the disease remitted, and ANCA of both IgM and IgG isotypes have been eluted from the kidneys of one patient at autopsy. This suggested that the IgM autoantibody might not only have determined the pattern of organ involvement, but also the severity of disease activity. A similar relationship of disease to isotype has been reported for Henoch-Schonlein purpura in adults (who have IgA ANCA) [9].

We have also studied the ANCA IgG subclass in patients at presentation and again in remission (yet still ANCA positive). Initially there was a predominance of ANCA of IgG3 isotype, but this later switched to IgG2 [10]. This is interesting, since IgG3 antibodies can fix complement and engage macrophages through receptors which IgG2 antibodies lack (complement and macrophages can substantially augment the inflammatory response once activated). Thus, these findings might explain why some patients in remission continue to have raised ANCA levels yet little disease activity.

Incidence of ANCA Positive Systemic Vasculitis

For the first time ANCA assays have provided a powerful diagnostic tool for the systemic vasculitides, which is not dependent on clinical interpretation. Our laboratory acts as a reference center for the population of East Anglia and this has allowed the incidence of ANCA positive disease to be estimated at 1:2,000, a level greater than for SLE and as high as that for rheumatoid arthritis. No doubt the tendency for vasculitis to present under any medical discipline, and the lack of a diagnostic laboratory test, has served to diminish estimates of its incidence.

Pathophysiological Role of ANCA

Whether ANCA fulfill a pathogenetic role is yet undecided. Levels of ANCA correlate with disease activity [6] and ANCA immunoglobulin can be eluted from vasculitic lesions and will bind to appropriate cells cultured in vitro [8,11]. Attempts to transfer disease to an experimental model have been frustrated by lack of a suitable recipient species (cross-reactive antigens are present only in baboons) and by the short time available, since serum sickness lesions, themselves vasculitic, develop from day 7 on. In a pilot study in baboons we did find a striking neutropenia in recipients given ANCA-rich immunoglobulin (C.M. Lockwood and C.B. Wilson, unpublished work).

This turned attention to in vitro effects of ANCA on neutrophil function, and on signal transduction in particular. We found that preincubation with ANCA markedly inhibited neutrophil activation brought about by agents such as phorbol myristate acetate (PMA), probably because ANCA can lead to sustained activation of polymorphs [12]. This is particularly interesting, since systemic vasculitis is hallmarked histologically by evidence of chronic polymorph activation, and argues for a direct role of ANCA in the disease process.

ANCA and Network Control of Immune Responses

If autoantibodies in patients with systemic vasculitis can mediate disease, then study of the regulation of these autoimmune responses may help to guide new strategies for treatment. The best understood immunological regulatory mechanisms involve control by way of a "network" of idiotypic anti-idiotypic reactions predicted by the "network theory" [13]. Idiotypic determinants have been characterized on autoantibodies occurring in different autoimmune diseases, and heterologous anti-idiotypic antibodies to those have been shown to have a regulatory effect in vitro [14]. The possibility that natural homeostatic mechanisms operate within the network framework has been supported by the finding that "normal" B cells possess the necessary genetic information to manufacture autoantibodies [15] and, that within the population of normal immunoglobulins, there exists a range of "natural" anti-idiotypic antibodies [16]. This has been exploited therapeutically for the treatment of a number of autoimmune diseases, best exemplified by spontaneous anti-factor VIII disease, where control of autoantibody formation has been shown to be explainable by idiotypic anti-idiotypic regulation [17]. It is of note that the treatment of choice for Kawasaki disease, an ANCA positive childhood vasculitis, is the administration of pooled normal immunoglobulin intravenously [18].

This has led us to study the properties of pooled immunoglobulins on ANCA reactions [19]. We have shown that $F(ab)_2$ of normal pooled immunoglobulin can inhibit binding of ANCA in vitro. The degree of inhibition ranged from 0%–100%, with up to 75% of a panel of 21 pretreatment ANCA positive sera being substantially inhibited by a single $F(ab)_2$ preparation of pooled immunoglobulin. Inhibitory reactivity was also found in remission sera, which were ANCA negative, including sera from patients whose remission occurred spontaneously. That this inhibition of binding fulfilled the criteria of idiotypic anti-idiotypic reactions was demonstrated by showing that the $F(ab)_2$ of affinity purified immunoglobulin reacted with, and was inhibited in its specific binding by, IgG from normal immunoglobulin. These experimental data have encouraged pilot studies of the use of pooled immunoglobulin for treatment of certain patients with systemic vasculitis.

Treatment of Systemic Vasculitis with Intravenous Immunoglobulin (IVIg)

We have treated four patients with pooled normal immunoglobulin given by intravenous infusion (Sandoglobulin, Sandoz, UK). All had ANCA positive vasculitis: for two this was the only treatment given, for the other two IVIg was given after failure

Table 2. Clinical and laboratory features of four patients treated with IVIg

Patient no.	Age	Sex	Diagnosis	Other treatment	Disease activity pre/post	CRP pre/post	Follow-ups (months)
1	62	F	WG	CP	2/0	148/10	6
2	57	M	WG	0	1/0	18/N	4
3	73	M	MP	0	1/0	N/N	11
4	61	M	MP	CP	1/0	N/N	5

C, cyclophosphamide; P, prednisolone; N, Normal (>6mg/100ml); CRP, C reactive protein; WG, Wegener's granulomatosis; MP, microscopic polyarteris

of conventional immunosuppressive drugs. The four patients were observed for a mean of three months before and six months after therapy. Clinical disease activity was recorded using a 2,1,0 scale (2, active disease requiring hospital or home care; 1, still symptomatic but institutionally independent; 0, remission); levels of ANCA (by radio-immunoassay) and C reactive protein (CRP) were measured serially. The potential efficacy of the Sandoglobulin was assessed by an in vitro test of inhibition of ANCA-binding activity. The clinical and laboratory data are shown in Table 2.

Clinical improvement was seen in all four patients, including the two resistant to standard therapy. After the IVIg, ANCA levels rose initially in all four patients, but in three then fell to levels substantially lower than pretreatment values, becoming undetectable in the fourth. Low levels of ANCA continued to be detectable, without overt evidence of disease, during follow-up in these three patients.

The numbers of patients studied so far is small but some points of interest emerge already. Firstly, clinical improvement occurred in all the patients treated and was maintained for periods of follow up ranging from four to eleven months (mean, six). Secondly, after the IVIg infusion ANCA levels rose transiently in all the patients, and remained detectable in three, without deleterious effect on the clinical outcome. The initial rise may have been due to displacement of ANCA from tissue-bound sites, since competitive inhibition of binding was demonstrated between the intravenous immunoglobulin (F(ab)$_2$ preparations) and the autoantibodies in each of the patients treated. It is equally possible that the persisting ANCA were from populations of autoantibodies bearing idiotypes not recognized by the normal pooled IgG and possibly not pathogenetically important. Thirdly, in the two untreated patients, in vitro tests of ANCA producing B cell activity indicated that in both patients this was abrogated after IVIg infusion, suggesting an immediate down regulation of autoantibody synthesis had been achieved (Mathieson et al., work in progress).

A Role for Plasma Exchange?

The balance of idiotypic and anti-idiotypic reactions appears symmetrical, but if ascendancy of one component could be promoted, then new strategies for therapy could be encouraged. Recently we have found that there is a difference in the isotype of the anti-idiotypic antibodies: a substantial proportion are IgM. IgM synthesis rates are markedly faster than those of IgG. Thus, depletion of all circulatory immunoglobulins by plasmapheresis might allow this desired alteration in homeostasis by virtue of the greater synthetic rate of IgM. In this context it is of interest that plasmapheresis has been shown to have an intrinsic benefit in treatment of patients with severe renal and systemic vasculitis (as tested in a randomized prospective controlled trial) [4].

Conclusions

It is now evident that autoimmune mechanisms may play an important role in systemic vasculitis, and their identification is useful for diagnosis and management of these disorders. Their further study may allow an understanding of the pathogenesis of these disorders and open up the prospects of new strategies for treatment. At the present time, one such strategy we are exploring involves a combination of treatment by plasma exchange followed by intravenous immunoglobulin infusion therapy.

References

1. Savage COS and Lockwood CM (1989) Autoantibodies in primary systemic vasculitis. In: Stollerman GH (ed) Advances in internal medicine, vol 35. Year Book Medical, Chicago, pp 73–92
2. Van der Woude FJ, Daha MR, Van Es LA (1989) The current status of neutrophil cytoplasmic antibodies. Clin Exp Immunol 78, 143–148
3. Katz P, Fauci AS (1981) Treatment of immune complex mediated diseases: corticosteroids and cytotoxic agents. In: Fauci AS (ed) Clinics in immunology, 1981. Saunders, Eastbourne, pp 415–431
4. Pusey CD, Lockwood CM (1985) Plasma exchange for glomerular disease. In: Robinson RR (ed) Nephrology, 1985. Springer, New York, pp 1474–1486
5. Davies DJ, Moran JE, Niall JF, Ryan GB (1982) Segmental necrotizing glomerulonephritis with antineutrophil antibody: possible arbovirus aetiology? Br Med J [Clin Res] 285:606
6. Van der Woude FJ, Rasmussen N, Lobatto S, Wiik A, Permin H, Van Es LA, Van der Giessen M, Van der Hem GK, The TH (1985) Autoantibodies against neutrophils and monocytes: tool for diagnosis and marker for disease activity in Wegener's granulomatosis. Lancet I:425–429
7. Savage COS, Winearls CG, Jones S, Marshall PD, Lockwood CM (1987) Prospective study of radioimmunoassay for antibodies against neutrophil cytoplasm in diagnosis of systemic vasculitis. Lancet I:1389–1393
8. Jayne DRW, Jones SJ, Severn A, Shaumack S, Murphy J, Lockwood CM (1989) Severe pulmonary haemorrhage and systemic vasculitis in association with circulating anti-neutrophil antibodies of IgM class only. Clin Nephrol 32:101–106
9. Van den Wall Bake AWL, Lobatto S, Jonges L, Daha MR, Van Es LA (1987) IgA antibodies directed against cytoplasmic antigens of polymorphonuclear leucocytes in patients with Henoch-Schonlein purpura. In: Mestecky J, et al. (eds) Recent advances in mucosal immunity: Part B, 1987. Plenum, London, p 1593
10. Jayne DRW, Lockwood CM (to be published) Subclass specificity of autoantibodies to neutrophil cytoplasm antigens in systemic vasculitis
11. Abbott F, Jones SJ, Lockwood CM, Rees AJ (1989) Autoantibodies to glomerular antigens in patients with Wegener's granulomatosis. Nephrol Dial Transpl 4:1–8
12. Lai KN, Lockwood CM (to be published) Down-regulation of signal transduction in human neutrophils by anti-neutrophil cytoplasm antibodies

13. Jerne NK (1974) Towards a network theory of the immune response. Ann Immunol (Paris) 125:373–389
14. Lockwood CM, Pye RJ (1990) Basic mechanisms in autoimmunity. In: Champion RH, Pye RJ (eds) Adv in dermatology, vol 8. Churchill Livingstone, Edinburgh, pp 71–84
15. Painter C, Monestier M, Bonin B, Bing CA (1986) Functional and molecular studies of V genes expressed in autoantibodies. Immunol Rev 94:75–98
16. Rossi F, Jayne DRW, Lockwood CM, Kazatchkine MD (to be published) Anti-idiotypes against anti-neutrophil cytoplasm antibodies in normal human polyspecific IgG for therapeutic use and in the serum of patients with systemic vasculitis in remission
17. Sultan Y, Rossi F, Kazatchkine MD (1987) Recovery from anti-VIII:C (anti-haemophilic factor) autoimmune disease dependent on generation of anti-idiotypes against anti-VIII:C autoantibodies. PNAS 84:828–830
18. Leung DYM, Burns JC, Neuburger M, Geha RS (1987) Reversal of lymphocyte activation in vivo in the Kawasaki syndrome by intravenous gamma globulin. J Clin Invest 79:468– 472
19. Rossi F, Jayne DRW, Lockwood CM. Kazatchkine MD (to be published) Anti-idiotypes against anti-neutrophil cytoplasmic antigen (ANCA) autoantibodies in normal human polyspecific IgG for therapeutic use and in the remission sera of patients with systemic vasculitis. Clin Exp Immunol

Therapeutic Trials in Lupus Nephritis

JAMES E. BALOW[1]

SUMMARY. Corticosteroids have had a profound effect on survival of patients with systemic lupus erythematosus. The salutary effects of these agents on lupus nephritis have been less satisfactory, from the perspective of both efficacy and long-term toxicity. Initial investigations of cytotoxic drugs in human lupus nephritis have been mostly contentious, while studies in murine lupus have demonstrated unequivocal advantages of cyclophosphamide over corticosteroids; increased longevity of the mice has been primarily due to control of nephritis by cyclophosphamide. The advantages of intermittent over continuous cyclophosphamide have been evident in the murine experiments and from experience in clinical oncology.

Controlled trials of corticosteroids, azathioprine and cyclophosphamide have demonstrated the best short-term control of the clinical signs of proliferative lupus nephritis in subjects under cyclophosphamide treatment. Studies of sustained treatment have documented long-term advantage of cyclophosphamide over prednisone in reducing clinical evidence of active nephritis, pathologic evidence of renal progression and the risk of developing end stage renal failure. Intermittent pulse cyclophosphamide has been demonstrated to have a better therapeutic index than conventional daily therapy.

Introduction

Among the numerous therapeutic advances in medicine and surgery achieved during the mid-twentieth century, corticosteroids played a key role in improved management of many of the critical components and complications of systemic lupus erythematosus. As longevity of lupus patients increased, nephritis became a central component of this disease. Lupus nephritis remains a pre-occupying concern of clinicians because its prevention is uncertain and treatment is controversial, usually com-

[1]National Institute of Health, Building 10, Room 9N222, Bethesda, MD 20892, USA

plicated, and often unsuccessful [1,2]. Moreover, patients who reach end stage renal failure as the result of lupus nephritis continue to have decreased longevity as a consequence of numerous systemic complications of lupus [3]. In the context of this historical background and of the therapeutic inadequacies, the rationale for continued pursuit of better techniques for management of lupus nephritis is self-evident.

Conventional Management of Lupus

The beneficial effects of corticosteroids on many of the systemic components of lupus have been so striking that controlled clinical trials have, by consensus, been considered superfluous. Although intellectually provocative, it is unlikely that prospective trials will ever be performed to document rigorously the superiority of corticosteroids over no immunosuppressive or anti-inflammatory treatment. Neither did knowledge of the short-term advantage of corticosteroids on the proliferative forms of lupus nephritis derive from prospective, controlled trials. The seminal observations of Pollak [4] and Baldwin [5] of the salutary effects of high-dose corticosteroids set the standards for therapy of lupus nephritis for several decades. Nonetheless, dissatisfaction with efficacy in many cases and with unacceptable toxicities in most cases fueled controversy about the use of prolonged high-dose corticosteroids and intensified the search for alternative treatments.

Experimental Aspects of Lupus

Lupus nephritis is the prototypical immune complex disease of the kidney. Lymphoid hyperplasia and spontaneous in vivo overactivity are nearly invariable and account for the exuberant production of polyclonal autoantibodies and immune complexes. Although a host of immunoregulatory disturbances surround the B lymphocyte excess, primary and secondary relationships among these immune system perturbations are nebulous [2]. Corticosteroids were shown experimentally to have a modest effect on B lymphocyte responses [6]. The search for agents which would more effectively suppress the excessive immune responses of lupus led investigators to the cytotoxic agents used in oncology. Among the chemotherapeutic drugs, cyclophosphamide was recognized to have a preferential effect on B lymphocyte responses [7].

Inbred stains of mice which exhibited immunological and clinical similarities to human lupus and which predictably succumbed from renal failure became invaluable resources for pilot studies of the effectiveness of cytotoxic drugs in lupus nephritis. Numerous controlled studies documented dramatic extensions of the longevity of these mice when treated with cytotoxic drugs [2,8]. Cyclophosphamide was among the most effective and high-dose intermittent pulse therapy appeared to have the highest therapeutic index [2].

Therapeutic Trials of Cytotoxic Drugs in Human Lupus Nephritis

Despite the encouraging results of treatment in the animal models of lupus nephritis, skepticism about their relevance to human disease prevailed. This was fueled by observations of serious drug-related morbidity in early (and often overzealous) clinical applications of cytotoxic drugs [9]. As clinical and laboratory experience accumulated, it appeared that a therapeutic window of efficacy and toxicity could be realized.

Controlled trials of cytotoxic drugs in patients with lupus nephritis were initiated around 1970. Azathioprine was shown in several early studies to have little advantage over corticosteroids alone [10,11,12]. Subsequent efforts began to focus on cyclophosphamide.

Studies at the Mayo Clinic [13] were designed to analyze the benefit of adding a brief course of daily oral cyclophosphamide to prednisone, while studies at the National Institutes of Health were designed to evaluate the effects of long-term cytotoxic drug therapy [14]. In the latter study, comparisons were made among patients treated with prednisone alone or prednisone plus azathioprine, cyclophosphamide, combined low-dose azathioprine and cyclophosphamide, or intermittent pulse cyclophosphamide. Both centers reported that the highest probabilities of stabilizing or improving clinical and laboratory signs of renal disease were observed in patients receiving cyclophosphamide in addition to prednisone. Follow-up renal biopsies obtained from patients in the National Institutes of Health studies showed that cytotoxic drug treatment protected against progressive renal damage more effectively than prednisone alone [15]. However, in the studies from both institutions, renal failure events were infrequent and no differences in risk of end stage renal failure among the treatment groups were discernible through the first five years of follow-up [13,14]. Understandably, the results of these studies provoked debate and controversy; the advantages of cyclophosphamide seemed modest and were of uncertain long-term value and the magnitude of delayed side-effects was unknown.

Extended follow-up of the patients in the Mayo Clinic trial failed to show a reduction of late renal failure events in patients who had received the initial short-course of cyclophosphamide [16]. On the other hand, after a median follow-up of seven years for the patients receiving long-term treatment in the National Institutes of Health studies, the risk of developing end stage renal failure was higher with prednisone alone than with intermittent pulse cyclophosphamide [14]. Also, treatment with daily oral cyclophosphamide or with daily low-dose combined cyclophosphamide and azathioprine has subsequently been shown to be more efficacious than prednisone, but consideration of high rates of side-effects of daily cytotoxic drugs led us to discontinue these therapeutic options despite their apparent efficacy. Intermittent pulse cyclophosphamide clearly had the highest therapeutic index among the options tested. Toxicity of the various regimens used in the studies at the National Institutes of Health has recently been reviewed [2,9]. Several recent reports have confirmed the efficacy of intermittent pulse cyclophosphamide for treatment of lupus nephritis [17,18] and of other systemic complications of lupus [19].

Other Therapeutic Options

Pulse methylprednisolone has been reported to be effective in management of lupus nephritis [20]. In a controlled trial currently being conducted at the National Institutes of Health, the hypothesis that intermittent pulse methylprednisolone is as efficacious as intermittent pulse cyclophosphamide is being tested in patients with severe proliferative lupus nephritis. In this study, 24 patients received monthly pulse methylprednisolone, 21 patients received monthly pulse cyclophosphamide for six months only, and 19 patients received monthly pulse cyclophosphamide for six months followed by quarterly pulse cyclophosphamide for an additional two years. Preliminary results show that patients receiving pulse methylprednisolone have the highest trend in risk of doubling their serum creatinine and of progressing to end stage renal failure. Long-term follow-up is in progress to provide valid statistically significant analysis.

Cyclosporine [21,22] and total lymphoid irradiation [23] have proven efficacious in lupus nephritis. No controlled clinical trials of these agents have been reported for treatment of human lupus nephritis.

Plasma exchange therapy has been utilized for a number of systemic complications of lupus. Controlled studies to date have not supported the benefit of plasma exchange therapy. In a double-blind study from the National Institutes of Health of real or sham procedure in patients with mild systemic lupus, little objective benefit of plasma exchange was found [24]. In a subsequent multi-centered study of patients with severe proliferative lupus nephritis, no difference in the rate of progression of renal disease was observed between the group of patients receiving immunosuppression alone and that receiving immunosuppression and adjunctive plasma exchange [25].

Novel Therapeutic Approaches to Lupus Nephritis

Controlled studies in murine lupus nephritis offer the promise of new and alternative approaches to the treatment of human disease. Monoclonal antibodies to subsets of T lymphocytes have been shown to prevent renal failure and prolong survival in animal models [26,27]. Similarly, exciting prospects for the use of biologic response modifiers, such as recombinant cytokines, appear to be ready for testing. Recombinant tumor necrosis factor has produced a salutary effect on murine lupus nephritis [28]. Preliminary data from human studies suggest that defective production of tumor necrosis factor may be genetically related to the predisposition for lupus [29].

Continued acquisition of insights into the multiplicity of immunologic disturbances contributing to the lupus syndrome may, in turn, lead to additional novel therapeutic options for management of patients with lupus nephritis.

References

1. Balow JE (1986) Lupus nephritis: natural history, prognosis and treatment. Clin Immunol Allergy 6:391–404
2. Balow JE, Austin HA III, Tsokos GC, Antonovych TT, Steinberg AD, Klippel JH (1987) Lupus nephritis. Ann Intern Med 106:79–94
3. Rosansky S, Eggers P (1987) Trends in the US end stage renal disease population: 1973–1983 Am J Kidney Dis 9:91–97
4. Pollak VE, Pirani CL, Kark RM (1961) Effect of large doses of prednisone on the renal lesions and life span of patients with lupus glomerulonephritis. J Lab Clin Med 57:495–511
5. Baldwin DS, Gluck MC, Lowenstein J, Gallo G (1977) Lupus nephritis: clinical course as related to morphologic forms and their transitions. Am J Med 62:12–30

6. Bach JF, Strom TB (1985) The mode of action of immunosuppressive agents. Elsevier, Amsterdam
7. Zhu LP, Cupps TR, Whalen G, Fauci AS (1987) Selective effects of cyclophosphamide therapy on activation, proliferation and differentiation of human B cells. J Clin Invest 79:1082–1090
8. Appleby P, Webber DG, Bowen JG (1989) Murine chronic graft-versus-host disease as a model of systemic lupus erythematosus: effect of immunosuppressive drugs on disease development. Clin Exp Immunol 78:449–453
9. Klippel JH (1990) Systemic lupus erythematosus: treatment-related complications superimposed on chronic disease. JAMA 263:1812–1815
10. Donadio JV Jr, Holley HE, Wagoner RD, Ferguson RH, McDuffie FC (1972) Treatment of lupus nephritis with prednisone and combined prednisone and azathioprine. Ann Intern Med 77:829–835
11. Decker JL, Klippel JH, Plotz PH, Steinberg AD (1975) Cyclophosphamide or azathioprine in lupus glomerulonephritis: a controlled trial: results at 28 months. Ann Intern Med 83:606–615
12. Hahn BH, Kantor, OS, Osterland CK (1975) Azathioprine plus prednisone compared with prednisone alone in the treatment of systemic lupus erythematosus. Ann Intern Med 83:597–605
13. Donadio JV Jr, Holley KE, Ferguson RH, Ilstrup DM (1978) Treatment of diffuse proliferative lupus nephritis with prednisone and combined prednisone and cyclophosphamide. N Engl J Med 299:1151–1155
14. Austin HA III, Klippel JH, Balow JE, leRiche NGH, Steinberg AD, Plotz PH, Decker JL (1986) Therapy of lupus nephritis: controlled trial of prednisone and cytotoxic drugs. N Engl J Med 314:614–619
15. Balow JE, Austin HA III, Muenz LR, Joyce KM, Antonovych TT, Klippel JH, Steinberg AD, Plotz PH, Decker JL (1984) Effect of treatment on the evolution of renal abnormalities in lupus nephritis. N Engl J Med 311:491–495
16. Donadio JV Jr, Holley KE, Ilstrup DN (1981) Adrenocorticoid and cyclophosphamide drug treatment of lupus nephropathy. In: Proc 8th Int Congress Nephrology, S. Karger, Basel, pp 643–648
17. McCune WJ, Golbus J, Zeldes W, Bohlke P, Dunne R, Fox DA (1988) Clinical and immunologic effects of monthly administration of intravenous cyclophosphamide in severe systemic lupus erythematosus. N Engl J Med 318:1423–1431
18. Lehman TJA, Sherry DD, Wagner-Weiner L, McCurdy DK, Emery HM, Magilavy DB, Kovalesky A (1989) Intermittent intravenous cyclophosphamide for lupus nephritis. J Pediatr 114:1055–1060
19. Boumpas DT, Barez S, Klippel JH, Balow JE (1990) Intermittent cyclophosphamide for the treatment of autoimmune thrombocytopenia in systemic lupus erythematosus. Ann Intern Med 112:674–677
20. Ponticelli C, Zucchelli P, Moroni G, Cagnoli L, Banfi G, Pascuali S (1987) Long-term prognosis of diffuse lupus nephritis. Clin Nephrol 28:263–271
21. Feutren G, Querin S, Tron F, Noel LH, Chatenoud L, Lesavre P, Bach JF (1986) The effects of cyclosporine in patients with systemic lupus. Transplant Proc 18:643–644
22. Mountz JD, Smith HR, Wilder RL (1987) CS-A therapy in MRL-lpr/lpr mice: amelioration of immunopathology despite autoantibody production. J Immunol 138:157–163
23. Strober S, Farinas MC, Field EH, Solovera JJ, Kiberd BA, Myers BD, Hoppe RT (1987) Lupus nephritis after total lymphoid irradiation: persistent improvement and reduction of steroid therapy. Ann Intern Med 107:689–690
24. Wei N, Klippel JH, Huston DP, Hall RP, Lawley TJ, Balow JE, Steinberg AD, Decker JL (1983) Randomized trial of plasma exchange in mild systemic lupus erythematosus. Lancet I:17–22

25. Lewis E, Lachin J (1987) Primary outcomes in the controlled trial of plasmapheresis therapy (PPT) in severe lupus nephritis (abstract). Kidney Int 31:208
26. Wofsy D, Seamon WE (1987) Reversal of advanced murine lupus in NZB/NZW F1 mice by treatment with monoclonal antibody to L3T4. J Immunol 138:3247–3253
27. Kelley VE, Gaulton GN, Ikegami H, Eisenbarth G, Strom TB (1988) Anti-interleukin 2 receptor antibody suppresses murine diabetic insulitis and lupus nephritis. J Immunol 140:59–61
28. Jacob CO, McDevitt HO (1988) Tumour necrosis factor-alpha in murine autoimmune lupus nephritis. Nature 331:356–358
29. Jacob CO, Fronek Z, Koo M, Hansen JA, McDevitt HO (1990) Heritable major histocompatibility complex class II-associated differences in production of tumor necrosis factor alpha: relevance to genetic predisposition to systemic lupus erythematosus. Proc Natl Acad Sci USA 87:1233–1237

Current Strategy of Management for Lupus Nephritis and Renal Vasculitis

Toshihiko Nagasawa[1]

Summary. Current strategy of management for lupus nephritis and renal vasculitis has been considered from clinical, morphologic, and immunologic points of view. In the immunologically active and rapidly progressive type of lupus nephritis, short-term intensive immunosuppressive therapy is recommended. However, in chronically ill patients with no flare-up of immunologic activity, long term corticosteroid administration is not recommended, especially in those patients with WHO type 5 histology. In rapidly progressive lupus nephritis, early initiation of hemodialysis is recommended, together with intensive immunosuppressive therapy, including plasma exchange. In patients on chronic hemodialysis without flare-up of immunologic activity (burning out systemic lupus erythematosus (SLE)), renal transplantation is indicated.

For the monitoring of immunosuppressive therapy in renal vasculitis, serial quantitative measurements of anti-neutrophil cytoplasmic antibodies are needed.

Introduction

Modern advances in intensive immunosuppressive therapy have remarkably prolonged the survival rates in patients with lupus nephritis (LN) and renal vasculitis (RV). However, associated with potent immunosuppressive therapy given for considerably long periods an increased number of patients with these diseases have lost their lives or have lost their ability to carry out daily life activities. Based on these facts, immunosuppressive therapy for LN and RV has been reconsidered from clinical, morphologic, and immunologic points of view. Also, modern management of end-stage renal failure in LN has been considered.

[1]The First Department of Internal Medicine, Kyorin University School of Medicine, 6-20-2 Shinkawa, Mitaka, Tokyo, 181 Japan

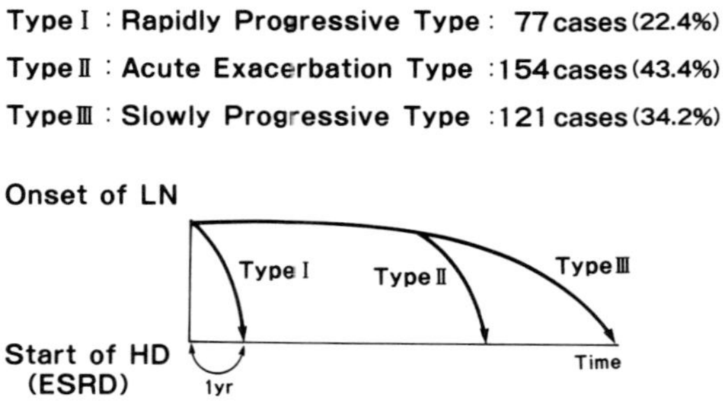

Fig. 1. Clinical courses to end-stage renal disease (*ESRD*) in patients with systemic lupus erythematosus (*SLE*) (n=352)

Clinical Studies of Lupus Nephritis

The clinical courses to end-stage renal disease (ESRD) of 352 patients with LN who began hemodialysis procedure (HD) were analyzed retrospectively. As shown in Fig. 1, the clinical courses to ESRD could be classified into 3 types. Within 1 year at most after the onset of LN 77 patients (22.4%) progressed very rapidly to ESRD (Type 1 LN). Suddenly, several years after the onset of LN 154 patients (43.4%) shifted to type 1 LN (Type 2 LN). In types 1 and 2 LN, extremely strong immunologic SLE activity appeared, together with rapidly progressive glomerulonephritis (RPGN). In addition to the immunologic activity, patients showed marked thrombocytopenia, which was found to be directly related to the causes of death, as shown in Table I. Types 1 and 2 LN are essentially the same except for the time difference in the occurrence of RPGN. In order to save lives, aggressive immunosuppressive therapy is indicated in these 2 types. In contrast to the patients with Types 1 and 2 LN, in 121 other patients (34.2%) the course to ESRD was very slow, without flare-up of clinical and immunologic SLE activities (Type 3 LN). In this type, long term corticosteroid (CS) administration and large doses of CS should be avoided to prevent the further progression of glomerular sclerosis due to the effects of CS.

Table 1. Lupus nephritis with Type I clinical course (n=10)

Case	Age/sex	Interval between the onset of LN to HD (Mo)	Thr $\times 10^4$	CH_{50} (U/ml)	a-DNA Ab (U/ml)	Outcome
1	16 F	3	5.6	<12	96	† (Cerebral bleeding)
2	17 F	3	9.0	<12	90	† (Sepsis)
3	23 F	2	4.5	12	100	† (Pulm. bleeding)
4	30 F	3	6.0	12	162	† (GI bleeding)
5	31 F	3	5.5	24	130	† (GI bleeding)
6	35 F	6	2.4	12	150	Maintenance HD
7	35 F	8	1.2	12	94	† (Cerebral bleeding)
8	37 F	3	2.6	12	110	Off HD
9	43 M	3	5.1	<12	113	† (GI bleeding)
10	44 F	6	9.6	<12	150	† (Sepsis)

Table 2. Survival rate of patients with lupus nephritis in whom progress to end-stage renal failure was regarded as "end point"

	5 Years		10 Years	
WHO other types	100	$P<0.05$	91.7±8.0	$P<0.05$
WHO type 4	75.8± 9.0		41.3±20.0	
Act-Sc<3.0	98.2± 2.0	$P<0.05$	91.9± 6.0	$P<0.05$
Act-Sc≥3.0	73.9±11.0		46.2±17.0	
Chr-Sc<1.7	98.0± 2.0	NS	89.5± 8.0	NS
Chr-Sc≥1.7	81.2± 9.0		54.2±17.0	
TI-Sc<1.8	93.5± 4.0	NS	75.3±10.0	NS
TI-Sc≥1.8	98.1± 4.0		58.9±15.0	

Act-Sc, activity score; Chr-Sc, chronicity score; TI-Sc, tubulointerstitial score

Morphologic Studies of Lupus Nephritis

One hundred and eighty-nine patients with LN were biopsied. Their types of WHO classification were as follows: type 1; 14 cases (7.4%), type 2; 40 cases (21.1%), type 3; 13 cases (6.9%), type 4; 67 cases (35.4%), and type 5; 55 cases (29.1%).

Survival rates 5 and 10 years after the biopsy are shown in Table 2. Significant differences were observed between WHO type 4 and the other types, and also between patients whose activity scores were less than and more than 3.0. These results indicate that WHO type 4 LN patients with activity scores over 3.0 should be carefully treated with relatively large doses of CS in order to avoid the transition from type 2 to type 1 LN. Also, the relationship between CS therapy and the sites of glomerular immune deposits was found to be important. As shown schematically in Fig. 2, it was possible to eliminate mesangial and subendothelial immune deposits by administration of large doses of CS over a relatively short period. However, it was not possible

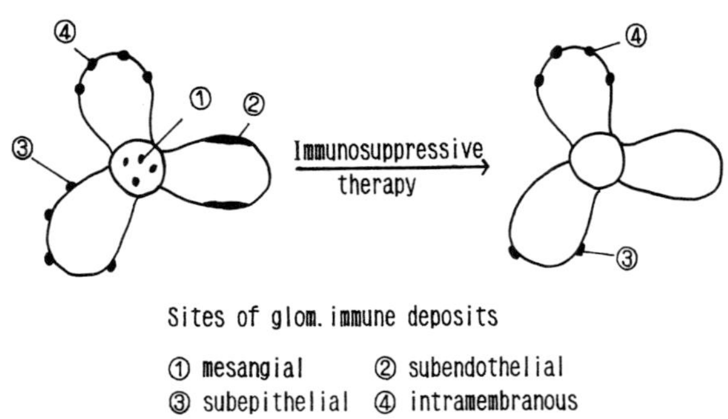

Fig. 2. Sites of glomerular immune deposits and immunosuppressive therapy

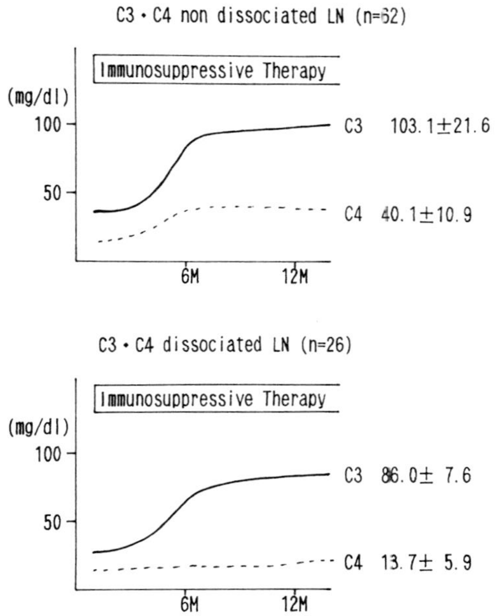

Fig. 3. Clinical course of lupus nephritis and complement ($n=88$)

to eliminate subepithelial and/or intramembranous immune deposits by administration of large doses of CS and/or by long-term CS administration. These results indicate that electron microscopic observation of renal biopsied sections is important not only for the diagnosis of WHO type classification and activity scores, but also in order to be able to judge whether or not large doses of CS and/or long term CS administration are indicated.

Immunologic Studies on Lupus Nephritis

When strong immunosuppressive therapy was given to patients with LN who had low serum levels of C3 and C4 before the start of therapy, levels returned to normal in considerable numbers of cases. However, there were some cases whose C3 levels returned to normal, while their C4 levels still remained low (Fig. 3). Renal involvement was compared in these 2 groups. As shown in Table 3, nephropathy occurred nearly equally in both groups. However, interestingly, there were no cases who developed RPGN (Types 1 or 2 LN) or chronic renal failure (CRF) (Type 3 LN)

Table 3. Dissociation of C3•C4 and lupus nephritis ($n=88$)

C3•C4 Dissociation	Presence ($n=26$)	Absence ($n=62$)
Nephropathy	20 (76.9%)	46 (74.2%)
Transition to RPGN	0	9 (14.5%)
Transition to CRF	0	12 (19.4%)
Death	0	7 (11.3%)

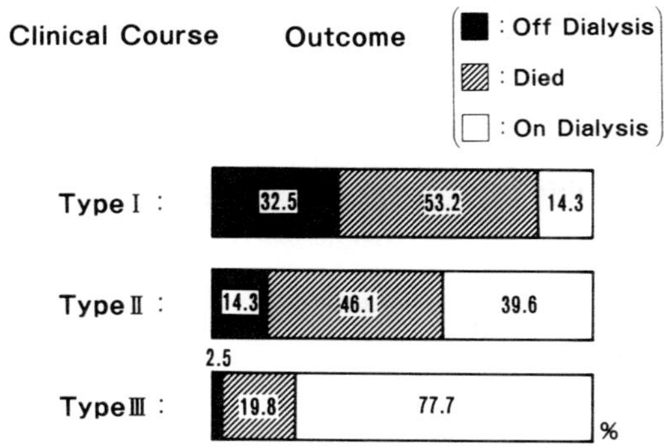

Fig. 4. Clinical courses to ESRD and outcome of hemodialysis (*HD*)

among the C3 and C4 dissociated patients. Also, there were no cases with WHO type 4 in this group, nor any with HLA DR 5, although the HLA-A, B, and C loci were not different in the 2 groups. These studies indicate that chronically ill LN patients with both C3 and C4 simultaneously normalized might still be at risk of transit from type 2 to type 1 LN, so they must be carefully followed-up.

Management of ESRD in LN

The outcome of 352 patients on HD is shown in Fig. 4. In type 1 LN, half of the patients died and one-third of the patients were able to come off HD. Plasma exchange and CS pulse therapy had excellent effects on "off dialysis," indicating that aggressive immunosuppressive therapy is still needed in type 1 LN in order to achieve "off dialysis" and to enable patients to return to type 3 LN (Table 4). The three main causes of death on HD were infections, bleeding, and heart failure. In those patients

Table 4. Treatment of systemic lupus erythematosus (SLE) at the start of hemodialysis (HD) and outcome of dialysis patients

	Outcome		
Treatment	Off dialysis	Died	On dialysis
Corticosteroids			
High dose oral	88.7	93.2	94.0
	NS (Off dialysis vs. Died)		
Corticosteroid pulse	69.8	36.1	27.5
	*** (Off dialysis vs. Died)		
Immunosuppressants	22.6	19.0	9.0
	NS (Off dialysis vs. Died)		
Plasma exchange	28.3	15.0	5.4
	* (Off dialysis vs. Died)		

(*$P<0.05$ ***$P<0.001$) %; NS, not significant

Table 5. ANCA titer and renal injury in Wegener's granulomatosis (WG)

Cases	ANCA titer (ELISA U/ml)	Proteinuria (mg/dl) Hematuria (1hpf)	S-Cr (mg/dl)	Renal histology
1. 51 ♂	860	260/Many	18.5	Cres. GN
2. 42 ♂	760	560/Many	0.6	Cres. GN
3. 29 ♂	750	70/Many	0.8	Seg. Necrot. GN
4. 38 ♀	730	160/10–20	1.3	Seg. Necrot. GN
5. 36 ♂	460	200/20–30	4.9	Cres. GN
6. 36 ♂	180	100/10–20	1.1	n.d.
7. 30 ♂	93	300/50–60	1.1	n.d.
8. 62 ♀	72	Negative	0.6	n.d.
9. 35 ♀	70	Negative	0.6	n.d.
10. 42 ♀	58	Negative	0.8	n.d.
11. 31 ♀	Negative	Negative	0.6	n.d.

ANCA, anti-neutrophil cytoplasmic antibody

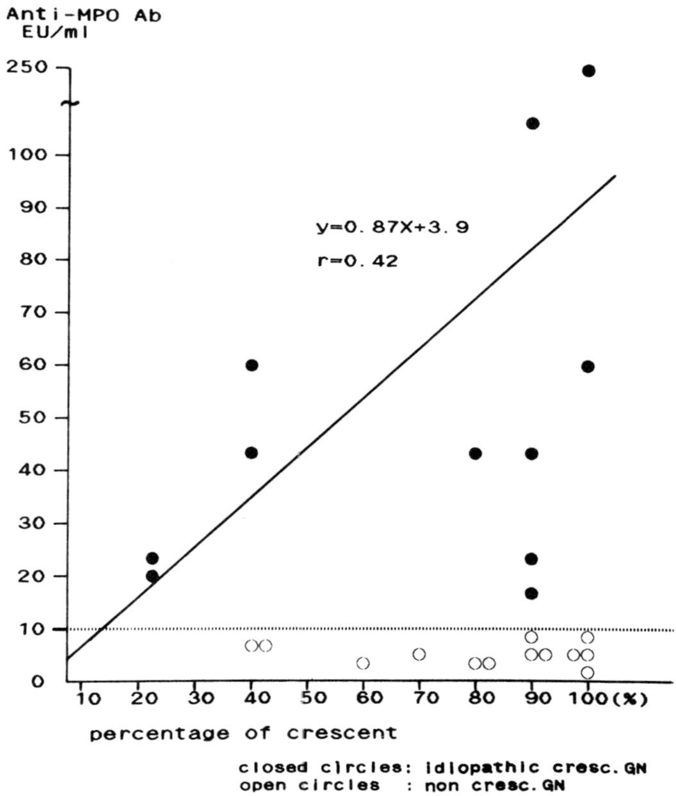

Fig. 5. Relationship between titers of anti-MPO antibodies and percentage of crescent formation

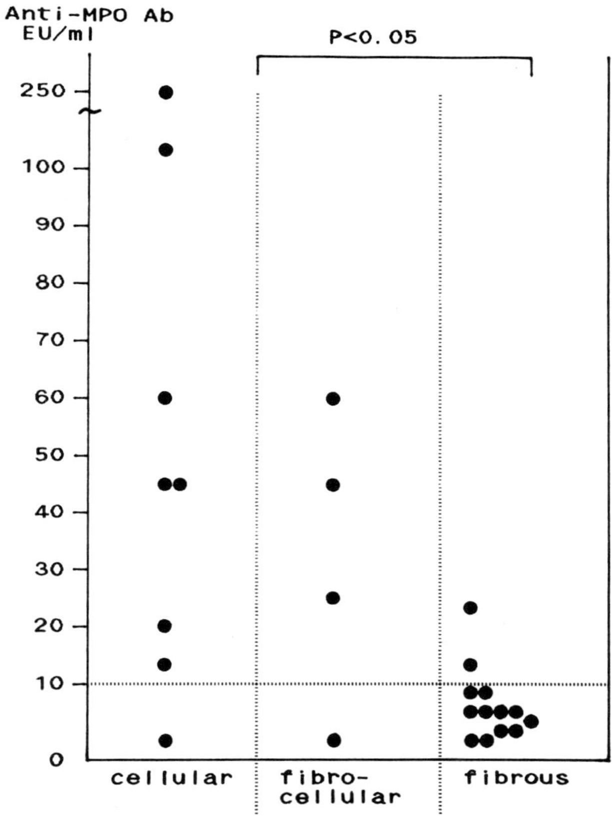

Fig. 6. Titers of anti-MPO antibodies and stage of crescent idiopathic crescentic GN

who had been on HD for less than 1 year, bleeding and heart failure had a high incidence. In type 1 LN patients especially, acute bleeding should be strictly controlled, since in these patients thrombocytopenia, as well as the influence of uremia, is the cause of bleeding.

In type 3 LN, the prognosis of patients on chronic HD was excellent. In nearly all of them immunologic and clinical SLE activities were burned out several years after beginning HD, suggesting that they were excellent candidates for renal transplantation. In fact, in Japan, a smaller number of patients received renal transplantation than in Western countries. However, these patients' long term prognosis, without LN relapse in the transplanted kidneys, are good.

Anti-Neutrophil Cytoplasmic Antibody (ANCA) and Renal Vasculitis

It is already well established that cytoplasmic ANCA is specific for Wegener's granulomatosis (WG) and that myeloperoxidase (MPO)-ANCA is specific for idiopathic crescentic glomerulonephritis (GN). Therefore, WG and idiopathic crescentic GN in Japan were examined for the presence of ANCA. As shown in Table 5, C-ANCA, examined by sandwich enzyme-linked immunoadsorbent assay (ELISA), was specifically positive in WG and its titer showed close correlation with the severity of renal injury. The same was true for anti-MPO antibody and idiopathic crescentic GN. As shown in Figs. 5 and 6, the percentages of the numbers of crescentic glomeruli and the stages of crescentic GN had close correlation with the titer of anti-MPO antibody. These results indicate that C- and MPO-ANCA should be used for monitoring WG and idiopathic crescentic GN immunosuppressive therapy.

In conclusion, when immunosuppressive therapy, especially CS therapy, is chosen for LN and RV patients the balance between its benefits and risks should be considered, utilizing new therapeutic indices, as described in this paper.

Renal Growth Factors

Chair: F. Gary Toback (USA)
Harry R. Jacobson (USA)

Expression of Growth-Related Genes in Human Fetal Kidney

PAUL R. GOODYER[1], JEHANE FATA[1], LOIS MULLIGAN[2], CYNTHIA G. GOODYER[3], HARVEY GUYDA[3], and DANIEL FISCHER[4]

SUMMARY. In early to midgestational human fetal life, branches of the ureteric bud begin to induce successive generations of nephrons from undifferentiated metanephric mesenchyme. Development of each evolving nephron is highly dependent on brisk, organized cell division. In order to identify molecular mechanisms potentially involved in fetal kidney growth, we screened a panel of fetal and adult kidneys for expression of 22 growth-related genes. Among the seven genes selectively expressed in fetal kidney, IGF-II, N-myc, and c-erbA have been investigated elsewhere. The "anti-oncogene", p53, and the homeobox gene, HHO.c13, are most likely involved in restriction of growth rather than in mitogenic events. The expression of epidermal growth factor (EGF) receptor in fetal kidney suggests a role for this pathway as an arbiter of rapid cell division. Using specific radioimmunoassays, we demonstrated that transforming growth factor (TGF)-Alpha peptide, but not EGF, was present in extracts of midgestation fetal kidney and amniotic fluid. Using the polymerase chain reaction, we identified TGF-Alpha messenger RNA (mRNA) in fetal kidney, indicating endogenous production of the peptide.

Introduction

Between the fifth and sixth weeks of human fetal life, undifferentiated metanephric mesenchyme is contacted by the ureteric bud (an outpouching of the Wolffian duct)

---

[1]Division of Pediatric Nephrology, McGill University-Montreal Children's Hospital Research Institute, Montreal, Quebec H3H 1P3, Canada
[2]Ludwig Cancer Institute, Royal Victoria Hospital, McGill University, Montreal, Quebec H3H 1P3, Canada
[3]Division of Pediatric Endocrinology, McGill University-Montreal Children's Hospital Research Institute, Montreal, Quebec H3K 1P3, Canada
[4]Nephrology Resident, Royal Victoria Hospital, McGill University, Montreal, Quebec H3H 1P3, Canada

resulting in induction of the first generation of nephrons [1]. Prior to induction, the metanephric tissue consists of loosely organized vimentin-positive cells proliferating in an extracellular matrix of fibronectin and collagens type I and III. As in the cells in Wilm's tumors, messenger RNA (mRNA) for insulin-like growth factor II is abundant [2]. Histologic observations indicate that clusters of metanephric cells condense at the point of contact with individual branches of the ureteric bud and then vesiculate to form S-shaped tubular structures [3]. The cells become polarized through laminin-mediated attachment to newly formed basement membrane, changes in cytoskeletal components, and increased lateral adhesion [1,4,5]. Recent work by Hastie et al. indicates that the committed cells of the emerging renal vesicle exhibit intense expression of the Wilm's tumor gene [3].

Induction of metanephric mesenchyme causes a shift in cellular phenotype, but it also initiates a phase of rapid cell division. It is intriguing to note that IGF-II mRNA is most intense in the undifferentiated cells of the metanephric mesenchyme rather than in the rapidly proliferating cells of the evolving nephron [6]. Little is known about the mitogenic signals which direct this proliferation, but it is clear that local regulatory events are involved. The nephron develops a primitive glomerulus at its proximal end through ingrowth of capillaries; fusion with the ureteric bud at its distal end achieves continuity with the bladder. Over the course of fetal life, successive branches of the ureteric bud penetrate nests of metanephric mesenchyme at the outer rim of the developing organ; tiers of newly formed units are layered upon deeper zones of the more advanced nephrons already producing fetal urine. By thirty-five weeks of gestation the ureteric bud stops dividing and the metanephric blastema involutes as the final generation of nephrons is formed.

In order to characterize the molecular mechanisms potentially responsible for the rapid growth of evolving nephrons, we probed a panel of human adult and fetal kidney RNAs with 23 known protooncogene probes. Among those genes expressed at especially high levels in fetal tissue was the EGF receptor. Further studies support the view that transforming growth factor-alpha (TGF-Alpha) is the most likely physiologic ligand for the EGF receptor in fetal kidney.

Materials and Methods

For Northern analyses, frozen tissues were pulverized on dry ice; total RNA was prepared by the guanidinium/cesium chloride gradient method [7]. For gene expression screening, 30 μg of total RNA was separated on 1% agarose/formaldehyde gels and was transferred to Hybond-N membranes (Amersham) using 20X SSC. The Northern blots were hybridized for 36 hours to [32P]-labelled probes (random oligonucleotide priming) in 50% formamide 40mM Na_2HPO_4 (pH=6.7), 5X SSC, 0.05% SDS, 0.02% PVP, 0.02% Ficoll, and 0.02% bovine serum albumin at 42°C. For detailed analysis of the EGF receptor, nitrocellulose Northern blots were hybridized overnight (55% deionized formamide, 5X SSC, 1X Denhardt's solution, 50 mM Na_2HPO_4, and 10% dextran sulfate at 42°C) to a [32-P]-labelled complementary DNA (cDNA) probe for the human EGF receptor (ATCC). The blots were washed and submitted to autoradiography.

For assay of transforming growth factor-alpha (TGF-Alpha), frozen kidney was pulverized on dry ice and homogenized in 5 volumes of buffer containing 20mM

TRIS (ph 7.4), 0.25M sucrose, 1mM phenylmethylsulfonylfluoride, and 0.1% Triton-X 100. TGF-Alpha was measured in amniotic fluid and tissue extracts in triplicate with the Biotope TGF-Alpha RIA kit (Biotope, Redmond, Washington) as previously described [8]. The kit utilizes antiserum raised against synthetic TGF-Alpha peptide (17 residues, 34–50) and gives linear displacement for human TGF-Alpha standard between 0.5–5 pmoles/ml, but does not recognize human EGF. Half-maximal competition is at 1.4 nM TGF-Alpha. Serial dilutions of kidney extracts or amniotic fluid samples produced displacement of TGF-Alpha tracer parallel to the standard curve; Triton X-100 buffer gave no displacement in the assay.

For assay of human EGF, tissues were prepared as above. EGF was measured by radioimmunoassay as described previously [9]. The antiserum used was raised in rabbits against recombinant human EGF (Amgen); it detects human EGF but not rat EGF or TGF-Alpha from either species. Half maximal competition is 0.3 nM.

Specific high-affinity EGF binding was performed as previously described [10]. Frozen tissues were homogenized in 5 volumes of buffer containing 20 mM TRIS (pH 7.4) and 0.25M sucrose. The homogenate was centrifuged twice at 500Xg, and the supernatant respun at 20,000Xg for 20 minutes to obtain a membrane pellet. Human EGF was iodinated by the chloramine T method and incubated (50000 CPM/assay) with 200–300 μg kidney membrane protein, or 100 μg placental membrane protein in 500 μl final volume of 25mM TRIS (pH 7.4)/10mM magnesium chloride buffer containing 1 mg/ml bovine serum albumin and 1 mg/ml bacitracin at 4°C. for 18 hours. Specific binding was estimated by comparing the fraction of total tracer bound in the presence or in the absence of excess unlabelled EGF (500ng/ml).

Results

Gene Expression in Fetal and Adult Kidney

The expression profile of 23 genes suspected of involvement in regulation of cell growth was assessed by Northern analysis, using a panel of total RNA samples (30 μg per lane) from human fetal ($n=11$) and adult kidneys ($n=4$). Fetal foot length was used to determine fetal age; the fetal samples ranged from 14–24 weeks gestation at 410 day intervals. For simplicity, semi-quantitative estimates of signal intensity for each gene were assigned to early (14–20 weeks) and mid (21–24 weeks) gestation fetal kidney samples and to the adult panel.

Of the 22 genes studied, 5 (NGF, IGF1, IL-2, c-ab1, and L-myc) were undetectable by Northern analysis in any of the fetal or adult kidney samples. Transcripts for 10 of the 22 genes (c-myc, c-raf, neu, TGF-B1, met, yes, sis, RB1, K-ras, H-ras) were detected in all samples, but the level of gene expression was equivalent in the early fetal, mid-fetal, and adult kidney groups. The expression pattern for the remaining 7 genes is summarized in Table 1. In each case, transcript was detected in fetal kidney but was much reduced or absent in adult kidney.

EGF Receptor

Among the genes selectively expressed in fetal kidney, the EGF receptor was chosen for further analysis. We noted that primary transcripts for the EGF receptor (9.4 and

Table 1. Summary of expression pattern for 7 of 22 genes studied

Gene	Gestational age 10–14 weeks	Fetal kidney 14–20 weeks	Adult kidney
IGF-II	+++	+++	–
EGF Receptor	+	+	–
N-myc	++	++	–
N-ras	++	+	+
c-erbA	++	++	±
HHO.c13	+	+	–
p53	++	+	±

5.6 kb) in fetal kidney RNA co-migrated with transcripts in mid-gestational human placenta but were absent in adult kidney; no unusual transcripts were seen. Specific high-affinity EGF binding in membrane fractions of fetal kidney was 2–5 times higher than in adult kidney, but was less than in mid-gestation placenta (Table 2).

TGF-Alpha and EGF

If the EGF receptor is to initiate mitogenic signals in fetal kidney, it must be activated by an appropriate ligand. Levels of TGF-Alpha and EGF peptides were assayed in detergent extracts of fetal kidney and amniotic fluid. As seen in Table 2, TGF-Alpha was detectable, by RIA, in fetal kidneys of 11–15 weeks gestation. In one pair of kidneys obtained at 7–8 weeks gestation, the level was significantly lower. TGF-Alpha was also present in all amniotic fluid samples tested (13–39 weeks gestation, n=20) (Table 3). Primer oligonucleotides, prepared from the published sequence for human TGF-Alpha, were used to convert TGF-Alpha mRNA in human fetal kidney total RNA to cDNA, using the reverse transcriptase reaction; this was followed by 25 cycles of PCR amplification. PCR products were dotted on nitrocellulose and identified with a cDNA probe for human TGF-Alpha. Significant TGF-Alpha expression was identified in all fetal kidneys (13–19 weeks gestation) tested (n=7).

Midgestational kidney extracts were also assessed for EGF content. In three fetal kidney samples, EGF was undetectable (lower limit of assay = 0.1 pmoles/ml). By contrast the extract from the normal kidney of an adult was 6 pmol/g. Significant levels of EGF in amniotic fluid were undetectable before 30 weeks gestation, when they began to rise (Table 3). At term, amniotic fluid EGF was still only 4% of the

Table 2. EGF binding, TGF-Alpha, and EGF in human fetal kidney

	Fetal	Adult
% EGF binding/200 μg protein	1.1 ± 0.1 (n=9)	0.3 (n=2)
pmoles TGF-Alpha/g wet weight	42.1 ± 1.4 (n=7)	ND
pmoles EGF/g wet weight	0.0 (n=3)	6.0 (n=3)

Table 3. TGF-Alpha and EGF in human amniotic fluid

Gestational age	TGF-Alpha (nM)	EGF (nM)
15–20 weeks ($n = 5$)	4.0 ± 0.3	< 0.05
20–25 weeks ($n = 5$)	6.1 ± 0.4	< 0.05
25–30 weeks ($n = 3$)	4.6 ± 0.5	< 0.05
30–35 weeks ($n = 2$)	2.5	< 0.05
35–40 weeks ($n = 5$)	3.9 ± 0.2	0.12 ± 0.04

level of TGF-Alpha. Although PCR amplification was not performed, EGF mRNA was identified in adult, but not in fetal kidney, by Northern analysis.

Discussion

In this report, we examined the expression profile of a panel of growth-related genes in human fetal kidney, in order to identify some which may be of particular importance to kidney development. As reported by others, we noted increased expression of IGF-II, N-myc, N-ras, and c-erbA (thyroxine receptor) in fetal kidney. The possible roles of these genes in kidney development have recently been reviewed [1]. The characteristics of the "anti-oncogene", p53, and the human homeobox gene, HHO.C13, suggest that their expression in human fetal kidney may be related to restrictions of cell division rather than to their acting as mitogenic signals. However, the increase in EGF receptor mRNA and the increase in EGF binding in midgestational renal tissue, compared to levels in the adult tissue, suggests that this receptor may be among the important mediators of rapid fetal kidney growth. Renal cells are known to proliferate in response to EGF in vitro [11].

Some controversy remains about whether fetal kidney can produce a physiologic ligand for the EGF receptor. Several groups have reported an EGF-like peptide in fetal kidneys of sheep and mice [12–14]; others have reported TGF-Alpha mRNA in fetal mouse [15], and in adult human [16] kidneys by Northern blotting. On the other hand, Han was unable to identify TGF-Alpha mRNA in fetal rat kidney [17] and Mydlo found none in normal adult human kidney by Northern blotting [18]. Using specific radioimmunoassays, we have demonstrated the presence of TGF-Alpha peptide, but not EGF, in extracts of human kidney and in amniotic fluid from early to mid-gestation. Using PCR amplification, we were able to demonstrate the presence of TGF-Alpha mRNA in fetal kidney, indicating endogenous synthesis there. We cannot rule out small quantities of renal EGF synthesis during fetal life, but the relative amounts of TGF-Alpha and EGF in amniotic fluid suggest that the former is the dominant physiologic EGF receptor ligand.

It is certain that the interaction between paracrine growth factors and critical nuclear transcription factors during renal development is extremely complex. Signals directing cell division must be exerted under tight spatial and temporal restrictions relevant to differentiation of the renal tubule. Nevertheless, efforts to identify the key molecular mechanisms involved in normal development are likely to shed light on the repair of renal injury in later life.

References

1. Bacallao R, Fine LG (1989) Molecular events in the organization of renal tubular epithelium: from nephrogenesis to regeneration. Am J Physiol 257:F913–F924
2. Paik S, Rosen N, Jung W, You JM, Lippman ME, et al. (1989) Expression of insulin-like growth factor II in RNA in fetal kidney and Wilm's tumor. Lab Invest 61:522–526
3. Hastie N, Pelletier J, et al. (to be published) Expression of a candidate Wilm's Tumour gene in human fetal tissues and Wilm's tumour. Nature
4. Ekblom M, Klein G, Mugrauer G, Fecker L, Deutzmann R, Trumph R, Ekblom P (1990) Transient and locally restricted expression of laminin A-chain in RNA by developing epithelial cells during kidney organogenesis. Cell 60:337–346
5. Klein G, Langegger M, Gordis C, Ekblom P (1988) Neural adhesion molecules during embryonic induction and development of the kidney. Develop 102:749–761
6. Han VKM, D'Ercole AJ, Lund PK (1987) Cellular localization of somatomedin (insulin-like growth factor) messenger RNA in the human fetus. Science 236:193–196
7. Goodyer PR, Langshur S, Fata J (1990) Renal synthesis of epidermal growth factor is unchanged by vitamin D deficiency. Can J Physiol Pharmacol 68:733–736
8. Goodyer PR, Fata J, Goodyer CG (to be published) Transforming growth factor-alpha and the ontogeny of epidermal growth factor receptors in rat kidney
9. Goodyer PR (1990) Excretion of epidermal growth factor-like material in acute Henoch-Schonlein purpura nephritis. Pediatr Nephrol 4:101–104
10. Goodyer PR, Fata J, Goodyer CG, Mulligan L, Guyda H (to be published) Transforming growth factor-alpha and epidermal growth factor receptor in human fetal kidney
11. Goodyer PR, Kachra Z, Bell C, Rozen R (1988) Renal tubular cells are potential targets for epidermal growth factor. Am J Physiol 255:F1191–F1196
12. Nexo E, Hollenberg MD, Figuerou A, Pratt RM (1980) Detection of epidermal growth factor-urogastrone and its receptor during fetal mouse development. Proc Natl Acad Sci (USA) 77:2782–2785
13. Freemark M, Comer M (1987) Epidermal growth factor (EGF)-like transforming growth factor (TGF) activity and EGF receptors in ovine fetal tissues: possible role for TGF in ovine fetal development. Pediatr Res 22:609–615
14. Twardzik Dr, Ranchalis JR, Todaro GJ (1982) Mouse embryos contain growth factors related to those from tumour cells. Cancer Res 42:590–593
15. Derynck R, Jarett JA, Chen EY, et al. (1985) Human transforming growth factor-beta complementary DNA sequence and expression in normal and transformed cells. Nature 316:701–705
16. Gomella LG, Sargent ER, Wade TP, Anglard P, Linehan WM, Kasid A (1989) Expression of transforming growth factor-alpha in normal human adult kidney and enhanced expression of transforming growth factors alpha and beta1 in renal cell carcinoma. Cancer Res 49:6972–6975
17. Han VKM, Hunter E III, Pratt RM, Zendegin JG, Lee DC (1987) Expression of rat transforming growth factor alpha in RNA during development occurs predominantly in the maternal decidua. Mol Cell Biol 7:2335–2343
18. Mydlo JH, Michaeli J, Cordon-Cardo C, Goldenberg AS, Heston WDW, Fair WR (1989) Expression of transforming growth factor alpha and epidermal growth factor receptor messenger RNA in neoplastic and nonneoplastic human kidney tissue. Cancer Res 49:3407–3411

Growth Hormone, Insulin-Like Growth Factor I, and Kidney

Marc R. Hammerman and Steven B. Miller

Summary. Insulin-like growth factor I (IGF I) exerts a variety of actions on kidney. To shed light upon its role in regulation of renal function and renal growth we have characterized its cellular biology in two parts of the nephron, proximal tubule and collecting duct. Receptors for IGF I are present in the basolateral membrane of the renal proximal tubular cell, but not in collecting duct. The peptide IGF I enhances gluconeogenesis in proximal tubule. IGF I is produced in collecting duct. Gene expression for IGF I in collecting duct is stimulated by both normal and supraphysiological levels of growth hormone (GH). Levels of IGF I in collecting duct are elevated in the setting of compensatory renal hypertrophy. IGF I of collecting duct origin could act as a paracrine growth factor in other portions of the nephron. IGF I may be causative of renal hypertrophy that occurs in the settings of hypersomatotropism and unilateral nephrectomy (compensatory hypertrophy).

Introduction

Insulin-like growth factor I (IGF I) is the predominant growth hormone (GH)-responsive IGF. It is present in circulation, where it can interact, as an endocrine hormone, with receptors present on the plasma membranes of a variety of cells. In addition, it is produced locally within a number of GH-sensitive tissues, where it acts as an autocrine or paracrine growth factor [1]. Kidney is a site of IGF I synthesis [2].

Receptors for IGF I have been described in renal glomerulus and proximal tubule [3,4]. IGF I is known to exert several actions on kidney. Administration of this peptide to rats [5] and humans [6] increases glomerular filtration rate and renal plasma flow. In addition, IGF I increases kidney size when infused directly into rats [7]. States of GH excess (hypersomatotropic states) are characterized by elevations of cir-

Renal and Endocrine Divisions, Departments of Internal Medicine and Cell Biology and Physiology, Washington University School of Medicine, St. Louis, MO 63110, USA

culating IGF I and are accompanied by hypertrophy of the renal glomerulus and proximal tubule [8]. Indeed, many actions of GH on renal size and kidney function appear to be mediated indirectly through stimulation of the synthesis and release of insulin-like growth factor I (IGF I).

In order to gain an understanding of the cellular biological mechanisms by which GH and IGF I regulate renal growth, renal metabolism, and renal function, we have characterized binding of, signal-transduction by, and metabolic actions of IGF I in proximal tubule, and IGF I gene expression in collecting duct. Our findings have shed new light on the GH-IGF I axis within the kidney.

Materials and Methods

The methodology used to generate data presented in this manuscript has been detailed elsewhere. Methods include measurement of ^{125}I-IGF I binding by rapid centrifugation and covalent crosslinking techniques [4], phosphorylation of canine renal proximal tubular basolateral membranes [9], measurement of gluconeogenesis in suspensions of canine renal proximal tubular segments [10], measurement of IGF I mRNA using a solution-hybridization, nuclease-protection assay [11], and measurement of IGF I of collecting duct origin using high performance liquid chromatography and radioimmunoassay [12]. A probe derived from a subclone of rat IGF I exon 3 was provided by Dr. Peter Rotwein, Washington University, St. Louis Mo. Recombinant bovine GH (bGH) was the gift of Monsanto Chemical Co., St. Louis Mo. Recombinant human IGF I (hIGF I) was purchased from Amgen Biologicals, Thousand Oaks CA.

Results

Renal Proximal Tubule

Receptors for IGF I are distributed asymmetrically in the plasma membrane of the renal proximal tubular cell, being localized predominantly on the basolateral side [4] (Fig. 1). In isolated proximal tubular basolateral membranes IGF I-stimulated phosphorylation of the beta subunit of its receptor can be demonstrated (Fig. 2), consistent with signal transduction being effected via this mechanism in proximal tubule, as it is in other IGF I-sensitive tissues [9]. In isolated proximal tubular segments IGF I stimulates gluconeogenesis (Fig. 3).

Renal Collecting Duct

Kidney is a site of GH-stimulated IGF I production [2]. We and other groups of investigators have shown that collecting duct is the site of IGF I synthesis within rat kidney [11–13]. IGF I has been localized to collecting duct by immunohistochemistry; IGF I mRNA is co-localized to this portion of the nephron [11] (Fig. 4). Administration of recombinant bovine GH (bGH) to normal [14] or hypophysectomized [11,15] rats results in enhanced immunostainable IGF I in collecting duct, as well as increased levels of IGF I mRNA.

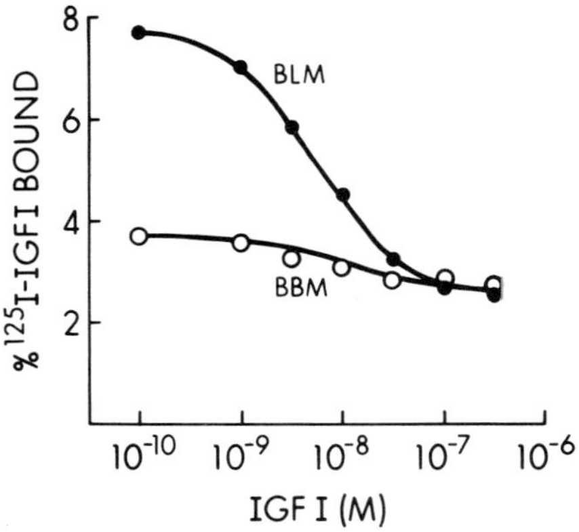

Fig. 1. Binding of ^{125}hI-IGF I to canine renal proximal tubular basolateral (*BLM*) and brush border membranes (*BBM*). Binding is expressed as % ^{125}I-IGF I bound

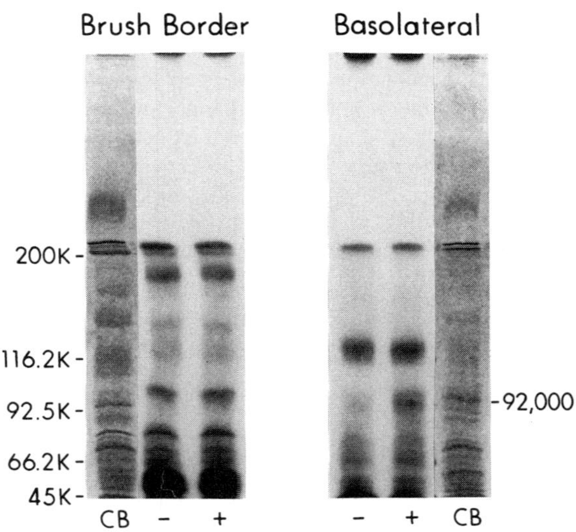

Fig. 2. IGF I-stimulated phosphorylation of canine renal proximal tubular brush border and basolateral membranes. Shown are Coomassie blue stained SDS-polyacrylamide gels (*CB*) and autoradiograms originating from proximal tubular brush border and basolateral membranes incubated without (-) or with (+) 10^{-6} M hIGF I prior to phosphorylation. Several M_r markers are shown. IGF I-stimulated phosphorylation of a 92000 M_r protein is demonstrable in basolateral membranes, but not in brush border membranes. (From [9] with permission)

Fig. 3. Stimulation of glucose production from gluconeogenic substrates by varying concentrations of hIGF I in suspensions of canine renal proximal tubular segments. (From [10] with permission)

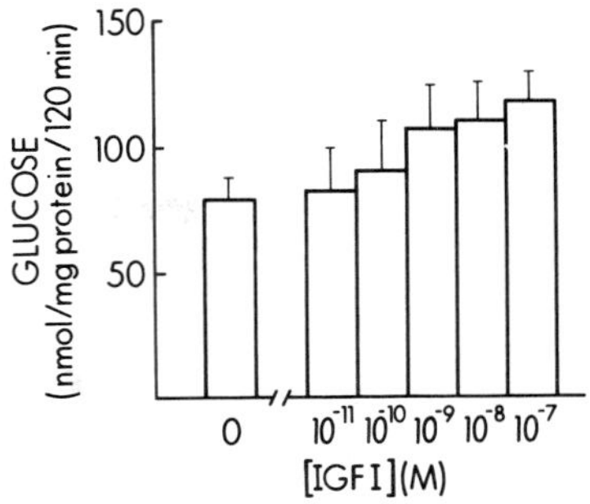

Incubation of collecting ducts isolated from rat kidney with bGH results in elevated levels of total IGF I extractable from total suspensions (cells plus media). In addition, GH enhances levels of IGF I present in extracellular suspending media [12] (Fig. 5). Prior to measurement by radioimmunoassay, IGF I of collecting duct origin (cdIGF I) is separated from IGF binding activity, using high performance liquid chromatography. It co-elutes with recombinant human ^{125}I-IGF I [12]. IGF I of collecting duct origin inhibits binding of ^{125}I-IGF I to the 135000 M_r alpha subunit of its receptor in canine proximal tubular basolateral membranes, identically to authentic human IGF I (hIGF I) (Fig. 6). Incubation of isolated collecting ducts with bGH elevates levels of IGF I mRNA in vitro (Fig. 7) [12]. These findings demonstrate that GH enhances IGF I gene expression via a direct action on renal collecting ducts.

Discussion

The Renal GH-IGF I Axis

The studies detailed above establish the potential for a GH-IGF I axis within kidney [16]. IGF I produced in isolated rat renal collecting ducts is released into extracellular

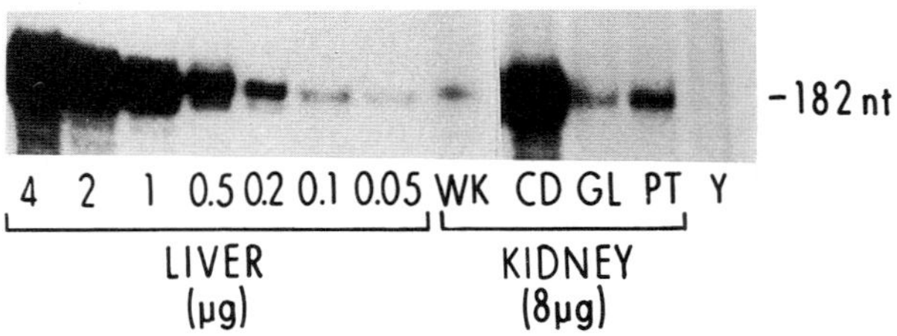

Fig. 4. Levels of IGF I mRNA in kidney. Shown is an autoradiogram depicting the results of a solution-hybridization nuclease-protection experiment using a ^{32}P-labeled rat IGF I exon 3 antisense probe (protected fragment = 182 nucleotides). Illustrated are protected RNA fragments from rat liver and from whole kidneys (*WK*), collecting duct (*CD*), glomeruli (*GL*), proximal tubule (*PT*), or yeast tRNA (*Y*). (Reproduced from the *Journal of Cell Biology* [11] by copyright permission of the Rockefeller University Press)

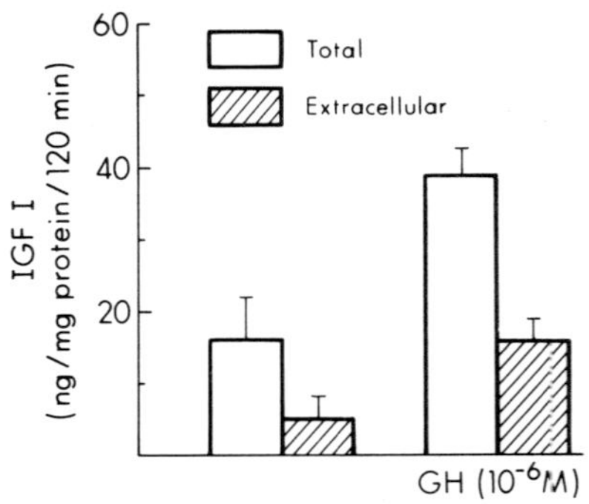

Fig. 5. Levels of immunoreactive IGF I present in whole collecting duct suspensions (*total*) and in extracellular media of the suspensions. Data are expressed ± SE of 3 experiments

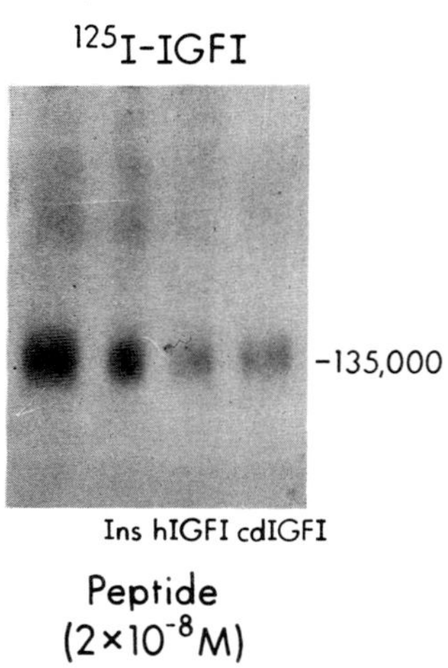

Fig. 6. Crosslinking of ^{125}I-hIGF I to canine renal proximal tubular basolateral membranes in the absence or presence of 2×10^{-8} M insulin (*Ins*), hIGF I or IGF I of collecting duct origin (*cdIGF I*). (From [12] with permission)

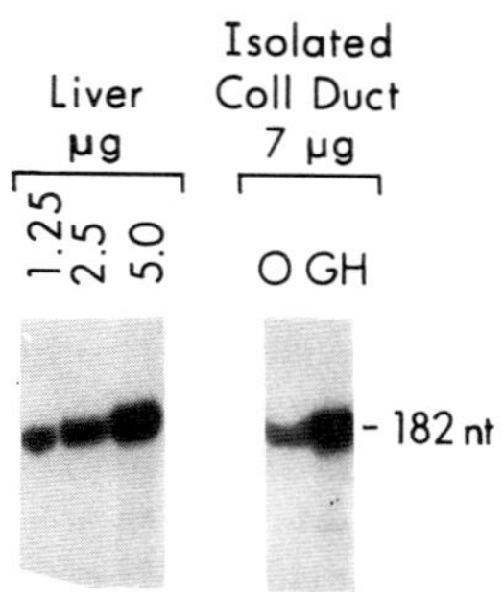

Fig. 7. Levels of IGF I mRNA in isolated rat renal collecting duct incubated with (*GH*) or without (*0*) 10^{-6} M bGH for 2 h. Shown is an autoradiogram depicting the results of a solution-hybridization nuclease-protection experiment conducted as described in Fig. 4. (From [12] with permission)

media. This is likely to reflect peptide secretion into renal tissue in vivo. Although IGF I can be detected in urine, its concentration is small (approximately 10^{-11} M) [17]. This suggests that IGF I is not secreted into the collecting duct lumen, but rather, exits from collecting duct across the basolateral membrane. Receptors for IGF I are not present in collecting duct [15]. Therefore IGF I produced there must act at other sites in kidney at which receptors are present, such as glomerulus and proximal tubule, where IGF I could function as a paracrine growth factor. IGF I produced in cortical collecting duct is located immediately adjacent to the basolateral membrane of the renal proximal tubular cell where IGF I receptors are present. IGF I produced in medullary collecting duct could reach the renal cortex via the ascending vasa recta, the walls of which are extensively fenestrated like those of renal capillaries. Indeed, segments of proximal tubule and other tubular structures in the outer stripe of medulla receive their blood supply from these vessels [16].

A role for renal IGF I as causative of the glomerular and proximal tubular hypertrophy that occurs in hypersomatotropic states and in compensatory renal hypertrophy is suggested by observations from several laboratories. First, IGF I may be the major stimulus for renal cellular growth in hypersomatotropic states such as acromegaly [8], since GH administered in vivo, or added to collecting ducts in vitro, enhances IGF I gene expression. Second, IGF I could function as a hypertrophic stimulus in compensatory renal hypertrophy. We [15] and other investigators [18,19] have demonstrated enhanced IGF I expression within kidney in the setting of compensatory growth.

Our knowledge of the GH-IGF I axis within kidney is incomplete. A number of important issues remain to be addressed. First, it is likely that factors in addition to GH affect IGF I gene expression in collecting duct. This is illustrated by the fact that the increase in renal IGF I that accompanies compensatory hypertrophy occurs in the hypopituitary state [18]. Second, the nature of feedback-loops for GH and IGF I in kidney is undefined. Third, sites of action for GH and IGF I, in addition to those that have been characterized, may exist along the nephron. In addition, interactions may occur between GH, IGF I, and other polypeptide growth factors within renal tissue. Future investigations will shed light on these and other important questions regarding the GH-IGF I axis in kidney.

Acknowledgments. We acknowledge the typing skills of Ms. Lynn Wesselmann. Contributions to the work upon which much of this review is based were made by Dr. Peter Bechtel, University of Illinois, Champaign-Urbana Ill.; Dr. James R. Gavin III, Oklahoma City Okla.; and Dr Jonathan Bortz, Dr. Rosemary Lajara, Dr. Peter Rotwein, Ms. Virginia Hansen, and Ms. Sharon Rogers, Washington University, St. Louis Mo. M.R. Hammerman was supported by N.I.H. grants DK-27600 and DK-09976 and by Grant 186270 from the Juvenile Diabetes Foundation. S. Miller was supported by N.I.H. training grant DK-07126.

References

1. Daughaday WH (1989) Growth hormone, normal synthesis, secretion, control, and mechanism of action. In: DeGroot LJ (ed) Endocrinology, vol 1. Saunders, Philadelphia, pp 318–329

2. D'Ercole JA, Stiles AD, Underwood LE (1984) Tissue concentrations of somatomedin C: further evidence for multiple sites of synthesis and paracrine or autocrine mechanisms of action. Proc Natl Acad Sci USA 81:935–939
3. Pillion DJ, Haskell JF, Meezen E (1988) Distinct receptors for insulin-like growth factor I in rat renal glomeruli and tubules. Am J Physiol 255:E504–E512
4. Hammerman MR, Rogers SA (1987) Distribution of IGF receptors in the plasma membrane of proximal tubular cells. Am J Physiol 253:F841–F847
5. Hirschberg R, Kopple JD (1989) Evidence that insulin-like growth factor I increases renal plasma flow and glomerular filtration rate in fasted rats. J Clin Invest 83:3267–3330
6. Guler HP, Schmid C, Zapf J, Froesch ER (1989) Effects of recombinant insulin-like growth factor I on insulin secretion and renal function in normal human subjects. Proc Natl Acad Sci USA 86:2868–2872
7. Guler HP, Zapf J, Schweiller E, Froesch ER (1988) Recombinant human insulin-like growth factor I stimulates growth and has distinct effects on organ size in hypophysectomized rats. Proc Natl Acad Sci USA 85:4889–4893
8. Gershberg H, Heinemann O, Stumpf HH (1957) Renal function studies and autopsy report in a patient with gigantism and acromegaly. J Clin Endocrinol Metab 17:377–385
9. Hammerman MR, Gavin JR III (1986) Binding of IGF I and IGF I-stimulated phosphorylation in canine renal basolateral membranes. Am J Physiol 251:E32–E41
10. Rogers SA, Karl IE, Hammerman MR (1989) Growth hormone directly stimulates gluconeogenesis in canine renal proximal tubule. Am J Physiol 257:E751–E756
11. Bortz JD, Rotwein P, DeVol D, Bechtel PJ, Hansen V, Hammerman MR (1988) Focal expression of insulin-like growth factor I in rat kidney collecting duct. J Cell Biol 107:811–819
12. Rogers SA, Miller SB, Hammerman MR (1990) Growth hormone stimulates IGF I gene expression in isolated rat renal collecting duct. Am J Physiol 259:F474–F479
13. Hansson HA, Nilsson A, Isgaard J, Billig H, Isaksson O, Skottner A, Andersson IK, Rozel B (1988) Immunohistochemical localization of insulin-like growth factor I in the adult rat. Histochemistry 89:403–410
14. Miller SB, Rotwein P, Bortz JD, Bechtel PJ, Hansen VA, Rogers SA, Hammerman, MR (1990) Renal expression of IGF I in hypersomatotropic states. Am J Physiol 259:F251–F257
15. Lajara R, Rotwein P, Bortz JD, Hansen VA, Sadow JL, Betts CR (1989) Dual regulation of insulin-like growth factor I expression during renal hypertrophy. Am J Physiol 257:F252–F261
16. Hammerman MR (1989) The growth hormone-insulin-like growth factor axis in kidney (editorial review). Am J Physiol 257:F503–F514
17. Hizuka N, Takano K, Tanaka I, Asakawa K, Miyakawa M, Horikawa R, Shizume K (1987) Demonstration of insulin-like growth factor I in human urine. J Clin Endocrinol Metab 64:1309–1312
18. Stiles AD, Sosenko RS, D'Ercole AJ, Smith BT (1985) Relation of kidney tissue somatomedin-C/insulin-like growth factor I to postnephrectomy renal growth in the rat. Endocrinology 117:2397–2401
19. Andersson GL, Skottner A, Jennische E (1988) Immunocytochemical and biochemical localization of insulin-like growth factor I in the kidney of rats before and after uninephrectomy. Acta Endocrinol (Copenh) 119:555–560

Epidermal Growth Factor and the Kidney

RAYMOND C. HARRIS[1]

Epidermal growth factor (EGF), a 53 amino acid polypeptide, with a molecular weight of 6045, is derived by proteolytic processing from a precursor (prepro-EGF) of 1207 amino acids in humans or 1217 amino acids in rodents [1,2]. PreproEGF is a membrane-spanning protein that contains a hydrophobic domain adjacent to the EGF moiety. EGF was originally isolated as the factor that stimulates precocious tooth eruption and eyelid opening in newborn mice; subsequently, it has been found to produce a wide variety of effects both in vitro and in vivo, including proliferation of cultured cells, acceleration of lung maturation, corneal healing, and inhibition of gastric acid secretion [1].

EGF binds to a 170 kilodalton plasma membrane receptor that contains intrinsic tyrosine kinase activity [2]. Binding of EGF to its receptor stimulates receptor autophosphorylation, as well as tyrosine phosphorylation of a number of other cellular proteins. Specific high affinity EGF receptors have been detected in cultured cells of epithelial, mesenchymal and endothelial origin. Receptors have also been detected in a variety of tissues, including kidney [3], breast [4], liver [5], and intestine [6]. EGF has been demonstrated to promote hyperplasia and maturation of the cells in the gastrointestinal epithelium [7], pancreas, and liver [8]. In addition to inhibition of gastric acid secretion, EGF also preserves the integrity of the intestinal epithelium and reduces ulceration [9]. Addition of EGF to cultured cells stimulates a number of intracellular responses including increased Na^+/H^+ antiport activity [10], activation of glycolysis [1], increased DNA, RNA, protein, and hyaluronic acid synthesis [1] and increased glucosamine incorporation in glycosaminoglycans [11].

In 1978, Delarco and Todaro described a peptide, released by retrovirally transformed fibroblasts, that bound to EGF receptors and promoted anchorage independent growth of normal rat kidney (NRK) cells in soft agar [12]. They termed this growth factor, transforming growth factor alpha (TGF-α). TFG-α possesses both structural and functional homology with EGF. Both TFG-α and EGF bind with simi-

[1]Vanderbilt University School of Medicine, Nashville, TN 37232, USA

lar affinity to the same receptor, and TFG-α binding will activate EGF receptor tyrosine kinase activity. Such observations raise the obvious possibility that "EGF receptors" may actually be targets for TFG-α and that EGF is one, possibly specialized, member of the family of TGF-α peptides. In many biological systems, the effects elicited by EGF and TGF-α are very similar, while in others, TGF-α appears quantitatively more potent than EGF.

Originally, EGF was detected in mouse submaxillary gland, the most abundant source of production in the rodent. Although levels of EGF are high in saliva, circulating blood levels are low [1]. Furthermore, in humans, EGF concentrations are much higher in serum than in plasma, and EGF in blood is not freely circulating but is associated with platelets [14]. Subsequent to its discovery in saliva, EGF has also been noted to be present in high (nanogram concentrations) in milk, urine, secretions of Brunner's glands [15], and in prostatic secretions [16]. Immunohistochemical localization in rodents has shown EGF to be present in submaxillary glands, exocrine glands of the gastrointestinal tract, and serous acini of the nasal cavity, as well as in kidney, further indicating the possible exocrine role for this peptide [17]. Urinary EGF, or urogastrone, is present in high concentrations in urine [18]. In humans, urinary EGF concentrations are 50–70 ng/mg creatinine.

A number of studies have indicated a renal source of urinary EGF. Urinary EGF/creatinine ratios are greater than one. Intravenously injected ^{125}I EGF is not detected in urine [19]. Following sialoadenctomy and duodenectomy, urinary EGF levels were unchanged [20], but following unilateral nephrectomy, urinary EGF levels fell to 50% of control, and did not increase over the subsequent 14 days [20,21]. In humans, urinary EGF levels have been demonstrated to be decreased in chronic renal failure of multiple etiologies [22]. In addition, in experimental renal failure induced by cis platinum [23] or ischemia [24], urinary EGF levels decreased markedly. However, Nielsen et al. have recently found that in isolated rabbit proximal tubules only 4% of filtered EGF is reabsorbed (compared to 73% for insulin) [25]. These authors also detected a small amount of apical secretion of EGF after presentation of EGF to proximal tubular basolateral membrane and suggested the possibility that a component of urinary EGF may originate from blood.

High concentrations of prepro-EGF mRNA have been found in the kidney [26]. In situ hybridization localization of prepro-EGF indicates the site of renal synthesis to be the thick ascending limb of Henle (TALH) and early distal convoluted tubule (DCT) [26]. Immunocytochemical and immunoelectron microscopic localization of EGF and preproEGF to cortical thick ascending limb and early distal convoluted tubule has been demonstrated. No staining of macula densa was observed [27,28].

The predicted structure of preproEGF suggests that it is a membrane protein, with an extracellular EGF moiety (amino acids 977-1029). The immunocytochemical identification of preproEGF in the TALH and DCT indicates that the protein is predominantly, if not exclusively, found anchored in the apical membrane [28]. This polarized distribution suggests that renal preproEGF may be acted upon by proteases in the tubular fluid and/or apical membrane and the derived EGF is released directly into the urine. The protease(s) responsible for processing of renal preproEGF have not been characterized. Arginine esterase, the protease responsible for cleaving submaxillary preproEGF, is not found in the kidney or in urine [29]. It has been suggested that the renal kallikrein or related enzymes may be responsible for cleavage of the precursor [30]. In addition to EGF, the EGF precursor contains other sequences homologous to EGF, as well as sequences homologous to atrial natriuretic factor precursor. Whether these sequences are processed to biologically active peptides is not known.

Processing of preproEGF may not be necessary for biological activity. Fibroblasts transfected with human preproEGF cDNA produce and secrete intact preproEGF, which binds to EGF receptors, activates EGF receptor tyrosine kinase and induces mitogenesis [31]. Since preproEGF appears to be an intrinsic membrane protein, and since it possesses homology to the low-density lipoprotein receptor, it has also been suggested that preproEGF may itself serve as a receptor for a yet unidentified ligand, but confirming evidence for this hypothesis has not been forthcoming.

The regulation of synthesis and release of renal EGF is not well understood. Unlike serum EGF, urinary EGF concentrations are higher in females than in males, and, unlike results in submaxillary gland, androgen administration to female mice increases neither preproEGF mRNA expression in the kidney nor urinary EGF levels [32]. In fact, estrogen administration increases urinary EGF levels in males [33]. Although human urinary EGF levels are not affected by menstrual cycle or oral contraceptives, pregnancy does induce a doubling of urinary EGF, with a peak at 20 weeks [34]. Chronic thyroxine and growth hormone administration also increase urinary EGF levels [35]. Evidence to date suggests that β-adrenergic stimulation increases, and β-adrenergic blockade decreases, urinary EGF levels, in contrast to salivary gland release, which is stimulated by a-adrenergic agonists [36].

In rat, EGF immunoreactivity in the kidney does not appear until after birth [37], although in human fetuses, EGF immunoreactivity is present from half-term onwards. Matilla et al. found that urinary EGF in humans was low at birth, rose progressively, peaked at two years of postnatal life (235 ng/mg creatinine), gradually fell to age 16 (30–60 ng/mg creatinine), and then remained stable until age 55, when it began to decline [38]. Urinary EGF levels are greater in term than in premature infants [39]. In contrast, in the rat embryo, TGF-α is present at days 8–10 but is not detectable near term (day 18) [40] . Similarly, fetal sheep kidney possesses high TGF-α activity [41], suggesting a role for this peptide in fetal renal development. Thus, it is likely that TGF-α is the physiologic ligand for the EGF receptors that have been detected in fetal kidney.

The physiologic roles of EGF produced in the kidney are not yet well understood. EGF may serve as a cytoprotective agent of the distal nephron, ureters, and bladder. It is of interest that EGF is produced in the TALH, a nephron segment just proximal to the nephron segments in which urinary acidification is accomplished; the collecting duct, ureters, and bladder are exposed to urine pH of as low as 4.5, as well as to a hypertonic mileau. There is evidence suggesting a role for EGF in modulation of growth and function of these distal structures. Specific, high affinity receptors have been demonstrated in microdissected cortical collecting ducts [42], cultured papillary collecting duct cells, and freshly isolated suspensions of papillary collecting ducts [43]. In isolated perfused cortical collecting ducts, EGF inhibits hydroosmotic conductivity [44], electrogenic Na reabsorption [45], and K secretion [46]. EGF has been shown to be mitogenic for cultured rabbit thick ascending limb and cortical collecting duct cells [47], cultured rat papillary collecting duct cells [43], and cultured bladder epithelial cells [48].

In addition to its mitogenic effects upon cultured papillary collecting duct cells, EGF increases arachidonate release and prostaglandin production in these cells [43].

The latter is of especial interest, since renal medullary prostaglandins have been implicated in solute and fluid reabsorption in this segment. Medullary interstitial cells, thought to be an important site of medullary arachidonate metabolism, also possess specific EGF receptors, and EGF is a potent mitogen for these cells [44]. In addition, EGF stimulates arachidonate release and prostaglandin production in MDCK cells, a cell line with many characterictics of distal nephron [45].

EGF is a potent mitogen for cultured rabbit [46] and rat [47] proximal tubule cells, as well as LLC-PKl cells, a cell line with many characteristics of proximal tubule [48]. In cultured rabbit proximal tubule cells, EGF also stimulates protein synthesis and S6 kinase activity [49]. In freshly isolated rat proximal tubule segments, EGF inhibits both basal and angiotensin-stimulated gluconeogenesis [50] and stimulates hexose monophosphate shunt activity [47] and protein synthesis [49].

Therefore, in cultured cells and isolated tubule segments, a number of potential tubular effects for EGF have been proposed. The unanswered question remains whether the EGF synthesized and secreted by the kidney serves a paracrine function in the kidney and/or in the lower urinary tract. As mentioned above, immunohistochemical studies localize preproEGF to the apical membrane of the thick ascending limb and distal convoluted tubule. However, studies to date suggest that EGF receptors are on basolateral membranes of polarized epithelia in the kidney. High affinity EGF binding was localized exclusively to basolateral membranes of proximal tubule of rat [50], rabbit [51], and mouse [52]. That the basolateral EGF binding represented binding to functional receptors was indicated by demonstration of EGF-mediated tyrosine kinase activity that was also localized to basolateral membranes [50]. Furthermore, all of the above-mentioned modulatory effects of EGF upon isolated perfused cortical collecting duct are induced only by administration of EGF to the basolateral membrane.

In spite of the apparent apical localization of preproEGF, it is possible that basolateral secretion of EGF does occur, thereby allowing access to receptors on adjacent tubules (which might include both proximal tubules as well as more distal tubule segments, given the topology of the cortex). Alternatively, EGF may be secreted into the lumen and then transcytosed in more distal nephron segments to the basolateral surface. In this regard, EGF is transcytosed from lumen to blood in the ileum of suckling mice [53]. However, in MDCK cells [54], transcytosis of EGF occurs only in the direction of basolateral to apical membrane.

It is also possible that under normal circumstances, the EGF produced in the kidney does not interact with EGF receptors in the kidney or the distal uroepithelium. However, following injury, either localized or general, intercellular tight junctions would be disrupted and EGF could traverse to the basolateral surfaces and interact with the EGF receptors located there. A potential role for EGF, in repair of renal tubules following injury, is suggested by the observations of the mitogenic effects of EGF on cells cultured from various tubule segments and by the indication that EGF serves to inhibit differentiated tubule functions (gluconeogenesis, salt and water reabsorption) either directly or through generation of prostaglandins. Since disruption of tight junctions (as well as loss of cell polarity) may occur following non-fatal cell injury, EGF may serve to inhibit the normal functioning of injured cells, thereby allowing repair and regeneration. A similar function for EGF in the bladder is suggested by the demonstration that only cells in the basal layer express EGF receptors [55].

These cells would not be exposed to urinary EGF unless there were injury and disruption of the superficial mucosa.

That EGF or TGF-α may play an important role in repair of renal injury is further suggested by recent studies of experimental tubular injury. In rat, following 50 minutes of unilateral renal ischemia induced by renal artery clamping, ^{125}I EGF binding increased, with the greatest relative increases seen in the cortex [24]. The increased binding was detectable at 24 hours following ischemia, and no change was noted in the contralateral, non-ischemic kidney. Similar findings have been reported in rabbit kidney following ischemia [56], and in rat kidney following folic acid administration [57]. Following ischemic renal injury in the rat, subcutaneous injection of EGF significantly accelerates ^{3}H thymidine incorporation and recovery of tubular function [58].

Although EGF and/or TGF-α may be important mediators of renal regeneration following acute tubular necrosis, EGF produced by the thick ascending limb/distal convoluted tubule is likely not involved. Following either cis-platinum renal toxicity [23] or ischemic tubular necrosis [24], both preproEGF mRNA levels and urinary EGF levels decrease and remain significantly depressed for up to 7 days. Whether this decrease in renal EGF production is a nonspecific result of cellular damage or whether it is a specific response to injury that is linked to the upregulation of receptors and increased sensitivity to EGF, remains to be determined. That renal EGF production decreased as a result of renal tubular damage was further suggested by the finding that in a series of patients with a variety of chronic renal diseases, urinary EGF excretion was depressed, and the relative decrease correlated with the decrease in renal function [22].

In contrast to renal regeneration, there is little current evidence suggesting a role for EGF in the mediation of compensatory hypertrophy. In cultured proximal tubule cells, the cells that undergo the greatest compensatory hypertrophy in vivo, EGF is a mitogenic rather than a hypertrophic agent. Following uninephrectomy, EGF receptors have been reported either to be unchanged [57], or to decrease slightly [59]. As previously mentioned, following unilateral nephrectomy, urinary EGF levels decrease by 50% and do not increase over the subsequent 14 days. However, immunolocalization studies indicate that EGF expression may be increased at 7, but not at 2 days, after contralateral nephrectomy [60]. Thus, the increases in expression of both EGF and insulin-like growth factor (IGF)-1 are not seen early after contralateral nephrectomy, during the period of greatest hypertrophy. Whether this late increase in growth factor expression serves a physiologic function in the growth process or is a response to the hypertrophy is unclear. A preliminary report by Uchida et al. has also suggested a role for serum EGF in renal hypertrophy. They found that sialoadenectomy inhibited compensatory hypertrophy following contralateral nephrectomy in mice, and that exogenous EGF administration overcame this inhibition [61].

In either streotpzotocin-induced or autoimmune diabetes mellitus, urinary EGF levels increase 4–9-fold, with partial normalization following insulin therapy [62]. Of interest, in mice with either streptozotocin-induced or genetic diabetes, submaxillary but not renal preproEGF mRNA expression was drastically reduced, with normalization following insulin therapy [63]. No role in either the hypertrophy or the glomerular pathology of diabetes has yet been attributed to EGF.

Preliminary evidence does suggest there may be a possible role for EGF/TGF-α in the mediation of the epithelial proliferation seen in cystic renal disease. In

C57BL/6J-cpk mice, which manifest an inheritable autosomal recessive form of polycystic kidney disease, with cystic dilatatior of the collecting duct, no renal preproEGF mRNA could be detected [64]. Furthermore, although submaxillary preproEGF mRNA was present in these animals, testosterone did not stimulate expression, suggesting the possibility of a systemic disorder in regulation of EGF production. Of interest, cyst fluid from these animals has been reported to contain high concentrations of EGF (60 ng/ml). Cyst fluid from humans with adult polycystic kidney disease has EGF concentrations higher than plasma but lower than urine (0.5 ng/ml) [65]. Whether EGF contributes to cyst development and/or growth in vivo, as has been recently suggested in a murine metanephric culture system [66], will have to be determined in further studies.

EGF and/or TGF-α may also be involved in modulation of glomerular hemodynamics, either under physiologic conditions or following inflammatory injury. Intrarenal infusion of EGF into rats [67] or sheep [68] produced decreases in renal blood flow and GFR. Micropuncture studies in rat indicated that EGF induced both afferent and efferent arteriolar vasoconstriction, as well as a profound fall in K_f [67]. That the fall in K_f was secondary to mesangial cell contraction was further suggested by identification of specific high-affinity EGF receptors on cultured rat mesangial cells, and demonstration that EGF stimulated Na^+/H^+ exchange and contraction of these cells [67]. In cultured mesangial cells, EGF has been demonstrated to activate phospholipase A_2 activity [69], to release arachidonic acid, and to increase prostaglandin production in synergism with phorbol esters or vasopressin [70]. Furthermore, following irreversible cyclooxygenase inactivation by aspirin, EGF stimulated synthesis of new cyclooxygenase in mesangial cells [71]. Therefore, it is possible that EGF or TGF-α may modulate glomerular prostaglandin production.

Recent studies have suggested a role for both cyclooxygenase and non-cyclooxygenase arachidonate metabolites in the mediation of EGF's renal hemodynamic effects [72]. In the presence of cyclooxygenase inhibition by ibuprofen, the vasoconstrictive effects of EGF were abolished. Instead, intrarenal EGF infusion led to both systemic and renal microcirculatory vasodilation. This vasodilatory effect was also suggested to be mediated by non-cyclooxygenase arachidonate metabolites, because pretreatment with the competitive inhibitor of arachidonate release, 5,8,11,14-eicosatetraynoic acid (ETYA), abolished the vasodilation. In the face of complete inhibition of arachdionate release, EGF was found to again induce mild vasoconstriction. That the non-cyclooxygenase arachidonate metabolites mediating the vasodilation were generated from metabolism by cytochrome P450 was suggested by studies demonstrating that ketoconazole, a relatively selective inhibitor of renal P450, also inhibited the above-described EGF-induced vasodilation. EGF-induced stimulation of P450 arachidonate metabolite production was suggested by the demonstration that in suspensions of isolated rat proximal tubules, EGF administration led to a 100% increase in endogenous epoxyeicosatrienoic acids (EETs) within 5 minutes [73].

Although circulating EGF levels in most mammals are low, platelets are known to contain EGF[14], as well as TGF-α [74]. In addition, activated macrophages synthesize and secrete TGF-α [75,76]. Therefore, during inflammatory injury, local glomerular concentrations of EGF and TGF-α may be high and play a role in mediating both acute alterations in renal hemodynamics and subsequent mesangial proliferation. The recent observations that transmembrane prepro TGF-α can bind to EGF receptors and stimulate acute signal transduction events without proteolytic cleavage and secretion [77,78] also raises the possibility that infiltrating cells could alter glomerular function even in the absence of peptide release. Mroczkowski et al. have also found that preproEGF expressed in a recombinant system does not require proteolytic processing in order to bind to EGF receptors and activate tyrosine kinase activity [31].

Although EGF and TGF-α modulate acute renal hemodynamic events and stimulate proliferation of mesangial cells in culture, studies of collagen production by cultured rat mesangial cells suggest that EGF does not promote increased mesangial matrix production, since EGF actually inhibits both basal [79] and retinoic acid-stimulated [80] production of collagen in mesangial cells. Stimulation of wound healing by epidermal growth factor is due to its stimulation of fibroblast proliferation, rather than stimulation of collagen production per se [81]. Since EGF and TGF-α are both potent mitogens for NRK cells, a fibroblast cell line derived from rat kidney, it is possible that under pathophysiologic conditions these peptides might also stimulate proliferation of renal fibroblasts in vivo and thereby increase cortical or medullary scarring.

In summary, the kidney is one of the major sites for EGF synthesis and urinary EGF levels are high. The expression of preproEGF mRNA and immunoreactive preproEGF and EGF are localized to the cells of the TALH and early DCT. A diverse number of potential responses to EGF and/or TGF-α have recently been described, including modulation of glomerular hemodynamics, renal metabolism, tubular transport functions, and eicosanoid synthesis. In addition, these growth factors have been shown to be potent mitogens in vitro for a variety of cell types in the kidney and they may play an important role in renal embryogenesis and repair following injury.

References

1. Carpenter G, Cohen S (1979) Epidermal growth factor. Annu Rev Biochem 48:193
2. Carpenter G (1987) Receptors for epidermal growth factor and other polypeptide mitogens. Annu Rev Biochem 56:881
3. Cohen S, Fava RA, Sawyer ST (1982) Purification and characterization of epidermal growth factor receptor/protein kinase from normal mouse liver. Proc Natl Acad Sci USA 79:6237
4. Taketani Y, Oka T (1983) Epidermal growth factor stimulates cell proliferation and inhibits functional differentiation of mouse mammary gland cells in culture. Endocrinology 133:871
5. Chabot JG, Walker P, Pelletier G (1986) Distribution of epidermal growth factor binding sites in the adult rat liver. Am J Physiol 250:G760
6. Scheving LA, Shiurba RA, Nguyen TD, Gray Gary M (1989) Epidermal growth factor receptor of the intestinal enterocyte. Localization to laterobasal but not brush border membrane. J Biol Chem 264:1735
7. Deminski AB, Johnson LR (1985) Effect of EGF on development of rat gastric mucosa. Endocrinology 116:90
8. Deminski A, Gregory H, Kontrutek S, Polanski M (1982) Trophic action of EGF on the pancreas and gastroduodenal mucosa in rats. J Physiol 325:35
9. Konturek SJ (1988) Role of epidermal growth factor in gastroprotection and ulcer healing. Scand J Gastroenterol 23:129

10. Moolenaar WH, Yarden Y, deLaat SW, Schlessinger J (1982) Epidermal growth factor induces electrically silent Na^{+} influx in human fibroblasts. J Biol Chem 275:8502
11. Lembach K (1977) Enhanced synthesis and extracellular accumulation of hyaluronic acid during stimulation of quiescent human fibroblasts by mouse epidermal growth factor. J Cell Physiol 89:277
12. DeLarco J, Todaro GJ (1978) Growth factors from murine sarcoma virus-transformed cells. Proc Natl Acad Sci USA 75:4001
13. Derynck R (1986) Transforming growth factor-a: Structure and biological activities. J Cell Biochem 32:293
14. Oka T, Orth DN (1983) Human plasma epidermal growth factor/β urogastrone is associated with blood platelets. J Clin Invest 72:249
15. Joh T, Itoh M, Katsumi K, Yokoyama Y, Takeuchi T, Kato T, Wada Y, Tanaka R (1986) Physiological concentrations of human epidermal growth factor in biological fluids: use of a sensitive enzyme immunoassay. Clin Chim Acta 158:81
16. Gregory H, Willshire IR, Kavanagh JP, Blacklock NJ, Chowdury S, Richards RC (1986) Urogastrone-epidermal growth factor concentrations in prostatic fluid of normal individuals and patients with benign prostatic hypertrophy. Clin Sci 70:359
17. Poulsen SS, Nexo E, Skov Olsen P, Hess J, Kirkegaard P (1986) Immunohistochemical localization of epidermal growth factor in rat and man. Histochemistry 85:389
18. Gregory H (1975) The isolation and structure of urogastrone and its relationship to epidermal growth factor. Nature 257:325
19. Kasselberg AG, Orth DN, Gray ME, Stahlman MT (1985) Immunocytochemical localization of human growth factor/urogastrone in several human tissues. J Histochem Cytochem 33:315
20. Skov Olsen P, Nexo E, Poulsen S, Hansen HF, Kirkegaard P (1984) Renal origin of rat urinary epidermal growth factor. Regul Pept 10:37
21. Harris RC, Gung A, Orth DN, Badr KF (1988) Effect of dietary protein and uninephrectomy on urinary epidermal growth factor excretion. FASEB J 2:1305A
22. Mattila A-L, Pasternack A, Viinikka L, Perheentupa J (1986) Subnormal concentrations of urinary epidermal growth factor in patients with kidney disease. J Clin Endocrinol Metab 62:1180
23. Safirstein R, Zelent AZ, Price PM (1989) Reduced renal prepro-epidermal growth factor mRNA and decreased EGF excretion in ARF. Kidney Int. 36:810
24. Safirstein R, Price PM, Saggi SJ, Harris RC (1990) Changes in gene expression after temporary renal ischemia. Kidney Int 37:1515
25. Nielsen S, Nexo E, Christensen EI (1989) Absorption of epidermal growth factor and insulin in rabbit renal proximal tubules. Am J Physiol 256:E55
26. Rall LB, Scott J, Bell GI, Crawford RJ, Penshcow JD, Niall HD, Coghlan JP (1985) Mouse prepro-epidermal growth factor synthesis by the kidney and other tissues. Nature 313:228
27. Salido EC, Barajas L, Lechago J, Laborde NP, Fisher DA (1986) Immunocytochemical localization of epidermal growth factor in mouse kidney. J Histochem Cytochem 34:1155
28. Salido EC, Yen PH, Shapiro LJ, Fisher DA, Barajas L (1989) In situ hybridization of prepro-epidermal growth factor mRNA in the mouse kidney. Am J Physiol F632
29. Drinkwater CC, Evans BA, Richards RI (1987) Mouse glandular kallikrein genes: identification and characterization of the genes encoding the epidermal growth factor binding proteins. Biochemistry 26:6750
30. Drinkwater CC, Evans BA, Richards RI (1988) Kallikreins, kinins and growth factor biosynthesis. Trends Biochem Sci 13:169
31. Mroczkowski B, Reich M, Chen K, Bell GI, Cohen S (1989) Recombinant human epidermal growth factor precursor is a glycosylated membrane protein with biological activity. Mol Cell Biol 9:2771

32. Perheentupa J, Lakshmanan J, Fisher DA (1985) Urine and kidney epidermal growth factor: ontogeny and sex difference in the mouse. Pediatr Res 19:428
33. Hoffmann GE, Rao CV, Brown MJ, Murray LF, Schultz GS, Siddiqi TA (1988) Epidermal growth factor in urine of nonpregnant women throughout pregnancy and at delivery. J Clin Endocrinol Metab 66:119
35. Mattila A-L, Perheentupa J, Salmi J, Miinikka L (1987) Human epidermal growth factor concentrations in urine, but not in saliva and serum, depend on thyroid state. Life Sci 41:2739
36. Olsen PS, Kirkegaard P, Poulsen SS, Nexo E (1985) Adrenergic effects on renal secretion of epidermal growth factor in the rat. Regul Pep 11:17
37. Raaberg L, Nexo E, Mikkelsen JD, Poulsen SS (1988) Immunohistochemical localisation and developmental aspects of epidermal growth factor in the rat. Histochemistry 89:351
38. Mattila A-L, Perheentupa J, Pesonen K, Viinikka L (1985) Epidermal growth factor in human urine from birth to puberty. J Clin Endocrinol Metab 61:997
39. Evans NJ, Rutter N, Gregory H (1986) Urinary excretion of epidermal growth factor in the newborn. Early Hum Dev 14:277
40. Lee DC, Rochford R, Todaro G, Villarreal LP (1985) Development expression of rat transforming growth factor alpha mRNA. Mol Cell Biol 5:3644
41. Freemark M, Comer M (1987) Epidermal growth factor (EGF)-like transforming growth factor (TGF) activity and EGF receptors in ovine fetal tissues: possible role for TGF in ovine fetal development. Pediatr Res 22:609
42. Rehda R, Lopez C, Breyer JA, Jacobson HR, Breyer MD (1989) Mapping of 125-I epidermal growth factor binding sites along the rabbit nephron. Kidney Int 35:319A
43. Harris RC (1989) Response of rat inner medullary collecting duct to epidermal growth factor. Am J Physiol 256:F1117
44. Breyer MD, Jacobson HR, Breyer JA (1988) Epidermal growth factor inhibits the hydroosmotic effect of vasopressin in the isolated perfused rabbit cortical collecting tubule. J Clin Invest 82:1313
45. Vehaskari VM, Hering-Smith KS, Moskowitz DW, Wiener ID, Hamm LL (1989) Effect of epidermal growth factor on sodium transport in the cortical collecting tubule. Am J Physiol 256:F803
46. Muto S, Furuya H, Tabei K, Asano Y (1990) Effect of epidermal growth factor on potassium transport in the rabbit cortical collecting duct. Kidney Int 37:568A
47. Wilson PD, Horster MF (1983) Differential response to hormones of defined distal nephron epithelia in culture. Am J Physiol 13:C166
48. Nissenkorn I, Mickey D, Soloway M (1982) Effect of media and growth promoters on in vitro cultivation of normal murine urinary bladder epithelium. J Urol 128:176
44. Breyer J, Harris RC (1988) EGF binds to specific EGF receptors and stimulates mitogenesis in renal medullary interstitial cells. Kidney Int 33:255A
45. Levine L, Hassid A (1977) Epidermal growth factor stimulates prostaglandin biosynthesis by canine kidney (MDCK) cells. Biochem Biophys Res Commun 76:1181
46. Norman J, Badie-Dezfooly B, Nord EP, Kurtz I, Schlosser J, Chaudhari A, Fine LG (1989) EGF-induced mitogenesis in proximal tubular cells: potentiation by angiotensin II. Am J Physiol 253:F299
47. Stanton RC, Seifter JL (1988) Epidermal growth factor rapidly activates the hexose monophosphate shunt in kidney cells. Am J Physiol 253:C267
48. Mullin JM, McGinn MT (1988) Epidermal growth factor-induced mitogenesis in kidney epithelial cells (LLC-PK1). Cancer Res 48:4886
49. Harris RC (1990) S6 kinase activity increases in cultured proximal tubule cells with epidermal growth factor and insulin and in renal cortex after uninephrectomy. Kidney Int 37:195A

50. Harris RC, Daniel TO (1989) Epidermal growth factor binding, stimulation of phosphorylation and inhibition of gluconeogenesis in rat proximal tubule. J Cell Physiol 139:383
51. Sack E, Talor Z (1988) High affinity binding sites for epidermal growth factor in renal membranes. Biochem Biophys Res Commun 154:312
52. Goodyer P, Kachra Z, Bell C, Rozen R (1988) Renal tubular cells are potential targets for epidermal growth factor. Am J Physiol 255:F1191
53. Gonnelia PA, Siminoski K, Murphy RA, Neutra MR (1987) Transepithelial transport of epidermal growth factor by absorptive cells of suckling rat ileum. J Clin Invest 80:22
54. Maratos-Flier E, Kao C-Y, Verdin E, King GL (1987) Receptor-mediated vectorial transcytosis of epidermal growth factor by Madin-Darby Canine Kidney Cells. J Cell Biol 105:1595
55. Neal DE, Marsh C, Bennett MK, Abel PD, Hall RR, Sainsbury JR, Harris AL (1985) Epidermal growth factor receptors in human bladder cancer: comparison of invasive and superficial tumours. Lancet I:366
56. Tsau YK, Norman JT, Fine LG (1989) Epidermal growth factor enhances renal regeneration and accelerates recovery from ischemic acute renal failure. Kidney Int 35:420A
57. Behrens MT, Corbin AL, Hise MK (1989) Epidermal growth factor receptor regulation in the rat kidney: two models of renal growth. Am J Physiol 257:F1059
58. Humes HD, Cieslinski DA, Coimbra TM, Messana JM, Calvao C (1989) Epidermal growth factor enhances renal tubule cell regeneration and repair and accelerates the recovery of renal function in postischemic acute renal failure. J Clin Invest 84:1757
59. Sack E, Arruda JAL, Talor Z (1989) EGF binding is decreased in compensatory renal hypertrophy. Kidney Int 35:319A
60. Jennische E, Andersson G, Hansson HA (1987) Epidermal growth factor is expressed by cells in the distal tubules during postnephrectomy renal growth. Acta Physiol Scand 129:449
61. Uchida S, Tsutsumi O, Hise MK, Oka T (1988) Role of epidermal growth factor in compensatory renal hypertrophy in mice. Kidney Int 33:387A
62. Hwang DL, Lev-Ran A, Tay YC, Chen CR, Dev N (1989) Epidermal growth factor excretion and receptor binding in diabetic rats. Life Sci 44:407
63. Kasayama S, Ohba Y, Oka T (1989) Epidermal growth factor deficiency associated with diabetes mellitus. Proc Natl Acad Sci USA 86:7644
64. Gattone VH, Fu-wen N, Andrews GK, Klein RM, Calvet JP (1989) Reduced ontogenic expression of epidermal growth factor (EGF) in a murine model of renal cystic disease. Kidney Int 35:311A
65. Moskowitz DW, Bonar SL, Marcus MD, Clayman RV, Avner ED (1989) Epidermal growth factor content of human and mouse (cpk) renal cysts. Clin Res 37:497A
66. Avner ED, Sweeney WE (1990) Epidermal growth factor induces hyperplastic tubular cysts and increased Na-K ATPase activity in vitro. Kidney Int 37:190A
67. Harris RC, Hoover RL, Jacobson HR, Badr KF (1988) Evidence for glomerular actions of epidermal growth factor in the rat. J Clin Invest 82:1028
68. Scoggins BA, Butkus A, Coghlan JP, Fei D, McDougall JG, Niall HD, Walsh JR, Wang X (1984) In vivo cardiovascular, renal and endocrine effects of epidermal growth factor in sheep. In: Labrie T, Prouix L (eds) Endocrinology. Elsevier, p 573
69. Margolis BL, Holub BJ, Troyer DA, Skorecki KL (1988) Epidermal growth factor stimulates phospholipase A2 in vasopressin-treated rat glomerular mesangial cells. Biochem J 256:469
70. Margolis BL, Bonventre JV, Kremer SG, Kudlow JE, Skorecki KL (1988) Epidermal growth factor is synergistic with phorbol esters and vasopressin in stimulating arachidonate release and prostaglandin production in renal glomerular mesangial cells. Biochem J 249:587

71. Harris RC, Badr KF (1990) Recovery of prostaglandin synthesis in rat glomerular mesangial cells after aspirin inhibition: induction of cyclooxygenase activity by serum and epidermal growth factor. Prostaglandins 39:213
72. Harris RC, Munger KA, Badr KF, Takahashi K (1990) Mediation of renal vascular effects of epidermal growth factor by arachidonate metabolites. FASEB J 4:1654
73. Capdevila JH, Harris RC, Karara A, Dishman E (1989) Characterization of the arachidonic acid epoxygenase reaction present in isolated rat kidney proximal tubule cells. Kidney Int 35:290A
74. Assoain RK, Grotendorst GR, Miller DM, Sporn MB (1984) Cellular transformation by coordinated action of three peptide growth factors from human platelets. Nature 309:804
75. Madtes DK, Raines EW, Sakariassen KS, Assoain RK, Sporn MB, Bell GJ, Ross R (1988) Induction of transforming growth factor-α in activated human macrophages. Cell 53:285
76. Rappolee DA, Mark D, Banda MJ, Werb Z (1988) Wound macrophages express TGF-α and other growth factors in vivo: Analysis by mRNA phenotyping. Science 241:708
77. Brachman R, Lindquist PB, Nagashima M, Kohr W, Lipari T, Napier M, Derynck R (1989) Transmembrane TGF-α precursors activate EGF/TGF-α receptors. Cell 56:691
78. Song ST, Winchell LF, McCune BK, Earp HS, Teixido J, Massague J, Herman B, Lee DC (1989) The TGF-α precursor expressed on the cell surface binds to the TGF receptor on adjacent cells, leading to signal transduction. Cell 56:495
79. Hoover RL, Harris RC, Haralson MA (1989) Effects of epidermal growth factor on collagen biosynthesis in cultured rat kidney mesangial cells. Kidney Int 35:349A
80. Haralson MA, DiMari SJ, Hoover RL, Harris RC (1990) Epidermal growth factor suppresses collagen biosynthesis in retinoic acid-treated cultured rat kidney mesangial cells. Kidney Int 37:195A
81. Laato M, Kahari V-M, Niinikoski J, Vuorio E (1987) Epidermal growth factor increases collagen production in granulation tissue by stimulation of fibroblast proliferation and not by activation of procollagen genes. Biochem J 247:385

Determinants of Autocrine and Paracrine Growth Factor Release by Kidney Epithelial Cells

F. Gary Toback, Sreedharan Kartha, and Margaret M. Walsh-Reitz[1]

Summary. During studies of mitogenic signal transduction mechanisms in nontransformed monkey kidney epithelial cells in culture, evidence for the release of autocrine and paracrine growth factors was obtained. Reduction of the K or Na concentration of the culture medium induced rapid release of novel growth-promoting activities, whereas addition of the mitogen, adenosine diphosphate, stimulated the appearance of a platelet-derived growth factor-like protein which could function in a paracrine manner. These cells constitutively release transforming growth factor β2, which acts as a negative autocrine growth factor. Thus, growth in culture appears to be regulated by the interplay of positive and negative autocrine growth factors and the responses of cell surface receptors and post-receptor events. Autocrine and paracrine growth factors released in response to alterations in the ionic and nutrient composition of the extracellular environment could play an important role in physiological and pathological states in the kidney.

Introduction

Few factors that regulate the growth of kidney epithelial cells have been defined. During the past decade, we have used a tissue culture model system to identify determinants of renal cell proliferation. Experiments were carried out using kidney epithelial cells of the nontransformed African green monkey (*Cercopithecus aethiops*) line, BSC-1. Although the growth of cells in culture may differ in certain respects from that in the intact organ, this approach eliminates many of the problems inherent in studies of growth in a tissue as complex as kidney. Studies were often carried out in quiescent, high-density cultures in order to simulate the low proliferative

[1]The University of Chicago, Department of Medicine, Chicago, IL 60637, USA

activity of kidney cells in vivo [1]. Under these conditions, the epithelial cell monolayer appears to form small domes (3 to 4 cells in size), which suggests that the cells carry out transepithelial transport.

Several determinants of growth regulation have been identified in BSC-1 cells [2]. These include growth factors and hormones in normal serum and their receptors on the cell surface, and low molecular weight nutrients. Specific growth-stimulatory molecules contained in serum include vasopressin, glucagon, and epidermal growth factor (EGF) [3]. The growth of BSC-1 cells in culture is also regulated by the cellular production of several inhibitors. These include lactate, ammonium ion, and a secreted protein which has an M_r of 25000 [4]. This inhibitor protein, which has been identified as transforming growth factor (TGF)-β2, is active at very low concentrations (1 ng/ml) on epithelial cells grown in culture, impedes exit of cells from the G_0/G_1 (resting) phase of the cell cycle, and can be overcome by the stimulatory action of serum or EGF [5]. We have reported that this protein appears to exert its growth inhibitory effect by interfering with cell Na flux [6]. Although the substratum upon which cells grow in culture is often considered a critical determinant of replication and differentiation [7], the contribution of collagen, fibronectin, and other extracellular factors to the growth of BSC-1 cells has not yet been defined in detail.

Growth Factors Isolated from Renal Tissue

While no growth factor specific to kidney has been described, several factors initially described in other types of cells have been identified in kidney tissue or have been shown to have actions on renal cells in culture. Growth factors isolated from kidney tissue include EGF, TGF-α and β, platelet-derived growth factor (PDGF), insulin-like growth factor (IGF)-I and II, acidic and basic fibroblast growth factor (FGF), and interleukin-1 [8]. EGF is found in abundance in urine and renal cyst fluid, and its precursor protein, preproEGF, is made by cells of the distal nephron in the mouse [9]. TGF-β1 has been isolated from bovine kidney, and TGF-β2 is an autocrine growth inhibitor for kidney epithelial cells in culture [6]. PDGF is produced by mesangial cells, stimulates mesangial cell contraction, and is an autocrine and paracrine mitogen for different types of renal cells [8]. IGF-I and II are probably synthesized in the kidney, although their physiologic functions in the organ are unknown. Both acidic and basic FGF are found in kidney and may play a role in angiogenesis during renal embryonic development [10].

The metabolism and excretion of growth factors in acute and chronic renal failure has not yet been studied in detail. Although most of the factors probably act locally, their presence has also been detected in the circulation and in urine. Some may be filtered at the glomerulus or may require intact tubular cells for degradation and might accumulate progressively in the extracellular fluid as glomerular and tubular function diminish. In this scenario, cells of the injured kidney could be exposed to abnormal concentrations of growth factors and thereby subjected to nonphysiologic growth-regulatory signals.

Initiation of DNA Synthesis and Multiplication is Induced in BSC-1 Cells Exposed to Altered Extracellular Concentrations of K or Na

Studies of renal epithelial cells in culture provided the first support for the hypothesis that cell proliferation can be induced by perturbations of the ionic environment. In 1980 it was shown that addition of NaCl to the culture medium of BSC-1 cells initiated DNA synthesis and induced cell multiplication in high-density, quiescent BSC-1 cells [1]. In 1983 a report from this laboratory demonstrated that BSC-1 cells exposed to a reduced concentration of K in the medium (control of 5.4 mM to 3.2 mM) exhibited accelerated growth analogous to that observed in kidneys of rats fed a K-deficient diet [11]. In addition, growth stimulation provoked by lowering the extracellular K concentration required a transient increase in intracellular Na content [12]. When this increment was prevented, low-K stimulation of cell multiplication was not observed. Since augmented influx of Na occurs during the onset of proliferation, one would expect that exposure of kidney cells to a reduced concentration of Na might inhibit mitogenesis. Contrary to this expectation, cell growth was stimulated when the concentration of the medium was reduced from 155 mM (control) to 130 mM [13]. It should be noted that the mitogenic effects in each condition cited above were shown not to be a consequence of increments or reductions in either the osmolality or the anion concentration of the culture medium. In summary, renal epithelial cells can respond to perturbations in the extracellular fluid concentration of K or Na by initiating DNA synthesis.

Reduced Extracellular Potassium Concentration Stimulates Growth of Renal Cells by an Autocrine Mechanism

More than fifty years ago, systemic K depletion, achieved experimentally by feeding rats a K-deficient diet, was found to induce kidney growth [14]. Sustained mild hypokalemia is associated with doubling of renal mass due to both hyperplasia and hypertrophy of kidney cells. An in vitro model to study this phenomenon became available when it was found that simply lowering the extracellular K concentration from 5.4 mM (control) to 3.2 mM in confluent cultures of BSC-1 cells induced accelerated growth [11]. Thus, these cells perceive a reduction in the K concentration of the medium as a mitogenic signal.

We tested the hypothesis that proliferation in response to low-K medium is mediated by release of a growth-promoting factor from the cells [15]. Low-K or control medium was conditioned by placing it on confluent cultures of BSC-1 cells. Growth-stimulating activity in low-K conditioned medium (CM) first appeared after 1 hour (Fig. 1, *a*) and was optimal when the K concentration during conditioning was 3.2 mM. Preliminary studies indicated that the growth factor(s) had an apparent M_r of 12000–30000, as determined by ultrafiltration and dialysis. The factor(s) is highly potent because it retains its stimulatory activity at dilutions greater than 1:1000. Its activity is destroyed by heating to 56°C for 30 minutes, but is stable at 4°C for at least 3 days. This activity differs from other previously described growth factors.

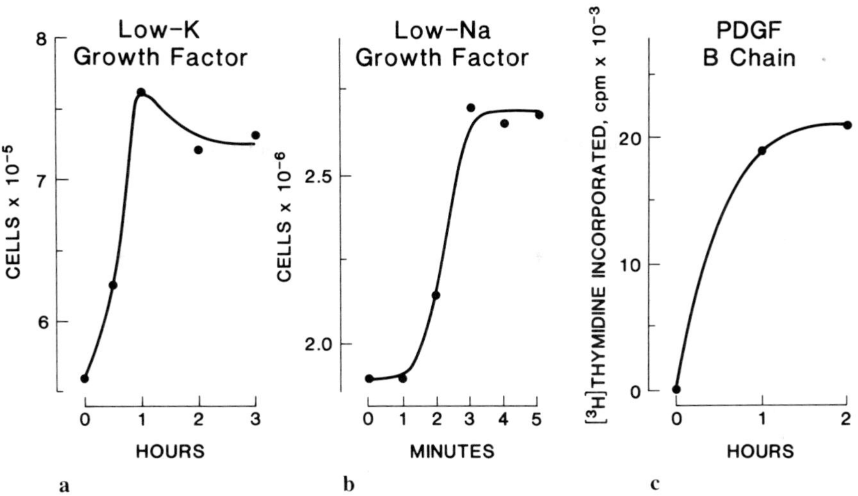

Fig. 1a-c. Release of autocrine and paracrine growth-promoting activities from BSC-1 cells exposed to low-K medium, low-Na medium, or adenosine diphosphate. **a** Appearance of growth-stimulating activity in low-K medium. Confluent, quiescent cultures of BSC-1 cells were exposed to medium containing 3.2 mM K and 0.01% calf serum for different periods of time and were collected. The K concentration of this low-K conditioned medium (*CM*) was adjusted to 5.4 mM by adding KCl. CM was filtered and its serum concentration was raised to 0.5%. Medium on fresh cultures was aspirated and replaced by the low-K CM. The effect of each medium on cell multiplication was assessed by counting the number of cells 3 days later. One hour of exposure of the cells to low-K CM was required to increase the growth-stimulating activity of this medium above that in control CM. **b** Appearance of growth-promoting activity in low-Na medium. At time 0, confluent cultures were exposed to low-Na medium (130 mM) containing 0.01% serum. At the times specified on the abscissa, the CM on the dish was collected. The Na concentration of this CM was adjusted to 155 mM by adding NaCl. CM was filtered and its serum concentration was raised to 0.5%. Medium on a fresh culture was aspirated and replaced by the low-Na CM. The number of cells per dish was counted 4 days later. Growth-promoting activity was maximal in low-Na CM after 3 minutes. **c** Release of PDGF-like mitogenic activity by ADP from high-density, quiescent cultures. BSC-1 cells were exposed to ADP for 1 or 2 hours, and CM was collected and assayed for its mitogenic activity in NRK fibroblasts. The stimulation of [^{3}H]thymidine incorporation into DNA was inhibited 85% by human anti-PDGF IgG. After 1 hour of exposure to ADP, PDGF-like activity was about 10-fold greater than that measured in control CM. (Data adapted from [13,15,27])

The growth-promoting activity in low-K CM can be antagonized by the addition of purified TGF-β2, the autocrine inhibitor of BSC-1 cell growth.

This study indicated that stimulation of renal epithelial cell growth induced by lowering the extracellular K concentration is associated with the appearance of a mitogenic factor(s) in the medium, and provided the first evidence that cell growth induced by an alteration in the ion concentration of the extracellular fluid could be mediated by an autocrine mechanism.

Lowering Extracellular Sodium Concentration Induces Renal Cell Growth and Production of Growth Factors

Since augmented influx of Na ions probably occurs during the onset of proliferation in virtually all mammalian cells [16], one would expect to find that exposure of BSC-1 cells to medium containing a reduced concentration of Na would inhibit mitogenesis. Surprisingly, we found that cell multiplication was stimulated when the Na concentration of the medium was reduced from 155 mM (control) to 130 mM [13]. The capacity of low-Na medium to enhance cell proliferation depended upon the decreased Na concentration, as growth stimulation was equivalent whether equimolar amounts of choline chloride or equiosmolar amounts of sucrose were used to replace NaCl deleted from the medium.

After exposure of confluent cultures to low-Na medium (130 mM) for only 3–5 minutes (Fig. 1, *b*), the cells released two growth-stimulatory factors (apparent M_r 6200 and 9000). Release was not dependent upon new protein synthesis, since it occurred in the presence of cycloheximide. The activity in CM was stable at 56°C for 30 minutes and was retained after freezing for many weeks. Treatment with trypsin abolished the growth-promoting effect, whereas treatment with dithiothreitol did not, which suggests that the low-Na growth factors are proteins that have no accessible disulfide bonds required for activity. The growth response to a reduction in extracellular Na concentration appears to be cell-type specific, since low-Na medium does not stimulate proliferation of fibroblasts. Release of growth factor activity is also cell-type specific, as CM from fibroblasts exposed to a reduced extracellular Na concentration is not stimulatory for epithelial cells. The low-Na growth factors appear to be chemically and functionally different from other known growth factors.

Low-K and Low-Na Growth Factors

The observations summarized above indicate that exposure of kidney epithelial cells to low-K or low-Na medium results in the rapid appearance of growth-promoting activities in the extracellular fluid. These autocrine products appear to differ in that (a) the apparent M_r of the growth factor(s) in low-K CM is 12000–30000, whereas those in low-Na CM are 6200 and 9000, (b) the low-K factor(s) first appears in the medium after 60 minutes, whereas the low-Na factors are detected as early as 3 minutes, and (c) the growth-stimulating effect of low-K CM is destroyed by heating at 56°C for 30 minutes, whereas the low-Na activity is stable under this condition.

The liberation of active factors by renal epithelial cells in culture suggests that kidney cells may respond similarly in vivo. Thus, modest reductions in the extracellular concentration of K and Na may result in the rapid appearance of physiological mediators that could communicate information to other cells along the nephron. These factors might act as messengers between glomerular and tubular cells in different parts of the nephron, in response to changes in peritubular or luminal ion concentrations. Although the factors released in response to low-K and low-Na media induce proliferation in cell culture, their physiologic role may be different in the intact kidney. Since many mitogens stimulate fluxes of ions and nutrients [16,17], one possible role could be to modify epithelial transport in response to changes in the extracellular environment. Release of autocrine or paracrine factors with this property suggests a previously undisclosed mechanism for regulation of ion and nutrient transport in adjacent and nonadjacent epithelial cells. Additional studies will be required to determine whether these factors contribute to the control of kidney epithelial cell growth and/or transport in vivo.

Transforming Growth Factor β2 Is a Negative Autocrine Growth Factor for Kidney Cells

The autocrine release of growth-inhibitory activity was inferred from observations made on crowded cultures of BSC-1 cells by Holley and co-workers in 1978 [4]. They noted stimulation of [^{3}H]thymidine incorporation into DNA when CM containing serum was aspirated and replaced with fresh serum-free medium. As no serum growth factors were added to the cells, it appeared that DNA synthesis was initiated by removal of a cell-derived growth inhibitor. Subsequent purification of this inhibitor protein indicated that it could arrest sparse cultures of growing cells in the G_1 phase of the cell cycle, but proliferation resumed when it was removed [6]. This reversible effect on cell growth, and the low concentration required for inhibition, suggested a physiological role for the inhibitor in the control of proliferation. In 1984, this growth inhibitor was shown to be biologically and chemically similar to TGF-β [18]. The complete amino acid sequence of the BSC-1 cell growth inhibitor has been determined from the nucleotide sequence of the cDNA, and has been shown to correspond to that of TGF-β2 [5].

In primary cultures of rabbit proximal tubular cells, TGF-β2 appears to transform a mitogenic stimulus into a hypertrophic one [19], and suggests that this negative autocrine growth factor could play a regulatory role in compensatory renal growth after uninephrectomy. Perhaps release of this protein by kidney cells in vivo converts what might otherwise have been a largely hyperplastic response into one that is expressed by an increase in renal mass that is 75% cell hypertrophy and 25% proliferation [20].

Purine Nucleotides Are Potent Mitogens for Renal Epithelial Cells and Stimulate Proto-oncogene Expression

During the course of a study to define the role of cAMP in kidney epithelial cell growth, we observed that exogenous adenosine 5′-monophosphate (AMP), used as a control, acted as a powerful mitogen [21]. Each of the adenine nucleotides was able to stimulate DNA synthesis in confluent cultures of BSC-1 cells. ADP and AMP were more potent mitogens than ATP or adenosine, or guanine or inosine and their nucleotides. Furthermore, ADP stimulated DNA synthesis 3-fold more than any known growth-promoting agent for BSC-1 cells. Importantly, ADP and AMP were mitogenic under serum-free conditions, and their stimulatory effects were apparently not mediated by cAMP-dependent mechanisms. In addition, known metabolites such as adenosine, hypoxanthine, or inosine did not appear to mediate ADP or AMP stimulation of DNA synthesis, because they were not as potent when added to the culture medium. Autoradiography of [^{3}H]thymidine-labeled cultures indicated that 6-fold more cells were synthesizing DNA. There was no detectable detachment of cells from the monolayer under these conditions. Finally, the mitogenic effect of ADP or AMP did not appear to be mediated through the adenosine receptor, because the predicted stimulation of DNA synthesis was observed in the presence of a large excess of theophylline or 5′-deoxy 5′-methylthioadenosine, which are potent adenosine receptor antagonists.

To explore the molecular mechanisms by which ADP exerts its mitogenic effect, we tested the hypothesis that stimulation of DNA synthesis in renal epithelial cells of the BSC-1 line is mediated by activation of proto-oncogenes. Transcripts of the c-Ha-*ras* proto-oncogene were identified in quiescent, high-density cells [22]. Addition of ADP to the culture medium stimulated expression by 4-fold. Maximal expression of c-*ras* was observed 12 hours following exposure to ADP, and preceded initiation of DNA synthesis. Expression of the c-*fos* and c-*myc* proto-oncogenes was not detected in unstimulated cells, but following exposure to ADP there was maximal accumulation of c-*fos* transcripts at 30 minutes and c-*myc* at 60 minutes.

We also evaluated the capacity of ADP to stimulate expression of the early growth response gene, Egr-1 [23]. ADP rapidly induced Egr-1 mRNA expression with a peak level about 10-fold higher than that attained for c-*fos*. Egr-1 mRNA induction occurred as early as 10 minutes following exposure of BSC-1 cells to ADP. This novel gene is also induced in serum-stimulated mouse fibroblasts, insulin-stimulated rat hepatoma cells, and phytohemagglutinin-stimulated human peripheral blood lymphocytes. Another early growth response gene, NAK1, the human homologue of mouse nur 77 and rat NGFI-B, also is induced by ADP [24]. NAK1 belongs to the superfamily of steroid and thyroid hormone and retinoic acid receptor genes. The expression of NAK1 is detected at 20 minutes, and is maximal after 1 hour of exposure to ADP. Genes which are activated rapidly and transiently are likely to be important in transduction of mitogenic signals and regulation of cell proliferation. The Egr-1 and NAK1 genes encode proteins with zinc-finger domains that could facilitate DNA binding [24,25]. These proteins are postulated to function as transcriptional regulators.

ADP stimulation of Egr-1, NAK1, and proto-oncogene expression occurred during the G_1 phase of the cell cycle because maximal expression of these transcripts was detected prior to the increment in DNA synthesis at 12–24 hours. These findings represent the first reported examples of enhanced expression of Egr-1, NAK1, c-*fos*, c-*myc*, c-Ha-*ras*, and transferrin receptor genes in stimulated, nontransformed epithelial cells.

Expression of 25 genes and proto-oncogenes, most of which contribute to growth control, were studied in BSC-1 cells in the absence and presence of ADP. The responses observed could be divided into four patterns, which are presented in Table 1; genes not constitutively expressed but induced by ADP, genes whose constitutive expression was enhanced or unaltered by the nucleotide, and genes that were neither constitutively expressed nor induced. It is possible that ADP represents a critical extracellular signal which activates genes such as Egr-1 and NAK1, which encode zinc-finger containing transcriptional regulatory proteins, and could in turn control induction of several other genes [24,25]. It is also of interest that ADP stimulates expression of the gene for TGF-β, which encodes a protein that inhibits growth of BSC-1 cells. Thus, ADP can mimic the action of a growth factor and stimulate

Table 1. Effect of ADP on gene expression in BSC-1 cells

Gene	Effect of ADP
Egr-1, NAK1, c-*fos*, c-*myc*	Expression induced
c-*Ha-ras*, c-*sis* (PDGF-B chain), TGF-β, transferrin receptor, fibronectin, plasminogen activator inhibitor	Constitutive expression enhanced
EGF receptor, β-actin, τ-actin, vimentin, cathepsin L, thymosin β_{10}	Constitutive expression unaltered by ADP
IGF-I, IGF-II, prepro EGF, TGF-α, PDGF receptor, PDGF-A chain, v-*src*, v-*fms*, v-*yes*	Genes not expressed or induced

expression of cell-cycle specific genes (Egr-1, NAK1, and proto-oncogenes), as well as the gene for TGF-β, whose expression could serve to limit cell proliferation by releasing a negative autocrine growth factor.

ADP Induces Release of PDGF-like Protein from Renal Epithelial Cells Which Could Act as a Paracrine Growth Factor

PDGF is produced by cells of mesodermal origin, such as fibroblasts and smooth muscle cells, and is released from platelets and macrophages during clotting and wound healing [26]. It is a mitogen for cells of mesenchymal origin, a chemoattractant for smooth muscle cells and monocytes, and a promoter of collagen, proteoglycan, and elastic fiber protein synthesis. PDGF is a dimeric glycoprotein of M_r 30000, comprised of A and/or B chains linked by disulfide bonds. It is most commonly found as a heterodimer (AB), although biologically active homodimers (AA and BB) have been described. The amino acid sequence of the B chain is nearly identical to the putative transforming protein of the simian sarcoma virus which is encoded by the v-*sis* oncogene; the cellular homologue is termed c-*sis*. Three classes of PDGF receptors have been defined, which are each comprised of two subunits located in the plasma membrane. During a study of ADP-induced gene expression, we showed that quiescent BSC-1 cells constitutively release PDGF-like activity [27]. The growth factor in BSC-1 CM was assayed for its mitogenic activity on NRK fibroblasts and its chemoattractant activity on bovine aortic smooth muscle cells. Both activities were found, and were blocked by human anti-PDGF IgG. The presence of a PDGF-like protein was unexpected because expression of PDGF was thought to be confined to cells of mesodermal origin [26]. The gene for the B chain of PDGF (c-*sis*) is constitutively expressed in these cells, whereas no PDGF A chain mRNA could be detected. Thus, the cells appear to synthesize and secrete a PDGF-like protein that is a BB homodimer. ADP increased by 3-fold the amounts of PDGF-B chain mRNA and secreted immunoreactive PDGF-like protein. Importantly, ADP rapidly induced release of PDGF-like activity, so that 1 hour after exposure of cells to the nucleotide, the amount of growth factor was increased by more than 10-fold (Fig. 1, *c*). TGF-β2 inhibited DNA synthesis in growing cultures and induced marked accumulation of c-*sis* RNA without a corresponding increase in released PDGF-like activity. Interestingly, BSC-1 cells do not exhibit a mitogenic response to authentic PDGF, nor do they express the gene encoding the PDGF receptor. These results imply that if PDGF-like protein is released by renal epithelial cells in vivo, it could

Table 2. Growth factors in renal physiology and pathology: possible roles

Embryonic growth and development of the kidney
Control of glomerular filtration and blood flow
Regulation of ionic and nutrient fluxes in tubular cells
Compensatory renal growth after uninephrectomy
Regeneration after acute renal failure
Proliferative glomerulonephritis
Cell proliferation in renal cystic diseases
Renal adenomas and adenocarcinomas

act by a paracrine mechanism to initiate proliferation of adjacent stromal (fibroblastic) and/or vascular (smooth muscle) cells within the organ.

Conclusions and Speculations

The studies described above indicate that brief alterations in the extracellular environment can signal release of physiological mediators from kidney epithelial cells of the BSC-1 line. The appearance of growth factors following reductions in the extracellular K or Na concentrations, within the physiological range, demonstrates the capacity of kidney cells to transduce changes in their ionic milieu into release of autocrine products. These growth factors could stimulate hypertrophic and/or proliferative cell growth, communicate information to other cells along the nephron, and/or facilitate adaptive changes in cell metabolism in response to the altered extracellular fluid composition. Thus, monkey renal epithelial cells can respond to extracellular ionic perturbations as do T-lymphocytes when presented with foreign antigens: they release polypeptide growth factors.

Infusion of adenine nucleotides can speed recovery of renal function and structure after ischemic, toxic, or obstructive injury [28]. The infused adenine nucleotides could exert their beneficial effects during renal regeneration by raising cell ATP content and thereby restoring the energy charge and metabolic integrity needed to carry out biosynthetic reactions [29,30]. The nucleotides could also stimulate DNA synthesis, and stimulate the release of growth-stimulating molecules which could accelerate the repair of sublethally-injured cells and the proliferation of new ones, thereby augmenting reepithelialization of the nephron. Provision of ADP stimulates release of PDGF-like protein by BSC-1 cells. If released from kidney cells in vivo, this growth factor could initiate proliferation of stromal and vascular cells by a paracrine mechanism at the site of renal injury. It should be noted that although BSC-1 cells are nontransformed they are immortal, so that their capacity to secrete growth factors in response to physiological signals may be one of the characteristics of their phenotype. Hence, caution should be used in extrapolating results obtained in these kidney epithelial cells in culture to renal tissue in vivo.

That autocrine and paracrine factors can be released by kidney cells in response to physiological and pathological signals suggests a previously unsuspected network of cell-to-cell communication within the organ. Growth factors may participate in many renal physiological and pathological processes, as suggested in Table 2. New research initiatives are needed to explore this heretofore unrecognized informational system, which, when defined in detail, could provide new insight into the normal regulation of renal function and the pathogenesis of kidney diseases.

Acknowledgments. Support for studies cited in the text was provided by National Institutes of Health Grants R01 DK39689, R01 DK18413, and R01 DK37227.

References

1. Toback FG (1980) Induction of growth in kidney epithelial cells in culture by Na^+. Proc Natl Acad Sci USA 77:6654–6656
2. Holley RW, Armour R, Baldwin JH, Brown KD, Yeh Y-C (1977) Density-dependent regulation of growth of BSC-1 cells in cell culture: control of growth by serum factors. Proc Natl Acad Sci USA 74:5046–5050
3. Walsh-Reitz MM, Toback FG (1983) Vasopressin stimulates growth of renal epithelial cells in culture. Am J Physiol 245:C365–C370
4. Holley RW, Armour R, Baldwin JH (1978) Density-dependent regulation of growth of BSC-1 cells in cell culture: growth inhibitors formed by the cells. Proc Natl Acad Sci USA 75:1864–1866
5. Hanks SK, Armour R, Baldwin JH, Maldonado F, Spiess J, Holley RW (1988) Amino acid sequence of the BSC-1 cell growth inhibitor (polyergin) deduced from the nucleotide sequence of the cDNA. Proc Natl Acad Sci USA 85:79–82
6. Walsh-Reitz MM, Toback FG, Holley RW (1984) Cell growth and net Na^+ flux are inhibited by a protein produced by kidney epithelial cells in culture. Proc Natl Acad Sci USA 81:793–796
7. Gospodarowicz D, Lepine J, Massoglia S, Wood I (1984) Comparison of the ability of basement membranes produced by corneal endothelial and mouse-derived endothelial PF-HR-9 cells to support the proliferation and differentiation of bovine kidney tubule epithelial cells in vitro. J Cell Biol 99:947–961
8. Mendley SR, Toback FG (1989) Autocrine and paracrine regulation of kidney epithelial cell growth. Annu Rev Physiol 51:33–50
9. Atkin BM, Franklin WA, Bell GI, Toback FG (1990) Macula densa cells of mouse kidney do not synthesize epidermal growth factor precursor mRNA. Nephron 54:313–317
10. Risau W, Ekblom P (1986) Production of a heparin-binding angiogenesis factor by the embryonic kidney. J Cell Biol 103:1101–1107
11. Walsh-Reitz MM, Toback FG (1983) Kidney epithelial cell growth is stimulated by lowering extracellular potassium concentration. Am J Physiol 244:C429–C432
12. Walsh-Reitz MM, Aithal HN, Toback FG (1984) Na regulates growth of kidney epithelial cells induced by lowering extracellular K concentration. Am J Physiol 247:C321–C326
13. Walsh-Reitz MM, Gluck SL, Waack S, Toback FG (1986) Lowering extracellular Na^+ concentration releases autocrine growth factors from renal epithelial cells. Proc Natl Acad Sci USA 83:4764–4768
14. Schrader GA, Prickett CO, Salmon WD (1937) Symptomatology and pathology of potassium and magnesium deficiencies in the rat. J Nutr 14:85–110
15. Mordan LJ, Toback FG (1984) Growth of kidney epithelial cells in culture: evidence for autocrine control. Am J Physiol 246:C351–C354
16. Koch KS, Leffert HL (1979) Increased sodium ion influx is necessary to initiate rat hepatocyte proliferation. Cell 18:153–163
17. Weber MJ, Evans PK, Johnson MA, McNair TF, Nakamura KD, Salter DW (1984) Transport of potassium, amino acids, and glucose in cells transformed by Rous sarcoma virus. Fed Proc 43:107–112

18. Tucker RF, Shipley GD, Moses HL, Holley RW (1984) Growth inhibitor from BSC-1 cells closely related to platelet type β transforming growth factor. Science 226:705–707
19. Fine LG, Holley RW, Nasri H, Badie-Dezfooly B (1985) BSC-1 growth inhibitor transforms a mitogenic stimulus into a hypertrophic stimulus for renal proximal tubular cells: relationship to Na^+-H^+ antiport activity. Proc Natl Acad Sci USA 82:6163–6166
20. Johnson HA, Vera Roman JM (1966) Compensatory renal enlargement. Hypertrophy versus hyperplasia. Am J Pathol 49:1–13
21. Kartha S, Toback FG (1985) Purine nucleotides stimulate DNA synthesis in kidney epithelial cells in culture. Am J Physiol 249:F967–F972
22. Kartha S, Sukhatme VP, Toback FG (1987) ADP activates protooncogene expression in renal epithelial cells. Am J Physiol 252:F1175–F1179
23. Sukhatme VP, Kartha S, Toback FG, Taub R, Hoover RV, Tsai-Morris C-H (1987) A novel early growth response gene rapidly induced by fibroblast, epithelial cell and lymphocyte mitogens. Oncogene Res 1:343–355
24. Nakai A, Kartha S, Sakurai A, Toback FG, DeGroot LJ (1990) A human early response gene homologous to murine nur77 and rat NGFI-B, and related to the nuclear receptor superfamily. Mol Endocrinol 4:1438–1443
25. Sukhatme VP, Cao X, Chang LC, Tsai-Morris C-H, Stamenkovich D, Ferreira P, Cohen D, Edwards S, Shows T, Curran T, Le Beau M, Adamson E (1988) A zinc finger encoding gene coregulated with c-*fos* during growth, differentiation and after cellular depolarization. Cell 53:37–43
26. Deuel TF, Pierce GF, Hsiu-Jeng Y, Shawver LK, Milner PG, Kimura A (1987) Platelet-derived growth factors/*sis* in normal and neoplastic cell growth. J Cell Physiol [Suppl] 5:95–99
27. Kartha S, Bradham DM, Grotendorst GR, Toback FG (1988) Kidney epithelial cells express the c-*sis* proto-oncogene and secrete PDGF-like protein: evidence for a paracrine mechanism. Am J Physiol 255:F800–F806
28. Siegel NJ, Gaudio KM (1988) Amino acids and adenine nucleotides in acute renal failure. In: Brenner BM, Lazarus JM (eds) Acute renal failure, 2nd edn. Churchill Livingstone, New York, pp 857–873
29. Weinberg JM, Humes HD (1986) Increases of cell ATP produced by exogenous adenine nucleotides in isolated rabbit kidney tubules. Am J Physiol 250:F720–F733
30. Mandel LJ, Takano T, Soltoff SP, Murdaugh S (1988) Mechanisms whereby adenine nucleotides improve rabbit renal proximal function during and after anoxia. J Clin Invest 81:1255–1264

Diabetic Nephropathy, from Hyperfiltration and Microproteinuria to ESRD: Perspective of Intervention

Chair: Carl E. Mogensen (Denmark)
Masaaki Arakawa (Japan)

Renal Hypertrophy and Hyperfunction in Experimental Diabetes

ALLAN FLYVBJERG[1]

SUMMARY. Induction of experimental diabetes causes a rapid increase in renal size, accompanied by parallel increases in total kidney RNA and protein, demonstrable 48–72 h after injection of streptozotocin. Within four days of diabetes the total glomerular volume increases by 30%, while tubules, which constitute the greater part of the kidney, grow relatively more slowly. However, the renal growth is apparent before any measurable kidney hyperfiltration. The diabetic renal hypertrophy is preceded by a rise in renal tissue concentration of insulin-like growth factor I (IGF-I), which reaches a peak 24–48 h after induction of diabetes. Strict insulin treatment abolishes both kidney IGF-I accumulation and kidney growth. Administration of a long-acting somatostatin analogue (Octreotide) has an equally inhibitory effect on kidney IGF-I and growth and this without affecting the metabolic control. This finding supports the hypothesis that IGF-I accumulation is a prerequisite for initial renal growth. Furthermore, the renal IGF-I concentration is linearly dependent on the prevailing blood glucose levels, as has been shown for renal growth. The mechanisms responsible for kidney IGF-I accumulation are discussed, including a presentation of results for kidney IGF-I receptor number and affinity, as well as renal IGF-I mRNA levels during initial diabetic hypertrophy. These results thus indicate that IGF-I may contribute to early kidney growth in experimental diabetes and it is noteworthy that six months treatment with Octreotide in diabetic rats reduces both long-term renal hypertrophy and urinary albumin excretion without altering the metabolic status or renal function, suggesting that growth factors may be involved in long-term renal changes as well.

Introduction

Several lines of evidence indicate that renal hypertrophy and hyperfiltration are characteristic and early manifestations of human and experimental diabetes which

[1]Medical Department M, (Diabetes and Endocrinology), Aarhus Kommunehospital, DK-8000 Aarhus C, Denmark

may contribute to the later development of diabetic nephropathy [1]. The renal hypertrophy and hyperfunction persist even in long-term diabetes and it is obvious that an understanding of the genesis of initial renal growth may throw light upon the changes in the sequence of events that eventually lead to late diabetic nephropathy. Furthermore, it is to be expected that a deeper insight into these early cellular pathogenetic events in the diabetic kidney may allow the design of specific antagonists, possibly useful for therapeutic manipulation in the treatment of diabetic patients.

In this review, the current knowledge of kidney growth, as observed in experimental diabetes in rats, is summarized. Firstly, the phenomenon is described according to the classical biochemical, morphological and functional changes. Secondly, various studies are reviewed concerning possible mechanisms behind renal hypertrophy, with the focus on recent facets of evidence for the significance of growth factors from our laboratories.

Biochemical, Morphological and Functional Changes Associated with Renal Hypertrophy in Experimental Diabetes

Induction of experimental diabetes causes a rapid increase in renal size, regularly occurring 48–72 h after the injection of streptozotocin (i.e., about 36 h after the onset of glucosuria), that is not due to accumulation of water, since the total kidney protein content rises in parallel to wet kidney weight [2]. The initial diabetic kidney growth is due to both cellular hypertrophy and hyperplasia. The first sign of growth is an increase in total RNA as early as 24–36 h after the onset of glucosuria [2] and about the same time the cellular pools of RNA precursors and the incorporation of orotate into uridine triphosphate are increased [3]. Shortly thereafter, an increased protein/DNA ratio is seen, indicating cellular hypertrophy, while total DNA is unchanged for the first four days [2]. By means of thymidine incorporation techniques it has been shown that the hyperplastic response is primarily located in the proximal and distal tubules, with almost no hyperplasia in the glomeruli [4].

The morphological features of the hypertrophying diabetic kidney have been studied both by light and electron microscopy and have revealed a non-uniform growth in its early stages, presenting an anatomical glomerulo-tubular imbalance. Within four days of streptozotocin diabetes the total glomerular volume increases by 30%, while tubules, which constitute the greater part of the kidney, grow relatively more slowly [5]. Whether this glomerulo-tubular imbalance is also reflected functionally is not clear at present. However, after a few weeks of diabetes the ratio between glomerular and tubular size returns to almost non-diabetic levels [5].

Several studies have shown that kidney function is increased in animals with a moderate degree of hyperglycemia, whereas in severely diabetic rats glomerular filtration rate (GFR) is similar to that in non-diabetic controls [6], as it is true for the degree of renal hypertrophy [7]. However, the exact relationship between increased renal mass and hyperfunction is controversial and only recently have studies appeared on this topic. Most studies of early diabetic renal abnormalities have been cross-sectional and confined to a well established diabetic state, whereas studies of the initial dynamic phase, during which kidney growth and hyperfunction evolve, have been largely ignored. It seems evident, however, from a recent paper by Cortes et al. [8] on the temporal relationship of renal growth and kidney function, that renal growth is apparent before any measurable kidney hyperfunction. When GFR was expressed per unit kidney weight, there was a significant decrease 48 h after induction of diabetes, indicating that it is unlikely that initial renal metabolic changes and hypertrophy are initiated by increased function and exaggerated work load [8].

On the Pathogenesis of Early Diabetic Renal Hypertrophy and Hyperfunction: The Possible Role of Growth Factors

The term "growth factor" is used as a generic designation for any substance capable of inducing cellular proliferation and/or differentiation. Certain growth factors extend the known hormone cascade beginning with the hypothalamic releasing factors flowing through the pituitary trophic hormones to endocrine gland hormones released into the circulation, and culminating with peripheral tissue growth. Some growth factors, however, do not mediate their actions as hormones because their effects are directly promoted through local paracrine/autocrine mechanisms.

Several lines of evidence suggest that *growth hormone (GH)* modulates renal function and size. GH-deficient patients tend to have abnormally low renal plasma flow (RPF) and GFR, both of which normalize after GH administration [9]. Hirschberg et al. [10] recently demonstrated that a single intramuscular injection of GH did not affect RPF and GFR acutely, but that it increased both functions within 24 h in parallel with the rise in serum *insulin-like growth factor I (IGF-I)*. These findings indicate that GH increases RPF and GFR indirectly through the growth factor IGF-I.

Hirschberg and Kopple [11] infused IGF-I in fasted, anesthetized rats for 20 min and found rises in RPF and GFR and a fall in renal vascular resistance lasting for 2 h. The effects of IGF-I were blocked by simultaneous infusion of indomethacin, while no blocking effect was found with somatostatin infusion, suggesting a role for eicosanoids in the action of IGF-I on the kidney. These acute studies point at a direct effect of IGF-I on kidney function, independent of primary changes in kidney size. In addition, recent studies have shown that IGF-I administration induces kidney growth in GH (and IGF-I) deficient rats within some days [12]. Thus, it can be concluded that IGF-I administration acutely increases kidney function and after some days also induces renal growth in rodents.

Although the mechanism of renal hypertrophy and hyperfiltration, as seen in the early phase after clinical onset of diabetes and in experimental diabetes is unknown, recent studies have suggested that GH and IGF-I may be involved. The increased plasma GH concentration in patients with type 1 diabetes has been suggested as the cause of the increased RPF and GFR. Christiansen et al. [13] showed that when GH was given subcutaneously twice daily (2 and 4 IU) to well-controlled C-peptide negative diabetic patients for a week to induce plasma levels similar to those found in diabetic patients in average to very poor metabolic control, small but significant increases in RPF and GFR were found. Whether this effect is mediated through IGF-I is, however, unknown.

In contrast to the well-established paradox that hyperglycemia (poor metabolic control) does not suppress, but augments GH secretion in diabetic patients, recent studies have shown that GH secretion in the streptozotocin diabetic rat is inhibited rather than

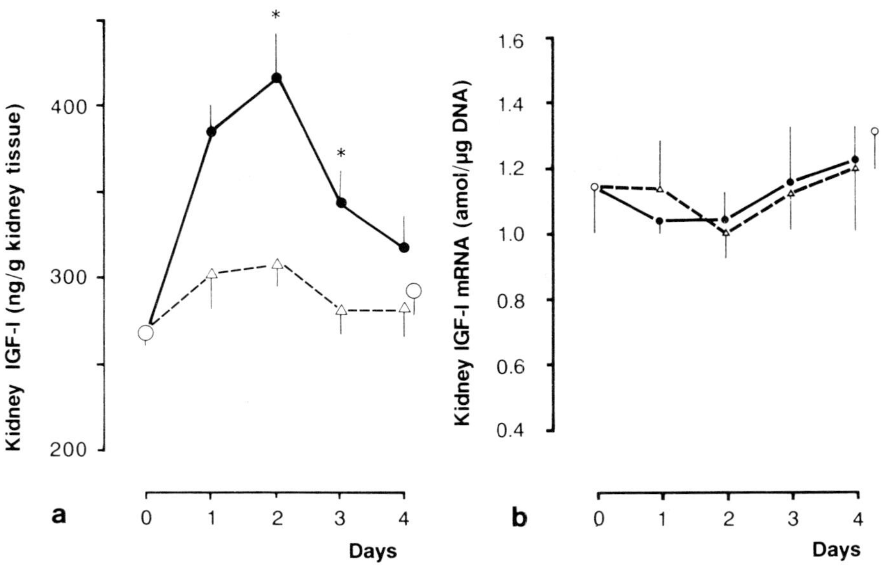

Fig. 1. Changes in **a** kidney insulin-like growth factor I (*IGF-I*) and **b** kidney IGF-I messenger RNA (*IGF-I mRNA*) in control (○), untreated diabetic (●——●), and insulin-treated diabetic rats (△---△) during the four days after induction of streptozotocin (*STZ*) diabetes. On day 0 STZ was injected i.v.; insulin treatment with a very long-acting, heat treated Ultralente Insulin was initiated after 18 h when all animals had blood glucose levels above 15 mmol/l. Insulin was given in an initial dose of 4–6 U, followed by 1-2 U daily thereafter depending on blood glucose values. Kidney IGF-I was measured by radioimmunoassay after previous extraction of the tissue in 1 mol/l acetic acid, while IGF-I mRNA was measured by solution-hybridization. *$P<0.05$ between untreated and insulin-treated diabetic animals. Values are mean ± SEM, n=6 for kidney IGF-I values and n=5 for kidney IGF-I mRNA. (Reproduced from [17] with permission)

paradoxically stimulated [14]. This observation would, at first glance, along with the observation that short-term GH-treatment of diabetic rats has no effect on the degree of renal growth [15], preclude a causal role for GH in diabetic renal hypertrophy. Very recently, however, we found that diabetic dwarf rats with an isolated GH-deficiency (i.e. with normal secretion of the other pituitary hormones) underwent a slower and lesser degree of initial renal hypertrophy when compared to diabetic controls with intact pituitary. Thus, these findings seem to indicate that the *lack* of GH or some GH-dependent factors (e.g., IGF-I or IGF-I binding proteins) attenuates diabetic renal growth in rats (A. Flyvbjerg et al., unpublished results, 1990).

In line with this observation it is interesting that the initial renal hypertrophy is preceded by a rise in extractable renal tissue concentration of IGF-I, which reaches a peak 24–48 h after the induction of diabetes (Fig. 1a) and returns to basal levels after about 4 days, and thus precedes the first demonstrable increase in kidney RNA, protein [16,17], function [8], and size (Fig. 2). The kidney IGF-I accumulation pattern parallels that of labelled thymidine incorporation into renal tubules [4], being in good accordance with a mitogenic effect of IGF-I and thus precedes the pronounced

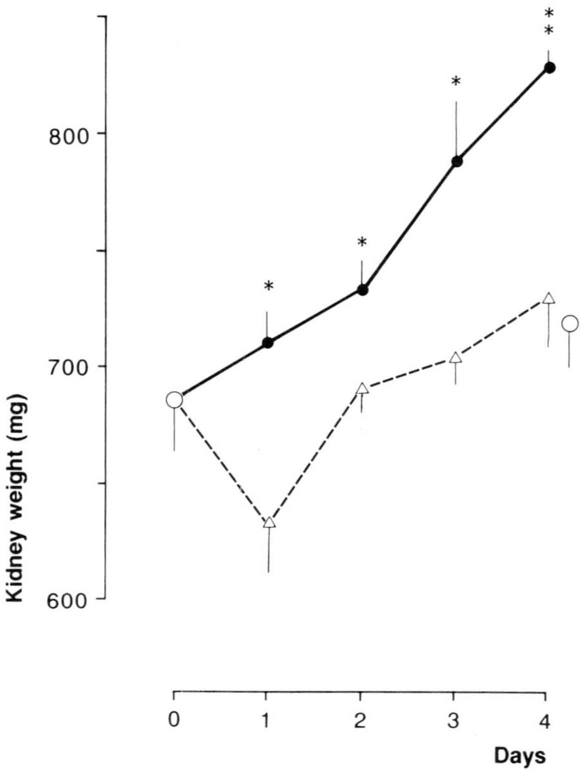

Fig. 2. Changes in kidney weight in streptozotocin-diabetic rats, untreated (●——●) and insulin-treated (△---△), over four days and in non-diabetic control rats on day 0 and 4 (0). Animals were treated as described in legend to Fig. 1. *P<0.05, **P<0.01 between untreated and insulin-treated diabetic animals. Values are given as mean ± SEM and every point represents 6 different animals. (Reproduced from [17] with permission)

hypertrophy of glomeruli [5]. Strict insulin treatment abolishes the increase in both kidney IGF-I and renal hypertrophy (Figs. 1a & 2), supporting the hypothesis of the involvement of this putative causal growth factor in renal hypertrophy and, furthermore, demonstrating that no toxic effect of streptozotocin is involved in the observed changes. Administration of a long-acting somatostatin analogue (Octreotide) has an equally inhibitory effect on kidney IGF-I accumulation and growth, and this without affecting the blood glucose levels, supporting the idea that renal IGF-I accumulation is a prerequisite for initial diabetic kidney growth [18]. It has previously been shown that diabetic kidney hypertrophy was linearly dependent on blood glucose levels one week after induction of diabetes [7]. Very recently it was shown that the degree of kidney IGF-I accumulation 48 h after injection with streptozotocin was directly proportional to the prevailing blood glucose in rats with graded severities of diabetes [19]. This adds weight to the hypothesis that renal IGF-I accumulation is promoted by the diabetic state in stimulating renal growth. The changes seen in kidney IGF-I and diabetic kidney growth have great similarities to those occurring in the remaining kidney after unilateral nephrectomy [16] and it is interesting therefore that induction of diabetes and unilateral nephrectomy combined in the same animal induce additive increase in both kidney IGF-I accumulation and renal enlargement [20].

It is still to be clarified how the increased IGF-I content arrives in the kidney, and thus whether it is due to increased uptake of circulating IGF-I or to increased local production. Traditionally, the liver has been considered to be the main site of IGF-I synthesis, mainly under the control of GH. However, the increase in kidney IGF-I after induction of moderate diabetes or after unilateral nephrectomy is accompanied by little or no change in hepatic or circulating levels of IGF-I [16–18]. Recent reports have shown the existence of distinct receptors for IGF-I in rat kidneys and we have recently shown that IGF-I receptor numbers and affinity in whole kidney homogenates, obtained from hypertrophying diabetic kidneys, are unchanged, suggesting that the increased kidney IGF-I concentration is not likely to be due to changes at receptor level [21]. Alternatively, sequestration of IGF-I within tubules and collecting ducts, or decreased breakdown of the peptide could be responsible for the IGF-I accumulation in the diabetic kidney.

By means of a sensitive solution-hybridization assay for the renal content of IGF-I messenger RNA (IGF-I mRNA), a marker of the cellular gene expression for IGF-I, changes in local kidney production of IGF-I were measured during the initial renal growth in diabetes (Fig. 1b). We found unaltered levels of IGF-I mRNA during the first four days after induction of diabetes, despite accumulation of IGF-I in the kidney (Fig. 1a); this thus seems to indicate that local production at transcriptional level is unchanged [17]. However, IGF-I accumulation in the diabetic kidney due to enhanced translatory regulation cannot be excluded, as has been suggested for IGF-I accumulation in unilateral nephrectomy [22].

The apparent dependence of diabetic renal hypertrophy on kidney IGF-I accumulation has been confirmed in a recent study [23], showing that renal hypertrophy in pre-pubertal rats is much slower than in post-pubertal, and that pre-pubertal rats have no significant increase in kidney IGF-I. This study was inspired by the fact that diabetic angiopathy takes a more benign course in pre-pubertal than in post-pubertal children. The reduced degree of renal hypertrophy in pre-pubertal animals seems to be independent of the presence of androgens, since castration does not attenuate the renotrophic activity of alloxan diabetes in mice [24].

Several observations on the streptozotocin rat model have suggested that increased intrarenal production of the vasodilating prostaglandins PGE_2 and PGI_2 may be involved in the early diabetic renal growth and hyperfiltration. Craven et al. [25] found that when indomethacin administration was begun concomitantly with induction of diabetes in rats, diabetic renal hypertrophy, hyperfiltration, and increased urinary prostaglandin excretion were all reduced, without affecting the metabolic state, when compared to untreated diabetic controls. By contrast, indomethacin treatment for three days in rats with diabetes which had lasted for four weeks, did not influence kidney size or function, indicating a possible role for prostaglandins in the very early renal changes in diabetic rats.

It may be hypothesized that blood glucose-dependent renal IGF-I accumulation, either directly or through eicosanoids, increases initial kidney growth and renal function. This is supported by the finding that indomethacin blocks both initial renal hypertrophy in experimental diabetes [25] and the IGF-I induced enhancement of renal function [11]. In addition, IGF-I is found to stimulate the synthesis of 6-keto PEG_{1a} and PEG_2 in cultured rat liver cells [26].

Altogether our studies indicate that IGF-I may contribute to early kidney growth in experimental diabetes, although the precise cellular mechanisms are a matter of debate. The suggested hypothesis deals with the possible contribution of IGF-I, at a very early stage, to a sequence of events that may lead to late diabetic nephropathy. A considerable amount of further information is of course required to elucidate whether or not IGF-I and other growth factors are also directly involved in the further development of diabetic renal disease. It is, however, intriguing that six months treatment with a long-acting somatostatin analogue (Octreotide) had effects on long-term kidney changes in streptozotocin diabetic rats, by reducing both long-term renal hypertrophy and urinary albumin excretion [27]. These effects were seen without any drug effects on metabolic control (blood glucose, Hgb_{A1c}, 24h glucose output) or renal function in diabetic animals; thus indicating that chronic administration of a "growth factor inhibitor" reduces certain functional abnormalities regarded to be prognostic of late diabetic kidney disease.

Acknowledgments. This manuscript reflects the contribution of co-workers in our own laboratories (Jan Frystyk, Klavs W. Hansen, Sally M. Marshall, Kirsten Nyborg, Ida B. Sillesen, Ole Thorlacius-Ussing, Hans Ørskov and Ruth Østerby) and our colleagues at Linköping University, Sweden (Hans J. Arnqvist and Karin E. Bornfeldt). The studies were supported by grants from the Danish Diabetes Association.

References

1. Mogensen CE, Christensen CK (1984) Predicting diabetic nephropathy in insulin-dependent patients. N Engl J Med 311:89–93
2. Seyer-Hansen K (1983) Renal hypertrophy in experimental diabetes. Kidney Int 23:643–646
3. Cortes P, Lewin NW, Dumler F, Rubenstein AH, Verghese CP, Venkatachalam KK (1980) Uridine triphosphate and RNA synthesis during diabetes-induced kidney growth. Am J Physiol 238:E349–E357
4. Rasch R, Rytter-Nørgaard JO (1983) Renal enlargement: Comparative autoradiographic studies of ^{3}H-thymidine uptake in diabetic and uninephrectomized rats. Diabetologia 25:280–287
5. Seyer-Hansen K, Hansen J, Gundersen HJG (1980) Renal hypertrophy in experimental diabetes. A morphometric study. Diabetologia 18:501–505
6. Hostetter TH, Troy JL, Brenner BM (1981) Glomerular hemodynamics in experimental diabetes. Kidney Int 19:410–415
7. Seyer-Hansen K (1977) Renal hypertrophy in experimental diabetes: Relation to severity of diabetes. Diabetologia 13:141–143
8. Cortes P, Dumler F, Goldman J, Levin NW (1987) Relationship between renal function and metabolic alterations in early streptozocin-induced diabetes in rats. Diabetes 36:80–87
9. Falkheden T, Wickbom I (1965) Renal function and kidney size following hypophysectomy in man. Acta Endocrinol (Copenh) 48:348–354
10. Hirschberg R, Rabb H, Bergamo R, Kopple JD (1989) The delayed effect of growth hormone on renal function in humans. Kidney Int 35:865–870
11. Hirschberg R, Kopple JD (1989) Evidence that insulin-like growth factor I increases renal plasma flow and glomerular filtration rate in fasted rats. J Clin Invest 83:326–330

12. Guler HP, Zapf J, Scheiwiller E, Froesch ER (1988) Recombinant human insulin-like growth factor I stimulates growth and has distinct effects on organ size in hypophysectomized rats. Proc Natl Acad Sci USA 85:4889–4893
13. Christiansen JS, Gammelgaard J, Frandsen M, Ørskov H, Parving HH (1982) Kidney function and size in insulin dependent diabetics before and during growth hormone administration for one week. Diabetologia 22:333–337
14. Robinson ICAF, Clark RG, Carlsson LMS (1987) Insulin, IGF-I and growth in diabetic rats (letter). Nature 326:549
15. Seyer-Hansen K, Gundersen HJG, Østerby R (1981) Acute renal hypertrophy in experimental diabetes: Lack of effect of growth hormone administration. Diabetologia 21:373–375
16. Flyvbjerg A, Thorlacius-Ussing O, Naeraa R, Ingerslev J, Ørskov H (1988) Kidney tissue somatomedin C and initial renal growth in diabetic and uninephrectomized rats. Diabetologia 31:310–314
17. Flyvbjerg A, Bornfeldt KE, Marshall SM, Arnqvist HJ, Ørskov H (1990) Kidney IGF-I mRNA in initial renal hypertrophy in experimental diabetes in rats. Diabetologia 33:334–338
18. Flyvbjerg A, Frystyk J, Thorlacius-Ussing O, Ørskov H (1989) Somatostatin analogue administration prevents increase in kidney somatomedin C and initial renal growth in diabetic and uninephrectomized rats. Diabetologia 32:261–265
19. Flyvbjerg A, Ørskov H (1990) Kidney tissue insulin-like growth factor I and initial renal growth in diabetic rats: Relation to severity of diabetes. Acta Endocrinol (Copenh) 122:374–378
20. Flyvbjerg A, Frystyk J, Marshall SM (1990) Additive increase in kidney insulin-like growth factor I and initial renal enlargement in uninephrectomized-diabetic rats. Horm Metab Res 22:516–520
21. Marshall SM, Korsgaard L, Flyvbjerg A, Frystyk J, Ørskov H (1990) Renal insulin-like growth factor I binding in experimental diabetes (abstract). Diabetologia 33:A148
22. Lajara R, Rotwein P, Bortz JD, Hansen VA, Sadow JL, Betts CR, Rogers SA, Hammerman MR (1989) Dual regulation of insulin-like growth factor I expression during renal hypertrophy. Am J Physiol 257:F252–F261
23. Bach LA, Jerums G (1990) Effect of puberty on initial kidney growth and rise in kidney IGF-I in diabetic rats. Diabetes 39:557–562
24. Broulik PD, Schreiber V (1982) Effect of alloxan diabetes on kidney growth in intact and castrated mice. Acta Endocrinol (Copenh) 99:109–111
25. Craven PA, Caines MA, DeRubertis FR (1987) Sequential alterations in glomerular prostaglandin and thromboxane synthesis in diabetic rats: Relationship to the hyperfiltration of early diabetes. Metabolism 36:95–103
26. Levine L, Xiao D, Fujiki D (1986) Comparisons of polytoxin or 12-O-tetradecanoylphorbol-13-acetate and recombinant human insulin-like growth factor I or insulin synergistically stimulates prostaglandin production in cultured rat liver cells and squirrel monkey aorta smooth muscle cells. Prostaglandins 31:669–681
27. Flyvbjerg A, Marshall SM, Frystyk J, Hansen KW, Østerby R, Harris AG, Ørskov H (1990) Six months Sandostatin treatment in diabetic rats: Effects on kidney growth and urinary albumin excretion (abstract). Diabetologia 33:A65

Renal Pathology in Insulin Dependent (IDDM) and Noninsulin Dependent Diabetes Mellitus (NIDDM)

Pascale H. Lane, S. Michael Mauer[1], and Michael W. Steffes[2]

Summary. Much has been learned in the last decade regarding the pathology of the kidney in insulin-dependent diabetes mellitus (IDDM) and noninsulin-dependent diabetes mellitus (NIDDM). The major pathologic changes of diabetes include thickening of all renal extracellular basement membranes and mesangial matrix, and mesangial cell expansion. Although much less is known regarding renal pathology in NIDDM compared to IDDM, most proteinuric patients with NIDDM have typical diabetic nephropathy while approximately 25% have another form of renal disease. Two renal lesions appear critical in diabetic nephropathy. Mesangial expansion out of proportion to the size of the glomerulus is closely and inversely related to measures of peripheral capillary wall filtration surface; this expansion is also closely related to clinical features of proteinuria, hypertension, and declining glomerular filtration rate (GFR). Arteriolar hyalinosis is related to global glomerulosclerosis and both are correlated with the clinical features of nephropathy. Renal extracellular basement membrane and matrix expansion appears to be secondary to increased production or decreased turnover, or both, of normal structural constituents of the kidney. Microalbuminuria in the "predictive range" is frequently accompanied by rising blood pressure and/or falling GFR and is associated with well-established structural lesions. Thus, microalbuminuria is a marker of quite advanced diabetic nephropathology. Further natural history studies of variables which might influence the rate of development of the earlier lesions of diabetic nephropathy are critical to our understanding of this important disorder.

Introduction

Diabetic nephropathy represents the single most important cause of renal failure in adults in the Western world, causing 25% of all new cases of uremia [1]. The peak

[1]Department of Pediatrics and [2]Department of Laboratory Medicine and Pathology, University of Minnesota, Minneapolis, MN 55455, USA

incidence for the development of clinical renal disease occurs after about 16 years of diabetes but does not reach zero even after 40 years of insulin-dependent diabetes mellitus (IDDM) [2]. Overall, approximately 35%–45% of patients with longstanding IDDM will ultimately develop nephropathy, defined as dipstick-positive proteinuria, hypertension, and falling GFR [2]. It has been recently shown that it is the IDDM patients with nephropathy who manifest virtually all of the increased mortality associated with type I diabetes [2], while those who escape nephropathy have a mortality rate which is little different from that of the background population [2]. Although it is commonly thought that nephropathy is more common in IDDM patients [3] more recent studies of diabetic Pima Indians suggest that the cumulative risk of nephropathy in these NIDDM patients is at least as high as in IDDM patients [4]. Perhaps these younger NIDDM Pima patients live long enough to manifest diabetic nephropathy while older age NIDDM patients more frequently die of other causes before nephropathy becomes clinically apparent.

General Pathological Findings in Diabetic Nephropathy

The glomerulus seems to be normal at the onset of IDDM, as shown by the early pioneering work of Østerby [5] and confirmed by our studies of identical twins discordant for IDDM [6]. In the latter studies the nondiabetic twins, presumably identical to their IDDM twins but for the presence of diabetes, all had normal glomerular structure. This indicated that the diabetic state is a necessary prerequisite for diabetic glomerulopathy to be expressed. Osterby demonstrated that glomerular basement membrane (GBM) thickening can be detected two years after onset of IDDM; mesangial expansion can be quantitated after 5 years of diabetes [5]. Ultimately, in those developing serious renal disease, the dominant pathologic process becomes that of diffuse mesangial expansion [7–9]. The Kimmelstiel-Wilson nodular lesion is the most marked pathologic expression of diabetic mesangial expansion. While specific for diabetes, only a minority of patients progressing to overt diabetic nephropathy have nodular glomerulosclerosis [10].

Other lesions commonly seen in the kidney of patients with type I diabetes include hyaline degenerative changes in the afferent and efferent glomerular arterioles, and exudative hyaline lesions (fibrin cap) in the subendothelial space and under the parietal layer of the epithelium along Bowman's capsule (capsular drop) [10]. The hyaline lesions in the glomerular arterioles may be early changes in the kidney in IDDM and may be important in promoting glomerular scarring (R.D. Harris et al., unpublished data). Capillary loops may develop microaneurysms. These microaneurysms may be the forerunners of Kimmelstiel-Wilson nodules [11]. Epithelial and endothelial cell structure are generally well preserved until late in the course of nephropathy [12,13]. Interstitial fibrosis [14] and tubular changes may also be seen as the disease progresses [6,15,16].

Much less work has been done on the description of the pathology of the kidney in NIDDM compared to work done in IDDM. Schmitz et al. have performed light microscopy studies indicating that mesangial expansion occurs in NIDDM patients [17]. However, detailed electron microscopic morphometric studies in these patients are lacking. It is also important to note that more than 25% of NIDDM patients with proteinuria may have a renal disease other than diabetic nephropathy [18]; while in our experience this occurs in fewer than 5% of proteinuric IDDM patients (unpublished data). Thus, it is not safe to assume that NIDDM patients with clinical renal disease have this on the basis of diabetic nephropathology. Studies indicate that the direct relationships between glycemic control and the risk of diabetic nephropathy known to be present in IDDM [19] hold for NIDDM (FC Goetz, unpublished data). Thus, the severity of the lesions of diabetic nephropathy, assessed by light microscopy studies from kidneys obtained at autopsy in NIDDM patients, were closely predicted by the level of the blood sugar at the time of diagnosis, as well as by the summed glucose values obtained during glucose tolerance testing, in these NIDDM patients (GC Goetz, unpublished data).

Accurate stereologic techniques have allowed quantitation of the structural changes of diabetic nephropathy [20,21]. This has facilitated correlation of these changes with renal function.

Structural-Functional Relationships in Diabetic Nephropathy

Glomerular Basement Membrane

Measurements of GBM width, using the orthogonal intercept method [20], demonstrate thickening in almost all long-standing IDDM patients [5,7]. This thickening, measurable after two years of diabetes [5,22], is generally uniform both within and between glomeruli. The nature of this thickening is not completely understood, but it primarily involves the lamina densa. Immunofluorescent studies by Falk et al. [23] have shown increased staining for normal GBM and tubular basement membrane (TBM), and mesangial matrix constituents, suggesting that increased production or decreased turnover, or both, result in the accumulation of renal extracellular matrix materials. Also, there is increased localization of plasma proteins in GBM as well as in other renal extracellular membranes in diabetes, including the tubular basement membrane (TBM) and Bowman's capsule; this is detectable by immunofluorescence microscopy [24,25]. There is evidence suggesting that this increased localization is related to the charge of the circulating molecules, since anionic proteins bind preferentially [26]. However, this binding is relatively irreversible, requiring harsh treatment with collagenase or acids to release the bound protein, so charge alone is unlikely to explain the phenomenon [25].

The width of the GBM correlates poorly with mesangial volume fraction and with the functional parameters of glomerular filtration rate (GFR) and hypertension [7]. However, there is a weak correlation of GBM width with urinary albumin excretion (UAE). Increased GBM width is a sensitive marker of the diabetic state [5,10,22]. In seven pairs of identical twins discordant for IDDM, only diabetic twins showed GMB thickening, demonstrating that the diabetic state is a prerequisite for expression of this abnormality [6]. The width of the TBM is also increased in IDDM patients [6]. This latter fact suggests that pressure and flows in the glomerular capillaries, normally much higher than those present in other capillaries, are not prerequisites for the development of renal extracellular basement membrane thickening in IDDM.

Mesangium

Shortly after the onset of IDDM the fraction of the glomerular tuft occupied by mesangium is normal, with roughly equal proportions of cells and matrix. After two to three years, matrix begins to accumulate [13,27], and mesangial expansion, out of proportion to any increase in glomerular volume (increased mesangial volume fraction or VvMes), may become quite marked after many years of diabetes [7,28]. Approximately two-thirds of this mesangial expansion is due to matrix accumulation, and the mesangium contains increased amounts of the usual matrix antigens [23], including smooth muscle antigens [29]. One-third of this mesangial expansion is due to cellular expansion. It is unclear if mesangial cell number is increased in the later stages of diabetic nephropathy, although the total number of cell nuclei per glomerulus is increased [28].

Mesangial expansion demonstrates important correlations with renal function in diabetic nephropathy [7]. There is a strong inverse correlation between mesangial volume fraction and GFR. This probably results from the expanding mesangium compromising the structure of contiguous glomerular capillaries. Thus, fractional mesangial volume is precisely and inversely related to the peripheral capillary filtration surface density [7]. This suggests that as the relative volume of the glomerulus occupied by mesangium increases, the relative peripheral capillary wall available for filtration decreases. Stronger support of this concept comes from the work of Ellis et al. [30], which is confirmed by the work of Østerby et al. [31], who showed that filtration surface per glomerulus is directly related to GFR.

Virtually all patients with marked mesangial expansion (specifically, a mesangial volume fraction >37%) have had more than 400 mg of albumin in their urine per 24 hours; all patients in this earlier study had hypertension [7]. Thus, severe mesangial expansion is closely associated with all of the manifestations of overt nephropathy: decreased GFR, proteinuria, and hypertension. More recent studies (unpublished data) indicate that about 20% of patients with overt nephropathy and marked mesangial expansion do not have hypertension. Further, hypertension can occur in IDDM patients with lesser degrees of mesangial expansion. When hypertension is present in a patient with IDDM, this is almost always associated with increased UAE and well-established glomerular lesions. Thus, in our experience, hypertension, without other features of overt diabetic nephropathy, is distinctly uncommon in IDDM patients (unpublished data).

It is important to discuss the relationships of microalbuminuria to the structural lesions of diabetic nephropathy. Using mesangial expansion as the key structural parameter [8], it was found that patients with longstanding IDDM and entirely normal renal function, as indicated by normal UAE, GFR, and blood pressure, have mesangial volume fractions ranging from normal to levels bordering on those regularly associated with overt nephropathy [32]. Patients with microalbuminuria, normal GFR, and normal blood pressure (UAE usually <45 mg/24 hours or 30 μg/minute) have mesangial volume fractions completely overlapping with those whose renal function is entirely normal [32]. Those IDDM patients with microalbuminuria, hypertension, and/or decreased GFR (UAE usually >45 mg/24 hours) have more advanced mesangial expansion [32]. Thus, normal UAE does not preclude the presence of important lesions, while microalbuminuria does not necessarily predict structural abnormalities. However, if other manifestations of overt nephropathy are present, then microalbuminuria indicates more advanced structural injury. In other words, microalbuminuria in the range regularly "predictive" of the later development of proteinuria is, in fact, a marker of well-established diabetic glomerulopathy.

Glomerular Arterioles

Hyaline changes, which can involve both the afferent and efferent glomerular arterioles, range in severity from the presence of small amounts of (PAS) positive translucent material under the elastic membrane of the arterioles to virtually complete replacement of the smooth muscle of the vessels by this material. Hyaline in these vessel walls, along the parietal layer of Bowman's capsule (capsular drop), and in the glomerular subendothelial space (fibrin cap) all appears to contain the same materials; immunoglobulins, fibrinogen, and complement, as well as other plasma proteins [37]. The pathogenesis of these lesions is unknown. We have recently found that the more advanced glomerular arteriolar lesions, defined as complete replacement of smooth muscle cells by hyaline, are directly correlated with greater numbers of globally sclerotic glomeruli [11]. This suggests that glomerular sclerosis in diabetic nephropathy may derive, in part, from vascular pathology. An additional mechanism of glomerular sclerosis in diabetes may be extreme mesangial expansion with consequent capillary closure [28].

Epithelial Cells

The epithelial cells in diabetic patients contain large numbers of mitochondria and ribosomes, extensive endoplasmic reticula and prominent Golgi apparatuses, these cells retain normal structure until overt proteinuria develops [12,13]. These findings could reflect an increased GBM synthetic activity, biochemical evidence for which has been presented [34]. Only in the later stages of diabetic nephropathy has measurable foot process expansion been observed [12], and we have also noted a parallel loss in filtration slit length density [35]. These changes occur in association with increased levels of UAE and suggest that these epithelial cell changes may be the consequence of the breakdown of the glomerular permselectivity barrier which develops as the disease enters its terminal stages consequent to decreased available filtration surface.

Endothelial Cells

Endothelial cell structure also appears to be well preserved in diabetic nephropathy in man, although in advanced stages with capillary closure and massive mesangial expansion, atrophic appearances have been described [36]. Scanning electron microscopy in alloxan diabetic rats has revealed subtle alterations in endothelial cell fenestrae [37]. To our knowledge, similar studies have not been reported in diabetic man.

Interstitium

Interstitial fibrosis is a concomitant of diabetic nephropathy. Bader et al. [14] have shown that there is an inverse relationship between morphometric measures of the severity of interstitial fibrosis and GFR. In our studies of structural-functional relationships [7] we found that mesangial expansion and expansion of the interstitium were covariables predicting GFR, but that the correlation was stronger with measures of the mesangium; interstitial measures did not improve the correlation of mesangium with GFR. Interstitial fibrosis correlated with mesangial expansion. Thus, in our view, interstitial expansion correlates with glomerular function through correlations with mesangial changes, but the mesangial changes are more likely to be the major cause of the glomerular dysfunction. However, the interstitial fibrosis which develops in relation to nephron death may be important in contributing to the pathologic process which characterize the end stage kidney.

Tubules

The Armanni-Ebstein lesion represents the accumulation of PAS positive glycogen in the epithelial cells of the loop of Henle, and in the distal convoluted tubule and collecting duct; this lesion occurs as a concomitant of poor glycemic control [38]. The thick ascending limb of the loop of Henle shows the most pronounced lesions. This is the location of the macula densa, which demonstrates other structural abnormalities as well [38]. Spaces between the macula densa cells show altered size and geometry; the basal contact area between these cells and the juxtaglomerular apparatus is increased by 38% in diabetic animals compared to controls. This area of the nephron is important in regulating glomerular blood flow and GFR via tubuloglomerular feedback. Thus, these abnormalities may play a role in hyperfiltration and other alterations of renal function [38].

A layered thickening and splitting of the tubular basement membrane and Bowman's capsule has been described [15,16]. As noted above, we have found that increases in tubular basement membrane width paralleled those observed in GBM and mesangium [6].

Glomerular Structure and Loss of Renal Function

It is our hypothesis that decreasing filtration surface is "viewed" by the kidney as would be a decrease in renal mass. This pathologic change, we suggest, stimulates adaptive hemodynamic responses [39] and, perhaps, other forces [40,41], resulting in disruption of permselectivity and production of proteinuria and the development of hypertension. This hypothesis argues that once the lesions of diabetes produce clinically detectable renal dysfunction, then the forces propelling the kidney toward its ultimate destruction become largely independent of the diabetic state and become similar to those of advanced renal injury in general.

Filtration surface is ultimately determined by the filtration area per glomerulus and by the number of glomeruli. Filtration area per glomerulus is inversely proportional to the fractional mesangial volume [7,30]. As the mesangium expands and occupies a greater proportion of the glomerular tuft, the capillary volume must decrease unless accompanied by expansion of the entire glomerular volume. If accumulation of mesangial material exceeds the ability of the glomerulus to hypertrophy, the capillary loops will ultimately close, resulting in a completely obliterated glomerulus. Thus, mesangial expansion may decrease functioning filtration surface, both by decreasing the surface per glomerulus and by decreasing the number of functioning glomeruli.

Glomerular numbers may be decreased by other mechanisms as well. Horlych et al. [42] demonstrated a nonrandom distribution of sclerotic glomeruli in a plane perpendicular to the surface of the kidney and, therefore, along the course of the interlobular arteries. As already mentioned, advanced glomerular arteriolar lesions are correlated with global glomerular sclerosis. Thus, vascular lesions may lead to a loss of functioning glomeruli.

Overt diabetic nephropathy progresses inexorably to uremia. Evidence that this stage is associated with advanced structural lesions is neither surprising nor helpful. No functional tests prior to this stage accurately indicate the severity of the underlying renal pathology. In patients with normal albumin excretion or microalbuminuria without hypertension or reduced GFR, we found no correlations between GBM thickness, mesangial volume fraction, or peripheral capillary filtration surface density and levels of UAE [32]. In fact, it is our view that microalbuminuria gains in strength as a "predictor" or serious diabetic renal disease primarily when associated with hypertension and/or with early reduction in GFR, that is, as one manifestation of already established, albeit subtle, clinical diabetic nephropathy [6,32].

Conclusions

There have been substantial advances in our understanding of diabetic nephropathy through the study of renal structure and function in diabetic patients. It is becoming clearer that the important processes driving the kidney toward its functional demise are matrix accumulation, which occurs in the mesangium, in other renal extracellular membranes, and in the interstitium, and hyaline changes, which occur in the glomerular arterioles. It is also clear that functional studies are not indicative of underlying renal pathology, except relatively late in the pathologic evolution when glomerular injury is already quite far advanced. Only carefully designed, quantitative, prospective studies of renal pathology, beginning early in the course of type I diabetes, can further clarify the relationship of structure and function with a variety of risk factors in the nephropathy of IDDM and NIDDM patients.

Acknowledgments. Supported in part by NIH grants AM13083 and AM20742 and by the Juvenile Diabetes Foundation International.

References

1. Rao TKS, Hirsh S, Avram MM, et al. (1980) Prevalence of diabetic nephropathy in Brooklyn. In: Friedman EA, L'Esperance FA Jr (eds) Diabetic renal-retinal syndrome. Grune and Strattan, New York, pp 205–207
2. Christiansen JS, Anderson AR, Koch Anderson J, et al. (1985) The natural history of diabetic nephropathy. Diabetic Nephro 4:104–106
3. Herman WT, Teutsch SM (1986) Renal disorders associated with diabetes mellitus. In: Friedman EA, L'Esperance FA Jr (eds) Diabetic renal-retinal syndrome. Grune and Stratton, New York, pp 9–52

4. Knowler WC, Kungelman CL (1988) Population comparisons of the frequency of diabetic nephropathy. In: Mogensen CE (ed) The kidney and hypertension in diabetes mellitus. Martinus Nijhoff, Boston, pp 25–32
5. Østerby R (1975) Early phases in the development of diabetic glomerulosclerosis. Acta Med Scand 574(Suppl 1):1–80
6. Steffes MW, Sutherland DER, Goetz FC, Rich SS, Mauer SM (1985) Studies of kidney and muscle biopsy specimens from identical twins discordant for type I diabetes mellitus. N Engl J Med 312:1282–1287
7. Mauer SM, Steffes MW, Ellis EN, Sutherland DER, Brown DM, Goetz FC (1984) Structural-functional relationships in diabetic nephropathy. J Clin Invest 74:1143–1155
8. Steffes MW, Østerby R, Chavers B, Mauer SM (1989) Mesangial expansion as a central mechanism for loss of kidney function in diabetic patients. Diabetes 38:1077–1081
9. Gellmann DD, Pirani CL, Soothill JF, et al. (1959) Structure and function in diabetic nephropathy. The importance of diffuse glomerulosclerosis. Diabetes 8:251–256
10. Mauer SM, Steffes MW, Brown DM (1981) The kidney in diabetes. Am J Med 70:603–612
11. Saito Y, Kida H, Takeda S, et al. (1988) Mesangiolysis in diabetic glomeruli: Its role in the formation of nodular lesions. Kidney Int 34:389–396
12. Farquhar MG, Hopper J, Moon HD (1959) Diabetic glomerulosclerosis: Electron and light microscopic studies. Am J Pathol 35:721–753
13. Østerby R (1972) The number of glomerular cells and substructures in early juvenile diabetes. Acta Pathol Microbiol Immunol Scand [A] 80:785–800
14. Bader R, Bader H, Grund KE, et al. (1980) Structure and function of the kidney in diabetic glomerulosclerosis: Correlations between morphologic and functional parameters. Pathol Res Pract 167:204–216
15. Sabour MS, MacDonald MK, Robson JS (1962) An electron microscopic study of the human kidney in young diabetic patients with normal renal function. Diabetes 11:291–295
16. Churg J, Dachs S (1966) Diabetic renal disease: Arteriosclerosis and glomerulosclerosis. Pathol Annu 1:148–171
17. Schmitz A, Gundersen HJG, Østerby R (1988) Glomerular morphology by light microscopy in non-insulin dependent diabetes—lack of glomerular hypertrophy. Diabetes 37:38–43
18. Parving H-H, Gall M-A, Skott P, Jorgensen HE, Jorgensen F, Larsen S (1990) Prevalence and causes of albuminuria in non-insulin dependent diabetic (NIDDM) patients. Kidney Int 37:243A
19. Krolewski AS, Warram JH, Christlieb AR, Busick EJ, Kahn CR (1985) The changing natural history of diabetic nephropathy. Am J Med 78:785–794
20. Jensen EB, Gundersen HJG, Østerby R (1979) Determination of membrane thickness distribution from orthogonal intercepts. J Microsc 115:19–33
21. Weiber ER (1979) Stereological methods: Practical methods for biological morphometry. Academic, London
22. Østerby R (1972) Morphometric studies of the peripheral glomerular basement membrane in early juvenile diabetes. II. Development of initial basement membrane thickening. Diabetologia 8:84–92
23. Falk RJ, Scheinman JI, Mauer SM, Michael AF (1983) Polyantigenic expansion of basement membrane constituents in diabetic nephropathy. Diabetes 32:34–39
24. Miller K, Michael AF (1976) Immunopathology of renal extracellular membranes in diabetes mellitus. Specificity of tubular basement membrane immunofluorescence. Diabetes 25:701–708
25. Michael AF, Brown D (1981) Increased concentration of albumin in kidney basement membranes in diabetes mellitus. Diabetes 30:843–846
26. Melvin T, Kim Y, Michael AF (1984) Selective binding of IgG4 and other negatively charged plasma proteins in normal and diabetic human kidneys. Am J Pathol 115:443–446

27. Østerby R (1973) A quantitative electron microscopic study of mesangial regions in glomeruli from patients with short-term juvenile diabetes mellitus. Lab Invest 29:99–110
28. Gundersen HJG, Østerby R (1977) Glomerular size and structure in diabetes mellitus. II. Late abnormalities. Diabetologia 13:43–48
29. Scheinman JF, Fish AJ, Michael AF (1974) The immunohistopathology of glomerular antigens: The GBM, collagen, and actomyosin antigens in normal and diseased kidneys. J Clin Invest 54:1144–1154
30. Ellis EN, Steffes MW, Goetz FC, Sutherland DER, Mauer SM (1986) Glomerular filtration surface in type I diabetes mellitus. Kidney Int 29:889–894
31. Østerby R, Parving H-H, Nyberg G, et al. (1988) A strong correlation between glomerular filtration rate and filtration surface in diabetic nephropathy. Diabetologia 31:265–270
32. Chavers BM, Bilous RW, Ellis EN, Steffes MW, Mauer SM (1989) Glomerular lesions and urinary albumin excretion in type I diabetes without overt proteinuria. N Engl J Med 320:966–970
33. Burkholder PM (1965) Immunohistopathologic study of localized plasma protein and fixation guinea pig complement in renal lesions of diabetic glomerulosclerosis. Diabetes 14:755–770
34. Walker F (1972) The origin, turnover, and removal of glomerular basement membrane. J Pathol 110:233–244
35. Elllis EN, Steffes MW, Chavers BM, et al. (1986) Foot process width (FP) and filtration slit (FS) length in diabetes mellitus (DM) (abstract). Kidney Int 29:273
36. Huang TW (1980) The nature of the basal lamina alterations in human diabetic glomerulosclerosis. Am J Pathol 100:225–238
37. Evan AP, Luft FC (1980) Effect of alloxan-induced diabetes on the glomerular filtration barrier of the rat. Renal Physiol 3:257–264
38. Rasch R (1988) Nonglomerular lesions in the diabetic kidney. In: Davison AM (ed) Nephrology: Proceedings of the Xth international congress of nephrology. Bailliere Tindall, London, pp 744–757
39. Hostetter TH, Olson JL, Rennke HG, et al. (1981) Hyperfiltration in remnant nephrons: A potentially adverse response to renal ablation. Am J Physiol 241:F85–F93
40. Klahr S, Schreiner G, Ichikawa I (1988) The progression of renal disease. N Engl J Med 318:1657–1666
41. Keane WF, Kasiske BL, O'Donnell MP (1988) Lipids and progressive glomerulosclerosis. Am J Nephrol 8:261–271
42. Horlyck A, Gundersen HJG, Østerby R (1986) The cortical distribution pattern of diabetic glomerulopathy. Diabetologia 29:146–150

The Proteinuric Phase of Diabetic Nephrology

Timothy W. Meyer[1]

Summary. In normal humans, very little protein is lost in the urine because the glomerular capillary wall imposes an efficient barrier to passage of macromolecules, excluding them from Bowman's space on the basis of both size and charge. Indeed, despite having an extraordinarily high permeability to water, the glomerular capillary wall, comprised of the fenestrated endothelial cells, basement membrane, and visceral epithelial cells with interdigitating podocytes, has a permeability to macromolecules which is among the lowest in the circulation. Leakiness of the glomerular capillary wall to proteins is the first sign of glomerular injury in diabetes and a reliable predictor of eventual renal failure in this disorder. Recent studies suggest, moreover, that antihypertensive therapies which reduce proteinuria will retard the progression of diabetic renal disease. This observation has provided a strong impetus to identify the mechanisms responsible for proteinuria in diabetic renal disease.

The Permeability of the Normal Glomerular Capillary Wall to Macromolecules

In order to discuss the mechanisms responsible for proteinuria in diabetic renal disease, it is necessary first to review current concepts of glomerular permeability to macromolecules. The principal basis on which the glomerular capillary wall excludes macromolecules from Bowman's space is *molecular size*. Molecules the size of inulin or smaller permeate the capillary wall as freely as water, but permeability decreases progressively with size for larger molecules, becoming very low as size nears that of serum albumin. Two methods have been employed to assess the size-selective properties of the glomerular capillary wall. The first method requires analysis of fluid samples collected from Bowman's space by micropuncture in

[1]Nephrology Division, Palo Alto Veterans Administration Medical Center, Palo Alto, CA 94304, USA

animals. The Bowman's space to plasma concentration ratio for a given protein then provides the fractional filtration or "sieving coefficient" (Θ) for that protein. The second method is based on measurement of the urinary clearance rates for intravenously infused test macromolecules [1]. This method avoids the difficulties encountered in analysis of small amounts of protein in tubule fluid samples, and can, moreover, be employed in human studies. The fractional clearance of a test macromolecule (M) is defined as the clearance of M divided by the glomerular filtration rate (GFR). When inulin is used to measure the GFR, the fractional clearance of a test macromolecule can be expressed as:

$$\text{Fractional clearance of M} = (U/P)_M/(U/P)_{In}$$

where $(U/P)_M$ and $(U/P)_{In}$ are the urine-to-plasma concentration ratios for the macromolecule M and for inulin. If, like inulin, the test macromolecule is neither reabsorbed nor secreted by the tubules, its fractional clearance will be equal to its fractional filtration by the glomerulus:

$$\text{Fractional clearance of M} = \Theta_M$$

The test substances most frequently employed to probe glomerular permeability to macromolecules have been the non-protein polymers dextran and polyvinylpyrrolidone [1]. These substances are available in a broad range of molecular sizes, appear not to be secreted or reabsorbed by renal tubules, and can be infused into humans. Results of studies in which dextran was used to assess the size-selectivity of the glomerular capillary wall are shown in Fig. 1. In these studies, dextran 40 was infused into 15 normal human volunteers [2,3]. Values for dextran fractional clearance (which are the same as values for the sieving coefficient, Θ) are plotted as a function of the Einstein-Stokes radii of the dextran molecules. A value of 1.0 on the y-axis represents equality of dextran and inulin clearances and indicates no measurable restriction to transport of dextran across the glomerular capillary wall when molecular radius is 20 Å or less. With increasing size, however, dextrans are progressively restricted, as indicated by a rapidly declining value for Θ. As indicated in Fig. 1, fractional clearances approach zero, indicating dextran impermeance in normal humans, when dextran radius exceeds 60 Å.

Theoretical studies employing mathematical models of solute transport through porous structures have shown that the size-selective properties of normal glomeruli, as exemplified in Fig. 1, can be accounted for by assuming that the glomerular capillary wall is permeated by numerous cylindrical pores with radius (r_o) ~55 Å [1–3]. It should be emphasized that structures of this size cannot be clearly distinguished even by the most sophisticated microscopic techniques, and that uniform cylindrical pores may not be a real feature of the glomerular capillary wall. Nevertheless, the assumption that the capillary wall is permeated by uniform pores accounts, with remarkable accuracy, for the dextran clearance profiles obtained in normal humans and animals. Theoretical analysis of dextran sieving curves based on this assumption thus provides a means to describe changes in glomerular size-selectivity associated with glomerular disease.

In addition to size, the glomerular capillary wall also excludes macromolecules from Bowman's space on the basis of *molecular charge*. The charge-selective proper-

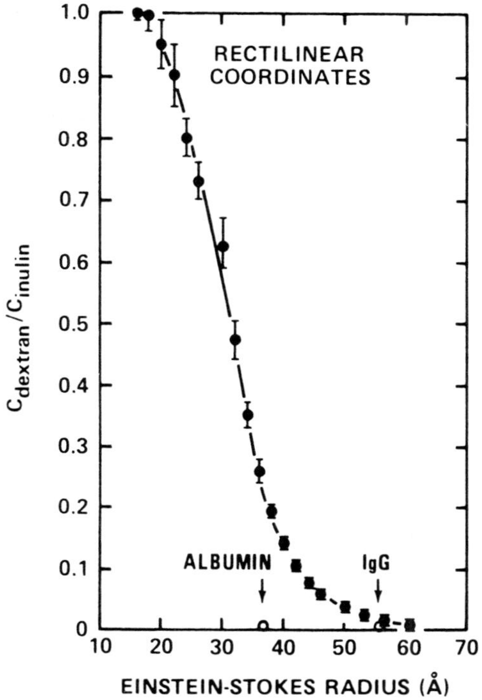

Fig. 1. The fractional dextran clearance profile of the normal glomerular capillary wall as determined in 15 healthy adult volunteers. Fractional dextran clearances are plotted as a function of the Einstein-Stokes radius of the dextran. The *vertical bars* represent 1 SEM. Data for albumin and IgG are illustrated for comparison. (Courtesy of B.D. Myers)

ties of the glomerular capillary wall have been most clearly demonstrated in animals, in which the clearances of charged and neutral test macromolecules can be directly compared. Bohrer et al. [4] showed that in normal rats the clearance of anionic dextran sulfate molecules is 10–50-fold lower than the clearance of neutral dextran molecules over the size range 26–42 Å. Further studies have shown that the capillary wall loses its ability to discriminate against anionic dextrans in rats with glomerular disease [5,6]. These results can be explained on the assumption that the normal glomerular capillary wall carries a fixed negative charge which is reduced by glomerular disease [7]. Presumably the glomerular capillary wall discriminates against anionic macromolecules in humans as it does it rats. Moreover, it is widely assumed that loss of capillary wall anionic charge contributes to proteinuria in human as well as in experimental glomerular disease. Because charged test macromolecules have not been available for human use, however, the contribution of reduced capillary wall charge to proteinuria in humans has not been quantified.

In addition to being determined by the intrinsic properties of the glomerular capillary wall, including size- and charge-selectivity, the glomerular filtration of macromolecules is determined by the *hemodynamic factors* which govern the GFR [2].

Thus proteinuria can be altered by hemodynamic events, such as changes in volume status or blood pressure, independent of any changes in capillary wall structure. The influence on macromolecule filtration of glomerular hemodynamic factors, which include the glomerular plasma flow rate, transcapillary hydraulic pressure, and the arterial plasma protein concentration, is complex and difficult to predict. In general, maneuvers which increase the filtration fraction while GFR remains constant may be expected to increase the glomerular filtration of macromolecules the size of albumin.

The Development of Proteinuria in Diabetic Renal Disease

Early "Functional" Proteinuria

During the first decade of diabetes, values for urinary albumin excretion rate (UAE) usually remain normal, averaging <10 mg/day. There are, however, at least two circumstances in which transient increases in UAE may be observed in patients with early diabetes. First, elevation of UAE may be observed during episodes of poor metabolic control [8]. Values for UAE in this setting usually remain <50 mg/day, but higher values have sometimes been recorded. Second, exercise may increase UAE to values as high as 500 mg/day in diabetic patients whose resting values for UAE are normal [9]. The mechanism(s) by which poor metabolic control and exercise increase filtration of albumin in diabetic patients have not been fully characterized. Poor metabolic control has been shown to increase the albumin excreting rate in patients with diabetes of only a few months duration, in whom defects in glomerular capillary wall structure presumably have not yet developed [8]. Albumin excretion rates are rapidly reduced following improvement in metabolic control and cessation of exercise, further suggesting that increased albumin filtration in these circumstances cannot be attributed to fixed defects in glomerular size- or charge-selectivity [8,9]. It thus seems likely that alterations in glomerular hemodynamic function cause transient increases in glomerular filtration of macromolecules early in the course of diabetes.

In patients with diabetes of several years duration, transient increases in UAE may result from the combination of altered glomerular hemodynamic function with early changes in glomerular capillary wall structure. In such patients, exercise may serve as a provocative test to reveal abnormalities in glomerular barrier function which are not apparent at rest [9]. It is not yet known, however, whether exercise-induced albuminuria, like resting "microalbuminuria," predicts development of clinical nephropathy in diabetes. At present, physicians should be aware of the effects of exercise and poor metabolic control on albumin filtration, chiefly in order to avoid over-interpretation of elevated values for UAE. As described by Viberti in this symposium, the diagnosis of "microalbuminuria" should be made only when urine specimens have been collected under well defined conditions, and should preferably be based on analysis of more than one urine sample.

Microalbuminuria

In clinical practice, the diagnosis of diabetic nephropathy has usually been established by the finding of "dipstick positive" proteinuria, representing an albumin excretion rate of approximately 500 mg/day. Recent studies, however, have emphasized the value of identifying patients with "microalbuminuria," usually defined as having albumin excretion rates in the range of 30–300 mg/day. Long term studies have shown that albumin excretion in such patients increases over several years to rates in excess of 500 mg/day. Development of this "clinical" level of albuminuria in turn reliably predicts the ultimate loss of kidney function in diabetic patients. The small defect in glomerular barrier function which causes "microalbuminuria" must therefore be regarded as the first sign of a pathological process which leads inexorably to renal failure.

The permselectivity defect(s) responsible for microalbuminuria have been difficult to identify because the macromolecule excretion rates, though abnormal, are still very low. It is important to note that excretion of proteins other than albumin is increased in patients with "microalbuminuria." Emphasis has been placed on albumin excretion because albumin is the predominant, and therefore the most easily measurable, protein in the urine as well as in the plasma. However, diabetic patients with values for UAE of 30–300 mg/day have been found also to exhibit increased excretion of IgG [10,11]. The finding of increased quantities of this large protein in the urine implies that a defect in glomerular size-selectivity contributes to proteinuria in patients with microalbuminuria. More rigorous proof that a defect in size selectivity contributes to early proteinuria in diabetes has been provided by a study showing that glomerular permeability to dextran molecules with radii of 50–60 Å is increased in type II diabetic patients with albumin excretion rates averaging <50 mg/day [12]. Given that a charge-selectivity defect accompanies the size-selectivity defect in diabetic patients with heavier proteinuria (see below), it seems likely that a charge-selectivity defect also accompanies the size-selectivity defect in diabetic patients with microalbuminuria. Attempts to identify a charge-selectivity defect early in the course of diabetic nephropathy, by comparing clearance values for IgG molecules with different isoelectric points, have yielded inconclusive results [11,13].

Clinical Proteinuria

The mechanisms responsible for proteinuria in diabetic patients with clinical nephropathy have been extensively investigated by Myers and coworkers [13–15]. These investigations have identified a size-selectivity defect, reflected by enhanced clearance of dextrans with radii of 50–60 Å, in diabetic patients with protein excretion which ranges from 300 mg/day to more than 10 g/day. To assess the magnitude of this size-selectivity defect, Myers and co-workers have employed a "heteroporous" model of the glomerular capillary wall [16]. The heteroporous model assumes that in injured, as in normal glomeruli, the major portion of the capillary wall is perforated by cylindrical pores of radius r_o. This model further assumes that a smaller portion of the capillary wall is permeated by "shunt" pores which are so large that they exhibit no size-selectivity. The portion of the capillary wall permeated by shunt pores denoted ω_o, as opposed to normal pores can be determined from dextran clearance profiles. Thus shunt parameter provides a quantitative measure of the magnitude of the size-selectivity defect in injured glomeruli.

Two important conclusions have so far emerged from the theoretical analysis of dextran clearance studies performed by Myers and co-workers in patients with diabetic renal disease [14,15]. First, these studies indicate that the magnitude of the "shunt" is sufficient to account for most of the protein excreted in the urine. Second, these studies have shown that the magnitude of the shunt increases as diabetic nephropathy advances. This latter finding has been most clearly demonstrated in a study in which dextran clearance studies were repeated at an interval of 24 months in ten patients with diabetic nephropathy [15]. During this interval, mean GFR decreased from 59 ± 9 to 34 ± 7 ml/min. Urinary excretion of albumin and IgG, however, did not change significantly. The finding that urinary protein excretion rates were maintained as the GFR fell clearly implies that fractional protein excretion rates increased over the course of the study. Dextran sieving studies revealed that this increase in fractional protein excretion was caused by a progressive impairment of glomerular size-selectivity, reflected by an increase in the shunt parameter ω_0 as renal disease advanced. It should be noted that, in patients with other glomerular diseases, proteinuria may also remain at high levels as GFR declines. Experimental studies suggest that these findings may reflect aggravation of glomerular barrier injury, associated with hypertrophy of remnant glomeruli when nephrons are lost in the setting of established nephrosis [17].

The heteroporous model of glomerular injury used by Myers and co-workers, though it provides a useful index of impaired size-selectivity, clearly provides an incomplete description of glomerular permeability to macromolecules in diabetic renal disease. If circulating macromolecules escaped injured glomeruli exclusively through a non-discriminatory shunt, the glomerular clearances of various proteins would be equal. Multiple studies have shown, however, that values for the fractional clearance of albumin are several-fold greater than values for the fractional clearance of IgG in patients with diabetic nephropathy [10,11,14,15]. The most likely explanation for this finding is that impairment of glomerular charge-selectivity accompanies impairment of glomerular size-selectivity in diabetic renal disease, so that glomerular permeability to albumin is increased relatively more than glomerular permeability to IgG. Studies employing charged test macromolecules have shown that charge-selectivity defects almost invariably accompany size-selectivity defects in animals with heavy proteinuria.

The Relation of Proteinuria to Altered Glomerular Structure in Diabetes

The structural changes responsible for increased glomerular permeability to proteins in diabetes remain largely unidentified. Research in this area has been hampered by limited access to renal tissue in diabetic humans and by difficulties in creating suitable animal models of diabetic renal disease.

Early morphologic studies identified *thickening of the basement membrane* as a regular feature of diabetic glomerular injury, and it was natural to assume that increased permeability to macromolecules might be caused by this change in glomerular capillary wall structure. Recent studies have shown, however, that urine albumin excretion rates are not correlated with glomerular basement membrane thickness in diabetic patients [18,19]. Marked basement membrane thickening has been observed in patients who have been diabetic for less than ten years and who have had albumin excretion rates only slightly above normal [19].

While proteinuria in diabetic renal disease cannot be attributed to glomerular basement membrane thickening per se, it may well be caused by associated changes in *basement membrane composition*. It has been suggested that glycosylation of basement membrane constituents increases the permeability of the basement membrane to macromolecules. This attractive hypothesis remains to be tested experimentally. Increased permeability of the glomerular capillary wall has also been attributed to altered synthesis of various basement membrane constituents. To date, the most extensively investigated of these basement membrane constituents has been *heparan sulfate proteoglycan* (HSPG). Because HSPG is highly anionic, it has been widely assumed that distribution of this substance within the glomerular basement membrane is largely responsible for maintenance of glomerular charge-selectivity. Functional studies have suggested that HSPG is also necessary for the maintenance of glomerular size-selectivity [20]. A relation between basement membrane HSPG content and albumin excretion rate, however, has not yet been demonstrated in diabetic animals or humans.

In addition to changes in basement membrane structure, proteinuria in diabetic renal disease may be related to changes in *epithelial cell structure*. As in other glomerular diseases, proteinuria in diabetic renal disease is associated with broadening and retraction of epithelial cell foot processes. Recent morphometric studies have demonstrated early broadening of epithelial cell foot processes in diabetic patients with albumin excretion rates of <1 g/day [21,22]. It is not known whether this change in epithelial cell structure represents a cause or a consequence of increased glomerular permeability to macromolecules.

Maneuvers which Reduce Proteinuria in Diabetic Renal Disease

The observation that proteinuria precedes loss of renal function in diabetic patients has led naturally to the assumption that maneuvers which reduce proteinuria will retard the progression of diabetic renal disease. Extensive clinical trials are required to establish the validity of this hypothesis. As described by Mauer in this symposium, morphometric studies suggest that the reduction of the GFR in diabetic nephrology is caused by progressive expansion of the glomerular mesangium. Since the mechanisms responsible for mesangial expansion may differ from those responsible for glomerular barrier dysfunction, it is not certain that all maneuvers which reduce proteinuria will prevent reduction of the GFR in diabetic patients.

Among therapies examined to date, *antihypertensive agents* have proven most effective in reducing proteinuria in patients with diabetic renal disease. Moreover, antihypertensive agents have the same effect on glomerular barrier function. Overall, studies to date suggest that albumin excretion rates are comparably reduced by regimens including converting enzyme inhibitors and beta adrenergic receptor blockers, while variable effects on albumin excretion rates have been observed with calcium channel antagonists.

The mechanisms by which antihypertensive agents improve glomerular barrier function in diabetic renal disease have not been fully elucidated. It has frequently been suggested that antihypertensive agents improve glomerular barrier function by lowering glomerular transcapillary hydraulic pressure, ΔP. A recent modification of this "hemodynamic" hypothesis suggests that antihypertensive agents improve

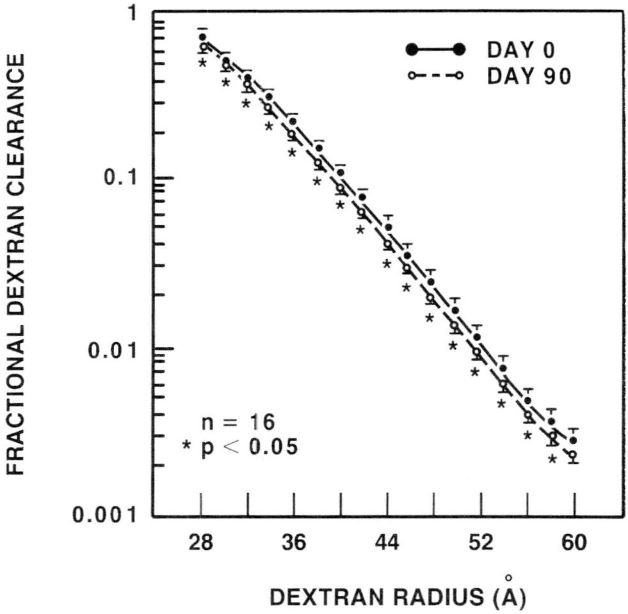

Fig. 2. The fractional dextran clearance profiles before (*day 0*) and after (*day 90*) converting enzyme inhibitor treatment in 16 diabetic patients with initial average proteinuria of 2.2 g/day. (From [26])

glomerular barrier function by reducing glomerular capillary wall tension, which is considered to be the product of ΔP and glomerular capillary radius. Studies in which converting enzyme inhibitor treatment was initiated at the outset of experimental diabetes are often cited in support of this hypothesis [25]. These studies have shown that continuous converting enzyme inhibitor treatment reduces ΔP and largely prevents development of albuminuria in diabetic rats. There is reason to question, however, whether lowering of capillary wall tension accounts for the beneficial effect of antihypertensive agents on glomerular barrier function in established diabetic nephropathy. A recent dextran clearance study suggests, alternatively, that converting enzyme inhibitor therapy may have a direct effect on glomerular capillary wall pore structure [26]. In this study, 16 diabetic patients with serum creatinine values < 2 mg/dl and proteinuria averaging 2.2 g/day were treated with a converting enzyme inhibitor for 90 days. Values for GFR remained stable during converting enzyme inhibitor treatment, while mean arterial pressure declined from 98 ± 3 to 92 ± 3 mmHg. As illustrated in Fig. 2, converting enzyme inhibitor treatment decreased fractional clearance values not only for large dextran molecules with radii of 50–60 Å, but also for dextran molecules with radii of 30–50 Å. This finding indicates that converting enzyme inhibitor therapy alters the structure of the capillary wall so as to shift the entire pore size distribution toward a lower value.

Other therapies which may reduce proteinuria in diabetic disease include *improved glycemic control* and *dietary protein restriction*. As described above, improved glycemic control has been shown to lower albumin excretion rates in patients with recent onset diabetes and poor initial glycemic control. The effect of rigorous glycemic control on albuminuria in patients with established diabetic renal disease is less well defined. Some, but not all, studies have shown that sustained normalization of blood glucose by insulin pump therapy reduces the albumin excretion rate in patients with microalbuminuria [27–29]. Viberti and coworkers [30] have shown, however, that long-term normalization of blood glucose neither reduces the protein excretion rate nor slows the progression of renal disease in diabetic patients with heavy proteinuria and reduction of the GFR. In contrast, dietary protein restriction has been shown to reduce the protein excretion rate in patients with established diabetic nephropathy [31].

Proteinuria in Type II Diabetes

Most of the studies described above have been performed in patients with type I diabetes. Available studies suggest, however, that the pattern of proteinuria is similar in type I and in type II diabetes [32–34]. One difference between the two conditions is that patients with type II diabetes may exhibit dipstick positive proteinuria at the time when diabetes is diagnosed [33,35,36]. Insulin resistance and hypertension may precipitate glomerular injury prior to development of overt hyperglycemia in these patients.

Acknowledgment. Supported by grants from the National Institutes of Health (DK35734) and the California Affiliate of the American Heart Association.

References

1. Deen WM, Bridges CR, Brenner BM (1983) Biophysical basis of glomerular permselectivity. J Membr Biol 71:1–10
2. Friedman S, Strober S, Field E, Silverman E, Myers BD (1984) Glomerular capillary wall function in human lupus nephritis. Am J Physiol 246 (Renal Fluid Electrolyte Physiol 15):F580–591
3. Shemesh O, Ross JC, Deen WM, Grant GW, Myers BD (1986) Nature of the glomerular capillary injury in human membranous glomerulopathy. J Clin Invest 77:868–877
4. Bohrer MP, Baylis C, Humes HD, Glassock RJ, Robertson CR, Brenner BM (1978) Permselectivity of the glomerular capillary wall: facilitated filtration of circulating polycations. J Clin Invest 61:72–78
5. Bohrer MP, Baylis C, Humes HD, Glassock RJ, Robertson CR, Brenner BM (1977) Mechanisms of the puromycin-induced defects in the transglomerular passage of water and macromolecules. J Clin Invest 60:152–161
6. Olson JL, Rennke HG, Venkatachalam MJ (1981) Alterations in the charge and size selectivity barrier of the glomerular filter in aminonucleoside nephrosis in rats. Lab Invest 4:271–279
7. Deen WM, Satvat B (1981) Determinants of the glomerular filtration of proteins. Am J Physiol 241 (Renal Fluid Electrolyte Physiol 10):F162–F170

8. Parving H-H, Noer I, Deckert T, Ervin PE, Nielsen SL, Lygsoe J, Mogensen CE (1976) The effect of metabolic regulation on microvascular permeability to small and large molecules in short-term juvenile diabetes. Diabetologia 12:161–166
9. Vittinghus E, Mogensen CE (1982) Graded exercise and protein excretion in diabetic man and the effect of insulin treatment. Kidney Int 21:725–729
10. Viberti G, Mackintosh D, Keen H (1983) Determinants of the penetration of proteins through the glomerular barrier in insulin-dependent diabetes mellitus. Diabetes 32(Suppl 2):92–95
11. Deckert T, Feldt-Rasmussen B, Djurup R, Deckert M (1988) Glomerular size and charge selectivity in insulin-dependent diabetes mellitus. Kidney Int 33:100–106
12. Loon N, Nelson R, Myers BD (1989) Glomerular barrier abnormality in new onset NIDDM in Pima Indians. Proceedings of the 22nd Annual Meeting of the American Society of Nephrology Washington, USA p 325A
13. Nakamura Y, Myers BD (1988) Charge selectivity of proteinuria in diabetic glomerulopathy. Diabetes 37:1202–1211
14. Friedman S, Jones HW III, Golbetz HV, Lee JA, Little HL, Myers BD (1983) Mechanisms of proteinuria in diabetic nephropathy II. Diabetes 32(Suppl 2):40–46
15. Tomlanovich S, Deen WM, Jones III HW, Schwartz HC, Myers BD (1987) Functional nature of glomerular injury in progressive diabetic glomerulopathy. Diabetes 36:556–565
16. Deen WM, Bridges CR, Brenner BM, Myers BD (1985) Heteroporous model of glomerular size selectivity: application to normal and nephrotic humans. Am J Physiol 249 (Renal Fluid Electrolyte Physiol 18):F374–F389
17. Meyer TW, Rennke HG (1988) Increased single-nephron protein excretion after renal ablation in nephrotic rats. Am J Physiol 255:F1243–F1248
18. Mauer SM, Steffes MW, Ellis EN, Sutherland DER, Brown DM, Goetz FC (1984) Structural-functional relationships in diabetic nephrology. J Clin Invest 74:1143–1155
19. Chavers BM, Bilous RW, Ellis EN, Steffes MW, Mauer SM (1989) Glomerular lesions and urinary albumin excretion in type I diabetes without overt proteinuria. N Engl J Med 320:966–970
20. Kanwar YS (1984) Biology of disease: Biophysiology of glomerular filtration and proteinuria. Lab Invest 51:7–21
21. Østerby R, Anderson AR, Gundersen HJ, Jorgensen HE, Mogensen CE, Parving HH (1984) Quantitative studies of glomerular ultrastructure in type I diabetics with incipient nephropathy. Diabetic Nephrol 3:95–100
22. Ellis EN, Steffes MW, Chavers B, Mauer SM (1987) Observations of glomerular epithelial cell structure in patients with type I diabetes mellitus. Kidney Int 32:736–741
23. Parving H-H, Andersen AR, Smidt UM, Hommel E, Mathiesen ER, Svendsen PA (1987) Effect of antihypertensive treatment on kidney function in diabetic nephropathy. Br Med J [Clin Res] 294:1443–1447
24. Parving H-H, Hommel E, Smidt UM (1988) Protection of kidney function and decrease in albuminuria by captopril in insulin dependent diabetics with nephropathy. Br Med J [Clin Res] 297:1086–1091
25. Zatz R, Dunn BR, Meyer TW, Anderson S, Rennke HG, Brenner BM (1986) Prevention of diabetic glomerulopathy by pharmacological amelioration of glomerular capillary hypertension. J Clin Invest 77:1925–1930
26. Morelli E, Loon N, Meyer TW, Peters W, Myers BD (to be published) Effects of converting enzyme inhibition on barrier function in diabetic glomerulopathy. Diabetes
27. Viberti GC, Pickup JC, Jarrett RJ, Keen H (1979) Effect of control of blood glucose on urinary albumin excretion and β_2-microglobulin in insulin-dependent diabetes. N Engl J Med 300:638–41
28. KROC Collaborative Study Group (1984) Blood glucose control and the evolution of

diabetic retinopathy and albuminuria: A preliminary multicenter trial. N Engl J Med 311:365–372
29. Feldt-Rasmussen B, Mathiesen ER, Hegedus L, Deckert T (1986) Kidney function during 12 months of strict metabolic control in insulin-dependent diabetic patients with incipient nephropathy. N Engl J Med 314:665–670
30. Viberti GC, Bilous RW, Mackintosh D, Bending JJ, Keen H (1983) Long-term correction of hyperglycemia and progression of renal failure in insulin dependent diabetes. Br Med J [Clin Res] 286:598–602
31. Anderson S (1990) Low protein diets and diabetic nephropathy. Semin Nephrol 10:287–293
32. Mogensen CE (1984) Microalbuminuria predicts clinical proteinuria and early mortality in maturity-onset diabetes. N Engl J Med 310:356–360
33. Ballard DJ, Humphrey LL, Melton III LJ, Frohnert PP, Chu C-P, O'Fallon WM, Palumbo PJ (1988) Epidemiology of persistent proteinuria in type II diabetes mellitus. Population-based study in Rochester, Minnesota. Diabetes 37:405–412
34. Kunzelman CL, Knowler WC, Pettitt DJ, Bennett PH (1989) Incidence of proteinuria in type 2 diabetes mellitus in the Pima Indians. Kidney Int 35:681–687
35. Fabre J, Balant LP, Dayer PG, Fox HM, Vernet AT (1982) The kidney in maturity onset diabetes mellitus. Kidney Int 21:730–738
36. Uusitupa M, Siitonen O, Penttila I, Aro A, Pyorala K (1987) Proteinuria in newly diagnosed type II diabetic patients. Diabetes Care 10:191–194

Management of Advanced Nephrotic Disease in Diabetics: Short-term and Long-term Effects of Angiotensin Converting Enzyme (ACE)-Inhibitors and a New Trial Using Camostat Mesilate

Yoshio Taguma, Mitsunobu Matsubara, Osamu Hotta, and Kosei Kurosawa[1]

Summary. Two studies of the management of nephrotic diabetics were performed. Captopril (37.5 mg/day, $n=16$), decreased urinary protein excretion from 9.6 ± 1.6 to 4.9 ± 1.0 g/day, $P<0.05$ (M $\pm$ SEM) and significantly decreased total cholesterol. No significant adverse effect was observed. Camostat mesilate (600 mg/day, $n=15$) decreased urinary protein from 4.8 ± 0.6 to 2.9 ± 0.4 ($P<0.01$). Elevated plasma fibrinogen level and noticeably enhanced urinary fibrin degradation product (FDP) excretion were also attenuated by this medication. No serious adverse effect was noted. These types of medication, particularly when combined, seemed promising for the treatment of nephrotic diabetics. The long-term effect of ACE-I was retrospectively analyzed in 56 azotemic diabetics, of whom almost all had noninsulin-dependent diabetes mellitus (NIDDM). The patients were divided into two groups (group A: treated with ACE-I, $n=27$; group B: without ACE-I, $n=29$). The inverse creatinine deteriorated by 0.023 per month in group B and by 0.012 in group A. Although the mean blood pressure was kept at a similar level, HBA1c differed significantly. In an additional study, ACE-I slowed the progression rate in 10 patients with nephrosclerosis. Taking these observations into consideration, it is suggested that ACE-I might slow the progression rate of advanced diabetic nephropathy.

Introduction

The management of diabetic patients with advanced nephropathy is not easy, because such patients tend to have the nephrotic syndrome and to have severe damage in many organs. This nephrotic syndrome is believed to accelerate the progression of nephropathy and to further accelerate damage in other organs. Consequently, it would be of great value to try and alleviate the massive proteinuria which is char-

[1]Department of Nephrology, Sendai Shakaihoken Hospital, 3-16-1 Tsutsumimachi Aobaku, Sendai, 981 Japan

acteristic of this condition. In this regard, we studied the effect of two kinds of drugs; captopril and camostate mesilate. We will discuss the advantages of these drugs in the treatment of advanced diabetic nephropathy.

Our greatest concern is whether or not long-term ACE-inhibition slows the progression rate of nephropathy. In order to investigate whether an ACE-inhibitor has such an effect, we retrospectively analyzed the clinical course of our patients with advanced diabetic nephropathy and hypertensive nephrosclerosis.

Methods

The Effects of Captopril on the Nephrotic Syndrome in Advanced Diabetic Nephropathy

This study was performed while patients were hospitalized. Sixteen NIDDM patients (8 men and 8 women, mean age of 49 years), were the subjects. All patients had azotemia and proliferative retinopathy. During the control period of more than two weeks, their hypertension was controlled by conventional antihypertensive drugs and their clinical variables were confirmed to be relatively constant. Thereafter, captopril, at 37.5 mg a day, was administered and the patients were observed for 8 weeks.

The Effects of Camostat Mesilate

This study was performed while patients were hospitalized. Fifteen patients (13 men and 2 women, mean age of 57 years) were the subjects. All patients had NIDDM and proliferative retinopathy; fourteen of them had azotemia. During the control period an ACE-inhibitor had been used to control their hypertension and massive proteinuria, and the clinical variables were confirmed to be almost constant. Thereafter, camostat mesilate, at 600 mg a day, was administered and the patients were observed for a minimum of 4 weeks.

The Long-term Effects of ACE-Inhibition

The clinical courses of 56 azotemic diabetics and 10 patients with hypertensive nephrosclerosis were analyzed. The azotemic diabetics were divided into two groups, according to whether or not ACE-inhibitors had been used. Twenty-seven patients (16 men and 11 women, mean age of 49), had been treated with an ACE-inhibitor for more than twelve months. In the remaining 29 patients (19 men and 10 women, mean age of 51), hypertension had been controlled using only conventional antihypertensive drugs. Patients who developed any acute complications were excluded from this study. Of the 56 patients, only two had insulin-dependent diabetes mellitus (IDDM).

The clinical courses of ten patients with hypertensive nephrosclerosis, who fell into the following category, were analyzed: azotemia was present at the initial point of observation, during the following twelve months no ACE-inhibitor was used, and thereafter we started administration of this drug. We examined the slopes of inverse creatinine in each period.

Table 1. The effects of captopril (37.5 mg a day) in 16 azotemic diabetics

		Before	After	
Urinary protein	(g/day)	9.6 ± 1.6	4.9 ± 1.0*	
Serum total protein	(g/dl)	5.8 ± 0.2	6.1 ± 0.2	ns
Serum total cholesterol	(mg/dl)	228 ± 13	177 ± 8**	
Serum creatinine	(mg/dl)	4.4 ± 0.5	4.6 ± 0.5	ns
Serum potassium	(mEq/L)	4.5 ± 0.1	4.7 ± 0.1	ns
Mean blood pressure	(mmHg)	108 ± 3	100 ± 4	ns
HBA1c	(%)	6.3 ± 0.4	5.9 ± 0.4	ns

Values are expressed as M ± SEM. $^{**}P < 0.01$, $^{*}P < 0.05$; ns, not significant

Results

The Effects of Captopril

Table 1 shows the result of this study. Urinary protein excretion of 9.6 grams a day decreased to about half by the end of the study. The increase in total protein concentration did not reach statistical significance, but the total cholesterol level decreased significantly. On the whole, neither serum creatinine nor serum potassium showed any significant increments. However, in one case acute worsening of azotemia was observed; this patient was excluded from the study. Mean blood pressure and level of HBA1c did not change significantly.

The Effects of Camostat Mesilate

Table 2 shows the result of this study. Urinary protein decreased significantly and serum albumin concentration increased. Serum creatinine was unchanged. Plasma fibrinogen concentration was abnormally high during the control period and fell to a normal level after this drug was administered. A large amount of urinary total-FDP, which is not excreted in the urine of healthy people, was observed during the control period, and decreased significantly after this drug was administered. In addition, no worsening in retinal hemorrhage was observed in any patient.

Table 2. The effects of camostat mesilate (600 mg a day) in 15 patients with advanced diabetic nephropathy

		Before	After	
Urinary protein	(g/day)	4.8 ± 0.6	2.9 ± 0.4**	
S-Albumin	(g/dl)	2.7 ± 0.2	2.9 ± 0.2**	
S-creatinine	(mg/dl)	3.8 ± 0.7	3.8 ± 0.1	ns
Plasma fibrinogen	(mg/dl)[a]	420 ± 42	307 ± 28**	
Urinary total-FDP	(μg/day)	26100 ± 9700	18100 ± 7100*	

[a]Normal range for plasma fibrinogen is 160–400 mg/dl.
Values are expressed as M±SEM. $^{*}P < 0.05$, $^{**}P < 0.01$; ns, not significant

Table 3. Profiles of our 56 patients with advanced diabetic nephropathy

I] Type of diabetes
IDDM 2 NIDDM 54
II] Historical data for 54 NIDDM patients
Proteinuria present at the onset/detection of diabetes
12 (22%)
Preceding hypertension
Present 26 (48%)
Absent 28 (52%)

Long-term Effects of ACE-inhibition

The profile of the 56 diabetic patients who were the subjects of this study are shown in Table 3. It seemed noteworthy that most of the patients were those with NIDDM, and that in about half of them, hypertension preceded diabetes. The patients' clinical courses were analyzed and they were divided into two groups according to whether or not an ACE-inhibitor had been used. Figure 1 shows the time course of inverse creatinine, mean blood pressure, and levels of HBA1c in these two groups. A regression line for the slope of inverse creatinine in each patient was drawn, and the calculated mean of this line was expressed for each group. The dots represent the mean values of each period of time for each group. The levels in mean blood pressure were kept at a similar range in the two groups, though the levels in HBA1c differed almost constantly throughout the observed period. Therefore, even though there was a significant difference in the deteriorating rate in renal function between these two groups, we should not draw a definite conclusion.

Figure 2 shows the time course of progression of 10 patients with hypertensive nephrosclerosis. During the first twelve months, when patients had been treated with conventional antihypertensive drugs, a further declining tendency in renal function was observed. The mean blood pressure tended to rise, and then, depending on the result, ACE-inhibitor was administered to each patient. During the following twelve months, the declining tendency seemed to disappear. The differences in the slopes of inverse creatinine during, before, and after ACE-inhibition, were statistically significant.

Discussion

Since we reported in 1985 that captopril had an effect on reducing massive proteinuria in advanced diabetic nephropathy patients some controversy was evoked [1]. But now it seems to be indisputable that ACE-inhibitors have a definite effect in reducing urinary protein excretion in various renal disorders [2,3]. This effect is thought to be brought about through attenuation of glomerular hyperfiltration. Glomerular hyperfiltration is suspected to be one of the factors responsible for the initiation and the progression of diabetic nephropathy [4]. Our result would be regarded as supporting evidence for this hypothesis.

In any type of renal disease, particularly in diabetes, the development of the nephrotic syndrome is considered to be an accelerating factor in the progression of

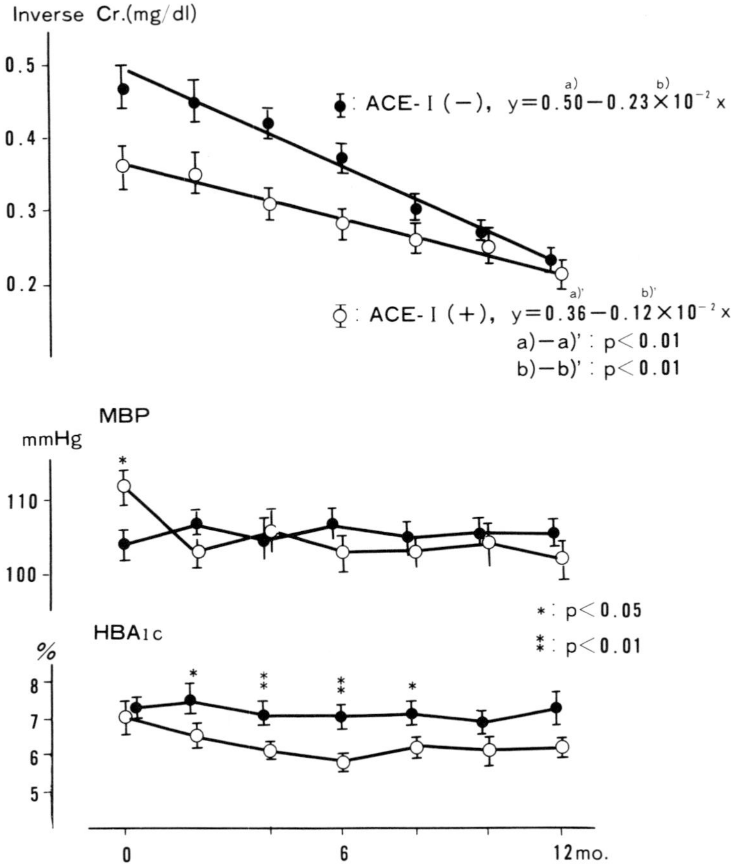

Fig. 1. Clinical course of azotemic diabetics treated with ACE-I (n=27) and without ACE-I (n=29). The *lines* drawn for the slope of inverse creatinine represent the calculated regression line for each group. The *dots* represent the mean values (M ± SEM) of each group in each time-period

nephropathy and in the damage in other organs [5]. Many factors other than hyperfiltration might also be responsible for the massive proteinuria which occurs in advanced diabetics [6], therefore, various therapeutic interventions would be necessary to alleviate this condition. At this juncture, we performed a new trial using camostat mesilate. Camostat mesilate is a derivative of gabexate mesilate, which is now used world-wide for the treatment of acute pancreatitis and disseminated intravascular coagulation. We recently found that use of this drug was advantageous in the treatment of heavy proteinuria in various nephropathies, including diabetic nephropathy [7,8]. The results of this study could be regarded as beneficial, in that massive proteinuria was reduced and also in that hypercoagulability was ameliorated. The long-term effects and the precise in vivo action of this drug remain to be elucidated. In any case, by using an ACE-inhibitor and camostat mesilate, we could

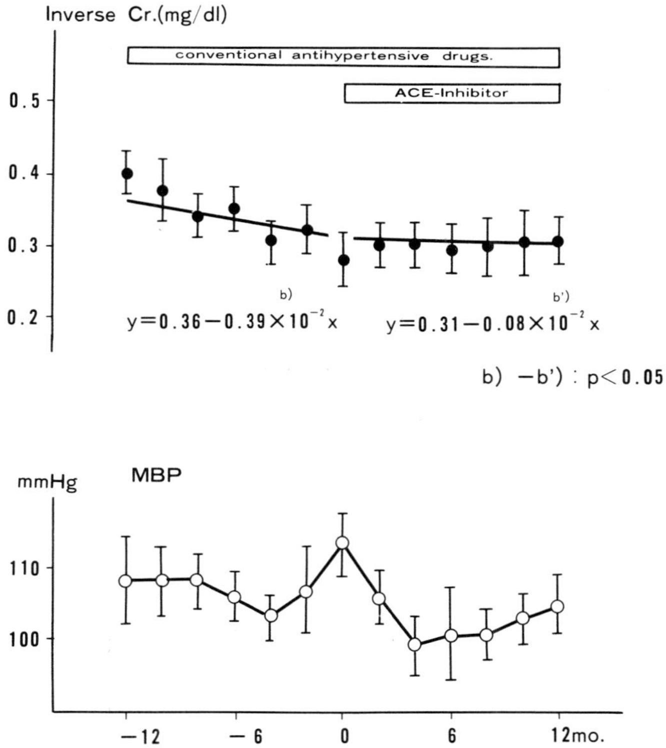

Fig. 2. Time course of progression before and after ACE-inhibition in 10 azotemic patients with hypertensive nephrosclerosis. The *lines* drawn for the slope of inverse creatinine represent the calculated regression line for each period. The *dots* represent the mean values of each time-period

alleviate the nephrotic syndrome in most patients with advanced diabetic nephropathy. Therefore, we may suppose that this combination therapy would be promising in improving the prognosis of these patients.

The pathogenesis of nephropathy in NIDDM is not clearly understood when compared to that in IDDM. The high prevalence rates, noted in our patients, of proteinuria and of hypertension preceding the detection of diabetes, seem to be one of the characteristics of NIDDM. This characteristic would be considered to be related to the concept of "insulin resistance" [8]. Another simpler explanation for this phenomenon is that, to some extent, arterionephrosclerosis precedes the development of diabetic glomerulosclerosis in some NIDDM patients. Figure 3 represents a schema of our line of thought in this direction. If we presume such a condition, we could expect to see similar effects of ACE-inhibitors in patients with hypertensive nephrosclerosis and in those with NIDDM. As was indicated by this study and by other researchers [9], an ACE-inhibitor slowed the progression rate in patients with hypertensive nephrosclerosis. Concerning advanced diabetic nephropathy, a similar beneficial effect, albeit not a definite one, was suggested by this study. Many factors might

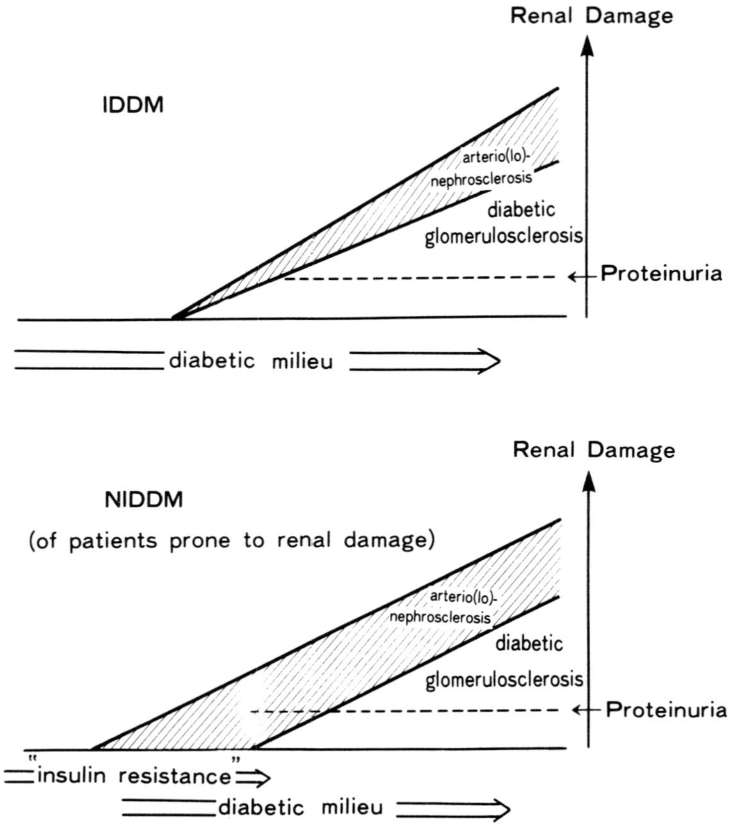

Fig. 3. A proposed schema of the pathophysiological alteration which takes place during the development of nephropathy in patients with IDDM and in NIDDM patients who are prone to renal damage

be responsible for the progression of diabetic glomerulosclerosis; ACE-inhibition alone would not be enough to stop the progression. We have to wait for future research before we can further improve the prognosis of advanced diabetic nephropathy.

Acknowledgment. We thank Ms Emiko Sakai for technical assistance.

References

1. Taguma Y, Kitamoto Y, Futaki G, Ueda H, Monma H, Ishizaki M, Takahashi H, Sekino H, Sasaki Y (1985) Effect of captopril on heavy proteinuria in azotemic diabetics. N Engl J Med 313:1617–1620
2. Hommel E, Parving HE, Mathiesen E, Edsberg B, Nielsen MD, Giese J (1986) Effect of captopril on kidney function in insulin-dependent diabetic patients with nephropathy. Br Med J [Clin Res] 293:467–470

3. Heeg JE, DeJong PE, Hem GK, Zeeum D (1987) Reduction of proteinuria by angiotensin converting enzyme inhibition. Kidney Int 32:78–83
4. Hostetter TH, Rennke HG, Brenner BM (1982) The case for intrarenal hypertension in the initiation and progression of diabetic and other glomerulopathies. Am J Med 72:375–380
5. Bernard DB (1982) Metabolic abnormalities in nephrotic syndrome: pathophysiology and complications. In: Brenner BM, Stein JH (eds) The nephrotic syndrome. Churchill Livingstone, New York, pp 85–120
6. Hostetter TH (1986) Pathogenosis of diabetic nephropathy. In: Mitch WE, Brenner BM, Stein JH (eds) The progressive nature of renal disease. Churchill Livingstone, New York, pp 149–166 (Contemporary issues in nephrology vol 14)
7. Matsubara M, Taguma Y, Kurosawa K, Hotta O, Suzuki K, Futaki G (1989) Effect of camostat mesilate on heavy proteinuria in various nephropathies. Clin Nephrol 32:119–123
8. Matsubara M, Taguma Y, Kurosawa K, Hotta O, Suzuki K, Ishizaki M (to be published) Effect of camostat mesilate for the treatment of advanced diabetic nephropathy. J Lab Clin Med
9. Reaven GM (1988) Role of insulin resistance in human disease. Diabetes 37:1595–1607
10. Jenkins AC, Dreslinski GR, Tardos SS, Groel JT, Fand R, Herczeg SA (1985) Captopril in hypertension: Seven years later. J Cardiovasc Pharmacol 7:S96–101

Transport of Organic Molecules

Chair: Karl J. Ullrich (FRG)
Takeshi Hoshi (Japan)

Transport of Organic Molecules

K.J. Ullrich[1]

Introduction

If we consider the transport processes in the proximal renal tubule, this symposium deals with the majority of transport agencies which are present there (Fig. 1): The transporter for glucose, luminally Na^+-dependent, contraluminally not so: the transporters for amino acids and for sulfate, again luminally Na^+-dependent, contraluminally not; Na^+-dependent transport processes for dicarboxylate at both cell sides; and then the two secretory systems a] for organic anions, contraluminally in exchange for α-ketoglutarate and luminally partially electrogenic, partially working as exchanger and b] for organic cations contraluminally driven by an electrogenic exchange and luminally driven by an H^+-organic cation antiport.

Since I personally have been working for eight years now with the stop flow peritubular capillary perfusion method to characterize contraluminal anion and cation transport systems, you expect at least a short message from me: As Fig. 2 shows, the *para*-aminohipporate (PAH) transporter likes substrates with a negative charge and a hydrophobic core. The negative charge may be one ionic negative charge or a partial negative charge. However, there can be a second ionic or partial negative charge. In each case a hydrophobic core is needed. When two ionic negative charges, or one ionic negative charge and a partial negative charge are 5-9 Å apart on a molecule, then the molecule is a substrate for the dicarboxylate transporter and if the negative charges are 3-7 Å apart then it is a substrate for the contraluminal sulfate/oxalate transporter. If the substrates for the dicarboxylate and sulfate transporter have, in addition, a hydrophobic core then they are also substrates for the PAH transporter. Thus, many substrates interact with two or with all three contraluminal anion transporters. The contraluminal organic cation transporter requires a positive ionic charge

[1]Max-Planck-Institut für Biophysik, 6000 Frankfurt 70, Federal Republic of Germany

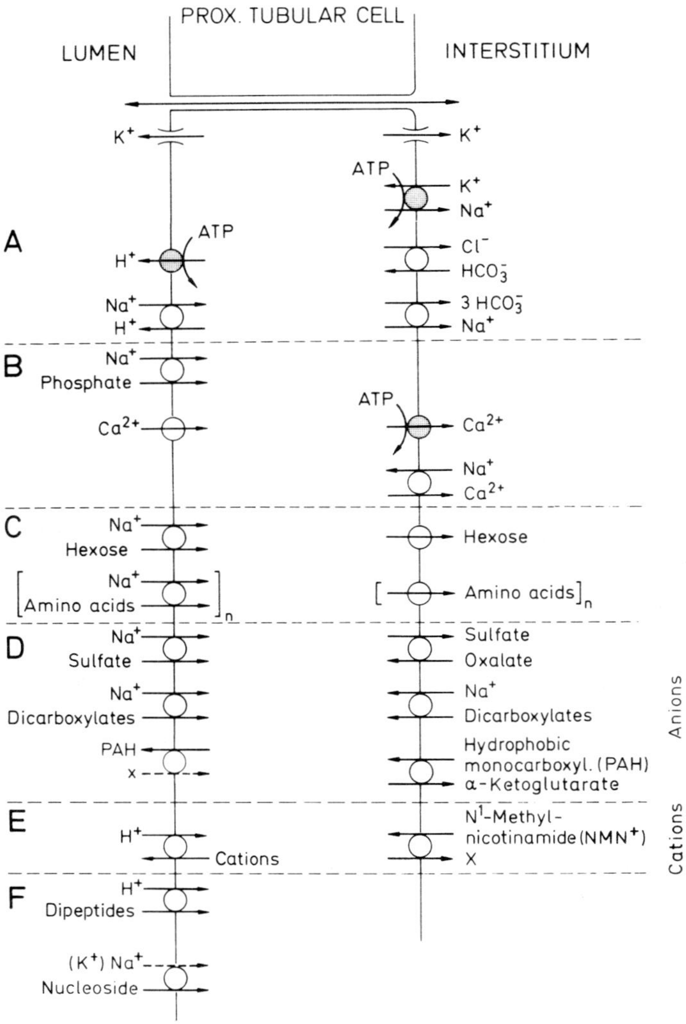

Fig. 1. Sidedness of the transport processes in the proximal renal tubule

and a hydrophobic core. If a substrate has two positive charges its interaction with the transporter is reduced.

Table 1 shows specific inhibitors of contraluminal anion and cation transport: The PAH transport, which has a K_m of 0.08 mmol/l, can be specifically inhibited by benzoylbutyrate, apalcillin, cyano-hydroxycinnamate and nitroazidophenyl-alanine with a K_i of 0.01–0.02 mmol/l. *Sulfate transport*, which has a rather high K_m of 1.4 mmol/l, can be specifically inhibited by thiosulfate, although the K_i, at 0.33 mmol/l, is also relatively high. *For dicarboxylate*, a specific substrate does not seem to exist. Thus, succinate and the best inhibitor, tetrafluorosuccinate, also interact

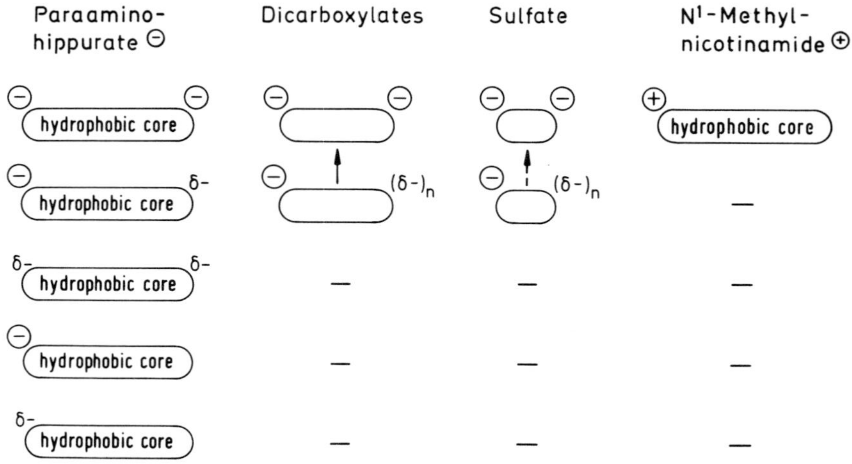

Fig. 2. Schematic specificity pattern of the PAH, dicarboxylate, and sulfate contraluminal organic anion transport systems, and the organic cation N[1]-methylnicotinamide transport system, in the proximal renal tubule

with the PAH transporter, although with a much higher K_i value, i.e., much lower affinity. Contraluminal transport for *N[1]-methylnicotinamide* (K_m 0.54 mmol/l) can be inhibited by a number of tetraalkylammonium compounds and methylnicotinamide analogues with a K_i around 0.1 mmol/l. Only one compound interacts much better than N[1]-methylnicotinamide: a heptafluorobutyroxy-analogue of N[1]-methylpyridinium.

Table 1. Specific inhibitors for contraluminal *anion and cation transport* in the proximal renal tubule (K_i and K_m in mmol/l)

	PAH $K_{i.PAH}$	Succinate $K_{i.Succ}$	Sulfate $K_{i.SO_4^{2-}}$
PAH	0.08 (K_m)	1.9	NS
Benzoylbutyrate	0.02	NS	NS
Apalcillin	0.02	NS	NS
2-Cyano-3-hydroxy-cinnamate	<0.01	NS	4.45
2-Nitro-4-azido-phenylalanine	<0.01	NS	NS
Sulfate	NS	NS	1.4 (K_m)
Thiosulfate	NS	NS	0.33
Succinate	1.3	0.09 (K_m)	NS
Tetrafluor-succinate	1.4	0.05	NS
		N[1]-methylnicotinamide $K_{i.NMN}$	
N[1]-Methylnicotinamide		0.54 (K_m)	
Tetraethylammonium Cl^-		0.07	
Tetrapropylammonium Cl^-		0.08	
Tetrabutylammonium Cl^-		0.09	
N′-Trifluoroethyl-N[1]-methylnicotinamide		0.14	
N[1]-Trifluorobenzyl-nicotinamide		0.12	
N[1]-Methyl-2-methyl-4-heptafluoro-butyroxy-pyridinium		0.02	

Table 2. Non-specific and relatively specific inhibitors of contraluminal *anion transport* in the proximal renal tubule (K_i and K_m in mmol/l)

	$K_{m,PAH}$ 0.08 / $K_{i,PAH}$	$K_{m,Succ}$ 0.09 / $K_{i,Succ}$	$K_{m,SO4^{2-}}$ 1.4 / $K_{i,SO4^{2-}}$
Probenecid	0.03	NS	7.9
Tienilic acid	0.01	NS	2.7
Indomethacin	0.05	NS	1.4
Diisothiocyanato-dihydrostilbene-disulfonate (H_2DIDS)	0.02	1.8	0.4
Eosinthiocyanate	0.04	0.75	0.19
8-Anilinonaphthalene-1 sulfonate (8-ANS)	0.04	0.5	0.09
Bromphenol-blue	0.13	2.5	0.11
Orange G	0.15	NS	0.02

You might have missed your favorite inhibitors for organic anion transport: probenecid, indomethacin, DIDS, and 8-ANS. As is evident from Table 2 they unfortunately interact not only with the PAH transporter with rather high affinity (low app. K_i values), but also with the sulfate transporter, and some interact with the dicarbosylate transporter. Fortunately the affinity of probenecid for the sulfate transporter is low, so that probenecid could be considered as a rather specific inhibitor for PAH transport. More care must be taken with indomethacin, DIDS, and the other compounds listed because their affinity for PAH and sulfate transport might be equal. At the bottom is Orange-G which has a 7 times higher affinity for sulfate than for PAH transport. Thus, at 0.01 mmol/l, Orange-G can be considered as a specific inhibitor for contraluminal sulfate transport.

Strategies for Evaluating the Molecular Structure of Membrane Transport Systems

Ernest M. Wright[1]

SUMMARY. The strategies that have been successfully employed to identify and characterize the brush border Na^+/glucose cotransporter are summarized. These include the use of photoaffinity and covalent reagents, expression cloning, polyclonal antibodies to defined domains of the predicted sequence, and cDNA probes. The successful application of these strategies to renal membrane proteins will significantly advance the study of transporters for organic molecules.

Introduction

Over the past 30 years much effort has been directed at describing the non-electrolyte transport across epithelial cells. The transport systems involved have been carefully delineated and characterized kinetically. Particular progress has been achieved in understanding the underlying role of Na^+ pumps in the active transport of organic molecules across epithelia. The renal Na^+/K-pump (Na/K-ATPase) has been isolated, purified, reconstituted, cloned, and sequenced. The availability of antibodies and cDNA probes for the α and β subunits has revolutionized research on Na/K pumps. The importance of the pump for the transport of organic molecules is that it provides the energy ($\Delta\ \bar{\mu}_{Na}$) for secondary active transport of many solutes.

In the case of organic substances, much less progress has been realized, and this is due to (1) the low amounts of transport proteins in epithelial membranes (typically less than 0.1% of the membrane protein) and the attendant difficulty in isolating and purifying rare hydrophobic membrane proteins; (2) the general absence of high affinity inhibitors and specific covalent probes. So, despite the fact that a dozen or so epithelial transporters have been described over the past 30 years, only a few have been identified, and only one has been cloned, sequenced, and expressed.

In this report I will describe the strategies that have been employed in the identification, characterization, and cloning of the intestinal brush border Na^+/glucose

[1]Department of Physiology, UCLA School of Medicine, Los Angeles, CA 90024-1751, USA

cotransporter. This is the archetypical eukaryote Na^+ cotransporter, and it has an advantage in that a high affinity competitive inhibitor, phlorizin, is available.

The first clues to the identity of the Na^+/glucose cotransporter came from a study by Semenza's group, using a H^3-azidophlorizin as a photoaffinity probe [1]. Despite a very high background incorporation of the label into brush border proteins, protection experiments with D-glucose and cold phlorizin revealed specific labeling of a 70–75 kDa polypeptide. This was subsequently confirmed by Semenza's group, using a monoclonal body [2], and by our group, using covalent group-specific reagents.

Our strategy with group-specific reagents was simply to screen reagents for their effect on Na^+/glucose cotransport in brush border vesicles, and then to attempt to protect against inhibiting reagents with Na^+ and D-glucose [3,4]. We first found that the lysine reagent phenylisothiocyanate (PITC) was a potent inhibitor and that the transporter was protected by the presence of Na^+ *and* D-glucose (or phlorizin). Neither Na^+ nor D-glucose alone protected, and the requirement for Na^+ and D-glucose was specific. The next step was to label the protein; the approach was, first, to react the membranes with PITC in the presence of Na^+ and D-glucose (to derivatize all exposed lysine residues), then to wash the membranes free of PITC, Na^+, and D-glucose, and finally, to label the membranes with a fluorescent PITC derivative (FITC). The brush borders were then subjected to SDS-PAGE analysis and the gel was sliced and assayed for FITC. We found a single band of protein, 70–75 kDa, labeled with FITC, and this labeling was blocked when the FITC labeling was conducted in the presence of Na^+ and D-glucose. Similar experiments carried out with tyrosine group-specific reagents, e.g., N-acetyl-imidazole, also labeled the 70–75 kDa band, and this was specifically blocked with physiological levels of Na^+. We concluded that lysines were near the D-glucose binding site and that tyrosine residues were near the Na^+ binding site on the polypeptide.

Using this differential labeling approach with fluorescent or non-fluorescent group-specific reagents, the Na^+/proline and Na^+/phosphate intestinal brush border cotransporters were identified as 100 kDa and 140 kDa polypeptides, respectively [5,6]. In principle, this approach can be employed to identify other intestinal and renal transport proteins. Given success in labeling membrane transporters, it should then be possible to isolate and purify the polypeptide to homogeneity. The intestinal Na^+/glucose cotransporter has been partially purified by chromatofocusing (pI ~ 5.3) [7]. More recently, it has apparently been purified to homogeneity in an active form, although no conventional purity criteria (e.g., amino acid composition, N-terminal microsequencing) have been presented [8].

Two successful studies have been reported in which Na^+-cotransporters were identified using functional assays. The brain Na/Cl/GABA-cotransporter was purified, using reconstitution of transport activity in liposomes as an assay [9], and this provided a reagent for the conventional molecular cloning of the GABA transporter cDNA [10]. An alternative approach, involving expression cloning, was employed by our group to identify the intestinal Na^+/glucose cotransporter [11]. The starting point was the observation that the rabbit intestinal Na^+/glucose cotransporter could be expressed in a functional form in *Xenopus* oocyte plasma membrane after the injection of intestinal mRNA. The mRNA was enriched by electrophoresis (in a 2.3 kb fraction), a cDNA library was made in an expression plasmid (Bluescript), and the clones were screened by injected RNA synthesized from the clones, using the T_3 and

T_7 promoters. A single 2.3 kb clone was isolated that coded for the classical Na^+/glucose cotransporter. The advantage of expression cloning is that a functional clone is isolated, which may be expressed (using a suitable vector) in cultured cells (oocytes, COS-7 cells, fibroblasts, etc.) [12].

The clone was sequenced and found to code for a 662 amino acid polypeptide with a predicted molecular weight of 73 kDa. The sequence showed no homology to any other eukaryote protein, but had high homology to the *E. coli* Na^+/protein cotransporters [13]. Again, in principle, this expression cloning strategy may be used to clone other transport proteins. So far, we have expressed renal transporters for lysine, alanine, phenylalanine, and succinate in oocytes, and found that all are coded by 2–3 kb RNA fractions [14]. The next step is to construct a cDNA library from this mRNA fraction and to screen the library.

Once a transporter has been cloned and sequenced, it is then possible to generate antibodies to the protein. Short peptides (10–20 residues), corresponding to specific domains on the predicted secondary structure of the cloned protein, can be synthesized and these are used to raise polyclonal antibodies. We have, so far, obtained two useful antibodies to the intestinal Na^+/glucose cotransporter (B.A. Hirayama, unpublished results). Using Western analysis, these antibodies have been found to recognize the cotransporter both in intestinal brush borders, from alligator to man, and in renal brush borders (pig, rabbit, human). These results have been confirmed using Northern analysis [15]. We have also used cDNA probes to isolate clones for the human intestinal [13] and rabbit renal [15] Na^+/glucose cotransporters.

In the case of the brush border Na^+/glucose cotransporter, we are now poised to map the human gene, examine the genetic defect in glucose-galactose malabsorption, and to probe the structure/function relations of the transport protein. We anticipate that similar biochemical and molecular approaches will be used to great advantage to unravel the secrets of organic solute transport by the kidney.

References

1. Hosang M, Vasella A, Semenza G (1981) Specific photoaffinity inactivation of the D-glucose transporter in small intestinal brush border membrane using new phlorizin analogues. Biochemistry 20:5844–5854
2. Schmidt UM, Eddy B, Frazer CM, Venter CJ, Semenza G (1983) Isolation of (a subunit of) the Na^+/D-glucose cotransporter(s) of rabbit intestinal brush border membranes using monoclonal antibodies. FEBS Lett 161:279–283
3. Peerce BE, Wright EM (1984) Sodium-induced conformational changes in the glucose transporter of intestinal brush borders. J Biol Chem 259:14105–14112
4. Peerce BE, Wright EM (1985) Evidence for tyrosyl residues at the Na^+ site on the intestinal Na^+/glucose cotransporter. J Biol Chem 260:6026–6031
5. Wright EM, Peerce BE (1984) Identification and conformational changes of the intestinal proline carrier. J Biol Chem 259:14993–14996
6. Peerce BE (1989) Identification of the intestinal Na^+/phosphate cotransporter. Am J Physiol 256:6645–6652
7. Peerce BE, Wright EM (1986) Distance between substrate sites on the glucose/glucose cotransporter by fluorescence energy transfer. Proc Natl Acad Sci USA 83:8092–8096
8. Peerce BE, Clarke RD (1990) Isolation and reconstitution of the intestinal Na^+/glucose cotransporter. J Biol Chem 265:1731–1736

9. Radian R, Bendahan A, Kanner BI (1986) Purification and identification of the functional sodium- and chloride-coupled γ-aminobutyric acid transport glycoprotein from rat brain. J Biol Chem 261:15437–15441
10. Guastella J, Nelson N, Nelson H, Czyzyk L, Keynan S, Miedel MC, Davidson N, Lester HA, Kanner BI (1990) Cloning and expression of a rat brain GABA transporter. Science 249:1303–1306
11. Hediger MA, Coady MJ, Ikeda TS, Wright EM (1987) Expression cloning and cDNA sequencing of the Na^+/glucose cotransporter. Nature 330:379–381
12. Birnir B, Lee H-S, Hediger MA, Wright EM (1990) Expression and characterization of the intestinal Na^+/glucose cotransporter in COS-7 cells. Biochim Biophys Acta 1048:100–104
13. Hediger MA, Turk E, Wright EM (1989) Homology of the human intestinal Na^+/glucose and *Escherichia coli* Na^+/proline cotransporters. Proc Natl Acad Sci USA 86:5748–5752
14. Coady MJ, Pajor AM, Toloza EM, Wright EM (1990) Expression of mammalian renal transporters in *Xenopus laevis* oocytes. Arch Biochem Biophys 283:130–134
15. Coady MJ, Pajor AM, Wright EM (1990) Sequence homologies amongst intestinal and renal Na^+/glucose cotransporters. Am J Physiol (Cell Physiol) 259:C605–C610

p-Aminohippurate Uptake Across the Basolateral Membrane of Rat Proximal Tubule Cells: Specificity and Mode of Energetization

GERHARD BURCKHARDT, CHRISTIANE SCHMITT, and KARL JULIUS ULLRICH[1]

SUMMARY. Uptake of [^{3}H]PAH (p-aminohippurate) across the basolateral membrane of rat proximal tubule cells was studied in intact kidneys and membrane vesicles to determine biologically and pharmacologically important substrates of the PAH transporter and its energization by ion gradients. Effective inhibition of in situ [^{3}H]PAH uptake by *trans*-2-decanoate, α-ketoglutarate, prostaglandin E_2, 11-dehydrocorticosterone, and dibutyryl cyclic GMP suggests an involvement of the PAH transporter in cellular entry and exit of metabolic products, selected hormones and second messengers. The high affinity for N-acetyl-, N-benzoyl-, N-acetylcysteine-, sulfate- and glucuronide-conjugates supports the role of the PAH transporter in renal excretion of metabolites. Among the drugs, apalcillin proved an inhibitor of high affinity (app. $K_{i,PAH}$ 0.02 mM) and selectivity for the PAH transporter. The nephrotoxic agents, ochratoxin A, orellanin, and β-amanitin, also inhibited in situ [^{3}H]PAH uptake indicating that their cellular uptake proceeds *via* the PAH transporter. In vesicles, glutarate and an out > in Na^+ gradient, but not a Na^+ gradient alone, drove uphill [^{3}H]PAH accumulation. Stimulation of [^{3}H]PAH uptake was half-maximal at 10.8 μM glutarate and 2.3 mM Na^+ with 3 Na^+ ions being involved. These results reflect the kinetic properties of the $(Na^+)_3$-dicarboxylate cotransporter and prove its role in uphill PAH transport. Glutarate/PAH exchange is electroneutral, suggesting either exchange of one glutarate for two PAH molecules, or the involvement of hitherto undefined ions in the exchange process. In conclusion, PAH uptake across the basolateral membrane occurs through exchange with α-ketoglutarate, which is itself intracellularly accumulated by the Na^+-coupled dicarboxylate transporter.

Introduction

The kidney has the capability to excrete a large number of endogenous and exogenous organic anions. Many of these compounds undergo filtration in the glomeruli and net

[1]Max-Planck-Institut für Biophysik, Kennedyallee 70, D-6000 Frankfurt 70, Federal Republic of Germany

secretion in the proximal tubules [1–3]. Secretion involves uptake of organic anions across the contraluminal (basolateral) membrane into the cell and exit from the cell into the tubulus lumen via the luminal (brush-border) membrane. Transport across the cell membranes in turn involves interaction of the anions with specialized transport systems. Using homologous series of substrates three organic anion transport systems with overlapping specificities have been found in the basolateral membrane of rat proximal tubule cells [4,5]: *First*, an anion exchanger accommodating sulfate, oxalate, HCO_3^-, and organic anions which bear two negative charges, or one negative and a partial negative charge, at less than 7 Å distance; *second*, a Na^+-coupled dicarboxylate transporter interacting with Krebs cycle intermediates as well as with organic anions carrying two negative charges, or one ionic and one partial negative charge, at 5–9 Å distance; *third*, the "*p*-aminohippurate (PAH) transporter" which accepts substrates with one or two partial, or one or two ionic negative charges at 6–10 Å distance and having a hydrophobic domain of at least 4 Å length.

Uptake of PAH across the basolateral membrane occurs "uphill" and requires energy. As reviewed recently [6] PAH uptake into renal cortical cells was impaired by anaerobic conditions, uncouplers of oxidative phosphorylation, lowering of temperature, addition of cyanide, as well as by removal of Na^+ or K^+, or addition of ouabain. Taken together these data suggested that intact metabolism is needed to create transmembrane gradients of Na^+ which drive uphill PAH transport presumably via a Na^+/PAH symporter. Pritchard [6,7] and Shimada et al. [8] suggested another mechanism for uphill transport of PAH. As indicated above, the basolateral membrane possesses a Na^+-coupled transport system for dicarboxylates. Since the PAH transporter shows affinity for some dicarboxylates too, both systems could cooperate through exchanging common substrates. Indeed, glutarate can be accumulated in basolateral membrane vesicles in the presence of an out > in gradient of Na^+, and can be subsequently exchanged for external labeled PAH. Thereby, the Na^+ gradient drives PAH uptake indirectly, i.e. via accumulation of glutarate, rather than by acting directly on the PAH transporter.

In this contribution we tested endogenous and pharmacologically important compounds as possible substrates of the PAH transporter, including those Krebs cycle intermediates that could serve for driving uphill PAH transport at the basolateral membrane. We also performed experiments with basolateral membrane vesicles to offer additional evidence for the involvement of the Na^+-coupled dicarboxylate transporter during PAH accumulation.

Methods

Experiments on the Intact Kidney

The details of measuring contraluminal influx of radioactively labeled substrates from the interstitium into the cells, and the mode of evaluating the transport parameters have been described elsewhere [9]. In essence, immediately after clamping the renal artery and vein, a blood capillary was punctured with an oil-filled sampling pipette. At 100–140 μm distance another blood vessel was impaled by a filling pipette containing tritiated PAH or methyl-succinate, and [^{14}C]inulin as a reference substance for estimation of the extracellular space. Besides 0.1 mM

[^{3}H]PAH, the solution in the filling pipette contained (in mM): 150 Na^+, 4 K^+, 154 gluconate, at pH 7.4. When dicarboxylate uptake was tested the filling pipette contained (in mM): 0.15 [^{3}H]-methyl-succinate, 136 Na^+, 4 K^+, 1.5 Ca^{2+}, 1 Mg^{2+}, 120 Cl^-, and 25 HCO_3^-, gassed with 95% O_2/5% CO_2. The test solutions were rapidly injected into the capillary and withdrawn after 2 s through the sampling pipette. The recovered radioactivity was determined by liquid scintillation counting. To screen for inhibitors of transport 1–10 mM of test anions were applied together with the labeled substrates. Using previously determined K_m values for PAH (0.08 mM [10]) an apparent K_i was determined from the degree of inhibition of contraluminal uptake, assuming competitive inhibition.

Experiments on basolateral membrane vesicles. Vesicles were prepared from the cortex of rat kidneys by the Percoll density gradient technique described by Scalera et al. [11]. They were preloaded with 150 mM KCl, 20 mM Hepes buffered with Tris to pH 7.4, adjusted to a protein concentration of 10 mg/ml, and stored in liquid nitrogen. For the experiment, 5 μl of vesicle suspension was added to 95 μl prewarmed (37°C) incubation medium containing (in mM) 0.05 [^{3}H]PAH, 150 NaCl, KCl, or tetramethylammonium chloride, respectively, and 20 Hepes/Tris, pH 7.4. Further additions are indicated in the legends. Uptake was stopped by addition of 1 ml ice-cold solution containing 150 mM NaCl, 20 mM Hepes/Tris, at pH 7.4, and separation of vesicles from the medium by rapid filtration. The radioactivity remaining with the vesicles on the filters was determined by liquid scintillation counting. The figures show means ± SD from 4–5 determinations.

Results and Discussion

At low concentrations, PAH is handled by a single transport system in the basolateral membrane, the PAH transporter (apparent K_m, 0.08 mM [10]). The interaction with the $(Na^+)_3$-dicarboxylate cotransporter is weak (inhibition of succinate uptake with an apparent K_i of 1.9 mM [12]) and that with the sulfate transporter not detectable [5]. Although a selective test anion, PAH is not the natural substrate of the PAH transport system. Searching for putative endogenous substrates we screened previously tested compounds for those having the highest affinities towards the PAH transporter. These compounds are listed in Table 1. Fatty acids such as, e.g., *trans*-2-decanoate, or dicarboxylates of intermediate chain length, e.g., α-ketoglutarate, interact strongly with the PAH transporter. Their affinity for the PAH transporter is nearly three times that of PAH. Comparably high affinities are displayed by hormones (prostaglandin E_2 and 11-dehydro-corticosterone) as well as by a derivatized second messenger, dbcGMP. The naturally occurring second messengers, cAMP and cGMP, also interact with the PAH transporter although with lower affinities (apparent K_i, 2.6 and 0.34 mM, respectively [13]). Another metabolite strongly inhibiting PAH transport is 3,7-diketo-cholate, an oxidized form of the unconjugated bile salt cholate. These results suggest that the PAH transporter may be involved in the exit and entry of fatty acids, some Krebs cycle intermediates, and, notably, the exit and entry of some hormones and second messengers. Whether the PAH transporter is thus involved in paracrine functions in the kidney and, possibly, in other cells remains an interesting question to be solved in the future.

Table 1. Biologically and pharmacologically important compounds which interact with the PAH transport system in the basolateral membrane

Compounds	$K_{i,PAH}$ (mM)
A. Metabolites and hormones	
Trans-2-decanoate	0.03
α-Ketoglutarate	0.03
Prostaglandin E_2	0.08
Dibutyryl-cyclic GMP	0.04
11-Dehydro-corticosterone	0.02
3,7-Diketo-cholate	0.17
B. Conjugates	
L-tryptophyl-L-tryptophan	0.21
N-α-acetyl-L-glutamate	0.17
N-α-benzoyl-D-glutamate	0.04
Pentachlorobutadienyl-L-cysteine	0.07
Pentachlorobutadienyl-N-acetyl-L-cysteine	0.07
Taurolithocholate-sulfate	0.17
Lithocholate-glucuronide	0.15
C. Drugs	
Probenecid	0.03
3,4-Dichlorophenoxy-acetate	0.03
Apalcillin	0.02
Cephodizime	0.22
Glycine-salicylate (salycuric acid)	0.03
Mercaptoethanedisulfide	0.25

The compounds listed have been tested as inhibitors of [^{3}H]PAH uptake in the intact kidney. (From [13,14,16,31,32])

Table 1, B, lists conjugates with high affinities for the PAH transporter. These consist of a dipeptide, N-acetylated and N-benzoylated L-glutamate, cysteine- and N-acetyl-cysteine-conjugates of pentachlorobutadiene, and the sulfate- and glucuronide-conjugates of litho- and taurolithocholate. It should be emphasized that the unconjugated compounds, L-tryptophan, L-glutamate, pentachlorobutadiene, lithocholate and taurolithocholate interact weakly or not at all with the PAH transporter [14,15] either because they are too hydrophilic (amino acids) or too hydrophobic. Therefore, conjugation plays an important role in rendering compounds acceptable for the PAH transporter and, thus, for their disposal by renal excretion. Among the drugs listed in Table 1, C, the antibiotic apalcillin may prove suitable to specifically inhibit the PAH transporter, since it displays a high affinity for this system and does not interact with the sulfate and dicarboxylate carriers [16].

Table 2 lists compounds which are known to damage proximal tubule cells. The metabolite of *Aspergillus* and *Penicillium* fungi, ochratoxin A, occurs as contaminant in grain and is involved in the development of Balkan nephritis [17]. Other nephrotoxic agents are the mushroom toxins, orellanin [18], and amanitin [19]. These toxins as well as the carcinogen, aflatoxin B_1, inhibit PAH uptake with apparent K_i values ranging between 0.02 and 2.3 mM, suggesting that these compounds enter proximal tubule cells and are accumulated to toxic levels by the PAH transporter. The primary location of lesions in proximal tubules is in accordance with this assumption.

Table 2. Interaction of nephrotoxic agents with the PAH transporter

Compounds	$K_{i,PAH}$ (mM)
Ochratoxin A	0.02
Aflatoxin B_1	0.41
Orellanin	0.13
α-Amanitin	2.3
β-Amanitin	0.7

Data for amanitins are from [14]; the other results are from unpublished observations

Since α-ketoglutarate inhibits [^{3}H]PAH uptake from the blood into the cell (cf Table 1) the ability of other Krebs cycle intermediates to interact with the PAH transporter was tested; the result is shown in Fig. 1, top. Only α-ketoglutarate strongly inhibits the PAH transporter. In contrast, all dicarboxylates proved to be efficient inhibitors of the Na^+-coupled dicarboxylate transporter, whereas the tricarboxylates, citrate and isocitrate, inhibit less (Fig. 1, bottom). Thus, of all the intermediates, α-ketoglutarate has a high affinity for both PAH and dicarboxylate transporter, and should therefore be suited to energize PAH uptake across the basolateral membrane. This was tested in the experiment for which results are shown in Fig. 2. Basolateral membrane vesicles were loaded with KCl and suspended at zero time in a buffer containing NaCl and [^{3}H]PAH without or with 10 μM glutarate. In the absence of glutarate, [^{3}H]PAH was not accumulated above the equilibrium value, indicating that the Na^+ gradient alone cannot drive uphill PAH uptake. In the presence of glutarate (or α-ketoglutarate [20]), however, PAH uptake was markedly stimulated and transiently exceeded the equilibrium value. This result, which is in agreement with our and Pritchard's earlier observations [7,8,20], indicates Na^+-coupled uptake of glutarate (or α-ketoglutarate) into the vesicles and subsequent exchange of intravesicular glutarate for extravesicular [^{3}H]PAH.

In order to substantiate the cooperation of Na^+-coupled dicarboxylate transporter and PAH/dicarboxylate exchanger, the effect of Li^+, which inhibits the dicarboxylate transporter was tested [12,21]. Li^+ had no effect on PAH/[^{3}H]PAH exchange but inhibited [^{3}H]PAH uptake driven by external glutarate and Na^+ [7,8]. This result indicates that glutarate is taken up by the Li^+-sensitive dicarboxylate transporter and subsequently exchanges for PAH via the Li^+-insensitive PAH transporter. A further argument for the involvement of the Na^+-coupled dicarboxylate transporter during PAH accumulation in basolateral membrane vesicles is provided by the results of the experiment shown in Fig. 3. Here, the dependence of [^{3}H]PAH uptake was tested as a function of glutarate and Na^+ concentration in the medium. At a fixed Na^+ concentration (150 mM) increasing glutarate concentrations caused an increasing stimulation of PAH uptake. Corrected for [^{3}H]PAH uptake observed in the absence of glutarate, this stimulation follows Michaelis-Menten kinetics, exhibiting an apparent K_m of 5.1 μM. In three experiments of this type, a mean K_m of 10.8 μM (SE 2.9) was found. This K_m value reflects the high affinity for its substrates of the dicarboxylate transporter in basolateral membrane vesicles [21,22]. At a fixed glutarate concentration (10 μM, Fig. 3, right panel), increasing Na^+ concentrations stimulate [^{3}H]PAH uptake. As opposed to glutarate, stimulation by Na^+ does not follow simple

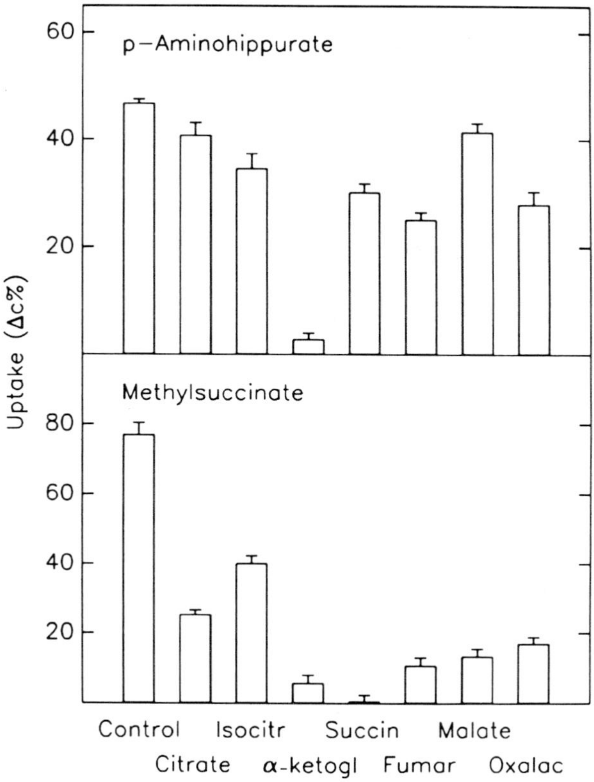

Fig. 1. Interaction of Krebs cycle intermediates with the renal contraluminal transporters for PAH and dicarboxylates. [^{3}H]PAH and [^{3}H]methyl-succinate uptake across the basolateral membrane was measured in the intact kidney. The indicated Krebs cycle intermediates were added at 10 mM concentration to the test solutions containing 0.1 mM [^{3}H]PAH (*top panel*) or 0.15 mM [^{3}H]methyl-succinate (*bottom panel*). Controls received the labeled substrates without added intermediates. The ordinate shows the decrease in [^{3}H]PAH and [^{3}H]methyl-succinate concentrations in the capillaries within 2 s incubation time. (Data from [12,31])

Michaelis-Menten kinetics. The data can, rather, be fitted to an equation taking the interaction of 3 Na^+ ions with the carrier into account [23]. A half-maximal effect of Na^+ is observed at 2.3 mM. The interaction of more than one sodium ion is typical for the dicarboxylate transporter; kinetic experiments and its electrogenicity [21,22] suggest that three sodium ions are cotransported with one doubly negatively charged dicarboxylate (surplus of one positive charge during cotransport). Taken together, the data shown in Fig. 3 reflect the properties of the $(Na^+)_3$-dicarboxylate cotransporter and thus prove its involvement in Na^+ and (α-keto)glutarate-stimulated [^{3}H]PAH uptake into basolateral membrane vesicles.

Next, we investigated whether the exchange of glutarate (two negative charges) for PAH (one negative charge) was electrogenic or electroneutral. As a control, we tested the influence of changes in membrane potential on PAH/[^{3}H]PAH exchange. Vesicles

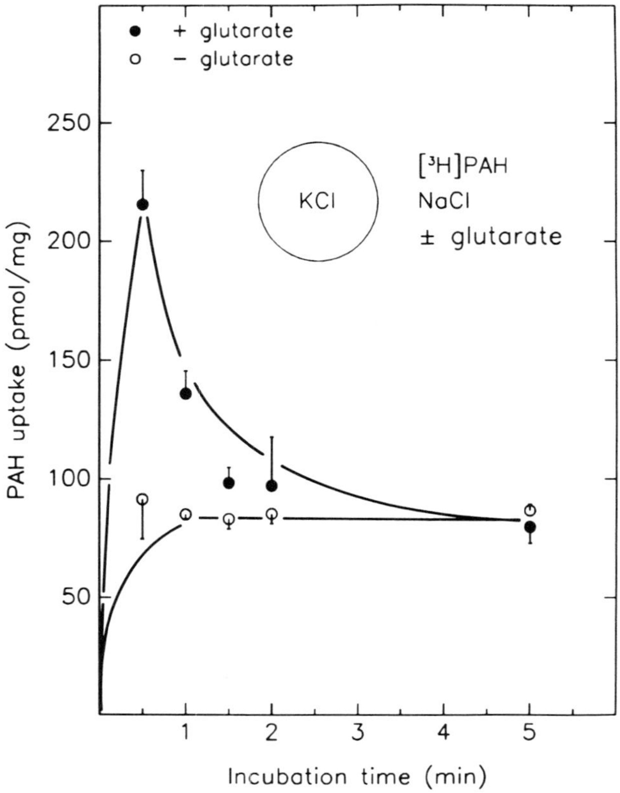

Fig. 2. Effect of glutarate and a Na^+ gradient on PAH uptake into rat renal basolateral membrane vesicles. The vesicles were loaded with KCl and suspended in buffers containing NaCl, 0.05 mM [^{3}H]PAH, and no (*open circles*) or 0.01 mM glutarate (*closed circles*). Uptake was terminated after the time periods indicated at the abscissa

were preloaded with KCl and either 1 mM PAH (for PAH/[^{3}H]PAH exchange) or 1 mM glutarate (for glutarate/[^{3}H]PAH exchange). At zero time the vesicles were diluted into media containing labeled PAH, the K^+ ionophor valinomycin, and either KCl or tetramethylammonium chloride (TMA Cl). In this setting, the imposition of an in > out K^+ gradient creates an inside negative K^+ diffusion potential. This potential does not influence PAH/[^{3}H]PAH exchange, as shown in Fig. 4, left panel (compare open bars with hatched bars). Surprisingly, the exchange of intravesicular glutarate for extravesicular [^{3}H]PAH was also not influenced by the K^+ diffusion potential, indicating an electroneutral exchange process (Fig. 4, right panel).

Electroneutral exchange can occur if one glutarate plus a proton is exchanged with PAH. In this case the hydrogen ion would compensate one negative charge of glutarate. Such an exchange should be favored by lowering pH, i.e., by increasing hydrogen ion concentration. Such a decrease in pH, however, rather decreased the rate of glutarate/PAH exchange (data not shown). Thus, we must assume that either

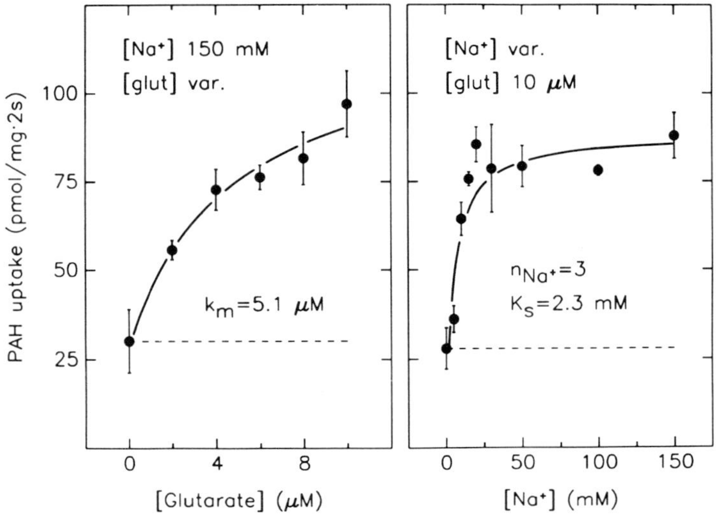

Fig. 3. Kinetics of cis-stimulation by glutarate and Na^+ of PAH uptake into basolateral membrane vesicles. *Left panel:* Vesicles loaded with KCl were added to media containing 150 mM NaCl, 0.05 mM [^{3}H]PAH, and 0–10 μM Na_2 glutarate. The curve fitted to the experimental results was calculated using a Michaelis-Menten equation with the parameters, K_m, 5.1 μM and V_{max}, 91.3 pmol/mg·2s. The dashed line shows [^{3}H]PAH uptake in the absence of glutarate. *Right panel:* Vesicles were suspended in buffers containing 0–150 mM NaCl, 150–0 mM tetramethylammonium Cl, 0.05 mM [^{3}H]PAH, and 0.01 mM glutarate. The curve was fitted to the data points considering the interaction of 3 Na^+ ions and using the kinetic parameters K_s 2.3 mM and V_{max} 60.1 pmol/mg·2s. The dashed line indicates [^{3}H]PAH uptake in the absence of Na^+

2 PAH molecules are exchanged for one glutarate, or that a hitherto unknown intravesicular (intracellular) cation or extravesicular (extracellular) anion is also involved in the exchange process.

Conclusions and Outlook

Experimental evidence indicates that uphill PAH uptake across the basolateral membrane of proximal tubule cells requires the cooperation of three transport systems. The (Na^+ + K^+)-ATPase maintains an out > in Na^+ gradient across the basolateral membrane and an in > out K^+ gradient, which in turn is responsible for the inside negative electrical potential difference across the basolateral membrane. The electrogenic $(Na^+)_3$-dicarboxylate cotransporter utilizes the electrochemical gradient for Na^+ ions for uptake and intracellular accumulation of α-ketoglutarate. In a final step, α-ketoglutarate exchanges for extracellular PAH (or other suitable organic anions). Thus, uphill PAH transport is indirectly energized by the Na^+ gradient (tertiary active transport). From our studies α-ketoglutarate seems to be the

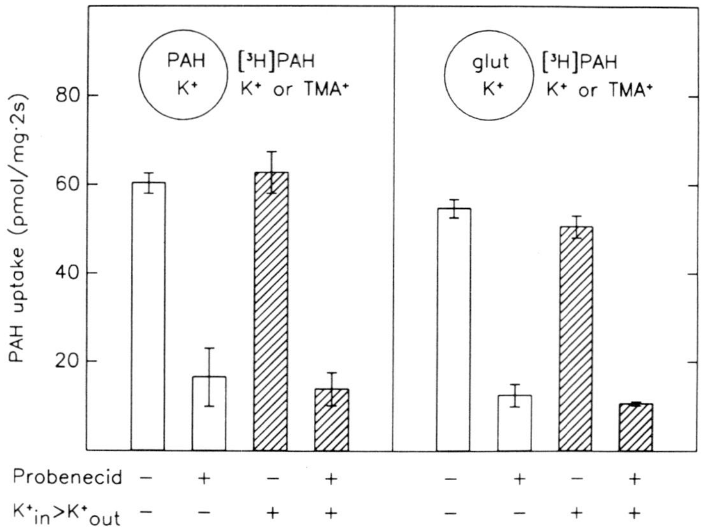

Fig. 4. Lack of effect of membrane potential on PAH/[^{3}H]PAH (*left*) and glutarate/[^{3}H]PAH exchange (*right*). Basolateral membrane vesicles were loaded with 150 mM KCl, either 1 mM PAH or glutarate, and suspended in 150 mM KCl or 150 mM tetramethylammonium (*TMA*$^+$) chloride ($K^+_{in} > K^+_{out}$) containing 5 μM valinomycin, 0.05 mM [^{3}H]PAH, and 0 or 1 mM probenecid. Uptake of [^{3}H]PAH was stopped after 2 s incubation time

only naturally occurring dicarboxylate which can be utilized in the coupled action of dicarboxylate and PAH transporters.

Data presented in this contribution suggest a physiologic role of the PAH transporter in translocation of long chain fatty acids, some steroid hormones and second messengers. The pharmacologically important role of this transport system relies on its ability to accept anionic xenobiotics and drugs and/or their metabolic products. The PAH transporter also plays an important pathophysiological role in cellular uptake and in the intracellular accumulation of toxic compounds which subsequently damage proximal tubule cells.

One of the questions remaining is the definition of PAH exit from the cell across the luminal membrane. Rabbit and pig proximal tubule cells possess in their brush-border membrane a conductive transport system for PAH [24,25]. Thereby, the inside electrical potential difference across this membrane can be utilized to drive PAH (and urate) out of the cell into the lumen. In brush-border membrane vesicles from rat and dog, however, a transport system has been found which can exchange PAH for succinate [26]. Since the rat renal brush-border membrane contains also a Na^+-coupled dicarboxylate transporter [27,28], PAH uptake would be favored rather than secretion, similar to the situation in the basolateral membrane. Net secretion may yet occur, due to different kinetic properties (affinities, maximal velocities) of the PAH transporters in the two membranes [29], or due to different substrate specificities, e.g., PAH/Cl^- and PAH/lactate exchange, in the brush-border [7,26,30], but not in the basolateral membrane. A detailed knowledge of organic anion uptake across the basolateral membrane and exit across the brush-border membrane may help in understanding and in preventing, the intracellular accumulation of nephrotoxic compounds.

Acknowledgments. The authors thank B. Moewes and G. Rumrich for their excellent technical assistance.

References

1. Despopoulos A (1965) A definition of substrate specificity in renal transport of organic anions. J Theor Biol 8:163–192
2. Møller JV, Sheikh MI (1983) Renal organic anion transport system: Pharmacological, physiological, and biochemical aspects. Pharmacol Rev 34:315–358
3. Weiner IM (1985) Organic acids and bases and uric acid. In: Seldin DW, Giebisch G (eds) The Kidney: Physiology and Pathophysiology. Raven, New York, pp 1703–1724
4. Fritzsch G, Rumrich G, Ullrich KJ (1989) Anion transport through the contraluminal cell membrane of renal proximal tubule. The influence of hydrophobicity and molecular charge distribution on the inhibitory activity of organic anions. Biochim Biophys Acta 978: 249–256
5. Ullrich KJ, Rumrich G (1988) Contraluminal transport systems in the proximal renal tubule involved in secretion of organic anions. Am J Physiol 254:F453–F462
6. Pritchard JB (1987) Luminal and peritubular steps in renal transport of *p*-aminohippurate. Biochim Biophys Acta 906:295–308
7. Pritchard JB (1988) Coupled transport of *p*-aminohippurate by rat kidney basolateral membrane vesicles. Am J Physiol 255:F597–F604
8. Shimada H, Moewes B, Burckhardt G (1987) Indirect coupling to Na^+ of *p*-aminohippuric acid uptake into rat renal basolateral membrane vesicles. Am J Physiol 253:F795–F801
9. Fritzsch G, Haase W, Rumrich G, Fasold H, Ullrich KJ (1984) A stopped flow capillary perfusion method to evaluate contraluminal transport parameters of methylsuccinate from interstitium into renal proximal tubular cells. Pflügers Arch 400:250–256
10. Ullrich KJ, Rumrich G, Fritzsch G, Klöss S (1987) Contraluminal para-aminohippurate transport in the proximal tubule of the rat kidney. I. Kinetics, influence of cations, anions, and capillary preperfusion. Pflügers Arch 409:229–235
11. Scalera V, Huang Y-K, Hildmann B, Murer H (1981) A simple isolation method for basallateral membranes from rat kidney cortex. Membr Biochem 4:49–61
12. Ullrich KJ, Fasold H, Rumrich G, Klöss S (1984) Secretion and contraluminal uptake of dicarboxylic acids in the proximal convolution of rat kidney. Pflügers Arch 400:241–249
13. Ullrich KJ, Rumrich G, Papavassiliou F, Klöss S, Fritzsch G (to be published) Contraluminal para-aminohippurate transport in the proximal tubule of the rat kidney. VII. Specificity: Cyclic nucleotides, eicosanoids. Pflügers Arch
14. Ullrich KJ, Rumrich G, Wieland Th, Dekant W (1989) Contraluminal para-aminohippurate transport in the proximal tubule of the rat kidney. VI. Specificity: Amino acids, their N-methyl-, N-acetyl and N-benzoylderivatives; glutathione- and cysteine conjugates, di- and oligopeptides. Pflügers Arch 415:342–350
15. Ullrich KJ, Rumrich G, Mark G, Dekant W (1990) Transformation and transport: How does metabolic transformation change the affinity for the renal contraluminal anion and cation transporters? In: International Symposium on "Renal Disposition and Nephrotoxicity of Xenobiotics." Toxicol Lett 53:19–27

16. Ullrich KJ, Rumrich G, Klöss S (1989) Contraluminal organic anion and cation transport in the proximal renal tubule: V. Interaction with sulfamoyl- and phenoxy diuretics, and with β-lactam antibiotics. Kidney Int 36:78–88
17. Cooper P (1979) The kidney and ochratoxin A. Food Cosmet Toxicol 17:406–408
18. Prast H, Pfaller W (1988) Toxic properties of the mushroom *Cortinarius orellanus (Fries)*. II. Impairment of renal function in rats. Arch Toxicol 62:89–96
19. Fiume L, Marinozzi V, Nardi F (1969) The effect of amanitin poisoning on mouse kidney. Br J Exp Pathol 50:270–276
20. Burckhardt G, Ullrich KJ (1989) Organic anion transport across the contraluminal membrane–dependence on sodium. Kidney Int 36:370–377
21. Burckhardt G (1984) Sodium-dependent dicarboxylate transport in rat renal basolateral membrane vesicles. Pflügers Arch 401:254–261
22. Wright SH, Wunz TM (1987) Succinate and citrate transport in renal basolateral and brush-border membranes. Am J Physiol 253:F432–F439
23. Wright SH, Kippen I, Wright EM (1982) Stoichiometry of Na^+-succinate cotransport in renal brush-border Membranes. J Biol Chem 257:1773–1778
24. Martinez F, Manganel M, Montrose-Rafizadeh C, Werner D, Roch-Ramel F (1990) Transport of urate and *p*-aminohippurate in rabbit renal brush-border membranes. Am J Physiol 258:F1145–F1153
25. Werner D, Martinez F, Roch-Ramel F (1990) Urate and *p*-aminohippurate transport in the brush border membrane of the pig kidney. J Pharmacol Exp Ther 252:792–799
26. Guggino SE, Martin GJ, Aronson PS (1983) Specificity and modes of the anion exchanger in dog renal microvillus membranes. Am J Physiol 244:F612–F621
27. Kahn AM, Branham S, Weinman EJ (1984) Mechanism of L-malate transport in rat renal basolateral membrane vesicles. Am J Physiol 246:F779–F784
28. Sheridan E, Rumrich G, Ullrich KJ (1983) Reabsorption of dicarboxylic acids from the proximal convolution of rat kidney. Pflügers Arch 399:18–28
29. Kinsella JL, Holohan PD, Pessah NI, Ross CR (1979) Transport of organic ions in renal cortical luminal and antiluminal membrane vesicles. J Pharmacol Exp Ther 209:443–450
30. Kahn AM, Aronson PS (1983) Urate transport via anion exchange in dog renal microvillus membrane vesicles. Am J Physiol 244:F56–F63
31. Ullrich KJ, Rumrich G, Fritzsch G, Klöss S (1987) Contraluminal para-aminohippurate transport in the proximal tubule of the rat kidney. II. Specificity: Aliphatic dicarboxylic acids. Pflügers Arch 408:38–45
32. Ullrich KJ, Rumrich G, Klöss S (1987) Contraluminal para-aminohippurate transport in the proximal tubule of the rat kidney. III. Specificity: monocarboxylic acids. Pflügers Arch 409:547–554

Organic Cation Transport in the Renal Brush-Border and Basolateral Membranes

KEN-ICHI INUI[1], MIKIHISA TAKANO, and RYOHEI HORI[2]

SUMMARY. To characterize the specific membrane events underlying the secretion of organic cations in the proximal tubules, the transport of tetraethylammonium (TEA), a prototype cation, has been studied, using brush-border and basolateral membrane vesicles isolated from rat renal cortex. TEA is transported across basolateral membranes via a carrier-mediated system, and this system is stimulated by an inside-negative membrane potential. The transport of TEA across brush-border membranes is driven by an H^+ gradient via an electroneutral H^+/organic cation antiport system. Aminocephalosporins such as cephalexin (an amphoteric molecule) share a common carrier transport system with TEA in brush-border membranes. The H^+/organic cation antiport system is very sensitive to pH (optimum pH 7.0), in contrast to organic anion and D-glucose transport systems. Sulfhydryl groups and histidine residues are essential for the H^+/organic cation antiport system in renal brush-border membranes.

Introduction

The function of the proximal tubule is to reabsorb solutes such as glucose and amino acids from the glomerular filtrate, and to secrete organic ions. Active secretion of organic ions in the proximal tubules is viewed as a means of eliminating many drugs and their metabolites from the body. The sequence of movement of organic ions is transport across basolateral membranes, accumulation in the cell, followed by efflux from the cell across brush-border membranes into the tubular fluid. Although the molecules secreted by the organic cation secretory mechanism have a variety of chemical structures, all contain a nitrogen atom carrying a positive charge at the

[1]Department of Hospital Pharmacy, School of Medicine, Tokyo Medical and Dental University, Bunkyo-ku, Tokyo, 113 Japan
[2]Department of Pharmacy, Kyoto University Hospital, Faculty of Medicine, Kyoto University, Sakyo-ku, Kyoto, 606 Japan

physiological pH. Numerous techniques have been used for studying the renal excretion of cations, including in vivo renal clearance and in vitro cortical slices. These techniques have generated a great deal of information about the overall sequence of events. However, it has been difficult to characterize the specific membrane events underlying the transepithelial transport of organic cations. In addition, transport studies with organic cations in intact tissues are limited because these compounds often lead to circulatory disturbances.

In recent years, a methodology has been developed for isolating the brush-border and basolateral membrane vesicles from renal cortex; the membrane vesicles have been used for the analysis of tubular transport of nutrients and organic ions in well-controlled conditions [1]. To obtain precise information about the mechanisms of tubular secretion of organic ions, we have studied the transport characteristics of p-aminohippurate (anion), tetraethylammonium (cation), and aminocephalosporin antibiotics (zwitterion) in brush-border and basolateral membranes. This article deals with the characteristics of organic cation transport systems in renal brush-border and basolateral membranes.

Organic Cation Transport Systems in Brush-Border and Basolateral Membranes

Brush-border and basolateral membrane vesicles were isolated from rat renal cortex by the methods of calcium precipitation and Percoll density gradient centrifugation, respectively [2].

To characterize organic cation transport systems, the uptake of tetraethylammonium, a prototype cation, was studied using brush-border and basolateral membrane vesicles [3]. In the concentration dependence of [^{3}H]tetraethylammonium uptake, the relationship between concentration and uptake rate was nonlinear in both membranes, providing evidence for saturability. After correction for the nonsaturable component, the kinetic values of K_m and V_{max} were 0.8 mM and 7.4 nmol/mg protein per min for brush-border membranes, and 2.5 mM and 5.6 nmol/mg protein per min for basolateral membranes, respectively. Vesicles preloaded with a high concentration of unlabeled tetraethylammonium showed enhancement of [^{3}H]tetraethylammonium accumulation by countertransport in brush-border and basolateral membranes. The countertransport effect, or trans-stimulation, is a criterion for carrier-mediated transport. These data suggest the contribution of a carrier-mediated transport system for tetraethylammonium in brush-border and basolateral membranes.

To obtain further information concerning the driving force of the transport, we studied the effect of various ionic conditions on the uptake of tetraethylammonium. Although ionic conditions had no effect on tetraethylammonium uptake in basolateral membranes, the presence of an outward sodium gradient stimulated the tetraethylammonium uptake by brush-border membrane vesicles; sodium chloride was inside the vesicles and potassium chloride was outside. Furthermore, by monitoring the changes in fluorescence of Acridine orange, we confirmed the intravesicular acidification of brush-border membrane vesicles with sodium inside and potassium outside. Therefore, the H^+ gradient was tested as to whether it could drive the active transport of tetraethylammonium.

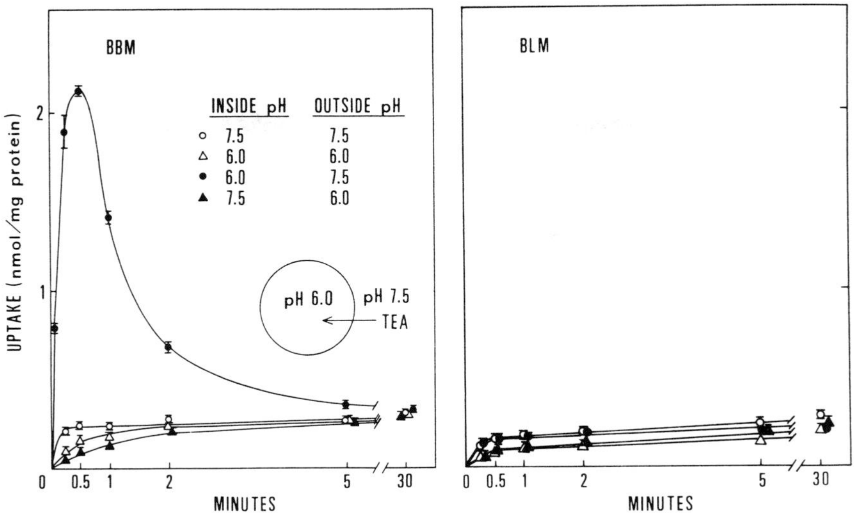

Fig. 1. Effect of H^+ gradient on tetraethylammonium (*TEA*) uptake by brush-border (*BBM*) and basolateral membrane (*BLM*) vesicles. (From [3] with permission)

Figure 1 shows the effect of H^+ gradient on tetraethylammonium uptake by brush-border and basolateral membrane vesicles [3]. In brush-border membranes, the presence of an outward H^+ gradient (inside pH 6.0, outside pH 7.5) induced a transient uphill transport of tetraethylammonium (overshoot phenomenon), while an inward H^+ gradient resulted in the lowest uptake. The final levels of uptake were all identical, indicating that the pH gradient did not affect vesicle size. In contrast, the H^+ gradient was ineffective in the transport of tetraethylammonium in basolateral membranes. These data strongly suggest that tetraethylammonium transport across brush-border membranes is driven actively by an outward H^+ gradient: that is, an H^+/organic cation antiport system.

It is important to clarify the role of membrane potential as a driving force in tetraethylammonium uptake by brush-border and basolateral membrane vesicles. To produce an inside-negative membrane potential, the potassium ionophore valinomycin was employed in the presence of an outward potassium gradient. Tetraethylammonium uptake by brush-border membrane vesicles was unaffected by valinomycin. In contrast, a valinomycin-induced inside-negative membrane potential significantly stimulated the initial rate of tetraethylammonium uptake by basolateral membrane vesicles.

These data suggest that tetraethylammonium is transported across basolateral membranes via a carrier-mediated system, which is stimulated by an inside-negative membrane potential. Tetraethylammonium transport across brush-border membranes is driven by an H^+ gradient via an electroneutral H^+/organic cation antiport system. These characteristics of an organic cation transport system are very different from those of an organic anion transport system [4–6].

Furthermore, the transport of other widely used drugs was examined in relation to the organic cation transport system. Cimetidine, a potent histamine H_2-receptor antagonist, is a weak organic base and its major route of elimination is in the urine. Cimetidine inhibited tetraethylammonium uptake by brush-border and basolateral membrane vesicles. In agreement with the tetraethylammonium transport mechanisms found in brush-border membranes, the presence of an outward H^+ gradient induced a marked stimulation of cimetidine uptake against its concentration gradient, and this concentrative uptake was inhibited by tetraethylammonium. These results suggest that cimetidine shares a common carrier system with tetraethylammonium in brush-border and basolateral membranes [7].

Aminocephalosporin antibiotics such as cephalexin are amphoteric molecules, having both amino and carboxyl groups, and, at physiological pH, are ionized mostly as zwitterions and anions. It has been thought that most cephalosporin antibiotics are actively secreted into the proximal tubules via an organic anion transport system. However, during the course of our studies of cephalosporin transport, we found that aminocephalosporins can be transported via H^+/organic cation antiport systems in renal brush-border membranes [8]. Cephalexin uptake by brush-border membrane vesicles was markedly stimulated in the presence of an outward H^+ gradient, and was inhibited in the presence of tetraethylammonium.

In addition, it was noted that apical membranes isolated from the LLC-PK_1 pig kidney epithelial cell line retained tetraethylammonium transport characteristics similar to those observed in renal brush-border membranes [9].

pH Sensitivity of the H^+/Organic Cation Antiport System in Renal Brush-Border Membranes

The time course of tetraethylammonium uptake was examined in the presence of various H^+ gradients, with a fixed extravesicular pH of 7.2 [10]. In spite of the increase of an outward H^+ gradient, the initial uptake rate of tetraethylammonium decreased at pH 5.7 and 5.2, compared with that at pH 6.2. These results suggest that pH, as well as an H^+ gradient, is an important factor in regulating the activity of the H^+/organic cation antiport system. To verify this possibility, we studied the pH profile of tetraethylammonium uptake by brush-border membrane vesicles in the absence of an H^+ gradient. As shown in Fig. 2, the uptake of tetraethylammonium for 30 s was maximum at pH 7.0, and at an acidic pH or an alkaline pH the uptake decreased [10]. However, the uptake for 30 min did not change in the indicated pH regions. Therefore, the inactivation was not considered to be due to the decrease in intravesicular space, but to the decrease in the activity of the H^+/organic cation antiport system.

We also examined the pH dependence of tetraethylammonium uptake by basolateral membrane vesicles compared with that in brush-border membranes. The uptake of tetraethylammonium for 30 s and 30 min did not change in the neutral pH regions, but decreased similarly in the acidic pH regions. Thus, the pH dependence of tetraethylammonium uptake in basolateral membranes was very different from that in brush-border membranes.

The uptake of tetraethylammonium, p-aminohippurate, and D-glucose in the absence of an H^+ gradient was compared at pH 6.0, 7.0, and 8.0. The transport of p-aminohippurate and D-glucose had no optimum pH in the range of 6.0–8.0. These results suggest that the H^+/organic cation antiport system, exclusively, is sensitive to pH, and is activated at pH 7.0.

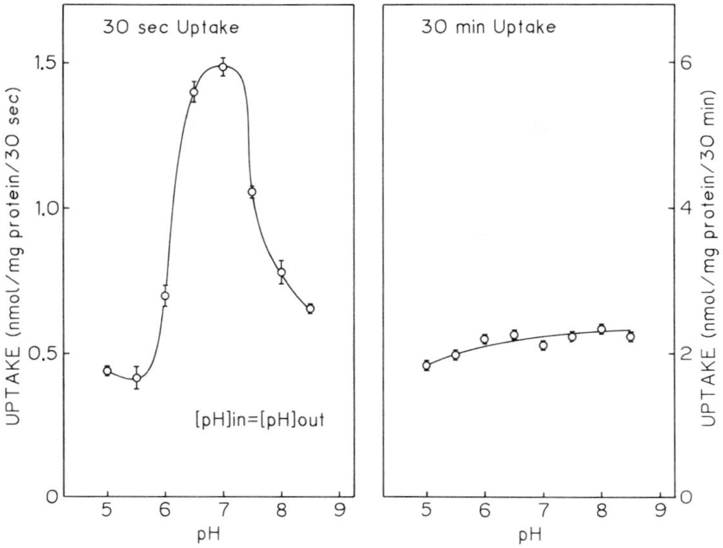

Fig. 2. pH Dependence of tetraethylammonium uptake by brush-border membrane vesicles (without H^+ gradient). (From [10] with permission)

For the kinetic parameters at an acidic pH, the K_m value increased significantly without any change in V_{max} value, compared with the values at pH 7.0. In contrast, at an alkaline pH, the V_{max} value decreased significantly without any change in K_m value. From these data, the activity of the H^+/organic cation antiport system was considered to be inhibited at an acidic pH due to the increase in K_m value, and was considered to be inhibited at an alkaline pH due to the decrease in V_{max} value.

Effect of Chemical Modifiers on the H^+/Organic Cation Antiport System

We examined the uptake of tetraethylammonium, in the absence of H^+ gradient, by brush-border membrane vesicles pretreated with p-chloromercuribenzene sulfonate (PCMBS), a sulfhydryl reagent, at various concentrations [11]. The initial rate of tetraethylammonium uptake decreased in a dose-dependent manner in the vesicles pretreated with PCMBS (IC_{50} = 38 μM). The inhibitory effect of PCMBS pretreatment was protected by preincubation with unlabeled tetraethylammonium.

The reversibility of the effect of PCMBS by subsequent treatment with thiols was examined. The inhibition of tetraethylammonium uptake was reversed almost to the control level by subsequent treatment of the vesicles with 10 mM dithiothreitol, glutathione, or cysteine. These results suggested that sulfhydryl reagent inhibits the transport of tetraethylammonium by specific interaction with the active sites of the carrier, and that sulfhydryl groups are essential as binding sites for substrate in the organic cation transport system in renal brush-border membranes. In the kidney,

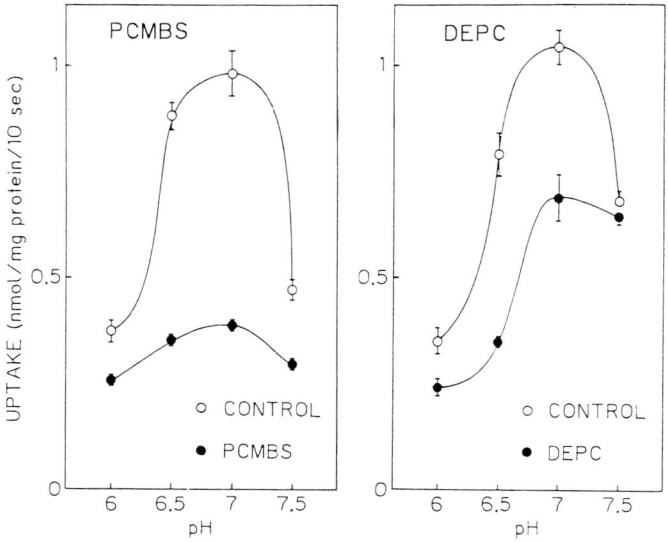

Fig. 3a,b. Tetraethylammonium uptake at various pH values by brush-border membrane vesicles pretreated with **a** p-chloromercuribenzene sulphonate (PCMBS) and with **b** diethyl pyrocarbonate (DEPC) (without H^+ gradient). (From [12] with permission)

glutathione is synthesized intracellularly and is translocated through the cell membranes. Therefore, endogenous thiols, such as glutathione and cysteine, may protect the functional sulfhydryl groups of the organic cation transport system against oxidative stress in vivo.

Furthermore, we studied the effect of diethyl pyrocarbonate (DEPC), a histidine modifying reagent, on the H^+/organic cation antiport system in brush-border membranes [12]. The overshoot uptake of tetraethylammonium was markedly inhibited by pretreatment of the vesicles with DEPC. We also examined tetraethylammonium uptake for 10 s and 30 min in the absence of an H^+ gradient using vesicles pretreated with DEPC. With DEPC pretreatment at concentrations of 0.01–1 mM, tetraethylammonium uptake for 30 min did not change but it decreased at higher concentrations. The uptake of tetraethylammonium for 10 s decreased in a concentration-dependent manner in vesicles pretreated with DEPC. The uptake decreased to 75% at 0.5 mM DEPC. These results indicate that DEPC directly inactivates the H^+/organic cation antiport system. The uptake of p-aminohippurate for 10 s and 30 min decreased when treated with DEPC only at the higher concentrations of 5 and 10 mM. Judging from the uptake for 30 min, the intravesicular space seemed to decrease when treated with 5 mM DEPC.

It has been reported that DEPC reacts not only with histidine residues, but also with sulfhydryl groups in some conditions, and that hydroxylamine can reverse the DEPC modification of histidine residues but not the DEPC modification of sulfhydryl groups. The inhibitory effect of DEPC pretreatment on tetraethylammonium uptake for 10 s was reversed significantly by subsequent treatment of the vesicles with 0.5 M hydroxylamine. However, there was no restoration of tetraethylammonium

Table 1. Characteristics of organic cation transport systems in renal brush-border and basolateral membranes

	Brush-border membrane	Basolateral membrane
Transport system	H^+/organic cation antiport	Carrier-mediated
Driving force	H^+ gradient	Membrane potential
Electrogenicity	Neutral	Electrogenic
Optimum pH	7.0	6.5 - 8.5
Functional moiety	Sulfhydryl groups	?
	Histidine residues	
	Carboxyl groups	
Substrate	Tetraethylammonium	Tetraethylammonium
	N^1-methylnicotinamde	N^1-Methylnicotinamide
	Cimetidine	Cimetidine
	Aminocephalosporins etc.	others

uptake on subsequent treatment with dithiothreitol, which could reverse the inhibition induced by PCMBS pretreatment. These results suggest that under the present experimental conditions DEPC reacted specifically with histidine residues, but not with sulfhydryl groups.

Figure 3 shows tetraethylammonium uptake, at various pH values, by brush-border membrane vesicles pretreated with DEPC and PCMBS [12]. Tetraethylammonium uptake for 10 s at pH 6.0–7.0, but not at pH 7.5, was inhibited by pretreatment with 1 mM DEPC (Fig. 3**b**), although the uptake for 30 min was not affected at various pH values by pretreatment with DEPC. In contrast, the uptake of tetraethylammonium for 10 s in the pH range used was inhibited by pretreatment with PCMBS (Fig. 3**a**). In the DEPC-pretreated vesicles, the V_{max} value of tetraethylammonium uptake at pH 7.0 decreased significantly without a change in the K_m value. Unlabeled tetraethylammonium had no protective effect on the inhibition of tetraethylammonium uptake by DEPC pretreatment. The data suggest that histidine residues in the carrier do not interact with the substrate, but may play a role in the regulation of H^+ transfer in this transport system.

Conclusion

Based on the data above, the characteristics of organic cation transport systems are summarized in Table 1. Tetraethylammonium is transported from blood to cell across basolateral membranes via a carrier-mediated system; this process is stimulated by the intracellular negative membrane potential. Tetraethylammonium transport from cell to urine across brush-border membranes is driven by an H^+ gradient via an electroneutral H^+/organic cation antiport system. The H^+ gradient can be created by a Na^+/H^+ antiport system and an ATP-driven H^+-pump in brush-border membranes. The H^+/organic cation antiport system in brush-border membranes is very sensitive to pH, in contrast to other transport systems in brush-border membranes and the organic cation transport system in basolateral membranes. Thus, pH is an important factor in regulating the activity of the H^+/organic cation antiport. Sulfhydryl groups and histidine residues are essential for the organic cation transport system in renal brush-border membranes. These studies provide new insight into our understanding of the regulatory mechanisms of organic cation transport in renal brush-border and basolateral membranes.

References

1. Murer H, Gmaj P (1986) Transport studies in plasma membrane vesicles isolated from renal cortex. Kidney Int 30:171–186
2. Inui K, Okano T, Takano M, Kitazawa S, Hori R (1981) A simple method for the isolation of basolateral plasma membrane vesicles from rat kidney cortex: Enzyme activities and some properties of glucose transport. Biochim Biophys Acta 647:150–154
3. Takano M, Inui K, Okano T, Saito H, Hori R (1984) Carrier-mediated transport systems of tetraethylammonium in rat renal brush-border and basolateral membrane vesicles. Biochim Biophys Acta 773:113–124
4. Hori R, Takano M, Okano T, Kitazawa S, Inui K (1982) Mechanisms of p-aminohippurate transport by brush-border and basolateral membrane vesicles isolated from rat kidney cortex. Biochim Biophys Acta 692:97–100
5. Inui K, Takano M, Okano T, Hori R (1986) Role of chloride on carrier-mediated transport of p-aminohippurate in rat renal basolateral membrane vesicles. Biochim Biophys Acta 855:425–428
6. Hori R, Takano M, Okano T, Inui K (1985) Transport of p-aminohippurate, tetraethylammonium and D-glucose in renal brush border membranes from rats with acute renal failure. J Pharmacol Exp Ther 233:776–781
7. Takano M, Inui K, Okano T, Hori R (1985) Cimetidine transport in rat renal brush border and basolateral membrane vesicles. Life Sci 37:1579–1585
8. Inui K, Takano M, Okano T, Hori R (1985) H^+ Gradient dependent transport of aminocephalosporins in rat renal brush border membrane vesicles: Role of H^+/organic cation antiport system. J Pharmacol Exp Ther 233:181–185
9. Inui K, Saito H, Hori R (1985) H^+ Gradient-dependent active transport of tetraethylammonium cation in apical-membrane vesicles isolated from kidney epithelial cell line LLC-PK_1. Biochem J 227:199–203
10. Maegawa H, Kato M, Inui K, Hori R (1988) pH Sensitivity of H^+/organic cation antiport system in rat renal brush-border membranes. J Biol Chem 263:11150–11154
11. Hori R, Maegawa H, Okano T, Takano M, Inui K (1987) Effect of sulfhydryl reagents on tetraethylammonium transport in rat renal brush border membranes. J Pharmacol Exp Ther 241:1010–1016
12. Hori R, Maegawa H, Kato M, Katsura T, Inui K (1989) Inhibitory effect of diethyl pyrocarbonate on the H^+/organic cation antiport system in rat renal brush-border membranes. J Biol Chem 264:12232–12237

Urate Transport in Mammalian Nephron

FRANÇOISE ROCH-RAMEL and DOMINIQUE WERNER[1]

SUMMARY. The differences in renal handling of urate by mammals are discussed, focusing on the main role played by the proximal tubule, which is responsible for urate secretion, as well as for most urate reabsorption. The membrane mechanisms involved in urate transport are different in urate reabsorbing and urate secreting species. Brush-border membranes of rats and dogs (urate reabsorbers) possess a urate/anion exchanger which accepts various organic anions as well as chloride, bicarbonate, and hydroxyl ions. Pigs and rabbits (urate secreters) do not possess this anion exchanger, but have a potential-dependent facilitated mechanism which favors urate efflux from cell to lumen. The basolateral membranes of rats (urate reabsorbers) have urate/chloride exchangers, whereas those of pigs (urate secreters) have urate/2-oxoglutarate exchangers, which, coupled to the activity of the sodium dicarboxylate cotransport, allows urate to concentrate into the cells.

Introduction

In man and closely related primates, uric acid is the end product of purine metabolism, whereas in other mammals, it is further broken down to allantoin by uricase, an enzyme which is missing in man. Due to lack of uricase activity, the plasma concentration of uric acid in man is higher than in other mammals [1]. In all mammals, urate, being little bound to plasma proteins, is freely filtered; it then undergoes transtubular bidirectional transport. Depending on the relative importance of the secretory and reabsorptive fluxes, urinary excretion exceeds filtered load (net secretion) or is smaller than filtered load (net reabsorption) [1]. Thus, large species differences have been observed, fractional excretion of urate (Curate/GFR) varying from about 10% in man to 100%–300% in pigs [1] (for a more complete report, see [2]).

[1]Institut de Pharmacologie de l'Université de Lausanne, CH-1005 Lausanne, Switzerland

Even within one species, important variations have been reported. For example, a few patients with hypouricemia were observed to excrete urate by net secretion [3]. Also, the case of the Dalmatian coach hound which, in contrast to mongrel dogs, excretes urate by net secretion, is well known [4]. Hereafter, we shall call mammalian species which excrete urate by net secretion, at normal or slightly elevated concentrations of urate in the plasma "urate secreters", and mammals which excrete less urate than is filtered, "urate reabsorbers."

Tubular Handling of Urate

The net transport of urate along the nephron was investigated in vivo, in tubular micropuncture experiments.

"Urate Reabsorbers"

In anesthetized non-diuretic rats, at endogenous plasma concentration of urate (35–60 μM), the fractional excretion of urate is about 30%. By using a sensitive and specific method for urate determination (high-performance liquid chromatography (HPLC) and amperometric detection), the fractional delivery of urate to the late proximal convoluted tubules was shown to be about 35%–50%, while that to the early distal tubules was close to 35% [5,6]. Most of the reabsorption appears thus to occur before the convoluted distal tubule. The same is true for deep nephrons, since fractional delivery of urate to Henle's loop of deep nephrons (micropuncture at the tip of the papilla) is about 35% [6]. The lower parts of the nephron are little permeable to urate (for review see [2]). For ethical reasons, tubular micropuncture experiments can obviously not be done in man. However, such experiments were performed on the Cebus monkey, a mammal which, as does man, excretes only a small fraction of the filtered load (about 3–4% in nondiuretic state) [7]. As in rats, urate reabsorption occurs mainly before early distal convolutions (Fig. 1). In mongrel dogs, also, proximal tubule is the main site of urate reabsorption [4].

"Urate Secreters"

In the pig, the fractional delivery of urate to proximal convoluted tubules largely exceeds the filtered load (Fig. 2), demonstrating net secretion along the convoluted proximal tubule [8]. In the Dalmatian coach hound, net secretion occurs mainly along the pars recta [4].

Characterization of Unidirectional Fluxes of Urate

The proximal tubule being the main site of urate transport, attempts have been made to characterize the secretory and reabsorptive fluxes by using in situ or in vitro tubular microperfusion techniques (for review, see [9]). In situ experiments were performed only in rats, a species in which the kidney can be immobilized well enough

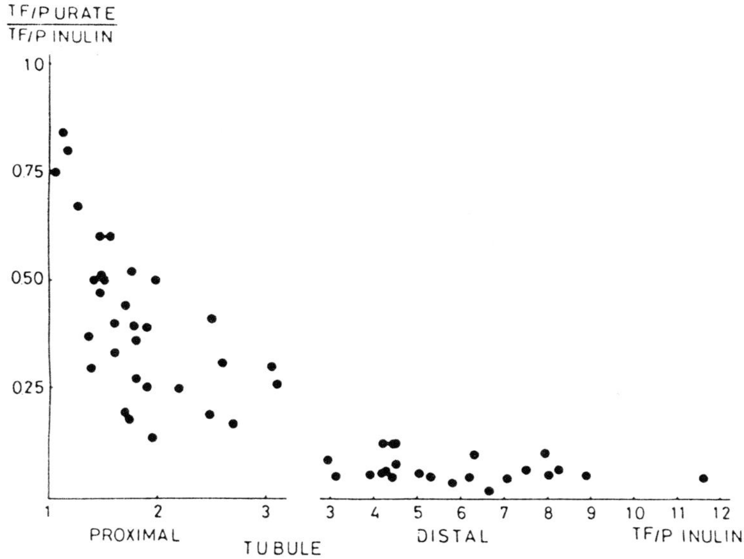

Fig. 1. Fractional deliveries of urate to proximal and distal tubules of Cebus monkeys. The fractional deliveries of urate ($TF/P_{urate}/TF/P_{inulin}$) to the sites of micropuncture are displayed as a function of TF/P_{inulin}. Mean endogenous urate concentration in the plasma was: 190 ± 30 μM. Fractional excretion of urate in the pelvic urine was: 3.3% ± 0.3% and that of water was: 1.4% ± 0.1%. At the end of the proximal convoluted tubule, about 75% of urate has already been reabsorbed as demonstrated by the low fractional delivery ($TF/P_{urate}/TF/P_{inulin} = 0.25$) to this site. At early distal convolutions, 90% of urate has been reabsorbed ($TF/P_{urate}/TF/P_{inulin} = 0.1$). TF/P_{urate}, ratio of urate concentrations in tubular fluid (*TF*) and in plasma (*P*); TF/P_{inulin}, ratio of inulin concentrations in TF and P. (From [7] with permission)

to allow microperfusion of tubular segments and of peritubular capillaries. In vitro perfusion experiments were performed on proximal tubules of rabbits and mice.

"Urate Reabsorbers" (Rats and Mice)

Reabsorption

In rats, it was clearly demonstrated that the reabsorption of urate is not directly coupled to that of sodium [10]. Urate reabsorption (see [9] for ref.) is saturable, but at rather high concentrations (about 0.5mM). It is inhibited by many organic anions, such as probenecid, pyrazinoate, furosemide, *para*-aminohippuric acid (PAH), as well as by SITS and DIDS when added to the tubular lumen (cis-inhibition) [9]. When added to the basolateral side by perfusion into peritubular capillaries, PAH stimulates urate reabsorption (trans-stimulation) [9], demonstrating that urate can be exchanged with PAH across the tubular epithelium. The characteristics of this exchange mechanism have been investigated independently in brush-border and basolateral membranes (see below).

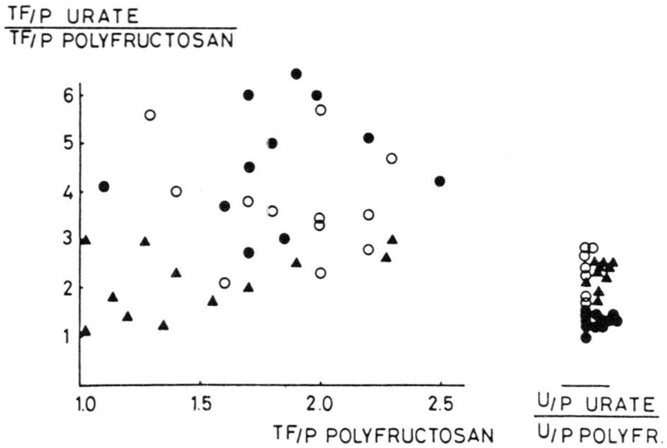

Fig. 2. Fractional excretion and fractional deliveries of urate to proximal tubules of pigs. The fractional deliveries of urate ($TF/P_{urate}/TF/P_{polyfructosan}$) to the sites of micropuncture in proximal tubules are displayed as a function of $TF/P_{polyfructosan}$ (polyfructosan is an analogue of inuline). Fractional excretion in pelvic urine is given by the $U/P_{urate}/U/P_{polyfructosan}$ ratio. Data are from 2 pigs, at endogenous concentration of urate in the plasma (3 μM, ●), 2 pigs at 21 μM (o), and 2 pigs at 95 μM (▲). At all plasma levels, fractional deliveries exceeded the filtration load ($TF/P_{urate}/TF/P_{polyfructosan} > 1$), demonstrating net secretion. (Data from [8] with permission)

Reabsorption was measured in vitro in mice proximal tubule [11]. As in rats, probenecid inhibits urate reabsorption when added to the lumen. It also inhibits reabsorption when added to the basolateral site (bathing medium) as it penetrates into the tubular lumen by secretion.

Secretion

In rats, in vivo tubular microperfusion demonstrated that the urate secretory flux is saturable. As for reabsorption, saturation is observed at rather high concentrations of urate (1 mM) (for ref., see [9]). When added to the peritubular site, probenecid and PAH inhibit secretion (cis-inhibition) [9]. When added to the lumen, PAH stimulates urate secretion (trans-stimulation). SITS, which inhibits anion exchangers, decreased the urate secretory flux when applied in the lumen or at the peritubular site [9].

"Urate Secreters" (Rabbits)

Reabsorption

In the rabbit, urate reabsorption was measured in the S_2 segments of proximal tubules, using in vitro microperfusion techniques. The reabsorptive flux was found to be of low magnitude, temperature independent [12], and not sensitive to probenecid [13]. Such data would suggest that reabsorption occurs by simple diffusion. However, as urate is not liposoluble, reabsorption by transcellular simple diffusion seems unlikely, although a facilitated transport has not been demonstrated.

Secretion

The secretory flux of urate was measured in all three proximal segments (S_1, S_2, S_3) of the rabbit. This flux can occur against an electrochemical gradient, is saturable, inhibitable by probenecid, and is larger in S_2 than in S_1 and S_3 segments [13]. PAH inhibits the cellular accumulation of urate in non-perfused proximal tubule, showing that these 2 organic anions compete for the same transporter at the basolateral membrane, i.e., for the first step of urate secretion. The intracellular concentration of urate can exceed that in the incubation medium, showing active transport at the basolateral membrane [14]. Similar data were obtained in non-perfused proximal tubules of pigs [15].

Transport of Urate in Membrane Vesicles

Brush-Border Membranes

"Urate Reabsorbers"

In contrast to other endogenous compounds such as aminoacids, lactate, and glucose, no sodium urate cotransport has been demonstrated in brush border membranes of urate reabsorbers [16,17]. This lack of direct sodium-urate cotransport is in agreement with in vivo findings, as reported above.

Blomstedt and Aronson [18] first demonstrated the presence of a mediated transport for urate in brush border membrane vesicles prepared from dog renal cortex, which allowed urate/OH^- exchange (or urate/H^+-cotransport). Thus, the imposition of an outwardly directed hydroxyl ion gradient (pH in = 7.5, pH out = 6) stimulates urate uptake into vesicles (Fig. 3). Further studies demonstrated that this transport mechanism is a urate-anion exchanger having affinity for a wide variety of anions, including chloride, lactate, succinate, etc. [19,20]. Another mechanism was also demonstrated, which is dependent on the activity of a membrane associated uricase [21].

"Urate Secreters"

Urate transport into brush-border membrane vesicles was investigated in rabbits and pigs, two urate secreters. In these "urate secreters" no urate-anion exchanger was demonstrated. However, another transport mechanism was observed. It was demonstrated in the pig [22] that urate uptake into (BBMV) vesicles was stimulated and exceeded chemical equilibrium when an electropositive intravesicular space was created by applying an inwardly directed potassium gradient in the presence of the potassium ionophore, valinomycin (Fig. 4). The same was observed in rabbits, although the stimulation was much smaller and no overshoot in concentration was observed [23]. PAH appears to share this transport mechanism with urate. It should be mentioned that in dogs and rats, the stimulation of urate uptake by the creation of an electropositive intravesicular space, per se, has not been specifically studied. It might be that part of the stimulation of urate uptake observed in the presence of a pH gradient might be due to an effect of potential [16,17].

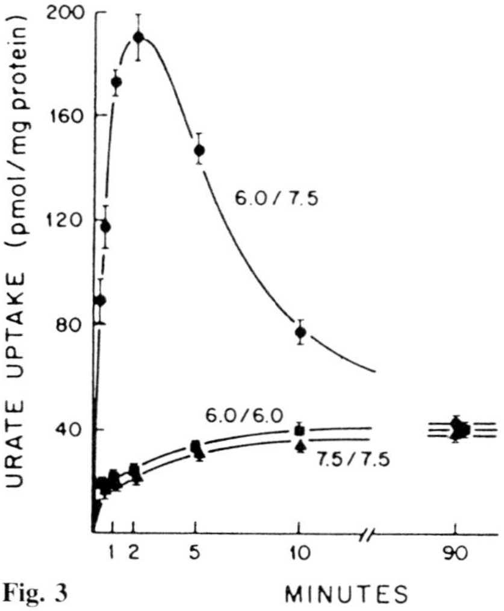

Fig. 3

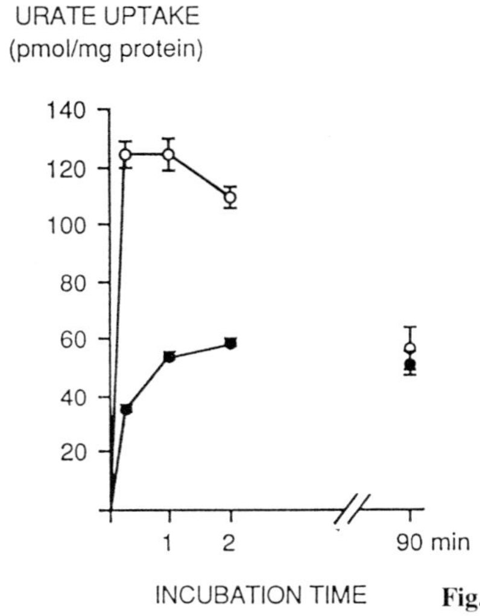

Fig. 4

Fig. 3. Effect of an outwardly directed hydroxyl ion gradient on urate uptake by dog brush-border membrane vesicles (BBMV). ▲, 7.5/7.5: Membrane vesicles were preincubated for 120 min at 20°C in 170 mM mannitol, 42 mM Tris, 67 mM Hepes, 36 mM K^+, and 18 mM sulfate at pH 7.5, and then uptake of 22 μM urate was assayed in the presence of 155 mM mannitol, 8 mM Tris, 13 mM Hepes, 104 mM K^+, 4 mM sulfate, and 52 mM phosphate at pH 7.5; ●, 6.0/7.5: Membranes were similarly preincubated at pH 7.5, but urate uptake was assayed in the presence of 200 mM mannitol, 8 mM Tris, 13 mM Hepes, 60 mM K^+, 4 mM sulfate, and 52 mM phosphate at pH 6.0; ■, 6.0/6.0: Membranes were preincubated in 200 mM mannitol, 42 mM Tris, 67 mM Hepes, and 18 mM sulfate at pH 6.0, and then urate uptake was assayed in the presence of 180 mM mannitol, 8 mM Tris, 13 mM Hepes, 60 mM K^+, 4 mM sulfate, and 52 mM phosphate at pH 6.0. Each point represents the mean ± SE for three determinations. (Data are reproduced from the *Journal of Clinical Investigation* by copyright permission of the American Society for Clinical Investigation [18])

Fig. 4. Effect of an electropositive intravesicular space on urate uptake by pig brush-border membrane vesicles (BBMV). BBMV (prepared as described in [22]) were suspended in 300 mM mannitol and 20 mM HEPES-Tris at pH 7.4, with 6.0–8.0 μg of valinomycin per mg of protein (electropositive intravesicular space: o) or with an equivalent volume of ethanol (control: ●), and then uptake of 46 μM [^{14}C] urate was assayed in the presence of 99 mM mannitol, 120 mM K^+ gluconate, and 20 mM HEPES-Tris at pH 7.4. Data represent the mean ± S.E. of three experiments

Basolateral Membranes

Urate transport into basolateral membrane vesicles has been studied in only two species: the rat (urate reabsorber) and the pig (urate secreter).

"Urate Reabsorbers"

In rat basolateral membrane, urate transport was shown to be mediated by a mechanism sensitive to probenecid and DIDS [24]. In addition, an outwardly directed chloride gradient resulted in an enhancement of urate uptake. This stimulation, which was not secondary to the creation of a chloride diffusion potential, is compatible with a chloride/urate exchange mechanism. This transport system, unlike the luminal exchanger, has no affinity for PAH. No sodium cotransport of urate was observed, urate uptake being not stimulated by applying an inwardly directed sodium gradient [24]. As in rat brush border membrane, a transport mechanism dependent on membrane associated uricase has also been reported in basolateral membrane [21].

"Urate Secreters"

Recently, in pig basolateral membrane vesicles obtained from renal outer cortex, we also found no *direct* coupling between sodium and urate. Thus, the replacement of 150 mM potassium from extravesicular medium by 150 mM sodium did not stimulate urate uptake. However, we observed that the presence of sodium in the extravesicular medium could influence urate uptake by an *indirect* effect. This effect is similar to that reported for PAH transport in rat basolateral membranes [25], i.e., the uptake occurs by the coupling of a sodium/dicarboxylate cotransport with a dicarboxylate/urate exchange [26]. The cis-addition of 150 μM 2-oxoglutarate to the extravesicular medium, in the presence of an inwardly directed sodium gradient, stimulated urate transport, compared to the control condition in the absence of 2-oxoglutarate [26]. Although of low magnitude, a concentrative urate uptake was observed. This stimulation was not the consequence of an ion diffusion potential, as a voltage clamp was applied. Thus, in the pig, the basolateral step of urate secretion might be, at least in part, mediated by the coupling of a sodium/2-oxoglutarate cotransport with a 2-oxoglutarate/urate exchange.

General Conclusions

Reabsorption and secretion in urate reabsorbers and secreters are summarized in Fig. 5.

Replaced in the intact proximal tubule, the physiological conditions are such that the urate/anion exchanger demonstrated in brush-border membranes of "urate reabsorbers" favors urate reabsorption, as evidenced by the low fractional delivery of urate to the late proximal tubule (see above). Urate entry into the cell might occur in exchange with bicarbonate or OH^-, as well as with cell metabolites such as succinate, pyruvate, or lactate, etc. The cellular efflux of urate might be facilitated at the basolateral membrane by an exchange with chloride (exchange with other anions has been little investigated).

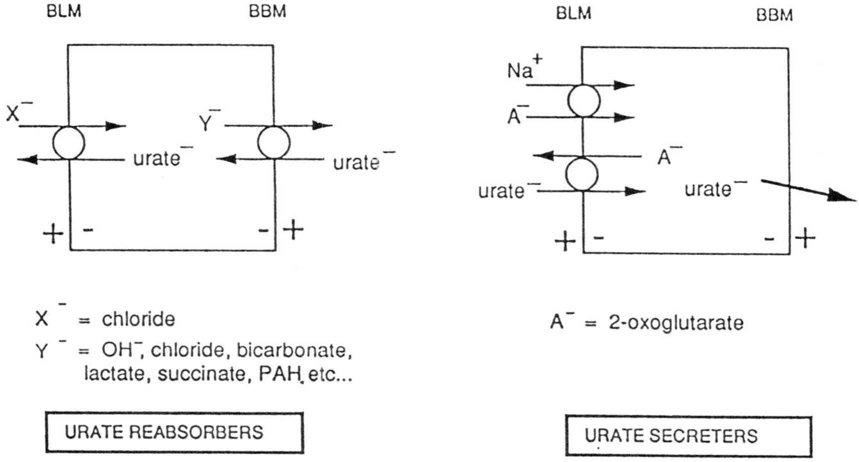

Fig. 5. Schematic representation of membrane mechanisms involved in urate transport BLM, basolateral membrane; BBM, brush-border membrane

The anion exchangers of each membrane can also allow the transport of urate in the secretory direction, depending on the anion present in the cell or in the lumen [20]. Anionic drugs, such as diuretics and uricosurics, might have affinity for the urate exchanger, and thus might favor reabsorption or secretion, depending on their concentrations in the lumen or in the blood capillaries.

In "urate secreters," the absence of the brush-border anion exchanger might explain the low rate of urate reabsorption. The mechanisms driven by electrical potential, demonstrated in pig and rabbit brush-border membranes, favor the efflux of urate into the lumen, which is positive compared to the cell. The physiological conditions are such that reabsorption is negligible. The anion exchanger present at the basolateral membrane, coupled to the activity of the Na^+/dicarboxylate cotransport, allows urate to concentrate into the cells.

References

1. Roch-Ramel F (1979) Renal excretion of uric acid in mammals. Clin Nephrol 12:1–6
2. Weiner IM (1979) Urate transport in the nephron. Am J Physiol 237:F85–F92
3. Sperling O (1989) Hereditary renal hypouricemia. In: Scriver CR, Beaudet AL, Sly WS, Valle D (eds) The metabolic basis of inherited disease, vol 1, 6th ed. McGraw-Hill, New York, pp 2605–2617
4. Roch-Ramel F, Wong NLM, Dirks JH (1976) Renal excretion of urate in mongrel and Dalmatian dogs: a micropuncture study. Am J Physiol 231:326–331
5. Roch-Ramel F, Granges F, Roth L, Widmer J, Weiner IM (1979/80) Renal handling of urate by nondiuretic and diuretic rats. HPLC-amperometric determination of urate concentrations. Renal Physiol 2:122–129
6. Frommer JP, Sheth AU, Senekjian HO, Babino H, Weinman EJ (1982) Free-flow micropuncture study of renal urate transport in the Munich-Wistar rat. Min Electrol Metab 7:324–330

7. Roch-Ramel F, Diezi-Chométy F, Roth L, Weiner IM (1980) A micropuncture study of urate excretion by Cebus monkeys employing high performance liquid chromatography with amperometric detection of urate. Pflugers Arch 383:203–207
8. Roch-Ramel F, White F, Vowles L, Simmonds HA, Cameron JS (1980) Micropuncture study of tubular transport of urate and PAH in the pig kidney. Am J Physiol 239:F107–F112
9. Kahn AM, Weinman EJ (1985) Urate transport in the proximal tubule: in vivo and vesicle studies. Am J Physiol 249:F789–F798
10. Kahn AM (1989) Indirect coupling between sodium and urate transport in the proximal tubule. Kidney Int 36:378–384
11. Lang F, Gstrein E, Geibel J, Rehwald W, Völkl H, Oberleithner H (1983) 605-redox microelectrodes for the continuous recording of organic substances in renal tubular fluid. Bioelectrochem. Bioenerg. 11:365–372
12. Senekjian HO, Knight TF, Weinman EJ (1981) Urate transport by the isolated perfused S_2 segment of the rabbit. Am J Physiol 240:F530–F535
13. Shimomura A, Chonko A, Tanner R, Edwards R, Grantham J (1981) Nature of urate transport in isolated rabbit proximal tubules. Am J Physiol 241:F565–F578
14. Schäli C, Roch-Ramel F (1980) Accumulation of [^{14}C]urate and [^{3}H]PAH in isolated proximal tubular segments of the rabbit kidney. Am J Physiol 239:F222–F227
15. Schäli C, Roch-Ramel F (1981) Uptake of [^{3}H]PAH and [^{14}C]urate into isolated proximal tubular segments of the pig kidney. Am J Physiol 241:F591–F596
16. Kahn AM, Aronson PS (1983) Urate transport via anion exchange in dog renal microvillus membrane vesicles. Am J Physiol 244:F56–F63
17. Kahn AM, Branham S, Weinman EJ (1983) Mechanism of urate and p-aminohippurate transport in rat renal microvillus membrane vesicles. Am J Physiol 245:F151–F158
18. Blomstedt JW, Aronson PS (1980) pH gradient-stimulated transport of urate and p-aminohippurate in dog renal microvillus membrane vesicles. J Clin Invest 65:931–934
19. Guggino SE, Martin GJ, Aronson PS (1983) Specificity and modes of the anion exchanger in dog renal microvillus membranes. Am J Physiol 244:F612–F621
20. Guggino SE, Aronson PS (1985) Paradoxical effects of pyrazinoate and nicotinate on urate transport in dog renal microvillus membranes. J Clin Invest 76:543–547
21. Abramson RG, King VF, Reif MC, Leal-Pinto E, Baruch SB (1982) Urate uptake in membrane vesicles of rat renal cortex: effect of copper. Am J Physiol 242:F158–F170
22. Werner D, Martinez F, Roch-Ramel F (1990) Urate and p-aminohippurate transport in the brush border membrane of the pig kidney. J Pharmacol Exp Ther 252:792–799
23. Martinez F, Manganel M, Montrose-Rafizadeh C, Werner D, Roch-Ramel F (1990) Transport of urate and p-aminohippurate in rabbit renal brush-border membranes. Am J Physiol 258:F1145–F1153
24. Kahn AM, Shelat H, Weinman EJ (1985) Urate and p-aminohippurate transport in rat renal basolateral vesicles. Am J Physiol 249:F654–F661
25. Shimada H, Moewes B, Burckhardt G (1987) Indirect coupling to Na^+ of p-aminohippuric acid uptake into rat renal basolateral membrane vesicles. Am J Physiol 253:F795–F801
26. Werner D, Roch-Ramel F (1990) Urate transport across the basolateral membrane of the pig renal proximal tubule (abstract). Experientia 46:A54

Pump, Leak and Metabolism: Postproximal Handling of Amino Acids in the Kidney

S. SILBERNAGL, M. GEKLE, K. VÖLKER[1], E. BRAUN, and W.H. DANTZLER[2]

SUMMARY. (1) During portal venous perfusion of the isolated non-filtering kidney of the toad (*Xenopus laevis*) with solutions containing 65 μM L-citrulline (L-Cit), urinary excretion of L-Cit was 2.25 nmol/2h. In the absence of NaCl or in the presence of 20 mM L-phenylalanine (L-Phe) in the perfusate, this value dropped to about 10% of the control value. The same was true for D-Cit excretion if L-Cit in the perfusate was replaced by D-Cit. Thus, secretory AA fluxes in the tubule seem to be carrier-mediated to at least 90%. (2) Rat kidney short loops of Henle were microperfused continuously in vivo et in situ with solutions containing ^{3}H-inulin and ^{14}C-amino acids. Fractional ^{14}C-reabsorption (FR) in the loop of Henle was high (glycine (Gly) 0.95; L-alanine (L-Ala) 0.97) at low concentrations (0.21 and 0.15 mM, respectively) but dropped to 0.24 (Gly) if 50 mM L-phenylalanine (L-Phe) or L-proline (L-Pro) was present. At 5 mM (L-arginine (L-Arg), L-glutamine (L-Glu) and at 50 mM (Gly, L-Phe, L-Pro), FR was 0.43, 0.74, 0.59, 0.50, and 0.18, respectively. At 0.6 mM, FR of L- and D-Ala was 0.97 and 0.84, respectively, but was 0.27 (L-Ala) and 0.74 (D-Ala) at 50 mM. The latter value dropped to 0.43 ($P<0.005$) in the presence of D-AA oxidase inhibitors. FR of ^{14}C-mannitol was 0.05 ± 0.07 SEM. In conclusion, resorptive fluxes in short loops of Henle are mediated by high-capacity carriers. For D-alanine, D-AA oxidase is a metabolic sink accelerating D-Ala resorption to a value higher than that for L-Ala. (3) Tissue serine concentrations in antidiuretic rat kidney are 2- to 30-fold (cortex to papilla) higher than in systemic plasma and 7- to 125-fold higher than in urine. The total intracellular AA concentration in the anti-diuretic papilla is > 100 mM contributing substantially to the intracellular osmolyte concentration.

[1]Department of Physiology, University of Würzburg, D-8700 Würzburg, Federal Republic of Germany

[2]Department of Physiology, University of Arizona, Tucson, AZ 85724, USA

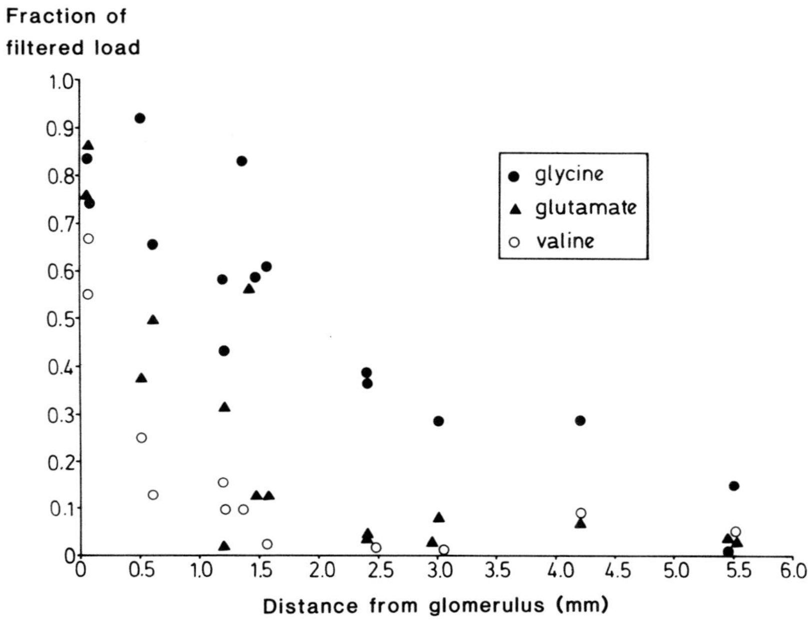

Fig. 1. Fractions of filtered loads of three amino acids found in samples collected by free-flow micropuncture along superficial proximal convoluted tubules of rat kidney. The mean endogenous plasma concentrations of glycine, glutamate, and valine during these experiments were 282, 117, and 278 μM, respectively. On the abscissa 5.5 mm represents the mean distance of the last accessible loop of the proximal convoluted tubule in 250 g rats

Introduction

It is well established that amino acids filtered at the glomerulus are reabsorbed rapidly along the proximal tubule (for review see [1]). With some exceptions, less than 1% of their filtered load is excreted in the final urine. Micropuncture data, obtained under endogenous free flow conditions, show that there are distinct values for the proximal reabsorption of different amino acids (see Fig. 1): Glycine is slowly reabsorbed, whereas more than 90% of the filtered load of glutamine [2], glutamate$^-$, valine (Fig. 1), and many other amino acids has already disappeared after about one fifth of the total length of the proximal tubule of these rats. The dots at the bottom of Fig. 1, however, show that the fractional delivery does not decrease further in this quasi-exponential manner. Depending on the amino acid, there is still some 2%–5% left even at a distance of 6 mm from the glomerulus. This phenomenon has been explained by the establishment of a pump-leak concentration in the later parts of the proximal tubule. "Pump" usually means secondary-active Na^+-Cotransport (dibasic amino acids may be an exception [3,4]), but what does "leak" mean? Is it a paracellular leak (see [5] and [1] for discussion) or do the amino acids use the brush-border carriers in the "wrong" direction if the transmembranal gradients toward the lumen are steep enough? This latter possibility is not unlikely, because many brush-border

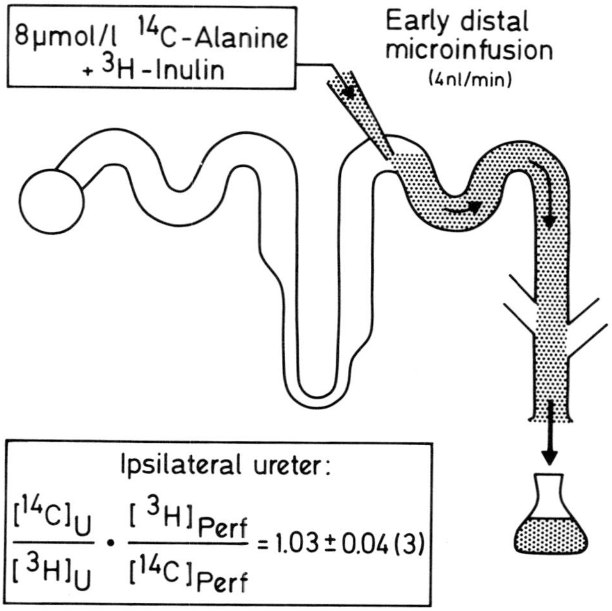

Fig. 2. Relative urinary recovery of ^{14}C-L-alanine microinjected into early superficial loops of distal convoluted tubules of rat kidney. The value does not differ significantly from that in Fig. 1, indicating that L-alanine does not leave the lumen in sections distal to the puncture site. Similar results have been obtained by Bergeron and Morel [8] for several other L-amino acids and by ourselves for D-alanine (S. Silbernagl et al. unpublished results)

membrane vesicle studies (see review in [1]) demonstrate that these carriers can be transstimulated. The first part of this study was designed to answer this question by investigating amino acid (citrulline) secretion in the non-filtering toad kidney.

What happens in the loop of Henle and in the distal nephron? As can be seen from Fig. 1, the fractional delivery of amino acids to the last accessible loop of the proximal convolution amounts to several percent, e.g., about 3% for alanine [6,7]; these values differ significantly from the fractional excretion of the respective amino acid (alanine 0.06–0.13% [6,7]). This may be explained by a high-affinity reabsorption and a relatively low leak of amino acids in the straight part of the proximal tubule, as shown with isolated perfused tubules (review, [5]). However, nearly the same amount (3%–4%) of filtered alanine was found in the superficial nephrons of the early distal tubule (short loops) [6,7]. Are amino acids reabsorbed in the distal nephron? The answer is "no" for superficial nephrons [7,8] (see Fig. 2), and "yes" for juxtamedullary nephrons [9,10]. In the second part of this study, we tested whether the zero net flux in the short loops of Henle was the result of opposed unidirectional fluxes of about the same size. As the answer to this question was "yes," we also characterized the unidirectional reabsorptive flux of several amino acids, including the D-isomer of alanine. In preliminary experiments we also measured the amino acid concentrations in six zones of the kidney situated between the cortex and the papilla to look for gradients that might favor one or the other of the unidirectional fluxes.

Methods

Isolated Perfused Non-Filtering Toad Kidney

Blood enters the toad kidney not only through the aorta but also through the portal vein [11]. We decapitated the toad (*Xenopus laevis*, male, 50–60 g BW), destroyed the spinal cord, opened the abdomen, and ligated all vessels to and from the kidney, except for the portal veins and the caval vein. We perfused the kidney only through the portal vein at a rate half as high as normal (2 ml/h into each portal vein). Under these conditions, venous volume recovery was 90%–100% and the inulin added to the perfusate did not reach the urine. Therefore, this preparation could be regarded as a non-filtering kidney, i.e., the perfusate reaches only the peritubular side of the tubule cells. Besides studying peritubular uptake and the metabolism of citrulline [12], we measured the urinary excretion of citrulline (column chromatography, see below) during perfusion of the kidneys with Ringer's solution containing inulin as well as citrulline and aspartate at the physiological concentrations of 65 and 35 µmol/l, respectively. p-Aminohippurate (2 mmol/l) was added to the perfusate in order to increase urinary flow.

Microperfusion of Short Loops of Henle

Male Wistar rats (200–250 g BW) were anesthetized with Inactin (120 mg/kg BW i.p.) and the left kidney was prepared and immobilized for micropuncture [13]. The perfusate, containing the ^{14}C-labelled amino acid and ^{3}H-inulin, was microperfused continuously in vivo et in situ [14] into the last accessible loop of the proximal convoluted tubule at a rate of 20 nl/min and was collected from the first accessible loop of the early distal convolution of the same nephron. Radioactivity was measured by liquid scintillation counting.

Measurement of Amino Acid Concentrations in Renal Tissue

In this preliminary experiment, a male antidiuretic Wistar rat (320 g BW) was anesthetized and the urinary bladder was punctured to obtain urine. The kidney was clamped, the hilus was cut, and, within about 5 s after clamping, the kidney was immersed in liquid nitrogen. Blood was obtained by subsequent heart puncture. Within several days, the kidney was warmed up to about −5°C and 6 pieces (10–40 mg each) were cut out (as shown in Fig. 3) in a cooled room. The frozen pieces were weighed (in preweighed vials) and were deep-frozen at −70°C. For amino acid determination, the cells of the tissue were destroyed by adding a buffer containing 1% Triton 100. After deproteinization with trichloracetic acid (100ml/l), amino acids were measured by ultramicro column chromatography (Kontron, Chromacon 500).

Results

Secretory Fluxes of Citrulline in the Toad Kidney

During perfusion of the toad kidney with a solution containing 65 µM L-citrulline, urinary excretion of this amino acid was about 2.5 nmol/2h (see Fig. 4). Replace-

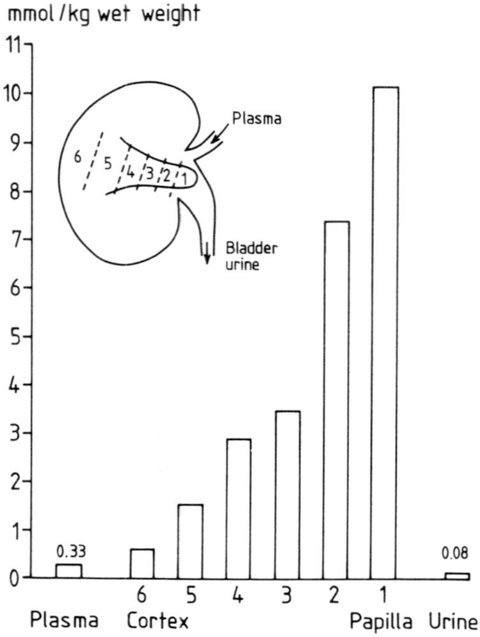

Fig. 3. Distribution of serine in kidney, systemic plasma, and bladder urine in one antidiuretic male rat of 326 g BW. Urine osmolality was 1400 mosm/l. A similar concentration gradient from cortex to papilla was found for all other amino acids. This results in a total amino acid concentration in the papilla (layer 1) of more than 100 mmol/kg wet weight

ment of NaCl with mannitol in the perfusate resulted in a dramatic drop of citrulline excretion to about 10% of the control value. Similarly, little excretion was found if 65 μM D-Citrulline was used or if 20 mM L-phenyl-alanine was added to the L-citrulline solution (see Fig. 4). These results clearly indicate that citrulline enters the urinary space nearly exclusively on a route which is stereospecific, inhibitable by another neutral amino acid, and Na(Cl)-dependent.

Unidirectional Amino Acid Fluxes in Short Loops of Henle in the Rat

As shown in Table 1, the radiolabels of glycine and L-alanine are nearly completely reabsorbed in the short loops of Henle if the initial concentration is small (0.21 and 0.15 mM, respectively), i.e., at about physiological concentrations. Fractional recovery is only 0.051 or 0.029, respectively, of the amount perfused. These non-reabsorbed fractions rise to 0.41 and 0.73, respectively, at the extremely high initial concentration of 50 mM; this indicates a significant but not full saturation of the reabsorptive process. Similar values are obtained with L-arginine, L-glutamate, L-phenylalanine and L-proline at high concentrations. As in the proximal convoluted tubule [1], L-proline and L-phenylalanine are potent inhibitors of glycine reabsorption (Table 1). At an initial concentration of 0.6 mM, D-alanine is reabsorbed more slowly than its L-isomer. This was to be expected. What is surprising, however, is

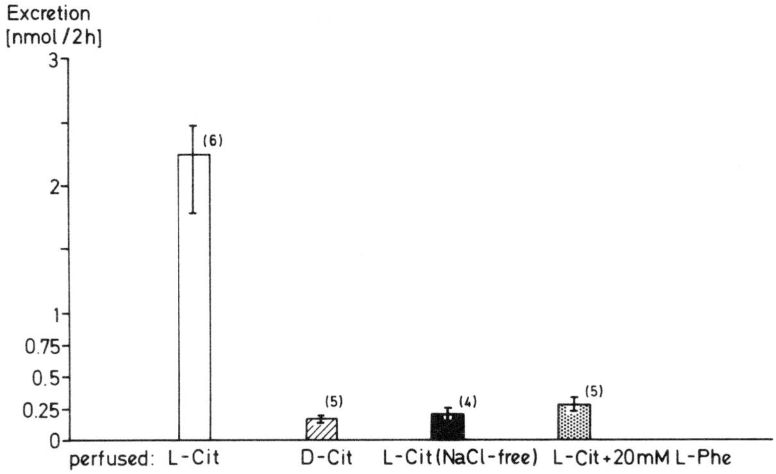

Fig. 4. Urinary excretion of L- and D-citrulline (*Cit*) during 2-hour portal-venous perfusion of isolated non-filtering kidneys of the toad (*Xenopus laevis*). The perfusion fluid contained L- or D-citrulline, respectively, in a concentration of 65 μM, i.e., the endogenous citrulline concentration that we found in the plasma of these toads. p-aminohippurate was added to the perfusate in order to increase urinary volume flow. Inulin was also added to the perfusion fluid. Under this condition, the absence of inulin in the urine proved the absence of glomerular filtration. The perfusion rate was 2 ml/h per portal vein. Phe, phenylalanine

that 84% of the D-alanine is reabsorbed. As 50 mM D-alanine inhibits the reabsorption of the radiolabel of 0.15 mM L-alanine (Table 1), this can be explained by assuming that the D-form is accepted by the carrier involved but possesses a lower affinity for it. It is even more surprising that, at high initial concentrations (50 mM), D-alanine is reabsorbed to a much greater extent (74%) than the L-form (27%) (see Table 1). This rapid reabsorption of D-alanine is partly blocked ($P < 0.005$) if benzoate and indole carboxylic acid are added to the perfusate (5 mM each). Both compounds are well-known inhibitors of D-amino acid oxidase [15], suggesting that this enzyme is involved in the quick removal of D-alanine from the tubule lumen.

Tissue Concentrations of Free Amino Acids in the Kidney

As described in the methods and as shown for serine in Fig. 3, overall amino acid concentrations (mmol/kg wet weight) are higher in the cortex than in the plasma. In the renal medulla the overall tissue concentration is even higher and increases further toward the papilla where the serine concentration amounts to more than 10 mmol/kg. In contrast, the urine (1400 mosm/kg H_2O), although excreted in the very neighborhood of the papillary tissue, contains only 0.08 mM serine. As all other amino acids measured in this experiment (data not shown) also show a high amino acid concentration gradient toward the papilla (papillary values in mmol/kg wet weight: taurine 4.7, aspartate$^-$ 8.8, threonine 7.5, glutamate$^-$ 14.0, etc.) they add up to a total

Table 1. Continuous microperfusion of the short loops of Henle of rat kidneys in vivo et in situ at a rate of 20 nl/min. ^{14}C-labeled amino acids, listed in the first row, and tritiated inulin were added to the perfusion fluid. Fractional delivery (*FD*) of the ^{14}C-label as compared to the ^{3}H-activity was determined in the collected samples. Fractional reabsorption, (1 − FD)

^{14}C-compounds (mM)	added (mM)	FD ± SEM (*n*)
L-arginine (5)	–	0.57 ± 0.05 (10)
L-glutamate (5)	–	0.26 ± 0.04 (14)
Glycine (0.21)	–	0.051 ± 0.006 (6)
Glycine (50)	–	0.41 ± 0.04 (9)
Glycine (0.21)	L-Phe (50)	0.76 ± 0.05 (9)
Glycine (0.21)	L-Pro (50)	0.76 ± 0.05 (9)
L-phenylalanine (50)	–	0.50 ± 0.10 (7)
L-proline (50)	–	0.82 ± 0.09 (5)
L-alanine (0.15)	–	0.029 ± 0.008 (6)
L-alanine (0.15)	D-Ala (50)	0.14 ± 0.03 (7)
L-alanine (0.6)	–	0.029 ± 0.009 (6)
D-alanine (0.6)	–	0.16 ± 0.03 (17)
L-alanine (50)	–	0.73[a] ± 0.03 (8)
D-alanine (50)	–	0.26* ± 0.04 (15)
D-alanine (50)	[b]	0.57 ± 0.08 (8)
Mannitol (0.68)	–	0.95 ± 0.07 (10)**

[a]More than 95% of this ^{14}C-activity was intact L-alanine
*Significantly different from the foregoing value ($P < 0.005$)
[b]The D-amino acid oxidase inhibitors benzoate and indole carboxylic acid (5 mM each) were added to the perfusate
**Not significantly different from one

amino acid tissue concentration in the papilla of about 100 mmol/kg wet weight. Within the cells, these concentrations should be even higher (see Discussion).

Discussion

Our microperfusion experiments show (Table 1) that the short loops of Henle have a very high capacity to reabsorb amino acids which may have escaped reabsorption in earlier parts of the proximal tubule or which may stem from intraluminal peptide degradation (review, [1]). The fact that net reabsorption in the short loops is zero [6,7] shows, however, that amino acids leak into the lumen to a great extent. The fact that citrulline virtually completely enters the lumen of the non-filtering tubule of the toad on a route which is stereospecific and Na(Cl)-dependent and can be inhibited by another neutral amino acid (Fig. 4) suggests that this entry is a transcellular pathway involving the well-known peritubular and luminal amino acid carriers in the "wrong" direction. Thus, a nonspecific leak does not play a significant role here, if no great differences can be assumed between the toad and rat kidney in this regard. This view is confirmed by the fact that the radiolabel of mannitol, which has a molecular size comparable to that of the amino acids, is not reabsorbed from the lumen of rat short loops of Henle to a significant extent (see Table 1).

If secretory fluxes of amino acids are mediated nearly exclusively by the membrane carriers of the tubule cells in humans also, the tubule defects in inherited specific hyperaminoacidurias have to be reconsidered. In some of these diseases ("classic" cystinuria, "acidic" hyperaminoaciduria), net secretion of cystine and "acidic" amino acids (glutamate$^-$ and aspartate$^-$), respectively, has been observed (review, [1]). Consequently, this would mean that amino acid binding and transport by the carriers involved are intact, as they are still able to transport in the "wrong" direction. What might be defective in the kidneys of these patients is the ability of the carrier to be energized by the sodium gradient which normally drives the secondary-active amino acid transport in the opposite direction. A defect at the Na^+-binding site of the carriers involved is one possible explanation. This hypothesis, however, needs to be tested in further studies.

Returning to the discrepancy between zero net flux and high unidirectional fluxes of amino acids in the short loops of Henle, it seems feasible that the unexpectedly high early distal amino acid recovery might be even higher if there were no potent reabsorptive pump mechanisms in the loops of Henle. Thus, the main business of these pump mechanisms may not be to reabsorb amino acids overflowing from the proximal convolution, but it may be, instead, to counteract the leak driven by the extremely high medullary amino acid concentrations found in this study (see Fig. 3). These tissue concentrations are most probably underestimated because the volume of the cortex, the outer stripe, and the inner medulla contains about 25% tubule lumina and collecting ducts [16], where the amino acid concentrations are relatively low and, therefore, do not contribute significantly to the overall amino acid concentration. Although luminal amino acid concentrations in the inner medullary sections of the long loops of Henle (as well as in inner medullary vasa recta) are higher than in the systemic plasma [10], they are still much lower than the values we found in the whole tissue: e.g., 0.6 –2 mM for serine (entire tissue 7–10 mM) or 0.1–0.3 mM for aspartate (whole tissue 6–8 mM). In view of the fact that the total concentration of amino acids found in the papillary tissue in this study (about 100 mM) is an underestimation of the intracellular concentration, amino acids seem to contribute quite significantly to the high osmolality in medullary cells during antidiuresis. (This 100 mM compares, e.g., with 65–110 mM glycerophosphorylcholine, 35–74 mM betaine and 60 mM sorbitol.)

Confirming earlier in vitro data obtained with luminal membrane vesicles of rabbit proximal tubules [17], our microperfusion data with L- and D-alanine show (see Table 1) that the D- and L-isomers of alanine seem to share one carrier in the wall of the loop of Henle, because (a) the D-alanine reabsorption rate is not very much different from that of the L-isomer and (b) the high concentrations of D-alanine inhibit reabsorption of the L-form to some extent. The result showing that, at high concentrations, the radiolabel of L-alanine is reabsorbed significantly more slowly than that of the D-form, could be explained by re-secretion of a (still radiolabelled) metabolite of L-alanine into the lumen. We therefore identified the compound to which the ^{14}C-label was bound in the collected samples of this series by combining column chromatography and scintillation counting. It turned out that more than 95% of the radiolabel represented L-alanine. This result shows that D-alanine is indeed reabsorbed faster than the L-form. The significant retardation of the reabsorption of D-alanine by D-amino acid oxidase inhibitors shows that D-alanine has access to this intracellular enzyme, which has been localized mainly in the straight part of the proximal tubule [18]. This phenomenon suggests that this enzyme provides a metabolic sink for D-alanine and also, perhaps, for other substrates of this enzyme. Besides other D-amino acids, glycine also belongs to this group.

Acknowledgments. We thank Ms. Olga Brokl for her great encouragement and support during the time S.S. spent his sabbatical in the lab at the University of Arizona. We also thank Ms. Margit Schulze for drawing the figures and Ms. Angelika Reuβ for secretarial help. Supported in part by NATO Collaborative Research Grant 0104/88 and by National Institute of Health Grant DK 16294.

References

1. Silbernagl S (1988) The renal handling of amino acids and oligopeptides. Physiol Rev 68:911–1007
2. Silbernagl S (1980) Tubular reabsorption of L-glutamine studied by free flow micropuncture and microperfusion of rat kidney. Int J Biochem 12:9–16
3. Schwegler JS, Heuner A, Silbernagl S (1989) Electrogenic transport of neutral and dibasic amino acids in a cultured opossum cell line (OK). Pflugers Arch 414:543–550
4. Schwegler JS, Schömig E, Heuner A, Silbernagl S (1990) Development of high-capacity, low-affinity L-arginine transport in a proximal tubular cell line during differentiation. In: Lubec G, Rosenthal GA (eds) Amino acids. Chemistry, biology and medicine. ESCOM, Leiden, pp 1017–1028
5. Schafer JA, Barfuss DW (1980) Membrane mechanisms for transepithelial amino acid absorption and secretion. Am J Physiol 238:F335–F346
6. Eisenbach GM, Weise M, Stolte H (1975) Amino acid reabsorption in the rat nephron. Free flow micropuncture study. Pflugers Arch 357:63–76
7. Günther R, Silbernagl S, Deetjen P (1979) Maleic acid induced aminoaciduria studied by free flow micropuncture and continuous microperfusion. Pflugers Arch 382:109–114
8. Bergeron M, Morel F (1969) Amino acid transport in rat renal tubules. Am J Physiol 216:1139–1149
9. Dantzler WH, Silbernagl S (1988) Amino acid transport by juxtamedullary nephrons: distal reabsorption and recycling. Am J Physiol 255:F397–F407
10. Dantzler WH, Silbernagl S (1990) Amino acid transport: microperfusion and micropuncture of Henle's loop and vasa recta. Am J Physiol 258:F504–513
11. Hayman JM Jr (1928) Notes on the arrangement of blood vessels of the frog's kidney together with some measurements of blood pressure in the renal portal and renal veins. Am J Physiol 86:331–339
12. Gekle M, Grimme M, Silbernagl S (1989) Peritubular transport, tubular metabolism, and transcellular secretion of L-citrulline in the isolated perfused kidney of the frog (*Xenopus laevis*). Kidney Int 36:311
13. Lang F, Greger R, Lechene C, Knox FG (1978) Micropuncture techniques. In: Martinez-Maldonado M (ed) Methods in pharmacology, renal pharmacology. Plenum, New York, pp 75–103
14. Sonnenberg H, Deetjen P (1964) Methode zur Durchströmung einzelner Nephronabschnitte. Pflugers Arch 278:669–674
15. Bartlett GR (1948) The inhibition of D-amino acid oxidase by benzoic acid and various monosubstituted benzoic acid derivatives. J Am Chem Soc 70:1010–1011
16. Pfaller W (1982) Structure function correlation in rat kidney. Quantitative correlation of structure and function in the normal and injured rat kidney. In: Pfaller W (ed) Advances in anatomy, embryology and cell biology, vol. 70. Springer, Berlin
17. Jessen H, Vorum H, Jørgensen KE, Sheikh MI (1988) Characteristics of D-alanine transport by luminal membrane vesicles from pars convoluta and pars recta of rabbit proximal tubule. Biochim Biophys Acta 942:262–270
18. Chan AWK, Perry SG, Burch HB, Fagioli S, Alvey TR, Lowry OH (1979) Distribution of two aminotransferases and D-amino acid oxidase within the nephron of young and adult rats. J Histochem Cytochem 27:751–755

Optical Techniques for Studying Kidney Cell Function

Chair: Walter F. Boron (USA)
Kenneth R. Spring (USA)

Optical Approaches for Studying Intracellular pH in Epithelial Cells

WALTER F. BORON[1]

Introduction

Ten years ago, the only practical approach for continuously monitoring intracellular pH (pH_i) in epithelial cells was to employ pH-sensitive microelectrodes with a recessed glass sensor [1]. Although these electrodes are extremely accurate and stable, they require skill to fabricate and use. Moreover, although they can be used with modestly small cells (e.g., amphibian proximal-tubule cells), the electrode response time increases with the sharpness of the electrode tip. In the ensuing years, the introduction of improved "proton cocktails" [2] for liquid-membrane electrodes has greatly simplified the preparation of pH-sensitive microelectrodes and, to a lesser extent, has increased the sharpness of their tips. Nevertheless, although it is relatively easy to use these pH-sensitive microelectrodes with amphibian renal tubules, it remains rather difficult to extend the technology to mammalian tubules. It is for this reason that we have devoted considerable effort during the past decade to developing three optical techniques for monitoring pH_i in isolated renal tubules and even in single cells. The first technique exploits photodiode array technology for measuring the absorbance spectrum of an intracellular pH-sensitive dye. It has been applied to isolated renal tubules from amphibians [3] and mammals [4], as well as to single cells [5]. The second technique is the use of an epifluorescence microscope to monitor the fluorescence of a pH-sensitive dye. Once again, this approach has been applied both to single cells [6] and to isolated mammalian tubules [7]. Finally, the approach on which we have devoted our most recent efforts is an extension of the earlier fluorescence technique in which the detector is an image-intensifier/TV-camera rather than a photomultiplier tube. Digital image processing makes it possible to monitor pH_i transients in multiple individual cells, or even in portions of a single cell.

[1]Department of Cellular and Molecular Physiology, Yale University School of Medicine, New Haven, CT 06510, USA

Before beginning a description of these techniques, I should make two points. First, the use of optical techniques for monitoring pH_i requires good dyes. In our absorbance measurements, we employ dimethylcarboxyfluorescein (Me_2CF). The dye is introduced into the cell by exposing the latter to a diacetate-ester derivative of Me_2CF. This ester is hydrolyzed intracellularly by native esterases, forming Me_2CF, which is relatively trapped inside the cell. Such ester derivatives of various fluorescein compounds were used to assess cell viability before it was recognized that these compounds could also be employed for measuring pH_i [8]. Probably the best of these fluorescein derivatives is 2,7-biscarboxyethyl-5(6)-carboxyfluorescein (BCECF); both it and its acetoxymethylester derivative were developed by Roger Tsien and his colleagues [9], who have pioneered several other dyes as well. The second point worth noting is that abandoning the microelectrode approach for optics has not come without a price: a loss of a continuous record of membrane voltage. The latter, which is a byproduct of every pH-sensitive microelectrode measurement, has proven extremely useful in characterizing electrogenic processes [10]. Thus, it would be desirable to supplement pH-sensitive dye measurements with either microelectrode or dye measurements of membrane voltage.

Absorbance Measurements

Theoretical Considerations

When a molecule absorbs a photon of energy $h\nu$, where h is Planck's constant and ν is the frequency, the molecule is raised to an excited state. The excited molecule can return to the ground state in any of three ways. First, through random collisions (*quenching*), it can transfer all or part of its excess energy to other molecules, which can in turn undergo a variety of reactions. Second, it can emit one or more photons. If the single emitted photon has the same wavelength as the exciting photo, the process is termed *resonance radiation*. If the emitted photon has less energy (i.e., a higher wavelength) than the exciting photon, the process is termed *fluorescence*. The remainder of the energy can be dissipated either by emitting another photon, or by transferring energy by random collisions. The third possible fate of an excited molecule is to fragment. Regardless of the mechanism by which the molecule returns to its ground state, the molecule must absorb light. The amount of absorbed light is termed the *absorbance*, which is defined as

$$A = -\log \frac{I}{I_o},$$

where A is the absorbance, I_o is the intensity of the beam of light as it enters the sample, I is the intensity as the light leaves the sample. According to Beer's law, the absorbance is proportional to the thickness of the sample (l) and the concentration of the molecule (c):

$$A = \varepsilon lc,$$

where ε is the *molar extinction coefficient*.

In general, ε is a function of wavelength (λ). For pH-sensitive dyes, such as Me_2CF, ε is also a function of pH. Thus, the shape of the absorbance spectrum is

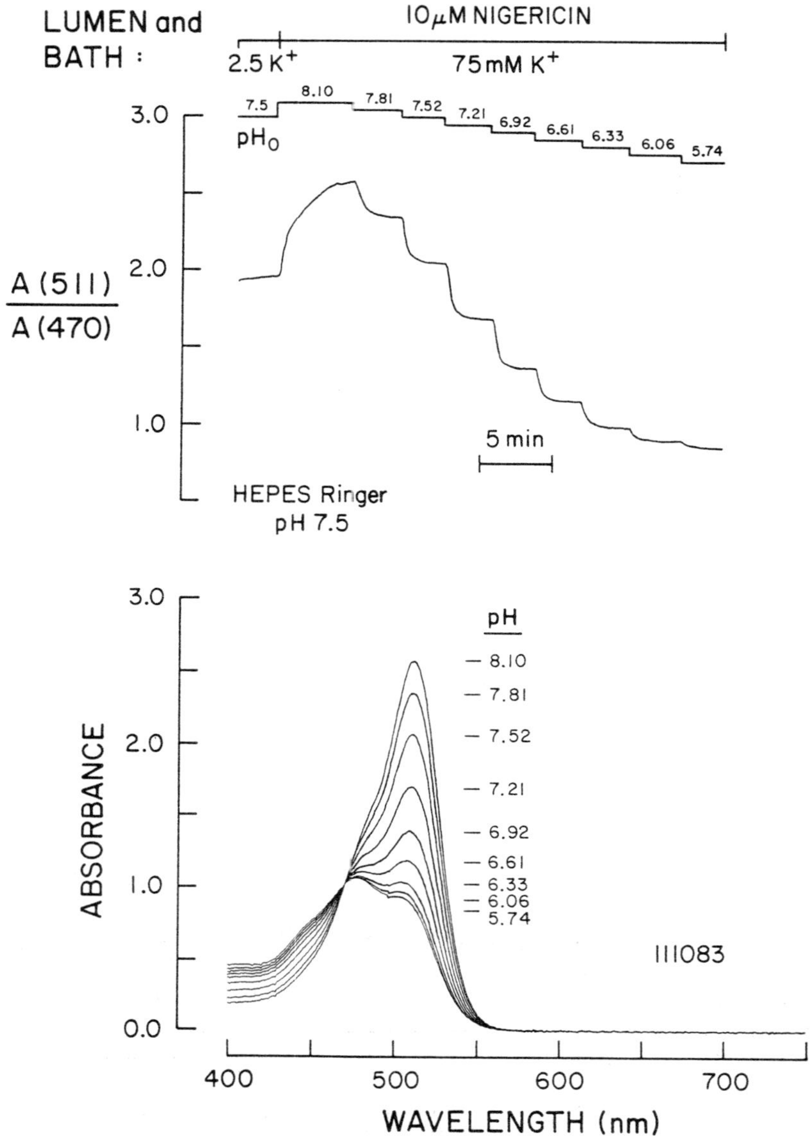

Fig. 1. pH dependence of the absorbance spectrum of in vitro dimethylcarboxyfluorescein. The data are normalized to unity at 470 nm, the isosbestic wavelength. The *inset* shows the ratio of absorbance at 505 nm (the peak) to that at 470 nm as a function of pH. (From [3] by permission of The Rockefeller University Press)

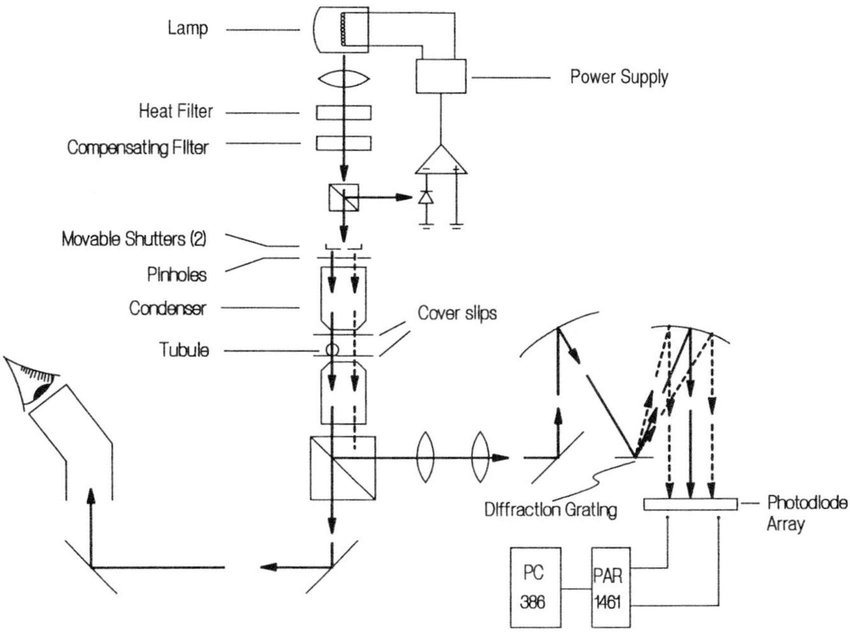

Fig. 2. Schematic diagram of the apparatus used in measuring the optical absorbance of pH sensitive dyes. In brief, white light is passed either next to (providing I_o) or through (providing I) an isolated tubule or a single cell. The intensity spectrum of this light is obtained by creating a spectrum with a diffraction grating, and focusing the spectrum on an array of 1024 photodiodes. The photon signal on each diode is read into the computer with 14-bit resolution (1 part in 16384). The absorbance spectrum is computed from the intensity spectra of the incident and transmitted light. (Redrawn from [3])

pH sensitive, as indicated in Fig. 1. Under the conditions employed in the experiment summarized in Fig. 1, the in-vitro absorbance of Me_2CF is most pH sensitive at a wavelength of 505 nm (the peak), and is not pH sensitive at all at 470 nm. Although it might be tempting to compute pH from the absorbance at the peak wavelength, this is not possible. *A* is not a unique function of pH; *A* is also dependent on *c* and *l*. If intracellular dye concentration changes during an experiment (it almost always drifts downward due to dye leakage and/or bleaching), or if the optical path length through the cell changes, *A* would change even if pH_i were to remain constant. A solution to this problem is to divide A_{505} by A_{470}, which has the effect of canceling out the contributions of *l* and *c*. A_{505} is chosen because this is the most pH sensitive wavelength. A_{470} is chosen for convenience because this value can be used to independently compute dye concentration, assuming that the path length and intracellular ε are known. However, it should be emphasized that in principle any pair of wavelengths could be used for computing the ratio. Some wavelength pairs are more sensitive to pH changes than others, but all provide an index of the pH-sensitive spectral shape change.

Measuring the Absorbance of an Intracellular pH Sensitive Dye

Fig. 2 is a schematic representation of the apparatus used in our laboratory to measure the absorbance of intracellular dyes. Me_2CF can be loaded into the cells as described above. The ionophore nigericin can be used in high-K^+ solutions to approximately clamp pH_i to pH_o, the limitations of which have been described previously [3]. When intracellular absorbance spectra are obtained, it is immediately obvious that intracellular Me_2CF behaves differently from the dye in the cuvette. As summarized in Fig. 3**a**, when both intra- and extracellular spectra are normalized to unity at 470 nm, the intracellular spectrum is shorter and broader. In addition, the peak absorbance of the intracellular spectrum is red shifted (i.e., shifted to higher wavelengths) by ~6 nm. When the A_{peak}/A_{470} ratios are compared as a function of pH (Fig. 3**b**), we see that the pK is shifted to more alkaline values by ~0.4 pH units. Some discrepancy between the spectral properties of intra- vs. extracellular dye can be accounted for by the higher concentrations of Me_2CF inside the cell. However, the majority is probably due to interactions of the dye with intracellular constituents. The combination of the red-shifted spectrum and the alkali-shifted calibration curve could lead to errors of as much as 0.5 pH units if extracellular calibration/spectral data were used to compute pH_i. Fig. 3 emphasizes the importance of obtaining intracellular calibration and spectral information.

Single-Cell Fluorescence Measurements

In our laboratory, we have found pH_i values derived from absorbance spectra of mammalian renal tubules to have outstanding signal to noise ratio. This is achievable because the cells are loaded with mM concentrations of the dye, and have a rather large total optical path length (through two cell layers). Although we have had some success in applying the absorbance approach to single LLC-PK1 cells in culture [5], the experiments are more difficult owing to the much smaller path length. Therefore, our group has explored methods for using the fluorescence excitation spectrum of fluoroscein dyes to compute pH_i, as previously employed by J. A. Thomas et al. [8]. The approach is to alternately excite the dye with light at a wavelength (e.g., 490 nM) at which the emitted fluorescent light (e.g., at 530 nm) is very pH sensitive, and at a wavelength at which the emitted light is less pH sensitive or even has the reverse pH sensitivity (e.g., 440 nm). The ratio I_{490}/I_{440} is thus very pH sensitive, but is relatively insensitive to parameters such as dye concentration.

Our apparatus, summarized in Fig. 4, is based on an inverted microscope with epi-illumination. A single cell or a small portion of a renal tubule typically is illuminated with a 10-μm diameter beam of 490-nm or 440-nm light. Light of the two wavelengths is generated by using a system of dichroic mirrors, band-pass filters and computer-controlled shutters. This is not the only approach for generating two wavelengths of light. Several laboratories select wavelengths by moving into the light path filters mounted on a linear or rotary actuator. In an ingenious approach introduced by Kurtz [11], light beams of the two desired wavelengths are chopped at different frequencies and then combined by a dichroic mirror, so that the preparation is simultaneously excited by light of the two different wavelengths. The emission-intensity data from the independent excitation wavelengths are extracted by using a

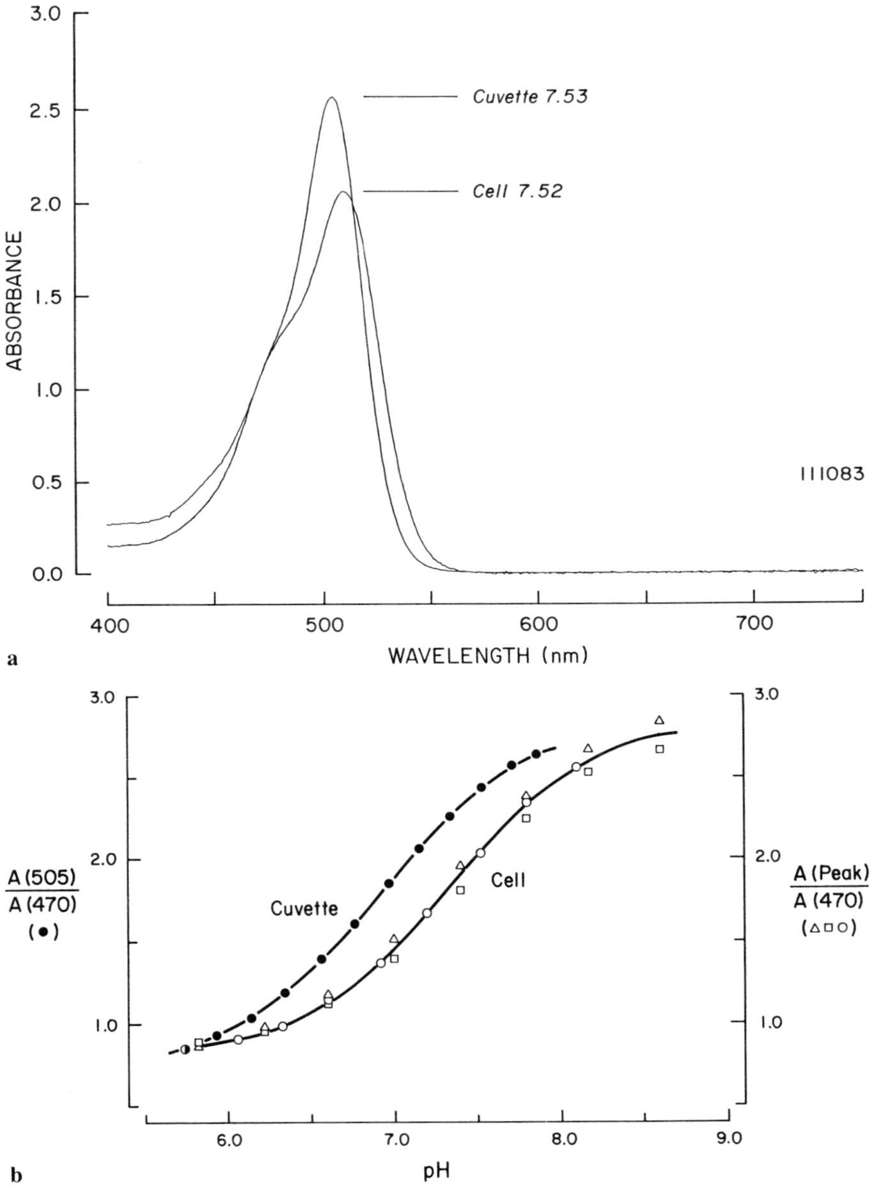

Fig. 3. Comparison of spectral properties of intra- and extracellular Me_2CF. **a** Comparison of absorbance spectra at a pH value of ~7.5. The curve labeled "cuvette" was obtained at a [Me_2CF] of 10 μM, that labeled "cell," at a [Me_2CF] in the mM range. **b** pH calibrations obtained from spectra similar to those shown in **a**. (From [3] by permission of The Rockefeller University Press)

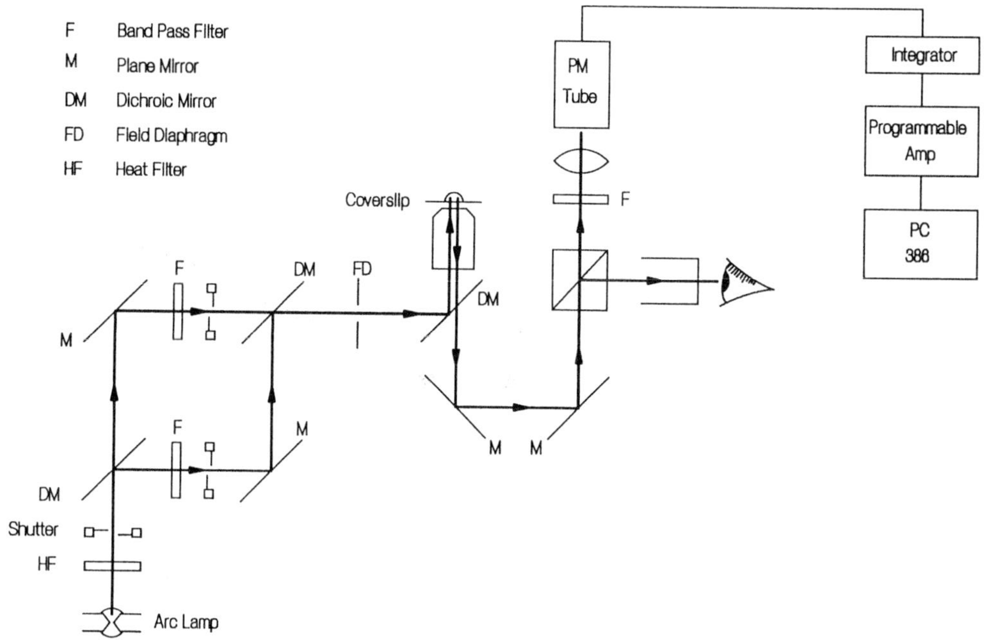

Fig. 4. Schematic diagram of the apparatus used in measuring the fluorescence excitation ratio of an intracellular dye. In brief, light from an arc lamp is split by a 470-nm short-pass dichroic mirror into one path that is filtered at 440 nm and another that is filtered at 490 nm. A series of computer-controlled shutters determines whether 440-nm light, 490-nm light or no light at all illuminates the cell(s) as a 10-µm beam on the microscope stage. The emitted light is filtered at 530 nm and sensed by a photomultiplier tube. (Redrawn from [6])

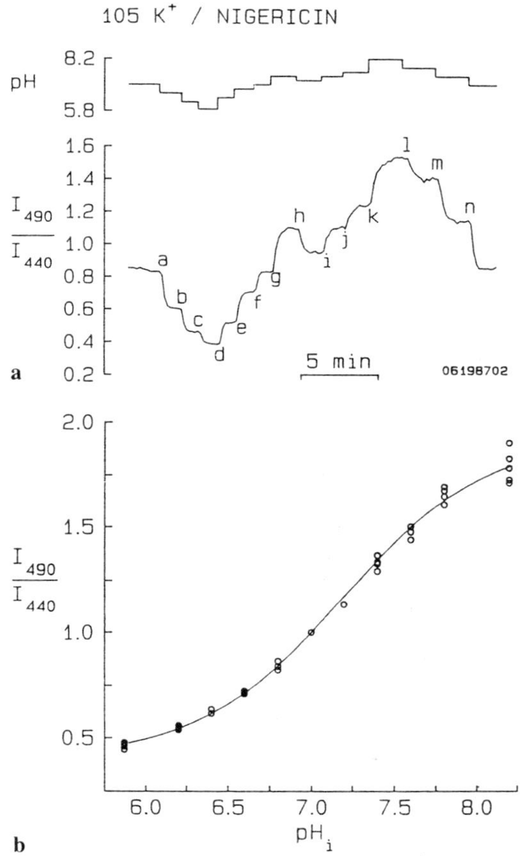

Fig. 5. Intracellular pH calibration of the fluorescence excitation ratio of BCECF. **a** Time course of I_{490}/I_{440} for a single renal mesangial cell exposed to high-K^+ solutions containing 10 μM nigericin, and titrated to various pH values, as indicated. **b** Summary of the pH dependence of I_{490}/I_{440} data from 6 experiments. The curve drawn through the points is the result of a non-linear least-squares curve fit, and has an apparent pK of 7.19. (From [6] by permission of The American Physiological Society)

lock-in amplifier. In our preliminary experiments, we found that two major problems were stray light and bleaching/photodynamic damage. We minimized bleaching/ photodynamic damage by keeping the cells in the dark for most of the time; a cell is typically illuminated with 440-nm light for 200 ms, 490-nm light for another 200 ms, and then is in the dark until another cycle begins. The fluorescence signal is optimized by programming the amplifier to adjust its gain to the magnitude of the expected signal at each of the two wavelengths. During the experiment, the operator monitors I_{440}, which is a good approximation of intracellular dye concentration, as well as the ratio I_{490}/I_{440}, which is an estimate of pH_i.

As is the case with absorbance experiments, it is essential to calibrate the dye inside the cell(s). A typical intracellular calibration experiment is shown in Fig. **5a**

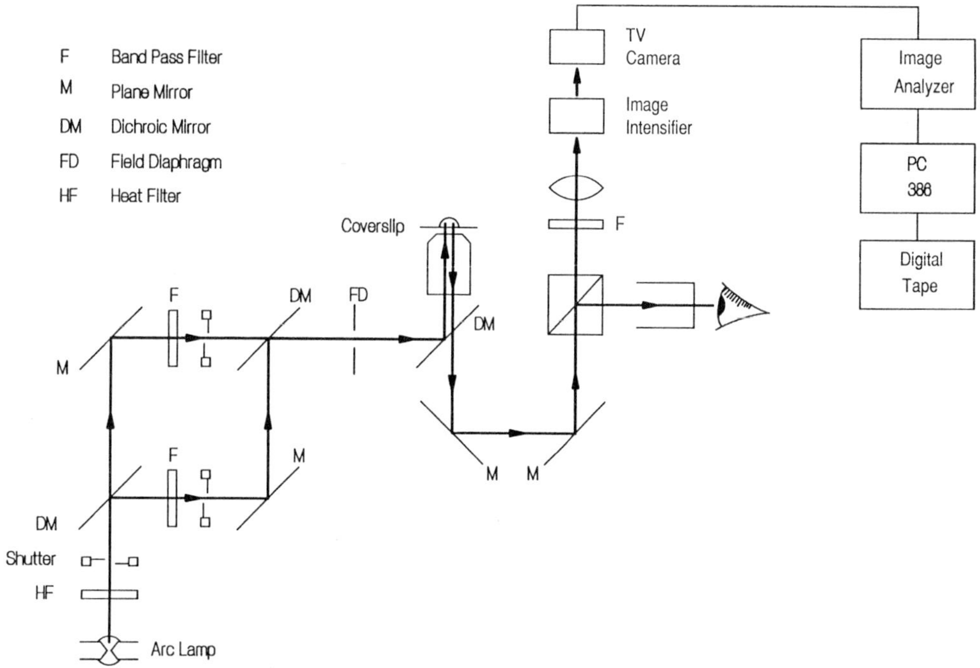

Fig. 6. Schematic diagram of the digital imaging system used in measuring the fluorescence excitation ratio of an intracellular dye. The apparatus is similar to that summarized in *Fig. 4*, except that the photomultiplier tube is replaced by an image intensifier and a television camera

for a single renal mesangial cell. The data from several cells is summarized in Fig. **5b**. We have used this fluorescence technique with single cultured cells of several different types [6,12], as well as with isolated rabbit proximal tubules [7].

Fluorescence Imaging

The approach outlined in the previous section provides the pH_i of a single cell or the average pH_i of a small group of cells. In a heterogeneous cell population, it would be advantageous to monitor, simultaneously, the pH_i of multiple cells. In addition, it might also be desirable to measure apparent pH_i values in different regions of a single cell. This can be achieved by imaging fluorescence signals, an approach used by others before us [13–18]. The approach used in our laboratory is similar to that used in single-cell fluorescence experiments, except that the photodetector is an image intensifier/television camera instead of a photomultiplier tube. In addition, we use a digital image processor to digitally analyze our fluorescence images. The apparatus is summarized in Fig. 6.

In preliminary experiments we found that, as expected, a major problem in imaging experiments was a shortage of photons at the pixel (picture element) level (Eisen and W. Boron, unpublished work). Because the limiting signal-to-noise ratio is proportional to the square root of the number of photons, the signal-to-noise ratio for a single pixel is extremely high [19]. However, we have found that if we group the pixels corresponding to a large part of a cell, the signal-to-noise ratio can approach that of the single-cell fluorescence technique, with a usable pH_i precision of ~ 0.02. We have employed digital analysis of fluorescence images to monitor pH_i transients with single osteoclasts (very large multinucleate cells), up to six simultaneous mesangial cells (moderately large cells, when in culture), and over 30 simultaneous MDCK cells (Eisen and W. Boron, unpublished work).

Acknowledgments. This work was supported by a grant from the NIH (DK30344). I acknowledge the dedicated efforts of Dr. J. Richard Chaillet and Mr. Andrey Yeatts, who developed the absorbance apparatus; Dr. Gregory Boyarsky, Dr. John P. Geibel, Mr. Andrey Yeatts and Mr. Vic Pantani, who developed the fluorescence apparatus; and Dr. Thomas D. Eisen and Mr. Duncan Wong, who developed the imaging system.

References

1. Thomas RC (1974) Intracellular pH of snail neurones measured with a new pH-sensitive glass microelectrode. J Physiol 238:159–180
2. Ammann D, Lanter F, Schulthess P, Shijo Y, Simon W (1981) Neutral carrier based hydrogen ion selective microelectrode for extra- and intracellular studies. Anal Chem 53:2267–2269
3. Chaillet JR, Boron WF (1985) Intracellular calibration of a pH-sensitive dye in isolated perfused salamander proximal tubules. J Gen Physiol 86:765–794
4. Nakhoul NL, Lopes AG, Chaillet JR, Boron WF (1988) Intracellular pH regulation in the S3 segment of the rabbit proximal tubule in HCO_3^--free solutions. J Gen Physiol 92:369–393

5. Chaillet JR, Amsler K, Boron WF (1986) Optical measurement of intracellular pH in single LLC-PK1 cells: demonstration of $Cl^-HCO_3^-$ exchange. Proc Natl Acad Sci USA 83:522–526
6. Boyarsky G, Ganz MB, Sterzel B, Boron WF (1988) pH regulation in single glomerular mesangial cells. I. Acid extrusion in absence and presence of HCO_3. Am J Physiol 255:C844–C856
7. Geibel JP, Giebisch G, Boron WF (1989) Basolateral sodium-coupled acid-base transport mechanisms of the rabbit proximal tubule. Am J Physiol 257:F790–F797
8. Thomas JA, Buchsbaum RN, Zimniak A, Racker E (1979) Intracellular pH measurements in Ehrlich ascites tumor cells utilizing spectroscopic probes generated in situ. Biochemistry 81:2210–2218
9. Rink TJ, Tsien RY, Pozzan T (1982) Cytoplasmic pH and free Mg^{+2} in lymphocytes. J Cell Biol 95:189–196
10. Boron WF, Boulpaep EL (1983) Intracellular pH regulation in the renal proximal tubule of the salamander: basolateral HCO_3^- transport. J Gen Physiol 81:53–94
11. Kurtz I (1987) Apical Na^+/H^+ antiporter and glycolysis-dependent H^+-ATPase regulate intracellular pH in the rabbit S3 proximal tubule. J Clin Invest 80:928–935
12. Boyarsky G, Ranson BR, Schlue W-R, Davis M (1989) Anomalous stimulation of pH regulation by ethylisopropyl amiloride in cultured mammalian astrocytes. Society for Neuroscience Abstracts 15:15
13. Ambler SK, Poenie M, Tsien RY, Taylor P (1988) Agonist-stimulated oscillations and cycling of intracellular free calcium in individual cultured muscle cells. J Biol Chem 263:1952–1959
14. Spring KR (1985) The study of epithelial function by quantitative light microscopy. Pflugers Arch 405:S23–S27
15. Kruskal BA, Shak S, Maxfield FR (1986) Spreading of human neutrophils is immediately preceded by a large increase in cytoplasmic free calcium. PNAS 83:2919–2923
16. Paradiso AM, Machen TE (1987) Digital image processing of intracellular pH in gastric oxyntic and chief cells. Nature 325:447–450
17. Negulescu PA, Harootunian A, Minta A, Tsien RY, Machen TE (1988) Intracellular sodium regulation in rabbit gastric glands determined using a fluorescent sodium indicator. J Gen Physiol 92:26a
18. Jacob R, Merritt JE, Hallam TJ, Rink TJ (1988) Repetitive spikes in cytoplasmic calcium evoked by histamine in human endothelial cells. Nature 335:40–45
19. Spring KR (To be published) Quantitative imaging at low light levels: differential interference contrast and fluorescence microscopy without significant light loss. Digitized Video Microscopy

Cell pH Regulation in Collecting Tubules

Michio Kuwahara, Sei Sasaki, and Fumiaki Marumo[1]

Summary. We measured the single cell pH of principal cells (PC) and intercalated cells (IC) in the outer stripe of the outer medullary collecting duct (OMCDo) of the rabbit using fluorescence ratio imaging.

1. It was suggested that single cell fluorescence measurement is influenced by fluorescence from neighboring, out-of-focus cells.
2. To minimize the effect of out-of-focus cells:
   a) in PC, a cell that is minimally surrounded by IC should be carefully selected.
   b) in IC, luminal dye loading is useful.
3. Using these techniques, HCO_3^--independent mechanisms of pHi regulation were examined. Our results suggest that:
   a) in PC, basolateral Na^+/H^+ exchange, and
   b) in IC, the luminal N-ethylmaleimide (NEM)- and N-N′-dicyclohexylcarbodiomide (DCCD)-inhibitable H^+ pump, and basolateral Na^+/H^+ exchange, contribute to cell pH regulation in rabbit OMCDo.

Introduction

A renal tubule is cylindrical in shape and contains hundreds of cells per mm of its length. It has been demonstrated that fluorescence measurement in a single cell in a three-dimensional tissue is influenced by fluorescence derived from surrounding out-of-focus cells [1]. Thus, to measure intracellular pH (pHi) of a single tubule cell accurately, special care should be taken to eliminate (or minimize) this "out-of-focus" effect.

The outer stripe of the outer medullary collecting duct (OMCDo) is one of the important sites of renal acidification [2,3]. In this segment HCO_3^- is absorbed con-

[1]Second Department of Internal Medicine, Tokyo Medical and Dental University, Tokyo, 113 Japan

sistently [3]. OMCDo consists of principal cells (PC) and intercalated cells (IC) [4–6]. Because there are morphological and functional differences between these two cell types [4–7], different mechanisms might be involved in pHi regulation. However, pHi regulation of individual cells in this segment has not been studied so far.

We measured single cell pHi of PC and IC in rabbit OMCDo, using fluorescence ratio imaging microscopy. In the first half of this paper, we describe detailed methods for pHi measurement in the tubule cell. In the latter half, we describe the HCO_3^--independent mechanisms of pHi regulation which were examined using these techniques.

Methods

Kidneys from Japanese white rabbits (2.0–2.5kg) were cut in coronal slices. Segments of OMCDo (300–600 um in length) were dissected and transferred to a thermo-regulated bath of 150ul volume. This bath was set on the stage of an inverted epifluorescence microscope (Olympus IMT-2, Japan) which was placed on a vibration-proof plate (Visolator, Meiritsu, Japan). After tubules were mounted between perfusion and holding pipettes, the lumen was perfused as described previously [8]. The perfusion rate was maintained at > 10nl/min. In some protocols, an isolated OMCDo was split with fine forceps along the long axis and a cell monolayer was made. The monolayer was also mounted between holding pipettes. The bath solution was pre-heated at 37°C and was exchanged at 10ml/min by gravity. The control perfusion and bath solutions were identical and contained (in mM) 134 NaCl, 5 KCl, 1.0 NaH_2PO_4, 1.2 $MgSO_4$, 1.0 $CaCl_2$, 5.5 glucose, 6.0 L-alanine, and 20 HEPES.

After tubules were perfused 20–30 min for equilibration, the acetoxymethyl derivative of 2′-7′-bis (carboxyethyl)-5(6)-carboxyfluorescein (BCECF-AM) was loaded to tubules from the lumen or the bath. For the luminal loading, tubules were perfused with 20–30 μM BCECF-AM for 15–20 min. For the basolateral loading, bath flow was stopped and tubules were bathed with 7–10 μM BCECF-AM for 15–20 min.

Tubule cells were viewed with a 40 × objective (Olympus DPlan Apo, Japan, NA=0.85) and a silicon-intensified target camera (Hamamatsu Photonics C2400-08H, Japan), and were displayed on a TV monitor with 483 × 512 pixels (SONY Trinitron PVM-1371Q, Japan). The final magnification on the TV monitor was 1400 ×. The area of each cell contained 800–2000 pixels at this magnification. One tubule image was recorded in 1/30 s and was stored in an image processor (ARGUS 100, Hamamatsu Photonics, Japan).

Fluorescence was excited using a 75-W xenon lamp. Excitation light was attenuated by neutral density filters. For pHi measurement with BCECF, 490 ± 10 nm and 440 ± 10 nm interference filters, a 520 nm dichroic mirror, a > 520 nm cut-on filter, and a 535 ± 6 nm bandpass filter were used. Background images were recorded before taking fluorescent images. Tubules were excited alternately at 490 and 440 nm by moving the interference filters placed on a computer-assisted slider. Each image was an average of 4 sequential 1/30 s images; a pair of images (490 and 440 nm excitation) were taken in 1s. After the background signal was subtracted, the 490 nm image was divided by the 440 nm image. For pHi measurement, a rectangular measuring area (15 × 15 pixels) was set on the center of each tubule cell. pHi was determined in 1–5 cells from one tubule.

The in vivo BCECF calibration curve was obtained by the nigericin high K^+ method [9]. The calibration solution contained (in mM) 105 KCl, 30 phosphate, 1.2 $MgSO_4$, 20 HEPES, 40 NMDG, 5.5 glucose, 6 alanine, 1.0 $CaCl_2$, and 10 μM nigericin. The solution pH was adjusted to 7 different pHs (pH 5.8 – 8.2) by KOH or HCl. The fluorescence ratios in PC were 0.68 ± 0.02 (means ± SE of 12 cells from 5 tubules) at pH 5.8; 0.86 ± 0.03 at pH 6.2; 1.04 ± 0.04 at pH 6.6; 1.35 ± 0.04 at pH 7.0; 1.73 ± 0.03 at pH 7.4; 2.03 ± 0.03 at pH 7.8; and 2.36 ± 0.04 at pH 8.2. The ratios in IC were higher than PC by 0.01 – 0.06 at any pH, although differences in values were not significant in these two cell types. Because the fluorescence ratio-pH relationship was approximately linear between pH 5.8 and 6.6 and between pH 6.6 and 7.8 in both PC and IC, linear conversion formulas (the ratio of 490/440 nm = a + b × pHi) were made separately for these two pH ranges. These calibrations were used to convert the ratios to pHi.

Because this study was focused on HCO_3^--independent mechanisms of pHi regulation, all experiments were performed in the absence of extracellular CO_2/HCO_3^-. pHi regulation processes were examined by analyzing the time course of pHi recovery from intracellular acid load, using the NH_4Cl pre-pulse technique [10]. Five to ten min after BCECF-AM removal, 20mM NH_4Cl was added to the bath (replaced by 20mM NaCl in the control solution) for 3min, and then NH_4Cl was rapidly removed. The time course of pHi was monitored at a 5 or 10 s interval. In response to NH_4Cl withdrawal, pHi decreased for 10–20s; this was followed by a gradual pHi recovery. pHi recovery rate (dpHi/dt, pHU/s × 10^3) was calculated from data points during 20s of the initial recovery phase. Similar experiments were carried out in the absence of Na^+ (replaced by $NMDG^+$). Acid loading was done by substituting 20mM $NMDG^+$ for NH_4^+. Data for pHi of 1–5 cells were obtained from one tubule.

The results are expressed as means ± SE. Student's *t*-test and an analysis of variance were used, when appropriate, to determine statistical significance. Values of $P<0.05$ were considered significant.

Results and Discussion

Measurement of Single Cell pHi

Because the OMCDo is cylindrical, a single cell fluorescence measurement would be affected by neighboring cells [1]. Before starting experiments with tubule cells, we tested this issue in our experimental system. A glass capillary of 5μm diameter (similar in size to a single cell in rabbit OMCDo) was filled with 200μM BCECF. The fluorescence intensity of this capillary sample was measured at various focus levels. When the focus was adjusted just at the level of the capillary, the fluorescence was detected virtually right on the sample (Fig. 1). This result indicates that the influence from neighboring cells could be negligible if fluorescence was measured in a flat sheet. Some protocols were performed with a cell monolayer made by splitting an isolated OMCDo (Fig. 2c). Fluorescence was also measured at 10μm, 20μm and 30μm above the capillary level (Fig. 1). Fluorescence was detected not only right above the sample but also around the sample. These results suggested

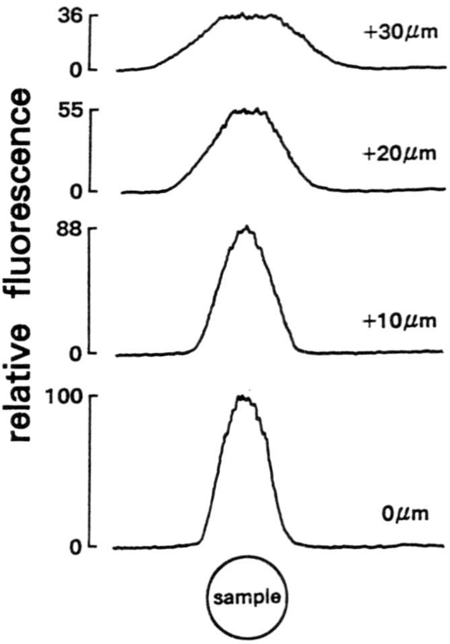

Fig. 1. Out-of-focus effect on fluorescence measurement. A glass capillary (5μm in diameter) was filled with 200μM BCECF and fluorescence was detected at various focus levels.

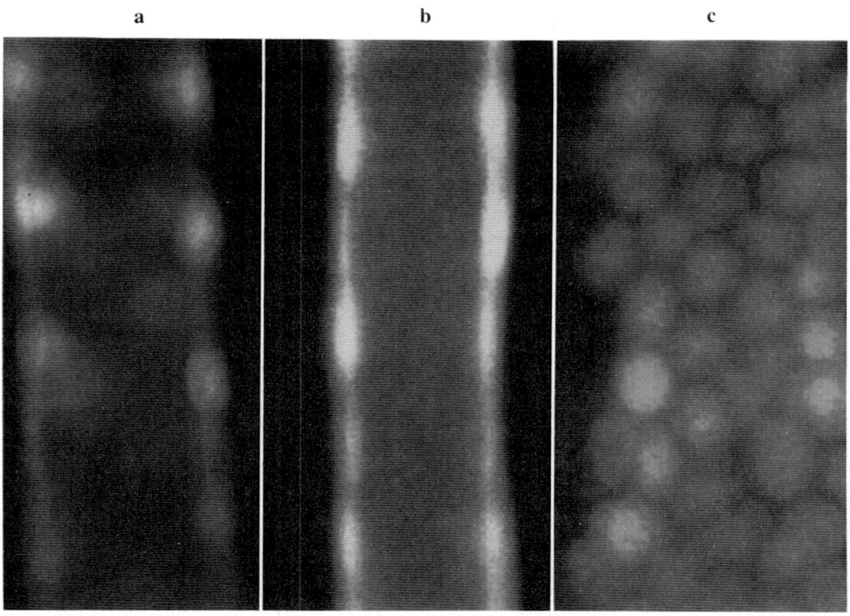

Fig. 2a-c. Fluorescent images of OMCDo perfused in vitro (400x). BCECF was loaded from the lumen (**a**) or the bath (**b**). **c** A fluorescent image of a cell monolayer that was made by splitting an isolated OMCDo. × 400

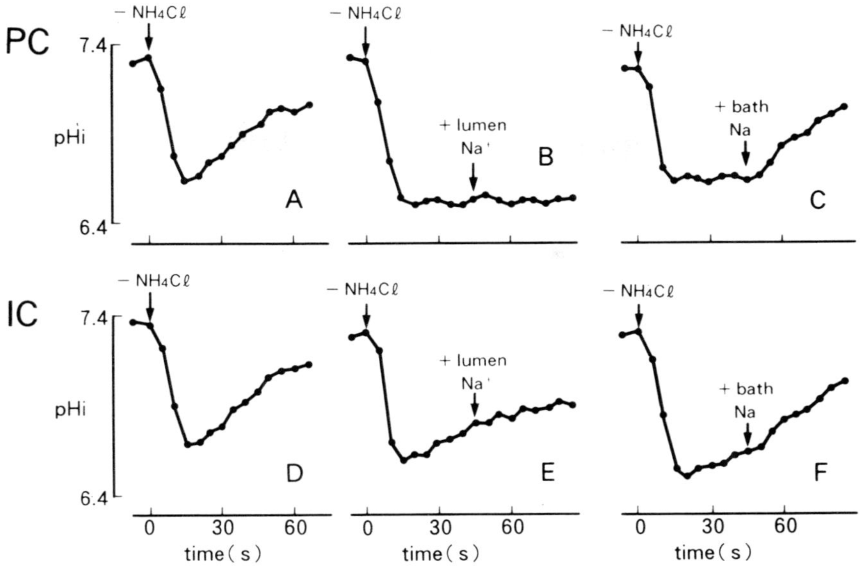

Fig. 3a-f. Time courses of pHi recovery from intracellular acid load in PC (**a-c**) and in IC (**d-f**) in the absence of extracellular HCO_3^-. NH_4Cl was removed from the bath at time zero. See text for details. PC, principal cells; IC, intercalated cells

that single cell fluorescence measurement in the intact tubule would be influenced by out-of-focus cells.

Cell identification was basically dependent on morphological criteria originally described in cortical collecting tubule (CCT) cells by Strange and Spring [11]. In most cases cells were identified without differential interference contrast optics. When BCECF was loaded from the lumen, only IC were intensely stained (Fig. 2a), a finding consistent with a recent report by Weiner and Hamm [12]. Because the fluorescence of PC was very weak, the interference from surrounding PC would be small. Thus, luminal loading was used in the pHi measurement of IC. In contrast, all cells were brightly stained with basolateral loading of BCECF (Fig. 2b). IC were slightly (<50%) brighter than PC. To avoid the influence of IC fluorescence in the pHi measurement of PC, we carefully chose PC that were minimally surrounded by IC (the ratio of the number of PC and IC is about 4:1 in OMCDo (see [4]). As will be shown later, pHi data obtained in intact tubule and monolayer preparations were in general quite similar for both PC and IC.

pHi Recovery from Intracellular Acid Load

To examine HCO_3^--independent mechanisms of pHi regulation, time courses of pHi upon acid load were observed in the absence of extracellular HCO_3^- (Fig. 3). Figs. 3a and 3d show experiments with monolayer cells. After NH_4Cl was removed from the bath at time zero, the pHi of PC (Fig. 3a) and IC (Fig. 3d) decreased promptly and recovered gradually thereafter. In PC dpHi/dt was 12.3 ± 0.9 (10 cells) and in IC it

lumial[Na^+]	135	0	135	0	0	0
bath[Na^+]	135	0	0	135	15	15

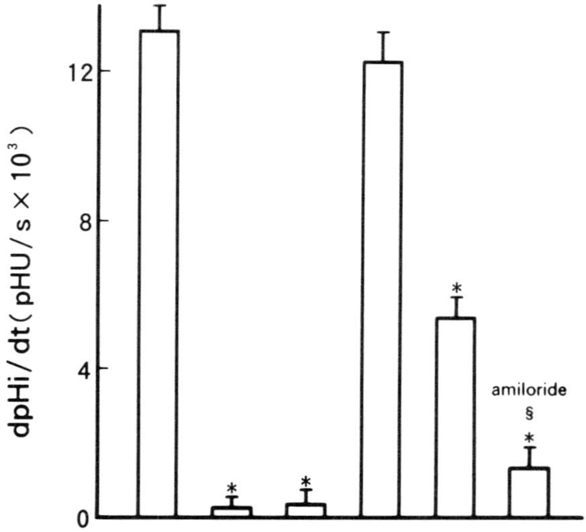

Fig. 4. pHi recovery rates (*dpHi/dt*) of PC at various [Na^+] (in mM). Each *bar* represents means ± SE of 10–21 cells from 4–11 tubules. amiloride; 1mM amiloride was added to the bath at the NH_4Cl removal. *$P < 0.001$ compared with the control, §$P < 0.01$ compared with the absence of amiloride

was 11.5 ± 1.0 (10 cells). Similar values of dpHi/dt were obtained in the intact tubule study (13.8 ± 0.7 in 15 PC; 12.7 ± 0.9 in 12 IC). The advantage of the experiment with the cell monolayer is that single cell fluorescent measurement would be free from the effect of ambient cells shown above. However, the localization (luminal or basolateral) of pHi regulation processes was not detected in this preparation because the solutions of both luminal and basolateral sides were altered simultaneously at bath fluid change. Thus most of the following experiments were performed in the intact tubule preparation.

Na^+ dependence was examined under nominally Na^+-free conditions. At NH_4Cl loading, Na^+ was eliminated from the lumen and the bath. pHi recovery was absent in PC (Figs. 3b and 3c). The addition of 135mM luminal Na^+ had no effect on the acidified pHi (Fig. 3b). pHi started to increase in response to 135mM bath Na^+ (Fig. 3c). A significant pHi recovery was observed in IC in the absence of Na^+ (Figs. 3e and 3f). Luminal Na^+ did not change dpHi/dt (Fig. 3e), whereas bath Na^+ further increased dpHi/dt (Fig. 3f). These results in PC and IC are summarized in Figs. 4 and 5, respectively.

Similar bath Na^+ effect was seen in the monolayer cells. In response to basolateral addition of Na^+, dpHi/dt increased from 0.6 ± 0.5 to 11.9 ± 1.5 in 15 PC, and from 9.1 ± 0.8 to 12.3 ± 0.9 in 11 IC.

To further examine the basolateral Na^+-dependent pHi recovery process, the effect of amiloride, a Na^+/H^+ exchanger inhibitor [13–16] was tested in PC. pHi recovery

lumial[Na⁺]	135	0	135	0	0	0	0	0
bath[Na⁺]	135	0	0	135	15	15	0	0

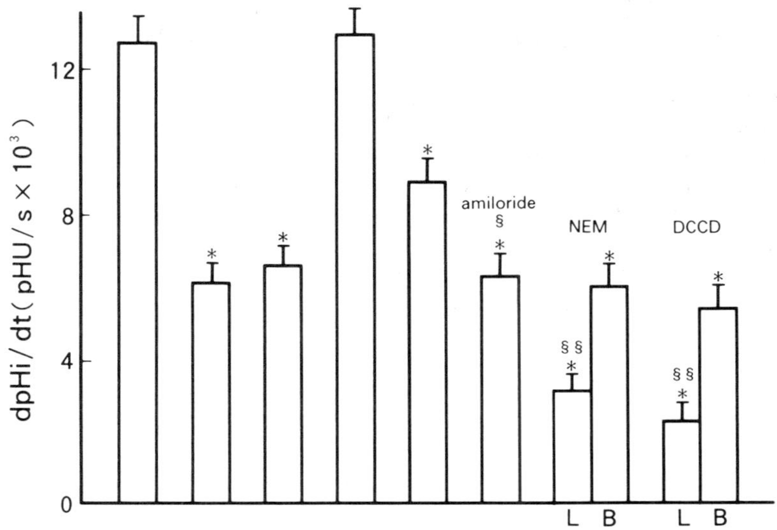

Fig. 5. pHi recovery rates (dpHi/dt) of IC at various [Na^+] (in mM). Each *bar* represents means ± SE of 8–24 cells from 4–12 tubules. Amiloride, 1mM amiloride was added to the bath at the NH_4Cl removal; NEM, DCCD 0.5mM NEM or DCCD was added to the lumen (*L*) or the bath (*B*) 10min before the experiment. *$P < 0.01$ compared with the control, §$P < 0.05$ compared with the absence of amiloride, §§$P < 0.01$ compared with the absence of H^+-ATPase inhibitor

induced by 15mM bath Na^+ was lower in the presence of 1mM basolateral amiloride (dpHi/dt = 1.4 ± 0.5) than in its absence (5.4 ± 0.5, $P<0.01$) (Fig. 4). A similar amiloride effect was seen on the bath Na^+-dependent pHi recovery in IC (Fig. 5). These results suggest the presence of a basolateral Na^+/H^+ exchanger in both PC and IC.

In the renal collecting duct, Chaillet et al. [13] first demonstrated the basolateral Na^+/H^+ antiporter in CCT. This antiporter has also been found in cultured inner medullary collecting duct (IMCD) cells [14,15] and in the inner stripe of OMCD (OMCDi) cells [16]. The physiological role of the peritubular Na^+/H^+ antiport in relation to transepithelial transport of H^+/HCO_3^- and other solutes is not clear at present. In contrast to findings in the basolateral membrane, evidence of the presence of luminal Na^+/H^+ was not detected, a finding consistent with previous studies in the collecting duct [13,17].

The pHi of IC consistently recovered from cellular acidification in the absence of Na^+ (Figs. 3 and 5). ATP-dependent H^+ secretion has been shown in collecting duct cells [2,14,18–20]. To determine whether H^+-ATPase is associated with the Na^+-independent pHi recovery, a known H^+-ATPase inhibitor, N-ethylmaleimide (NEM) [21–23] was added at 0.5 mM to the lumen or the bath 10 min before the experiment. The results are summarized in Fig. 5. In the presence of bath NEM dpHi/dt (6.1 ± 0.5, 10 cells) was not significantly different from dpHi/dt in its absence (6.4 ± 0.3, 24 cells). In contrast, dpHi/dt was significantly lower in the presence of luminal NEM (3.3 ± 0.6, 11 cells). Similar results were obtained with another H^+-ATPase inhibitor, N,N′-dicyclohexylcarbodiomide (DCCD) [21,24] at 0.5 mM (Fig. 5). These results suggest that a luminal H^+-ATPase is involved in Na^+-independent pHi recovery in IC. Our finding supports the view that most of the IC in rabbit OMCDo are type A [8,25]. Our finding is also compatible with the recent work done by Brown et al. [26], in which the luminal membrane of IC in OMCDo was heavily labeled with antibodies to bovine kidney H^+ pump.

Luminal 0.5 mM NEM or DCCD did not totally inhibit the Na^+-independent pHi recovery of IC (Fig. 5). This result shows the possibility of the presence of another pHi recovery process besides that of H^+-ATPase. In fact, Wingo [27] has recently shown functional evidence for the presence of omeprazole-sensitive, NEM-insensitive H^+-K^+-ATPase in the rabbit OMCDi. We did not test this possibility in the present study.

Acknowledgments. The authors thank Dr. Tomita for encouragement of this work. The authors are grateful to Miss Mayumi Mirokuji for her excellent secretarial assistance.

This work was supported by a Grant-in-Aid from the Ministry of Education, Science, and Culture, Japan.

References

1. Agard DA, Hiraoka Y, Shaw P, Sedat JW (1989) Fluorescence microscopy in three dimensions. In: Taylor DL, Wang Y-L (eds) Methods in Cell Biology, vol 30. Fluorescence microscopy of living cells in culture, part B. Academic Press, pp 379–398
2. Schwartz GJ, Al-Awqati Q (1985) Carbon dioxide causes exocytosis of vesicles containing H^+ pumps in isolated perfused proximal and collecting tubules. J Clin Invest 75:1638–1644
3. McKinney TD, Davidson KK (1987) Bicarbonate transport in collecting tubules from outer stripe of outer medulla of rabbit kidneys. Am J Physiol 253 (Renal Fluid Electrolyte Physiol 22):F816–F822
4. LeFurgey A, Tisher CC (1979) Morphology of rabbit collecting duct. Am J Anat 155:111–124
5. Kaissling B, Kriz W (1979) Structural analysis of the rabbit kidney. Adv Anat Embryol Cell Biol 56:1–123
6. Ridderstrale Y, Kashgarian M, Koeppen B, Giebisch G, Stetson D, Ardito T, Stanton B (1988) Morphological heterogeneity of the rabbit collecting duct. Kidney Int 34:655–670
7. Koeppen BM (1986) Conductive properties of the rabbit outer medullary collecting duct: outer stripe. Am J Physiol 250 (Renal Fluid Electrolyte Physiol 19):F70–F76
8. Kuwahara M, Sasaki S, Marumo F (to be published) Intracellular pH regulation in rabbit outer medullary collecting duct cells: mechanisms and localization of HCO_3^--independent processes. Am J Physiol
9. Thomas JA, Buchsbaum RN, Zimniak A, Racker E (1979) Intracellular pH measurements in Ehrlich ascites tumor cells utilizing spectroscopic probes generated in situ. Biochemistry 18:2210–2218
10. Roos A, Boron WF (1981) Intracellular pH. Physiol Rev 61:296–434
11. Strange K, Spring KR (1987) Cell membrane water permeability of rabbit cortical collecting duct. J Membr Biol 96:27–43

12. Weiner ID, Hamm LL (1989) Use of fluorescent dye BCECF to measure intracellular pH in cortical collecting tubule. Am J Physiol 256 (Renal Fluid Electrolyte Physiol 25):F957–F964
13. Chaillet JR, Lopes AG, Boron WF (1985) Basolateral Na-H exchange in the rabbit cortical collecting tubule. J Gen Physiol 86:795–812
14. Kleinman JG, Blumenthal SS, Weissner JH, Reetz KL, Lewand DL, Mandel NS, Mandel GS, Garanics JC, Cragoe EJ Jr (1987) Regulation of pH in rat papillary tubule cells in primary culture. J Clin Invest 80:1660–1669
15. Wall SM, Muallem S, Kraut JA (1987) Detection of a sodium-hydrogen antiporter in cultured rat renal papillary collecting duct cell. Am J Physiol 253 (Renal Fluid Electrolyte Physiol 22):F889–F895
16. Breyer MD, Jacobson HR (1989) Regulation of rabbit medullary collecting duct pH by basolateral Na^+/H^+ and Cl^-/base exchange. J Clin Invest 84:996–1004
17. McKinney TD, Burg MB (1978) Bicarbonate absorption by rabbit cortical collecting tubules in vitro. Am J Physiol 234 (Renal Fluid Electrolyte Physiol 3):F141–F145
18. Graber ML, Bengele HH, Schwartz JH, Alexander EA (1981) pH and PCo_2 profiles of the rat inner medullary collecting duct. Am J Physiol 241 (Renal Fluid Electrolyte Physiol 10):F659–F668
19. Prigent A, Bichara M, Paillard M (1985) Hydrogen transport in papillary collecting duct in rabbit kidney. Am J Physiol 248 (Cell Physiol 17):C241–C246
20. Zeidel ML, Silva P, Seifter JL (1986) Intracellular pH regulation and proton transport by rabbit renal medullary collecting duct cells: role of plasma membrane proton adenosine triphosphatase. J Clin Invest 77:113–120
21. Gluck S, Al-Awqati Q (1984) An electrogenic proton-translocating adenosine triphosphatase from bovine kidney medulla. J Clin Invest 73:1704–1710
22. Kaunitz JD, Gunther RD, Sachs G (1984) Characterization of an electrogenic ATP and chloride-dependent proton translocating pump from rat renal medulla. J Biol Chem 260:11567–11573
23. Ait-Mohamed AK, Marsy S, Barlet C, Khadouri C, Doucet A (1986) Characterization of N-ethylmaleimide-sensitive proton pump in the rat kidney: localization along the nephron. J Biol Chem 261:12526–12533
24. Stone DK, Xie X-S, Wu LT, Racker E (1984) Proton translocating ATPases of clathrin-coated vesicles, renal medulla, and Ehrlich ascites tumor cells. In: Forte JG, Warnock DG, Rector FC Jr (eds) Hydrogen transport in epithelia. John Wiley and Sons, New York, pp 219–230
25. Schwartz GJ, Satlin LM, Bergmann JE (1988) Fluorescent characterization of collecting duct cells: a second H^+-secreting type. Am J Physiol 255 (Renal Fluid Electrolyte Physiol 24):F1003–F1014
26. Brown D, Hirsch S, Gluck S (1988) Localization of a proton-pumping ATPase in rat kidney. J Clin Invest 82:2114–2126
27. Wingo CS (1989) Active proton secretion and potassium absorption in the rabbit outer medullary collecting duct: functional evidence for proton-potassium-activated adenosine triphosphatase. J Clin Invest 84:361–365

Ultramicro-Analysis of Tubular Fluid by Continuous-Flow Methodology

MARK A. KNEPPER[1]

SUMMARY. The measurement of net transepithelial fluxes in isolated perfused tubule experiments requires highly sensitive analytical methods, capable of precise determination of solute concentrations in 1–30 nanoliter samples of collected fluid. The continuous-flow approach to ultramicro-analysis of small aqueous samples, developed by Vurek in the early 1980s, has provided the sensitivity, precision, and speed necessary to dramatically enhance the efficiency of transepithelial flux measurements in isolated perfused tubules. The instruments used, a continuous-flow colorimeter and a continuous-flow fluorometer, are extremely versatile, allowing measurement of any of the major osmotically-active components of either plasma or urine in nanoliter volume samples. Specifically, these two instruments have been used to measure chloride, bicarbonate, sodium, potassium, ammonium, urea, creatinine, glucose, raffinose, lactate, calcium, magnesium, phosphate, and acetaminophen concentrations in 1–30 nanoliter samples with a coefficient of variation in the range 2%–4%. This paper reviews the design and application of these continuous-flow instruments.

Introduction

In vitro perfusion of renal tubules, a technique developed by Burg and his colleagues in the late 1960s [1], remains one of the mainstays of renal physiological research. This technique has allowed detailed investigation of the transport properties of renal tubule segments not accessible to micropuncture and other in vivo approaches. Furthermore, the ability to maintain well-controlled conditions in isolated perfused tubule experiments, free of the complexity of the normal in vivo environment, has led to substantial progress in the understanding of transport processes and their control, even in renal tubule segments that can be studied in vivo.

[1]Laboratory of Kidney and Electrolyte Metabolism, National Heart, Lung and Blood Institute, National Institutes of Health, Bethesda, MD 20892, USA

Table 1. Ultramicroanalytical methods using the continuous-flow colorimeter

Solute	Chemistry	Detection limit (pmol)	Coefficient of variation[a]	Reference
Chloride	Ferric thiocyanate	5	2%–3%	[8]
Sodium	Macrocylic ionophore	57	3%–5%	[5]
Potassium	Macrocylic ionophore	8	3%–5%	[5]
Creatinine	Alkaline picrate	2	2%–3%	[9]
Calcium	Methylthymol blue	1	3%–4%	[2]
Magnesium	Calmagite	0.2	2%–3%	[3]
Phosphate	Ammonium molybdate	1	3%–4%	[3]
Acetominophen	Sodium nitrate	2	4%–5%	[10]

[a]Standard deviation divided by mean for 4–5 repeat determinations using as standards the usual range of sample sizes from isolated perfused tubule collections

Measurement of transepithelial fluxes in isolated perfused tubules generally requires the collection and analysis of the fluid exiting the tubule lumen. Depending on the flow rates required to measure the appropriate fluxes, the volumes of the collected samples typically range from 2–100 nl. Success in such studies has required the availability of precise methods for the analysis of these small tubule fluid samples. In the early years of isolated perfused tubule studies, most flux measurements were achieved using radio-isotopic tracers. This approach yields unidirectional solute fluxes, i.e., bath-to-lumen or lumen-to-bath fluxes. Estimates of net fluxes from radio-isotopic flux measurements have usually been achieved by subtracting one unidirectional flux from the other. The precision of such net flux measurements is therefore somewhat limited. Consequently, renal physiologists began very early to search for sensitive ultramicroanalytical methods capable of measuring solute concentrations in nanoliter volume fluid samples, thus permitting direct determination of net solute fluxes. In the early 1980s, Vurek introduced a new "continuous-flow" approach for the ultramicroanalysis of tubule fluid samples [2–4]. This approach has dramatically broadened the utility of the isolated perfused tubule technique. Vurek's continuous-flow approach has been further developed to allow the determination, in nanoliter-range samples, of concentrations of virtually all of the osmotically-important solutes normally present in urine or plasma [5] (Tables 1 and 2).

The continuous-flow method is diagrammed in Fig. 1. It consists of four elements. A *reagent reservoir* contains the appropriate reagent to allow conversion of the target

Table 2. Ultramicroanalytical methods using the continuous-flow fluorometer

Solute	Enzyme(s)	Detection limit (pmol)	Coefficient of variation[a]	Reference
Ammonium	Glutamic dehydrogenase	0.50	3%–5%	[7]
Urea	Urease/glutamic dehydrogenase	0.25	3%–5%	[11]
Bicarbonate	PEP carboxylase/malic dehydrogenase	0.50	3%–5%	[12]
Glucose	Hexokinase/glucose-6-phosphate dehydrogenase	0.25	3%–5%	–
Lactate	Lactic dehydrogenase	0.25	4%–6%	[13]
Raffinose	Galactosidase/galactose dehydrogenase	0.75	4%–5%	[14]

[a]Standard deviation divided by mean for 4–5 repeat determinations using as standards the usual range of sample sizes from isolated perfused tubule collections

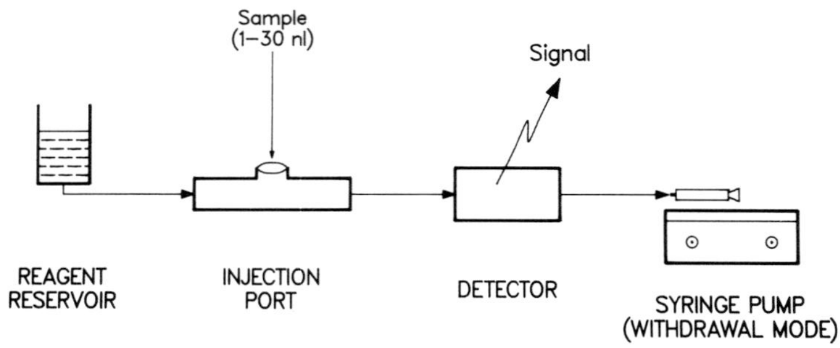

Fig. 1. *General scheme for continuous-flow instruments.* Typically, one to thirty nanoliter samples are injected into the flowing reagent stream. The appropriate chemical reaction occurs while the injected sample flows toward the detector to form a colored or fluorescent product. The detector is either a miniature colorimeter (Fig. 2) or a miniature fluorometer (Fig. 3). (From [4] with permission)

substance into a colored or fluorescent product. A precision *syringe pump* fitted with a Teflon-tipped gas tight syringe draws the reagent through the *injection port* and the *detector element* at a constant rate. Typically a 1–30 nanoliter volume sample is injected into the flowing reagent stream via the injection port. The appropriate color-producing or fluorescence-producing chemical reaction takes place as the sample bolus flows toward the detector. The detector element is essentially a scaled-down colorimeter or fluorometer, capable of accurately measuring either the absorbance or the fluorescence of the reaction product. It contains a sensitive photo-detector, either a silicon photodiode [6] or a photomultiplier tube [7], which converts an optical signal to an electronic signal (see below). Generally, the output is available within 2–5 minutes of sample injection, allowing measurements to be made as the samples are collected from the perfused tubules.

In the following sections, we discuss first the design and application of the continuous-flow *colorimeter*. Then, we describe the design and application of the continuous-flow *fluorometer*.

Continuous-Flow Colorimeter

Figure 2 is a diagram of the detector element for the continuous-flow colorimeter [5]. The cuvet is a U-tube fashioned from a small-bore glass capillary which is connected to the injection port at one end and the syringe pump at the other. An incandescent lamp containing a built-in lens is oriented so as to send a beam of broad-spectrum light along the shaft of the cuvet. Thus, when the colored reaction product flows into the cuvet, light is absorbed, resulting in a measurable reduction in the amount of light exiting the cuvet. The emerging light is filtered by an appropriate band-pass interference filter that passes only the wavelengths corresponding to the absorption maximum of the reaction product. The optical signal is measured using a sensitive silicon photodiode. A simple electronic circuit utilizing a low cost operational amplifier is used to convert the change in resistance of the photodiode to an amplified voltage

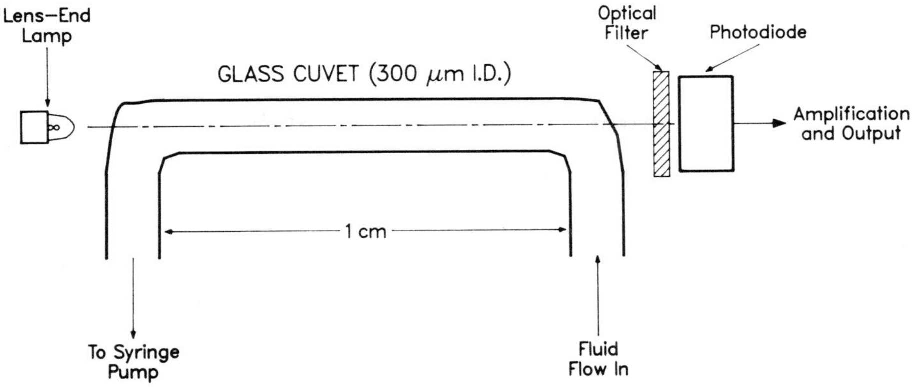

Fig. 2. *Detector system for ultramicro-colorimeter.* The colored reaction product flows through the light path, decreasing the amount of light impinging on the silicon photodiode. (From [4] with permission)

signal [6]. The output can then be read out on a linear chart recorder or can be fed to an analog-to-digital converted to allow a computer to carry out digital filtering and peak integration [5].

As described in Table 1, the continuous-flow colorimeter has been used successfully for the ultramicro-analysis of several solutes including chloride, sodium, potassium, creatinine, calcium, magnesium, phosphate, and acetaminophen. These methods have allowed the detection of as little as 5–10 pmol of some solutes, while at the same time affording a high degree of precision. When working in the optimal range of sample sizes (generally about 5–10 fold above the detection limit), the coefficient of variation (standard deviation/mean ×100%) for repeat injections of standards is generally in the range 2%–3%. Reaction times vary among the assay methods, ranging from a virtually instantaneous reaction for the magnesium method to about 10 minutes for the sodium method. Most of the reactions are complete within 3–4 minutes, allowing samples to be injected into the apparatus as they are collected from the perfused tubule. It is relatively easy to switch from the analysis of one solute to the analysis of another within 5–10 minutes by changing the reagent in the reagent reservoir and replacing the optical filter with the appropriate one to match the absorbance spectrum of the reaction product.

Continuous-Flow Fluorometer

Figure 3 is a diagram of the detector element for the continuous-flow fluorometer. As with the colorimeter, the fluorometer cuvet is a small-bore U-tube connected at one end to the injection port and at the other end to the withdrawal pump. Ultraviolet excitation light from a Hg-Xe lamp is delivered to the cuvet via a fused-silica optical fiber inserted into the side of the cuvet. The fluorescent reaction product is excited as it passes through the cuvet, resulting in an emission signal proportional to the amount of fluorescent material. The emitted light is filtered by an appropriate long-

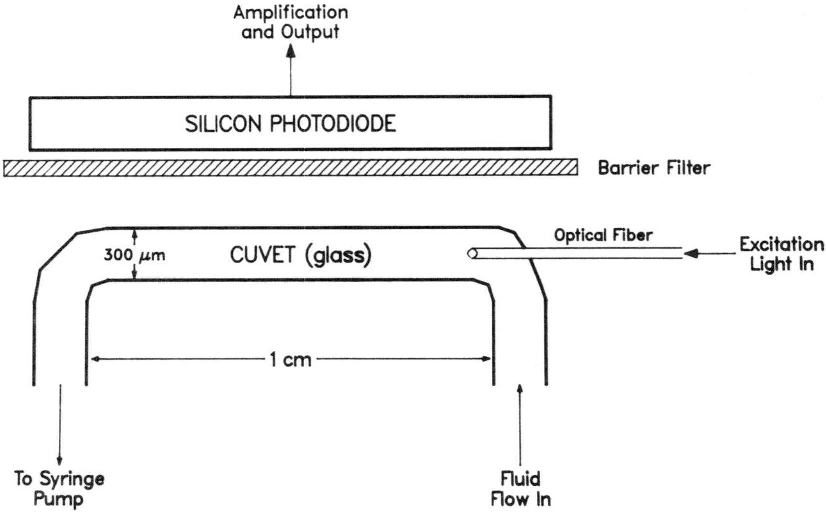

Fig. 3. *Detector system for ultramicro-fluorometer.* The fluorescent reaction product (generally NADH) flows past the tip of a fused-silica optical fiber carrying ultraviolet excitation light from a Mercury-Xenon lamp. The emitted light passes through a barrier filter to impinge on a silicon photodiode

pass optical filter and impinges on a silicon photodiode. Amplification of the photodiode output and processing of the amplified signal is accomplished in a manner nearly identical to the approach used for the continuous-flow colorimeter.

As described in Table 2, the continuous-flow fluorometer has been used successfully for the ultramicroanalysis of several solutes including ammonium, urea, bicarbonate, glucose, lactate, and raffinose. All of these methods depend on the use of various dehydrogenase enzymes, which catalyze oxidation-reduction reactions coupled to the simultaneous reduction of NAD or oxidation of NADH. Since NADH is fluorescent and NAD is not, the enzyme-catalyzed chemical reactions result in either an increase or a decrease in the fluorescent signal, which is proportional to the amount of the substrate injected into the reagent stream. Thus, a variety of substances can be assayed with a single instrument that measures the concentration of NADH, simply by changing the enzymes that are placed in the reagent stream. Because fluorescence measurements are intrinsically more sensitive that absorbance measurements, the methods shown in Table 2 have detection limits considerably lower than those shown in Table 1 (generally less than 1 pmol). When working in the optimal range of sample sizes (generally about 5–50 fold above the detection limit), the coefficient of variation (standard deviation/mean $\times 100\%$) for repeat injections of standards is generally in the range 3%–4%. The reaction time depends on the amount of enzyme added to the reagent stream. Generally, it is possible to add enough enzyme to enable the appropriate chemical reaction to go to completion within 2 minutes of injection, permitting samples to be run every 2–3 minutes. Consequently, as for the colorimetric methods, it is generally feasible to analyze tubule fluid samples during the course of a perfused tubule experiment. Because the specificity of the fluorescent assay depends only on the enzymes that are placed in the reagent reservoir, the same instrument can be used for the measurement of any of the solutes shown on Table 2.

Discussion

The continuous-flow methods discussed in this paper afford the investigator an unprecedented degree of precision in the analysis of 1–30 nanoliter volume tubule fluid samples. A coefficient of variation in the range 2%–4% is typical when the instruments are set up to measure quantities of solutes in the optimal range (generally 5–10 times greater than the detection limit). This high degree of reproducibility is the consequence of the mechanical simplicity of the instruments; the only moving mechanical component is the stepping-motor syringe pump which, when used with a clean gas-tight syringe, can produce extremely steady flow rates through the instruments. The method is quite insensitive to the injection technique, allowing even inexperienced operators to attain a high degree of reproducibility.

The continuous-flow techniques are very rapid. The collected fluid samples can generally be injected directly into the instrument immediately after collection and the output is available within 2–5 minutes of injection. Consequently, the investigator obtains immediate feedback which allows him to adjust the rate of tubule perfusion or other conditions to optimize the accuracy of flux measurements. With other assay methods (radio-isotope measurement and older chemical analytical techniques) it was generally necessary to accumulate samples during experiments and to complete the measurements either later in the day or overnight. Because of the speed and simplicity of the measurements, the efficiency of the isolated perfused tubule technique has improved, i.e., we are generally able to obtain a greater yield of successful experiments.

The continuous-flow methods are also very inexpensive to run. Most of the reagents needed for the assays are available commercially as relatively inexpensive analytical kits. Because of the small volume of reagent needed (2–4 ml per day), one kit often lasts several weeks or months. The instruments are now commercially available for under $6000 (Sewell Machine Shop, Birmingham, Ala.). Several tubule perfusion laboratories in the United States and Japan are presently using either the commercial version of the continuous-flow instruments or custom-built instruments made locally.

The continuous-flow instruments described in this paper have been divided into two classes (colorimetric and fluorometric) depending on the type of detector utilized. Other types of continuous-flow instruments can be devised based on other methods of detection. For example, Garvin [15] has recently introduced a continuous-flow method for measuring potassium using a potassium-selective electrode as the detection element.

References

1. Burg MB, Grantham JJ, Abramow M, Orloff J (1983) Preparation and study of fragments of single rabbit nephrons. Am J Physiol 210:1293–1298

2. Vurek GG (1981) Calcium measurement: picomole quantitiation by continuous-flow colorimetry. Anal Biochem 114:288–293
3. Vurek GG (1981) Flow-through nanocolorimeter for measurement of picomole amounts of magnesium and phosphate. Anal Letters 14:261–269
4. Vurek GG (1982) Nanoliter-volume flow-through fluorometer. Anal Chem 54:840–842
5. Terada Y, Knepper MA (1989) Continuous-flow quantitation of Na^+ and K^+ in nanoliter samples using chromogenic macrocyclic ionophores. Am J Physiol 257:F893–F898
6. Vurek GG, Knepper MA (1982) A colorimeter for measurement of picomole quantities of urea. Kidney Int 21:656–658
7. Good DW, Vuek GG (1983) Picomole quantitation of ammonia by flow-through fluorometry. Anal Biochem 130:199–202
8. Star RA, Burg MB, Knepper MA (1985) Bicarbonate secretion and chloride absorption by rabbit cortical collecting ducts. J Clin Invest 76:1123–1130
9. Knepper MA, Good DW, Burg MB (1985) Ammonia and bicarbonate transport by rat cortical collecting ducts perfused in vitro. Am J Physiol 249:F870–F877
10. Chou C-L, Sands JM, Nonoguchi H, Knepper MA (1990) Concentration dependence of urea and thiourea transport in rat inner medullary collecting duct. Am J Physiol 258:F486–F494
11. Sands JM, Knepper MA (1987) Urea permeability of mammalian inner medullary collecting duct system and papillary surface epithelium. J Clin Invest 79:138–147
12. Star RA (1990) Quantitation of total carbon dioxide in nanoliter samples by flow-through fluorometry. Am J Physiol 258:F429–F432
13. Bagnasco S, Good D, Balaban R, Burg M (1985) Lactate production in isolated segments of the rat nephron. Am J Physiol 248:F522–F526
14. Garvin JL, Burg MB, Knepper MA (1985) Ammonium replaces potassium in supporting sodium transport by the Na^+-K^+-ATPase of renal proximal straight tubules. Am J Physiol 249:F785–F788
15. Garvin JL (1989) Picomole quantitation of potassium using a continuous-flow apparatus. Kidney Int 36:726–729

Optical Methods for Quantifying Cell Volume Changes in Isolated Nephron Segments

KEVIN STRANGE[1]

SUMMARY. Animal cell volume is determined by extracellular and intracellular solute content. Measurements of cell volume changes induced by osmotic, ionic, electrophysiological and/or pharmacological manipulations can therefore provide important and often unique insights into membrane solute and water transport properties. In addition, volume measurements allow the elucidation of cell volume regulatory mechanism. The purpose of this brief review article is to describe the requirements for measuring volume changes in isolated nephron segments and to illustrate the types of questions that can be addressed using this powerful approach.

Introduction

Water is in thermodynamic equilibrium across animal cell membranes and cell volume is therefore determined by extracellular and intracellular solute content. This fundamental characteristic can be exploited as an experimental tool. Measurements of cell volume changes induced by osmotic, ionic, electrophysiological, and/or pharmacological manipulations provide important and often unique insights into membrane solute and water transport properties. The purpose of this article is to describe briefly the requirements for measuring volume changes in isolated nephron segments and to illustrate the types of questions that can be addressed using this powerful approach. For a more extensive discussion of the use of optical techniques to study epithelial function, the reader is referred to a recent excellent review by Foskett [1].

MacRobbie and Ussing [2] were the first to employ cell volume measurements to study epithelial function. These investigators monitored experimentally-induced changes in the thickness of isolated frog skin by light microscopy and demonstrated that the mucosal and serosal membranes were permeable to NaCl and KCl, respec-

[1]The Children's Hospital, Division of Nephrology, Harvard Medical School, Boston, MA 02115, USA

tively, and that the mucosal membrane was the site of antidiuretic hormone (ADH) action. The capacity of epithelial cells to regulate their volume following osmotic perturbations was also revealed in these early studies. In the late 1970s and early 1980s, Spring and co-workers established the technical and conceptual foundations necessary for rapid and continuous volume measurements in living epithelial cells using high resolution differential interference contrast (DIC) microscopy, video recording methods, and computer image processing techniques [3].

The development of the isolated perfused tubule preparation by Burg and co-workers [4] revolutionized renal physiology and provided the first step toward utilizing volume measurements to study nephron cell function. In a very general sense, observations of cell volume are an inherent component of all perfusion studies. Because of the small size of nephron segments, tubule perfusion is necessarily done under microscopic examination. As such, cell volume changes during experimental manipulations have frequently been reported, beginning with the earliest in vitro studies. For example, Burg et al. [5] noted that addition of glucose and alanine to the luminal perfusate caused marked cell swelling in the proximal convoluted tubule. These studies provided direct evidence for the existence of apical organic solute transport pathways in this nephron segment.

The earliest measurements of nephron cell volume were carried out using conventional brightfield microscopy and photography or measuring devices such as reticules and image-splitting eyepieces. A major advance was made when DIC microscopy was applied to in vitro perfusion methods. Horster and Gundlach [6] were the first to utilize this approach, noting that it generated images with high resolution and contrast, provided optical sectioning capabilities, and allowed for rapid recording of morphology changes. Shortly thereafter, video enhancement and recording methods were combined with both DIC and conventional brightfield microscopy to quantify rapid, experimentally-induced changes in nephron cell volume [7–8].

Video Methods for Measuring Cell Volume

There are many methods for measuring cell volume in both fixed and living tissues. For the purposes of this review, however, I will restrict my discussion of methodology to video techniques combined with light microscopy. Video methods allow the continuous monitoring of rapid cell volume changes and low cost video recording and analysis equipment is now readily available and commonplace in many research laboratories. The advantages afforded by combining video technology with the light microscope are numerous and include image contrast enhancement, ease and speed of data storage and playback, and the ability and ease of digitizing images for processing and analysis.

Two main approaches for quantifying renal tubule cell volume changes by video methods have been taken. In nephron segments composed of a single cell type, tubule length and inner and outer diameter are measured. The tubule geometry is approximated as a cylinder and total epithelial volume is calculated (e.g., [9–10]). This method has three potential sources of error. First, it is assumed that changes in interspace volume do not occur or do not contribute significantly to total epithelial volume. In most nephron segments this assumption is valid, but it should be assessed for each experimental situation. As discussed by Strange and Spring [11], failure to correct for interspace distension has caused significant overestimates of cell swelling during ADH-induced water flow in the cortical collecting tubule (CCT). Second, changes in tubule length accompanying volume perturbations need to be monitored and corrected for, or volume perturbations should be minimized so that length changes do not occur. With respect to the latter approach, a number of investigators have reported that small volume changes have no effect on tubule length [9]. Third, Kirk et al. [9] have noted that significant curvature of the apical surface will invalidate the assumption of a cylindrical tubule geometry. This error has been assessed in the proximal straight tubule [9] and medullary thick ascending limb [10] and found to be less than 1% of the measured cell volume.

Tubule length and diameter can be measured manually from recorded video images using precision calipers [12]. Individual video fields have been analyzed by this method, providing for a maximum image acquisition rate of 60 images/s. Welling et al. [12] have claimed that this method can detect tubule diameter changes of 0.05 μm. Tubule diameters have also been measured by digitizing video images and tracing tubule inner and outer borders using a computer-generated cursor and image analysis software [9–10]. This approach is capable of detecting volume changes of approximately 2% [13].

A fully automated procedure for monitoring cell volume has been described by Whittembury and co-workers [7,14]. In this approach, perfused or nonperfused tubules are imaged so that the video scan lines are oriented perpendicular to the longitudinal tubule axis. For on-line volume determinations, high contrast tubule images are generated by vital staining of the cells or by addition of dye (FDC green) to the perfusate, followed by suitable filtering of the transmitted light. Each video scan line is converted to a binary signal by one or two analog comparators with appropriate threshold settings. Measurement of the duration of binary pulses passing through the cellular or luminal compartment is a measurement of the cell and lumen diameter, respectively. This method can analyze 50–60 images/s and can detect a 1% change in tubule diameter.

For heterogeneous nephron segments such as the CCT, it is necessary to quantify volume changes at the single cell level. Cells can be imaged either en face or in the lateral tubule wall [8]. In both cases it is essential to use DIC microscopy to generate high contrast images and to be able to visualize lateral, apical, and basal cell borders.

Imaging in the en face mode allows the determination of cell volume directly by optical sectioning methods [8]. In this approach, high numerical aperture objective and condenser lenses are used to obtain high resolution in the vertical axis (i.e., shallow depth-of-field). The microscope is step focused through the cell, either manually or under computer control by a stepping motor. At the bottom of the cell and at predetermined levels of focal displacement, video images are recorded. The cross-sectional area of each optical "slice" of the cell is then determined at a later time by tracing the cellular outline on a video monitor with a planimeter [15] or with a computer-generated cursor and image analysis software [16]. Cell volume is calculated from the area measurements and the known distance between each image [16].

Optical sectioning has been used to monitor cell volume in the rabbit CCT [16]. In this nephron segment, minimum volume changes of only 5%–7% can be detected with this method and approximately 2–4 seconds are required to complete an optical sectioning scan of a single cell [8,16]. Because of the high cellular surface area-to-

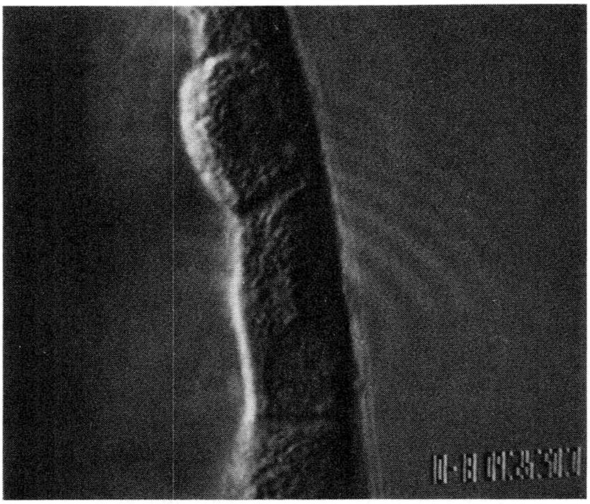

Fig. 1. Video-enhanced DIC image of a principal (*bottom cell*) and an intercalated cell in the lateral wall of the rabbit CCT. Apical surface is to the *left*

volume ratio of most mammalian nephrons, experimentally-induced volume changes can often be complete in less than 1 second (e.g., [16]; Fig. 2). Thus, optical sectioning does not have sufficient speed and resolution to detect initial rates of cell volume change under many experimental conditions. The preferred approach for monitoring the volume of single nephron cells is to image random cellular cross sections in the lateral tubule wall (see Fig. 1). Lateral wall images can be recorded at video framing rates (i.e., 30 images/s). Images are digitized at a later time and cellular outlines are traced on a television monitor with a computer-generated cursor and image analysis software. Relative volume changes are quantified by monitoring changes in cross-sectional area (see [8] for a detailed discussion). Minimum volume changes of 2%–3% can be detected by this approach [16].

Optical and Video Equipment Requirements

The minimum requirements for video quantification of cell volume include a microscope, a video camera, and a measuring system. For tubule perfusion studies, an inverted microscope with a focusable nosepiece is essential. We have used the Nikon Diaphot (Nikon Inc., Garden City, New Jersey) extensively for our studies of the CCT. Optical component micromanipulators are used to mount tubule perfusion V-tracks (White Instrument Co., Suitland, Md.) directly to the microscope stage (see [8,16]), which is equipped with a low-mounted coaxial control arm. This arrangement allows the entire tubule to be scanned simply by translating the stage in the x and y directions.

For many types of volume measurements, the microscope must be equipped with DIC optics. The merits of various DIC systems have been described in detail previously [17]. Our studies of the CCT have utilized calcite polarizer and analyzer prisms (Zeta International Corp., Mt. Prospect, Ill.), a quartz ¼ wave plate (Esco Products Inc., Oak Ridge, N.Y.), and matched Wollaston prisms (Carl Zeiss Inc., New York, N.Y.; see [8] for details). Tubules are imaged using a Zeiss Neofluar 63X (1.25 N.A) lens as the objective and a Leitz 32X (0.4 N.A.) lens as the condenser.

A wide variety of high resolution, research-grade video cameras are readily available from a number of different manufacturers. Inoue has discussed in detail the numerous considerations that go into the choice of a camera for a given microscopy application [17]. For measurements of cell volume, tube-type cameras are generally preferred because of their higher resolution compared to most solid-state imagers. Our studies of the CCT have utilized a Dage camera (Model NC-65S; Dage-MTI Inc., Michigan City, Ind.) equipped with a Newvicon tube. This camera has low geometric distortion, a horizontal resolution of approximately 800 lines, adequate sensitivity for brightfield illumination, electronic magnification capability (Insta-View option), and automatic gain and black level control. It is advantageous to use cameras that allow manual control over gain and black levels for certain types of volume measurements such as the real-time area-tracker described by Whittembury and coworkers [7,14].

The quality of incoming video images can be significantly improved by edge enhancement using a differentiating circuit (e.g., Model IV-530; FOR-A Corp., West Newton, Mass.) or digital image processing. This is particularly useful when DIC microscopy is employed. Some camera systems can be purchased with built-in analog edge enhancement features (e.g., Dage-MTI).

Additional hardware needed for quantifying cell volume changes is dependent on the type of measuring system utilized. The real-time area-tracker method [7] requires construction of an analog image processing circuit. Lindemann has described this circuitry in detail and has published the necessary circuit diagrams [14]. All other methods require the recording of video images for later analysis. Currently, we use an optical disc recorder (Model TQ-2028F; Panasonic Industrial Co., Secaucus, N.J.), which is capable of recording video images in real-time with a horizontal resolution of 450 lines. Video tape recorders can also be employed, but they should be research or broadcast quality instruments with high resolution and they should allow for frame-by-frame analysis of images. In the stop frame mode, the images must be free of excessive jitter, particularly if computer digitization and analysis is to be used.

Image acquisition and analysis systems have undergone tremendous development during the last 10 years. Complex image processing algorithms can now easily be carried out on a personal computer (PC). My laboratory has extensively utilized IBM-AT and compatible machines. A wide variety of high quality data acquisition and image digitizing hardware and software is available for these instruments. We quantify cell volume changes off-line at a data analysis station separate from the experimental setups. Recorded video images are digitized using an image processing computer board with 512 × 512 × 8-bit resolution (Model FG-100-AT; Imaging Technology Inc., Woburn, Mass.). Cell borders are traced on a high resolution video monitor (Model 8831; Aydin Controls, Fort Washington, Pa.) using a 12 × 12 inch graphics tablet (SummaSketch; Summagraphics Corp., Fairfield, Conn.).

An important consideration in the development of a cell volume measuring system is the type of image analysis software that will be employed. Custom programming can be done by the user, or commercial software can be purchased. Numerous PC-based software packages are available that provide an extensive array of menu-driven image processing routines. For volume measurements, where the user is digitizing and tracing a large number of sequential video images, menu-driven software can be tedious to use. The software package purchased should include the capability to develop custom programs via macro routines or by providing the source code to image processing algorithms. If macros are used, the program should allow easy retrieval and storage of data in ASCII format.

General Experimental Requirements

It is necessary to rigorously fulfill several experimental requirements when cell volume changes are used to characterize epithelial membrane water and solute transport. First, the preparation must have good mechanical stability to prevent shifts in focal position during volume measurements. Second, unstirred layers must be minimized and/or corrected for in data analysis. Third, bath and perfusate composition changes need to be made at rates significantly faster than the time constant of the solute and/or water flow under study. Fourth, the image acquisition and recording system utilized must have sufficient spatial and temporal resolution so that initial rates of volume change can be quantified.

For our studies of the CCT, we designed and constructed a rapid laminar flow bath chamber [8]. This chamber provides excellent mechanical stability and allows for peritubular solution changes with half-times of 50–60 ms. Peritubular unstirred layer thickness, measured by observing the flow pattern of latex beads and liposomes, is less than the thickness of the basal lamina. A recent modification of this chamber design allows simultaneous electrophysiological and optical measurements [19].

Apical unstirred layers in isolated nephron segments are negligible due to the small luminal diameter and the laminar flow characteristics of the perfusate. Rapid changes in perfusate composition can be carried out using double barrelled pipets, a retractable pipet assembly, or a conventional exchange pipet arrangement (reviewed in [8]).

Cell Membrane Water Permeability

One of the earliest applications of cell volume measurements in the isolated nephron was the determination of apical and basolateral membrane water permeability. Membrane water flow is characterized by making “step” changes in extracellular osmolality and then monitoring the initial rate of cell swelling or shrinkage (Fig. 2). Water permeability (L_p) is calculated according to the equation,

$$J_v = L_p \, \sigma \, \Delta \pi$$

where J_v is the rate of cell volume change (i.e., rate of transmembrane water flow), σ is the solute reflection coefficient and $\Delta\pi$ is the experimentally-induced osmotic pressure difference.

Determination of apical or basolateral L_p in the nephron is complicated by water flow across the opposing membrane [16]. Water flow needs to be blocked at the

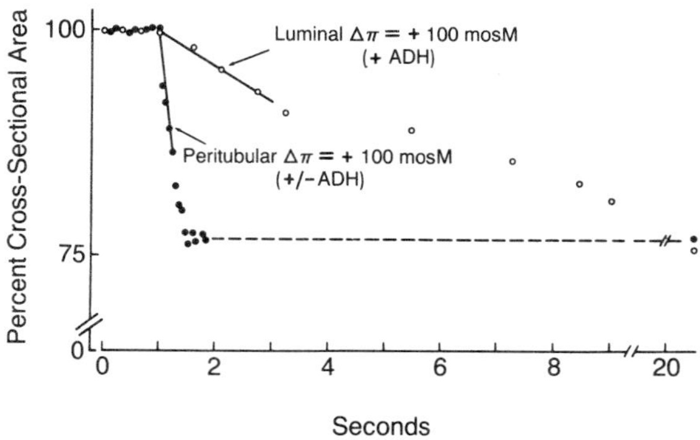

Fig. 2. Volume changes in rabbit CCT principal cells induced by raising luminal or peritubular osmolality from 290 mOsm to 390 mOsm. Luminal osmolality was changed shortly after replacing the peritubular bath with silicone oil [16]. Rates of volume change reflect the total water permeability of each membrane. ADH, antidiuretic hormone

opposing membrane if it has an L_p similar to or greater than the membrane under study. This is usually done by replacing the bath or perfusate with oil [7,16].

Measurement of membrane water permeability is crucial for understanding the routes and mechanisms of transepithelial water flow. Video measurements of membrane L_p (e.g., [12,20]) and solute reflection coefficients [21] have been carried out in the proximal tubule. These studies have demonstrated that both the apical and basolateral membranes of this nephron segment have extremely high water permeabilities and that high rates of transcellular water reabsorption can be driven by osmotic gradients of less than 1–2 mOsm. Recent investigations also indicate that the paracellular pathway may play a significant role in proximal tubule water reabsorption [20]. Guggino et al. [15] measured membrane L_p values in the *Amphiuma* distal tubule and demonstrated that the apical membrane is a major barrier to water flow. This is a result of both an intrinsically low apical bilayer L_p and a greatly reduced apical membrane surface area. Strange and Spring [16] measured water permeability in the rabbit CCT and demonstrated directly that the apical membrane was the site of ADH action and was rate limiting for water reabsorption. In addition, these investigators demonstrated that apical and basolateral membranes had similar *intrinsic* water permeabilities in the presence of ADH. The basolateral membrane, however, had a much higher *total* L_p (see Fig. 2) due to a greatly amplified surface area. This asymmetry has important physiological consequences; it prevents excessive cell swelling and intracellular dilution during ADH-stimulated water reabsorption [11].

Transepithelial Solute Transport Pathways

Optical methods have been particularly powerful in defining solute transport pathways in perfused nephron segments. For example, Guggino et al. [15] demonstrated that ouabain-induced cell swelling in *Amphiuma* distal tubule could be blocked by

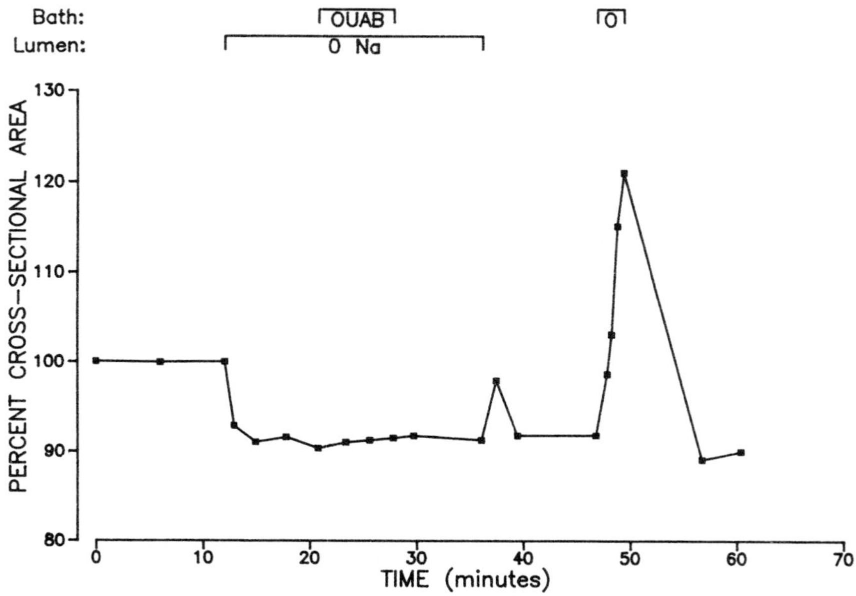

Fig. 3. Effects of luminal Na^+ removal on ouabain (*Ouab*)-induced swelling in a rabbit CCT principal cell [25]

luminal furosemide, suggesting that apical $Na^+/K^+/2Cl^-$ cotransport was the major pathway for cellular NaCl entry. Sun et al. [22] have recently shown that ouabain-induced swelling in the mouse medullary thick ascending limb is blocked by luminal Na^+ removal or furosemide addition, but is unaffected by luminal K^+ deletion. When the tubules were treated with ADH, however, removal of luminal K^+ dramatically inhibited ouabain-swelling. These results indicate that in the unstimulated tubule the apical cotransporter functions in a NaCl uptake mode. ADH modifies the pathway to become K^+-dependent and function as a $Na^+/K^+/2Cl^-$ cotransporter. In mineralocorticoid-treated CCT, ouabain causes rapid swelling in principal cells ([23]; Fig. 3). This swelling is inhibited by luminal Na^+ removal (Fig. 3) or by addition of low concentrations of amiloride, indicating that the major pathway for cellular Na^+ uptake is via apical amiloride-sensitive channels. Luminal Cl^- removal or addition of Cl^- transport inhibitors in the CCT causes significant principal cell shrinkage and also inhibits ouabain-swelling [23]. These results argue for the presence of an apical Cl^- transport pathway and suggest that this cell type plays a role in Cl^- reabsorption. Volume measurements in the rabbit proximal convoluted tubule have indicated the presence of apical Na^+/H^+ and Cl^-/formate exchangers that mediate transepithelial NaCl movement [24].

Basolateral solute transport pathways have also been elucidated by volume measurements. For example, Strange [19] recently demonstrated that peritubular K^+ elevation causes rapid swelling in CCT principal cells, which is completely blocked by bath Cl^- removal or addition of 5.0 mM Ba^{2+} (Fig. 4). These and previous results [23]

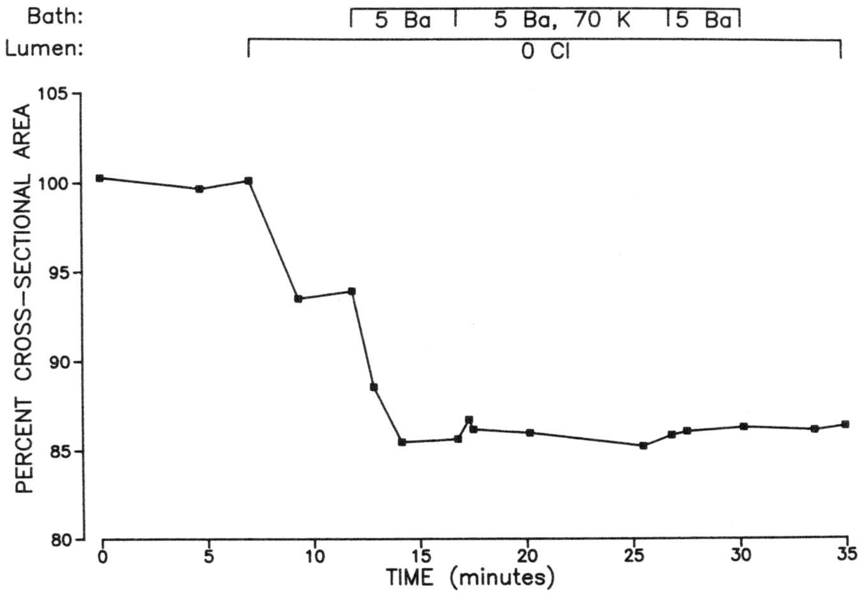

Fig. 4. Effects of 5.0 mM $BaCl_2$ on K^+-induced swelling in a principal cell of a CCT dissected from a desoxycorticosterone acetate (DOCA)-treated rabbit. Principal cells normally swell at a rate of 106%/min when peritubular K^+ concentration is raised from 5 mM to 70 mM [19]. As shown here, this swelling is completely blocked by peritubular $BaCl_2$. The cell shrinkage observed during Ba^{2+} addition most likely reflects inhibition of conductive, basolateral K^+ entry in the presence of continued basolateral and/or apical net solute efflux (discussed in [19])

indicate that the major pathways for basolateral K^+ movement are via the Na^+ pump and K^+ channels.

Studies of Cell Heterogeneity

Cell volume measurements are particularly valuable for defining the functional properties of specific cell types in heterogeneous epithelia. This approach was first used by O'Neil and Hayhurst [25] to study the rabbit CCT. These investigators observed that passage of current pulses across the epithelium had no effect on intercalated cell volume, but caused significant swelling in principal cells. Current-induced swelling could be blocked by luminal amiloride and Ba^{2+}, indicating the presence of apical Na^+ and K^+ channels in this cell type. Similar findings have been made using ouabain-induced cell swelling measurements [23]. Volume measurements by Strange and Spring [16] demonstrated that the apical membrane of both the CCT principal and intercalated cell has an extremely low L_p under resting conditions. Furthermore, their results demonstrated directly that ADH increases the water permeability of this membrane in principal and possibly in intercalated cells. In the *Amphiuma* distal tubule, Guggino [26] noted the presence of two populations of cells that exhibit distinctly different rates of swelling when bath K^+ was elevated. Electrophysiological measurements demonstrated that cells with the highest rate of swelling also had a high basolateral conductance to K^+ and Cl^-. The cells with the lower rate of swelling, however, were poorly conductive to these ions, suggesting the presence of an electroneutral basolateral KCl entry pathway. Measurements of the volume of macula densa cells in the cortical thick ascending limb have demonstrated the presence of an apical furosemide-sensitive NaCl cotransport process [27]. Finally, studies of hypertonic volume regulation in the CCT have revealed the presence of two physiologically distinct populations of intercalated cell [16]. One cell type shows almost complete volume recovery following shrinkage while the other has no hypertonic volume regulatory capabilities. The relationship between these physiological characteristics and the so-called type "A" and type "B" intercalated cell morphology and function is unknown.

Cell Volume Regulation

Renal tubule cells are normally faced with constant challenges to their volume and ionic composition. In medullary nephron segments, extracellular osmolality fluctuates with the diuretic state of the animal, leading to cell swelling or shrinkage. Variations in transcellular transport rates can also lead to cell volume changes. For some time, it has been clear that renal tubule cells respond to such volume perturbations by activating volume regulatory solute loss or accumulation pathways. The development and utilization of optical methods for quantifying cell volume have been essential in understanding the mechanisms by which this occurs. A lengthy discussion of volume regulation, however, is not warranted here. Interested readers should consult the recent review by Montrose-Rafizadeh and Guggino [28] and several articles published elsewhere in these proceedings (see List of Contributors).

Future Perspectives

Optical technology continues to evolve at a rapid pace. The development of higher resolution television monitors, recording devices, and digitization hardware may significantly improve the quality of nephron cell video images and be of value in cell volume studies. Utilization of so-called ultrathin optical sectioning techniques [18] may also enhance image quality. The combination of fluorescence and brightfield microscopy will allow simultaneous [29] or rapid, sequential [30] imaging of cell volume and fluorescent probes for membrane potential and intracellular ions. This, in turn, will provide a detailed understanding of the driving forces, ionic fluxes, and intracellular messengers involved in nephron salt and water transport and cell volume regulation.

References

1. Foskett JK (1990) Optical studies of ion and water transport in single cells. In: Foskett JK, Grinstein S (eds) Noninvasive techniques in cell biology. Wiley-Liss, New York, pp 237–272

2. MacRobbie EAC, Ussing HH (1961) Osmotic behaviour of the epithelial cells of frog skin. Acta Physiol Scand 53:348–365
3. Spring K (1985) The study of epithelial function by quantitative light microscopy. Pflugers Arch 405:S23–S27
4. Burg MB (1972) Perfusion of isolated renal tubules. Yale J Biol Med 45:321–326
5. Burg M, Patlak C, Green N, Villey D (1976) Organic solutes in fluid absorption by renal proximal convoluted tubules. Am J Physiol 231:627–637
6. Horster M, Gundlach H (1979) Application of differential interference contrast with inverted microscopes to the in vitro perfused nephron. J Micro 117:375–379
7. Whittembury G, Lindemann B, Carpi-Medina P, Gonzalez E, Linares H (1986) Continuous measurements of cell volume changes in single kidney tubules. Kidney Int 30:187–191
8. Strange K, Spring KR (1986) Methods for imaging renal tubule cells. Kidney Int 30: 192–200
9. Kirk KL, Schafer JA, DiBona DR (1987) Cell volume regulation in rabbit proximal tubule perfused in vitro. Am J Physiol 252:F922–F932
10. Hebert SC, Sun A (1988) Hypotonic cell volume regulation in mouse medullary thick ascending limb: effects of ADH. Am J Physiol 255:F962–F969
11. Strange K, Spring KR (1987) Absence of significant cellular dilution during ADH-stimulated water reabsorption. Science 235:1068–1070
12. Welling LW, Welling DJ, Ochs TJ (1983) Video measurements of basolateral membrane hydraulic conductivity in the proximal tubule. Am J Physiol 245:F123–F129
13. Kirk KL, Dibona DR, Schafer JA (1984) Morphologic response of the rabbit cortical collecting tubule to peritubular hypotonicity: quantitative examination with differential interference contrast microscopy. J Membr Biol 79:53–64
14. Lindemann B (1984) Real-time area-tracker records cellular volume changes from video images. Rev Sci Instrum 55:1788–1790
15. Guggino WB, Oberleithner H, Giebisch G (1985) Relationship between cell volume and ion transport in the early distal tubule of the *Amphiuma* kidney. J Gen Physiol 86:31–58
16. Strange K, Spring KR (1987) Cell membrane water permeability of rabbit cortical collecting duct. J Membr Biol 96:27–43
17. Spring KR (1985) The study of epithelial function by quantitative light microscopy. Pflugers Arch 405:S23–S27
18. Inoue S (1986) Video microscopy. Plenum, New York
19. Strange K Volume regulatory Cl^- loss following Na^+ pump inhibition in CCT principal cells. Am J Physiol, in press
20. Carpi-Medina P, Whittembury G (1988) Comparison of transcellular and transepithelial water permeabilities (P_{os}) in the isolated proximal straight proximal tubule (PST) of the rabbit kidney. Pflugers Arch 412:66–74
21. Welling LW, Welling DJ, Ochs TJ (1987) Video measurement of basolateral NaCl reflection coefficient in proximal tubule. Am J Physiol 253:F290–F298
22. Sun A, Grossman EB, Lombardi M, Hebert SC (to be published) Vasopressin alters the mechanism of apical Cl^- entry from Na:Cl to Na:K:2Cl cotransport in mouse medullary thick ascending limb
23. Strange K (1989) Ouabain-induced cell swelling in rabbit cortical collecting tubule: NaCl transport by principal cells. J Membr Biol 107:249–261
24. Schild L, Aronson PS, Giebisch G (1990) Effects of apical membrane Cl^- formate exchange on cell volume in rabbit proximal tubule. Am J Physiol 258:F530–F536
25. O'Neil RG, Hayhurst RA (1985) Functional differentiation of cell types of cortical collecting duct. Am J Physiol 248:F449–F453
26. Guggino WB (1986) Functional differentiation in the early distal tubule of the *Amphiuma* kidney: evidence for two modes of Cl^- and K^+ transport across the basolateral cell membrane. Am J Physiol 250:F430–F440

27. Gonzalez E, Salomonsson M, Muller-Suur C, Persson AEG (1988) Measurements of macula densa cell volume changes in isolated and perfused rabbit cortical thick ascending limb. I. Isosmotic and anisosmotic cell volume changes. Acta Physiol Scand 133:149–157
28. Montrose-Rafizadeh C, Guggino WB (1990) Cell volume regulation in the nephron. Annu Rev Physiol 52:761–772
29. Foskett JK (1988) Simultaneous Nomarski and fluorescence imaging during video microscopy of living cells. Am J Physiol 255:C566–C571
30. Spring KR (to be published) Differential interference contrast and fluorescence microscopy without significant light loss. In: Herman B, Jacobsen K (eds) Optical microscopy in biology. Alan R. Liss, New York

Management of Childhood Nephrotic Syndrome

Chair: Alan M. Robson (USA)
Sunao Maki (Japan)

Steroids and Cytotoxic Drugs in the Treatment of Minimal Change Nephrotic Syndrome

JOHANNES BRODEHL[1]

SUMMARY. Treatment of minimal change nephrotic syndrome has 3 aims: to induce remission, to prevent relapses, and to avoid side-effects. Initial treatment with prednisone should be intensive, because it can be shown that the more intense the initial treatment, the lower the relapse rate thereafter. Therefore, it is recommended to extend the initial treatment to 6 weeks of continuous prednisone and 6 weeks alternate-day prednisone. Relapses do not respond better to intensified treatment and, therefore, should be treated in a standard way. Alkylating drugs are indicated in frequent relapser and steroid dependent cases who have developed steroid-toxicity. Drug of choice is cyclophosphamide, which should be given for 8 weeks in cases without steroid-dependency, and for 12 weeks in steroid-dependent cases.

Introduction

Minimal change nephrotic syndrome (MCNS) is the most frequent type of idiopathic nephrotic syndrome in childhood. It is briefly defined as a nephrotic syndrome of unknown etiology with a characteristic course, responsiveness to glucocorticoids, alkylating agents, and cyclosporine A, a high tendency to relapse, an absence of progressive renal deterioration, and a minimal morphological finding by light- and immunomicroscopy. There is much evidence that the disease is of pathoimmunological origin [1]. The association of MCNS with allergy and with genetic markers of immune responsiveness, as well as the excellent response of proteinuria to immunosuppressive agents has suggested a causal relationship between the immunological and the renal abnormality. However, the exact nature of this relationship is still uncertain.

[1]Medizinische Hochschule Hannover, Kinderklinik, Abteilung Pädiatrische Nephrologie, D-3000 Hannover 61, Federal Republic of Germany

Treatment

The treatment of MCNS has a threefold aim: (1) a remission should be induced as soon as possible, since the nephrotic state is associated with a high rate of dangerous and even fatal complications, such as infections, thromboembolism and vascular collapse. (2) Relapses of the nephrotic syndrome should be prevented as much as possible, since each relapse endangers the patient by new complications and side-effects of treatment. (3) The treatment should avoid side-effects as much as possible, since the disease can run a long relapsing course, which could potentiate the side-effects.

Glucocorticoids have been used for more than 40 years in the treatment of MCNS and are generally considered to be the drug of first choice. The steroid derivative most widely used is prednisone. Therefore, the following statements will be related to prednisone exclusively. There are no convincing data available which can claim that other derivatives of glucosteroids are more advantageous than prednisone or prednisolone in the treatment of MCNS.

Initial Treatment

The initial attack of MCNS is very sensitive to prednisone, as shown from the data of the International Study of Kidney Disease in Children (ISKDC) [2]. Ninety-three percent of cases with MCNS responded to an eight week course of prednisone, which means that almost 72% of all children with the nephrotic syndrome were steroid-responsive (Table 1). Of all other histological categories of the nephrotic syndrome, only focal global glomerulosclerosis (FGGS) exhibited a similar high response rate, while all other categories did not respond to prednisone, i.e., remained steroid-resistant.

The response to prednisone does not occur very promptly; it takes a delay time of one to two weeks before a urinary remission can be observed [3]. In the cooperative study of the Arbeitsgemeinschaft für Pädiatrische Nephrologie (APN) urinary remission was defined as the disappearance of significant proteinuria (< 4 mg/m2/h) for at least 3 consecutive days under prednisone treatment. After 8 days, 50% of cases had urinary remission; the great majority had urinary remission after 14 days. A

Table 1. Steroid response in children with the nephrotic syndrome (ISKDC 1981)

Histopathological category	Number patients = n	Responder n	Responder (%)	Percentage of ΣN
MCNS	363	338	(93.1)	71.8%
FGGS	8	6	(75.0)	1.3%
DMH	9	5	(55.6)	1.1%
FSGS	37	11	(29.7)	2.3%
PROLIF GN	12	3	(25.0)	0.6%
MPGN	29	2	(6.9)	0.4%
Miscellaneous	13	3	(23.0)	0.6%

ISKDC, International study of kidney disease in children; *MCNS*, minimal change nephrotic syndrome; *FGGS*, focal global glomerulosclerosis; *DMH*, diffuse mesangial hypercellularity; *FSGS*, focal segmental glomerulosclerosis; *PROLIF GN*, proliferative glomerulonephritis; *MPGN*, membrano proliferative glomerulonephritis

Table 2. Initial prednisone treatment in children with N.S. (studies of APN)

	Continuous 60 mg/m2/per day	Alternate–day 40 mg/m2/per 48 h days
Long	42	42
Standard	28	28
Short	14 ± 6	16 ± 8

complete remission was defined as the normalization of serum albumin (≥ 35 g/l), it followed the urinary remission after two further weeks of treatment. Thus, a complete remission in children with MCNS, i.e., the first stated aim of treatment, could be achieved after 4 weeks of prednisone treatment.

The question is whether four weeks of prednisone in the initial treatment are enough to achieve the second aim of therapy, i.e., the prevention of subsequent relapses. In order to test the efficacy of the initial treatment the APN conducted comparative, randomized trials with 3 types of initial treatment: the short versus standard regimen [3], and the standard versus long treatment (Arbeitsgemeinschaft für Pädiatrische Nephrologie 1990, unpublished). The duration and dosage of prednisone treatment are shown on Table 2. In the short regimen 81% of patients experienced a relapse within the first 12 months after cessation of continuous prednisone; in the standard regimen 61% experienced such relapses, and in the long regimen only 36% experienced these relapses (Table 3). Not only the number of patients with relapses, but also the number of relapses which occurred in these patients, was highest after the short treatment. This is recognizable by the percentage of patients defined as infrequent relapsers (less than 2 relapses within 6 months) and frequent relapsers (≥ 2 relapses within 6 months). More than twice as many of the patients became frequent relapsers after the short than after the long therapy (Table 3). Thus, the risk of becoming a frequent relapser is much higher after a short than after a long regimen of initial treatment.

In actuarial life table analysis for 24 months the difference between the three initial prednisone treatment groups becomes quite obvious (Fig. 1). The cumulative percentage of patients in sustained remission is highest after long treatment, and significantly lower after short treatment, while the standard treatment lies in between.

From the results it is obvious that the intensity of the initial treatment has a decisive influence on the subsequent rate of relapse. The more intense the initial prednisone treatment is, the lower the relapse rate thereafter, and the longer the subsequent remission will last.

Table 3. Percentage of patients with relapses within 12 months after cessation of continuous initial prednisone therapy

Regimen		Total patients	Infrequent relapsers	Frequent relapsers	Both
Long	(12w)	33	21%	15%	36%
Standard	(8w)	66	44%	17%	61%
Short	(4w)	32	47%	34%	81%

(from Arbeitsgemeinschaft für Pädiatrische Nephrologie 1990)

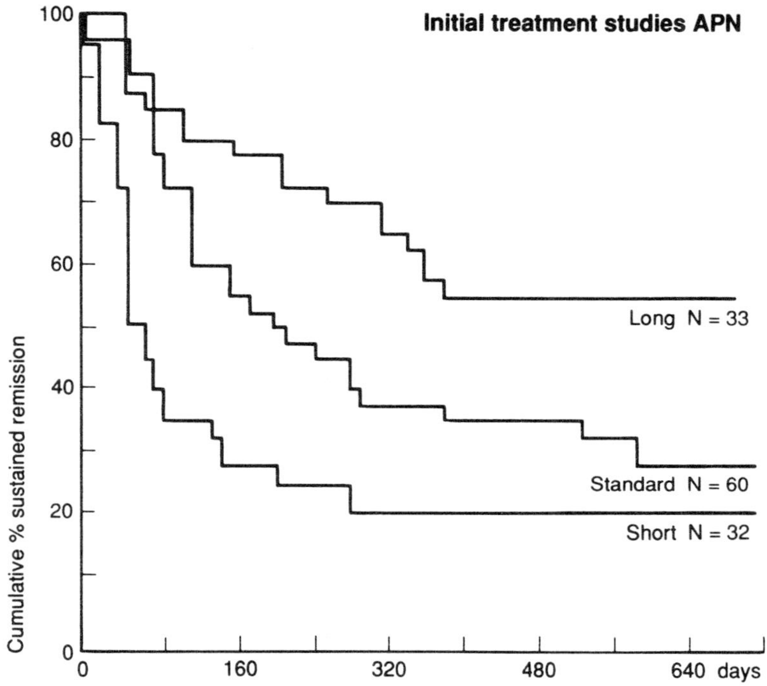

Fig. 1. Cumulative percentage of patients with sustained remission after 3 different prednisone regimens of initial treatment. Long, 12 weeks; standard, 8 weeks; and short, 4 weeks. (Preliminary data from Arbeitsgemeinschaft für Päediatrische Nephrologie)

It should be pointed out that this phenomenon can be only observed after the initial attack. If a relapse occurs, it usually is as steroid responsive as the initial attack. However, the length of the treatment and the dosage of prednisone no longer has any influence on the subsequent relapse rate [3,4]. This is shown in Table 4, which compares the mean duration of remissions after the initial attack and after the first and second relapse in those patients who relapsed [3]. There was a significantly longer remission after standard treatment of the initial attack than after short treatment. However, there were no differences after the relapse treatment, whether this was short or standard.

Table 4. Mean duration of remission after initial attack and relapses (APN 1988)

	Short prednisone therapy	Standard prednisone therapy	Significance*
Days after			
initial attack (SD)	79 (74)	169 (143)	P = 0.004
first relapse (SD)	58 (34)	84 (57)	ns
second relapse (SD)	66 (36)	61 (46)	ns

*Mann-Whitney test; ns, not significant
APN Arbeitsgemeinschaft für Päediatrische Nephrologie

Table 5. Side effects of initial prednisone treatment (APN 1990)

	Standard (8 w)		Long (12w)	
	n = 33	(%)	n = 32	(%)
Steroid-Cushing	11	(33)	11	(34)
Steroid-Cushing with striae	2	(6)	6	(19)
Hypertrichosis	2	(6)	6	(19)
Psycho-emot. disturbances	2	(6)	3	(9)
Path.slit lamp	2/15	(13)	0/9	(0)
Other	3	(9)	1	(3)

Other, convulsions, pseudomotor cerebri, hypertension, thromboembolism, severe infection, osteochondritis etc
APN, Arbeitsgemeinschaft für Päediatrische Nephrologie

Thus, the second aim of MCNS treatment, i.e., the prevention of relapses, is approached best with an intensification of the initial treatment. However, before a definitive recommendation for the initial treatment can be issued, one has to evaluate the side-effects of the treatment according to the third aim of treatment, i.e., the avoidance of side-effects of drugs. It is self evident that the side-effects of steroids will increase, along with the dosage and length of treatment. Well known side-effects of steroids are cushingoid appearance, striae, hypertension, osteoporosis, cataracts, and, especially in children, growth retardation and psychosocial disturbances. The APN study, therefore, tried to evaluate the side-effects of long-prednisone treatment as compared with the standard treatment. The results are listed in Table 5. From these data it was concluded that the risk of a 12-week prednisone course is not essentially higher than that of an 8-week course. The members of APN, therefore, believed that the advantages of a prolonged initial prednisone treatment outweighed the risks, and therefore recommended the 12-week prednisone course for the initial treatment (Table 6). Since there was no benefit from a prolonged prednisone treatment of a relapse, the recommendation for relapse therapy remains the same as that proposed some years ago [5].

The majority of children with MCNS can be managed by this procedure. There are, however, a few who are, or become, steroid resistant, and others who turn out to be frequent relapsers or steroid-dependent.

Steroid-Resistant MCNS

Initial steroid resistance in MCNS is rare (see Table 1). Even if there is no remission after 8 weeks of prednisone treatment, there is still a good chance that prolonged

Table 6. Recommended treatment for initial attack and relapse of nephrotic syndrome in children (APN 1990)

Initial:	Continuous **prednisone** 60 mg/m2 per day in 3 divided doses (not more than 80 mg/day) for 6 weeks followed by alternate-day **prednidsone** 40 mg/m2 per 48h for 6 weeks
Relapse:	Continuous **prednisone** 60 mg/m2 per day in 3 divided doses (not more than 80 mg/day) until urine protein free for 3 days followed by alternate-day **prednisone** 40 mg/m2 per 48h for 4 weeks

APN, Arbeitsgemeinschaft für Päediatrische Nephrologie

Table 7. Steroid resistance of children with MCNS. Percentage of total cases according to histological subcategories (ISKDC 1981)

	Weeks after initial prednisone			
Subcategory	8	26	52	104 (n)
Nil	4.7	1.4	0.9	0.9 (2)
FGO	7.8	3.3	2.2	2.2 (2)
MMT	6.3	6.3	0.0	0.0 (0)
FTC	14.3	10.7	3.6	0.0 (0)
MMH	14.8	14.8	7.4	7.4 (2)
DMH	45.5	18.2	9.1	9.1 (1)
Total	31/383 =8.1%	16/383 =4.2%	8/383 =2.1%	7/383 =1.8%

ISKDC, International Study of Kidney Disease in Children
Abbreviations for subcategories of minimal change nephrotic syndrome (*MCNS*): Nil, nil - disease; FGO, focal global obsolescence; MMT, mild mesangial thickening; FTC, focal tubular changes; MMH, mild mesangial hypercellularity; DMH, diffuse mesangial hypercellularity

treatment with steroids or the addition of a cytotoxic agent can produce a final remission. As can be seen in Table 7, almost all subcategories of MCNS responded to treatment after 2 years, and only 7 cases out of 383 were left unresponsive to treatment [6]. It is, therefore, our policy in histologically proven cases of MCNS, after an 8–12 week course of prednisone, to continue immunosuppressive treatment, either with a combination of prednisone plus cyclophosphamide, or with a combination of prednisone plus cyclosporine A. To our knowledge, there are no controlled studies available which could indicate which type of treatment would be superior.

Frequent Relapsing and Steroid-Dependent MCNS

The rate at which children with MCNS will become frequent relapsers or steroid-dependent is partially determined by the initial treatment, as described above. There are no serological, laboratory, or morphological criteria which could be predictive of the future course of the disease. It is, therefore, necessary to conduct the treatment in a standardized way because this is the only way which helps to classify the patient according to the severity of the disease.

We speak of a frequent relapser without steroid dependency as a patient who responds initially to prednisone, but has two relapses within six months of his initial response, or 4 relapses within a one year period, without fulfilling the criteria of steroid-dependency [7]. The criterion for steroid-dependency is fulfilled when two consecutive relapses occur during the standard relapse therapy or within 14 days after cessation of steroid therapy—which then is called "fast relapse"—or when 2 out of 4 relapses in a period of 6 months are fast relapses.

Children with frequent relapses or steroid dependency are endangered by steroid toxicity, since steroids have to be administered for long periods and in high doses. Review of the literature reveals that in larger series of steroid treated children with glomerulopathies, more than 5% of patients died due to steroid complications, and not because of the renal disease [8]. Therefore, in the cases of frequent relapse and steroid-dependency an alternative immunosuppressive treatment is mandatory.

It has been known for many years that such alkylating substances as nitrogen mustard, cyclophosphamide, and chlorambucil are effective in MCNS. The majority of physicians prefer cyclophosphamide, since its longlasting toxicity within the immunosuppressive therapeutic range seems to be less than that of chlorambucil. Therefore, most experience has been accumulated with cyclophosphamide.

In our experience cyclophosphamide is indicated in children with frequent relapses or with steroid dependency who develop signs of steroid toxicity due to prolonged steroid application, and in children in whom a steroid contraindication exists, as in diabetes mellitus. The action of cyclophosphamide can be described thus [9]:

1) Cyclophosphamide induces remissions of MCNS in all patients who respond to steroids.
2) In addition, cyclophosphamide is also effective in some cases of steroid-resistant MCNS.
3) The time sequence until remission is achieved is somewhat slower than after steroids.
4) Remissions after cyclophosphamide are often long-lasting, even if cyclophospha-mide is administered in steroid-induced remission.
5) The subsequent relapse rate is dependent on dosage and/or on length of cyclophosphamide treatment.

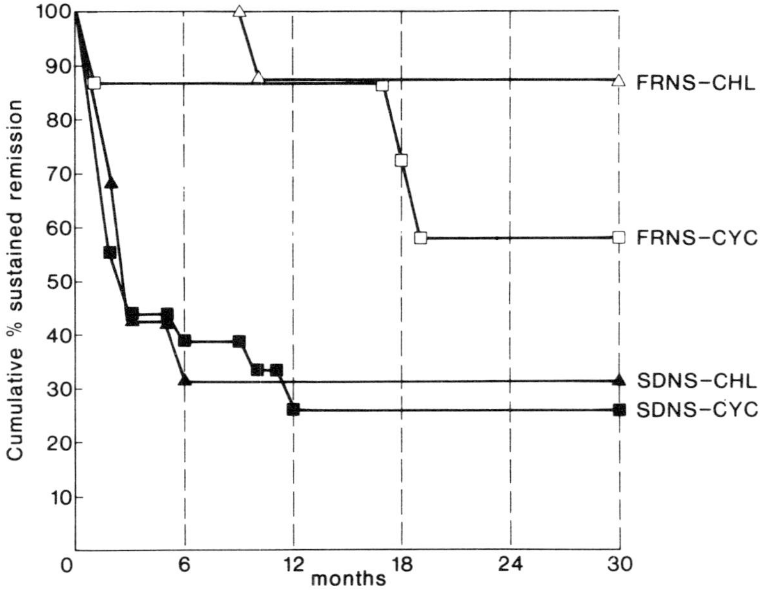

Fig. 2. Cumulative percentage of sustained remission in frequent relapser (*FRNS*) and steroid depender (*SDNS*) treated either with chlorambucil (*CHL*) or cyclophosphamide (*CYC*). (Data from [7])

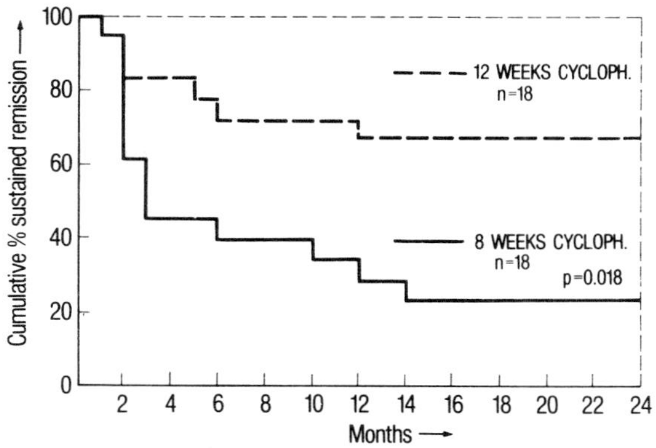

Fig. 3. Cumulative percentage of sustained remission in steroid-dependent minimal change nephrotic syndrome (*MCNS*): comparison of eight weeks with 12 weeks treatment with cyclophosphamide after 2 years. (From [10] with permission)

6) The efficacy of cyclophosphamide in repeated courses is uncertain (beware side-effects!).

The Arbeitsgemeinschaft für Pädiatrische Nephrologie has compared the efficacy of cyclophosphamide with that of chlorambucil in nephrotic children with and without steroid dependency [7]. It was shown that cyclophosphamide in a dosage of 2 mg/kg per day was as effective as chlorambucil in a dosage of 0.15 mg/kg per day. Both drugs were administered for 8 weeks after remission had been induced by prednisone therapy. Children with frequent relapses, but without steroid dependency, gained so much from the treatment that about 70% of them remained in prolonged remission thereafter. In contrast, steroid-dependent cases did not gain enough from the treatment, since only 30% remained in prolonged remission (Fig. 2).

Therefore, in a further study, the steroid-dependent children were treated with cyclophosphamide for 12 weeks instead of 8 weeks [10]. By this it was shown that the percentage of patients with long-lasting remissions was increased to 70% (Fig. 3). Remissions usually persisted for at least 5 years, as a follow-up study determined [11]; no serious side-effects were observed. The cumulative dosage of cyclophosphamide amounted to 168 mg/kg, which is below the known toxic threshold for gonadal toxicity in prepubertal boys [12].

Immunosuppressive Action

Both steroids and alkylating substances are immunosuppressive agents, for which, however, the exact pharmacomechanism in MCNS is not known. Steroids interfere with gene transcription through binding of the glucocorticoid receptors to regulating DNA sequences, thereby abrogating gene expression of important monokines [13]. They obviously suppress the secretion of IL1, IL6, and IL8 [14], mainly in monocytes. It is not known whether this mechanism is responsible for the antiproteinuric effects in MCNS.

Table 8. Comparison of prednisone and cyclophosphamide in the treatment of MCNS

	Prednisone	Cyclophosphamide
Delay time until antiproteinuric effect	7–14	14–21 days
Dose-response	yes	yes
Additive effect	yes	yes
Sustained effect after discontinuation	no	yes
Effective in repeated courses	yes	no

MCNS, minimal change nephrotic syndrome

Alkylating substances are antimitotic. By alkylating DNA they cause nuclear damage which is irreversible and results in cytotoxicity. The whole range of lymphocytes is susceptible to cyclophosphamide, the descending order of sensitivity being suppressor T cells, B cells, helper T cells, and cytotoxic T cells [15, 16]. Whether functional changes of lymphocytes are induced by cyclophosphamide is not yet known.

If one compares the in vivo effects of both immunosuppressive substances in children with MCNS, one recognizes similarities and dissimilarities. These are shown in Table 8. Cyclophosphamide needs a little more time than steroids to produce urinary remission. Both substances exhibit additive effects, and it is noteworthy that cyclophosphamide can exert its longlasting effect even in the prednisone-induced remission state. While prednisone has no longlasting effect, i.e., it does not protect against relapses after discontinuation, this is not the case with cyclophosphamide. In this respect cyclophosphamide is superior to prednisone. Finally, prednisone is effective in repeated courses, while cyclophosphamide is probably not. However, because of the gonadal toxicity, this has not been extensively tested.

Conclusion

From the findings of multicenter studies the recommendation for immunosuppressive treatment of children with MCNS today is as follows:

1) The initial attack needs an intensive steroid treatment: prednisone 60 mg/m2 per day for 6 weeks, followed by alternate-day 40 mg/m2 per 48 h for 6 weeks.
2) Relapses should receive a standardized treatment: prednisone 60 mg/m2 per day until urine is protein free for 3 days, followed by 40 mg/m2 per 48h for 4 weeks. This should be repeated in cases of infrequent relapse.
3) Frequent relapses and steroid dependency with steroid-toxicity should receive alkylating drug treatment: cyclophosphamide 2 mg/kg per day for 8 weeks in frequent relapsers; for 12 weeks in steroid-dependency.
4) Frequent relapsers, after cyclophosphamide, should receive treatment with cyclosporine A 100–150 mg/m2 per day for 6–12 months or more.

References

1. Schnaper HW (1989) The immune system in minimal change nephrotic syndrome. Pediatr Nephrol 3:101–110

2. International Study of Kidney Disease in Children (1981) The primary nephrotic syndrome in children. Identification of patients with minimal change nephrotic syndrome from initial response to prednisone. J Pediatr 98:561–564
3. Arbeitsgemeinschaft für Pädiatrische Nephrologie (1988) Short versus standard prednisone therapy for initial treatment of idiopathic nephrotic syndrome in children. Lancet I:380–383
4. Arbeitsgemeinschaft für Pädiatrische Nephrologie (1979) Alternate day versus intermittent prednisone in frequently relapsing nephrotic syndrome. Lancet I:401–403
5. Brodehl J, Krohn HP, Ehrich JHH (1982) The treatment of minimal change nephrotic syndrome (lipoidnephrosis): cooperative studies of the Arbeitsgemeinschaft für Pädiatrische Nephrologie (APN). Klin Pädiatr 194:162–165
6. International Study of Kidney Disease in Children (1981) Primary nephrotic syndrome in children: clinical significance of histopathologic variants of minimal change and of diffuse mesangial hypercellularity. Kidney Int 20:765–771
7. Arbeitsgemeinschaft für Pädiatrische Nephrologie (1982) Effect of cytotoxic drugs in frequently relapsing nephrotic syndrome with and without steroid dependence. N Engl J Med 306:451–454
8. Brodehl J (1986) Nephrotic syndrome in children: diagnosis and treatment. World Pediatrics and Child Care 1:9–18
9. Brodehl J (1989) Effective drugs for MCNS and their implications on the pathophysiology. VIII Congress of Int Pediatr Nephrology Association. Pediatr Nephrol 3:C74
10. Arbeitsgemeinschaft für Pädiatrische Nephrologie (1987) Cyclophosphamide treatment of steroid dependent nephrotic syndrome: comparison of eight weeks with 12 weeks course. Arch Dis Child 62:1102–1106
11. Krohn HP, Brodehl J (1986) Cytotoxic drug study I of the APN: 5 years follow-up. Helv Paediatr Acta 41:107
12. Etteldorf JN, West CD, Pitcock JA, Williams DL (1976) Gonadal function, testicular histology and meiosis following cyclophosphamide therapy in patients with nephrotic syndrome. J Pediatr 88:206–212
13. Beato M (1989) Gene regulation by steroid hormones. Cell 56:335–344
14. Zanker B, Walz G, Wieder KJ, Strom TB (1990) Evidence that glucocorticosteroids block expression of the human interleukin-6 gene by accessory cells. Transplantation 49:183–185
15. Balow JZ, Hurley DL, Fauci AS (1975) Cyclophosphamide expression of established cell-mediated immunity. J Clin Invest 56:65–70
16. Feehally J, Beattle TJ, Brenchley PEC, Coupes BM, Houston IB, Mallick NP, Postlethwaite RJ (1984) Modulation of cellular immune function by cyclophosphamide in children with minimal change. N Engl J Med 310:415–420

New Therapies for the Treatment of Idiopathic Nephrotic Syndrome

Patrick Niaudet, Michel Broyer, and Renée Habib[1]

Summary. The treatment of children with idiopathic nephrotic syndrome who have multiple relapses or who are steroid-resistant is a difficult issue. Alkylating agents are often proposed but they have several side effects, including gonadal toxicity, which limit their use. Treatment with levamisole may be efficient in steroid-dependent patients, allowing prednisone to be tapered or stopped in approximately 50% of cases. Cyclosporine has proved to be effective in 85% of steroid-dependent patients, but most patients relapse when cyclosporine is tapered or withdrawn. Thus, in these patients, cyclosporine may be required for long periods of time. Conversely, cyclosporine alone is less effective in steroid-resistant patients, as only 28% of these patients respond to the treatment. Cyclosporine in association with prednisone may be a better alternative as, in our experience, 14 out of 31 patients went into remission with such treatment. It should be stressed that response to cyclosporine is better correlated with initial steroid responsiveness than with histological category. Eighteen out of 43 patients with serial renal biopsies developed significant tubulo interstitial lesions which could be attributable to cyclosporine nephrotoxicity. The risk of developing chronic nephrotoxicity appears to be higher in steroid-resistant patients. Cyclosporine nephrotoxicity is not related to the duration of treatment and may develop in patients with normal renal function.

Introduction

Idiopathic nephrotic syndrome (INS), the most common glomerular disease in children, is defined by the combination of nephrotic syndrome and minimal change glomerular disease with foot process fusion seen on electron microscopy. No immunoglobulin deposits are seen on immunofluorescence. However, in some cases,

[1]Service de Néphrologie Pédiatrique and INSERM U192, Hôpital Necker Enfants Malades, 75743 Paris, France

diffuse mesangial proliferation or focal and segmental glomerulosclerosis may be seen on light microscopy and sometimes immunofluorescence reveals mesangial IgM or, less frequently, IgA deposits. Although several authors consider that minimal change disease, focal and segmental glomerulosclerosis, diffuse mesangial proliferation, and IgM nephropathy are distinct entities as the response to treatment and the clinical course can be different, there is in fact a clinical overlap between the different anatomical entities and INS should rather be considered as a syndrome with different clinical and histologic variants [1].

The clinical experience shows that the response to steroid therapy carries greater prognostic weight than the histological features seen on initial biopsy. In the vast majority of childhood cases (90%), INS is steroid-responsive but 60% of these steroid responders relapse as soon as steroid therapy is withdrawn or when the dosage is decreased. This constitutes steroid-dependent INS, the severity of which lies less in the risk of developing end stage renal failure, which is a very rare outcome, than in the complications of treatment. When the level of steroid therapy required to maintain remission is too high, the side effects force one to resort to other drugs such as immunosuppressive agents that are themselves not without risk.

In 10% of cases, INS is steroid-resistant. The severity of this condition lies essentially in the risk of developing end stage renal failure, which occurs in about half of the cases.

Alkylating agents, which achieve long lasting remission, have been used for some 20 years in INS [2]. The majority of studies have concentrated on their use in steroid-dependent patients and in relapsing steroid-responders. Their efficacy has been clearly demonstrated in such cases. The duration of remission depends on the severity of the disease and the duration of treatment. The limitation on longer use of alkylating agents lies in their long-term toxic effects, in particular the risks of cancer and leukemia and, in boys, the gonadal toxicity. The efficacy of alkylating agents in steroid-resistant INS is more open to question.

In this paper we will discuss the other therapeutic approaches besides corticosteroids and alkylating agents, that have been proposed for patients with INS, namely levamisole and cyclosporine.

Levamisole

Levamisole is an anthelmintic which has immunostimulatory activity in different experimental systems. It was first used by Tanphaichitr et al. [3] in 7 children with steroid-responsive nephrotic syndrome; the treatment induced a remission within 6 months in all of them. Mehta et al. [4] treated 25 children with relapsing steroid-responsive nephrotic syndrome; 13 of them went into remission and 12 went into partial remission. Mongeau et al. [5] found that levamisole was able to reduce the mean dose of prednisone by 60% and the monthly relapse rate from 0.35 to 0.13. Our experience concerns 71 patients with steroid-dependent nephrotic syndrome who were treated with levamisole given twice weekly at a dose of 2.5 mg/kg while the dose of prednisone was gradually decreased. Prednisone could be stopped without relapse in 17 patients (24%) on levamisole. In 32 patients (45%), prednisone therapy could be reduced but not withdrawn. In the remaining 22 patients (31%) prednisone could not be tapered. The majority of the children in whom levamisole had been effective relapsed after the treatment was stopped.

Cyclosporine and Steroid-Dependent INS

Cyclosporine, an immunosuppressive drug introduced in organ transplantation more than a decade ago, was found to be effective in the treatment of patients with idiopathic nephrotic syndrome by Meyrier et al. [6] and by Hoyer et al. [7]. In children, Hoyer et al. [7] treated five steroid-dependent patients who all responded to cyclosporine with fewer relapses and with reduced prednisone requirements. Capodicasa et al. [8] treated six steroid-dependent patients; in 5 of them cyclosporine induced long lasting remissions. Tejani et al. [9] treated 13 steroid-dependent children for eight weeks. Eleven patients remained in remission for over nine months after discontinuation of therapy.

Our experience concerns 45 patients with steroid-responsive and steroid-dependent INS. Histological examination of renal biopsy specimens obtained before initiation of cyclosporine therapy showed minimal change disease in 40 cases, diffuse mesangial proliferation in 2 cases, and focal and segmental glomerulosclerosis in 3 cases. The 45 steroid-responders had had their last relapse while receiving alternate-day prednisone within 3 months preceding cyclosporine treatment. They received cyclosporine for periods of at least 3 months. Fifteen patients were receiving daily prednisone treatment and 27 were receiving alternate-day prednisone when cyclosporine therapy was started. Three patients were no longer receiving prednisone.

Thirty-six of the 45 patients either went into remission or did not relapse at all during the period of full-dose cyclosporine, despite the fact that prednisone treatment was withdrawn. Among the 36 patients, 3 were protein-free at last examination, but they were still receiving cyclosporine. Thirty-three patients relapsed: 23 relapsed while receiving cyclosporine at tapering doses varying between 0.7 and 6.6 mg/kg; 10 patients relapsed 7–120 days after withdrawal of cyclosporine therapy. Cyclosporine was ineffective in 2 patients, who relapsed as soon as alternate-day prednisone therapy was started. The remaining 7 patients relapsed at withdrawal of prednisone treatment, and the association of cyclosporine with low-dose prednisone allowed remission to be maintained.

Between 1985 and 1989, the French Society of Pediatric Nephrology performed an open randomized controlled study which compared the efficacy and the tolerance of cyclosporine with those of chlorambucil in children with steroid-dependent nephrotic syndrome and signs of steroid toxicity. Forty children, 9 girls and 31 boys, were entered in the study. Twenty children received cyclosporine at an initial dose of 6 mg/kgBW; the dose was adjusted to obtain trough plasma levels of between 50 and 150 ng/ml (radio-immunoassay (RIA), polyclonal antibodies). After 3 months, cyclosporine was tapered off within the next 3 months. Twenty children received chlorambucil 0.2 mg/kgBW during 6–8 weeks, with a cumulative dosage of 8 mg/kg, a dose which avoids gonadal toxicity. The two groups did not show significant differences concerning the proportion of girls and boys, the age at onset of the disease, the duration of disease, the number of relapses and the histology (minimal change disease (MCD), focal and segmental glomerulosclerosis (FSGS), diffuse mesangial proliferation (DMP)).

Among the 20 patients who received cyclosporine, 2 relapsed before prednisone withdrawal, 9 relapsed after prednisone withdrawal, at doses of cyclosporine ranging from 0.9 to 8.5 mg/kg (mean 4.15 mg/kg), 8 relapsed 1 week–7 months after cyclosporine withdrawal, and only one patient remained in remission 18 months after cyclosporine withdrawal.

Among the 20 patients who received chlorambucil, 4 patients relapsed before prednisone withdrawal, 10 relapsed within 34 months after prednisone withdrawal, and the remaining 6 patients were still in remission 21–42 months after chlorambucil treatment.

In summary, cyclosporine made it possible to stop prednisone in 18 out of 20 children, but subsequent relapses occurred in 17 of the children during the tapering phase or after withdrawal of cyclosporine. Conversely, chlorambucil allowed the withdrawal of prednisone in 16 out of 20 patients, but 10 of these patients experienced further relapses. At last follow-up, after 21–42 months, 30% of the patients who received chlorambucil and only 5% of the patients who received cyclosporine were still in remission.

Cyclosporine and Steroid-Resistant INS

Cyclosporine has been given to children with steroid-resistant idiopathic nephrotic syndrome in several uncontrolled studies. Capodicasa et al. reported that 2 of 4 patients treated with a combination of cyclosporine and prednisone went into remission [8]. Similarly, Brandis et al. [10] found a beneficial effect of cyclosporine given alone in 4 patients. Conversely, Waldo and Kohaut [11] reported partial remission among 6 treated children, while Brodehl et al. [12] found 2 partial remissions out of 7 cases and Tejani et al. [9] reported 3 remissions out of 7 cases.

We treated 14 steroid-resistant patients, including 11 early non-responders and 3 late non-responders. Only one patient, a late non-responder, went into complete remission on cyclosporine alone, while a partial and transient remission was observed in 4 patients. The remaining 9 patients failed to respond to cyclosporine. Cyclosporine in association with prednisone induced a remission in 2 out of 4 patients.

This observation led us to start an open trial with the French Society of Pediatric Nephrology on the effect of cyclosporine in association with prednisone [13]. Thirty one patients, 13 girls and 18 boys, aged 1 month–14.3 years at onset of the disease and in whom renal biopsy had shown MCD in 19 cases and FSGS in 12 cases, received cyclosporine (150–200 mg/m^2) in combination with daily prednisone (30 mg/m^2) for one month and with alternate day prednisone, 30 mg/m^2, for 5 months thereafter. Fourteen patients (45%) went into complete remission, nine of them during the first two months of the treatment. Three patients had a partial remission and 14 failed to respond to the treatment. Interestingly, the response to cyclosporine and prednisone was not correlated with the histopathological findings, since among the 14 patients who responded to the treatment, 9 had MCD and 5 FSGS, whereas among the 14 patients who failed to respond 9 had MCD and 5 had FSGS.

Nephrotoxicity of Cyclosporine

Among the side effects of cyclosporine, nephrotoxicity is the most worrying. Nephrotoxicity is generally evidenced by deterioration of renal function. In idiopathic nephrotic syndrome, renal insufficiency may occur during a relapse or as end stage renal failure develops in steroid-resistant patients. In patients treated with cyclosporine, it may be difficult to determine to what extent deterioration of renal function is due to drug-induced nephrotoxicity or to renal insufficiency due to the renal disease itself. Furthermore, the two events may be superimposed on one another.

We observed an impairment of renal function in 10 patients. Four out of the 45 steroid-dependent patients had a transient increase in serum creatinine levels. The increase occurred during a relapse in 3 patients with low cyclosporine trough levels. In the other patients, the increase in plasma creatinine levels completely reversed after withdrawal of cyclosporine therapy. Six out of the 14 steroid-resistant patients had an impairment of renal function. This impairment was transient, with complete recovery in 4 of the patients. In two patients, the impairment in renal function was only partially reversible and deteriorated further following withdrawal of cyclosporine therapy.

In order to better evaluate the eventual nephrotoxicity of cyclosporine in these patients with INS, we undertook a prospective study concerning 43 patients in whom at least two renal biopsies were performed, including one before initiation of cyclosporine. Thirty seven patients were steroid-dependent and six were steroid-resistant. Initial biopsy had shown minimal change disease (MCD) in 34 patients (32 steroid-dependent and 2 steroid-resistant), diffuse mesangial proliferation (DMP) in 2 steroid-dependent patients, and focal and segmental glomerulosclerosis (FSGS) in 7 patients (3 steroid-dependent and 4 steroid-resistant). Cyclosporine was efficient in 33 steroid-dependent patients and in 3 steroid-resistant patients (29 MCD, 2 DMP, and 5 FSGS). The second renal biopsy was performed after a 2–20 month cyclosporine treatment period. The lesions observed on these biopsies were classified as follows: Grade 0 included 16 patients, all steroid-dependent, who had no modification of renal parenchyma. Grade I was diagnosed in 11 patients, 10 steroid-dependent and 1 steroid-resistant, who showed scattered atrophic tubules; grade II was diagnosed in 11 patients, 10 steroid-dependent and one steroid-resistant, who showed several foci of atrophic tubules within stripes of interstitial fibrosis; and grade III was diagnosed in 5 patients (1 steroid-dependent and 4 steroid-resistant) in whom confluent areas of interstitial fibrosis with atrophic or collapsed tubules were observed. A third biopsy was obtained in 13 patients, after 11–37 months of cyclosporine therapy. Of the 5 patients with grade 0 on second biopsy, 3 remained grade 0 and 2 progressed to grade I. Of the 5 patients with grade I, 3 remained grade I and 2 progressed to grade II. Finally, the 3 patients with grade II progressed to grade III. Among the 43 patients, only 3 showed an impairment of renal function which, in two of them, was reversible. This study shows that cyclosporine nephrotoxicity is not related to the duration of treatment. The risk of developing chronic nephrotoxicity appears to be higher in steroid-resistant patients than in steroid-dependent ones. Histological signs of nephrotoxicity can develop in patients with normal renal function. Renal biopsy seems, therefore, the only way of detecting patients who develop cyclosporine nephrotoxicity.

References

1. Habib R, Churg J (1984) Minimal change disease, mesangial proliferation glomerulonephritis and focal sclerosis: individual entities or a spectrum. In: RR Robinson (ed) Nephrology. Springer, New York, pp 634–644

2. Niaudet P, Habib R, Gagnadoux MF, Tête MJ, Broyer M (1988) Treatment of severe childhood nephrosis. In: Grunfeld JP, Bach JF, Crosnier J, Funk-Brentano JL, Maxwell MH (eds) Advances in nephrology. Year Book Medical, pp 151–172
3. Tanphaichitr P, Tanphaichitr D, Sureesatanan J (1980) Treatment of nephrotic syndrome with levamisole. J Pediatr 96:490–493
4. Mehta K, Ali U (1987) New approach to relapsing nephrotic syndrome. Pediatr Nephrol 1:C46
5. Mongeau JG, Robitaille PO, Roy F (1988) Clinical efficacy of levamisole in the treatment of primary nephrosis in children. Pediatr Nephrol 2:398–401
6. Meyrier A, Simon P, Perret G, Condamin-Meyrier MC (1986) Remission of idiopathic nephrotic syndrome after treatment with cyclosporine A. Br Med J [Clin Res] 292:789–793
7. Hoyer PF, Krull F, Brodehl J (1986) Cyclosporine in frequently relapsing minimal change nephrotic syndrome. Lancet II:385
8. Capodicasa G, De Santo NG, Nuzzi F, Giordano C (1986) Cyclosporine A in nephrotic syndrome of childhood. A 14 month experience. Int J Pediatr Nephrol 7:69–72
9. Tejani A, Butt K, Trachtman H, Suthanthiran M, Rosenthal CJ, Khawar MR (1988) Cyclosporine A induced remission of relapsing nephrotic syndrome in children. Kidney Int 33:729–734
10. Brandis M, Burghard R, Leititis J, Zimmerhackl B, Hildebrandt F, Helmcher U (1988) Cyclosporine A for treatment of nephrotic syndrome. Transplant Proc 20 (Suppl 4):275–279
11. Waldo FB, Kohaut EC (1987) Therapy of focal segmental glomerulosclerosis with cyclosporine A. Pediatr Nephrol 1:180–182
12. Brodehl J, Hoyer PF (1989) Cyclosporin in idiopathic nephrotic syndrome of children. Am J Nephrol 9 (Suppl 1):61–64
13. Niaudet P, the French Society of Pediatric Nephrology. (to be published) Steroid resistant idiopathic nephrotic syndrome and cyclosporine. Nephron

Nephrotic Syndrome in Japan and Other Asian Countries – Epidemiology and Treatment

Kazuo Yoshioka and Sunao Maki[1]

Epidemiology

Nephrotic syndrome (NS) is a common form of childhood renal disease in Asian, as well as in Western, countries. According to the multicenter clinical study on the epidemiology of NS in Japan [1,2], approximately 9000 children with renal disease were seen as in- or out-patients over the two-year period between 1984 and 1985. Of these patients, 14% had NS. Steroids were first used to treat the patients with primary NS, and 90% of the patients responded well, but subsequent relapse during steroid therapy, or shortly after stopping the therapy, was noticed in 33% of the patients. Proteinuria persisted in 9%. Renal biopsy was done on a quarter of the patients who showed good response to steroids, including frequently relapsing patients, and on 80% of the children who showed poor response to, or resistance to, steroids. Under these circumstances, minor abnormalities and diffuse mesangial proliferation were often seen in patients who responded well to steroids. Patients who responded poorly to steroids or were resistant to steroid therapy were prone to show diffuse mesangial prolification, focal segmental sclerosis, and membranoproliferative glomerulonephritis. Approximately 10% of the patients in this group had minor lesions. The majority of primary NS patients in Korea (Dr. KW Ko, Seoul, 1990, personal communication) and in China (Dr. P. Wang, Beijing, 1990, personal communication) had minimal change disease and proliferative glomerulonephritis. Focal segmental sclerosis was diagnosed in a significant number of Korean patients.

Initial Corticosteroid Therapy

Most of the children with primary NS responded well to corticosteroids, but many of them experienced subsequent relapses. In order to prevent frequent relapse, and to

[1]Department of Pediatrics, Kinki University, Osaka-sayama, 589 Japan

find a more effective and safer treatment, Dr. Ueda and coworkers in Japan compared two initial steroid therapy regimens, a long-term tapering regimen and a short-term intermittent regimen [3]. The latter was originally proposed by ISKDC. Dr. Ueda and coworkers found that the numbers of patients who had a relapse within 6 months after terminating initial therapy and the numbers of patients with frequent relapses or steroid-dependence were significantly higher in the group treated with the short-term intermittent protocol. They concluded that the long-term tapering regimen was safe and preferable, and that this regimen had a favorable effect on the subsequent clinical course of this disease. Currently, in Japan, this long-term prednisolone therapy is commonly used to treat children with NS. This is also the case in Korea and in China. According to our own experience, 4% of primary NS patients did not show any response to the initial oral prednisolone, but they successfully responded to intravenous methylprednisolone "pulse" therapy.

Cyclophosphamide Therapy

Hitherto, children classified as frequently relapsing NS patients were treated with repeated courses of steroids. When steroid toxicity developed, cytotoxic drugs were used. Cyclophosphamide therapy, for 8 weeks, was generally chosen. Several studies, and our own experience, have shown that a period of 8 weeks is not sufficient to reduce the relapse. We examined the relationship between duration of remission and the age when cyclophosphamide therapy began. There was a significant correlation between relapse within 2 years and age when cyclophosphamide was given. In other words, cyclophosphamide therapy, at a dosage of 3 mg/kg per day for 8 weeks, was not effective, particularly in young children.

We prospectively compared three different durations of cyclophosphamide administration. Group A was of 8-weeks duration, Group B, 10 weeks, and Group C, 12 weeks (Table 1). The patients also received a small dosage of prednisolone during the therapy. There was no difference between the three groups in age at onset of NS, age at entry to study, relapse rate during 1 year before the treatment, and duration of follow-up. Renal histology was either minimal change or mesangial proliferation. These factors were not significantly different between the groups. Figure 1 shows the

Table 1. Frequently relapsing nephrotic syndrome. Cyclophosphamide treatment 3 mg/kg per day

	Group A (8 weeks)	Group B (10 weeks)	Group C (12 weeks)
Total dose (mg/kg)	168	210	252
No. of patients	20	16	8
Male/female	14/6	12/4	7/1
Age when nephrotic syndrome diagnosed (year)	6.7 ± 3.7	6.5 ± 3.7	6.3 ± 3.3
Age at entry to study (year)	9.5 ± 4.2	9.1 ± 3.9	9.1 ± 3.9
Renal history			
Minimal change	13	15	6
Mesangial proliferation	7	1	2
Duration of follow-up (month)	111 ± 48	95 ± 47	71 ± 47

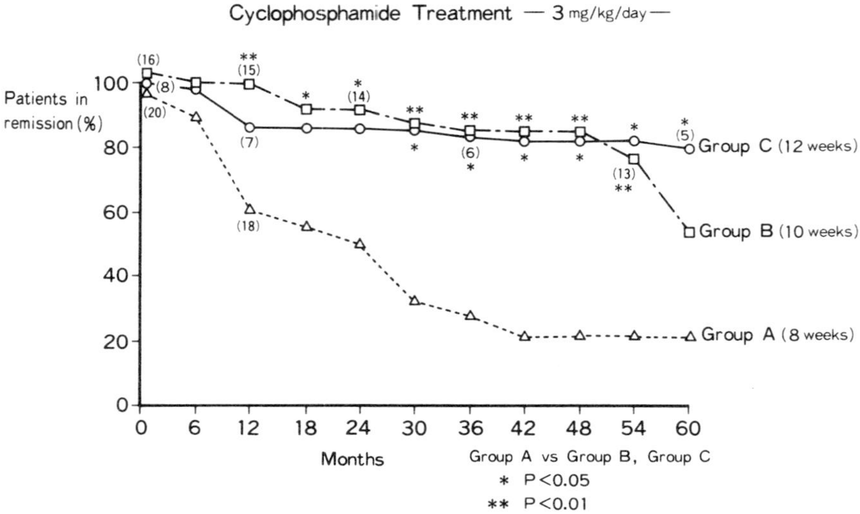

Fig. 1. Frequently relapsing nephrotic syndrome

rate of remission in the three groups. Significant difference between Group A and Group B was found at 12 months and subsequently. The difference between Group A and Group C was significant at 30 months and subsequently. There was no difference between Group B and Group C. No severe toxic effects of cyclophosphamide was observed during the treatment and the follow-up period. However, transient adverse effects, such as alopecia, leucocytopenia, gastrointestinal symptoms, mild elevation of transaminases, or hemorrhagic cystitis, developed in about 60% of the patients. The incidence of these complications was similar in the three groups. There was no correlation between the lowest leukocyte count and the remission period. Taken together, these observations suggest the efficacy and safety of the 10-week regimen. Toxicity to gonads should be monitored for long periods, even though such toxicity is difficult to assess.

Cyclosporin Therapy

Cyclosporin (CsA) therapy has recently been introduced into the treatment program for frequently relapsing NS patients. Several previous studies have shown the efficacy and minimal nephrotoxicity of CsA in nephrotic patients. In Japan, a clinical trial, comparing high and low doses of CsA in frequently relapsing NS patients, was recently carried out. When patients relapsed, CsA at 5 mg/kg per day (high dose) and 2.5 mg/kg per day (low dose) was begun. These dosages were administered for 6 months. Steroid therapy, similar to that given at the previous relapse, was given. Trough levels of CsA were monitored in whole blood and were adjusted to the optimal range of 100–500 ng/ml by polyclonal antibody radio-immunoassay (RIA) and 50–200 ng/ml by monoclonal antibody RIA.

Table 2. Cyclosporin therapy

	Frequently relapsing NS		Steroid-resistant NS	
Histology	High	Low	High	Low
Minimal change	12	8	7	4
Proliferative GN	1	1	6	2
Membranous nephropathy	0	0	0	3
Membranoproliferative GN	0	0	2	6
Focal segmental sclerosis	2	0	5	3
Biopsy, not done	9	10	1	0
Total	24	19	21	18

NS, nephrotic syndrome; GN, glomerulonephritis

Twenty four children received high doses of CsA, and 19 received low doses. Renal histology of the patients is shown in Table 2. Age, sex, duration of NS, relapse rate, and dosage of steroids used during the 6 months before CsA treatment were similar in the two groups. Relapse rate per patient decreased significantly after the therapy, when compared with the rates 6 months before and after starting CsA therapy (Fig. 2). A high dose of CsA significantly reduced the total dosage of steroids (Fig. 3), but a low dose of CsA did not significantly change the steroid dosage, because relapse occurred occasionally during low dose therapy.

In order to investigate whether CsA is effective on steroid-resistant NS, a multicenter study was also conducted. Again, high and low doses were used for 6 months. The histological classification of the patients is listed in Table 2. A high dose of CsA decreased proteinuria significantly 12 and 24 weeks after beginning the therapy (Fig. 4). In these patients, creatinine clearance did not change significantly.

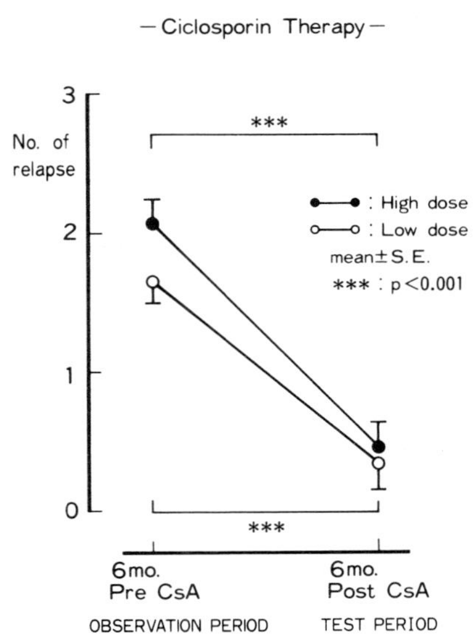

Fig. 2. Frequently relapsing nephrotic syndrome

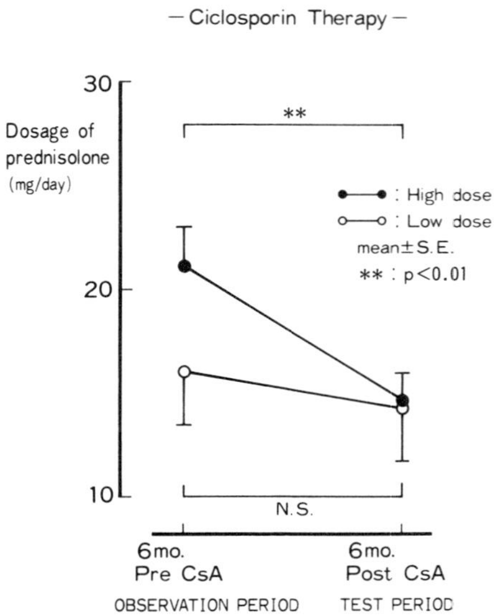

Fig. 3. Frequently relapsing nephrotic syndrome

Side effects of CsA, such as elevation of serum alkaline phosphatase, hypertension, hirsutism, and gastrointestinal symptoms, were observed frequently. Hypertension was controlled by decreasing the dose of CsA or by temporary administration of a Ca channel blocker. Renal function was temporariliy impaired in 3 (12%) patients with steroid-resistant NS. Most patients with frequently relapsing NS who were treated

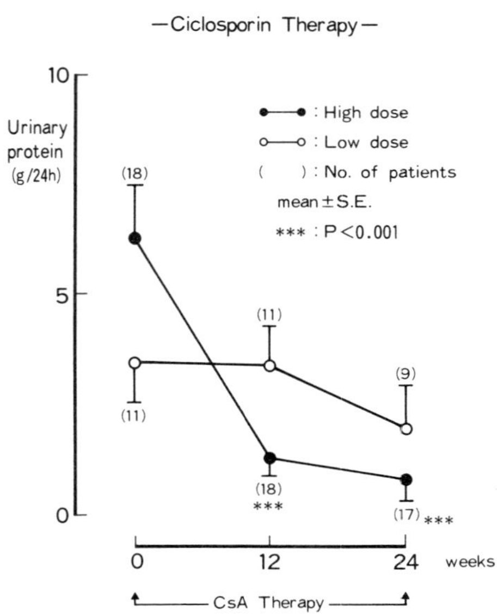

Fig. 4. Steroid-resistant nephrotic syndrome

with CsA relapsed shortly after the therapy had ended. Steroid-resistant patients obviously needed long-term CsA therapy.

In order to find out how long we can use CsA in nephrotic patients without causing nephrotoxicity, we are currently studying one-year CsA treatment. Our subjects are children with frequently relapsing NS, who have had severe steroid toxicity and have previously been treated with cyclophosphamide. In a total of 12 children, 5 mg/kg per day of CsA was administered with steroids. Trough levels of CsA were carefully monitored at least once a month. Significant decreases in the relapse rate and in the total dosage of steroids were observed. After CsA treatment, we biopsied four patients, and the results were compared with the biopsy findings which had been done prior to the therapy. In three out of four patients, no alterations suggesting CsA nephrotoxicity were found. In one patient with minimal glomerular changes, hypertrophy of the juxtaglomerular apparatus was observed in approximately half of the glomeruli. This patient was hypertensive at the beginning of CsA therapy, but he became normotensive thereafter. Renal function, urinary and serum Na concentration, and aldosterone and angiotensin II levels were normal at the time of biopsy. Plasma renin activity was slightly elevated. Taken together, these observations suggest that CsA therapy is effective and favorable for children, not only for those with frequently-relapsing NS, but also for those with steroid resistant NS. However, we need to conduct more research on this type of new therapy before we can use it for long periods with minimal CsA toxicity.

Acknowledgment. We appreciate the collaboration offered by Dr. K.W. Ko (Seoul National University, Children's Hospital, Korea) and Dr. P. Wang (First Hospital, Beijing Medical School, China) and permission to present CsA studies done by Dr. S. Tojo.

References

1. Kitagawa T, Sakai T (1985) Multicenter study on epidemiology of childhood renal diseases. In: Ishimaru T (ed) Annual report on study of prevention and treatment of childhood chronic renal diseases, pp 282–286
2. Kitagawa T, Sakai T (1986) Multicenter study on epidemiology of childhood renal diseases. In: Ishimaru T (ed) Annual report on study of prevention and treatment of childhood chronic renal diseases, pp 314–319
3. Ueda N, Chihara M, Kawaguchi S, Niinomi Y, Nonoda T, Matsumoto J, Ohnishi M, Yasaki T (1988) Intermittent versus long-term tapering prednisolone for initial therapy in children with idiopathic nephrotic syndrome. J Pediatr 112:122–126

Treatment of Childhood Steroid-Resistant Focal Segmental Glomerulosclerosis with Pulse Methylprednisolone and Alkylating Agents*

STANLEY A. MENDOZA[1], VIVIAN M. REZNIK[1], WILLIAM R. GRISWOLD[1], ALAN M. KRENSKY[2], PETER D. YORGIN[2], and BRUCE M. TUNE[2]

SUMMARY. In children, steroid-resistant nephrotic syndrome due to focal segmental glomerulosclerosis (FSGS) is frequently a progressive condition resulting in end-stage renal disease in spite of treatment. For the past several years, the Pediatric Nephrology services at the University of California, San Diego and Stanford University Schools of Medicine have treated these patients with a protocol involving infusions of high doses of methylprednisolone (MP), often in combination with oral alkylating agents. Twenty-three children have been treated in this manner with a follow-up of 55 ± 6 months. Thirteen of these children are in complete remission. Five have minimal to moderate proteinuria. Four children remain nephrotic. Each of these children has a normal glomerular filtration rate. One child developed chronic renal failure and subsequently died while on dialysis. These results appear better than those in previous series of children with FSGS. A controlled, multi-center trial of this protocol has been proposed.

Introduction

Focal segmental glomerulosclerosis (FSGS) is a cause of steroid-resistant nephrotic syndrome and chronic renal failure in childhood [1–7]. The incidence of renal failure is 20%–40% by 5 years after the onset of FSGS and increases further after 10 years. FSGS is the most common form of glomerular disease leading to chronic renal failure in children [8] and is seen in 10%–20% of children requiring dialysis or renal transplantation [9]. In recent years, the Pediatric Nephrology services at the Stanford and University of California, San Diego Schools of Medicine have treated these children

[1]Department of Pediatrics, University of California, San Diego, La Jolla, CA 92093, USA
[2]Department of Pediatrics, Stanford University School of Medicine, Stanford, CA, USA
*A manuscript describing this series of patients at a somewhat earlier time has been accepted for publication in *Pediatric Nephrology*

with a protocol involving intravenous infusions of high doses of MP, often in association with oral alkylating agents. Results of this treatment on the first seven patients have been described [10]. We now report the outcome of the first 23 patients treated with this protocol and followed for 55 ± 6 months.

Methods

Each of the patients included in this report presented with the nephrotic syndrome. The patients remained nephrotic after 4–8 weeks of treatment with oral prednisone at a dose of 2 mg/kg per day. Because of the steroid-resistance, a renal biopsy was done on each patient and was read as focal segmental glomerulosclerosis. The patients were 7.6 ± 0.95 years old at the time of entry into the protocol. Sixteen of the patients were male; seven were female. Eighteen of the children were steroid-resistant at the time of initial presentation (primary steroid-resistance); five initially responded to oral steroids, but were resistant later (secondary steroid-resistance).

Since this is a retrospective study, there were minor differences in the protocol from patient to patient. The protocol which was used most often is shown in Table 1. In some cases, the initial six MP infusions were given while the child was hospitalized. In most cases, all of the infusions were given by a nephrology nurse in an outpatient setting. If the patients either failed to respond to the initial 10 weeks of MP infusions or improved and later relapsed, they were restarted at the beginning of the MP protocol and given an 8–12 week course of therapy with an oral alkylating agent (cyclophosphamide 2 mg/kg per day or chlorambucil 0.2 mg/kg per day). Fifteen patients had at least one course of alkylating agent therapy. Seven patients received more than one course of treatment with alkylating agents. In general, multiple courses of alkylating agent therapy were given when a patient improved with the first course and subsequently relapsed.

The patients were seen frequently while they were receiving MP and/or alkylating agent therapy. In addition to routine clinical evaluation, serum creatinine concentrations and ratios of the concentrations of protein and creatinine in the urine were obtained. The glomerular filtration rate [GFR] was estimated using the height formula [11,12]. An estimated GFR greater than 80 ml/min per 1.73 m^2 was interpreted as normal. The magnitude of proteinuria was assessed by comparing the urinary concentrations of protein, in mg/dl, and creatinine, in mg/dl [13,14]. A urinary protein/creatinine ratio ≤ 0.20 was considered to be normal; a ratio of 0.21–0.5 was

Table 1. Usual FSGS protocol

Week	Methylprednisolone	Prednisone
1	30 mg/kg every other day X3	None
2	30 mg/kg every other day X3	None
3–10	30 mg/kg weekly	2 mg/kg qod (every other day)
11–18	30 mg/kg every other week	2 mg/kg qod
19–52	30 mg/kg monthly	2 mg/kg qod
53–78	30 mg/kg every other month	2 mg/kg qod

Methylprednisolone is then discontinued and oral prednisone tapered and discontinued

Table 2. Status of FSGS patients after 55 ± 6 months

In remission	13 (56.5%)
Minimal proteinuria	3 (13.1%)
Moderate proteinuria	2 (8.7%)
Nephrotic syndrome	4 (17.4%)
Renal failure	1 (4.4%)

called minimal proteinuria; a ratio of 0.51–2.0 was interpreted as moderate proteinuria; a ratio > 2.0 was seen in children with nephrotic levels of proteinuria. Data are presented as Mean ± SD.

Results

We have treated 23 patients with steroid-resistant nephrotic syndrome and biopsy-proven FSGS with MP infusions. The status of these patients at their most recent follow-up is summarized in Table 2. The mean follow-up is 55 ± 6 months. Twenty-two patients had a normal estimated GFR. One child progressed to end-stage renal failure (ESRD) and subsequently died. Thirteen patients were in complete remission (after 21–100 months). These patients were receiving no treatment when last seen. Three patients had minimally elevated urine protein excretion; 2 had moderately elevated urinary protein excretion without edema; and 4 children continued to have nephrotic levels of proteinuria. Three of these four nephrotic children had a urinary protein excretion at the time of their most recent follow-up which was more than 50% lower than that obtained before starting the MP protocol. The fourth child with persistent nephrotic levels of proteinuria had no change in his urinary protein excretion following MP therapy.

Side effects of the MP therapy have been acceptable to date, although no information is available regarding long-term side effects, such as sterility and oncogenesis. Five patients developed small cataracts which did not interfere with vision while receiving this treatment. In one child, the cataract improved after he went into remission and treatment was discontinued. In most children, growth during MP therapy was similar to the pretreatment growth rate. However, four children had significant growth retardation while receiving frequent MP infusions, alternate day oral prednisone, and several courses of treatment with oral alkylating agents. Eventually, each of these children went into remission. One of these patients subsequently had a period of "catch-up" growth. The other three remain growth-retarded. A number of children reported nausea during the MP infusions. This was particularly common when the interval between infusions was one month or longer. Four patients developed hypertension which required treatment during the MP protocol. The hypertension was easily controlled and resolved as the interval between MP infusions increased. Other complications of high dose steroid therapy such as striae, aseptic necrosis of the femoral head, diabetes, and pancreatitis were not observed.

No major adverse effects of alkylating agent therapy were observed in these patients. Three patients developed transient leukopenia during alkylating agent therapy, which led to an interruption of the treatment. In each case, the course of alkylating agent therapy was completed after the white blood count returned to normal.

Although fatal infections have been reported in patients treated with MP [15], we have not noted an increased incidence of serious infections in the FSGS patients treated with this protocol. Four of these patients had had an episode of bacterial peritonitis or sepsis before starting MP. Two patients had peritonitis while on this treatment. In addition, one patient had herpes zoster and another patient had cellulitis of the leg while receiving MP. Each patient recovered from his/her infection uneventfully.

Discussion

The prognosis of children with FSGS is poor [16]. It is estimated that 10%–20% of children who progress to dialysis or transplantation have FSGS [9]. In fact, FSGS is the most common form of glomerular disease leading to chronic renal failure in children [8]. In addition, there is a significant risk of recurrence of FSGS following renal transplantation [8,9,16].

In some series of children with FSGS, the prognosis of primary steroid-resistant patients and late steroid non-responders was equally poor [2,4]. Other authors have reported that FSGS patients with primary steroid-resistance progress to renal failure faster than late non-responders [5]. Eighteen of our 23 patients had primary steroid-resistance; 5 had secondary steroid-resistance. The numbers are too small to assess possible differences in outcome between primary and secondary steroid-resistant FSGS patients treated in this way.

The effect of alkylating agents in steroid-resistant FSGS is somewhat controversial. Several groups, including the International Study of Kidney Disease in Children, reported that cyclophosphamide does not improve the outcome in steroid-resistant children with FSGS [17,18]. In contrast, it has been reported that many children with FSGS and steroid-resistant nephrotic syndrome have a partial response to cyclophosphamide, which leads to an improved prognosis [19]. Recently, there has been interest in the use of cyclosporine A in the treatment of FSGS. Preliminary results with this agent have been disappointing, although somewhat variable [20–24].

We have reported previously that the initial response to the treatment of steroid-resistant nephrotic syndrome and FSGS with MP infusions appeared to be favorable [10]. Seven patients had been treated; disappearance of edema and improvement in serum and urine chemistries occurred within a short time after beginning MP therapy.

After a follow-up period of 55 $\pm$ 6 months, 56.5% of our 23 patients are in complete remission, 13.1% have minimal proteinuria, 8.7% have moderate proteinuria with no edema or hypoproteinemia, 17.4% remain nephrotic, and only one child [4.4%] developed ESRD. In Table 3, the outcome of our prednisone-resistant patients is compared with the outcome in other series of children with FSGS; series which include both prednisone-responsive and prednisone-resistant patients. Our patients had a strikingly lower incidence of ESRD and a markedly higher incidence of remission of their renal disease.

Side effects of the MP therapy have not been severe. We have not seen cardiac arrhythmias following MP infusions, but these have been reported by others [25,26]. We have seen a mild anaphylactoid reaction to MP [27] in a patient receiving the drug for a different reason, and we are aware of one child with FSGS who had an allergic reaction to intravenous MP (N.J. Siegel, personal communication).

Table 3. Outcome of FSGS in children in current and previous series

Series	No. patients	Follow-up (months)	ESRD or death	Remission
Habib [1]	64	61	31.2%	20.3%
Ito [28]	27	73	29.6%	N.S.
Arbus [4]	32	56	53.1%	N.S.
SPNSG [2]	75	57	21.0%	11.0%
Tejani [5]	24	114	62.5%	N.S.
Ellis [29]	32	62	37.5%	18.8%
Cameron [6]	12	N.S.	75.0%	0
Current series	23	55	4.4%	56.5%

N.S., Not stated in the manuscript; SPNSG, Southwest Pediatric Nephrology Study Group

In conclusion, this group of children with FSGS has done remarkably well following treatment with intravenous MP. The outcome of the patients in this study appears to be better than the outcome in each series of children with steroid-resistant nephrotic syndrome and FSGS of which we are aware. The authors are organizing a multi-center, randomized, controlled clinical trial of this protocol.

References

1. Habib R (1973) Focal glomerular sclerosis. Kidney Int 4:355–361
2. Southwest Pediatric Nephrology Study Group (1985) Focal segmental glomerulosclerosis in children with idiopathic nephrotic syndrome. A report of the Southwest Pediatric Nephrology Study Group. Kidney Int 27:442–449
3. Kohaut EC, Singer DB, Hill LL (1976) The significance of focal glomerular sclerosis in children who have nephrotic syndrome. Am J Clin Pathol 66:545–550
4. Arbus GS, Poucell S, Bacheyie GS, Bauman R (1982) Focal segmental glomerulosclerosis with idiopathic nephrotic syndrome: Three types of clinical response. J Pediatr 101: 40–45
5. Tejani A, Nicastri AD, Sen D, Chen CK, Phadke K, Adamson O, Butt KM (1983) Long-term evaluation of children with nephrotic syndrome and focal segmental glomerular sclerosis. Nephron 35:225–231
6. Cameron JS, Turner DR, Ogg CS, Chantler C, Williams DG (1978) The long-term prognosis of patients with focal segmental glomerulosclerosis. Clin Nephrol 10:213–218
7. Halevy J, Hayslett JP (1986) Clinical features and course of focal glomerulosclerosis. In: Mitch WE, Brenner BM, Stein JH (eds) The progressive nature of renal disease. Churchill Livingstone, New York, pp 189–201
8. Fine R (1987) Renal transplantation in children. Nephron 47:81–86
9. Broyer M, Gagnadoux MF, Guest G, Beurton D, Niaudet P, Habib R, Busson M (1987) Kidney transplantation in children: results of 383 grafts performed at Enfants Malades Hospital from 1973 to 1984. Adv Nephrol 16:307–333
10. Griswold WR, Tune BM, Reznik VM, Vazquez M, Prime DJ, Brock P, Mendoza SA (1987) Treatment of childhood prednisone-resistant nephrotic syndrome and focal segmental glomerulosclerosis with intravenous methylprednisolone and oral alkylating agents. Nephron 46:73–77
11. Schwartz GJ, Haycock GB, Edelmann CM Jr, Spitzer A (1976) A simple estimate of glomerular filtration rate in children derived from body length and plasma creatinine. Pediatrics 58:259–63

12. Schwartz GJ, Feld LG, Langford DJ (1984) A simple estimate of glomerular filtration rate in full-term infants during the first year of life. J Pediatr 104:849–854
13. Houser M (1984) Assessment of proteinuria using random urine samples. J Pediatr 104:845–849
14. Ginsberg JM, Chang BS, Matarese RA, Garella S (1983) Use of single voided urine samples to estimate quantitative proteinuria. New Engl J Med 309:1543–1546
15. Kozeny G, Quinn J, Bansal V, Vertuno L, Hano E (1987) Pneumocystis carinii pneumonia: a lethal complication of "pulse" methylprednisolone therapy. Int J Artif Organs 10(5):304–306
16. Sheldon CA, McLorie GA, Churchill BM (1987) Renal transplantation in children. Pediatr Clin North Am 34:1209–1232
17. International Study of Kidney Disease in Children (1982) Cyclophosphamide therapy in focal segmental glomerular sclerosis: A controlled clinical trial. Pediatr Res 16:320A
18. Mongeau J-G, Corneille L, Robitaille P, O'Regan S, Pelletier M (1981) Primary nephrosis in childhood associated with focal glomerular sclerosis: Is long-term prognosis that severe? Kidney Int 20:743–746
19. Geary DF, Farine M, Thorner P, Baumal R (1984) Response to cyclophosphamide in steroid-resistant focal segmental glomerulosclerosis: a reappraisal. Clin Nephrol 22:109–113
20. Trompeter RS (1987) Steroid resistant nephrotic syndrome: A review of the treatment of focal segmental glomerulosclerosis (FSGS) in children. In: Murakami K, Kitagawa T, Yabuta K, Sakai T (eds) Recent advances in pediatric nephrology. Elsevier Science, Amsterdam, pp 363–371
21. Tejani A, Butt K, Trachtman H, Suthanthiran M, Rosenthal CJ, Khawar MR (1988) Cyclosporine A induced remission of relapsing nephrotic syndrome in children. Kidney Int 33:729–734
22. Waldo FB, Kohaut EC (1987) Therapy of focal segmental glomerulosclerosis with cyclosporine A. Pediatr Nephrol 1:180–182
23. Niaudet P, Habib R, Tete M-J, Hinglais N, Broyer M (1987) Cyclosporin in the treatment of idiopathic nephrotic syndrome in children. Pediatr Nephrol 1:566–573
24. Brodehl J, Hoyer PF, Oemar BS, Helmchen U, Wonigeit K (1988) Cyclosporine treatment of nephrotic syndrome in children. Transplant Proc 20:269–274
25. Ueda N, Yoshikawa T, Chihara M, Kawaguchi S, Niinomi Y, Yasaki T (1988) Atrial fibrillation following methylprednisolone pulse therapy. Pediatr Nephrol 2:29–31
26. Bocanegra TS, Castaneda MO, Espinoza LR, Vasey FB, Germain BF (1981) Sudden death after methylprednisolone pulse therapy. Ann Intern Med 95:122
27. Preuss L (1985) Allergic reactions to systemic glucocorticoids: A review. Ann Allergy 55:772–775
28. Ito H, Yoshikawa N, Aozai F, Hazikano H, Sakaguchi H, Akamatsu R, Matsuo T, Matsuyama S (1984) Twenty-seven children with focal segmental glomerulosclerosis: Correlation between the segmental location of the glomerular lesions and prognosis. Clin Nephrol 22:9–14
29. Ellis D, Kapur S, Antonovych TT, Salcedo JR, Yunis EJ (1978) Focal glomerulosclerosis in children: Correlation of histology with prognosis. J Pediatr 93:762–768

Ca, Pi, PTH, and Vitamin D

Chair: Keith A. Hruska (USA)
Mordecai M. Popovtzer (Israel)

Towards Structural Identification of the Na^+/P_i-Cotransport System

HEINI MURER, ANDREAS WERNER, FRANÇOIS WUARIN,
STEPHAN J. RESHKIN, AND JÜRG BIBER[1]

SUMMARY. During the last several years different strategies have been developed for a structural identification of the renal proximal tubular Na^+/P_i-cotransport system. Such approaches can be related to the use of either "specific" (e.g., competitive) or "unspecific" inhibitors (e.g., amino-acid group-specific reagents) in combination with substrate protection and to labeling via specific cellular regulatory pathway (e.g., protein-phosphorylation or protein-turnover). As an additional strategy, expression cloning may be used for structural identification of Na^+/P_i-cotransport. Finally, the "functional" apparent molecular mass of the protein-complex(es) involved in Na^+/P_i-cotransport can be determined by radiation inactivation (target size) analysis.

Introduction

Renal proximal tubular phosphate reabsorption is under the control of a variety of hormonal and non-hormonal factors; the regulatory mechanisms seem, ultimately, to affect an apically located Na^+/P_i-cotransport system (for review see: [1–5]). Inhibition by parathyroid hormone (PTH) is the best studied example of hormonal control mechanisms; increases in Na^+/P_i-cotransport activity in response to low phosphate intake or to an increased phosphate demand may be examples of "non-hormonal" control mechanisms [1–5]. Over the years, rather specific regulatory cascades have been postulated to be involved, e.g., in PTH-dependent control (i.e., phosphorylation mechanisms) or in adaptive control (de novo synthesis or change in membrane fluidity) of Na^+/P_i-cotransport. Obviously, without structural identification of the Na^+/P_i-cotransport system, a detailed study of specific cellular mechanisms involved in the regulation of Na^+/P_i-cotransport is rather difficult and would provide only a working hypothesis which would remain to be proven.

[1]Department of Physiology, University of Zürich, Winterthurerstrasse 190, CH - 8057 Zürich, Switzerland

In this report we will briefly summarize present "knowledge" of the structural identity of the Na^+/P_i-cotransport system. Several very different approaches will be discussed, for which detailed descriptions of the methods will be not be included; the reader is referred to the original literature.

Experiments Involving Reconstitution and/or Measurements of Phosphate-Binding/Transport

Solubilization of brush border membrane proteins and protein separation followed by reconstitution into artificial lipid bilayers provided some evidence for a hydrophobic peptide ("phosphorin") which showed P_i-transport properties [6–9]; however, these activities were not Na^+-dependent processes [9], i.e., a participation in Na^+/P_i-cotransport was not documented. Similar phenomena were also reported for a protein of 155 kDa molecular weight, which under denaturing conditions shows a molecular weight of 70 kDa. P_i-binding to this protein was saturable (K_D = 10 µM) as was Na^+-binding (K_D = 7.5 mM); however, an effect of Na^+ on P_i-binding was not shown [10]. In all of the above-mentioned studies the basic function, i.e., N^+-gradient-dependent transport of P_i, was not documented; except for the observation, in a report by Kinne and Faust [11], of a small effect of a Na^+-gradient on P_i-uptake into liposomes which had been reconstituted from solubilized unfractionated brush border membrane protein and lipids isolated from renal cortex.

Experiments Using "Specific" or "Unspecific" Inhibitors

Phosphonoformic acid (PFA) is a competitive ("specific") inhibitor of Na^+/P_i-cotransport (e.g., [12]); this fact could offer the possibility of identifying the transporter in purification/separation experiments, as well as in affinity labeling/purification experiments [13,14]. However, until now this approach has not yet provided information on the molecular identity of the Na^+/P_i-cotransport system. We would like to add here some potential problems which could occur in the use of PFA as a ligand in experiments aiming to purify Na^+/P_i-cotransport: 1] the amount of "specific" Na^+-dependent, P_i-protectable PFA-binding is rather high and simple calculations assuming a molecular weight of 50–100 kDa (see below) for the Na^+/P_i-cotransport system would suggest that a rather high percentage of total brush border membrane protein is related to this transport activity; 2] recently it was shown that sulfate and phosphate interact with the same PFA-binding sites, documenting a lack of specificity of PFA-binding [15]. Furthermore, PFA also inhibits Na^+-dependent sulfate transport in brush border membrane vesicles [15].

As "unspecific" inhibitors, two amino acid group-specific reagents were used. Phenylglyoxal has been used to inhibit renal Na^+/P_i-cotransport, indicating the involvement of functionally important arginine groups; no attempts using phenylglyoxal for structural identification have been reported [16]. In our laboratory, we have found that N-acetylimidazole was able to inhibit P_i-transport via Na^+/P_i-cotransport in a P_i protectable manner; subsequently it was possible to label membrane proteins by this procedure. It was concluded that proteins of 31, 53, 105, and/or 107 kDa may be important in mediating Na^+/P_i-cotransport across apical membranes of PTH-sensitive renal epithelial cells, i.e., OK cells [17], and rat renal proximal tubular cells (F. Wuarin, J. Biber, and H. Murer, unpublished work).

It should be mentioned that recent work on intestinal Na^+/P_i-cotransport using FITC-labeled phenylglyoxal or N-acetylimidazole provided evidence for an involvement of a 130 kDa protein in transmembrane transport of P_i in small intestine [18]. However, in view of the fundamental differences in kinetic behavior and regulatory control of intestinal vs renal Na^+/P_i-cotransport it cannot, a priori, be assumed that these transport pathways are structurally related [19].

Labeling Via Cellular Regulatory Pathways

In an attempt to identify the Na^+/P_i-cotransport system or proteins involved in its control, experiments on in situ labeling of apical membrane proteins either by PTH-dependent phosphorylation reactions, or on ^{35}S-L-methionine incorporation during phases of protein synthesis-dependent increases in Na^+/P_i-cotransport activity were also performed in OK cells. In the phosphorylation experiment a 105 kDa integral membrane protein turned out to be preferentially marked by high and low PTH concentrations as well as by pharmacological kinase A- and kinase C-activation ([120], SJ Reshkin, F Wuarin, and H Murer, manuscript in preparation). During protein synthesis-dependent increases in Na^+/P_i-cotransport (PTH removal and P_i-deprivation) preferential incorporation of radioactivity occurred in specific integral membrane proteins (J. Biber and H. Murer, manuscript in preparation). Further work on these proteins will determine at which level they are involved in Na^+/P_i-cotransport and/or its regulation.

Identification of Na^+/P_i-Cotransport via Expression Cloning

The only brush border membrane cotransport system which has been structurally identified up to now, the Na^+/D-glucose-cotransport system, was "obtained" by expression cloning using *Xenopus laevis* oocytes as an expression system [21]. In our laboratory we have applied a similar strategy for identification of the Na^+/P_i-cotransport system. A first success was the identification of a mRNA fraction from rabbit kidney cortex and OK cells which led, after injection into oocytes, to an increased Na^+/P_i-cotransport activity with kinetic properties similar to the transport pathway in the brush border membrane [22]. After cDNA-synthesis and insertion into a pBluescript-plasmid we could identify a single clone which, after in vitro mRNA transcription, produced a stimulation of Na^+/P_i-cotransport activity in mRNA-injected *Xenopus laevis* oocytes; the kinetics of expressed transport activity were different from the intrinsic activity of oocytes and similar to that in brush border membrane transport. The deduced amino acid sequence shows 489 amino acid residues and several putative transmembrane spanning regions (A. Werner, J. Biber and H. Murer, manuscript in preparation; M. Moore, N. Mantei, and G. Semenza, manuscript in preparation). On the basis of these results we conclude that we have cloned the renal proximal tubular brush border membrane Na^+/P_i-cotransporter.

Target-Size Analysis Na^+/P_i-Cotransport

Béliveau and his colleagues have determined the functional molecular weight (target size) of a protein complex apparently involved in Na^+/P_i-cotransport. Based on radiation inactivation analysis they concluded that a protein complex with an apparent molecular mass of 205 ± 36 kDa was involved in Na^+/P_i-cotransport [23]. For phosphate-protectable, Na^+-dependent PFA-binding the apparent molecular mass was 130 kDa [23]; as indicated above, it is not known at present whether PFA-binding and Na^+/P_i-cotransport activity are related properties [15].

Recently, a target size analysis of Na^+-dependent D-glucose transport has been reported for intestinal [24] and renal brush border membranes [25]; the apparent molecular mass was found to be 290 kDa for Na^+-dependent D-glucose transport in both membrane preparations. Taken together with the predicted molecular mass of 73 kDa from the cloning experiments, the suggestion was made that Na^+-dependent D-glucose transport operates as a homotetramer [21,24]. By analogy, the predicted molecular mass, around 50–60 kDa obtained for the Na^+/P_i-cotransport from our cloning experiment (A. Werner, J. Biber and H. Murer, manuscript in preparation; M. Moore, N. Mantei, and G. Semenza, manuscript in preparation), together with the target size of 205 ± 36 kDa [23,25] would suggest that N^+/P_i-cotransport also functions as a homotetramer.

Conclusions

In recent years renal proximal tubular Na^+/P_i-cotransport and its regulation based on analysis of function, i.e., transport activity, has been studied extensively. For a more precise analysis of Na^+/P_i-cotransport activity and its regulation a structural identification of the Na^+/P_i-cotransport system is mandatory. Different indirect and direct approaches, aiming for such identification, have been developed; none of these strategies have led to identification of the Na^+/P_i-cotransport system, although candidate-proteins for participation in Na^+/P_i-cotransport and/or its regulation could be identified. Recent progress in expression cloning has resulted in the identification of a 498 amino acid residue membrane protein which fulfills several criteria of being the renal proximal tubular Na^+/P_i-cotransport system. Thus, we hope that the availability of probes on the nucleic acid and protein level opens a new area in the study of renal Na^+/P_i-cotransport and its regulation.

Acknowledgments. The financial support of the Swiss National Science Foundation (Grant No. 3.851.088), the "Stiftung für wissenschaftliche Forschung an der Universität Zürich," the "Hartmann Müller Stiftung," the "Geigy-Jubiläumsstiftung" and the "Sandoz Stiftung" are gratefully acknowledged.

References

1. Biber J (1989) Cellular aspects of proximal tubular phosphate reabsorption. Kidney Int 36:360–369
2. Bonjour JP, Caverzasio J (1984) Phosphate transport in the kidney. Rev Physiol Biochem Pharmacol 100:161–214

3. Dennis VW (to be published) Phosphate homeostasis. In: Windhager EE, Giebisch G (eds) American Physiological Society, Bethesda (Handbook of Physiology)
4. Gmaj P, Murer H (1986) Cellular mechanisms of inorganic phosphate transport in kidney. Physiol Rev 66:36–70
5. Murer H, Biber J (to be published) Renal tubular phosphate transport: Cellular mechanisms. In: Seldin DW, Giebisch G (eds) The kidney. Raven, New York
6. Kessler RJ, Fanestil DD (1981) Identification of a phosphate-binding proteolipid in kidney brush border. In: Bronner F, Peterlik M (eds) Calcium and phosphate transport across biomembranes. Academic, New York, pp 123–126
7. Kessler RJ, Vaughn DA, Fensetil DD (1982) Phosphate-binding proteolipid from brush border. J Biol Chem 257:14311–14317
8. Kessler RJ, Vaughn DA (1984) Divalent metal is required for both phosphate transport and phosphate binding to phosphorin, a proteolipid isolated from brush-border membrane vesicles. J Biol Chem 259:9059–9063
9. Schaeli C, Vaughn DA, Fanestil DD (1986) Reconstitution of the partially purified renal phosphate (P_i) transporter. Biochem J 235:189–197
10. Debiec H, Lorenc R (1988) Identification of Na^+, P_i-binding protein in kidney and intestinal brush-border membranes. Biochem J 225:185–191
11. Kinne R, Faust RG (1977) Incorporation of D-glucose, L-alanine- and phosphate-transport systems from rat renal brush-border membranes into liposomes. Biochem J 168:311–314
12. Szczepanska-Konkel M, Yusufi ANK, Van Scoy M, Webster SK, Dousa TP (1986) Phosphonocarboxylic acids as specific inhibitors of Na^+-dependent transport of phosphate across renal brush border membrane. J Biol Chem 261:6375–6383
13. Lin JT, Dousa TP (to be published) Determination of Na^+-P_i symporters in solubilized renal brush border membranes (BBM) by ^{14}C-phosphonoformic acid (PFA) binding. Kidney Int 37:459
14. McKenna CE, Pham P, Hoppe A, Rassier ME, Dousa TP (to be published) Alpha-halophenyl (phosphonomethyl)-phosphinates as specific inhibitors of Na^+-P_i cotransport across renal BBM. Kidney Int 37:460
15. Tennenhouse HS, Lee J (to be published) Sulfate inhibits ^{14}C-phosphonoformic acid binding to renal brush-border membranes. Am J Physiol
16. Strevey J, Brunette MG, Béliveau R (1984) Effect of arginine modification on kidney brush border membrane transport activity. Biochem J 223:793–802
17. Wuarin F, Wu K, Murer H, Biber J (1989) The Na/P_i cotransporter of OK cells: Reaction and tentative identification with N-acethylimidazole. Biochim Biophys Acta 981: 185–192
18. Peerce BE (1989) Identification of the intestinal Na-phosphate cotransporter. Am J Physiol 256:G645–G652
19. Danisi G, Murer H (to be published) Inorganic phosphate absorption in small intestine. In: M Field (ed) American Physiological Society, Bethesda (Handbook of Physiology)
20. Reshkin SJ, Wuarin F, Biber J, Murer H (1990) Parathyroid hormone induced alterations of apical membrane protein content and phosphorylation in opossum kidney cells. J Biol Chem 265:15261–15266
21. Hediger MA, Coady MJ, Ikeda TS, Wright EM (1987) Expression cloning and cDNA sequencing of the Na^+/glucose cotransporter. Nature 330:379–381
22. Werner A, Biber J, Forgo J, Palacin M, Murer H (1990) Expression of renal transport systems for inorganic phosphate and sulphate in *Xenopus laevis* oocytes. J Biol Chem 265:12331–12336
23. Béliveau R, Jette M, Demeule M, Potter M, Lee J, Tennenhouse HS (to be published) Different molecular size for Na^+-dependent phosphonoformic acid binding and phosphate transport in renal brush-border membrane vesicles. Biochim Biophys Acta

24. Stevens BR, Fernandez A, Hirayama B, Wright EM, Dempner ES (1990) Intestinal brush border membrane Na^+/glucose cotransporter functions in situ as a homotetramer. Proc Natl Acad Sci USA 87:1456–1460
25. Béliveau R, Demeule M, Ibnoul-Khatib H, Bergeron M, Beauregard G, Potier M (1988) Radiation-inactivation studies on brush-border-membrane vesicles. General considerations, and application to the glucose and phosphate carriers. Biochem J 252:807–813

Insulin-Like Growth Factor I (IGF-I), Possible Mediator of the Stimulatory Effects of Growth Hormone on Renal Phosphate Transport and 1,25-Dihydroxyvitamin D3 Production

J. Caverzasio, C. Montessuit, and J.-P. Bonjour[1]

Introduction

Inorganic phosphate (Pi), which is a limiting factor in the stimulation of DNA synthesis by mitogenic agents [1], is an essential determinant of cellular growth and replication. In vivo, the level of extracellular Pi and thereby the amount of Pi available for cellular metabolism and growth, is mainly determined and regulated by the tubular reabsorption of Pi. This process is markedly influenced by the growth rate of the organism [2–4]. Thus, both the tubular reabsorption and the plasma concentration of Pi are maintained at a higher level in young growing, as compared to adult, individuals [2–4]. Likewise, tubular Pi reabsorption is lower in hypophysectomized than in intact counterparts [5]. Studies with brush border membrane vesicles isolated from rat renal cortex indicate that growth-related change in the tubular handling of Pi can be expressed at the level of the luminal membrane of the proximal tubule [6]. The mechanism responsible for this growth related enhancement in the tubular reabsorption of Pi is still not known. Growth hormone (GH) itself has been logically considered as a putative mediator. Indeed, a stimulation of the tubular capacity to reabsorb Pi, as assessed by determining the maximal rate of Pi reabsorption per unit volume of glomerular filtrate (maxTRPi/mlGFR or TmPi/GFR), can be observed both in human subjects and in experimental animals chronically treated with GH (7–9). Increased TmPi/GFR is also found in active acromegaly with excessive secretion of GH [2]. However, in animal experiments acute administration of GH failed for hours to stimulate the renal transport of Pi [10]. This lag time in the renal response suggested [11] that GH-induced stimulation of the tubular transport of Pi could, like other growth-related effects, be mediated by insulin-like growth factor I (IGF-I) [12,13]. Growth hormone can increase the circulating level of IGF-I, probably by enhancing its hepatic production [14]. Besides this classical endocrine pathway,

[1]Division of Clinical Pathophysiology, Department of Medicine, University Hospital of Geneva, CH-1211 Geneva 4, Switzerland

GH enhances the content of IGF-I in various tissues, suggesting the existence of autocrine and/or paracrine mechanisms [15]. Receptors specific for IGF-I have been identified in basolateral membranes of renal proximal tubules [16]. Therefore, change in the plasma level and/or in the renal production of IGF-I could mediate the effect of GH on the tubular transport of Pi. Interestingly, in many growth-related or GH-dependent physiological or pathophysiological conditions, changes in TmPi/GFR are associated with parallel alterations in the plasma level of 1,25-dihydroxyvitamin D3 (1,25(OH)2D3), a hormone implicated in the homeostasis of Pi [17–18]. As mentioned below, the mechanism responsible for this most intriguing parallelism could be IGF-I.

Stimulatory Effect of IGF-I in Vitro on Sodium-Dependent Pi Transport in Cultured Kidney Cells

In a first series of experiments [19] we speculated whether IGF-I could exert a direct effect on renal Pi transport. In order to examine this question we used kidney epithelial cell cultures, which have been shown to be an adequate system for in vitro study of the mechanisms regulating the renal transport of Pi [20–22]. The effect of recombinant IGF-I on Pi transport was studied in cultured opossum kidney (OK) epithelia. The results indicated that IGF-I (5.10^{-10} to 10^{-7} M) induced a dose-related stimulation of the Na-dependent Pi transport (NaPiT). A maximal response was observed at 10^{-7} M (IGF-I 1.64 ± 0.12; vehicle 0.90 ± 0.02 nmol/mg protein per 4 min, $P < 0.001$). Kinetic analysis of the stimulatory effect of IGF-I on NaPiT indicated an increase in Vmax and no change in Km. Insulin also stimulated NaPiT in OK epithelia, but only at concentrations about 2 orders of magnitude higher than IGF-I. The effect of IGF-I on NaPiT was detectable in less than 30 min, with a maximal response occurring after 4–5 h. The effect was selective for NaPiT, since the Na-dependent alanine transport was not affected by IGF-I. Inhibition of protein synthesis by either cycloheximide or cordycepin markedly attenuated the stimulatory effect of IGF-I on NaPiT. Cellular cAMP content was not modified by the growth factor. These results indicated that IGF-I selectively increases NaPiT through a mechanism that appears to involve de novo protein synthesis. These observations suggested that growth and growth hormone related stimulation of renal Pi transport could be mediated by IGF-I [19].

Stimulatory Effect of IGF-I in Vivo on Tubular Pi Transport and on Plasma 1,25(OH)2D3

In a second series of experiment [23], the influence of recombinant human IGF-I on renal Pi transport and on plasma 1,25(OH)2D3 was examined in hypophysectomized (HPX) rats. Infused by miniosmotic pump at a dose of 10 μg/h for 6 days, IGF-I significantly increased max TRPi/mlGRF: IGF-I 3.50 ± 0.16; vehicle 2.78 ± 0.14 μmol/mlGFR, $P < 0.005$. In brush border membrane vesicles isolated from renal cortex of HPX rats, the Na-dependent Pi transport was stimulated by IGF-I. Neither the Na-dependent glucose transport nor that of alanine was affected by the growth factor. Thus, as in OK epithelial culture [19], the in vivo effect of IGF-I on the Pi transport system localized in the luminal membrane of the proximal tubule cannot be ascribed to an unspecific alteration in the driving force generated by the transmembrane sodium gradient [23]. The stimulatory effect of IGF-I on maxTRPi/mlGFR was also expressed in thyroparathyroidectomized (TPTX) HPX rats (IGF-I 5.20 ± 0.29; vehicle 3.88 ± 0.37 µmol/mlGFR, $P < 0.025$). The increase in renal Pi transport was associated with a marked stimulation of plasma 1,25(OH)2D3 (IGF-I 409 ± 23; vehicle 208 ± 22 pmol/l, $P < 0.001$). As previously reported for GH, IGF-I also increased GFR and reduced urinary sodium excretion [23].

Thus, administration of IGF-I to HPX rats mimics the stimulatory effect of GH on maxTRPi/mlGFR and on plasma 1,25(OH)2D3. As described for GH [3], the IGF-I induced change in maxTRPi/mlGFR is mediated by a PTH independent mechanism and is expressed at the level of the luminal membrane of proximal tubules [24]. The fact that IGF-I simultaneously increases renal Pi transport and plasma 1,25(OH)2D3 levels raises the question of whether this peptide hormone might play a key role in Pi homeostasis in physiological and pathological conditions other than those associated with changes in growth and/or circulating GH. Parallel PTH-independent changes in renal Pi reabsorption and in plasma 1,25(OH)2D3 levels have been observed in many experimental and clinical conditions, particularly in relation to alterations in the Pi supply and demand of the organism [17,18,25]. From these results, obtained both in vitro [19] and in vivo [23], it is tempting to speculate that IGF-I, or an homologous protein, might be the common mediator influencing both the renal reabsorption of Pi and the production of 1,25(OH)2D3, which are two essential controlling elements of Pi homeostasis. The question arises as to whether the stimulatory effect of IGF-I on renal Pi transport could be directly mediated by the plasma level elevation of 1,25(OH)2D3. As mentioned in several reviews, a direct physiological role of 1,25(OH)2D3 on the renal transport of Pi has not been established, particularly in vitamin D-repleted animals [25–27]. According to the experimental conditions [25–29], 1,25(OH)2D3 has been shown variously to stimulate or to decrease the renal transport of Pi. Thus the possibility that 1,25(OH)2D3 could contribute to the stimulatory effect of IGF-I on tubular Pi reabsorption appears to be unlikely.

Conclusion

IGF-I stimulates the renal tubular transport of Pi and elevates the plasma level of 1,25(OH)2D3 in hypophysectomized rats. These findings and the results obtained in opossum cultured epithelia suggest that IGF-I mediates the renal effect of GH on tubular Pi transport. Thus, IGF-I might play an important role in the control of Pi economy, particularly in relation to growth.

Acknowledgments. Recent studies quoted in this report [19,23] were supported by the Swiss National Science Foundation (Grant No 3200-025.535) and by Ciba-Geigy, Basel, Switzerland.

References

1. Becker MA, Rozengurt E (1982) Inorganic phosphate is necessary for the stimulation of DNA synthesis in Swiss 3T3 cells by pure mitogenic agents. Exp Cell Res 139:431–436
2. Corvilain J, Abramow M (1972) Growth and renal control of plasma phosphate. J Clin Endocrinol Metab 34:452–459
3. Caverzasio J, Bonjour JP, Fleisch H (1982) Tubular handling of Pi in young growing and adult rats. Am J Physiol 242:F705–F710
4. Kiebzak, GM, Sacktor B (1986) Effect of age on renal conservation of phosphate in the rat. Am J Physiol 251:F399–F407
5. Caverzasio J, Faundez R, Fleisch H, Bonjour JP (1981) Tubular adaptation to Pi restriction in hypophysectomized rats. Pflugers Arch 392:17–21
6. Caverzasio J, Murer H, Fleisch H, Bonjour JP (1982) Phosphate transport in brush border membrane vesicles isolated from renal cortex in young growing and adult rats, comparison with whole kidney data. Pflugers Arch 394:217–221
7. Corvilain J, Abramow M (1962) Some effects of human growth hormone on renal hemodynamics and tubular Pi transport in man. J Clin Invest 41:1230–1235
8. Corvilain J, Abramow M (1964) Effect of growth hormone on tubular transport of Pi in normal and parathyroidectomized dogs. J Clin Invest 43:1608–1612
9. Hammerman MR, Karl IE, Hruska KA (1980) Regulation of canine renal vesicle Pi transport by growth hormone and parathyroid hormone. Biochim. Biophys. Acta 603:322–335
10. Westby GR, Goldfarb S, Goldberg M, Agus ZS (1977) Acute effects of bovine growth hormone on renal calcium and phosphate excretion. Metabolism 26:525–530
11. Ritz E, Kreusser W, Bommer J (1980) Effects of hormones other than parathyroid hormone on renal handling of phosphate. In: Massry SG, Fleisch H (eds) Renal handling of phosphate. Plenum, New York, pp 137–195
12. Froesch ER, Schmid C, Swander J, Zapf J (1985) Actions of insulin-like growth factors. Annu Rev Physiol 47:443–467
13. Underwood LE, D'Ercole AJ, Clemmons DR, Van Wyk J (1986) Paracrine functions of somatomedins. Clin Endocrinol Metab 15:59–77
14. Schalch DS, Heinrich UE, Draznin B, Johnson CJ, Miller LL (1979) Role of the liver in regulatory somatomedin activity: hormonal effects on the synthesis and release of insulin-like growth factor and its carrier protein by the isolated perfused rat liver. Endocrinology 104:1143–1151
15. D'Ercole AJ, Stiles AD, Underwood LE (1984) Tissue concentrations of somatomedin C: further evidence for multiple sites of synthesis and paracrine or autocrine mechanisms of action. Proc Natl Acad Sci USA 81:935–939
16. Hammerman MR, Gavin III JR (1986) Binding of IGF-I and IGF-I stimulated phosphorylation in canine renal basolateral membranes. Am J Physiol 251:E32–E41
17. Bonjour JP, Caverzasio J, Mühlbauer R, Trechsel U, Troehler U (1982) Are 1,25(OH)2D3 production and tubular phosphate transport regulated by one common mechanism which would be defective in X-linked hypophosphatemia rickets? In: Vitamin D, chemical, biochemical and clinical endocrinology of calcium metabolism. Walter de Gruyter, Berlin, pp 427–433
18. Lyles KW, Hasley DL, Friedman NE, Lobaugh B (1988) Correlations of serum concentrations of 1,25-dihydroxyvitamin D, phosphorus and parathyroid hormone in tumoral calcinosis. J Clin Endocrinol Metab 67:88–92
19. Caverzasio J, Bonjour JP (1989) Insulin-like growth factor I stimulates Na-dependent Pi transport in cultured kidney cells. Am J Physiol 257:F712–F717
20. Caverzasio J, Brown CDA, Biber J, Bonjour JP, Murer H (1985) Adaptation of phosphate transport in phosphate deprived LLC-PK1 cells. Am J Physiol 248:F122–F127

21. Caverzasio J, Rizzoli R, Bonjour JP (1986) Sodium-dependent phosphate transport inhibited by parathyroid hormone and cyclic AMP production in opossum kidney cell line. J Biol Chem 261:3233–3237
22. Malmström K, Murer H (1986) Parathyroid hormone inhibits phosphate transport in OK cells but not in LLC-PK1 and JTC-12P3 cells. Am J Physiol 251:C23–C31
23. Caverzasio J, Montessuit C, Bonjour JP (1990) Stimulatory effect of insulin-like growth factor-I on renal Pi transport and plasma 1,25-dihydroxyvitamin D3. Endocrinology 127:453–459
24. Hammerman MR, Karl IE, Hruska KA (1980) Regulation of canine renal vesicle Pi transport by growth hormone and parathyroid hormone. Biochim. Biophys. Acta 603:322–335
25. Bonjour JP, Caverzasio J (1984) Phosphate transport in the kidney. Rev Physiol Biochem Pharmacol 100:162–164
26. Knox FG, Haramati A (1984) Renal regulation of phosphate excretion. In: Seldin DW, Giebisch G (eds) Physiology and pathology of electrolyte metabolism. Raven, New York
27. Avioli LV (1980) Effects of vitamin D and its metabolites on renal handling of phosphate. In: Massry SG, Fleisch H (eds) Renal handling of phosphate. Plenum, New York, pp 197–207
28. Liang CI, Barnes J, Balakir R, Cheng L, Sacktor B (1982) In vitro stimulation of phosphate uptake in isolated chick renal cells by 1,25-dihydroxycholecalciferol. Proc Natl Acad Sci USA 79:3532–3536
29. Kurnik BRC, Hruska KA (1984) Effects of 1,25-dihydroxycholecalciferol on phosphate transport in vitamin D-deprived rats. Am J Physiol 247:F177–F182

Parathyroid Hormone Receptor Coupling to Phospholipase C is an Alternate Pathway of Signal Transduction in the Bone and Kidney

KEITH HRUSKA, ROBERT DUNLAY, ROBERTO CIVITELLI, AKIMITSU MIYAUCHI, CONSTANTA VICTORIEA DOBRE, and AJAY GUPTA[1]

SUMMARY. The parathyroid hormone (PTH) receptor is coupled via guanine nucleotide-binding regulatory proteins (G proteins) to adenylate cyclase and phospholipase C (PLC). Activation of PLC with the subsequent hydrolysis of phosphatidylinositol 4,5-bisphosphate produces inositol 1,4,5-trisphosphate (IP_3) and diacylglycerol (DAG). Generation of IP_3 leads to the release of intracellular calcium stores, which produce an increase in the intracellular calcium concentration. DAG activates protein kinase C (PKC). Both IP_3 metabolites and PKC play roles in returning the intracellular calcium concentration back to base line, by sequestering calcium within intracellular organelles and by stimulating the movement of calcium from the intracellular to the extracellular compartment. PKC appears to be important in the development of desensitization and down-regulation of the PTH receptor to PTH. Activation of PLC may be important in modulating the well-known effects of PTH on bone and kidney, and also less well-known actions, such as the role of PTH as an osteoblast and chondrocyte growth factor.

Introduction

Parathyroid hormone (PTH) is responsible for maintenance of calcium homeostasis and normocalcemia. Secretion of PTH is stimulated or suppressed by perturbations in the serum calcium level. The calciotropic effects of PTH are mediated primarily by the kidneys, where calcium resorption and phosphate excretion are increased, and by bone, where PTH-stimulated resorption releases calcium to the extracellular fluid.

Binding of PTH to its receptors on the plasma membranes of target cells leads to guanine nucleotide binding protein (G protein) regulated enhancement of enzyme activities which, in turn, generates second messengers that regulate cellular functions. Among the enzymes activated by PTH-receptor binding is adenylate cyclase.

---

[1]Department of Medicine (Nephrology), Jewish Hospital/Washington University, St. Louis, MO 63110, USA

The result is an increase in the intracellular concentration of 3′5′ cyclic adenosine monophosphate (cAMP), the classic second messenger for PTH. The final step in this sequence of events is phosphorylation of regulatory proteins by cAMP dependent protein kinases [1,2].

Recently, new mechanisms for generation of intracellular signals by the PTH-receptor have been identified. The best documentation of these is PTH activation of phospholipase C activity. In this report we will discuss our data regarding PTH mediated formation of second messengers by polyphosphoinositide hydrolysis; the possible role of G proteins in regulating this reaction; and the biologic effects of activating this system. Although PTH effects have been described in many organs, we will concentrate on its principal target tissues—bone and kidney.

Polyphosphoinositides and G Proteins

Phosphatidylinositol (PI) is formed in the plasma membrane from phosphatidic acid (PA) and inositol (Fig. 1). Stimulated by phosphatidylinositol kinase, PI then undergoes sequential phosphorylation to form phosphatidylinositol 4,5 bisphosphate (PIP_2). Initiation of signal transduction through the phospholipase C (PLC) system begins with agonist binding to its receptor, which, through a G protein (Gp), activates phospholipase C and leads to the hydrolysis of PIP_2. PIP_2 hydrolysis results in production of inositol 1,4,5 triphosphate (IP_3) and diacylglycerol (DAG). IP_3 acts through a specific receptor on the endoplasmic reticulum or calcisome, leading to opening of a Ca^{2+} channel and release of calcium stores—the phase I response. This produces an immediate and transient elevation of cytosolic Ca^{2+} ($[Ca^{2+}]_i$) which can be observed in the absence of extracellular Ca^{2+} [3,4]. Phosphorylation of the 4 and 5 positions of inositol is necessary for the interaction of IP_3 with the Ca^{2+} channel and the immediate production of a calcium transient [5]. The increase in $[Ca^{2+}]_i$ activates calmodulin-dependent protein kinases [6]. The $[Ca^{2+}]_i$ is rapidly lowered by calcium\magnesium adenosine triphosphatases (Ca\Mg\ATPase), Ca^{2+} pumps which serve to transport Ca^{2+} uphill from the cytosol to the extracellular fluid and into the endoplasmic reticulum [7]. IP_3 disappears rapidly with a $t^1/_2$ of about four seconds; at least two relevant metabolism routes are available. First, IP_3 can undergo sequential dephosphorylation [8] to IP, and finally, to inositol, which may be recycled into PI. Alternatively [9], IP_3 can be phosphorylated to an intermediate compound, inositol 1,3,4,5 tetrakisphosphate (I 1,3,4,5 P_4), which then undergoes dephosphorylation to form inositol 1,3,4 trisphosphate (I 1,3,4 P_3). Both I 1,3,4,5 P_4 and I 1,3,4 P_3 may function as messengers in Ca^{2+} entry and Ca^{2+} release (see below). Note that in either degradation route the first dephosphorylation involves removal of a phosphate from either the 4 or 5 position. This precludes further stimulation of the endoplasmic reticulum receptor mediating the phase I response.

DAG remains within the plane of the plasma membrane, where it activates protein kinase C (PKC), which is translocated from the cytosol to the plasma membrane as a result of the increase in $[Ca^{2+}]_i$ during phase I [10]. In addition to DAG and calcium, PKC activity also requires the presence of phosphatidylserine. Characterization of the functions of PKC has been facilitated by the use of phorbol esters, which activate the enzyme in the presence of calcium. PKC phosphorylates various target proteins, including receptors, and also provides negative feedback to the polyphos-

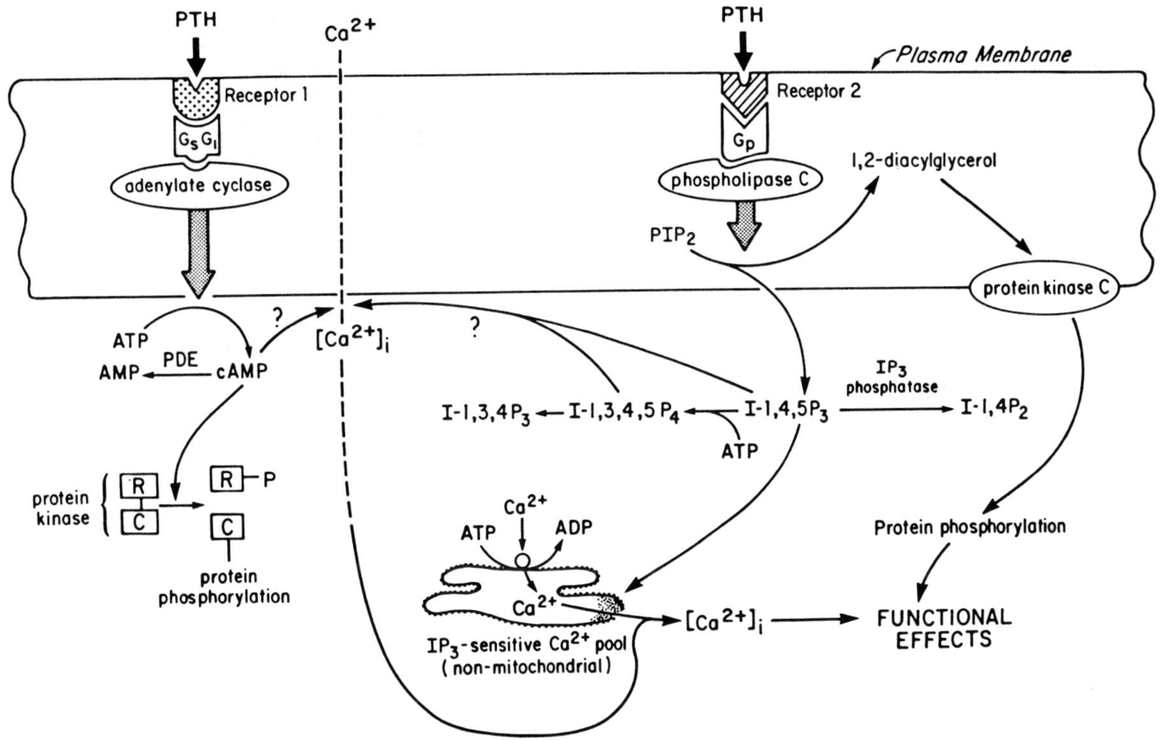

Fig. 1. Schematic concepts of parathyroid stimulated signal transduction in target cells based on a two receptor model (reproduced with permission from Dunlay and Hruska AJP 258:F223, 1990)

phoinositide cascade by phosphorylation of PLC, thus inhibiting the hydrolysis of PIP_2 [11]. Stimulation of PKC with phorbol esters increases the formation of PIP_2, as well as that of PA [12,13]. PKC also acts to decrease the elevated $[Ca^{2+}]_i$ found during the primary response by accelerating the exit of calcium across the plasma membrane [14].

During phase II, enhanced entry of calcium from the extracellular fluid replenishes intracellular calcium stores. I 1,3,4,5 P_4, as well as I 1,3,4 P_3, has been reported to facilitate this process [15]. A model proposed by Putney [16] requires no mediator; he suggests that depletion of calcium from the endoplasmic reticulum adjacent to the plasma membrane leads to calcium entry from the extracellular fluid without any change in the overall $[Ca^{2+}]_i$. Ongoing investigations should soon provide a better understanding of the phase II response.

G proteins are heterotrimers first described in association with receptors coupled to adenylate cyclase. They were initially characterized as either cholera (G stimulatory, Gs) or pertussis (G inhibitory, Gi) toxin sensitive [17]. The alpha subunit (M_r 39-52000) confers specificity for receptors and effectors. Upon receptor occupancy, the alpha subunit releases GDP, binds GTP, and dissociates from the beta and gamma subunits. The alpha subunit possesses intrinsic GTP hydrolytic activity, and interacts with its target effector protein until GTP is hydrolyzed to GDP; then, the heterotrimer reassembles. The G protein associated with PLC (Gp) is pertussis toxin sensitive in some, but not all, cells [6,18]. Gp appears to enhance PLC activity, but the exact mechanism by which this enhancement occurs is uncertain. The recent demonstration by Mattera et al. [19] that alpha subunits stimulatory for adenylate cyclase can also activate voltage regulated calcium channels has added greater complexity to the area of G protein regulation, as previously an alpha subunit had been thought to interact with only one effector protein. In recent years, several low molecular weight G proteins have been described, and their role requires further elucidation. We (Gupta and Hruska, submitted) have recently demonstrated several low molecular weight GTP-binding proteins in the microsomes of the proximal tubule. Their molecular weights range between 21 and 29 $\times 10^3$ daltons. One is a botulinum toxin substrate, possibly rho and another is a ral. We are testing the hypothesis that PTH may stimulate binding of one of these low molecular weight G proteins to the PTH receptor, thus serving to amplify the number of potential signals emanating from a receptor class.

The Kidney

Parathyroid hormone increases turnover of phosphatidylinositol and the polyphosphoinositides, PIP and PIP_2 [20,21]. The effect is also associated with increased turnover of diacylglycerol and phosphatidic acid, indicating that the Pi cycle has been activated. The stimulus begins with hydrolysis of PIP_2, which is detectable within seconds and maximal by 10 seconds [12]. The effect of PTH to reduce PIP_2 levels is overcome by phosphorylation of PI and PIP within 5 minutes. The product of PIP_2 hydrolysis, inositol 1,4,5 trisphosphate (IP_3) is detectably increased by 5–10 seconds of stimulation by parathyroid hormone (Fig. 2) [12]. IP_3 is rapidly phosphorylated to IP_4, which is then acted upon by a phosphatase to produce I 1,3,4 P_3. The production of I 1,3,4 P_3 accounts for the sustained elevation in IP_3 levels for several minutes after PTH stimulation. These actions of parathyroid hormone have

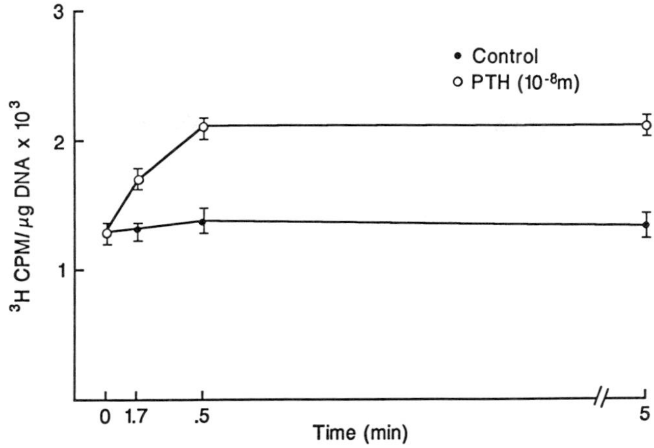

Fig. 2. Effect of parathyroid hormone on IP_3 production in opossum kidney (*OK*) cells. The initial effect represents an increase in I 1,4,5 P_3 which subsides within 1 min. The sustained elevation is due to I 1,3,4 P_3 which is produced by phosphatase activity on I 1,3,4,5 P_4 which is, in turn, a product of I 1,4,5 P_3 phosphorylation. I 1,3,4 P_3 has a longer half life than I 1,4,5 P_3, but its biologic role in the kidney is unclear. CPM, counts per minute

been observed in proximal kidney cells, in the primary cultures of the canine proximal tubule, and in basolateral membranes of the proximal tubular cells isolated from tubular segments in vitro. The dose response curve demonstrates a threshold at 10^{-10} M and a half-maximal effect at 10^{-9} M (Fig. 3).

The increase in IP_3 levels is associated with release of calcium from IP_3-sensitive intracellular stores and with the production of a rapid transient increase in $[Ca^{2+}]_i$. Parathyroid hormone also stimulates calcium entry across the plasma membrane, which contributes to the transient elevation in $[Ca^{2+}]_i$ following hormonal stimulation [22,3,4]. The mechanism of PTH-stimulated calcium entry is independent of the membrane potential and insensitive to Ca^{2+} channel antagonists. Data from isolated membrane vesicles suggest that the parathyroid hormone-stimulated Ca^{2+} entry is related to a receptor-operated Ca^{2+} channel, or is through a second-messenger-operated Ca^{2+} channel stimulated by IP_3 [23,24].

Activation of phospholipase C by parathyroid hormone in the basolateral membrane of the proximal tubule also results in the production of diacylglycerol. Measurement of DAG indicates a difference in the time course of stimulus, compared to IP_3 production. This may suggest that part of the DAG is derived from an effect of parathyroid hormone on phosphatidylcholine-specific phospholipase C, or possibly on phosphatidylethanolamine-specific phospholipase C. These studies will require further analysis. It is also possible that the observed increase in phosphatidic acid is derived from the stimulation of phospholipase D. This also requires further analysis.

The biologic effects of activation of the Ca^{2+} message system in the proximal tubule have been incompletely investigated. We have shown that parathyroid hormone produces dramatic shortening and rarefaction of proximal tubule and microvilli within one minute, with recovery after 5 minutes [25]. The effect of parathyroid hormone on brush border topography was associated with disappearance of micro-

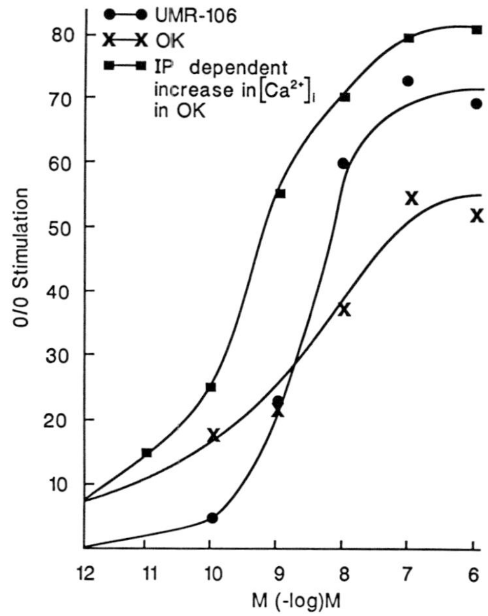

Fig. 3. Dose response of PTH stimulated IP_3 production in opossum kidney (*OK*) cells, UMR-106-01 cells, and IP_3 dependent stimulation of $[Ca^{2+}]_i$ in OK cells. $[Ca^{2+}]_i$ is a more sensitive measure of PTH stimulation of PLC activity than direct measurement of IP_3 production (reprinted with permission from Dunlay and Hruska AJP 258:F223, 1990)

villar core filaments, and it was abolished by a calmodulin inhibitor. Staining F-actin revealed that parathyroid hormone produced fragmentation of stress fibers.

Parathyroid hormone also stimulates proximal tubular gluconeogenesis; this effect is dependent upon $[Ca^{2+}]_i$ and can be stimulated by Ca^{2+} without participation of other second messengers, i.e., cAMP [26]. Stimulation of gluconeogenesis was observed with additions of parathyroid hormone, angiotensin-II and phenylephrine, all of which stimulated Ca^{2+} transients and whose gluconeogenic effect was inhibited by maptam, which prevented the production of the transient elevations in $[Ca^{2+}]_i$. Thus, elevations in $[Ca^{2+}]_i$ were a sufficient stimulus for glucose production and were also necessary for the effects of other second messengers.

The major effect of parathyroid hormone in the proximal tubule is inhibition of Na-dependent phosphate cotransport. The phosphaturic action of PTH is associated with an increase in intracellular cAMP and phosphorylation of proteins in the brush border membrane [2]. Recent studies [27] indicate that activation of protein kinase C may also participate in the inhibition of Na-dependent phosphate cotransport.

When two clones of opossum kidney cells were compared for their response to PTH [28] intriguing results were observed. Both clones (H and P) exhibited similar PTH binding and adenylate cyclase activation. However, the H clone was unresponsive to PTH when analyzed for stimulation of transient elevations in cytosolic calcium. On the other hand, PTH stimulated the P clone cells to produce IP_3 and elevate cytosolic calcium. The up-slope of these transient elevations in cytosolic calcium was

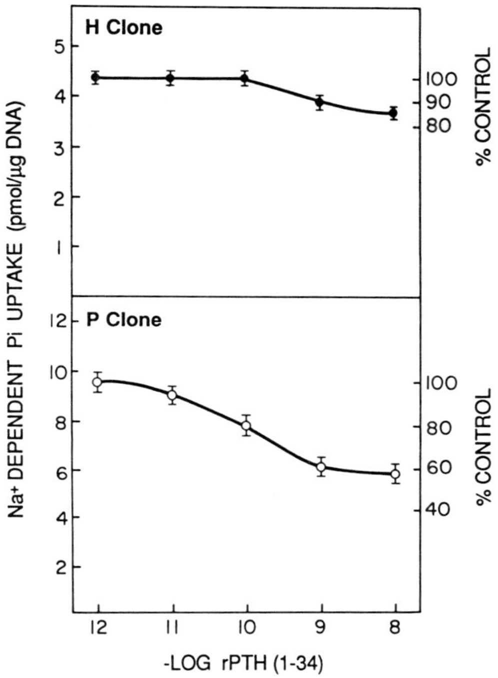

Fig. 4. Effect of PTH on Na^+-Pi co-transport in OK clones (*OKP* and *OKH*). Experimental conditions: 1.5×10^4 cells/well of 12 well clusters, grown to confluency in DMEM with 7% fetal bovine serum; 72 h on serum-free DMEM; 4 hrs preincubation with rPTH-(1-34). ^{32}P uptake was performed in uptake buffer containing 0.1 mM Pi and 150 mM Na^+. Means ± SE of five experiments in triplicate are presented (reprinted with permission from [28])

due in part to inositol trisphosphate-stimulated release of cytosolic calcium (Fig. 3). When sodium-dependent phosphate transport activity was analyzed in these two clones of opossum kidney cells, the H clone was nearly insensitive to the effects of PTH, while the P clone was extremely sensitive [28]. Half-maximal inhibition of phosphate transport was produced by 10^{-10} M PTH in P clone cells, similar to the half-maximal ability of PTH to stimulate increases in cytosolic calcium (5×10^{-10} M). This represents a greater concordance of the dose response curves for a biologic function and second messenger generation for the calcium message system than for stimulation of cAMP production. However, recent studies indicate that threshold levels of cAMP generation may represent sufficient levels to saturate protein kinase A. Nevertheless, in the opossum kidney cells, absence of PTH response to inhibition of phosphate transport was associated with absence of PTH-stimulated phospholipase C activity.

Thus, the mechanism of PTH-generated signal transduction in the renal tubule require further study. It is clear that multiple second messages are generated by the occupancy of the PTH receptor. The exact functional role of these messages should be elucidated in the future.

Bone

We have recently shown that parathyroid hormone increases $[Ca^{2+}]_i$ in a number of osteoblast-like cells, including the UMR-106 cell line, the ROS 17/2.8 cell line, and normal rat and human osteoblasts [29,30]. The effects have been confirmed in several laboratories [31,32]. We have shown that the Ca^{2+} transient stimulated by PTH is, in part, dependent upon Ca^{2+} release of IP_3-sensitive stores, and is, in part, due to both dihydropyridine-sensitive and -insensitive Ca^{2+} entry mechanisms. We have recently demonstrated the presence of L-type Ca^{2+} channels and non-specific stretch-activated cation channels in the plasma membrane of UMR-106 cells, which may be regulated by parathyroid hormone [33].

As expected from the nature of the transient elevation of $[Ca^{2+}]_i$ produced in osteoblast-like cells, we were able to demonstrate that parathyroid hormone elevated IP_3 production in the UMR-106 cells [29]. The effect was associated with increases in inositol 1,4,5 P_3, inositol 1,3,4 P_3, and inositol 1,3,4,5 teterakisphosphate. The effect was dose-dependent with the threshold dose being 10^{-10} M. It was pertussis toxin insensitive, similar to the opossum kidney cell where the PTH effect was also pertussis toxin insensitive [28,29].

In the plasma membrane of the UMR-106, we have characterized a phosphatidylinositol-specific phospholipase C activity which is stimulated by guanine nucleotides and is Ca^{2+} independent [34]. The characteristics of this PIP_2-specific phospholipase C suggest that it is the enzyme recoupled to the PTH receptor through G proteins. Recent investigations by Farndale et al. [35] and Babich [23] support these conclusions. Other studies have also indicated that PTH stimulates protein kinase C and its translocation to the plasma membrane [36].

The biologic effects of the parathyroid hormone-stimulated activation of the Ca^{2+}-protein kinase C message system in the regulation of bone remodeling are unclear. Parathyroid hormone induces both bone resorption and bone formation. The initial effect of parathyroid hormone on the osteoblast is to induce cell contraction, and this is likely to involve Ca^{2+} [22]. Parathyroid hormone also decreases osteoblast collagen production and may increase collagenase production. Parathyroid hormone stimulation of collagenase production can be demonstrated in UMR-106 cells, and in these cells, a participation of the Ca^{2+} message system in collagenase production has been demonstrated [37].

Conclusion

The available evidence indicates that the polyphosphoinositide pathway is stimulated in mediating the actions of PTH in both the kidneys and in bone. Many important issues remain, including: 1) characterization of the G protein modulating PLC activation in response to PTH binding to its receptor; 2) the possibility that different subclasses of PTH receptors coupled to different G proteins and effector proteins exist. Alternatively, if only one type of PTH receptor is found, activation of multiple G proteins or association with multiple effector proteins could explain the diverse messages produced by PTH.

Acknowledgments. This work was supported by NIH grants AR39561, AR32087, and DK09976 and a grant from the Shriner's Hospital (St. Louis Division).

References

1. Cochet C, Gill GN, Meisenhelder J, Cooper JA, Hunter T (1984) C-kinase phosphorylates the epidermal growth factor receptor and reduces its epidermal growth factor-stimulated tyrosine protein kinase activity. J Biol Chem 259:2553–2558
2. Hammerman MR, Hruska KA (1982) Cyclic AMP dependent protein phosphorylation in canine renal brush border membrane vesicles is associated with decreased phosphate transport. J Biol Chem 257:992–999
3. Hruska KA, Goligorsky M, Scoble J, Tsutsumi M, Westbrook S, Moskowitz D (1986) The effects of parathyroid hormone on cytosolic calcium in renal proximal tubular primary cultures. Am J Physiol 251:F188–F198
4. Prentki M, Wollheim CB, Lew PD (1984) Calcium homeostasis in permeabilized human neutrophils. J Biol Chem 259:13777–13782
5. Burgess GMK, Irvine RF, Berridge MJ, McKinney JS, Putney JW (1984) Actions of inositol phosphates on Ca pools in guinea-pig hepatocytes. Biochem J 224:741–746
6. Cohen P (1988) Protein phosphorylation and hormone action. Proc R Soc Lond [Biol] 234:115–144
7. Carafoli E (1987) Intracellular calcium homeostasis. Annu Rev Biochem 56:395–433
8. Connoly TM, Bross TE, Majerus PW (1985) Isolation of a phosphomonoesterase from human platelets that specifically hydrolyzes the 5-phosphate of inositol 1,4,5-triphosphate. J Biol Chem 260:7868–7874
9. Irvine RF, Letcher AJ, Heslop JP, Berridge MJ (1986) The inositol tris\tetrakisphosphate pathway-demonstration of Ins 1,4,5 3-kinase activity in animal tissues. Nature 320: 631–634
10. Nishizuka Y (1984) The role of protein kinase C in cell surface signal transduction and tumour promotion. Nature 308:693–698
11. Berridge M (1987) Inositol triphosphate and diacylglycerol: Two interacting second messengers. Annu Rev Biochem 56:159–193
12. Hruska KA, Moskowitz D, Esbrit P, Civitelli R, Westbrook S, Huskey M (1987) Stimulation of inositol triphosphate and diacylglycerol production in renal tubular cells by parathyroid hormone. J Clin Invest 79:230–239
13. Taylor MV, Metcalfe JC, Hesketh TR, Smith GA, Moore JP (1984) Mitogens increase phosphorylation of phosphoinositides in thymocytes. Nature 312:462–465
14. Lagast H, Pozzan T, Waldvogel FA, Lew PD (1984) Phorbol myristate acetate stimulates ATP-dependent calcium transport by the plasma membrane of neutrophils. J Clin Invest 73:878–883
15. Irvine RF, Moor RM (1986) Micro-injection of inositol 1,3,4,5 tetrakisphosphate activates sea urchin eggs by a mechanism dependent on external calcium. Biochem J 240:917–920
16. Putney JW (1986) A model for receptor-regulated calcium entry. Cell Calcium 7:1–12
17. Stryer L (1986) G proteins: A family of signal transducers. Annu Rev Cell Biol 2:391–419
18. Fain JN, Wallace MA, Wojcikiewicz RJH (1988) Evidence for involvement of guanine nucleotide binding regulatory proteins in the activation of phospholipase by hormones. FASEB J 2:2569–2574
19. Mattera R, Graziano M, Yatani A, Zhou Z, Graf R, Codina J, Birnbaumer L, Gilman AG, Brown AM (1989) Splice variants of the alpha subunit of the G protein Gs activate both adenylyl cyclase and calcium channels. Science 243:804–807
20. Bidot-Lopez P, Farese R, Sabir M (1981) Parathyroid hormone and adenosine-3′,5′-monophosphate acutely increase phospholipids of the phosphatidate-polyphosphoinositide pathway in rabbit kidney cortex tubules *in vitro* by a cycloheximide-sensitive process. Endocrinology 108:2078–2081
21. Meltzer V, Weinreb S, Bellorin-Font E, Hruska KA (1982) Parathyroid hormone stimulation of renal phosphoinositide metabolism is a cyclic nucleotide independent effect. Biochim Biophys Acta 712:258–267

22. Goligorsky MS, Loftus D, Hruska KA (1986) Cytoplasmic Ca^{2+} in individual proximal tubular cells in culture: effects of parathyroid hormone. Am J Physiol 251:F938–F944
23. Scoble JE, Mills S, Hruska KA (1985) Calcium transport in canine renal basolateral membrane vesicles. J Clin Invest 75:1096–1105
24. Scoble JE, Civitelli R, Hruska KA (1988) Evidence for receptor operated Ca^{2+} chennels in basolateral membranes (BLM) of proximal tubular cells (PTC): Effects of inositol 1,4,5-trisphosphate (IP_3). Kidney Int 33:171A
25. Goligorsky MS, Menton DN, Hruska KA (1986) Parathyroid hormone-induced topography and cytoskeleton in cultured renal proximal tubular cells. J Membr Biol 92:151–162
26. Goligorsky MS, Osborne D, Howard T, Hruska KA, Karl IE (1987) Hormonal regulation of gluconeogenesis in cultured proximal tubular cells: role of cytosolic calcium. Am J Physiol 253:F802–F809
27. Cole JA, Forte LR, Eber S, Thorne PK, Poelling RE (1988) Regulation of sodium-dependent phosphate transport by parathyroid hormone in opossum kidney cells: Adenosine 3′,5′-monophosphate-dependent and -independent mechanisms. Endocrinology 122: 2981–2989
28. Miyauchi A, Dobre V, Rickmeyer M, Cole J, Forte L, Hruska KA (1990) Stimulation of transient elevations in cytosolic Ca^{2+} is related to inhibition of Pi transport in OK cells. Am J Physiol 259:F485–493
29. Civitelli R, Reid IR, Westbrook S, Avioli LV, Hruska KA (1988) PTH elevates inositol polyphosphates and diacylglycerol in a rat osteoblast-like cell line. Am J Physiol 255: E660–E667
30. Reid IR, Civitelli R, Halstead LR, Avioli LV, Hruska KA (1987) Parathyroid hormone acutely elevates intracellular calcium in osteoblastlike cells. Am J Physiol 252:E45–E51
31. Lowik CWGM, van Leeuwen JM, van der Meer JK, van Zeeland BAA, Scheven JPTM, Herrmann-Erlee MPM (1985) A two-receptor model for the action of parathyroid hormone on osteoblasts: a role for intracellular free calcium and cAMP. Cell Calcium 6:311–326
32. Yamaguchi DT, Hahn TJ, Iida-Klein A, Kleeman CR, Muallem S (1987) Parathyroid hormone-activated calcium channels in an osteoblast-like clonal osteosarcoma cell line. J Biol Chem 262:7711–7718
33. Duncan R, Misler S (1989) Voltage-activated and stretch-activated Ba^{2+} conducting channels in an osteoblast-like cell line (UMR 106). Elsevier Sci Pubs 251:17–21
34. Suzuki Y, Hruska KA, Reid I, Alvarez UM, Avioli LV (1989) Characterization of phospholipase C activity of the plasma membrane and cytosol of an osteoblast-like cell line. Am J Med Sci 296:135–144
35. Farndale RW, Sandy JR, Atkinson SJ, Pennington SR, Meghji S, Meikle MC (1988) Parathyroid hormone and prostaglandin E2 stimulate both inositol phosphates and cyclic AMP accumulation in mouse osteoblast cultures. Biochem J 252:263–268
36. Abdul-Badi A, Jueppner H, Westerberg D, Potts JT, Segre GV (1989) Parathyroid hormone causes translocation of protein kinase-C from cytosol to membranes in rat osteosarcoma cells. Endocrinology 124:1107–1113
37. Civitelli R, Hruska KA, Jeffrey JJ, Kahn JJ, Avioli LV, Partridge NC (1989) Second messenger signaling in the regulation of collagenase production by osteogenic sarcoma cells. Endocrinology 124:2928–2933
00. Cockroft S, Stutchfield J (1988) G-proteins, the inositol lipid signalling pathway, and secretion. Philos Trans R Soc Lond [Biol] 320:247–265
00. Babich M, King KL, Nissenson RA (1989) G protein-dependent activation of a phosphoinositide-specific phospholipase C in UMR-106 osteosarcoma cell membranes. J Bone Mineral Res 4:549–556

The Effects of Parathyroid Hormone (PTH) on Ca Transport

YUSUKE TSUKAMOTO[1]

SUMMARY. Parathyroid hormone (PTH) stimulates active Ca^{2+} reabsorption in the distal convoluted tubule of the rat and in the cortical connecting tubule, distal convoluted tubule, and granular portion of the cortical collecting tubule of the rabbit. The dominant mechanism of Ca^{2+} reabsorption in the proximal tubules is passive diffusion via the paracellular pathway and PTH does not stimulate this Ca^{2+} transport. The distal tubules are equipped with molecular mechanisms which favor active transcellular Ca^{2+} transport. $1,25(OH)_2D_3$ dependent calcium binding protein (CaBPr) facilitates Ca^{2+} diffusion in the cytosolic space and increases the supply of the Ca^{2+} pump. PTH regulates the Ca^{2+} pump directly by increasing the affinity for cytosolic Ca^{2+} and by facilitating Ca^{2+} extrusion from the cell. Lack of CaBPr makes the proximal tubule less capable of transcellular Ca^{2+} reabsorption.

Introduction

Parathyroid hormone (PTH) regulates various cellular functions other than Ca^{2+} transport in the kidney [1]. Firstly, PTH reduces the glomerular capillary ultrafiltration coefficient (Kf) and then decreases the glomerular filtration rate (GFR). PTH inhibits the Na/Pi antiporter at the brush-border membrane of proximal tubules and causes phosphaturia. PTH also inhibits the Na/H antiporter in this nephron to cause bicarbonaturia. PTH also alters water transport by acting as a partial agonist to ADH within the papillary collecting duct [2].

Other than participating in mineral transport, PTH also participates in the regulation of metabolism in the kidney. PTH stimulates 1δ-hydroxylation of $25(OH)D_3$ and increases the production of $1,25(OH)_2D_3$ in proximal tubular cells [3]. Gluconeo-

[1]Department of Medicine, Kitasato University School of Medicine, 1–15–1 Kitasato, Sagamihara, Kanagawa, 228 Japan

genesis is also stimulated by PTH in the proximal tubules and this stimulation is mediated by the Ca^{2+} messenger system [4].

These multifunctional aspects of PTH make the study of PTH regulation of renal calcium handling rather difficult. Furthermore, renal calcium transport mechanisms are not yet fully understood, either. A tremendous number of variable factors influence renal Ca^{2+} transport mechanisms. This is the reason why I would like to start this review with renal Ca^{2+} transport mechanisms. I believe this first part of the review makes the interpretation of PTH action on Ca^{2+} transport much easier and more comprehensive.

Calcium Transport Along the Nephron

In the case of interpretation of individual investigations, one should be aware of species difference. Rat and rabbit are frequently employed for this kind of study. In every species, the major part of Ca^{2+} reabsorption by the kidney takes place in the proximal tubules. In this segment, 60% of the filtered Ca^{2+} is reabsorbed. The paracellular permeability of Ca^{2+} in this segment is very high and is similar to the one for Na^+ [5]. Na^+ and water reabsorption through the paracellular pathway give enough energy as a solvent drug to carry a bulk of Ca^{2+} via the paracellular pathway. A Ca^{2+} concentration which is higher in the lumen than in the plasma at the end of rabbit S2 segment, and a positive lumen membrane potential favor the passive paracellular diffusion of Ca^{2+} in this segment. Ng et al. [6] concluded that virtually no portion of Ca^{2+} transport is operated by active transcellular reabsorption in rabbit proximal convoluted tubules. However, this conclusion does not completely agree with the results obtained from rats. Although paracellular passive diffusion accounts for a major portion of Ca^{2+} reabsorption in the rat proximal tubule, the active transcellular pathway accounts for about 25% of total reabsorption [7]. Bomsztyk [8] demonstrated that lumen HCO_3^- stimulates active transcellular Ca^{2+} reabsorption in the absence of net water movement, a process linked to tubule fluid acidification in rat proximal tubules.

In the rabbit straight proximal tubule, 10% of filtered Ca^{2+} is reabsorbed. Rouse et al. [9] showed that Ca^{2+} is actively transported against the electrochemical gradient in this segment. This Ca^{2+} reabsorption was inhibited by cooling and not by oubain, suggesting that the Na^+/Ca^{2+} exchange at the basolateral membrane did not operate this active transport. In contrasts, Sacks and Bourdeau concluded that diffusion is the primary mechanism in this section [10,11]; high transepithelial Ca^{2+} permeability in this segment is compatible with this result.

In the rabbit, Henle's loop, from the thin descending to the thin ascending limb, was found to be relatively impermeable to Ca^{2+} and no significant transport was found [9,12]. Then, beginning from the medullary thick ascending limb, the tubules become very permeable to Ca^{2+}. However, in the thick ascending limb of the rabbit Ca^{2+} transport is heterogenous. In the medullary segment, it is passive and paracellular, inhibited by furosemide [13]. In the cortical segment, however, Ca^{2+} transport appears to be a mixture of both active transcellular and passive paracellular types [13,14]. The passive component of Ca^{2+} transport in cortical thick ascending limb is driven by the lumen-positive transepithelial potential generated by active Cl^- transport [14].

In the distal convoluted tubules of the rat and in the cortical connecting tubule and the granular portion of the cortical collecting tubule of the rabbit, approximately 10% of the filtered Ca^{2+} is reabsorbed. These portions of the nephron, including the cortical thick ascending limb, are believed to be the main regulatory sites of renal Ca^{2+} reabsorption both in rabbit and in rat [15–19]. Ca^{2+} reabsorption in these segments has to be carried out against an electrochemical gradient; apparently the active transcellular pathway is dominant. In the rat, the distal tubule is morphologically heterogeneous. The early distal tubule consists mainly of distal convoluted tubule cells with a few intercalated cells; the late distal tubule consists of intercalated cells, connecting tubule cells, and principal cells [20]. Thiazide diuretics, which are known to be hypocalciuric, act preferentially on early distal tubules [21]. Thiazide inhibits Na^+ reabsorption and increases Ca^{2+} reabsorption in this segment, then dissociation of Ca^{2+} and Na^+ transport occurs. It is known that amiloride, another diuretic known to be an inhibitor of the Na^+/H^+ antiporter and the Na^+/Ca^{2+} exchanger, has an additive hypocalciuric effect on thiazide. However, this action of amiloride has been noted in late distal tubules [21]. This finding suggests that in the distal tubule the Ca^{2+} transport mechanism is heterogeneous; varying in type between the early and late portion or among different cell types. Actually, vitamin D-dependent calcium binding protein (CaBPr) and Ca pump have been located in the principal cells of rat kidney [22].

The last part of the nephron has not been studied extensively. In the light portion of the cortical collecting tubule of the rabbit, epithelial Ca^{2+} permeability is extremely low [19]. In the rat inner medullary collecting duct, Ca^{2+} transport is Na^+-independent and inhibited by verapamil, suggesting voltage-dependent passive diffusion [23].

Effect of PTH on Ca^{2+} Transport Along the Nephron

It is now clear that PTH stimulates active Ca^{2+} reabsorption in the distal nephron. It has been determined that PTH stimulates Ca^{2+} reabsorption in the cortical thick ascending limb [13,14,24] and cortical connecting tubules [24] of the rabbit, and in the distal convoluted tubules of the rat [18]. These are also the nephron segments in which active transport is the dominant mechanism of Ca^{2+} reabsorption. PTH-dependent adenylate cyclase activity is rich in these nephron segments [24] and the stimulation of Ca^{2+} transport is mediated via c-AMP in these segments. The hormonal regulation of Ca^{2+} transport is heterogenous along the thick ascending limb of the rabbit. Suki et al. demonstrated that calcitonin stimulates Ca^{2+} transport in the medullary part, whereas PTH stimulates Ca^{2+} transport in the cortical part of the thick ascending limb [13]. Besides PTH and calcitonin, glucagon has also been reported to stimulate both Ca^{2+} and Mg^{2+} reabsorption in the rat superficial distal convoluted tubule in which glucagon-dependent adenylate cyclase activity is rich [18].

PTH-dependent adenylate cyclase activity also locates in the proximal tubule in both rabbit and rat, although the activity is lower than that in the distal nephron [24]. It is still a matter of controversy whether PTH stimulates Ca^{2+} transport in the proximal tubule. In the 1970s, three studies reported different results of PTH action. Agus et al. [25] and Sutton et al. [26] reported that PTH inhibited both Ca^{2+} and Na^+ reabsorption proportionally in the proximal tubule of both normal and thyroparathyroidectomized (TPTX) dogs. In contrast, micropuncture technique revealed a 10%

increment of Ca^{2+} reabsorption with no augmentation of water movement induced by PTH infusion into the TPTX hamster [27]. In the rabbit, there is virtually no component of active Ca^{2+} transport in proximal convoluted tubule. However, an active transport might be operated to some extent in the rat proximal convoluted tubule. Although PTH could stimulate these active Ca^{2+} transports, it is very hard to determine whether this is true behind the large storm of passive Ca^{2+} flux associated with water and Na^+ reabsorption.

Cellular Mechanism of Renal Ca^{2+} Transport and the Role of PTH

When Ca^{2+} is reabsorbed from the ultrafiltrate to blood through the transcellular pathway, at least 3 modulators must exist. The first one is the barrier in the luminal plasma membrane which controls Ca^{2+} entry into the cell; the second one is the carrier or storage organelles which transfer and store Ca^{2+} in the cytosolic space; the third one is the barrier in the basolateral membrane which controls Ca^{2+} exit from the cell. When Ca^{2+} enters the cell through the luminal membrane, Ca^{2+} can be passively transported according to the favorable electrochemical gradient in both distal and proximal tubules. PTH has been shown to stimulate Ca^{2+} binding to the brush-border membrane, through the phosphorylation of phospholipids via a c-AMP-dependent pathway [28]. This phosphorylation is accompanied by the inhibition of Na^+/Pi cotransport in the proximal tubule [29]. In the distal nephron, the presence of a calcium channel on the luminal membrane has been investigated by using the fluorescent Ca^{2+} indicator, fura-2. In this study, Taniguchi et al. suggested that the voltage-independent calcium channel regulated passive Ca^{2+} entry in the rat cortical collecting tubules [30].

In contrast to its entry on the luminal side, Ca^{2+} must exit from the cell through the basolateral membrane against the electrochemical gradient. Ca^{2+} has to be pumped out by an active transport mechanism at this side of the plasma membrane. Two active transporters are identified in the basolateral membrane; the Na^+/Ca^{2+} exchanger and the ATP-dependent Ca^{2+} pump. Na^+/Ca^{2+} exchange is a secondary active transport, driven by the Na^+ gradient generated by (Na^+ +K^+)-ATPase. Recently, Ramachandran and Brunette [31] found that the Na^+/Ca^{2+} exchanger is located exclusively in the distal tubule of the rabbit. This exchanger transports Ca^{2+} very fast, in the order of seconds. This is an electrogenic and voltage-dependent process the same as the one found in excitable tissues [32]. Findings on the affinity that the Na^+/Ca^{2+} exchanger has for Ca^{2+} vary between studies. Jayakumar [33] and Scoble [34] reported 8 μM for rat and 10 μM for dog. This does not agree with the cytosolic Ca^{2+} concentration if this is the system for Ca^{2+} extrusion. In contrast, Van Heeswijk and Van Os reported 0.2 μM for the rat [35]. Although Van Os insisted that the difference in results could be attributed to the difference in Ca^{2+}-buffering systems employed, we also obtained a value similar to that of Jayakumar's study, using the EGTA buffer system which was also employed by van Heeswijk et al. In contrast to the different values found for Ca^{2+} affinity, all studies agree on the value for $[Na^+]_{0.5}$, which is around 15 mM [33]. This value is within the range of cytosolic Na^+ concentration. These studies strongly suggest that the Na^+/Ca^{2+} exchanger operates symmetrically in the kidney in the same way as it does in the heart sarcolemma. The Na^+/Ca^{2+} exchanger may be the system which operates Ca^{2+} entry most of the time.

Even if the Na^+/Ca^{2+} exchanger operates to extrude Ca^{2+} out of the cell, the capacity of this transporter is only 20% that of the ATP-dependent Ca^{2+} pump. This makes us believe that the ATP-dependent Ca^{2+} pump is the main system for the Ca^{2+} exit through the basolateral membrane. In the kidney, the ATP-dependent Ca^{2+} pump was first studied in the basolateral membrane vesicles of rat kidney cortex [36]. For a long time, it has been believed that this preparation of basolateral membrane vesicles originated from the proximal tubules. However, it has been found that the renal cortex contains not only PTH-dependent adenylate cyclase activity, but also ADH-dependent activity which locates only in the distal tubules [33]. Recently, we succeeded in obtaining the basolateral membrane vesicles separately, from proximal tubules and from distal tubules [37]. As a result, ATP-dependent Ca^{2+} pump activity in the tubules can be kinetically separated. The affinity of the Ca^{2+} pump is much higher in the distal tubules ($Ca^{2+}=44.8$ nM) than in the proximal tubules ($Ca^{2+}=80.4$ nM). Vmax is higher in the proximal tubules (9.18 nmol $^{45}Ca^{2+}$/min per mg) than in the distal tubules (3.26 nmol $^{45}Ca^{2+}$/min per mg). These Ca^{2+} pumps are apparently stimulated in a different fashion by PTH. Selective parathyroidectomy decreased the Vmax of the Ca^{2+} pump in the proximal tubules while it decreased the affinity of the Ca^{2+} pump in the distal tubules (unpublished data). The kinetic character of the Ca^{2+} pump is very suitable for active Ca^{2+} reabsorption in the distal tubules, because very high Ca^{2+} affinity forces the pump to operate continuously.

The molecular characteristics of the distal tubular cells strongly suggest that this segment is the main site of the regulation of Ca^{2+} transport by active transcellular Ca^{2+} reabsorption. The critical molecular difference between the proximal and distal tubules is that the latter possess $1,25(OH)_2D_3$-dependent CaBPr but the former do not [22]. Bronner [38] postulated that, in the presence of CaBPr, Ca^{2+} can diffuse in the cytosolic space without being trapped by calcium storage organelles at a speed 30 times faster than in the absence of this protein. For effective transcellular Ca^{2+} reabsorption, the Ca^{2+} extrusion pump at the basolateral membrane cannot work efficiently without a continuous supply of the substrate, Ca^{2+}. Kumar found that both the Ca^{2+} pump and CaBPr are located in the same cell, the principal cell of human distal tubules; this finding also supports the cooperative function of these two mechanisms [22]. Proximal tubule lacks this CaBPr, which makes transcellular Ca^{2+} movement least effective and indicates that it cannot be the dominant mechanism of Ca^{2+} reabsorption. Thus, the molecular findings strongly support the physiological findings.

From these results, I would like to propose a molecular mechanism for Ca^{2+} reabsorption and regulation by PTH. This is shown in Fig. 1. In the proximal tubules, most Ca^{2+} reabsorption takes place by a passive diffusion mechanism via the paracellular pathway. Neither PTH nor $1,25(OH)_2D_3$ directly regulates this passive diffusion. However, there is an influence of PTH on the Ca^{2+} flow indirectly, through water movement. In the rat, transcellular active transport also participates in a small proportion of Ca^{2+} reabsorption. There is a possibility that PTH might stimulate this active transport by increasing the Vmax of Ca^{2+} pump activity at the basolateral membrane. However, the capacity of this active transport is much less than the capacity of the active transport in the distal tubules, which possesses CaBPr. The distal tubules definitely have the main role in the regulation of Ca^{2+} reabsorption in the kidney. PTH stimulates 1δ-hydroxylation of $25(OH)D_3$ at the proximal tubules, and then the increased $1,25(OH)_2D_3$ level stimulates CaBPr production in the principal cell of the distal nephron. CaBPr facilitates Ca^{2+} diffusion inside the cell and increases the

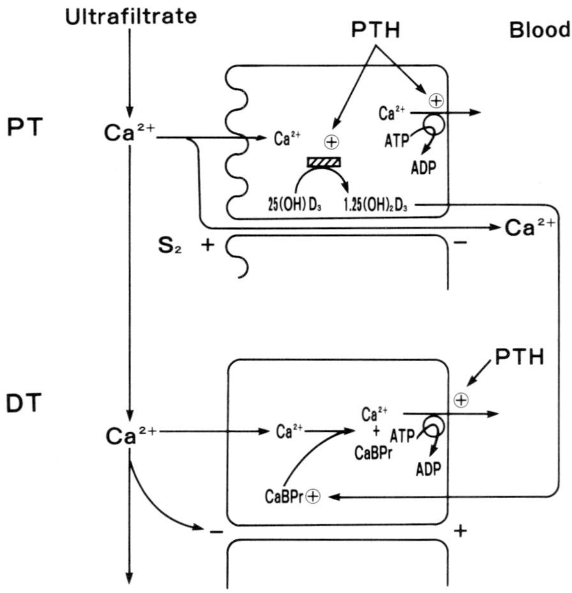

Fig. 1. Hypothesis for the molecular mechanisms of renal Ca^{2+} reabsorption and the effects of PTH

supply of Ca^{2+} to the Ca^{2+} pump. Then, the Ca^{2+} pump, whose affinity is stimulated by PTH, pumps an increased amount of Ca^{2+} out of the cell. Studies of molecular mechanisms support this hypothesis. However, we still lack direct investigation of the sequential movement of Ca^{2+} in native tubular cells, results of which could confirm this hypothesis.

References

1. Sutton RAL, Dirks JH (1986) Calcium and magnesium: Renal handlings and disorders of metabolism. In: Brenner BM, Rector FC Jr (eds) The kidney, 3rd edn. WB Saunders, Philadelphia, pp 551–618
2. Carney SL, Dirks JH (1988) Effect of parathyroid and antidiuretic hormone on water and calcium permeability in the rat collecting duct. Miner Electrolyte Metab 14:142–145
3. Kawashima H, Kurikawa K (1983) Unique hormonal regulation of vitamin D metabolism in the mammalian kidney. Miner Electrolyte Metab 9:227–235
4. Goligorsky MS, Osborne D, Howard T (1987) Hormonal regulation of gluconeogenesis in cultured proximal tubular cells: role of cytosolic calcium. Am J Physiol 253:F802–F809
5. Bomsztyk K, Wright FS (1982) Kidney Int 21:269–275
6. Ng RCK, Rouse D, Suki WN (1984) Calcium transport in the rabbit superficial proximal convoluted tubule. J Clin Invest 74:834–842
7. Ullrich KJ, Rumrich G, Kloss S (1976) Active Ca^{2+} reabsorption in the proximal tubule of the rat kidney. Dependence on sodium and buffer transport. Pflugers Arch 364:223–228

8. Bomsztyk K, Calaib MB (1988) Bicarbonate absorption stimulates active calcium absorption in the rat proximal tubule. J Clin Invest 81:1455–1461
9. Rouse D, Ng RCK, Suki WN (1979) Calcium transport in the pars recta and thin descending limb of Henle of the rabbit, perfused in vitro. J Clin Invest 65:37–42
10. Bourdeau JE (1986) Calcium transport across the pars recta of cortical segment 2 proximal tubules. Am J Physiol 251:F718–F724
11. Sacks P, Bourdeau JE (1989) Ca^{2+} absorption in the pars recta of cortical S2 rabbit proximal tubules: role of diffusion. Am J Physiol 257:F262–F267
12. Rocha AS, Magaldi JB, Kokko JP (1977) Calcium and phosphate transport in isolated segments of rabbit Henle's loop. J Clin Invest 59:975–983
13. Suki WN, Rouse D, Ng RCK, Kokko JP (1980) Calcium transport in the thick ascending limb of Henle. Heterogeneity of function in the medullary and cortical segments. J Clin Invest 66:1004–1009
14. Bourdeau JE, Burg MB (1980) Effect of PTH on calcium transport across the cortical thick ascending limb of Henle's loop. Am J Physiol 239:F121–F126
15. Suki WN, Rouse D (1981) Hormonal regulation of calcium transport in thick ascending limb renal tubules. Am J Physiol 241:F171–F174
16. Imai M (1981) Effects of parathyroid hormone and N_6,O_2-dibutyryl cyclic AMP on Ca^{2+} transport across the rabbit distal nephron segments perfused in vitro. Pflugers Arch 390:145–151
17. Shareghi GR, Stoner LC (1978) Calcium transport across segments of the rabbit distal nephron in vitro. Am J Physiol 235:F367–F375
18. Bailly C, Roinel N, Amiel C (1985) Stimulation by glucagon and PTH of Ca and Mg reabsorption in the superficial distal tubule of the rat kidney. Pflugers Arch 403:28–34
19. Bourdeau JE, Hellstrom-Stein RJ (1982) Voltage-dependent calcium movement across the cortical collecting duct. Am J Physiol 242:F285–F292
20. Kaissling B (1982) Structural aspects of adaptive changes in renal electrolyte excretion. Am J Physiol 243:F211–F226
21. Costanzo LS (1985) Localization of diuretic action in microperfused rat distal tubules: Ca and Na transport. Am J Physiol 248:F527–F535
22. Borkes JL, Caride A, Verma AK, Penniston JT, Kumar R (1989) Plasma membrane calcium pump and 28-kDa calcium binding protein in cells of rat kidney distal tubules. Am J Physiol 257:F842–F849
23. Magaldi AJ, van Baak AA, Rocha AS (1989) Calcium transport across rat inner medullary collecting duct perfused in vitro. Am J Physiol 257:F738–F745
24. Morrel F (1981) Sites of hormone action in the mammalian nephron. Am J Physiol 240:F159–F164
25. Agus ZS, Gardner LB, Beck LH, Goldberg M (1973) Effects of parathyroid hormone and renal tubular reabsorption of calcium, sodium, and phosphate. Am J Physiol 224:1143–1148
26. Sutton RAL, Wong NLM, Dirks JH (1976) Effects of parathyroid hormone on sodium and calcium transport in the dog nephron. Clin Sci Mol Med 51:345–351
27. Harris CA, Burnatowska MA, Seely JF, Sutton RAL, Quamme GA, Dirks JH (1979) Effects of parathyroid hormone on electrolyte transport in the hamster nephron. Am J Physiol 236:F342–F348
28. Hruska KA, Mills SC, Khalifa S, Hammerman MR (1983) Phosphorylation of renal brush border membrane vesicles. J Biol Chem 258:2501–2507
29. Hammerman MR, Hruska KA (1982) Cyclic AMP-dependent protein phosphorylation in canine renal brush-border membrane vesicles is associated with decreased phosphate transport. J Biol Chem 257:992–999
30. Taniguchi S, Marchetti J, Morel F (1989) Cytosolic free calcium in single microdissected rat cortical collecting tubules. Pflugers Arch 414:125–133

31. Ramachandran C, Brunette MG (1989) The renal Na^{+}/Ca^{2+} exchange system is located exclusively in the distal tubule. Biochem J 257:259–264
32. Eisner DA, Lederer WJ (1985) Na-Ca exchange: stoichiometry and electrogenicity. Am J Physiol 248:C189–C202
33. Jayakumar A, Cheng L, Liang CT, Sacktor B (1984) Sodium gradient-dependent calcium uptake in renal basolateral membrane vesicles. Effect of parathyroid hormone. J Biol Chem 259:10827–10833
34. Scoble JE, Mills S, Hruska KA (1985) Calcium transport in canine renal basolateral membrane vesicles. J Clin Invest 75:1096–1105
35. Van Heeswijk MPE, Geertsen JAM, Van Os CH (1984) J Membr Biol 79:19–31
36. Gmaj P, Murer H, Kinne R (1979) Calcium ion transport across plasma membranes isolated from rat kidney cortex. Biochem J 178:549–557
37. Tsukamoto Y, Saka S, Saitoh M, Sugimura K (1990) Heterogeneity of calcium pump activity in proximal and distal tubules of rat kidney (abstract) Kidney Int 37:2471
38. Bronner F, Stein WD (1988) CaBPr facilitates intracellular Ca diffusion for Ca pumping in distal convoluted tubule. Am J Physiol 255:F558–F562

The Biology of Vitamin D-Dependent Calcium Binding Proteins

Rajiv Kumar[1]

Summary. Vitamin D-dependent calcium binding protein (CaBPs) are widely dispersed in many tissues that play an important role in calcium translocation. They are vitamin D-dependent in most tissues except for those in the central nervous system. The calcium binding proteins are co-localized with calcium pumps in many Ca^{2+} transporting tissues.

Introduction

Vitamin D_3, via its active metabolite $1,25(OH)_2D_3$, plays a crucial role in the active absorption of Ca in the intestine, the mobilization of bone and soft tissue Ca, the maintenance of normal serum Ca and phosphorus concentrations, and the normal mineralization of bone [1–5]. Although the hormone may not directly alter mineralization, many direct effects of the hormone on bone cell activity have been noted [4–14]. In vitro, $1,25(OH)_2D_3$ promotes differentiation and inhibits the growth of various cell lines. It also diminishes the secretion of interleukin 2 from mitogen-stimulated lymphocytes in vitro and alters monocyte and macrophage function.

In the intestine, $1,25(OH)_2D_3$ brings about this effect, at least in part, by a receptor-mediated mechanism that influences the expression of various genes in the nucleus [1–5]. Receptors for the hormone have been characterized with respect to their physical characteristics, ligand-binding properties, and amino acid sequences [6–8]. Protein synthesis is important in bringing about the actions of $1,25(OH)_2D_3$ in the intestine, although contrary views exist [4]. Intestinal lipid metabolism, cyclic nucleotide levels, and the uptake of Ca by Golgi and endoplasmic reticulum are altered by $1,25(OH)_2D_3$ [4]. Extensive work has been performed by us and others concerning the metabolic events that control the tissue levels and metabolism of

[1]Nephrology Research Unit, Departments of Medicine, Biochemistry, and Molecular Biology, Mayo Clinic/Foundation, Rochester, MN 55905, USA

$1,25(OH)_2D_3$ [3]. Thermodynamic considerations in the transepithelial movement of Ca have been reviewed by Wasserman and recently discussed by us [4,9]. The transport of Ca across the enterocyte requires energy and sodium ions. The entry of Ca into the enterocyte is down a concentration and electrical gradient and, while it is facilitated by vitamin D, it does not require the expenditure of energy. The energy-requiring step is at the basolateral membrane, where Ca is pumped up a concentration and electrical gradient, most likely by a Ca-pumping ATPase.

Vitamin D-Dependent Calcium Binding Proteins

Physiology and Structure of CaBPs

In the intestine, $1,25(OH)_2D_3$ increases, and sometimes decreases, the synthesis of various proteins and alters the activity of various enzymes [1–5]. In some instances, these changes are related to active intestinal Ca transport in vivo. The most notable of the proteins whose synthesis is altered by $1,25(OH)_2D$ is vitamin D-dependent CaBP [1–5,10–13]; the appearance of the protein in the intestine is temporally related to increases in calcium transport. Careful experiments have shown that CaBP is regulated by vitamin D in intestinal tissue and that it does not act merely as a Ca buffer [12]. Recent work has shown that CaBP plays a role in the diffusion of Ca across the cellular compartment [14]. There is some evidence that CaBP may interact with the plasma membrane Ca pump in order to increase the movement of Ca from within the cellular compartment into the extracellular fluid space; while this is an attractive hypothesis, work from several laboratories, including our own, has shown that this may not be the case [16–17]. Concentrations of CaBP in tissues are regulated by both transcriptional and non-transcriptional mechanisms [18–21]. It is clear that CaBP concentrations in tissues are controlled in large part by transcriptional mechanisms—hence it is likely that $1,25(OH)_2D_3$-specific promoter or enhancer elements are present either proximal (5′) to the transcription start site or within the gene itself.

There is considerable information about the structure of CaBPs and their distribution in tissues. As noted in Table 1, CaBP exists in two forms [5,13,18,22]. There is an ~9 kDa CaBP present in the intestine and placenta of mammalian tissues; it is also found in mouse kidney. In addition, an ~28 kDa CaBP is present in the intestine and in other tissues of avian species, and in the brain and distal tubule of mammalian species. The amino acid sequences of porcine, murine, and a truncated form of bovine intestinal CaBP have been determined by Edman degradation [22–27]. The sequence of rat intestinal CaBP has been deduced from the sequence of a cDNA clone [28]. Recently, we determined the sequence of a full-length cDNA clone of bovine intestinal CaBP and demonstrated that the protein encoded by this cDNA was three amino acids longer than that of the truncated protein whose sequence had been determined earlier by Edman degradation [23]. The truncated form arises due to the action of trypsin on a lysine-lysine bond present between amino acids 3 and 4 of the protein. Chick intestinal 28 kDa CaBP has been sequenced by us and by Wasserman using protein sequencing techniques [24,25]. Its amino acid sequence has been derived from the sequence of appropriate cDNA clones [26]. In addition, we have recently determined the sequence of appropriate cDNA clones [26]. In addition, we have recently determined the sequence of rat brain 28-kDa CaBP from the sequence

Table 1. Tissue and species distribution of calbindin-D. (From (5) with permission of the American Physiological Society)

Species and tissue	Approximate molecular weight (kDa)	Cross-reacts with antisera prepared to calbindin-D from
Chicken		
Intestine	28	–
Kidney	28	Chicken intestine, human kidney
Uterus	28	Chicken intestine
Hypothalamus	ND	Chicken intestine
Bone	34	Chicken intestine
Brain	28	Chicken intestine
Pancreas	28	Chicken intestine, human kidney
Blood	ND	Chicken intestine
Parathyroid	ND	Chicken intestine
Adrenal	ND	Chicken intestine
Esophagus	ND	Chicken intestine
Testes	ND	Chicken intestine
Mouse		
Yolk sac	10.05	Rat intestine
Kidney	25 and 10	Human cerebellar, mouse intestine, rat intestine
Intestine	9–10	Rat intestine
Placenta	ND	Rat intestine
Uterus	ND	Rat intestine
Pig		
Intestine	9–13	–
Kidney	12 and 25	Pig intestine
Blood	ND	Pig intestine
Liver	12	Pig intestine
Pancreas	12	Pig intestine
Thyroid	12	Pig intestine
Human		
Intestine	10–28	Chicken intestine, human kidney
Brain	28	Chicken intestine
Kidney	28	Chicken intestine

of appropriate cDNA clones. Others have determined the sequences of the human 27–28 kDa CaBP gene, the chicken 28 kDa CaBP gene, and the rat 9 kDa CaBP gene [29]. All the data concerning the structure of these proteins demonstrates that they are related to other calcium binding proteins of the troponin-C superfamily of proteins.

Biophysical Properties of CaBPs

Recently, several laboratories, including our own, have examined the biophysical properties of CaBPs in order to obtain information on the manner in which they bind Ca and in order to bind insights into how they might act as trigger proteins or facilitate the movement of calcium across cells. The 9 kDa bovine intestinal CaBP binds 2 moles of Ca, whereas the chick intestinal CaBP binds 4 moles of Ca per mole of protein [22]. The 9 kDa and 28 kDa vitamin D-induced CaBPs bind Ca within E-F hand structures. These structures consist of helix-loop-helix structures that were initially described by Kretsinger and his colleagues [22]. The 9 kDa CaBP has two E-F hand structures whereas the 28 kDa CaBP has six. Moffat and colleagues have determined the 3-dimensional x-ray crystal structure of the 9 kDa CaBP.

We examined the mechanism of Ca and lanthanide binding of the 28 kDa CaBP [30]. We demonstrated that the chick intestinal CaBP binds 3 moles of terbium with high affinity, another mole of terbium with relatively high affinity, and several other molecules of terbium with low affinity. Ca binding occurs at two classes of sites; furthermore, the protein undergoes a conformational change upon binding Ca. We have also demonstrated similar conformational changes with human kidney CaBP. Similar Ca^{2+}-dependent conformation changes have been noted with the porcine 9 kDa CaBP. Recently, we examined the Ca binding properties of the rat brain 28 kDa CaBPs in E. coli and purified it and three mutants. We have shown that both the mutants which lack either one or two E-F hands bind Ca in a manner similar to that of the full-length protein. Considerable work, however, needs to be done in defining the precise stoichiometry of Ca binding in the full-length and mutant forms of CaBP. Recently, Forsen and Grundstrom have examined the biophysical properties of mutated forms of the 9 kDa CaBP using NMR and other methods. We have also used NMR techniques in order to examine the NMR characteristics of the 28 kDa CaBP. We have confirmed, by NMR, that the conformation of these CaBPs is controlled by Ca.

References

1. DeLuca HF (1988) The vitamin D story: a collaborative effort of basic science and clinical medicine. FASEB J 2:224–236
2. Minghetti PP, Norman AW (1988) 1,25$(OH)_2$-vitamin D_3 receptors: gene regulation and genetic circuitry. FASEB J 2:3043–3053
3. Kumar R (1984) The metabolism of 1,25-dihydroxyvitamin D_3. Physiol Rev 64:478–504
4. Kumar R (1986) The metabolism and mechanism of action of 1,25-dihydroxyvitamin D_3. Kidney Int 30:793–803
5. Gross MD, Kumar R (1990) Physiology and biochemistry of vitamin D-dependent calcium binding proteins. Am J Physiol 259:F195–F205
6. Pike JW, Sleator NM, Haussler MR (1987) Chicken intestinal receptor for 1,25-dihydroxy-vitamin D_3. Immunologic characterization and homogeneous isolation of a 60000-dalton protein. J Biol Chem 25:262:1305–1311
7. Baker AR, McDonnell DP, Hughes M, Crisp TM, Mangelsdorf DJ, Haussler MR, Pike JW, Shine J, O'Malley BW (1988) Cloning and expression of full-length cDNA encoding human vitamin D receptor. Proc Natl Acad Sci USA 85:3294–3298
8. Pierce EA, Dame MC, DeLuca HF (1987) Size and charge of the functional 1,25-dihydroxyvitamin D (receptor) in porcine intestine. J Biol Chem 262:17092–17099
9. Wasserman RH, Fullmer CS, Shimura F (1984) Calcium absorption and the molecular effects of vitamin D_3. In: Kumar D (ed) Martinus Nijhoff, Hingham, pp 233–257
10. Wasserman RH, Corradino RA, Taylor AN (1968) Vitamin D-dependent calcium-binding protein. Purification and some properties. J Biol Chem 243:3978–3986
11. Response to some physiological and nutritional variables. J Biol Chem 243:3987–3993
12. Bar A, Hurwitz S (1979) Relationship of intestinal and plasma calcium binding protein to intestinal calcium absorption. FEBS Lett 102:79–81
13. Thomasset M, Parkes CO, Cuisinier-Gleizes P (1982) Rat calcium-binding proteins: distribution, development, and vitamin D dependence. Am J Physiol 243:E483–E488

14. Feher JJ, Fullmer CS, Fritzsch GK (1989) Comparison of the enhanced steady-state diffusion of calcium by calbindin-D9K and calmodulin: possible importance in intestinal calcium absorption. Cell Calcium 10:189–203
15. Morgan DW, Welton AF, Heick AE, Christakos S (1986) Specific in vitro activation of Ca, Mg-ATPase by vitamin D-dependent rat renal calcium binding protein (calbindin D_28K). Biochem Biophys Res Commun 138:547–553
16. Walters JR (1989) Calbindin-D9K stimulates the (calcium) pump in rat enterocyte basolateral membranes. Am J Physiol 256:G124–G128
17. Ghijsen WEJM, Van Os CH, Heizmann CW, Murer H (1986) Regulation of duodenal Ca^{2+} pump by calmodulin and vitamin D-dependent Ca^{2+}-binding protein. Am J Physiol 251:G223–G229
18. Christakos S, Gabrielides C, Rhoten WB (1989) Vitamin D-dependent calcium binding proteins: chemistry, distribution, functional considerations, and molecular biology. Endocr Rev 10:3–26
19. Varghese S, Deaven LL, Huang YC, Gill RK, Iacopino AM, Christakos S (1989) Transcriptional regulation and chromosomal assignment of the mammalian calbinding-D28k gene. Mol Cell Endocrinol 3:495–502
20. Clemens TL, McGlade SA, Garrett KP, Craviso GL, Hendy GL (1989) Extracellular calcium modulates vitamin D-dependent calbindin-D28k gene expression in chick kidney cells. Endocrinology 124:1582–1584
21. Dupret JM, Brun P, Perret C, Lomri N, Thomasset M, Cuisinier-Gleizes P (1987) Transcriptional and post-transcriptional regulation of vitamin D-dependent calcium-binding protein gene expression in the rat duodenum by 1,25-dihydroxycholecalciferol. J Biol Chem 262:16553–16557
22. Gross M, Kumar R (1987) The physiology and biochemistry of vitamin D-dependent calcium binding proteins. In: Spelsberg TC, Kumar R (eds) Sterol/steroid hormone action. Martinus Nijhoff, Hingham, pp 371–394
23. Kumar R, Wieben E, Beecher SJ (1989) The molecular cloning of the complementary deoxyribonucleic acid for bovine vitamin D-dependent calcium-binding protein: structure of the full-length protein and evidence for homologies with other calcium-proteins of the troponin-C superfamily of proteins. Mol Cell Endocrinol 3:427–432
24. Tsarbopoulos A, Gross M, Kumar R, Jardine I (1989) Rapid identification of calbindin-D28k cyanogen bromide peptide fragments by plasma desorption mass spectrometry. Biomed Environ Mass Spectrom 18:387–393
25. Fullmer CS, Wasserman RH (1987) Chicken intestinal 28-kilodalton calbindin-D: complete amino acid sequence and structural considerations. Proc Natl Acad Sci USA 84:4772–4776
26. Hunziker W (1986) The 28-kDa vitamin D-dependent calcium-binding protein has a six-domain structure. Proc Natl Acad Sci USA 83:7578–7582
27. Hunziker W, Schrickel S (1988) Rat brain calbinding D28: six domain structure and extensive amino acid homology with chicken calbindin D28. Mol Cell Endocrinol 2:465–473
28. Desplan C, Heidmann O, Lillie JW, Auffray C, Thomasset M (1983) Sequence of rat intestinal vitamin D-dependent calcium-binding protein derived from a cDNA clone. Evolutionary implications. J Biol Chem 258:13502–13505
29. Minghetti PP, Cancela L, Fujisawa Y, Theofan G, Norman AW (1988) Molecular structure of the chicken vitamin D-induced calbindin-D28k gene reveals eleven exons, six Ca^{2+}-binding domains, and numerous promoter regulatory elements. Mol Cell Endocrinol 2:355–367
30. Gross MD, Nelsestuen GL, Kumar R (1987) Observations on the binding of lanthanides and calcium to vitamin D-dependent chick intestinal calcium-binding protein. Implications regarding calcium-binding protein function. J Biol Chem 262:6539–6545

Cystic Diseases of the Kidney

Chair: Jean-Pierre Grünfeld (France)
Eiji Higashihara (Japan)

Control of Renal Cyst Formation and Enlargement

Jared J. Grantham[1]

Summary. Evidence is presented to indicate that renal cysts derived in a collagen matrix in vitro from primary cultures of human cortex and from an established cell line (MDCK) are subject to growth regulation by peptide mitogens (EGF and insulin) and by agents of the adenylyl cyclase signal transduction system. The findings are consonant with recent evidence obtained by direct measurement of fluid transport in liver and kidney cysts of humans with autosomal dominant polycystic kidney disease and support the hypothesis that these potential regulatory mechanisms may participate in the initiation and expansion of cysts.

Introduction and Discussion

Although renal cysts come in different shapes and sizes, recent work leads to the conclusion that when encountered in hereditary and acquired disorders they have certain key elements in common: 1) Cysts evolve from renal tubules; they may arise in fetal kidneys or in otherwise fully mature and well-differentiated renal tubules [1]. 2) Enlargement involves the proliferation of epithelial cells that comprise the wall of the cyst [2], the accumulation of fluid within the cavity formed by the increase in cyst wall area [3], and the remodeling of the extracellular matrix and the interstitium adjacent to the enlarging cysts [4].

We have become accustomed to viewing renal cysts in two general contexts: 1) acquired and 2) hereditary. Acquired cysts develop in renal tubules that have no genetic history of de novo cyst formation, whereas dominant and recessive mutations cause cysts to form with regularity in the renal tubules of susceptible individuals. Acquired cysts can be formed by feeding animals selected chemicals, or they can be formed as a consequence of a severe reduction in the number of functioning nephrons [5]. The maintenance of acquired cysts appears to require the sustained stimulation

[1]University of Kansas Medical Center, Kansas City, KS 66103, USA

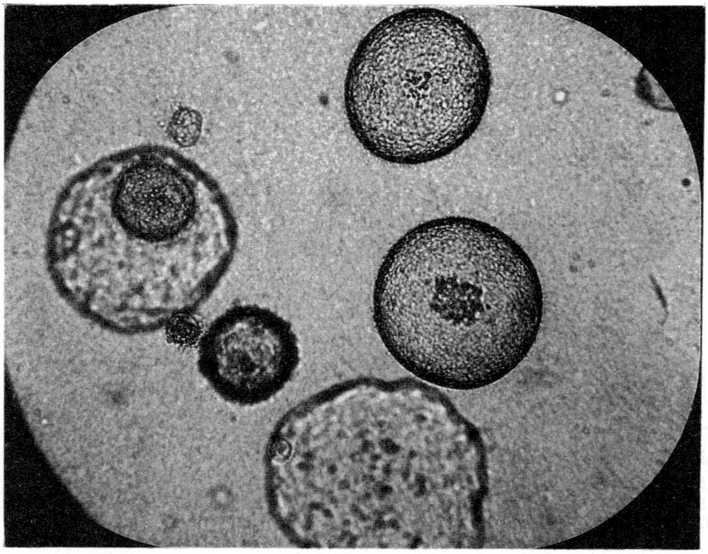

Fig. 1. Madin Darby Canine Kidney (*MDCK*) cysts in hydrated gel of Type 1 collagen. Largest cyst is 367 μm in diameter

of cyst-building forces, since the cysts can be diminished in size by withholding the cystsogen, or by transplanting a functioning kidney [6]. Acquired cystic disease can also be accelerated by increasing the number of inflammatory cells in the kidneys [7].

The highly variable clinical course of autosomal dominant polycystic kidney disease (ADPKD) and autosomal recessive polycystic kidney disease (ARPKD), also suggests that non-genetic factors may have a commanding role in determining the expression of these diseases in the kidneys.

Renal cysts appear to be neoplastic but otherwise differentiated tissue masses that derive from one or more tubule epithelial cells in a segment of renal tubule [8]. Renal cysts are distinguished from solid tumors by the sustained sequestration of fluid within the cavity formed by the orderly expansion of the intact monolayer of epithelial cells. Abnormal proliferation of epithelial cells may be initiated by inherited or acquired factors that interfere with the normal control of cell division. Once cysts are initiated, hormonal, autocrine, or paracrine factors may promote the expansion of both hereditary and acquired cysts by accelerating the rate of cell proliferation and net transepithelial fluid secretion.

In recent studies, my collaborators and I have searched for some of the potential factors that may contribute to the initiation and progressive enlargement of hereditary and acquired cysts [9–14]. We have used two types of in vitro cells to evaluate the roles of mitogens and fluid transport agonists. Madin Darby Canine Kidney (MDCK) cells are a continuous line of epithelial cells that retain certain differentiated features of the distal tubule. When cultured within a matrix of gelled collagen, MDCK cells develop cysts that enlarge progressively [15]. We have examined these cells as a model of cysts with a genetic abberation in the control of cell division (Fig. 1). This *genetic cyst model*

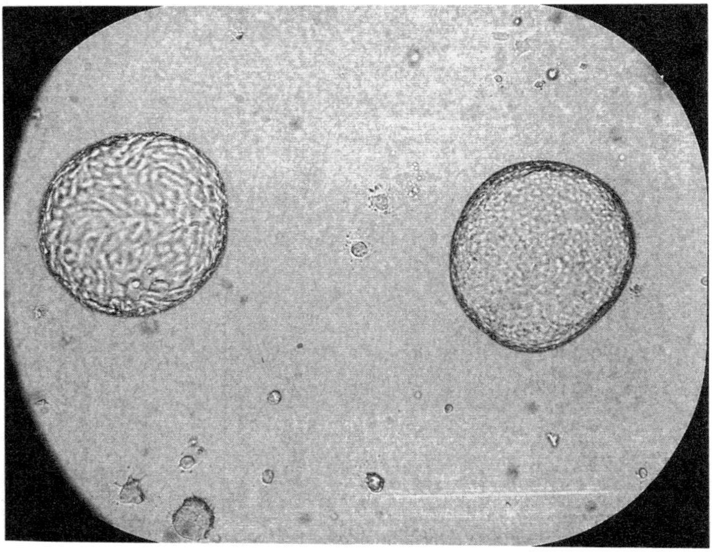

Fig. 2. Normal human kidney (*NHK*) cysts in hydrated gel of Type 1 collagen. Largest cyst is 417 μm in diameter

mimics the autosomal dominant and recessive types of PKD which are caused by mutated DNA. By contrast, we have used primary cultures of human renal cortex to study cyst biogenesis in cells with a normal genetic history with respect to cyst formation. When passaged into a collagen matrix and fed with certain growth factors, human cortex cells form cysts that resemble those observed in the MDCK cell cultures (Fig. 2). We have used the normal human kidney cortex cells (NHK) as an *acquired cyst model*.

Cultures of MDCK and NHK cysts within collagen matrix have been used to assess the impact of exogenous agents on the induction and formation of cysts.

MDCK

In defined medium, MDCK cells embedded in collagen matrix induce cyst formation when they are treated with agonists of the adenylyl cyclase signal transduction pathway [9–14]. Epidermal growth factor (EGF), a renal cell mitogen, does not increase the rate of MDCK cyst formation, but these same cells form cysts when fed with fetal calf serum.

NHK

Only when they are treated with EGF and insulin do NHK cells form cysts [14]. Transferrin and selenium promote cyst growth, but are not essential for cysts to form. Fetal calf serum does not initiate cyst formation. Agonists of the adenylyl cyclase signal transduction pathway also increase the rate of NKH cyst expansion in collagen matrix.

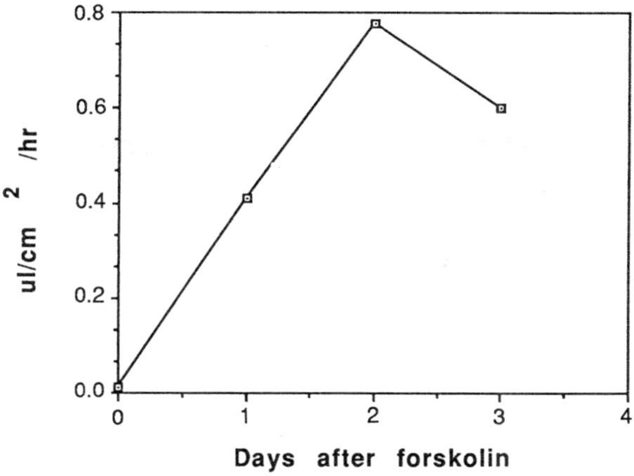

Fig. 3. Effect of forskolin (10^{-5} M) on the rate of net fluid secretion across monolayers of normal human kidney (*NHK*) cells

The formation and expansion of cysts in collagen matrix requires the highly coordinated organization of proliferating cells. Studies of MDCK cells indicate that each cyst derives from a single cell that divides repeatedly, i.e., each cyst represents the clonal growth of a solitary cell [15]. The matrix is critical in determining the type of cyst that will be formed and in determining the polarity of the cells. MDCK cells grown in type 1 collagen have orthodox polarity; however, cysts grown in agarose gels or in suspension culture have reversed polarity, and the Na+K, ATPase is deposited within the apical, rather than within the basolateral plasma membranes [15–17]. The expansion of MDCK cysts in type 1 collagen gel (orthodox polarity) depends in the last analysis on the rate of cell *proliferation* in the cyst wall and on the rate of fluid *secretion* into the cyst cavity. Cyclic AMP agonists stimulate the proliferation of MDCK cells [10,13]. Although the effect of cAMP on the proliferation of NHK cells has not been tested directly, the expansion of the cyst wall area after cAMP stimulation is consistent with stimulation of cell proliferation.

Evaluation of the role of net fluid secretion on the rate of cyst expansion has required a different technical approach. To determine net fluid secretion directly, we grew MDCK and NHK cells on collagen-coated permeable membranes that permitted the collection of fluid which was secreted under a layer of mineral oil directly onto the apical surface of the cells [10,11,13,14]. Monolayers of MDCK cells showed marked stimulation of net fluid secretion when treated with cAMP agonists, but not when treated with EGF and insulin. By contrast, NHK cells revealed marked stimulation of net fluid secretion by EGF and insulin, and the cAMP agonists (Fig. 3). These findings indicate that activation of the adenylyl cyclase signal transduction pathway may promote cyst enlargement by accelerating the rate of net fluid secretion into the cysts. Recent studies indicate that secretin, a hormone that stimulates cyclic AMP production in biliary epithelium, increases the rate of fluid secretion into hepatic and renal cysts of patients with polycystic kidney disease [18].

We have not explicitly determined the extent to which net fluid secretion and cell proliferation are linked in the process of cyst expansion, but simple observation of the increased proliferative response of cells grown on monolayers precludes net fluid accumulation as an explanation for the stimulation of cell growth by cAMP. In addition, cell proliferation can be uncoupled from net fluid secretion by treatment with ouabain [9]. This glycoside, which blocks net fluid secretion, inhibits the enlargement of cysts, but the cells continue to proliferate, leading to solid tumor masses. Such findings would support the view that *cell proliferation* and *fluid secretion* are not obligatorily tied together, and while both protagonists of cyst formation and enlargement appear to be regulated by cAMP, ultimate control of each function may not be conducted through the same effector mechanism.

The foregoing considerations have led to the formulation of an *hypothesis* to explain the progressive enlargement of renal cysts induced by either hereditary or acquired etiologies:

It is hypothesized that cell proliferation and net fluid secretion within established cysts are regulated by a common signal transduction mechanism, the adenylyl cyclase pathway. Mutations in genes which control rate limiting processes in this pathway may alter the sensitivity to surface membrane receptor-mediated agonists, which, at normal levels, may induce cyst formation in hereditary states. In renal tubule cells which lack mutations, autocrine or paracrine mitogens may induce the formation of cysts which expand in response to receptor-mediated cyclase agonists.

References

1. Evan AP, McAteer JA (1990) Cyst cells and cyst walls. In: Gardner KD, Bernstein J (eds) The Cystic Kidney. Kluwer, Highman, pp 21–42
2. Grantham JJ, Geiser JL, Evan AP (1987) Cyst formation and growth in autosomal dominant polycystic kidney disease. Kidney Int 31:1145–1152
3. Grantham JJ (1983) Polycystic kidney disease: A predominance of giant nephrons. Am J Physiol 23:526–529
4. Carone FA, Makino H, Kanwar YS (1988) Basement membrane antigens in renal polycystic disease. Am J Pathol 130:466–471
5. Grantham JJ, Levine E (1985) Acquired cystic disease: Replacing one kidney disease with another. Kidney Int 28:99–105
6. Ishikawa I (1990) Acquired renal cystic disease. In: Gardner KD, Bernstein J (eds) The Cystic Kidney. Kluwer, Highman, pp 351–377
7. Gardner KD Jr, Evan AP, Reed WP (1986) Accelerated renal cyst development in deconditioned germ-free rats. Kidney Int 29:1116–1123
8. Grantham JJ (1990) Polycystic kidney disease: Neoplasia in disguise. Am J Kidney Dis 15:110–116
9. Grantham JJ, Uchic M, Cragoe EJ Jr, Kornhaus J, Grantham JA, Donoso V, Mangoo-Karim R, Evan AP, McAteer J 1989 Chemical modification of cell proliferation and fluid secretion in renal cysts. Kidney Int 35:1379–1389
10. Mangoo-Karim R, Uchic M, Lechene C, Grantham JJ (1989) Renal epithelial cyst formation and enlargement in vitro: Dependence on cAMP. Proc Natl Acad Sci USA 86:6007–6011
11. Mangoo-Karim R, Uchic M, Grant M, Shumate WA, Calvet JA, Park CH, Grantham JJ (1989) Renal epithelial fluid secretion and cyst growth: the role of cyclic AMP. FASEB J 3:2629–2632

12. Grant M, Cragoe EJ, Grantham JJ (1990) Arginine vasopressin stimulates net fluid secretion in a cyst-forming epithelium (MDCK). Kidney Int 37:581
13. Neufeld TJ, Grantham JJ (1990) Epidermal growth factor initiates and cyclic AMP promotes the formation and progressive enlargement of human renal epithelial cysts in vitro. Clin Res 38:444A
14. McAteer JA, Evan AP, Gardner KD (1987) Morphogenetic clonal growth of kidney epithelial cell line MDCK. Anat Rec 217:229–239
16. Wang AZ, Ojakian GE, Nelson WJ (1990) Steps in the morphogenesis of a polarized epithelium 1. Uncoupling the roles of cell-cell and cell-substratum contact in establishing plasma membrane polarity in multicellular epithelial (MDCK) cysts. J Cell Sci 95:137–151
17. Wang AZ, Ojakian GK, Nelson WJ (1990) Steps in the morphogenesis of a polarized epithelium 11. Disassembly and assembly of plasma membrane domains during reversal of epithelial cell polarity in multicellular epithelial (MDCK) cysts. J Cell Sci 95:153–165
18. Everson GT, Emmett M, Brown WR, Redmond P, Thickman D (1990) Functional similarities of hepatic cystic and biliary epithelium: Studies of fluid constituents and in vivo secretion in response to secretin. Hepatology 11:557–656

Inflammatory Mediators in the Progression of Renal Cystic Disease

KENNETH D. GARDNER JR.[1], JANET S. BURNSIDE[1], LAWRENCE W. ELZINGA[2], and RICHARD M. LOCKSLEY[3]

SUMMARY. The possibility that cytokines are present and active in polycystic kidneys was raised by two observations: (i) Endotoxin potentiates cyst formation in the kidneys of germfree rats fed nordihydroguaiaretic acid. (ii) Some cyst fluids are mitogenic for mouse thymocytes. Analyses of fluids from 13 individuals with symptomatic autosomal dominant polycystic kidney disease have detected interleukin-1β, tumor necrosis factor α, interleukin-2, stromelysin, and prostaglandin E_2, evidence which not only indicates that interleukin-1β is present but which also supports the likelihood of its biological activity in cyst fluids. The findings provide support for a hypothesis that cytokines participate in the morbidity and/or pathogenesis of autosomal dominant polycystic kidney disease.

Introduction

Two recent, fundamental observations in our laboratory directed our attention to the possibility that cytokines are active in the setting of polycystic kidney disease. One involves the antioxidant nordihydroguaiaretic acid (NDGA), which injures kidney cells [1]. When NDGA is fed to normal rats, cysts form in the animals' kidneys [1]. The effects of NDGA are progressive and evolve over weeks to months. When NDGA is fed to germfree rats, it has little effect on renal morphology unless the rats are exposed to endotoxin. Then, renal cyst formation is dramatic and explosive, even when the animals are maintained under sterile conditions [2]. In this particular model, cysts develop within days after exposure to lipopolysaccharide. The progres-

[1]Department of Medicine, University of New Mexico School of Medicine, Albuquerque, NM 87131, USA
[2]Oregon Health Sciences Center, Portland, OR 97201, USA
[3]University of California, San Francisco, CA 94143, USA

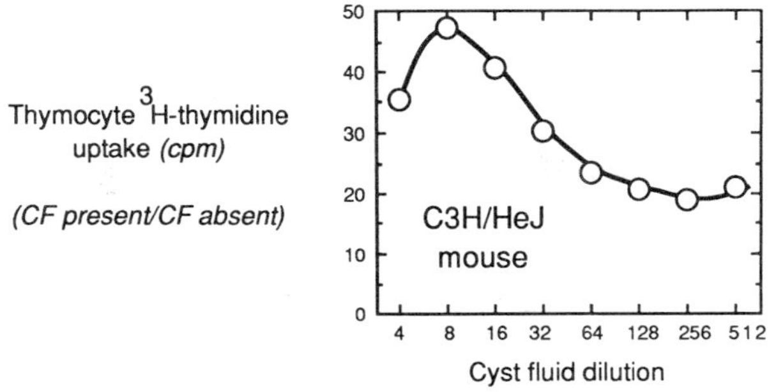

Fig. 1. Mitogenic response of mouse thymocytes to cyst fluid from a polycystic kidney. *Circles* represent means of three determinations. An almost 50-fold increase over baseline thymidine incorporation is evident at the 1:8 dilution. CPM, counts per minute; CF, cyst fluid

sion of the lesion relates directly to the numbers of circulating and infiltrating inflammatory cells.

The second observation is shown in Fig. 1. Fluid drawn from some cysts of human polycystic kidneys induces a proliferative response among thymocytes of the endotoxin-insensitive C3H/HeJ mouse [3]. Such a response is presumptive evidence that cytokine-like substances are present [4,5].

Cytokines are pluripotent proteins [4,5] which are produced by nucleated cells. They act locally and transiently and are present at sites of inflammation and immunologic injury. For example, they may be found in the synovial fluid of acute rheumatoid arthritis and in cerebrospinal fluid during bacterial meningitis. Cytokines mediate the effects of endotoxin [5,6]. Cytokines are mitogenic for mouse thymocytes in comitogen assays [3,7]. One of the best studied cytokines is the monokine, interleukin-1 (IL-1) [5]. IL-1 is relevant to the kidney. It is made by glomerular mesangial cells [8]; it inhibits sodium, glucose, and amino acid transport by renal tubules in vivo [9–11] and it stimulates prostaglandin E_2 (PGE_2) production by papillary collecting duct cells in vitro [12]. IL-1 exists in two forms, IL-1α and IL-1β.

Methods and Results

In order to detect cytokines in cyst fluids we used the enzyme-linked immunoabsorbent assay (ELISA). The sandwich ELISA is highly specific and is a standard technique for the detection of cytokines in biological fluids [13]. An IL-1β-specific commercial ELISA was utilized to assay for IL-1β in most of the 104 aerobic culture-negative fluid samples that had been aspirated from 13 patients with symptomatic autosomal dominant polycystic kidney disease (ADPKD) [14]. Four individuals were female, nine were male. Their ages ranged from 31–54 years. Their renal function, as evaluated by serum creatinines, extended from normal to endstage disease.

Immunoreactive IL-1β concentrations in cyst fluids ranged from 0 to more than 400 pg/ml. The higher concentrations were equal to those that are found in the synovial fluid of rheumatoid arthritics with acute disease [15]. Of 102 fluid samples, roughly one-third contained no IL-1β, one-third contained IL-1β in low concentra-

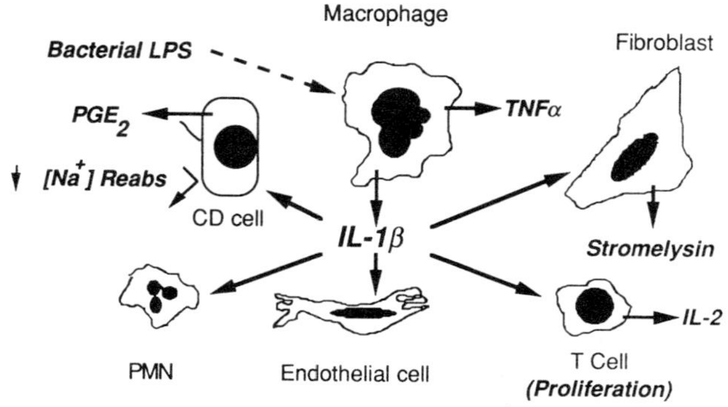

Fig. 2. Cartoon of cellular interactions. Effects of IL-1β on selected target cells are shown in *italics*. All but the reduced reabsorption of sodium by collecting duct cells have been demonstrated in vitro. PMN, polymorphonuclear neutrophils; CD, collecting duct; LPS, lipopolysaccharide (endotoxin)

tions (< 20 pg/ml), and one-third contained IL-1β in relatively high concentrations (> 20 pg/ml). We concluded that immunoreactive IL-1β is present in most cyst fluids of polycystic kidneys.

It remained to be demonstrated that this immunoreactive IL-1β was active biologically. In order to establish bioactivity, we sought evidence of some of the known second-order effects that IL-1 provokes among other cells.

A scheme of IL-1 interactions, as they relate to this study, is shown in Fig. 2. Bacterial lipopolysaccharide (endotoxin) stimulates macrophages to produce and release IL-1 and tumor necrosis factor. Macrophage IL-1, in turn, may stimulate fibroblasts to produce stromelysin [16,17], induce T-cells to proliferate and to produce IL-2 [7], cause endothelial cells and polymorphonuclear leukocytes to become activated [5], and incite cells of the papillary collecting duct to increase their production of PGE_2 [12] and, in vivo, to reduce their reabsorption of sodium [10–11]. The first evidence of bioactivity that we sought was documentation of the proliferative response of T-cells to cyst fluid. We used thymocyte comitogen assays.

In contrast to the sandwich ELISA, thymocyte comitogen assays are not specific [18]. Mouse thymocytes are exposed to fluids suspected of containing mitogenic substances in the presence of a comitogen such as phytohemagglutinin or concanavalin A. Thymidine incorporation is taken as a measure of thymocyte proliferation. The assays are not specific because other cytokines are mitogenic and because IL-1 bioactivity may be inhibited by specific inactivators. The results of these assays, unlike those of the ELISA, represent only presumptive evidence of cytokine presence. We recorded bioassay results in terms of a *stimulation index*: the ratio of counts per minute of tritiated thymidine incorporated by thymocytes in the presence versus the absence of cyst fluid. We defined a *mitogenic fluid* as one with a *stimulation index* greater than unity.

Two-thirds of the cyst fluids were mitogenic (Fig. 3), some provoking upwards of a 50-fold increase in thymocyte proliferation (Fig. 3a). There was no correlation between stimulation indices and IL-1β concentrations. However, most mitogenic

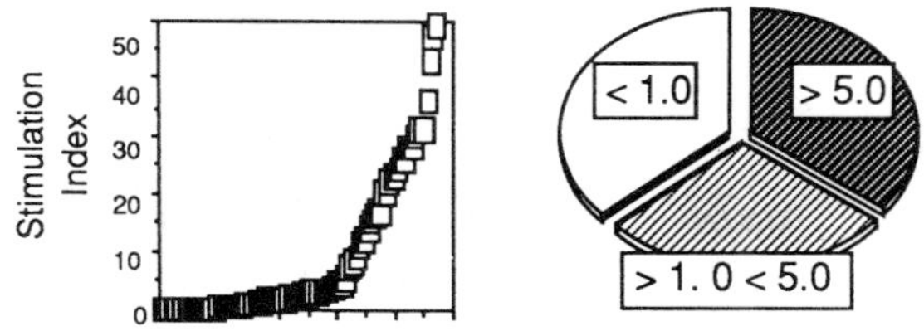

Fig. 3a,b. Mitogenic response to cyst fluids. **a** Range of stimulation indices among 102 tested fluids **b** Responses grouped by degree of response

fluids were fluids that contained immunoreactive IL-1β ($\chi^2 = 3.87$; $P < 0.05$). Fewer mitogenic fluids had no IL-1β, and IL-1β was present in some non-mitogenic fluids. The observation that a significant majority of fluids that were mitogenic also contained immunoreactive IL-1β implied to us that some, at least, of the immunoreactive IL-1β that we detected by ELISA was active biologically.

We continued to search for evidence which would support bioactivity by performing three additional ELISAs and a radioimmunoassay. We assayed cyst fluids for IL-2, stromelysin, tumor necrosis factor alpha (TNFα), and PGE_2, all demonstrated in vitro to be products of specific IL-1β-stimulated cells (Fig. 2). In addition, we tested fluids for bacterial lipopolysaccharide and related the findings to IL-1β concentrations in the same fluids. Finally, we related the concentrations of immunoreactive IL-1β to the concentrations of sodium in the same cyst fluids.

Immunoreactive IL-2 was present in 7 of 23 fluids. Its concentrations were higher in the presence than in the absence of IL-1. They correlated significantly with those of IL-1β ($r = 0.65$; $P < 0.05$). This was the result anticipated had thymus-derived cells been present in or near cysts and responded to an IL-1β signal in vivo.

Immunoreactive stromelysin (kindly assayed by MW Lark and LA Walakovits, Merck Sharp and Dohme Research Laboratories, Division of Merck and Co., Inc., Rahway, NJ, USA) was present in 18 of 23 fluids, in concentrations ranging from 0–55 ng/ml. Its mean concentration was higher, but insignificantly so, in IL-1β-containing fluids. While stromelysin concentrations did not correlate directly with those of IL-1β, we found that when fluids were grouped in relation to their IL-1β immunoreactivity, significantly more fluids contained IL-1β and stromelysin together ($\chi^2 = 5.901$; $P < 0.05$).

Both TNFα (assayed by ELISA) and PGE_2 (assayed by radioimmunoassay) were detected in a majority of fluids. While concentrations did not correlate with those of IL-1β, mean concentrations of both TNFα and PGE_2 were higher, albeit insignificantly so, in the presence than in the absence of IL-1β.

Bacterial lipopolysaccharide (LPS) was detected in 8 of 41 fluids. The mean concentration of IL-1β was higher in LPS positive fluids, but again the difference was not statistically significant.

The findings, in the form of mean index and concentration differences, are summarized in Fig. 4. Fluids containing immunoreactive IL-1β were more apt to cause T-cells to proliferate. They also were associated with higher mean concentrations of IL-2, stromelysin, TNFα, and PGE_2. Finally, the mean concentration of IL-1β was

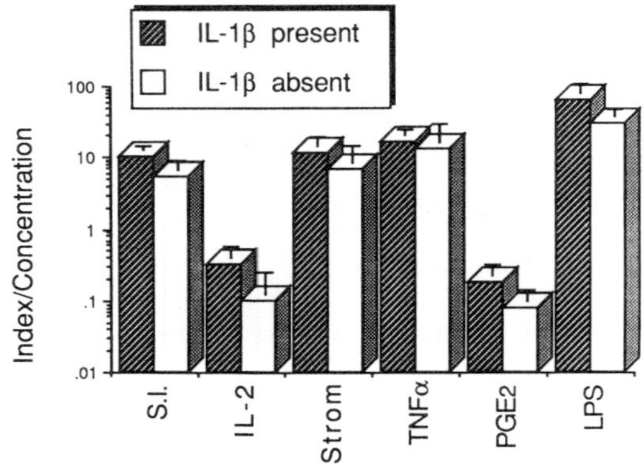

Fig. 4. Mean (±SE) differences (log scale) in index/concentrations between fluids with and fluids without immunoreactive IL-1β. Greater mitogenicity (*S.I.*); and higher concentrations of IL-2, stromelysin, (*strom*) tumor necrosis factor α, (*TNF*α) and PGE_2 were found among fluids with IL-1β; a greater mean concentration of IL-1β was recorded among endotoxin-positive (*LPS*) fluids

higher among fluids in which bacterial lipopolysaccharide was detected. Except for the concentration of IL-2 and stromelysin, mean differences between fluids with and without IL-1β were not statistically significant. Means, however, were always greater in IL-1β-containing fluids (Fig. 4), a direction of difference that was predicted by experimental experience (Fig. 2). This is, given its consistency here in six of six independent trials, statistically significant ($P < 0.02$; one tail).

Discussion

We concluded from our observations that IL-1β is present and is biologically active in cyst fluids from polycystic kidneys. The findings raised the question of what role IL-1β and/or other cytokines might play in the morbidity or pathogenesis of ADPKD.

It is not likely that IL-1β is responsible for the salt wasting that is sometimes associated with cystic kidney disease [19]. We found no relationship between the concentrations of sodium and IL-1β. Thus, we found no evidence that intraluminal IL-1β influences sodium concentrations in, and presumably net sodium reabsorption from, cyst fluids. Accordingly, we cannot implicate intraluminal IL-1β activity in the salt wasting of renal cystic disease.

A more likely role for cytokines relates to pain. Of the 13 subjects from whom our fluids came, 11 had painful polycystic kidneys and were undergoing therapeutic cyst aspiration and decompression [14]. We cannot rule out the possibility that cytokines, such as IL-1β and TNFα, are involved in the renal pain of polycystic kidney disease.

A second plausible possibility of a role for cytokines is in the remodeling that characterizes the polycystic kidney. Cystic nephrons are remodeled nephrons. Stromelysin is a metalloproteinase known to participate in the remodeling of joints in rheumatoid arthritis [16,17]. Stromelysin degrades collagen IV and proteoglycan, two components of renal tubular basement membrane, whose abnormalities have long been implicated in the pathogenesis of polycystic kidney disease [20]. Thus, activation of the cytokine cascade in genetically predisposed individuals may account for the dilation of nephrons and the formation of cysts in kidneys which, ultimately, we come to recognize as polycystic kidneys.

Conclusion

This study has shown that cytokines, specifically IL-1β, TNFα, and IL-2, are present in the cyst fluids of polycystic kidneys. The study has provided strong presumptive evidence that the IL-1β in cyst fluid is active biologically. Given the known consequences of cytokine activity at other sites of disease, it must be considered likely that cytokines participate in the morbidity and pathogenesis of autosomal dominant polycystic kidney disease.

References

1. Gardner KD Jr, Evan AP (1984) Cystic kidneys: An enigma evolves. Am J Kidney Dis 3:403–413
2. Gardner KD Jr, Reed WP, Evan AP, Zedalis J, Hylarides MD, Leon AA (1987) Endotoxin provocation of experimental renal cystic disease. Kidney Int 32:329–334
3. Ryan JL, Glode LM, Rosenstreich DL (1979) Lack of responsiveness of C3H/HeJ macrophages to lipopolysaccharide: The cellular basis of LPS-stimulated metabolism. J Immunol 122:932–935
4. Balkwill FR, Burke F (1989) The cytokine network. Immunol Today 10:299–304
5. Fibbe WE, Schaafsma MR, Falkenburg JHF, Willemze R (1989) The biological activities of interleukin-1. Blut 59:147–156
6. Richardson RP, Rhyne CD, Fong Y, Hesse DG, Tracey KY, Marano MA, Lowry SF, Antonacci AC, Calvano SE (1989) Peripheral blood leukocyte kinetics following in vivo lipopolysaccharide (LPS) administration to normal human subjects. Ann Surg 210:239–245
7. Kaye J, Gillis S, Mizel SB, Shevach EM, Malek TR, Dinarello CA, Lachman LB, Janeway CA Jr (1984) Growth of a cloned helper T cell line induced by a monoclonal antibody specific for the antigen receptor: Interleukin 1 is required for the expression of receptors for interleukin 2. J Immunol 133:1339–1345
8. Lovett DH, Ryan JL, Sterzel RB (1983) A thymocyte-activating factor derived from glomerular mesangial cells. J Immunol 130:1796–1801
9. Kohan DE, Schreiner GF (1988) Interleukin 1 modulation of renal epithelial glucose and amino acid transport. Am J Physiol 254:F879–F886
10. Caverzasio J, Rizzoli R, Dayer J-M, Bonjour J-P (1987) Interleukin-1 decreases renal sodium reabsorption: possible mechanism of endotoxin-induced natriuresis. Am J Physiol 252:F943–F946
11. Beasley D, Dinarello CA, Cannon JG (1988) Interleukin-1 induces natriuresis in conscious rats: Role of renal prostaglandins. Kidney Int 33:1059–1065
12. Kohan DE (1989) Interleukin-1 regulation of prostaglandin E_2 synthesis by the papillary collecting duct. J Lab Clin Med 114:717–723

13. Herbelin A, Nguyen AT, Zingraff J, Urena P, Descamps-Latscha B (1990) Influence of uremia and hemodialysis on circulating interleukin-1 and tumor necrosis factor α. Kidney Int 37:116–125
14. Bennett WM, Elzinga L, Golper TA, Barry JM (1987) Reduction of cyst volume for symptomatic management of autosomal dominant polycystic kidney disease. J Urol 137:620–622
15. Smith MD (1989) Cytokines in synovial fluid in rheumatoid arthritis. J Rheumatol 16:706
16. Case JP, Lafyatis R, Remmers EF, Kumkumian GK, Wilder RL (1989) Transin/stromelysin expression in rheumatoid synovium. Am J Pathol 135:1055–1064
17. Teahan J, Harrison R, Izquierdo M, Stein RL (1989) Substrate specificity of human fibroblast stromelysin. Hydrolysis of substance P and its analogues. Biochemistry 28:8497–8501
18. Hurme M (1988) Both interleukin 1 and tumor necrosis factor enhance thymocyte proliferation. Eur J Immunol 18:1303–1306
19. Gardner KD Jr (1988) Cystic kidneys. Kidney Int 33:610–621
20. Carone FA, Hollenberg PF, Makamura S, Punyarit P, Glogowski W, Flouret G (1989) Tubular basement membrane change occurs pari passu with the development of cyst formation. Kidney Int 35:1034–1040

Extrarenal Manifestations of Autosomal Dominant Polycystic Kidney Disease

DOMINIQUE CHAUVEAU, YVES PIRSON[2], DOMINIQUE DROZ, JOSEPH ROSENFELD[3], and JEAN-PIERRE GRÜNFELD[1],

SUMMARY. Among extrarenal manifestations of autosomal dominant polycystic kidney disease (ADPKD), liver abnormalities are the most frequent and intracranial aneurysms, the most severe. Liver cysts develop later than renal cysts, and are more prevalent in females, most particularly in those who have had multiple pregnancies. The treatment of massive polycystic liver is difficult. In very rare families, congenital hepatic fibrosis may be associated with ADPKD. Rupture of an intracranial aneurysm (ICA) is a life-threatening complication. The mean age at rupture is 39 years. This accident may occur in normotensive patients with normal renal function. Routine screening is indicated when there is a positive family history of ICA or when there has been a previous accident of ICA rupture.

Introduction

Extrarenal manifestations in autosomal dominant polycystic kidney disease (ADPKD) encompass both cystic changes, among which liver involvement predominates, and non-cystic changes, including intracranial aneurysms, other cardiovascular lesions, and possible abdominal hernias and colon diverticulosis. Extrarenal involvement may expose ADPKD patients to life-threatening complications, such as rupture of an intracranial aneurysm or severe liver cyst function.

In this review, we will focus mainly on recent data on liver abnormalities, intracranial aneurysms, and mitral-valve prolapse. These manifestations raise not only clinical problems of dealing with their detection and management, but also pathophysiological issues, with regard to the relation between the mechanisms

[1]Département de Néphrologie, Hôpital Necker, 75015 Paris, France
[2]Service de Néphrologie, Cliniques Universitaires Saint-Luc, 1200 Brussels, Belgium
[3]Beilinson Medical Center, Tel Aviv University Medical School, Tel Aviv, Israel

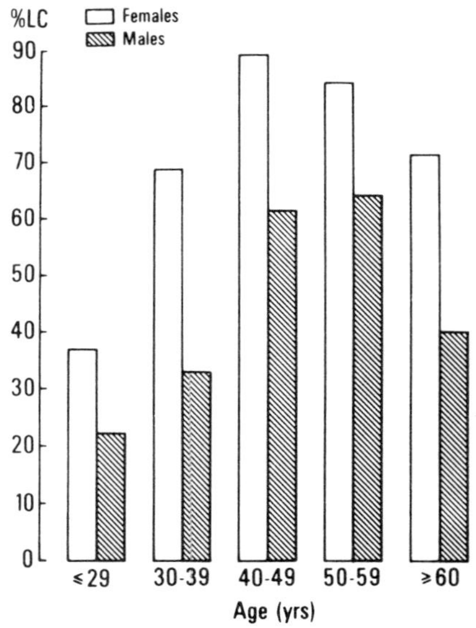

Fig. 1. Prevalence of liver cysts (*LC*) as detected by ultrasonography in 120 non-hemodialyzed ADPKD patients according to age and sex. (From [1] with permission)

involved in renal cyst formation and those implicated in the development of these extrarenal lesions.

Liver Involvement

Liver cysts are frequently found in ADPKD, and their ultrasonographic demonstration may be helpful for diagnosis. The prevalence of liver cysts increases with age and is higher in female patients. In both sexes, liver cysts develop later than kidney cysts. Approximately 70% of ADPKD patients aged 60 years or more have liver cysts detected by ultrasonography [1]. In autopsy series, liver cysts were found in about 90% of cases [1,2]. Liver cysts develop earlier in women than in men (Fig. 1) [1]. Similar findings were reported by Kaehny et al. [3] in patients aged less than 50 years; women had a higher prevalence of, and more numerous liver cysts than men, regardless of age and renal function. Females with liver cysts had had more pregnancies than those without liver cysts. These data suggest that the female hormonal environment may trigger or accelerate the expression and development of the liver cystic process.

Liver cysts are thought to result from progressive dilatation of von Meyenburg's complexes (or biliary microhamartomas). These complexes are considered to represent the remnants of embryonic bile ductules which were formed in excess and did not involute after failing to establish a connection with canaliculi and interlobular bile ducts [1]. This view has recently been challenged by Ramos et al. [2]. These authors showed that microhamartomas were not observed in young patients and that their number or detectability increased with age. This was in striking contrast to results found by Karhunen [4]. In addition, biliary microhamartomas may contain bile-like material. Ramos et al. indicate that, initially, microhamartomas and microcysts may be connected to biliary canaliculi, whereas later, larger cysts become disconnected. Ramos et al. also suggest that epithelial hyperplasia is crucial in the formation of both liver and kidney cysts [2].

Cystic fluid results from secretion by the biliary-type epithelium of the cyst. The electrolyte composition of hepatic cyst fluid is similar to that of serum. Organic anions normally transported by hepatocytes are not transported into liver cysts. Both IgA and secretory components, and high glutamyltranspeptidase concentrations, are found in cyst fluid. The cyst secretion rate can be stimulated by intravenous administration of secretin, a hormone known to induce secretion by normal biliary epithelium [5]. This suggests that, conversely, somatostatin may decrease the liver cyst fluid formation rate.

The incidence of liver cyst complications has long been underestimated. These complications occur mainly in dialyzed or renal transplanted patients. Liver cyst infections are the most frequent complications (see review in [6]). Cholangiocarcinoma develops in very rare cases, as in other biliary diseases with bile duct proliferation, such as Caroli's disease [1]. Massive polycystic liver, which predominates in women, may be the source of severe discomfort and digestive disorders. The management of such patients is difficult. Cyst fenestration and segmental hepatic resection have recently been advocated [7].

In addition to cysts, other hepatobiliary changes may occasionally be encountered in ADPKD patients. Idiopathic dilatation of intrahepatic [8,9], or extrahepatic (J.P. Grünfeld unpublished cases), biliary tract has been observed. Congenital hepatic fibrosis (diffuse biliary fibroadenomatosis associated with enlarged fibrotic portal spaces), which is responsible for portal hypertension, is the characteristic liver lesion in autosomal recessive polycystic kidney disease (PKD). Rare cases of ADPKD with congenital hepatic fibrosis have, however, been reported. Four families with this association have recently been investigated by Cobben et al. [10]. The liver disease may have a slow rate of progression. Close linkage between the disease allele and DNA markers on the short arm of chromosome 16 has been demonstrated. In these families, the renal lesion is clearly transmitted in an autosomal dominant pattern, whereas congenital hepatic fibrosis has not been found to be vertically transmitted [10]. Several hypotheses have been considered, including the coexistence of the dominant ADPKD mutant gene and of the autosomal recessive PKD mutant gene in these kindreds.

Intracranial Aneurysms

The coexistence of ADPKD and ruptured intracranial aneurysm (ICA) was first reported in 1901 by Borelius (Lund) in a 38-year-old "Kavallerie-Offizier" [11]. In 1904 Dunger first emphasized this association and reported rupture of ICA in a 54-year-old woman with ADPKD whose daughter had died at the age of 26 from a pontine hemorrhage, which may have been due to a ruptured ICA [12]. Dunger therefore probably observed the first ADPKD family with clustering of ICA.

Information on the prevalence and complications of ICA in ADPKD may be found in previous papers [13,14,15]. Cases of subarachnoid hemorrhage have been reported in which no aneurysm was found [13]. Intracranial hemorrhage may occur in patients who are unaware of having ADPKD [16].

Intracranial aneurysms occur in the general population with an incidence of 1.2% to 7.8%. The role of inborn defects in the arterial wall has been put forward, since ICA may be associated with various inherited disorders (type IV Ehlers-Danlos syndrome, Marfan's syndrome, pseudoxanthoma elasticum and ADPKD); a large number of familial cases of ICA, not associated with a recognized inherited disorder have been reported, including eight identical twins who had aneurysms at the same site or at the mirror site [17]. Lozano and Leblanc have analyzed the data from 243 aneurysms in 177 patients from 74 families. They concluded that familial ICAs rupture at a smaller size and when the patient is younger (mean age of 42.3 years versus 51.4 years) than do cases of sporadic aneurysms. There is a similar sex distribution, a similar incidence of multiple aneurysms, and a similar incidence of females over males with multiple aneurysms. Anterior communicating artery aneurysms occur less often in familial than in sporadic cases [17].

It would be of interest to know the epidemiology of ICAs in ADPKD. No large study is so far available. In a Concerted Action of the European Economic Community, we have initiated a cooperative effort on this topic. In a preliminary survey made in France, Belgium and Switzerland, we collected data on 46 patients with ruptured ICA and ADPKD. The age distribution of these patients was similar to that found by Lozano and Leblanc in familial intracranial aneurysms not associated with other inherited defects; the mean age at rupture was 39 years. Approximately 30% of the patients were normotensive and 21 had normal renal function at rupture; only 2 were in end-stage renal failure. Thus, ICA rupture may occur in young patients, and in the absence of hypertension and/or renal function impairment.

Familial clustering of ICA in ADPKD has already been emphasized by others (see [6]). In our study, precise information was available in 37 families: "proven" ICA and "possible" ICA were found in 3 and 7 cases, respectively, i.e., an overall prevalence of 27%. Of note, Torres et al. found a positive family history of ICA in 32% of patients with symptomatic ICA and ADPKD. It should be stressed, however, that a similar positive family history of ICA was detected in 11% of asymptomatic ADPKD patients with negative routine screening for ICA [18].

Intracranial aneurysms are progressive in ADPKD, and a new ICA may develop after successful surgical cure of a rupture accident [19]. We have observed such occurrence in three patients, with the two ICA rupture episodes separated by an interval of from 7–13 years. Madonick et al. (cited in [13]) reported one case in which two episodes of subarachnoid hemorrhage had occurred, with recovery for five years.

The limitations of routine screening for occult ICAs in ADPKD have been extensively discussed by Levey et al. [15]. Using cranial computed tomography and magnetic resonance imaging, Torres et al. recently performed a prospective study in 96 ADPKD patients without central nervous system involvement. They detected no definite ICA [20]. This confirms that routine screening is not rewarding and probably not indicated. In contrast, screening is indicated in the following circumstances: when there is a positive family history of ICA, a previous accident of ICA rupture, and perhaps before major elective surgery, or in high-risk occupations. The best means of screening and the rate of re-screening remain to be determined in ADPKD patients at high risk for ICA.

Mitral Valve Prolapse

Hossack et al. [21] were the first to draw attention to the high prevalence of mitral-valve prolapse in ADPKD patients. Using echocardiography, they studied 163 patients with ADPKD, 130 unaffected family members, and 100 control subjects. In these three groups, the prevalence of mitral-valve prolapse was 26, 14, and 2%, respectively. There was no clear predominance in ADPKD females. A higher prevalence of mitral incompetence, aortic incompetence, tricuspid incompetence and tricuspid valve prolapsus was also found in the ADPKD patients [21]. This association has some clinical implications. As mitral valve prolapse may be complicated by cerebral embolization, this should be considered in the differential diagnosis of cerebrovascular accident in ADPKD patients. In addition, bacterial endocarditis may complicate mitral valve prolapse. Among non-ADPKD patients with this abnormality, those with systolic bruit and leaflet thickening are more prone to develop endocarditis than those without these features. Endocarditis complicating mitral valve prolapse must therefore be considered in ADPKD patients with fever [6].

Of interest, mitral-valve prolapse is a complication of some inherited connective tissue disorders – such as Marfan's syndrome, Ehlers-Danlos syndrome, osteogenesis imperfecta, and the joint hypermobility syndrome – some of which are also diseases predisposing to ICAs (see above). In addition, primary mitral valve prolapse, unassociated with other symptoms of connective tissue disease, can appear as an inherited autosomal dominant trait, a condition also found in familial intracranial aneurysms (see above). Complete concordance in monozygotic twins has been reported. The expression of the diseases is affected by sex, the incidence being higher in females [22]. In three such families, the segregation of the genes encoding the major fibrillar collagens present in valve tissue, collagens I and III, was analyzed by use of restriction enzyme site variants as genetic markers. The primary gene locus for mitral-valve prolapse is not linked to either of the two collagen I loci nor, probably, to the collagen III locus [22].

Other cardiovascular abnormalities, including abdominal aortic aneurysms and annuloaortic ectasia, have been found in ADPKD [6,21]. Dissection of the ascending thoracic aorta has recently been reported in an ADPKD patient after kidney transplantation; the condition required resection and insertion of a teflon graft [23]. This complication again underlines some analogy with Marfan's syndrome. The basic defect predisposing to cardiovascular abnormalities in ADPKD remains, however, unknown. Recent findings by Powell et al., showing that there is a familial tendency to abdominal aortic aneurysm, might be relevant [24]. These authors have shown that genetic variation in the haptoglobin and cholesterol ester protein genes (located on the *long* arm of chromosome 16) appears to influence dilatation of the abdominal aorta. It might be of interest to test this hypothesis in ADPKD patients with intracranial or abdominal aortic aneurysm.

Acknowledgments. We thank Doreen Broneer for her invaluable secretarial assistance, and we thank all the nephrologists who participated in the study on intracranial aneurysms in ADPKD.

References

1. Grünfeld JP, Albouze G, Jungers P, Landais P, Dana A, Droz D, Moynot A, Lafforgue B, Boursztyn E, Franco D (1984) Liver changes and complications in adult polycystic kidney disease. Adv Nephrol 14:1–20
2. Ramos A, Torres VE, Holley KE, Offord KP, Rakela J, Ludwig J (1990) The liver in autosomal dominant polycystic kidney disease. Arch Pathol Lab Med 114:180–184
3. Kaehny WD, Manco-Johnson M, Johnson M, Tangel DJ, Gabow PA (1988) Influence of sex on liver manifestations of autosomal dominant polycystic kidney disease (ADPKD). Kidney Int 33:196
4. Karhunen PJ (1986) Adult polycystic liver disease and biliary microhamartomas (von Meyenburg's complexes). Acta pathol Microbiol Immunol Scand [A] 94:397–400
5. Everson GT, Emmett M, Brown WR, Redmond P, Thickman D (1990) Functional similarities of hepatic cystic and biliary epithelium: Studies of fluid constituents and in vivo secretion in response to secretin. Hepatology 11:557–565
6. Pirson Y, Grünfeld JP (to be published) Autosomal-dominant polycystic kidney disease. In: Cameron JS, Davison AM, Grünfeld JP, Kerr DNS, Ritz E (eds) Oxford Textbook of Clinical Nephrology. Oxford University Press, Oxford
7. Newman KD, Torres VE, Rakela J, Nagorney DM (1990) Treatment of highly symptomatic polycystic liver disease: preliminary experience with a combined hepatic resection fenestration procedure. Ann Surg 212:30–37
8. Terada T, Nakanuma Y (1988) Congenital biliary dilatation in autosomal dominant adult polycystic disease of the liver and kidneys. Arch Pathol Lab Med 112:1113–1116
9. Jordan D, Harpaz N, Thung SN (1989) Caroli's disease and adult polycystic kidney disease: a rarely recognized association. Liver 9:30–35
10. Cobben JM, Breuning MH, Schoots C, ten Kate LP, Zerres K (to be published) Congenital hepatic fibrosis in adult polycystic kidney disease. Kidney Int
11. Borelius J (1901) Zur Genese und klinischen Diagnose der polycystischen Degeneration der Nieren. Nord Med Arkiv I:1–13
12. Dunger R (1904) Zur Lehre von der Cystenniere, mit besonderer Berücksichtigung ihrer Heredität. Beitr Path Anat 35:445–509
13. Brown RAP (1951) Polycystic disease of the kidneys and intracranial aneurysms: The etiology and interrelationship of these conditions: Review of recent literature and report of seven cases in which both conditions coexisted. Glasgow Med J 32:333–348
14. Bigelow NH (1953) The association of polycystic kidneys with intracranial aneurysms and other related disorders. Am J Med Sci 225:485–494
15. Levey AS, Pauker SG, Kassirer JP (1983) Occult intracranial aneurysms in polycystic kidney disease. When is cerebral arteriography indicated? N Engl J Med 308:986–994
16. Ryu SJ (1990) Intracranial hemorrhage in patients with polycystic kidney disease. Stroke 21:291–294
17. Lozano AM, Leblanc R (1987) Familial intracranial aneurysms. J Neurosurg 66:522–528
18. Torres VE, Forbes GS, Wiebers DO, Erickson SB, Smith LH (1987) Value of routine screening for intracranial aneurysms in autosomal dominant polycystic kidney disease. Xth International Congress of Nephrology, London, p 45
19. Chauveau D, Sirieix ME, Schillinger F, Legendre C, Grünfeld JP (1990) Recurrent rupture of intracranial aneurysms in autosomal dominant polycystic disease. Br Med J 301:966–967
20. Torres VE, Wiebers DQ, Forbes GS (1990) Cranial computed tomography and magnetic resonance imaging in autosomal dominant polycystic kidney disease. JASN 1:84–90
21. Hossack KF, Leddy CL, Johnson AM, Schrier RW, Gabow PA (1988) Echocardiographic findings in autosomal dominant polycystic kidney disease. N Engl J Med 319:907–912

22. Wordsworth P, Ogilvie D, Akhras F, Jackson G, Sykes B (1989) Genetic segregation analysis of familial mitral valve prolapse shows no linkage to fibrillar collagen genes. Br Heart J 61:300–306
23. Fitzpatrick PM, Torres VE, Charboneau W, Offord KP, Holley KE, Zincke H (1990) Long-term outcome of renal transplantation in autosomal dominant polycystic kidney disease. Am J Kidney Dis 15:1535–543
24. Powell JT, Bashir A, Dawson S, Vine N, Henney AM, Humphries SE, Greenhalgh RM (1990) Genetic variation on chromosome 16 is associated with abdominal aortic aneurysm. Clin Sci 78:13–16

Malignancy and Cystic Disease

Isao Ishikawa[1]

Summary. The natural history of acquired renal cystic disease (ARCD) has started to become clear over the last 10 years. It is known, for example, that the longer the duration of hemodialysis, the more numerous are the cysts that develop, and that male dialysis patients with the disease tend to reveal more extensive cystic degeneration than do female dialysis patients. In addition, it has been shown that acquired cystic disease regresses after successful renal transplantation. A 10-year prospective study by the present authors has revealed that the incidence of renal cell carcinoma in dialysis patients is one in 249 patient-years. The study also shows that there are two types of renal cell carcinoma in dialysis patients; one occurring in older patients after a short time on hemodialysis and involving fewer renal cysts, and the other, which occurs with extensive cyst formation, in relatively young patients after long-term dialysis. In the latter condition particularly, the development of cysts is closely related to the development of renal malignancy. Thus, there is much circumstantial evidence for a causal relation between acquired renal cystic disease and renal cell carcinoma, however, as yet, there is no direct proof of this via molecular biological and other techniques.

Introduction

Acquired renal cystic disease involves the bilateral development of multiple renal cysts in uremic patients with an initial cyst-unrelated renal disease [1]. Dunnill et al. [2] have pointed out that the major complications of this acquired cystic disease are renal cell carcinoma and hemorrhage due to cyst rupture; the incidence of renal cell carcinoma has been shown, in a previous summary of the literature, to be high [1]. The pathologic investigation by Dunnill et al. [2] indicates that the label acquired

[1]Division of Nephrology, Department of Internal Medicine, Kanazawa Medical University, Uchinada, Kahoku, Ishikawa, 92002 Japan

cystic disease of the kidney may encompass a whole spectrum from cyst to adenoma to renal cell carcinoma. Similarly, Hughson et al. report that atypical cysts may be seen in cases of these kidney disorders. These observations suggest that epithelial hyperplasia or proliferation is a likely complication of acquired cystic disease of the kidney [3].

Therefore, we evaluated the incidence of renal cell carcinoma during a 10-year prospective study, and undertook a series of nationwide questionnaire studies on renal malignancy in hemodialysis patients. Moreover, in this paper we review recent developments concerning acquired cystic disease and renal cell carcinoma in dialysis patients.

Natural History of Acquired Renal Cystic Disease

Acquired renal cystic disease is characterized by the bilateral development of multiple cysts in kidneys that are uremic or have sustained nephron loss. This disease appears typically in long-term hemodialysis or in continuous ambulatory peritoneal dialysis (CAPD) patients [1,4]. However, acquired cysts may also appear in native kidneys in predialysis periods or at times of poor graft function [5]. The incidence of acquired cystic disease is 7%–26% in predialysis periods, 35.2%–79.3% in dialysis patients [1,2,6,7], 35% in CAPD patients, [8] and 33% in pediatric dialysis patients [9].

The most important risk factor associated with acquired cystic disease is the duration of uremia or duration of dialysis [1]. The longer either has been present, the more severe the cystic changes that appear in the kidneys. Usually, the original kidney disease causing uremia or chronic renal failure is unrelated to the development of acquired cysts [2], however, every end-stage renal disease has a potential link with cyst formation; even in cases of graft failure where acquired cysts develop in the transplanted kidney, more severe cystic changes may appear in the native kidney [5]. In our study, the incidence of acquired cysts was 43.7% in all dialysis patients and 90% in those on hemodialysis for more than 10 years [1].

A second major variable influencing the onset and proliferation of acquired cysts is the patient's sex [1]. Male patients on dialysis developed more of these acquired cysts and displayed greater kidney enlargement due to cystic changes than did female patients in this study (Fig. 1). In 1979, the mean bilateral kidney volume was 80.5 $\pm$ 32.3 ml (mean $\pm$ SD) in male patients and 66.4 $\pm$ 32.3 ml in female patients after a mean hemodialysis duration of 3.3 years. Ten years later, these values had increased to 207 $\pm$ 189.7 ml and 86.3 $\pm$ 55.8 ml, respectively [10]. These figures represent a 2.7 $\pm$ 1.7-fold enlargement of male kidneys during the 10 year period, but only a slight, statistically insignificant, increase in female kidney size.

Recently, several reports have been published concerning the development of acquired cysts in patients on CAPD [4,8]; they have quoted incidences of acquired cysts [4,8] and renal cell carcinoma [11] in CAPD patients, similar to those mentioned above. However, the exact difference between hemodialysis patients and CAPD patients in severity of acquired cystic disease is not known.

Figure 2 illustrates a third factor affecting the development of acquired cystic disease—successful renal transplantation [12]. During a serial study in recipients with good graft function, the mean volume of bilateral native kidneys of 14 patients subjected to hemodialysis for more than 3 years was found to be 82.1 $\pm$ 56.4 ml

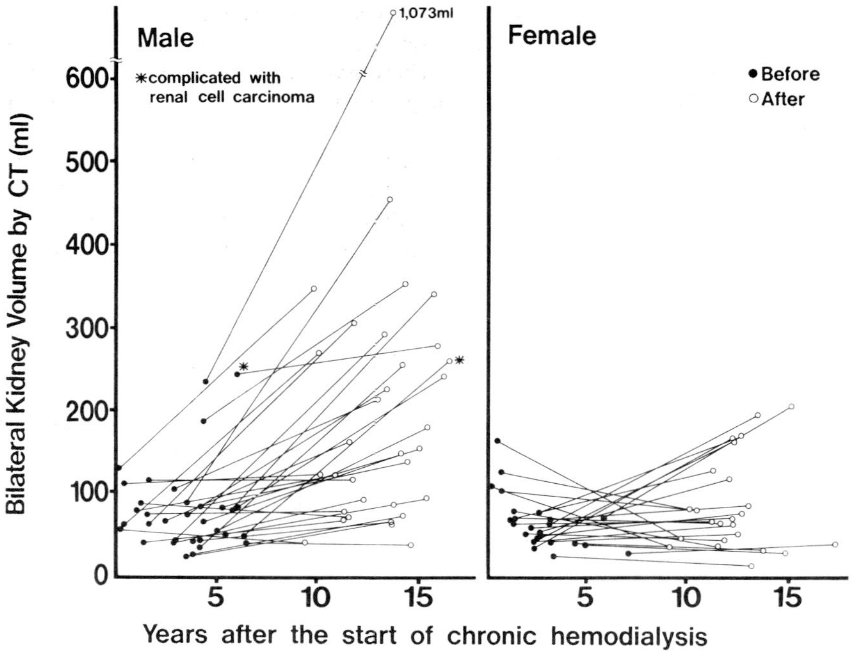

Fig. 1. Ten year follow up study of bilateral kidney volume in hemodialysis patients. The mean kidney volume in male patients after 10 years of follow up increased significantly due to acquired cysts. CT, computerized tomography. From [10] with permission)

prior to kidney transplant; however, this decreased to 42.9 ± 10.8 ml within 1–3 months of surgery, to 35.6 ± 5.9 ml within 1 year, and to 33.8 ± 10.0 ml within 3 years. The rate of kidney shrinkage was greater in patients with more extensive cyst formation (Fig. 2). In another study, the overall incidence of cystic transformation after renal transplantation was calculated to change from 36.1% (base line study) to 42.6% (follow up study) [Ishikawa I, unpublished data]. Thus, the incidence of patients with renal cysts is slightly less in allograft recipients than in hemodialysis patients; however, severity of cystic transformation and change in the kidney volume (as a likely reflection of changes in both cyst size and number) both differ in the two treatment groups. The native kidneys following transplantation are severely atrophic and have only one, or a few visible, cysts, a situation entirely different from that seen in hemodialysis patients.

The mechanism accounting for such rapid regression of acquired cysts after transplantation is not clear; however it may be very important in leading us to an understanding of the pathogenesis of acquired cystic disease. One explanation could be that the disappearance of uremic growth factor after transplantation [12,13] may bring about cyst regression. Another possibility is that the reduction of osmotic load to the remaining glomeruli and/or the improvement of transepithelial sodium movement may cause filtered fluid to diminish, and hence the cysts to reduce in size and number. On the other hand, this regression of acquired cysts is one line of evidence that they are induced "acquired" in nature.

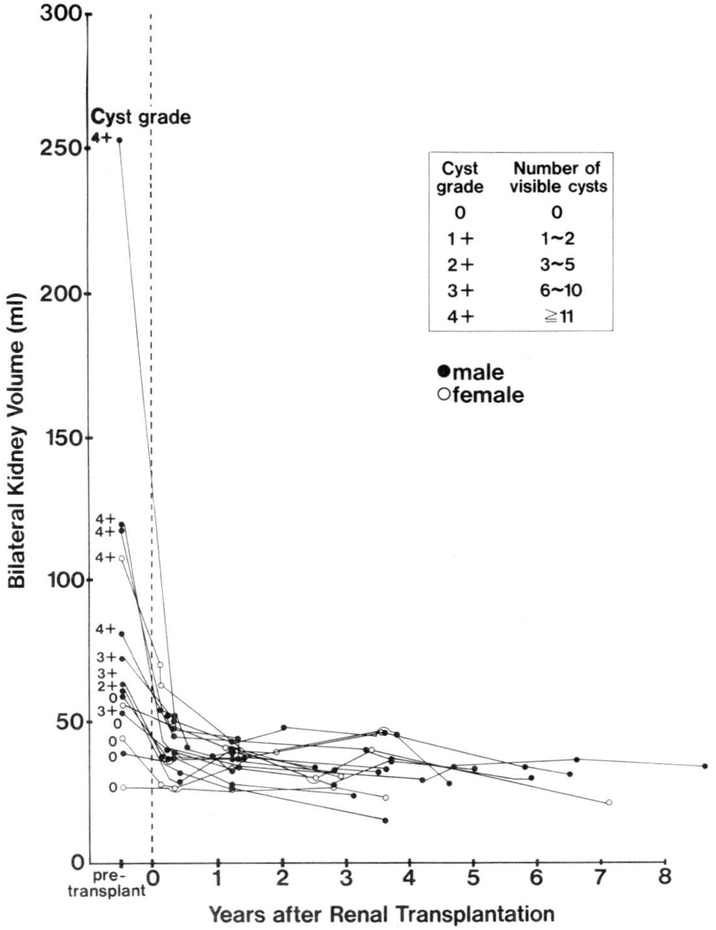

Fig. 2. Volume of native kidneys after renal transplantation. After successful transplantation, mean kidney volume decreases due to the regression of acquired cysts

Characteristics of Renal Cell Carcinoma in Dialysis Patients

It has been suggested that the prevalence of renal cell carcinoma in dialysis patients is 1.4%–2.0% [1], or 7–40 times higher than in the general population. However, some authors [8,11,12] are skeptical of this reported high incidence because the figures were obtained by investigators with high levels of interest in renal cell carcinoma and so may be subject to bias.

In our ten year prospective study of 96 patients begun in 1979, one renal cell carcinoma was detected in 249 patient-years [10]. Over the entire patient-time dialysis period, there were 6 renal cell carcinomas in 1,070 patient-years (1/178 patient-years). The incidence was higher in male patients (1/140 patient-years) than in

Table 1. Renal cell carcinoma in hemodialysis patients (questionnaire studies[a] performed in Japan)

Number of renal cell carcinoma cases	364
male	299(82.1%)
female	65(17.9%)
Mean age (years)	51.2±11.6[b]
Mean duration of hemodialysis (months)	90.8±55.8
Presence of ARCD (%)	276/350(78.9%)
Number of patients with metastases (%)	61/346(17.6%)

[a]results of the past five questionnaires, performed in 1982, 1984, 1986, 1988, and 1990
[b]mean ± SD
ARCD, acquired renal cystic disease

female patients (1/369 patient-years). This indicates that the incidence of renal cancer in dialysis patients is then 57–134 times higher than the 3–7 per 100000 persons per year seen in the general population. These figures may be applicable only to Japanese patients, since differences in the rates of several cancers have been observed between Japan and the United States. However, the incidence of renal cell carcinoma in Japan is lower than that in the US and Europe, although the incidence of chronic glomerulonephritis is higher in Japan. There are a large number of transplant patients in the US and Europe and many hemodialysis patients in Japan, the latter being screened quite well for renal cell carcinoma.

Table 1 illustrates sex differences in the occurrence of renal cell carcinoma, male cases outweighing female ones by 299 to 65 (82.1% were male patients). Mean age of these patients was 51.2 ± 11.6 years, which is significantly younger than in the general population (64 ± 12 years). One of the other characteristics of renal cell carcinoma as a complication of acquired cysts is that it occurs at higher rates in patients that have been hemodialyzed for longer duration: a survey of the literature reveals a prevalence of 1.5% among all dialysis patients and 5% in those with a greater than 10 year history of dialysis (1). For Japan, questionnaire studies performed by us indicate that the mean duration of hemodialysis was 90.8 ± 55.8 months (Table 1). Thus, it seems at present that there are 2 types of renal cell carcinoma in dialysis patients [15], one afflicting younger people on long-term dialysis and characterized by extensive cystic formation (Figs. 3 and 4), and the other developing in older patients with a short history of dialysis and manifesting few or no cysts. This is illustrated in Fig. 3.

Recently Chung-Park et al. [16] have described renal cell carcinomas in end stage kidney disease before dialysis treatment [16]. In addition, cases of renal malignancy occurring prior to and after dialysis treatment have been collected by the Japanese Society of Dialysis Therapy (1988). This research has shown that malignancy is most common within 1 year before and after the start of dialysis therapy. It may be that a state of immunodeficiency due to uremia causes malignancy, with the treatment modality, whether hemodialysis or CAPD, apparently unrelated to tumor development. There is no relation between the original disease and the incidence of renal cell carcinoma. The incidence of autosomal dominant polycystic kidney disease (ADPKD) was not high, however, and analgesic nephropathy was not evident in our study.

The effect of renal transplantation on the development of renal cell carcinoma in dialysis patients has been investigated previously [Ishikawa I, to be published, 1991].

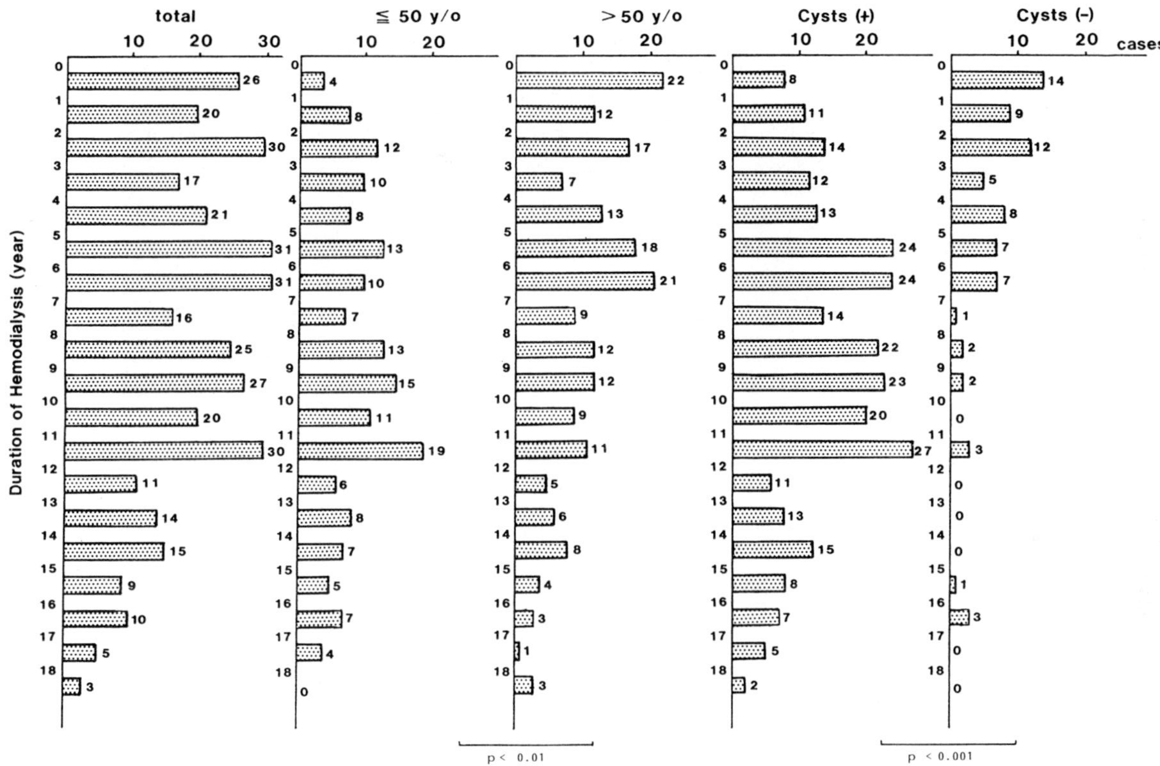

Fig. 3. Patients with renal cell carcinoma ranked (*vertically*) according to duration of hemodialysis (*years*) and (*horizontally*) according to age (*below and above 50 years old (y/o)*) as well as according to the *presence* or *absence* of cysts (+) or (−)

a b c d e f

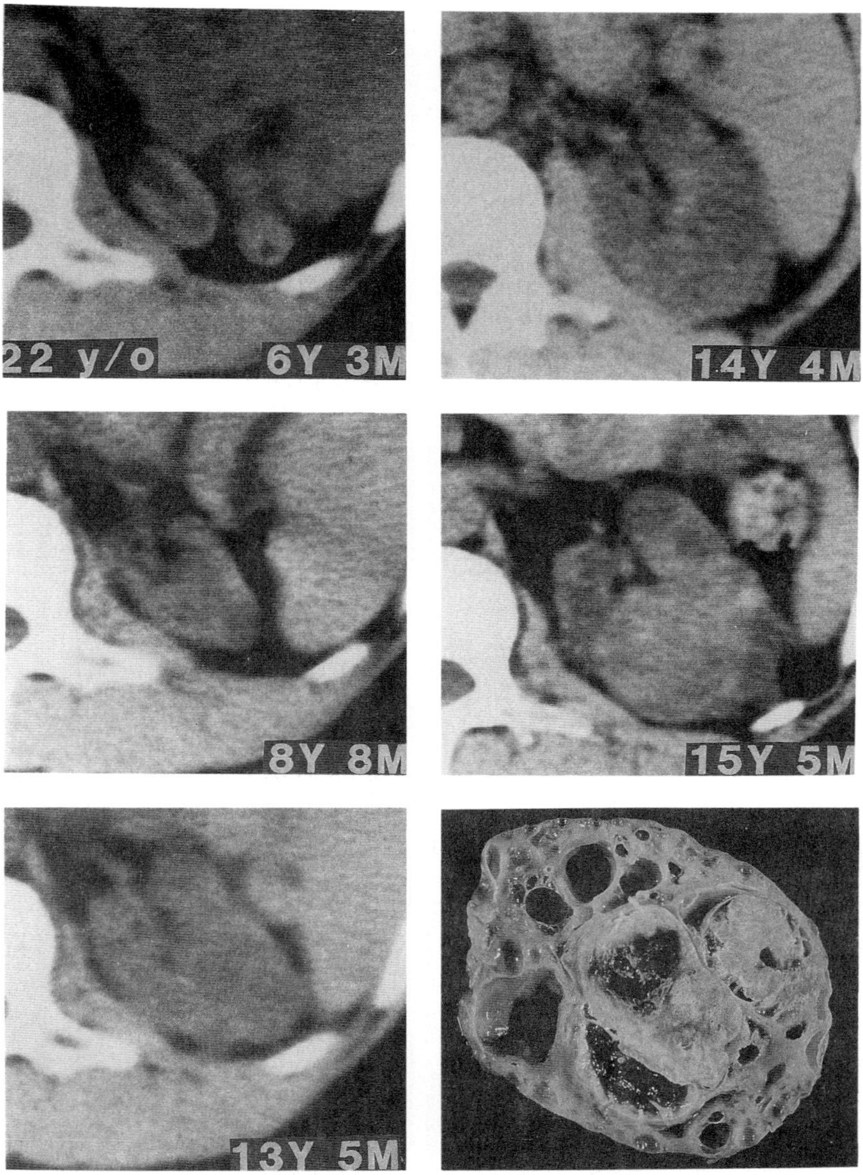

Fig. 4a-f. Development of renal cell carcinoma and acquired renal cysts in long-term hemodialysis patients. The mean kidney size increased over time due to acquired cysts. No trace of renal tumor was noted at 14 years and 4 months of hemodialysis (**d**). A renal tumor 4.5 cm in diameter and surrounded by multiple cysts was seen at 15 years and 5 months (**e**). From [10] with permission)

Acquired cyst regression following transplantation [13] tends to favor the view that the incidence of renal cell carcinoma decreases after such surgery, however, there is no direct evidence for this at present. Rather, Penn and Brunson [17] report a high incidence of renal cell carcinoma after transplantation, especially where cyclosporine is used. These authors list 101 cases with another 16 case reports. We observed one 39 year-old male patient, who was diagnosed as having a 2.4 cm diameter renal cell carcinoma 8 years and 4 months after successful renal transplantation [Ishikawa I, to be published, 1991], but serial CT scans suggested it to have been present before the operation. Therefore, not all renal cell carcinomas diagnosed after transplantation necessarily developed postoperatively, and in fact Noronha et al. point out that there is a low prevalence of metastasizing renal cell carcinomas in transplant recipients [18]. However, a number of case reports do not support this observation [19].

In Japan, as of 1990, 4 cases of renal cell carcinoma have been diagnosed after renal transplantation from 6176 patients, and 364 cases have been diagnosed during hemodialysis from populations of 88553 patients, respectively, undergoing each treatment modality. Since the number of allograft recipients is growing steadily, the question of whether or not the incidence of this cancer decreases after transplantation has become very important.

The biological activity of renal cell carcinomas in dialysis patients is open to question [20]. In a small study, Hughson et al. reported a metastatic rate of 27%, while our own questionnaire survey led us to a figure of 61 patients out of 346 (17.6%) with renal cell carcinoma. Though there are some limitations to questionnaire studies, the following figures were derived: 36 of the 61, 32 male and 4 female patients, displayed extensive acquired cysts, had a mean duration of hemodialysis of 117.1 $\pm$ 48.5 months, and a mean age of 55.9 $\pm$ 11.1 years; and 20 of the 61 showed no or few cysts, had a mean age of 58.6 $\pm$ 37.6 years, and a mean duration of hemodialysis of 50.6 $\pm$ 37.6 months. Tumor size was 6.8 $\pm$ 3.7 cm in the former group and 7.9 $\pm$ 4.5 cm in the latter. The mean duration of hemodialysis is, therefore, significantly longer in cases of metastatic renal cell carcinoma where cystic alteration is extensive than in those cases where there are no or few cysts. It should be noted that reports of metastatic renal cell carcinoma have been increasing recently [21,22].

On the other hand, Hughson et al. describe this tumor as a pathologist's tumor, while other researchers state that they have never seen a metastatic renal cell carcinoma in dialysis patients [8,12,20]; for example, Katz et al. find no such cancer in 353 people undergoing dialysis [8]. Nevertheless, the combination of renal cell carcinoma with acquired renal cystic disease was observed in 276/350 cases (78.9%) in our questionnaire studies.

Evidence for a Causal Relationship Between Acquired Cysts and Renal Cell Carcinoma

Gibson [23] describes four types of relationship between cyst and renal cell carcinoma; (1) chance occurrence of the two diseases together, (2) cystic degeneration or regression or healing of renal cell carcinoma, (3) a tumor originating within a cyst (rare), which we deal with here, and (4) a cyst originating distal to a tumor.

In dialysis patients, there is some circumstantial evidence that a causal link exists between acquired cysts and renal tumors. Extensive cystic transformation often accompanies renal cell carcinoma, and both acquired cystic disease and renal cell carcinoma develop more often in male patients than in female patients. Also, this form of carcinoma occurs in dialysis patients at a relatively younger age than in the general population. Therefore, young male patients with long-term hemodialysis and extensive cystic changes tend to have renal cell carcinoma as a complication [15]. Further support for a causal relation between acquired cysts and renal cell carcinoma is provided by the pathological observation that acquired cystic disease of the kidney often involves a continuum from epithelial hyperplasia to cyst, to atypical cyst, to adenoma and adenocarcinoma [2]. Such pathologic changes have been described by many investigators. Experiments with transgenic mice have proven that epithelial hyperplasia [3] leads directly to cyst and adenoma formation [24].

The origin of renal tumors and of epithelial cells lining the cysts is mainly the proximal tubules; immunohistochemical examination, using lectin [25], together with the study of hippuran excretion have shown that epithelial cells lining cyst walls are derived mainly from proximal tubular cells; Noronha et al. [18] have reported that both cytokeratin and vimentin are stained in microadenomas (therefore, epithelium lining atypical cysts in dialysis patients shows active proliferation). However, there is no direct proof for a causal relationship between acquired cysts and renal tumors, i.e., that acquired cysts cause renal tumors or that cyst walls change to become malignant. It is also probable that the tubular epithelium in acquired cystic kidneys, proliferating either due to ischemia [26] or environmental factors [14], is closely related to the development of renal cell carcinoma, while there is a morphologic gradation from atypical cyst to carcinoma in patients with phacomatosis (atypical cysts and renal cell carcinomas exhibit similar DNA indices and euploidy). In general, it seems evident that acquired cystic kidney demonstrates high proliferative activity that is likely to result in cyst, adenoma, and adenocarcinoma formation.

The mechanisms responsible for the initiation and development of these cysts and tumors have yet to be elucidated; in future investigations we intend to shed light on this area using cytogenetic or molecular biological techniques, such as those used by Vogelstein et al. in their study of chromosomal abnormalities in the progression of colonic polyposis to metastatic adenocarcinoma of the colon [27]. Furthermore, renal cyst growth factor needs to be investigated more thoroughly [28,29].

Screening for Acquired Cysts and Renal Cell Carcinoma

Many, but not all, investigators agree that screening for renal cell carcinoma is necessary. It is also generally agreed that CT scanning is better for this purpose than sonographic examination [30]; however, 60% of cysts are usually smaller than 0.2cm, which is far beyond the detection capability of either of these procedures.

Some conservative investigators point out that patients with end stage renal disease already have a markedly reduced life expectancy and, since the true outcome of acquired cystic disease is not yet known, these investigators are reluctant to apportion resources for screening [31]. Results from our 10 year follow-up and questionnaire studies in Japan lead us to contest this viewpoint; we feel that periodic screening of long-term dialysis patients may be useful for detection of small renal cell carcinomas. Yearly CT screening of patients, especially males, on hemodialysis is highly advisable, and should begin the year treatment starts. The relatively low incidence of renal cell carcinoma in female dialysis patients and in transplant recipients with good graft function suggests that biannual screening would be sufficient in such cases, providing that the prevalence of rapidly growing cancer is proven to be low. The only drawback of screening is, as usual, cost.

References

1. Ishikawa I (1990) Acquired renal cystic disease. In: Gardner KD Jr, Bernstein J (eds) The Cystic Kidney. Kluwer, Dordrecht, pp 351–377
2. Dunnill MS, Millard PR, Oliver D (1977) Acquired cystic disease of the kidneys: A hazard of long-term intermittent maintenance haemodialysis. J Clin Pathol 30:868–877
3. Bernstein J, Evan AP, Gardner KD Jr (1987) Epithelial hyperplasia in human polycystic kidney diseases: Its role in pathogenesis and risk of neoplasia. Am J Pathol 129:92–101
4. Ishikawa I, Moncrief JW, Aguirre F, Brindley BW, Mott CL (1984) Acquired cystic kidney disease in continuous ambulatory peritoneal dialysis patients. In: Maekawa M et al. (eds) Machine free dialysis for patient convenience. ISAO, Cleveland, pp 131–133
5. Ishikawa I, Shikura N, Kitada H, Yuri T, Shinoda A, Nakazawa T (1989) Severity of acquired renal cysts in native kidneys and renal allograft with long-standing poor function. Am J Kidney Dis 14:18–24
6. Grantham JJ, Levine E (1985) Acquired cystic disease: Replacing one kidney disease with another. Kidney Int 28:99–105
7. Gardner KD Jr (1984) Acquired renal cystic disease and renal adenocarcinoma in patients on long-term hemodialysis. New Engl J Med 310:390
8. Katz A, Sombolos K, Oreopoulos DG (1987) Acquired cystic disease of the kidney in association with chronic ambulatory peritoneal dialysis. Am J Kidney Dis 9:426–429
9. Leichter HE, Dietrich R, Salusky IB, Foley J, Cohen AH, Kangarloo H, Fine RN (1988) Acquired cystic kidney disease in children undergoing long-term dialysis. Pediatr Nephrol 2:8–11
10. Ishikawa I, Saito Y, Shikura N, Kitada H, Shinoda A, Suzuki S (1990) Ten-year prospective study on the development of renal cell carcinoma on the development of renal cell carcinoma in dialysis patients. Am J Kidney Dis 16:452–458
11. Fallon B, Williams RD (1989) Renal cancer associated with acquired cystic disease of the kidney and chronic renal failure. Semin Urol 7:228–236
12. Endreny R (1990) Acquired cystic disease. Nephron 55:222
13. Ishikawa I, Yuri T, Kitada H, Shinoda A (1983) Regression of acquired cystic disease of the kidney after successful renal transplantation. Am J Nephrol 3:310–314
14. Grantham JJ (1990) Polycystic kidney disease: Neoplasia in disguise. Am J Kidney Dis 15:110–116
15. Ishikawa I, Shinoda A (1983) Renal adenocarcinoma with or without acquired cysts in chronic hemodialysis patients. Clin Nephrol 20:321–322
16. Chung-Park M, Parveen T, Lam M (1989) Acquired cystic disease of the kidneys and renal cell carcinoma in chronic renal insufficiency without dialysis treatment. Nephron 53: 157–161
17. Penn I, Brunson ME (1988) Cancers after cyclosporine therapy. Transplant Proc 20: 885–892
18. Noronha IL, Ritz E, Waldherr R, Stein G, Fassbinder W (1989) Renal cell carcinoma in dialysis patients with acquired renal cysts. Nephrol Dial Transplant 4:763–769
19. Ludmerer KM, Kissane JM (1988) Clinicopathologic conference. A new chest mass in a 49-year-old man with a transplanted kidney. Am J Med 84:121–128
20. Miller LR, Soffer O, Nassar VH, Kutner MH (1989) Acquired renal cystic disease in end-stage renal disease: an autopsy study of 155 cases. Am J Nephrol 9:322–328

21. MacDougall ML, Welling LW, Wiegmann TB (1987) Renal adenocarcinoma and acquired cystic disease in chronic hemodialysis patients. Am J Kidney Dis 9:166–171
22. Almirall J, Mallofre C, Campistol JM, Montoliu J, Ribalta T, Revert L (1989) Metastatic renal cell carcinoma in hemodialysis patient with acquired renal cystic disease. Nephron 52:96–97
23. Gibson TE (1954) Interrelationship of renal cysts and tumors: report of 3 cases. J Urol 71:241–252
24. MacKay K, Striker LJ, Pinkert CA, Brinster RL, Striker GE (1987) Glomerulosclerosis and renal cysts in mice transgenic for the early region of SV40. Kidney Int 32:827–837
25. Ishikawa I, Horiguchi T, Shikura N (1989) Lectin peroxidase conjugate reactivity in acquired cystic disease of the kidney. Nephron 51:211–214
26. Cohen EP, Elliott WC (1990) The role of ischemia in acquired cystic kidney disease. Am J Kidney Dis 15:55–60
27. Vogelstein B, Fearon ER, Hamilton SR, Kern SE, Preisinger AC, Leppert M, Nakamura Y, White R, Smits AMM, Bos JL (1988) Genetic alterations during colorectal-tumor development. New Engl J Med 319:525–532
28. Marcus MD, Seline P, Long S, Torrence RJ, Huang JS, Clayman RV (1989) Characterization of a renal cyst growth factor (RCGF). J Urol 141:294A
29. Klotz L, Kulcarni C, Mills G (1989) Analysis of a human renal cell growth factor present in sera of patients with end stage renal disease. J Urol 141:297A
30. Taylor AJ, Cohen EP, Erickson SJ, Olson DL, Foley WD (1989) Renal imaging in long-term dialysis patients: a comparison of CT and sonography. AJR 153:765–767
31. Mindell HJ (1989) Imaging studies for screening native kidneys in long-term dialysis patients. AJR 153:768–769

Continuous Ambulatory Peritoneal Dialysis (CAPD)

Chair: Karl D. Nolph (USA)
Yoshindo Kawaguchi (Japan)

Overview of Continuous Ambulatory Peritoneal Dialysis – 1990

KARL D. NOLPH[1]

SUMMARY. As of early 1990, the number of patients maintained on chronic peritoneal dialysis world-wide approached 50,000. In the United States, approximately 80% were on continuous ambulatory peritoneal dialysis (CAPD) while 15% used cycler techniques such as continuous cyclic peritoneal dialysis or nightly peritoneal dialysis. In other countries, the percentage of patients on chronic peritoneal dialysis on CAPD is presumably even higher. Studies from North America, Europe, and Australia-New Zealand all agree that mortalities on CAPD and hemodialysis are not significantly different if populations with similar characteristics are compared. Technique survivals have tended to be lower in CAPD than in hemodialysis, even with population adjustments. Differences in technique survival can, in part, be attributed to the tendency for patients to transfer from CAPD to hemodialysis after severe or frequent peritonitis. However, evidence continues to accumulate from multiple countries that disconnect devices, such as the Y-set, can reduce the rate of peritonitis to less than one episode per 20 patient months. As peritonitis rates decrease, transfer rates decrease and technique survival improves. In some Y-set populations, technique survivals similar to hemodialysis have been reported. Current research interests in CAPD are focused on improved catheters, exit site care, verification that CAPD may preserve GFR better than hemodialysis, manipulation of lymphatic absorption to enhance ultrafiltration, more sophisticated models of peritoneal transport, improved control of calcium and phosphorus without aluminum, and individualization of peritoneal dialysis prescriptions to assure adequacy.

[1]Department of Medicine, University of Missouri, MA436 Health Sciences Center, VA Hospital and Dalton Research Center, Columbia, MO 65212, USA

Demographics

As of early 1990, there were near 50,000 patients world-wide maintained on chronic peritoneal dialysis (A. Holden, Baxter Healthcare, personal communication). In the United States, there were about 19,000 patients on chronic peritoneal dialysis, with approximately 85% of these on continuous ambulatory peritoneal dialysis (CAPD). The other 15% utilized cycler techniques, such as continuous cyclic peritoneal dialysis (CCPD) and nightly peritoneal dialysis.

In an industrial survey of the USA, Europe, Japan, Latin America, South America, and the Far East, the overall population on chronic peritoneal dialysis was found to have grown an average of 13% during calendar year 1989, while the hemodialysis population grew an average of 7% during the same period (A. Holden, Baxter Healthcare, personal communication).

On a worldwide basis, it's estimated that near 13% of dialysis patients are maintained on chronic peritoneal dialysis (mainly CAPD) while 87% are on chronic hemodialysis. This distribution varies markedly from country to country, however. For example, in the United States, the percentage is estimated to be near 17%, while in the United Kingdom, the percentage on chronic peritoneal dialysis is near 45%–50%. In the USA, there are larger PD programs in centers where 39% of the dialysis population is on chronic peritoneal dialysis; also, the percentage of patients on chronic peritoneal dialysis is higher in the midwest than in other sections of the country.

The increasing role of CAPD/CCPD in the United States is reported in the 1989 Annual Data Report of the United States Renal Data System [1]. An increase in the percentage of patients being treated by CAPD/CCPD from 1980 to 1987 is documented. These therapies were used in the 1984 cohort of patients with polycystic kidney disease to a slightly greater extent than in the 1984 cohort with other forms of primary renal disease. This suggests that there are very few patients with polycystic kidney disease that cannot tolerate peritoneal dialysis because of the space occupied by the enlarged kidneys. Near one-third of new end stage renal disease patients in the USA are thought to have diabetic nephropathy and this is reflected in increasing percentages of diabetic patients on all forms of dialysis. In the 1984 cohort, white patients were more likely to be treated with CAPD/CCPD than blacks. Percentages of patients on CAPD/CCPD are much higher in the pediatric population than in the adult population.

Patient Survivals

Numerous comparisons of patient survival on CAPD and hemodialysis have been published [2–6]. All agree that age and the presence or absence of diabetes mellitus are major determinants of mortality on chronic dialysis therapy. Comparisons of CAPD and hemodialysis must be of similar populations or must use statistical tools to correct for the distribution of these and other risk factors. Either by direct comparison of similar populations or by statistical adjustments, mortality rates for CAPD and hemodialysis populations appear to be essentially identical. Some of the reports have suggested even lower mortalities with CAPD in the elderly [5,6]. In the recent report from Australia/New Zealand, lower mortality rates with CAPD were found in diabetics [5].

Technique Survivals–the Impact of Falling Peritonitis Rates

Until recently, most comparisons of technique survivals between CAPD and hemodialysis have shown better results with hemodialysis [3,5,6]. Technique survival refers to percentages of patients, by actuarial analysis, still on dialysis and still on their original dialysis treatment. Death, kidney transplantation, or recovery of renal function are considered losses to risk and not dropout events. A technique failure mainly implies transfer to another mode of dialysis. Many factors may contribute to decisions to transfer, such as development of visual difficulties, severe arthritis, or stroke. Failure to control serum concentrations of nitrogenous metabolites or failure to control edema are rare reasons for transfer (probably less than 2% of patients). Doubtful patients are often given a trial on CAPD, since the training period is short and they can be promptly transferred if things do not go well. Although this can account for CAPD transfers, in part, it allows some doubtful patients to succeed and be offered the benefits of the home therapy. Severe or frequent peritonitis is probably the main reason for the lower technique survival rates with CAPD than with hemodialysis. Registry data from North America and Canada suggest that peritonitis can account for over 30% of transfers from CAPD to hemodialysis [3,7]. However, since those reports were made, peritonitis rates have been decreasing in Europe, Canada, and the United States with the use of disconnect devices such as the Y-set [8,9]. Rates of less than one episode every 20 months are frequently reported. In a population of patients on CAPD for over five years with the Y-set, 49% were still peritonitis-free after five years [4]. Technique survivals similar to those of hemodialysis are reported in such programs. One Italian center using the Y-set has reported technique survivals that are actually better than those on hemodialysis [9]. A multicenter study in the USA has been monitoring technique survivals and has shown improved technique survivals in more recently trained patient cohorts [10].

Peritoneal Membrane Stability

Numerous studies have demonstrated preservation of peritoneal membrane function over many years [4,11,12]. The use of dialysis solutions containing lactate (rather than acetate), the rapid diagnosis and treatment of peritonitis with early catheter removal in refractory cases, and the avoidance of chlorhexidine as an antiseptic have dramatically decreased the incidence of peritoneal sclerosis in countries where it was previously observed [13]. Over time, many patients show some increase in peritoneal permeability and an increased need for more hypertonic exchanges. Such changes may be associated with submesothelial fibrosis, loss of microvilli, and patchy mesothelial denudation [14–16]. Such changes do not seem to progress, however, to advanced peritoneal sclerosis and appear to be compatible with long-term peritoneal dialysis treatment of 10 years or more.

The Manipulation of Ultrafiltration

The major osmotic agent for peritoneal dialysis is still glucose. There was an interest in large molecular weight polymers as potentially slowly-absorbed osmotic agents, but these were found to be absorbed at higher rates than predicted, presumably by convection through subdiaphragmatic lymphatics [17–19]. Solutions containing glucose polymers that are nearly iso-osmotic with plasma are under investigation, but the accumulation of maltose and serum with such solutions mandates additional studies before they are used widely [18].

Net ultrafiltration is reduced substantially by fluid reabsorption through the subdiaphragmatic lymphatics [17]. The addition of agents such as neostigmine and phosphatidylcholine to peritoneal dialysis solution has decreased lymphatic absorption and increased net ultrafiltration [20,21].

Does CAPD Preserve Residual Renal Function Better than Hemodialysis?

In chronic peritoneal dialysis patients, as in chronic hemodialysis patients, residual renal function tends to decline, but there is increasing evidence that residual renal function may be better preserved in patients on chronic peritoneal dialysis [22–25], although additional studies are needed to verify these preliminary observations. There are possible mechanisms to explain such differences, such as (1) the undesirable effects of recurring hypotension and renal ischemia on hemodialysis and (2) the release, during hemodialysis, of cytokines which damage residual renal tissue.

Peritoneal Dialysis Prescriptions to Achieve Adequacy

In our center, we try to provide each patient with at least 40–50 liters of creatinine clearance per week per 1.73 M^2 body surface area. This total clearance represents the sum of dialysis clearance and the residual renal clearance. Patients are classified by the peritoneal equilibration test as high transporters, high average transporters, low average transporters, or low transporters [26]. Although high transporters have high clearances, they also have rapid glucose absorption, early loss of the osmotic gradient for ultrafiltration, and low drainage volumes. They often do better on short cycle techniques, such as nightly intermittent peritoneal dialysis or daytime ambulatory peritoneal dialysis without a nocturnal exchange. Low transporters have poor clearances and good drain volumes. They often need large volume exchanges or more than four exchanges per day to maintain the weekly clearances in the desired range.

The development of edema or an increase in serum creatinine concentration, in our experience, more often reflects the effects of a decline in residual renal function than a change in peritoneal membrane transport. It is important to adjust the peritoneal dialysis prescription to maintain adequate balance of sodium and water and to maintain total clearances in the desirable range as patients lose their residual renal function [27].

The peritoneal dialysis prescription can also be adjusted to provide a targeted weekly urea clearance [28]. The weekly urea clearance is usually normalized to total body water. This urea kinetic modeling approach to CAPD was a major focus of many presentations at the 10th Annual Peritoneal Dialysis Conference in Dallas, Texas, in February of 1990. Based on studies now available and to be published in the Proceedings of this meeting, it would seem desirable to aim for a dietary protein intake of 1.0–1.2 per kg of ideal body weight and a total weekly urea clearance (the sum of dialysis clearance and residual renal function) of at least 1.4 times the volume of total body water. Recommendations for a minimum value for this ratio at the present time range from 1.4 to 2.2. Clinical studies now underway may allow us to target the minimum value recommended more precisely.

CAPD usually provides weekly clearances which are only 50%–60% of those provided by standard three-times-per-week hemodialysis therapy [29]. The peak concentration hypothesis proposes that much higher weekly urea clearances are needed with an intermittent therapy such as hemodialysis in order to maintain the serum urea concentration at all times below or equal to the steady state concentration of CAPD. If hemodialysis therapy three times per week were to provide an overall weekly urea clearance only equal to that of CAPD, the serum urea nitrogen concentration would be above the steady state CAPD value for significant portions of the time, especially on the day before each treatment. If peak concentrations of small molecular weight solutes correlate with uremic symptomatology, then intermittent therapies have an inherent need to provide higher clearances than continuous therapy. This hypothesis has been invoked to explain why lower urea clearances on CAPD appear adequate to alleviate clinical symptoms apparently as well as hemodialysis. It is important to remember that control of serum urea nitrogen concentration alone is not an adequate index of dialysis adequacy; the serum urea nitrogen concentration must be considered in relationship to dietary protein intake and the protein catabolic rate.

Short cycle clearances can be increased 10%–20% using cyclers that incorporate the new tidal peritoneal dialysis approach [30,31]. Tidal peritoneal dialysis cycles frequent volumes, usually of 1000–1500 ml, on top of an indwelling reservoir of 1000–1500 ml. This maintains better solution-membrane contact and delays complete drainage until the end of the total treatment. With complete drainage techniques at the end of every cycle, there are periods during the treatment when very little fluid remains in the peritoneal cavity, resulting in an inherent inefficiency.

There is good evidence that attention to peritoneal dialysis prescriptions and anticipation of changes as residual renal function declines can reduce unnecessary dropout from CAPD programs [27].

Peritoneal Dialysis Access

It is my impression that one of the most important developments in peritoneal catheters has been the permanent bend or "Swan Neck" configuration [32]. At the April 1990 meeting of the American Society for Artificial Internal Organs in Washington, D.C., Dr. Twardowski reviewed experiences with the Missouri Swan Neck Catheter that will be published in the upcoming Transactions. Catheter survivals are better than those reported with other types of catheters and are better than our experiences with other types of catheters at the University of Missouri. Complications, such as exit-cuff extrusion, catheter tip migration, and refractory exit-site infections, seem to have been drastically reduced.

General Comments

I have given brief overviews of the status of chronic peritoneal dialysis worldwide in 1990 and associated areas of interest. Other speakers in this session will address some of these topics in more detail and will address some other areas of interest that I have not mentioned.

Dr. Rippe will update our understanding of the Kinetics of Peritoneal Transport. Dr. Keshaviah will go into more detail on the comparison of the adequacy of CAPD and hemodialysis. Dr. Khanna will expand on the manipulation of lymphatics to control net ultrafiltration. Dr. Maiorca will update the findings with the Y-set. Dr. Gokal will review the current approach to control of serum calcium and serum phosphorus concentrations on CAPD with minimal exposure to aluminum.

References

1. United States Renal Data System 1989 Annual Report, The National Institutes of Health, National Institute of Diabetes and Digestive and Kidney Diseases, August 1989. Bethesda, MD.
2. Nolph KD (1988) Comparison of continuous ambulatory peritoneal dialysis and hemodialysis. Kidney Int 33:S123
3. Nolph KD (1990) Clinical results with peritoneal dialysis – registry experiences. In: Twardowski ZJ, Nolph KD, Khanna R, Stein J (eds) Contemporary issues in nephrology: peritoneal dialysis. Churchill-Livingston, New York, pp 127–144
4. Maiorca R, Cancarini GC, Camerini C, Brunori G, Manili L, Movilli E, Feller P, Mombelloni S (1989) Is CAPD competitive with haemodialysis for long-term treatment of uraemic patients? Nephrol Dial Transpl 4:244–253
5. Disney APS (1989) Twelfth Report of the Australia and New Zealand combined Dialysis and Transplant Registry. Queen Elizabeth Hospital, Woodville, South Australia
6. Maiorca R, Vonesh E, Cancarini GC, Cantaluppi A, Manili L, Brunori G, Camerini C, Feller P, Strada A (1988) A six-year comparison of patient and technique survivals in CAPD and HD. Kidney Int 34:518–524
7. Lindblad AS, Novak JW, Nolph KD (1989) Continuous ambulatory peritoneal dialysis in the USA – final report of the National CAPD Registry 1981–1988. Kluwer, Dordrecht
8. Canadian CAPD Clinical Trials Group (1989) Peritonitis in CAPD: a multi-center randomized clinical trial comparing the Y-connector disinfectant system to standard systems. Perit Dial Int 9:159–163
9. Caballi PL, Viglino G, Goia F, Cottino R, Mariano F, Gandolfo C (1989) CAPD versus hemodialysis: seven years of experience. Adv Perit Dial 5:52–55
10. Holden A, Gaumer G (1987) Best demonstrated practices program promoting CAPD patient retention in the United States. Advances in CAPD. Proceedings of the seventh annual CAPD conference, Kansas City, United States, 3:186–191
11. Krediet RT, Arisz L (1989) Fluid and solute transport across the peritoneum during CAPD. Perit Dial Int 9:15–25
12. Park MS, Lee J, Lee MS, Baick SH, Hwang SD, Lee HB (1989) Peritoneal solute clearances after four years of continuous ambulatory peritoneal dialysis (CAPD). Perit Dial Int 9:75–78
13. An International Cooperative Study Third Report with 40 participating centers (1985) A Survey of ultrafiltration in continuous ambulatory peritoneal dialysis. In: Khanna R, Nolph KD, Prowant B, Twardowski ZJ, Oreopoulos DG (eds) Advances in continuous ambulatory

peritoneal dialysis. Proceedings of the fifth annual CAPD conference, Kansas City, United States. Toronto Press, Toronto, pp 79–86
14. Dobbie JW (1989) Morphology of the peritoneum in CAPD. Blood Purif 7:74
15. Dobbie JW (1989) Monitoring peritoneal histopathology in peritoneal dialysis: the role of a biopsy registry. Dial Transplant 18:319–325, 335
16. Pollock CA, Ibels LS, Eckstein RP, Graham JC, Caterson RJ, Mahony JF, Ross Sheil AG (1989) Peritoneal morphology on maintenance dialysis. Am J Nephrol 9:198–204
17. Mactier RA, Khanna R (1989) Absorption of fluid and solute from the peritoneal cavity: theoretic and therapeutic implications and applications. Trans Am Soc Artif Intern Organs 35:122–131
18. Mistry CD, Gokal R (1989) Alternative osmotic agents. Blood Purif 7:109–114
19. Henderson IS (1989) Composition of peritoneal dialysis solutions: potential hazards. Blood Purification 7:86–94
20. Mactier RA, Khanna R, Moore H, Twardowski ZJ, Nolph KD (1988) Pharmacological reduction of lymphatic absorption from the peritoneal cavity increases net ultrafiltration and solution clearances in peritoneal dialysis. Nephron 50:229–232
21. Mactier RA, Khanna R, Twardowski ZJ (1988) Influence of phosphatidylcholine on lymphatic absorption during peritoneal dialysis in the rat. Perit Dial Int 8:179–186
22. Rottembourg J, Issad B, Gallego JL, Degoulet P, Aime F, Gueffaf B, Legrain M (1982) Evolution of residual renal function in patients undergoing maintenance haemodialysis or continuous ambulatory peritoneal dialysis. Proc Eur Dial Transplant Assoc 19:397–401
23. Rottembourg J, Issad B, Poignet JL, Strippoli P, Balducci A, Slama G, Gahl GM (1983) Residual renal function and control of blood glucose levels in insulin dependent diabetic patients treated by CAPD. In: Keen H, Legrain M (eds) Prevention and treatment of diabetic nephropathy. Lancaster, Boston, pp 339–359
24. Cancarini GC, Brunori G, Camerini C, Brasa S, Manili L, Maiorca R (1986) Renal function recovery and maintenance of residual diuresis in CAPD and hemodialysis. Perit Dial Bull 6:77–79
25. Lysaght M, Vonesh E, Ibels L, Lindholm B, Nolph KD, Pollock C, Prowant B, Farrell P (1989) Decline of residual renal function in hemodialysis and CAPD patients: a risk adjusted growth function analysis. Nephrol Dial Transpl 4:499
26. Twardowski ZJ (1989) Clinical value of standardized equilibration tests in CAPD patients. Blood Purif 7:95–108
27. Twardowski ZJ, Khanna R, Nolph KD (1987) Peritoneal dialysis modifications to avoid CAPD drop-out. Advances in continuous ambulatory peritoneal dialysis. Proceedings of the seventh annual CAPD conference. Kansas City, United States. 3:171–178
28. Lysaght MJ, Pollock CA, Hallet MD, Ibels LS, Farrell PC (1989) The relevance of ureal kinetic modeling to CAPD. Trans Am Soc Artif Intern Organs 35:784–790
29. Keshaviah PR, Nolph KD, Van Stone JC (1989) The peak concentration hypotheses: a urea kinetic approach to comparing the adequacy of CAPD and hemodialysis. Perit Dial Int 9:257–260
30. Twardowski ZJ (1989) New approaches to intermittent peritoneal dialysis therapies. In: Nolph K (ed) Peritoneal dialysis, 3rd edn. Kluwer, Dordrecht, pp 133–151
31. Twardowski ZJ (1990) Dialysis adequacy and new cycler techniques. In: Twardowski ZJ, Nolph KD, Khanna R, Stein JH (eds) Peritoneal dialysis. Churchill-Livingston, New York, pp 67–100
32. Khanna R (1990) Peritoneal dialysis access. In: Twardowski ZJ, Nolph KD, Khanna R, Stein JH (eds) Peritoneal dialysis. Churchill-Livingston, New York, pp 101–126

Understanding the Kinetics of Peritoneal Transport

BENGT RIPPE[1], GUNNAR STELIN[1], and BÖRJE HARALDSSON[1,2]

SUMMARY. In this article we describe the characteristics of peritoneal barrier exchange in terms of a three-pore model of membrane permselectivity. The peritoneal membrane is thus simulated to have a large number of small pores of radius 40–55 Å, a small number of large pores of radius 200–300 Å, and an abundance of transcellular pores of radius 4–5 Å. According to this model, solutes < 25 Å in radius were found to be permeating across the peritoneal membrane mainly by means of diffusion across the small pores, whereas solutes larger than 40 Å were found to reach the peritoneal cavity exclusively by unidirectional convection through the large pores. In addition, water was simulated to be partly transported through the transcellular "ultrapores," which are not accessible to hydrophilic solute permeation. Small solute absorption from the peritoneal cavity was found to occur by diffusion across small pores. However, molecules larger than 30 Å in radius (Mol. weight > 30000) seemed to be absorbed from the peritoneal cavity exclusively via non-size-selective lymphatic drainage. Applying the three-pore model to literature peritoneal equilibration test (PET) data, solute mass transfer area coefficients (PS) appeared to be higher during the first 30 mins of dwell time than subsequently. Reductions in solute PS-values with dwell time are discussed in terms of a progressively increasing impact of interstitial "unstirred layers" on small solute permeation over the course of the cycle.

Introduction

Water and solutes exchanging between the blood and the peritoneal cavity have to permeate at least three serial morphological barriers: 1] the walls of the mesenteric and peritoneal capillaries, 2] the peritoneal interstitium, and 3] the highly permeable mesothelium. In addition, "unstirred layers" in the peritoneal dialysate and/or in the interstitium contribute to the peritoneal barrier characteristics, at least with respect

[1]Dept of Nephrology, Sahlgrenska Hospital, S-413 45 Göteborg, Sweden
[2]Dept of Physiology, University of Göteborg, S-400 33 Göteborg, Sweden

to small solute exchange. Conceivably, however, the capillary walls would be the principal barrier determining transperitoneal fluid and solute exchange, and we have tested the validity of this assumption.

Functional Ultrastructure of Peritoneal Capillary Walls

Peritoneal capillaries belong to the continuous type, as found in, e.g., muscle, heart, and skin. With respect to transcapillary solute exchange, continuous microvascular walls show a bimodal size selectivity. Functionally they behave as membranes having a large number of "small pores" (radius 40–60 Å), accounting for 90%–95% of the total hydraulic conductance (UF-coefficient), and a very small number (1 part per 5000–15000 small pores) of "large pores" (radius 200–300 Å), accounting for 5%–10% of the UF-coefficient [1–2]. Morphologically the small pores correspond to the clefts (slits) between individual endothelial cells. While lipid-soluble species (e.g., O_2 and CO_2) can permeate the endothelial cell membrane proper, the intercellular clefts are the major exchange routes for water and small solutes. These clefts have a complex structure, but small solutes and water can pass from the capillary lumen to the interstitium via tortuous spaces within the clefts, here created by an irregular labyrinth of cell-to-cell adhesion lines [3]. The average cleft width appears to be 200 Å, except for a few "restricted" portions being 70–80 Å in width.

The exact morphological counterpart to the large pores, allowing albumin and larger proteins to filter between plasma and interstitium, has not yet been identified. Large pores may be represented either by interendothelial "gaps," similar to the mentioned clefts but wider, or, less likely, by channels formed by fused plasmalemmal vesicles. Recent evidence strongly indicates that vesicular transport (transcytosis) is not the likely morphological candidate for the large pores [4].

To describe both solute and fluid transfer across vascular walls, capillary physiologists have long proposed the existence of a third exchange route between blood and tissue, namely a transcellular (ultra-small pore) pathway (radius 4–5 Å), accounting for 1%–7% of the total capillary hydraulic conductance [1,5,6]. Hence, the classical two-pore model of vascular permeability may actually be regarded as a "three-pore" model [1].

Two-Pore Model of Peritoneal Exchange

We have tested the hypothesis that the walls of the microvessels in the blood-peritoneal barrier are the major determinants of transperitoneal exchange. Thus, we have determined the blood-peritoneal clearances of several endogenous substances in patients undergoing continuous ambulatory peritoneal dialysis (CAPD), and we have analyzed the data according to current concepts in microvascular physiology.

Measurements were performed in the early phase of 1.36% Dianeal dwells when intraperitoneal (i.p.) solute concentrations were near zero. Transperitoneal "unidirectional" clearances were assessed as transperitoneal mass transfer per time unit (during 10–15 min) as divided by the mean solute concentration gradient through the peritoneal membrane. Data were analyzed according to recent developments of the two-pore theory [2] and according to non-linear solute flux formalism [7], employing current hydrodynamic theories to describe restricted diffusion [6] and reflection coefficients [8] in cylindrical pores.

The first step of a two-pore analysis of membrane transport involves the partitioning of *net* transmembrane filtration flow (J_v) into the separate *partial* volume flows occurring through the small pores (radius 40–60 Å) and the large pores (radius 200–300 Å), respectively. How to do that from J_v, utilizing measured clearances of at least two solutes larger than 50 Å in radius (in order to obtain the large volume flow), has been described previously [2]. Note that regardless of the direction of the net transmembrane fluid transport, there is always blood-peritoneal filtration across large pores, since the "effective" colloid osmotic pressure gradient across these pores is very low (near zero). It is also worth noting that protein transport across large pores is always convective (filtrative) for normal capillary pressures [2,4].

When experimental unidirectional clearance data from patients in CAPD, obtained at a net blood-peritoneal volume flow of 1 ml/min [9], were adapted to the two-pore model of membrane permselectivity as outlined above [10], we obtained a small pore radius (r_s) of 47±1.02 Å (±SE) and a large pore radius (r_L) of 305±41 Å. The so-called "unrestricted total pore area over unit diffusion path length" ($A_o/\Delta x$) became 45000±2300 cm, while the large pore volume flow was 0.052±0.006 ml/min. The fractional UF-coefficient (L_pS) accounted for by large pores (denoted α_L) was estimated to be 0.055. This "simple" two pore model was found to comply very well with a majority of previously published peritoneal solute flux data obtained in CAPD patients and in animal models [10].

Three-Pore Model of Peritoneal Permselectivity

When modelling fluid transport across microvascular walls, capillary physiologists conventionally take into account a so-called "transcellular" fluid conductive pathway, or "ultra-small pore" pathway, accounting for 1%–5% [6] of L_pS, besides the small and large pores [1,5,6]. Thus, we have extended our analysis to comprise all three fluid conductive pathways existing in microvascular membranes. In this extended analysis we also included the impact of peritoneal lymphatic drainage upon net transperitoneal fluid transfer (J_v). Furthermore, we assumed that the transperitoneal glucose concentration gradient (ΔC_g) generates the major crystalloid osmotic pressure gradient determining the peritoneal fluid shifts (J_V). Partitioning of fluid fluxes between the three sets of pores in this analysis was performed according to:

$$J_{v_n} = \alpha_n\, L_pS\, (\Delta P - \sigma_{prot,n}\, \Delta\pi + \Delta C_g\, R\, T\, \sigma_{g,n}) \qquad (1)$$

Here "n" refers to either small pores (s), large pores (L), or transcellular pores (c). α stands for *fractional*, and L_pS for *total* peritoneal hydraulic conductance (UF-coefficient), while RT is the product of the gas constant and the temperature in degrees Kelvin. σ[3] refers to the osmotic "reflection coefficient" for either total pro-

[3] σ denotes the fraction of the *ideal* solute osmotic pressure gradient (exerted across a semipermeable membrane), which is operative across a leaky membrane. σ equals 1 for a semipermeable membrane, from which the molecule is totally reflected; σ equals zero if the membrane is freely permeable to the solute

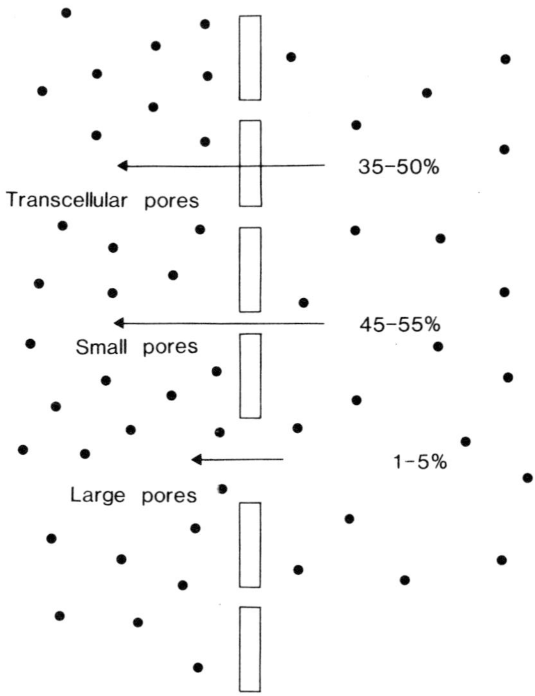

Fig. 1. The partitioning of transperitoneal fluid flows between the different peritoneal pathways, as modelled for a large glucose osmotic gradient across the peritoneal membrane. In this simulation the transcellular pores account for only 1.5% of the total peritoneal ultrafiltration (*UF*)-coefficient

tein (prot) or for glucose (g). ΔP represents the hydrostatic pressure gradient existing between the peritoneal capillaries and the peritoneal fluid and $\Delta\pi$ the transperitoneal colloid osmotic pressure gradient. The difference between the two major "Starling forces," ($\Delta P - \Delta\pi$), was set to ≈ -12 mmHg, whereas L_pS was set to 0.08 ml/min per mm Hg [10]. Reflection coefficients for glucose and albumin (total protein) were modelled by the Drake and Davis equation [8] using the pore radii determined in our previous two-pore analysis. Thus, the tentative small pore radius was set to 47 Å and the large pore radius to 300 Å. The fractional small pore and large pore L_pS values (α_s and α_L) were set to 0.930 and 0.055, respectively.

We were surprised to find that if α_c was only 0.015–0.02, then approximately *one half* of the peritoneal fluid filtration was found to occur transcellularly, when peritoneal fluid transport was induced by a large glucose osmotic pressure gradient [10]. This is illustrated in Fig. 1. This offers an explanation for the fact that small solute sieving coefficients (Φ), as measured for large glucose induced ultrafiltration rates, are close to 0.5–0.6 during peritoneal dialysis, and not near unity, as predicted by the strict two-pore theory.

The total fluid filtration occurring across the peritoneal membrane ($J_{V_{tot}}$) is obtained by summing up the partial small pore, large pore, and transcellular volume flows (J_{V_S}, J_{V_L} and J_{V_c}, respectively):

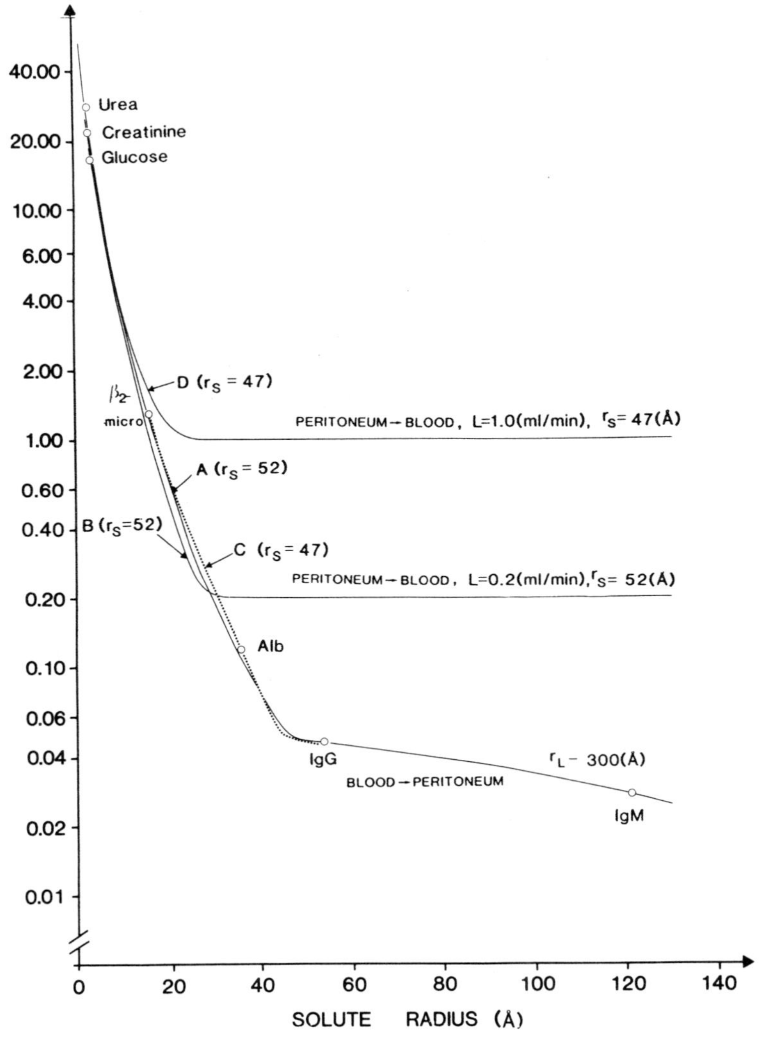

Fig. 2. Semi-log plot of simulated solute clearance as a function of mol. radius, employing the parameters fitting to the data of Rippe et al. [9], as indicated in the figure. Curves *A* and *B* represent clearances simulated for a peritoneal lymph flow of 0.2 ml/min and curves *C* and *D* for a lymph flow of 1.00 ml/min. Curves *A* (r_s = 52) and *C* (r_s = 47) and simulated for transport in the direction from the blood to the peritoneal cavity, whereas curves *B* and *D* show solute clearance vs solute radius for transport occurring in the opposite direction due to transcapillary and lymphatic absorption. (Reprinted from *Kidney International* with permission [10])

$$J_{V_{tot}} = J_{V_S} + J_{V_L} + J_{V_c} \tag{2}$$

Furthermore, the *net* intraperitoneal volume alteration is described by

$$J_V = J_{V_{tot}} - L \tag{3}$$

where L stands for the lymphatic flow from the peritoneal cavity.

For the three-pore model, and for a $J_{V_{tot}}$ of 1.20 ml/min (occurring for a ΔC_g of 34 mmoles/l) and L = 0.2 (ml/min) [11], the small pore volume flow (J_{V_S}) is only 0.471 ml/min, using the parameters presented above, and *not* 1.148 (1.20 minus 0.052) ml/min, as would be predicted by the simple two-pore theory. This reduction in calculated volume flow across the small pores causes the small pore radius estimate to increase in the three-pore analysis. In all other respects the two analyses presented are identical.

Figure 2 represents a semi-log plot of "unidirectional" solute clearance (approximately equalling "mass transfer area coefficients" for small solutes) as a function of molecular radius [10]. Curves are simulated to fit experimental data [9] for transport both in the blood-peritoneal (curves A and C) and peritoneal-to-blood direction (curves B and D), and for a peritoneal lymph flow being set to 0.2 ml/min [11] (curves A and B) and to 1 ml/min [12] (curves C and D).

Transport of small solutes seemed to occur by restricted diffusion through "small pores" of radius ≈ 52 Å for L = 0.2 (ml/min), or of radius 47 Å for L being set to 1.00 ml/min, whereas the large macromolecules, IgG and IgM, appeared to have reached the peritoneal cavity by unidirectional convection (directed from the blood to the peritoneal cavity) through large pores of radius ≈ 300 Å.

Note the assymmetry of peritoneal transport! According to the model, solutes larger than 30 Å in radius are absorbed from the peritoneal cavity due to non-size-selective convection by lymphatic drainage. Thus, there is no local back transport of large solutes to plasma by direct diffusion across blood capillary walls. Note also the large difference between the unidirectional clearance (mass transfer area coefficient) of urea (29 ml/min) and the blood-peritoneal clearance of albumin (0.1 ml/min), the urea/albumin clearance ratio being near 300! In comparison, the ratio of the *free* diffusion coefficients for urea/albumin is 14. Indeed, transperitoneal transport of albumin must occur by *restricted* and not by free diffusion/convection.

Understanding the Kinetics of Solute Equilibration Between Blood and Peritoneal Cavity

Analyses of transperitoneal solute equilibration, as measured, e.g., in peritoneal equilibration tests (PETs), are complicated by the fact that fluid and solute transport occur simultaneously. Furthermore, only approximately one half of the net volume flow carries solute, namely J_{V_S}. Thus, i.p. solute concentrations are affected by dilution. Setting L = 0.2 (ml/min) [11] and employing the assumptions for the three-pore model outlined above, the relationship between J_{V_S} and J_V was previously derived to be approximately [10]:

$$J_{V_S} = 0.649\, J_V - 0.178 \tag{4}$$

The combined diffusive and convective solute transport, in terms of "unidirectional clearance" (Cl) during a relatively short time period $(t_1 - t_2)$, may be obtained as outlined above, i.e., as solute flux divided by the transperitoneal solute concentration, or as

$$Cl = \frac{\overline{V_D}}{t_2 - t_1} \ln \frac{(C_B - C_{D_1})}{(C_B - C_{D_2})} \tag{5}$$

where $\overline{V_D}$ is the mean intraperitoneal (i.p.) volume during the measurement, C_B is the blood concentration of solute and C_{D_1} and C_{D_2} are the i.p. solute concentrations at time t_1 and t_2, respectively (cf [10]).

The solute mass transfer area coefficient (PS) may now be solved from the so-called non-linear flux equation (6) as arranged for "unidirectional" transport, i.e.:

$$PS = J_{V_s} (1 - \sigma_s) \Big/ \ln \left\{ \frac{Cl}{Cl - J_{V_s} (1 - \sigma_s)} \right\} \tag{6}$$

Here the subscript "s" stands for "small pores," and hence, σ_s denotes the small pore solute reflection coefficient (being of the order of 0.02 for small solutes), whereas all other factors have been defined above. Note also that J_{V_S} is the *small pore* volume flow.

We have employed equations 4, 5, and 6 to calculate PS values from PET data previously published [13]. PS was determined sequentially for various time intervals (30–60 min) of the PET cycle, and likewise, sequential values for $\overline{V_D}$ were obtained from an arbitrary function determining the i.p. dialysate volume vs time relationship (cf [14]):

$$V_t = V_o + a_1 (1 - e^{-kt}) - a_2 t \tag{7}$$

Here V_t represents the i.p. dialysate volume as a function of time. V_o is i.p. volume at time zero, and a_1, a_2, and k are some arbitrary coefficients that determine the change occurring in V_t over dwell time [14]. The parameters a_1, a_2, and k were fitted to the average drained volume vs time data published by Twardowski et al. [13] for 22.5 per cent Dianeal in PET tests. The following parameter values were selected: $V_o = (2050 + 300)$ (ml) (instilled volume + residual volume), $k = 0.01$ (min^{-1}), $a_1 = 700$ (ml), and $a_2 = 1.25$ (ml/min). The arithmetic mean value of intraperitoneal volume obtained at t_1 and t_2 in each interval, as calculated according to equation 7, was employed for $\overline{V_D}$.

Figure 3 displays PS values for creatinine, as calculated from published PET data [13] (mean value curve, curve depicting PET data being + 1 SD "above mean" and − 1 SD "below mean," respectively) according to equations 4–7, for 0–30 min, 1–2 h and 3–4 h. Note that PS values for 0–30 min seem to be higher than subsequent values. This may, at least partly, explain why the "initial clearance" data determined by Rippe et al. [9] during the "early" phase (0–30 min) of the dwell are much higher than the average PS values obtained from all the PETs analyzed here for creatinine. Alternatively, our previous investigation [9] comprises a subpopulation of CAPD patients with unusually high solute clearances. However, there are good reasons to believe that the impact of interstitial factors, such as "unstirred fluid layers," may increase with dwell time and lower the "apparent" PS progressively over the dwell.

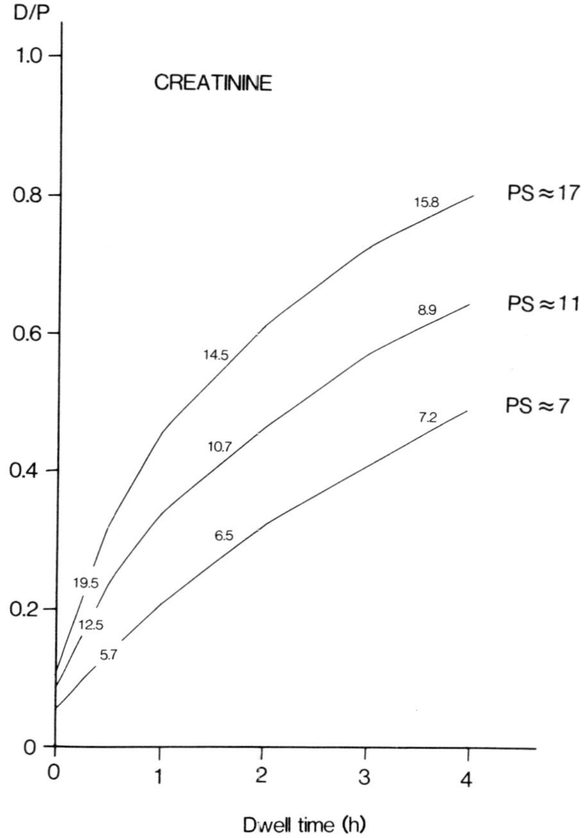

Fig. 3. Dialysate to plasma creatinine concentration ratios (*D/P*), vs dwell time in a population studied by Twardowsky et al. [13] using the "peritoneal equilibration test" as introduced by these authors. PS values calculated according to eqs. 4–7 are indicated in the Fig. for 0–30 min, 60–120 min and 180–240 min, the other calculated results being left out (for didactic reasons). Average approximate PS values calculated for all sequential determinations in each curve are shown *to the right*. Only average D/P vs time curve (*middle curve*) and curves designating D/P vs time relationships being +1 SD "above mean" (*upper curve*) and −1 SD "below mean" (*lower curve*), respectively, are depicted in this figure

This is probably because the large ("stirring") peritoneal ultrafiltrate (UF) flows, existing initially, will gradually "dissipate" with cycle time.

Lymph Flow From the Peritoneal Cavity in CAPD

The parameters determining the intraperitoneal dialysate volume (V(t)) vs time curve (cf eq. 7) may be interpreted into meaningful phenomenological coefficients; this is discussed at some length elsewhere [14]. Concerning the parameter a_2 of equation 7, which represents the fluid absorption occurring from the peritoneal cavity to the blood when all major *crystalloid* osmotic concentration gradients have come to equilibrium, it has been most controversial whether a_2 is mainly accounted for by lymphatic drainage or by fluid absorption through the capillary walls [11]. We have shown previously [14] that a_2 can be described by:

$$a_2 = - L_pS (\Delta P - \sigma_{prot} \Delta\pi_{prot}) + L \quad (8)$$

The numerical value for the expression within the parenthesis is approximately −10 to −11 mmHg. Hence, setting L_pS to 0.08 ml/min per mmHg, as employed above, and a_2 to 1.2–1.3 ml/min, as usually measured for dwell times exceeding 5–6 hours, yields a lymphatic flow (L) of 0.4–0.5 ml/min. Thus, fluid absorption from the peritoneal cavity must occur due to *both* lymphatic flow *and* due to osmotic fluid transport directly into the capillaries [15]. There may, however, be situations when lymphatic absorption is the predominating peritoneal fluid absorptive mechanism. Normally *far from all* of the peritoneal fluid absorption would be lymph flow.

Concluding Remarks

In conclusion, the exchange characteristics of the peritoneal membrane can be adequately described by a three-pore model of membrane selectivity. In this respect the “peritoneal membrane” mimics the continuous capillary wall. Thus, the capillary walls in the peritoneum are likely to be the principal structures determining the blood-peritoneal exchange.

Acknowledgments. This study was supported by grants Nos. 8285 and 8796 from the Swedish Medical Research Council.

References

1. Taylor AE, Granger DN (1984) Exchange of macromolecules across the microcirculation. In: Renkin EM, Michel CC (eds) The cardiovascular system. Am Physiol Soc, pp 467–520 (Handbook of physiology, Sect 2, vol IV)
2. Rippe B, Haraldsson B (1987) Fluid and protein fluxes across small and large pores in the microvasculature. Application of two-pore equations. Acta Physiol Scand 131:411–428
3. Bundgaard M (1984) The three-dimensional organization of tight junctions in a capillary endothelium revealed by serial-section electron microscopy. J Ultrastruct Res 88:1–17
4. Rippe B, Haraldsson B (1987) How are macromolecules transported across the capillary wall? News Physiol Sci 2:135–138
5. Crone C, Levitt DG (1984) Capillary permeability to small solutes. In: Renkin EM, Michel CC (eds) The Cardiovascular System. Am Physiol Soc, pp 411–466 Handbook of physiology, sect 2, vol IV
6. Curry FE (1984) Mechanics and thermodynamics of transcapillary exchange. In: Renkin EM, Michel CC (eds) The Cardiovascular System. Am Physiol Soc, pp 309–374 (Handbook of physiology, sect 2, vol IV)
7. Patlak CS, Goldstein DA, Hoffman JF (1963) The flow of solute and solvent across two-membrane system. J Theor Biol 5:425–442

8. Drake R, Davis E (1978) A corrected equation for the calculation of reflection coefficients. Microvasc Res 15:259
9. Rippe B, Stelin G, Ahlmén J (1981) Basal permeability of the peritoneal membrane during continuous ambulatory peritoneal dialysis (CAPD). In: Gahl GM, Kessel M, Nolph KD (eds) Advances in peritoneal dialysis. Proceedings of the 2nd International Symposium on Peritoneal Dialysis. Excerpta Medica, Amsterdam, pp 5–9
10. Rippe B, Stelin G (1989) Simulations of peritoneal solute transport during CAPD. Application of two-pore formalism. Kidney Int 35:1234–1244
11. Rippe B, Stelin G, Ahlmén J (1986) Lymph flow from the peritoneal cavity in CAPD patients. In: Maher JF, Winchester JF (eds) Frontiers in peritoneal dialysis. Field, Rich, New York, pp 24–30
12. Nolph KD, Mactier RA, Khanna R, Twardowski ZJ, Moore H, McGary T (1987) The kinetics of ultrafiltration during peritoneal dialysis: the role of lymphatics. Kidney Int 32:219
13. Twardowski ZJ, Nolph KD, Khanna R (1987) Peritoneal equilibration test. Perit Dial Bull 7:138–147
14. Stelin G, Rippe B (1990) A phenomenological interpretation of the variation in dialysate volume with dwell time in CAPD. Kidney Int 38:465–472
15. Flessner MF, Dedrick RL, Rippe B (1989) Peritoneal tissue and capillary absorption vs. peritoneal lymphatic transport. (letter). ASAIO Trans 35:178–180

Comparing the Adequacy of Continuous Ambulatory Peritoneal Dialysis (CAPD) and Hemodialysis

PRAKASH KESHAVIAH[1] and KARL NOLPH[2]

SUMMARY. Inadequate dialysis is easier to define and recognize than adequate dialysis. With hemodialysis, values of the Kt/V urea index <0.8 (K:clearance, t:treatment time and V:volume of urea distribution), are associated with significant morbidity. For the standard continuous ambulatory peritoneal dialysis (CAPD) regimen (2 L × 4 exchanges/day), the Kt/V for the week is ~1.5 or ~0.5 for a thrice weekly comparison to hemodialysis. Patients on CAPD do not exhibit the morbidity associated with the same low values of Kt/V in hemodialysis. According to the recently formulated peak concentration, because hemodialysis is an intermittent therapy with peaks and troughs of serum urea concentrations, a higher Kt/V is required to match peak serum urea concentrations to the steady state CAPD concentration. Urea kinetic calculations based on this hypothesis suggest weekly Kt/V values for CAPD <1.2 may be associated with inadequate dialysis, values >1.7 being the minimum recommended for adequacy. Pilot clinical studies in 19 patients demonstrate agreement with urea kinetic model predictions concerning the relationship between blood urea nitrogen (BUN), Kt/V and protein catabolic rate. In 74% of the clinical observations there was agreement between assessment of adequacy with Kt/V and a clinical assessment score used at the University of Missouri. Lack of agreement in the remaining observations is being investigated.

Introduction

Adequacy of dialysis eludes a clear-cut definition but inadequate dialysis is more readily defined and recognized. The National Cooperative Dialysis Study (NCDS) [1] established clearly that a high degree of morbidity was evident when the small

[1]Baxter Clinical Engineering Laboratory, Renal Division, Baxter Healthcare Corporation, Minneapolis, MN 55404, USA
[2]University of Missouri, Columbia, MO 65212-0001, USA

Table 1. Calculation of Kt/V index for CAPD

	Definition of KT/V
Hemodialysis	K = Urea clearance
	T = Treatment time
	V = Volume of urea distribution determined from urea kinetics
C.A.P.D.	$KT = (V)_{drained} \times (D/P)_{ratio}$
	V = Volume of urea distribution ($\approx$ total body water)
	V estimated from sex, age, height, and weight
	Typical KT/V Calculation for CAPD
	Regimen: 4 exchanges/day
	$V_{dialysate} = 2 \times 4$ l, $V_{uf} = 1.5$ l
	$\because$ $V_{drained} = 8 + 1.5 = 9.5$ l
	$D/P = 0.9$
	$\because$ $KT = 0.9 \times 9.5 = 8.55$
	$V = 40$ l (B.wt = 70 kg)
	$\because$ $(KT/V)_{day} = 8.55 / 40 = 0.21$
	$(KT/V)_{H.D.equiv} = 0.21 \times 7 / 3 = 0.49$

marker solute urea was not adequately removed, resulting in high time averaged urea concentrations. Further analysis of this data resulted in the formulation of the Kt/V index [2], K being the dialyzer urea clearance (ml/min), t the treatment time (min) and V the volume of urea distribution (ml), which is commonly considered to be equal to total body water. Analysis of the NCDS and prior literature indicates that the Kt/V urea index provides a good definition of the lower limits of the hemodialysis therapy prescription. At Kt/V levels of ~ 0.5, frank uremic symptoms such as anorexia, nausea, insomnia and pericarditis were noted by Dyck et al. [3]. In the NCDS, Groups II and IV were dialyzed at Kt/V levels of ~ 0.6 and had a high degree of morbidity manifested as medical withdrawals, hospitalizations and death. The underlying medical problems were similar to those observed in the Dyck study. At Kt/V levels of ~0.7, Teschan et al. [4] observed neurobehavioral abnormalities characterized by slowing of the EEG. In both the Dyck and Teschan studies, alleviation of symptoms was noted when Kt/V was increased to ~1.0. In the NCDS, in Groups I and III, the Kt/V was >0.8 and in these groups a smaller percentage of therapy failures was noted. While none of these short-term studies define the optimal therapy prescription, they clearly delineate inadequate dialysis prescriptions as those with Kt/V < 0.8.

The purpose of this paper is to examine the applicability of the Kt/V urea index to CAPD, a therapy that is different from hemodialysis in several respects. The calculation of the Kt/V index for CAPD is quite different from that for hemodialysis, as shown in Table 1. The sample calculation (based on no residual renal function) indicates that for the typical CAPD regimen of 4 exchanges of 2 L each per day with 1.5 L of ultrafiltration and average peritoneal permeability characteristics, the Kt/V for the average 70 kg patient will be only 0.21 per day or 0.49 for an equivalent thrice weekly schedule comparable to hemodialysis. The additional contributions of residual renal function to the thrice weekly Kt/V index will be approximately 0.08

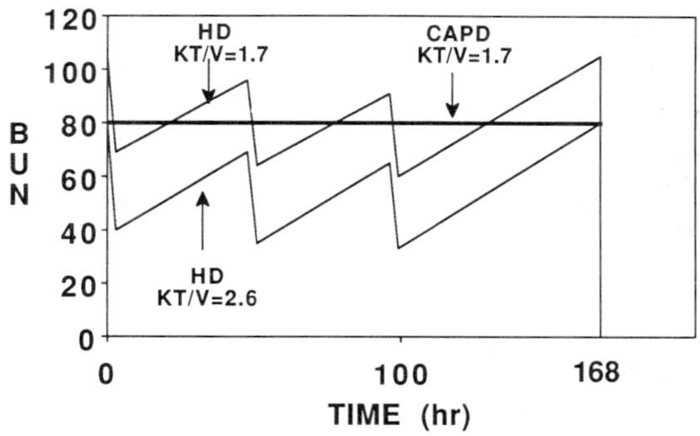

Fig. 1. The weekly blood urea nitrogen (BUN) profile for hemodialysis (HD) and CAPD at the same level of Kt/V = 1.7 and the effect of increasing the Kt/V for hemodialysis from 1.7 to 2.6 to make the peak concentration equal to the steady-state CAPD concentration

for each ml/min of residual urea clearance. So assuming a residual urea clearance of 2 ml/min, the thrice weekly equivalent Kt/V index for CAPD will still be only 0.65, a value similar to that of Groups II and IV of the NCDS. The percentage of patients failing therapy in these groups was of the order of 60%. Such a high degree of morbidity is not commonly observed with the standard CAPD regimen. This, therefore, poses a serious challenge to the validity of the Kt/V index for characterizing the adequacy of CAPD.

Background

As stated earlier, CAPD differs from hemodialysis in several respects. For example, the natural peritoneal membrane has permeability characteristics that are very different from those of conventional cellulosic hemodialysis membranes. The peritoneal membrane is less permeable than cellulosic membranes for small solutes such as urea but is more permeable than cellulosic membranes for larger solutes such as inulin and Beta-2 microglobulin. Those who subscribe to the middle-molecule hypothesis will see in this seeming invalidity of the Kt/V index a reaffirmation of their faith in middle molecules. However, the search for middle molecules, undertaken over more than a decade by well-qualified investigators using sophisticated detection tools, has been unsuccessful.

There is another slightly different hypothesis that can be put forward, based on the differences in permeability of the peritoneal and cellulosic membranes. This hypothesis is that while urea is not toxic per se, it is a surrogate for other toxic solutes that are associated with protein catabolism and urea generation. The relationship between the removal of urea and these toxic catabolites of protein depends on the permeability characteristics of the membrane. As the CAPD membrane is different, the scaling factors between urea removal and these unknown protein catabolites may be different between CAPD and hemodialysis.

While one cannot rule out the above hypotheses based on membrane permeability differences, an alternative hypothesis based on another important difference between CAPD and hemodialysis will be considered. This important difference is that while CAPD is a steady state continuous therapy, hemodialysis is an intermittent therapy characterized by peaks and troughs of serum urea concentrations. Application of the single pool urea kinetic model to these two therapies provides some interesting insights. At the same level of Kt/V, the steady state serum urea concentration with CAPD is almost identical to the time averaged serum urea concentration achieved with hemodialysis. However, because of the intermittent nature of hemodialysis, for approximately half the hours of the week, the serum urea concentration is above this time-averaged correlation (Fig. 1). According to the recently formulated peak concentration hypothesis (5), if the peak concentration is better correlated with uremic toxicity than the mathematically derived abstraction called the time averaged concentration, the hemodialysis Kt/V has to be increased substantially in order to bring the hemodialysis peak concentration down to the steady state CAPD concentration. In other words, serum urea concentration related equivalence between CAPD and hemodialysis is not achieved at the same Kt/V, but may require a higher Kt/V for hemodialysis in order to compensate for the intermittent nature of the therapy. Using the urea kinetic model and the peak concentration hypothesis, Keshaviah et al. [5] have estimated that a Kt/V value of 0.55 for CAPD is equivalent to a value of 1.0 for hemodialysis and that a Kt/V value of approximately 0.4 for CAPD is equivalent to the hemodialysis value of 0.6, a level of Kt/V at which significant morbidity was evident in the NCDS. Converting the Kt/V thrice weekly equivalents to a Kt/V value for the whole week on CAPD, we get a lower bound of 1.2 for inadequate dialysis and a value of 1.7 and above for short-term adequacy. The range from 1.2 to 1.7 represents the transition from inadequate to adequate dialysis according to the peak concentration hypothesis.

Clinical Study

A pilot clinical study in 19 patients was undertaken at the University of Missouri to test the peak concentration hypothesis. The results of this study were presented in some detail at the 10th Annual Conference on Peritoneal Dialysis at Dallas (1990) and will appear in the transactions of the meeting [6]. A brief summary of the results is presented here.

The demographics of the patients studied are presented in Table 2. The patients studied are representative of the typical CAPD population in the United States. The relationship between the steady state serum urea concentration and the weekly Kt/V for urea is shown in Fig. 2. The solid lines represent the theoretical relationship

Table 2. Patient demographics

	Mean	Range
Age (years)	52	(30–75)
Body weight (kg)	71	(44–94)
B.S.A. (M^2)	1.81	(1.41–2.21)
Months on dialysis	30	(1–94)
Residual kidney fn. (ml/min) (average of residual urea and creatinine clearances)	2.1	(0–10.1)

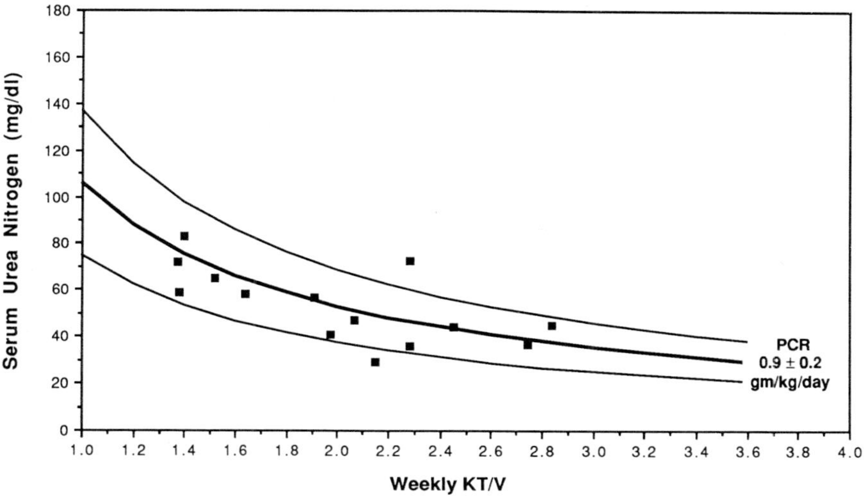

Fig. 2. The steady-state serum urea nitrogen concentration of CAPD (n= 14) plotted against the Kt/V urea with the theoretical relationship derived from urea kinetics for PCR = 0.9 ± 0.2 gm/kg per day superimposed

derived from single pool urea kinetics for a protein catabolic rate (PCR) of 0.9 ± 0.2 gm/kg per day. Of the 19 patients, 14 had a PCR within this range and their data is superimposed on the theoretical predictions of Fig. 2. As is evident from this figure, there is a fairly close match between the experimental measurements and theory. The calculation used for the PCR is based on the relationship of Randerson [7] presented in Table 3. The correlation between the calculated PCR and the dietary protein intake based on a 3 day diet history is shown in Fig. 3. The correlation coefficient for the line of best fit is 0.55, suggesting a fairly strong correlation between the two. A paired t-test revealed no significant difference between the calculated PCR and the dietary protein intake. Three other methods for calculating the PCR in CAPD patients were investigated and yielded similar results to the Randerson formulation.

While the above data confirm the applicability of the urea kinetic model to CAPD, the specific question about CAPD adequacy and Kt/V needs to be addressed. In order to examine this, a clinical assessment score developed at the University of Missouri was used as a clinical indicator of adequacy that could be correlated to the Kt/V measurement. Details of this assessment score are presented in Table 4. With this 12 parameter score, 36 is a perfect score. A score of 23 or less represents inadequate

Table 3. Calculation of PCR for CAPD

PCR (gm/day) = 10.76 (G_{un} + 1.46)
Urea nitrogen generation rate $G_{un\ (mg/min)} = (V_d \times D_{un} + V_u \times U_{un})/t$
Where V_d and V_u are dialysate and urine volumes respectively (ml), D_{un} and U_{un} are dialysate and urine urea nitrogen concentrations respectively, (mg/dl) and t is the collection time (min)

(Adapted from [7])

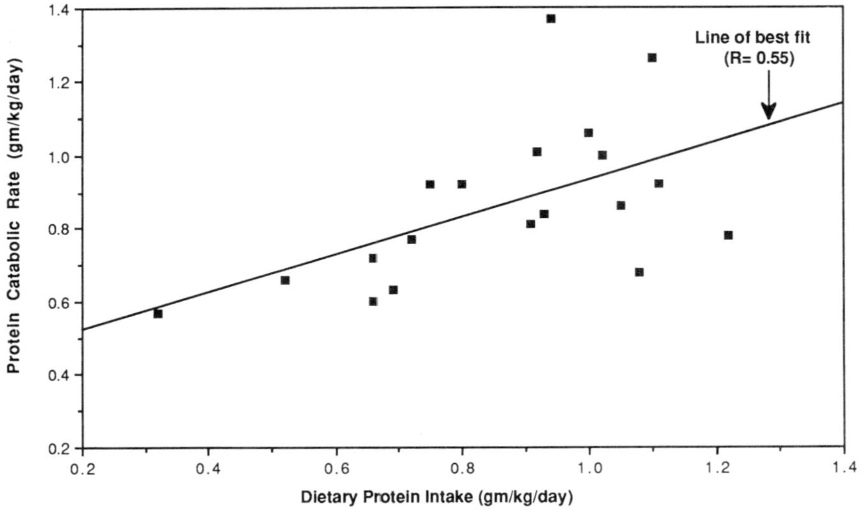

Fig. 3. Correlation between the calculated protein catabolic rate (*PCR*) and the dietary protein intake

therapy, 23–39 is a transitional zone and a score above 29 indicates adequate therapy. The weekly Kt/V ranges derived from the peak concentration hypothesis are <1.2 connoting inadequate dialysis, 1.2–1.7 being a transition, and >1.7 being adequate. Figure 4 shows the domains defined by the clinical assessment in conjunction with the weekly Kt/V. There are thus 3 boxes – inadequate, transitional, and adequate dialysis. The clinical measurements of the assessment score and Kt/V are super-

Table 4. Clinical assessment score

	Frequent	Occasional	No problem
Insomnia	1	2	3
Weakness	1	2	3
Dysgeusia	1	2	3
Anorexia	1	2	3
Nausea	1	2	3
Vomiting	1	2	3
Fluid balance	1	2	3
Blood pr. control	1	2	3
	Score 1	Score 2	Score 3
Albumin (gm/dl)	< 3.0	3.0 -3.4	> 3.4
Hct (%)	<20	20–24	>24
Crt. Lean Body Mass (mg/dl per cm ht.)	> 0.10 ↓	0.08–0.10 → (Non-ideal)	< 0.08 ↑ (or ideal)

Inadequate	< 23 points
Marginal	23–29 points
Adequate	29–36 points

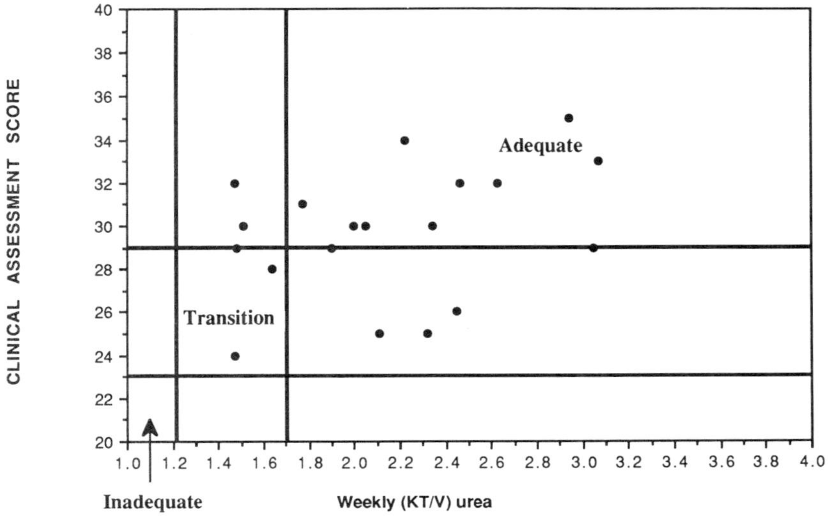

Fig. 4. Plot of the clinical assessment score vs Kt/V urea superimposed on the domains of inadequate, transitional, and adequate dialysis, derived from the intersections of the clinical assessment and Kt/V ranges

imposed on these domains in Fig. 4. Note that none of the patients falls into the inadequate domain. Of the 19 patients, 14 (74%) fall into the appropriate domain boxes. Of the remaining 5, 2 have adequate clinical scores but a low Kt/V (transitional) and 3 have low scores (transition zone) but an adequate Kt/V. It is reasonable to consider the clinical assessment to be the cumulative result of therapy prescription characterized by the Kt/V. Therefore, if a patient is treated with a low Kt/V, it may take several months before the effects of the underdialysis are manifested clinically and measurable as a lower assessment score. Of the two patients with a low Kt/V, one has been on CAPD for only 9 months. It would be interesting to note the time course of the clinical assessment score in this patient. In the 3 patients whose assessment score was low despite an adequate Kt/V, some of the symptoms noted may be unrelated to underdialysis and may have a different etiology. Of the 14 patients who fell into the appropriate domains, 3 were judged to be in the transitional zone by both the clinical assessment and the Kt/V. The therapy prescription in these patients is being increased and the assessment score will be followed to see if it moves upward into the zone of adequacy.

Conclusion

It appears that the urea kinetic model developed for hemodialysis can be applied to CAPD to provide some meaningful insights. The relationship between serum urea concentration, Kt/V and PCR matches the model predictions. The clinical data indicate that patients on CAPD whose Kt/V is much lower than that required for hemodialysis appear to be doing well by clinical assessment criteria. The correlation between clinical assessment and the Kt/V is strong but needs further refinement. The peak concentration hypothesis is an interesting attempt at unifying the comparative bases for adequacy of hemodialysis and CAPD. Its validity has not yet been completely established and awaits further study.

References

1. Lowrie EG, Laird NM, Parker TF, et al. (1981) Effect of the hemodialysis prescription on patient morbidity. N Engl J Med 20:1176–1181
2. Gotch F, Sargent JA (1985) A mechanistic analysis of the National Cooperative Dialysis Study (NCDS). Kidney Int 28:526–534
3. Dyck PJ, Johnson WJ, Lambert EH, O'Brien PC, Daube JR, Oviatt KF (1979) Comparison of symptoms, chemistry, and nerve function to assess adequacy of hemodialysis. Neurology 29:1361–1368
4. Teschan PE, Ginn HE, Bourne JR, Ward JW, Schaffer JD (1983) A prospective study of reduced dialysis. ASAIO J 6:108–122
5. Keshaviah PR, Nolph KD, Van Stone JC (1989) The peak concentration hypothesis: A urea kinetic approach to comparing the adequacy of continuous ambulatory peritoneal dialysis (CAPD) and hemodialysis. Perit Dial Int 9:257–260
6. Keshaviah PR, Nolph KD, Prowant B, Moore H, Ponferrada L, Van Stone J, Twardowski ZJ, Khanna R (1990) Defining Adequacy of CAPD with Urea Kinetics. Adv Perit Dial 6:173–177
7. Randerson DH, Chapman GV, Farrell PC (1981) Amino acid and dietary status in long-term CAPD patients. In: Atkins RC, Farrell PC, Thomson N (eds) Peritoneal dialysis, pp 179–191

Pharmacological Alteration of Ultrafiltration

RAMESH KHANNA, KARL D. NOLPH, and ZBYLUT J. TWARDOWSKI[1]

SUMMARY. Several pharmacological agents have shown a potential for enhancing ultrafiltration in experimental settings during peritoneal dialysis exchanges. Knowledge of ultrafiltration kinetics has improved our understanding of how and at what site these agents are effective in enhancing ultrafiltration. Of all the agents discussed, only phosphatidylcholine, which presumably acts at multiple sites, has shown promise of clinical application. It has several potential advantages. First, phosphatidylcholine is a normal constituent of peritoneal fluid and its addition may help restore and maintain normal peritoneal physiology. Secondly, by reducing intraperitoneal fluid absorption, phosphatidylcholine may decrease dialysate glucose absorption and allow a decrease in the dialysis solution glucose load. Thirdly, studies have indicated that phosphatidylcholine can greatly enhance net ultrafiltration in patients with poor ultrafiltration capacity. Further studies are indicated to clearly define the patients who are likely to benefit from the use of this agent during peritoneal dialysis.

Background

Glucose is an effective osmotic agent for ultrafiltration during peritoneal dialysis. However the use of glucose has been associated with numerous undesirable metabolic effects; this has led to the search for alternative osmotic agents. An average CAPD patient typically absorbs 100–150 grams of glucose per day during the course of CAPD therapy. This inevitable high carbohydrate absorption predisposes to undesirable metabolic problems such as obesity, hypertriglyceridemia, and premature atherosclerosis. In addition, higher doses of insulin required to maintain the blood sugar at normal levels in diabetics may cause hyper-insulinemia, which in healthy persons has been shown to be a risk factor for atherosclerotic heart disease

[1]Department of Medicine, Division of Nephrology, School of Medicine, University of Missouri-Columbia, Columbia, MO 65212, USA

[1,2]. To obviate the undesirable metabolic consequences of glucose absorption, efforts have been made in the past to substitute glucose with alternative osmotic agents such as xylitol [3], amino acids [4], gelatin [5], polyglucose [6], and glycerol [7]. However, none of the agents tried have the favorable therapeutic profile of glucose. Either because of prohibitive cost, or because of an unacceptable toxicity profile, the use of these agents as osmotic agents has been limited. One to two percent amino acid mixtures in the dialysis solution have been used effectively to induce ultrafiltration in nondiabetic CAPD patients [4]. Also, the absorbed amino-acids cause significant increases in the total body nitrogen and transferrin, reduce the inevitable glucose load, and lower serum triglyceride levels. Use of such mixtures in diabetic CAPD patients has the potential to reduce may of the undesirable effects of glucose. However, their effectiveness over long periods has not been established. Furthermore, the high cost of amino-acid mixtures is a major limiting factor. Glycerol-containing dialysis solution has been used successfully in diabetic CAPD patients. This agent was well tolerated by the patients, was non-toxic to the peritoneal membrane, did not cause hepato-toxicity, and did not increase protein losses in the dialysate [7]. Blood sugar was easily controlled with insulin. Some patients did develop signs and symptoms of hyperosmolality. However, glycerol showed no benefits over glucose because it delivered similar total caloric loads and the problem with hyperlipidemia was unaltered. Thus, for now, glucose still remains the least toxic osmotic agent for use in peritoneal dialysis. Also, many non-osmotic pharmacological agents have been shown in experimental settings to enhance net ultrafiltration, by modifying the forces of ultrafiltration kinetics while glucose was still used as the osmotic agent (in concentrations equal to or less than those conventionally used in clinical settings). This concept has lead to the identification of several more pharmacological agents which could be used to enhance ultrafiltration —still using glucose as the osmotic agent while reducing the glucose load per exchange. This review will describe those pharmacological agents known to cause such ultrafiltration enhancement and their mechanisms of action.

Forces That Govern Fluid Transport Across the Peritoneal Membrane

Under physiological conditions there is a continuous leakage of ultrafiltrate from the capillaries into the peritoneal cavity. The fluid transport across the peritoneum is believed to be governed by the hydrostatic and colloid osmotic pressures in the capillaries and interstitium [8]. The hydrostatic pressure in the capillaries tends to force fluid and its dissolved substances through the capillary pores into the interstitial spaces, particularly from the proximal capillaries. This process is aided by the colloidal pressure and the relatively low hydrostatic pressure in the interstitial spaces. Under physiological conditions, in the tissues around the peritoneal cavity, the net hydrostatic pressure across the capillary membrane is greater than the net colloid osmotic pressure of plasma and interstitial proteins, causing net transmembrane pressure to favor ultrafiltration from the capillary lumen into the surrounding interstitium. This outward net driving pressure causes continuous leakage of ultrafiltrate out of the capillaries. It is this ultrafiltrate that becomes interstitital free fluid.

Lymph is derived from this interstitial fluid. The exact proportions of this fluid reabsorbed in lymphatics, distal capillaries, and venules in the peritoneum are unknown. Small amounts of this fluid constantly enter the peritoneal cavity, probably to lubricate the mesothelial surface of the organs that protrude into the cavity. Turnover is maintained by the continuous uptake of this fluid by the subdiaphragmatic lymphatics.

Kinetics of Ultrafiltration During Peritoneal Dialysis

During peritoneal dialysis, in order to induce ultrafiltration, glucose is added to dialysis solution at concentrations that greatly exceed the plasma concentration. This concentration difference creates a large driving force for ultrafiltration to occur from the interstitium and the capillary blood. When 2 liters of dialysis solution containing glucose are introduced into the peritoneal cavity during peritoneal dialysis, the forces that normally are operative across the capillary are modified in favor of enhanced ultrafiltration into the peritoneal cavity. For example, the net osmotic pressure difference across the peritoneum contributed by glucose when using dialysis fluid containing 4.25% dextrose is 210 mosm/kg H_2O (3990 mm Hg). Because of the relatively low reflection coefficient for glucose across the peritoneal membrane, this potential osmotic force is not fully manifested. Glucose is fairly rapidly absorbed across the peritoneal membrane into the capillaries. Therefore, transcapillary ultrafiltration is maximum at time zero and decreases exponentially as the dialysate glucose concentration is dissipated by a combination of dilution due to ultrafiltration and transperitoneal glucose absorption. As osmotic and solute equilibrium is approached, transcapillary ultrafiltration rate becomes equal to reabsorption rate and peak ultrafiltration volume is observed.

Fluid and solute absorption from the peritoneal cavity may occur by way of distal capillaries, venules, or lymphatics. The driving force for capillary and venular uptake is the net sum of hydrostatic and osmotic pressure gradients across the membrane. Peritoneal lymphatics continuously absorb intraperitoneal fluid by convective flow, mainly via the specialized end lymphatics located on the under surface of the diaphragm [9–12]. The physiologic role of the peritoneal lymphatics is to act as a one-way pathway for returning excess intraperitoneal fluid and proteins to the systemic circulation. Under normal conditions, there is a balance between the rate of ultrafiltration and lymph drainage, which allows for only a small volume of isosmotic fluid to be maintained within the peritoneal cavity.

The measured net ultrafiltration volume at the end of each exchange equals the dialysate drain volume minus the infusion volume, but physiologically this represents the difference between cumulative net transcapillary ultrafiltration into the peritoneal cavity and the total lymphatic drainage out of the peritoneal cavity over the dwell time. The term "net transcapillary ultrafiltration" refers to the total net influx of fluid from the peritoneal capillaries and interstitium into the peritoneal cavity in response to the osmotic pressure of the dialysis solution. The resultant net influx of fluid would equal measured net ultrafiltration if it were not for the constant drainage via the peritoneal lymphatics. Depending on the glucose concentration used and the peritoneal membrane transport rates, peak intraperitoneal volume is observed at about 2–6 h into the dwell, when the lymph flow rate equals the transcapillary ultrafiltration rate. From then on, the intraperitoneal volume will start decreasing when the lymph flow rate (which is nearly constant) exceeds the transcapillary ultrafiltration rate (which declines due to the gradual dissipation of the glucose osmotic gradient). Glucose equilibrium is achieved after peak volume, perhaps as late as 6–8 h after the infusion. Transcapillary ultrafiltration, though at a very low rate, continues beyond osmolar equilibrium. The likely reasons for the continued ultrafiltration are two-fold: persistent glucose disequilibrium even though osmotic equilibrium is achieved, and the sum effect of Starling's forces, favoring movement of fluid out of the capillary. Any persistent glucose gradient can still generate a net osmotic pressure since the reflection coefficient for glucose is greater than that for electrolytes and urea. Equilibrium is achieved before glucose equilibrium, in part because of electrolyte sieving and the low electrolyte content of ultrafiltrate. Hydrostatic pressure in peritoneal capillaries may also contribute to continued transcapillary ultrafiltration in the presence of osmotic equilibrium and even total equilibrium for all solutes.

Studies done in CAPD patients have shown that a 2 liter volume of 2.5% dextrose dialysis solution, when infused and permitted to dwell for 4 hours in the peritoneal cavity, causes about 500–800 ml of cumulative net transcapillary ultrafiltration [13]. During the same period, cumulative absorption from the sub-diaphragmatic lymphatics would be about 350 ml. Thus, the net measured ultrafiltration would be appreciably reduced to 150–450 ml. In short-dwell exchanges, net transcapillary ultrafiltration exceeds lymphatic absorption, so the reduction in the dialysate drain volume due to lymphatic drainage is relative minor.

Pharmacological Enhancement of Ultrafiltration

There are a number of potential sites where pharmacological agents could act to enhance ultrafiltration during peritoneal dialysis (Table 1). The agents can be divided into those which primarily act to enhance transcapillary ultrafiltration and those which mainly reduce lymphatic absorption.

Drugs that Enhance Transcapillary Ultrafiltration

Theoretically transcapillary ultrafiltration can be enhanced by drugs which either modify the forces acting across the peritoneal membrane or alter membrane mass transfer area coefficients.

Modification of Forces Across Peritoneal Membrane

Increasing the capillary hydrostatic pressure, lowering the capillary oncotic pressure, or reducing the interstitial hydrostatic pressure, singly or in combination, could accentuate the balance of forces which, under physiological conditions, favor ultrafiltration out of capillary lumen. In experimental settings, except for dopamine, vasoactive agents in general have failed to increase capillary hydrostatic pressure at the peritoneal level [14–20]. The capillary hydrostatic pressure in the body is not easily altered, due to the phenomenon of capillary flow autoregulation (the systemic arterial pressure can be changed over a wide range, and the blood flow and perfusion

Table 1. Potential sites where pharmacological agents could act to enhance ultrafiltration during peritoneal dialysis

A. Drugs that enhance transcapillary ultrafiltration	
1. Modification of forces across peritoneal membrane	2. Alter resistance sites
a. Raise capillary hydrostatic pressure	a. Increase hydraulic permeability
Dopamine	Secretin
L-epinephrine	Puromycine
b. Lower capillary oncotic pressure	Amphotericin B
Hypoproteinemia	Verapamil
c. Reduce interstitial hydrostatic pressure	$1,25(OH)_2D_3$
???	b. Reduce stagnant fluid film layer (surfactants)
d. Generate osmotic pressure gradient	Chlorpromazine
	Docusate sodium
	Phosphatidylcholine
	Furosemide
B. Drugs that reduce lymph flow	**C. Drugs that improve mechanics of flow**
Close stomata:	Reduce/dissolve fibrin heparin
Neostigmine	Heparin
Phosphatidylcholine	Streptokinase
	Urokinase
	Lessen catheter compression laxatives

pressures through the tissue capillaries will remain almost unaltered). Supportive evidence for the autoregulation is seen in the settings of hypotension and hypothermia, in which peritoneal transport rates of solutes and water are only modestly decreased. Vasodilator and vasopressor therapies in these situations do not significantly alter the peritoneal transport rates [14,15]. L-norepinephrine decreases solute clearances without change in ultrafiltration [21,22]. Administration of intravenous or intraperitoneal dopamine during a peritoneal dialysis exchange increases both solute and water transport. This is unaffected by the simultaneous administration of propranolol, is decreased by phentolamine, and is abolished by haloperidol, a dopamine receptor competitor [22,23]. Since the predominant effect of dopamine at the microcirulatory level is shown to be venular constriction, in contrast to L-epinephrine [24], the augmented ultrafiltration probably results from an increased net capillary hydrostatic pressure [21]. Neither dopamine nor L-norepinephrine have been found clinically usable because of their widespread unwanted actions elsewhere in the body.

Hypoproteinemia results in a lowered oncotic pressure and contributes to the generation of ascites in certain disease conditions. In those CAPD patients who are severely malnourished with very low plasma protein and albumin concentrations, enhanced ultrafiltration rates have been observed. Such a phenomenon, however, is unlikely to provide a therapeutic role in the manipulation of ultrafiltration in clinical situations.

There is as yet no practical method to lower interstitial fluid pressure during a peritoneal dialysis exchange. This approach, therefore, is clinically not used in CAPD patients.

Osmotic pressure generation with alternative non-glucose osmotic agents has had limited success; as discussed above an agent with a therapeutic profile comparable to glucose has not been found.

Thus, in experimental settings, several pharmacological agents have been shown to enhance transcapillary ultrafiltration by modifying forces which function across the peritoneal membrane under physiological conditions. But clinically useful agents other than non-glucose osmotic agents have not been, as yet, identified.

Agents that Modify the Membrane Resistance Sites

Major increases in membrane permeability, such as those which occur with peritonitis, may enhance glucose uptake, cause rapid loss of the osmotic gradient, and decrease net ultrafiltration. Investigators have searched for agents that increase hydraulic permeability without major changes in glucose absorption. Theoretically, this could be made possible by increasing the number or size of very tiny pores available for water transport.

Solutes and fluid must cross resistance sites in moving from peritoneal capillaries into the peritoneal dialysis solution [25]. These sites include stagnant fluid films in the capillary, the endothelial cell layer, the capillary endothelial basement membrane, the interstitium, the mesothelial cell layer, and the stagnant fluid films in the peritoneal cavity. Modification in one or more sites is referred to as alteration in hydraulic permeability.

The hydraulic permeability of rabbit mesentery has been significantly altered with the gastrointestinal hormone, secretin, and the aminonucleoside, puromycin, when applied from the vascular side only [26]. These agents significantly augment osmotically induced water flux. Amphotericin B, when applied from the serosal side, presumably by creating channels in biological membranes for solute and water, increases ultrafiltration rate more than 70% compared to control without changing the osmotic gradient [27]. Because of the short half life and/or serious toxic side effects, these agents have not found clinical application in peritoneal dialysis.

The calcium channel blocker, Verapamil, after a few months of therapy in CAPD patients with reduced ultrafiltration capacity, has been shown to cause significant increases in the drainage volume [28]. In addition, when verapamil was used in these patients for up to 6 months, they showed a progressive decrease in intracellular calcium, secretory product interferon-Y and interleukin-1 in the peritoneal lymphocytes and macrophages. Based on these observations, the authors proposed that increases in the concentrations of lymphokines in the peritoneal cavity probably stimulate fibroblastic proliferation, resulting in peritoneal structural and functional alterations with a change in peritoneal hydraulic permeability. Verapamil presumably reverses these trends.

The stagnant dialysis fluid films in the peritoneal cavity and the resistance site overlying the mesothelial cell layer have been modified by drugs with surfactant properties. The peritoneal effluent in CAPD patients was reported to contain a phospholipid surface active material, identified on thin layer chromatography as positively charged phosphatidylcholine [29]. Peritoneal physiology may be altered in CAPD patients by the constant removal of phosphatidylcholine and other phospholipids in the dialysis effluent [29]. Phospholipid concentrations in the dialysate effluent are significantly reduced after long-term CAPD and during peritonitis [30]. The prominence of intracellular synthetic organelles in the mesothelium from CAPD patients may reflect increased production of phosphatidylcholine in an attempt to compensate for constant losses in the dialysate [30,31]. The poor ultrafiltration capacity in such patients is greatly improved with the addition of 50 mg/l of phosphatidylcholine to the infused dialysis solution, despite the likelihood of co-existing alterations in the integrity, and perhaps in the surface anionic charge of the mesothelium [31–33]. The observed net increase in the ultrafiltration and solute clearances with the addition of phosphatidylcholine to the infused dialysis solution has been attributed to its surface tension lowering properties [26,30]. It is believed that surfactants increase ultrafiltration by narrowing the stagnant dialysate layers over the mesothelium and by creating a water repellent lining on the surface of the peritoneum. Since glucose absorption from the dialysate does not increase during exchanges with phosphatidylcholine [30,34], it is proposed that the thinning of fluid films over the mesothelium causes unidirectional enhancement of peritoneal transport from the peritoneal microcirculation to the dialysis solution. Since the original studies of Di Paolo et al. [30], several recent studies have either confirmed [35,36] or refuted [37,38] the observation of enhanced ultrafiltration, with the use of either oral or intraperitoneal phosphatidylcholine administration. Our studies in rats [36] have confirmed enhanced ultrafiltration with phosphatidylcholine, but we have proposed an additional mechanism for its action, which will be discussed more in the section on reduced lymphatic absorption from the peritoneal cavity (see below).

Intraperitoneal chlorpromazine (2 mg/l dialysis solution), another surfactant, was reported to increase ultrafiltration and solute clearance rates more than 50% in 12 patients on CAPD [39]. These changes were unaccompanied by any changes in the dialysate osmolality or protein concentration. This agent was also shown to lower dialysate surface tension in vitro and was hence postulated to alter the thickness of the stagnant fluid films and to enhance water flux across the peritoneum.

Agents that Reduce Lymph Flow From the Peritoneal Cavity

We have previously shown that cumulative lymphatic absorption from the peritoneal cavity significantly reduces net ultrafiltration and solute clearances during long-dwell exchanges in man [13] and rat [40]. Most lymphatic drainage from the peritoneal cavity occurs by convective transport via the subdiaphragmatic stomata [9–12]. Fixed contraction of these stomata, which has been observed with intraperitoneal infusion of cholinergic drugs [41], also ought to reduce lymphatic absorption of intraperitoneal fluid [12,42]. Neostigmine, a quaternary ammonium carbamyl ester anticholinesterase agent, has been used therapeutically in myasthenia gravis and paralytic ileus [43]; it was shown to enhance net ultrafiltration in rats during a peritoneal dialysis exchange using 2.5% dextrose dialysis solution [44]. The enhancement of ultrafiltration was achieved by a reduction in cumulatiave lymphatic absorption, and was achieved without an increase in total capillary ultrafiltration during the dwell time. Likewise, solute clearances were augmented with neostigmine, primarily due to the increase in dialysate drain volume without a change in dialysate to serum solute ratios. Despite the impressive ultrafiltration enhancement during glucose ultrafiltration, neostigmine, because of its cumulative systemic toxicity, is clinically unusable for the long-term peritoneal dialysis patient. The effect of phosphatidylcholine in enhancing ultrafiltration during a peritoneal dialysis exchange in the rat was shown to be similar to that of neostigmine [44]. Besides the surfactant properties discussed earlier, based on our rat studies, phosphatidylcholine causes reduction of lymph flow during a peritoneal dialysis exchange in the rat. This lymph flow reducing property of phosphatidylcholine may be related to one of the following two mechanisms: 1) It has a cholingeric effect when taken systemically. This cholinergic effect [45–50] has been the biochemical basis of its reported beneficial effects when large doses were given to patients with tardive dyskinesia [51–53], Friedreich's ataxia [54], Alzheimer's disease [55], and memory and mood disorders [56–59]. Our rat studies suggest that, similarly to neostigmine, the cholinergic effects of phosphatidylcholine, when given intraperitoneally, cause the subdiaphragmatic stomata to contract and reduce lymph flow. The uptake of Indian ink by the lymphatics of rats who received dialysis exchanges without phosphatidylcholine, and the lack of uptake in rats treated with phosphatidylcholine are supportive of this hypothesis [36]. 2) Alternatively, another presumptive mode of action of phosphatidylcholine relates to its charge effect. The high density anionic charges on the lymphatic endothelium and, to a lesser extent, the microvilli and intercellular clefts of the subdiaphragmatic mesothelium, may play a role in the resorption of intraperitoneal fluid into the interstitium or lymphatics by a mechanism of charges repelling one another in such a way as to favor open stoma [60]. Positively charged choline may bind to and negate the surface anionic charge thereby reducing the functional patency of the intercellular channels between mesothelial and endothelial cells [36]. This hypothesis is supported by the observation that the cationic dye, alcian blue, abolishes the effect of phosphatidylcholine on isolated membranes in vitro [61]. The optimal conditions necessary for phosphatidylcholine (PC) to be effective are unclear at this time. Is it effective only when PC is deficient in phospholipid content? What concentration in the dialysis solution is required for it to be clinically useful? Is oral administration as effective as ip administration? These are some of the questions that need to be answered before it would prove to be clinically usable.

Drugs that Improve Mechanics of Flow

Mechanical problems resulting in slow drainage are often associated with build up of a residual volume. This may enhance reabsorption and/or dilute infused glucose concentrations and thereby decease daily net ultrafiltration.

Use of heparin in the dialysis solution improves drainage and reduces residual volume in patients who are prone to form fibrin, especially during peritonitis. Intraperitoneal heparin, up to a dose of 5000 units/2 l dialysis solution, causes very little activity in the plasma [62]. A slightly higher concentration of antithrombin in dialysate at the end of 4 hour dwell time is sufficient to inhibit fibrin formation in heparinized dialysis solution [63]. Despite the lack of evidence for other mechanisms of action for heparin at the membrane level, some believe it enhances ultrafiltration due to a charge effect.

Constipation frequently leads to poor drainage. Laxatives, by relieving constipation, improve drainage simply by reducing external pressure on the intraperitoneal segment of the catheter.

References

1. Stout RW (1979) Diabetes and atherosclerosis–The role of insulin. Diabetologia 16:141
2. Zavaroni A, Bonora E, Pagliara M, Dall'Aglio E, Luchetti L, Buonanno G, Bonati PA, Bergonzani M, Gnudi L, Passeri M, Reaven G (1989) Risk factor for coronary artery

disease in healthy persons with hyperinsulemia and normal glucose tolerance. N Engl J Med 320:702–706
3. Bazzato G, Coli U, Landini S (1982) Xylitol and low doses of insulin: New perspectives for diabetic uremic patients on CAPD. Perit Dial Bull 2:161
4. Williams FP, Marliss EB, Anderson GH, et al. (1982) Amino acids absorption following intraperitoneal administration in CAPD patients. Perit Dial Bull 2:124
5. Twardowski ZJ, Khanna R, Nolph KD (1986) Osmotic agents and ultrafiltration in peritoneal dialysis. Nephron 42:93
6. Mistry CD, Mallick NP, Gokal R (1986) The use of large molecular weight glucose polymer as an osmotic agent in CAPD. In: Khanna R, Nolph KD, Prowant BF, Twardowski ZJ, Oreopoulos DG (eds) Advances in continuous ambulatory peritoneal dialysis. Peritoneal Dialysis Bulletin, Toronto, pp 7–11
7. Matthys E, Dolkart R, Lameire N (1987) Extended use of a glycerol containing dialysate in the treatment of diabetic CAPD patients. Perit Dial Bull 7:10
8. Guyton AC (1981) The lymphatic system, interstitial fluid dynamics, edema, and pulmonary fluid. Textbook of medical physiology, 6th edn. Saunders, Philadelphia, pp 370–380
9. Courtice FC, Simmonds WJ (1954) Physiological significance of lymph drainage of the serous cavities and lungs. Physiol Rev 34:419–448
10. Von Recklinghausen F (1863) Zur Fettresorption. Arch Patholog Anat Physiol Klin Med 26:172
11. Khanna R, Mactier R, Twardowski ZJ, Nolph KD (1986) Peritoneal cavity lymphatics. Perit Dial Bull 6:113–121
12. Raybuck HE, Allen L, Harms WS (1960) Absorption of serum from the peritoneal cavity. Am J Physiol 119:1021–1024
13. Mactier RA, Khanna R, Twardowski ZJ, Nolph KD (1987) Contribution of lymphatic absorption to loss of ultrafiltration and solute clearances in CAPD. J Clin Invest 80:1311–1316
14. Patton JF, Doolittle WH, Hamlet MP (1974) Peritoneal clearance of urea and potassium following experimental hypothermia. J Appl Physiol 36:403–406
15. Greene JA, Lapco L, Weller JM (1970) Effect of drug therapy of hemorrhagic hypotension on kinetics of peritoneal dialysis in the dog. Nephron 7:178–183
16. Surdiel LG, Castillo D, Martin-Malo A (1985) Effect of verapamil and prostaglandin E_1 on peritoneal membrane transport (abstract). Proc Eur Dial Transplant Assoc, p 95
17. Nolph KD, Ghods AJ, Van Stone J, et al. (1976) The effects of intraperitoneal vasodilator on peritoneal clearances. Trans Am Soc Artif Intern Organs 22:586–594
18. Wideroe TE, Smeby LC, Dahl K, et al. (1988) Definitions of differences and changes in peritoneal membrane transport properties. Kidney Int 33:S107–113
19. Grzegorzewska A, Grala T, Alexiewicz J (1984) Effect of intraperitoneal administration of furosemide and sodium nitroprusside on the elimination of water, sodium and potassium during peritoneal dialysis. Pol Arch Med Wewn 71:281–291
20. Panasiuk E (1985) Effect of sodium nitroprusside, furosemide and dopamine on the efficiency of peritoneal dialysis. Pol Arch Med Wewn 74:316–326
21. Hirszel P, Lasrich M, Maher JF (1979) Divergent effects of catecholamines on peritoneal mass transport. Trans Am Soc Artif Intern Organs 25:110
22. Hirszel P, Lasrich M, Maher JF (1979) Augmentation of peritoneal mass transport by dopamine: Comparison with norepinephrine and evaluation of pharmacologic mechanisms. J Lab Clin Med 94:747
23. Chan MK, Varghese Z, Baillod RA, et al. (1980) Peritoneal dialysis: effect of intraperitoneal dopamine. Dial Transplant 9:380
24. Goldberg LI (1972) Cardiovascular and renal actions of dopamine; potential clinical applications. Pharmacol Rev 24:1
25. Nolph KD, Miller F, Rubin J, et al. (1980) New directions in peritoneal dialysis concepts and applications. Kidney Int 18:S111–S116

26. Maher JF, Hirszel P, Lasrich M (1979) The effects of gastrointestinal hormones on transport by peritoneal dialysis. Kidney Int 16:130
27. Maher JF, Hirszel P, Bennett RR, et al. (1984) Amphotericin B selectively increases peritoneal ultrafiltration. Am J Kidney Dis 4:285–288
28. Lamperi S, Carozzi S, Nasini MG (1987) Calcium antagonists improve ultrafiltration in patients on continuous ambulatory peritoneal dialysis. Trans Am Soc Artif Intern Organs 33:657–663
29. Grahame GR, Torchia MG, Dankewich KA, et al. (1985) Surface-active material in peritoneal effluent of CAPD patients. Perit Dial Bull 5:109
30. DiPaolo N, Buoncristiani U, Capotundo L, et al. (1986) Phosphatidylcholine and peritoneal transport during peritoneal dialysis. Nephron 44:365
31. Dobbie JW, Zaki M, Wilson L (1981) Ultrastructural studies on the peritoneum with special reference to chronic ambulatory peritoneal dialysis. Scott Med 26:213–223
32. Di Paolo N, Sacchi G, De Mia M, et al. (1986) Morphology of the peritoneal membrane during peritoneal dialysis. Nephron 44:204–211
33. Verger C, Brunschvigg O, Le Carpentier Y, et al. (1981) Structural and ultrastructural peritoneal membrane changes and permeability alterations during CAPD. Proc Eur Dial Transplant Assoc 18:199–203
34. Breborowicz A, Sombolos K, Rodela H, et al. (1987) Mechanism of phosphatidylcholine action during peritoneal dialysis. Nephron 7:6
35. Chan H, Abraham G, Oreopoulos DG (1989) Oral lecithin improves ultrafiltration in patients on peritoneal dialysis. Perit Dial Int 9:203–205
36. Mactier RA, Khanna R, Twardowski ZJ, Moore H, Nolph KD (1988) Influence of phosphatidylcholine on lymphatic absorption during peritoneal dialysis in the rat. Perit Dial Int 8:179–186
37. De Vecchi A, Castelnovo C, Guerra L, et al. (1989) Phosphatidylcholine administration in continuous ambulatory peritoneal dialysis (CAPD) patients with reduced ultrafiltration. Perit Dial Int 9:207–210
38. Di Paolo B, Chakrabarti, Maher JF (1989) Phosphatidylcholine does not affect peritoneal transport of intact rabbits. Perit Dial Int 9:211–213
39. Indraprasit S, Sooksriwongse C (1985) Effect of chlorpromazine on peritoneal clearances. Nephron 40:341–343
40. Nolph KD, Mactier RA, Khanna R, et al. (1987) Kinetics of peritoneal ultrafiltration: the role of lymphatics. Kidney Int 32:219–226
41. Tsilibary EC, Wissig SL (1983) Lymphatic absorption from the peritoneal cavity: regulation of patency of mesothelial stomata. Microvasc Res 25:22–39
42. Lill SR, Parsons RH, Bohac I (1979) Permeability of the diaphragm and fluid resorption from the peritoneal cavity in the rat. Gastroenterology 76:997–1001
43. Koelle GB (1975) Anticholinesterase agents. In: Goodman LS, Gilman A (eds) The pharmacological basis of therapeutics, 5th edn. Macmillan, New York, pp 445–466
44. Mactier RA, Khanna R, Moore H, Twardowski ZJ, Nolph KD (1988) Pharmacological reduction of lymphatic absorption from the peritoneal cavity increases net ultrafiltration and solute clearances in peritoneal dialysis. Nephron 50:229–232
45. Cohen EL, Wurtman RJ (1975) Brain acetylcholine: Increase after systemic choline administration. Life Sci 16:1095–2000
46. Hambrich DR, Chippendale TJ (1977) Regulation of acetylcholine synthesis in nervous tissue. Life Sci 20:1465–1478
47. Hirsch MJ, Ulus IH, Wurtman RJ (1976) Elevation of brain and adrenal acetylcholine levels and of adrenal tyrosine hydroxylase activity following administration of choline via stomach tube. Neurosci Abstr 1:765
48. Cohen EL, Wurtman RJ (1976) Brain acetylcholine: control by dietary choline. Science 191:561–562

49. Morley BJ, Robinson GR, Brown GB, et al. (1977) Effect of dietary choline on nicotinic acetylcholine receptors in brain. Nature 266:848–859
50. Ulus IH, Wurtman RJ (1976) Choline administration: activation of tyrosine hydroxylase in dopaminergic neurons of rat brain. Science 194:1060–1061
51. Fann WE, Lake CR, Gerber CT, et al. (1974) Cholinergic suppression of tardive dyskinesia. Psychopharmacologia 37:101–107
52. Growdon JH, Gelenberg AJ, Doller J, et al. (1978) Lecithin can suppress tardive dyskinesia. N Engl J Med 297:524–527
53. Jackson IV, Davis LG, Cohen RK, et al. (1981) Lecithin administration in tardive dyskinesia: Clinical and biomedical correlates. Biol Psychiatry 16:85–89
54. Pentland B, Martyn CN, Steer CR, et al. (1981) Lecithin treatment in Friedreich's ataxia. Br Med J [Clin Res] 282:1197–1198
55. Etienne P, Gauthier S, Dastoor D, et al. (1979) Alzheimer's disease: clinical effect of lecithin treatment. In: Barbeau A (ed) Nutrition and the brain. Raven, New York, pp 389–396
56. Drachman DA, Sahakian BJ (1979) Effects of cholinergic agents on human learning and memory. In: Barbeau A (ed) Nutrition and the brain. Raven, New York, pp 351–366
57. Sitaram N, Weingartner H, Christian Gillin J (1979) Choline chloride and arecoline: Effects on memory and sleep in man. In: Barbeau A (ed) Nutrition and the brain. Raven, New York, pp 367–376
58. Harris CM, Davis JM, Janowsky DS (1979) Use of cholinergic drugs in mental illness. In: Barbeau A (ed) Nutrition and the brain. Raven, New York, pp 397–408
59. Tamminga CA, Nutt JG (1979) Cholinergic influences on affect. In: Barbeau A (ed) Nutrition and the brain. Raven, New York, pp 409–416
60. Leak LV (1986) Distribution of cell surface charges on mesothelium and lymphatic endothelium. Microvasc Res 31:18–30
61. Breborowicz A, Sombolos K, Rodela H, Oreopoulos DG (1987) Mechanism of phosphatidylcholine action during peritoneal dialysis. Perit Dial Bull 7:6–9
62. Gries E, Paar D, Graben N, Bock KD (1986) Intraperitoneal fibrin formation and its inhibition in CAPD. Clin Nephrology 26:209–212

The Impact of the Y-System and Low Peritonitis Rate on CAPD Results

R. Maiorca, G.C. Cancarini, L. Manili, C. Camerini, and G. Brunori

Summary. The impact of peritonitis rate on continuous ambulatory peritoneal dialysis (CAPD) results was evaluated in 288 patients. Of these 288 patients 186 used a Y-connector with an in-line disinfectant (Y-system) from the same firm; 142 patients used this system from the beginning of their first treatment. The Y-system was confirmed to be an effective means of preventing peritonitis episodes, with 50% of patients being peritonitis-free after 3 and a half years (5 months for the standard set). A minority of patients had had 2 (7%) or 3 or more (9%) peritonitis episodes after a follow-up of 290 patient-years (19% and 33% after 77 patient-years, on the standard set).

Peritoneal function (ultrafiltration volume and peritoneal equilibration tests), peripheral neural function (motor nerve conduction velocity), and several laboratory data (blood urea nitrogen (BUN), serum creatinine, hemoglobin, total proteins, albumin, transferrin, pseudocholinesterase, cholesterol, triglycerides), some of them indicative of nutritional status, did not appear to be affected by peritonitis frequency. Serum beta-2m also was not influenced by the rate of peritonitis.

An influence of peritonitis frequency on patient survival was seen only after excluding patients who died before having a peritonitis episode. In the entire population, causes other than peritonitis were of major importance for patient survival. Peritonitis almost completely accounted for the greater drop-out rate from the CAPD technique than from the hemodialysis (HD) technique. A low rate of peritonitis, such as that obtained with the Y-system, appears to be important for improving CAPD results.

Introduction

As is well known, the Y-system consists of a Y-shaped connector filled with a disinfectant during the dwell-time and flushed before filling the peritoneal cavity [1].

Institute of Nephrology, University of Brescia, 25100, Brescia, Italy, and Division of Nephrology, Spedali Civili, 25100, Brescia, Italy

This system, suggested by Buoncristiani et al. some years ago [2], has been shown in controlled studies [1,3] to reduce peritonitis frequency better than any other method [4]. In this paper, the results obtained in a single institution with a large experience of the Y-system are analyzed in order to evaluate the impact of the low peritonitis rate on CAPD results.

Patients and Methods

Overall CAPD experience at the Institute of Nephrology of the University of Brescia includes 288 patients, in part new patients and in part patients coming from other treatments, using other connection systems. Of these 288 patients, 186 were put on Y-solution transfer sets purchased from one firm. Of these, 142 were new patients. For these 186 patients, in 3479 patient-months, we had 104 peritonitis episodes, with an incidence of 1 every 33.4 patient-months. All our experience with the standard set was in the first years of our use of CAPD, because after the good results obtained with the Y-set, all our patients were put on this connector. However, the peritonitis incidence recently reported in the literature with standard sets [4] is the same as our former results.

Routine methods were used for biochemical tests, and radio-immunoassay (RIA) was used for β2-microglobulin. Motor nerve conduction velocity was measured on the external sciatic popliteal nerve.

Statistics: patient and method survivals were calculated and compared according to Peto et al. [5,6]. Analysis of variance and multiple regression analysis were done with Statworks from Cricket Software.

Results

Peritonitis Frequency on Y and Standard Connectors

Peritonitis incidence has changed over the years, from a minimum of 1 episode every 23 patient-months to 1 every 64 patient-months, with the usual incidence being over 30. In our experience the 50% patient probability of remaining peritonitis free was 5 months on the standard set and 3 and half years on the Y-system. On the standard set, the probability of having the second and the third peritonitis episode was about the same as for the first (50% after 6 months), whereas on the Y-system, the 50% probability of having the second episode after the first was 1.5 years and, for the third episode, was 6 months (Fig. 1). Actually, for our 142 patients who had begun on the Y-system, after a follow-up of 290 patient-years, only 9% had had three or more peritonitis episodes, a figure to be compared to the 33% for the standard set after a follow-up of 77 patient-years.

Patient and Technique Survival

To better evaluate the impact of the low peritonitis rate on CAPD results we examined our entire group of 288 patients, treated from the start of our experience by CAPD. These were in large part new patients, but also included patients switched from other

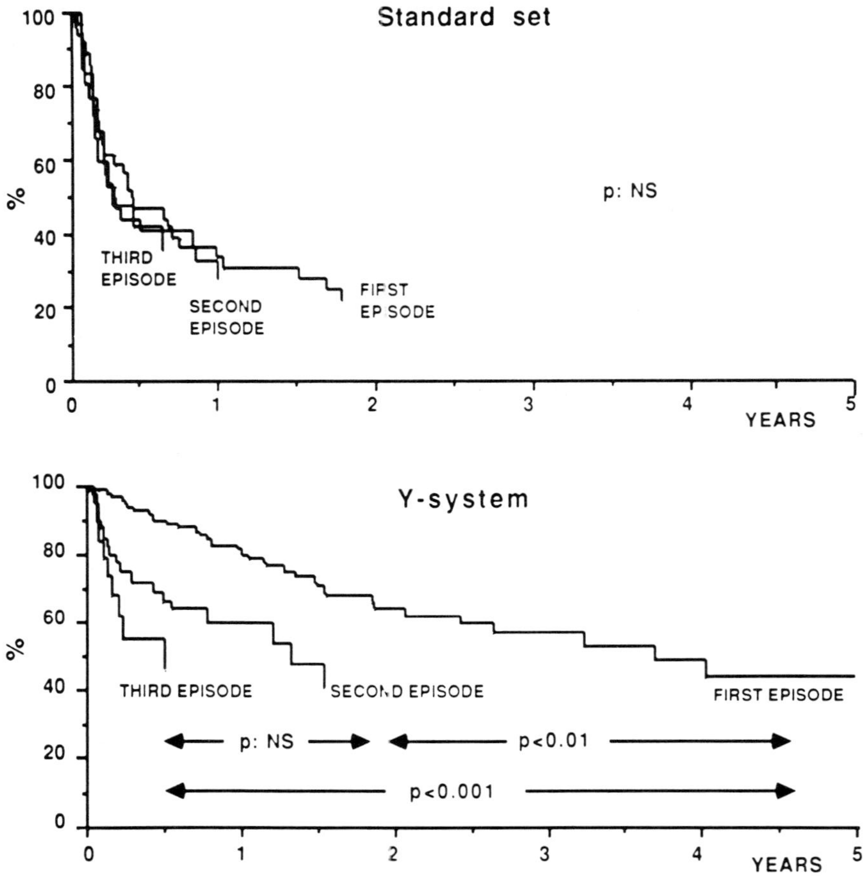

Fig. 1. Probability of remaining peritonitis-free for new patients on the Standard-set (*upper panel*) and the Y-system (*lower panel*)

treatments, and put on standard and on the Y-set; this last Y-set included Y-connectors and solutions of two different brands. Patients were divided into 4 groups, one with no peritonitis episodes; one with fewer than 0.5; one group with up to 1; and one group with more than 1 peritonitis episode per year. Number and mean age of

Table 1. Groups of patients according to peritonitis rate

Group	Peritonitis rate (episode/year)	Number of patients	Mean age at start (M±SD)	Months on CAPD (M±SD)
1	No. episodes	131	61 ± 13	16 ± 15
2	<0.5	33	60 ± 11	61 ± 25
3	0.5–1	53	61 ± 14	43 ± 24
4	>1	71	60 ± 16	25 ± 23

Table 2. Causes of death in patients divided according to peritonitis rate. Events/100 patients per year

Cause of death	Group 1	Group 2	Group 3	Group 4
Cardiac	10.11	3.59	1.57	6.04
Vascular	3.93	2.39	1.57	1.34
Infectious	1.68	0	1.57	1.34
Peritonitis	0	0	2.09	3.36
Cachexia	1.12	0.60	0.52	0.67
Dementia	1.12	0.60	0	0.67
Malignancy	3.37	0	1.05	1.34
Liver diseases	0	0.60	0.52	2.63
Other	1.12	1.20	0.53	1.34

patients and follow-up for each group are given in Table 1. Table 2 shows the incidence of every cause of death in the groups with different rates of peritonitis. Those patients who were more seriously ill died from their associated illnesses in the first months of treatment, before they arrived at a first peritonitis episode. The mortality rate was maximal for patients with cardio-vascular disease and malignancy. In this group and in the one with a very low peritonitis rate, which included the great majority of patients treated with the Y-system, there were no deaths because of peritonitis. In the groups with high peritonitis rates, death was due to cardio-vascular causes, liver disease, and other causes as well as to peritonitis. Among the liver disease patients, the percentages with cirrhosis, were 5%, 9%, 7%, and 13%, for the four groups, respectively. Finally, there was no relationship between other infections or cachexia-dementia or other causes of death and the peritonitis rate.

Excluding patients who had no peritonitis episodes, life table analysis of patient survival showed different survival curves for the three groups of patients with different peritonitis rates (Fig. 2). The difference was significantly different only between the groups with very low and very high peritonitis rates. Patients with more than 1

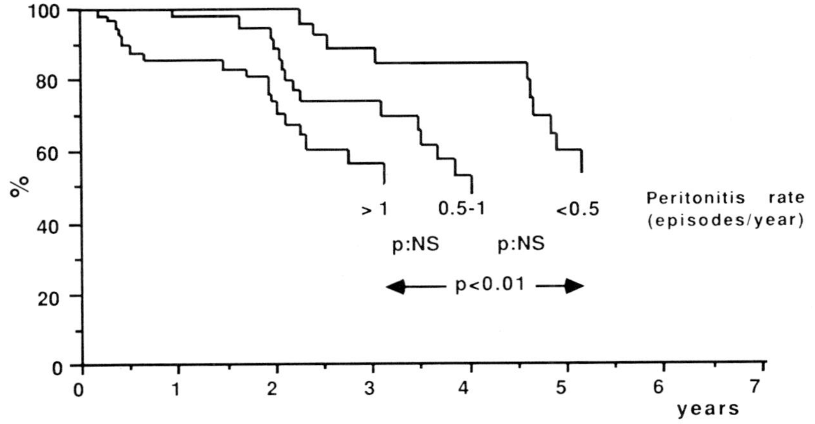

Fig. 2. Patient survival, according to peritonitis rate

Table 3. Causes for drop-out of patients divided according to peritonitis rate. Events/100 patients per year

Cause of CAPD failure	Group 1	Group 2	Group 3	Group 4
Poor compliance	1.68	0	0	1.34
Inadequate ultrafiltration	1.68	0	0	0
Poor biochemical control	1.12	0.60	0	0.67
Patient choice	3.37	0	0.52	0
Catheter/abdominal wall related	0.56	0.60	0.52	0.67
Clinical	1.12	0	0	4.03
Peritonitis	0	0	2.09	6.04
Other	0.56	0	0	0

peritonitis episode per year seem to have a definitely greater probability of death than patients with fewer than 0.5 episodes per year.

In the same patients, causes of drop-out were examined according to peritonitis rate (Table 3). A large number of drop-outs were in the first group, patients who changed methods before having a peritonitis episode. The causes were poor compliance, inadequate ultrafiltration (UF) or biochemical control, and, less important, other clinical reasons (metabolic, others). In the groups with more than 0.5 peritonitis episodes per year, peritonitis and other problems related to the catheter and to the abdominal well were the most frequent causes for leaving the method, with a low incidence of other causes.

True *technique survivals*, obtained by treating those patients who had died, had transplants, or had recovered renal function as lost to follow-up in the analysis, were high for patients with up to 1 peritonitis episode per patient-year, but were significantly worse for patients with more than 1 peritonitis episode per patient-year. The difference was statistically significant only between patients with fewer than 0.5 episodes per year and patients with more than 1 episode per year (Fig. 3).

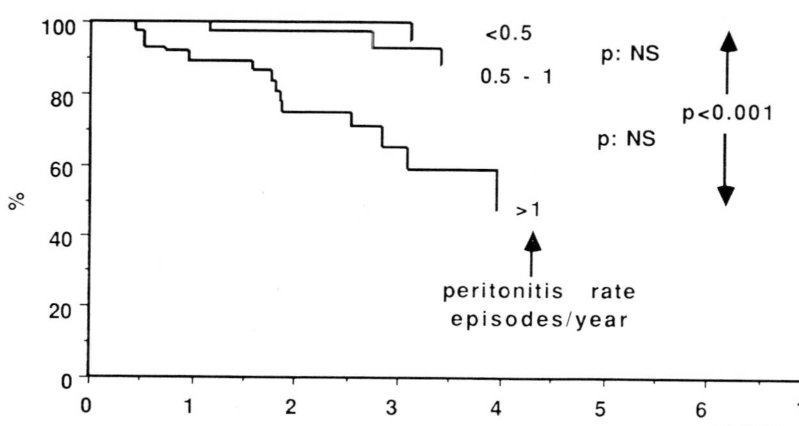

Fig. 3. True technique survival (only CAPD failure considered as final event), according to peritonitis rate

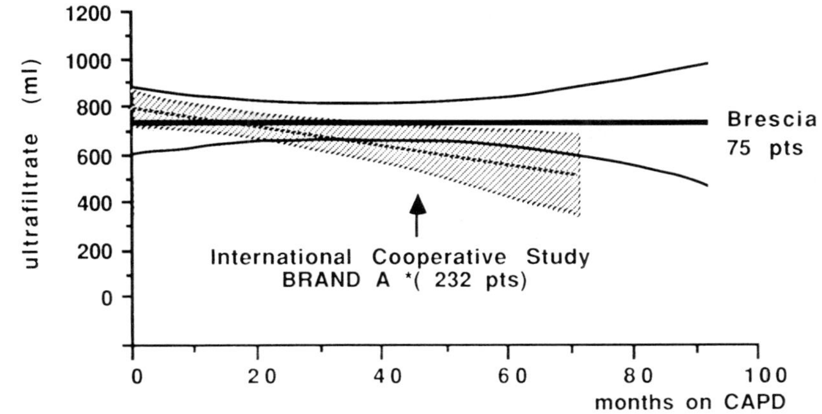

Fig. 4. Trend of ultrafiltration volume over time on CAPD. Comparison between the results of the International Cooperative Study and data of our center

Peritoneal Function

Of our CAPD Y-patients 71 were studied with peritoneal equilibration tests, performed with 2 liters 4.25% glucose and a dwell-time of 4 hours. Mean CAPD duration was 25 months, with a mean number of 0.8 peritonitis episodes during this time.

We found no relationship between glucose absorption, or creatinine transfer, or drainage volume and the number of peritonitis episodes, incidence of peritonitis episodes, or time on CAPD.

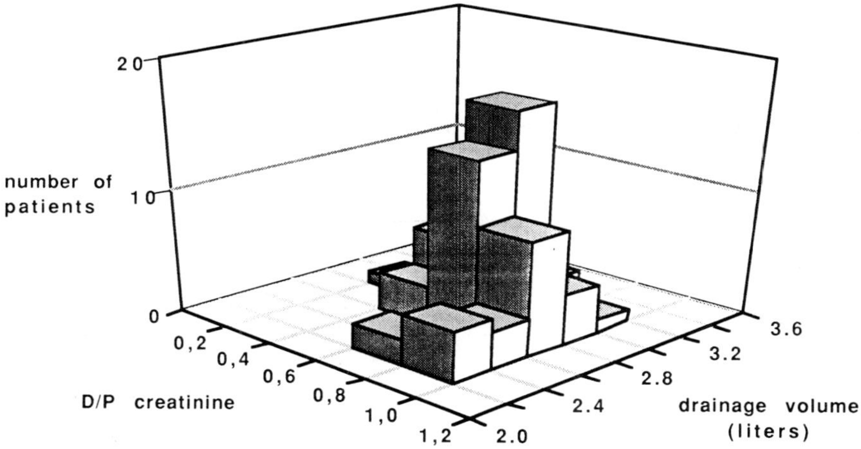

Fig. 5. Seventy-one patients on CAPD. (D/P) creatinine and drainage volume after a 4-hour dwell with 4.25% glucose, two liter bag

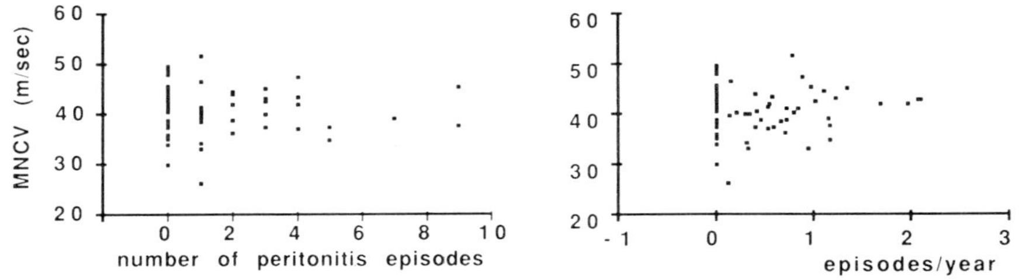

Fig. 6. Motor nerve conduction velocity (*MNCV*) versus number of peritonitis episodes and peritonitis rate

In the International Cooperative Study published in 1984 [7] the relationship between ultrafiltrate volume with 4.25% glucose bags and time on CAPD was investigated in a large number of patients. In that study, the ultrafiltered volume appeared to become smaller as time on treatment lengthened. Such a negative relationship was not apparent in our patients, all on the Y-system, who were followed up until more than 90 months of treatment (Fig. 4). In our series only a very few cases had low, but still sufficient, drainage volumes or low solute transfer (Fig. 5). In no cases were the two indexes of peritoneal function associated, as has been seen in the severe peritoneal malfunction which evolves in sclerosing encapsulating peritonitis. Actually, in the 142 new patients put on the Y-set, we have so far observed only 1 patient with inadequate ultrafiltration and 2 patients with poor biochemical control. In our overall experience with 288 patients, we have had 3 cases (1%) with inadequate ultrafiltration and 4 cases (1.4%) with poor biochemical control. In no case have we had sclerosing encapsulating peritonitis.

Metabolic and Nutritional Data

The influence of peritonitis rate on some biochemical tests was investigated in 108 unselected patients with a mean age of 63±13 years, who had been on CAPD for 28±25 months (range 4–100). In the analysis of variance, we found no relationship between incidence of peritonitis and BUN, serum creatinine, hemoglobin, serum

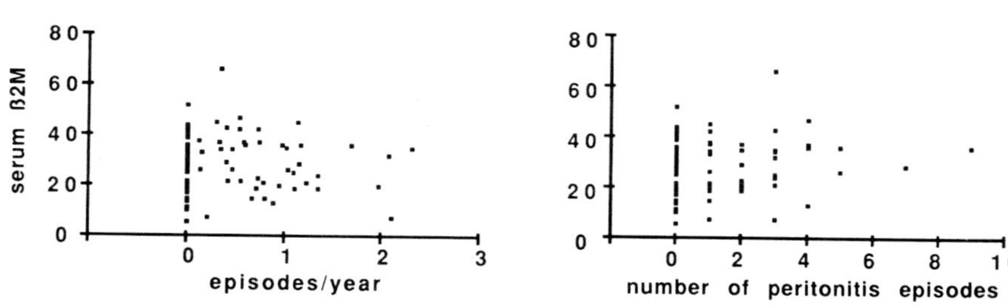

Fig. 7. Serum β2-microglobulin (*Serum β2M*) concentration versus peritonitis rate and number of peritonitis episodes

Table 4. Multiple regression analysis of variables that might affect serum β2-microglobulin concentration

Independent variables:	*P*
Age	0.338
Time of CAPD	0.830
Number of peritonitis episodes	0.593
Peritonitis rate	0.487
Residual urinary volume	<0.001

protein levels (total proteins), albumin, transferrin, pseudocholinesterases, cholesterol, or triglycerides.

Conduction velocity in a motor nerve, the external sciatic-popliteal nerve, did not change as a function of the number of peritonitis episodes or as a function of their frequency (Fig. 6). We also found no relationship between number and frequency of peritonitis episodes and serum level of beta-2 microglobulin (Fig. 7). The only independent variable that clearly influenced the serum beta-2m level in CAPD was the residual urinary volume (Table 4, Fig. 8), that is, the residual renal function.

Discussion

The peritonitis free survival curve was much better with the Y-system than with the standard set for the first two peritonitis episodes, but the intervals between the second and the third peritonitis episodes were the same for the standard and the Y-set. Interpretation of these data is difficult. One possible explanation might be that after the first episodes some changes, such as non-apparent tunnel infections, or intracatheter bacterial slime, or other changes, also immunological factors, intervene to make new peritonitis episodes more likely. Another possibility is that the Y-system

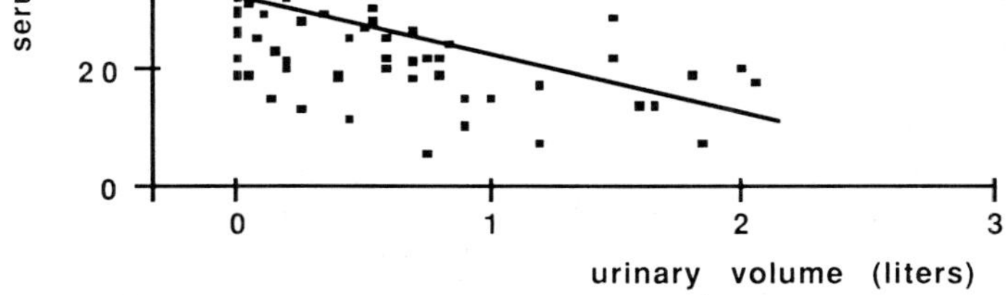

Fig. 8. Relationship between residual urinary volume (*r*) and serum β2-microglobulin (*Serum β2M*) concentration

reveals one population of patients for whom the Y-system is ineffective. As mentioned above, the Y-system cannot prevent hematogenic peritonitis, or peritonitis from bowel infections or from exit-site or tunnel infections. From the clinical point of view it is important to realize that the Y-system becomes of little help when three or more peritonitis episodes follow. In these patients, who are only a minority of the population on the Y-system (9% in our experience with 142 patients with a follow-up of 3479 patient-months), substitution of the catheter or a change to hemodialysis might be taken into consideration. Also, methods that might re-establish the preventive efficacy of the Y-system, for instance fibrinolytic, or other treatment, should be tested.

The impact of the peritonitis rate on patient survival is difficult to assess because of the interference caused by the frequent cardiovascular and neoplastic deaths which occurred even before the appearance of the first peritonitis episode. Excluding the first group of patients who did not have any peritonitis episodes, we can see that patient mortality increased with peritonitis frequency. Patients in the different peritonitis rate groups had the same mean age, so the differences in survival were not due to patient age at the beginning of CAPD. Since cardiac and liver disease are, with peritonitis, the main causes of death in the higher peritonitis rate group, the question arises whether cardiac and hepatic patients are more prone to peritonitis or whether high peritonitis frequency can worsen the prognosis for these patients. Presumably, both statements are right. A high peritonitis rate does not cause an increased death rate from cachexia: so the increased loss of proteins during peritonitis seems to be without consequence for patient survival.

Obviously, the peritonitis rate influences method survival, but a high percentage of drop-outs happen before the appearance of the first peritonitis episode, due to patient choice, or poor compliance, or inadequate peritoneal function, or due to clinical reasons. It is interesting to note, as we documented in a multicenter study (accepted for publication on Pent. Dial. Intern.) of 480 patients on CAPD and 373 on HD, that if we exclude peritonitis as a cause for dropping-out, the relative risk of leaving CAPD is lowered from 1.8 to 1.1, very close to that for hemodialysis, set at 1.

Peritonitis frequency does not affect peritoneal function; this was also assessed by Stablein et al. [9], for the large series of the National Institutes of Health (NIH) Registry. In our patients there was seldom need to change method because of inadequate peritoneal function, and in no case was there an association of low solute transport with low ultrafiltration. Contrary to what was observed in the International Cooperative Study [7], in our patients there was no trend to reduced peritoneal ultrafiltration volume with time. The good prognosis for long term function in CAPD patients on the Y-system is supported by the absence, in our patients, of cases of sclerosing encapsulating peritonitis.

The lack of any relationship between incidence of peritonitis and some protein indexes seems to point out that, within the limits of our experience and of such an evaluation, the peritonitis rate does not significantly affect nutritional status. Also, as shown before, the percentage of deaths due to malnutrition did not differ between CAPD and HD. In former studies [10,11] we showed that protein levels remained stable on CAPD for 4 years and more. As regards the relationship between peritonitis and beta-2M serum levels, our observations seem to indicate that a high peritonitis rate is not a sufficient stimulus to persistently increase the synthesis of this molecule, which is so deeply involved in uremic amyloidosis.

Conclusions

Our experience with the Y-system is largely reassuring, in that it shows that this method can avoid some important side-effects of CAPD. Under our conditions, peritoneal function, neuropathy, nutritional status, and beta-2m levels do not appear to be affected by peritonitis frequency. An influence of peritonitis rate on patient survival can be seen only after excluding patients who died before having a peritonitis episode; in the entire population, causes other than peritonitis are of major importance for patient survival. Peritonitis almost completely accounts for the greater drop-out rate from the CAPD technique than from the HD technique. A low peritonitis rate, such as that obtained with the Y-system, appears to be important for improving CAPD results.

References

1. Maiorca R, Cantaluppi A, Cancarini GC, et al. (1983) Prospective controlled trial of a Y-connector and disinfectant to prevent peritonitis in continuous ambulatory peritoneal dialysis. Lancet II:642–644
2. Buoncristiani U, Bianchi P, Cozzari M, et al. (1980) A new safe simple connection system for CAPD. Int J Nephrol Urol Androl 1:50–53
3. Canadian CAPD Clinical Trials Group (1989) Peritonitis in continuous ambulatory peritoneal dialysis. Randomized clinical trial comparing the Y connector disinfectant system to standard systems. Perit Dial Int 9:159–164
4. Maiorca R, Cancarini GC, Camerini C (1989) Prevention of peritonitis during CAPD: special precautions and use of connection systems. In: Andreucci VE (ed) Vascular and peritoneal access for dialysis. Kluwer Academic, Boston, pp 333–355
5. Peto R, Pike MC, Armitage P, et al. (1976) Design and analysis of randomized clinical trials requiring prolonged observation of each patient. Part 1. Br J Cancer 34:585–621
6. Peto R, Pike MC, Armitage P, et al. (1977) Design and analysis of randomized clinical trials requiring prolonged observation of each patient. Part 2. Br J Cancer 35:1–39
7. A survey of ultrafiltration in continuous ambulatory peritoneal dialysis. An international cooperative study. Second Report. (1984) Perit Dial Bull 4:137–142
8. Dasgupta MK, Ulan RA, Bettcher KB, et al. (1986) Effect of exit site and peritonitis on the distribution of biofilm encased adherent bacterial microcolonies (BABM) on Tenckhoff catheters in patients undergoing continuous ambulatory peritoneal dialysis. In: Khanna R, Nolph KD, Prowant B, Twardowski Z, Oreopoulos DG (eds) Advances in continuous ambulatory peritoneal dialysis 1986. Peritoneal Dialysis Bulletin, Toronto, pp 102–109
9. Stablein DM, Nolph KD, Lindblad AS (1989) Timing and characteristics of multiple peritonitis episodes: a report on the National CAPD Registry. Am J Kidney Dis 14:44–49
10. Maiorca R, Cancarini G, Manili L, et al. (1988) CAPD is a first class treatment: results of an eight-year experience with a comparison of patient and method survival in CAPD and hemodialysis. Clin Nephrol 30:S3–S7
11. Maiorca R, Cancarini GC, Camerini C, et al. (1989) Is CAPD competitive with Haemodialysis for long-term treatment of uraemic patients? Nephrol Dial Trans 4:244–253

Calcium, Phosphorus, Aluminum, and Bone Disease in Continuous Ambulatory Peritoneal Dialysis (CAPD) Patients

R. GOKAL and A. HUTCHISON[1]

SUMMARY. In patients on continuous ambulatory peritoneal dialysis (CAPD), factors that influence calcium balance include calcium intake and net dialysis mass transfer; the latter is positive into the patient, when a current dialysate calcium content of 1.75 mmol/l in dialysis fluid containing 1.36% glucose is used. However, if calcium salts are to be used as phosphate binders, then the risk of hypercalcemia is markedly increased; this can be avoided by lowering the dialysate calcium to 1.25 mmol/l. Using calcium carbonate at meal times, both as a calcium supplement and as an oral phosphate binder, high normal ionized calcium levels are readily achieved. Appropriate dietary phosphate binding in the gut is also achieved (1000 mg phosphate intake and 300 mg dialysate clearance, results in need to bind 700 mg in the gut), while serum phosphate levels are maintained at around 1.5 mmol/l. With this sort of control, serum parathyroid hormone (PTH) levels decline, with significant improvement in the high turnover hyperparathyroid bone disease (osteitis fibrosa) as well as in vitamin D osteomalacia. The pathogenesis of the recently described non-aluminum aplastic bone disease is unknown, but may be related to "severe" PTH reduction and hypercalcemia. The major source of aluminum intoxication is the use of aluminum containing phosphate binders; this can now be totally avoided, thus reducing the risk considerably.

Introduction

Renal osteodystrophy is a virtually universal complication of renal failure. It encompasses the histological lesions of osteitis fibrosa and mild hyperparathyroidism (high bone turnover), and the histological lesions of osteomalacia, aplastic bone disease and mixed lesions (low bone turnover). The pathogenetic mechanisms for the above are complex, but include the interrelationship between calcium and phosphate,

[1]Manchester Royal Infirmary, Manchester, M13 9WL, UK

parathyroid hormone (PTH), vitamin D, and aluminum metabolism. The use of CAPD in the management of end stage renal failure further affects these interrelationships in a variable manner. Over the last ten years the use of CAPD has increased dramatically [1], and considerable knowledge has been gained in this area, enabling the development of a rational approach to the prevention and treatment of renal osteodystrophy during CAPD [2].

Calcium and Phosphate Metabolism

Using a dialysate calcium content of 1.75 mmol/l and a glucose concentration of 1.36%, there is net mass calcium transfer into the patient. However, the reported literature shows a wide disparity in calcium balances. Calcium balance was positive (84–300 mg/day) in two studies where ionized calcium levels were not measured [3,4], while Delmez et al. [5] showed that the transfer of calcium was not only dependent on the ionized serum calcium level but also on the ultrafiltration rate and volume. Thus, a 1.36% glucose solution resulted in a 10 mg calcium uptake into the patient but hypertonic 3.86% glucose solution led to a net loss of 20 mg of calcium. A negative balance resulted from the use of dialysate calcium of 1.5 mmol/l [6] but a positive balance resulted when a level of 2.0 mmol/l was used [7]. In reality, while there is this conflict, total serum and ionized calcium levels are readily normalized upon commencing CAPD in new patients [2]. However, in order to suppress PTH overactivity, the desired ionized calcium level appears to be at the upper limit of normal [8], and to achieve this, a high intake of calcium may be necessary. This factor has to be balanced with the risk of hypercalcemia resulting from high oral calcium intake and the use of 1.75 mmol/l dialysate calcium. This approach does need considerable modification in view of the need to lower serum phosphate levels and the danger of using aluminum free phosphate binders.

While the hyperphosphatemia of renal failure is rapidly improved by CAPD, serum phosphate fails to normalize on CAPD therapy. The obligatory intake of phosphate is about 1000 mg/day, with only 300 mg removed through dialysis. This leaves about 700 mg to be bound and removed fecally [5]. Assuming 50% gut absorption, a considerable phosphate load would result, which would lead to hyperphosphatemia. This condition plays a key role in the development of secondary hyperparathyroidism. The need for an appropriate and effective phosphate binding agent is paramount.

Calcium Carbonate as Phosphate Binder and Low Dialysate Calcium

Hyperphosphatemia has been traditionally managed with aluminum-containing phosphate binders such as aluminum hydroxide. Although these agents are effective as phosphate binders, they lead to an accumulation of aluminum in the body; over a prolonged period of time this can result in vitamin D refractory osteomalacia, microcytic anemia, and dialysis encephalopathy [9]. Hence, there is continued interest in developing alternative but effective non-toxic phosphate binders.

In 1966 Clarkson et al. [10] reported that high calcium carbonate intake resulted not only in a positive calcium balance, but also in reduced gastrointestinal absorption of phosphate. Subsequent reports have shown calcium carbonate to be an effective phosphate binder. However, hypercalcemia, with the risk of metastatic calcification, is the most common side effect [11,12]. Additional problems occur with compliance, gastrointestinal symptoms, and preparation and timing of administration.

If calcium carbonate is to be used as the sole phosphate binder, then in order to achieve fecal phosphate excretion of 700 mg, as Sheikh et al. [13] have shown, 6.25 gm calcium carbonate (2500 mg elemental calcium) is required. Assuming 25% calcium absorption, a considerable amount of calcium would be taken in and hypercalcemia would result. An attractive way to reduce this risk would be to adjust and lower dialysate calcium. Martis et al. [14] have calculated, on theoretical grounds, that a dialysate concentration of 1.25 mmol/l would allow the use of oral calcium carbonate without the risk of hypercalcemia. Our own experience in Manchester, in a group of new CAPD patients using this low calcium dialysis fluid, shows that effective phosphate binding can be achieved (serum levels of about 1.5 mmol/l readily achieved) with the use of a mean daily dose of 10 gm calcium carbonate (Calcichew) given at meal times. No significant hypercalcemia resulted and there was a concomitant decrease in PTH [15]. Similar results have been reported by Hercz et al. [16] who used 1 mmol/l calcium solution in hypercalcemia CAPD patients who had low turnover aplastic bone disease.

Current evidence would suggest that a lower dialysate calcium is essential if the large doses of calcium carbonate needed for phosphate binding are to be used in place of aluminum hydroxide.

Vitamin D and Parathyroid Hormone

The levels of 1,25 dihydroxyvitamin D3 are generally reported to be low in CAPD patients, but levels of 25 hydroxyvitamin D3 are usually normal at the start of therapy, then decline with time [17] or remain stable [7]. This discrepancy may be related to the amount of sunlight exposure [18] and availability of adequate amounts of parent vitamin D [7]. The role of routine vitamin D supplementation is not clear and the danger of hypercalcemia and hyperphosphatemia does mean that this therapy should be based on clinical indications of hypocalcemia and hyperparathyroid bone disease. The intraperitoneal route of administration has evoked some interest; this route raised ionized calcium levels with PTH suppression greater than that obtained with an increased dialysate calcium of 2 mmol/l [7]. In addition, Carozzi et al. [19] have shown that low dialysate calcium level and 1,25 dihydroxyvitamin D3 given intraperitoneally can enhance peritoneal macrophage and antimicrobial function in CAPD.

Even though CAPD removes substantial quantities of PTH (mainly in the form of carboxyterminal fragments), interpreting the results on CAPD has been difficult. The steady decline in PTH with time in some reports [17,18] has not been confirmed by others [6]. However, suppression of high PTH activity may only be brought about by high normal serum ionized calcium levels, in conjunction with normal phosphate levels, suggesting a higher set point than expected for calcium regulated PTH secretion [8].

Recently, Hercz et al. [16] described a non aluminum aplastic bone lesion. In these patients, who were hypercalcemic, PTH levels were "low" (2–3 × normal); on correction of the hypercalcemia with low dialysate calcium the PTH levels rose. This phenomenon raises the question of the role of "low" serum PTH levels in the pathogenesis of the aplastic bone disease. It would be interesting to see further studies in this area. This also raises the issue of how low the PTH level can fall before the aplastic lesion is manifest.

Aluminum Metabolism

Oral ingestion of aluminum containing phosphate binders is the main source of aluminum in CAPD patients, now that manufacturers are able to produce fluids with levels well below 10 μg/l. After 2–3 years on CAPD a significant elevation of serum aluminum (30–40 μg/l) was found in patients who had intermittent aluminum exposure [17]; however those with no aluminum exposure at all were able to maintain levels within the normal range [20].

Although the number of cases of aluminum related osteomalacia (low turnover aplastic bone disease) is small in patients on CAPD [16], this may well increase with prolonged use of aluminum containing phosphate binders. However, now that calcium salts are becoming the major form of phosphate binders (used in conjunction with low dialysate calcium solution) the problem of aluminum related toxicity should diminish into oblivion.

The problems of assessing the total tissue load of aluminum are enormous. Channon et al. [21] showed a good correlation between bone aluminum content and total dose of aluminum prescribed, but showed a poorer correlation between bone aluminum and serum aluminum levels; the latter almost certainly reflect recent exposure to aluminum. The desferrioxamine test has not proven to be a reliable indicator, either of tissue stores or of the development of osteomalacia [22]. In practical terms serum aluminum levels of >50 μg/l (in the absence of recent aluminum exposure) may be cause for concern; levels of >100 μg/l need action which may necessitate therapy with desferrioxamine, which is given intravenously or intraperitoneally [23]. The ultimate diagnostic tool for tissue load may reside in bone histology and bone content of aluminum. For those patients with aluminum toxicity, the use of desferrioxamine has caused a significant rise in hemoglobin and has increased the effectiveness of recombinant human erythropoietin therapy.

Avoidance of aluminum as a phosphate binder appears to be of paramount importance. This is now possible; caution should be exercised in the use of calcium citrate as a phosphate binder. This compound does enhance aluminum absorption and should be avoided.

Renal Bone Disease

There have not been enough studies done on sufficiently large numbers of patients, observed for sufficient lengths of time, to enable firm conclusions to be drawn on the aforementioned interrelationships and on the measures to be used on renal osteodystrophy in CAPD patients. Some reports support the view that careful management can prevent or ameliorate symptomatic hyperparathyroid bone disease [17,18,24], while other reports show no change [25,26], or even deterioration [6,27,28]. These conflicting reports reflect the heterogeneity of patients and their management. However, several recent studies have shown improved control of renal osteodystrophy under CAPD as compared to the control under hemodialysis [29–31].

The major concern of late has been a report on the fairly high incidence of the new histological entity of aplastic, or low turnover, bone disease unrelated to aluminum (Hercz et al. [16]). In a cross-sectional study of both hemodialysis and CAPD patients ($n-260$), nearly 50% of the biopsies showed an aplastic histopathological change; of these, roughly a third had less than 5% aluminum staining. Interestingly, PTH levels were significantly lower in these patients when compared to levels in those patients with normal or high bone turnover. When the patients with less than 5% aluminum staining were switched to a low dialysate calcium the PTH levels increased, escaping the seemingly suppressant effect of an elevated dialysate calcium. These findings raise interesting questions, not only about the pathogenesis of this entity, but also about its significance, its management, and the level of PTH to aim for–should that be important. These are important issues which will be answered only with long term careful observation, now that aluminum can be eliminated as a source of histological aluminum-related osteomalacia.

Overall, it seems that parathyroid bone disease can be ameliorated on CAPD, as can vitamin D related osteomalacia.

In conclusion, it seems that when serum PTH declines with time there is a concomitant improvement in osteitis fibrosa. Suppression of PTH is unlikely, unless a high serum ionized calcium level is achieved together with a normal phosphate level. Non-aluminum related osteomalacia at the start of CAPD invariably improves. Aluminum related aplastic bone disease remains a potential problem, which needs to be minimized by avoiding aluminum containing phosphate binders; however, this disease can be treated with desferrioxamine. There is still considerable debate about the role of vitamin D therapy in the prevention of renal osteodystrophy. What seems to be crucial is the need for maintaining high normal serum ionized calcium levels and normal phosphate levels; this can be only achieved by low calcium concentration in the peritoneal dialysis fluid, coupled with high oral intake of calcium carbonate; in this setting vitamin D analogues may be useful in healing bone, but a role for prophylactic vitamin D cannot be justified. The newly emerging non-aluminum related aplastic bone disease is interesting; its pathogenesis is unclear, as is its significance. Further understanding of this entity may well modify our approach to managing CAPD patients with renal bone disease. Recommendations for managing patients are included in Table 1.

Table 1. Recommendations for managing ROD in CAPD patients

1. Dietary phosphate reduction within 1–1.2 g/kg protein intake
2. Use of $CaCO_3$ (with meals) as phosphate binder–serum phosphate 1.5 mmol/l
3. Serum ionized Ca–upper limit of normal
4. Use of low dialysate Ca (1.25 mmol/l) to achieve 2 and 3
5. Routine vit D unnecessary; based on overt bone disease
6. Monitor PTH. How low PTH?–to avoid aplastic bone disease
7. Monitor aluminum–bone biopsy, serum levels persistently 100 μg/l–use DFO

ROD, renal osteodystrophy; DFO, desferrioxamine

Acknowledgments. Our sincere thanks to Kerry Hulme for typing the manuscript.

References

1. Gokal R (1987) Continuous ambulatory peritoneal dialysis (CAPD) – 10 years on. Q J Med 63:465–472
2. Gokal R (1988) Renal osteodystrophy and aluminum bone disease in CAPD patients. Clin Nephrol 30(Suppl 1):564–567
3. Blumenkrantz M, Kopple J, Moran J, Coburn JW (1982) Metabolic balance studies and dietary protein requirements in patients undergoing CAPD. Kidney Int 21:849–864
4. Parker A, Nolph KD (1980) Magnesium and calcium transfer during CAPD. Trans Am Soc Artif Intern Organs 26:194–196
5. Delmez JA, Slatopolsky E, Martin KJ, Gearing BJ, Harter HR (1982) Minerals, Vitamin D and parathyroid hormone in CAPD. Kidney Int 21:362–367
6. Digenis G, Khanna R, Pierratos A, Meema H, Rabinovich S, Petit J, Oreopoulos D (1983) Renal osteodystrophy in patients managed by CAPD for more than 3 years. Perit Dial Bull 3:81–86
7. Delmez JA, Dougan S, Gearing BK, Rothstein M, Windus D, Rapp N, Slatopolsky E (1987) The effects of intraperitoneal calcitriol on calcium and parathyroid hormone. Kidney Int 31:795–799
8. Slatopolsky E, Martin KJ, Morrissey JJ, Hruska KA (1985) Parathyroid hormone alterations in chronic renal failure. In: Robinson RR (ed) Nephrology, vol II. Springer, New York, pp 1292–1304
9. Wills MR, Savory J (1983) Aluminum poisoning: Dialysis encephalopathy, osteomalacia and anaemia. Lancet II:29–34
10. Clarkson EM, McDonald SJ, deWardener HE (1966) The effect of a high intake of calcium carbonate in normal subjects and patients with chronic renal failure. Clin Sci 30:425–438
11. Stein HD, Yudis M, Sirota RA (1987) Calcium carbonate as a phosphate binder. N Engl J Med 315:609–610
12. Slatopolsky E, Weerts C, Lopex-Hilker S, Norwood K, Zinc M, Winders D, Delmez J (1986) Calcium carbonate as a phosphate binder in patients with chronic renal failure undergoing dialysis. N Engl J Med 315:157–161
13. Sheikh MS, Maguire JA, Emmett M (1989) Reduction of dietary phosphorus absorption by phosphate binders. A theoretical in vitro and in vivo study. J Clin Invest 83:66–73
14. Martis L, Serkes KD, Nolph KD (1989) Calcium carbonate as a phosphate binder: is there a need to adjust peritoneal dialysate calcium concentrations for patients using $CaCo_3$? Perit Dial Int 9:325–328
15. Hutchison A, Gokal R (to be published) Low calcium dialysis fluid and oral calcium carbonate in CAPD. Nephrol Dial Transpl
16. Hercz G, Pei Y, Manueal A (1990) Aplastic osteodystrophy without aluminum in dialysis patients (abstract). Kidney Int 37:449
17. Gokal R, Ramos JM, Ellis HA, Parkinson I, Sweetaman V, Dewar J, Ward MK, Kerr D (1983) Histological renal osteodystrophy and 25 hydroxycholecalciferol and aluminum levels in patients on CAPD. Kidney Int 23:15–21
18. Cassidy M, Owen JP, Ellis HA, Dewar J, Robinson CJ, Wilkinson R, Ward MK, Kerr DNS (1985) Renal osteodystrophy and metastatic calcification in long term CAPD. Q J Med 213:29–48
19. Carozzi S, Nassini M, Schelotto C, Cavelgia P, Santoni O, Barocci S, Versace F, Cantaluppi A, Salit M, Lamperi S (1989) Ca# and function in CAPD. In: Khanna et al. (eds) Peritoneal dialysis bull, Toronto pp 103–110

20. Gokal R (to be published) Peritoneal Dialysis. In: Davidson et al. (eds) Oxford Textbook of Nephrology. Oxford University Press, Oxford
21. Channon SM, Arfeen S, Ward MK (1988) Long term accumulation of aluminium in patients with renal failure. Trace Elements in Medicine 5:154–157
22. Millinar DS, Nebeker H, OHS, Sherrard D, Andrers D, Alfrey AC, Coburn J (1984) Desferrioxamine infusion tests for diagnosis of aluminium osteomalacia. Kidney Int 30:944–948
24. Rahman R, Heaton A, Goodship T, Rodger R, Tapson J, Sellars L, Ellis H, Wilkinson R, Ward MK (1987) Renal osteodystrophy in patients on CAPD: A five year study. Perit Dial Bull 7:1–4
25. Delmez J, Fallon MD, Bergfeld MA, Gearing BK, Dougan CS, Teitelbaum S (1986) CAPD and Bone. Kidney Int 30:379–384
26. Nilsson P, Danielsson BG, Grefberg N, Wide L (1985) Secondary hyperparathyroidism in diabetic and non diabetic patients in long term CAPD. Scand J Urol Nephrol 19:59–65
27. Kurtz SB (1985) Clinical parameters of renal bone disease: a comparison of CAPD and haemodialysis. Dial Transplant 14:30–36
28. Bucciante G, Biachi ML, Valenti G (1984) Progress of renal osteodystrophy during CAPD. Clin Nephrol 6:279–283
29. Shusterman NH, Wasserstein AG, Morrison G, Audet P, Fallon M, Kaplan F (1987) Controlled study of renal osteodystrophy in patients undergoing dialysis. Improved response to CAPD compared with hemodialysis. Am J Med 82:1148–1156
30. Zuccelli P, Catizone L, Casanova S, Fusarole L, Fabri L, Ferran G (1984) Renal osteodystrophy in CAPD patients. Min Electrol Metab 10:326–332
31. Ramsey M, Tapson J, Ward MK (1989) Comparison of renal osteodystrophy between hemodialysis and CAPD (abstract). Perit Dial Int 9(Suppl 1):208

Autacoids and the Kidney

Chair: Raymond Ardaillou (France)
Keishi Abe (Japan)

Oxidant Mechanisms in Glomerulonephritis

SUDHIR V. SHAH[1]

SUMMARY. Several lines of evidence derived from both in vitro and in vivo studies suggest an important role for reactive oxygen metabolites and glomerular pathophysiology. Both leukocytes and glomeruli have been shown to increase the generation of reactive oxygen metabolites in response to a wide variety of stimuli. Reactive oxygen metabolites generated enzymatically or by stimulated neutrophils have been shown to affect several biological processes of potential importance in glomerular injury, including glomerular basement degradation, eicosanoid synthesis, cyclic nucleotide metabolism, and glomerular ADPase activity. Scavengers of reactive oxygen metabolites have been shown to reduce proteinuria in several leukocyte-dependent and leukocyte-independent models of glomerular disease. Taken together, these studies suggest an important role of reactive oxygen metabolites in glomerular disease.

Introduction

Despite extensive investigation, the mechanisms that ultimately cause the functional and morphological changes in glomerular diseases (one of the commonest causes of end stage renal disease), remain poorly understood. A large body of evidence accumulated over the last decade indicates that partially reduced oxygen metabolites are important mediators of ischemic, toxic, and immune-mediated tissue injury [1–3]. In this review, I will introduce the term reactive oxygen metabolites, and then present the available evidence in support of the role of reactive oxygen metabolites in glomerular disease.

Oxygen normally accepts four electrons and is converted directly to water. However, partial reduction of oxygen can and does occur in biological systems, leading to

[1]Tulane University School of Medicine, Department of Medicine, Section of Nephrology, New Orleans, LA 70112, USA

the generation of partially reduced and potentially toxic reactive oxygen metabolites. Thus, when oxygen accepts one electron, superoxide anion, a free radical is generated.

$$O_2 \xrightarrow{e^-} O_2^- \xrightarrow{e^-} H_2O_2 \xrightarrow{e^-} HO\cdot \xrightarrow{e^-} H_2O$$

When oxygen accepts two electrons either directly or by the dismutation of superoxide, hydrogen peroxide is formed. Further reduction of oxygen leads to the generation of highly reactive hydroxyl radical. These oxygen metabolites, including the free radical species, superoxide and hydroxyl radical, and other metabolites such as hydrogen peroxide and hypohalous acids (derived from myeloperoxidase-hydrogen peroxide-halide system) are often collectively referred to as reactive oxygen metabolites.

Several human and experimental glomerulonephritides are characterized by the infiltration of glomeruli by neutrophils and/or monocytes. The importance of leukocytes as mediators of glomerular injury has been delineated in experiments in which selective depletion of neutrophils or monocytes led to amelioration of the glomerular injury. In many other common forms of glomerular diseases (for example, minimal change disease, membranous nephropathy) leukocytes do not play an important role in the glomerular injury. Evidence in support of the role of reactive oxygen metabolites in leukocyte-dependent and leukocyte-independent glomerular disease will be considered separately.

Role of Reactive Oxygen Metabolites in Leukocyte-Dependent Glomerular Disease

Although glomerular injury has been attributed to the release of enzymes from leukocytes, studies from other tissues and recent studies related to glomerular injury indicate that neutrophil-derived reactive oxygen metabolites are also important in tissue injury. Neutrophils and monocytes/macrophages exhibit a burst of oxidative metabolism (respiratory burst) with marked increase in oxygen uptake and the generation of reactive oxygen metabolites in response to plasma membrane perturbation by a variety of soluble and particulate stimuli [3]. Phagocytosis, per se, is not essential to trigger the oxidative burst; pertubation of the plasma membrane appears to be the critical event. Of particular interest is the demonstration that several immune reactants such as serum treated zymosan, a C_3b receptor stimulus, heat aggregated IgG, an Fc receptor stimulus, immune complexes, and complement components, have all

Table 1. Potential sources of reactive oxygen metabolites

Cells	Stimuli
Neutrophils Monocytes	A wide variety of soluble and particulate stimuli, including immune complexes, complement components, and ANCA
Glomeruli Mesangial Cells	Phorbol myristate acetate, zymosan, trypsin, chymotrypsin, PAF, immune complexes, MAC, TNF, and Adriamycin

PAF, platelet aggregation factor; MAC, membrane attack complex; TNF, tumor necrosis factor; ANCA, antineutrophil cytoplasmic autoantibodies

Table 2. Effect of reactive oxygen metabolites on biological processes relevant to glomerular pathophysiology

Reactive oxygen metabolites generated enzymatically or by stimulated neutrophils:

- Increase glomerular eicosanoid synthesis [1]
- Increase glomerular cyclic AMP content [6]
- Participate in GBM degradation [5]
- Reduce glomerular ADPase activity [14]

been shown to trigger the oxidative burst [3]. Of interest, in a recent study it was shown that antineutrophil cytoplasmic autoantibodies (ANCA), which are present in the circulation of most patients with pauci-immune necrotizing vasculitis and pauci-immune crescentic glomerulonephritis, significantly increased the generation of superoxide by neutrophils [4]. Thus, stimulated neutrophils or monocytes are potential sources of reactive oxygen metabolites in leukocyte-dependent glomerular injury.

Superoxide and hydrogen peroxide appear to be the primary species generated; these may then play a role in the generation of additional and more reactive oxidants, including the hydroxyl radical and hypochlorous acid. The direct interaction between superoxide and hydrogen peroxide is rather slow and it has been postulated that in biological systems a trace metal, such as iron, participates in the reaction commonly referred to as the metal-catalyzed Haber-Weiss reaction. This reaction may be summarized as follows:

$$\begin{array}{l} Fe^{3} + O_2^- \rightarrow Fe^{2} + O_2 \\ Fe^{2} + H_2O_2 \rightarrow Fe^{3} + OH^- + HO\cdot \\ \hline O_2^- + H_2O_2 \rightarrow O_2 + OH^- + HO\cdot \end{array}$$

It must be pointed out that while several studies have clearly documented the generation of a potent oxidizing species in the presence of a metal, the possibility that the oxidant may not be hydroxyl radical has been recently raised. Additional reactive oxygen metabolites can be formed, as a result of the metabolism of hydrogen peroxide by neutrophil- and macrophage-derived myeloperoxidase (MPO), to produce high reactive toxic products, including hypochlorous acid.

$$H_2O_2 + Cl^- \xrightarrow{MPO} HOCl + H^+$$

Other hypohalous acids may also be generated, for example, generation of hypobromous acid by eosinophils has recently been reported. Human neutrophils have also

Table 3. In vivo evidence for the role of reactive oxygen metabolites in neutrophil dependent glomerular injury

Scavengers of reactive oxygen metabolites reduce proteinuria in:

- Neutrophil-dependent glomerular injury induced by phorbol myristate acetate and cobra venom factor [8]
- Complement and neutrophil-dependent heterologous phase of anti-GBM antibody disease [12,13]

Infusion of myleo-peroxidase-hydrogen peroxide causes significant proteinuria, endothelial cell swelling, and marked cell foot process effacement. Four to ten days later a marked proliferative glomerular lesion develops [9]

Table 4. In vivo evidence for the role of reactive oxygen metabolites in neutrophil independent glomerular injury

Scavengers of reactive oxygen metabolites reduce proteinuria in:
- Puromycin aminonucleoside model of minimal change disease [20–22]
- Passive Heymann nephritis model of membranous nephropathy [18]
- Cationized gamma globulin-induced immune complex glomerulonephritis [19]

been reported to generate long-lived oxidants (half-life approximately 18 hours) with characteristics similar to N-chloramines.

It is generally accepted that leukocytes cause proteinuria (a hallmark of glomerular diseases) by damaging the glomerular basement membrane (GBM) which serves as the major ultrafiltration barrier to restrict the entry of proteins into the urinary space. Recently, the degradation of the GBM by stimulated neutrophils was shown to be due to the activation of a latent metalloenzyme (most likely gelatinase) by hypochlorous acid or a similar oxidant generated by the myleoperoxidase-hydrogen peroxide-halide system [5]. In addition, several recent studies have shown that oxidants could contribute to GBM damage by increasing its susceptibility to proteolytic damage and by inactivating the alpha-1-proteinase inhibitor (the primary regulator of neutrophil elastase) thus allowing the released elastase to more readily inflict damage to the extracellular matrix. Prevention of proteinuria by catalase in neutrophil-dependent glomerulonephritides suggests that the oxidative mechanism for GBM degradation described above may be quite relevant to leukocyte-dependent glomerular injury.

While the critical role played by leukocytes in proteinuria is generally accepted, infiltrating leukocytes in proliferative glomerulonephritides may also modulate the inflammatory response and glomerular function by altering glomerular metabolism. Reactive oxygen metabolites generated by the xanthine-xanthine oxidase system or by stimulated neutrophils have been shown to increase cyclic AMP content [1,6] and to enhance the synthesis of prostaglandin E_2 (PGE_2), prostaglandin $F_{2\alpha}$ ($PGF_{2\alpha}$), 6 keto$PGF_{1\alpha}$ (the stable metabolite of prostacyclin), and TXB_2 (the stable metabolite of thromboxane) by glomeruli [1]. Thus, by affecting glomerular cyclic nucleotides and/or eicosanoid synthesis, reactive oxygen metabolites may play an important modulatory role in glomerular pathophysiology. In addition, reactive oxygen metabolites affect biological pathophysiology in other tissues relevant to glomerular pathophysiology. For example, several interactions between reactive oxygen metabolites and platelets (which have been postulated to be important in the development of local glomerular injury) have recently been described, infusion of myeloperoxidase-hydrogen peroxide in the renal artery caused glomerular injury that was associated with marked influx of platelets in the glomerular capillaries [7].

Support for the role of reactive oxygen metabolites generated by neutrophils in glomerular injury has been recently obtained from several in vivo studies. Infusion of phorbol myristate acetate (PMA) (a well known potent activator of leukocytes) or infusion of cobra venom factor in the renal artery caused significant proteinuria which was prevented by catalase (which destroys hydrogen peroxide) and neutrophil depletion [1,8]. These studies indicate that hydrogen peroxide and/or its metabolites generated by the neutrophils can cause proteinuria. Johnson et al. reasoned that hydrogen peroxide-mediated injury may involve the myeloperoxidase-hydrogen peroxide-halide system [7]. They demonstrated that infusion of myeloperoxidase followed by infusion of hydrogen peroxide in a chloride-containing solution into the renal artery in rats results in significant proteinuria [9] and four to ten days later, results in the development of a marked proliferative glomerular lesion [7]. In addition, halogenation (as measured by the incorporation of ^{125}I) in glomeruli and GBM was demonstrated in an in situ model of neutrophil-mediated immune complex glomerulonephritis [10]. These studies indicate the activation of myeloperoxidase-hydrogen peroxide-halide in a model of neutrophil-mediated immune complex glomerulonephritis, and indicate that the myeloperoxidase-hydrogen peroxide-halide system is capable of inducing glomerular injury that results in proteinuria.

In addition to increased glomerular permeability, the other common manifestation of glomerular disease is an alteration in glomerular function. Rehan et al. observed that PMA infusion or infusion of cobra venom factor reduced the whole kidney glomerular filtration rate (GFR) by about 50%–90% but catalase (in doses that reduced the proteinuria) did not prevent the fall in GFR [8]. In contrast, Yoshioka et al. have reported that unilateral infusion of PMA led to a fall in the single nephron GFR and evoked a profound constrictive response in the glomerular microcirculation which was prevented by neutrophil depletion or pre-treatment with catalase [11].

One of the best characterized models of complement- and neutrophil-dependent glomerular injury is the heterologous phase of anti-GBM antibody disease. In this model of neutrophil-dependent glomerular injury, treatment with catalase markedly reduced the proteinuria, whereas superoxide dismutase had no protective effect [12]. In another study, dimethylthiourea, a potent hydroxyl radical scavenger, or deferoxamine, an iron chelator, significantly attenuated proteinuria in the complement- and neutrophil-dependent heterologous phase of anti-GBM antibody disease in rabbits [13]. Although the role of iron is not completely understood, the protective effect of iron chelators has been generally taken as evidence for the participation of hydroxyl radical in tissue injury, because iron is critical in the generation of hydroxyl radical (via the Haber-Weiss reaction). Taken together, the studies with PMA, cobra venom factor, and studies in the heterologous phase of anti-GBM antibody disease, demonstrate that reactive oxygen metabolites generated by activated neutrophils play an important role in altering glomerular permeability.

It has been suggested that glomerular ADPase is of major importance in preventing intra-glomerular thrombus formation in experimental glomerulonephritis [14]. These membrane associated enzymes are apparently highly susceptible to reactive oxygen metabolites [15]. Recently it was shown that there is a marked decrease in the activity of these enzymes in two models of glomerulonephritis (anti-GBM and anti-Thy1) which are characterized by the influx of polymorphonuclear neutrophils [14]. Additionally, scavengers of oxygen metabolites prevented the decrease in glomerular ADPase, suggesting a role of reactive oxygen metabolites in the reduction of glomerular ADPase activity [14].

Neutrophil-Independent Glomerular Injury

In proliferative glomerulonephritis, the infiltrating neutrophils and monocytes are potential sources for reactive oxygen metabolites. But what about the non-proliferative glomerulonephritides? Because of the presence of phagocyte-like cells in the glomerulus (particularly mesangial cells) it was postulated that glomerular cells, like other phagocytic cells, would also generate reactive oxygen metabolites in response to a plasma membrane perturbation. In response to PMA, rat glomeruli showed a marked chemiluminescence response, a sensitive measure of the generation of reactive oxygen metabolites by phagocytic cells [16]. In a subsequent study, chymotrypsin or trypsin were shown to markedly increase light emission from the glomeruli. Neutral proteases from infiltrating leukocytes and/or from renal tissue have been shown to be released in glomerular diseases; these results which show the generation of chemiluminescence in response to neutral proteases suggest a potential mechanism for the production of reactive oxygen metabolites in glomerular diseases. In addition to these studies with freshly isolated glomeruli, several investigators have demonstrated the ability of mesangial cells to generate superoxide and hydrogen peroxide in response to a variety of stimuli, including opsonized zymosan, immune complexes, membrane attack complex, and platelet activating factor [1,17]. Thus, the ability of glomerular cells to generate reactive oxygen metabolites in response to plasma membrane perturbation appears to be well established. In addition, as described below, enhanced intracellular generation of reactive oxygen metabolites (for example, hypoxanthine-xanthine oxidase) may also be relevant to glomerular pathophysiology.

The ability of glomerular cells to generate reactive oxygen metabolites suggests that reactive oxygen metabolites may be important mediators of glomerular injury in glomerular diseases that lack infiltrating leukocytes. Passive Heymann nephritis, induced by a single intravenous injection of anti-Fx1A, is a complement-dependent and neutrophil-independent model of glomerular disease that resembles membranous nephropathy in humans. Shah reported that superoxide dismutase or catalase (native or polyethylene glycol-coupled) did not affect the anti-Fx1A-induced proteinuria. In contrast, scavengers of hydroxyl radical, and an iron chelator, deferoxamine, markedly reduced the proteinuria [18]. The protective effects of both the hydroxyl radical scavengers and an iron chelator suggest a role of the hydroxyl radical in passive Heymann nephritis. Similarly, Sedor et al. have reported that two hydroxyl radical scavengers significantly reduced the proteinuria in cationized gamma globulin-induced immune complex glomerulonephritis, a complement- and neutrophil-independent model of membranous nephropathy [19]. Taken together, these studies suggest an important role for hydroxyl radical in animal models of membranous nephropathy.

A single intravenous injection of puromycin aminonucleoside (PAN) results in marked proteinuria and glomerular morphological changes that are similar to minimal change disease in humans. Recently, Diamond et al. postulated that the glomerular injury associated with PAN was mediated by oxygen free radical generation, since hypoxanthine, an intermediate metabolite of PAN, can serve as a substrate for superoxide anion production via the xanthine oxidase system [20]. They reported that allopurinol (an inhibitor of xanthine oxidase) and superoxide dismutase were protective in PAN-induced nephrotic syndrome, suggesting a role for xanthine oxidase generated superoxide anion in this model of minimal change disease [20]. Beaman et al. confirmed the protective effect of superoxide dismutase and, in addition, reported that proteinuria was significantly reduced in rats receiving polyethylene glycol (PEG)-catalase, suggesting a role for both hydrogen peroxide and superoxide anion in this model of glomerular disease [21]. Superoxide anion and hydrogen peroxide may interact (with iron as catalyst) to generate the hydroxyl radical. Several studies have, in fact, shown that enhanced generation of hydrogen peroxide and superoxide anion is accompanied by enhanced generation by hydroxyl radical (or a similar highly oxidizing species). Thakur et al. reported the protective effect of two hydroxyl radical scavengers and an iron chelator, implicating hydroxyl radical in PAN-induced nephrotic syndrome [22].

Conclusions

Reactive oxygen metabolites have been implicated in the development of tissue injury in an increasing number of diseases. While it is currently popular to incriminate oxygen metabolites as ultimate injurious agents, given the complexity and multifaceted nature of inflammation, the cooperative and sometimes complex interaction between different injurious mechanisms appears much more likely. The interaction between proteases and oxidants in the degradation of GBM is just one example of this. Nonetheless, the existence of a sufficient body of in vitro and in vivo information allows us to postulate that reactive oxygen metabolites appear to be important mediators in glomerular pathophysiology.

References

1. Baud L, Aradillou R (1986) Reactive oxygen species: production and role in the kidney. Am J Physiol 251:F765–F776
2. Cross CE, Halliwell B, Borish ET, Pryor WA, Ames BN, Saul RL, McCord JM, Harman D (1987) Davis Conference: Oxygen radicals and human disease. Ann Intern Med 107:526–545
3. Fantone JC, Ward PA (1982) Role of oxygen-derived free radicals and metabolites in leukocyte-dependent inflammatory reactions. Am J Pathol 107:397–418
4. Falk FJ, Terrell RS, Charles LA, Jennette JC (1990) Anti-neutrophil cytoplasmic autoantibodies induce neutrophils to degranulate and produce oxygen radicals in vitro. Proc Natl Acad Sci USA 87:4115–4119
5. Shah SV, Baricos WH, Basci A (1987) Degradation of human glomerular basement membrane by stimulated neutrophils: Activation of metalloproteinase/s by reactive oxygen metabolites. J Clin Invest 79:25–31
6. Basci A, Wallin JD, Shah SV (1987) Effect of stimulated neutrophils on cyclic nucleotide content in isolated rat glomeruli. Am J Physiol 252:F429–F436
7. Johnson RJ, Guggenheim SJ, Klebanoff SJ, Ochi RF, Wass A, Baker P, Schulze M, Couser WG (1988) Morphologic correlates of glomerular oxidant injury induced by the myeloperoxidase-hydrogen peroxide-halide system of the neutrophil. Lab Invest 5:294–301
8. Rehan A, Wiggins RC, Kunkel RG, Till GO, Johnson KJ (1986) Glomerular injury and proteinuria in rats after intrarenal injection of cobra venom factor. Am J Pathol 123:57–66
9. Johnson RJ, Couser WG, Chi EY, Adler S, Klebanoff SJ (1987) New mechanism for glomerular injury. Myeloperoxidase hydrogen peroxide-halide system. J Clin Invest 79:1379–1387
10. Johnson RJ, Klebanoff SJ, Ochi RF, Adler S, Baker P, Sparks L, Couser WG (1987) Participation of the myeloperoxidase-H_2O_2-halide system in immune complex nephritis. Kidney Int 32:342–349

11. Yoshioka T, Badr KR, Ichikawa I (1988) Reactive oxygen species (ROS) mediate the reduction in ultrafiltration coefficient (Kf) and increase in efferent arteriolar resistance induced by activated polymorphonuclear leukocytes (PMN) (abstract). Kidney Int 33:369
12. Rehan A, Johnson KJ, Wiggins RC, Kunkel RG, Ward PA (1984) Evidence for the role of oxygen radicals in acute nephrotoxic nephritis. Lab Invest 51:396–403
13. Boyce NW, Holdsworth SR (1986) Hydroxyl radical mediation of immune renal injury by desferrioxamine. Kidney Int 30:813–817
14. Poelstra K, Hardonk MJ, Koudstaal J, Bakker WW (1990) Intraglomerular platelet aggregation and experimental glomerulonephritis. Kidney Int 37:1500–1508
15. Bakker WW, Baller JFW, Hardonk MJ (1987) Decrease of glomerular ATP-ase activity induced by adriamycin is mediated by oxygen free radical species (abstract). Kidney Int 31:1045–1046
16. Shah SV (1981) Light emission by isolated rat glomeruli in response to phorbol myristate acetate. J Lab Clin Med 98:46–57
17. Adler S, Baker PJ, Johnson RJ, Ochi RF, Pritzl P, Couser WG (1986) Complement membrane attack complex stimulates production of reactive oxygen metabolites by cultured rat mesangial cells. J Clin Invest 77:762–767
18. Shah SV (1988) Evidence suggesting a role for hydroxyl radical in passive Heymann nephritis in rats. Am J Physiol 254:F337–F344
19. Sedor J, Emancipator S, Rahman M (1987) Hydroxyl radical (OH) scavengers ameliorate proteinuria in immune complex glomerulonephritis (IC-GN) (abstract). Proceedings of the Xth international congress of nephrology July 26–31, 1987. p 404
20. Diamond JR, Bonventre JV, Karnovsky MJ (1986) A role for oxygen free radicals in aminonucleoside necrosis. Kidney Int 29:478–483
21. Beaman M, Birtwistle R, Howie AJ, Michael J, Adu D (1987) The role of superoxide anion and hydrogen peroxide in glomerular injury induced by puromycin aminonucleoside in rats. Clin Sci 73:329–332
22. Thakur V, Walker PD, Shah SV (1988) Evidence suggesting a role for hydroxyl radical in puromycin aminonucleoside-induced proteinuria in rats. Kidney Int 34:494–499

Mechanisms of the Biological Effects of Eicosanoids in the Glomerulus

PAOLO MENÈ, ANNA TARANTA, FRANCESCO PUGLIESE, GIULIO A. CINOTTI[1], and ANGELA D'AGOSTINO[2]

SUMMARY. Human glomerular mesangial cells respond to stimulation by vasoconstrictor eicosanoids, such as thromboxane A_2 (TxA_2), with a rapid and sustained elevation of cytosolic Ca^{2+} ($[Ca^{2+}]_i$), followed by enhanced Na^+/H^+ exchange activity. These early ionic signals are accompanied by immediate and persistent membrane depolarization, triggered by enhanced Cl^- conductance. Depolarization is independent of extracellular Na^+, while the amplitude of the $[Ca^{2+}]_i$ transient is regulated by transmembrane Na^+ gradients via a Na^+/Ca^{2+} exchanger. The exchanger is, in turn, activated by a TxA_2 mimetic, suggesting its homeostatic role in controlling $[Ca^{2+}]_i$ of activated cells. Enhanced cycling of intracellular ions is followed within three hours of stimulation with a TxA_2 mimetic by complex changes in the pattern of cellular proteins, with enhanced expression of membrane and cytosolic proteins of approximate MW 38–53 Kda and 125–200 Kda, in the presence or absence of serum, respectively. Regulation of human mesangial cell function and structure by vasoconstrictor eicosanoids in culture may reflect a critical role of these compounds in renal pathophysiology.

Introduction

Glomerular cells metabolize arachidonic acid (AA) to a vast group of biologically active eicosanoids, i.e., 20 C atom unsaturated lipids [1,2]. Only recently, along with some of their biologic effects functional receptors for eicosanoids have been described in cultured cells of glomerular origin [3–5]. Eicosanoids can therefore be regarded as glomerular autacoids, or compounds with a site of action on the same cells, or cells contiguous to those that produce them. The implications of these obser-

[1]Cattedra di Nefrologia Medica, 2a Clinica Medica, Policlinico Umberto I, Viale del Policlinico, 00161 Rome, Italy

[2]Istituto di Istologia ed Embriologia generale, University "La Sapienza," 00161 Rome, Italy

vations are several-fold: first, glomerular eicosanoids may participate in the autocrine and paracrine regulation of intrinsic glomerular cells; second, eicosanoids could mediate cell-to-cell communication between glomerular cells and blood-borne cells; and third, enhanced AA metabolism in renal inflammation may contribute to functional changes of glomerular cells [1,6].

We have undertaken an investigation of the intracellular mechanisms which lead to responses of glomerular cells to eicosanoids. Employing cultured human mesangial cells, we have demonstrated that two families of receptors for eicosanoids can be distinguished, on the basis of their coupling with intracellular signalling mechanisms. A first group of receptors is linked to a phospholipase C, and mediates contraction of smooth muscle-like mesangial cells [4,5]. Typical responses to thromboxane A_2 (TxA_2), prostaglandin $F_{2\alpha}$ ($PGF_{2\alpha}$), and leukotrienes C_4/D_4 (LTC_4, LTD_4) include phosphoinositide breakdown, accumulation of water-soluble inositol phosphates, and the release of intracellularly stored Ca^{2+} [4,5]. These agents also activate Na^+/H^+ exchange, which results in cytosolic alkalinization in the absence of HCO_3^- [4,7]. Since Na^+/H^+ exchange is promoted by a number of activators of protein kinase C, it is possible that vasoconstrictor eicosanoids also enhance translocation of this cytosolic enzyme to the plasma membrane [8]. These signals trigger modest proliferation of G_0/G_1-arrested cells, while they modulate proliferation initiated by peptide growth factors [9]. Vasodilator eicosanoids such as PGI_2—or prostacyclin—and PGE_2 activate adenylate cyclase, thus leading to enhanced formation of cyclic adenosine 3,5-monophosphate (cAMP) [3,10]. Stimulation of this pathway leads to relaxation of the cells, refractoriness to contractile stimuli, and a substantial inhibition of mitogen-stimulated proliferation [9,10]. Some overlap exists between these signalling mechanisms, with certain PGs capable of activating both vasoconstrictor and vasodilator receptors, such as is the case with PGE_2 [5]. Discrete receptors appear to exist for the various eicosanoids, although competitive binding and displacement have been shown, consistent with most other biologic systems sensitive to eicosanoids [5].

Phospholipase C activation is only one early step in the complex cellular responses of cultured human mesangial cells to the vasoconstrictor eicosanoid, TxA_2. In the present study, we briefly review both the early effects of TxA_2 on ion transport mechanisms, and later functional changes, revealed by regulation of the cellular synthesis of protein.

Materials and Methods

Cell Culture

Human mesangial cells were cultured from glomerular explants isolated by sequential sieving from histologically normal nephrectomy specimens. Cells were characterized and grown as described [5,11]. Culture medium was RPMI 1640 supplemented with 17% fetal bovine serum (FBS, Gibco, Paisley, U.K.), 5 ug/ml human recombinant insulin (Novo, Copenhagen, Denmark), and 10 ug/ml ceftriaxone (Roche, Basel, Switzerland). Confluent monolayers from four independent cell lines in passages 2–15 were used.

Measurement of Cytosolic Free Ca^{2+} ($[Ca^{2+}]_i$)

$[Ca^{2+}]_i$ was measured by a modification of previously described fluorimetric techniques [4,5]. Confluent monolayers on plastic Aclar coverslips (Allied Engineered Plastics, IL) were grown for 24 h in serum-free RPMI 1640 medium and were then loaded with 1 uM fura-2 (Molecular Probes, Eugene, OR) for 40 min at 37°C [12]. The cells were then incubated for a further 20 min in fluoroprobe-free medium, and were then placed on ice until assayed. Measurements were performed at 37°C in Krebs-Hensleit-based solutions buffered with 20 mM HEPES. Whenever appropriate, Na^+ was replaced isoosmotically with choline chloride or n-methyl-D-glucamine chloride. The coverslips were inserted into thermostatically controlled quartz cuvettes in a Perkin-Elmer LS5B spectrofluorometer fitted with stirring equipment. Ca^{2+}-dependent fluorescence was measured with excitation/emission wavelengths set at 339/500 nm, respectively. The recordings were calibrated with standard formulae by saturation of $[Ca^{2+}]_i$ with 15–40 uM ionomycin, followed by chelation to minimal fluorescence with 7.5 mM EGTA + 60 mM Tris base [12,13].

Measurement of Membrane Potential (E_m)

E_m was measured in bis-(1,3-diethylthiobarbiturate)-trimethineoxonol (bisoxonol, Molecular Probes, Eugene, Ore.)-equilibrated suspensions [14]. Confluent monolayers grown in 750 ml tissue culture flasks (Becton & Dickinson, Lincoln Park, N.J.) were released by brief trypsinization (3 min, 0.05% trypsin + 0.02% Na-ethylenediamine-tetraacetate, GIBCO, Paisley, United Kingdom), followed by gentle scraping in serum-free RPMI 1640 supplemented with neutralizing amounts of soybean trypsin inhibitor (1:3 trypsin/inhibitor, w/w, Fluka, Buchs, Switzerland). The cells were spun for 10 min at 900 g and the pellet was resuspended in the appropriate experimental solutions at a final density of 2×10^6 cells/ml. Bisoxonol was then added to 1 ml of the cell suspension under continuous stirring in the fluorometer, to a final concentration of 0.2 uM. Equilibration of bisoxonol was achieved within 2–5 min, as indicated by stable fluorescence readings at 540/580 nm excitation/emission wavelengths. Slits were 5/10 nm, respectively. Calibration of E_m-dependent fluorescence was performed in the presence of the monovalent cation ionophore, gramicidin D, 0.2 uM. Its addition determined rapid hyperpolarization of the cells, reflected by a downward shift of fluorescence. Graded additions of extracellular Na^+ progressively depolarized the cells, as revealed by a linear increase of fluorescence in the range of calculated E_m values between −50 and 0 mV. E_m in the presence of gramicidin D was calculated by the equation $E_m = -59 \log [K^+ + Na^+]_i / [K^+ + Na^+]_e$, assuming $[K^+ + Na^+] = 140$ mM [15,16]. The fluorescence readings at various imposed E_m were employed to draw a standard curve, to which recordings from experiments on aliquots of the same cell preparation were normalized. Choline (as the Cl salt) was employed for replacement of Na^+ in Na^+-free experiments, while gluconate (as the Na^+, K^+, and Ca^{2+} salts) was employed for Cl^- replacement.

Metabolic Labelling and Fluorography of Cellular Proteins

Confluent monolayers were grown in 250 or 750 ml tissue culture flasks in the continuous presence of FBS, or in the absence of FBS, for 72 h after reaching confluence. The monolayers were incubated for 1 h in methionine-free Dulbecco's modified minimal essential medium (DMEM), followed by labelling with 15 uCi/ml [^{35}S]-methionine in methionine-free DMEM for 4 h. At the end of labelling, monolayers were scraped off the flasks in 20 ml total Ca^{2+}, Mg^{2+}-free phosphate buffer saline (PBS) supplemented with 3 mM ethylenediaminotetraacetic acid (EDTA). Cells were spun at 500 g for 10 min, resuspended in 1 ml 10 mM Tris-HCl solution containing 2 mM polymethylsulfonate, and homogenized with 10 strokes of a Teflon pestle. Cell homogenates were spun at 3000 g for 20 min to eliminate nuclei, then at 12000 g for 30 min to discard mitochondria. The resulting supernatant was run at 100000 g for 60 min, to yield a membrane protein pellet and a cytosolic protein supernatant. Aliquots of the two preparations were TCA-precipitated for total protein assay, by a modification of Lowry's technique [17], and counted for total radioactivity by liquid scintillation spectrometry. The remaining sample material was subjected to sodium dodecylsulfate gel electrophoresis (SDS-PAGE) with a modification of Laemmli's technique [18], followed by fluorography.

Results

Short-Term Effects of TxA_2

Stimulation of human mesangial cells with the TxA_2 mimetic, U-46619 (Upjohn, Kalamazoo, Mich.), induces a rapid, partially reversible increase of $[Ca^{2+}]_i$. These

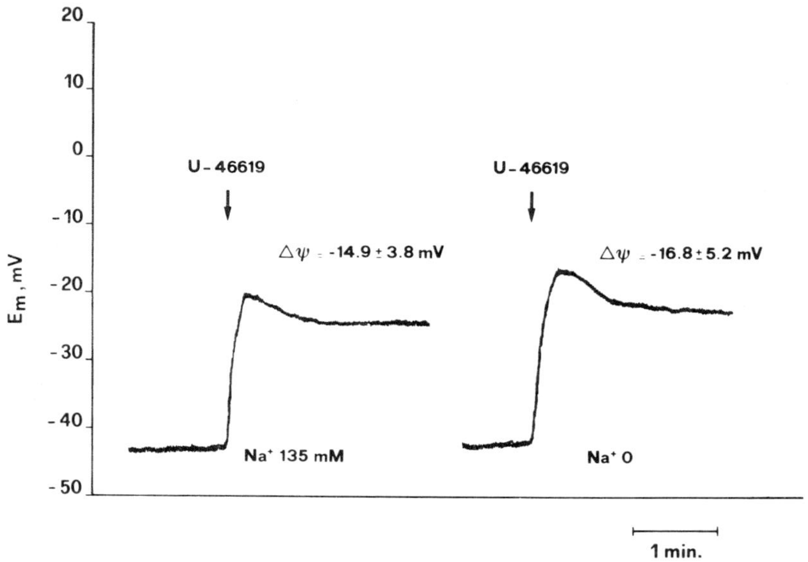

Fig. 1. Effects of the TxA_2 mimetic U-46619, 1 uM, on membrane potential (E_m) of cultured human mesangial cells bathed in 135 mM Na^+ solution (*left*), or Na^+-free, choline chloride solution (*right*). Mean depolarization in mV ± SE from $n = 5$ experiments on *top of each graph*

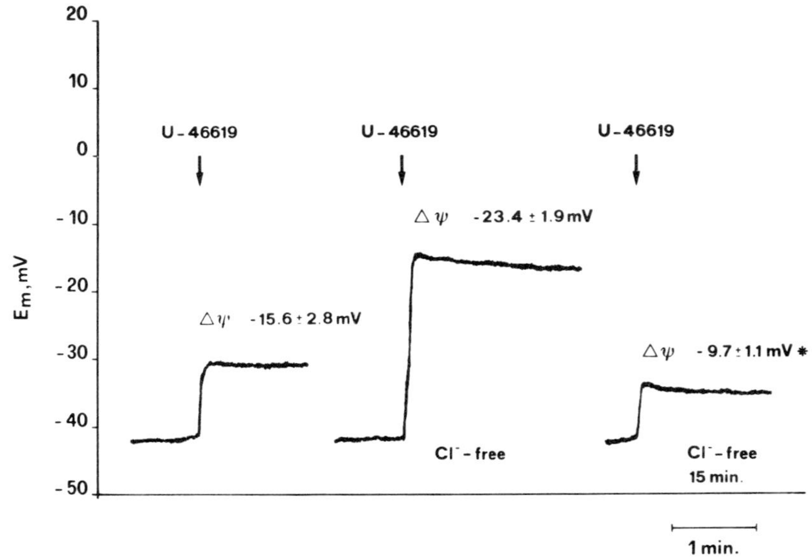

Fig. 2. Effects of 1 uM U-46619 on membrane potential (E_m) of cultured human mesangial cells. *Left*, 135 mM Na^+ solution; *middle*, acute exposure to Cl^--free solution; *right*, cells preincubated for 15 min in Cl^--free solution. Mean depolarization in mV ± SE from $n=5$–8 experiments on *top of each graph*. $^*P<0.05$ vs Cl^- solution, one-way analysis of variance

effects are paralleled by transient cytosolic acidification and followed by enhanced Na^+/H^+ antiport activity, unmasked by HCO_3^- removal from the bathing solution [7]. We asked whether enhanced ion fluxes, i.e., Ca^{2+} and Na^+ entry, result in, or are to any extent related to, perturbation of E_m. Cells loaded with the lipophilic anion, bisoxonol, were rapidly depolarized by application of U-46619, as revealed by an immediate increase of fluorescence due to internalization of the dye (Fig. 1). Depolarization was dose-dependent, persistent both in Na^+-containing and Na^+-free solutions, and was therefore unrelated to Na^+ influx (Fig. 1). Since Ca^{2+} influx would not account for the observed large changes of E_m, we turned to Cl^- as the major anion potentially responsible for depolarization. Acute isoosmotic replacement of Cl^- with gluconate, which by itself did not depolarize the cells, magnified the depolarizing response to U-46619, presumably by facilitated efflux of Cl^- (Fig. 2). Conversely, cells incubated in Cl^--free solution for 15 min at 37°C displayed marked inhibition of depolarization, consistent with Cl^- depletion. This indicates that TxA_2, in a manner similar to that of arginine vasopressin (AVP, not shown), enhances a Cl^- conductance in human mesangial cells, thus leading to depolarization of the plasma membrane. In turn, depolarization is possibly responsible for the opening of voltage-gated Ca^{2+} channels, thus contributing to the rise of $[Ca^{2+}]_i$ brought upon by the eicosanoid.

Other pathways of Ca^{2+} influx exist, however, in these cells. We have recently obtained evidence for a Na^+/Ca^{2+} exchange mechanism in cultured human mesangial

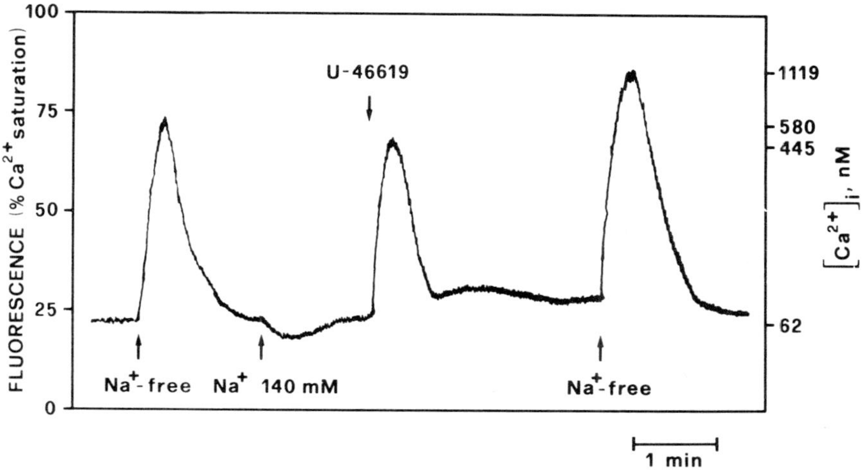

Fig. 3. Effects of rapid Na^+ removal (Na^+-free) on $[Ca^{2+}]_i$ of fura-2-loaded monolayers of cultured human mesangial cells. Note enhancement of the effects of repeated Na^+ removal, following stimulation of the same monolayer with 1 uM U-46619. Continuous fluorescence monitoring representative of $n=6$ experiments

cells. As shown in Fig. 3, abrupt withdrawal of extracellular Na^+, by replacing the bathing solution with isoosmotic choline or n-methyl-D-glucamine chloride solutions, stimulates a rapid rise of $[Ca^{2+}]_i$, resulting from Ca^{2+} influx. Evidence for this pathway includes suppression of the $[Ca^{2+}]_i$ response in EGTA-containing solutions, lack of sensitivity to blockers of voltage-operated Ca^{2+} channels, inhibition by amiloride, enhancement by Na^+-loading the cells with ouabain, and the action of the Na^+ ionophores, monensin and gramicidin [19]. Following the initial influx of Ca^{2+}, exposure of the cells to 1 uM U-46619 in Na^+ solution markedly enhanced the $[Ca^{2+}]_i$ response to a second removal of Na^+ in the same monolayer. In $n=5$ experiments, U-46619 increased the peak $[Ca^{2+}]_i$ response to Na^+ removal from 1009 ± 142 to 1442 ± 247 nM ($P < 0.05$ by unpaired analysis of variance). Conversely, the amplitude of the $[Ca^{2+}]_i$ spike in response to 1 uM U-46619 was significantly enhanced in Na^+-free solutions, from 688 ± 220 to 1152 ± 123 nM ($P < 0.01$ by unpaired analysis of variance, $n=5$). This implies that (1) Na^+/Ca^{2+} exchange contributes to the efflux of Ca^{2+} upon stimulation of mesangial cells by vasoconstrictor eicosanoids, and (2) activation of this exchanger by TxA_2 may serve homeostatic functions, modulating the amplitude of the $[Ca^{2+}]_i$ transient.

Long-Term Effects of TxA_2

Activation of these early signals translates into later functional changes. We and others have previously described the antagonism between adenylate cyclase-and phospholipase C-transduced eicosanoids on the contraction and proliferation of mesangial cells [9,10]. We have now undertaken a study of the effects of TxA_2 on

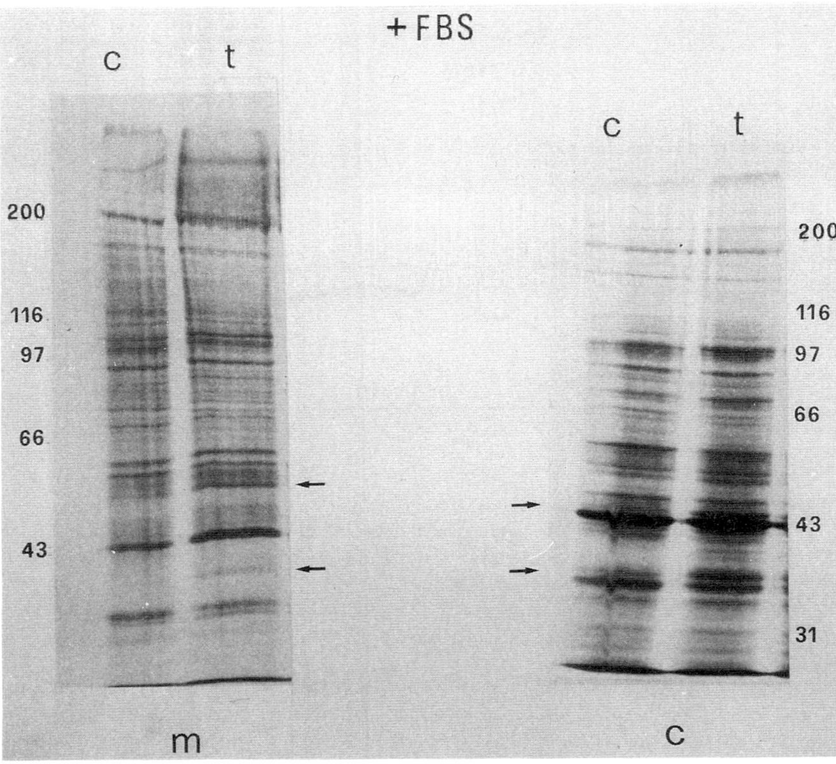

Fig. 4. Effects of U-46619 on protein synthesis of cultured human mesangial cells proliferating in response to 17% fetal bovine serum (*FBS*). SDS-PAGE of membrane-associated (*m*) and cytosolic (*c*) [^{35}S]-methionine-labelled proteins, 24-h incubation with 1 uM U-46619 (*t*) vs control (*c*). Representative fluorography of $n=4$ experiments

protein synthesis of confluent monolayers of human mesangial cells. Both types of cells maintained in the presence of FBS, i.e., cycling cells, and quiescent cells after 72 h in the absence of FBS, responded to acute (4 h) and chronic (24 h) exposure to 1 μM U-46619 with typical changes of the pattern of protein synthesis. Despite a modest, non-significant reduction of total [^{35}S]-methionine incorporation into cell proteins during 24-h incubations with U-46619 (membrane proteins $-6 \pm 13\%$ and $-136 \pm 113\%$, cytosolic proteins $-11 \pm 20\%$ and $-57 \pm 55\%$, w/ and w/FBS, respectively; % of control ± SE, $n=4$), increased expression of membrane and cytosolic proteins of approximate MW 38–53 Kda in the presence of FBS (Fig. 4), as well as membrane proteins of MW 125–200 Kda in the absence of FBS, indicated specific induction of multiple transcripts by TxA_2. While identification of such proteins is in progress, these results are consistent with modulation of mesangial cell phenotype by TxA_2, with possible differentiation and expression of specialized functions.

Discussion

Human mesangial cells respond to stimulation by vasoconstrictor eicosanoids with multiple functional changes, reflecting activation of specific receptors. We herein report that a TxA_2 mimetic acutely depolarizes the cells, presumably by promoting a Cl^- current. The process is independent of extracellular Na^+, and may lead to initiation of Ca^{2+} influx, with resulting sustained elevations of $[Ca^{2+}]_i$. Similar findings have been reported with fluorimetric and electrophysiological techniques in rat mesangial cells exposed to peptide vasoconstrictors [15,20,21]. In turn, the Ca^{2+} signalling pathway is markedly altered by removal of extracellular Na^+, which magnifies the stimulatory effects of the TxA_2 mimetic, as well as the effects of other vasoconstrictors (not shown). Na^+ removal unmasks the presence of a mechanism linking Ca^{2+} and Na^+ fluxes, namely a Na^+/Ca^{2+} exchanger. This transporter is acutely activated by TxA_2, as revealed by the larger amplitude of the $[Ca^{2+}]_i$ spike in cells prestimulated by U-46619. This activation may result from (i) synergism with TxA_2–promoted discharge of Ca^{2+} from internal stores, (ii) Na^+-loading via Na^+/H^+ exchange, with resulting increased Na^+ export via Na^+/Ca^{2+} exchange, or (iii) Ca^{2+} or protein kinase C direct effects on the exchanger. In general, enhancement of the antiporter by phospholipase C agonists may represent a homeostatic mechanism modulating the $[Ca^{2+}]_i$ surges. Evidence for such Na^+/Ca^{2+} exchange mechanisms has been presented for several smooth muscle cell lines, although differences exist in their regulation and sensitivity to vasoconstrictors [22–24]. The presence of a Na^+/Ca^{2+} exchanger in cultured mesangial cells strengthens the belief that these cells structurally and functionally resemble smooth muscle [25]. From these experiments, one may conclude that vasoconstrictor eicosanoids promote a resetting of ion balance across the plasma membrane, taking place within seconds to a few minutes. The process is followed by functional changes including contraction, interference with cell proliferation, and complex alterations of protein synthesis. This last aspect is particularly interesting, in view of the stimulation of specific protein synthesis, even though total protein synthesis is substantially unchanged, both in the presence and in the absence of FBS. This phenomenon is consistent with a substantial lack of stimulation or inhibition of cell growth, previously described by us in quiescent and cycling cells, respectively [9]. On the other hand, stimulation of certain protein products points to structural modifications of the cells, which may acquire a differentiated phenotype upon exposure to vasoconstrictor eicosanoids. Clearly, further work is required in order to identify the proteins induced by TxA_2, as well as their location and function. This may lead to significant progress in our understanding of the pathophysiologic role of eicosanoids in the kidney.

Acknowledgments. We are indebted to Ms. Stefania De Grossi, Ms. Tiziana Menna and Mr. Salvatore Greci for expert technical assistance. These studies were partially funded by grants from the Ministry of Education of Italy (quota 40% and 60%).

References

1. Dunn MJ (1983) Renal prostaglandins. In: Dunn MJ (ed) Renal Endocrinology. Williams and Wilkins, Baltimore, pp 1–74

2. Ardaillou N, Hagege J, Nivez MP, Ardaillou R, Schlondorff D (1985) Vasoconstrictor-evoked prostaglandin synthesis in cultured human mesangial cells. Am J Physiol 248 (Renal Fluid Electrolyte Physiol 17):F240–F246
3. Friedlander G, Chansel D, Sraer J, Bens M, Ardaillou R (1983) PGE_2 binding sites and PG-stimulated cyclic AMP accumulation in rat isolated glomeruli and glomerular cultured cells. Mol Cell Endocrinol 30:201–214
4. Simonson MS, Menè P, Dubyak GR, Dunn MJ (1988) Identification and transmembrane signaling of leukotriene D_4 receptors in human mesangial cells. Am J Physiol 255:C771–C7805
5. Menè P, Dubyak GR, Abboud HE, Scarpa A, Dunn MJ (1988) Phospholipase C activation by prostaglandins and thromboxane A_2 in cultured mesangial cells. Am J Physiol 255:F1059–F1069
6. Menè P, Cinotti GA (1989) Paracrine and autocrine functions of glomerular mesangial cells. J Endocrinol Invest 12:497–509
7. Menè P, Dubyak GR, Scarpa A, Dunn MJ (1991) Regulation of cytosolic pH of cultured mesangial cells by prostaglandin $F_{2\alpha}$ and thromboxane A_2. Am J Physiol 260 (Cell Physiol 29)
8. Nishizuka Y (1986) Studies and perspectives of protein kinase C. Science 233:305–312
9. Menè P, Abboud HE, Dunn MJ (1990) Regulation of human mesangial cell growth in culture by thromboxane A_2 and prostacyclin. Kidney Int 38:232–239
10. Menè P, Dunn MJ (1988) Eicosanoids and control of mesangial cell contraction. Circ Res 62:916–925
11. Striker GE, Killen PD, Farin FM (1980) Human glomerular cells in vitro: isolation and characterization. Transplant Proc 12:88–99
12. Grynkiewicz G, Poenie M, Tsien RY (1985) A new generation of Ca^{2+} indicators with greatly improved fluorescence properties. J Biol Chem 260:3440–3450
13. Cobbold PH, Rink TJ (1987) Fluorescence and bioluminescence measurement of cytoplasmic free calcium. Biochem J 248:313–328
14. Waggoner AS (1979) The use of cyanine dyes for the determination of membrane potentials in cells, organelles, and vesicles. Methods Enzymol 55:689–695
15. Kremer SG, Breuer WV, Skorecki KL (1989) Vasoconstrictor hormones depolarize renal glomerular mesangial cells by activating chloride channels. J Cell Physiol 138: 97–105
16. Rink TJ, Montecucco C, Hesketh TR, Tsien RY (1980) Lymphocyte membrane potential assessed with fluorescent probes. Biochim Biophys Acta 595:15–30
17. Markwell MK, Haas SM, Bieber LL, Tolbert NE (1978) A modification of the Lowry procedure to simplify protein determination in membrane and lipoprotein samples. Anal Biochem 87:206–210
18. Laemmli UK (1970) Cleavage of structural proteins during the assembly of the head of bacteriophage T4. Nature 227:680–685
19. Menè P, Pugliese F, Cinotti GA (1990) Na^+/Ca^{2+} exchange in cultured human mesangial cells (abstract). Kidney Int 37:210
20. Okuda T, Yamashita N, Kurokawa K (1986) Angiotensin II and vasopressin stimulate calcium-activated chloride conductance in rat mesangial cells. J Clin Invest 78:1443–1448
21. Okuda T, Kojima I, Ogata E, Kurokawa K (1989) Ambient Cl^- ions modify rat mesangial cell contraction by modulating cell inositol trisphosphate and Ca^{2+} via enhanced prostaglandin E_2. J Clin Invest 84:1866–1872
22. Vigne P, Breittmayer J-P, Duval D, Frelin C, Ladzunski M (1988) The Na^+/Ca^{2+} antiporter in aortic smooth muscle cells. Characterization and demonstration of an activation by phorbol esters. J Biol Chem 263:8078–8083

23. Smith JB, Zheng T, Smith L (1989) Relationship between cytosolic free Ca^{2+} and Na^+/Ca^{2+} exchange in aortic muscle cells. Am J Physiol 256 (Cell Physiol 25):C147–C154
24. Aaronson PI, Benham CD (1989) Alterations in $[Ca^{2+}]_i$ mediated by sodium-calcium exchange in smooth muscle cells isolated from the guinea-pig ureter. J Physiol (Lond) 416:1–18
25. Menè P, Simonson MS, Dunn MJ (1989) Physiology of the mesangial cell. Physiol Rev 69:1347–1424

The Functional Significance of Lipoxygenase Products of Arachidonic Acid in the Glomerular Microcirculation

KAMAL F. BADR and KIHITO TAKAHASHI[1]

SUMMARY. Intrarenal administration of Lipoxin A_4 (LXA_4) results in vasodilatory responses, but reduces the ultrafiltration coefficient, K_f. LipoxinA_4 competes for the ^{3}H-Leukotriene D_4 (LTD_4) binding to rat mesangial cells and stimulates inositol trisphosphate ($INsP_3$) formation from these cells. Reversal of stereochemical orientation of the polar substituents at C5 and C6 from S,R to R,S in both LTD_4 and LXA_4 abolishes both homologous and heterologous competition for ^{3}H-LTD_4 binding to mesangial cells and leads to total loss of biologic activity. Taken together, these data provided evidence for the involvement of a common recognition site mediating the actions of these two eicosanoids on mesangial cells. Cyclooxygenase inhibition reversed the vasodilatory action of LXA_4, suggesting that LXA_4-mediated increases in RPF were due to the secondary release of vasodilatory cyclooxygenase products. Intrarenal arterial administration of other lipoxins, LXB_4 and 7-cis, 11-trans LXA_4, induced vasoconstriction. Administration of the last named lipoxin which has a configuration at C5 and C6 identical with that of LTD_4, resulted in systemic and renal effects similar to those of LTD_4, suggesting that these actions resulted from activation of LTD_4 receptor-coupled responses.

Introduction

The functional significance of lipoxygenase metabolites of arachidonic acid in glomerular inflammation has been increasingly recognized. We have previously shown that intrarenal arterial infusion of Leukotriene D_4 (LTD_4) resulted in vasoconstriction [1], while that of Lipoxin A_4 (LXA_4) induced vasodilatory responses [2]. However, interestingly, both compounds reduced the glomerular capillary ultrafiltration coefficient, K_f, which is currently considered to result from the con-

[1]Division of Nephrology, Vanderbilt University School of Medicine, Nashville, TN 37232, USA

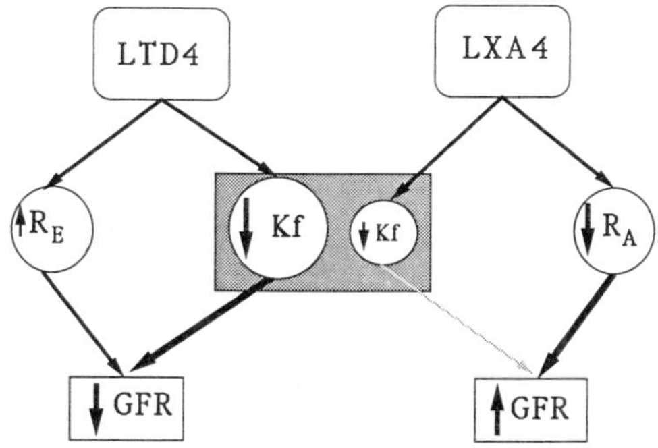

Fig. 1. Summary of LTD_4 and LXA_4-induced changes in glomerular dynamics. LTD_4 reduces GFR as a result of combined reductions in glomerular plasma flow [induced mainly by an increase in efferent arteriolar resistance (R_E)] and ultrafiltration coefficient, K_f. On the other hand, LXA_4 reduces selectively afferent (R_A), but not efferent arterial resistance, thereby leading to increases in glomerular plasma flow and net transcapillary hydraulic pressure difference. This results in an increase in GFR, an effect partially offset by a simultaneous fall in K_f

certed contractile action of smooth muscle-containing glomerular mesangial cells; this action thereby reduces the total glomerular capillary surface area available for filtration [3] (Fig. 1). Recently, we have characterized the binding of LTD_4 to rat mesangial cells and its intracellular signal transduction pathways [4]. Because LTD_4 and LXA_4 share a common orientation of polar substitutes at the C5 and C6 positions (5S, 6R), and this stereochemical configuration is an absolute requirement for the biological activity of these eicosanoids [5], we investigated whether LXA_4-induced falls in K_f were in part due to its action on the mesangial cell LTD_4 receptors. In addition, we

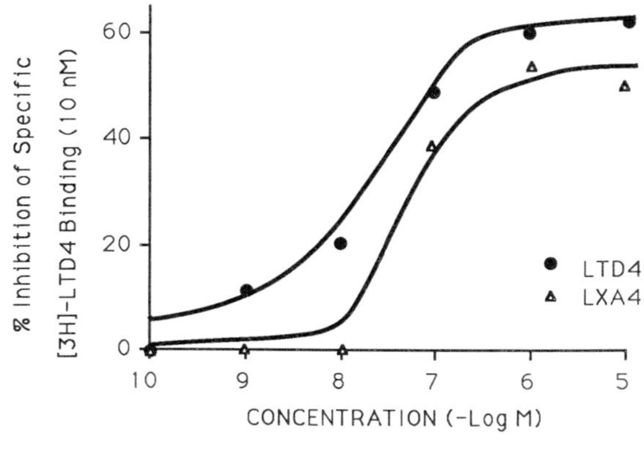

Fig. 2. Percent inhibition of ^3H-LTD_4 (10 nM) binding to rat glomerular mesangial cells by LTD_4 (●) and LXA_4 (Δ). Each point represents the mean of four experiments performed in duplicate. (From [5])

investigated the mechanism of LXA_4-induced vasodilatation, and, in view of expanding interest in other lipoxins, the effects of LXB_4 and a newly discovered biologically active isomer of LXA_4, 7-cis, 11-trans LXA_4, [6] on the renal vasculature.

Methods

All micropuncture studies were performed on Inactin-anesthetized male Munich-Wistar rats, weighing 200-230 g, which were prepared for micropuncture according to protocols previously described [1]. A 30-gauge needle was placed at the root of the left renal artery; through this were infused all the compounds tested in this study. Homologous rat plasma was administered i.v. to maintain euvolemia. Studies of ^{3}H-LTD_4 binding were performed routinely at 4°C on mesangial cells grown to confluence in 24-well cluster dishes. The formation of $InsP_3$ in ^{3}H-inositol labelled mesangial cells, in response to either LTD_4 or LXA_4, was measured by separating ^{3}H-$InsP_3$ by anion-exchange column chromatography by Berridge's method [7].

Results and Discussion

Intrarenal arterial administration of LXA_4 (0.75 µg/kg/min) induced significant increases in single nephron glomerular filtration rate (SNGFR) and plasma flow (Q_A) from 38.4±1.7 to 45.5±3.0 nl/min ($P<0.05$) and from 95±6 to 127±9 nl/min ($P<0.05$), respectively. The increase in Q_A was due to a selective fall in preglomerular resistance (R_A) from 2.55±0.16 to 1.75±0.20 10^{10} dyn.s.cm^{-5} ($P<0.05$), while postglomerular resistance (R_E) was unchanged: from 1.70±0.22 to 1.50±0.08 10^{10} dyn.s.cm^{-5}. The constancy of R_E coupled with the increase in Q_A, leads to an increase in the ultrafiltration pressure difference, ΔP. These increases in Q_A and ΔP were jointly responsible for the observed increase in SNGFR. However, the latter effect was partially offset by a concomittant significant reduction in K_f, which fell from 0.060±0.013 to 0.033±0.005 nl/(s.mmHg) ($P<0.05$).

To investigate the mechanism of the LXA_4-mediated fall in K_f, we performed competitive binding inhibition studies. Competitive binding inhibition showed that the addition of unlabelled LXA_4 competed with ^{3}H-LTD_4 in binding to mesangial cells. Half-maximal inhibition of binding by LXA_4 was at 100 nM compared to 10 nM for the homoligand. This degree of ^{3}H-LTD_4 binding inhibition was equivalent to that seen with LTE_4, and several orders of magnitude greater than that of the biologically inactive 5R, 6S isomers of LTD_4 and LXA_4 (Fig. 2). Furthermore, five seconds after addition of LXA_4 (1, 10, 50 and 100 nM) to mesangial cells labelled with ^{3}H-inositol, low but significant increases [46±14% ($P<0.05$), 50±21% ($P<0.05$), 44±22% ($P<0.05$), and 45±26% ($P<0.05$), respectively] were observed in radioactive counts (cpm). These increases, corresponding to inositol trisphosphate ($InsP_3$) formation by these cells, were noted to be more than those in vehicle-treated samples. Incubation of mesangial cells with the LTD_4 receptor antagonist, SKF 104353 (100 nm) abolished the LXA_4-induced stimulation of ^{3}H-$InsP_3$ formation in these cells. Addition of 10 and 50 nM LTD_4 to these cells was associated with 146±20% ($P<0.01$) and 106±13% ($P<0.005$) increases, respectively, in ^{3}H-$InsP_3$ counts compared to the controls; values significantly greater than

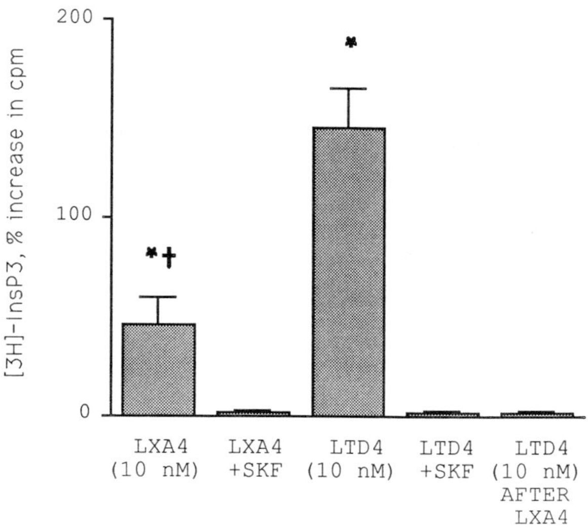

Fig. 3. $InsP_3$ formation in rat mesangial cells in response to LXA_4 and LTD_4 and its complete abolition in the presence of 100-fold concentration of SKF 104353 (SKF). The *far right column* depicts the abrogation of LTD_4-induced stimulation of $InsP_3$ formation by preexposure of the cells to 100 nM LXA_4 for 10 min. *, $P<0.01$ versus vehicle-stimulated controls. †, $P<0.05$ versus LTD_4 alone. (From [5])

those for LXA_4 ($P<0.05$). Incubation of mesangial cells with SKF 104353 in a concentration 100-fold that of the ligand, followed by addition of LTD_4, was associated with total abrogation of the LTD_4-induced stimulation of ^3H-$InsP_3$ formation in these cells. And similarly, preincubation of these cells with LXA_4 (100 nM) for 10 min before adding 10 nM LTD_4 completely prevented LTD_4-induced $InsP_3$ generation (Fig. 3). Taken together, these data provide evidence for the involvement of a common recognition site which mediates the actions of these two eicosanoids on mesangial cells.

Intrarenal arterial infusion of LTD_4 (0.5, 7.0, 14.0 and 20.0 μg/kg/min) was associated with dose-dependent reductions in GFR and RPF. Mean percent falls in GFR/RPF during LTD_4 infusion were 27/24, 25/40, 70/65, 73/70 at the doses above, respectively. However, administration of these doses of LTD_4 in the presence of LXA_4 (1.0 μg/kg/min) was associated with marked blunting of LTD_4-induced reduction in GFR, but no such blunting occurred in RPF. Mean percent falls in GFR/RPF during LTD_4 infusion in the presence of LXA_4 were 9/20, 11/37, 42/51, and 50/68 at the doses above, respectively. The relative protection given by LXA_4 against the GFR-depressant action of LTD_4, despite the absence of any modification of the potent vasoconstrictor actions of LTD_4, is interpreted as LXA_4-mediated prevention of the LTD_4-induced fall in K_f. These data support our in vitro finding, which showed competition by LXA_4 for LTD_4 receptors on mesangial cells.

To elucidate the mechanism for LXA_4-induced vasodilatation, we investigated the effect of cyclooxygenase inhibition in vivo on the renal action of LXA_4, in the light of lipoxin-induced prostaglandin release from bronchial and vascular tissues [8,9]. In non-cyclooxygenase-inhibited rats, LXA_4, infused into the left renal artery at 1.0 and 2.0 μg/kg per min led to dose-dependent increases in RPF and GFR. In the presence of the cyclooxygenase inhibitor, ibuprofen (20 mg/kg i.v.), these responses were reversed. Thus, these data suggested that LXA_4-mediated increases in RPF were due to the secondary release of vasodilatory cyclooxygenase products.

To investigate the effects of lipoxin B_4 and 7-cis, 11-trans LXA_4 on renal functions, we performed clearance studies by infusing these compounds into the left renal artery. The infusion of lipoxin B_4 (2.0 μg/kg per min) had no effect on systemic arterial pressure and hematocrit, whereas this compound induced a mild but significant decrease in GFR and RPF. The GFR decreased from 0.75 to 0.67 ml/min ($P<0.05$) and the RPF decreased from 4.20 to 3.66 ml/min ($P<0.05$). Filtration fraction was unchanged, due to the similar magnitude of GFR and RPF reductions. While modest in magnitude, these changes were notable in that they were opposite in nature to those observed in response to LXA_4. The infusion of 7-cis, 11-trans LXA_4 (1.0 μg/kg per min) induced an increase in hematocrit and in systemic arterial pressure, as well as inducing dramatic reductions in GFR and RPF, which were similar to those induced by Leukotrien C_4 and D_4 [1,10].

Because of the identical configuration, at C5 and C6 of 7-cis, 11-trans LXA_4 and LTD_4, it is reasonable to postulate that the systemic and renal action of 7-cis, 11-trans LXA_4 results from the activation of LTD_4 receptor coupled responses. The mechanism for the activity of LXB_4 remains unclear. In view of previous reports suggesting the secondary release of other eicosanoids by lipoxins in vitro [8,9], possible mechanisms could include interactions with other eicosanoids.

References

1. Badr KF, Brenner BM, Ichikawa II (1987) Effects of leukotriene D_4 on glomerular dynamics in the rat. Am J Physiol 22:F239–F243
2. Badr KF, Serhan CN, Nicolaou KC, Samuelsson B (1987) The action of lipoxin-A on glomerular microcirculatory dynamics in the rat. Biochem Biophys Res Commun 145:408–414
3. Harris RC, Hoover RL, Jacobson HR, Badr KF (1988) Evidence for glomerular actions of epidermal growth factor in the rat. J Clin Invest 82:1028–1039
4. Badr KF, Mong S, Hoover RL, Schwarzberg M, Ebert J, Jacobson HR, Harris RC (1989) Leukotriene D_4 binding and signal transduction in rat glomerular mesangial cells. Am J Physiol 26:F280–F287
5. Badr KF, Deboer DK, Schwarzberg M, Serhan CN (1989) Lipoxin A_4 antagonizes cellular and in vivo actions of leukotriene D_4 in rat glomerular mesangial cells: Evidence for competition at a common receptor. Proc Natl Acad Sci USA 86:3438–3442
6. Nicolaou KC, Marron BE, Veale CA, Webber SE, Dahlen SE, Samuelsson B, Serhan CN (1989) Identification of a novel 7-cis-11-trans-lipoxin A_4 generated by human neutrophils: total synthesis, spasmogenic activities and comparison with other geometric isomers of lipoxins A_4 and B_4. Biochem Biophys Acta 1003:44–53
7. Berridge MJ (1984) Inositol trisphosphate and diacylglycerol as second messengers. Biochem J 220:345–360
8. Dahlen SE, Frazen L, Raud J, Serhan CN, Westlung P, Wikstrom E, Bjorck T, Matsuda H, Webber SE, Veale CA, Puustinen T, Haeggstrom J, Nicolaou KC, Samuelsson B (1988) Actions of lipoxin A_4 and released compounds in smooth muscle preparations and on the

microcirculation in vivo. In: Wong WY-K, Serhan CN (eds) Lipoxins: Biosynthesis, Chemistry and Biological activities. Plenum, New York, pp 107–130

9. Brezinski ME, Gimbrone MA JR, Nicolaou KC, Serhan CN (1989) Lipoxins stimulate prostacyclin generation by human endothelial cells. FEBS Lett 245:162–172
10. Badr KF, Baylis C, Peffer JM, Peffer MA, Soberman RJ, Lewis RA, Austen KF, Corey EJ, Brenner BM (1984) Renal and systemic hemodynamic responses to intravenous infusion of leukotriene C_4 in the rat. Circ Res 54:492–499

Activation by Adenosine of Cultured Mesangial Cells: Receptors Involved and Intracellular Mechanisms

Ana Olivera, Manuela Tomás[1], and José M. López-Novoa[2]

SUMMARY. We studied the effects of the adenosine (ADO) analogues R-PIA (A1 agonist) and NECA (A2 agonist) on cAMP production and calcium inflow in cultured rat mesangial cells (MC). NECA, 10^{-6} M overstimulated cAMP content, and this effect was inhibited by the selective A_1 antagonist PD115199 (AT_2, 10^{-6} M). R-PIA 10^{-6} M, decreased cAMP content in forskolin-stimulated MC and this effect was blocked by the selective A_2 antagonist PD116948 (AT_2, 10^{-6} M). In addition, 10^{-6} M R-PIA + 10^{-6} M AT_2 increased ^{45}Ca-uptake after 30 s of stimulation, whereas 10^{-6} M NECA + 10^{-6} M AT_1 mediated a reduction in ^{45}Ca uptake in MC. Adenosine 10^{-4} M induced an increase in cAMP levels in forskolin-stimulated MC and an increase in $^{45}Ca^{2+}$ uptake. Neither AT_2 nor AT_1 affected ADO-induced cAMP production in forskolin-stimulated MC, but this effect was inhibited by 10^{-4} M theophylline. ADO-induced $^{45}Ca^{2+}$ uptake stimulation was inhibited by AT_2, unlike the effect shown with R-PIA. This effect was also inhibited by AT_1. These data demonstrate in a functional way the existence of A_1 and A_2 type receptors in cultured rat mesangial cells. Activation of the A_1-type stimulates calcium entry and inhibits cAMP generation. In contrast, activation of the A_2-type stimulates cAMP generation and inhibits calcium entry. Adenosine stimulates both cAMP generation and calcium uptake, but these actions do not seem to be mediated by the A_1 or A_2 receptors present in mesangial cells.

Introduction

Adenosine (ADO) has been shown to mediate a large number of physiological responses in cells from different tissues. Two specific cell surface receptors for

[1]Fundación Jimenez Diaz, Consejo Superior de Investigaciones Cientificas, Madrid, Spain
[2]Department of Physiology and Pharmacology, Faculty of Medicine, University of Salamanca, Avenida del Campo Charro s/n, 37007-Salamanca, Spain

adenosine have been classically described, on the basis of their ability to stimulate (A_2 ADO receptor) or inhibit (A_1 ADO receptor) membrane adenylate cyclase [1,2]. Synthesis of ADO derivatives with differential effects on adenylate cyclase activity has been developed in recent years. This has permitted a characterization of ADO receptor subtypes by additional pharmacological criteria [3]. Although A_1 or A_2 ADO receptors have been characterized, in most cells, some investigators have suggested the existence of a third ADO receptor, in order to explain some ADO-induced effects that cannot be attributed to activation of A_1 or A_2 subtypes [4–6].

Adenosine and the Kidney

In the kidney, ADO produces a wide range of responses, including a transient reduction of renal blood flow and a persistent decrement of glomerular filtration rate [7–9], inhibition of renin secretion [10,11], and some direct effect on renal tubules [12]. The two receptors defined for ADO have been identified in several renal structures and cells [12–14].

Freissmuth et al. described both A_1 and A_2 ADO receptors in rat isolated glomeruli [13], but the distribution of these receptors in the different glomerular cell types remains to be elucidated. We have previously demonstrated that ADO is able to contract rat mesangial cells in culture, probably through an A_1 ADO receptor [15]. Another set of experiments performed in our laboratory also suggests the existence of a functional A_2 receptor. Preincubation of MC with 10^{-6} M NECA, a potent A_2 agonist, partially blocked Angiotensin II-induced MC contraction (data not shown). Although all these data seem to indicate the existence of both A_1 and A_2 receptors in MC, we performed a further characterization of ADO receptors in these cells.

Functional Identification of A_1 and A_2 Receptors by the Effects of Adenosine Agonist on cAMP Levels

We studied the effects of the ADO analogues R-PIA and NECA on cAMP production. Mesangial cells were prestimulated for 5 min with 5 μM forskolin to augment cyclase activity. This methodological approach is frequently used to make agonist-induced effects, especially the inhibitory ones, on adenylate cyclase more evident.

After 2 minutes of incubation, 10^{-6} M NECA overstimulated intracellular cAMP content, whereas 10^{-6} M R-PIA decreased cAMP content in forskolin-stimulated MC (Fig. 1). The stimulation induced by NECA was inhibited only in the presence of the selective A_2 antagonist PD115199 [19] (AT_2, 10^{-6} M), whereas the inhibition of cAMP production was blocked in the presence of the A_1 antagonist PD115948 [20] (AT_1, 10^{-6} M) (Fig. 1). The contrasting effects of the agonists on cAMP content, the inhibition of these effects by the respective antagonists, and the direction of the change suggest that A_1 and A_2-like ADO receptors, linked by adenylate cyclase exist in MC.

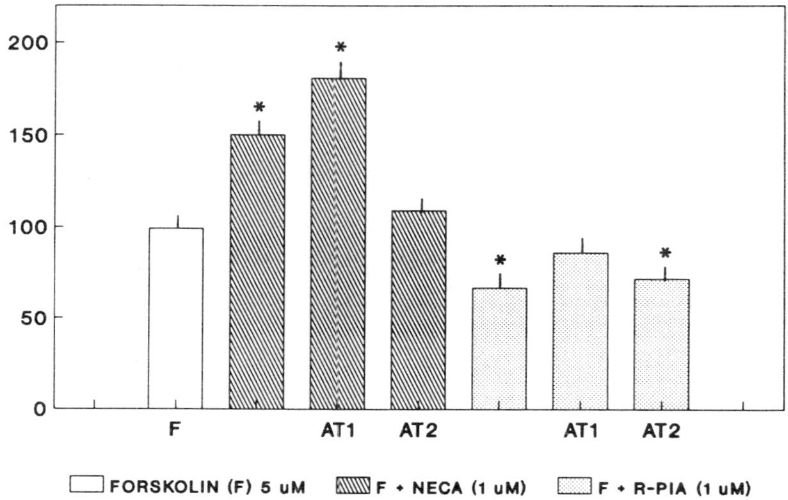

Fig. 1. Effect of the ADO agonists NECA (A_2) and R-PIA (A_1) and the selective antagonists PD 116948 (AT_1, 1 μM) and PD 115199 (AT_2, 1 μM) on cAMP intracellular content in Forskolin-pre-stimulated mesangial cells after 2 min of incubation. cAMP was extracted from the cells with ethanol, samples were dried and cAMP was determined by a specific RIA. Data are mean ± SEM of at least 12 determinations. *Asterisks* represent significant differences ($P < 0.05$) with respect to F-treated MC, RIA, radio-immunoassay

Effects of the Agonists on $^{45}Ca^{2+}$ Uptake

Adenylate cyclase is not the only effector system that has been described to be modulated by ADO receptors. For instance, ADO can modify calcium currents in several cell types [21–23]. As mesangial cell contraction induced by ADO seems to be dependent on extracellular calcium [15], we also decided to study the effect of preferential activation of A_1 or A_2 receptors on ^{45}Ca uptake in these cells.

The A_1 agonist R-PIA (10^{-6} M) increased ^{45}Ca-uptake after 30 s of stimulation, whereas the potent A_2 agonist NECA (10^{-6} M) mediated a reduction in ^{45}Ca uptake that did not reach statistical significance (Fig. 2). Since ADO agonists, specially NECA, are not absolutely selective for one or another kind of ADO receptor [3], we tried to further characterize NECA's actions by blocking the opposite receptors with the selective ADO antagonists PD116948 (A_1, 10^{-6} M) and PD115199 (AT_2, 10^{-6} M). Blockade of the A_2 receptor with AT_2 potentiated the increase of $^{45}Ca^{2+}$-uptake induced by the preferential activation of the A_1 receptor by R-PIA. On the other hand, blockade of the A_1 receptor with AT_1 potentiated the tendency of NECA to decrease $^{45}Ca^{2+}$ uptake in MC (Fig. 2).

Thus we can identify two subtypes of ADO receptors in MC, with opposite effects on cAMP production and on $^{45}Ca^{2+}$ uptake, i.e., and R-PIA-activable ADO receptor that mediates a reduction of cAMP levels and an increase in $^{45}Ca^{2+}$ uptake, which can then be defined as an A_1-like receptor, and a NECA-activable ADO receptor that

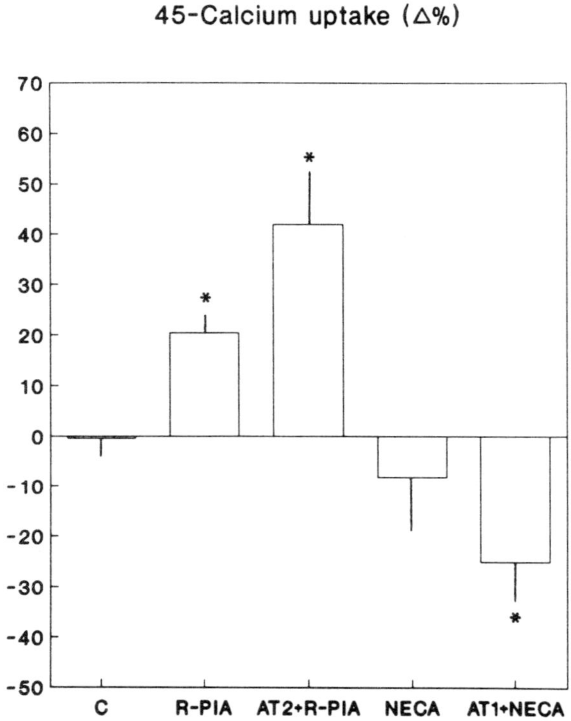

Fig. 2. Effect of the ADO agonists NECA (A_2, 1 μM) and R-PIA (A_2, *1* μM) alone or together with the selective antagonists of the opposite receptors PD 116948 (AT_1, 1 μM) and PD 115199 (AT_2, 1 μM) on ^{45}Ca uptake by mesangial cells. When corresponded, cells were preincubated with the antagonists for 10 min, and were then incubated in the presence of the isotope and the agonists for 30 s. Intracellular ^{45}Ca content was measured by liquid scintillation counting. Data are mean ± SEM of at least 12 determinations. *Asterisks* represent significant differences ($P < 0.05$) with respect to basal uptake

produces an increase in cAMP levels and a decrease on $^{45}Ca^{2+}$ uptake, which can then be defined as an A_2-like ADO receptor.

Effects of Adenosine on cAMP Production and on $^{45}Ca^{2+}$ Uptake: Possibility of a Third Adenosine Receptor

Once we had defined A_1 and A_2-like ADO receptors in MC, we studied the effects of ADO both on cAMP levels and on $^{45}Ca^{2+}$ uptake, and on $^{45}Ca^{2+}$ uptake, and we tried to characterize the receptor involved in these responses.

Adenosine 10^{-4} M induced, as did NECA, an increase in cAMP levels in forskolin-stimulated MC (Fig. 3) and, as did R-PIA, an increase in $^{45}Ca^{2+}$ uptake (Fig. 4). To characterize the receptor involved in ADO responses we studied the effects of the selective antagonists on the actions of ADO.

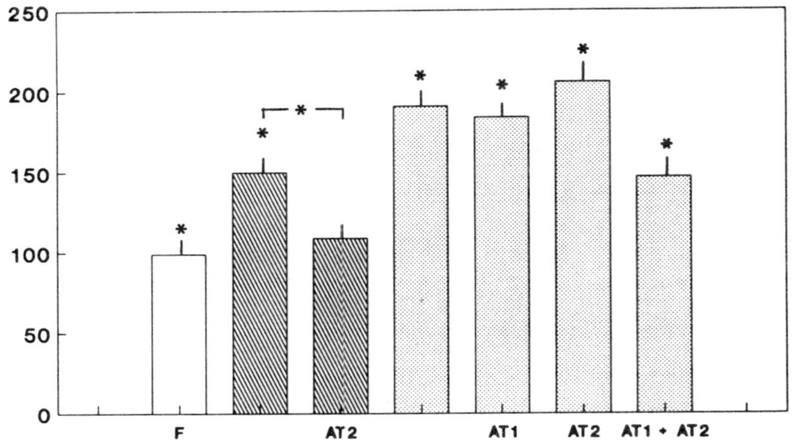

Fig. 3. Effect of the selective antagonists PD 116948 (*AT_1*, 1 μM) and PD 115199 (*AT_2*, 1 μM) on the 10^{-4} M adenosine-induced increase in cAMP intracellular content in forskolin-prestimulated mesangial cells (*MC*) after 2 min of incubation. Data of NECA and NECA + AT_2 are also shown for comparison. Methods as in Fig. 1. Data are mean ± SEM of at least 12 determinations. *Asterisks* represent significant differences ($P < 0.05$) with respect to f-treated MC

Effects on cAMP

Comparing the effect of ADO with the effects of the analogues on cAMP production, it would seem very likely that ADO action on cAMP production was mediated through the activation of an A_2 receptor. If this is right, blockade of the A_2 receptor should inhibit the ADO-induced stimulatory effect, as was observed with NECA. However, neither A_2 nor A_1 selective ADO antagonists affected the ADO-induced increase in cAMP content in forskolin-stimulated MC, and only the combination of A_1 and A_2 antagonists partially inhibited this increase (Fig. 3). The effects of ADO are mediated by a surface receptor, since 10^{-4} M theophylline (THEO) inhibited the increase in cAMP induced by ADO within 5 min of incubation (C: 11.4 ± 2.8, THEO: 13.1 ± 2.7; ADO: 25.32 ± 5.4, $P<0.05$ with respect to the control of cAMP content; THEO+ ADO: 15.07 ± 2.7, NS), but these results do not support the involvement of a receptor such as that activated by NECA.

Effects on $^{45}Ca^{2+}$ Uptake

The comparison of the effect of ADO and its analogues on $^{45}Ca^{2+}$ uptake would lead us to the conclusion that an A_1 receptor should be involved in the ADO-mediated stimulation of $^{45}Ca^{2+}$ uptake. However, the relatively selective antagonist A_2, instead of potentiating the effect of ADO, as we had observed with R-PIA, completely inhibited the $^{45}Ca^{2+}$ uptake stimulated by ADO (Fig. 4). This effect was also inhibited

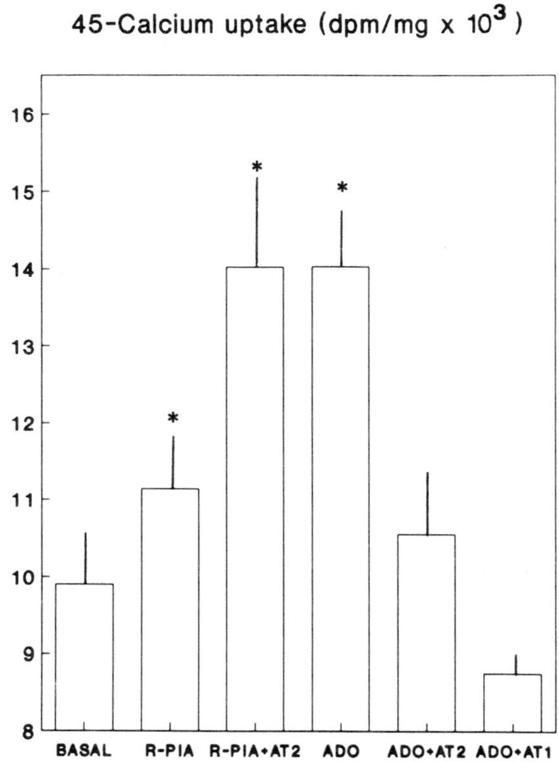

Fig. 4. Effect of the selective antagonists PD 116948 (*AT_1*, 1 μM) and PD 115199 (*AT_2*, 1 μM) on the 10^{-4} M adenosine-induced increase in ^{45}Ca uptake after 30 min of incubation. Data of R-PIA and R-PIA + AT_2 are also shown for comparison. Methods as in Fig. 3. Data are mean ± SEM of at least 12 determinations. *Asterisks* represent significant differences ($P < 0.05$) with respect to basal uptake

by the A_1 antagonist. So we have to discard again the involvement of a typical A_1 ADO receptor for explaining the effects of ADO on $^{45}Ca^{2+}$ uptake.

Considering all the effects which ADO has on cAMP formation and on $^{45}Ca^{2+}$, we should suggest either that 1) a third receptor for ADO exists, whose functional activity does not fit the pharmacological criteria usually accepted, or that 2) simultaneous occupation of A_1 or A_2 receptors by ADO synergizes both the A_2-mediated cAMP response and the A_1-mediated calcium influx response.

Some investigators have found actions of ADO that cannot be explained as a result of the activation of either of the described A_1 or A_2 ADO receptors [4–6,24], and the existence of another kind of ADO receptor with different binding [6] and pharmacological [4] properties to those of A_1 and A_2 receptors has been suggested. Our results could well be more evidence for the existence of a third kind of receptor for ADO. However, it is also possible that a synergism between A_1 and A_2 receptors occurs in the activator responses when both are equally occupied by ADO. In this regard, we have demonstrated that simultaneous addition of R-PIA and NECA to the cells enhanced R-PIA-induced stimulation of calcium entry, and accelerated NECA-induced stimulation of cAMP production (results not shown). An effect similar to this has been found in parathyroid acinar cells in which occupation of α and β adrenergic receptors by norepinephrine evoked a secretory response greater than the sum of the responses elicited by each adrenergic receptor separately [25].

For these reasons, we think that occupation of A_1 and A_2 sites in high proportion may induce a conformational or aggregatory receptor state that makes possible a special coupling to transduction systems different from that produced by activation of each receptor individually. Another possibility may be that when both receptors are equally occupied, there exists a synergism in the cross talk between the cAMP and Ca^{2+} messenger systems which potentiate calcium entry and cAMP production, respectively, and mask negative responses. Cyclic AMP has been shown to phosphorylate calcium channels [26] and to stimulate calcium entry [27]. In addition, Ca^{2+} has also been shown to activate adenylate cyclase in some cells [28].

It is worth noting that the effects of the high affinity antagonists on cAMP and on $^{45}Ca^{2+}$ uptake differ, i.e., both of them failed to inhibit ADO-induced increases in cAMP, whereas both of them completely inhibited ADO-induced stimulation of $^{45}Ca^{2+}$ uptake. This could be interpreted as a different coupling effectiveness to the transduction systems of each second messenger. The distortion induced by the selective antagonists in the binding of ADO can affect in a distinct way the coupling to calcium channels and to adenylate cyclase, because of the different threshold of each effector. Another explanation could be a model in which simultaneous activation of both receptors changes their spatial conformation, creating a pore for calcium as a part of the molecule. The antagonists A_1 and A_2 would not displace ADO binding (they do not modify the increase of cAMP levels), but would occupy main domains for the functionality of the pore (they inhibit calcium uptake).

Conclusions

The experiments shown above demonstrate in a functional way the existence of A_1 and A_2 type receptors in cultured rat mesangial cells. These receptors have contrasting effects on cAMP generation and calcium uptake. Activation of the A_1-type stimulates calcium entry and inhibits calcium entry. Adenosine stimulates both cAMP generation and calcium uptake, but these effects do not seem to be mediated by the A_1 or A_2 receptors present in mesangial cells. All these results may implicate a very complex regulation of adenosine metabolism in glomeruli or in the mesangium and also a complex role for adenosine in mesangial cells.

References

1. Londos C, Cooper DMF, Wolff J (1980) Subclasses of external adenosine receptors. Proc Natl Acad Sci USA 77:2551–2554
2. Shimizu H (1983) Adenosine receptors associated with the adenylate cyclase system. In: Daly JW, Kuroda Y, Phillis JW, Shimizu H, Ui M (eds) Physiology and pharmacology of adenosine derivates. Raven, New York, pp 31–40

3. Bruns RF, Daly JW, Snyder SH (1983) Adenosine receptor binding: structure-activity analysis generates extremely potent xanthine antagonists. Proc Natl Acad Sci USA 80:2077–2080
4. Belloni FL, Belardinelli L, Halperin C, Hintze TH (1989) An unusual receptor mediates adenosine-induced SA nodal bradycardia in dogs. Am J Physiol 256:H1553–H1564
5. Arend LJ, Burnatowska-Hledin MA, Spielman WS (1988) Adenosine receptor-mediated calcium mobilization in cortical collecting tubule cells. Am J Physiol 255:C581–C588
6. Chin JH, Delorenzo RJ (1986) A new class of adenosine receptors in brain. Characterization by 2-chloro[^{3}H]-adenosine binding. Biochem Pharmacol 35:847–856
7. Hall JE, Granger JP (1986) Renal hemodynamics and arterial pressure during chronic intrarenal adenosine infusion in conscious dogs. Am J Physiol 250:F32–F39
8. Osswald H, Spielman WS, Knox FG (1978) Mechanisms of adenosine-mediated decreases in glomerular filtration rate in dogs. Circ Res 43:465–469
9. Churchill PC, Bidani A (1987) Renal effects of selective adenosine receptor agonists in anesthesized rats. Am J Physiol 252:F299–F303
10. Arend L, Haramati A, Thompson CI, Spielman W (1987) Adenosine-induced decrease in renin release: dissociation from hemodynamic effects. Am J Physiol 247:F447–F452
11. Tagawa H, Vander AJ (1970) Effect of adenosine compounds on renal function and renin secretion in dogs. Circ Res 26:327–338
12. Arend LJ, Sonnenburg WK, Smith WL, Spielman WS (1987) A_1 and A_2 adenosine receptors in rabbit cortical collecting tubule cells. J Clin Invest 79:710–714
13. Freissmuth M, Hausleithner V, Tuisl E, Nanoff C, Schutz W (1987) Glomeruli and microvessels of the rabbit kidney contain both A_1 and A_2 adenosine receptors. Naunyn Schmiedebergs Arch Pharmacol 335:438–444
14. Palacios JM, Fastbom J, Wiederhold KH, Probst A (1987) Visualization of adenosine A1 receptors in the human and the guinea-pig kidney. Eur J Pharmacol 138:273–276
15. Olivera A, Lamas S, Rodriguez-Puyol D, Lopez-Novoa JM (1989) Adenosine induces mesangial cell contraction by an A_1-type receptor. Kidney Int 35:1300–1305
16. Fredholm BB, Jonzon B, Lindstrom K (1983) Adenosine receptor mediated increases and decreases in cyclic AMP in hippocampal slices treated with forskolin. Acta Physiol Scand 117:461–463
17. Jonzon B, Nilson J, Fredholm BB (1985) Adenosine receptor-mediated changes in cyclic AMP production and DNA synthesis in cultured arterial smooth muscle cells. J Cell Physiol 124:451–456
18. Darfler FJ, Maham LC, Koachman AM, Insel PA (1982) Stimulation by Forskolin of intact S49 Lymphoma cells involves the nucleotide regulatory protein of adenylate cyclase. J Biol Chem 257:11901–11907
19. Bruns RF, Fergus JH, Badger EW, Bristol JA, Santay LA, Hays SJ (1987) PD 115,199: an antagonist ligand for adenosine A_2 receptors. Naunyn Schmiedebergs Arch Pharmacol 335:64–69
20. Haleen SJ, Steffen RP, Hamilton HW (1987) PD 116,948, a highly selective A_1 adenosine receptor antagonist. Life Sci 40:555–561
21. Cerbai E, Klöckner U, Isenberg G (1988) Ca-antagonistic effects of adenosine in guinea pig atrial cells. Am J Physiol 255:H872–H878
22. Fenton RA, Bruttig SP, Rubio R, Berne RM (1982) Effect of adenosine on calcium uptake by intact and cultured vascular smooth muscle. Am J Physiol 242:H797–H804
23. Ramagopal MV, Mustafa SJ (1988) Effect of adenosine and its analogues on calcium influx in coronary artery. Am J Physiol 255:H1492–H1498
24. Ribeiro JA, Sebastiao AM (1986) Adenosine receptors and calcium: basis for proposing a third (A_3) adenosine receptor. Prog Neurobiol 26:179–209

25. McKinney JS, Desole MS, Rubin RP (1989) Convergence of cAMP and phosphoinositide pathways during rat parotid secretion. Am J Physiol 257:C651–C657
26. Nunoki K, Florio V, Catteral WA (1989) Activation of purified calcium channels by stoichiometric protein phosphorylation. Proc Natl Acad Sci USA 86:6816–6820
27. Bourdeau JE, Eby BK (1990) Cyclic AMP-stimulated rise in rabbit connecting tubules: role of peritubular Ca. Am J Physiol 258:F751–F755
28. Alkon DL, Rasmussen H (1988) A spatial-temporal model of cell activation. Science 239:998–1005

Interactions Between Glomerular Autacoids

Raymond Ardaillou, Laurent Baud, Nicole Ardaillou, and Dominique Chansel[1]

SUMMARY. Cell-cell interaction occurs in glomeruli via locally formed messengers acting in the vicinity of their sites of synthesis (autacoids). One autacoid from a given cell may act on a second autacoid at the stage of its synthesis or at successive steps of its cellular mode of action: by binding to receptors, by formation of second messengers, or by action on final biological effects. Various examples of modified synthesis are presented. Hydrogen peroxide (H_2O_2) produced by macrophages increases prostaglandin synthesis in glomerular cells; macrophages coincubated with glomeruli produce more prostaglandins than could be expected from the amounts synthesized separately by both preparations. The latter effect is due to the stimulation of macrophages by hydroperoxyeicosatetraenoic acids (HPETEs) of glomerular origin and is associated with the binding of stimulated macrophages to glomeruli. Macrophages also release interleukin-1 and tumor necrosis factor (TNF) which increase ecto 5′-nucleotidase expression and PGE_2 production in mesangial cells, PGE_2 in turn limiting TNF production. Alternatively, autacoids interact at the stage of their cellular effects. For example, H_2O_2 reduces the number of TNF receptors via inhibition of their synthesis and cyclic GMP-producing agonists inhibit angiotensin II (AII)-stimulated intracellular calcium concentration. PGE_2 inhibits LTD_4- or TNF-induced cell proliferation and AII-stimulated mesangial cell contraction. PGE_2-stimulated renin synthesis by mesangial cells is inhibited by 12-HETE. These different examples indicate that: Interaction between glomerular resident cells and blood-borne cells is bidirectional; regulatory loops occur frequently; final effects may imply cascade reactions, and autacoids often act synergistically. Any therapeutical approach will have to take into consideration the multiplicity of autacoids and their interactions.

Introduction

Autacoids are mediators which act at or near their sites of synthesis. Glomerular autacoids may originate from the resident glomerular cells or bone marrow-derived

[1]INSERM U64, Hôpital Tenon, 4 rue de la Chine, 75020 Paris Cedex 20, France

cells including monocyte-macrophages, polymorphonuclear leukocytes, and platelets invading the glomerular capillaries. Autacoids are not specific to the glomerulus and belong to a variety of chemical species, essentially reactive oxygen species, metabolites of arachidonic acid (prostaglandins and products of lipoxygenase), bioactive phospholipids such as platelet activating factor, cytokines and growth factors, proteolytic enzymes, products of local autocrine and paracrine systems such as angiotensin II, endothelin, bradykinin, adenosine, and finally, the recently discovered endothelium-derived relaxing factor identified as nitric oxide. These various autacoids interact in different ways and behave as messengers between two cells. Schematically, one autacoid from a given cell may act on the synthesis of a second autacoid in another cell or modify the mode of action of a second autacoid in its target cells. In the latter hypothesis, the effect may occur at different steps of the cellular mode of action: binding to receptors, formation of second messengers, or during final biological events. We should like, in this short review, to give examples of these different processes of interaction and to draw some general conclusions about the mechanism of glomerular injury and its therapeutical approach.

Interactions Between Two Autacoids at the Stage of Synthesis

The most studied of these interactions have been those between macrophages and isolated glomeruli or macrophages and mesangial cells. Macrophages are known to be the source of a variety of mediators, particularly metabolites of arachidonic acid, reactive oxygen species and cytokines [1]. The role of macrophages in both human and experimental glomerulonephritis has been advanced for the following reasons: Circulating monocytes infiltrate the glomerulus. They migrate into the subendothelial area, the mesangial matrix and the urinary space and undergo transformation into macrophages [2]; a close temporal relationship has been observed between macrophage accumulation and proteinuria [3]; monocyte depletion, as well as administration of a macrophage antiserum, [4] inhibits the progression of glomerular injury.

We have demonstrated in several studies [5,6] that during interaction between glomerular and bone marrow-derived cells, changes occur in arachidonate (C20:4) metabolism. We investigated the conversion of ^3H C20:4 into hydroxyeicosatetraenoic acids (HETE) and prostaglandins (PG) by isolated glomeruli and macrophages from rats, separately and in combination. As demonstrated by high performance liquid chromatography (HPLC), glomeruli converted C20:4 predominantly to lipoxygenase products, mainly 12-HETE, and to a lesser extent, to PG, mainly PGE_2 and $PGF_{2\alpha}$. Resident macrophages converted C20:4 to equivalent amounts of HETE and PG, mainly 12-HETE and 6 keto-$PGF_{1\alpha}$. When macrophages and glomeruli were studied in combination, a striking interaction was detected in both pathways of C20:4 metabolism. Production of 6 keto-$PGF_{1\alpha}$ was stimulated and considerable amounts of PGD_2, TXB_2 and hydroxyheptadecatrienoic acid (HHT), another product of thromboxane synthetase activity, were also produced (Fig. 1). Total 12-HETE production was unchanged. When a lipid extract of glomeruli, containing oxygenated metabolites of C20:4, was added to macrophages, there was stimulation of both the lipoxygenase (12- and 15-HETE) and cyclooxygenase (TXB_2 and 6 keto-$PGF_{1\alpha}$) production. Similar results were obtained by direct addition to macrophages of 12-

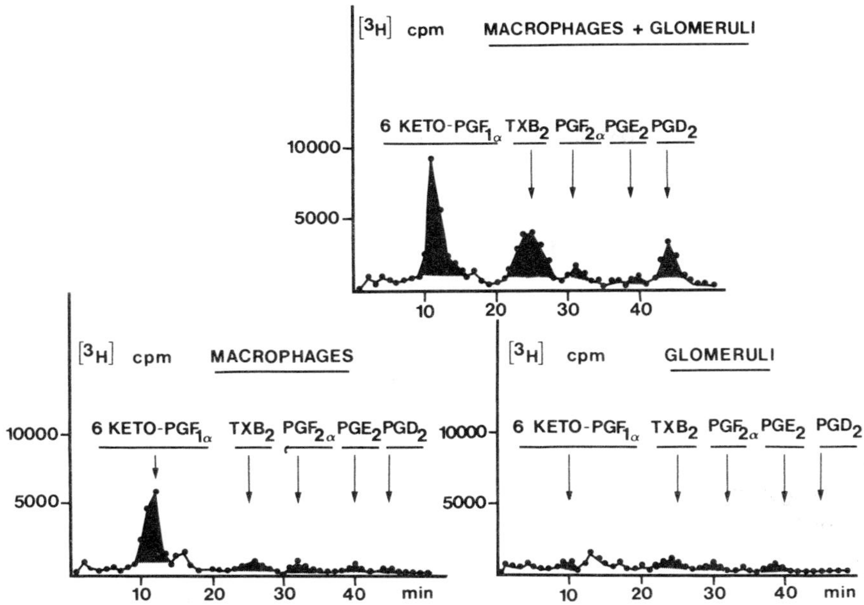

Fig. 1. High performance liquid chromatography profile of cyclooxygenase products synthesized by macrophages and glomeruli, alone and in combination. (From [5] with permission)

HPETE, which suggests that this metabolite was the agent present in the lipidic glomerular extract which was responsible for macrophage activation. When, in contrast, a lipid extract from macrophages was added to glomeruli, 12-HETE production by glomeruli was almost completely abolished. Thus, the unchanged total 12-HETE production obtained by coincubated glomeruli and macrophages resulted from its increased production by macrophages and its decreased production by glomeruli. We have also evaluated, in vitro, the role of lipoxygenase products of glomeruli origin in the attachment of rat macrophages to glomeruli [6]. We found that ^{3}H-uridine labeled macrophages bound to isolated glomeruli. Binding was related to the glomerular protein and macrophage concentrations, temperature, and time of incubation, and was a saturable process. Macrophage adherence depended on glomerular lipoxygenase activity, but not on glomerular cyclooxygenase activity, since preincubation of glomeruli with nordihydroguaiaretic acid inhibited this phenomenon. Preincubation with indomethacin was ineffective.

Macrophages also release reactive oxygen species which may stimulate arachidonic acid metabolism in isolated glomeruli. Indeed, rat glomeruli incubated in the presence of enzymatically generated superoxide anion ($O_2^{\cdot-}$) synthesized PGE_2, $PGF_{2\alpha}$, 6 keto-$PGF_{1\alpha}$, and TXB_2 in greater amounts than under control conditions [7]. Inhibition of this effect by catalase and the direct stimulatory effect of H_2O_2 itself suggested that H_2O_2 was the by-product responsible. The increase in PG synthesis in response to H_2O_2 was due to activation of glomerular phospholipase. The same stimulatory effect of H_2O_2 on PGE_2 synthesis has also been found in rat cultured mesangial cells [8]. As in the glomeruli, catalase was inhibitory. We have also shown that rat cultured mesangial cells produced H_2O_2 and O_2^- in response to particulate (opsonized zymosan) or soluble (platelet activating factor) stimuli [9]. Therefore, reactive oxygen species released either by infiltrating inflammatory cells or by resident glomerular cells may modulate immune-inflammatory events within the glomerulus and modify the glomerular microcirculation via PG synthesis. Because PGE_2 and PGI_2 stimulate adenylate cyclase and endogenous cyclic AMP production in murine [10] as well as in human [11] glomerular cells, the effect of reactive oxygen species on glomerular cyclic AMP has also been studied. Shah demonstrated that enzymatically produced O_2^- and H_2O_2 stimulated cyclic AMP synthesis in glomeruli and that this effect was suppressed in the presence of cyclooxygenase inhibitors, which confirmed its dependence on PG synthesis [12].

Macrophages are the source of a number of cytokines, particularly interleukin-1 (IL-1) and tumor necrosis factor (TNF). We have demonstrated that human recombinant TNFα stimulated the production of PG by cultured rat mesangial cells [13]. This effect was demonstrable from 5 hours, was dose-dependent, and affected the synthesis of PGE_2, $PGF_{2\alpha}$ and 6 keto-$PGF_{1\alpha}$ (Fig. 2). It required both RNA and protein synthesis but was not associated with a modification of cell proliferation, at least in cycling cells. TNF also stimulated cyclic AMP levels in mesangial cells. Indomethacin suppressed the effect of TNF on PG but only reduced that effect on cyclic AMP, indicating that PG production mediates, only in part, the increase in cyclic AMP. In the presence of indomethacin, TNF was mitogenic, which confirms that in this system, as in others, [14] PGE_2 production inhibits cell proliferation. TNFα also increased PGE_2 synthesis in human mesangial cells. IL-1 exhibited a similar effect both in rat [15] and human [16] mesangial cells. Using a L-929 fibroblast lytic assay, we showed that TNF was also synthesized by rat mesangial cells [17]. TNF biological activity was detectable only when mesangial cells were exposed to bacterial lipopolysaccharide for periods longer than one hour. PGE_2 produced in the presence of TNF in turn regulated TNF synthesis in a negative feed-back manner. Indeed, lipopolysaccharide caused a dose-dependent increase of PGE_2 synthesis by mesangial cells; treatment with indomethacin promoted suppression of PGE_2 production together with an increase of TNF synthesis. Addition of PGE_2 or 8 bromo-cyclic AMP induced similar dose-dependent reductions of TNF synthesis. Thus the inhibitory effect of PGE_2 probably required, in part, the accumulation of cyclic AMP. These events provide an example of a loop between two autacoids, with TNF stimulating the synthesis of PGE_2 and PGE_2 in turn limiting that of TNF.

We have been interested in the effect of cytokines on ecto 5′-nucleotidase expression in mesangial cells and thereby on their role in the control of local adenosine production. First, we demonstrated that a macrophage-conditioned medium produced a dose-dependent increase of mesangial ecto 5′-nucleotidase activity. A similar effect was observed in cocultures of rat mesangial cells and peritoneal macrophages [18]. The effect of the macrophage-conditioned medium was apparent after 24h and increased with time. Stimulation of ecto 5′-nucleotidase activity by the macrophage-conditioned medium was inhibited by cycloheximide, which, together with the necessary lag-time suggested that protein synthesis was required. Because the macrophage-conditioned medium contained high concentrations of IL-1 and TNF, we investigated whether or not these cytokines were responsible for this effect. We found that IL-1β and TNFα stimulated mesangial cell 5′-nucleotidase activity in a

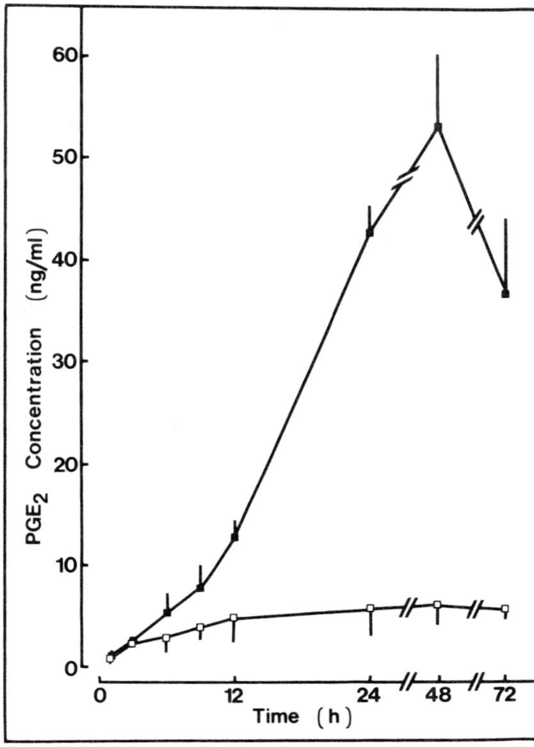

Fig. 2. Time-course of PGE_2 release from rat mesangial cells incubated without, (unfilled squares) and with, (filled squares) 100 ng/ml TNF. (From [13] with permission)

dose-dependent manner after a treatment of 24h. Maximum increases reached 4.5 times and 1.7 times basal values for IL-1β (20 U/ml) and TNFα (25 ng/ml), respectively. The effect of both cytokines was additive. Stimulation of 5′-nucleotidase by IL-1β and TNFα was specific, as had been observed with the macrophage-conditioned medium, since the activity of another ectoenzyme, Mg^{2+}-ATPase, was unchanged. Cycloheximide suppressed the cytokine-dependent increase of 5′-nucleotidase activity. Cyclooxygenase inhibitors such as indomethacin and ibuprofen inhibited approximately 50% of the effects of both cytokines. Their inhibitory effect was abolished in the presence of PGE_2. In addition, PGE_2 itself produced a dose-related (0.1 - 10 μM) increase of 5′-nucleotidase activity with a maximum of 2.2 times basal values. PGE_2 operated likely via cyclic AMP synthesis since 8-bromo cyclic AMP, a permeant analogue of cyclic AMP, was also active [19]. Taken together, these results indicate that IL-1, essentially, and TNFα, to a lesser extent, regulate 5′-nucleotidase expression in the plasma membrane of cultured mesangial cells and that their effect depends in part on PGE_2 synthesis. The enzyme 5′-nucleotidase plays a key role in the synthesis of adenosine from nucleotides. Therefore, factors controlling its expression may influence the local production of adenosine, which displays both powerful vasoactive and antiinflammatory properties. The effect of IL-1 on adenosine is an example of a cascade reaction, implying successively, PGE_2, cyclic AMP, and adenosine.

The role of platelets in glomerular injury has also been advanced, essentially because they represent the main site of synthesis of thromboxane which is considered to be a noxious agent in the development of glomerular injury. We have shown that platelets could be activated by saturated fatty acids of glomerular origin [20]. Initially, we demonstrated that when a tracer dose of ^3H C20:4 was added to a mixture of human glomeruli and platelets, a striking increase in ^3H TXB_2 production was observed. It was verified, by aspirin pretreatment, that platelets were responsible for the excess of TXB_2 generated and that the stimulus was of glomerular origin. When TXB_2 generated from endogenous C20:4 was measured by radioimmunoassay in coincubated cells, a dramatic increase of this metabolite was detected. We found that the factors responsible for this stimulation were present in the lipidic extract of glomeruli and corresponded to saturated and monounsaturated fatty acids (C14:0, C16:0, C18:0, and C18:1). An exogenous supply of the same synthetic acids produced the same stimulatory effect. The question of whether this glomerulus-platelet interaction also occurs in vivo cannot be answered easily. It is possible that injured glomerular cells with membrane disturbances may release these fatty acids together with the procoagulant factor which plays a role in the formation of thrombi. We also found this procoagulant factor in the glomerular supernatant in vitro.

Interactions at the stage of synthesis may also correspond to a sharing of substrate between two cell types. This process has been described between polymorphonuclear leukocytes and platelets. For example, 12-HETE synthesized by platelets is further hydroxylated in leukocytes into 12,20 diHETE or 5,12 diHETE by the ω-lipoxygenase and the 5 lipoxygenase present in the latter cell type [21]. It is also admitted that endothelial cells utilize platelet endoperoxides to produce PGI_2 [22]. Such interactions may also occur within the glomerular capillaries.

Interactions Between Two Autacoids at the Stage of Binding to Surface Receptors or Second Messenger Formation

Many agents induce the simultaneous production of cytokines and reactive oxygen species by macrophages and mesangial glomerular cells. This led us to examine whether cell sensitivity to TNF might also be regulated by reactive oxygen species [23]. When L-929 fibroblasts, which represent a TNF-sensitized murine cell line, were exposed simultaneously to TNF and H_2O_2 (100 to 500 μM), the cytotoxic activity of TNF was inhibited by up to 67%. This inhibition was also effective when the cells were pretreated with H_2O_2, but not when TNF alone was preexposed to H_2O_2. These data suggest that H_2O_2 altered the cell sensitivity to TNF without modifying the activity of the TNF molecule. Maximum loss of cell sensitivity to TNF occurred after 30 min preexposure to 500 μM H_2O_2; complete restoration of TNF sensitivity was obtained within 12h following H_2O_2 removal. Restoration required protein synthesis, as demonstrated by the suppressive effect of actinomycin D. The inhibitory effect of H_2O_2 was suppressed by catalase, but was unaffected by the scavengers of hydroxyl radical ($OH^{\cdot}$) and hypochlorous acid

(O Cl^-), suggesting that H_2O_2 itself, and not one of its metabolites, was responsible for this inhibition. Binding experiments of ^{125}I-TNF to L-929 fibroblasts revealed that the mechanism whereby H_2O_2 affected cell sensitivity to TNF involved the reduction, by about 50%, of the density of TNF receptors. There was no change in TNF affinity for its receptors. Moreover, H_2O_2 did not affect the rate of degradation of TNF, and only slightly increased the degree of internalization of ^{125}I-TNF receptors. Therefore the effectiveness of H_2O_2 appears to be mediated at the TNF receptor level. Another example of interaction between two autacoids at the receptor level is the demonstration by Badr et al. [24] that lipoxin A_4 (LXA_4) antagonizes the in vivo and cellular actions of leukotriene D_4 (LTD_4) in rat glomerular mesangial cells, via competition at a common receptor. Evidence was obtained from the inhibition of binding of [^{3}H] LTD_4 to mesangial cells in the presence of LXA_4, the prevention – by LXA_4 – of LTD_4-induced inositol trisphosphate generation, and the blockade of LXA_4-induced inositol trisphosphate stimulation by a LTD_4 receptor antagonist.

It is also possible for an autacoid to modify the effect of a second autacoid at the stage of the production of its second messenger. An example is the control that cyclic GMP-producing mediators exert on the effects of such vasoconstrictory agents as angiotensin II, or endothelin, on vascular smooth muscle cells. It has been shown that endothelial cells released a relaxing factor different from the other well known vasodilatory agents, PGI_2 and adenosine. This factor was named endothelium-derived relaxing factor; it has been identified as nitric oxide. It originates from L-arginine and stimulates the soluble guanylate cyclase of the adjacent smooth muscle cells [25]. Thus, it could counteract the vasoconstriction induced by angiotensin II or endothelin by decreasing the intracellular concentration of calcium, via stimulation of cyclic GMP production. This hypothesis would be in accordance with the demonstration by Hassid [26] that atrial natriuretic factor, another activator of guanylate cyclase, is an endogenous antagonist of calcium-mediated processes.

Interactions Between Two Autacoids at the Stage of Biological Effect

Finally, one autacoid may act on the target cell of a second autacoid at the stage of biological effect. For example, PGE_2 inhibits LTD_4- or TNF-induced cell proliferation and AII-stimulated mesangial cell contraction. We have shown that LTC_4 and LTD_4 promoted the proliferation of human glomerular epithelial cells [27] and of fibroblasts [14]. Human glomerular epithelial cells synthesize little PG, whereas fibroblasts produce large amounts of PGE_2. We demonstrated that, in the latter cell line, the mitogenic effect of sulfidopeptide leukotrienes was apparent only in the presence of cyclooxygenase inhibitors. Under these conditions, LTD_4 promoted proliferation of growing cells as well as of quiescent cells. Interestingly, LTD_4 and LTC_4 did not modify PGE_2 production by fibroblasts, thus showing no evidence for a negative feed-back loop. Similarly, the mitogenic effect of TNF on rat mesangial cells occurred only when PGE_2 synthesis was inhibited [28]; the mitogenic effect of IL-1 was suppressed in the presence of PGE_2 [29]. These latter examples are associated with negative feed-back loops, since both cytokine stimulate the synthesis of PGE_2 in mesangial cells [13,19].

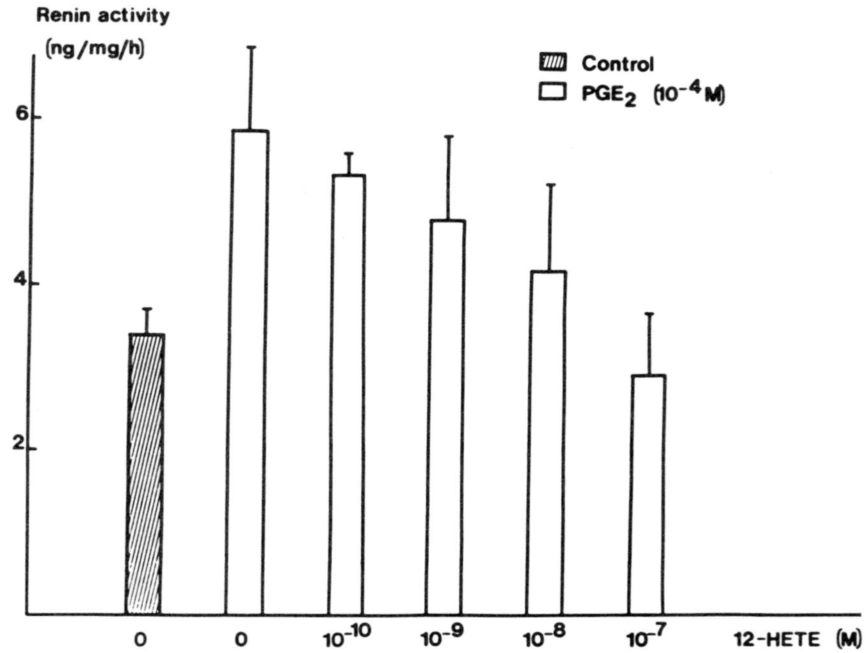

Fig. 3. Effect of increasing doses of 12-HETE on PGE_2-simulated renin activity produced by human cultured mesangial cells. (From [11] with permission)

AII can be considered as a glomerular autacoid which is generated locally by juxtaglomerular or glomerular renin and the converting enzyme of the vascular endothelial cells. AII stimulated PG synthesis by isolated glomeruli [30] and murine [31] or human [32] mesangial cells. In the human mesangial cell preparation, threshold stimulation was observed at around 10 pM AII. Schlondorff et al. [28] have proposed that AII preferentially, but not exclusively, stimulates a phosphatidylinositol specific phospholipase C. This results in the formation of diacylglycerol which could serve as an intermediate in the release of arachidonic acid. Phospholipase A_2 activation could also occur as a consequence of the increase in intracellular calcium concentration and of the phosphorylation of lipocortin by a diacylglycerol-sensitive protein kinase C. The arachidonate released in response to AII is tightly coupled to cyclooxygenase and thus transformed into PG. AII, after binding to specific receptors, also produces contraction of isolated glomeruli via contraction of mesangial cells. Scharschmidt et al. [33] have demonstrated that glomerular vasoreactivity has great sensitivity to AII with a threshold dose of 0.01 pM. The maximum surface area decrease was 20% and occurred at 0.1 nM AII. These authors showed that the dose-effect curve was displaced toward the left (lower concentrations of AII) in the presence of indomethacin and towards the right (higher concentrations of AII) in the presence of arachidonic acid or PGE_2. The mechanism of the inhibitory effect of PGE_2 is mediated by cyclic AMP. PGE_2 stimulates adenylate cyclase activity and increases the cellular content in cyclic AMP, which in turn activates protein kinase A. Activation of protein kinase A produces phosphorylation of myosin light chain kinase and, as a consequence, decreases its affinity for the calcium-calmodulin complex, resulting in inhibition of cell contraction. In this schema, PGE_2 acts as a self-induced inhibitor of AII.

Mediators other than PGE_2 may also act to modulate the effects of autacoids at the stage of their biological effects. We have demonstrated that the stimulatory effect of PGE_2 on renin production by human mesangial cells was inhibited by 12-hydroxyeicosatetraenoic acid (12-HETE) between 0.1 and 100 nM [11]. Extracellular and intracellular renin were affected similarly. The effects of 15-hydroxyeicosatetraenoic acid (15-HETE), 12-hydroperoxyeicosatetraenoic acid (12-HPETE), and 15-hydroperoxyeicosatetraenoic acid (15-HPETE) were the same as those of 12-HETE (Fig. 3). We hypothesized that in this system, as in others [34], the lipoxygenase products inhibited diacylglycerol kinase, which could result in an increase of diacylglycerol concentration and stimulation of protein kinase C. Such stimulation has been shown to be associated with the inhibition of renin production [35].

Conclusions

It is possible to draw general conclusions from these various examples of interaction between glomerular autacoids. First, it is clear that interactions are not only represented by the effects which autacoids from blood-borne cells have on glomerular resident cells. The reverse also occurs frequently. In addition, there are interactions between different types of blood cells and between different types of glomerular cells. In particular, the role of mesangial cells, which are proinflammatory cells, has now been extensively demonstrated. These cells, in addition to their smooth muscle cell-like properties, possess many characteristics resembling those of macrophages. Therefore, they release a variety of autacoids which act both on the other glomerular resident cells and on the circulating blood cells they can attract in the glomeruli. A second conclusion is that of the frequency of cross-talks between different pathways. PGs play a major role in these cross-talks as agents of regulatory feed-back loops. In particular, PGs inhibit vasoconstriction and cell proliferation which are often promoted by the same compounds. Cross-talks between pathways may also result in synergy between the effects of both autacoids. This has been well demonstrated between cytokines, particularly between IL-1 and TNF. Finally, the most characteristic feature of these interactions between autacoids is their complexity. This complexity has several consequences: A single autacoid is not responsible for a pathological effect. Therefore the question is: What kinds of autacoids exist, how do they interact, and what is the sequence of the reactions? The answer to the last question is essential for a therapeutical approach. Autacoids have several cellular sources, but what their relative parts are and what cells must be the targets for drugs, have still to be established. The mechanism of the toxicity of autacoids is, for the most part, unknown. In the cascade of reactions between the response of the initial mediator to glomerular injury and the production of the agents which cause proteinuria, the main event—which must be the target of treatment—is still often unknown. A given autacoid may be blocked either at the stage of its synthesis by synthesis inhibitors, or at the stage of its effects by antagonists. Ideal drugs should be specific to an autacoid, devoid of toxicity, easily administrable, and efficient, both extra- and intracellularly.

References

1. Takemura R, Werb Z (1984) Secretory products of macrophages and their physiological functions. Am J Physiol 246: C1–C9
2. Holdsworth SR, Neale TJ, Wilson CB (1980) The participation of macrophages and monocytes in experimental immune complex glomerulonephritis. Clin Immunol Immunopathol 15: 510–524
3. Schreiner GF, Cotran RS, Pardo V, Unanue ER (1978) A mononuclear cell component in experimental immunological glomerulonephritis. J Exp Med 147: 369–384
4. Holdsworth SR, Neale TJ, Wilson CB (1981) Abrogation of macrophage-dependent injury in experimental glomerulonephritis in the rabbit. Use of an antimacrophage serum. J Clin Invest 68: 686–698
5. Sraer J, Baud L, Bens M, Podjarny E, Schlondorff D, Ardaillou R (1984) Glomeruli cooperate with macrophages in converting arachidonic acid to prostaglandins and hydroxyeicosatetraenoic acids. Prostaglandins Leukotrienes Med 13: 67–74
6. Baud L, Sraer J, Delarue F, Bens M, Balavoine F, Schlondorff D, Ardaillou R, Sraer JD (1985) Lipoxygenase products mediate the attachment of rat macrophages to glomeruli in vitro. Kidney Int 27: 855–863
7. Baud L, Nivez MP, Chansel D, Ardaillou R (1981) Stimulation by oxygen radicals of prostaglandin production by rat renal glomeruli. Kidney Int 20: 332–339
8. Sedor JR, Abboud HE (1985) Hydrogen peroxide stimulates PGE_2 synthesis by cultured rat mesangial cells (Abstract). Kidney Int 29: 291
9. Baud L, Hagege J, Sraer J, Rondeau E, Perez J, Ardaillou R (1983) Reactive oxygen production by cultured rat glomerular mesangial cells during phagocytosis is associated with stimulation of lipoxygenase activity. J Exp Med 158: 1836–1852
10. Friedlander G, Chansel D, Sraer J, Bens M, Ardaillou F (1983) PGE_2 binding sites and PG-stimulated cyclic AMP accumulation in rat isolated glomeruli and glomerular cultured cells. Mol Cell Endocrinol 30: 201–214
11. Chansel D, Béa ML, Ardaillou R (1989) Modulation of renin synthesis by lipoxygenase products in cultured human mesangial cells. Mol Cell Endocrinol. 62: 263–271
12. Shah SV (1984) Effect of enzymatically generated reactive oxygen metabolites on the cyclic nucleotide content in isolated rat glomeruli. J Clin Invest 74: 393–401
13. Baud L, Perez J, Friedlander G, Ardaillou R (1988) Tumor necrosis factor stimulates prostaglandin production and cyclic AMP levels in rat cultured mesangial cells. FEBS Lett 239: 50–54
14. Baud L, Perez J, Denis M, Ardaillou R (1987) Modulation of fibroblast proliferation by sulfidopeptide leukotrienes: effect of indomethacin. J Immunol 138:1190–1195
15. Lovett DH, Resch K, Gemsa D (1987) Interleukin 1 and the glomerular mesangium II Monokine stimulation of mesangial cell prostanoid secretion. Am J Pathol 129: 543–551
16. Topley N, Floege J, Wessel K, Hass R, Radeke AH, Kaever V, Resh K (1989) Prostaglandin E_2 production is synergistically increased in cultured human glomerular mesangial cells by combinations of IL-1 and tumor necrosis factor α. J Immunol 143: 1989–1995
17. Baud L, Oudinet JP, Bens M, Noe L, Peraldi MN, Rondeau E, Etienne J, Ardaillou R (1989) Production of tumor necrosis factor by rat mesangial cells in response to bacterial lipopolysaccharide. Kidney Int 35: 1111–1118
18. Stefanovic V, Savic V, Vlahovic P, Ardaillou N, Ardaillou R (1989) Macrophages selectively stimulate ecto 5′-nucleotidase activity of cultured mesangial cells. Kidney Int 36: 249–256
19. Savic V, Stefanovic V, Ardaillou N, Ardaillou R (1990) Induction of ecto 5′-nucleotidase of rat cultured mesangial cells by interleukin 1β and tumour necrosis factor α. Immunology 70:321–326

20. Sraer J, Wolf C, Oudinet JP, Bens M, Ardaillou R, Sraer JD (1987) Human glomeruli release fatty acids which stimulate thromboxane synthesis in platelets. Kidney Int 32: 62–68
21. Marcus AJ, Broekman MJ, Safier LB, Ullman HL, Islam N (1982) Formation of leukotrienes and other hydroxyacids during platelet-neutrophil interactions in vitro. Biochem Biophys Res Commun 109: 130–137
22. Schafer AI, Crawford DD, Gimbrone MA (1984) Unidirectional transfer of prostacyclin endoperoxides between platelets and endothelial cells. J Clin Invest 73: 1105–1112
23. Baud L, Affres H, Perez J, Ardaillou R (1990) Reduction in tumor necrosis factor binding and cytotoxicity by hydrogen peroxide. J Immunol 145:556–560
24. Badr KF, DeBoer DK, Schwartzberg M, Serhan CN (1989) Lipoxin A_4 antagonizes cellular and in vivo actions of leukotriene D_4 in rat glomerular mesangial cells: Evidence for competition at a common receptor. Proc Natl Acad Sci USA 86: 3438–3442
25. Förstermann U, Mulsch A, Bohme E, Basse R (1986) Stimulation of soluble guanylate cyclase by an acetylcholine-induced endothelium-derived factor from rabbit and canine arteries. Circ Res 58: 531–538
26. Hassid A (1986) Atriopeptin II decreases cytosolic free Ca in cultured vascular smooth muscle cells. Am J Physiol 251: C681–C686
27. Baud L, Sraer J, Perez J, Nivez MP, Ardaillou R (1985) Leukotriene C_4 binds to human glomerular epithelial cells and promotes their proliferation in vitro. J Clin Invest 73: 374–377
28. Perez J, Baud L, Ardaillou R (1989) Tumor necrosis factor stimulates prostaglandin, cyclic AMP and DNA synthesis by cultured rat mesangial cells. Kidney Int 35: 318 (Abstr.)
29. Stahl RAK, Thaiss F, Kahf S, Shaw A, Schoeppe W (1989) Cyclooxygenase inhibition enhances rat interleukin 1β-induced proliferation of rat mesangial cells in culture (abstract). Kidney Int. 35: 320
30. Schlondorff D, Rocznick S, Satriano JA, Folkert WW (1980) Prostaglandin synthesis by isolated rat renal glomeruli: effect of angiotensin II. Am J Physiol 239: F486–F495
31. Sraer J, Foidart J, Chansel D, Mahieu P, Ardaillou R (1980) Prostaglandin synthesis by rat isolated glomeruli and glomerular cultured cells. Int J Biochem 12: 203–207
32. Ardaillou N, Nivez MP, Schlondorff D, Ardaillou R (1985) Vasoconstrictor-evoked prostaglandin synthesis in cultured human mesangial cells. Am J Physiol 248: F240–F246
33. Scharschmidt LA, Lianos E, Dunn MJ (1983) Arachidonate metabolites and the control of glomerular function. Fed Proc 42: 3058–3063
34. Setty YBN, Graeber JE, Stuart J (1987) The mitogenic effect of 15- and 12-hydroxyeicosatetraenoic acid on endothelial cells may be mediated via diacylglycerol kinase inhibition. J Biol Chem 262: 17613–17622
35. Kurtz A, Pfeilschifter J, Hutter A, Bührle C, Nobiling R, Taugner R, Hackenthal E, Bauer C (1986) Role of protein kinase C in inhibition of renin caused by vasoconstrictors. Am J Physiol 250: C563–C571

Ion Channels of the Kidney

Chair: Rainer Greger (FRG)
Mamoru Fujimoto (Japan)

Ion Channels in the Mammalian Nephron

R. GREGER, E. SCHLATTER, M. BLEICH[1], and H. GÖGELEIN[2]

SUMMARY. After the initial description of ion channels by patch clamp analysis in cultured cell lines derived from renal epithelia some 7 years ago, much progress has been made in the application of this technique to primary cultures of renal cells of defined origin, and to intact and even to in vitro perfused renal tubules. The present brief overview will focus mostly on data derived from intact tubules; the emphasis will be on the most recent data on ion channel regulation. Comparison to data obtained from cultured cells reveals that there are distinct differences between various preparations. Furthermore, in patch clamp experiments, several types of ion channels have been found which are probably not relevant for the normal function of the intact tubule cell. Conversely, some of the conductance properties of the intact cell are not recovered by corresponding ion channels in patch clamp experiments. Much further work and new methods will be required to reconstitute the conductance properties of the intact tubule from the findings in single ion channels.

Ion Channel Properties of Renal Epithelia

The renal tubules possess various K^+ channels, non-selective cation channels, Cl^- channels and Na^+ channels. In the following we will address only some of these channels and we refer the reader to recent, more general reviews on this topic [1–7].

Patch Clamp Studies in Cell Cultures of Renal Origin

The easiest way to study tubule cells by the patch clamp technique is to use established cell lines such as Mardin-Darby Canine Kidney (MDCK) cells, opossum

[1]Albert-Ludwigs-Universität Freiburg, Hermann-Herder-Straße 7, D 7800 Freiburg, Federal Republic of Germany
[2]Pharma-Forschung, Hoechst AG, D 6230 Frankfurt/Main 80, Federal Republic of Germany

kidney cells, etc. One example will be discussed in this volume by Ohno-Shosaku. These kinds of studies have been very helpful in the detailed description of the properties of several types of channels [3] and in the study of hormonal control of the maxi K^+-channel [2].

Primary cell cultures offer the advantage that they resemble the properties of native tissue more closely than do cultured cell lines. In cultures from the proximal tubule, several types of K^+-channels and non-selective cation channels have been reported [8–10]. Some of this work will be discussed in this volume by Poujeol. A recent review of ion channels in the proximal tubule by one of the authors of this study [11] reveals that most of the channels reported in these studies (except for the maxi K^+-channel) correspond well with those found in the isolated perfused proximal tubule [12].

In cultures of thick ascending limb cells maxi K^+-channels have been found [13] and described in much detail, regarding inhibitors [14–16]. As will be shown below, this type of K^+-channel is *not* responsible for K^+ recycling across the luminal membrane. It appears to be activated by cell volume increase [17]; this will be discussed by Guggino in this volume. In the isolated thick ascending limb segment other K^+-channels have been found [18,19], (also c.f. below).

Primary cultures of collecting ducts obtained from collecting duct-"anlagen" have been examined in much detail [20,21]. Nonselective cation channels with small to intermediate conductance, and small and large K^+ channels have been found, but the Na^+-channel, which has been described in much detail in studies with isolated collecting ducts [22], could not be identified at the single channel level. The authors conclude that the Na^+ channel might have a conductance of <5pS in their preparation and might therefore be difficult to detect in single channel studies [21]. In primary cultures of inner medullary collecting duct a non-selective cation channel with intermediate conductance has been found. This channel was claimed to be sensitive to amiloride with a reasonable K_D [23]. It should be noted, however, that the amiloride inhibition was only deduced from unpaired observations. In intercalated cells from cortical collecting duct, excision activated Cl^- channels [24] with a large conductance of around 300 pS have been found [24a].

Patch Clamp Analysis of Single Channel Properties of Isolated Nephron Segments

Several approaches have been developed to study the single channel properties of isolated tubules. In one approach the tubule is cut open and the luminal cell membrane becomes accessible to the patch pipette [25]. In another approach the tubules are treated with the collagenase, the basement membrane is destroyed, and the basolateral membrane can be studied [26,27]. We have developed a method in which the tubule segment is perfused in vitro [28,29]. The free end of the tubule is then accessible to the patch electrode which can then be pressed against the lateral membrane of the free end of the tubule, hence enabling one to study the properties of the basolateral membrane. Alternatively, the patch pipette is inserted into the lumen and a recording is made from the luminal membrane. The free tubule end can be immobilized by another suction pipette which is attached to one edge. With this technique we have studied rabbit, rat, and mouse tubule segments of the proximal nephron [30–32], the thick ascending limb of the loop of Henle [18,33,34], and the cortical collecting duct [35]. In our experience mouse and rat tubules are more suited for this method, because they are easier to tear at one end and the lumen of this end can be held wide open. The disadvantage of this method is its complexity. It is rather difficult to insert the patch pipette into the lumen without touching any structure before pressing the pipette against the luminal surface of the cell to be studied. Furthermore, only lateral membranes of the torn end can be studied; it is tacitly assumed that the properties of these lateral membranes resemble those of the basolateral membrane of the remainder of the tubule. In our experience, this assumption seems to be correct. The advantages of this method can be summarized as follows: The tubule lumen perfusate is under experimental control. The tubule is in exactly the same state as that from which we have other pertinent information on its function and properties. Another relevant methodological detail is the fact that all our experiments, unlike those in most other studies, were carried out at 37°C.

Properties and Regulation of Ion Channels in the Proximal Tubule

This issue has been reviewed recently [11,12]. In the luminal membrane of rabbit and mouse proximal tubule a K^+ channel with 33–63 pS was found. This channel was found in cell attached patches, indicating that it is present on cells with physiologically low cytosolic Ca^{2+} activities. It is highly selective for K^+ over Na^+. This channel requires further examination. In the luminal membrane of S_3-segments of the rabbit a Na^+ channel with around 12 pS conductance was found in cell attached and in cell excised patches [31]. This channel could be inhibited from the cytosolic side by high concentrations of amiloride. We have argued that the right shift in the dose response curve was due to the fact that amiloride had to cross the membrane and to enter the patch pipette before it inhibited this channel from its binding site on the outside mouth of the channel.

In the basolateral (c.f. lateral, above) membrane two types of K^+ channels have been found in rabbit S_2 and S_3 segments. Both were of intermediate conductance (36 and 46 pS, respectively) [36]. The larger channel was seen more frequently. It had flicker type kinetics with burst appearance. It was present in cell attached patches, and it was shown to be Ca^{2+} independent in excised patches. In fact, it was perfectly activated in seemingly Ca^{2+} free solutions. This channel showed an increasing open state probability with increasing depolarization of the clamp voltage. With respect to its conductance and Ca^{2+} insensitivity, this channel is comparable to the K^+ channel present in the luminal membrane of the thick ascending limb of rabbit [19] and rat [18] (also c.f. below).

In addition to these K^+ channels we found a non-selective cation channel in the basolateral membrane of rabbit S_2 and S_3 segments. We have seen this channel in cell attached and in cell excised patches. With identical solutions on both sides the channel had a linear current voltage relation with a mean conductance of 24 pS. This channel was Ca^{2+} sensitive and it required some 10^{-5} mol/l Ca^{2+} for its activation [37]. It was non-selective in the sense that it did not discriminate between Na^+ and K^+ [11]. It was inhibited reversibly by stilbenes such as 4-acetamido-4′-isothiocyanostilbene-2,2′ disulfonic acid (SITS) and by diphenylamino-2-carboxylate. This type of channel has been found in many other preparations of the thick ascending limb, collecting duct-"anlagen," and the cortical collecting duct [18,21,35,38], and it cannot be entirely excluded that it is the same channel as that found in cultures of inner medullary collecting duct [23]. We still have no firm information on the function of this channel in the intact cell.

Properties and Regulation of Ion Channels in the Thick Ascending Limb of the Loop of Henle

The luminal membrane of this nephron segment contains a K^+ conductance through which K^+ recycles into the lumen. A few years ago it was speculated that this conductance corresponded to a Ca^{2+} sensitive maxi K^+ channel [39]. This was, however, highly unlikely since this type of channel required rather high cytosolic Ca^{2+} activity to become activated [13]. These data were obtained in cell cultures of chicken kidney cells and, later, in cell cultures from rabbit thick ascending limb. More recently, we and others have reexamined this issue and have tested the properties of the luminal membrane of thick ascending limbs of rabbit [19] and rat [18]. In cell attached patches we did not find the above maxi K^+ channel but found, rather, an intermediate conductance (60 pS) K^+ channel [18,33,34]. The most intriguing properties of this channel are its control by cytosolic pH, Ca^{2+} and ATP. An example of this channel is shown in Fig. 1. It is apparent from this figure that the open probability of this channel is reduced markedly when cytosolic pH falls just slightly below the normal value. The sensitivity towards cytosolilc pH is very steep. Comparable observations have been made in the diluting segment of amphibian kidney [40], reinforcing the similarity of the thick ascending limb and other diluting segments. Figure 1 shows that this channel in the thick ascending limb has a Ca^{2+} sensitivity which is opposite to that found for the maxi K^+ channel. Low Ca^{2+} increases, and high Ca^{2+} reduces, the open state probability. This effect is not very marked for physiological cytosolic Ca^{2+} activities [41]. A comparable Ca^{2+} effect has been noted in the basolateral K^+ channel of the rectal gland of *Squalus acanthias* [42]. Ca^{2+} insensitivity of a K^+ channel in the luminal membrane of the rabbit thick ascending limb has been noted in another study [19]. Inhibition of K^+ channels by ATP was first noted in the pancreas [43], and is now known to occur in a variety of K^+ channels in skeletal and heart muscle [44,45]. Recently, ATP inhibition was also reported for a Ca^{2+} activated K^+ channel in the amphibian diluting segment and in respiratory cells [46,47]. It is likely that the ATP sensitivity of K^+ channels and non-selective cation channels [38,48] is much more common than is recognized at this stage. Unlike the maxi K^+ channel, this smaller K^+ channel is not inhibited by charybdotoxin [34]. This fits well with the finding that charybdotoxin, when added to the luminal perfusate, has no effect on the equivalent short circuit current in isolated in vitro perfused rabbit thick ascending limb segments (unpublished work). The sensitivities of this kind of K^+ channel to other blockers are summarized in Table 1. None of the blockers used is characteristic in a qualitative sense for this type of channel, and none of the known toxins (apamin, dendrotoxin, or charybdotoxin) inhibits. In our study we found no other type of channel in the luminal membrane, even in the presence of high Ca^{2+} on the cytosolic side. Hence, we believe that more but increased cytosolic Ca^{2+} is necessary for the activation of the maxi K^+ channel in our preparation of the thick ascending limb.

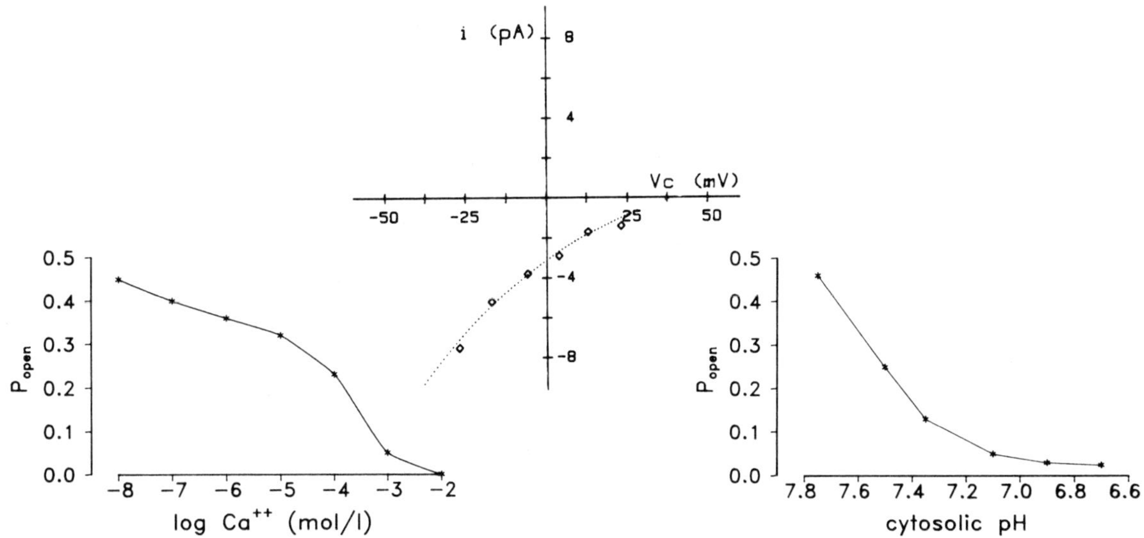

Fig. 1. K^+-channel in the luminal membrane of a rat thick ascending limb. Excised inside/out patch. Pipette KCl, Bath NaCl. The current-voltage (i/V_c) relation was fitted by the Goldman-Hodgkin-Katz equation. The conductance at 0 mV clamp voltage was around 60 pS. *Lower left panel:* The open state probability (p_{open}) of this channel is plotted against the cytosolic Ca^{2+} activity. Clamp voltage 0 mV. Note that p_{open} was reduced with increasing Ca^{2+}. *Lower right panel:* The open state probability of this channel as a function of the cytosolic pH. Note that p_{open} is reduced sharply with acid pH

Table 1. Inhibitors of the K^+ channel of the luminal membrane of rat thick ascending limb. The concentrations refer to half maximal inhibition (IC_{50} in mmol/l)

Substance	Side of action	IC_{50}	Type of block
H^+	cytosolic	pH 7.4	P_0 reduced
Ba^{2+}	cytosolic	0.1	P_0 reduced
Ca^{2+}	cytosolic	0.1	P_0 reduced
Mg^{2+}	cytosolic	5.0	P_0 reduced
Rb^+	both sides	>50, estimate	P_0 reduced
Cs^+	both sides	<50, estimate	P_0 reduced
NH_4^+	both sides	<50, estimate	P_0 reduced
Choline	both sides	~50	current amplitude reduced
TEA	outside	<1	P_0 reduced
	cytosolic side	>10	Current amplitude reduced
lidocain	both sides	10	flicker block
quinine	both sides	0.01	flicker block
quinidine	both sides	0.01	flicker block
verapamil	both sides	0.01	flicker block
diltiazem	both sides	0.1	flicker block

TEA, tetraethylammonium

In the basolateral (cf lateral above) membrane Cl^- channels of intermediate conductance were found in cell attached patches [33]. These channels had a mean conductance of 41 pS for positive and 31 pS for negative clamp voltages in excised patches with identical NaCl solutions on both sides of the channel. The open state probability was increased with depolarization of the clamp voltage. These channels were inhibited reversibly by the Cl^- channel blocker 5-nitro-2-(3-phenylpropylamino)-benzoate (NPPB). An example of this kind of channel is shown in Fig. 2. It has been shown that this channel is a weak outward rectifier [24]. The effect of NPPB was entirely reversible. As in other Cl^- channels, NPPB induced a flicker type block [49,50]. In another study [51], a similar channel was noted in the basolateral membrane of collagenase treated non perfused mouse thick ascending limb segments; it was reported that this channel was found more frequently after pretreatment with forskolin and 8-Br-cAMP.

We [33] and others [26] have found a non-selective cation channel with a mean conductance of 20–30 pS in the basolateral membrane of the thick ascending limb of rat and mouse. This channel requires high cytosolic Ca^{2+} activity to become activated. It is apparently inhibited by ATP [38]. As in the case of the proximal tubule, we have no firm indication of the physiological role of this channel (c.f. above).

Properties and Regulation of Ion Channels in the Distal Tubule

Recently, using distal convoluted tubules from rabbit kidneys treated with collagenase, K^+ channels were found in the basolateral membrane [27]. These channels had conductances in the range of 50 and 60 pS; they were inhibited by Ba^{2+}. Apart from the finding that the open state probability was not strongly altered with varying clamp voltages, little is known at this stage about these two types of K^+ channels.

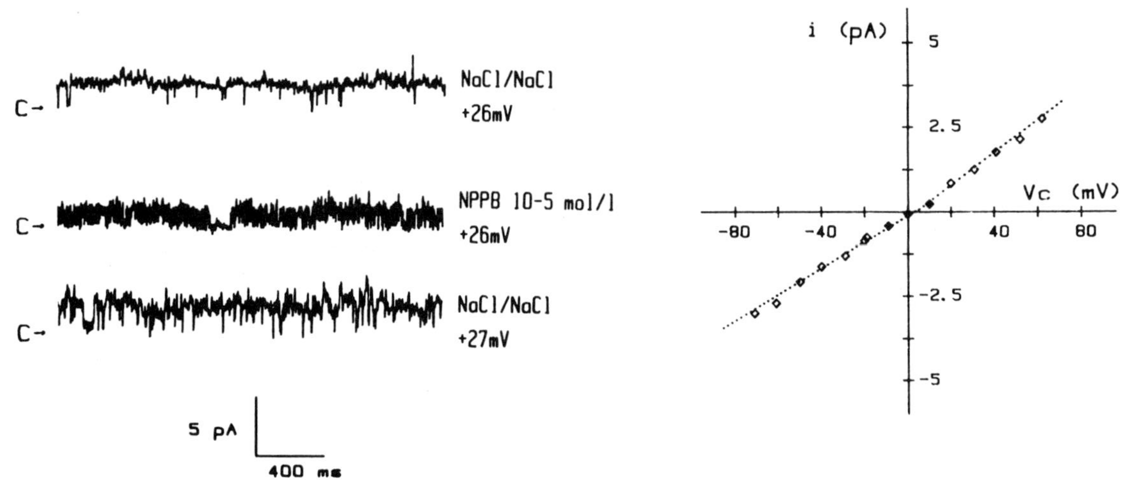

Fig. 2. Cl^- channels in the basolateral membrane of a rat thick ascending limb. Excised inside/out patch. Pipette and bath NaCl. *Left panel:* Typical recording and effect of 5-nitro- 2-(3-phenylpropylamino)-benzoate (*NPPB*). *C*→ denotes the closed state of this channel. Note the flicker block induced by NPPB. *Right panel:* Current-voltage relationship (i/V_c) of this channel

Properties and Regulation of Ion Channels in the Collecting Duct

Amiloride sensitive Na^+ channels in the luminal membrane of isolated cortical collecting ducts of Na^+ deprived rats have been reported previously [52,53]. These channels were localized in the principal cell; they had a small conductance of 5 pS. They were not directly regulated by cytosolic Ca^{2+}, but they showed increased open state probability with alkaline versus acid pH on the cytosolic side [53]. On the basis of the voltage dependent block of these Na^+ channels by impermeant ions, a model for this channel has recently been proposed [54]. This channel is permeable for H^+, Li^+, and Na^+, but is impermeable for K^+, guanidinium ions, and tetraethylammonium. Comparable channels have been found in pilot experiments in the luminal membrane of isolated in vitro perfused rat cortical collecting ducts [35]. It is not quite clear whether the Na^+ channel of this membrane can also occur with an even smaller conductance. This might explain the difficulty of finding this channel (reported in several studies [21], [25], and found in our own unpublished work). One alternative approach to dealing with this problem is the use of whole cell patch clamp analysis. This approach has been used recently [55], and an amiloride sensitive conductance increased by low Na^+ diet has been identified.

Besides these Na^+ channels, K^+ channels have been found in several studies in the luminal membrane of cortical collecting ducts of rabbit [25] and rat [35,56,57]. The channel found in the rabbit had an intermediate conductance and was Ca^{2+} dependent [25]. In the rat [35,57] the Ca^{2+} dependent channel belongs to the maxi K^+ channel family. Much knowledge has recently been gained concerning the properties of this channel. It seems unlikely that the channel is responsible for K^+ secretion in this nephron segment. We found this channel only very rarely in cell attached patches when the cells were depolarized by high extracellular K^+ concentrations. The finding that this channel coexists with Na^+ channels in the same cell membrane indicates that the channel is also localized in the principal cell [35]. The same channel has also been observed in cultures of collecting duct-"anlagen" [20]. We and others have found yet another K^+ channel in the same cell membrane. This channel had a small to intermediate conductance of some 20–35 pS. It was Ca^{2+} independent and may be controlled by cytosolic pH. A recording of this K^+ channel is shown in Fig. 3. In this figure the small and the large K^+ channel were present in the same membrane patch. It is highly likely that K^+ secretion occurs via this small conductance K^+ channel. This small channel has also been noted in experiments with collecting duct-"anlagen" [21]. Much more work is needed to characterize this channel in more detail.

A few Cl^- channels were noted in our studies on the luminal membrane of the rat cortical collecting duct [35]. Again, this matches well with previous studies in collecting duct-"anlagen" [21]. This Cl^- channel had an intermediate conductance of 20–60 pS and was inhibited by NPPB. We have no indication of the function of this channel, nor do we know whether it occurs in intercalated or in principal cells.

Conclusion

The present short review indicates that our knowledge of ion channels in renal tubules is still far from complete. The problems are manifold: 1) Several cell membranes have not been looked at with sufficient thoroughness. One such example is the lumi-

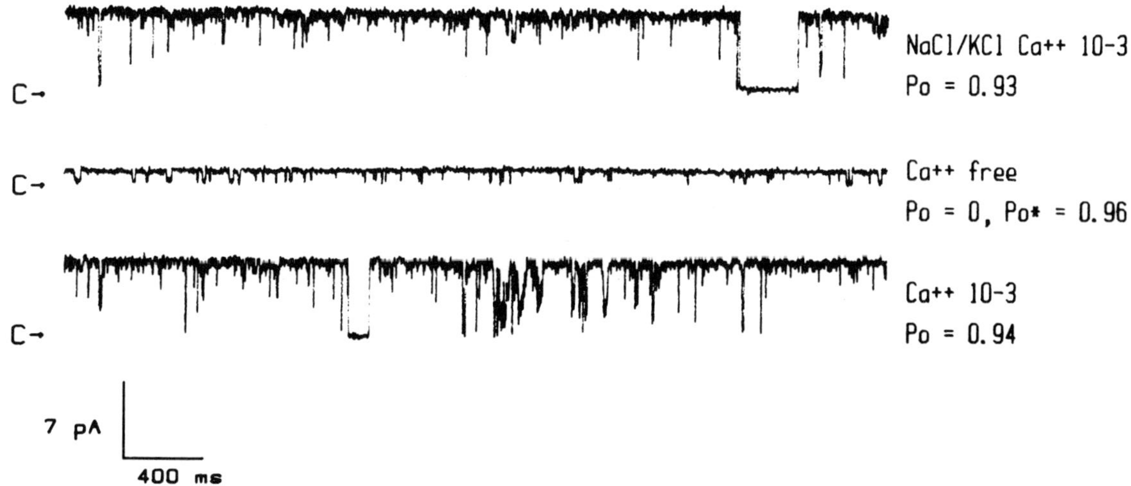

Fig. 3. Coexisting small and large K^+-channels in the luminal membrane of a rat cortical collecting duct. Inside/out patch. Pipette NaCl, bath KCl. Typical traces at 0 mV clamp voltage. *C*→ indicates the zero current level. Note that the large (maxi) K^+-channel is inhibited in Ca^{2+}-free solution (*middle trace*). Now the small K^+-channel, which, upon close inspection, is also hidden in the *upper* and *lower trace*, becomes clearly apparent. P_0 and P_0* denote the open state probability of the large and small K^+-channel, respectively

nal membrane of the proximal tubule. Other nephron segments are entirely empty spots on our map. 2) Analysis of the basolateral membrane is complicated by the fact that pretreatment with collagenase is required. Analysis of the properties of the lateral membrane at the torn end of the tubule makes the assumption that this membrane has properties identical with those of the basolateral membrane. 3) Several channels, such as the non-selective cation channel and the maxi K^+ channel, have been found in many excised patches of several nephron segments. These channels probably do not function in the normal cell and are activated under circumstances which are, so far, not clearly understood. 4) Other channels, which we know are present in a given membrane, are difficult to demonstrate by single channel analysis. One such example is the Na^+ channel in the collecting duct. Another example is the Ca^{2+}-channel in the luminal membrane of the thick ascending limb. 5) Culture techniques have made an important contribution to our current understanding of single channel properties in renal epithelia. Unfortunately, only with much caution can such data be extrapolated to the intact tubule. 6) The method of single channel analysis has an "analytical window" through which we view the conductance properties of a given membrane. With a time resolution in the 1 kHz range, only channels with open states lasting for around 1 ms will be detectable. Furthermore, the noise band of current traces filtered at 1 kHz is usually of the order of 0.3–0.5 pA. Any channel with a conductance <5 pS will have a current amplitude of <0.5 pA if the driving force is as high as 100 mV, and will therefore be difficult to detect. 7) That ion channels which operate on the cell are inactivated by the excision procedure cannot be excluded. These channels could therefore only be described in cell attached and possibly in whole cell recordings. Much more work and probably new techniques will be required to provide us with a more complete understanding of the function of ion channels in renal tubules.

Acknowledgments. This work was supported by Deutsche Forschungsgemeinschaft Gr 480/10 Schl 277/2-1.

References

1. Greger R, Gögelein H (1987) K^+ conductive pathways in the nephron. Kidney Int 31:1055–1064
2. Lang F, Friedrich F, Schobersberger W, Jungwirth A, Ritter M, Steidl M, Weiss H, Wöll E, Tschernko E, Paulmichl R, Hallbrucker C (1990) Ion channels in Mardin-Darby canine kidney cells. Renal Physiol Biochem 13:82–93
3. Kolb HA (1990) Ion channels in opossum kidney cells. Renal Physiol Biochem 131:26–36
4. Gögelein H (1988) Chloride channels in epithelia. Biochim Biophys Acta 947:521–547
5. Hunter M, Kawahara K, Giebisch G (1988) Calcium-activated epthelial potassium channels. Min Electrol Metab 14:48–57
6. Garty H, Benos DJ (1988) Characteristics and regulatory mechanisms of the amiloride-blockade Na^+ channel. Physiol Rev 68:309–373
7. Hunter M (1990) Patch clamp studies of the amphibian nephron. Renal Physiol Biochem 13:94–111
8. Parent L, Cardinal J, Sauve R (1988) Single-channel analysis of a K channel at basolateral membrane of rabbit proximal convoluted tubule. Am J Physiol 254:F105–F113

9. Merot J, Bidet M, Le Maout S, Tauc M, Poujeol P (1989) Two types of K^+ channels in the apical membrane of rabbit proximal tubule in primary culture. Biochim Biophys Acta 978:134–144
10. Merot J, Bidet M, Gachot B, Le Maout S, Tauc M, Poujeol P (1988) Patch clamp study on primary culture of isolated proximal convoluted tubules. Pflugers Arch 51:61
11. Gögelein H (1990) Ion channels in mammalian proximal renal tubule. Renal Physiol Biochem 13:8–25
12. Gögelein H, Greger R (1988) Patch clamp analysis of ionic channels in renal proximal tubules. In: Davison AM (ed) Proceedings of the Xth international congress of nephrology. Baillere Tindall, London, pp 159–178
13. Guggino SE, Guggino WB, Green N, Sacktor B (1987) Ca^{2+}-activated K^+ channels in cultured medullary thick ascending limb cells. Am J Physiol 252:C121–C127
14. Cornejo M, Guggino SE, Sastre A, Guggino WB (1989) Isomeric yohimbine alkaloids block calcium-activated K^+ channels in medullary thick ascending limb cells of rabbit kidney. J Mem Biol 107:25–33
15. Cornejo M, Guggino SE, Guggino WB (1987) Modification of Ca^{2+}-activated K^+ channels in cultured medullary thick ascending limb cells by N-bromoacetamide. J Membr Biol 99:147–155
16. Cornejo M, Guggino SE, Guggino WB (1989) Ca^{2+}-activated K^+ channels from cultured renal medullary thick ascending limb cells: effects of pH. J Membr Biol 110:49–55
17. Taniguchi J, Guggino WB (1989) Membrane stretch: a physiological stimulator of Ca^{2+}-activated K^+ channels in thick ascending limb. Am J Physiol 257:F347–F352
18. Bleich M, Schlatter E, Greger R (1990) The luminal K^+ channel of the thick ascending limb of Henle's loop. Pflugers Arch 415:449–460
19. Wang W, White S, Geibel J, Giebisch G (1990) A potassium channel in the apical membrane of rabbit thick ascending limb of Henle's loop. Am J Physiol 258:F244–F253
20. Gitter AH, Beyenbach KW, Christine CW, Gross P, Minuth WW, Frömter E (1987) High-conductance of K^+ channel in apical membranes of principal cells cultured from rabbit renal cortical collecting duct anlagen. Pflugers Arch 408:282–290
21. Laskowski FH, Christine CHW, Gitter AH, Beyenbach KW, Gross P, Frömter E (1990) Cation channels in the apical membrane of collecting duct principal cell epithelium in culture. Renal Physiol Biochem 13:70–81
22. Palmer LG, Frindt G (1986) Epithelial sodium channels: characterization by using the patch-clamp technique. Fed Proc 45:2708–2712
23. Light DB, McCann FV, Keller TM, Stanton BA (1988) Amiloride-sensitive cation channel in apical membrane of inner medullary collecting duct. Am J Physiol 255: F278–F286
24. Kunzelmann K, Pavenstädt H, Greger R (1989) Properties and regulation of chloride channels in cystic fibrosis and normal airway cells. Pflugers Arch 415:172–182
24a. Light DB, Schweibert EM, Fejes-Toth G, Naray-Fejes-Toth A, Karlson KH, McCann F, Stanton B (1990) Chloride channels in the apical membrane of cortical collecting duct cells. Am J Physiol 268:F273–F280
25. Hunter M, Lopes AG, Boulpaep E, Giebisch GH (1986) Regulation of single potassium ion channels from apical membrane of rabbit collecting tubule. Am J Physiol 251:F725–F733
26. Teulon J, Paulais M, Bouthier M (1987) A Ca^{2+}-activated cation-selective channel in the basolateral membrane of the cortical thick ascending limb of Henle's loop of the mouse. Biochim Biophys Acta 905:125–132
27. Taniguchi J, Yoshitomi K, Imai M (1989) K^+ channel currents in basolateral membrane of distal convoluted tubule of rabbit kidney. Am J Physiol 256:F246–F254
28. Burg M, Grantham J, Abramow M, Orloff J (1966) Preparation and study of fragments of single rabbit nephrons. Am J Physiol 210(6):1293–1298

29. Greger R, Hampel W (1981) A modified system for in vitro perfusion of isolated renal tubules. Pflugers Arch 389:175–176
30. Gögelein H, Greger R (1984) Single channel recordings from basolateral and apical membranes of renal proximal tubules. Pflugers Arch 401:424–426
31. Gögelein H, Greger R (1986) Na^+ selective channels in the apical membrane of rabbit late proximal tubule (pars recta). Pflugers Arch 406:198–203
32. Gögelein H, Greger R, Schlatter E (1987) Potassium channels in the basolateral membrane of the rectal gland of *Squalus acanthias*. Regulation and inhibitors. Pflugers Arch 409:107–113
33. Greger R, Bleich M, Schlatter E (1990) Ion channels in the thick ascending limb of Henle's loop. Renal Physiol Biochem 13:37–50
34. Greger R, Bleich M, Schlatter E (to be published) Ion channel regulation in the thick ascending limb of the loop of Henle. Kidney Int
35. Schlatter E, Bleich M, Greger R (1989) Properties of the luminal K^+-channel of isolated perfused cortical collecting ducts (CCT) of the rat (abstract). Proc Am Soc Nephrol 22nd annual meeting, Washington DC, 374A
36. Gögelein H, Greger R (1987) Properties of single K^+ channels in the basolateral membrane of rabbit proximal straight tubules. Pflugers Arch 410:288–295
37. Gögelein H, Greger R (1986) A voltage dependent ionic channel in the basolateral membrane of late proximal tubules of the rabbit kidney. Pflugers Arch 407:S142–S148
38. Paulais M, Teulon J (1989) A cation channel in the thick ascending limb of Henle's loop of the mouse kidney: inhibition by adenine nucleotides. J Physiol 413:315–327
39. Guggino SE, Suarez-Isla BA, Guggino WB, Sacktor B (1985) Forskolin and antidiuretic hormone stimulate a Ca^{2+}-activated K^+ channel in cultured kidney cells. Am J Physiol 249:F448–F455
40. Hunter M, Oberleithner H, Henderson RM, Giebisch G (1988) Whole-cell potassium currents in single early distal tubule cells. Am J Physiol 255:F699–F703
41. Nitschke R, Fröbe U, Greger R (1991 in press) ADH increases cytosolic Ca^{2+}-activity in isolated perfused rabbit thick ascending limb via a V1 receptor. Pflugers Arch
42. Greger R, Gögelein H, Schlatter E (1987) Potassium channels in the basolateral membrane of the rectal gland of the dogfish (*Squalus acanthias*). Pflugers Arch 409:100–106
43. Cook DL, Hales CN (1984) Intracellular ATP directly blocks K^+ channels in pancreatic B-cells. Nature 311:271–273
44. Stanfield PR (1987) Nucleotides such as ATP may control the activity of ion channels. Trends Neurosci 10:335–339
45. Noma A (1983) ATP-regulated K^+ channels in cardiac muscle. Nature 305:147–148
46. Hunter M, Giebisch G (1988) Calcium-activated K-channels of amphibiuma early distal tubule: inhibition by ATP. Pflugers Arch 412:331–333
47. Kunzelmann K, Pavenstädt H, Greger R (1989) Characterization of potassium channels in respiratory cells II. Inhibitors and Regulation. Pflugers Arch 414:297–303
48. Petersen OH, Gallacher DV (1988) Electrophysiology of the pancreatic and salivary acinar cells. Annu Rev Physiol 50:65–80
49. Hayslett JP, Gögelein H, Kunzelmann K, Greger R (1987) Characteristics of apical chloride channels in human colon cells (HT_{29}). Pflugers Arch 410:487–494
50. Dreinhöfer J, Gögelein H, Greger R (1988) Blocking kinetics of Cl^- channels in colonic carcinoma cells (HT_{29}) as revealed by 5-nitro-2-(3-phenylpropylamino)-benzoic acid (NPPB). Biochim Biophys Acta 959:135–142
51. Paulais M, Teulon J (1990) cAMP-activated chloride channel in the basolateral membrane of the thick ascending limb of the mouse kidney. J Membr Biol 113:253–260
52. Palmer LG, Frindt G (1986) Amiloride-sensitive Na channels from the apical membrane of the rat cortical collecting tubule. Proc Natl Acad Sci USA 83:2767–2770
53. Palmer LG, Frindt G (1987) Effects of cell Ca and pH on Na channels from rat cortical collecting tubule. Am J Physiol 253:F333–F339

54. Palmer LG (1990) Epithelial Na channels: the nature of the conducting pore. Renal Physiol Biochem 13:51–58
55. Frindt G, Sackin H, Palmer LG (1990) Whole-cell currents in rat cortical collecting tubule: low-Na diet increases amiloride-sensitive conductance. Am J Physiol 258:F562– F565
56. Frindt G, Palmer LG (1987) Ca-activated K channels in apical membrane of mammalian CCT, and their role in K secretion. Am J Physiol 252:F458–F467
57. Frindt G, Palmer G (1989) Low-conductance K channels in the apical membrane of the rat cortical collecting tubule. Am J Physiol 256:F143–F151

Single Sodium Channels in the Apical Membrane of Proximal Tubule Cells in Culture

EMILE L. BOULPAEP and ROSEMARIE DRAKE-BAUMANN[1]

SUMMARY. Isolated proximal tubule cells of Ambystoma kidney were grown in primary cultures to confluence. Using the patch clamp technique single Na^+ channels were found in the apical membrane of the proximal tubule cells. In control conditions in the cell attached configuration these Na^+ channels showed a single channel conductance of 3 to 4 pS (referred to symmetrical 100 mM Na) and were highly selective. In the presence of 10 μM amiloride added to the pipette solution there was an increased number of transitions without complete block, and the single channel conductance, referred to symmetrical 100 mM Na, increased to 10–13 pS. In control conditions the probability of opening increased with hyperpolarization of the membrane patch. In the presence of amiloride open probability decreased with hyperpolarization. Analysis of open and closed time constants revealed a single open and closed time constant in control conditions, but multiple time constants after the addition of amiloride. It is concluded that the apical membrane of the amphibian proximal tubule has a subtype of Na^+ channels whose properties differ, qualitatively and quantitatively, from other epithelial sodium channels.

Introduction

Multiple transport systems account for the translocation of sodium from the ultrafiltrate in the lumen of the proximal tubule to the cytoplasm of the cell. In isolated tubule preparations of Ambystoma [1], the following Na transporters have been identified at the level of the apical cell membrane: rheogenic Na^+/glucose symport [2] Na^+/aminoacids symport [2], electroneutral Na^+/lactate$^-$ symport [3], and electroneutral Na^+-H^+ antiport [4]. No evidence has been found for $Na^+/K^+/2Cl^-$ symport [5,6] or Na^+/Cl^- symport [5,6]. In the presence of ultrafiltrate-like solutions, a major

[1]Department of Cellular and Molecular Physiology, Yale University School of Medicine, 333 Cedar Street, New Haven, CT 06510, USA

moiety of Na uptake from lumen to cell is mediated by Na^+/substrate cotransport [2]. However, in the absence of Na^+/substrate symport and of Na^+-H^+ antiport, apical Na entry was detected from changes in intracellular Na activity measured with ion-selective microelectrodes, indicating the presence of conductive Na channels at the luminal membrane [5]. Following preferential reabsorption of organic substrates and HCO_3^- in early proximal tubule, Na channels may thus contribute appreciably to Na entry at the end of the proximal tubule.

In rabbit, late proximal tubule Na channels have been reported by patch-clamping of the microvillar surface [7], but baseline tracings were too noisy to record channel activity at normal resting potentials. Moreover, the effect of amiloride was examined only from the cytoplasmic side of the membrane patch [7].

Patch clamping of the apical surface of dissected proximal tubules is not readily feasible, in view of the presence of numerous tall microvilli. Confluent monolayers of epithelial cells offer free access to the apical membrane. We have developed primary cultures of salamander proximal tubule cells and have characterized the ultrastructural and electrophysiological properties as representative of proximal tubule function in situ [8].

Typical epithelial sodium channels have been described by patch-clamping of apical membranes in models of Na^+ absorbing "tight" epithelia such as A6 cells [9,10] and rat cortical collecting tubules [11–14]. The present study attempts, first, to identify the presence of Na^+ channels in apical membranes of cultured salamander proximal tubule cells using the patch clamp technique, and second, to establish whether these channels have properties identical to classical epithelial sodium channels.

Procedure

Confluent cultures of Ambystoma proximal tubule cells grown for two to three weeks on permeable supports were used. All patch clamp recordings were performed on the apical cell membrane in the cell-attached configuration. Patch pipettes were filled either with a control solution containing Na^+ 100 mM, K^+ 2.44 mM, Mg^{2+} 1 mM, Ca^{2+} 0.9 mM, Cl^- 89.68 mM, HCO_3^- 10 mM, HPO_4^{2-} 0.56 mM, $H_2PO_4^-$ 0.14 mM, SO_4^{2-} 0.5 mM, pyruvate$^-$ 4.3 mM, and glucose 1.9 mM, or with a low chloride solution containing Na^+ 100 mM, K^+ 2.44 mM, Ca^{2+} 1.8 mM, Cl^- 6.0 mM, and cyclamate$^-$ 95 mM. In addition, each solution was buffered with 10 mM Hepes acid titrated to pH 7.45 with NaOH. The bath contained the culture medium with an electrolyte composition similar to the pipette control solution.

Proximal Tubule Apical Na^+ Channels

With symmetrical control 100 mM Na^+ solutions in pipette and bath, spontaneous activity of inward currents of small amplitude was noted at the resting membrane potential, i.e., when the clamp voltage of the pipette V_{pip} was held at 0 mV (Fig. 1). Channel openings and closings lasted for intervals ranging from about 10 ms–1 second.

Hyperpolarization of the membrane patch with more negative values of $-V_{pip}$ enhanced the amplitude of the inward current. At depolarized membrane patch

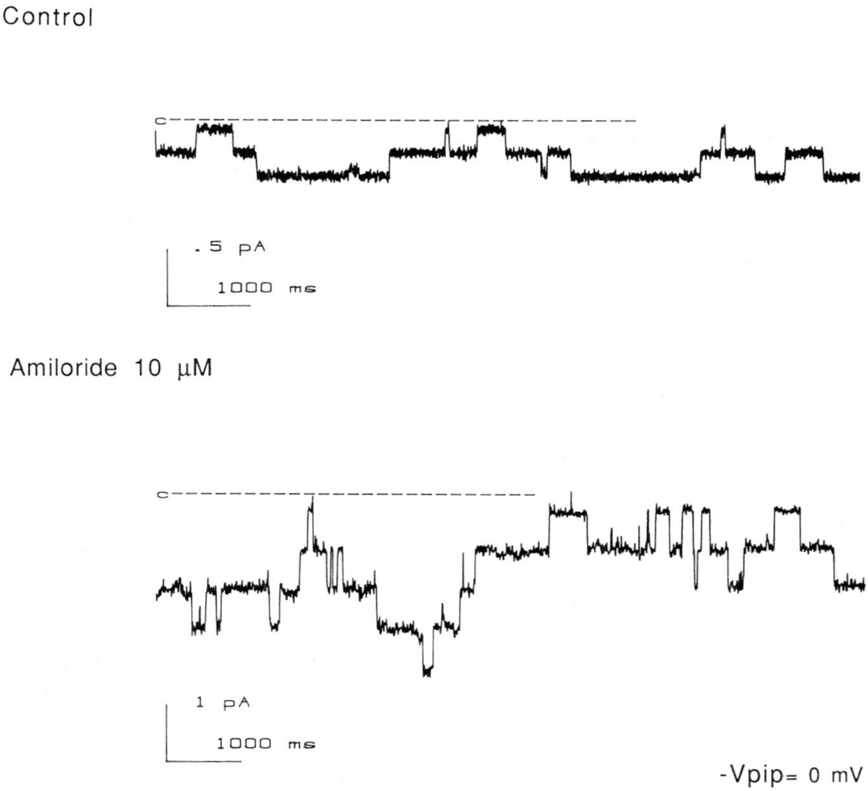

Fig. 1. Patch clamp recordings of apical sodium channels from cultured Ambystoma proximal tubule cells. Single channel currents were recorded in cell-attached configuration with 100 mM Na^+ in the pipette solution and bath. *Upper tracings* are the control condition. At least two channels are present in the patch. *Lower tracings* are obtained in the presence of 10 µM amiloride. At least four channels are present in the patch. Both recordings were obtained at resting membrane potential, i.e. $-V_{pip} = 0$ mV. Note the different current scale for the two records

potentials ($-V_{pip} = +$) outward currents could not be resolved. Often multiple channels per patch were observed, up to 7 channels in a single patch. The top part of Fig. 1 shows a patch with at least two channels.

Using current amplitude histograms of the current measured at different pipette potentials, single channel current amplitudes were plotted against $-V_{pip}$ potentials of $+40$ to -100 mV. The experimental current-voltage relations were adequately fitted by theoretical Goldman curves predicted for a perfectly selective Na^+ channel under the asymmetric Na concentrations prevailing across the membrane patch. The theoretical curves extrapolated to a reversal potential of $+93$ mV, assuming a membrane potential of -50 mV (Drake-Baumann R. et al., to be published) [8] and a E_{rev} for Na^+ of $+ 43$ mV calculated from an intracellular Na activity of 19 mM. Single channel conductance g_{Na}^* for a symmetrical 100 mM Na^+ concentration, as obtained from the Goldman equation, ranged from 3–4 pS.

Single channel conductance for Na^+ in the Ambystoma proximal tubule compares closely with the conductance of classical epithelial Na^+ channels, e.g., the apical Na channel in rat cortical collecting tubule [11] and the low conductance highly selective channel of A6 cells [15–18]. However, the g_{Na}^* of Na^+ channels in the amphibian proximal tubule is less than the values reported for Na^+ channels in mammalian proximal tubules, such as rabbit straight proximal segments [7] and rat proximal tubules [19]. Our Na channels also have a lower conductance than the high conductance non-selective Na^+ channel in A6 cells [15,16,20], and the Na^+ channel in LLC PK1 cells [21].

Amiloride Effect on Proximal Tubule Apical Na^+ Channels

When the pipette solution contained 100 mM Na^+ and 10 μM amiloride and the bath contained 100 mM Na^+, the spontaneous activity of inward currents at the resting membrane potential exhibited no closure of the channel, but exhibited frequent brief interruptions, as shown in the lower part of Fig. 1. In the example of Fig. 1, the patch contained at least 4 channels and it is clear that 10 μM amiloride did not suppress the single channel currents, but altered its kinetics. At hyperpolarized potentials the frequency of interruptions was even more pronounced.

Current amplitude histograms were obtained and single channel currents were plotted against $-V_{pip}$ potentials of +70 to −100 mV. These current-voltage relations were adequately fitted by theoretical Goldman curves predicted for a perfectly selective Na^+ channel; which also extrapolated to the theoretical reversal potential of +93 mV. Thus, amiloride does not alter the high selectivity of the Na^+ channel. However, a striking observation is that, in the presence of amiloride, single channel conductance g_{Na}^* for a symmetrical 100 mM Na^+ concentration, as obtained from the Goldman fits, rose to values of 10–13 pS/channel. Note the difference in current amplitude scale in the upper and lower portion of Fig. 1.

There is no precedent in the literature for the higher single channel conductance in amiloride treated patches. It is known that A6 cells exhibit both unselective high conductance (7–10 pS) channels and highly selective low conductance (4–5pS) channels [9]. Several arguments plead against the existence of two populations of channels in the amphibian apical membrane. First, in control conditions, high conductance channels were never observed. Second, in amiloride-treated membranes, low conductance channels were never seen. Third, there is no indication for the occurrence of highly selective as well as unselective channels, since the current-voltage relationships of both control and amiloride-treated channels extrapolated well to a reversal potential predicted for an ideal high Na^+ selectivity. We conclude that the amphibian proximal tubule Na^+ channel is an isoform of the classical epithelial channel with a qualitatively different amiloride response.

Voltage-Dependence of Channel Activity

The open probability was studied on recordings obtained from single-channel and multi-channel patches. Open probability was calculated as the product nP_o, where n = number of channels and P_o is the single channel open probability. To permit com-

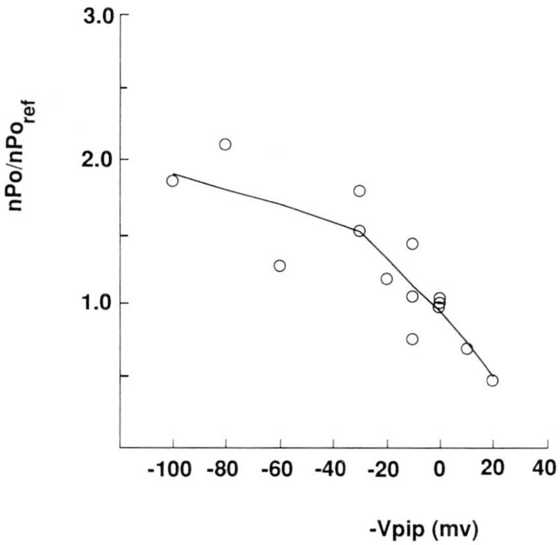

Fig. 2. Normalized open probability nP_o/nP_{oref} values in spontaneously active channels, at various pipette potentials where the normal resting potential at $-V_{pip} = 0$ mV is the reference potential

parison of the open probability from patches containing a different number of channels n, the nP_o values were normalized to a reference value nP_{oref} which was the value of P_o at the resting potential when $-V_{pip} = 0$. Fig. 2 shows the ratio nP_o/nP_{oref} for a spontaneously active Na^+ channel in the 100 mM Na control conditions. There was a moderate rise in open probability with hyperpolarization of the patch membrane. The data in Fig. 2 were fitted by Lowess fits, indicating a maximum rate of voltage dependence in the range of $-V_{pip}$ +20 mV to −30 mV. From fitting the data of Fig. 2 to a Boltzmann equation it was possible to conclude that the gating charge for the opening for the Na^+ channel did not appreciably depart from 1.

There is conflicting evidence in the literature regarding the voltage dependence of epithelial Na^+ channels. The voltage dependence in Fig. 2 is of the same shape and sign as in the apical Na^+ channel of the rat cortical collecting tubule [14]. However, in the highly selective Na^+ channels of A6 cells there appears to be no clear voltage-dependence [17], whereas the non-selective Na^+ channels in A6 cells [9] appear to have a voltage dependence of a sign opposite to our proximal tubule Na^+ channels.

The voltage dependence of Ambystoma apical Na^+ channels was drastically different in the presence of amiloride. Fig. 3 illustrates that the addition of 10 μM amiloride reversed the sign of the voltage dependence. In Fig. 3 hyperpolarization of the patch pipette reduced the nP_o/nP_{oref} of the sodium channel, as opposed to the increase of nP_o/nP_{oref} seen above in the absence of amiloride. The curve in Fig. 3 is a Lowess fit and shows the highest sensitivity of open probability to potential in the range of $-V_{pip} = 0$ to −60 mV. Alternatively, fitting the data to a Boltzmann equation showed that the gating charge for the voltage dependence of amiloride block does not differ from 1.

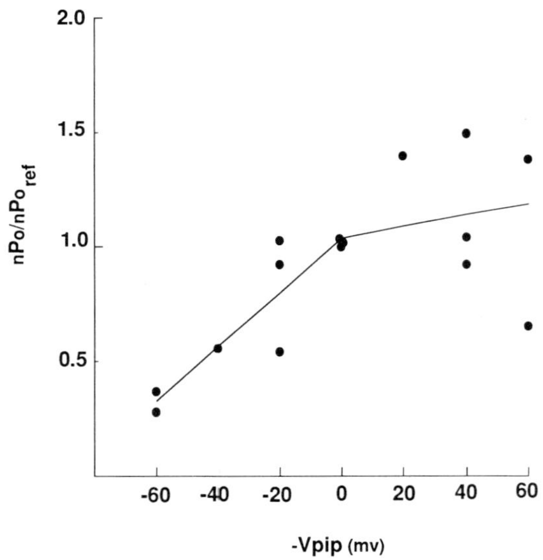

Fig. 3. Normalized open probability nP_o/nP_{oref} values in the presence of 10 μM amiloride, at various pipette potentials where the normal resting membrane potential at $-V_{pip} = 0$ mV is the reference potential

Voltage-dependent amiloride block of Na channels is well known to exist in A6 cells [20], in inner medullary collecting duct, [22] and "tight" epithelia [23]. The voltage dependence of amiloride blocking is thought to result from the position of the amiloride binding site in the channel, such that the cationic guanidinium group of amiloride senses the transmembrane electrical field.

Kinetics of Single Channels

Using a threshold analysis program [24] open and closed time durations were tabulated. From histograms of dwell time distributions plotted on a logarithmically binned time axis, a number of open and closed time components could be resolved, using the maximum likelihood method to fit a probability density function [25].

In control conditions, at a holding potential of $-V_{pip} = -60$ mV, only a single open time constant $\tau_{ol} = 312$ ms was calculated, as well as a single closed time constant of $\tau_{cl} = 289$ ms. However, in the presence of 10 μM amiloride at a holding potential of $-V_{pip} = -60$ mV, two open time constants τ_o were noted: flickery openings with a $\tau_{ol} = 0.3$ ms and longer openings with a time constant of $\tau_{o2} = 152$ ms. The longer time constant was, however, much shorter than the open time constant in control conditions. Examination of the closed time events during amiloride inhibition revealed four time constants τ_c. These were a rapid flickery block with time constants $\tau_{cl} = 0.32$ ms and $\tau_{c2} = 3.7$ ms; a third time constant $\tau_{c3} = 113$ ms was shorter than that of the single closed time constant observed in control channels; a fourth component, $\tau_{c4} = 813$ ms resulted from long closures or a blocked state condition.

Physiological Role of Proximal Tubule Na^+-Channels

Na^+ entry from apical bath to cell through conductive channels is not inhibited by amiloride in isolated perfused Ambystoma proximal tubules [5]. The present study reports responses to amiloride which are qualitatively and quantitatively different from other epithelial channels. Although flickering and the addition of several closed time constants was induced by amiloride in the amphibian proximal tubule, the time-averaged mean open probability was not significantly reduced after amiloride. This observation, when combined with the increased single channel conductance of amiloride-treated channels, most likely explains why macroscopic membrane conductance and transmembrane conductive fluxes are not inhibited by amiloride in intact proximal tubules.

The relative contribution of Na^+ uptake derived from the activity of Na^+ channels, as opposed to other Na^+ transporters, is an important issue in the overall regulation of proximal sodium handling. Two properties may converge to achieve powerful regulation. First, rheogenic symporters, such as rheogenic Na^+/glucose symport [2], induce a depolarization of the apical membrane as Na^+ ions enter the cell. Second, the present study shows that the probability of opening of Na^+ channels is very dependent on potential. It is therefore likely that regulatory feedback results from the interaction of these two properties. As long as glucose or other organic substrates are present, the apical membrane potential depolarizes as a result of rheogenic symport activity and the Na^+ channels should be closed. However, in the absence of these organic substrates, the apical membrane should hyperpolarize and the Na^+ channels should open.

Acknowledgments. This work was supported by grants DK-13844 and DK-17433 from the National Institute of Diabetes and Digestive and Kidney Diseases.

References

1. Sackin H, Boulpaep EL (1981) Isolated perfused salamander proximal tubule: methods, electrophysiology and transport. Am J Physiol 241:F39–F52
2. Morgunov N, Boulpaep EL (1987) Electrochemical analysis of renal Na^+-glucose cotransport in salamander proximal tubules. Am J Physiol 252:F154–F169
3. Siebens AW, Boron WF (1987) Effect of electroneutral luminal and basolateral lactate transport on intracellular pH in salamander proximal tubules. J Gen Physiol 90:799–831
4. Boron WF, Boulpaep EL (1983) Intracellular pH regulation in the renal proximal tubule of the salamender: Na-H exchange. J Gen Physiol 81:29–52
5. Abdulnour-Nakhoul S, Boulpaep EL (1986) Apical membrane transport mechanisms for Na entry in Ambystoma kidney proximal tubule. Kidney Int 29:403
6. Abdulnour-Nakhoul S, Boulpaep EL (1988) Chloride transport mechanisms linked to sodium in Ambystoma proximal tubule. Kidney Int 33:423
7. Gogelein H, Greger R (1986) Na^+ selective channels in the apical membrane of rabbit late proximal tubules. Pflugers Arch 406:198–203
8. Drake-Baumann R, Maunsbach A, Boulpaep EL (to be published) Primary cultures of Ambystoma proximal tubule cells: ultrastructure and electrophysiology. Am J Physiol
9. Eaton DC, Hamilton KL (1988) The amiloride-blockable sodium channel of epithelial tissue. In: Toshio Narahashi (ed) Ion channels vol 1. Plenum, New York, pp, 151–282

10. Garty H, Benos DJ (1988) Characteristics and regulatory mechanisms of the amiloride-blockable Na+ channel. Physiol Rev 68:309–373
11. Palmer LG, Frindt G (1986) Amiloride-sensitive Na channels from apical membrane of the rat cortical collecting tubule. Proc Natl Acad Sci USA 83:2767–2770
12. Palmer LG, Frindt G (1987) Effect of cell Ca and pH on Na channels from rat cortical collecting tubule. Am J Physiol 253:F333–F339
13. Palmer LG (1987) Ion selectivity of epithelial Na channels. J Membr Biol 96:97–106
14. Palmer LG, Frindt G (1988) Conductance and gating of epithelial Na channels from rat cortical collecting tubule. J Gen Physiol 92:121–138
15. Sariban-Sohraby S, LaTorre R, Burg M, Olans L, Benos D (1984) Amiloride-sensitive epithelial Na+ channels reconstituted into planar lipid bilayer membranes. Nature 308:80–82
16. Olans L, Sariban-Sohraby S, Benos DJ (1984) Saturation behavior of single amiloride-sensitive Na+ channels in planar lipid bilayers. Biophys J 46:831–835
17. Hamilton KL, Eaton DC (1986) Single channel recordings from two types of amiloride sensitive epithelial Na+ channels. Membr Biochem 6:149–171
18. Hamilton KL, Eaton DC (1986) Regulation of single sodium channels in renal tissue: a role in sodium homeostasis. Fed Proc 45:2713–2717
19. Marom S, Dagan D, Winaver J, Palti Y (1989) Brush-border membrane cation conducting channels from rat kidney proximal tubules. Am J Physiol 257:F328–F335
20. Hamilton KL, Eaton DC (1985) Single-channel recordings from amiloride-sensitive epithelial sodium channel. Am J Physiol 249:C200–C207
21. Moran A, Moran N (1984) Amiloride-sensitive channels from LLC-PK1 apical membranes. Fed Proc 43A:447
22. Light DB, McCann FV, Keller TM, Stanton BA (1988) Amiloride-sensitive cation channel in apical membrane of inner medullary collecting duct. Am J Physiol 255:F278–F286
23. Palmer LG (1984) Voltage-dependent block by amiloride and other monovalent cations of apical Na channels in the toad urinary bladder. J Membr Biol 80:153–165
24. Colquhoun D, Sigworth F (1983) Fitting and statistical analysis of single-channel records. In: Sackmann B, Neher E (eds) Single Channel Recording. Plenum, New York, pp 191–264
25. Sigworth FJ, Sine SM (1987) Data transformations for improved display and fitting of single-channels dwell time histograms. Biophys J 52:1047–1054

Regulation of K^+ Channels in Proximal Tubules: Studies in Opossum Kidney Cells

TAKAKO OHNO-SHOSAKU, TAKAHIRO KUBOTA, YOSHIAKI MORI, JUN YAMAGUCHI, and MAMORU FUJIMOTO[1]

SUMMARY. Using the patch clamp technique, we examined the properties of an inwardly rectifying K^+ (K_{in}) channel, which contributes greatly to an overall K^+ conductance in opossum kidney (OK) cells. The K_{in} channel was sensitive to Ba^{2+} and quinine, less sensitive to tolbutamide, and insensitive to tetraethylammonium (TEA). Experiments with inside-out patches demonstrated that the activity of K_{in} channels was regulated by intracellular Mg^{2+} and ATP. The K_{in} channel was inactivated by Mg^{2+} and reactivated by Mg-ATP, via a process requiring hydrolysis of ATP. The inactivation/reactivation of the K_{in} channel is suggested to be due to a dephosphorylation/phosphorylation of the channel protein. Intracellular pH also influenced the activity of K_{in} channels. The activity was low at acid pH and high at alkaline pH, presenting a sigmoidal pH-dependence with a half-maximum activation at pH 7.5. The pH-effects could be attributed to a combination of two different processes: one, a simple binding of H^+ to the channel protein, and the other, a H^+-induced inactivation of the channel, probably due to a dephosphorylation of the channel protein. These results suggest that under physiological conditions the K^+ conductance of OK cell membranes is controlled by intracellular Mg^{2+}, ATP, and pH.

Introduction

Electrophysiological studies with conventional microelectrodes have demonstrated the presence of K^+ conductive pathways in the basolateral membrane of proximal tubules [1]. The evidence so far suggests that the properties of the K^+ conductance are subject to regulation, although the precise mechanisms are still unknown. The purpose of this study is to detect the intracellular factors regulating the K^+ conductance, using the patch clamp technique, which enables us to examine the direct effects of intracellular factors on single K^+ channels.

[1]Department of Physiology, Osaka Medical College, Takatsuki, Osaka, 569 Japan

Cultured opossum kidney (OK) cells [2] have been used as a model system for proximal tubular epithelia [3,4], since they retain some physiological functions of proximal tubules [5,6]. We have already found an inwardly rectifying K^+ channel in this cell line [7], which contributes largely to the overall K^+ conductance. In the following pages, the activity of the K^+ channel, controlled by intracellular Mg^{2+}, ATP, and pH, will be demonstrated. Some of the results have been reported previously [7,8].

Materials and Methods

Cell Culture

OK cells were cultured in Dulbecco's modified Eagle's medium, supplemented with 10% fetal bovine serum, at 37°C in 5% CO_2. For patch-clamp experiments, the cells were harvested from confluent monolayers with trypsin, and were then incubated in the above culture medium for 4–8 hours before use. All experiments were performed at room temperature.

Electrical Recordings

Patch-clamp experiments were performed according to the method of Hamill et al. [9]. Electrical measurements and data analysis were made as described previously [8]. The composition of the solutions used in this study is given in Table 1. Patch pipettes were filled with either a 3 mM adenosine triphosphate (ATP) solution for whole-cell and outside-out patch experiments, or a K-rich solution for inside-out patch experiments. The pH values of ATP-free and 3 mM ATP solutions were adjusted to the desired levels with KOH or HCl, while the free Ca^{2+} concentration was held constant at either 10^{-8} M in ATP-free solutions or 3×10^{-7} M in 3 mM ATP solutions. The free Ca^{2+} concentration was calculated using the absolute values of the stability constants of ethylene bis(oxyethylenenitrilo)tetra-acetic acid (EGTA) for binding of Ca^{2+}, Mg^{2+}, and H^+ [10]. Values for the potential represent the voltages at the cytoplasmic side of the membrane with respect to the extracellular side. Currents flowing from the cytoplasmic side to the extracellular side were defined as outward and are shown as upward deflections in the figures.

Table 1. Compositions of bath solutions (in mM)

	NaCl	KCl	$MgCl_2$	$CaCl_2$	EGTA	HEPES	KOH	Na_2ATP	Glucose
Na-rich solution	140	5	1	2		10			10
K-rich solution		145	1			10			
Mg^{2+}-, ATP-free solution		115		3	10	5	30		
ATP-free solution		115	1	3	10	5	30		
1 mM ATP solution		115	2	3	10	5	30	1	
3 mM ATP solution		115	4	3	10	5	30	3	

The pH was adjusted to 7.3 with KOH, NaOH or HCl. HEPES, hydroxyethylpiperazine ethanesulfonic acid

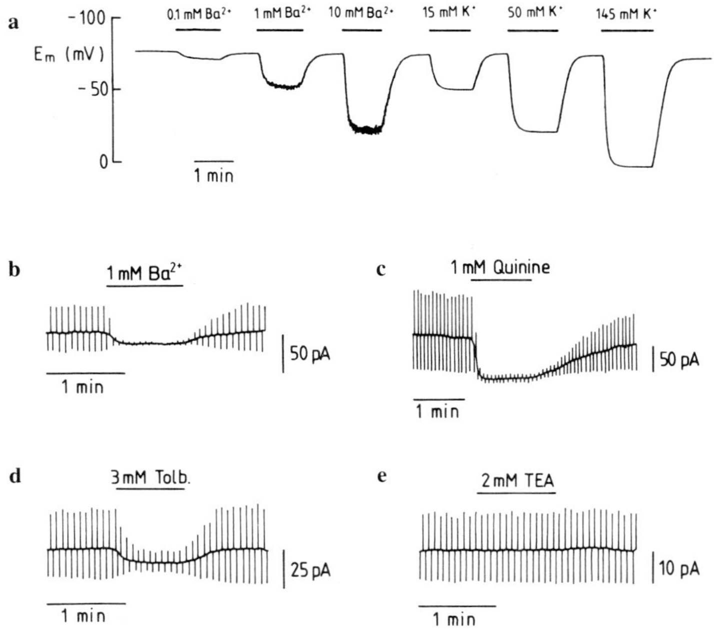

Fig. 1a-e. Whole-cell recordings of OK cells at the current-clamp mode (**a**) or the voltage-clamp mode (**b-e**). The bath contained a Na-rich solution with or without K^+ channel inhibitor, or a solution with the indicated K^+ concentration, which was made by replacing an appropriate amount of NaCl with KCl in a Na-rich solution. **a** The current was clamped at zero. **b-e** The membrane potential was clamped at −70 mV, and positive and negative voltage pulses of 10 mV were alternately applied to the membrane. The amplitude of the current deflection induced by a voltage pulse reflects a membrane conductance. Tolb., tolbutamide; TEA, tetraethylammonium

Results and Discussion

Whole-Cell Recordings

The electrical properties of the cell membranes were examined using the whole-cell configuration. The membrane potential was measured at the current-clamp mode, and the membrane conductance was measured by applying voltage pulses at the voltage-clamp mode. In a Na-rich solution the membrane potential was -69.4 ± 1.5 mV ($n=16$). Ba^{2+}, a K^+ channel blocker, depolarized the membrane in a dose-dependent manner (Fig. 1a). The membrane potential was greatly affected by changes in K^+ concentration of the bath solution, indicating a K^+-selective property of the cell membrane. The cell membrane conductance was 1.38 ± 0.33 nS ($n=53$) in a Na-rich solution, and was effectively inhibited by 1mM Ba^{2+} (Fig. 1b). The effects of other K^+ channel inhibitors were also examined (Fig. 1c-e). Quinine (1 mM) inhibited conductance as well as Ba^{2+}, whereas 2 mM TEA was without effect. Tolbutamide (3 mM), which is known to inhibit ATP-sensitive K^+ channels at

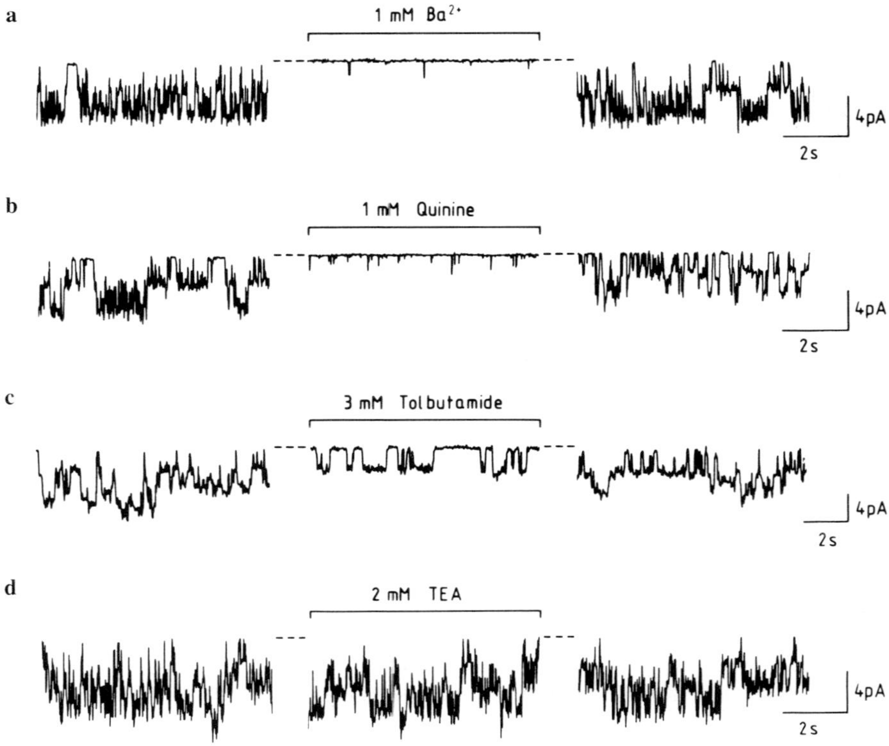

Fig. 2a-d. Effects of K^+ channel inhibitors on K_{in} channels. These records were obtained from inside-out patches. The patch membrane potential was clamped throughout at −50 mV. The bath contained a 3 mM ATP solution with or without K^+ channel inhibitor

micromolar levels, inhibited the conductance only partially. These results indicate that the membranes of OK cells are K^+-selective and have a large K^+ conductance, which is inhibited by Ba^{2+} and quinine, but not by TEA.

Single-Channel Recordings

In order to find the K^+ channels responsible for membrane K^+ conductance, single-channel recordings were carried out. In cell-attached patches, an inwardly rectifying K^+ (K_{in}) channel [7] was most frequently observed. Since the other K^+ channels were rarely observed in cell-attached patches, we concluded that the K_{in} channel contributed most to the membrane K^+ conductance in OK cells. This conclusion was further supported by other experiments, in which the effects of K^+ channel inhibitors were tested with outside-out patches. As shown in Fig. 2, the K_{in} channel was inhibited strongly by Ba^{2+} and quinine, partially by tolbutamide, and was not inhibited by TEA. The sensitivities to these inhibitors were the same as those of the K^+ conductance of the cell membranes.

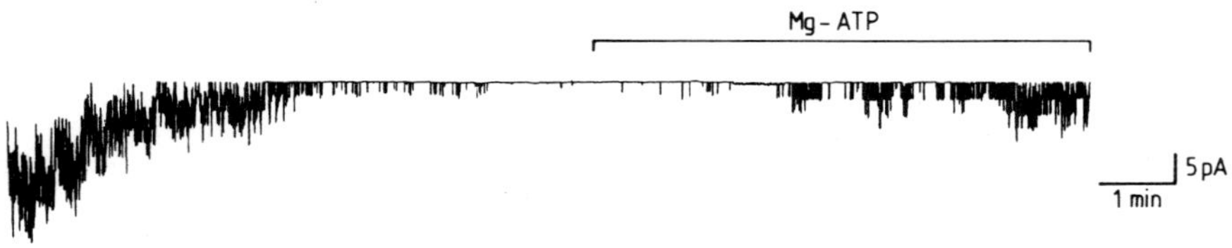

Fig. 3. Effects of intracellular Mg^{2+} and ATP on K_{in} channels. This record was obtained from an inside-out patch. The patch membrane was excised from the cell (at the left margin of the trace) in an ATP-free solution containing 1 mM Mg^{2+}, and then the internal surface of the patch membrane was exposed to 1 mM ATP solution. The patch membrane potential was clamped throughout at −50 mV

Effects of Mg^{2+} and ATP

The activity of K_{in} channels was stable in cell-attached patches. After excision of membrane patches from the cells (inside-out patches), however, channel activity declined with time ("run-down") in the absence of ATP (Fig. 3). This run-down was prevented by removal of Mg^{2+} from the bath solution, indicating that the run-down was due to a Mg^{2+}-induced inactivation of the channel. The channels inactivated by Mg^{2+} were reactivated by addition of ATP to the bath solution containing Mg^{2+}. The channel could not be reactivated by ATP in the absence of Mg^{2+}, or by AMPPNP, a nonhydrolyzable ATP analog, even in the presence of Mg^{2+}. Thus, the activity of K_{in} channels may be controlled by intracellular Mg^{2+} and ATP, probably via a dephosphorylation/phosphorylation process of the channel protein.

Effects of pH

The effects of pH on the K_{in} channel were examined, using excised patches. Changes in extracellular pH did not significantly affect the activity of the channel (Fig. 4a).

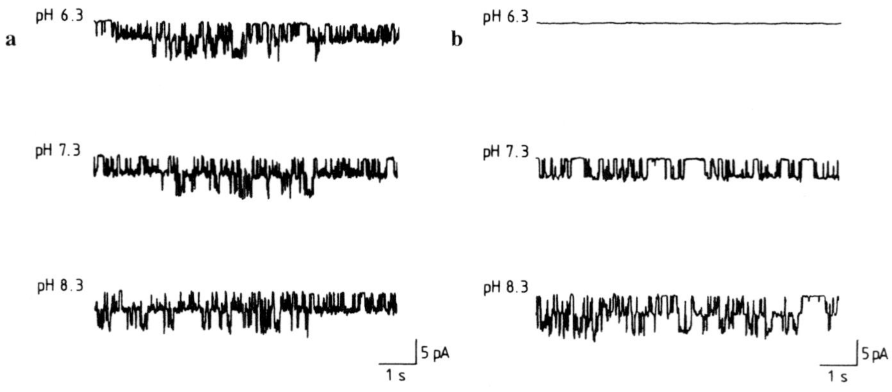

Fig. 4a,b. Effects of extracellular and intracellular pH on K_{in} channels. These traces were obtained from an outside-out (**a**) or an inside-out (**b**) patch. The patch membrane potential was clamped throughout at −50 mV. The bath contained a K-rich (**a**) or an ATP-free (**b**) solution adjusted to the indicated pH level

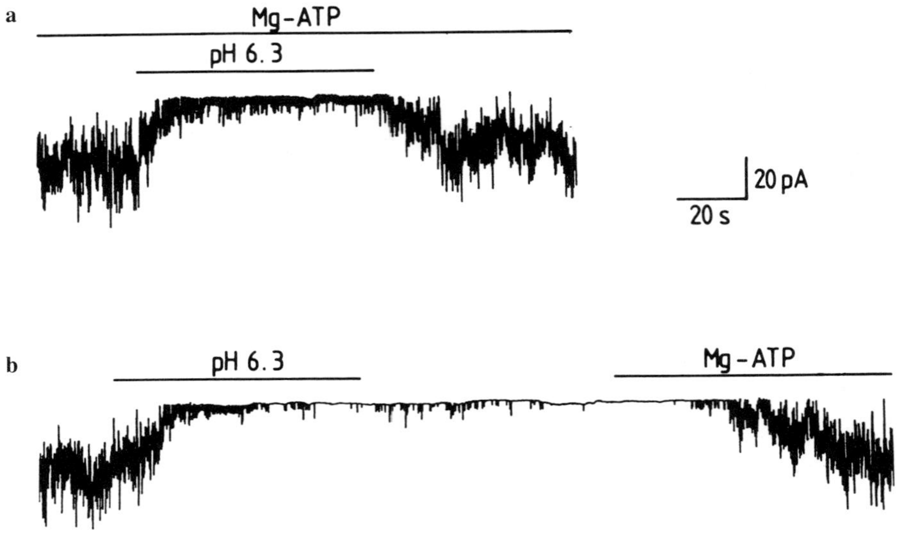

Fig. 5a,b. Effects of acid pH on K_{in} channels in the presence (**a**) or absence (**b**) of Mg-ATP. These records were obtained from an inside-out patch. **a**, the bath pH was changed from 7.3 to 6.3 by bath perfusion with 3mM ATP solutions for a given period of time. **b**, the bath pH was changed from 7.3 to 6.3 by bath perfusion with ATP-free solutions. After returning the pH to 7.3, ATP and Mg^{2+} were applied by perfusion with a 3mM ATP solution (pH 7.3)

On the other hand, changes in intracellular pH influenced channel activity remarkably (Fig. 4b). The channel was inhibited by acid pH and activated by alkaline pH.

The activating effects of alkaline pH were fully reversible, irrespective of the presence or absence of Mg-ATP. However, the inhibitory effects of acid pH were reversible only in the presence of Mg-ATP (Fig. 5a). In the absence of Mg-ATP, channel activity was not restored after returning the pH to 7.3 (Fig. 5b). This result indicates that H^+ inactivates the channels. The inactivated channels could be reactivated by adding Mg-ATP to the bath solution (Fig. 5b). All these findings would suggest that two different processes may be involved in the pH-effects: one, a protonation/deprotonation of the channel protein, and the other, a H^+-induced inactivation of the channel, which is probably caused by a dephosphorylation of the channel protein.

A Model of Channel Regulation

Figure 6 illustrates our model of channel regulation. According to this model, the K_{in} channel can be in four different states: one open state, where the channel protein is phosphorylated and deprotonated, and three closed states which are dependent on protonation and dephosphorylation of the protein. The transition from the open state to a closed state is considered to occur via dephosphorylation or protonation of the channel protein. The dephosphorylation process is promoted by Mg^{2+} and H^+, and the phosphorylation requires Mg-ATP. The observation that the channels inactivated by Mg^{2+} and H^+ in the absence of ATP were reactivated by Mg-ATP is consistent with this

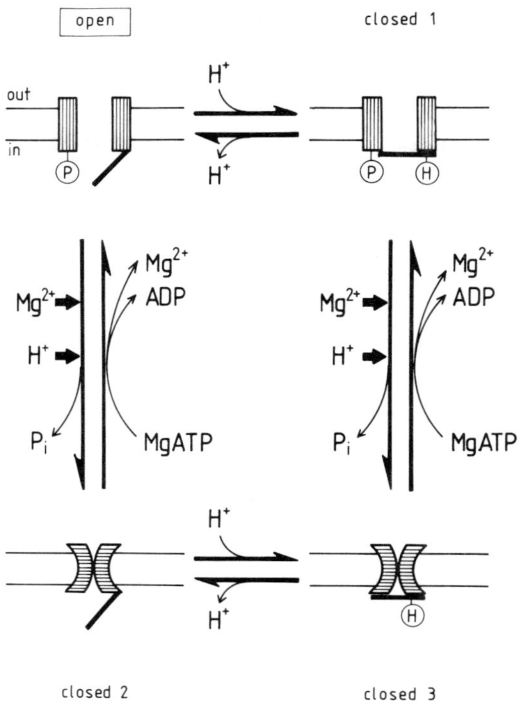

Fig. 6. A schematic model of regulation of the K_{in} channel

model. In the presence of Mg-ATP, the channel protein remains phosphorylated, because of continuous phosphorylation by Mg-ATP. Thus, this model can also explain the results which show that the pH-effects were fully reversible in the presence of ATP.

Acknowledgments. The authors are grateful to Dr. M. Fukase (Kobe Univ.) for providing us with OK cells, and to Drs. K. Kotera, N. Hagiwara and M. Kubokawa in our laboratory for their help, advice and encouragement in carrying out these experiments.

This work was supported by Grants-in-Aid for Scientific Research from the Ministry of Education, Science and Culture, Japan, and by a grant from The Salt Science Foundation to Prof. Mamoru Fujimoto (390B-4, 1990).

References

1. Giebisch G, Aronson PS (1986) The proximal nephron. In: Andreoli TE, Hoffman JF, Fanestil DD, Schults SG (eds) Physiology of membrane disorders. Plenum, New York, pp 669–700
2. Koyama H, Goodpasture C, Miller MM, Teplitz RL, Riggs AD (1978) Establishment and characterization of a cell line from the American opossum (*Didelphys virginiana*). In Vitro 14:239–246

3. Miller RT, Pollock AS (1987) Modification of the internal pH sensitivity of the Na^+/H^+ antiporter by parathyroid hormone in a cultured renal cell line. J Biol Chem 262:9115–9120
4. Ubl J, Murer H, Kolb H-A (1988) Ion channels activated by osmotic and mechanical stress in membranes of opossum kidney cells. J Membr Biol 104:223–232
5. Cole JA, Eber SL, Poelling RE, Thorne PK, Forte LR (1987) A dual mechanism for regulation of kidney phosphate transport by parathyroid hormone. Am J Physiol 253:E221–E227
6. Malmström K, Stange G, Murer H (1987) Identification of proximal tubular transport functions in the established kidney cell line, OK. Biochim Biophys Acta 902:269–277
7. Ohno-Shosaku T, Kubota T, Yamaguchi J, Fukase M, Fujita T, Fujimoto M (1989) Reciprocal effects of Ca^{2+} and Mg-ATP on the 'run-down' of the K^+ channels in opossum kidney cells. Pflügers Arch 413:562–564
8. Ohno-Shosaku T, Kubota T, Yamaguchi J, Fujimoto M (1990) Regulation of inwardly rectifying K^+ channels by intracellular pH in opossum kidney cells. Pflügers Arch 416:138–143
9. Hamill OP, Marty A, Neher E, Sakmann B, Sigworth FJ (1981) Improved patch-clamp technique for high-resolution current recording from cells and cell-free membrane patches. Pflügers Arch 391:85–100
10. Martell AE, Smith R (1977) Critical stability constants, vol 1. Other organic ligands. Plenum, New York

Regulation of K^+ Channels in the Thick Ascending Limb

WILLIAM B. GUGGINO[1]

SUMMARY. The apical K^+ conductance in the thick ascending limb (TAL) is important in the recycling of the K^+ which enters via the apical Na/K/Cl cotransport; in generating the positive transepithelial potential; and in the reabsorption of Na^+ across the paracellular pathway. Two types of K^+ channels have been identified in the apical membrane of the TAL. One group of K^+ channels is inhibited by ATP [1–3]; these are referred to as the ATP-sensitive channels. A second group is Ca^{2+}-activated [4–12]; because of their relatively large single channel conductance, they have been called Ca^{+2}-activated, maxi-K^+ channels. In this review, the properties and modulators of these groups of channels and their physiological role in TAL function are discussed.

Introduction

The TAL of the kidney reabsorbs NaCl, preferentially to water diluting tubular fluid [14]. The reabsorption of NaCl by this segment occurs via a combination of transcellular and paracellular routes. NaCl is taken into the cell across the apical cell membrane via a triple Na/K/2Cl cotransporter which is present in parallel with an apical K^+ conductance. This apical K^+ conductance functions to recycle the K^+ out of the cell across the apical cell membrane. Several transporters are present in the basolateral cell membrane, including the Na/K pump, a K^+ conductance, a K/Cl cotransporter, and a Cl^- conductance. These basolateral transporters function to move Na^+ and Cl^- out of the cell and to recycle the K^+ which moves into the cell via the Na/K pump (see Fig. 1).

The arrangement of an apical cell membrane, which is almost exclusively K^+ conductive and a basolateral cell membrane, which is conductive to both Cl^- and K^+ is an important feature of the thick ascending limb. This arrangement of conductances

[1]Department of Physiology, the John Hopkins University, Baltimore, MD 21205, USA

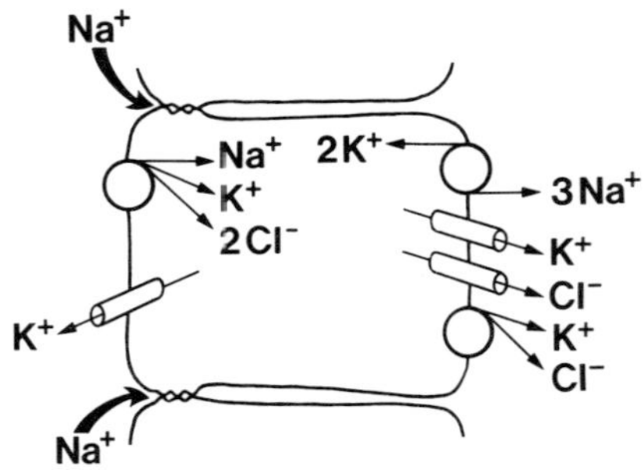

Fig. 1. A model of transcellular and paracellular ion transport in the thick ascending limb and the amphibian diluting segments. (Adapted from [14])

generates a lumen positive transepithelial potential, which, combined with a highly Na^+ conductive paracellular shunt pathway, allows about half of the Na^+ reabsorbed by the thick ascending limb to cross the paracellular pathway. This is an efficient mechanism, because for every Na^+ that is reabsorbed via a transcellular route an additional Na^+ is reabsorbed via a paracellular pathway. Because the Na/K pump is the major source of energy for the reabsorption of solutes by the thick ascending limb, this increased efficiency doubles the amount of Na^+ which is reabsorbed per turnover of the pump (see [14] for a review).

Several investigators have focussed attention on the biophysics and regulation of ion channels in the apical cell membrane of the thick ascending limb [1–12]. Most have utilized the path clamp technique, whereas others have isolated apical membrane vesicles to study the properties of the apical K^+ conductance, using radiolabelled K^+ or Rb^+ fluxes. These studies have been performed on rat or rabbit TAL cells, purified apical membranes, cultured medullary thick ascending limb (MTAL) cells, and amphibian diluting segments. The diluting segment is the amphibian homologue of the mammalian thick ascending limb.

Types of Potassium Channels in the Thick Ascending Limb

There are two classes of K^+ channels present in the apical cell membrane of the TAL and the diluting segment. The first group contains the ATP-sensitive K^+ channels (Fig. 2a). These channels have been observed primarily in both cell attached and excised patches of the apical cell membranes of freshly isolated TAL cells. The open probability of the channels is high in unstimulated cells (Fig. 2a). ATP-sensitive K^+ channels display inward rectification and a higher single channel conductance when current is carried into the cell than when current moves in the outward direction (Fig. 2b). The ATP-sensitive channels in the rat medullary thick ascending limb [1] have a higher single channel conductance (60 pS for inward current; 31 pS for outward current) than those in the rabbit [3] cortical thick ascending limb (22 pS for inward current; 10 pS for outward current). There are additional differences. The rabbit channel is not sensitive to either pH or Ca^{2+}, whereas the open channel probability of the rat channel is reduced by increasing H^+ or Ca^{2+} concentrations on the intra-

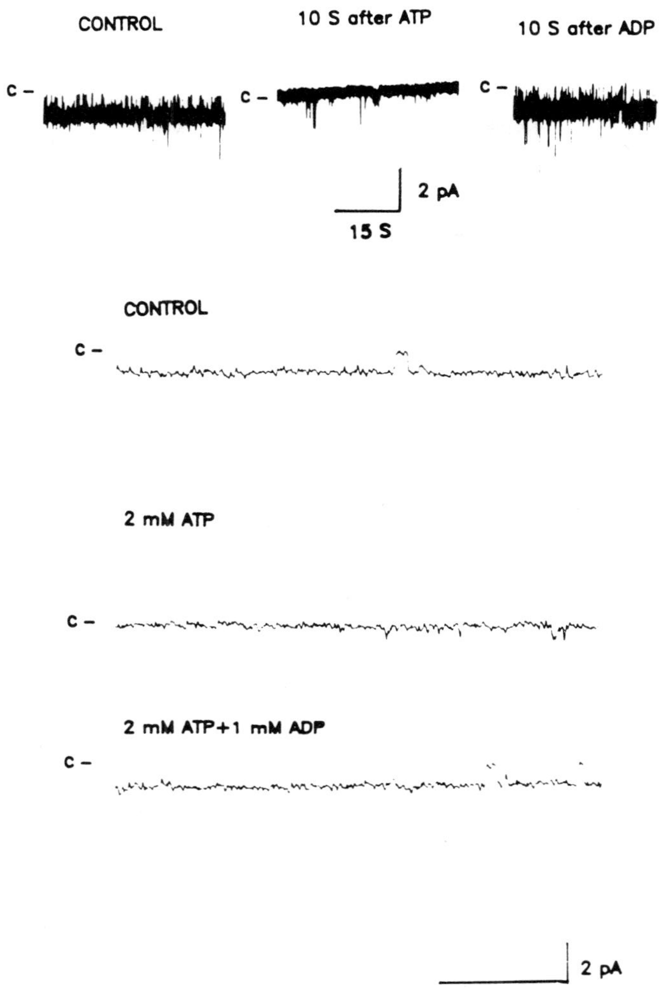

Fig. 2a. Inside-out patch at 33–37°C of the apical cell membrane of the rabbit TAL. Note that in control the channel is mostly in the open state; 1 mM ATP blocks the channel and 2 mM ADP reverses the effect. Recorded at 25 mV transmembrane potential (with respect to a bath ground). (Adapted from [3] with permission)

cellular face of the channel. The reason for these differences between the channels is not understood.

When exposed to millimolar amounts of ATP on the cytoplasmic face of the membrane in an excised patch configuration, channel open probability decreases dramatically, suggesting that ATP blocks these channels (Fig. 2a). The blocking effect of ATP can be reversed by addition of millimolar amounts of ADP. Thus, hormonal control of these channels depends heavily upon the metabolic state of the thick ascending

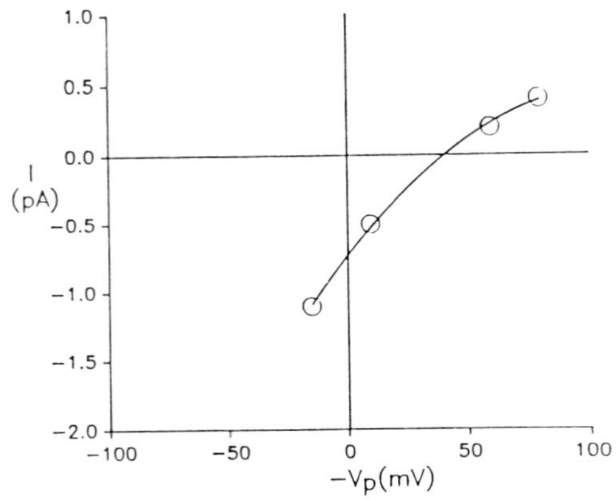

Fig. 2b. Current versus voltage relationship of ATP-dependent K^+ channel in a cell attached patch of the rabbit TAL. (Adapted from [3] with permission)

limb cell. At high transport rates it is expected that Na/K pump activity is high and ATP concentrations are low. In this transport state, the channel will spend most of the time in the open configuration. If these channels are present in the apical cell membrane in large numbers, at lower levels of ATP, the channels would be expected to contribute significantly to apical K^+ recycling.

A second group of channels found in the thick ascending limb and diluting segments includes the Ca^{2+}-activated K^+ channels (see Fig. 3a). These channels are activated by increasing concentrations of Ca^{2+} on the intracellular face of the membrane (Fig. 3b). In contrast to the ATP-sensitive channels, the Ca^{2+}-dependent channels have a linear conductance over a wide range of voltages. They usually have a large single channel conductance of 100–200 pS.

Ca^{2+}-activated K^+ channel activity is voltage dependent, with positive voltages increasing and negative voltages decreasing, open probability. However, voltage does not directly affect the channel gating mechanism. Instead, voltage affects gating by influencing Ca^{2+} binding [4]. Ca^{2+}-activated K^+ channel activity is also decreased at acid pH (see Fig. 3b). Again, the effect of increased hydrogen ion concentration is not direct, instead it decreases Ca^{2+} binding to the gating mechanism. Finally, in one study, ATP has been shown to inhibit Ca^{2+}-activated K^+ channel activity in the diluting segment [9].

Two factors are thought to increase Ca^{2+}-activated K^+ channel activity in physiological conditions: antidiuretic hormone and membrane stretch induced by cell swelling. In the next two sections, I will focus specifically on these two mechanisms.

Hormonal Stimulation of Calcium-Activated Potassium Channels

An increase in net NaCl reabsorption by the thick ascending limb must involve increases in rates of transport through both the cotransporter and the apical K^+ conductance (see Fig. 1). One factor which is known to increase NaCl reabsorption in

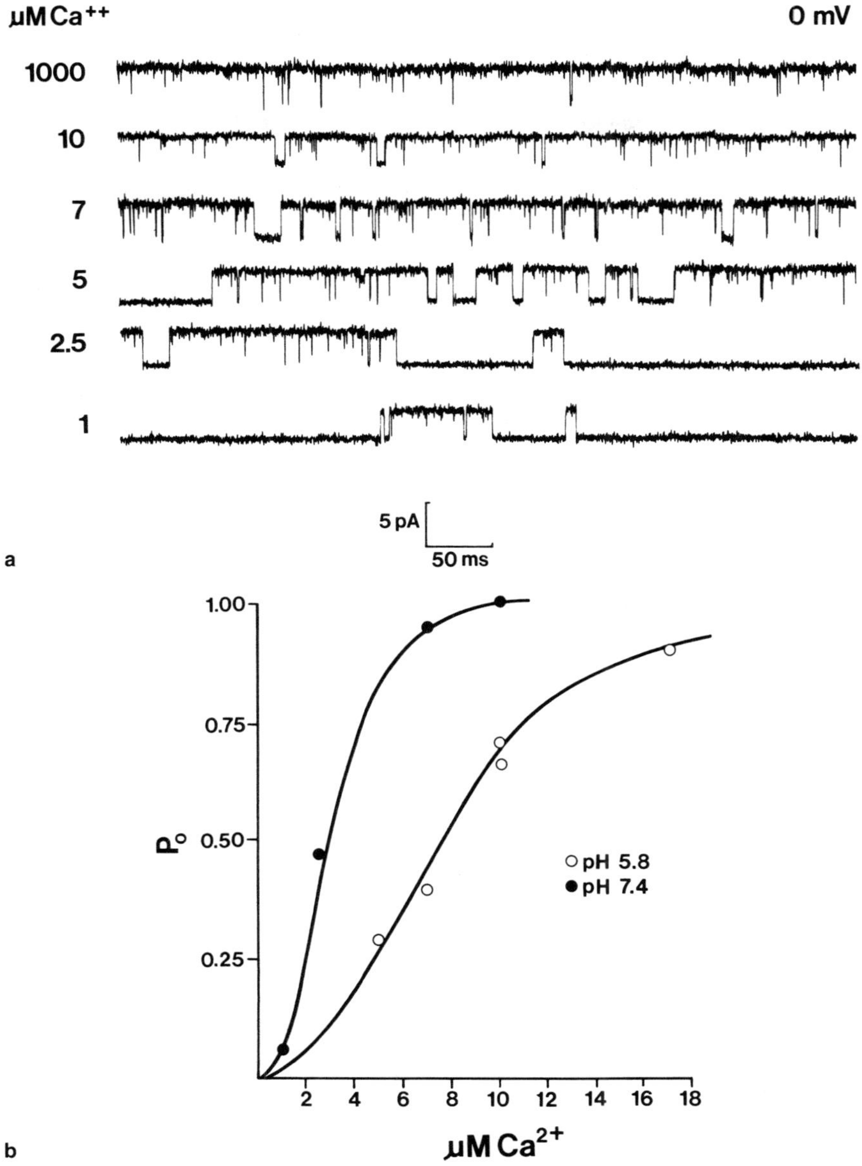

Fig. 3a. Ca^{2+} dependence of a K^+ channel in the apical cell membrane of cultured thick ascending limb cells. The tracing is from an excised patch clamped at 0 mV. Ca^{2+} was varied on the intracellular face of the channel. **b.** Open probability versus Ca^{2+} of channels in an excised patch clamped at 0 mV. The channel spends about half of the time in the open state at 3 µM Ca^{2+} at pH 7.4 but is at almost 10 µM Ca^{2+} at pH 5.8. (Reproduced from [4])

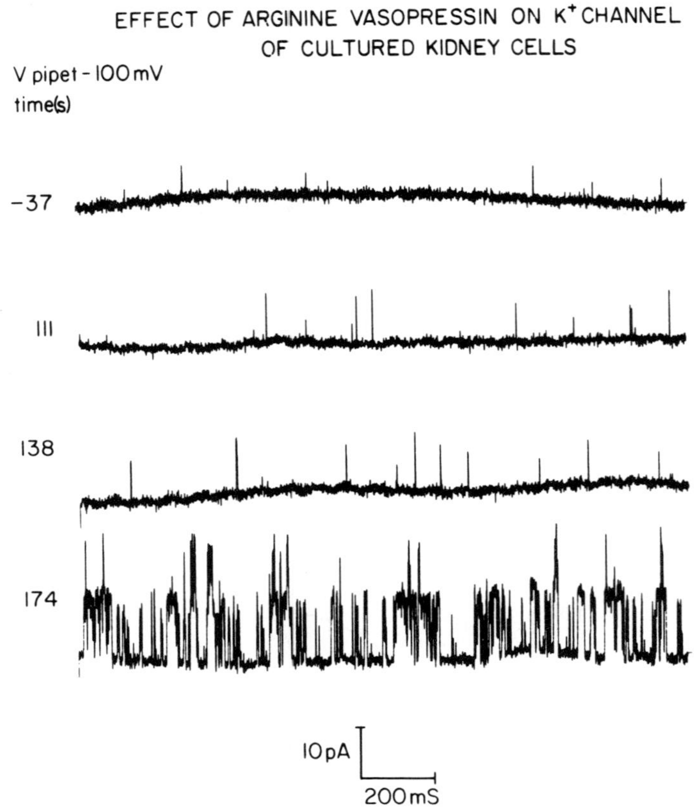

Fig. 4. The effect of arginine vasopressin (*ADH*) on a cell-attached patch held at 100 mV. *Top trace* shows that channel activity is low before ADH. *Lower traces* show the times for maximal increase in open probability to occur. (Reproduced from [8])

the mouse medullary TAL is arginine vasopressin ADH (see [15]). In cell attached patches of primary cultures of chick kidney cells, application of ADH increases Ca^{2+}-activated, maxi K^+ channel activity several-fold (see Fig. 4). Forskolin also activates maxi-K^+ channels in these cells. Since the major action of forskolin is to increase adenylate cyclase activity, the activation of Ca^{2+}-activated K^+ channels is probably via an increase in cAMP. Since ADH produces its effect through an increase in cAMP [16], it is safe to conclude that the ADH-induced increase in Ca^{2+}-activated K^+ channel activity occurs via an increase in cAMP levels. Although the final steps in the cascade by which ADH leads to an increase in channel activity are not known, experiments in isolated and purified apical cell membranes suggest that cAMP-dependent phosphorylation of the channel may play a role in activating Ca^{2+}-activated K^+ channels in this segment [11,24].

For example, Ca^{+2}activated K^+ channels can be purified from apical membranes of the mammalian thick ascending limb, using a calmodulin-affinity column [11]. These

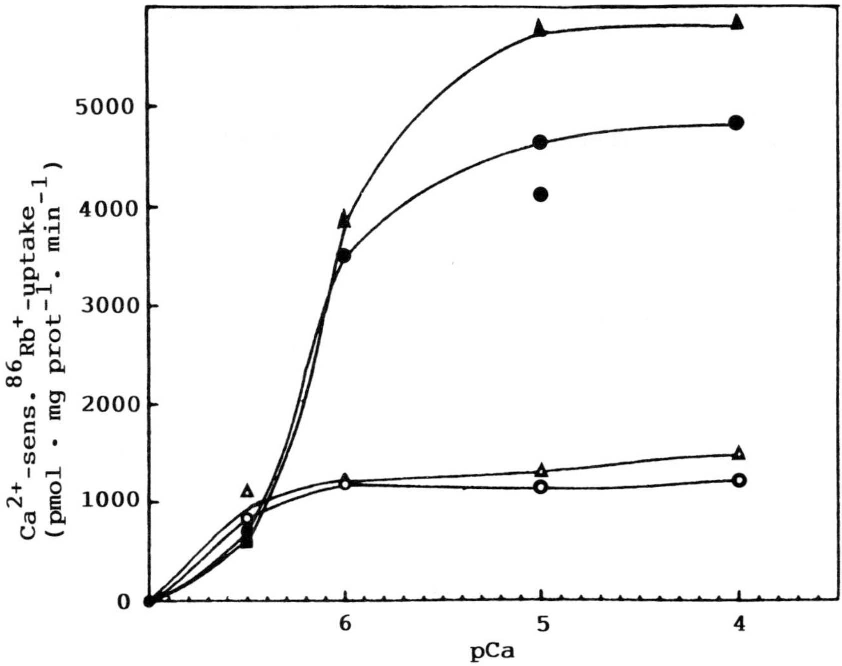

Fig. 5. $^{86}Rb^+$ uptake after phosphorylation of purified K^+ channel protein in reconstituted vesicles (▲, ●) compared to uptake without phosphorylation (△, ○). K^+ channel was purified on a calmodulin affinity column and reconstituted into phospholipid vesicles. Uptake was measured at different Ca^{2+} concentration. Uptake was also measured in the presence (▲, △) and absence (●, ○) of 0.1 μM calmodulin. (Reproduced from [11] with permission)

channels can also be reconstituted into phospholipid vesicles. Phosphorylation in this configuration by cAMP-dependent kinase stimulates by several-fold the maximum activity of Ca^{2+}-activated K^+ channels (Fig. 5). Interestingly, calmodulin by itself stimulates channel activity and is required for the phosphorylation-induced activation to occur. Since the activity of calmodulin is Ca^{2+}-dependent andADH is known to cause an increase in intracellular Ca^{2+} in cultured cells, stimulation of Ca^{2+}-activated K^+ channels by ADH may involve the actions of Ca^{2+}, both through calmodulin and cAMP-dependent phosphorylation.

Stimulation of Calcium-Activated Potassium Channels in Hyposmotic Solutions

Epithelial cells in the kidney medulla must maintain their volume despite large changes in extracellular osmolalities which occur during the diuretic versus antidiuretic state [see 13]. Thick ascending limb cells in isolated and perfused mouse tubules and in a cloned MTAL rabbit cell line regulate volume when exposed to hypotonic solutions [20]. In most kidney cells, K^+ efflux during volume regulation occurs via K^+ channels. There is evidence that Ca^{+2}-activated K^+ channels participate in regulatory volume decrease in hyposmotic solutions [12,18–21].

For example, in a cell attached patch configuration, stretching the cell membrane of cultured MTAL cells, by applying negative pressure to the patch pipette, causes a large increase in Ca^{+2}-activated K^+ channel open probability (see Fig. 6a). This effect is dependent upon extracellular Ca^{2+}, because removal of Ca^{2+} from only the pipette solution eliminates this effect of membrane stretch. Ca^{+2}-activated K^+ channels are not intrinsically stretch sensitive. For example, Ca^{+2}-activated K^+ channels are activated by membrane stretch only in the intact cell but not in excised patches.

Membrane stretch is expected to occur when cells swell following exposure to hyposmotic solutions. Figure 6b shows that exposing cultured medullary thick ascending limb cells to hyposmotic solutions causes a large increase in Ca^{+2}-activated K^+ channel open probability recorded in cell attached patches. This increase in open probability does not occur in the absence of extracellular Ca^{2+}.

These observations following membrane stretch or exposure to hyposmotic solutions suggest that membrane stretch acts to increase the influx of Ca^{2+} via stretch-sensitive Ca^{2+} channels. This influx of Ca^{2+} either raises intracellular Ca^{2+} directly or stimulates internal release. It is the increased intracellular Ca^{2+} which increases the open probability of Ca^{+2}activated K^+ channels in the apical cell membrane. The increase in Ca^{+2}activated K^+ channel open probability would result in enhanced K^+ loss from the cell. An enhanced K^+ loss, accompanied by anion, would be important for the volume regulatory processes of the thick ascending limb cell to occur. Similar activation of Ca^{2+}-activated K^+ channels by stretch has also been demonstrated in opossum kidney cells [21], in choroid plexus [18], and in *Necturus* proximal tubule cells [19]. In choroid plexus and *Necturus* proximal tubule, stretch is thought to act directly to increase Ca^{2+} influx, while in opossum kidney, Ca^{2+} is released from intracellular stores. The widespread occurrence of this Ca^{2+}-dependent stretch mechanism in different cell types suggests that maxi-K^+ channels may play an important role in volume regulation in hyposmotic solutions.

A rise in intracellular Ca^{2+} has been observed in cultured MTAL cells exposed to hyposmotic solutions (Figs. 7a and b). For example, exposure of cultured MTAL cells to hyposmotic solutions causes a maximal increase in intracellular Ca^{2+} in 40–60 seconds, followed by a decline toward baseline values (Fig. 7a). In hyposmotic solutions (42% decrease of osmolality), intracellular Ca^{2+} concentration increases from 163.5 ± 11.6nM (n=22) to a peak value of 738.6 ± 65.8 nM (n=22) at a rate of 12.5 $\pm$ 1.4nM/s (n=20). Intracellular Ca^{2+} concentration then decreases and reaches a value of 479.9 ± 43.4nM (n=21) at 200 seconds. Verapamil and nifedipine in the hyposmotic solution inhibit the increase of intracellular Ca^{2+} in a dose dependent manner (Fig. 7b). This sensitivity of Ca^{2+} influx to Ca^{2+} channel inhibitors such as verapamil and nifedipine [22] suggests that Ca^{2+} channels in either the apical or basolateral cell membrane of cultured MTAL cells are activated by stretch in hyposmotic solutions.

Thus, the simplest model of volume regulation in MTAL cells involves swelling which activates a nifedipine- and verapamil-sensitive Ca^{2+} channel. Increased entry through Ca^{2+} channels increases intracellular Ca^{2+} and thereby stimulates apical Ca^{2+}-activated K^+ channels to release cellular K^+. However, several pieces of information taken together show that the mechanism of activation of Ca^{2+}-activated K^+

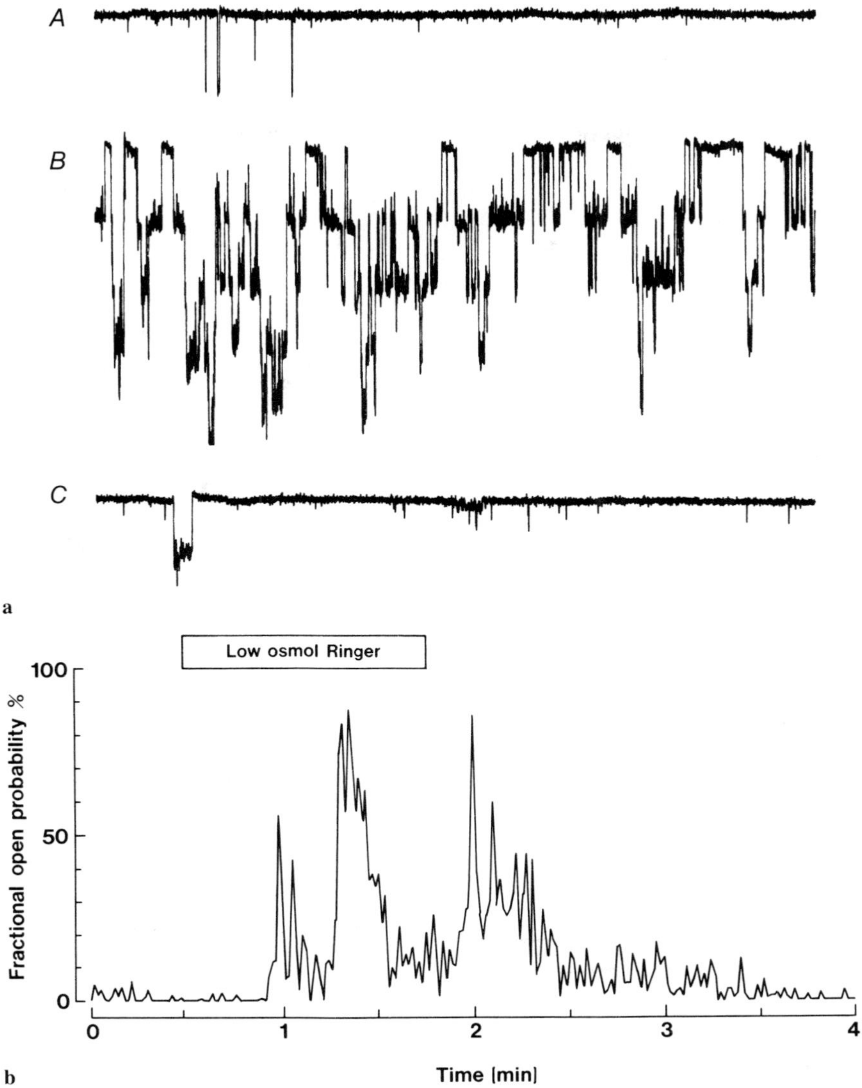

Fig. 6a. Negative pressure activation of K^+ channels in apical cell membrane of an MTAL cell. Tracing from a cell attached patch clamped at 0 mV. *A* was recorded before, *B* during, and *C* following application of −40 cm water of negative pressure. Suction increased the open probability from 0.1 to 89%. **b** Time course of low osmotic pressure activation. Osmolalities of the control and low osmotic Ringer were 293 and 219, respectively. Data were obtained from a cell attached patch at 0 mV. (Reproduced from [12])

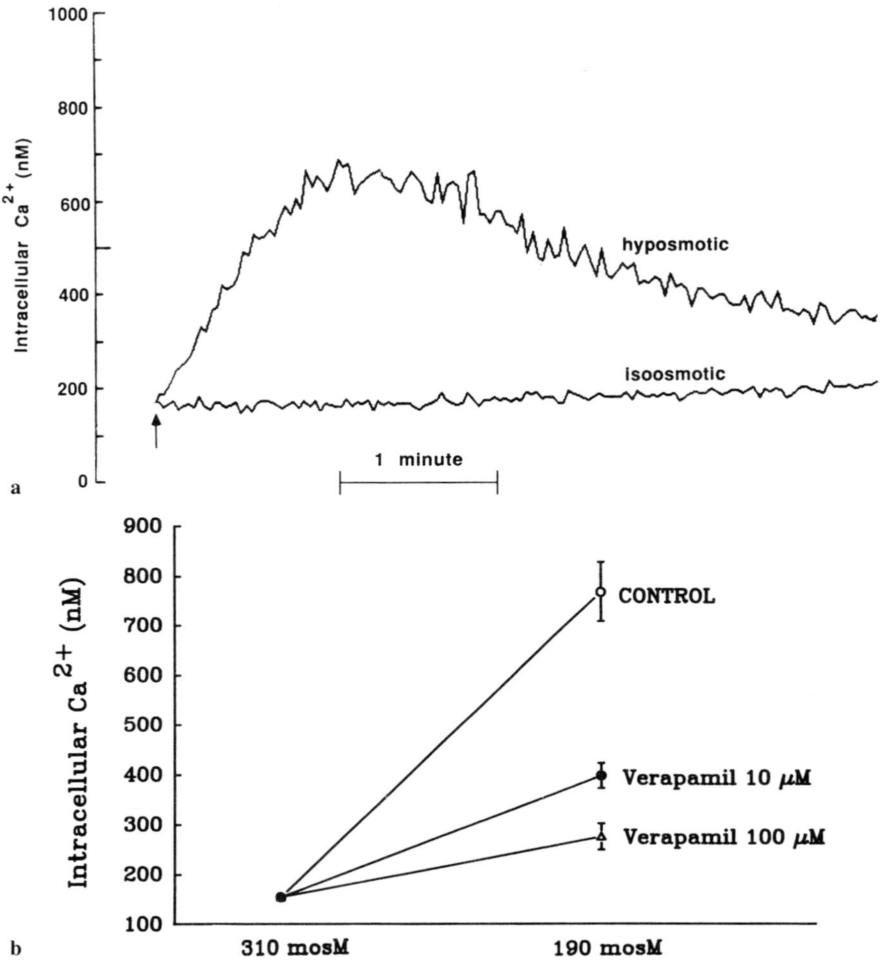

Fig. 7a. Measurements of intracellular Ca^{2+} in hyposmotic and isosmotic solutions. Aliquots of suspended MTAL cells were loaded with Fura-2 and fluorescence measured in an SLM-500C fluorometer. At the *arrow*, cells were exposed to either control isosmotic (315 mosmol/kg H_2O, *lower tracing*) or hyposmotic (180 mosmol/kg H_2O, *upper tracing*) medium. **b** Effect of verapamil on the hyposmotic-induced increase in intracellular Ca^{2+}. Peak increases of intracellular Ca^{2+} concentration in hyposmotic media were measured. The cells were exposed to hyposmotic medium (180 mosmol/kg H_2O) in the presence or the absence of two different concentrations of verapamil. The maximum increase of intracellular Ca^{2+} in these different conditions was measured. (Reproduced from [20])

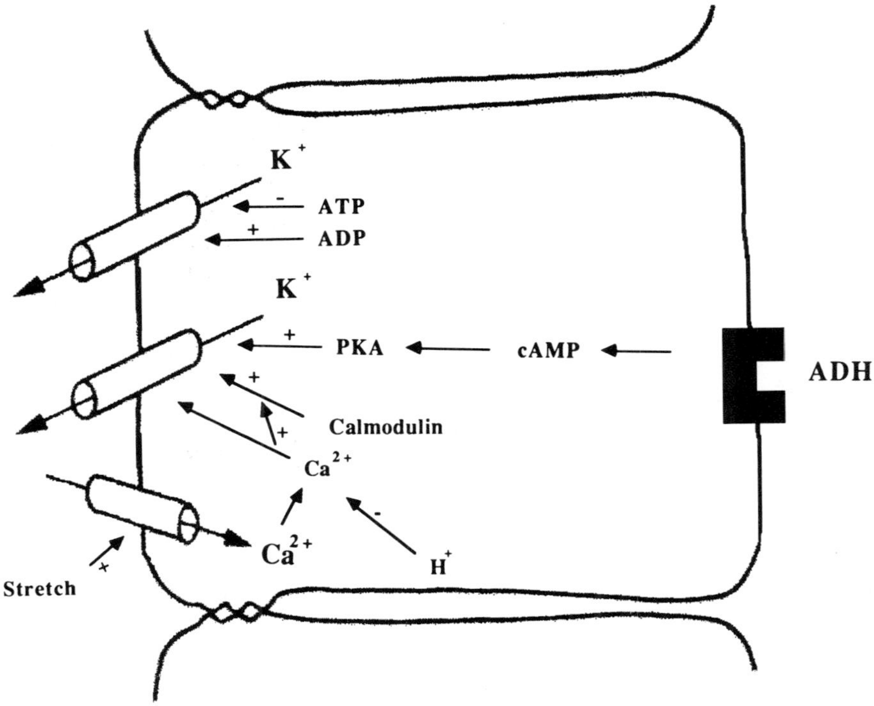

Fig. 8. Model of K+ channel regulation in the thick ascending limb. Three channels are depicted, *from upper to lower*: an ATP sensitive K+ channel; a Ca^{+2}-activated K+ channel; and a Ca^{2+} channel. For convenience the Ca^{2+} channel is located in the apical cell membrane, but direct evidence is not available for the exact location of the verapamil-sensitive Ca^{2+} entry pathway. (Model is a summary of data from [1–12] and [20–25]) ADH, arginine vasopressin

channels may be more complex. For example, in MTAL cells, one limitation of this hypothesis is an apparent discrepancy in the amount of Ca^{2+} released by hypotonicity versus the amount required to activate K^+ channels. Open probability curves for Ca^{2+}-activated K^+ channels in excised patches from MTAL cells show that these channels require 3uM Ca^{2+} to spend about half of the time in the open state (see Fig. 3b). However, exposure of cells to a change in osmolality that is known to stimulate Ca^{2+}-activated K^+ channels in cell attached patches increases intracellular Ca^{2+} to only 400 nM. The channels would be expected to be mostly closed at 400 nM Ca^{2+}. As described below, at least two possible explanations could account for this apparent discrepancy.

First, stimulation of Ca^{+2}-activated K^+ channels in hyposmotic solutions may not be driven directly via an increase in intracellular Ca^{2+}. For example, as mentioned above, Ca^{+2}-activated K^+ channels purified from the apical cell membrane of thick ascending limb are stimulated by calmodulin and protein kinase A (see Fig. 5). It is possible that an increase in intracellular Ca^{2+} in hyposmotic solutions activates calmodulin, which in turn stimulates Ca^{+2}-activated K^+ channels. Alternatively, hyposmotic solutions could cause a phosphorylation of the channel or an associated regulatory protein (perhaps via a Ca^{2+}-dependent kinase) which may cause activation of the channel.

Second, it is possible that the increase in intracellular Ca^{2+} in MTAL cells exposed to hyposmotic solutions is not uniform throughout the cell. The local Ca^{2+} concentration near the plasma membrane could be high enough to activate Ca^{2+}-activated K^+ channels. Recently, a restricted volume in cardiac cells, of only 0.3% of the total volume of the cell, has been hypothesized to exist near the plasma membrane [23]. If such a restricted volume of even 10% exists in intact MTAL cells, then the apparent rise of 400 nM could represent a 4uM increase in a local area near the plasma membrane.

Review

Two classes of K^+ channels have been identified in the apical cell membrane of the thick ascending limb. One class is inwardly rectifying and inhibited by ATP. ATP-sensitive channels have a high open probability in resting thick ascending limb cells and are probably involved in generating the resting apical K^+ conductance. A second class contains the large conductance, maxi K^+ channels. These channels have a very low open probability at resting levels of cell Ca^{2+}, but are stimulated by ADH and by hyposmotic solutions. Ca^{+2}-activated K^+ channels in the TAL are mediated by intracellular Ca^{2+}, pH, calmodulin, and PKA-mediated phosphorylation (Fig. 8). Clearly, K^+ channels in the apical cell membrane are highly regulated, which is important both for net transepithelial NaCl reabsorption and for volume regulation.

Acknowledgments. This work was supported by NIH grant DK 32753. Thanks to Dr. C. Montrose-Rafizadeh and Zeitlin for editorial comments on the manuscript.

References

1. Bleich M, Schlatter E, Greger R (1990) The luminal potassium channel of the thick ascending limb of Henle's loop. Pflugers Arch 415:449–460
2. Greger R, Bleich M, Schlatter E (1990) Ion channels in the thick ascending limb of Henle's loop. Renal Physiol Biochem 13:37–50
3. Wang W, White S, Geibel J, Giebisch G (1990) A potassium channel in the apical membrane of rabbit thick ascending limb of Henle's loop. Am J Physiol 258:F244–F253
4. Cornejo M, Guggino SE, Guggino WB (1989) Calcium-activated potassium channels from cultured renal medullary thick ascending limb cells:effects of pH. J Membr Biol 110:49–55
5. Cornejo M, Guggino SE, Guggino WB (1989) Calcium-activated potassium channels from cultured renal medullary thick ascending limb cells: effects of pH. J Membr Biol 110:49–55
6. Guggino SE, Guggino WB, Green N, Sacktor B (1987) Blocking agents of calcium activated potassium channels in cultured medullary thick ascending limb cells. Am J Physiol 252:C128–C137
7. Guggino SE, Guggino WB, Green W, Sacktor B (1987) Calcium-activated potassium channels in cultured medullary thick ascending limb cells. Am J Physiol 252:C121–C127

8. Guggino SE, Suarez-Isla BA, Guggino WB, Sacktor B (1985) Forskolin and antidiuretic hormone stimulate a calcium-activated potassium channel in cultured kidney cells. Am J Physiol 249:F448–F455
9. Hunter M, Giebisch G (1988) Calcium-activated potassium channels of Amphiuma early distal tubule: inhibition by ATP. Pflugers Arch 412:331–333
10. Hunter M, Kawahara K, Giebisch G (1988) Calcium-activated epithelial potassium channels. Min Electrol Metab 14:48–57
11. Klaerle DA, Jorgensen PL (1988) Role of calcium-activated potassium channel in regulation of NaCl reabsorption in thick ascending limb of Henle's loop. Comp Biochem Physiol [A] 90:757–765
12. Taniguchi T, Guggino WB (1989) Membrane stretch: a physiological stimulator of calcium-activated potassium channels in thick ascending limb. Am J Physiol 257:F347–F352
13. Montrose-Rafizadeh C, Guggino WB (1990) Cell volume regulation in the nephron. Annu Rev Physiol 52:761–72
14. Guggino WB, Oberleithner H, Giebisch G (1988) The amphibian diluting segment. Am J Physiol 254:F615–F627
15. Hebert SC, Andreoli TE (1984) Control of NaCl reabsorption in the thick ascending limb. Am J Physiol 246:F745–F756
16. Handler JS, Orloff J (1981) Antidiuretic hormone. Annu Rev Physiol 43:611–624
17. Hebert SC, Sun A (1988) Hypotonic cell volume regulation in mouse medullary thick ascending limb: effects of ADH. Am J Physiol 255:F962–F969
18. Christensen O (1987) Mediation of cell volume regulation by Ca^{2+} influx through stretch-activated channels. Nature 330:66–68
19. Filipovic D, Sackin H (to be published) Stretch-activated calcium currents in renal proximal tubule. Am J Physiol
20. Montrose-Rafizadeh C, Guggino WB (to be published) Role of potassium and calcium channels in volume regulation by rabbit medullary thick ascending limb vesicles. Am J Physiol
21. Ubl J, Murer H, Kolb H-A (1988) Hypotonic shock evokes opening of Ca^{2+}-activated K channels in opossum kidney cells. Pflugers Arch 412:551–553
22. Hosey MM, Lazdunski M (1988) Calcium channels: molecular pharmacology, structure and regulation. J Membr Biol 104:81–105
23. Lederer WJ, Niggli E, Hadley RW (1990) Sodium-calcium exchange in excitable cells: fuzzy space. Science 248:283
24. Reeves WB, McDonald GA, Mehta P, Andreoli TE (1989) Activation of potassium channels in renal medullary vesicles by cAMP-dependent protein kinase. J Membr Biol 109:65–72
25. Hunter M, Oberleithner H (1988) Whole-cell potassium currents in single early distal tubule cells. Am J Physiol 255:F699–F703

Ion Channels in the Distal Convoluted Tubule in Primary Culture

JEAN MEROT, MICHEL TAUC, MICHEL BIDET, and PHILIPPE POUJEOL[1]

SUMMARY. Cortical distal bright convoluted tubules (DCTb) were microdissected from rabbit kidneys and cultured in a hormonally-defined medium. The cultured cells grew as a monolayer and retained the morphological and biochemical characteristics of the original tubule. The cultured epithelia developed a transepithelial potential of 3.11 ± 0.53 mV that was oriented negatively towards the apical compartment. The apical membrane of the cells exhibited a sodium conductance sensitive to 10^{-6} M amiloride and 10^{-7} M phenamil and a small K^+ conductance which was blocked by 5 mM Ba^{2+}. The basolateral membrane was highly permeable to K^+. Patch clamp analysis conducted on the apical membrane of the cells revealed the presence of three types of ionic channel. The first was a small conductance cation channel (3 pS), sensitive to phenamil, which resembled the Na^+ channel, but the specificity of which seemed to be altered in excised configuration. The second was a non selective cation channel, it did not discriminate between Na^+ and K^+ and had a conductance of 20.5 pS. It was strongly voltage-dependent and required a high calcium concentration (1 mM) to its cytoplasmic face. The last channel was a small conductance highly selective K^+ channel (8 pS). These three channels could account for the macroscopic Na^+ and K^+ conductances found in the apical membrane of rabbit DCTb in primary culture.

Introduction

The study of the physiological properties of distal nephron segments is difficult owing to the presence of different cell types along this structure. In the rabbit, the very early distal tubule (bright part DCTb) contains only one cell type and the transi-

[1]Département de Biologie, Service de Biolgie Cellulaire, Centre d'Etudes Nucléaires de Saclay, 91191 Gif sur Yvette Cedex, France

tion to the following segment is sharp. However, probably due to the difficulties of gaining access to this segment in vivo and of microdissecting it without collagenase, little is known about the ionic channels present in the apical membrane. Cell culture technique provides a potential means of overcoming some of these problems. Thus, to investigate the properties of DCTb, we developed primary cultures of a well-defined nephron segment. The monolayers exhibited a transepithelial voltage, oriented negatively toward the apical membrane, which was inhibited by amiloride, phenamil, and 5 mM Ba^{2+} applied on the apical side. This confirms the results reported in DCTb perfused in vitro [1] and indicates that both Na^+ and K^+ conductances exist in the apical membrane. Patch clamp analysis reveals the existence of several types of channels which could well account for the macroscopic conductance of the apical membrane.

Materials and Methods

Primary Cultures

The primary cell culture technique has been described in detail in previous papers [2–4]. The cortical fragments of early distal convoluted tubule (bright part) of 4–5 week-old New Zealand rabbit kidneys were carefully dissected under sterile conditions. The kidneys were cut into small pyramids which were incubated in a dissection medium containing 0.1 mg/ml collagenase (Cooper, USA). The tubules were seeded in collagen-coated culture wells filled with primary culture medium composed of equal mixtures of Dulbecco's modified Eagle medium (DMEM) and HAM F12 (Gibco) containing 15 mM $NaHCO_3$, 20 mM HEPES (pH 7.5), 2 mM glutamine, 5 μg/ml insulin, 5.10^{-8} M dexamethasone, 10 ng/ml EGF, 5 μg/ml transferrin, 3.10^{-8} M sodium selenite, 10^{-8} M triiodothyronine, 100 U/ml penicillin, and 100 μg/ml streptomycin. Cultures were maintained at 37°C in 5% CO_2 – 95% air water saturated atmosphere. The medium was changed 4 days after seeding and every 2 days thereafter. The antibiotics were definitively removed from the medium after the first rinsing. The culture chamber was custom made. A polycarbonate filter formed the bottom of the cylinder and was coated with rat tail collagen. The surface available for tubular growth was 0.2 cm^2.

Electrophysiological Study

Vt was measured on 15–20-day-old cultures grown on permeable chambers by recording the difference between two calomel electrodes connected to the bathing solution by KCl-saturated Agar bridges (Keitley 601 electrometer). The basal side was grounded. The transepithelial resistance (Rt) was estimated by applying square-current pulses (1.5 μA, 2 sec duration) through Ag-AgCl electrodes and measuring Vt changes with electrodes placed as near as possible to the epithelium surface. Vt was measured with RPMI medium (Gibco) bathing apical and basolateral compartments. Rt measurements were corrected for series resistances measured after removing the cells from the support at the end of the experiment. All the experiments were performed at room temperature.

Patch Clamp Experiments

The single channel recordings were made on the apical membrane of 15–20-day-old cultured cells grown on a permeable support. Patch pipettes were made in two steps from hematocrit capillaries, using a vertical puller, coated with Sylgard 184 and fire polished immediately before using. Pipettes filled with NaCl solution had a resistance of 5–10 MΩ. Seals between 10 and 50 gigaΩ were achieved by applying a slight suction when the pipette was lowered onto the cell. Channel currents were recorded with RK 300 patch clamp amplifier (Biologic, France), stored on digital audio tapes using a DTR 1200 recorder (Biologic, France), and visualized on a digital oscilloscope (Nicolet Instruments, Madison, Wis., USA). For consistency throughout the paper the potential is defined as the potential on the cytoplasmic face of the membrane relative to the pipette. In cell-attached experiments, the intracellular potential that contributes to the actual membrane potential was assumed to be −60 mV. On the recordings given in the Figures, upward deflections represent currents of positive charge moving from the cell interior to the pipette. All experiments were performed at room temperature.

Data Analysis

Channel current amplitudes were measured by replaying the tape onto a digital oscilloscope (Nicolet Instruments, Madison, Wis., USA). The current-voltage (I/V) relations of the channels were constructed from the average amplitude of 10–20 well defined transitions between closed and open current levels at each applied potential.

Solutions

In patch clamp experiments the NaCl solution contained (in mM): 140 NaCl, 5 KCl, 1 $CaCl_2$, 1 $MgCl_2$, 5 glucose, and 10 HEPES, at pH 7.4. The KCl solution contained (in mM): 140 KCl, 5 NaCl, 1 $MgCl_2$, and 10 HEPES, at pH 7.2. The calcium concentration, (10^{-5} or 10^{-3} M), was adjusted by the addition of $CaCl_2$. In Cl^- free solution 140 mM NaCl was replaced by 70 mM Na_2SO_4. In Na^+ free solution 140 mM NaCl was replaced by 140 mM choline chloride.

Calculations

The values are presented as means ± SE. Student's t test was employed to determine statistical significances of differences.

Results

Electrophysiological Studies

The cultures growing on permeable chambers reached the edges of the culture wells (0.63 cm^2) 15–20 days after seeding. They had a transepithelial potential that was oriented negatively towards the apical surface of the monolayer (Vt = −3.11 ± 0.53 mV, n=9). The apical and basolateral ionic membrane conductances of the cells were assessed by examining the effects of different ionic channel blockers and solutions on Vt. When applied on the apical side of the monolayer the diuretic amiloride (10^{-6} M) induced, within 1 second, a sharp depolarization (Vt = -0.43 ± 0.08 mV, $n=9$). Vt returned to its control value when amiloride was rinsed out. Phenamil (10^{-7} M), a specific epithelial sodium channel blocker, inhibited the Vt (-0.22 ± 0.11 mV, $n=8$) when applied on the apical side of the culture. As for amiloride, the effect was completely reversible. Addition of both drugs on the basolateral side of the cultured DCTb remained without significant effect on Vt. On the apical membrane, the application of 5 mM Ba^{2+} hyperpolarized the Vt (Vt = -6.9 ± 2.3 mV, $n=7$), whereas 10 mM tetraethylammonium (TEA) did not modify Vt. At the basolateral face of the monolayer, KCl solution or 1 mM Ba^{2+} induced a strong depolarization of Vt.

Patch Clamp Experiments

Gigaseals were obtained in 50% of the trials. In the cell attached mode only 10% of the patches contained channel activity. At least three different channels were characterized during the experimental series.

Poorly Selective Na^+ Channel

Cell Attached Configuration

The predominant ion channel recorded in the cell attached mode had a low conductance and a slow open kinetic. An example of this, when pipette and bath contained the NaCl solution, is given in Fig. la. At resting membrane potential (Vm = -60 mV or Vp = 0) channel currents were directed from the pipette to the cell interior. The current amplitude was small (0.15 pA) and increased when the membrane potential was hyperpolarized from -80 to -120 mV. The current voltage relation for these experiments is shown in Fig. 1b. For membrane potentials between -140 and -40 mV, the relation was linear and the mean channel conductance was 3.0 ± 0.1 pS, ($n=5$). Due to the very low current flowing through the channel, it was impossible to detect a significant activity above -40 mV. Moreover, at high positive membrane potential, channel openings were never recorded. Similar data were obtained when the NaCl solution in the pipette was replaced by Na_2SO_4 solution (Fig. 1b). In a series of experiments we perfused both sides of the culture while the patch was in the cell-attached configuration with the tetramethylammonium (TMA)Cl solution, keeping the NaCl solution in the pipette. This maneuver induced, in some cases, an increase of channel activity. Figure 2b is an example of single channel records showing the appearance of inward current events after 3 minutes TMACl exposure. Histograms of currents amplitude shown in Fig. 2b demonstrate the increase in the channel openings at resting membrane potential (Vm = -60 mV, Vp = 0 mV). In this typical experiment the open probability increased from 0.03 to 0.6. From the I/V relationship after exposure to TMACl, the mean conductance was 6.70 ± 1.7 pS ($n=3$).

Excised Patch Configuration

In order to investigate the ionic selectivity of the channel, experiments were performed on excised patches. Inside-out patches were made from cell attached configurations. At first, the patch was studied with NaCl solution in the pipette and in the

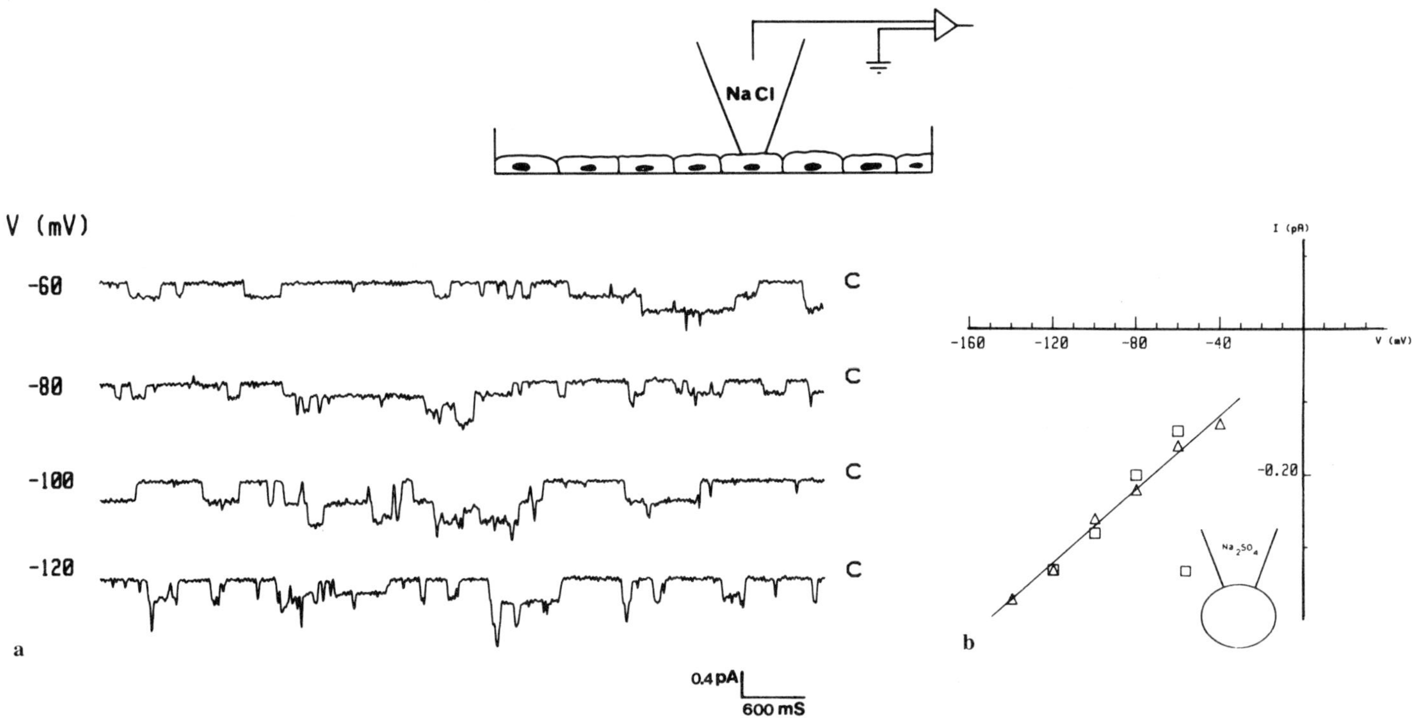

Fig. 1a. Single channel current recordings in a cell-attached patch. Channel openings are *downward*. The pipette and the bath contained NaCl solution. The membrane holding potentials are indicated on the *left of each recording*. *C* on the *right* of the *recordings* indicates the closed state of the channel. **b** current-voltage (I/V) relationships of the channel in the cell-attached condition ($n=5$). The pipette and the bath contained the same solution as in **a** (Δ) or contained 70 mM Na_2SO_4 (□)

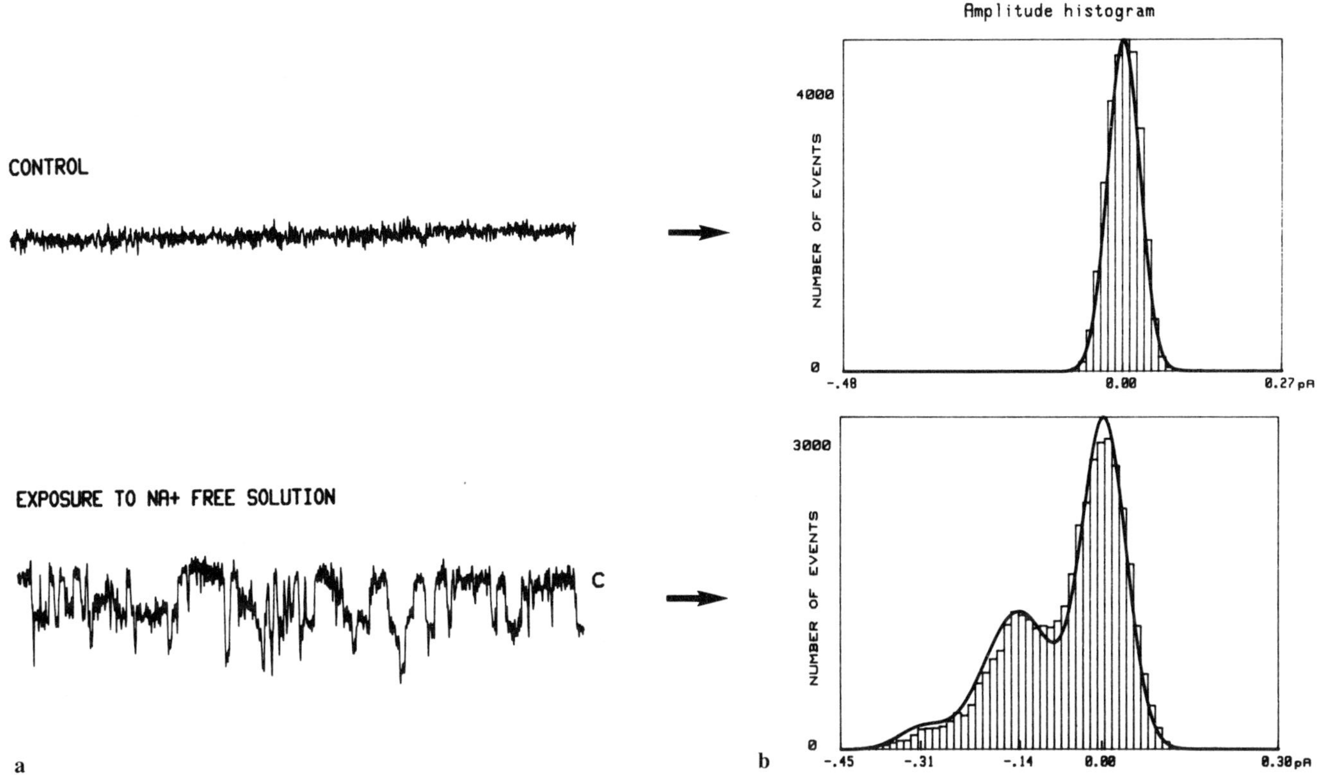

Fig. 2a,b. Effect of external sodium removal on the activity of poorly selective sodium channel, recorded in cell attached configuration. **a** The membrane potential was −60 mV (Vp = 0 mV) and the channel openings were *downward deflections*. **b** Current amplitude histograms plot channel events frequency versus amplitude (*pA*). Control histogram (*upper*) with the sodium solution in the bath shows that the channel was in closed state (0 pA). After replacing the tetramethylammonium sodium bath by $(TMA)^+$, channel activity appeared in the patch membrane (*lower*)

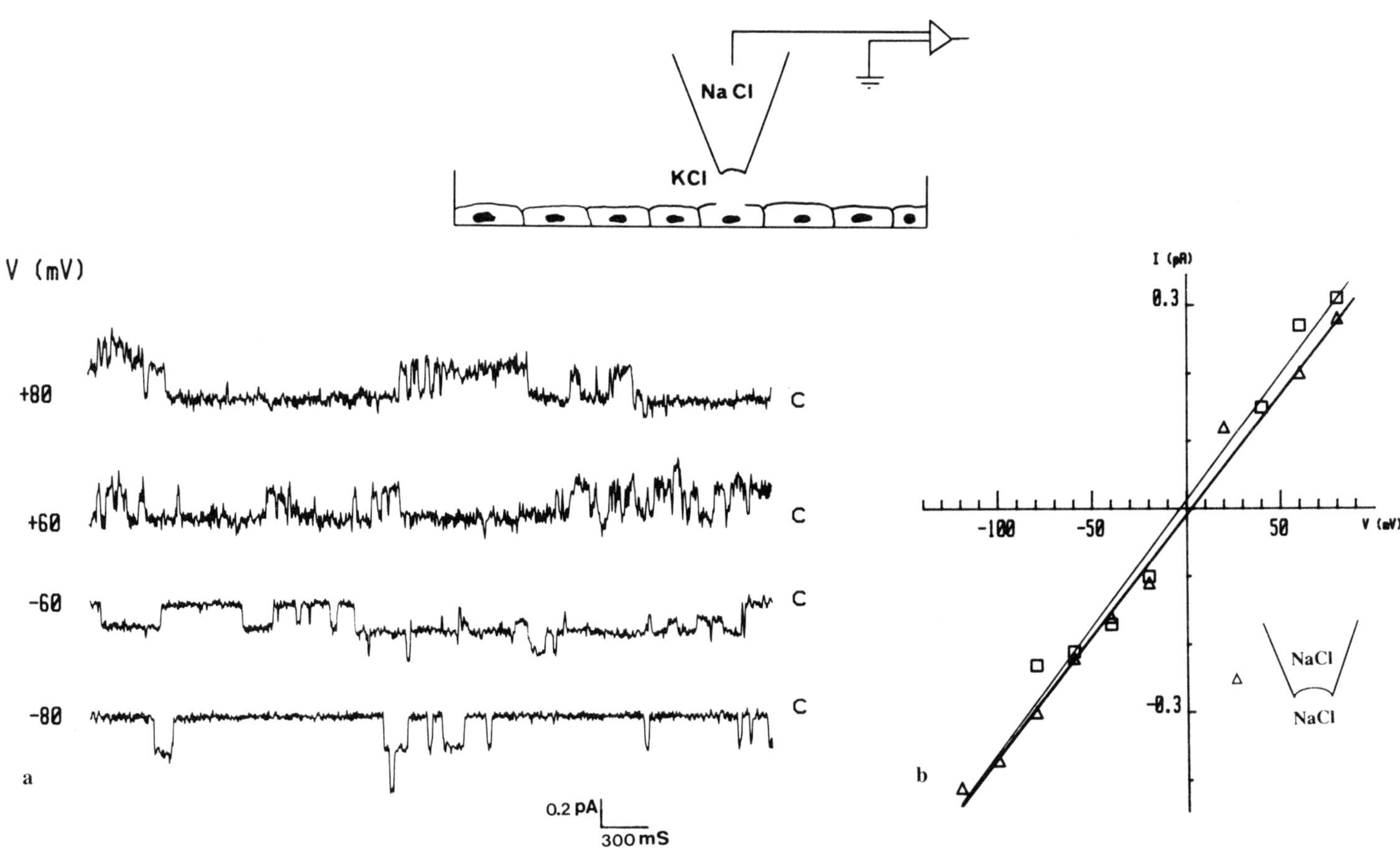

Fig. 3a. Single channel current recordings of the poorly selective sodium channel in an inside-out patch. The pipette contained NaCl soludion and the bath contained KCl solution. Membrane holding potentials are given on the *left* of the recordings. *C* indicates the closed state of the channel. **b** current-voltage (I/V) relationships of the channel in the excised patch. The pipette and the bath contained NaCl solution (Δ, n=5). The bath solution was replaced by KCl solution (□, n=5)

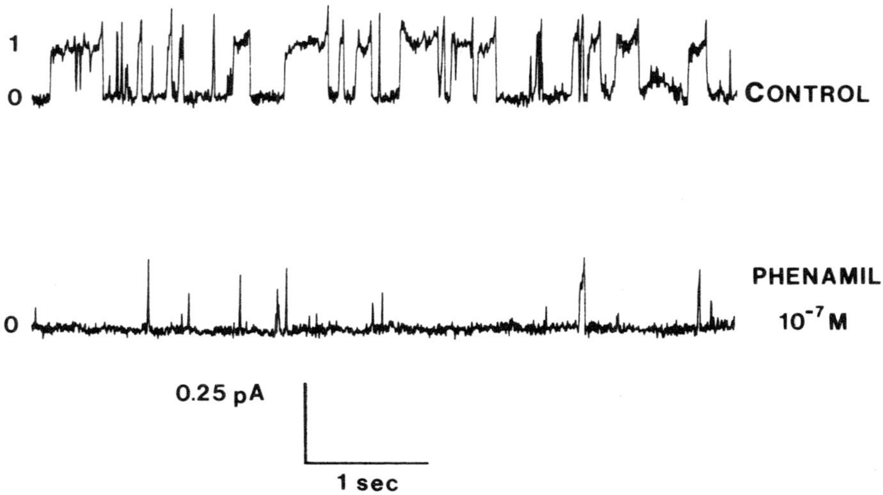

Fig. 4. Effect of 10^{-7} M phenamil applied on the cytosolic side of an inside-out excised patch. The membrane holding potential was +80 mV. The pipette contained NaCl solution and the bath contained KCl solution. The recordings represented three different experiments

bath and the I/V curves were constructed, then the cytoplasmic NaCl solution was replaced by KCl solution. Figure 3a illustrates the single channel currents recorded in KCl solution. At −60 and −80 mV holding potentials, the channel openings were downward deflections. Positive membrane potentials increased the noise of the recording and often broke the seal. The channel openings were upward directed and the current amplitude was near that measured at negative potentials. The I/V relationship was linear with a 0 mV reversal potential, and the channel conductance was 3.8 ± 0.2 pS (n=5). These values were not significantly different from those obtained when the bath contained the NaCl solution (Fig. 3b). The data indicate a low selectivity for Na^+ over K^+ ions.

The effect of phenamil on channel activity was tested from the cytosolic side of the inside-out patches (Fig. 4). Addition of 10^{-7} M phenamil almost completely inhibited the channel openings.

Non Selective Cationic Channel

Another type of ionic channel was observed in excised inside-out patches, although no channel activity was recorded in the cell attached condition. Typical channel current recordings are presented in Fig. 5a, where the pipette contained the NaCl solution and the bath the KCl solution. The channel openings are upward at negative holding membrane potentials (−40, −80 mV), and downward at positive potentials. The I/V relationship of the channel in these experiments was linear (Fig. 5b) and a channel conductance of 22.9 ± 1.2 pS (n=5) was calculated from the slope of the straight line. The current reversal potential was not different from 0 mV. Since the equilibrium potentials for Na^+, K^+, and Cl^- were +84, −84, and 0 mV respectively,

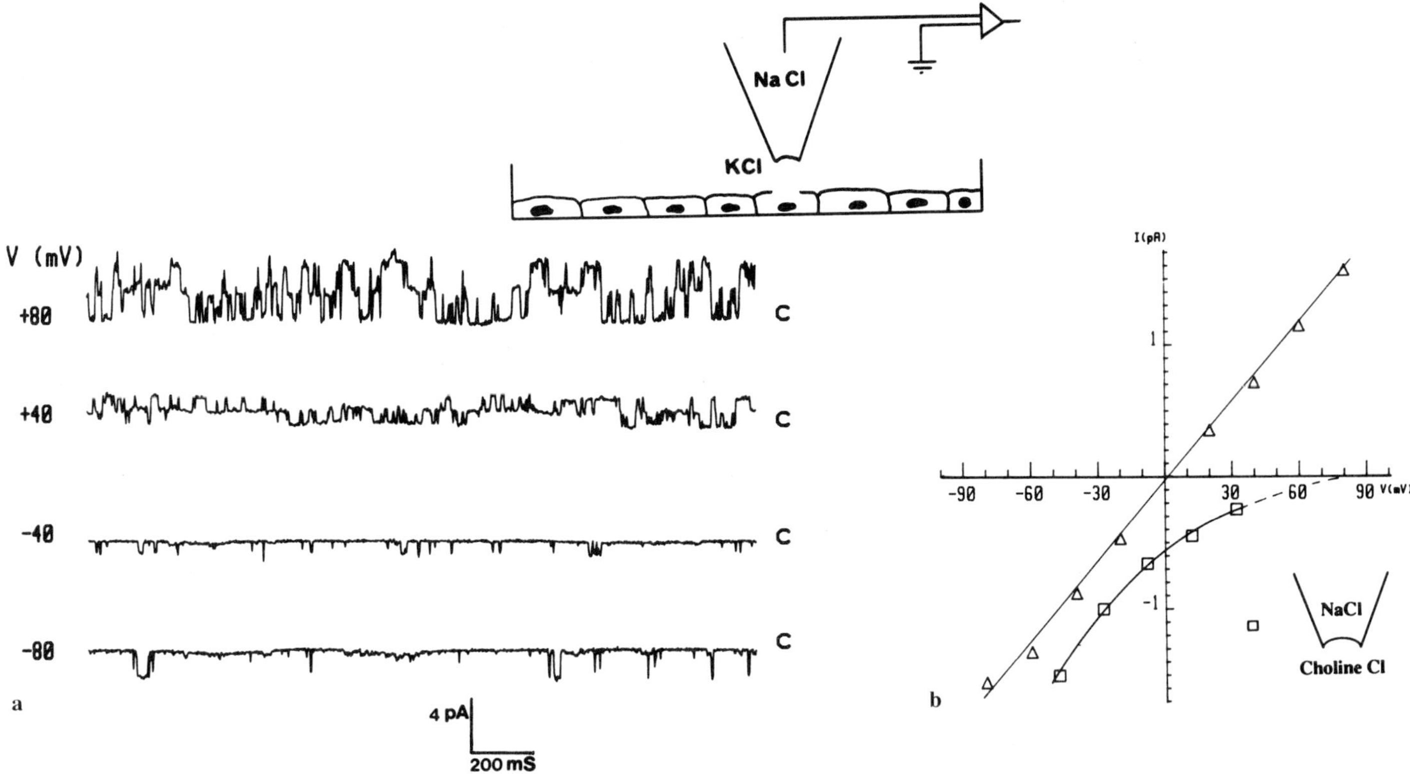

Fig. 5.a. Single channel current recordings of the non-selective cationic channel in an excised inside-out patch. The pipette contained NaCl solution and the bath contained KCl solution. The different membrane holding potentials are indicated on the *left* of each recording. *C* indicates the closed state of the channel. **b** current-voltage (I/V) relationships of the channel in different conditions. (Δ) corresponds to experiments in which pipette and bath contained the same solutions as in **a** (□) represents experiments in which the bath contained a choline chloride solution

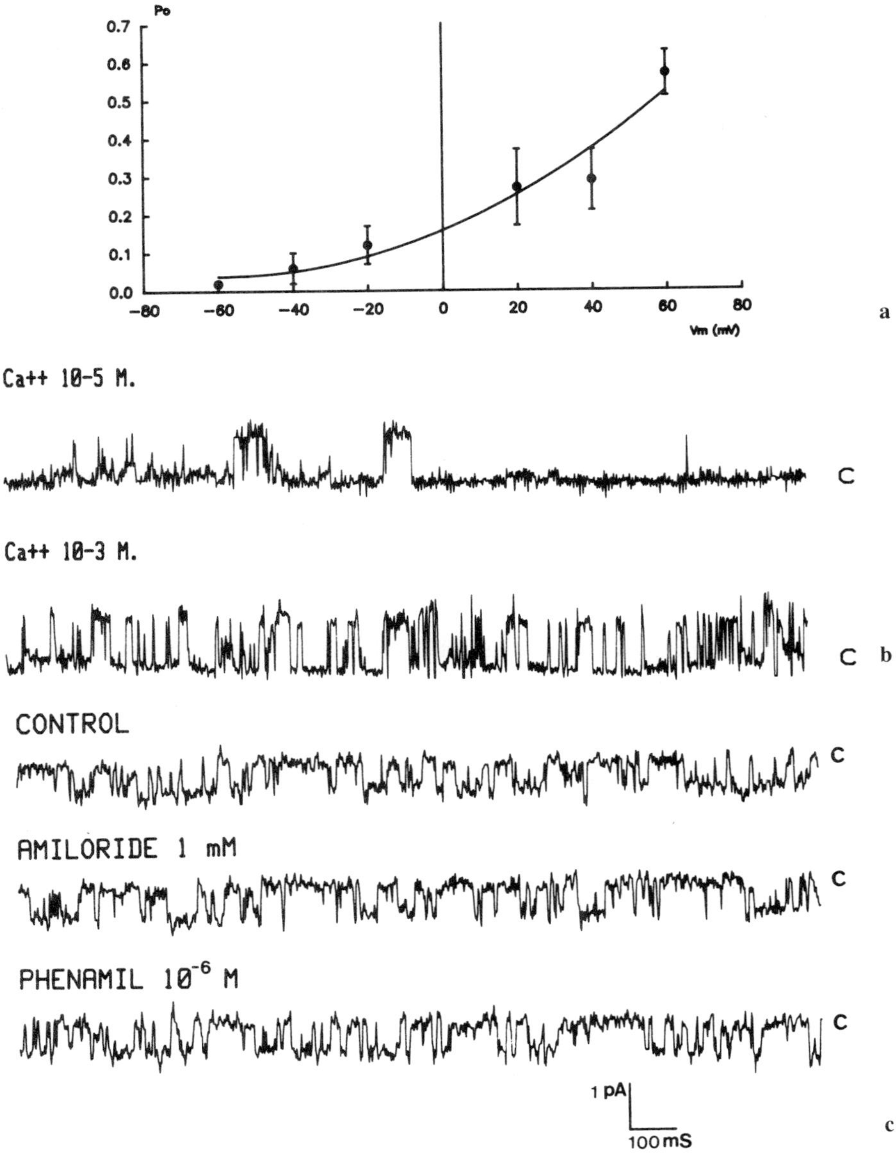

Fig. 6.a. Open probability of the non-selective cationic channel versus membrane holding potentials. The data were fitted according to exponential function. **b** Effect of cytosolic calcium concentration on non-selective cationic channel activity. The pipette contained NaCl solution and the bath contained KCl solution with two different Ca^{2+} concentrations. The membrane holding potential was +60 mV and the channel openings were *upward* deflections. **c** Effects of amiloride and phenamil on non-selective cationic channel recorded on an inside-out excised patch. The pipette contained NaCl solution and the bath contained KCl solution. The membrane holding potential was −60 mV and the channel openings were *downward* deflections. *C* indicates the closed state of the channel

the channel must either not have discriminated between Na^+ and K^+ or must have been Cl^- selective. To investigate these possibilities, the KCl in the bath was replaced by 140 mM Na gluconate. Because this maneuver did not significantly modify the reversal potential (data not given) we concluded that the channel was cationic and did not discriminate between Na^+ and K^+. In contrast, replacement of bath NaCl solution by choline chloride modified the I/V relationship, since a Goldman type rectification for Na^+ ions was observed. In this condition, the maximal channel conductance was 22.4 pS and the reversal potential obtained by extrapolation of the I/V curve was 80 mV.

The channel activity was clearly voltage-dependent. As illustrated in Fig. 6a, the opening probability was an exponential function of the membrane potential. Another characteristic of the channel is the high calcium concentration needed on the cytoplasmic side for its activation. Figure 6b illustrates an experiment in which a patch was excised in a KCl solution containing 10 μM calcium. Only one channel of low activity was observed: increasing the calcium concentration to 1 mM enhanced the channel activity. To test whether the non selective cation channels might correspond to the poorly selective Na^+ channel described above, we applied high amiloride concentration or 10^{-7} M phenamil on the cytoplasmic face of an inside-out excised patch. Neither drugs inhibited the channel (Fig. 6c).

K^+ Channels

In excised patch experiments, we recorded a K^+ channel, although no activity was found in the cell attached configuration. Figure 7a shows the single channel currents when the pipette contained the NaCl solution and the bath contained KCl solution. At 0 mV holding potential, the channel openings were upwardly directed and might have corresponded to K^+ currents, since Na^+ currents would have produced downward deflections and Cl^- was at the electrochemical equilibrium. The I/V relationship was linear (Fig. 7b) and the extrapolated reversal potential was -76 ± 9 mV ($n=3$) (Fig. 7b), indicating a high selectivity for K^+ over Na^+ ions (pK/pNa = 65). Figure 7c shows that the addition of 1 mM barium to the cytosolic side of the patch completely blocked the channel activity recorded at 0 mV.

Discussion

In an attempt to further understand the function of DCTb, we undertook primary cultures of microdissected nephron segments. Most of the morphological, biochemical and antigenic properties of DCTb in primary culture have been described in detail in a previous paper [4]. Monitoring the transepithelial voltage and resistance showed that Vt was inhibited by the diuretic drug amiloride at low concentration. This effect was rapid and completely reversible. It indicates the existence of a Na^+ channel in the apical membrane of DCTb in culture [5], a hypothesis confirmed by experiments using phenamil. Phenamil is a derivative of amiloride, which is the most potent known inhibitor of the epithelial Na^+ channel [6,7]. With regard to the K^+ movements, barium applied apically hyperpolarized the Vt, showing a small K^+ conductance at this level. In contrast, barium applied to the basolateral side of the monolayer strongly depolarized the Vt, as did KCl perfusion. Thus our data are quite in agree-

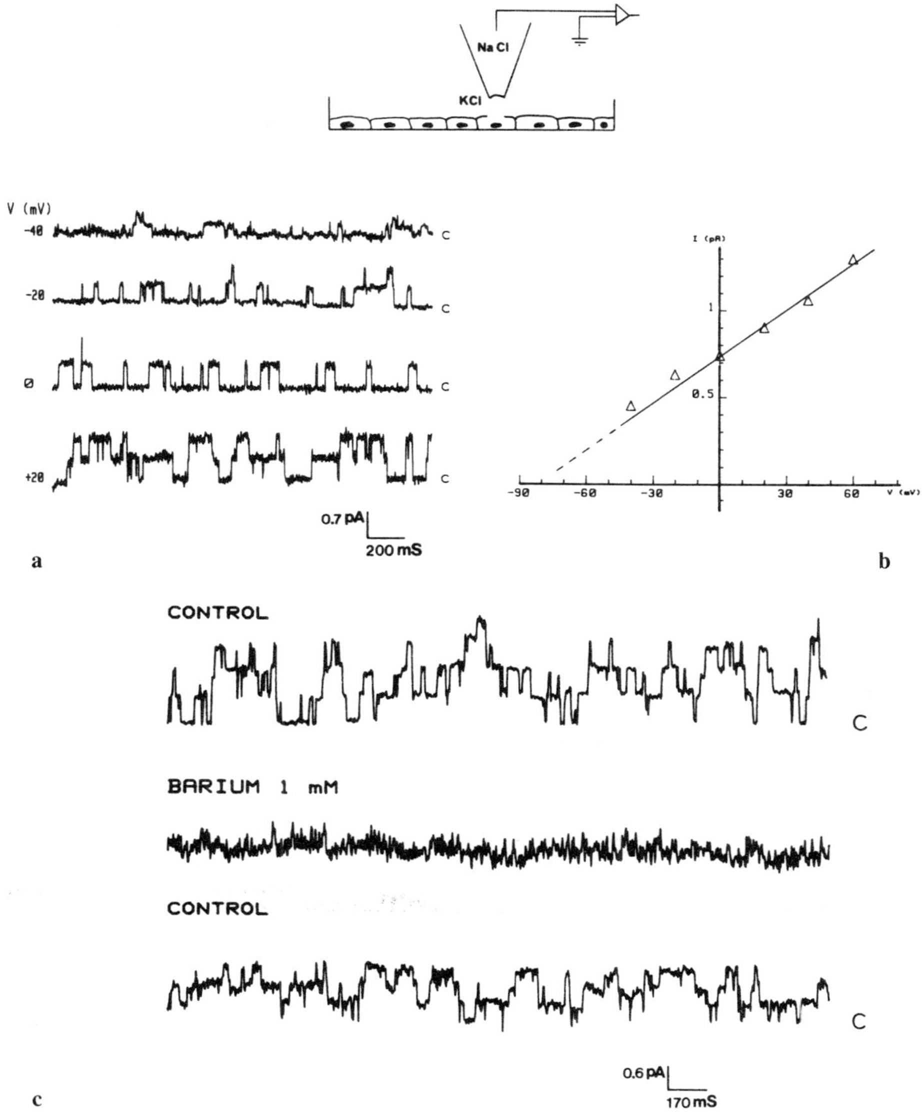

Fig. 7.a. Single K^+ channel currents recorded in an inside-out excised patch. The pipette contained NaCl solution and the bath contained KCl solution. Membrane holding potentials are given on the *left* of the *recordings*. *C* indicates the closed state of the channel. **b** current-voltage (I/V) relationship of the channel in excised patches ($n=3$). The pipette and the bath contained the same solution as in **a**. **c** Effect of barium on K^+ channel currents recorded in an inside-out patch. The pipette contained NaCl solution and the bath contained KCl solution with or without 1 mM barium. The membrane holding potential was 0 mV and the channel openings were *upward* deflections

ment with those reported by Yoshitomi et al. [8] on in vitro microperfused rabbit DCT. Single channel analysis performed on the apical membrane revealed the existence of various ionic channels, one of which was recorded in the cell attached configuration. It was a small conductance channel (3 pS) and the data lead us to conclude that in this configuration the current was probably carried by Na^+ ions. However, when the patches were excised from the membrane, the channel also allowed K^+ to pass. The gating properties (data not shown) and the conductance of this channel were not modified by the excision process. Moreover, phenamil (10^{-7} M) completely inhibited the channel openings, although the current flowing through the channel was K^+ current (Fig. 4). According to Palmer and Frindt [9], in the rat collecting duct, Na^+ channels have a low conductance but have a very high Na^+ selectivity. However, conditions could exist where this selectivity may be impaired. Thus, it appears that the ionic selectivity of Na^+ channels could depend on the culture conditions [10] and/or on the lipidic environment of the channel itself [11]. Moreover, a process of degradation by proteolytic enzymes could also explain the loss of selectivity of some Na^+ channels [12]. In cell attached experiments we have observed that the replacement of external Na^+ by TMA induced the appearance of channel activity. For the moment we have no further indication regarding the ionic selectivity of this channel. However, in the light of experiments performed by Ling and Eaton [131], this channel could correspond to a Na^+ channel which was masked by the Na^+ self-inhibition phenomenon. In addition to this channel species, the apical membrane contained another channel which did not discriminate between Na^+ and K^+. Its gating behavior, conductance, and low Ca^{2+} sensitivity were very similar to those reported for the Ca^{2+} sensitive cation channel in various tissues [3,14,15]. In the cultured DCTb we, unfortunately, never demonstrated the channel in the cell-attached configuration. Paulais et al. [16] have recently shown that a Ca^{2+} activated non specific cation channel is present in the basolateral membrane of the mouse cortical thick ascending limb (cTAL). Moreover, another type of non selective cation channel was recorded in the basolateral membrane of the rabbit proximal tubule [17], so the channel could exist in the intact structure. We have already found a non selective cation channel in the apical membrane of each of the nephron segments that we have cultured, i.e., proximal convoluted tubule [3], cortical thin ascending limb [18], and cortical collecting tubule [19]. As in the present study, this channel was never sensitive to amiloride or phenamil. Light et al. [20], on the other hand, observed an amiloride sensitive non specific cation channel in the apical membrane of inner medullary collecting duct in primary culture. Thus the question arises whether there are several kinds of non-specific cation epithelial channels. In the excised configuration we also found a low conductance high selective K^+ channel, which showed some analogies with that described in the apical membrane of rabbit [21] and rat [22] cortical collecting tubule.

In conclusion, the present study demonstrates that the electrophysiological properties of DCTb can profitably be investigated in primary culture. The action of amiloride and phenamil in depolarizing the Vt indicates the presence of a Na^+ conductance in the apical membrane of DCTb in culture. By using the patch clamp technique we identified a channel which could account for the Na^+ conductance, although we were not able to establish its selectivity with certainty. We also recorded a non selective cation channel, the exact role of which remains to be determined. Nevertheless, since we have shown that 10^{-6} M amiloride blocked 85% of the Vt, it is possible that the remaining 13% would be due to sodium transport via the non-selective channel which is insensitive to amiloride. On the other hand, the low conductance K^+ channel that we have demonstrated in the apical membrane could mediate K^+ secretion in DCTb. Such a secretion has now been demonstrated by Shimizu et al. in microperfused DCTb [1].

References

1. Shimizu T, Yoshitomi K, Taniguchi J, Imai M (1989) Effect of high NaCl intake on Na^+ and K^+ transport in the rabbit distal convoluted tubule. Pflugers Arch 414:500–508
2. Tauc M, Merot J, Bidet M, Koechlin N, Gastineau M, Othmani L, Poujeol P (1989) Antigenic expression of aminopeptidase M, dipeptidyl-peptidase IV and endopeptidase by primary cultures from rabbit kidney proximal tubule. Histochemistry 91:17–30
3. Merot J, Bidet M, Gachot B, Le Maout S, Tauc M, Poujeol P (1988) Patch clamp study on primary culture of isolated proximal convoluted tubules. Pflugers Arch 413:51–61
4. Merot J, Bidet M, Gachot B, Le Maout S, Koechlin N, Tauc M, Poujeol P (1989) Electrical properties of rabbit early distal convoluted tubule in primary culture. Am J Physiol 257:F288–F299
5. Garty H, Benos DJ (1988) Characteristics and regulatory mechanisms of the amiloride-blockable Na^+ channel. Physiol Rev 68:309–373
6. Barbry P, Frelin C, Vigne P, Cragoe ED, Lazdunski M (1988) ^{3}[H]Phenamil, a radiolabelled diuretic for the analysis of amiloride-sensitive Na^+ channels in kidney membranes. Biochem Biophys Res Commun 135:25–32
7. Garvin JL, Simon SA, Cragoe EJ, Mandel LJ (1985) Phenamyl: an irreversible inhibitor of sodium channels in the toad urinary bladder. J Membr Biol 87:45–54
8. Yoshitomi K, Shimizu T, Taniguchi J, Imai M (1989) Electrophysiological characterization of rabbit distal convoluted tubule cell. Pflugers Arch 414:457–463
9. Palmer LG, Frindt G (1986) Amiloride sensitive Na channels from the apical membrane of the rat collecting tubule. Proc Natl Acad Sci USA 83:2767–2770
10. Hamilton KL, Eaton DC (1986) Regulation of single sodium channels in renal tissue: a role in sodium homeostasis. Fed Proc 45(12):2713–2717
11. Sariban-Sohraby S, Latorre R, Burg M, Olans L, Benos D (1984) Amiloride-sensitive Na channels reconstructed into planar lipid bilayer membranes. Nature 308:80–82
12. Kolb HA, Brown CDA, Murer H (1986) Characterization of a Ca-dependent maxi K channel in the apical membrane of a cultured renal epithelium (JTC-12 P3). J Membr Biol 92:207–215
13. Ling BN, Eaton DC (1989) Effects of luminal Na^+ on single Na^+ channels in A6 cells, a regulatory role for protein kinase C. Am J Physiol 256:F1094–F1103
14. Fichtner H, Frobe U, Busse R, Kolhardt M (1987) Single non selective cation channels and Ca^{2+}-activated K^+ channels in aortic endothelial cells. J Membr Biol 98:125–133
15. Yellen G (1982) Single Ca^{2+}-activated nonselective cation channels in neuroblastoma. Nature 296:357–359
16. Paulais M, Teulon J (1989) A cation channel in the thick ascending limb of Henle's loop of the mouse kidney: inhibition by adenine neucleotides. J Physiol 413:315–327
17. Gögelein H, Greger R (1986) A voltage dependent ionic channel in the basolateral membrane of late proximal tubules of the rabbit kidney. Pflugers Arch 407:S142–S148
18. Merot J, Bidet M, Gachot B, Tauc M, Poujeol P (1988) Patch clamp characterization of K^+ and non selective channels in the apical membrane of rabbit early distal convoluted tubule in primary culture. Act Physiol Pharmacol Bulg 14:102(A)
19. Merot J, Bidet M, Tauc M, Poujeol P (1987) Etude des canaux ioniques dans des cultures primaires de différents segments de néphron de lapin. J Physiol (Paris) 82(3):63(A)

20. Light DB, McCann FV, Keller TM, Stanton BA (1988) Amiloride-sensitive cation channel in apical membrane of inner medullary collecting duct. Am J Physiol 255:F278–F286
21. Koeppen BM, Beyenbach KW, Helman SI (1984) Single channel currents in renal tubules. Am J Physiol 247:F380–F384
22. Frindt G, Palmer LG (1989) Low-conductance K channels in apical membrane of rat cortical collecting tubule. Am J Physiol 256:F143–F151

Index

B

D

F

H

I

M

O

T

Nephrology

This congress has been executed with the grant of the Commemorative Association for the Japan World Exposition.

Nephrology VOLUME I

PROCEEDINGS OF THE
XIth INTERNATIONAL CONGRESS OF NEPHROLOGY

Editor
Michinobu Hatano

Associate Editors
Nishio Honda · Hyoe Ishikawa · Kenkichi Koiso
Kiyoshi Kurokawa · Tadao Niijima
Nobuhiro Sugino · Susumu Takahashi

With 253 Figures

Springer-Verlag
Tokyo Berlin Heidelberg
New York London Paris
Hong Kong Barcelona

Editor

MICHINOBU HATANO, M.D., Professor of Medicine, Director, Department of Internal Medicine, Nihon University School of Medicine, Tokyo, Japan

Associate Editors

NISHIO HONDA, Tokyo Senbai Hospital, Tokyo
HYOE ISHIKAWA, Nara Medical University, Nara
KENKICHI KOISO, The University of Tsukuba, Ibaraki
KIYOSHI KUROKAWA, University of Tokyo, Tokyo
TADAO NIIJIMA, Tokyo Seamen's Medical College, Tokyo
NOBUHIRO SUGINO, Tokyo Women's Medical College, Tokyo
SUSUMU TAKAHASHI, Nihon University, Tokyo

ISBN 4-413-70074-9 Springer-Verlag Tokyo Berlin Heidelberg New York
ISBN 3-540-70074-9 Springer-Verlag Berlin Heidelberg New York Tokyo
ISBN 0-387-70074-9 Springer-Verlag New York Berlin Heidelberg Tokyo

Library of Congress Cataloging-in-Publication Data
International Congress on Nephrology (11th: 1990: Tokyo, Japan); Nephrology: proceedings of the XIth International Congress of Nephrology/editors, Michinobu Hatano: associate editors, Nishio Honda...[et al.]. p. cm. Congress held in Tokyo, Japan, July 15-20, 1990. Includes bibliographical references. Includes index. ISBN 4-431-70074-9. – ISBN 3-540-70074-9. – ISBN 0-387-70074-9. 1. Kidneys – Diseases – Congresses. 2. Nephrology – Congresses. 3. Kidney Diseases – congresses. 4. Nephrology – congresses. I. Hatano, Michinobu, 1926- . II. Honda, Nishio. III. Title. [DNLM: WJ 300 I59n 1990]. RC902.A2I56 1990. 616.6'1 –dc20. DNLM/DLC. for Library of Congress 91-4651

Typesetting: Publishers Service of Montana, Bozeman, Montana
Printing and binding: Sanbi Printing, Tokyo

Foreword

The proceedings of the XIth International Congress of Nephrology held in Tokyo in 1990, form the most international and complete document of the present state of basic and clinical science in nephrology. In addition, they document the progress made in this field during the 3 years since the London Congress. The result is nothing short of impressive. The material presented by the invited lecturers and the participants of the symposia all show a remarkable pattern; not only the "height" of the science, but also the depth of the specialized knowledge, both prerequisites of excellency in science, which do not necessarily imply narrowness of outlook. On the contrary, this written document of the Tokyo Congress is a witness to the enormous progress made over the last few years in communication between basic scientists and clinical scientists.

The International Society of Nephrology is a fine example of how fruitful and productive this interaction can be, if it is conducted with the desire to understand each other. The members of the Scientific Program Committee of the Tokyo Congress are to be congratulated, not only for a thoughtful and well designed program, but also for carefully selecting those speakers who, besides their own contribution to nephrological science, also have the talent of being able to communicate with a large, international audience. In particular, I would like to express my deep appreciation to the editors of the Proceedings for their commitment and industriousness which made it possible for this publication to appear so soon after the Congress.

Since the first Congress of the International Society of Nephrology in Evian in 1960, nephrologists have witnessed a phenomenal increase in knowledge, a progress which still continues and will do so in the future. The present proceedings are a snapshot of this process. The counterpoint to the intellectual challenge of acquiring deeper understanding is the duty and promise to utilize that understanding for the benefit of our patients.

KLAUS THURAU, M.D.
President,
International Society of Nephrology
(1987–1990)

Preface

The XIth International Congress of Nephrology was held in Tokyo, Japan from July 15–20, 1990.

Since the first congress in Evian, France in 1960, this is the first time that this prestigious congress has been held in Asia. Therefore, enthusiastic expectations were held by nephrologists not only in Japan but also throughout the world.

In organizing the congress under the estimable guidance of Prof. Klaus Thurau, President of the International Society of Nephrology, the ISN Executive Committee and the International Advisory Committee, Prof. Michinobu Hatano, Chairman of the local organizing committee as well as the organizing committee made every effort to make the congress a success.

Over three thousand participants from 71 countries attended the congress. These included 1,470 participants from Japan, 472 from the United States, 150 from France, and 128 from Italy. We were particularly pleased to welcome eight representatives from Czechoslavakia as well as an increased participation from other eastern European countries, the Soviet Union, and China. Forty-nine delegates from Taiwan were also in attendance.

The opening ceremony was held at the New Takanawa Prince Hotel in the presence of the Crown Prince, whose address noted that progress in nephrology would contribute greatly to the welfare of patients worldwide.

The scientific program consisted of 15 state-of-the-art lectures, 36 symposia, 11 workshops, 256 oral and 1,778 poster presentations. Following the advice of the ISN Executive Committee, the Scientific Program Committee encouraged the presentation of clinical and research papers at the same time in each session. This ensured that throughout the scientific program, discussions were constructive, and this helped to make the congress both stimulating and fruitful.

A total of 12 ISN satellite symposia, 4 overseas and 8 in Japan, were also held. The specific topics discussed at each symposium, combined with sightseeing tours at each site, contributed greatly to exchanges of both friendship and information.

Finally, we would like to express our sincere thanks and appreciation to the ISN Committee and all the participants of the congress.

Kenzo Oshima, M.D.
President

Yawara Yoshitoshi, M.D.
Vice-President

Yasushi Ueda, M.D.
Vice-President

Hiroshi Abe, M.D.
Vice-President

XIth International Congress of Nephrology

Organized by:	The Organizing Committee of the XIth International Congress of Nephrology
Under the Auspices of:	International Society of Nephrology
Sponsored by:	Japanese Society of Nephrology The Kidney Foundation, Japan
In Cooperation with:	The Japanese Association of Medical Science Japan Medical Association The Japanese Urological Association The Japan Society for Transplantation Japanese Society for Artificial Organs Japanese Society for Dialysis Therapy The Japanese Society of Pediatric Nephrology Japan Incorporated Medical Association for Dialysis
Supported by:	Ministry of Education, Science and Culture Ministry of Health and Welfare Science Council of Japan Tokyo Metropolitan Government

The International Society of Nephrology

Executive Committee 1987–1990

Klaus Thurau	FRG	President
Donald W. Seldin	USA	Past President
Roscoe R. Robinson	USA	President Elect
John Stewart Cameron	UK	Vice-President
Claude Amiel	France	Secretary-General
Robert W. Schrier	USA	Treasurer
Thomas E. Andreoli	USA	Editor, Kidney International

Advisory Committee for the 1990 Congress

Klaus Thurau	FRG	Chairman
Robert C. Atkins	Australia	
Claude Amiel	France	
John Stewart Cameron	UK	
Jared James Grantham	USA	
Roscoe R. Robinson	USA	

Nominating Committee

Paul Michielsen	Belgium	President
Franklin H. Epstein	USA	
Gerhard Giebisch	USA	
Richard J. Glassock	USA	
Colin I. Johnston	Australia	
Norman F. Jones	UK	
Franciszek Kokot	Poland	
Jean-Philippe Mery	France	
Jose C. Pena	Mexico	
Mordecai M. Popovtzer	Israel	
Yawara Yoshitoshi	Japan	

Management Committee

Klaus Thurau	FRG	President
Roscoe R. Robinson	USA	President Elect
Claude Amiel	France	Secretary-General
Robert W. Schrier	USA	Treasurer
Thomas E. Andreoli	USA	Editor, Kidney International
Saulo Klahr	USA	Councillor
D. Keith Peters	UK	Councillor

Council

Stephen Angielski	Poland
Robert C. Atkins	Australia
Knut Auklund	Norway
Vittorio Bonomini	Italy
Barry M. Brenner	USA
Giuseppe D'Amico	Italy
Vincent W. Dennis	USA
John H. Dirks	Canada
Evert J. Dorhout Mees	The Netherlands
Carl W. Gottschalk	USA
Jean-Pierre Grünfeld	France
Jean Hamburger	France
Klaus Hierholzer	FRG
David N.S. Kerr	UK
Saulo Klahr	USA
Robert T. McCluskey	USA
Gerhard Malnic	Brazil
D. Keith Peters	UK
Hidekazu Shigematsu	Japan
Jay Stein	USA
Nobuhiro Sugino	Japan
Guillermo Whittembury	Venezuela

XIth International Congress Officers

President	Kenzo Oshima
Vice Presidents	Yawara Yoshitoshi Yasushi Ueda Hiroshi Abe

Organizing Committee

Chairman	Michinobu Hatano
Secretary-General	Susumu Takahashi

Members

Yoshio Aso	Tadashi Miyahara
Toshiyuki Furukawa	Toshihiko Nagasawa
Kohei Hara	Mitsuharu Narita
Nishio Honda	Hiromi Nihira
Takeshi Hoshi	Tadao Niijima
Kazunari Iidaka	Teruo Omae
Hyoe Ishikawa	Zensuke Ota
Chuichi Kawai	Fuminori Sakai
Teruo Kitagawa	Takao Sonoda
Kenkichi Koiso	Nobuhiro Sugino
Kiyoshi Kurokawa	Shizuo Tojo
Sunao Maki	

Scientific Program Committee

Chairmen — Nobuhiro Sugino, Nishio Honda

Executive Secretary — Kiyoshi Kurokawa

Members

Akitoshi Ando
Kikuo Arakawa
Masaaki Arakawa
Hitoshi Endou
Mamoru Fujimoto
Gerhard Giebisch
Takashi Harada
Eiji Higashihara
Kazunari Iidaka
Masashi Imai
Hiroshi Kida
Hikaru Koide
Kenkichi Koiso
Shozo Koshikawa
Akio Koyama
Kenji Maeda
Sunao Maki
Koichi Matsumoto
Toshihiko Nagasawa
Mitsumasa Nagase
Yasushi Nakamoto
Hiroshi Nihei
Michio Odaka
Hiroyuki Ohi
Yoshimasa Orita
Kazuo Ota
Hideto Sakai
Osamu Sakai
Tadasu Sakai
Takao Saruta
Hidekazu Shigematsu
Kenjiro Yamamoto
Nobuyuki Yoshizawa

Fund Raising Committee

Chairmen — Tadao Niijima, Hyoe Ishikawa

Members

Keishi Abe
Yoshio Aso
Tohru Azuma
Kohei Hara
Yoshihei Hirasawa
Hiroshi Kida
Joichi Kumazawa
Yuji Nagura
Zensuke Ota
Tsutomu Sanaka
Takao Sonoda
Naohiko Ueda

Finance Committee

Chairman — Kenkichi Koiso

Members

Hiroshi Kawamura
Gengo Osawa

Contents of Volume I

State of the Art Lectures

Symposia

Immunological and Cellular Mechanisms of Glomerulonephritis

Role of Potassium in Acid-Base Disturbances

Role of Kidney in the Pathogenesis of Hypertension

Cellular and Integrative Functions of the Juxtaglomerular Apparatus

Systemic Dysfunctions in Renal Failure and Their Management

ATPases of the Kidney

Vitamin D and Uremic Bone Disease

AIDS/AIDS – Nephropathy

Cyclosporine Nephrotoxicity: From Experimental Animal to Clinical Practice

Cell Volume Regulation in Health and Disease

Mechanisms of Renal Cell Injury of Acute Renal Failure

Cellular and Integrative Regulation of Renal Circulation

Dietary Factors and Progression of Chronic Renal Failure

Renal Diseases in Asia

Pathobiology of Glomerular and Tubular Basement Membranes

Contents of Volume II

Symposia

Cytokines, Mitogens and Their Receptors on Glomerular Cells

Frontiers of Research on Natriuretic Peptides

Polarity of Tubular Epithelia

Masugi Memorial Symposium: Experimental Nephritis and Its Contribution to Nephrology

Nephrolithiasis: New Ideas in Pathophysiology, New Facts in Therapy

Molecular Action of Diuretics

Cystic Diseases of the Kidney

Continuous Ambulatory Peritoneal Dialysis (CAPD)

Autacoids and the Kidney

Ion Channels of the Kidney

List of Contributors

For contributors' addresses see chapter opening pages

State-of-the-Art Lectures

Pathogenesis of Glomerulonephritis – 1990

ROBERT C. ATKINS

Chair: Yasushi Ueda

Pathogenesis of Glomerulonephritis – 1990

ROBERT C. ATKINS[1]

SUMMARY. Recent advances in our understanding of the pathogenesis of glomerulonephritis are reviewed, focusing on evidence for the importance of the role of sensitized T cells and/or activated macrophages in causing glomerular injury, either directly, or via production of cytokines capable of modulating the normal biosynthetic and proliferative activities of intrinsic glomerular cells. In addition, recent data on the hitherto unrecognized importance of interstitial mononuclear cell infiltration to the progression of renal injury and declining function in glomerulonephritis is discussed. Insights gained from these developing areas of nephrologic research suggest important new approaches to the understanding and improved therapy of glomerulonephritis.

Introduction

Glomerulonephritis has long been considered to result from activation of immune mechanisms. This was first recognized at the turn of the century, and the concept of induction of glomerular injury by immune mechanisms leading to glomerulonephritis still pertains today. The evidence for human glomerular disease being immunologically induced stems, in part, from the localization of immune reactants within glomeruli. The understanding of its immune pathogenesis, as originally proposed by Dixon [1,2] has served us well over the ensuing years, although the linear staining of anti-GBM antibody and the classic deposits of circulating immune complexes within glomeruli may well represent opposite poles of a spectrum of antibody localization, rather than discrete disease entities [3].

Probably most glomerulonephritides, apart from those initiated by an exogenous antigen, such as in post-infectious glomerulonephritis, result from an auto-immune

[1]Department of Nephrology, Prince Henry's Hospital, Monash Medical Centre, Melbourne, Victoria 3004, Australia

reaction to self antigen. Autoimmune mechanisms and their relationship to the kidney have been recently reviewed [4]. Renal damage in glomerulonephritis is caused by immune products which are derived from B or T lymphocytes activated by the nominal antigen [5]. Details of humoral immunity and glomerulonephritis, a field which has historically been the subject of intense study, were recently reviewed [6,7]. The role of sensitized T-cells has not been completely assessed, but we now know that these cells do contribute to the inflammatory process [8–10]. Over the past few years there has been an increasing awareness of the contribution to the glomerular nephritic process by both intrinsic glomerular cells and infiltrating glomerular leucocytes. The cytokine interrelationships of these cells and the balance of their effects are just beginning to be unravelled. Such studies, using approaches made possible by the recent technical advances in cell and molecular biology, have considerably changed research direction in glomerulonephritis over the past few years. This chapter will review three areas where recent work has resulted in conceptual advances in the understanding of the pathogenesis of glomerulonephritis:

1. The role of T-cells and monocytes in glomerular injury.
2. The contribution of intrinsic glomerular cells to the glomerulonephritis process.
3. Involvement of the interstitium in the initiation and evolution of glomerulonephritis.

The Role of T Lymphocytes and Monocytes in Glomerular Injury

T Lymphocytes

Over the past 10 years, evidence for the initiation of glomerular injury by sensitized T cells has been convincingly demonstrated in several models. Initial experiments by Bhan and co-workers demonstrated, both in anti-GBM and in immune complex models of glomerulonephritis, that adoptive transfer of sensitized T lymphocytes produced mild proliferative glomerulonephritis [11]. Further evidence of the capacity of sensitized T cells to induce glomerular injury was provided by Bolton et al. Chickens were depleted of B cells by bursectomy, and an auto-immune glomerulonephritis of varying histologic severity, including, in some cases, glomerulonephritis with crescent formation was induced by injection of heterologous glomeruli in Freund's adjuvant [12,13]. Injury was associated with the presence of intraglomerular T cells, and was also induced in naive chickens by transfer of T cells from affected, but not control, hosts. The fact that T cell depleted nude mice cannot be induced to produce a crescentic glomerulonephritis due to anti-GBM disease also supports the concept that T cells are involved in the genesis of this type of experimental glomerulonephritis [14].

Studies using monoclonal antibodies as specific markers of lymphocyte subsets have demonstrated that in experimental anti-GBM disease, glomerular accumulation of T cells precedes monocyte infiltration and glomerular injury [15]. Such T cells produce the lymphokine, migration inhibition factor [16], and express receptors for interleukin-2 (IL-2 (IL-2R)) [17], indicating their functional activation.

Two recent studies have demonstrated that a proliferative glomerulonephritis can also be induced, in the absence of antibody, by cellular immune responses to exogenous antigens which lodge in the glomeruli. Otie et al. [18] immunized rats with the hapten TNP; this produced sensitized T cells as demonstrated by a local delayed-type hypersensitivity (DTH) reaction to injected antigen, 7 days after immunization. When the hapten was coupled to cationized albumin and injected into the renal arteries of sensitized rats, a proliferative glomerulonephritis with proteinuria developed, without evidence of antibody involvement. Rennke et al. [19] also reported induction of a crescentic glomerulonephritis with marked interstitial involvement in a similar model, using a different antigen. In addition to producing crescentic nephritis after renal artery infusion, transfer of sensitized T cells to naive recipients, followed by antigen injection into the renal artery, produced a focal crescentic glomerulonephritis. Together with the work of Bhan et al. and Bolton et al., these studies provide impressive evidence that T cells alone can induce proliferative crescentic glomerulonephritis in a variety of experimental models of glomerulonephritis.

The evidence for T cell directed glomerulonephritis in human disease is understandably more circumstantial. It has been known for many years that there are no glomerular immune humoral reactants detected in 20% of patients with glomerulonephritis, suggesting a possible cellular causation. Circulating T cells have been shown to be sensitized to renal antigens in some forms of human glomerulonephritis [20]. In addition, intraglomerular T cells have recently been demonstrated in crescentic glomeruli [21–24], and within glomeruli of patients with aggressive proliferative glomerulonephritides such as lupus nephritis and cryoglobulinemic glomerulonephritis [25]. Such T cells are almost certainly functionally active in proliferative and/or crescentic glomerulonephritis, as shown by their association with monocytes and fibrin, the other components of cell mediated immunity [26], and their expression of IL-2R [24].

Though the types of human glomerulonephritis and the extent to which cell mediated immunity is involved remain uncertain, the findings of activated T cells within damaged glomeruli, in conjunction with the mounting experimental evidence cited above, suggests that T cells probably participate in aggressive proliferative glomerular injury in human disease. However, it is likely that both antibody mediated and T cell directed cellular immune mechanisms are involved in many immune mediated glomerulonephritides, and future studies will have to delineate these initiator and effector mechanisms more clearly.

How T cells induce glomerular damage is, as yet, unknown. However, they could recruit and activate monocytes within glomeruli by cell mediated immune mechanisms, as in the classic delayed type hypersensitivity reaction. T cells may also cause damage by production and release of various cytokines, which can cause direct cell injury, or can stimulate intrinsic glomerular cells to proliferate and secrete inflammatory mediators. Direct damage to glomerular cells by cytotoxic T cells may also occur, although there is currently no evidence to support or refute this point [9,10].

Monocytes/Macrophages

Monocytes contribute to glomerular hypercellularity in both human and experimental glomerulonephritis [8,10]. Early workers used ultrastructural examination to demonstrate the presence of monocytes within glomeruli of rabbits with experimental anti-GBM disease [27]. Subsequently, using various identification techniques such as glomerular culture, enzyme histochemistry, and monoclonal antibody analysis, intraglomerular monocytes were demonstrated in experimental anti-GBM disease, immune complex disease, lupus nephritis, and focal glomerular sclerosis [10,28,29].

The presence of monocytes in diseased human glomeruli was first described by Jones in 1951 [30]. We initially used glomerular culture to quantitate macrophages within glomeruli from patients with crescentic glomerulonephritis [31], but with the use of specific monoclonal antibodies and sensitive immunohistochemical labelling techniques it became feasible to compare the degree of macrophage involvement among the various human glomerular nephritides [8,32,33]. Thus, from these and other studies, it is now apparent that macrophages are found within glomeruli in many forms of proliferative glomerulonephritis, but especially in crescentic disease (of all etiologies), and in post-infectious, cryoglobulinemic, and diffuse lupus nephritis [21–23,25,32–35].

Macrophages can be recruited to glomeruli in several ways [10]. Monocyte accumulation and activation can result from elaboration of cytokines by sensitized T cells, by Fc receptor binding to glomerular deposits of immunoglobulin [36], via surface receptors for activated complement components, or in response to chemotactic fragments of fibrin and its degradation products [37]. In addition, glomerular endothelial leucocyte adhesion molecules are transiently induced in response to stimulation by endotoxin or cytokines, such as IL-1 or TNF [38,39], and such a mechanism could be responsible for macrophage entrapment within inflamed glomeruli.

Once localized to glomeruli, macrophages produce inflammatory mediators such as reactive oxygen species [40], thromboxane A2 [41], and IL-1 [29,42]. Indeed, increased IL-1 production from glomeruli from patients with glomerulonephritis was recently reported, suggesting that this cytokine may be important in the pathogenesis of human disease as well [43]. Moreover, in addition to its well-known pro-inflammatory effects, IL-1 is now known to directly affect tubular transport mechanisms [44].

Macrophage induced fibrin deposition via activation of the extrinsic pathway of coagulation was shown in experimental disease [10,45]. The association of glomerular macrophages expressing the pro-coagulant tissue factor with fibrin deposition within glomeruli suggests that this may also be a mechanism of macrophage induced injury in patients with proliferative glomerulonephritis [26,46]. Macrophages are also involved in the generation of crescents, the presence of which usually signifies extensive renal damage and a poor prognosis [10,47].

Cytokines produced by macrophages can induce other complex alterations in the normal physiology of intrinsic glomerular cells [48]. Recently, additional evidence for this interaction of inflammatory and intrinsic glomerular cells was demonstrated in rats with accelerated anti-GBM nephritis by Matsumoto and Hatano [42]. Glomerular monocytes were eliminated by treatment with anti-macrophage serum, causing a reduction in mesangial cell numbers and IL-1 production from isolated glomeruli, and diminished proteinuria. One interpretation of these results is that macrophage-produced IL-1 stimulates mesangial cell proliferation. This explanation is further supported by experiments studying progressive glomerulosclerosis in rats, where the numbers of glomerular macrophages and mesangial cells were progressively reduced, in conjunction with decreasing production of glomerular IL-1, as the disease evolved [29].

Thus, there is ample evidence for T-cell directed mechanisms of injury, together with macrophage participation, in experimental and human glomerulonephritis, although the unravelling of the complex interplay of the initiation and mediation of glomerular injury, by cytokine cell to cell signalling, is just beginning.

Contribution of Intrinsic Glomerular Cells to the Glomerulonephritic Process

Though proliferation of intrinsic glomerular cells is one of the key histologic features for the diagnosis and classification of glomerulonephritis, just how and why these cells proliferate beyond the normal level is unknown. Few studies determining the actual increased cell numbers of the intrinsic glomerular types in the various forms of glomerulonephritis are available [49,50]. One of the major changes in recent thinking has been the realization that intrinsic glomerular cells respond to various stimuli, not as passive targets nor as innocent bystanders, but with specific structural and metabolic changes which can directly influence evolution of the glomerular inflammatory process. It is now realized that the three intrinsic glomerular cells – mesangial, endothelial, and epithelial cells – are potentially all capable of exhibiting an active role in the initiation and progression of glomerulonephritis. Studies of the complex interplay between glomerular cells, both in normal and in diseased states, has just begun.

The technical ability to obtain these cells as pure isolates in culture, thereby enabling controlled manipulation of their properties, has led to intensive study of their in vitro properties over the past few years [51,52]. There is now a considerable literature, especially relating to the properties of mesangial cells, reflecting the relative ease of their isolation and homogenous culture, compared to the other glomerular cell types. Mesangial cells are increasingly thought to play a significant pathophysiologic role, because of their pivotal position within the glomerulus, surrounded by matrix, yet directly accessible to the plasma, and with actions ranging from regulation of glomerular blood flow to modulation of matrix production.

Mesangial Cells

The mesangial cell is a pluripotential cell with many features of a smooth muscle cell. The properties of mesangial cells have been identified, largely using mesangial cells cultured in vitro. Such studies have shown that mesangial cells contract in response to vasoactive amines and peptides, proliferate in response to inflammatory agents such as cytokines and growth factors, complement, immune complexes, and endotoxin, and secrete many factors, including cytokines, matrix proteins, bioactive lipids, and enzymes [51,52]. However, since many of the characteristics demonstrated using cultured mesangial cells vary considerably depending upon the culture conditions, great care must be exercised when extrapolating from in vitro mesangial cell properties to an assumed function in vivo.

In vitro, the cytokines IL-1, IL-6, prostaglandin F (PGF), and epidermal growth factor (EGF) induce mesangial cell proliferation, whereas proliferation is inhibited by transforming growth factor (TGF) beta and gamma interferon (Kakazaki and Kraft, Atkins 1990, unpublished observations). Likewise, lipids produced by mesangial cells, such as platelet activating factor, induce mesangial cell proliferation, whereas the prostaglandins inhibit proliferation. Similarly, addition of some matrix proteins, such as fibronectin, stimulate proliferation of cultured mesangial cells, but others, like heparan sulfate, inhibit this effect. Clearly, this balance between proliferation and its inhibition could be easily perturbed during the inflammation process and, depending on the dominance of the various inflammatory mediators, could result in either mesangial proliferation and/or sclerosis.

Mesangial cells produce a host of secreted substances in culture. These products are produced under "normal" culture conditions and may be further increased by immune and other stimuli. These secretory products include cytokines: interleukin-1 (IL-1), interleukin-6 (IL-6), tumor necrosis factor (TNF), transforming growth factor beta (TGF-B), and epidermal growth factor (EGF); enzymes, such as neutral proteinase and collagenase; bioactive lipids, such as the prostaglandins and platelet activating factor; and matrix proteins including Collagen III, IV and V, fibrinectin, laminin, and heparan sulfate [51,52,59].

Since mesangial cells both make and respond to various cytokines, the concept of mesangial cell auto-regulation was introduced, by Sterzel and Lovett, particularly in regard to IL-1 production [48]. These workers suggested that the perpetuation of mesangial cell activity by the breakdown in this auto-regulation might be one reason for the progression of mesangial glomerular sclerosis following cessation of the initial glomerular insult, in some forms of glomerulonephritis.

Additional evidence for such a concept was the demonstration that IL-6 is an autocrine growth factor for mesangial cells. Horii et al. demonstrated that mesangial cells in culture produced IL-6, and IL-6 itself induces a dose-dependent proliferation of rat mesangial cells in culture [60]. This group further showed that IL-6 was present within glomeruli of patients with proliferative glomerulonephritis, but not in normal glomeruli or in glomeruli from patients with minimal change glomerulonephritis, and that IL-6 urinary excretion was raised only in patients with proliferative glomerulonephritis. By inference, these results suggest that unregulated production of IL-6, presumably by mesangial cells, is a factor in progressive mesangial dysfunction in proliferative types of glomerulonephritis. This would also support the findings that IL-6 transgenic mice develop mesangial proliferative glomerulonephritis [61].

Another cytokine, TGF beta, also promotes mesangial matrix accumulation in experimental glomerulonephritis [62]. In rat mesangial injury induced by anti-thymocyte serum, cultured nephritic glomeruli produced increased amounts of TGF beta and matrix proteins. Normal rat mesangial cells in culture increased proteoglycan production when stimulated by TGF-beta or conditioned media from these nephritic glomeruli. These changes were blocked by anti-TGF serum. The time-course of matrix accumulation in these animals paralleled TGF-beta mRNA expression in glomeruli. These results suggest that TGF beta has a central role in the accumulation of pathological extracellular matrix and raises the possibility that therapy to regulate TGF beta action might be salutary.

Endothelial Cells in Glomerulonephritis

Normal glomerular endothelial cells have complex functions, including growth, permeability, maintenance of an anti-coagulant state, and matrix production; these functions may be modified following interactions with circulating leucocytes. Most studies of endothelial cells in culture have relied on non-glomerular endothelial cells. However, recently, glomerular endothelial cells have been grown and sustained in culture [63,64], and hence the relevance of many of the properties of activated endothelial cells determined so far may soon be examined using glomerular endothelial cells.

With immune stimulation, cultured non-renal endothelial cells produce cytokines and vasoactive lipids, express leucocyte adhesion and HLA molecules, promote procoagulant activity, and undergo changes in their cell structure [39]. Proliferation of these cells is enhanced by the cytokines IL-1, TNF, PGF, and EGF, and inhibited by TGF beta and gamma interferon. Hence, as for mesangial cells, these cytokines appear to closely regulate proliferation, and this balance between competing agents may be disrupted in disease states.

No studies are, as yet, available concerning isolated glomerular endothelial cells. However, incubation of isolated human glomeruli with endotoxin or with cytokines such as IL-1 and tumor necrosis factor (TNF) induces leucocyte adhesion molecules [38]. Similarly, such cytokines induce glomerular endothelial expression of procoagulant molecules [38] and downregulation of endothelial thrombomodulin expression [53]. Moreover, infusion of TNF into rabbit causes glomerular endothelial damage [54], downregulation of thrombomodulin expression, and induction of fibrin deposition, features which are also found in experimental anti-GBM disease [53]. Hence, initial studies indicate that cytokines do have in vivo effects similar to those induced in culture, and which may be relevant to the glomerulonephritic inflammatory process. These observations raise the potential for therapy by specific blocking of cytokine actions.

Epithelial Cells and Glomerulonephritis

Role in Membranous Nephropathy

For many years idiopathic membranous nephropathy in humans was considered a classic immune complex nephropathy, caused by deposition of circulating immune complexes. However, evidence now suggests that membranous glomerulonephritis is the result of an autoimmune response to native renal epithelial cell antigens. Intensive study of Heymann's nephritis, induced by immunization of rats with brush border antigen FXIA, has changed our concept of the pathogenesis of membranous nephritis. Heymann nephritis, both passive and active, mimics human membranous nephropathy and was originally also thought to be due to deposition of circulating immune complexes. The antigen responsible for Heymann's nephritis, gp330 (recently sequenced and found to be homologous with the low density lipoprotein receptors [55], occurs both within cells of the proximal tubule and in the coated pits of glomerular epithelial cells [56]. Moreover, antibodies to epithelial cell antigens can redistribute antigens at the surface of human and monkey glomerular epithelial cells in vitro, in vivo, and ex vivo [57]. Furthermore, specific membrane proteins were detected in immune deposits of patients with membranous nephropathy [58]. Hence, these suggest that human membranous nephritis, like Heymann's nephritis in rats, is due to the formation of auto-antibodies to epithelial cell antigens, resulting in in-situ immune complex formation.

Modulation of Epithelial Cell Growth In Vitro

Both human and animal glomerular epithelial cells can now be reproducibly grown in culture, using special culture media, and their response to, and production of, inflammatory mediators are currently being assessed [63,65,66]. Glomerular epithelial cells in vitro proliferate in response to leukotrienes, thrombin, and EGF, and this proliferation is inhibited by heparan sulfate and transforming growth factor beta [66]. Based on these initial experiments, matrix proteins and inflammatory cytokines, such as EGF and TGF-b, may exert a regulatory influence on epithelial cell proliferation.

Epithelial Cells and Glomerular Crescent Formation

Crescent formation occurs in a heterogenous group of glomerulonephritides, but generally indicates an increased severity of disease and is frequently associated with a poorer outcome. Langhans originally proposed that proliferating glomerular epithelial cells formed the crescent, and this view became widely accepted [67]. However, numerous experimental and human studies [10,47] have now demonstrated that monocytes are also intimately involved in crescent formation. Thus, it is now generally accepted that both monocytes and epithelial cells contribute to crescent formation, and in fact the composition appears to depend upon the age of the crescent [68] and the integrity of Bowman's capsule [69]. Indeed, there is a prominent interstitial periglomerular infiltration of leucocytes associated with crescentic glomerulonephritis, and it may be that many of the leucocytes entering Bowman's space enter from the interstitium, as well as via the capillary tuft, perhaps in response to fibrin [10,47].

The mechanism leading to the migration of monocytes is only partially understood, and is almost certainly multifactorial, yet a recent study has again highlighted the importance of fibrin in this regard. Zoja et al. [70] showed that recombinant plasminogen activator, which causes lysis of fibrin clots by activating plasminogen to plasmin, markedly reduced glomerular fibrin deposition and crescent formation, and also prevented deterioration of renal function in rabbit nephrotic nephritis. Since fibrin is only one determinant of crescent formation, and can itself result from macrophage activation and initiation of the extrinsic pathway of coagulation, interpretation of these results may be complex [46]. Nevertheless, such studies emphasize the many complex interrelationships potentially active between inflammatory cells and mediators, intrinsic glomerular cells, particularly parietal and visceral epithelial cells, and the coagulation system.

With regard to further analysis of mononuclear cell involvement in crescentic glomerulonephritis, we have recently noted that with the advent of crescent formation in IgA nephropathy, there is increased T-cell and monocyte activation, particularly in the interstitium, and a decrease in renal function [24]. Indeed, our most recent studies of leucocyte composition of crescents, in 34 patients, have demonstrated that leucocytes make up some 80% of the cells in active cellular crescents; the majority of these leucocytes are monocytes, though a few T-cells and IL-2R+ mononuclear cells, as yet unidentified further, are present. In contrast, in inactive, sclerosed crescents, the proportion of leucocytes was reduced to about 20% of total cells, emphasizing the potential importance of cellular immune activation in crescent formation [71].

Involvement of the Interstitium in the Initiation and Evolution of Glomerulonephritis

In trying to understand the relationship between alteration of glomerular structure and decreased function in glomerulonephritis, the paradox arises that glomerular morphological changes do not correlate with renal functional impairment, whereas the interstitial changes do [72]. We demonstrated a relationship between a decreasing glomerular filtration rate and the intensity of interstitial leucocytic infiltration in 145 patients with glomerulonephritis [33]. This interstitial leucocytic infiltration was prominent in all forms of glomerulonephritis except minimal change glomerulonephritis, and its density reflected the severity of the underlying glomerular disease. The infiltrate was similar in composition to that seen in acute interstitial allograft rejection, as well as interstitial nephritis, consisting predominantly of T lymphocytes and macrophages, and with a notable absence of B cells. About 50% of T cells were of the CD4+ phenotype, and the ratio of CD4+ to CD8+ cells remained relatively constant within the varying disease types. The interstitial infiltrate increased in intensity with increasing degree of morphological evidence of glomerular injury, contained immune activated mononuclear cells expressing IL-2R, and activated macrophages producing the procoagulant tissue factor. A relationship between the glomerular crescentic activity and interstitial leucocyte infiltration was demonstrated in human IgA disease [24], whereby greater interstitial infiltration of leucocytes occurred in biopsies from patients with glomerular crescents. The number of T-cells and monocytes were greater in crescentic disease, and a higher proportion of mononuclear cells, approximately 20%, expressed IL-2R. Other recent studies have also examined the interstitial leucocytic infiltrate [73,74] and the degree of interstitial leucocytic infiltration has been shown to be a good predictor of clinical progression, including cases of membranous nephritis [75], IgA disease [76,77], and lupus nephritis [25,78,79], providing additional credence to the importance of the interstitial events in progression of glomerulonephritis.

The relationship between glomerular and interstitial leucocyte involvement was studied experimentally, using both immune and non-immune models of glomerulonephritis. In accelerated anti-GBM disease, leucocytes appeared, within 15 minutes of disease induction, in the glomerulus and surrounding the afferent and efferent arterioles of the periglomerular stalk. These cells consisted of both T lymphocytes and monocytes, and over the ensuing days accumulated and encircled the glomerulus before spreading throughout the interstitium by day 7. However, the leucocyte profile differed between glomerulus and interstitium, the glomerular leucocytes consisting mainly of monocytes, whereas the periglomerular and interstitial cells consisted of approximately 50% monocytes and 50% T lymphocytes [17]. This rapid localization of leucocytes around hilar vessels, which occurred in the absence of local immunoglobulin deposition and concurrently with the glomerular leucocyte ingress, may provide a route for cytokine dispersal from the inflamed glomerulus and mesangium into the interstitial and other cortical areas.

An interstitial infiltrate was also present in a "non-immune" model of progressive focal glomerulosclerosis induced in rats by the concomitant injection of aminonucleoside and protamine sulfate [80]. Prednisolone treatment begun 10 days after the instigation of the disease produced a significant improvement in renal function, corresponding to a decrease in severity of the interstitial changes, decrease in the relative interstitial volume, and reduction in leucocyte infiltration, yet without any glomerular alteration in sclerosis or leucocyte infiltration. This study further suggests that glomerular filtration rate and disease progression is more dependent on changes in the interstitium than in the glomerulus. Both studies are consistent with a hypothesis that infiltration of leucocytes into the interstitium in glomerulonephritis, of whatever etiology, determines evolution of the disease. Other recent studies have also evaluated the significance of the interstitial component in "non-immune" renal disease and the importance of interstitial macrophages and T cells in mediation of injury, including effects on tubular transport mechanisms [44,81].

Hence, though the pathogenesis of these interstitial changes and their relationship to the primary glomerular disease is currently uncertain, it could well be that the interstitial changes in glomerulonephritis may progress, regardless of the type of initial glomerular insult, perhaps due to cellular immune mechanisms. This interstitial leucocyte infiltration could result from classic T-cell directed cellular immunity to planted or unmasked tubular antigens. It might be the consequence of non-antigenic specific leucocyte accumulation following cytokine dispersal from injured glomeruli. Interstitial leucocytic accumulation could also follow increased expression of leucocyte adhesion molecules. Cytokine mediated upregulation of ICAM-1 in lupus nephritis in mice, which could well promote such leucocyte attraction to the interstitium, has recently been described [82]. Whatever the etiology, the interstitial component in glomerulonephritis has clinical implications for estimation of progression of disease and for therapy. Further understanding of the pathogenesis of the interstitial component of glomerulonephritis will perhaps lead to more specific therapy by targeting of the mediator systems involved. Such a therapeutic approach is vital for the current clinical situation, where the nephrologist is frequently faced with a disease which is ongoing, an initiating antigen which is unknown, and mediators which are obscure.

Concluding Remarks

Progress in our understanding of the pathogenesis of glomerulonephritis has occurred in recent years in incremental steps. Re-analysis of familiar animal models of glomerulonephritis, using monoclonal antibodies to markers of immune activation; widescale culture and passage of isolated glomerular cells (mesangial, epithelial, but still only with difficulty, endothelial cells) and their use in studies of proliferation, matrix production, and the effects of recombinant proteins, especially cytokines; and detailed clinicopathologic studies of biopsies from patients with glomerulonephritis have all contributed to this progress. However, the challenge remains to convert recent advances in basic cellular and molecular biology into clinically relevant, meaningful, and cost-effective applications. Meeting this challenge will require the clinician to become more conversant with the seemingly difficult, and increasingly complex, developments in biologic research, and the basic scientist to ask, and attempt answers to, clinically relevant questions. Nevertheless, the accelerating pace of development in nephrologic research, set against the ongoing revolution in biology brought about by the advent of monoclonal antibodies, and, more recently, molecular biology, is likely to yield quantum leaps in our understanding of the pathogenesis of glomerulonephritis.

References

1. Dixon FJ (1968) The pathogenesis of glomerulonephritis. Am J Med 44:493–494
2. Wilson CB, Dixon FJ (1986) The renal response to immunological injury. In: Brenner BJ, Rector FC (eds) The kidney, 3rd edn. WB Saunders, Philadelphia, pp 800–889
3. Bruijn JA, Hoedemaeker PJ, Fleuren GJ (1989) Pathogenesis of anti-basement membrane glomerulopathy and immune-complex glomerulonephritis: dichotomy dissolved. Lab Invest 61:480–488
4. Oliviera DBG, Peters DK (1989) Autoimmunity and the kidney. Kidney Int 35:923–928
5. Kelly CJ, Haverty T, Neilson EG (1988) Control of the nephritogenic immune response. In: Wilson CB (ed) Immunopathology of renal disease, vol 18. Churchill Livingstone, New York, pp 35–56
6. Wilson CB (1988) Antibody reactions with native or planted glomerular antigens producing nephritogenic immune deposits or selective glomerular cell injury. In: Wilson CB (ed) Immunopathology of renal disease, vol 18. Churchill Livingstone, New York, pp 1–34
7. Brentjens JR, Andres G (1989) Interaction of antibodies with renal cell surface antigens. Kidney Int 35:954–968
8. Atkins RC, Holdsworth SR, Hancock WW, Thomson NM, Glasgow EF (1982) Cellular immune mechanisms in human glomerulonephritis: The role of mononuclear leucocytes. Springer Semin Immunopathol 5:269–296
9. McCluskey RT, Bhan AK (1986) Cell mediated immunity in renal disease. Hum Pathol 17:146–153
10. Atkins RC, Holdsworth SR (1988) Cellular mechanisms of immune glomerular injury. In: Brenner and Stein (eds) Cellular mechanisms of injury in GN. Churchill Livingstone, New York, pp 111–135
11. Bhan AK, Schneeberger EE, Collins AB, McCluskey RT (1978) Evidence for a pathogenic role of a cell-mediated immune mechanism in experimental glomerulonephritis. J Exp Med 148:246–260
12. Bolton WK, Tucker FL, Sturgill BC (1984) New avian model of experimental GN consistent with mediation by cellular immunity. J Clin Invest 73:1263–1276
13. Bolton WK, Chandra M, Tyson TM, Kirkpatrick PR, Sadovnic MJ, Sturgill BC (1988) Transfer of experimental glomerulonephritis in chickens by mononuclear cells. Kidney Int 34(5):598–610
14. Okada K, Otie T, Kihara I, Morita T, Yamamoto T (1982) Masugi nephritis in the nude mice and their normal littermates. Acta Pathol Jpn 32:1
15. Tipping PG, Neale TJ, Holdsworth SR (1985) T lymphocyte participation in antibody-induced experimental glomerulonephritis. Kidney Int 27:530–537
16. Boyce NW, Tipping PG, Holdsworth SR (1986) Lymphokine (MIF) production by glomerular T-lymphocytes in experimental glomerulonephritis. Kidney Int 30:673
17. Lan HY, Paterson DJ, Atkins RC (1989) Evolving pattern of the interstitial leucocyte infiltrate in experimental anti-GBM glomerulonephritis (abstract). Kidney Int 36:1176
18. Otie T, Shimuzu F, Kagami S, Morioka T (1989) Hapten-specific cellular immune response producing glomerular injury. Clin Exp Immunol 76(3):463–468
19. Rennke HG, Klein PS, Mendrick DL (1990) Cell-mediated Immunity (CMI) in hapten-induced interstitial nephritis and glomerular crescent formation in the rat (abstract). Kidney Int 37:428
20. Rocklin R, Lewis E, David J (1970) In-vitro evidence for cellular hypersensitivity to glomerular-basement-membrane antigens in human glomerulonephritis. N Engl J Med 283:497–501
21. Nolasco FEB, Cameron JS, Hartley B, Coelho RA, Reuben R (1987) Intraglomerular T cells and monocytes in nephritis: study with monoclonal antibodies. Kidney Int 31:1160–1166

22. Bolton WK, Innes DJ, Sturgill BC, Kaiser DL (1987) T Cells and macrophages in rapidly progressive glomerulonephritis: clinicopathological correlations. Kidney Int 32:869–876
23. Muller GA, Muller CA, Markovic-Lipkovski J, Kilper RB, Risler T (1988) Renal major histocompatibility complex antigens and cellular components in rapidly progressive glomerulonephritis identified by monoclonal antibodies (with 1 color plate). Nephron 49:132–139
24. Li HL, Hancock WW, Hooke DH, Dowling JP, Atkins RC (1990) Mononuclear cell activation and decreased renal function in IgA nephropathy with crescents. Kidney Int 37: In Press
25. Castiglione A, Bucci A, Fellin G, D'Amico G, Atkins RC (1988) The relationship of infiltrating renal leucocytes to disease activity in lupus and cryoglobuilinaemic glomerulonephritis. Nephron 50:14–23
26. Neale TJ, Tipping PG, Carson SD, Holdsworth SR (1988) Participation of cell-mediated immunity in deposition of fibrin in glomerulonephritis. Lancet II(8608):421–424
27. Shigematsu H (1970) Glomerular events during the initial phase of rat Masugi nephritis. Virchows Arch [Cell Pathol] 5:187
28. Boyce NW, Holdsworth SR, Dijkstra CD, Atkins RC (1987) Quantitation of intraglomerular mononuclear phagocytes in experimental glomerulonephritis in the rat using specific monoclonal antibodies. Pathology 19:290–293
29. Matsumoto K, Atkins RC (1989) Glomerular cells and macrophages in the progression of experimental focal and segmental glomerulosclerosis. Am J Pathol 134(4):933–945
30. Jones DB (1951) Inflammation and repair of the glomerulus. Am J Pathol 27:991–1009
31. Atkins RC, Glasgow EF, Holdsworth SR, Matthews FE (1976) The macrophage in human rapidly progressive glomerulonephritis. Lancet I:830–832
32. Hooke DH, Hancock WW, Gee DC, Kraft N, Atkins RC (1984) Monoclonal antibody analysis of glomerular hypercellularity in human glomerulonephritis. Clin Nephrol 22(4):163–168
33. Hooke DH, Gee DC, Atkins RC (1987) Leukocyte analysis using monoclonal antibodies in human glomerulonephritis. Kidney Int 31:964–972
34. Magil AB, Wadsworth LD, Loewen M (1981) Monocytes and human renal glomerular disease. A quantitative evaluation. Lab Invest 44:23–33
35. D'Amico G, Colasanti G, Ferrario F, Sinico RA (1989) Renal involvement in essential mixed cryoglobulinemia. Kidney Int 35:1004–1014
36. Holdworth SR (1983) Fc dependence of macrophage accumulation and subsequent injury in experimental glomerulonephritis. J Immunol 130:735–739
37. Holdsworth SR, Thomson NM, Glasgow EF, Atkins RC (1979) The effect of defibrination on macrophage participation in rabbit nephrotoxic nephritis: Studies using glomerular culture and electromicroscopy. Clin Exp Immunol 37:38–43
38. Hancock WW, Cotran RS (1987) Induction of activation antigens on human glomerular endothelium by interleukin 1 (IL-1), interferon-gamma (IFN-g) and endotoxin (LPS) (abstract). Kidney Int 31:322
39. Cotran RS, Pober JS (1989) Effects of cytokines on vascular endothelium: their role in vascular and immune injury. Kidney Int 35:969–975
40. Boyce NW, Tipping PG, Holdsworth SR (1989) Glomerular macrophages produce reactive oxygen species in experimental glomerulonephritis. Kidney Int 35:778–782
41. Cook HT, Smith J, Salmon JA, Cattell V (1989) Functional characteristics of macrophages in glomerulonephritis in the rat: 02-generation, MHC class II expression, and eicosanoid synthesis. Am J Pathol 134:431–437
42. Matsumoto K, Hatano M (1989) Production of interleukin-1 in glomerular cell cultures from rats with nephrotoxic serum nephritis. Clin Exp Immunol 75:123–128
43. Matsumoto K, Dowling J, Atkins RC (1988) Production of Interleukin-1 in glomerular cell cultures from patients with rapidly progressive crescentic glomerulonephritis. Am J Nephrol 8:463–470

44. Schreiner GF, Kohan DE (1990) Regulation of renal transport processes and hemodynamics by macrophages and lymphocytes. Am J Physiol 258:F761–767
45. Tipping PG, Lowe MG, Holdsworth SR (1988) Glomerular macrophages express augmented procoagulant activity in experimental fibrin-related glomerulonephritis in rabbits. J Clin Invest 82(4):1253–1259
46. Hancock WW, Atkins RC (1985) Activation of coagulation pathways and fibrin deposition in human glomerulonephritis. Semin Nephrol 5:69–75
47. Atkins RC, Thomson NM (1988) Rapidly progressive glomerulonephritis. In: Schrier RW, Gooschalk CW (eds) Diseases of the kidney, vol 2. Little, Brown, Boston, pp 1903–1927
48. Sterzel RB, Lovett DH (1988) Interactions of inflammatory and glomerular cells in the response to glomerular injury. In: Wilson CB (ed) Immunopathology of renal disease, vol 18. Churchill Livingstone, New York, pp 137–173
49. Atkins RC, Glasgow EF, Holdsworth S, Thomson NM, Hancock WW (1980) Tissue culture of isolated glomeruli from patients with glomerulonephritis. Kidney Int 17(4):515–527
50. Sterzel RB, Pabst R, Kregeler M, Perfetto M (1982) The temporal relationship between glomerular cell proliferation and monocyte infiltration in experimental glomerulonephritis. Virchows Arch [Cell Pathol] 38:337–350
51. Mene P, Simonson MS, Dunn MJ (1989) Physiology of the mesangial cell. Physiol Rev 69:1347–1424
52. Hawkins NJ, Wakefield D, Charlesworth JA (1990) The role of mesangial cells in glomerular pathology. Pathology 22
53. Hancock WW (to be published) IL-1 and TNF depress glomerular endothelial thrombomodulin expressin in vitro and in vivo. Kidney Int
54. Bertani T, Abbate M, Zoja C, Corna D, Perico N, Ghezzi P, Remuzzi G (1989) Tumor necrosis factor induces glomerular damage in the rabbit. Am J Pathol 134:419–430
55. Raychowdhury R, Hiles JL, McCluskey RT, Smith JA (1989) Autoimmune target in Heymann nephritis is a glycoprotein with homology to the LDL receptor. Science 244(4909): 1163–1165
56. Kerjaschki D (1990) The pathogenesis of membranous glomerulonephritis: from morphology to molecules. Virchows Arch [Cell Pathol] 58:253–271
57. Fukatsu A, Yuzawa Y, Olson L, Miller J, Andres G (1989) Interaction of antibodies with human glomerular epithelial cells. Lab Invest 61:389–403
58. Kerjaschki D (1989) Kinetics of immune deposits in membranous nephropathy. Kidney Int 35:1423
59. Hancock WW, Kraft N, Clarke F, Atkins RC (1984) Production of monoclonal antibodies to fibronectin, type IV collagen and other antigens of the human glomerulus. Pathology 16:197–206
60. Horii Y, Muraguchi A, Iwano M, Matsuda T, Hirayama T, Yamada H, Fujii Y, Dohi K, Ishikawa H, Ohmoto Y, Yoshizaki K, Hirano T, Kishimoto T (1989) Involvement of IL-6 in mesangial proliferative glomerulonephritis. J Immunol 143(12):3949–3955
61. Suematsu S, Matsuda T, Aozasa K, Akira S, Nakano N, Ohno S, Miyazaki JI, Yamamura KI, Hirano, T, Kishimoto T (1989) IgGl plasmacytosis in interleukin 6 transgenic mice. Proc Natl Acad Sci USA (Immunol) 86:7547–7551
62. Okuda S, Languino LR, Ruoslanti E, Border WA (to be published) Elevated expression of transforming growth factor-beta and proteoglycan production in experimental glomerulonephritis: possible role in expansion of the mesangial extracellular matrix. J Clin Invest
63. MacKay K, Striker LJ, Elliot S, Pinkert CA, Brinster RL, Striker GE (1988) Glomerular epithelial, mesangial and endothelial cell lines from transgenic mice. Kidney Int 33:677–684
64. Ballerman BJ (1989) Regulation of bovine glomerular endothelial cell growth in vitro. Am J Physiol 256(1 Pt 1):C182–C189
65. Quigg RJ, Abrahamson DR, Cybulsky AV, Badalamenti J, Minto AW, Salant DJ (1989) Studies of antibodies to cultured rat glomerular epithelial cells. Subepithelial immune deposit formation after in vivo injection. Am J Pathol 134(5):1125–1133

66. Adler S, Chen X, Eng B (1990) Control of rat glomerular epithelial cell growth in vitro. Kidney Int 37:1048–1054
67. Langhans T (1979) Über die Veränderungen der Glomeruli bei der Nephritis nebst einigen Bemerkungen über die Enstshung der Fibrinzylinder. Arch Pathol Physiol Klin Med 76:85
68. Hancock WW, Atkins RC (1984) Cellular composition of crescents in human rapidly progressive glomerulonephritis identified using monoclonal antibodies. Am J Nephrol 3:177–181
69. Boucher A, Droz D, Adafer E, Laure-Helene N (1987) Relationship between the integrity of Bowman's capsule and the composition of cellular crescents in human crescentic glomerulonephritis. Lab Invest 56(5):526–533
70. Zoja C, Corna D, Macconi D, Zilio P, Bertani T, Remuzzi G (1990) Tissue plasminogen activator therapy of rabbit nephrotoxic nephritis. Lab Invest 62(1):34–40
71. Li HL, Hancock WW, Dowling JP, Atkins RC (to be published) IL-2R mononuclear cell (MNC) composition of crescents in human crescentic glomerulonephritis (CGN) (abstract). Kidney Int
72. Risdon RA, Sloper JC, DeWardner HE (1968) Relationship between renal function and histological changes found in renal biopsy specimens from patients with persistent glomerulonephritis. Lancet II:363–366
73. D'Amico G (1988) Role of interstitial infiltration of leukocytes in glomerular diseases. Nephrol Dial Transplant 3(5):596–600
74. Markovic-Lipkovski J, Muller CA, Risler T, Bohle A, Muller GA (1990) Association of glomerular and interstitial mononuclear leukocytes with different forms of glomerulonephritis. Nephrol Dial Transplant 5:10–17
75. Alexopoulos E, Seron D, Hartley RB, Nolasco F, Cameron JS (1989) Immune mechanisms in idiopathic membranous nephropathy: the role of the interstitial infiltrates. Am J Kidney Dis 13(5):404–412
76. Sabadini E, Castiglione A, Colasanti G, Ferrario F, D'Amico G (1988) Characterisation of interstitial infiltrating cells in Berger's disease. Am J Kidney Dis 12:307–315
77. Alexopoulos E, Scron D, Hartley RB, Nolasco F, Cameron JS (1989) The role of interstitial infiltrates in IgA nephropathy: a study with monoclonal antibodies. Nephrol Dial Transplant 4:187–195
78. D'Agati UD, Appel GA, Estes D, Knowles DM, Pirani CL (1986) Monoclonal antibody identification of infiltrating mononuclear leucocytes in lupus nephritis. Kidney Int 30:573–581
79. Alexopoulos E, Seron D, Hartley RB, Cameron JS (1990) Lupus nephritis: correlation of interstitial cells with glomerular function. Kidney Int 37:100–109
80. Saito T, Atkins RC (1990) Contribution of mononuclear leucocytes to the progression of experimental focal glomerular sclerosis. Kidney Int 37:1076–1083
81. Schreiner GF, Harris KP, Purkerson ML, Klahr S (1988) Immunological aspects of acute ureteral obstruction: immune cell infiltrate in the kidney. Kidney Int 34(4):487–493
82. Wuthrich RP, Jeunikar AM, Takei F, Glimcher LH, Kelley VE (1990) Intercellular adhesion molecule-1 (ICAM-1) expression is unregulated in autoimmune murine lupus nephritis. Am J Pathol 136:441–450

Functional Morphology of the Nephron

C. Craig Tisher, Kirsten M. Madsen, and Jill W. Verlander

Chair: Wilhelm Kriz

Functional Morphology of the Nephron

C. Craig Tisher, Kirsten M. Madsen, and Jill W. Verlander[1]

Introduction

The mammalian nephron is composed of the renal corpuscle (commonly referred to as the "glomerulus") and the renal tubule. The tubular component of the nephron is traditionally divided into three functional regions: the proximal tubule, the thin limb, and the distal tubule. Strictly speaking, the collecting duct system is not part of the nephron since its embryonic derivation is from the ureteric bud rather than the metanephric mass. However, physiologists and anatomists now view the collecting duct as an integral portion of the nephron regardless of its embryonic origin.

During the past two decades a variety of investigative techniques have allowed scientists to more precisely define the structural and functional properties of the nephron. This effort received a major impetus with the development of the isolated perfused tubule technique, by Burg and his colleagues [1], which permitted examination of the functional properties of individual segments of the renal tubule under carefully controlled and defined experimental conditions. Concurrently, Morel [2] and Garg et al. [3] developed and adapted analytical biochemical techniques to measure enzyme activities in individually dissected segments of the renal tubule. Simultaneously, morphologists took advantage of improved methods of tissue preservation that made it possible to examine the renal tubule in greater detail, at both the cellular and subcellular level. The more recent availability of monoclonal and polyclonal antibodies directed against specific transport and structural proteins located in the kidney has allowed investigators to locate not only the segment of the renal tubule involved in a particular transport event, but also the exact cell(s) and often the precise subcellular location of a specific transport function. Currently under development are methods of in situ hybridization which permit scientists to examine gene expression and regulation in individual components of the nephron, at both the light microscopic and electron microscopic level.

[1]Laboratory of Experimental Morphology, Division of Nephrology, Hypertension and Transplantation, University of Florida College of Medicine, Gainesville, FL 32610, USA

The results of all of these technologies have underscored the fact that major structural and functional axial heterogeneity exists in the entire renal tubule. This review will focus on specific structural-functional relationships in the distal tubule and collecting duct, since it is in these regions of the renal tubule where the greatest progress has been made in the past few years in correlating structure with function.

Distal Tubule

Structure

Anatomically, the distal tubule consists of three distinct segments: the thick ascending limb (TAL) of Henle's loop, the macula densa, and the distal convoluted tubule (DCT). The macula densa actually represents a specialized segment of the TAL and will not receive further comment in this review. There is an abrupt transition from the TAL to the DCT, approximately 90–100 μm beyond the region of the macula densa. The DCT resembles the TAL by light microscopy, but major differences have been identified between these two segments ultrastructurally and functionally. Both the TAL and the DCT possess extensive invaginations of the basolateral membrane and lateral interdigitations between adjacent cells. Numerous elongate mitochondria in close apposition to the plasma membrane are present within the interdigitating processes, a feature that is common to epithelia involved in active solute transport. The cells of the DCT are generally taller and their nuclei are located in a more apical position than those of the TAL.

Thick Ascending Limb

Based on the location within the kidney, the TAL can be divided into two segments: the medullary and cortical TAL. Structural and functional differences exist between these two segments. Cells forming the inner stripe TAL measure 7–8 μm in height, but the height decreases progressively in the outer medullary and cortical TAL, finally reaching values of 2 μm in the rabbit and 5 μm in the rat [4]. The decrease in height is associated with a decrease both in the relative volume of mitochondria and in the surface area of the basolateral plasma membrane per millimeter of tubule length. However, because of an increase in lateral interdigitations in the apical region of the cells and an increase in the number of luminal surface microprojections, there is a significant increase in the surface area of the apical plasma membrane as the cortical TAL ascends toward its parent glomerulus [4]. The invaginations of the basolateral membrane, which are extensive throughout the TAL, form lateral cell processes that are oriented mainly parallel to the long axis of the cells and perpendicular to the long axis of the tubule. Some years ago we observed with scanning electron microscopy that cells of the medullary TAL had very few apical lateral interdigitations and a relatively smooth luminal surface, while in the cortical TAL apical lateral interdigitations were more prominent and the cells were covered by extensive luminal microprojections [5]. The functional significance of these two cell configurations, if any, remains to be established.

Immunocytochemical studies reveal the presence of Na,K-ATPase [6] and Tamm-Horsfall protein in this region of the nephron. Recent results from our own laboratory demonstrate the presence of a serotonin receptor, 5-HT_{1A}, in the basolateral plasma membrane of the medullary and cortical TAL of both rat and human kidney (J.R. Raymond, C.C. Tisher 1990, unpublished observations).

Distal Convoluted Tubule

This region of the distal tubule corresponds to the "early distal tubule" described in the micropuncture literature. In both the rat and the rabbit the DCT measures 1 mm in length. The cells in this region are considerably taller than those of the TAL, especially the cortical TAL, and in contrast to the cortical TAL, there are no extensive apical lateral interdigitations. Surface microprojections are prominent, especially in the rabbit DCT. Basolateral invaginations of the plasma membrane extend two-thirds to three-fourths of the distance from the base to the apex of the cell and contain elongate mitochondria. Numerous small vesicles are located above the nucleus in the apical region of the cell. In the rat, intercalated cells begin to appear in the terminal portion of the DCT near the connecting segment, a transition region located between the DCT and the collecting duct.

Immunocytochemical studies have identified Na,K-ATPase in this segment of the distal tubule [6], and we have recently observed the presence of the 5-HT_{1A} serotonin receptor in the basolateral membrane of DCT cells (J.R. Raymond, C.C. Tisher 1990, unpublished observations). In contrast to its presence in the TAL, there is no evidence for the presence of Tamm-Horsfall protein in the DCT.

Structural-Functional Relationships

The distal tubule is involved in ion transport, including monovalent ions such as sodium, potassium, and chloride and divalent ions, including calcium and magnesium. There is also evidence for proton and ammonium ion transport in this region of the nephron. Na,K-ATPase provides most of the energy for these transport events and abundant levels of activity of this ATPase have been measured in both the TAL and the DCT.

Thick Ascending Limb

A major function of the TAL is the maintenance of a hypertonic medullary interstitium and the delivery of a dilute tubular fluid to the DCT. This is accomplished by the active reabsorption of NaCl, a process driven by the Na, K-ATPase pump that is located along the basolateral membrane of the cell [6]. Greger et al. [7] have demonstrated that throughout the TAL of the rabbit, NaCl reabsorption is mediated by a sodium-potassium-chloride (Na^+-K^+-2 Cl^-) cotransport mechanism. Hebert et al. [8] have shown that the mouse medullary TAL possesses a similar transport mechanism.

Excellent correlations exist between the morphologic, biochemical, and physiologic characteristics of the TAL. For instance, the basolateral membrane area of the medullary TAL is greatest in the inner stripe [4], and it is in this segment of the TAL that Na,K-ATPase activity is the highest [9]. In addition, isolated perfused tubule studies have revealed a greater capacity for NaCl reabsorption in the medullary than the cortical TAL [10]. The cortical TAL is capable of maintaining a steeper concentration gradient for NaCl, which results in a lower concentration of this solute in the tubular fluid, and a lower fluid osmolality [11]. It is interesting to speculate that the more complicated apical lateral interdigitations between the cells of the cortical TAL, that result in an increase in the luminal surface area, may be responsible in some manner for this physiological characteristic.

Several hormones operating through activation of the adenylate cyclase system influence the function of the TAL. For instance, vasopressin stimulates NaCl reabsorption in the medullary TAL of the mouse [8] and rat [12], but not the rabbit [12], and biochemical studies have shown vasopressin stimulation of adenylate cyclase activity in the mouse and rat medullary TAL, but little in the rabbit. In contrast, there is no evidence for either vasopressin-stimulated NaCl transport or increased adenylate cyclase activity in the cortical TAL. Chronic administration of vasopressin to rats with hereditary hypothalamic diabetes insipidus leads to hypertrophy of the medullary TAL [13], presumably the result of enhanced NaCl transport, while acute vasopressin administration stimulates NaCl reabsorption in isolated perfused medullary TAL segments from the same animals [14]. These data suggest a role for vasopressin in the maintenance of a hypertonic medullary interstitium through regulation of NaCl transport by the medullary TAL.

We have demonstrated a decrease in cell height and an increase in surface area of the basolateral membrane in cells of the medullary TAL in drug-induced hypothyroidism in rats, which could be prevented by treatment with thyroid hormone [15,16]. Since hypothyroidism is associated with a decrease in adenylate cyclase activity, these morphological changes may be the result of impairment in vasopressin-stimulated ion transport.

Distal Convoluted Tubule

This segment of the distal tubule is actively involved in NaCl transport, although the exact transport mechanism, while incompletely understood, probably differs from the Na^+-K^+-$2Cl^-$ cotransport mechanism that is characteristic of the TAL. The morphology of the DCT is greatly affected by the delivery of NaCl to this segment. For instance, Kaissling et al. [17,18] have demonstrated that in rabbits fed a high sodium, low potassium diet there is an increase in the surface area of the basolateral plasma membrane of DCT cells and an increase in Na,K-ATPase activity. Furthermore, chronic administration of a loop diuretic is associated with a significant increase in cell height and basolateral membrane area in rat DCT cells [18]. In our own laboratory we have demonstrated that chronic bumetanide administration in the rat is associated with hypertrophy of the DCT only when animals receive augmented NaCl in their drinking water (K.M. Madsen, W.J. Welch, K. Jin 1990, unpublished observations), thus providing additional evidence that the morphologic and biochemical alterations described previously with a loop diuretic are quite likely due to enhanced NaCl delivery to the DCT.

Connecting Segment

Structure

This region of the renal tubule represents the transition from the DCT to the initial portion of the cortical collecting duct, commonly referred to as the initial collecting tubule (ICT). In superficial nephrons there is a direct one on one transition, whereas in mid-cortical and juxtamedullary nephrons connecting tubules join to form arcades that actually ascend in the cortex before joining an ICT. In most species, including humans and rats, the connecting segment is not well defined because of extensive intermingling of cells from the DCT and the ICT. This gives rise to a very gradual transition, which contrasts with the transition in the rabbit, where there is a well-defined connecting tubule (CNT) composed of two cell types, CNT cells and intercalated cells. In the rat kidney, the transition region is composed of four cell types—DCT cells, CNT cells, intercalated cells, and principal cells. The CNT cell which is characteristic of this region is intermediate in its ultrastructural appearance between the DCT cell and the principal cell and features a combination of basolateral interdigitations and true basal infoldings of the plasma membrane. Mitochondria, though prominent, are less numerous than in the cells of the DCT.

The intercalated cells vary greatly in their appearance in the same species and between species. For instance, in the rabbit CNT a black and a gray form have been described, both of which are rich in mitochondria [19]. The latter, however, possesses more tubulovesicular profiles in the apical cytoplasm. We have described two types of intercalated cells, type A and type B, in this region and throughout the cortical collecting duct of the rat (Fig. 1a, b) [20]. The type A cells in the rat resemble the gray intercalated cells of the rabbit.

Structural-Functional Relationships

High levels of parathyroid hormone—and isoproterenol-dependent adenylate cyclase activity—have been measured in the rabbit CNT [2], but there is no stimulation of this second messenger by vasopressin, nor is there any physiologic or morphologic evidence for increased water permeability in response to this hormone [21].

Both morphologic and physiologic data have identified a role in potassium secretion for the connecting segment [22,23] which, at least in part, is under the control of mineralocorticoids. Potassium secretion is decreased in the superficial distal nephron (which includes the DCT, the connecting segment, and the ICT) in adrenalectomized rats [24], and morphologic studies performed in the same segments reveal a decrease in the surface area of the basolateral membrane of principal cells of the ICT, which is a site of Na,K-ATPase activity [25]. The chronic administration of aldosterone can prevent the decrease in basolateral membrane area and larger doses will actually increase the surface area of the basolateral membrane of principal cells. Potassium loading, which stimulates aldosterone secretion, exerts a similar effect in both rats and rabbits. Potassium secretion in the late distal tubule (including the connecting segment and ICT) is increased and the surface area of the basolateral membrane is also increased in both principal cells and CNT cells [17,26].

Cortical Collecting Duct

Structure

Generally we divide the cortical collecting duct (CCD) into two major segments—the ICT and the medullary ray portion. Taken together, the connecting segment and the ICT of superficial nephrons constitute the so-called "late" distal tubule, which has

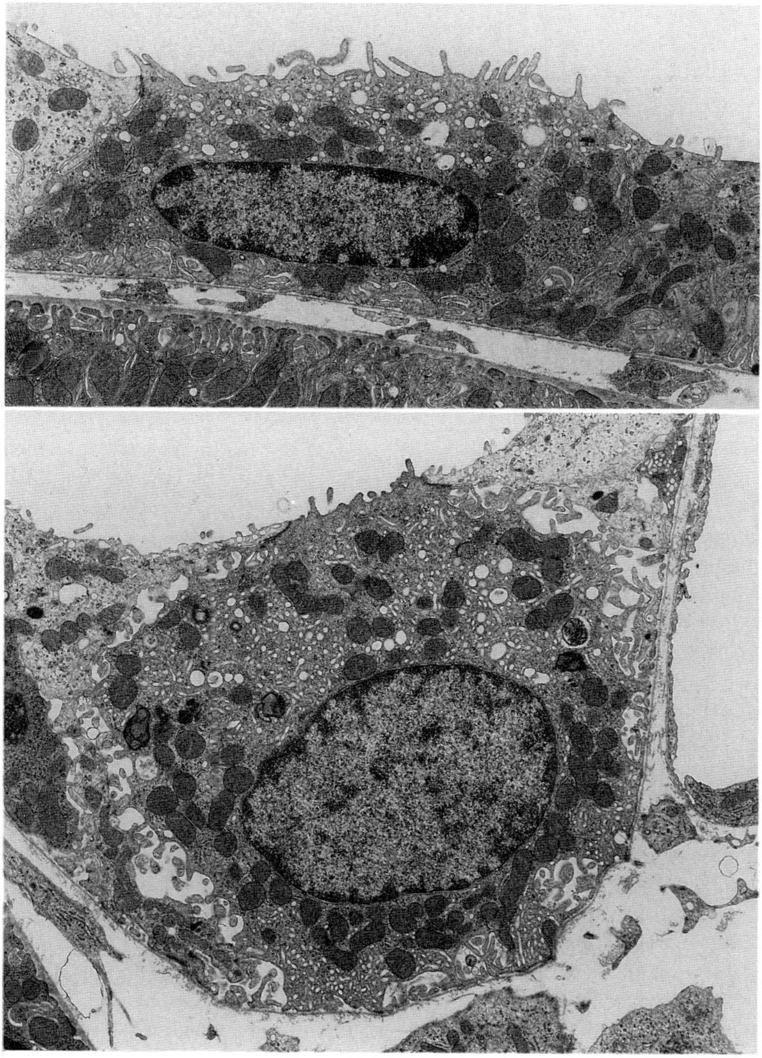

Fig. 1a,b. Electron micrographs from rat CCD illustrating the differences in structure of: **a** the type A intercalated cell, × 6370 and **b** the type B intercalated cell, × 5400

been studied extensively by renal micropuncturists. The medullary ray portion of the CCD is commonly used in isolated perfused tubule experiments. This region contains both intercalated cells, which in the rat and rabbit contribute from 37% to 39% of the total cell population, and principal cells. No major differences in the overall morphology of the principal cell have been reported to exist in the various regions of the CCD. However, it has become increasingly evident that structural as well as functional heterogeneity exists in the intercalated cells in the CCD.

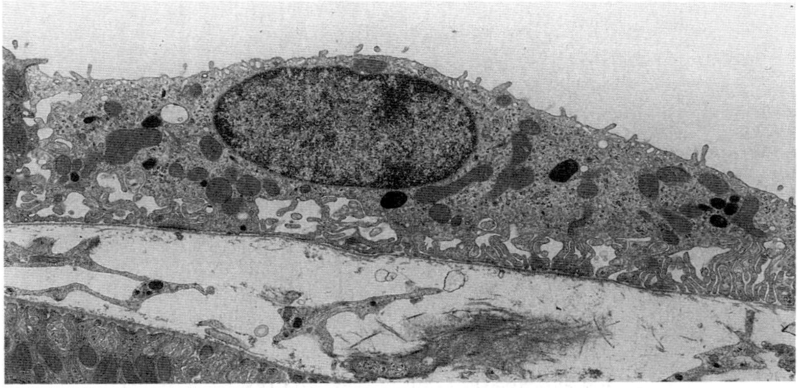

Fig. 2. Electron micrograph from rat CCD depicting the characteristic appearance of a principal cell, × 5200

Principal cells exhibit extensive infoldings of the basal plasma membrane, but lack lateral interdigitations (Fig. 2). The cells contain relatively few mitochondria, which are scattered randomly through a light staining cytoplasm. The luminal surface is covered with a few blunt microvilli and has a single centrally-positioned cilium.

Studies from our laboratory [20] and by other investigators [19] have identified at least two distinct populations of intercalated cells throughout the CCD. Type A intercalated cells, which are believed to be involved in proton secretion, are more common in the early portion of the ICT, whereas type B intercalated cells increase in number as the collecting duct approaches the medullary ray. With scanning electron microscopy it has been possible to identify distinct surface patterns for each cell type (Fig. 3). Type A cells are generally covered with microplicae, while type B cells exhibit microvilli. Microplicae are especially prominent in those cells located in the connecting segment and early ICT, but tend to be less extensive on type A cells in the medullary ray. In the rabbit, some intercalated cells have either microplicae or microvilli, but the majority exhibit both.

Transmission electron microscopy has revealed distinct differences in the appearance of these two forms of intercalated cells in the CCD (Fig. 1a, b) [20]. Type A cells have a cytoplasm that is rich in mitochondria and polyribosomes. Tubulovesicular membrane structures are extensive in the apical cytoplasm. Prominent studs are present on the cytoplasmic surface of many of the tubulovesicular structures and along the apical, but not the basolateral plasma membrane. The cytoplasm of the type B cells is generally more electron dense and, in addition to an extensive population of polyribosomes and mitochondria, contains numerous vesicular structures throughout the cell. In contrast to type A cells, the vesicles in these cells are generally smooth on the cytoplasmic surface and lack studs. Occasional studs have been observed on the cytoplasmic surface of the basolateral, but not the apical plasma, membrane of type B intercalated cells.

Immunocytochemical studies from our laboratory [27] and by other investigators have revealed striking differences between type A and type B intercalated cells in the CCD. For instance, we have demonstrated that antibodies against band 3 protein, an

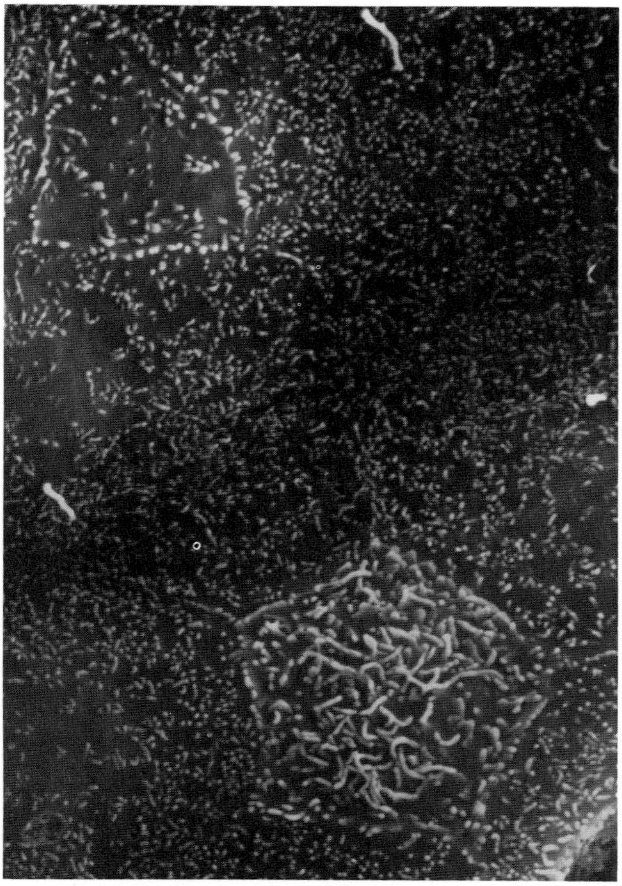

Fig. 3. Scanning electron micrograph from rat CCD illustrating the luminal surface of a type B intercalated cell (*upper left*) and a type A intercalated cell (*lower right*). Principal cells are covered with short, blunt microvilli and possess a single centrally-positioned cilium, × 9000

anion transporter involved in HCO_3-Cl exchange, bind to the basolateral membrane of type A cells (Fig. 4), but fail to label type B cells. Recently, it has been observed that antibodies against H-ATPase bind to tubulovesicular structures and the apical plasma membrane of type A cells (Fig. 5a) and to cytoplasmic vesicles and the basolateral plasma membrane of type B cells (Fig. 5b) [28].

Both types of intercalated cells in the rat and the rabbit have been found to possess high levels of carbonic anhydrase activity when subjected to the appropriate immunocytochemical procedures [29]. However, we have demonstrated recently that major differences do exist in the amount and distribution of carbonic anhydrase II immunoreactivity between these two populations of intercalated cells [30]. When we used a rabbit polyclonal antibody directed against mouse erythrocyte carbonic anhydrase II in combination with a horseradish peroxidase detection procedure, immuno-

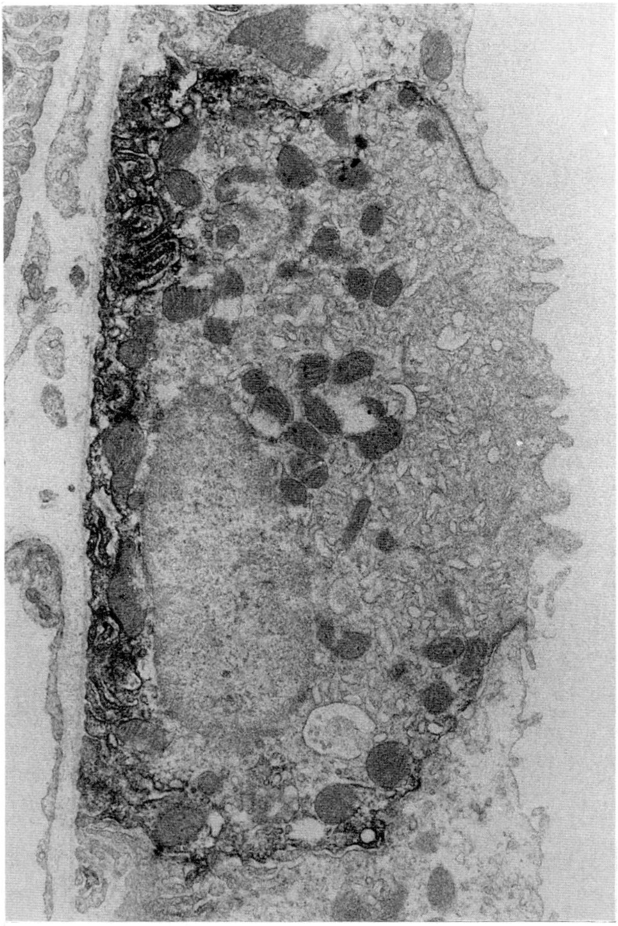

Fig. 4. Electron micrograph of type A intercalated cell from rat CCD, depicting localization of antibodies to band 3 protein along the basolateral plasma membrane of a type A intercalated cell, using an immunoperoxidase technique, × 12740

staining was strikingly more pronounced in type A than in type B cells (Fig. 6). In the former, the staining was especially prominent over the apical region, whereas type B cells had weak diffuse staining throughout the cytoplasm. In addition, the densely staining A cells had a spider-like cell configuration, while the type B cells were round or ovoid in appearance. Thus, this immunocytochemical reaction provides an excellent marker to separate type A from type B intercalated cells by both light and electron microscopy in the rat. The findings provide additional evidence that at least two distinct populations of intercalated cells exist in the CCD, populations that are morphologically, as well as functionally, distinct.

Wingo et al. [31], working in our laboratory, have recently published immunocytochemical evidence for the presence of H-K-ATPase activity in the intercalated

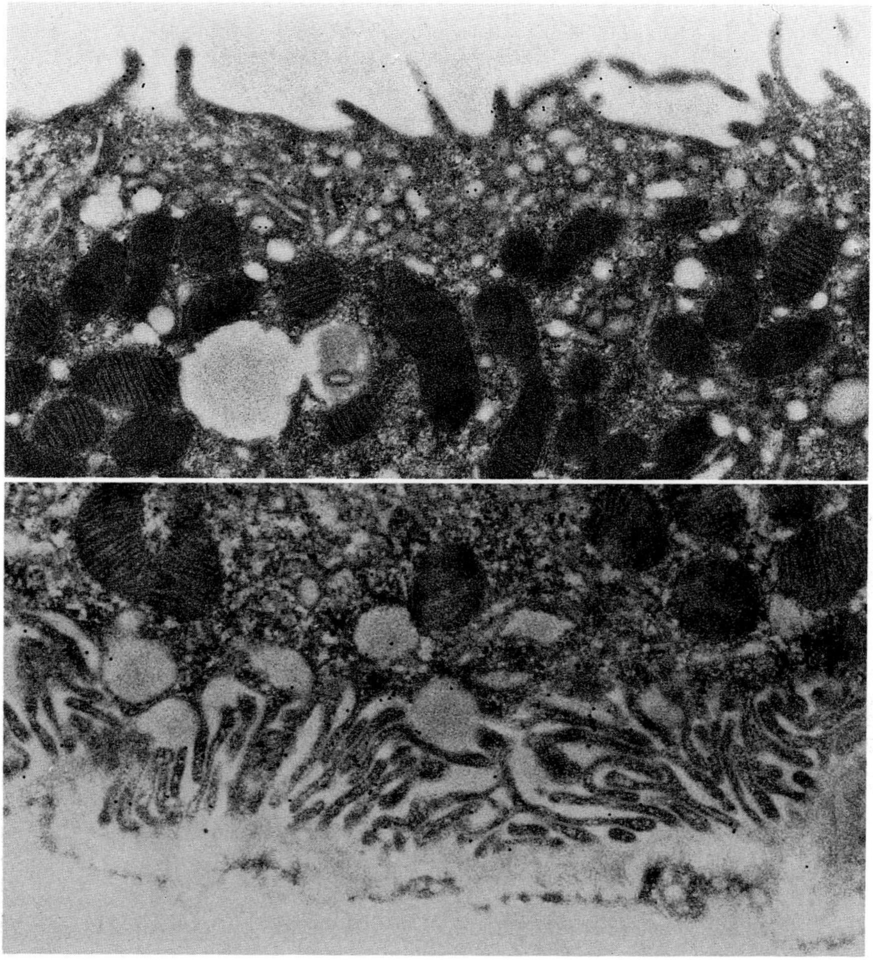

Fig. 5a,b. Electron micrographs from rat CCD depicting localization of antibodies against H^+-ATPase: **a** along the luminal membrane and apical tubulovesicles in a type A intercalated cell, × 21060 and **b** along the basolateral membrane of a type B intercalated cell, × 19840

cells of the CCD and the outer medullary collecting duct (OMCD) of the rat and rabbit. Using a mouse monoclonal antibody against hog gastric H-K-ATPase that did not cross react with either Na,K-ATPase or H-ATPase, Wingo and coworkers found diffuse cytoplasmic staining, indicative of H-K-ATPase immunoreactivity, to be present in intercalated cells in the CCD and OMCD of rat and rabbit. In all segments except the rat CCD, the percentage of H-K-ATPase immunoreactive cells corresponded to the percentage of intercalated cells. However, in the rat, only 23% of the cells were reactive, which is less than the percentage of intercalated cells in this segment of the collecting duct. It is possible that, in the rat, only type A intercalated cells

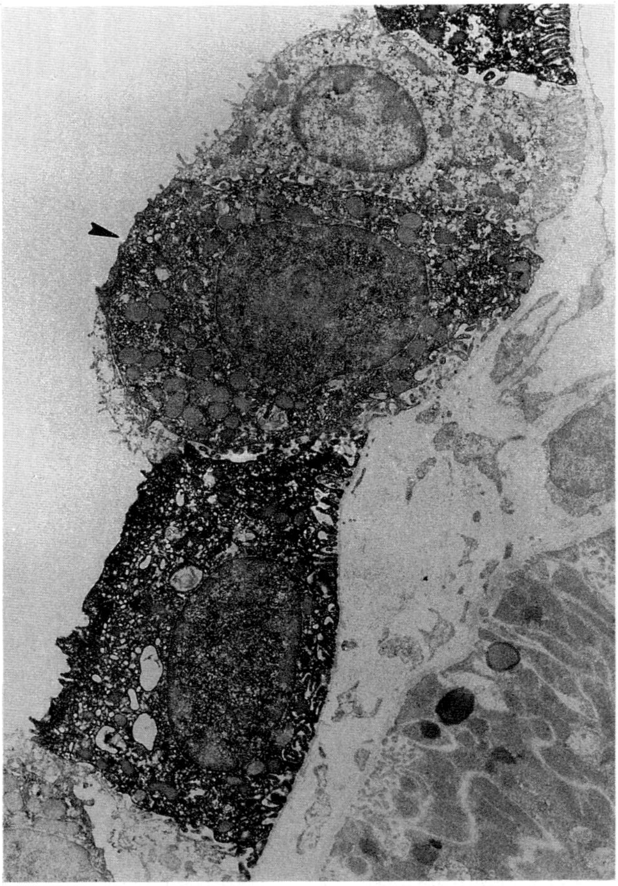

Fig. 6. Electron micrograph of rat CCD, depicting the localization of carbonic anhydrase II immunoreactivity in intercalated cells. Note that the intensity of staining is much greater in type A than in type B (*arrowhead*) cells. The principal cells have only faint staining for carbonic anhydrase II immunoreactivity, × 5250

possess H-K-ATPase activity, or that some intercalated cells did not have sufficient activity to be detected by the immunocytochemical method that was employed.

Structural-Functional Relationships

There is both structural and functional evidence that the ICT is involved in potassium secretion [23], hydrogen ion secretion, and vasopressin-induced water reabsorption. The ICT behaves in a manner similar to that of the connecting segment with respect to potassium secretion. Stanton and co-workers [26] have provided convincing evidence that chronic potassium loading, which stimulates aldosterone secretion, is associated with both an increase in potassium secretion in the so-called "late" distal tubule and with proliferation of the basolateral membrane of principal cells in the ICT. Moreover, in adrenalectomized rats these same cells exhibit a decrease in surface area of the basolateral membrane [25], and potassium secretion is impaired [24]. These defects can be either reversed or prevented with aldosterone administration [24,25]. Thus, the principal cells appear to be responsible for mineralocorticoid-dependent potassium secretion in the ICT.

Hydrogen ion secretion also appears to be a function of the ICT. Evidence from micropuncture studies has documented the presence of proton secretion in superficial distal tubules of acid-loaded rats [32]. We have observed a striking increase in the surface density of type A intercalated cells in both the ICT and the medullary ray portion of the CCD of the rat with acute respiratory acidosis [20].

The entire collecting duct, including the ICT, plays an important role in urine dilution and concentration. With vasopressin stimulation the apical membrane of the principal cells becomes permeable to water, due to the insertion of water channels [33]. Early morphologic studies from our laboratory [34] demonstrated that vasopressin-induced osmotic water reabsorption is associated with swelling of the principal cells and with intercellular space dilatation. In the absence of the hormone these morphologic features of transepithelial water flow are not observed.

Many of the structural-functional relationships described in the ICT are also present in the CCD. For instance, physiologic studies performed in the isolated perfused rabbit CCD have demonstrated that mineralocorticoids stimulate potassium secretion [35]. Biochemical studies have documented increased levels of Na,K-ATPase activity following mineralocorticoid administration in the CCD of both the rat [36] and the rabbit [3]. Morphologists have demonstrated a significant increase in the surface area of the basolateral plasma membrane of principal cells in the CCD of rabbits treated with deoxycorticosterone acetate [37] or fed a diet high in potassium and low in sodium [17]. In addition, optical and microelectrode studies have demonstrated that principal cells, but not intercalated cells, possess a barium-sensitive potassium conductance in the luminal membrane, thus providing further evidence that the principal cell is involved in potassium secretion [38,39]. These morphologic, physiologic, and biochemical data all suggest that the principal cells in the CCD are responsible for mineralocorticoid-stimulated potassium secretion in association with sodium reabsorption.

As described briefly in an earlier section, there is considerable structural and functional evidence that type A intercalated cells are involved in proton and bicarbonate transport. Depending on the physiologic condition of the animal, the CCD can either reabsorb or secrete bicarbonate. Using the isolated perfused tubule technique it has been found that the rabbit CCD dissected from normal and acid-loaded rabbits reabsorbs bicarbonate [40,41]. In contrast, CCD from bicarbonate-loaded rabbits [42] or rabbits treated with deoxycorticosterone [43] secretes bicarbonate. Furthermore, CCD from rats receiving an ammonium chloride load reabsorbs bicarbonate, while CCD dissected from rats receiving either deoxycorticosterone [44] or a bicarbonate load [45] secretes bicarbonate.

Morphologic studies performed in our laboratory by Verlander et al. [20] have demonstrated that, in the rat CCD, type A intercalated cells respond to acute respiratory acidosis with an increase in the apical or luminal membrane area, secondary to fusion of tubulovesicular structures, normally located in the apical cell cytoplasm, with the luminal plasma membrane. We and others [28], using immunocytochemical

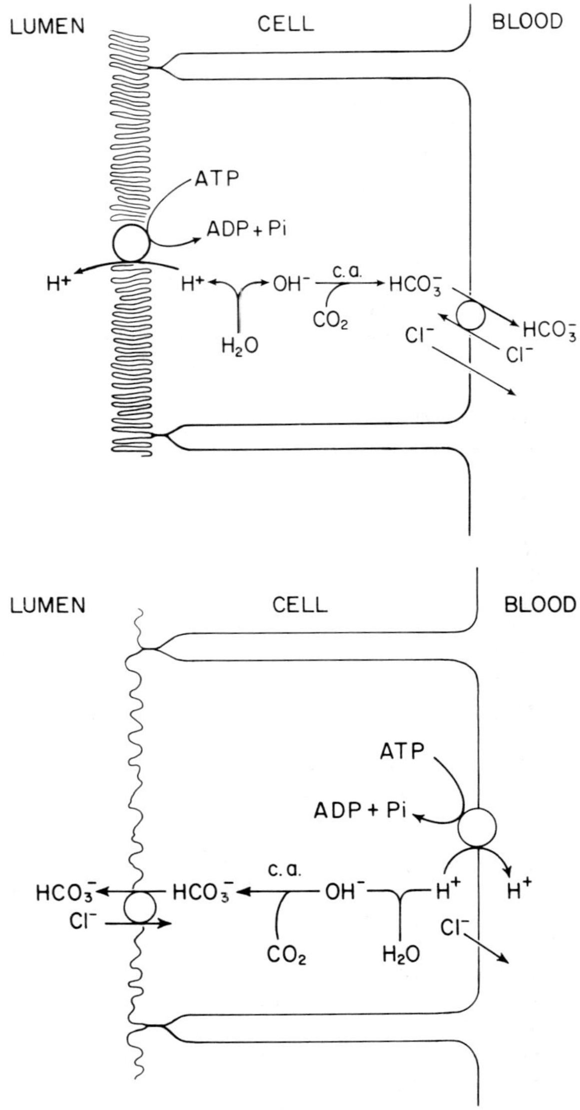

a

b

Fig. 7a,b. Functional characteristics of: **a** type A intercalated cell and **b** type B intercalated cell in the rat CCD. c.a., carbonic anhydrase

techniques, have demonstrated the presence of an H-ATPase in the tubulovesicular structures, and it is this transporter that is believed to be inserted into the luminal membrane of the type A intercalated cell in response to the need to secrete protons. There is also histochemical and immunocytochemical evidence for the presence of carbonic anhydrase II throughout the cytoplasm of both types of intercalated cells

[29,30,46]. We [27] and other investigators [47] have demonstrated that antibodies against erythrocyte band 3 protein, an anion transporter responsible for Cl-HCO_3 exchange, are located along the basolateral plasma membrane of type A intercalated cells. Thus, type A cells possess a Cl-HCO_3 exchanger to permit bicarbonate reabsorption, an H-ATPase to effect secretion of protons at the luminal surface, and carbonic anhydrase activity within the cytoplasm to catalyze the hydration of CO_2 to form hydroxyl ions and protons. This mechanism for proton secretion and bicarbonate reabsorption in the type A cells is illustrated in Fig. 7a.

Evidence is accumulating that type B intercalated cells are involved in bicarbonate secretion. As noted in an earlier section, CCD from both rats and rabbits secretes bicarbonate, following a bicarbonate load [42,45] or deoxycorticosterone treatment [43,44]. Functional studies employing fluorescent pH-sensitive probes have provided evidence for a Cl-HCO_3 exchange process across the luminal plasma membrane of peanut lectin-positive cells in the rabbit CCD, which correspond to type B intercalated cells in the rat. All intercalated cells in the rat and rabbit, including type B cells, are immunoreactive for carbonic anhydrase II [30]. There is additional immunocytochemical evidence for the presence of H-ATPase activity distributed diffusely in the cytoplasm or in the basal region of the type B cells. We have preliminary evidence from our laboratory suggesting that stimulation of bicarbonate secretion leads to an increase in both the volume of B cells and their basolateral plasma membrane area [48]. We have also observed that the type B intercalated cells decrease in size in chronic metabolic acidosis. Thus, type B cells appear to play a significant role in regulating bicarbonate secretion under the appropriate experimental conditions, as illustrated in Fig. 7b.

The presence of H-K-ATPase immunoreactivity in the rat and rabbit CCD [31] raises the distinct possibility that intercalated cells are also involved in the reabsorption of potassium in exchange for protons. This possibility will be explored in greater detail in the section on the OMCD that follows.

Outer Medullary Collecting Duct

Structure

The OMCD has two distinct segments, the $OMCD_o$, located in the outer stripe and the $OMCD_i$, located in the inner stripe of the outer medulla. In both segments in the rat, intercalated cells constitute approximately 36%–40% of the cells, with the percentage remaining representing principal cells [49]. In the rabbit, however, there is a gradual decrease in the number of intercalated cells along the entire OMCD, where they represent approximately 18% of the total cell population [50]. In the rat, the overwhelming majority of intercalated cells in the outer stripe, and essentially all intercalated cells in the inner stripe, resemble the type A cells in the CCD. Tubulovesicular membrane structures, often possessing studs on their cytoplasmic surface, are extensive throughout the apical cytoplasm, and micro-projections, so-called microplicae that are appreciated best with scanning electron microscopy, are extensive on the luminal membrane surface. The cytoplasmic surface of the luminal plasma membrane is, also, often studded. Rod-shaped particles have been described with freeze-fracture in the luminal membrane of these cells [51], but their relationship, if any, to the studs on the cytoplasmic side of the apical cell membrane remains unclear.

The principal cells in the OMCD resemble those located in the CCD, although some differences have been described. The basal infoldings of the former are less extensive and they have fewer organelles.

Immunocytochemical studies have documented that antibodies against band 3 protein, the anion transporter involved in Cl-HCO_3 exchange, bind along the basolateral membrane of all intercalated cells in the rat and rabbit OMCD. Antibodies against H-ATPase bind to tubulovesicular structures and to the apical membrane of these same intercalated cells [46], which are also positive for carbonic anhydrase II immunoreactivity. Finally, as noted in an earlier section, Wingo et al. [31] have demonstrated H-K-ATPase immunoreactivity in all intercalated cells in the OMCD of both the rat and the rabbit.

Structural-Functional Relationships

Physiologic, biochemical, and morphologic studies all provide evidence that the OMCD is a major site of proton secretion in the distal nephron. Proton secretion, measured as bicarbonate reabsorption, is well documented in the isolated perfused $OMCD_i$ dissected from the kidneys of both normal and acidotic rabbits [41]. This electrogenic sodium-independent process that is mineralocorticoid-sensitive [52] resembles the acidification process described in the turtle urinary bladder. Studies in both the turtle urinary bladder [53] and the bovine renal medulla [54] have led to isolation of an H-ATPase believed to be responsible for this electrogenic hydrogen-translocating process. Studies employing a fluorescent pH-sensitive dye, performed first in the turtle urinary bladder [55] and later in the rabbit $OMCD_i$ [56], demonstrated that an increase in the ambient carbon dioxide caused a simultaneous increase in hydrogen ion secretion and release of fluorescent vesicle contents from mitochondria-rich and intercalated cells, respectively. Based on the findings in the turtle, it was suggested that proton secretion is regulated by exocytotic insertion of H-ATPase into the luminal membrane of the mitochondria-rich cell [55]. Subsequent morphologic data supported this hypothesis by demonstrating that stimulation of proton secretion in the turtle urinary bladder caused an increase in surface area of the luminal membrane and a decrease in the volume density of apical vesicles in mitochondria-rich cells [57]. Studies from our own laboratory [58,59] demonstrated significant ultrastructural changes in OMCD intercalated cells of rats with either acute respiratory acidosis or chronic metabolic acidosis, suggesting that the intercalated cells are responsible for proton secretion in the OMCD. These morphologic changes with acidosis included an increase in the surface density and surface area of the luminal plasma membrane and a simultaneous decrease in the number of tubulovesicular membrane profiles in the apical cell region. The stud-like structures located on the cytoplasmic surface of the tubulovesicular profiles were transferred to the cytoplasmic surface of the luminal membranes. On the basis of these observations, we suggested that membrane containing a proton pump was inserted into the luminal membrane when hydrogen ion secretion was stimulated. Immunocytochemical studies by Brown et al. [28], using the immunogold technique, were reproduced later in our own laboratory and have demonstrated H-ATPase immunoreactivity within the tubulovesicular structures and along the luminal cell membrane of intercalated cells. Antibodies against band 3 protein, the Cl-HCO_3 exchanger, have been demonstrated along the basolateral membrane of these same cells [27]. As noted in an earlier section, the intercalated cells also possess a high level of immunoreactivity to carbonic anhydrase II [30]. Thus, intercalated cells in the OMCD resemble the type A cells in the CCD and appear capable of secreting protons.

Biochemical, physiologic, and morphologic studies have provided evidence for the presence of an H-K-ATPase in the CCD and OMCD, which is believed to be involved in the reabsorption of potassium in exchange for protons. K-ATPase activity that is ouabain-insensitive, but inhibited by omeprazole and SCH 28080 has been described in individual segments of the CCD and OMCD in both rat [60] and rabbit [60,61]. Wingo [62] has provided physiologic evidence for active potassium reabsorption and proton secretion that is also inhibited by omeprazole, a known inhibitor of gastric H-K-ATPase, in the isolated OMCD dissected from rabbits on a potassium restricted diet. Immunocytochemical studies by Wingo et al. [31] have identified H-K-ATPase immunoreactivity in all intercalated cells in the OMCD of both the rat and the rabbit. Taken together, these data provide strong support for an additional mechanism for acid secretion by the collecting duct, in which protons are exchanged for potassium in the intercalated cell, a process similar to that present in the parietal cell of the gastric mucosa.

Acknowledgments. The authors acknowledge the technical assistance of James K. Cannon, Frederick Kopp, and Wendy L. Wilber, and the secretarial support of Deborah S. Malis. The authors also thank Dr. W. Fischlschweiger, Director of the Electron Microscope Facility of the College of Dentistry at the University of Florida, where the electron microscope studies were performed.

This work was supported, in part, by National Institutes of Health Grant DK-28330.

References

1. Burg MB, Grantham J, Abramow M, Orloff J (1966) Preparation and study of fragments of single rabbit nephrons. Am J Physiol 210:1293–1298
2. Morel F (1981) Sites of hormone action in the mammalian nephron. Am J Physiol 240: F159–F164
3. Garg LC, Knepper MA, Burg MB (1981) Mineralocorticoid effects of Na-K-ATPase in individual nephron segments. Am J Physiol 240:F536–F544
4. Kone BC, Madsen KM, Tisher CC (1984) Ultrastructure of the thick ascending limb of Henle in the rat kidney. Am J Anat 171:217–226
5. Allen F, Tisher CC (1976) Morphology of the ascending thick limb of Henle. Kidney Int 9:8–22
6. Kashgarian M, Biemesderfer D, Caplan M, Forbus B (1985) Monoclonal antibody to Na,K-ATPase: immunocytochemical localization along nephron segments. Kidney Int 28:899–913
7. Greger R, Schlatter E, Lang F (1983) Evidence for electroneutral sodium chloride cotransport in the cortical thick ascending limb of Henle's loop of rabbit kidney. Pflugers Arch 396:308–314
8. Hebert SC, Culpepper RM, Andreoli TE (1981) NaCl transport in mouse medullary thick ascending limbs. I. Functional nephron heterogeneity and ADH-stimulated NaCl cotransport. Am J Physiol 241:F412–F431
9. Garg LC, Mackie S, Tisher CC (1982) Effect of low potassium diet on Na^+-K^+-ATPase in rat nephron segments. Pflugers Arch 394:113–117

10. Rocha AS, Kokko JP (1973) Sodium chloride and water transport in the medullary thick ascending limb of Henle. Evidence for active chloride transport. J Clin Invest 54:612–623
11. Burg MB, Green N (1973) Function of the thick ascending limb of Henle's loop. Am J Physiol 224:659–668
12. Sasaki S, Imai M (1980) Effects of vasopressin on water and NaCl transport across the in vitro perfused medullary thick ascending limb of Henle's loop of mouse, rat, and rabbit kidneys. Pflugers Arch 383:215–221
13. Bouby N, Bankir L, Thinh-Trang-Tan MM, Minuth WW, Kriz W (1985) Selective ADH-induced hypertrophy of the medullary thick ascending limb in Brattleboro rats. Kidney Int 28:456–466
14. Work J, Galla JH, Booker B, Schafer JA, Luke R (1985) Effect of ADH on chloride reabsorption in the loop of Henle of Brattleboro rats. Am J Physiol 249:F698–F703
15. Davis RG, Madsen KM, Fregly MJ, Tisher CC (1983) Kidney structure in hypothyroidism. Am J Pathol 113:41–49
16. Bentley AG, Madsen KM, Davis RG, Tisher CC (1985) Response of the medullary thick ascending limb to hypothyroidism in the rat. Am J Pathol 120:215–221
17. Kaissling B, LeHir M (1982) Distal tubular segments of the rabbit kidney after adaptation to altered Na- and K-intake. I. Structural changes. Cell Tissue Res 224:469–492
18. Kaissling B, Bachmann S, Kriz W (1985) Structural adaptation of the distal convoluted tubule to prolonged furosemide treatment. Am J Physiol 248:F374–F381
19. Kaissling B, Kriz W (1979) Structural analysis of the rabbit kidney. Adv Anat Embryol Cell Biol 56:1–123
20. Verlander JW, Madsen KM, Tisher CC (1987) Effect of acute respiratory acidosis on two populations of intercalated cells in the rat cortical collecting duct. Am J Physiol 253:F1142–F1156
21. Imai M (1979) The connecting tubule: a functional subdivision of the rabbit distal nephron segments. Kidney Int 15:346–356
22. Kaissling B (1982) Structural aspects of adaptive changes in renal electrolyte excretion. Am J Physiol 243:F211–F226
23. Wright FS, Giebisch G (1978) Renal potassium transport: contributions of individual nephron segments and populations. Am J Physiol 235:F515–F527
24. Field MJ, Stanton BA, Giebisch GH (1984) Differential acute effects of aldosterone, dexamethasone, and hyperkalemia on distal tubular potassium secretion in the rat kidney. J Clin Invest 74:1792–1802
25. Stanton B, Janzen A, Klein-Robbenhaar G, De Fronzo R, Giebisch G, Wade J (1985) Ultrastructure of rat initial collecting tubule. Effect of adrenal corticosteroid treatment. J Clin Invest 75:1327–1334
26. Stanton BA, Biemesderfer D, Wade JB, Giebisch G (1981) Structural and functional study of the rat distal nephron: effects of potassium adaptation and depletion. Kidney Int 19:36–48
27. Verlander JW, Madsen KM, Low PS, Allen DP, Tisher CC (1988) Immunocytochemical localization of band 3 protein in the rat collecting duct. Am J Physiol 255:F115–F125
28. Brown D, Hirsch S, Gluck S (1988) An H^+-ATPase in opposite plasma membrane domains in kidney epithelial cell subpopulations. Nature 331:622–624
29. Brown D, Kumpulainen T, Roth J, Orci L (1983) Immunohistochemical localization of carbonic anhydrase in postnatal and adult rat kidney. Am J Physiol 245:F110–F118
30. Kim J, Tisher CC, Linser PJ, Madsen KM (1990) Ultrastructural localization of carbonic anhydrase II in subpopulations of intercalated cells of the rat kidney. J Am Soc Nephrol 1:245–256
31. Wingo CS, Madsen KM, Smolka A, Tisher CC (1990) H-K-ATPase immunoreactivity in cortical and outer medullary collecting duct. Kidney Int 38:985–990
32. Lucci MS, Pucacco LR, Carter NW, DuBose TD (1982) Evaluation of bicarbonate transport in rat distal tubule: effects of acid-base status. Am J Physiol 243:F335–F341

33. Strange K, Willingham MC, Handler JS, Harris HW, Jr (1988) Apical membrane endocytosis via coated pits is stimulated by removal of antidiuretic hormone from isolated, perfused rabbit cortical collecting tubule. J Membr Biol 103:17–28
34. Woodhall PB, Tisher CC (1973) Response of the distal tubule and cortical collecting duct to vasopressin in the rat. J Clin Invest 52:3095–3108
35. O'Neil RG, Helman SI (1977) Transport characteristics of renal collecting tubules: influences of DOCA and diet. Am J Physiol 233:F544–F558
36. Mujais SK, Chekal MA, Jones WJ, Hayslett JP, Katz AI (1984) Regulation of renal Na-K-ATPase in the rat: role of the natural mineralo- and glucocorticoid hormones. J Clin Invest 73:13–19
37. Wade JB, O'Neil RG, Pryor JL, Boulpaep EL (1979) Modulation of cell membrane area in renal collecting tubules by corticosteroid hormones. J Cell Biol 81:439–445
38. O'Neil RG, Hayhurst RA (1985) Functional differentiation of cell types of cortical collecting duct. Am J Physiol 248:F449–F453
39. Muto S, Giebisch G, Sansom S (1987) Effects of adrenalectomy on CCD: evidence for differential response of two cell types. Am J Physiol 253:F742–F752
40. McKinney TD, Burg MB (1978) Bicarbonate absorption by rabbit cortical collecting tubules in vitro. Am J Physiol 234:F141–F145
41. Lombard WE, Jacobson HR, Kokko JP (1983) Bicarbonate transport in cortical and outer medullary collecting tubules. Am J Physiol 244:F289–F296
42. McKinney TD, Burg MB (1978) Bicarbonate secretion by rabbit cortical collecting tubules in vitro. J Clin Invest 61:1421–1427
43. Star RA, Burg MB, Knepper MA (1985) Bicarbonate secretion by rabbit cortical collecting ducts. Role of chloride/bicarbonate exchange. J Clin Invest 76:1123–1130
44. Knepper MA, Good DW, Burg MB (1985) Ammonia and bicarbonate transport by rat cortical collecting ducts perfused in vitro. Am J Physiol 249:F870–F877
45. Atkins JL, Burg MB (1985) Bicarbonate transport by isolated perfused rat collecting ducts. Am J Physiol 249:F485–F489
46. Lonnerholm G, Ridderstrale Y (1980) Intracellular distribution of carbonic anhydrase in the rat kidney. Kidney Int 17:162–174
47. Schuster VL, Bonsib SM, Jennings ML (1986) Two types of collecting duct mitochondria-rich (intercalated) cells: lectin and band 3 cytochemistry. Am J Physiol 251:C347–C355
48. Tisher CC, Verlander JW, Madsen KM, Galla JH, Luke RG, Bonduris D (1989) Morphological findings in rat collecting duct during chloride-depletion metabolic alkalosis. Kidney Int 35:464A
49. Hansen GP, Tisher CC, Robinson RR (1980) Response of the collecting duct to disturbances of acid-base and potassium balance. Kidney Int 17:326–337
50. Le Furgey A, Tisher CC (1979) Morphology of rabbit collecting duct. Am J Anat 155:111–124
51. Stetson DL, Wade JB, Giebisch G (1980) Morphologic alterations in the rat medullary collecting duct following potassium depletion. Kidney Int 17:45–56
52. Stone DK, Seldin DW, Kokko JP, Jacobson HR (1983) Mineralocorticoid modulation of rabbit medullary collecting duct acidification. A sodium-independent effect. J Clin Invest 72:77–83
53. Gluck S, Kelly S, Al-Awqati Q (1982) The proton-translocating ATPase responsible for urinary acidification. J Biol Chem 257:9230–9233
54. Gluck S, Al Awqati Q (1984) An electrogenic proton-translocating adenosine triphosphatase from bovine kidney medulla. J Clin Invest 73:1704–1710
55. Gluck S, Cannon C, Al-Awqati Q (1982) Exocytosis regulates urinary acidification in turtle bladder by rapid insertion of H^+ pumps into the luminal membrane. Proc Natl Acad Sci USA 79:4327–4331
56. Schwartz GJ, Al-Awqati Q (1985) Carbon dioxide causes exocytosis of vesicles containing H^+ pumps in isolated perfused proximal and collecting tubules. J Clin Invest 75:1638–1644

57. Stetson DL, Steinmetz PR (1983) Role of membrane fusion in CO_2 stimulation of proton secretion by turtle bladder. Am J Physiol 245:C113–C120
58. Madsen KM, Tisher CC (1983) Cellular response to acute respiratory acidosis in rat medullary collecting ducts. Am J Physiol 245:F670–F679
59. Madsen KM, Tisher CC (1984) Response of intercalated cells of rat outer medullary collecting duct to chronic metabolic acidosis. Lab Invest 51:268–276
60. Doucet A, Marsy S (1987) Characterization of K-ATPase activity in distal nephron: stimulation by potassium depletion. Am J Physiol 253:F418–F423
61. Garg LC, Narang N (1988) Ouabain-insensitive K-adenosine triphosphatase in distal nephron segments of the rabbit. J Clin Invest 81:1204–1208
62. Wingo CS (1989) Active proton secretion and potassium absorption in the rabbit outer medullary collecting duct: functional evidence for H-K-ATPase. J Clin Invest 84:361–365

Function of Thin Segments of Henle's Loop

MASASHI IMAI, KOJI YOSHITOMI, YOSHIAKI KONDO,
JUNICHI TANIGUCHI, CHIZUKO KOSEKI, TAISUKE ISOZAKI,
KAORU TABEI, and SHIGERU KOYAMA

Chair: Donald W. Seldin

Function of Thin Segments of Henle's Loop

Masashi Imai[1], Koji Yoshitomi[1], Yoshiaki Kondo[2], Junichi Taniguchi[3], Chizuko Koseki[3], Taisuke Isozaki[4], Kaoru Tabei[1], and Shigeru Koyama[1]

Introduction

It is well known that the renal medulla plays an important role in the generation of concentrated urine, which is critical in the maintenance of body fluid osmolality. Since the proposal of the operation of countercurrent systems in the renal medulla by Kuhn and his associates [1–3], it has been widely accepted that the loop structures of the nephron in the renal medulla are essential for the generation and maintenance of a steep osmotic gradient along the axis of the renal medulla. However, the detailed mechanisms by which a steep osmotic gradient is generated by the countercurrent multiplication system remain to be established.

Micropuncture studies on exposed renal papilla of rodents have established essential characteristics of the loop of Henle [4]. The luminal fluid in the descending limb of Henle's loop is concentrated as it flows down toward the papillary tip, whereas the fluid in the ascending limb is diluted as it flows upward. The observations that the fluid in the ascending limb is relatively hypotonic as compared to that in the descending limb [5] are compatible with the view that the countercurrent multiplication system operates in the loop of Henle. Although the in vitro microperfusion studies of thin loop segments in renal papillary slices shed light on the membrane properties of the thin loop segments [6], detailed mechanisms of water and ion transport are unknown.

The in vitro microperfusion technique developed by Burg et al. [7] provides a useful tool with which to examine detailed transport properties across those nephron segments which are inaccessible by conventional micropuncture techniques. More

[1]Department of Pharmacology, Jichi Medical School, Minamikawachi, Kawachi, Tochigi, 329-04 Japan
[2]Department of Pediatrics, Tohoku University, Sendai 980, Japan
[3]Departments of Molecular Physiology and Cell Biology, National Cardiovascular Center, Osaka, 565 Japan
[4]Department of Internal Medicine, Hamamatsu University School of Medicine, Hamamatsu, 431-31 Japan

recently, technical advances have allowed us to apply intracellular impalement of microelectrodes or fluorescent dye technique on the in vitro microperfused thin loop segments, thereby providing information on the cell membrane properties of these segments.

In addition to operating the urine concentrating mechanism, the renal medulla also contributes to renal handling of potassium and regulation of acid-base balance. The purpose of the present communication is to review the works in which characteristics of water and ion transport across these segments have been studied by in vitro microperfusion and to discuss their functional significance, with respect to the three distinct but inter-related functions of the renal medulla; namely, the urine concentrating mechanism, K^+ recycling, and regulation of acid-base balance.

Morphology of Henle's Loop

The thin loop segments belong to the intermediate segments [4]. They include descending thin limb for the short-looped nephron (short descending limb, SDL), and descending (long descending limb, LDL) and ascending thin limbs (ATL) for the long-looped nephron. Since comprehensive reviews on the morphological features of the thin loop segments have been reported [4,8,9], we will briefly mention only the essential features which are relevant for understanding the function of the thin loop segments (Fig. 1).

Architectural Organization

The descending limb and the ascending limb of Henle's loop do not necessarily make a simple countercurrent contact with each other. Rather, they a have complicated architectural organization, with vascular bundles and capillary networks supplied from the vasa rectae. The renal medullary vasculatures originate from efferent arterioles of the juxtamedullary glomeruli. A group consisting of arteriole and venous vasa recta constitutes a vascular bundle in the outer medulla. In some species, several vascular bundles are combined to make a giant bundle [4,8,9]. It should be emphasized that blood of the venous vasa recta of the vascular bundle is supplied mainly from the capillary network in the inner medulla. In contrast, blood supplied to the outer medulla returns directly to the interlobular vein. Such distinct separation of blood supply, between outer and inner medulla, must have some physiological significance.

In most animal species, the descending limbs of the long-looped nephron are distributed in the interbundle regions, and appear to be separated from the vascular bundles by interpositioned thick ascending limbs [4,8,9]. In marked contrast, the descending limbs of the short-looped nephron have much closer contact with the vascular bundles [4,8,9]. However, there are some species differences in the pattern of the contact of the SDL with the vascular bundle. The pattern can be classified into three types. In the first type, the SDL distributes within the vascular bundle. In this type, the SDL clearly constitutes a countercurrent system with the ascending vasa recta. The segments of SDL in *Psammomys* [10], *Meriones* [11], *Perognathus* [12], and mice [13] belong to this type. In the second type, the SDL distributes around the vascular bundle. The SDL of the rat belongs to this type [14]. In the third type, the SDL distributes in the interbundle region. The SDLs of rabbits and hamsters belong

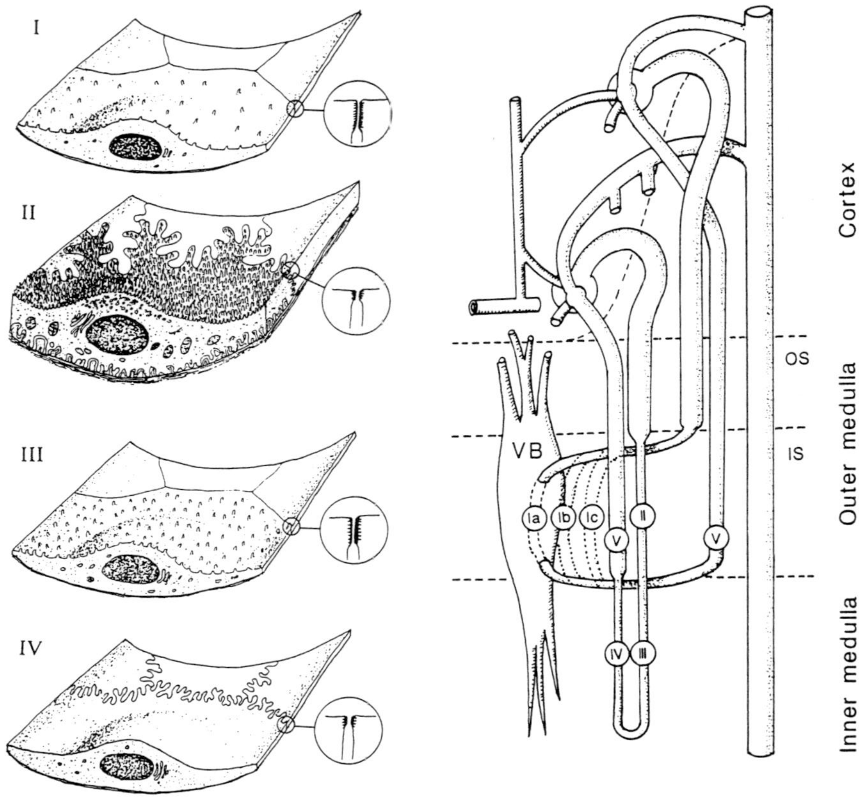

Fig. 1. Epithelial morphology and architectural organization of thin loop segments. I, Short looped descending limb (*SDL*); II, Upper portion of long-looped descending limb (*LDLu*); III, Lower portion of long-looped descending limb (*LDLl*); IV, Ascending thin limb (*ATL*). OS, outer stripe; IS, inner stripe; VB, vascular bundle. Figures in circles represent magnification of morphology of tight junctions

to this type [15,16]. Although it is not a general rule, there is a tendency that the species having closer contact of SDL with the vascular bundle have higher urine concentrating capacity.

Epithelial Morphology

With the exception of the rabbit, there are considerable heterogeneities in the morphology of the descending limb. Heterogeneity exists not only between short and long-looped nephrons (internephron heterogeneity), but also within the same long-looped nephron (intranephron or axial heterogeneity). These heterogeneities are prominent in rodent kidneys [4,8]. The short loop descending limb (SDL) consists of simple and flat epithelia (type I cells). The microvilli of the luminal membrane are not well developed. Only scarce organelles are present in cytoplasm. The apposition to the neighboring cells is simple and lacks interdigitation. The tight junctions are deep and contain several ramified junctional strands. These features are representative for tight epithelia.

In contrast, the morphology of the epithelia in the upper portion of the long-loop descending limb (LDLu) is more complicated [4]. The LDLu consists of the most elaborate cells, which have abundant microvilli in the apical membrane, are rich in cytoplasmic mitochondria, and have meticulously developed interdigitation with neighboring cells (Type II cells). The basal infolding of LDLu is also well developed. The tight junctions are very shallow, having only one or two junctional strands. These features are representative for leaky epithelia. Along the axis of the long-looped nephron, epithelial morphology changes gradually, with the height of epithelia becoming shorter. Qualitative changes in morphology occur somewhere near the border of the outer and inner medulla, but the position of the transition varies among nephrons. Sometimes the transition occurs in inner medulla.

The morphology of the lower portion of the long-loop descending limb (LDLl) is very similar to that of the SDL (Type III cell).

Functions of the Descending Limb

Water Permeability

Early micropuncture studies in exposed renal papilla of rats and hamsters have demonstrated that tubular fluid to plasma (TF/P) inulin concentration is about 11[17,18]. This value indicates that a considerable amount of water is absorbed along the descending limb, because TF/P inulin concentration in the latest part of the superficial proximal tubule is 5–6.

By perfusing the descending limb of tissue slices of rat renal papilla, Morgan and Berliner [6], demonstrated that the diffusional water permeability was high in the descending limb. Kokko [19] reported that the rabbit descending limb perfused in vitro exhibited high osmotic water permeability. This finding was later supported by several investigators [20,21].

In spite of the considerable heterogeneity of the epithelial morphology between SDL and LDLu, as mentioned above, both segments are highly permeable to water [22]. Although water permeability tended to be higher in the LDLu than in the SDL, because of the considerable scatter of the data, they were not significantly different.

Mechanism of Water Transport

Miwa and Imai [20] reported that in the rabbit descending thin limb, the osmotic water permeability was 56 times greater than the diffusional water permeability. This large difference in two parameters for water permeability could only be explained by the hypothesis that water is transported, at least in part, through a water channel having a single file mechanism, which has also been postulated to exist in two other water permeable nephron segments, namely vasopressin stimulated collecting duct [23] and proximal tubules [24].

More recently, Imai et al. [25] examined the mechanism of water transport across the hamster LDLu in more detail. Osmotic water permeability of the hamster LDLu

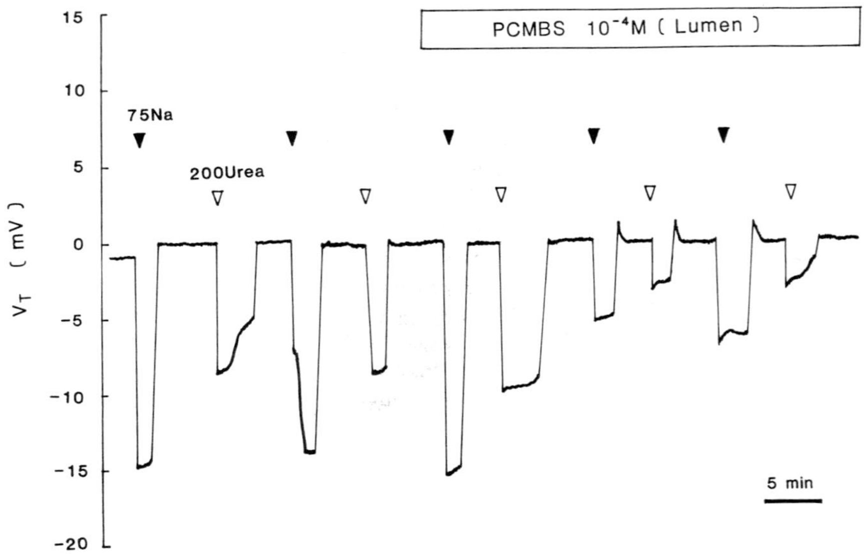

Fig. 2. A representative study showing that parachloromercuri-benzene sulfonate (*PCMBS*) inhibits both NaCl diffusion voltage and streaming voltage, induced by a urea osmotic gradient in hamster LDLu. (From [25])

was 26 times higher than diffusional water permeability. They showed that parachloro-mercuribenzene sulfonate (PCMBS), which is known to be an inhibitor of the water channel, decreased both diffusional and osmotic water permeabilities of the hamster LDLu. Additional evidence which supports the existence of a water channel is the low activation energy for diffusion of water. Diffusional water permeability of the LDLu was measured at various temperatures, and apparent activation energy was calculated according to the following equation:

$$ln\ (P_{dw}) = -K_A/T + C$$

where P_{dw} is diffusional water permeability, K_A is activation energy, T is absolute temperature, and C is a constant value. Apparent activation energy thus calculated was 3.16 kCal/mol, a low value compatible with a channel mechanism for water transport.

The water channel of the LDLu has a unique characteristic in that it is also permeable to cations. As will be discussed in the next section, the LDLu is highly permeable to cations. Part of the cation selective permeability is mediated by the water channel. This view was supported by the observation that PCMBS reduced streaming potential, as well as NaCl diffusion potential, as shown in Fig. 2 [25]. To rule out the possibility that PCMBS also acts on the tight junction to inhibit paracellular cation conductance, we examined the effect of PCMBS on another nephron segment which is known to have a cation selective paracellular pathway, but is impermeable to water. The medullary thick ascending limbs of hamsters were chosen for this purpose. In the presence of 0.1 mM furosemide, reduction of NaCl concentration in the bath by a

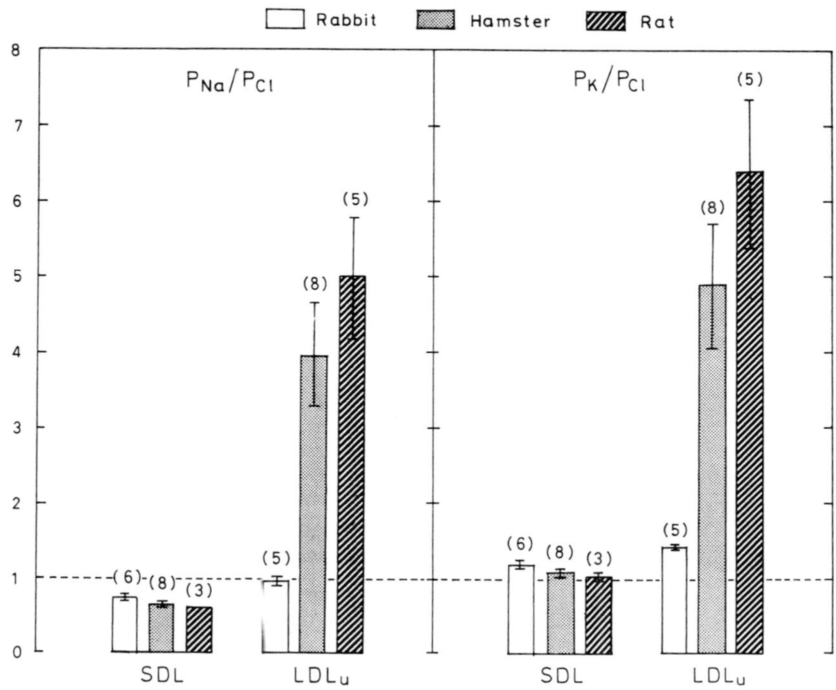

Fig. 3. Internephron heterogeneity and species differences of relative Na/Cl and K/Cl permeabilities, determined by diffusion voltage. (From [26])

half caused negative deflection of transepithelial voltage (V_T). However, addition of PCMBS to the lumen did not affect the diffusion voltage. This suggests that PCMBS does not affect paracellular cation selective conductance.

Solute Permeabilities

Heterogeneity of Ion and Urea Permeability

As suggested by the heterogeneity of epithelial morphology, it is possible that there is intranephron, as well as internephron, heterogeneity with respect to ion permeability properties. We have performed a series of studies, in which internephron heterogeneity and species differences were examined [22,26]. From the deflection of V_T when the composition of the bathing fluid was varied, we calculated the relative permeabilities of Na^+/Cl^- and of K^+/Cl^- in descending limbs of hamsters, rats, and rabbits.

The results are summarized in Fig. 3. In hamsters and rats, both P_{Na}/P_{Cl} and P_K/P_{Cl} are very much higher in the LDLu than in the SDL. This is definite evidence that there is internephron heterogeneity between the descending limbs of long-looped and short-looped nephrons. The data of this figure also show that there is species difference in the internephron heterogeneity: in contrast to the cases of hamsters and rats, no striking difference in relative ion permeability was observed in rabbits.

Table 1. Transport parameters of the hamster thin loop segments

Parameters	SDL	LDLu	LDLl	ATL
Pf (10^{-3} cm/s)	285	403	390	3
P_{Na} (10^{-5} cm/s)	4.2	5.0	3.5	87.6
P_{Cl} (10^{-5} cm/s)	1.3	4.2	n.d.	196.0
P_K (10^{-5} cm/s)	n.d.	85.4	n.d.	n.d.
P_{urea} (10^{-5} cm/s)	7.4	1.5	13.5	18.5
σ NaCl	n.d.	0.83	0.99	n.d.
σ KCl	n.d.	0.81	n.d.	n.d.
σ urea	n.d.	0.95	0.97	n.d.

SDL, short descending limb; LDLu, upper portion of long descending limb; LDLl, lower portion of long descending limb; ATL, ascending thin limb. Pf, osmotic water permeability; n.d., not determined

The relative permeabilities shown in Fig. 3 do not necessarily indicate absolute ion permeabilities. In addition, electrophysiological measurements do not provide permeability values for non-ionic solutes. It is important to know urea permeability, especially in the segments of the renal medulla. Therefore, we measured Na^+, Cl^-, and urea permeabilities in SDL and LDLu of hamsters, by using ^{22}Na, ^{36}Cl, and ^{14}C-urea, respectively. As summarized in Table 1, Na^+ and Cl^- permeabilities were higher in LDLu, whereas urea permeability was higher in SDL. It should be noted that permeability for Na was 10 times higher than that for Cl^-. This value is higher than the value of 4 for the P_{Na}/P_{Cl} ratio, calculated from diffusion voltage. One possible explanation for this discrepancy is that there is an electroneutral process for Na^+ transport, which is distinct from a cation selective ionic diffusion process. However, no one has ever tested this possibility.

In addition to internephron heterogeneity, there is an axial heterogeneity in the permeability properties of the long-looped descending limb. As was expected from the morphological transition of epithelia along the axis of the long-loop descending limb [27], we demonstrated that the characteristic of preferential Na^+ permeability in LDLu diminished along the descending limb. Such transition occurred at various levels of the renal medulla. The transport parameters of the lower portion of long loop descending limb (LDLl) are essentially the same as those of SDL. In other words, the segment is less permeable to Na^+ and moderately permeable to urea.

Selectivity of Ion Permeability

As mentioned above, LDLu of hamster is more permeable to Na^+ than to Cl^-; it is of interest to know whether the permeability of this segment is specific for Na^+ or not. Tabei and Imai [28] examined relative ion permeabilities of hamster LDLu by observing V_T deflection upon ion substitution (biionic diffusion voltage). The sequence of relative permeabilities of cation to Cl^- were: 8.89 for NH_4^+, 7.07 for K^+, 6.70 for Rb^+, 5.88 for Na^+, 5.76 for Cs, and 4.19 for Li^+. On the other hand, relative permeabilities of anions to Cl^- were: 1.16 for NO_3^-, 0.80 for Br^-, and 0.58 for acetate. These findings indicate that this segment is permeable to cations in general.

Transepithelial Resistance and Paracellular Pathway

In accordance with species differences in ion permeability properties, the transepithelial resistance of the descending limb also differs between rabbits and hamsters.

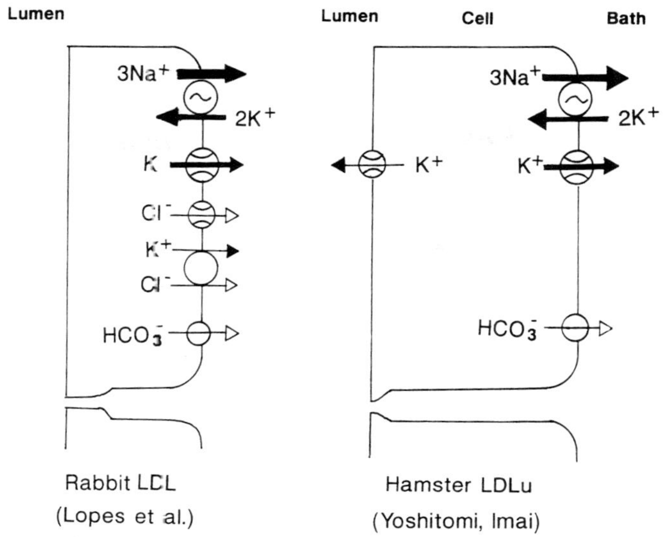

Fig. 4. Cell model for descending limb of rabbit, deduced from study of cell volume regulation and from electrophysiological study. (*left*, from [30], *right*, from [29])

Abramow and Orci [21] reported that in rabbit descending limb, transepithelial resistance (R_T) was 600 ohm cm^2. In contrast, Yoshitomi and Imai [29] found that R_T of hamster LDLu was 18 ohm cm^2.

Although, as discussed earlier, cation selective permeability is accounted for, in part, by the water channel associated with cation selective conductance, the contribution of the paracellular pathway should be also considered. This idea is supported by the observation that NaCl diffusion voltage was symmetrical when the direction of the concentration gradient was reversed [28]. A preliminary study by Koyama, Yoshitomi, and Imai further supported this view. They observed that protamine inhibited NaCl diffusion voltage, as well as transepithelial conductance. These effects were reversed by heparin. Along with other observations, they estimated that about 50% of the transepithelial resistance was accounted for by paracellular shunt resistance.

Transcellular Pathway

Lopez et al. [30] have conducted a very elegant study to clarify the mechanisms of ion transport across basolateral membrane of rabbit descending limb. They studied the ion transport mechanisms responsible for cell volume regulation of this segment. Based on ion substitution studies, they proposed a cell model, depicted in Fig. 4.

We have recently succeeded in impaling the epithelia of hamster LDLu [29]. Our current cell model, deduced from an electrophysiological mean, is also depicted in Fig. 4 for comparison. In steady state, basolateral membrane voltage (V_B) was -18 ± 2 mV ($n=55$). Because the basolateral membrane was depolarized by 40 mV by the action of ouabain, it is probable that the Na^+/K^+ pump may contribute to the generation of V_B.

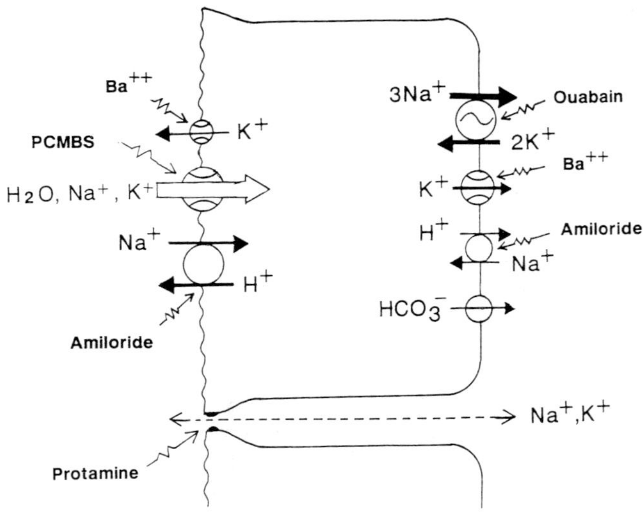

Fig. 5. Cell model of hamster LDLu based on pHi measurement and electrophysiological study

In addition to an ouabain sensitive pump, barium sensitive high K^+ conductance also exists in the basolateral membrane. This conclusion was based on the observations that the increase in K^+ concentration in the bath, from 5 to 50 mM, or application of 2 mM $BaCl_2$ to the bath, depolarized basolateral membrane by 36 mV or 46 mV, respectively. The electrophysiological method is insufficient for evaluating whether neutral carrier, such as K^+-Cl^- or Na^+-K^+-$2Cl^-$, cotransport exists in the basolateral membrane.

With regard to anion conductance, we could demonstrate a small, but significant, V_B deflection upon reduction of bath HCO_3^- from 25 to 2.5 mM, which became more prominent when K^+ conductance was suppressed by Ba^{2+}. On the other hand, we could not obtain definite evidence for the presence of Cl^- conductance. However, because of the technical difficulty in demonstrating a small Cl^- conductance, we cannot exclude such a possibility.

In the apical membrane, there is a small K^+ conductance. Increase in lumen K concentration, from 5 to 50 mM, or luminal addition of 2 mM $BaCl_2$, caused the apical membrane to depolarize by 10 mV or 8 mV, respectively. Thus, along with nonselective cation conductance associated with the water channel, there are significant ion conductances in the apical membrane. However, fractional apical membrane resistance was relatively high, at 0.92 [29].

H^+ Transport

Kurtz [31] reported for the first time that in rabbit descending limb, Na^+/H^+ antiporters exist in both apical and basolateral membranes. Independently, Koseki et al. [32] also reported that Na^+/H^+ antiporters exist in apical and basolateral membranes of hamster LDLu. They further showed that lumen pH, as determined by fluorescence of free BCECF, became acid when luminal flow was stopped by obstruction of tubular outflow. Under this condition, addition of ouabain to the bath

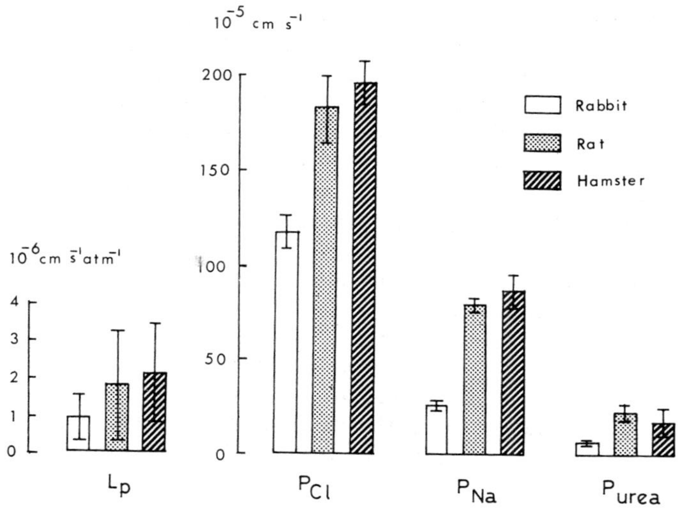

Fig. 6. Permeability properties of the ATL of rabbits, rats, and hamsters

dissipated the pH gradient, indicating that the generation of pH gradient is mediated by a process of luminal H^+ transport, secondarily driven by Na^+/K^+ pump in the basolateral membrane, possibly Na^+/H^+ antiporter.

Under the stopped flow condition, abrupt changes in bath pH caused rapid parallel changes in luminal pH, indicating that this segment is also highly permeable to proton. Therefore, it is suggested that the transepithelial pH gradient across this segment is maintained by a strong secondarily active H^+ secretory mechanism, which is associated with a leak of H^+, probably through the paracellular pathway.

Cell Model of LDLu

Based on our observations, which were the result of various approaches, we constructed a cell model, as in Fig. 5. The Na^+/K^+ pump in the basolateral membrane provides the driving force for Na^+/H^+ antiporters in both basolateral and apical membranes. Along with the presence of HCO_3^- conductance in the basolateral membrane, the LDLu may play a significant role in the acidification of tubular fluid. The existence of K^+ conductance in the apical membrane may, in part, account for K^+ recycling, which is known to occur along the descending limb [33].

Functions of the Ascending Thin Limb

Water and Solute Permeabilities

Water and solute permeabilities of the ascending thin limb (ATL) have been reported for rabbits, rats, and hamsters [34–40]. The data are summarized in Fig. 6. Osmotic water permeability of the ATL is very low. Diffusional water permeability was also shown to be low in the ATL of rabbits and hamsters.

On the other hand, the ATL is highly permeable to Na^+ and to Cl^-, but less permeable to urea. In contrast to the descending limb, permeability properties are essentially the same among various species, including rabbits, rats, and hamsters [34–36]. It should be noted that Cl^- permeability is extremely high in all species.

When a segment of ATL was perfused with a solution having identical composition to the bathing fluid, neither V_T nor net solute absorption was demonstrated. Bidirectional fluxes for ^{22}Na, ^{36}Cl, or ^{14}C urea from lumen-to-bath and from bath-to-lumen were identical [34]. These findings are compatible with the view that the ATL has no detectable net transport capacity. The transport parameters of the ATL, as mentioned above, indicate that Na^+, Cl^-, and urea are transported across this segment by purely passive mechanisms.

Mechanisms of Cl^- Transport

Because Cl^- permeability of the ATL is extremely high, it has been postulated that there are some special mechanisms which accelerate Cl^- transport across this segment.

Evidence for Facilitated Cl^- Transport

Imai and Kokko [35] proposed that Cl^- transport across the rabbit ATL was mediated by facilitated diffusion. This proposition was based on the following three major observations. First, ^{36}Cl flux from the lumen-to-bath exhibited a tendency for saturation as Cl^- concentration was increased. On the other hand, the ^{22}Na flux increased as a linear function of Na^+ concentration. Second, the Cl^- flux was inhibited by Br^-. The inhibitory effect of Br^- was greater when Cl^- concentration was low, suggesting that the inhibition of Cl^- flux by Br^- was roughly competitive in nature. Third, when Ussing's flux ratio analysis was performed, by measuring bidirectional ^{36}Cl fluxes at various diffusion V_T, the flux ratio for Cl^- clearly deviated from the line predicted for simple passive diffusion. These findings suggest that Cl^- transport is mediated by some processes which require interactions of Cl^- with membranes. From these observations, however, we cannot specify the exact mechanism of Cl^- transport.

Effects of Anion Transport Inhibitors

In an attempt to specify the mechanism of Cl^- transport across the ATL, we observed the effects of various anion transport inhibitors on Cl^- transport in the hamster ATL.

Stilbene disulfonate derivatives, such as 4,4′-dithiocyanostilbene-2,2′-disulfonic acid (DIDS) or 4-acetamido-4′-isothiocyanostilbene-2,2′-disulfonic acid (SITS), are known to be highly specific inhibitors for the Cl^-/HCO_3^- antiporter in the red blood cell, the band 3 protein. The apparent high specificity, however, depends on the fact that in red blood cells this is the only protein which is exposed to the cell surface [41]. Therefore, in other biological membranes, their inhibitory effects are not limited to the Cl^-/HCO_3^- antiporter. In the renal tubule they also inhibit Na^+-$3HCO_3^-$ flux. Thus, possible contributions of the K^+-Cl^-, or the Na^+-K^+-$2Cl^-$ cotransporters could be rejected.

Because a transmural NaCl concentration gradient causes diffusion voltage [34–40], the Cl^- transport in the ATL is conductive in nature. Although electrogenic

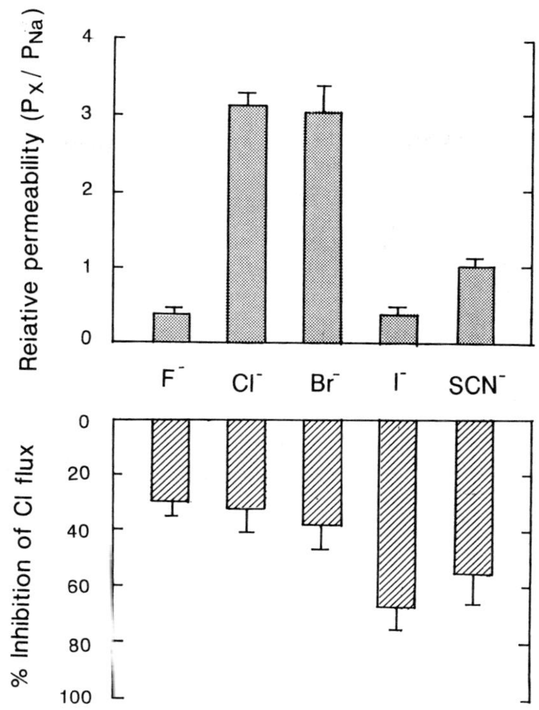

Fig. 7. Halogen permeabilities relative to Cl^-, measured by simple salt dilution voltage. (*upper panel*), and inhibition of 36Cl flux by halogens (*lower panel*). (Data from Isozaki et al., [62])

antiport or cotransport cannot be ruled out, the mechanisms coupled with major ions, such as HCO_3^-, Na^+, and K^+ are excluded. Thus, by exclusion, we reached the conclusion that a Cl^- channel is the most plausible mechanism for Cl^- transport across the ATL.

Halogen Selectivity

Recently, Isozaki et al. [62] examined the selectivity of ion permeation across the ATL by measuring the single salt dilution voltage. Figure 7 summarizes halogen permeabilities of this segment, with reference to Na^+. It is clear that this segment is highly permeable to Br^-, as well as to Cl^-, but less permeable to I^- and to F^-. By using ^{36}Cl and ^{125}I, we measured permeability for Cl^- and I^- simultaneously, and confirmed that permeability for Cl^- was 6 times higher than that for I^-.

Because Imai and Kokko [35] had previously reported that Br^- inhibited Cl^- flux, we examined whether other halogens have a similar effect or not. The inhibitory effects of the respective halogens (50 mM) are also shown in Fig. 7. As can be seen in this figure, all halogens and SCN^- showed some inhibitory effects. It should be noted that iodine is the most potent inhibitor among these ions, in spite of its low permeability.

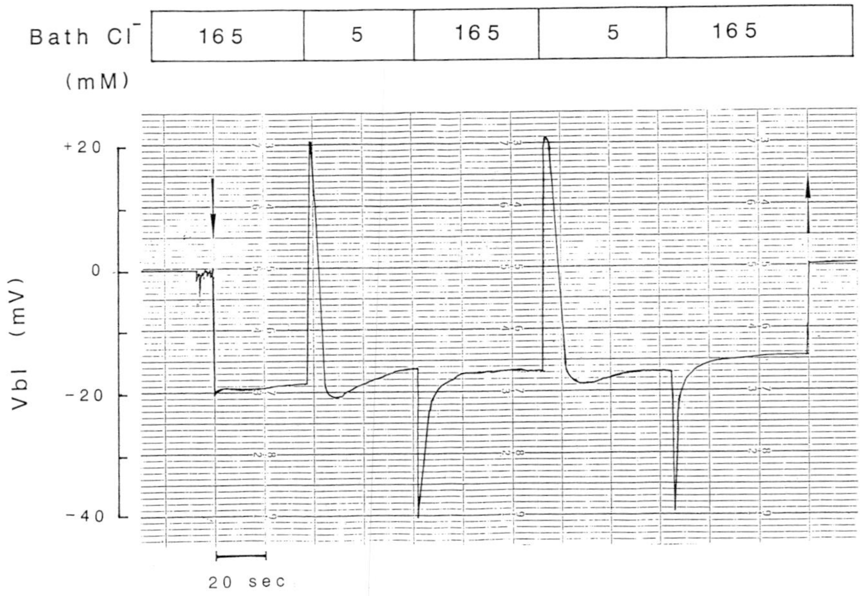

Fig. 8. A representative recording of the basolateral membrane voltage of hamster ATL, showing that Cl^- conductance is present in the basolateral membrane. (From [47])

These observations suggest that the putative Cl^- channels in the ATL have binding sites which are common to all halogens, but that only Cl^- and Br^- are permeable.

Route of Cl^- Conductance

It is most difficult to answer the question whether Cl^- is transported across the transcellular, or the paracellular route, However, success in cell puncture with conventional electrodes by Imai et al. [48] provided a definite answer to this question. In 18 successful impalements V_B was revealed to be -24.5 ± 1.5 mV. As shown in Fig. 8, an abrupt decrease in Cl^- concentration in the bath caused transient positive spiky deflection of V_B, indicating that there is a Cl^- conductance in the basolateral membrane. The rapid dissipation of the voltage may reflect the fact that Cl^- concentration in the cell is rapidly equilibrated with that in ambient solution. When luminal Cl^- concentration was decreased, the apical membrane voltage was also deflected. Thus, Cl^- conductances exist in series in the apical, as well as in the basolateral, membrane.

Regulation of Cl^- Conductance

Because ion channels, in general, are composed of protein, factors which modulate protein conformation may affect the functions of channels. Therefore, we examined the effects of pH, Ca^{2+}, and SH reagents on Cl^- conductance in the hamster ATL [38,39,48].

Effects of pH

It is well-known that many ion channels are affected by pH. Usually, acidification of ambient fluid is associated with a decrease in ion transport or conductance. Kondo et al. [38] found that acidification of the bathing fluid sharply decreased relative Cl^- conductance, as well as Cl^- flux, in the hamster ATL. The P_{Cl}/P_{Na} ratios calculated from salt diffusion voltage were functions of the pH of the bathing or luminal fluid. The affinities for H^+ binding were pH 5.78 and pH 6.31 at the luminal and the basolateral side, respectively. The slope of Hill's plot was greater than 2, suggesting that there are at least two proton binding sites, or that the proton binding exhibits positive cooperativity.

Effects of Ca^{2+}

Ca^{2+} is also known to regulate various channels, including the Cl^- channel [49]. The Cl^- conductance of the ATL is also regulated by ambient Ca^{2+}: a decrease in Ca^{2+} is associated with a decrease in Cl^- conductance [39]. Ca^{2+} and proton have mutual interaction in modulating Cl^- conductance in the ATL. The mode of the interaction is the uncompetitive type.

Effects of Sulfhydryl Reagents

Kondo and Imai [50] reported that treatment of the ATL with glutaraldehyde selectively inhibited Cl^- conductance. Glutaraldehyde is known to cross-link both sulfhydryl and amino groups. Therefore, it is possible that one of these groups of amino acids in the protein moiety of the putative channel may play a critical role in the conductive pathway for Cl^-. We observed the effects of various SH inhibitors [48], including PCMBS, maleimide, and N-ethyl maleimide (NEM). All these agents showed irreversible inhibitory effects on the Cl^- conductance of the ATL.

During the course of this study, we noticed that NEM exhibited a unique dual action on Cl^- conductance (Fig. 9). Although an initial application of NEM caused a small suppression of Cl^- conductance, elimination of NEM caused further sharp decrease in the conductance, suggesting that NEM caused an irreversible inhibition. However, to our surprise, a second addition of NEM stimulated the conductance. This stimulatory effect of NEM was prevented by dithiothreitol, indicating that the effect is also due to modification of the SH site. The stimulatory effect of NEM was reversible. It was also prevented by NPPB [40], suggesting that the Cl^- channel is stimulated by NEM. These observations clearly show that there are at least two distinct regulatory sites, having SH groups, associated with the Cl^- channel.

Loci of the Action of Regulating Factors

Because there are two regulatory sites in the channel, as discussed above, we wished to know the modes of action of pH, Ca^{2+}, and various transport inhibitors with special reference to these two regulatory sites.

First, we examined whether the stimulatory effect of NEM could be preserved under conditions where the Cl^- conductance was inhibited by either low pH or nominally free Ca^{2+} [48]. The experimental protocols were as follows. We observed NaCl

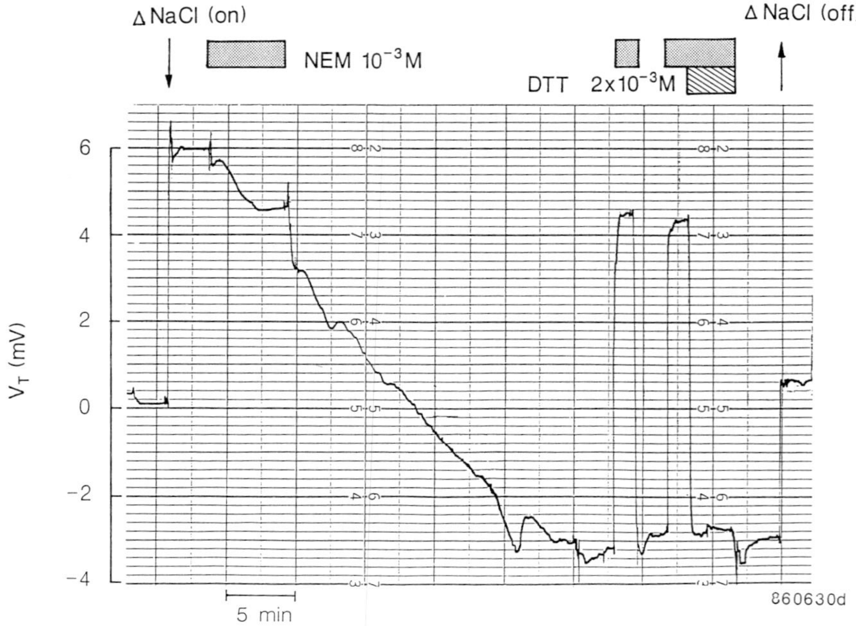

Fig. 9. A representative recording of NaCl diffusion voltage in hamster ATL, showing the dual action of NEM. NEM, N-ethylmaleimide; DTT, dithiothreitol. (From [48])

diffusion voltage as a measure of Cl^- conductance, and the suppressive effects of bath pH 5.8 on the diffusion voltage were observed before and after administration of 1 mM NEM to the bath. After washing NEM from the bath, we observed the stimulatory effect of NEM by applying it again. The stimulatory effect of NEM was also examined when bath pH was 5.8. As for recovery data, the same challenge was repeated, while bath pH was changed to 7.4 again. A similar protocol was conducted, using Ca^{2+}-free bath solution instead of acid pH. The results are summarized in Fig. 10. As clearly shown in this figure, the stimulatory effect of NEM was suppressed markedly when the bath pH was acid, whereas the effect was not prevented by nominally free Ca^{2+}. These observations suggest that the inhibitory site of H^+ is located distal to the NEM-stimulating site. On the other hand, the calcium-stimulated site seems to be independent from the NEM-stimulating site.

By using similar protocols, we also examined the sites of action of other inhibitors, such as DIDS and phloretin. The results are summarized in Fig. 11. As shown in the left panel, addition of 1mM DIDS to the bath markedly decreased the diffusion voltage, reflecting the suppression of Cl^- conductance. Under this condition, addition of 1mM NEM caused a stimulatory effect of the same magnitude as that of the second challenge of NEM. On the other hand, in the presence of 1mM phloretin, NEM did not exert any stimulatory effect, as shown in the right panel. These observations support the view that the site of action of DIDS may be the same site at which SH reagents show an irreversible inhibitory effect, whereas the site of action of phloretin is distal to the stimulatory site of NEM.

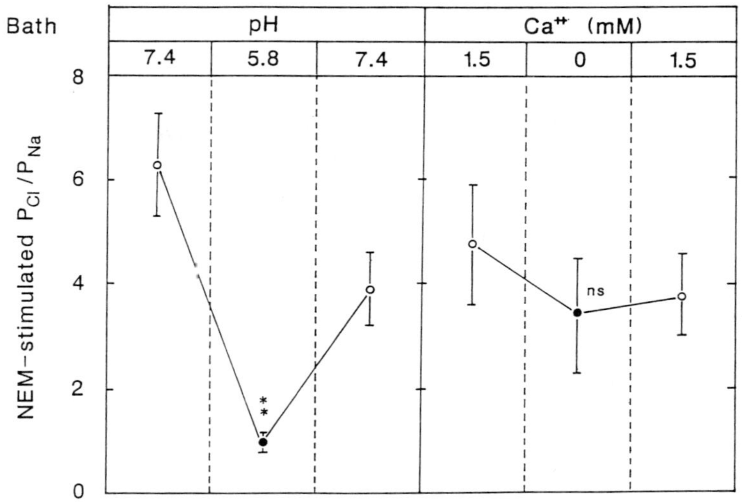

Fig. 10. Effects of pH or Ca^{2+} on N-ethylmaleimide (*NEM*)-stimulated relative Cl^- conductance, as measured by NaCl diffusion voltage. (Data from M. Imai et al. [48])

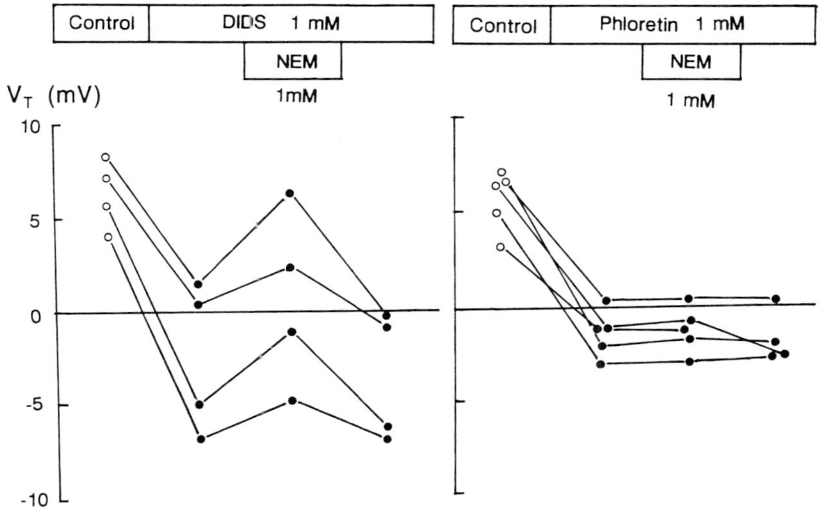

Fig. 11. Effects of DIDD or phloretin on N-ethylmaleimide (*NEM*)-stimualted relative Cl^- permeability in hamster ATL

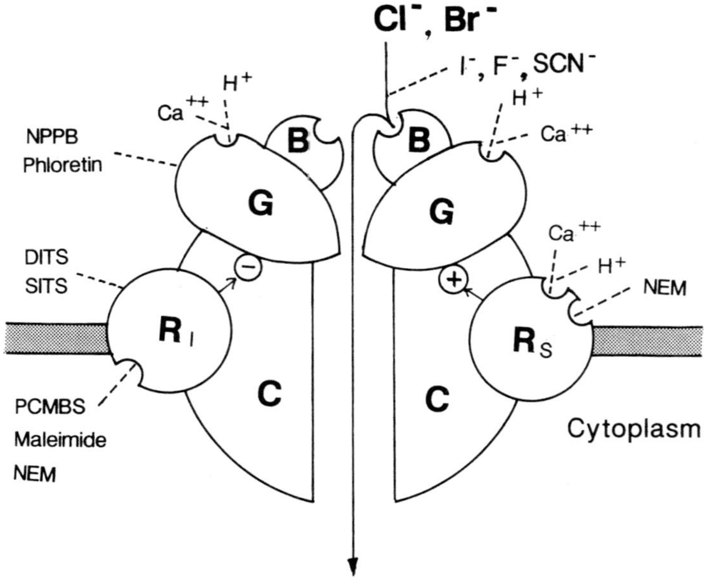

Fig. 12. Conceptual model of the putative Cl⁻ channel in the ATL. B, binding sites; C, channel; G, gates or filters; Ri, inhibitory regulation; Rs, stimulatory regulation

Conceptual Model of the Cl⁻ Channel

Based on the facts discussed above, we constructed a conceptual model for the putative Cl⁻ channel in the ATL, as shown in Fig. 12. The channel is supposed to have binding sites (B) to halogens in general. However, only Cl⁻ and Br⁻ can pass through the channel, probably because there is a barrier or filter in the channel to determine ion selectivity. As in many other ion channels, there may be a gate (G). H^+, NPPB, and phloretin may act on this gate or on the halogen binding sites to inhibit Cl⁻ conductance. The gating mechanism may be regulated by two distinct sites having SH groups, inhibitory (R_i) and stimulatory (R_S) sites. NEM is highly specific to the latter. DIDS may act on R_i. The stimulatory site of Ca^{2+} may be distinct from that of NEM. Although we admit that this model is much too speculative, we hope that it might provide a working hypothesis, which should be challenged in the future.

Physiological Significance of the Functions of Thin Loop Segments

As a summary of this review, we would like to discuss the physiological significance of thin loop segments very briefly, with reference to three distinct, but somehow interrelated, functions: i.e., 1) the urine concentrating mechanism, 2) K^+ recycling, and 3) urine acidification.

Urine Concentrating Mechanism

It is needless to say that the thin loop of Henle plays an integral part in the countercurrent multiplication system in the renal medulla. Our data clearly show that there is no appreciable active NaCl transport which is sufficient to generate a transepithelial NaCl gradient. Rather, we have strong evidence in support of the view that Cl^- is transported across the ATL by a special passive mechanism, possibly a Cl^- channel. In this regard, the passive diffusion model proposed by Kokko and Rector [51] and by Stephenson [52] may still be relevant. However, computer analysis, based on the transport parameters of the descending limb, showed that, against the hypothesis of the passive model, a significant amount of urea is accumulated in the fluid of the descending limb [53,54]. This would hamper the operation of the proposed single effect in the ATL. This situation is unrelated to species difference or to the inter- and intranephron heterogeneity of the descending limb.

Therefore, it is necessary to develop a new version of the passive model, which allows diffusion of both NaCl and urea out of the ATL. We have previously proposed that a single effect could be operating between the compartments of the ATL, the inner medullary collecting duct (IMCD), and capillary networks, if we assume that the low reflection coefficient for urea in the IMCD constitutes an initial driving force which generates a single effect [55]. Although there are considerable disputes about the exact value of the reflection coefficient for urea in the IMCD [56,57], there is no doubt that the osmotic work across the IMCD is operated by the two-solute model [56]. Thus, all passive models should incorporate this single effect. In addition, the special architectural organization of the tubulo-vascular arrangement should also be considered. The internephron heterogeneity in solute permeability properties may be essential for such a three dimensional model. We assume that the SDL may play an important role in the medullary recycling of urea. Furthermore, we should also consider the fact that the blood supply of the outer and inner medullar is strictly separate.

K^+ Recycling

K^+ reabsorbed in the medullary collecting duct is secreted again into the loop of Henle [33]. It is widely accepted that this K^+ recycling occurs somewhere in the proximal straight tubule or in the descending limb of Henle's loop [33]. The high K^+ permeability in the LDLu may indicate that this segment plays an important role in this phenomenon. In fact, the computer simulation done by Taniguchi et al. [54] supported this hypothesis. Although the high permeability for K^+ in this segment may be mainly accounted for by the leaky paracellular shunt pathway, the existence of K^+ conductance in the apical membrane of the LDLu may also be favorable for the secretion of K^+ across this segment.

Urine Acidification

We found that the LDLu has a high capacity for the secretion H^+ and that it maintains a transmural pH gradient, even though the segment is highly permeable to proton. The physiological significance of the proton secretion is unknown at the present time, because pH in the bend of the loop became less acidic, as compared to the end proximal tubular fluid pH [58]. Therefore, proton secretion in the LDLu may not be directly related to final urine pH. However, it should be noted that Henle's loop may play an important role in the accumulation of ammonia in the renal medulla [59]. Buerkert et al. [60] demonstrated that, in the rat, ammonia secretion occurs somewhere along the proximal straight tubule or descending limb. Good, Knepper, and Burg [61] demonstrated that NH_4^+ is reabsorbed as an ionic form in the thick ascending limb, via Na^+-K^+-$2Cl^-$ cotransport system. These observations are in accordance with the hypothesis that ammonia is accumulated in the renal medulla through the countercurrent multiplication system. Kurtz [31] speculated that acidification of the luminal fluid in the LDLu would shift more of the luminal ammonia to the NH_4^+ form, decrease the luminal NH_3, and would thus favor the non-ionic diffusion of NH_3 into the lumen. Furthermore, it is important to note that the LDLu in hamster is highly permeable to NH_4^+ [28]. Therefore, ionic diffusion, possibly via the paracellular shunt pathway, may also contribute to the medullary recycling of ammonia.

References

1. Kuhn W, Ryffel K (1942) Herstellung konzentrierter Lösungen aus verdünnten durch blosse Membranwirkung. (Ein Modelversuch zur Funktion der Niere). Hoppe Seylers Z Physiol Chem 276:145–178
2. Wirz H, Hargitay B, Kuhn W (1951) Lokalization des Konzentrierungsprozesses in der Niere durch direkte Kryoskopie. Helv Physiol Pharmacol Acta 9:196–207
3. Kuhn W, Ramel L (1959) Aktiver Salztransport als möglicher (und warscheinlicher) Einzeleffekt bei der Harnkonzentrierung in der Niere. Helv Chim Acta 42:628–660
4. Jamison RL, Kritz W (1982) Urinary concentrating mechanism. Structure and function. Oxford, New York
5. Jamison RL, Bennett CM, Berliner RW (1967) Countercurrent multiplication by the thin loops of Henle. Am J Physiol 212:357–366
6. Morgan T, Berliner RW (1968) Permeability of loop of Henle, vasa recta, and collecting duct to water, urea and sodium. Am J Physiol 215:108–115
7. Burg M, Grantham J, Abramow M, Orloff J (1966) Preparation and study of fragments of single rabbit nephrons. Am J Physiol 210:1293–1298
8. Kritz W (1981) Structural organization of the renal medulla: comparative and functional aspects. Am J Physiol 241:R3–R16
9. Bankir L, De Rouffignac C (1985) Urinary concentrating ability: insight from comparative anatomy. Am J Physiol 249:R643–R666
10. Kaissling B, de Rouffignac C, Barrett JM, Kriz W (1975) The structural organization of the kidney of the desert rodent *Psammomys obesus*. Acta Embryol 148:121–143
11. Kriz W, Dietrich J, Hoffman S (1968) Aufbau der Gefassbündel im Nierenmark von Wüstenmäusen (abstract). Naturwissenschaften 50:40
12. Dietrich HJ, Barrett JM, Kriz W, Bulhoff JP (1975) The ultrastructure of thin loop limbs of the mouse kidney. Anat Embryol (Berl) 147:1–13
13. Kriz W, Koepsell H (1974) The structural organization of the mouse kidney. Z Anat Entwicklungsgesch 144:137–163
14. Kritz W, Schnermann J, Koepsell H (1972) The position of short and long loops of Henle in the rat kidney. Z. Anat Entwicklungsgesch 138:301–309
15. Bachman S, Kriz W (1982) Histotopography and ultrastructure of the thin limbs of the loop of Henle in the hamster. Cell Tiss Res 225:111–127
16. Kaissling B, Kritz Z W (1975) Structural organization of the rabbit kidney. Adv Anat Embryol Cell Biol 148:121–143

17. Gottschalk CW, Lassiter WE, Mylle M, Ullrich K, Schmidt-Nielsen B, O'Dell R, Pehling G (1963) Micropuncture study of composition of loop of Henle fluid in desert rodents. Am J Physiol 204:532–535
18. Jamison RL (1968) Micropuncture study of segments of thin loops of Henle in the rat. Am J Physiol 215:236–242
19. Kokko JP (1970) Sodium and water transport in the descending limb of Henle. J Clin Invest 49:1838–1846
20. Miwa T, Imai M (1983) Flow dependent water permeability of the rabbit descending limb of Henle's loop. Am J Physiol 245:F743–F754
21. Abramow M, Orci L (1980) On the "tightness" of the rabbit descending limb of the loop of Henle, physiological and morphological evidence. Int J Biochem 12:23–27
22. Imai M, Hayashi M, Araki M (1984) Functional heterogeneity of the descending limbs of Henle's loop. I. Internephron heterogeneity in the hamster kidney. Pflugers Arch 402:385–392
23. Hebert SC, Andreoli TE (1980) Interactions of temperature and ADH on transport processes in cortical collecting tubules. Am J Physiol 238:F470–F480
24. Berry CA (1985) Characteristics of water diffusion in the rabbit proximal convoluted tubule. Am J Physiol 249:F729–F738
25. Imai M, Yasoshima K, Yoshitomi K (1990) Mechanism of water transport across the upper portion of the descending thin limb of long-looped nephron of hamsters. Pflugers Arch 415:630–637
26. Imai M (1984) Functional heterogeneity of the descending limbs of Henle's loop. II. Interspecies difference among rabbits, rats, and hamsters. Pflugers Arch 402:393–401
27. Imai M, Taniguchi J, Yoshitomi K (1988) Transition of permeability properties along the descending limb of long-loop nephron. Am J Physiol 254:F323–F328
28. Tabei K, Imai M (1986) Permselectivity for cations over anions in the upper portion of the descending limbs of Henle of long loop nephron isolated from hamsters. Pflugers Arch 406:279–384
29. Yoshitomi K, Imai M (1990) Electrophysiological study of the upper part of long descending thin limb (LDLu) (abstract). Kidney Int 37:576A
30. Lopez AG, Amzel LM, Markakis K, Guggino WB (1988) Cell volume regulation by the thin descending limb of Henle's loop. Proc Natl Acad Sci USA 85:2873–2877
31. Kurtz I (1988) Apical and basolateral Na^+/H^+ exchange in the rabbit outer medullary thin descending limb of Henle: Role in intracellular pH regulation. J Membr Biol 106: 253–260
32. Koseki C, Matsushima Y, Yoshitomi K, Imai M (1989) Regulation of intracellular pH (pHi) in the upper part of descending limb of long-looped nephron (LDLu): a fluorometric study (abstract). Kidney Int 35:457
33. Jamison RL, Work J, Schafer JA (1982) New pathways for potassium transport in the kidney. Am J Physiol 242:F297–F312
34. Imai M, Kokko JP (1974) Sodium chloride, urea and water transport in the thin ascending limb of Henle. Generation of osmotic gradient by passive diffusion of solutes. J Clin Invest 53:393–402
35. Imai M, Kokko JP (1976) Mechanism of sodium and chloride transport in the thin ascending limb of Henle. J Clin Invest 58:1054–1061
36. Imai M (1977) Function of the thin ascending limb of Henle of rats and hamsters perfused in vitro. Am J Physiol 232:F201–F209
37. Kondo Y, Yoshitomi K, Imai M (1987) Effects of anion transport inhibitors and ion substitution on Cl^- transport in TAL of Henle's loop. Am J Physiol 253:F1206–F1215
38. Kondo Y, Yoshitomi K, Imai M (1987) Effect of pH on Cl^- transport in TAL of Henle's loop. Am J Physiol 253:F1216–F1222
39. Kondo Y, Yoshitomi K, Imai M (1988) Effect of Ca^{2+} on Cl^- transport in thin ascending limb of Henle's loop. Am J Physiol 254:F232–F239

40. Isozaki T, Yoshitomi K, Imai M (1989) Effects of Cl^- transport inhibitors on Cl^- permeability across hamster ascending thin limb. Am J Physiol 257:F92–F98
41. Wieth JO, Brahm J (1985) Cellular anion transport. In: Seldin DW, Giebisch G (eds) The kidney. Physiology and pathophysiology. Raven, New York, pp 49–89
42. Boron WF, Boulpaep EL (1983) Intracellular pH regulation in the renal proximal tubule of the salamander. Basolateral HCO_3^- transport. J Gen Physiol 81:53–94
43. Yoshitomi K, Frömter E (1984) Cell pH of rat proximal tubule in vivo and the conductive nature of peritubular HCO_3^- (OH^-). Pflugers Arch 402:300–305
44. Nelson DJ, Tang JM, Palmer LG (1984) Single-channel recordings of apical membrane chloride conductance in A6 epithelial cells. J Membr Biol 80:81–89
45. Brahm J, Wieth JO (1977) Separate pathways for urea and water and for chloride for chicken erythrocytes. J Physiol (Lond) 266:727–749
46. Wangemann P, Witter M, Di Stefano A, Englert HC, Lang HJ, Schlatter E, Greger R (1986) Cl^- channel blockers in the thick ascending limb of the loop of Henle. Structure activity relationship. Pflugers Arch 407:S128–S141
47. Yoshitomi K, Kondo Y, Imai M (1988) Evidence for conductive Cl^- pathways across the cell membranes of the thin ascending limb of Henle's loop. J Clin Invest 82:866–871
48. Imai M, Kondo Y, Koseki C, Yoshitomi K (1988) Dual effect of N-ethylmaleimide on Cl^- transport across the thin ascending limb of Henle's loop. Pflugers Arch 411:520–528
49. Marty A, Tan VP, Trautmann A (1984) Three types of calcium-dependent channel in rat lacrimal glands. J Physiol (Lond) 357:293–325
50. Kondo Y, Imai M (1987) Effects of glutaraldehyde on renal tubular function. II. Selective inhibition of Cl^- transporter in the hamster thin ascending limb of Henle's loop. Pflugers Arch 408:484–490
51. Kokko JP, Rector F Jr (1972) Countercurrent multiplication without active transport in inner medulla. Kidney Int 2:214–223
52. Stephenson JL (1972) Central core model of the renal counterflow system. Kidney Int 2:85–94
53. Pennel JP, Lacy FB, Jamison R (1974) An in vivo study of the concentrating process in descending limb of Henle's loop. Kidney Int 5:337–347
54. Taniguchi J, Tabei K, Imai M (1987) Profiles of water and solute transport along the descending limb: analysis by mathematical model. Am J Physiol 252:F393–F402
55. Imai M, Taniguchi J, Tabei K (1987) Function of thin loops of Henle. Kidney Int 31:565–579
56. Imai M, Taniguchi J, Yoshitomi K (1988) Osmotic work across inner medullary collecting duct accomplished by difference in reflection coefficients for urea and NaCl. Pflugers Arch 412:557–567
57. Chou CL, Sands JM, Nonoguchi H, Knepper MA (1990) Urea gradient-associated fluid absorption with urea =1 in rat terminal collecting duct. Am J Physiol 258:F1173–F1180
58. DuBose TD Jr, Lucci MS, Hogg RJ, Puccaco LR, Kokko JP, Carter NW (1983) Comparison of acidification parameters in superficial and deep nephron in rats. Am J Physiol 244:F479–F503
59. Good D, Knepper MA (1985) Ammonia transport in the mammalian kidney. Am J Physiol 248:F459–F471
60. Buerkert J, Martin DT (1982) Ammonia handling by superficial and juxtamedullary nephrons in the rat: evidence for an ammonia shunt between the loop of Henle and the collecting duct. J Clin Invest 70:1–12
61. Good DW, Knepper MA, Burg MB (1984) Ammonia and bicarbonate transport by thick ascending limb of rat kidney. Am J Physiol 247:F35–F44
62. Isozaki T, Yoshitomik K, Imai M (in press) Selective ion permeability across thin limb of Henle's loop: interaction of Cl^- and other halogens with anion antiport system. Kidney Int

IgA Nephropathy: Recent Views on Pathogenesis and Treatment

Hideto Sakai

Chair: J. Stewart Cameron

IgA Nephropathy: Recent Views on Pathogenesis and Treatment

HIDETO SAKAI[1]

SUMMARY. In many parts of the world, IgA nephropathy is one of the most common types of glomerulonephritis. The aim of this lecture is to summarize recent views on the pathogenesis of this disease and to evaluate current treatment in various countries.

The pathogenesis of IgA nephropathy has been investigated primarily in human patients because of the lack of appropriate animal models. It is generally agreed that IgA nephropathy is mediated by circulating IgA-dominant immune complexes which are deposited in the glomeruli. The formation of IgA-dominant immune complexes is likely to be enhanced by genetic factors which promote in vivo production of IgA. The enhancement of IgA production in this disease leads to the formation of various IgA-class autoantibodies. Nonimmunological factors, including various mediators, blood coagulation, and hemodynamic alterations, may cause exacerbation of this disease.

No specific treatment is known to improve the clinical course of IgA nephropathy. Current treatment is aimed at preserving renal functions and stabilizing associated symptoms such as hypertension. The selection of treatment protocols depends on the histopathological findings of renal biopsy specimens, which, so far, provide the most reliable parameters for predicting the prognosis in each patient. The drugs most widely used for treatment of IgA nephropathy are antiplatelet agents. Administration of corticosteroids is more effective for the preservation of renal function in patients with moderate levels of proteinuria than in those with severe proteinuria. Other types of treatment have not been evaluated by multi-center, double-blind studies. Despite relatively high rates of recurrence, transplantation is not contraindicated in the treatment of patients with IgA nephropathy.

---

[1]Division of Nephrology and Metabolism, Department of Internal Medicine, School of Medicine, Tokai University, Isehara, Kanagawa, 259-11 Japan

Introduction

IgA nephropathy was first reported by Berger and Hinglais [1] in 1968. It is now well known that this disease is one of the most common types of primary glomerulonephritis in many parts of the world. Prognosis of IgA nephropathy is not so benign as initially thought, and approximately 10%–20% of patients with this disease will eventually shift to end-stage renal disease [2]. Specific treatment is currently not available for IgA nephropathy because of lack of knowledge of the precise mechanism of the development and exacerbation of this disease. The aim of this lecture is to summarize recent views on the pathogenesis of this disease and to evaluate current treatment in various countries. The term, "IgA nephropathy," in this lecture is limited to primary IgA nephropathy, because mesangial deposits of IgA are observed in various other diseases [3].

Pathogenesis

Clinical Features

The pathogenesis of IgA nephropathy has been investigated primarily in human patients because of the lack of appropriate animal models. Analysis of clinical features is therefore important in the elucidation of the mechanisms which might be related to the development of this disease.

Age and Sex

It is well known that IgA nephropathy is common in young males, although the age distribution, as well as the ratio of male to female patients with this disease, differs in different countries around the world [2]. The reason for the dominance of IgA nephropathy is unknown. The hyperfunction of IgA-producing B lymphocytes, to be discussed later, might be related to age and to some sex hormones, but there is no direct evidence to support this hypothesis.

Proteinuria and Hematuria

Persistent proteinuria and microscopic hematuria, associated with sporadic macroscopic hematuria, are the main clinical symptoms of IgA nephropathy. It is generally accepted that massive proteinuria is a sign of poor prognosis, although the clinical significance of macroscopic hematuria is yet to be clarified. The precise mechanism which induces occasional macroscopic hematuria is presently unknown.

Persistent Deposition of IgA1 in the Glomeruli

Preponderant deposition of IgA in the mesangial areas, as well as in other parts of the glomeruli, is the major immunohistopathological finding of IgA nephropathy. Intraglomerular deposition of IgA persists for several years or more in the majority of adult patients and in many pediatric patients. An increasing body of evidence suggests that the source of the intra-glomerular IgA is circulating IgA-dominant immune complexes. The reasons for this assumption are as follows: (a) IgA and C3 coexist in the glomerular mesangial areas, as shown by immuno-fluorescence [4], (b) electron-dense deposits are observed in the same area [4], (c) IgA and/or C3 are also observed in the vascular walls of subcutaneous or intramuscular vessels [5], (d) IgA-dominant immune complexes in the circulation are detected by several different techniques [6], (e) IgA nephropathy recurs frequently in allografted kidneys [7], and (f) glomerular IgA disappears rapidly from kidneys with IgA nephropathy when kidneys are transplanted in patients without IgA nephropathy [8].

In most countries, the subclass of IgA deposited in the glomeruli is now regarded as IgA1. The dominance of IgA2 was initially reported by a French group [9], but a subsequent study using monoclonal antibodies indicated that IgA1 is the dominant subclass of intraglomerular IgA [10]. The origin of these IgA1 antibodies is presently unknown. The monoclonarity of intraglomerular IgA was suggested by the dominance of the lambda light chain [11], but deviation in the kappa/lambda ratio has not been confirmed in most countries. It is generally agreed that IgA deposited in the glomeruli does not possess a secretory component. As far as the size and charge of intraglomerular IgA are concerned, anionic polymeric IgA is the dominant molecule, at least in IgA which is deposited in the mesangial areas. In mesangial IgA eluted by acid buffer, the presence of the J chain [12] and molecules of dimeric or even larger size [13], together with relatively negative charge [14], supported the above-mentioned physicochemical characteristics of mesangial IgA. Recently, it was suggested that subepithelial accumulation of proteinaceous materials from the mesangium might result in the degeneration and exfoliation of podocytes, followed by formation of segmental extracapillary lesions or adhesion to Bowman's capsule [15]. In order to elucidate the physicochemical characteristics and clinicopathological significance of IgA in various parts of the glomeruli in this disease, further studies are warranted. The origin of intraglomerular IgA is not fully clarified, but circulating IgA-dominant immune complexes are highly likely to be the source of such IgA, as indicated by the high rate of recurrence of this disease in cadaveric allografted kidneys [7], and the rapid disappearance of IgA from kidneys with IgA nephropathy in recipients with other renal diseases [8]. That these IgA antibodies are not anti mesangial cells and/or their matrix is indicated by the lack of binding of acid-eluted IgA, from renal biopsy specimens of patients with IgA nephropathy, with normal human renal tissues. In situ deposition of some antigen in the glomeruli prior to recurrence of IgA deposition is unlikely, since IgA deposition recurs as early as within one hour.

Geographical Heterogeneity

Immediately after the first report of IgA nephropathy [1], a marked geographical heterogeneity was observed in the prevalence of this disease. IgA nephropathy is frequent in southern European countries such as France, Italy, and Spain, as well as in the Asian-Pacific region, including China, Korea, Singapore, Australia, and Japan [2]. In contrast, this disease is relatively rare in the countries of northern Europe, and in North America and Africa [2]. The differences in the incidence of this disease might be due to racial, rather than environmental, factors, indicated by its heterogenous prevalence in multi-ethnic countries. For example, in the United States, IgA nephropathy is frequent in at least some tribes of American Indians [16], but shows a low incidence in Blacks [17]. There is no clear relationship between IgA nephropathy and HLA antigens [18]. The significance of the alteration in phenotypes of C3 [19] and C4 [20] in the pathogenesis of this disease is presently unknown.

Familial Increase in IgA Production

There has been an increasing number of reports showing the presence of familial increase of both in vivo and in vitro IgA production in this disease. Such familial increase in IgA production suggests the presence of an IgA-specific high responder which might be influenced by some genetic aberrations.

Familial Increase of In Vivo IgA Production

It is well known that more than half of the patients with IgA nephropathy show increased levels of serum IgA. The increased levels of serum IgA were shown to contain a large amount of polymeric IgA1 [21], and isoelectric analysis showed that these larger IgA molecules were negatively charged [22]. It was therefore suggested that the IgA whose levels are increased in the circulation has some common denominators with the IgA in the glomeruli of patients with IgA nephropathy. Increased levels of serum IgA were also observed in some relatives of patients with IgA nephropathy, with or without association of increased levels of IgA-bearing B cells in peripheral blood [23]. Increased levels of peripheral blood IgA-bearing B cells were also confirmed in Spain [24]. The origin of these IgA-bearing B cells in the circulation is presently obscure. However, distribution of isotypes in immunoglobulin-bearing cells in the tonsils from patients with IgA nephropathy [25] was very similar to that observed in peripheral blood, suggesting that some antigenic stimulation in the upper respiratory tract might induce the increased levels of IgA-bearing B cells, which subsequently migrate into the circulation. The increased infiltration of IgA-bearing B cells into tissues was also observed in biopsied specimens of episcleritis in some patients [26], suggesting the presence of systemic vasculitis in this disease.

Familial Increase of In Vitro IgA Production

Familial increase of IgA production has been observed not only in vivo, but also in vitro [27]. It is a matter of controversy, however, whether such an increase is observed in cultures with or without addition of pokeweed mitogens. Details of the references on this aspect have been reviewed elsewhere [28], but it is difficult to compare the results of studies on cell cultures in various laboratories, because of heterogeneity, not only in culture systems, but also in populations of patients examined. The size and subclass of IgA produced in cultured lymphocytes were, at least in patients if not in their relatives, similar to those of IgA deposited in the glomeruli, i.e., polymeric [29] IgA1 [30]. Therefore, it is postulated that IgA-bearing B cells in the circulation might be related to intraglomerular IgA.

Polyclonal Activation of IgA-Producing B Cells

The increased levels of serum IgA observed in patients with IgA nephropathy and in their relatives are probably due to polyclonal IgA, since monoclonal IgA is not found in these subjects. To further confirm this possibility, the kappa/lambda ratio of serum IgA, IgA-bearing B cells, and IgA produced by cultured B cells was examined in patients and their relatives [31]. The results obtained clearly showed that there was no deviation in the kappa/lambda ratio for any of these IgA antibodies. Furthermore, immunization, both of patients with IgA nephropathy [32] and of some of their relatives [31], induced not only an increase in IgA class anti influenza virus antibody, but also an increase in IgA class rheumatoid factor. These results suggested that antigenic stimulation of patients and their families induced not only increases in antigen-specific IgA antibodies, but also simultaneous increases in nonspecific IgA antibodies. These increases in nonspecific IgA antibodies might be responsible for the increase of serum levels of IgA in some patients and their relatives.

Emergence of Various Autoantibodies

Recently, the emergence of various kinds of autoantibodies has been noted in patients with IgA nephropathy, and also, sometimes, in their relatives. These autoantibodies include structural proteins of the glomeruli, such as nuclear protein [33] and collagen [34], and rheumatoid factors [35,36], as well as anti idiotype antibodies [37] and anti $F(ab')_2$ antibodies [38]. The polyclonal expansion of IgA-producing B cells might be responsible for the emergence of these autoantibodies. It is interesting to note that the majority of these antibodies was not restricted to the IgA class but included IgG and IgM to some extent. The polyclonal expansion of B cells in patients with IgA nephropathy might involve various isotypes, although the dominant class was IgA. Furthermore, serum titers of anti nuclear protein in relatives correlated significantly with the severity of tissue damage in renal biopsy specimens from patients [39]. The mechanism of this correlation is presently unknown, but familial increase in autoantibodies might be related to heterogeneous deposition of IgA in the glomeruli, followed by tissue damage caused by complement activation. As of the time of this writing, however, there is no direct evidence showing the deposition of autoantibodies in the glomeruli of patients with IgA nephropathy. In addition, the emergence of autoantibodies in relatives produces the new question of why these relatives do not seem to have renal diseases, at least as judged by urinalysis without renal biopsy.

Mechanism of Polyclonal Activation of IgA-Producing B Cells

Because IgA is a highly T cell-dependent antibody, altered T cell function has been suspected as a mechanism inducing polyclonal activation of IgA-producing B cells [40]. Decrease in IgA-specific suppressor T cell activity has been observed in patients [41] and in some of their relatives [42]. The decrease in such suppressor T cells was, however, a secondary phenomenon due to activation of IgA-producing B cells, since there was no abnormality in IgA-specific suppressor T cell activity in an identical twin sister of a patient with IgA nephropathy [41]. As far as helper T cells are concerned, there was an elevation in the $CD_4^+/CD8^+$ ratio [43], as well as an increase in IgA-specific helper T cells which have receptors for the Fc portion of IgA (FcαR) (i.e., Tα cells) [44]. The effect of Tα cells on IgA-producing B cells is a matter of controversy. There have been a series of reports showing that both T α cells and FcαR have an inhibitory action in cultures of IgA-producing B cells [45]. The reason for this dichotomy is presently unknown, but addition of IgA to culture systems might induce such inhibitory effects, since all studies showing the inhibitory effects of Tα cells used in vitro addition of IgA, while the studies of helper effects used IgA-free culture media. At least one of the T cell subsets which induce polyclonal activation of IgA-producing B cells is that of IgA-specific switch T cells which specifically convert IgM-producing B cells to IgA-producing B cells. Such IgA-specific switch T cells were first reported by Kawanishi and his associates [46], using a T cell clone from murine Peyer's patches. Subsequently, peripheral blood T cells with FcαR and CD4 antigen (i.e., Tα4 cells) were demonstrated to have IgA-specific switch activity, and these Tα4 cells were significantly increased in patients with IgA nephropathy [47]. Peripheral blood Tα4 cells were also increased in relatives of patients with IgA nephropathy [48], suggesting that these T cells might be responsible for polyclonal activation of IgA-producing B cells in families of patients with this disease.

Isotype switching of immunoglobulins is mediated by the switch region of genes located immediately before heavy chain regions. In the case of IgA, two switch regions (i.e., Sα1 and Sα2) have been recognized to correspond with two subclasses of IgA (i.e., IgA1 and IgA2). The relationship between Tα4 cells and these switch regions is presently unknown, but presumably some cytokines influence these switch regions. Polymorphism of the Sα1 region was reported in European patients with IgA nephropathy [49], while polymorphism of the Sα2 region was observed in Japanese patients [50]. It is presently unknown how these polymorphisms in the switch region induce dominant production of IgA1.

Cytokines responsible for IgA-specific switch activity have not been identified in humans. Interleukin 2 (IL-2), IL-4, IL-5, and IL-6 were proved to induce the expansion of precommitted IgA-producing B cells, but do not induce de novo switch activity. Transforming growth factor β (TGFβ) was demonstrated to be a prospective IgA-specific switch factor in mice [51], but preliminary studies failed to confirm activity in humans (unpublished data).

Impaired Catabolism of IgA

Intraglomerular deposition of IgA in patients with IgA nephropathy might be associated with impaired catabolism of IgA. Decreased function of the reticuloendothelial system [52], as well as the macrophage-monocyte system [53], has been reported. Emergence of blocking factors against Fc receptors has also been reported [54]. It is, however, premature to conclude that impaired clearance is the primary cause of intraglomerular deposition of IgA in this disease, since evidence is lacking for a relationship between the degree of clinical activity of IgA nephropathy, and the degree of impairment in the clearance system.

Search for Antigens

Antigens responsible for the development of IgA nephropathy have been investigated, because this disease is presumed to be mediated by IgA-dominant immune complexes. Numerous candidates for such antigens have been reported, but, in the author's opinion, these candidates should satisfy the following two requirements: (a) the antigen should be observed at the same location as the majority of IgA deposited in the glomeruli, and (b) the antigen should be specifically bound with IgA eluted from the glomeruli of many patients with IgA nephropathy. Elevation of serum antibody titers is not sufficient to prove the pathogenic role of that antigen, because non-specific elevation of various IgA antibodies is likely to be due to polyclonal expansion of IgA-producing B cells in this disease. Presently, there is no antigen which completely satisfies the two requirements listed above. However, a few candidates for such antigens meet these requirements at least partially.

Virus-Like Antigens in the Upper Respiratory Tract

This candidate can satisfy the above requirement (b), but it is not yet proven whether it can meet requirement (a). Many patients with IgA nephropathy show exacerbation of proteinuria and/or hematuria after episodes of upper respiratory infection. It was demonstrated that epithelial cells obtained from the upper respiratory tract showed specific binding with 125-I labelled IgA eluted from the same or allogenic patients with IgA nephropathy [55]. Subsequently, an antigenic substance from the upper respiratory tract was cultured successively in human fibroblasts, suggesting that these antigens were virus-like materials [55]. Recently, polyclonal rabbit antisera against these antigens were produced, and these antisera showed specific binding with the mesangial areas of many patients with IgA nephropathy, without cross reactions with any serum proteins [56]. Further studies, using specific antisera, are warranted in order to identify these virus-like antigens.

Soybean Protein

This candidate satisfies the above requirement (a) but so far it is not known whether soybean protein binds specifically with IgA eluted from the glomeruli of many patients with IgA nephropathy. Various environmental antigens have been observed in some patients with IgA nephropathy, and soybean protein was one of these antigens [57]. The specificity of antisera against soybean has been evaluated, and this antigen was observed in as many as 75% of patients with IgA nephropathy [58]. A combination of several different monoclonal antibodies is required to identify these food antigens in the glomeruli of patients with this disease.

Exacerbating Factors in IgA Nephropathy

Various factors not specific to IgA nephropathy, but more ubiquitous in many renal diseases, have been found to exacerbate this disease. From the clinical standpoint, these factors are important in the management of patients with IgA nephropathy.

Activation of Complement

It has long been a matter of controversy whether IgA-dominant immune complexes in the glomeruli of patients with IgA nephropathy activate the complement component. Recently, however, there is an increasing body of evidence showing the activation of complement, including alternate pathways [59], and evidence showing that the membrane attack complex (MAC) [60] occurs in the glomeruli of patients with IgA nephropathy.

Infiltration of Phagocytic Cells

It is well known that intraglomerular infiltration of phagocytic cells induces progression of tissue damage in many renal diseases. Until recently, however, there has been no evidence showing whether such a phenomenon occurs in IgA nephropathy. Kincaid-Smith et al. [61] reported that polymorphonuclear cells and monocytes infiltrated into the glomeruli of many patients with IgA nephropathy; they thus showed that this phenomenon actually occurred in this disease.

Role of Cytokines

Various cytokines have been demonstrated to induce proliferation of mesangial cells in vitro. Recently, Horii et al. [62], using transgenic mice, demonstrated that interleukin 6 (IL-6) has a potent capacity to proliferate mesangial cells not only in vitro, but also in vivo. They also showed a significant increase in the urinary levels of IL-6 in patients with IgA nephropathy, further suggesting the exacerbating role of IL-6 in this disease.

Blood Coagulation in the Glomeruli

It is well known that intraglomerular coagulation impairs local blood flow and thus causes deterioration of renal functions. The clinical effects of antiplatelet agents such as dipyridamole have been established since the early 1970s [63], and these drugs are now most commonly used for the treatment of IgA nephropathy in many countries.

Hypertension and Microvascular Lesions

Systemic hypertension, with and without associated intraglomerular hypertension, is known as the major factor in the progression of renal dysfunction. The exacerbating roles of hypertension and microvascular lesions have been shown to be related to the progression of IgA nephropathy [64].

Summary of Proposed Pathogenesis

Figure 1 summarizes a proposed model of the pathogenesis of IgA nephropathy. The initial events leading to the development of IgA nephropathy seem to be mediated by various kinds of IgA-dominant immune complexes, which might be induced by some antigenic stimulation in genetic high responders of IgA production. The later events are common in various renal diseases and presumably contribute to the progression of renal damage in this disease.

Treatment

Selection of Therapy

There is no specific treatment for IgA nephropathy. The aim of current treatment is to preserve renal functions and to stabilize associated symptoms such as hypertension. The selection of therapy depends on the prediction of prognosis of individual

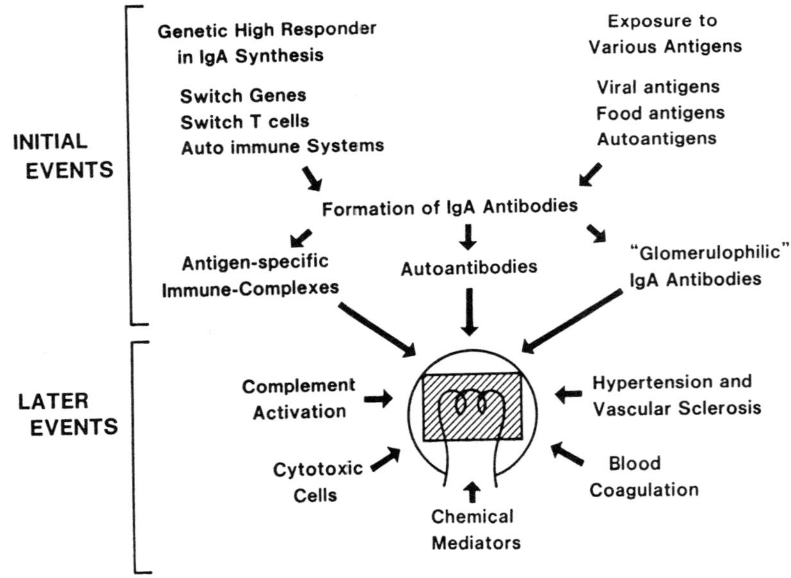

Fig. 1. Pathogenesis of IgA nephropathy (model proposed in 1990). (From [80] with permission)

patients. With respect to parameters for the prediction of prognosis, there are two major streams: (a) one which evaluates multiple factors, including severity of glomerular lesions, proteinuria of more than 2g/day, hypertension, age of more than 35 at onset, and male sex [65], and (b) one which evaluates the single most reliable parameter, which is the severity of glomerular lesions [66]. The common denominator between these two streams is the histopathological findings in renal biopsy specimens. The prognosis of almost all adult patients and the majority of pediatric patients can be predicted by histological findings at the time of the first biopsy, because there will not be much deviation in the degree of tissue damage after the diagnosis. Most institutions around the world classify the histological lesions into several categories, e.g., minimal, slight, moderate, and advanced. No drug therapy is required for the treatment of patients with minimal to slight degree of damage because, with a few exceptions in pediatric patients, most of them remain unchanged during periodic checks. In patients with advanced IgA nephropathy, there is no effective method of preventing renal failure. Therefore, these patients should avoid vigorous immunosuppressive treatment in order to preserve their general condition in preparation for hemodialysis or allotransplantation. However, all these minimal, slight, and advanced patients need to be treated by appropriate diet, adequate degree of restriction of physical activity, and maintenance of general condition, such as control of hypertension. In addition to this general therapy, administration of drugs will be required in patients with a moderate degree of IgA nephropathy. The prognosis of patients in this category is heterogeneous, but drug therapy is required in all of them because of the lack of a reliable method of predicting their individual prognoses.

Drugs Evaluated by Double Blind Studies

As of the time of this writing, only two drugs have been evaluated by multi-center double-blind studies. These studies, however, were performed in Japan and there are no reports in English. Sixty mg/day of trimetazidine hydrochloride (t.i.d., p.o.) [67] and 300 mg/day of dilazep hydrochloride (t.i.d., p.o.) [68] were found to be effective in the improvement and reduction of proteinuria. One of these drugs, dilazep hydrochloride, has been approved by the Ministry of Health and Welfare of Japan as a drug for treatment of IgA nephropathy. However, double-blind administration of these drugs was performed for only six months, followed by two year follow-ups. Longer periods of double-blind studies were not feasible, for ethical reasons.

Drugs Evaluated by Multi-Center Studies

In many countries, dipyridamole has a relatively long history of use for treatment of IgA nephropathy, but so far no double-blind study has been performed; only multi-center open studies have been performed since 1970 [63]. The clinical effects of these anti platelet agents, i.e., trimetazidine dihydrochloride, dilazep hydrochloride, and dipyridamole, are regarded as similar, although precise scientific comparisons have never been made.

Previously, corticosteroids were used in patients with IgA nephropathy associated with severe proteinuria. Recent studies have shown, however, that steroids are effective in maintaining renal functions in patients with moderate degrees of glomerular lesions associated with a moderate degree of proteinuria, i.e., less than 2 g/day [69]. Similar results have been obtained in an on-going research project of the Ministry of Health and Welfare of Japan (Professor M. Narita, personal communication). In order to establish guidelines for the selection of patients for steroid therapy, further evaluation is warranted.

Drugs and Other Treatment Still in the Experimental Stage

In many countries, nonsteroidal anti inflammatory drugs have been used in patients with various types of chronic glomerulonephritis, but there have been no large-scale studies of this type of drug [70]. Drug-induced gastric irritation and possible increase in serum creatinine levels are still being debated.

The effects of other drugs which interfere with the blood coagulation system have been reported. Defibrination of intraglomerular fibrin deposits by urokinase effected significantly better preservation of renal function for three years, when compared with antiplatelet agents [71]. Use of antiallergic drugs is potentially interesting because of the possible role of allergic reactions in the pathogenesis of IgA nephropathy [72]. Other drugs, such as low dose dopamine [73], danazol [74], and eicosapentaenoic acid [75], showed some limited effects, and further confirmation is warranted.

Coppo et al. [76] have advocated plasmapheresis in the treatment of progressive IgA nephropathy. The experience of Australian groups suggested, however, that this treatment may alter the course of the disease only while treatment continues [77].

Allotransplantation in patients with IgA nephropathy is known to show recurrence rates of more than 50%, but the prognosis of recurrent IgA nephropathy has been regarded as relatively benign [78]. Recently, there have been a few reports showing

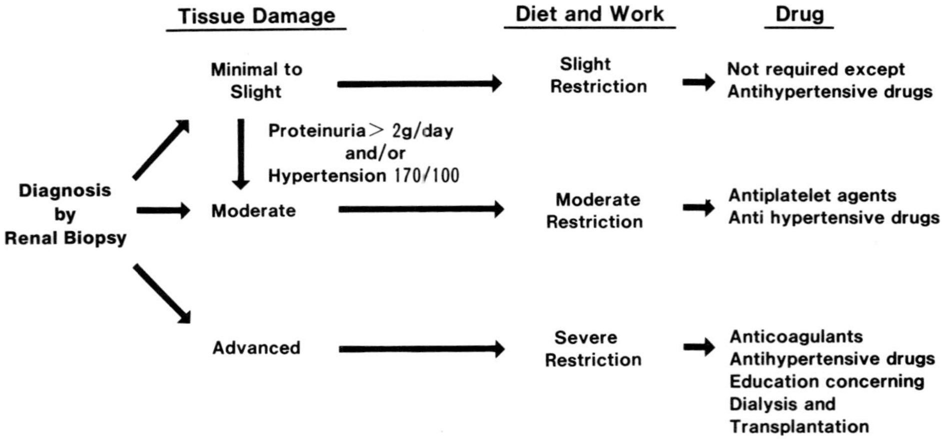

Fig. 2. Treatment of IgA nephropathy (model proposed in 1990)

the progression of recurrent IgA nephropathy to end stage renal disease [79]. However, the rates of progression in transplant patients are relatively low and thus transplantation is not prohibited in the treatment of patients with IgA nephropathy.

Summary of Proposed Treatment

Figure 2 summarizes treatment protocols from recent reports. Selection of treatment should be based on the degree of tissue damage in renal biopsy specimens, although the presence of massive proteinuria and/or hypertension influences the evaluation. Restriction of diet and daily activities will be routine procedure. No drugs are required for patients with a minimal to slight degree of tissue damage. Antiplatelet agents are the drugs of choice in moderate IgA nephropathy. Preservation of general condition and appropriate education are required in patients with severe IgA nephropathy, together with treatment by anticoagulants such as warfarin. Administration of antihypertensive drugs is mandatory if persistent high blood pressure is observed in patients at any stage of IgA nephropathy.

References

1. Berger J, Hingalis N (1968) Les dépôts intercapillaires d'IgA-IgG. J Urol (Paris) 74:694–695
2. D'Amico G (1985) Idiopathic IgA mesangial nephropathy. Nephron 41:1–13
3. Clarkson AR (1987) IgA nephropathy: history, classification, and geographic distribution. In: Clarkson AR (ed) IgA Nephropathy. Martinus Nijhoff, Boston, pp 1–8
4. Berger J (1969) IgA glomerular deposits in renal disease. Transplant Proc 1:939–944
5. Lamperi S, Carozzi S (1979) Skin-muscle biopsy in patients with various nephropathies. Nephron 24:46–50
6. Hall RP, Stachura I, Cason J, Whiteside TL, Lawley TJ (1983) IgA-containing circulating immune complexes in patients with IgA nephropathy. Am J Med 74:56–63

7. Berger J, Yaneva H, Nabarra B, Barbanel C (1975) Recurrence of mesangial deposition after renal transplantation. Kidney Int 7:232–241
8. Sanfilippo F, Croker BP, Bollinger RB (1982) Fate of four cadaveric donor renal allografts with mesangial IgA nephropathy. Transplantation 33:370–376
9. André C, Berthoux FC, André F, Gillon J, Genin C, Sabatier J-C (1980) Prevalence of IgA2 deposits in IgA nephropathies. N Engl J Med 303:1343–1346
10. Conley ME, Cooper MD, Michael AF (1980) Selective deposition of IgA1 in IgA nephropathy, anaphylactoid purpura nephritis, and systemic lupus erythematosus. J Clin Invest 66:1432–1436
11. Lai K-N, Chan KW, Lai FM-C, Ho CP, Yan KW, Lam CWK, Vallnce-Owen J (1986) The immunochemical characterization of the light chains in the mesangial IgA deposits in IgA nephropathy. Am J Clin Pathol 85:548–551
12. Komatsu N, Nagura H, Watanabe K, Nomoto Y, Kobayashi K (1983) Mesangial deposits of J-chain linked polymeric IgA nephropathy. Nephron 33:61–64
13. Tomino Y, Sakai H, Miura M, Endoh M, Nomoto Y (1982) Detection of polymeric IgA in glomeruli from patients with IgA nephropathy. Clin Exp Immunol 49:419–425
14. Monteiro RC, Halbwachs-Mecarelli L, Roque-Barreira MC, Noel L-H, Berger J, Lesavre P (1985) Charge and size of mesangial IgA in IgA nephropathy. Kidney Int 28:666–671
15. Shigematsu H, Kobayashi Y, Hiki Y (1990) Paramesangial destructive lesions in immunoglobulin A nephritis. Ultrastruct Pathol 14:129–139
16. Smith SM, Tung KS (1985) Incidence of IgA-related nephritis in American Indians in New Mexico. Hum Pathol 16:181–184
17. Jennette JC, Wall SD, Wilkman AS (1985) Low incidence of IgA nephropathy in blacks. Kidney Int 28:944–950
18. Egido J, Julian BA, Wyatt RJ (1987) Genetic factors in primary IgA nephropathy. Nephrol Dial Transpl 2:134–142
19. Wyatt RJ, Julian BA, Galla JH, McLean R (1984) Increased frequency of C3 fast alleles in IgA nephropathy. Disease Markers 2:419–428
20. McLean RH, Wyatt RJ, Julian BA (1984) Complement phenotypes in glomerulonephritis: increased frequency of homozygous null C4 phenotypes in IgA nephropathy and Henoch-Schonlein purpura. Kidney Int 26:855–860
21. Valentijn RM, Radl J, Haaijman JJ, Vermeer BJ, Weening JJ, Kaufmann RH, Daha MR, van Es LA (1984) Circulating and mesangial secretory component-binding IgA1 in primary IgA nephropathy. Kidney Int 26:760–766
22. Harada T, Hobby P, Courteau M, Knight JF, Williams DG (1989) Charge distribution of plasma IgA in IgA nephropathy. Clin Exp Immunol 77:211–214
23. Sakai H, Nomoto Y, Arimori S, Komori K, Inouye H, Tsuji, K (1979) Increase of IgA-bearing peripheral blood lymphocytes in families of patients with IgA nephropathy. Am J Clin Pathol 72:452–456
24. Garcia-Hoyo R, Lozano L, Egido J (1987) Immune abnormalities of IgA in six families with IgA nephropathy. In: McGhee JR, Mestecky J, Ogra PL, Beinenstock J (eds) Recent advances in mucosal immunology, Part B. Plenum, New York, pp 1499–1505
25. Béné M-C, Faure G, de Ligney BH, Kessler M, Duheille J (1983) IgA nephropathy: quantitative immunohistomorphometry of the tonsilar plasma cells evidences an inversion of the IgA versus IgG secreting cell membrane. J Clin Invest 71:1342–1347
26. Béné M-C, de Ligney BH, Sirbat D, Faure G, Kessler M, Duheille J (1984) IgA nephropathy: dimeric IgA-secreting cells are present in episcleral infiltrate. Am J Clin Pathol 82:608–611
27. Waldo FB, Beischel L, West CD (1986) IgA synthesis by lymphocytes from patients with IgA nephropathy and their relatives. Kidney Int 29:1229–1233
28. Sakai H (1987) Lymphocyte function in IgA nephropathy. In: Clarkson AR (ed) IgA nephropathy. Martinus Nijhoff, Boston, pp 176–187

29. Egido J, Blasco R, Sancho J, Lozano L, Anchez-Crespo M, Hernando L (1982) Increased rates of polymeric IgA synthesis by circulating lymphoid cells in IgA mesangial glomerulonephritis. Clin Exp Immunol 47:309–316
30. van den Wall Bake AWL, Daha MR, van der Ark A, Hiemstra PS, Radl J, van Es LA (1988) Serum levels and in vitro production of IgA subclasses in patients with primary IgA nephropathy. Clin Exp Immunol 74:115–120
31. Sakai H, Nomoto Y, Tomino Y, Endoh M, Miura M, Suga T (1987) Increases of in vitro and in vivo production of polyclonal IgA in patients and their family members with IgA nephropathy. In: McGhee JR, Mestecky J, Ogra PL, Beinenstock J (eds) Recent advances in mucosal immunology, Part B. Plenum, New York, pp 1507–1514
32. Endoh M, Suga T, Miura M, Tomino Y, Nomoto Y, Sakai H (1984) In vivo alteration of antibody production in patients with IgA nephropathy. Clin Exp Immunol 57:564–570
33. Nomoto Y, Suga T, Miura M, Nomoto H, Tomino Y, Sakai H (1986) Characterization of an acidic nuclear protein recognized by autoantibodies in sera from patients with IgA nephropathy. Clin Exp Immunol 65:513–519
34. Cederholm B, Wieslander J, Bygren P, Heinegard D (1986) Patients with IgA nephropathy have circulating anti-basement membrane antibodies reacting with structures common to collagen I, II, and IV. Proc Natl Acad Sci USA 83:6151–6155
35. Endoh M, Suga T, Sakai H (1985) IgG, IgA, and IgM rheumatoid factors in patients with glomerulonephritis. Nephron 39:330–335
36. Sinico RA, Fornasieri A, Oreni N, Benuzzi S, D'Amico G (1986) Polymeric IgA rheumatoid factor in idiopathic IgA mesangial nephropathy (Berger's disease). J Immunol 137:536–541
37. Gonzalez-Cabrero J, Egido J, Mampaso F, Rivas MC, Hernando L (1989) Characterization of circulating idiotypes containing immune complexes and their presence in the glomerular mesangium in patients with IgA nephropathy. Clin Exp Immunol 76:204–209
38. Schena FP, Pastore A, Ludovico N, Sinico RA, Benuzzi S, Montinaro V (1989) Increased serum levels of IgAl-IgG immune complexes and anti-F(ab')$_2$ antibodies in patients with primary IgA nephropathy. Clin Exp Immunol 77:15–20
39. Nomoto Y, Miura M, Suga T, Endoh M, Tomino Y, Sakai H (1984) Cold reacting antinuclear factor (ANF) in families of patients with IgA nephropathy. Clin Exp Immunol 58:63–67
40. Elson CO (1983) T cell specific for IgA switching and for IgA B-cell differentiation. Immunol Today 4:189–190
41. Sakai H, Nomoto Y, Arimori S (1979) Decrease of IgA-specific suppressor T cell activity in patients with IgA nephropathy. Clin Exp Immunol 38:243–248
42. Egido J, Blasco RA, Sancho J, Hernando L (1985) Immunological abnormalities in healthy relatives of patients with IgA nephropathy. Am J Nephrol 5:14–20
43. Chatenoud L, Bach M-A (1981) Abnormalities of T-cell subsets in glomerulonephritis and systemic lupus erythematosus. Kidney Int 20:267–274
44. Sakai H, Endoh M, Tomino Y, Nomoto Y (1982) Increase of IgA specific helper Tα cells in patients with IgA nephropathy. Clin Exp Immunol 50:77–82
45. Yodoi J, Adachi M, Noro N (1987) IgA-binding factors and Fc receptors for IgA: comparative studies between IgA and IgE Fc receptor systems. Int Rev Immunol 2:117–141
46. Kawanishi H, Saltzman LE, Strober W (1983) Mechanism regulating IgA class-specific immunoglobulin production in murine gut-associated lymphoid tissue. 1. T cells derived from Peyer's patches that switch sIgM cells to sIgA B cells in vitro. J Exp Med 157:433–450
47. Sakai H, Miyazaki M, Endoh M, Nomoto Y (1989) Increase of IgA-specific switch T cells in patients with IgA nephropathy. Clin Exp Immunol 78:378–382
48. Miyazaki M (to be published) Abnormalities of cellular immunity in patients with IgA nephropathy and their relatives. Jpn J Med

49. Demaine AG, Rambausek M, Knight JF, Williams DG, Welsh KI, Ritz E (1988) Relation of mesangial IgA glomerulonephritis to polymorphism of immunoglobulin heavy chain switch region. J Clin Invest 81:611–614
50. Miyazaki M (1990) Heterogeneity of the Sα2 region—increased frequency of the heterozygous switch region of IgA2 in patients with IgA nephropathy. In: Sakai H, Sakai O, Nomoto Y (eds) Pathogenesis of IgG nephropathy. HBJ Japan, Tokyo, pp 65–80
51. Coffman RL, Lebman DA, Shrader B (1989) Transforming growth factor β specifically enhances IgA production by lipopolysaccharide-stimulated murine B lymphocytes. J Exp Med 170:1039–1044
52. Bannister KM, Hay J, Clarkson AR, Woodroffe AJ (1984) Fc specific reticulo-endothelial clearance in SLE and glomerulonephritis. Am J Kidney Dis 3:287–292
53. Roccatello D, Coppo R, Piccoli G (1984) Monocyte macrophage system function in primary IgA nephropathy. Contrib Nephrol 40:130–136
54. Roccatello D, Coppo R, Piccoli G, Cordonnier D, Martina G, Rollino C, Picciotto G, Sena LM, Amoroso A (1985) Fc receptors blocking factors in IgA nephropathies. Clin Nephrol 23:159–168
55. Tomino Y, Sakai H, Miura M, Suga T, Endoh M, Nomoto Y, Umehara K, Hashimoto K (1985) Specific binding of circulating IgA antibodies in patients with IgA nephropathy. Am J Kidney Dis 3:149–153
56. Eguchi K, Sakai H, Endoh M, Nomoto Y (1990) Specific antisera against pharyngeal antigens in patients with IgA nephropathy. In: Sakai H, Sakai O, Nomoto Y (eds) Pathogenesis of IgA nephropathy. HBJ Japan, Tokyo, pp 231–246
57. Russell MW, Mestecky J, Julian BA, Galla JH (1986) IgA-associated renal disease: antibodies to environmental antigens in sera and deposition of immunoglobulins and antigens in glomeruli. J Clin Immunol 6:74–78
58. Sato M, Kojima H, Takayama K, Koshikawa S (1988) Glomerular deposition of food antigens in IgA nephropathy. Clin Exp Immunol 73:295–299
59. Wyatt RJ, Kanayama Y, Julian BA, Negoro M, Sugimoto S, Hudson EC, Curd JG (1987) Complement activation in IgA nephropathy. Kidney Int 31:1019–1023
60. Rauterberg EW, Lieberknecht H-M, Wingen A-M, Ritz E (1987) Complement membrane attack (MAC) in idiopathic IgA-glomerulonephritis. Kidney Int 31:820–829
61. Kincaid-Smith P, Nicholls K, Birchall I (1989) Polymorphs infiltrate glomeruli in mesangial IgA glomerulonephritis. Kidney Int 36:1108–1111
62. Horii Y, Iwano M, Suematshu S, Matsusaka T, Matsuda T, Muraguchi A, Yamamoto T, Miyazaki J, Yamamura K, Ishikawa H, Hirano T, Kishimoto T (1990) Interleukin-6 is a growth factor for mouse mesangial cells. In: Sakai H, Sakai O, Nomoto Y (eds) Pathogenesis of IgA nephropathy. HBJ Japan, Tokyo, pp 127–143
63. Kincaid-Smith P, Laver MC, Fairley KF (1970) Dipyridamole and anticoagulants in renal disease due to glomerular and vascular lesions. A new approach to therapy. Med J Aust 1:145–151
64. Katafuchi R, Vamvakas E, Neelakantappa K, Baldwin DS, Gallo GR (1990) Microvascular disease and the progression of IgA nephropathy. Am J Kidney Dis 15:72–79
65. Droz D (1987) IgA nephropathy: clinicopathological correlations. In: Clarkson AR (ed) IgA nephropathy. Martinus Nijhoff, Boston, pp 97–107
66. D'Amico G, Minetti L, Ponticelli C, Fellin G, Ferrario F, Barbiano di Belgioioso G, Duca G (1986) Prognostic indicators in idiopathic IgA mesangial nephropathy. Q J Med New Series 59:363–378
67. Tojo S, Narita M, Miyahara T, Sakai O, Ohono J, Soeda N, Honda N, Nagase M, Sibata M, Orita Y, Ishikawa H, Hara K, Sakuma A (1985) Manseishikyuutaijinen ni taisuru trimetazidine dihydrochloride no rinshokoka. Jin to Toseki 19:1367–1380
68. Tojo S, Honda N, Sibata M, Narita M, Miyahara T, Sakai O, Katoh E, Kida H, Orita Y, Ishikawa H, Hara K, Tanaka T, Takasaki H (1986) Manseishikyuutaijinen ni taisuru AS-05 (Dilazep) no rinshoukouka. Jin to Toseki 20:289–313

69. Kobayashi Y, Hiki Y, Tateno S, Fujii K, Kurokawa A (1990) Indication of steroid therapy in IgA nephropathy (abstract). Proceedings of the XIth international congress of nephrology, July 15–20 1990. Springer, Tokyo Berlin Heidelberg
70. Laurent J, Belghiti D, Bruneau C, Lagrue G (1987) Diclofenac, a nonsteroidal anti-inflammatory drug, decreases proteinuria in some glomerular diseases: A controlled study. Am J Nephrol 7:198–202
71. Miura M, Endoh M, Nomoto Y, Sakai H (1989) Long-term effect of urokinase therapy in IgA nephropathy. Clin Nephrol 32:209–216
72. Sato M, Takayama K, Kojima H, Koshikawa S (1990) Sodium cromoglycate therapy in IgA nephropathy: a preliminary short-term trial. Am J Kidney Dis 15:141–146
73. Beukhof HR, ter Wee PM, Sluiter WJ, Donker AJM (1985) Effect of low-dose dopamine on effective renal plasma flow and glomerular filtration rate in 32 patients with IgA nephropathy. Am J Nephrol 5:267–270
74. Tomino Y, Sakai H, Miura M, Suga T, Endoh M, Nomoto Y (1984) Effect of danazol on solubilization of immune deposits in patients with IgA nephropathy. Am J Kidney Dis 4:135–140
75. Hamazaki T, Tateno S, Shishido H (1984) Eicosapentaenoic acid and IgA nephropathy. Lancet I:1017–1018
76. Coppo R, Basolo B, Giachino O, Rocatelli D, Lajola D, Mazzucco G, Amore A, Piccoli G (1985) Plasmapheresis in a patient with rapidly progressive idiopathic IgA nephropathy: removal of IgA-containing immune complexes and clinical recovery. Nephron 40:488–490
77. Clarkson AR (1987) The treatment of IgA nephropathy. In: Clarkson AR (ed) IgA nephropathy. Martinus Nijhoff, Boston, pp 214–224
78. Berger J, Noel L, Nabarra B (1984) Recurrence of mesangial IgA nephropathy after renal transplantation. Contrib Nephrol 40:195–197
79. Brensilver JM, Mallat S, Scholes J, McCabe R (1988) Recurrent IgA nephropathy in living-related donor transplantation: recurrence or transmission of familial disease? Am J Kidney Dis 12:147–151
80. Sakai H (1990) Pathogenesis of IgA nephropathy. Japn J Clin Immunol 13:307–319

Pathophysiology of Obstructive Nephropathy

SAULO KLAHR

Chair: Shaul G. Massry

Pathophysiology of Obstructive Nephropathy

SAULO KLAHR[1]

SUMMARY. The effects of obstructive uropathy on renal function are the consequence of a variety of factors with complex interactions. Obstruction of the urinary tract decreases glomerular filtration rate (GFR) and renal plasma flow, and modifies tubular function. The decrease in GFR and plasma flow is mediated, in part, by the vasoconstrictors angiotensin II and thromboxane A_2.

A significant infiltration of leukocytes occurs in the kidney following obstruction; furthermore, by abolishing this infiltrate the renal function of the post-obstructed kidney is significantly improved. This indicates that leukocytes have an important role in modulating renal hemodynamics after release of obstruction, whose pathophysiology must now be considered to include an immunological component. Further work is required to define the mechanisms whereby macrophages can influence renal function and to define how the kidney can recruit these cells in such large numbers following obstruction.

Abnormalities in renal tubule function are common in urinary tract obstruction. The major alterations appear to be located in distal segments of the nephron. There is decreased ability to concentrate the urine, the reabsorption of sodium and water is altered, and the secretion of hydrogen and potassium is impaired.

Effects of Obstruction on the Kidney

Urinary tract obstruction has diverse effects on renal function in humans. There is a marked reduction in renal blood flow and glomerular filtration rate, and there are significant changes in renal tubular function [1]. Partial chronic obstruction of the urinary tract can cause progressive atrophy and destruction of nephrons, which may lead to chronic renal insufficiency. Unilateral complete obstruction of urine flow

[1]Renal Division, Department of Medicine, Washington University School of Medicine, St. Louis, MO 63110, USA

may be well tolerated for several days; however, if the obstruction persists for more than a week, permanent damage ensues. By the end of three weeks of complete obstruction, recovery of function is usually nil. On the other hand, acute complete bilateral obstruction results in renal failure. Because obstruction is generally a reversible cause of kidney failure, early and accurate diagnosis and prompt treatment are vital to the preservation and restoration of renal function [1].

The clinical manifestations of urinary tract obstructions vary [1]. Complete bilateral obstruction of urine flow is manifested as anuria. Partial obstruction can cause: 1) fluctuating urine output, alternating from oliguria to polyuria; 2) urinary tract infection, usually refractory to treatment; 3) abdominal or flank pain; or 4) unexplained acute or chronic renal failure. Obstruction always must be included in the differential diagnosis of acute renal failure, especially when urine output fluctuates or anuria occurs suddenly.

Pathophysiology of Obstructive Nephropathy

The effects of obstructive uropathy on renal function are the consequence of a variety of factors with complex interactions [2]. Obstruction of the urinary tract has marked effects on glomerular filtration, renal blood flow, and tubular function (see Fig. 1). Studies in experimental animals, using clearance and micropuncture techniques, have examined mainly the effect of acute short-term obstruction of the urinary tract on renal function. The effects of prolonged partial obstruction on renal function are less well characterized.

The Effects of Obstruction on Glomerular Filtration Rate

Glomerular filtration rate decreases progressively after the onset of complete ureteral obstruction [3]. The maintenance of some glomerular filtration following ureteral obstruction is presumably due to: a) the reabsorption of solutes and water along the nephron; b) the ability of the renal tract to dilate; and c) an alteration in renal hemodynamics.

Ureteral obstruction decreases glomerular filtration rate in rats, rabbits, and dogs [2]. After the onset of obstruction, the increased intraureteral pressure is transmitted upward, leading to increased intratubular pressure without a comparable quantitative increase in intraglomerular capillary hydrostatic pressure, resulting in a lower net filtration pressure across the glomerular capillary wall [3]. This appears to be the major factor responsible for the decrease in GFR after the onset of obstruction [3]. However, after 24 hours of obstruction, proximal intratubular pressure returns to normal, or below normal, values in animals with unilateral ureteral obstruction. In animals with bilateral ureteral obstruction, intratubular pressure also decreases, but remains above normal after 24 hours of obstruction [4]. At this time interval both renal plasma flow and intraglomerular capillary pressure are decreased. The decrease in intraglomerular capillary pressure after 24 hours of obstruction accounts for most of the fall in net filtration pressure and diminished single nephron GFR seen in animals with unilateral ureteral obstruction.

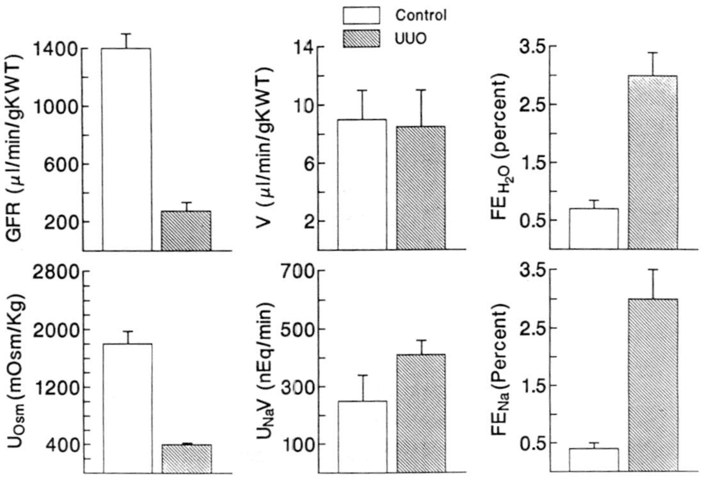

Fig. 1. Renal function after relief of unilateral ureteral obstruction (*UUO*) of 18 hours duration in 6 rats. Values are the mean ± SE for the control untouched kidney (□ and the post-obstructed kidney (▩). Both inulin clearance (*GFR*) and urine osmolality (U_{osm}) were significantly lower in the post-obstructed kidney than in the control kidney. There were no significant differences in urine flow (*V*) or absolute sodium excretion ($U_{Na}V$) between the two kidneys. Fractional sodium and water excretion were significantly greater in the post-obstructed kidney than in the control

The decrease in total renal blood flow, due to both afferent and efferent arteriolar vasoconstriction, is accompanied by a fall in plasma flow per nephron, which contributes to the decrease in GFR [2,3]. With acute ureteral obstruction, the decrement in GFR exceeds the fall in renal plasma flow, resulting in a decrease in filtration fraction. This suggests that renal vasoconstriction alone does not account completely for the fall in GFR. Indeed, after relief of obstruction, the ultrafiltration coefficient (K_f) is decreased. This decrement in K_f may be due to a decrease in the total glomerular surface area available for filtration or to a change in the intrinsic permeability characteristics of the glomerular capillary wall. With short-term obstruction (24 hours) total kidney GFR decreases more than single nephron GFR, due to a decrease in the total number of filtering nephrons. Hence, the fall in GFR in acute obstruction is due to a decrement in single nephron GFR and a decrease in the total number of filtering nephrons [2].

Renal Hemodynamics in Animals with Unilateral or Bilateral Ureteral Obstruction

The renal hemodynamics of animals with unilateral or bilateral ureteral obstruction differ [2,3]. Whereas, at 24 hours after unilateral ureteral ligation in rats, the decrease in single nephron GFR is due almost exclusively to a fall in intraglomerular capillary pressure, in rats with bilateral ureteral obstruction both a decrease in intraglomerular capillary pressure and a persistent elevation of intratubular pressure account for the decrease in net filtration pressure. Furthermore, the number of filtering nephrons is greater in animals with bilateral obstruction than in those with unilateral obstruction after 24 hours of ureteral ligation [5]. The mechanisms responsible for these hemodynamic differences between unilateral and bilateral ureteral obstruction have not been elucidated. It has been reported that the levels of circulating atrial peptide, a potent vasodilator, are higher in rats with bilateral ureteral obstruction than in rats with unilateral ureteral obstruction [6]. Atrial peptide causes pre-glomerular vasodilatation and post-glomerular vasoconstriction and has been demonstrated to increase K_f in the isolated perfused glomerular preparation. In addition, the administration of exogenous atrial peptide increases GFR following release of unilateral or bilateral ureteral obstruction [6,7]. Since atrial peptide antagonizes the vasoconstrictive effects of angiotensin II, it is probable that, in vivo, the elevated levels of endogenous atrial peptide in animals with bilateral ureteral obstruction minimize the vasoconstriction that occurs, as compared to animals with unilateral ureteral obstruction.

Role of Vasoactive Compounds

Two major vasoconstrictors, angiotensin II and thromboxane A_2, have a role in the decrease in plasma flow per nephron and in single nephron GFR seen in obstruction [8]. Inhibition of thromboxane A_2 synthesis in rats with ureteral obstruction increases plasma flow per nephron, through decreased vasoconstriction of both afferent and efferent arterioles [8]. Thromboxane may also decrease K_f through mesangial cell contraction [9] and a decrease in the glomerular surface area available for filtration. Although infusion of angiotensin II into normal animals increases net filtration pressure, presumably due to greater vasoconstriction of the efferent than the afferent arteriole, blockade of angiotensin II formation after relief of obstruction increases GFR [8]. This increase in GFR may be due to a greater filtering surface area, since angiotensin II causes mesangial cell contraction [2] and therefore can reduce the total glomerular capillary area available for filtration. In addition, angiotensin II decreases plasma flow per nephron, which also contributes to the fall in single nephron GFR. The central and critical role of these two vasoconstrictors in modulating post-obstructive renal hemodynamics is illustrated (see Fig. 2) by the fact that rats pretreated with both an angiotensin converting enzyme inhibitor and a thromboxane synthase inhibitor prior to obstruction, demonstrate almost normal renal function after release of the obstruction [7].

Vasodilatory prostaglandins such as PGE_2 and prostacyclin, which are produced in increased amounts by the obstructed kidney, may prevent further decrements in GFR by antagonizing the vasoconstrictive effects of thromboxane A_2 and/or angiotensin. Indeed, it has been demonstrated that after release of obstruction in rats, administration of inhibitors of the cyclooxygenase, in the setting of prior inhibition of the thromboxane synthase, leads to a marked decrease in whole kidney GFR and in renal plasma flow [8].

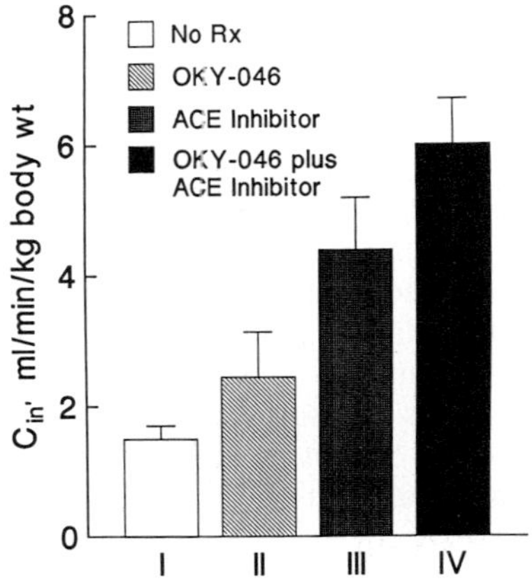

Fig. 2. Inulin clearance values measured 3–4 hours after unilateral release of bilateral ureteral obstruction of 24 h duration in four groups of rats. Values for inulin clearance were significantly greater in rats of group II (pretreated with an inhibitor of thromboxane synthesis), in rats of group III (pretreated with an inhibitor of the angiotensin converting enzyme), and in rats of group IV (treated with both a thromboxane synthase inhibitor and an inhibitor of the angiotensin converting enzyme (*ACE*), as compared to rats of group I, which were untreated. Notice that the values for inulin clearance in rats of group III are significantly higher than those in group II ($P < 0.01$), and that the combination of the ACE inhibitor and OKY-046 resulted in the highest values of GFR observed after release of obstruction (group IV). (From [7])

Effects of Obstruction on Renal Plasma Flow

After ureteral ligation, there is an initial increase in renal blood flow, which peaks at 2–3 hours after the onset of obstruction. Subsequently, renal blood flow decreases so that by 5 hours after the onset of obstruction the values are comparable to those seen prior to obstruction [1,2]. Intrinsic myogenic changes in the afferent arteriole, occurring as a consequence of ureteral obstruction, may account for the decrease seen in blood flow. It has been suggested also that the initial increase in renal blood flow to the obstructed kidney is mediated by prostaglandins, presumably prostacyclin [1,2]. Indeed, blockade of prostaglandin synthesis with cyclooxygenase inhibitors completely prevents the increase in ipsilateral blood flow that occurs with obstruction. Also, the exogenous infusion of PGI_2 (prostacyclin) increases blood flow in the obstructed kidney of animals pretreated with cyclooxygenase inhibitors. The increased release of prostaglandins during the initial period of obstruction depends on the de novo synthesis of key enzymes involved in the synthesis of eicosanoids. The activities of both cyclooxygenase and phospholipase A_2 are increased in the obstructed kidney. We have found increased activity of a phosphoethenolamine-specific phospholipase A_2 in isolated glomeruli of rats with ureteral obstruction. This enzyme may be responsible for the release of arachidonic acid from the phospholipid pool. Arachidonic acid in turn serves as the substrate for the synthesis of prostaglandins. The mechanism by which obstruction increases the synthesis and activity of the cyclooxygenase and phospholipase A_2 enzymes is unknown.

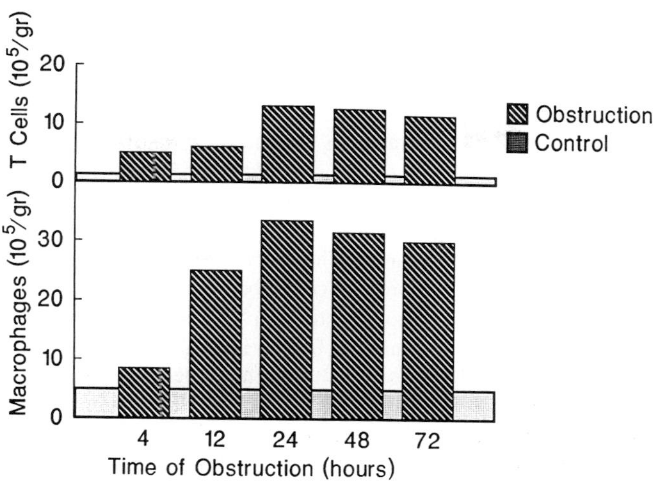

Fig. 3. The T lymphocyte (*upper panel*) and macrophage (*lower panel*) content, expressed as 10^5 cells per gram tissue, of the obstructed kidneys (▧) of rats at different time intervals after the initiation of unilateral obstruction. Control (■) values represent normal kidneys from non-obstructed littermates. Results are expressed as mean ± SE. (From [12])

With more prolonged obstruction, a progressive decrease in renal blood flow occurs, such that by 24–48 hours after the onset of obstruction, renal plasma flow is only 30%–40% of the values obtained prior to ureteral ligation [1,2]. In addition, 12–24 hours after the onset of obstruction there is a marked increase in the synthesis of thromboxane A_2 by the kidney. Thromboxane A_2 is a powerful vasoconstrictor, which may be responsible, in part, for the increased renal vascular resistance and decreased renal blood flow observed at later stages of obstruction [1,2].

Role of Infiltrating White Blood Cells in the Decrement in GFR and Renal Plasma Flow

In the 1970s it was found that a proliferation of interstitial fibroblasts and an infiltration of mononuclear cells occurred in the renal parenchyma of rabbits with chronic ureteral obstruction [10]. Subsequently, this leukocyte infiltrate was linked to the increase in prostaglandin E_2 production by the chronically hydronephrotic rabbit kidney [11]. It was also postulated, but not proven, that the infiltration of the renal parenchyma by mononuclear cells may underlie the augmented release of thromboxane A_2 and prostaglandin E_2 in response to bradykinin or endotoxin [11].

We have examined the initial phases of cell infiltration in a model of acute ureteral obstruction [12]. We found that a leukocyte influx is one of the earliest responses of the kidney to ureteral obstruction. The infiltrate was observed within 4 hours of obstruction, but its peak response occurred at 24 hours, after which a plateau was observed (Fig. 3). The leukocytes did not appear to represent a destructive infiltrate. They formed distinctive rings around tubular cells, particularly in distal tubules [12].

It is known that normal kidneys have small numbers of resident leukocytes, predominantly macrophages, in the renal cortex, mainly in the glomeruli. The normal medulla is completely devoid of resident leukocytes. In obstruction, however, the medulla is also infiltrated by mononuclear cells, to an extent comparable to that of the cortex. This leukocyte infiltration of the interstitium of the obstructed kidney was associated with a relative depletion of resident macrophages from the glomeruli. The fate of these glomerular leukocytes, which are resident mesangial macrophages, has not been elucidated. The mononuclear cell infiltrate present in the obstructed kidney consists mainly of macrophages. The second most abundant leukocytes are T lymphocytes of the cytotoxic suppressor cell subclass (see Fig. 3). The fact that T lymphocytes of the helper type do not constitute a significant portion of the infiltrate, despite the fact that they predominate in the peripheral circulation, suggests some degree of selectivity. B-lymphocytes are not present in the renal interstitium. Neutrophils are also absent from this infiltrate.

The infiltrate is slowly reversible, requiring several days after release of obstruction to revert to near normal levels [12]. Two days after release of obstruction, the macrophage content of the cortical interstitium appeared to increase modestly and then to fall to near normal levels by six days after release of the obstruction. In contrast, the T lymphocytes in the cortex diminish rapidly, to less than 20% of their values, during obstruction and two days after release of the ureteral ligation, with a further decrement noted four days later. However, a small increase in both cell populations, as compared to normal kidneys, was noted as long as a week after release of obstruction.

We also examined the functional significance of this leukocyte infiltration. The kinetics of arrival of the macrophages and leukocytes correlates temporally with the decline in glomerular filtration rate. As mentioned above, following the onset of obstruction there is an initial increase in renal blood flow, mediated by prostaglandins, which declines after 4 hours. At 24 hours, values for renal plasma flow are between 40%–70% of those observed prior to obstruction. The mechanism underlying this progressive vasoconstriction appears to be augmented production of thromboxane A_2. The chronically obstructed kidney displays an enhanced ability to metabolize arachidonic acid [1,2,11], and thromboxane synthase activity is increased. Inhibition of thromboxane synthase dramatically improves post-obstructive renal hemodynamics and partially reverses the renal vasoconstriction that occurs with acute ureteral obstruction [7,8].

To examine the potential role of the infiltrating cells in the decrease in GFR and renal plasma flow seen with ureteral obstruction, we studied rats that underwent total body radiation prior to ureteral obstruction [13]. Irradiation abolished the leukocyte infiltration observed in the kidney after 24 hours of obstruction. Irradiation had no effect on renal morphology or function in normal rats. In contrast, elimination of the infiltrate by prior irradiation of the rats with bilateral ureteral obstruction decreased thromboxane B_2 excretion in the urine and significantly improved renal hemodynamics in the post-obstructed kidney [13]. This implies that the infiltrating leukocytes contribute to the hemodynamic changes observed in the post-obstructed kidney. We propose that the leukocytic infiltrate is, in part, responsible for the decline in GFR and renal plasma flow seen after obstruction, possibly via the production of vasoactive prostanoids such as thromboxane A_2. Indeed, it is of note that renal plasma flow, which increases for the first few hours after obstruction, only begins to decline at about 4 hours after obstruction, at a time when the leukocyte infiltrate is becoming evident.

Eliminating the leukocyte infiltrate from the renal parenchyma does not, however, return the function of the post-obstructed kidney to normal. This suggests that leukocyte-independent mechanisms are also present. It is also clear that the elimination of the infiltrating macrophages by prior irradiation does not reduce the excretion of thromboxane B_2 in the urine to baseline levels. This is consistent with obstruction causing enhanced production of this vasoactive prostanoid by structures intrinsic to the kidney, such as glomerular epithelial or mesangial cells [14]. Such leukocyte independent sources of thromboxane A_2 may also be capable of modulating renal hemodynamics [1,2].

We have found recently that glomeruli isolated from animals with bilateral ureteral obstruction produce greater quantities of prostaglandin E_2 (PGE_2), 6-keto $PGF_{1\alpha}$, the stable metabolite of prostacyclin, and thromboxane B_2, the stable metabolite of thromboxane A_2, than glomeruli isolated from kidneys of normal animals [14]. Since there is a depletion of endogenous macrophages from the glomeruli of the obstructed kidney, it is clear that the increased synthesis of thromboxane B_2 by isolated glomeruli is related to its production by an intrinsic glomerular cell. Most likely this reflects increased production of thromboxane A_2 by mesangial cells, although this has not been established in the obstructed model. In addition, we found that this increased synthesis of prostanoids by isolated glomeruli was restored to levels comparable to those seen in normal kidneys when the animals were pretreated with an ACE inhibitor prior to the onset of ureteral obstruction [14]. This suggests that endogenous angiotensin II has an important role in the increased synthesis of prostanoids found in isolated glomeruli from rats with bilateral ureteral obstruction. The most likely explanation for these results may be a marked stimulation of phospholipase A_2 and/or cyclooxygenase by angiotensin II in glomeruli from rats with bilateral ureteral obstruction. Therefore, the increased thromboxane excretion in the urine of animals with bilateral ureteral obstruction may have two origins: increased production by intrinsic glomerular cells, as well as production by macrophages that invade the renal parenchyma during obstruction.

Although the available data indicate that leukocytes may promote, or directly contribute to, a locally enhanced production of thromboxane A_2, it has not been established whether or not other substances or factors released by infiltrating macrophages modulate epithelial cell function. What contribution, if any, the accompanying suppressor T lymphocytes present in the infiltrate make to the renal response to obstruction requires further characterization. Finally, the nature of the stimulus coupling urinary tract obstruction to the appearance of a leukocyte infiltrate in the renal parenchyma has not been completely defined. Initial experiments indicate the release of a chemoattractant substance by the obstructed kidney. The nature of this chemoattractant agent has not been completely elucidated, although preliminary observations suggest that it is a lipid substance [15].

Polymorphonuclear leukocytes and monocytes are present in the renal interstitium of rabbits subjected to three days of ureteral obstruction. The obstructed kidney, when perfused ex vivo, exhibits an exaggerated increase in the elaboration of eicosanoids in response to bradykinin and the chemotactic peptide, N-formilmethionil-leucil-phenylalanine. Essential fatty acid deficiency (i.e., deprivation of ω-6-fatty acids) attenuated the elaboration of eicosanoids by the obstructed kidney perfused ex vivo. It also prevented the increase in the activities of microsomal cyclooxygenase and thromboxane synthase seen after three days of ureteral occlusion. Fatty acid deficiency also attenuated the influx of macrophages into the kidney, an effect that was attributed to inhibition of the synthesis of leukotriene B_4, which is a known chemoattractant for monocytes [16].

The long-term effects of this immunological infiltrate on renal function and structure remain to be defined. However, focal segmental glomerulosclerosis is a common histological finding in patients with ureteropelvic obstruction [17]. This focal segmental glomerulosclerosis was present in areas closely associated with intense interstitial and periglomerular inflammation. It could be envisioned that growth factors released by invading leukocytes have a role in the development and progression of fibrotic and sclerotic changes that occur in the chronically obstructed kidney [18]. It is, therefore, likely that the cellular infiltrate may contribute to the renal damage and to the progressive decrease in renal function observed with chronic urinary tract obstruction.

Recovery of Renal Function after Release of Ureteral Obstruction

The extent to which GFR recovers after release of ureteral obstruction depends on the duration of the obstruction. This has been studied in both the dog and the rat. In the dog, serial measurements of GFR have been made after one week of complete ureteral obstruction [1,2]. Assuming the glomerular filtration rate for each kidney was half that of the whole animal prior to ureteric ligation, immediately after release of the obstruction GFR averaged 25% of ipsilateral control values and 16% of the concurrent values for the contralateral kidney, the latter having undergone a compensatory increase in function. Follow-up studies revealed an increase in the GFR of the obstructed kidney and a decline in the GFR of the normal kidney, with values stabilizing at 2 months. In no case was there complete functional recovery of the obstructed kidney, and at 2 years the GFR of the experimental kidney remained 50% below the simultaneous value obtained for the contralateral kidney. These changes in glomerular filtration rate were paralleled by decrements in effective renal plasma flow, as assessed by the clearance of paraaminohippurate, consequently filtration fraction did not change.

In the rat, a permanent decrease in GFR occurs if ureteral obstruction is present for more than 72 hours [9]. Complete recovery of glomerular filtration rate is seen 7–9 days after release of shorter periods (less than 30 hours) of obstruction [2,3]. Although this would suggest that short-term obstruction is completely reversible and that most of the decrease in GFR is functional, there is evidence to suggest that the "normalization" in filtration rate may not be a consequence of a homogenous recovery in the single nephron GFR (SNGFR) of all nephrons. In post-obstructed kidneys calculations of total glomerular filtration rate, based on determinations of surface nephron SNGFR, yielded values that were greater than those obtained from clearance measurements [1,2]. This may be explained by the fact that, using Hansen's technique, 40% of superficial nephrons (those accessible to micropuncture) were found to be filtering immediately following release of the obstruction, whereas only 12% of juxtamedullary nephrons were filtering, suggesting a selective loss of juxtamedullary nephrons [1,2]. Subsequent studies indicated that 3–6 hours after release of unilateral ureteral obstruction of 24 hours duration, GFR values are one-sixth of those observed prior to ligation of the ureter. With time there is an increase in the GFR, such that by days 14 and 60 after the release of obstruction, values for GFR in the post-obstructed kidney are comparable to those in the contralateral untouched kidney [19]. However, when SNGFR and the number of filtering nephrons were determined, using a modification of Hansen's technique, a decrease in the total number of filtering nephrons was found in the post-obstructed kidney, such that only 85% of the nephrons in this kidney were filtering, compared to 100% in the contralateral kidney. The normalization of whole kidney GFR was therefore at the expense of hyperfiltration (increase in SNGFR) in the remaining functional nephrons, and there was a permanent decrement in the total number of functional nephrons. The mechanism responsible for this permanent loss of nephrons following ureteral obstruction remains to be defined, as does its long-term significance in terms of the development of chronic renal failure in patients with obstructive uropathy.

Alterations in Tubular Function

Abnormalities in renal tubule function are common in urinary tract obstruction [1,2]. The major alterations appear to be located in distal segments of the nephron. There is a concentrating defect, the reabsorption of sodium and other solutes such as phosphorus, magnesium and calcium is altered, and the secretion of hydrogen and potassium is impaired.

Sodium and Water Reabsorption

The absolute amount of sodium excreted by the post-obstructed kidney after release of unilateral ureteral obstruction differs little from that excreted by the contralateral untouched kidney [1,2]. However, fractional sodium excretion is greater in the post-obstructed kidney, due to the marked fall in GFR. In addition, fractional water excretion is increased and the ability to concentrate the urine is markedly impaired, with a maximal osmolality of 300–400 mOsm reported in the rat [1,2,20]. Micropuncture experiments after release of unilateral ureteral obstruction in rats have shown that fractional reabsorption of salt and water is increased in proximal segments of surface nephrons of the post-obstructed kidney [20]. This contrasts with the marked decrease in salt and water reabsorption in juxtamedullary nephrons [20]. Calculations, based on analysis of fluid collected from the bend of the loop of Henle in the post-obstructed kidney, suggest a marked decrease in salt and water reabsorption in proximal segments of juxtamedullary nephrons. In addition, due to a decrease in medullary tonicity, related at least in part to decreased reabsorption of sodium chloride in the thick ascending limb during obstruction, there is a marked fall in the abstraction of water from the descending limb which traverses the medulla [20]. As a consequence, water delivery to the bend of the loop of Henle of juxtamedullary nephrons is significantly increased in the post-obstructed kidney, when compared with the contralateral kidney of the same animals. Despite a decrease in the filtered load of sodium in the post-obstructed kidney, the absolute excretion of this cation is comparable to that in the contralateral control kidney. This is, presumably, due to decreased sodium reabsorption in the proximal tubule and thick ascending limb of juxtamedullary nephrons [21]. The increased excretion of water may be related not only to decreased reabsorption in juxtamedullary nephrons, but also to a marked decrease in the response to antidiuretic hormone at the level of the cortical collecting duct. Indeed, it has been demonstrated that water permeability, in response to an osmotic gradient and antidiuretic hormone, is markedly decreased in in vitro perfused cortical collecting tubules isolated from kidneys of rabbits obstructed for 4 or 24 hours [21,22].

Following relief of obstruction, the ability to concentrate the urine is impaired to a greater extent than the ability to dilute the urine. Dilution of the urine occurs mainly in the thick ascending limb of Henle's loop, due to greater reabsorption of solute than water in this nephron segment. The differential impairment of concentration and dilution suggests that factors other than decreased reabsorption of solute by the thick ascending limb of Henle have a role in the concentrating defect. One such factor may be the relative increase in papillary blood flow in obstruction, which, combined with an overall decrease in glomerular filtration rate in deep nephrons, would lead to solute depletion in the medullary interstitium.

In summary, decreases in medullary tonicity are, presumably, due to: 1) decreased removal of solute from the thick ascending limb of Henle's loop; 2) decrease in the total number of juxtamedullary nephrons; 3) washout of solutes from the medulla, due to increased medullary blood flow; and 4) decreased hydrosmotic response of the cortical collecting duct to antidiuretic hormone. All these factors contribute to the concentrating defect seen after release of obstruction.

The quantitative excretion of sodium and water is somewhat different after unilateral release of bilateral ureteral obstruction. In this setting, sodium and water reabsorption in proximal segments of surface nephrons is decreased, in contrast with the increased reabsorption observed after release of unilateral ureteral obstruction. Consequently, after unilateral release of bilateral ureteral obstruction, proximal delivery of salt and water to more distal segments is augmented. Part of this increased natriuresis and diuresis could be attributed to urea excretion [23]. Urea retained during the period of bilateral obstruction is excreted in the urine after release of obstruction and acts as an osmotic agent, promoting salt and water excretion. However, the osmotic diuresis due to urea does not account quantitatively for all the natriuresis and diuresis seen after relief of bilateral obstruction [23]. Therefore, other factors may be important. Recent observations indicate that the plasma levels of atrial peptide are elevated in animals with bilateral ureteral obstruction, but not in those with unilateral ureteral obstruction. Indirect evidence, using heparin, which has been shown to antagonize some of the biological effects of atrial peptide, indicates that atrial peptide may play a role in the increased natriuresis and diuresis observed after relief of bilateral ureteral obstruction [6]. Data in patients also indicate that the levels of atrial peptide are increased in obstruction and that these plasma levels decrease after relief of obstruction.

Defective Urinary Acidification

Acid excretion is impaired after release of bilateral or unilateral ureteral obstruction in both humans and experimental animals [1,2]. Falls and Stacy noted a urine pH of 7.2 and bicarbonate wasting in a patient with post-obstructive diuresis in a solitary kidney. This patient also did not acidify his urine adequately after ammonium chloride loading. Following recovery of renal function the acidification defect disappeared. This patient had decreased proximal reabsorption of bicarbonate during the post-obstructive diuresis. However, most studies suggest that a distal renal tubular acidosis with inability to lower the urine pH to normal minimum values in response to acidemia is much more common in patients with urinary tract obstruction [1,2]. This acidifying defect seems to be reversible in the majority of patients. However, in certain patients the acidifying defect may persist. Berlyne found that after a brief ammonium chloride load 6 of 7 patients with chronic hydronephrosis could not acidify their urine to pH values below 5.3. However, in two patients the acidification defect was corrected several weeks following relief of obstruction. Better et al. described urine pHs of 6.5–7.5 in the post-obstructed kidney of a patient with complete unilateral ureteral obstruction of three months' duration. After ammonium chloride loading, the urine pH from the post-obstructed kidney fell from 6.7 to 5.7, while the contralateral kidney had a normal response.

An acidifying defect similar to that seen in humans can be elicited after ureteral obstruction in both the rat and the dog [1,2]. In this setting, urine pH from the post-obstructed kidney of rats was greater than 7 and was not influenced by an acid load. Bicarbonate titration studies and micropuncture studies revealed no decrease in proximal reabsorption of bicarbonate after release of unilateral ureteral obstruction, when compared to sham-operated animals. In the post-obstructed kidney, urine pCO_2 values remained low after bicarbonate loading. These data suggest that the acidifying defect observed after release of unilateral ureteral obstruction is due either to decreased hydrogen secretion in the distal tubule of surface nephrons and the collecting duct, or to marked alterations in the reabsorption of bicarbonate in juxtamedullary nephrons. Laski and Kurtzman [24], using perfused nephron segments from rabbits with ureteral obstruction, found a decrease in JT_{CO_2} that was detected earlier in perfused medullary collecting duct segments. Only later was there a slight fall in JT_{CO_2} in cortical segments. These data suggest that the initial defect in acidification occurs in medullary segments. Sabbatini and Kurtzman [25], using an indirect method, have evaluated the activity of H-ATPase in microdissected segments of rat nephrons obtained 24 hours after the onset of urinary tract obstruction. In animals with acute ureteral obstruction, NEM-sensitive ATPase activity was markedly reduced. In the cortical collecting duct, NEM-sensitive ATPase activity fell significantly, but to a lesser degree than was observed in the medullary collecting duct. If, indeed, NEM-sensitive ATPase is an adequate measure of hydrogen ATPase, this finding suggests that in obstruction there is an abnormality in acidification in the cortical collecting duct, but that the major defect in acidification is located at the level of the medullary collecting duct.

Using monoclonal antibodies to the 31 kilodalton subunit of the hydrogen ATPase, Purcell and associates [26] have demonstrated a decrease in the apical staining for hydrogen ATPase in intercalated cells of rats with ureteral obstruction. This decrease in staining suggests a loss, or removal, of hydrogen ATPase from the apical border of intercalated cells during the period of obstruction. Three–five days after release of obstruction of 24 h duration, the staining for hydrogen ATPase in the apical border was normal; this was accompanied by values of urine pH in the post-obstructed kidney similar to those observed in the contralateral untouched kidney. These data, then, would suggest that a decreased number of hydrogen ATPase pumps in the apical surface of intercalated cells are responsible for the acidifying defect that occurs with ureteral obstruction. The mechanism underlying the removal of H^+ pumps from the apical membrane of acid-secreting cells remains to be determined.

Abnormal Potassium Excretion

Hyperkalemic distal renal tubular acidosis has also been found in patients with chronic obstructive uropathy [27]. At all levels of glomerular filtration rate, the fractional excretion of potassium was less in patients with obstructive uropathy than in patients with comparable degrees of renal insufficiency due to a garden variety of renal diseases. Hyperkalemic-hyperchloremic acidosis has been described in a series of patients with urinary tract obstruction [27]. Three major mechanisms were uncovered that may explain the development of hyperkalemic-hyperchloremic acidosis in individuals with obstructive uropathy: 1) a selective deficiency of aldosterone secretion, probably secondary to diminished production of renin by the kidney, hyporeninemic hypoaldosteronism; 2) a defect in renal hydrogen secretion, with inability to lower urine pH maximally in the presence of systemic acidosis and decreased urinary excretion of both ammonium and titratable acid (type IV distal renal tubular acidosis); and 3) a combination of these two defects. It is possible that part of the defect may relate to a decreased sensitivity of the distal tubule to the kaliuretic effect of aldosterone. Batlle and coworkers [27] have suggested that a defect in sodium reabsorption in the distal nephron results in a decrease in the intraluminal negative potential difference. This voltage-dependent defect could contribute to the diminished secretion of both hydrogen ion and potassium. This defect, of course, may be due, in part, to an altered response to the action of aldosterone of this nephron segment during obstruction.

Pathological Changes in the Obstructed Kidney and Mechanisms of Nephron Destruction

Complete ureteral occlusion produces progressive dilatation of the renal pelvis during the first few weeks. There is perirenal and periureteral edema. The kidney weight increases due to edema, although the renal tissue, per se, atrophies. After 4–8 weeks, parenchymal weight decreases, due to atrophy which is greater than the intrarenal edema. The obstructed kidney appears dark blue with scattered areas of ischemia, wedges of congestion, necrosis, and some frank infarcts [1].

The microscopic changes of hydronephrosis have been studied in experimental animals. During the first few days after the onset of obstruction, there is flattening of the papilla with pronounced dilatation of the distal nephron [1,28]. The proximal tubules initially undergo dilatation and then slowly atrophy [1,28]. After the first week of obstruction, the dilated collecting tubules also show atrophy and necrosis. By two weeks, there is progressive dilatation of the collecting and distal tubules and atrophy of the proximal tubule epithelial cells. After 4 weeks of obstruction, there is a 50% decrease in the medullary thickness, with continued atrophy and dilatation of distal and collecting tubules. The cortex is thinner with marked atrophy of the proximal tubules. After 8 weeks of obstruction, only a thin parenchymal strip remains, consisting primarily of connective tissue and small sclerotic glomeruli.

Proliferation of medullary interstitial cells has been noted by the fifth day of obstruction [10]. There are also chronic interstitial inflammatory changes, which are more severe than glomerular changes. Ultimately, however, glomeruli become hyalinized in a pattern not dissimilar from that seen in nephrosclerosis. It should be emphasized, however, that chronic obstruction results predominantly in an interstitial disease, with relative preservation of glomerular structures.

Recently, Tanner and Evan [29] have examined glomerular and proximal tubular morphology after single nephron obstruction, utilizing a wax block. The anatomical changes found after obstruction of single nephrons resembled those seen after ureteral obstruction. There was nephron atrophy and there were glomerular changes. The latter developed at a later time than the tubular changes. The major glomerular abnormalities, after one month of obstruction, were reduced diameter, decreased number and size of capillaries, fusion of epithelial cell foot processes, thickened basement membrane of Bowman's capsule, and periglomerular fibrosis. The changes seen in the proximal tubule with prolonged single nephron blockade or urinary tract obstruction include a loss of apical microvilli, decreased cell height, simplification of basolateral membranes, and a reduction in the number of mitochondria. There is widening of the interstitial space and thickening of the tubular basement membrane. When single nephrons were obstructed, the morphological changes were circumscribed to that nephron and no ultrastructural abnormalities were seen in adjacent nephrons. After one day of obstruction, the morphological changes seen in the tubule upstream or downstream to the block were quite different. Severe injury occurred in downstream segments, whereas changes in upstream segments were modest. These differences in morphology may be due to the interruption of tubule fluid flow to the downstream segments.

The mechanisms underlying the development of nephron atrophy and nephron destruction following urinary tract obstruction have not been established, but three interrelated changes may have a role: 1) decreased blood flow; 2) disuse atrophy; and 3) infiltration of the renal parenchyma by leukocytes.

When single nephrons are obstructed, glomerular blood flow to such nephrons decreases. Glomerular blood flow decreases by 35% after 24 h of obstruction and by 70% after one week of obstruction [29]. Similar changes in blood flow are observed in animals with ureteral obstruction. Blood flow to the kidney is markedly decreased after one month of obstruction. The markedly decreased size of the glomerulus at this time is consistent with a pronounced decrease in perfusion. Increased local production of angiotensin II and thromboxane A_2 may play a role in the decreased blood flow to the glomerulus [1,2,14]. Peritubular capillary flow may be reduced with prolonged tubule obstruction and may contribute to the morphological changes. However, Tanner and Evan [29] did not observe cell necrosis, which is commonly seen with severe ischemia. On the other hand, the metabolic demands of the obstructed tubule may be less, due to a decrease in the filtered load of sodium as GFR declines. Therefore, the oxygen supply to a blocked nephron might be adequate for its metabolic needs. A reduction in blood flow alone may not be sufficient to account for the development of nephron atrophy.

Disuse atrophy [28] may account, at least in part, for the involution of the glomerular and tubular units. If the filtered load decreases, the tubular transport of solutes and water falls. The decreases in cell size and number of mitochondria are consistent with a decrease in tubular transport of solutes. The potential mechanisms linking changes in renal tubular transport to changes in cell structure are unknown.

Invading leukocytes may also play a role in the morphological changes observed. As early as a few hours after obstruction, T lymphocytes and macrophages are present in the kidney [12]. Tanner and Evan [29] also observed neutrophils and lymphocytes in the glomerulus and near the tubules during single nephron obstruction. Cells were associated only with blocked nephrons. The stimulus causing accumulation of inflammatory cells is not known. It may be related to the release of a chemoattractant by the kidney. The presence of inflammatory cells with urinary tract obstruction is characteristic of this disorder. Such cells, particularly macrophages, are known to release proteases, other enzymes, and cytokines, and to produce oxygen derived free radicals [30]. These and other chemical agents may damage the nephron. Stimulated macrophages produce increased amounts of thromboxane A_2 and other prostanoids, which can also affect blood flow [30]. Infiltrating leukocytes may stimulate the proliferation of fibroblasts and cause increased deposition of collagen and mucopolysaccharides in the interstitium. This may increase the diffusion distances between tubular cells and capillaries, causing impaired oxygen delivery to the tubular cells and subsequent tubule atrophy [28]. Therefore, infiltrating leukocytes may have an important role in the nephron atrophy that occurs with prolonged urinary tract obstruction.

Acknowledgments. The original work cited in this manuscript was supported by U.S.P.H.S. NIDDK Grants DK-09976, DK-07126, and DK-40321.

The author thanks Ms. Pat Verplancke for her assistance in the preparation of this manuscript.

References

1. Klahr S, Harris KPG (to be published) Obstructive nephropathy. In: Seldin DW, Giebisch G (eds) The kidney, 2nd Edn. Raven, New York
2. Klahr S, Harris KPG, Purkerson ML (1988) Effects of obstruction on renal function. Pediatr Nephrol 2:34–42
3. Wright FS (1982) Effects of urinary tract obstruction on glomerular filtration rate and renal blood flow. Semin Nephrol 2:5–16
4. Dal Canton A, Corradi A, Stanziale R, Maruccio G, Migone L (1979) Effects of 24-hour ureteral obstruction on glomerular hemodynamics in rat kidney. Kidney Int 15:457–462
5. Buerkert J, Martin D (1983) Relation of nephron recruitment to detectable filtration and recovery of function after release of ureteral obstruction. Proc Soc Exp Biol Med 173: 533–540
6. Purkerson ML, Blaine EH, Stokes TJ, Klahr S (1989) Role of atrial peptide in the natriuresis and diuresis that follows relief of obstruction in the rat. Am J Physiol 256:F583–F589
7. Purkerson ML, Klahr S (1989) Prior inhibition of vasoconstrictors normalizes GFR in postobstructed kidneys. Kidney Int 35:1305–1314
8. Yarger WE, Shocken DD, Harris RH (1980) Obstructive nephropathy in the rat: possible roles for the renin-angiotensin system, prostaglandins, and thromboxanes in postobstructive renal function. J Clin Invest 65:400–412
9. Mene P, Dunn MJ (1986) Contractile effects of TxA_2 and endoperoxide analogues on cultured rat glomerular mesangial cells. Am J Physiol 251:F1029–F1035

10. Nagle RB, Johnson ME, Jervis HR (1976) Proliferation of renal interstitial cells following injury induced by ureteral obstruction. Lab Invest 35:18–22
11. Okegawa T, Jonas PE, DeSchryver K, Kawasaki A, Needleman P (1983) Metabolic and cellular alterations underlying the exaggerated renal prostaglandin and thromboxane synthesis in ureter obstruction in rabbits. Inflammatory response involving fibroblasts and mononuclear cells. J Clin Invest 71:81–90
12. Schreiner G, Harris KPG, Purkerson ML, Klahr S (1988) The immunological aspects of acute ureteral obstruction: Immune cell infiltrate in the kidney. Kidney Int 34:487–493
13. Harris KPG, Schreiner GF, Klahr S (1989) Effect of leukocyte depletion on the function of the postobstructed kidney in the rat. Kidney Int 36:210–215
14. Yanagisawa H, Morrissey J, Morrison AR, Klahr S (1990) Role of angiotensin II in eicosanoid production by isolated glomeruli from rats with bilateral ureteral obstruction. Am J Physiol 258:F85–F93
15. Rovin BH, Harris KPG, Morrison A, Klahr S, Schreiner GF (1990) Renal cortical release of a specific macrophage chemoattractant in response to ureteral obstruction. Lab Invest 63:213–220
16. Spaethe SM, Freed MS, De Schryver-Kecskemeti K, Lefkowith JB, Needleman P (1988) Essential fatty acid deficiency reduces the inflammatory cell invasion in rabbit hydronephrosis resulting in suppression of the exaggerated eicosanoid production. J Pharmacol Exp Ther 245:1088–1094
17. Steinhardt GF, Ramon G, Salinas-Madrigal L (1988) Glomerulosclerosis in obstructive uropathy. J Urol 140:1316–1318
18. Davis BB, Thomason D, Zenser TV (1983) Renal disease profoundly alters cortical interstitial cell function. Kidney Int 23:458–464
19. Bander SJ, Buerkert JE, Martin D, Klahr S (1985) Long-term effects of 24-hour unilateral ureteral obstruction on renal function in the rat. Kidney Int 28:614–620
20. Yarger WE, Buerkert J (1982) Effect of urinary tract obstruction on renal tubular function. Semin Nephrol 2:17–30
21. Hanley MJ, Davidson K (1982) Isolated nephron segments from rabbit models of obstructive nephropathy. J Clin Invest 69:165–174
22. Campbell HT, Bello-Reuss E, Klahr S (1985) Hydraulic water permeability and transepithelial voltage in the isolated perfused rabbit cortical collecting tubule following acute unilateral ureteral obstruction. J Clin Invest 75:219–225
23. Purkerson ML, Klahr S (1984) Protein intake conditions the diuresis seen after relief of bilateral ureteral obstruction in the rat. Proc Soc Exp Biol Med 177:62–68
24. Laski ME, Kurtzman NA (1989) Site of the acidification defect in the post-obstructed collecting tubule. Miner Electrolyte Metab 15:195–200
25. Sabatini S, Kurtzman NA (1990) Enzyme activity in obstructive uropathy: basis for salt wastage and the acidification defect. Kidney Int 37:79–84
26. Purcell H, Harris KPG, Lim I, Klahr S, Gluck S (1989) Mechanisms of the acidifying defect after release of unilateral ureteral obstruction (abstract) Kidney Int 35:461
27. Batlle DC, Arruda JAL, Kurtzman NA (1981) Hyperkalemic distal tubular renal acidosis associated with obstructive uropathy. N Engl J Med 304:373–380
28. Møller JC, Jorgensen TM, Mortensen J (1986) Proximal tubular atrophy: qualitative and quantitative structural changes in chronic obstructive nephropathy in the pig. Cell Tiss Res 244:479–491
29. Tanner GA, Evan AP (1989) Glomerular and proximal tubular morphology after single nephron obstruction. Kidney Int 36:1050–1060
30. Nathan CR (1987) Secretory products of macrophages. J Clin Invest 79:319–326

Very Long-Term Dialysis

Yoshihei Hirasawa

Chair: Belding H. Scribner

Very Long-Term Dialysis

Yoshihei Hirasawa[1]

In this presentation, I would like to report our clinical results of long-term dialysis and discuss present problems. In the past 24 years, 1650 patients have been treated chronically by dialysis in our hospitals and satellite hospitals; 480 patients have died. The cumulative survival rate was 62% in the 10th year after starting dialysis therapy and 50% in the 20th year after starting dialysis therapy.

The main causes of death were cardiac (33%), infectious (21%), cerebro-vascular (18%), gastrointestinal (8%), and malignant (7%) diseases. The death rate due to cerebro-vascular disease and cancer increased in patients who had been on dialysis for longer than 10 years. Reflecting the progress of therapy, the survival rate in young patients has risen remarkably in the past 10 years.

Therapeutic progress has overcome many complications that occur frequently in patients receiving long-term dialysis treatment. These complications are hepatitis, pericarditis, peripheral neuropathy, dialysis hypersensitivity (ethylene oxide allergy), aluminum intoxication, and others. Recently, rHuEOP treatment of anemia has also been achieved.

However, it became clear that dialysis amyloidosis, a new complication, was occurring frequently in long-term dialysis patients. Among our patients, carpal tunnel syndrome and arthropathy, deriving from dialysis amyloidosis, began to appear from about the 8th year of dialysis therapy, and the complication rate rose with prolongation of dialysis, reaching about 50% in the 20th year of therapy.

In order to prevent dialysis amyloidosis, in the past 5 years we have performed hemodialysis with endotoxin-free bicarbonate-dialysate and with dialyzers which we have found to be extremely effective in the elimination of B_2 microglobulin (B_2M). Endotoxin concentration in dialysate was always below 20pg/ml, and the highest levels of serum β_2M of the patients were maintained within 20–40mg/l. It is interesting to note that in the last two years a decrease has been observed in the incidence of carpal tunnel syndrome, bone cyst formation, and arthropathy.

[1]Shinrakuen Hospital, 1–27 Nishi Ariake-machi, Niigata, 950–21 Japan

The pathogenesis of dialysis amyloidosis is unknown, therefore long-term observation is necessary to judge whether or not these measures are useful. If the correction of hyper β_2 microglobulinemia is effective in the prevention of dialysis amyloidosis, the administration of hemofiltration (HF) or hemodiafiltration (HDF) would be significant, and the development of on line HF or HDF would be an important factor.

In spite of the administration of active vitamin D, an increase in the incidence rate of secondary hyperparathyroidism has been observed in long-term dialysis patients. About 60% of our patients who had been on dialysis treatment for over 10 years had an abnormal rise of serum parathyroid hormone, and about 10% of those patients underwent parathyroidectomy. Pulse therapy with $1{,}25(OH)_2D_3$ was effective against hyperparathyroidism in many patients. However, it was often difficult to proceed with this therapy because of the development of hypercalcemia.

A better method for prevention of hyperparathyroidism would be the clinical administration of a drug that has a suppressive action on the parathyroid without enhancing hypercalcemia. Further, the development of a phosphate-binder that does not cause hypercalcemia is important.

Acceleration of vascular caldification is a conspicuous phenomenon in long-term dialysis patients. Since the cause of vascular calcification is assumed to be partly related to a disorder of Ca and P metabolism, the progress of therapy against secondary hyperparathyroidism may decrease the incidence of vascular calcification.

At present, 328 patients (127 in our hospital and 201 in our satellite hospitals) are being treated by dialysis which has lasted over 10 years. Twenty-six of them have a dialysis history of over 20 years, and 138 of them have been on dialysis for 15–20 years. Of these 328 patients, 40.5% are receiving night-time dialysis, 50.5% are on day-time dialysis, and 9.0% are on dialysis during hospitalization, due to complications. Almost all patients on night-time dialysis are engaged in full-time occupations. About half of the patients on day-time dialysis work as housewives or have part-time jobs.

Although some problems remain to be solved, I believe that we have been able to achieve excellent results through dialysis treatment, in terms both of prolongation of life and of rehabilitation.

Mechanisms of Na^+, Cl^-, and HCO_3^- Transport in the Proximal Tubule

PETER S. ARONSON

Chair: Gerhard Giebisch

Mechanisms of Na^+, Cl^-, and HCO_3^- Transport in the Proximal Tubule

Peter S. Aronson[1]

Introduction

The general purpose of this lecture/chapter is to provide an overview of the mechanisms mediating Na^+, Cl^-, and HCO_3^- transport in the proximal tubule of the mammalian kidney. Because this topic is so broad, attention will be focussed on four main issues concerning transport across the membranes of the proximal tubule cell: 1) mechanisms of acid secretion across the luminal membrane; 2) mechanisms of base exit across the basolateral membrane; 3) mechanisms of Cl^- entry across the luminal membrane; and 4) mechanisms for Cl^- exit across the basolateral membrane. For each of these topics, the properties of the major transport pathways determined largely (but not exclusively) on the basis of studies on isolated membrane vesicles will be correlated with the physiological roles of these same pathways as determined on the basis of studies on the intact tubule. Finally, a summary attempting to integrate these subcellular mechanisms into the overall functioning of the intact proximal tubule will be presented. Literature citations will be representative, rather than comprehensive, due to the time/space limitations imposed on this lecture/chapter.

Mechanisms of Acid Secretion Across the Luminal Membrane

The first mechanism to be described that was capable of mediating the uphill secretion of H^+ across the luminal membrane of the proximal tubule cell was Na^+-H^+ exchange, which was demonstrated by Murer et al. in brush border membrane vesicles isolated from rat renal cortex [1]. We confirmed the presence of a Na^+-H^+ exchanger in rabbit renal brush border membrane vesicles [2], and then used this experimental preparation to define several properties of this transport system [2–8].

[1]Section of Nephrology, Department of Medicine, Yale School of Medicine, New Haven, CT 06510, USA

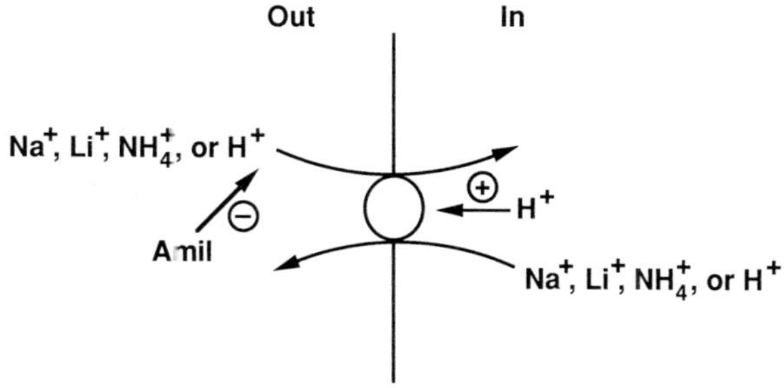

Fig. 1. Schematic model of the Na^+-H^+ exchanger. Amil, amiloride

We found that Li^+ and NH_4^+ competitively inhibited Na^+ uptake, suggesting that these cations might also be substrates for transport by this pathway [3,8]. Indeed, we demonstrated that in addition to Na^+-H^+ exchange, the system could also mediate Li^+-H^+ exchange, Na^+-Na^+ exchange and Na^+-NH_4^+ exchange [2,3,7]. External H^+ could compete for binding with external Na^+, Li^+, and NH_4^+ [7]. Amiloride was identified as an inhibitor of this pathway [2,4,8] that competed at the external site shared by Na^+, Li^+, and H^+ [4,7,8]. Internal H^+, in addition to serving as a substrate for transport, was found to be a potent allosteric activator of the Na^+-H^+ exchanger [6].

Taken together, our studies supported the model illustrated in Fig. 1, indicating that the Na^+-H^+ exchanger behaves as if it could bind any one of four cations – Na^+, H^+, Li^+, or NH_4^+ – on one side of the membrane and exchange the cation for any one of the same four cations on the opposite side of the membrane. The model also indicates that external amiloride acts as a competitive inhibitor and that internal H^+ acts as an allosteric activator. This model predicts at least two transport modes – namely, external Na^+ for internal H^+ exchange, and external Na^+ for internal NH_4^+ exchange – whereby the Na^+-H^+ exchanger could mediate secondary active acid secretion across the luminal membrane driven by the inward Na^+ gradient that is normally present due to the active extrusion of Na^+ across the basolateral membrane via the Na^+, K^+-ATPase.

Since the initial description of the Na^+-H^+ exchanger, additional mechanisms for acid secretion across the luminal membrane of the proximal tubule cell have been

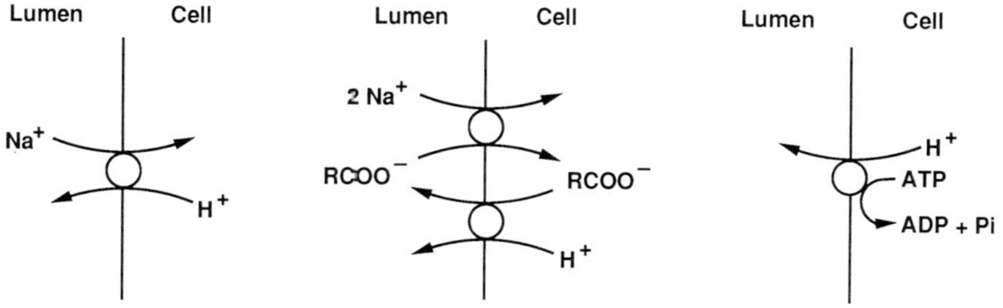

Fig. 2. Mechanisms of acid secretion across the luminal membrane of the proximal tubule cell

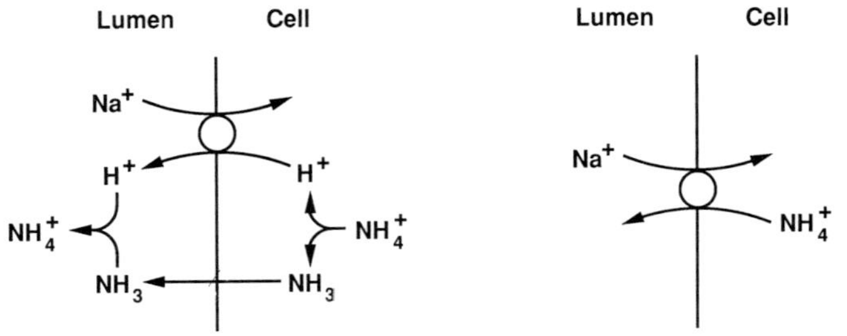

Fig. 3. Possible mechanisms of NH_4^+ secretion across the luminal membrane of the proximal tubule cell

described, as illustrated in Fig. 2. A Na^+-cotransport system for the secondary active reabsorption of monocarboxylates like lactate was first described by Barac-Nieto and Kinne in renal brush border membrane vesicles [9]. When we found that the brush border membrane also contained a separate pathway mediating H^+-organic anion cotransport (indistinguishable from organic anion-OH^- exchange) [10,11], we postulated that Na^+-coupled monocarboxylate uptake followed by H^+-coupled monocarboxylate backflux might be a mechanism for uphill H^+ secretion [12]. That such a mechanism could actually mediate acid extrusion from the proximal tubule cell was demonstrated by Nakhoul and Boron [13]. However, the contribution of this mechanism to transtubular acid secretion under physiologic conditions could not be detected by Geibel and coworkers [14].

The existence in brush border membrane vesicles of an ATPase activity that might be involved in acid-base transport was first reported by Kinne-Saffran and Kinne [15]. Controversy persisted as to whether this activity was mitochondrial or endosomal, rather than brush border, in origin. However, Burkhardt and colleagues have recently provided strong evidence that a H^+-ATPase coexists on the brush border membrane with the Na^+-H^+ exchanger [16].

What is the relative proportion of acid secretion that is mediated by Na^+-H^+ exchange versus the H^+-ATPase in the intact proximal tubule under physiologic conditions? Multiple studies have shown that $\geq 80\%$ of acid secretion in the proximal tubule is Na^+-dependent and/or dependent on operation of the Na^+, K^+-ATPase [12], seeming to argue that the Na^+-H^+ exchanger mediates almost all of proximal tubule acid secretion. But, given the recent evidence that base exit from the proximal tubule cell is Na^+-dependent (see below), this argument is no longer valid. Therefore, Preisig et al. reevaluated the role of the Na^+-H^+ exchanger in mediating proximal tubule acidification by comparing the inhibition of Na^+-H^+ exchange with the inhibition of HCO_3^- reabsorption by amiloride and an amiloride analog in the microperfused rat proximal tubule [17]. These workers concluded that Na^+-H^+ exchange mediates approximately 2/3 of proximal tubule HCO_3^- reabsorption, with the remainder mediated by a Na^+-independent, amiloride-insensitive mechanism, most likely the H^+-ATPase.

There are two potential mechanisms by which the Na^+-H^+ exchanger could participate in mediating NH_4^+ secretion in the proximal tubule, as illustrated in Fig. 3. First, by virtue of its being the principal pathway for active H^+ secretion across the luminal membrane, the Na^+-H^+ exchanger would acidify the lumen, thereby providing a favorable gradient for secretion of NH_4^+ by nonionic diffusion of NH_3. Second, as predicted by the membrane vesicle studies described above [3], the Na^+-H^+ exchanger might be capable of mediating direct Na^+-NH_4^+ exchange. Nagami has recently provided important evidence supporting the concept that direct Na^+-NH_4^+ exchange via the Na^+-H^+ exchanger contributes importantly to net secretion of NH_4^+ produced in proximal tubule cells [18]. He measured total NH_4^+ production and the portion of the produced NH_4^+ that was actually secreted into the lumen of isolated and perfused proximal tubules of the mouse. When operation of the Na^+-H^+ exchanger was inhibited by changing the luminal perfusate to one containing a reduced Na^+ concentration and amiloride, total NH_4^+ production was unchanged, but luminal NH_4^+ secretion was virtually abolished. Additional experiments demonstrated that this inhibition of luminal NH_4^+ secretion by inhibiting the function of the Na^+-H^+ exchanger could not be attributed to a change in luminal pH secondarily affecting nonionic diffusion of NH_3. Thus, these data strongly supported the notion that direct Na^+-NH_4^+ exchange can occur on the Na^+-H^+ exchanger, as predicted by the vesicle studies.

Mechanisms of Base Exit Across the Basolateral Membrane

Boron and Boulpaep identified a stilbene-sensitive, electrogenic Na^+-HCO_3^- cotransport system that mediates the coupled transfer of Na^+, HCO_3^- and net negative charge across the basolateral membrane of the isolated, perfused proximal tubule of the salamander [19]. We confirmed the presence of this transporter in basolateral membrane vesicles isolated from the rabbit renal cortex [20], and then used this experimental preparation to define several properties of this transport system [20–23].

One issue we examined was the stoichiometry of the Na^+-HCO_3^- cotransporter [21]. When the membrane potential is approximated by the Nernst potential for K^+, as in the presence of the K^+ ionophore valinomycin, equilibrium thermodynamics predicts that the Na^+-HCO_3^- cotransport system should come to equilibrium and mediate no net flux when:

$$\frac{[Na^+]_i}{[Na^+]_o} = \left(\frac{[HCO_3^-]_o}{[HCO_3^-]_i}\right)^{\mathbf{n}} \left(\frac{[K^+]_o}{[K^+]_i}\right)^{\mathbf{n}-1}$$

where **n** is the HCO_3^-:Na^+ stoichiometry [21]. Our experimental approach was to impose transmembrane Na^+, HCO_3^-, and K^+ gradients of varying magnitude and direction, and then to measure the net flux of Na^+ over the subsequent short interval. In this way, we could determine the conditions for equilibrium of the transport system and thereby calculate **n**. The data indicated that the stoichiometry of the Na^+-HCO_3^- cotransporter is 3 HCO_3^-:Na^+, or a thermodynamically equivalent process. Studying rat proximal tubules by in situ microperfusion, Yoshitomi et al. also estimated that the HCO_3^-:Na^+ stoichiometery is 3:1, based on comparison of the fall in both intracellular Na^+ activity and intracellular pH that occurred in response to a sudden reduction of peritubular HCO_3^- concentration [24].

It should be emphasized that although the preceding results were consistent with a cotransport stoichiometry of 3 HCO_3^- per Na^+, they were equally consistent with

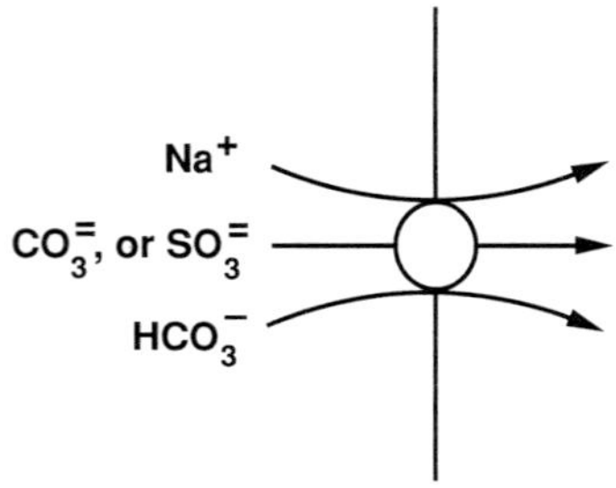

Fig. 4. Schematic model of the Na^+-HCO_3^- cotransporter

any transport process in which there is the net transfer of 3 equivalents of base, 1 Na^+, and 2 negative charges per transport event. Therefore, the purpose of the next series of experiments was to define the actual ionic mechanism of the Na^+-HCO_3^- cotransport system [22]. We found that the rate of Na^+ influx into basolateral membrane vesicles was stimulated as a function of [CO_3^{2-}] at constant [HCO_3^-], suggesting that CO_3^{2-} is a substrate for the Na^+-HCO_3^- cotransporter. The presence of a divalent anion site was confirmed by the finding that SO_3^{2-} but not SO_4^{2-} could compete with CO_3^{2-} and could itself be cotransported with Na^+. Importantly, Na^+-SO_3^{2-} cotransport was demonstrable only in the presence of HCO_3^-, indicating that in addition to the divalent anion site there must be a HCO_3^- site whose occupancy is mandatory for operation of the transport system. As illustrated in Fig. 4, the results of these experiments suggested that CO_3^{2-} can interact with the Na^+-HCO_3^- cotransporter at a site shared by SO_3^{2-}, and that HCO_3^- interacts at a separate site. Electrogenic cotransport of 3 equivalents of base per Na^+ would then occur by 1:1:1 coupled fluxes of Na^+, CO_3^{2-}, and HCO_3^-.

The exquisite HCO_3^- dependence of this transporter suggested to us that there might be an important interaction between carbonic anhydrase and the Na^+-HCO_3^- cotransporter. We therefore examined whether inhibition of carbonic anhydrase with acetazolamide would affect operation of the Na^+-HCO_3^- cotransporter in basolateral membrane vesicles [23]. We found that concentrations of acetazolamide up to 0.6 mM added to the external solution and preloaded into the vesicles had virtually no effect when Na^+ influx was measured in the presence of a directly imposed inward HCO_3^- gradient. This result indicated that carbonic anhydrase is not directly involved in mediating transport through the Na^+-HCO_3^- cotransporter. We then tested whether carbonic anhydrase in the basolateral membrane vesicles could be rate limiting for Na^+-HCO_3^- cotransport under conditions where HCO_3^- was being generated or consumed.

In the presence of a CO_2/HCO_3^- buffer system, but in the absence of an initial HCO_3^- gradient, Na^+ influx was stimulated by an outward NH_4^+ gradient. This stimulation of Na^+ influx by an outward NH_4^+ gradient was significantly inhibited by 0.6 mM acetazolamide, suggesting that acetazolamide blocked the ability of the NH_4^+ gradient to generate an inward HCO_3^- gradient. In the presence of an inward HCO_3^- gradient, Na^+ influx was inhibited by an inward NH_4^+ gradient. The magnitude of this inhibition of Na^+ influx was reduced by 0.6 mM acetazolamide, suggesting that acetazolamide blocked the ability of NH_4^+ to collapse the inward HCO_3^- gradient. Similarly, Na^+ influx in the presence of an inward HCO_3^- gradient was

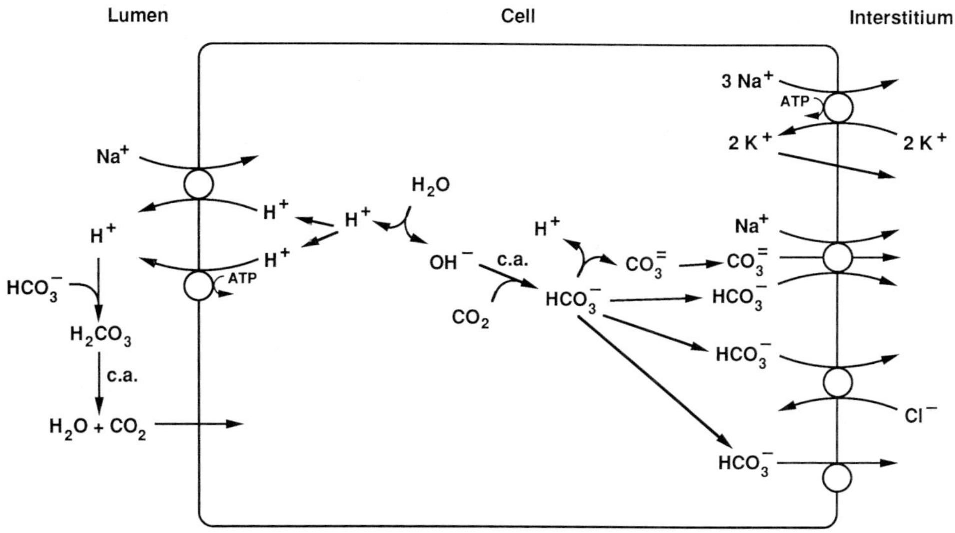

Fig. 5. Model of the proximal tubule cell emphasizing possible mechanisms of base exit across the basolateral membrane. c.a., carbonic anhydrase

inhibited by an outward acetate gradient, and this inhibition was reduced by acetazolamide. Thus, acetazolamide caused either inhibition or stimulation of Na^+ uptake depending on the conditions with respect to pH and HCO_3^- gradients. These results indicated that the operation of the Na^+-HCO_3^- cotransporter is markedly, although indirectly, dependent on the activity of carbonic anhydrase.

The physiological role of the Na^+-HCO_3^- cotransporter in the process of proximal tubule acidification is illustrated in Fig. 5. Secretion of H^+ across the luminal membrane occurs principally by Na^+-H^+ exchange with an additional contribution from a H^+-ATPase. Secretion of H^+ via recycling of monocarboxylates is not shown. It should be emphasized that membrane vesicle studies have clearly shown that both the Na^+-H^+ exchanger and the H^+-ATPase can operate in the absence of CO_2/HCO_3^-. Thus, the effect of luminal membrane H^+ secretion is to split water and liberate OH^- in the cell. As just discussed, the Na^+-HCO_3^- cotransporter can transport base only in the form of HCO_3^- and CO_3^{2-}, which are generated within the cell or at the basolateral membrane by the action of carbonic anhydrase. Thus, the essential role of intracellular and/or basolateral membrane carbonic anhydrase is to convert OH^- to the forms of base that can exit the cell via the Na^+-HCO_3^- cotransporter. This leads to the prediction that inhibition of carbonic anhydrase should prevent base exit.

The stoichiometry of the Na^+-HCO_3^- cotransporter is important for understanding why this system normally functions in the direction of mediating base exit from the cell. Under physiologic conditions, a large Na^+ gradient is directed inward across the basolateral membrane; the pH and HCO_3^- concentration in the cell are slightly lower than in the interstitial fluid. Thus, inward Na^+, HCO_3^-, and CO_3^{2-} gradients favor this transport system operating in the inward direction. But the fact that two negative charges are transported per transport cycle makes it possible for the normal inside-negative membrane potential membrane to drive efflux against the inward Na^+, HCO_3^-, and CO_3^{2-} gradients [24]. This membrane potential is in turn due to the outward K^+ gradient and high K^+ conductance of the basolateral membrane.

Other possible mechanisms of base exit across the basolateral membrane are also illustrated in Fig. 5. Simple conductive OH^- or HCO_3^- exit not coupled to Na^+ appears to contribute negligibly to base exit [25]. On the other hand, studies from a number of laboratories have indicated that significant Cl^--HCO_3^- exchange also takes place at the basolateral membrane of the proximal tubule cell [25].

How important is Cl^--HCO_3^- exchange vs Na^+-HCO_3^- cotransport as a mechanism of base exit? The rate of Na^+-HCO_3^- cotransport can be assessed by studying the effect on intracellular pH of acutely lowering basolateral Na^+ concentration in the absence of Cl^-. This should result in a rapid acidification of intracellular pH if Na^+-HCO_3^- cotransport is a major pathway for base exit across the basolateral membrane. On the other hand, the rate of Cl^--HCO_3^- exchange can be assessed by taking away all Cl^- and then studying the effect on intracellular pH of acutely adding Cl^- back to the basolateral solution. This should result in a rapid efflux of HCO_3^-, causing acidification of intracellular pH if Cl^--HCO_3^- exchange is a major pathway for base efflux across the basolateral membrane. Experiments of this type were carried out by Alpern and Chambers in the rat proximal tubule [26]. Lowering basolateral Na^+ caused a much greater drop in intracellular pH by operation of the Na^+-HCO_3^- cotransporter, compared to the very small effect of peritubular Cl^- in causing intracellular acidification by operation of the Cl^--HCO_3^- exchanger. Thus, these studies indicated that Na^+-HCO_3^- cotransport is far and away the predominant mechanism for base exit across the basolateral membrane of the proximal tubule cell. Recent evidence suggests that Cl^--HCO_3^- exchange may play a more important role in mediating base exit across the basolateral membrane in the S_3 segment of the proximal tubule [27].

Given that Na^+-HCO_3^- cotransport is the predominant mechanism of base exit through most of the proximal tubule, is its operation dependent on a functional interaction with carbonic anhydrase as predicted by the membrane vesicle studies? This issue was studied by Sasaki and Marumo [28]. These workers measured intracellular pH and stimulated efflux of HCO_3^- through the Na^+-HCO_3^- cotransporter by either lowering peritubular HCO_3^- or by lowering peritubular Na^+. In both cases, the operation of the Na^+-HCO_3^- cotransporter, as reflected by its causing intracellular acidification, was markedly inhibited by acetazolamide. These findings confirm the vesicle studies, indicating an important role for cytoplasmic and/or basolateral membrane carbonic anhydrase in providing transportable substrate, namely HCO_3^- and CO_3^{2-}, for the Na^+-HCO_3^- cotransport system.

Mechanisms of Cl^- Entry Across the Luminal Membrane

As will be discussed in more detail later, there is a passive driving force for Cl^- reabsorption via the paracellular pathway all along the proximal tubule. However, studies from a number of laboratories have indicated that there must also be a component of

Fig. 6. Model of NaCl entry across the luminal membrane by Cl^--formate exchange in parallel with Na^+-H^+ exchange and nonionic diffusion of formic acid

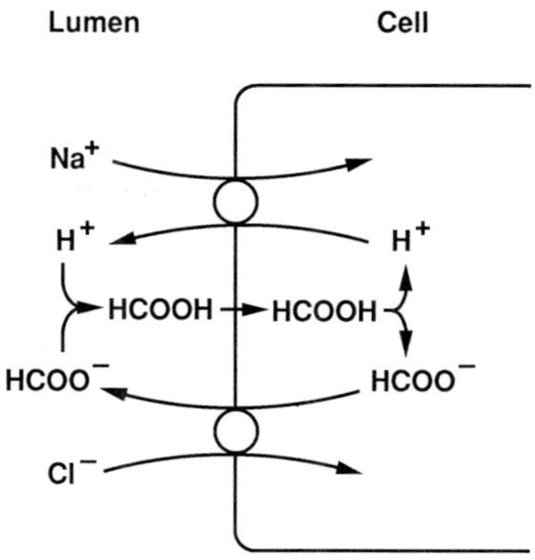

transcellular Cl^- reabsorption as well [29]. Because intracellular Cl^- in the proximal tubule cell is above electrochemical equilibrium, Cl^- entry must occur by an uphill mechanism.

Using rabbit brush border membrane vesicles we could find no evidence for Na^+-Cl^- or Na^+-K^+-$2Cl^-$ cotransport [30] as found in other nephron segments. We therefore tested for the presence of anion exchange processes that might account for uphill Cl^- transport across the luminal membrane [31]. We initially tested whether outward gradients of HCO_3^-, or well-known organic anions like acetate, would stimulate Cl^- uptake, compared to the inert anion gluconate. Disappointingly, we found that outward gradients of neither HCO_3^- nor acetate were particularly effective in stimulating Cl^- uptake. Surprisingly, an outward gradient of formate caused a much more appreciable stimulation of Cl^- uptake, suggesting the presence of a Cl^--formate exchange process. Confirming the presence of a Cl^--formate anion exchanger, we found that imposing an outward Cl^- gradient stimulated the uphill transport of formate. An outward Cl^- gradient did not stimulate the uptake of acetate, confirming the selectivity of this transport process for formate.

Clearly, given the low concentrations (0.2–0.5 mM) of formate found in biological fluids, not much Cl^- could be reabsorbed in exchange for formate unless there was a mechanism to recycle formate across the luminal membrane. Since formate was known to cross lipid bilayers fairly well by nonionic diffusion, we proposed the model illustrated in Fig. 6 for the role of Cl^--formate exchange in mediating Cl^- entry across the luminal membrane. According to this model, H^+ secretion, which largely occurs by Na^+-H^+ exchange, would generate an inward H^+ gradient across the luminal membrane. This would then drive filtered formate into the cell by nonionic diffusion of formic acid. In the more alkaline environment of the cell, the formic acid would dissociate to form H^+ and formate. The resulting outward formate gradient could then drive uphill Cl^- uptake by Cl^--formate exchange. Formate would continually recycle by nonionic diffusion; the net process is formate-catalyzed NaCl entry.

This model makes several testable predictions. First, if the Na^+-H^+ exchanger is blocked with amiloride, adding back luminal Cl^- to a Cl^--free luminal solution should cause cell acidification by the parallel operation of Cl^--formate exchange and nonionic diffusion of formic acid. Indeed, if Cl^--formate exchange, rather than

Cl^--HCO_3^- exchange, is the predominant mechanism for Cl^--base exchange across the luminal membrane, the effect of luminal Cl^- on intracellular pH should be much greater in the presence of formate than in its absence. This prediction was tested in the rabbit proximal tubule by Baum [32]. He found that intracellular pH significantly acidified when Cl^- was added to the lumen in the presence of formate, consistent with the operation of Cl^--formate exchange in parallel with nonionic diffusion of formic acid. In contrast, the effect of Cl^- on intracellular pH was very much smaller in the absence of formate. Thus, Cl^--formate exchange is the major pathway for luminal membrane Cl^--base exchange, as predicted by the vesicle studies.

Given that Cl^--formate exchange is the major pathway for Cl^--base exchange, does it actually result in physiologically significant NaCl transport into and across the cell? One manifestation of increased NaCl entry across the luminal membrane would be an increase in cell volume. We tested this prediction in isolated and perfused proximal tubules of the rabbit [33]. In the absence of Cl^-, adding a phyisological concentration of formate to the luminal perfusate (0.5 mM) induced a small increase in cell volume, presumably due to uptake of Na^+-formate by nonionic diffusion of formic acid in parallel with Na^+-H^+ exchange. In the presence of Cl^-, formate induced a much larger increase in cell volume, as predicted if formate catalyzes NaCl entry across the brush border membrane. Accordingly, this experiment suggested that a physiological formate concentration actually can induce significant net NaCl entry across the luminal membrane of the proximal tubule cell.

But does this NaCl entry across the luminal membrane, induced by formate, actually stimulate transtubular NaCl transport? To answer this question, we measured Jv, the rate of volume reabsorption, under conditions of low HCO_3^-, where Jv would reflect the rate of isotonic NaCl reabsorption in isolated perfused proximal tubules of rabbit [34]. We found that adding physiological formate concentrations to the lumen and bath caused a significant and reversible stimulation of Jv, indicating that Cl^--formate exchange actually does contribute importantly to transtubular Cl^- reabsorption. Acetate could not mimic the effect of formate, confirming the selectivity for formate determined in the vesicle studies. However, a significant Jv was observed even in the absence of added formate, despite the symmetrical conditions with no measurable transtubular potential difference, and thus no passive driving force for Cl^- reabsorption. This suggested either that the tubule may produce formate endogenously, or that additional pathways for Cl^- entry across the luminal membrane must exist.

We therefore screened for additional anion exchange modes of Cl^- transport [35]. When outward gradients of various organic anions were tested for their ability to stimulate ^{36}Cl uptake, we found that only oxalate significantly stimulated Cl^- uptake. Imposing a large outward Cl^- gradient stimulated the uphill accumulation of oxalate, confirming the presence of a Cl^--oxalate exchange process. In contrast, an outward Cl^- gradient had virtually no effect on SO_4^{2-} uptake, and an outward SO_4^{2-} gradient had minimal effect on Cl^- uptake, confirming that SO_4^{2-} does not share this pathway.

However, an outward SO_4^{2-} gradient stimulated uphill oxalate uptake, and an outward oxalate gradient stimulated uphill SO_4^{2-} uptake, indicating the presence of another anion exchange pathway, shared by oxalate and SO_4^{2-}, that was similar to, if not identical with, that present in basolaeral membrane vesicles [36]. These and additional studies led us to conclude that at least three distinct anion exchangers were present on the brush border membrane of the proximal tubule, as illustrated in Fig. 7.

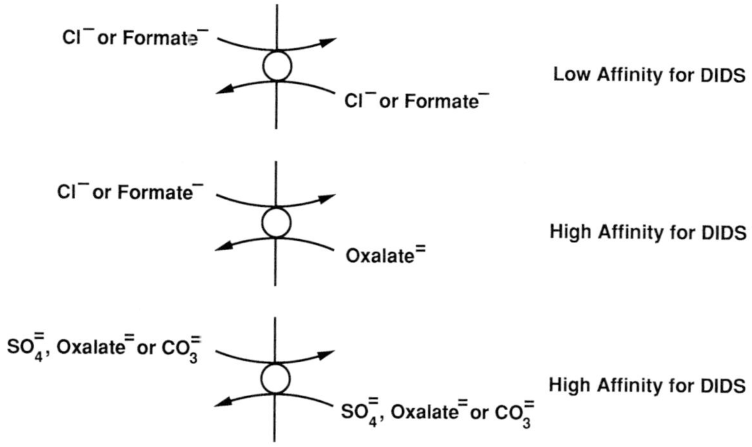

Fig. 7. Summary of properties of three luminal membrane anion exchangers

One exchanger, the Cl^--formate exchanger, can perform electroneutral monovalent anion exchange using formate or Cl^- as substrates, but has little or no affinity for divalent anions such as oxalate or SO_4^{2-}. This system is sensitive to inhibition only by relatively high, near mM, concentrations of disulfonic stilbenes like DIDS. A separate transporter, the Cl^--oxalate exchanger, can exchange the monovalent anion Cl^- or formate for oxalate but cannot exchange monovalent anions for each other or for SO_4^{2-}. By virtue of exchanging a monovalent for a divalent anion, this system is electrogenic. The Cl^--oxalate exchanger is sensitive to relatively low micromolar concentrations of DIDS. Finally, a third anion exchanger was present that could exchange any pair of divalent anions among SO_4^{2-}, oxalate, and CO_3^{2-}. This system was electroneutral, had no affinity for Cl^-, and was highly sensitive to inhibition by DIDS.

The possible role of the Cl^--formate exchanger in mediating Cl^- entry across the brush border membrane has already been discussed. For Cl^--oxalate exchange to likewise contribute importantly to luminal Cl^- entry, there would need to be a mechanism present to recycle oxalate from lumen to cell. There are at least two possible mechanisms by which this third exchanger, the SO_4^{2-}-oxalate-CO_3^{2-} exchanger, could serve that function, as shown in Fig. 8. First, consider that every two cycles of the Na^+-H^+ exchanger would generate an intracellular CO_3^{2-}. The resulting outward gradient of CO_3^{2-} could drive uphill oxalate uptake via CO_3^{2-}-oxalate exchange. The resulting outward oxalate gradient could then drive Cl^- entry via Cl^--oxalate exchange. In this scheme, oxalate would recycle, and the net effect would be Na^+-coupled Cl^- entry with a 2 Na^+:Cl^- stoichiometry.

Alternatively, the process of Na^+-SO_4^{2-} cotransport known to be present in the brush border membrane [37] leads to the cell uptake of SO_4^{2-} and the generation of an outward SO_4^{2-} gradient. This outward SO_4^{2-} gradient could then drive oxalate uptake via SO_4^{2-}-oxalate exchange. The resulting outward oxalate gradient could then drive Cl^- entry via Cl^--oxalate exchange. Again, oxalate would recycle, and the net effect

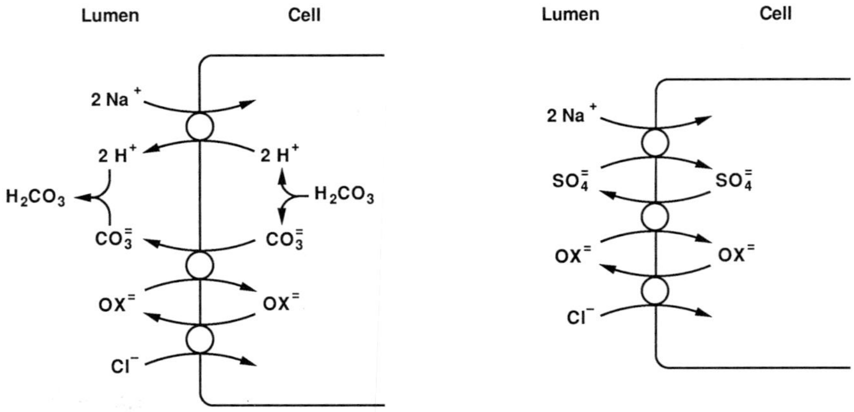

Fig. 8. Possible mechanisms for Cl$^-$ entry across the luminal membrane by Cl$^-$-oxalate exchange

would be Na$^+$-coupled Cl$^-$ entry with a 2 Na$^+$:Cl$^-$ stoichiometry. These potential mechanisms have not yet been tested in the intact tubule.

Mechanisms of Cl$^-$ Exit Across the Basolateral Membrane

At least three different mechanisms for Cl$^-$ exit across the basolateral membrane have been proposed, as illustrated in Fig. 9. One possibility is Cl$^-$ exit through a Cl$^-$ conductive pathway not coupled to the movement of any other ions. Since Cl$^-$ is above electrochemical equilibrium in the proximal tubule cell, there is a passive driving force favoring Cl$^-$ exit through any such Cl$^-$ conductance present in the basolateral membrane. Studies from several groups have suggested that the Cl$^-$ conductance of the basolateral membrane of the proximal tubule cell is negligibly small and cannot contribute significantly to Cl$^-$ exit [38–40]. However, recent electrophysiologic studies by Welling and O'Neill [41], and our measurements of KCl movement across the basolateral membrane as manifested by cell volume changes [42], have suggested that the basolateral membrane Cl$^-$ conductance is volume-activated. The increased cell volume induced by formate, as discussed above,

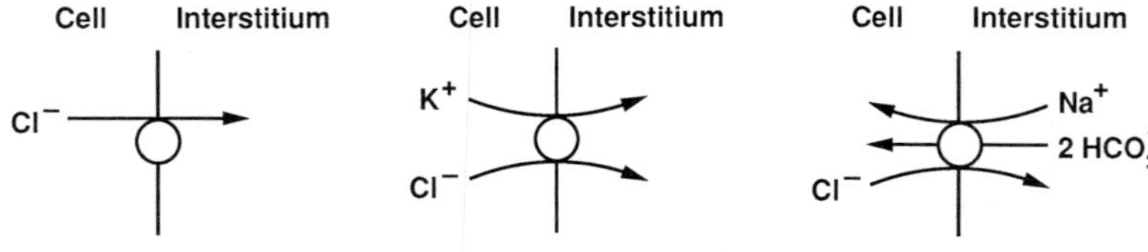

Fig. 9. Possible mechanisms of Cl$^-$ exit across the basolateral membrane of the proximal tubule cell

might then activate the Cl^- conductance so that it becomes a major mechanism for Cl^- exit under physiologic conditions.

Alternatively, studies by Sasaki and co-workers have indicated that two electroneutral mechanisms, namely K^+-Cl^- cotransport and Na^+-dependent Cl^--HCO_3^- exchange, are present at the basolateral membrane of the rabbit proximal straight tubule [40,43]. Similar evidence has been presented by Ishibashi, Rector, and Berry for the rabbit proximal convoluted tubule [44]. These workers found that changes in peritubular K^+ caused changes in intracellular Cl^- activity as predicted for a K^+-Cl^- cotransport process. Membrane vesicle studies have conflicted concerning the presence of K^+-Cl^- cotransport [45,46]. Under physiologic conditions, the electrochemical gradients for both K^+ and Cl^- are directed outward across the basolateral membrane so that this pathway will mediate Cl^- efflux.

Intracellular Cl^- was also found to respond to changes in peritubular Na^+ and HCO_3^- consistent with the presence of a Na^+-dependent Cl^--HCO_3^- exchanger [43,44]. Membrane vesicle studies have conflicted concerning the presence of Na^+-dependent Cl^--HCO_3^- exchange [20,46,47]. This is a transport process that moves Na^+ and two equivalents of base in one direction, in exchange for Cl^- in the opposite direction. Under physiologic conditions, the inward Na^+ gradient would provide the driving force for this system to operate in the direction shown. How much of Cl^- exit occurs by this or any other pathway is at present not clear and is a topic of active investigation in several laboratories.

Summary of Proximal Tubule Transport Processes

The principal mechanisms for transcellular Na^+, Cl^-, and HCO_3^- transport in the mammalian proximal tubule are illustrated in Fig. 10. The most important primary active transport process is, of course, the Na^+ pump, which uses the free energy of ATP hydrolysis to extrude Na^+ and take up K^+ across the basolateral membrane. Most of the K^+ taken up by the pump recycles out across the basolateral membrane. The resulting inward Na^+ gradient is then used to drive the cotransport systems for organic solutes such as glucose and amino acids. There are really multiple distinct cotransport sytems that are lumped together in Fig. 10 only for simplicity. Sugars and amino acids driven into the cell by Na^+ cotransport exit passively across the basolateral membrane. The current of Na^+ across the cell associated with Na^+ cotransport of organic solutes generates a lumen-negative transtubular potential difference in the early proximal tubule that drives a small amount of passive Cl^- reabsorption through the paracellular pathway [48].

H^+ is secreted largely by Na^+-H^+ exchange, with some additional contribution from the H^+-ATPase and possibly from recycling of monocarboxylates, a mechanism that is not illustrated. The HCO_3^- formed in the cell exits largely via Na-HCO_3^- cotransport, with perhaps a small contribution from Cl^--HCO_3^- exchange, that becomes more appreciable relative to Na^+-HCO_3^- cotransport in S_3. The overall process of acidification results in HCO_3^- reabsorption. In addition to the well-known role of luminal membrane carbonic anhydrase, intracellular and/or basolateral carbonic anhydrase is critically important for presenting base in a transportable form to the base exit mechanisms, particularly the Na^+-HCO_3^- cotransporter.

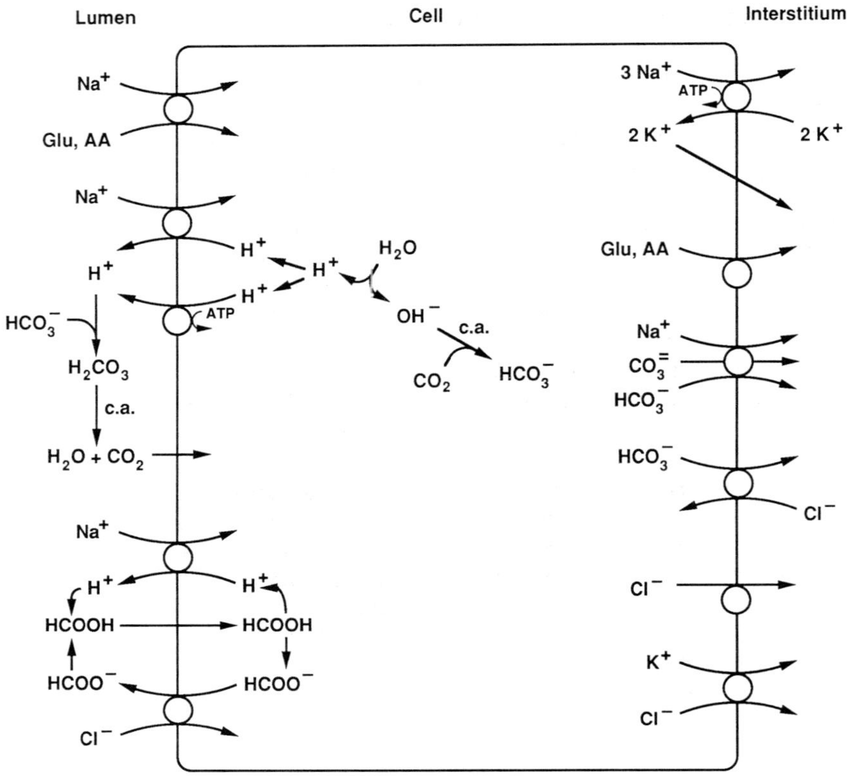

Fig. 10. Summary of the principal mechanisms for transcellular Na^+, Cl^- and HCO_3^- transport in the proximal tubule. c.a., carbonic anhydrase; AA, amino acid; Glu, glucose

In the early proximal tubule there is probably very little Cl^- transport via the Cl^--formate exchanger, because the luminal pH is not yet acid enough to permit efficient recycling of formic acid. In studies not discussed above, we found that NaCl transport catalyzed by formic acid recycling can occur in S_1, but depends critically on an acid luminal pH [34]. However, as acidification and HCO_3^- reabsorption proceed along the course of the proximal tubule, the lumen pH does become more acid, formic acid recycling would be facilitated, and Na^+-Cl^- entry via the Cl^--formate exchanger would then occur in parallel with the Na^+-H^+ exchanger. Whether other luminal membrane pathways, such as Cl^--oxalate exchange, which is not illustrated here, contribute to Cl^- entry is not known. The relative contributions of various Cl^- exit mechanisms are also unclear. It is possible that due to the increased cell volume resulting from Na^+-coupled organic solute entry and from formate-induced NaCl entry, the basolateral Cl^- conductance becomes sufficiently activated to mediate an important fraction of Cl^- exit. Alternatively, Cl^- exit may be largely by K^+-Cl^- cotransport, or by the Na^+-dependent Cl^--HCO_3^- exchanger that is not illustrated.

In any event, one consequence of the luminal pH dependence of Na^+-Cl^- transport via the formate-dependent mechanism may be the preferential HCO_3^- reabsorption that occurs in the early proximal tubule. The resulting isotonic water reabsorption causes luminal Cl^- concentration to rise. An outward Cl^- concentration gradient then develops across the proximal tubule. Passive resorption of Cl^- can then occur through the paracellular pathway, generating a lumen-positive transtubular potential difference that can drive a component of passive Na^+ reabsorption as well [48]. The net effect of this additional passive NaCl reabsorption is to increase the amount of total Na^+ and Cl^- that can be reabsorbed per ATP hydrolyzed by the Na^+, K^+-ATPase.

It should be clear that the Na^+-H^+ exchanger plays a critical role in mediating both HCO_3^- and Cl^- reabsorption in the proximal tubule. For this reason, considerable recent attention has focussed on the regulation of Na^+-H^+ exchange activity in the proximal tubule by hormones and neurotransmitters involved in Na^+ and volume homeostasis, such as angiotensin II, alpha adrenergic agonists, and dopamine.

Acknowledgment. Work in the author's laboratory has been supported by NIH Grants DK-33793 and DK-17433.

References

1. Murer H, Hopfer U, Kinne R (1976) Sodium/proton antiport in brush-border-membrane vesicles isolated from rat small intestine and kidney. Biochem J 154:597–604
2. Kinsella JL, Aronson PS (1980) Properties of the Na^+-H^+ exchanger in renal microvillus membrane vesicles. Am J Physiol 238:F461–F469
3. Kinsella JL, Aronson PS (1981) Interaction of NH_4^+ and Li^+ with the renal microvillus membrane Na^+-H^+ exchanger. Am J Physiol 241:C220–C226
4. Kinsella JL, Aronson PS (1981) Amiloride inhibition of the Na^+-H^+ exchanger in renal microvillus membrane vesicles. Am J Physiol 241:F374–F379
5. Kinsella JL, Aronson PS (1982) Determination of the coupling ratio for Na^+-H^+ exchange in renal microvillus membrane vesicles. Biochim Biophys Acta 689:161–164
6. Aronson PS, Nee J, Suhm MA (1982) Modifier role of internal H^+ in activating the Na^+-H^+ exchanger in renal microvillus membrane vesicles. Nature 299:161–163
7. Aronson PS, Suhm MA, Nee J (1983) Interaction of external H^+ with the Na^+-H^+ exchanger in renal microvillus membrane vesicles. J Biol Chem 258:6767–6771
8. Mahnensmith RL, Aronson PS (1985) Interrelationships among quinidine, amiloride and lithium as inhibitors of the renal Na^+-H^+ exchanger. J Biol Chem 260:12586–12592
9. Barac-Nieto M, Murer H, Kinne R (1980) Lactate-sodium cotransport in rat renal brush border membranes. Am J Physiol 239:F496–F506
10. Blomstedt JW, Aronson PS (1980) pH gradient-stimulated transport of urate and para-aminohippurate in dog renal microvillus membrane vesicles. J Clin Invest 65:931–934
11. Guggino SE, Martin GJ, Aronson PS (1983) Specificity and modes of the anion exchanger in dog renal microvillus membrane vesicles. Am J Physiol 244:F612–F621
12. Aronson PS (1983) Mechanisms of active H^+ secretion in the proximal tubule. Am J Physiol 245:F647–F659
13. Nakhoul NL, Boron WF (1988) Acetate transport in the S3 segment of the proximal tubule and its effect on intracellular pH. J Gen Physiol 92:395–412
14. Geibel J, Giebisch G, Boron WF (1989) Effects of acetate on luminal acidification processes in the S3 segment of the rabbit proximal tubule. Am J Physiol 257:F586–F594

15. Kinne-Saffran E, Kinne R (1974) Presence of bicarbonate-stimulated ATPase in the brush border microvillus membrane of the proximal tubule. Proc Soc Exp Biol Med 146:751–753
16. Turrini F, Sabolic I, Zimolo Z, Moewes B, Burckhardt G (1989) Relation of ATPases in rat renal brush-border membranes to ATP-driven H^+ secretion. J Membr Biol 107:1–12
17. Preisig PA, Ives HE, Cragoe EJ Jr, Alpern RJ, Rector FC Jr (1987) Role of the Na^+/H^+ antiporter in rat proximal tubule bicarbonate absorption. J Clin Invest 80:970–978
18. Nagami GT (1988) Luminal secretion of ammonia in the mouse proximal tubule perfused in vitro. J Clin Invest 81:159–164
19. Boron WF, Boulpaep EL (1983) Intracellular pH regulation in the renal proximal tubule of the salamander. Basolateral HCO_3^- transport. J Gen Physiol 81:53–94
20. Grassl SM, Aronson PS (1986) Na^+/HCO_3^- cotransport in basolateral membrane vesicles isolated from rabbit renal cortex. J Biol Chem 261:8778–8783
21. Soleimani M, Grassl SM, Aronson PS (1987) Stoichiometry of Na^+-HCO_3^- cotransport in basolateral membrane vesicles isolated from rabbit renal cortex. J Clin Invest 79:1276–1280
22. Soleimani M, Aronson PS (1989) Ionic mechanism of Na^+-HCO_3^- cotransport in rabbit renal basolateral membrane vesicles. J Biol Chem 264:18302–18308
23. Soleimani M, Aronson PS (1989) Effects of acetazolamide on Na^+-HCO_3^- cotransport in basolateral membrane vesicles isolated from rabbit renal cortex. J Clin Invest 83:945–951
24. Yoshitomi K, Burckhardt B-Ch, Frömter E (1985) Rheogenic sodium-bicarbonate cotransport in the peritubular cell membrane of rat renal proximal tubule. Pflugers Arch 405:360–366
25. Preisig PA, Alpern RJ (1989) Basolateral membrane H-OH-HCO_3 transport in the proximal tubule. Am J Physiol 256:F751–F765
26. Alpern RJ, Chambers M (1987) Basolateral membrane Cl/HCO_3 exchange in the rat proximal convoluted tubule. J Gen Physiol 89:581–598
27. Kurtz I (1989) Basolateral membrane Na^+/H^+ antiport, Na^+/base cotransport, and Na^+-independent Cl^-/base exchange in the rabbit S_3 proximal tubule. J Clin Invest 83:616–622
28. Sasaki S, Marumo F (1989) Effects of carbonic anhydrase inhibitors on basolateral base transport of rabbit proximal straight tubule. Am J Physiol 257:F947–F952
29. Schild L, Giebisch G, Karniski L, Aronson PS (1986) Chloride transport in the mammalian proximal tubule. Pflugers Arch 407(Suppl 2):S156–S159
30. Seifter JL, Knickelbein R, Aronson PS (1984) Absence of Cl-OH exchange and Na-Cl cotransport in rabbit renal microvillus membrane vesicles. Am J Physiol 247:F753–F759
31. Karniski LP, Aronson PS (1985) Chloride/formate exchange with formic acid recycling: a mechanism of active chloride transport across epithelial membranes. Proc Natl Acad Sci USA 82:6362–6365
32. Baum M (1988) Effect of luminal chloride on cell pH in rabbit proximal tubule. Am J Physiol 254:F677–F683
33. Schild L, Aronson PS, Giebisch G (1990) Effects of apical membrane Cl^--formate exchange on cell volume in rabbit proximal tubule. Am J Physiol 258:F530–F536
34. Schild L, Giebisch G, Karniski LP, Aronson PS (1987) Effect of formate on volume reabsorption in the rabbit proximal tubule. J Clin Invest 79:32–38
35. Karniski LP, Aronson PS (1987) Anion exchange pathways for Cl^- transport in rabbit renal microvillus membranes. Am J Physiol 253:F513–F521
36. Kuo S-M, Aronson PS (1988) Oxalate transport via the sulfate-HCO_3 exchanger in rabbit renal basolateral membrane vesicles. J Biol Chem 263:9710–9717
37. Lücke H, Stange G, Murer H (1979) Sulfate-ion/sodium-ion cotransport by brush-border membrane vesicles from rat kidney cortex. Biochem J 182:223–229
38. Bello-Reuss E (1982) Electrical properties of the basolateral membrane of the straight portion of the rabbit proximal renal tubule. Am J Physiol 326:49–63
39. Cardinal J, Lapointe J-Y, Laprade R (1984) Luminal and peritubular ionic substitutions

and intracellular potential of the rabbit proximal convoluted tubule. Am J Physiol 247:F352–F364

40. Sasaki S, Ishibashi K, Yoshiyama N, Shiigai T (1988) KCl cotransport across the basolateral membrane of rabbit renal proximal straight tubule. J Clin Invest 81:194–199
41. Welling PA, O'Neill RG (1990) Cell swelling activates basolateral Cl and K conductances in rabbit proximal tubule. Am J Physiol 258:F951–F962
42. Schild L, Aronson PS, Giebisch G (to be published) Basolateral transport pathways for K^+ and Cl^- in the rabbit proximal tubule: effects on cell volume. Am J Physiol
43. Sasaki S, Yoshiyama N (1988) Interaction of chloride and bicarbonate transport across the basolateral membrane of rabbit proximal straight tubule. Evidence for sodium coupled chloride/bicarbonate exchange. J Clin Invest 81:1004–1011
44. Ishibashi Y, Rector FC Jr, Berry CA (1990) Chloride transport across the basolateral membrane of rabbit proximal convoluted tubules. Am J Physiol 258:F1569–F1578
45. Eveloff J, Warnock DG (1987) K-Cl transport systems in rabbit renal basolateral membrane vesicles. Am J Physiol 252:F883–F889
46. Grassl SM, Holohan PD, Ross CR (1987) Cl^--HCO_3^- exchange in rat renal basolateral membrane vesicles. Biochim Biophys Acta 905:475–484
47. Chen P-Y, Verkman AS (1988) Sodium-dependent chloride transport in basolateral membrane vesicles isolated from rabbit proximal tubule. Biochemistry 27:655–660
48. Rector FC Jr (1983) Sodium, bicarbonate, and chloride absorption by the proximal tubule. Am J Physiol 244:F461–F471

Biology of Acid-Base Transport in Distal Urinary Epithelia

PHILIP R. STEINMETZ

Chair: Claude Amiel

Biology of Acid-Base Transport in Distal Urinary Epithelia

PHILIP R. STEINMETZ[1]

SUMMARY. The biology of acid-base transport in distal urinary epithelia is reviewed under four headings: 1) The major function of urinary acidification is based in α intercalated cells or carbonic anhydrase cells. The α cells secrete H^+ into the urinary compartment by means of a vacuolar H^+-ATPase located at the apical cell membrane. Structure-function studies reveal that the number of pumps in an apical membrane position varies with acid-base conditions via a mechanism of exocytosis and endocytosis. The basolateral membrane of the α cell contains Cl-HCO_3 exchangers, which closely resemble the red cell band 3 protein, and parallel conductive Cl channels. The high transport rates achieved by α cells appear to be a function of the efficient packing of H^+-ATPase molecules in the apical membrane. 2) The function of bicarbonate secretion is confined to a small population of β intercalated cells and is less well understood. β cell function is observed in turtle urinary bladder and in the cortical segments of the mammalian collecting duct. The apical membrane of the β cell contains a Cl-HCO_3 exchanger that differs from the basolateral one of the α cell. Transport is driven by a basolateral H^+-ATPase. 3) The sodium transporting cells of the distal nephron usually contain basolateral Na/H antiporters involved in the regulation of intracellular pH. In some segments an apical Na/H antiporter may contribute to vectorial H^+ secretion. 4) Overall acid-base transport in the distal nephron is a complex function of the geometry of the transporting systems and the availability of proton acceptors.

Introduction

The last decade has seen rapid expansion of our understanding of acid-base transport in the kidney: perfusion studies of tubule segments, studies of individual cell types by electrophysiologic and fluorescence techniques, structure-function studies of

[1]Division of Nephrology, University of Connecticut School of Medicine, Farmington, CT 06032, USA

model epithelia of turtle and toad bladder and of mammalian collecting duct (CD), and, most recently, immunocytochemical studies of transport proteins and purification and cDNA cloning of several major transporters. We have characterized many new acid-base transporters and we have learned about the remarkable diversity of structure and function along the nephron.

For this lecture I focus on urinary acidification by the tight urinary epithelia of the distal nephron and of the turtle and toad bladder, which are responsible for the final regulation of H^+ excretion and which are equipped to maintain steep pH gradients and to respond to acid-base changes and to hormonal control. At one time during the early years of nephrology, the great "black box" period of kidney physiology, it was thought that there was *one* major mechanism for proximal HCO_3 reabsorption and *one* for distal acidification.

Now we know all too well how several hundred million years of evolution have left us with great complexity, reflecting a long history of adaptations to new demands. On the *one hand* we have learned to accept this complexity, on the other we keep encountering some remarkably similar arrangements in the cellular organization of acid-base transporter, and we find that the transport proteins being used have barely changed over more than a hundred million years and that the same transporters are used in different cells, tissues, and species. A good transporter will be used over and over again. Therefore we can still come up with general models for the major transport functions. For example, the major system for distal urinary acidification is contained in the α type intercalated or carbonic anhydrase-rich cells of turtle bladder and of collecting duct. In some segments these α cells function as pure H^+ secretors. Much has been learned about the acid-base transporters at their apical and basolateral cell membranes and about the organization and regulation of H^+ secretion. The first part of this review will be devoted to this system. The next part will deal with the so-called β cell system, which is less well understood and is confined to only a small population of cells in turtle bladder and to only one segment, the cortical segment, in the rabbit CD. This HCO_3-secreting cell population is quite interesting, even if it is not always operative. The third topic deals with the acid-base function of the Na-transporting cells, such as the principal cells (PC) and inner medullary collecting duct (IMCD) cells. Here, we have to distinguish between "housekeeping" functions and net transepithelial transport of acid or base. By looking at the prototypes of these functions I hope to avoid generating a long catalogue of different transport systems in different places of the nephron. At the end, I shall present a brief survey of the regulation of the major acid-base transporters and the importance of proton acceptors in net acid excretion.

α Cell Function of H^+ Secretion

Physiologic Studies in Turtle Bladder

The initial studies of the flat sheet preparation of turtle urinary bladder reflected, primarily, the function of H^+ secretion in the α type carbonic anhydrase cells. The epithelium was treated as a black box. Physiologic studies revealed that H^+ secretion is *not directly* dependent on Na transport. There is only indirect electrical coupling, so that H^+ secretion is accelerated by lumen-negative PD. Serosal addition of HCO_3

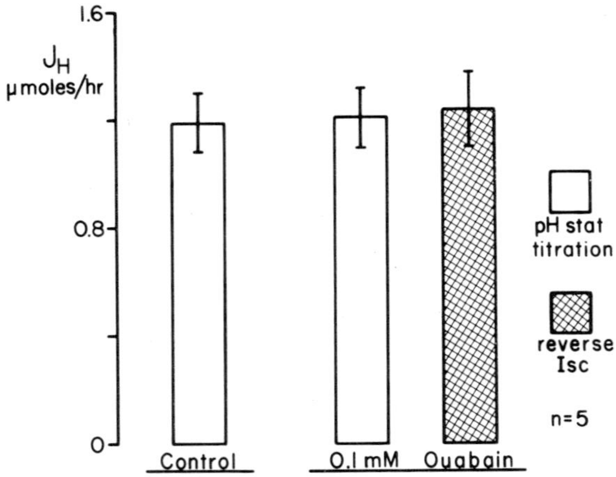

Fig. 1. Failure of ouabain to inhibit H^+ secretion (J_H) at constant p CO_2. The reverse short-circuit current (*Isc*) is approximately equal to the pH state rate. (From [8] with permission)

caused a marked reduction in net acid secretion if Cl^- was present in luminal solution. The discovery of an electroneutral Cl-HCO_3 exchange transport system complicated the model system for some time until this complication itself became the subject of study, i.e., the existence of two polarities of acid-base transport in the same epithelium.

Figure 1 shows that H^+ secretion in the short-circuited state is unaffected by inhibition of Na^+ transport. In fact, the Isc in presence of ouabain is equivalent to the pH stat rate, indicating that all of the H^+ secretion occurs with transfer of charge. In support for the electrogenicity of H^+ secretion is, also, the fact that H^+ secretion is not dependent on the presence of other electrolytes: Na^+ and K^+ are not required. Cl^- is required in trace amounts only on the serosal side, presumably for the exit step of HCO_3^-.

H^+ secretion continues under anaerobic conditions. In the absence of O_2 the transport of H^+ becomes critically dependent on glucose as a substrate. It turns out that H^+ transport is tightly coupled to metabolism. In this example, two H^+ are transported for each lactate produced anaerobically and this stoichiometry is preserved when the transport rate is manipulated by inhibitors or an opposing electrochemical potential gradient for protons. These studies [1], and others by Beauwens and Al Awqati [2], indicate that the apical cell membrane is very tight to H^+ ions. In contrast, the basolateral cell membrane has a very high HCO_3^- permeability.

Structure-Function Studies Reveal Different Cell Types

The studies by Rosen [3], Husted et al. [4], and Stetson and Steinmetz [5,6] led first to the distinction between granular and carbonic anhydrase-rich (CA) cells and, later, to the distinction of α and β type CA cells in turtle bladder. Gluck et al. [7] described the stimulation of exocytosis by CO_2, which could account for the remarkable apical area changes of the CA cells reported by Husted et al. [4]. The reader is referred

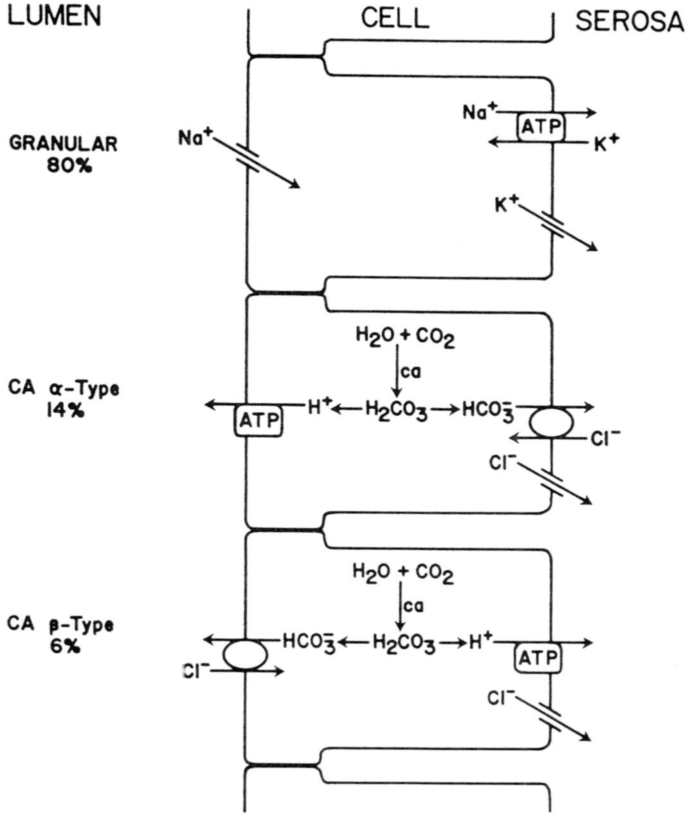

Fig. 2. The major cell types correspond to major transport functions in turtle urinary bladder and, probably, in certain other tight urinary epithelia, such as the cortical segment of the collecting duct (CD). CA, carbonic anhydrase. (From [8] with permission)

to references [5,6,8] for a more detailed description of the structure-function studies that form the basis for the three cell types shown in Fig. 2. These cell types are comparable to those of the cortical collecting duct (CCD).

The cell type constituting the majority is the granular or principal cell, which absorbs Na and is capable of secreting K in the cortical segment. The acid-base functions of this cell appear to be confined to intracellular pH regulatioin. It has a Na/H antiporter in the basolateral membrane (not shown), which probably does not participate in vectorial transport. The next cell type is the α CA cell which, in turtle bladder, makes up about 14% of total cell number. It is common in the outer medullary collecting duct (OMCD), where it is the only type of acid-base transporting cell. In the absence of Na^+ transport this cell dominates the transport functions of turtle bladder and OMCD. It produces a lumen positive PD, is inhibited by acetazolamide, and has a remarkable apical membrane that can be expanded by fusion of subapical membrane vesicles or shrunk by retrieval of apical membrane and formation of reserve

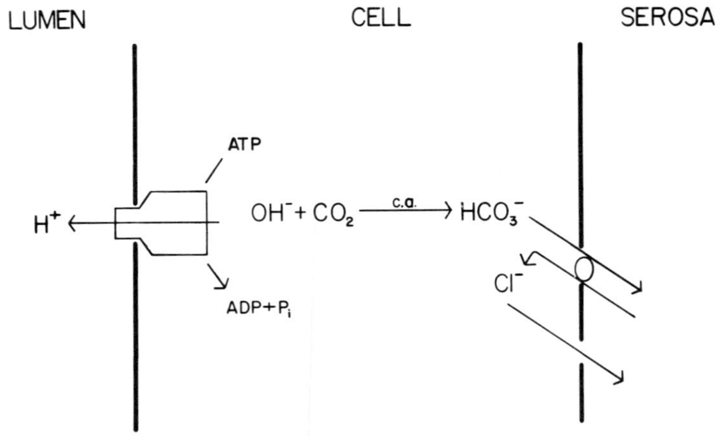

Fig. 3. Double membrane model of the α-type carbonic anhydrase (*c.a.*) or intercalated cell of tight urinary epithelia

vesicles. It contains cytoplasmic CA which catalyzes the formation of HCO_3^- behind the H^+ pump. This HCO_3^- exits the cell via a Cl-HCO_3 exchanger that is inhibited by the disulfonic stilbenes, as mentioned before. This anion exchanger is closely related to the band 3 protein of the red cell, as shown by the immunocytochemical studies of Drenckhahn and his associates [9].

The third cell type is the β cell. There is considerable evidence that it is involved in HCO_3^- secretion. It has basolateral studs and rod-shaped particles and, in the rat, the basolateral regions react with antibodies against H^+-ATPase. Under ordinary conditions, the Cl-HCO_3 exchange transport by the β cells is electroneutral, a one for one exchange. The basolateral H^+-ATPase is thought to be the primary active transport process. A parallel Cl^- conductance permits the overall exchange to operate electroneutrally. The apical Cl-HCO_3 exchanger, however, fails to react with red cell band 3 antibodies and is not easily inhibited by disulfonic stilbenes. Hence, it differs substantially from the basolateral exchanger of the cells. I shall come back to the β cell later. For now, we may conclude that the functions of Na^+ absorption, H^+ secretion and HCO_3^- secretion are based in different cell types in turtle bladder and in certain segments of CD.

Organization of α Cell: Apical Membrane

Figure 3 is focussed on the α cell: this is the double membrane model. H^+ transport by the apical pump is tightly coupled to ATP hydrolysis. The work of Dixon and Al Awqati [10] in turtle bladder was based on this coupling and first suggested that the pump of urinary acidification was a reversible H^+-translocating ATPase. Subsequent studies, by Gluck and his associates, in turtle bladder and bovine medulla have led to characterization of the ATPase as an electrogenic H^+-ATPase that is inhibited by NEM and DCCD and that differs from the mitochondrial ATPase. Immunoaffinity purification of the bovine ATPase by Gluck and Caldwell [11] has defined the

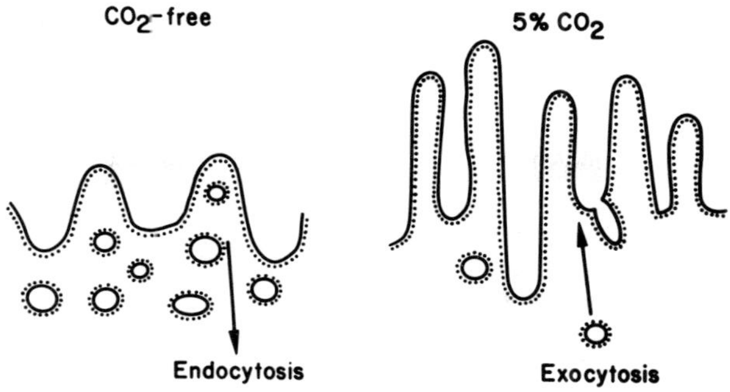

Fig. 4. Schematic representation of apical membrane coated with studs. CO_2 stimulation of H^+ secretion is associated with expansion of the apical area of α cells, by a mechanism of exocytosis

ATPase as a vacuolar H^+-ATPase with a molecular weight of about 580000 dalton and about 10 different subunits. Immunocytochemical studies with antibodies against the 70 and 56 kD subunits of the H^+-ATPase demonstrate that the ATPase is localized at the cytoplasmic regions below the apical microplicae, where high magnification electron microscopy reveals a stud-like coating of the cytoplasmic leaflet of the apical membrane [12,13]. The studs are stalked spheres about 10 nM long and about 9 nM in their widest diameter. The new lines of evidence now available strongly suggest that the studs correspond to the catalytic units of the H^+-ATPase molecules.

In Fig. 4 the response of the "studded" apical membrane to CO_2 is shown. In turtle bladder, the apical membrane of the microplicae and the membrane vesicles have roughly the same density of studs. In the absence of CO_2 (left), the apical membrane is shrunk and there are many membrane vesicles coated with studs in the cytoplasm. The pumps are in a reserve position and don't contribute to transepithelial transport. If CO_2 is added, these vesicles fuse with the apical membrane in a matter of minutes, expand the apical surface, and increase the number of pumps in position. This expansion was quantitated by morphometric measurements by Stetson and Steinmetz [6].

The planar surface area of individual α cells increased from 28 $\pm$ 2 to 65 $\pm$ 4 μm^2 after CO_2 addition. The degree of folding also increased, so that the total folded area increased more than fourfold. These comparisons were made in paired bladder halves fixed in Ussing chambers after H^+ secretion rates had been measured. The density of rod-shaped particles (RSP) on freeze fracture replicas of the apical membrane was also determined. In turtle and toadbladder, as well as in the CD, RSPs are seen in the same cell membranes and membrane vesicles as the studs. The two, however, are observed with different techniques and represent different structures. The studs appear to represent catalytic units of the H^+ ATPase within the cytoplasm and the RSP are a linear array of 2 or 3 spherical units representing intramembrane components, possibly transmembrane components of the ATPase. Hence, a RSP may represent 2 or 3 pumps or a multiple thereof. Since we had estimated the total area of apical membrane and had freeze fracture studies of several α cell apical membranes at low and high CO_2, we estimated the total number of RSP and compared it with the total H^+ transport rates for the same tissues. Because of the small sample of α cell

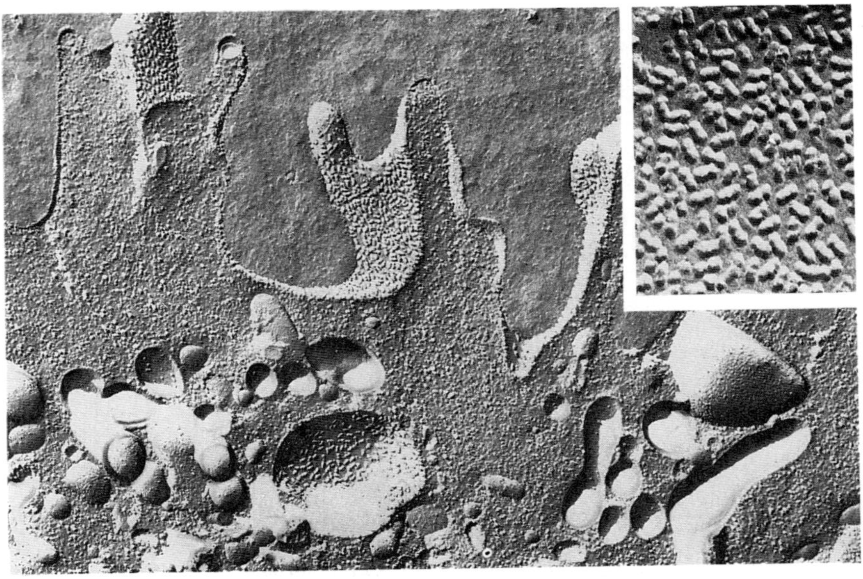

Fig. 5. Freeze-fracture electron micrograph of the apical membrane of an α-type carbonic anhydrase cell. Numerous *rod-shaped particles* are shown on the protoplasmic phase of apical microplicae and certain cytoplasmic vesicles. *Inset* reveals higher magnification of rod-shaped particles. (From [5] with permission)

fractures we couldn't be sure that CO_2 increased the density of RSP, but it was clear that the total area and the total number of RSP in an apical position was increased about five-fold, while the transport rate increased nine-fold. Taken together, these studies suggest that a large part, about 60%, of the CO_2 induced increase in H^+ secretion is accounted for by an increased number of pumps at the apical membrane of the α cells.

Figure 5 shows a freeze fracture surface of the apical cell membrane of an α cell. Note numerous RSP on the protoplasmic face. Each RSP consists of 2 or 3 spherical subunits of 12 nM diameter (Inset). A major question is how RSPs on freeze fracture relate to studs on transmission electron microscopy (TEM). The simplest arrangement would be that in which each spherical subunit in a RSP was linked to a cytoplasmic stud. On the average, there were about 3000 RSP/μm^2 or 7500 spherical subunit/μm^2. This estimate is not very different from that made by Brown, Hartwig, and Gluck [12] in α cells of toadbladder, for studs. These authors used a rapid freezing method, in which they sheared away the apical membrane of the cytoplasm and obtained a beautiful view of the studs on the cytoplasmic side of the membrane. They found a density of studs in toadbladder of about 16000/μm^2, which is about twice the density of the spherical subunits in RSP. Whether the spherical subunits are linked to one or two studs, and whether they actually represent transmembrane channels or some other structural characteristic of the way pumps are packed in the membrane, is not known.

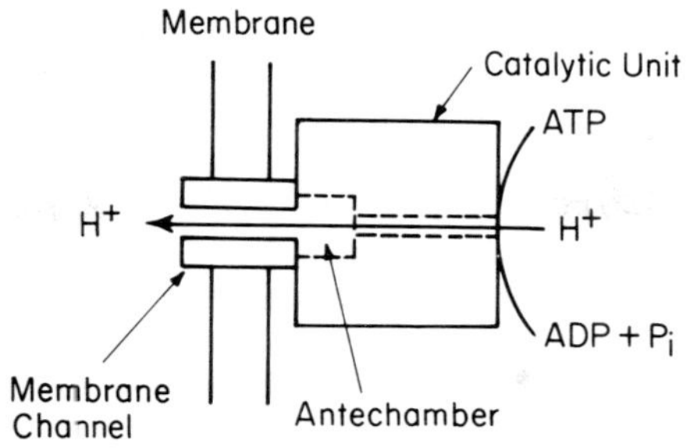

Fig. 6. A physiologist's working model for an ATP-driven proton pump. The pump complex consists of a membrane channel and a catalytic unit, linked via an antechamber that serves as a buffer compartment. (From [15] with permission)

In the near future these questions may be resolved by means of high resolution electron microscopy. According to our estimates, the average transport rate per RSP in turtle bladder at room temperature was 200 protons per s, or 80 per spherical subunit. That would be 80 or 40 per s per pump, depending on the number of pumps associated.

To return to the double membrane model of the αcell. The primary active transport step at the apical membrane is a H^+-ATPase. Based on the monomer assumption of 2 1/2 studs per RSP, the pump number at the apex of an αcell varies between 1 1/2 million and 6 million, as a function of CO_2 tension. Changes in pump number constitute a major way of regulating the transport rate. Aside from the H^+ pumps, there are few transporters or channels detectable in the apical cell membrane under ordinary conditions. Old studies on the coupling between transport and metabolism in bladder and more recent electrophysiologic studies, carried out in the outer medullary collecting duct by Koeppen [14], indicate that the apical membrane is very tight to ions, including protons.

As a result of this tightness, the rate of H^+ secretion (J_H) during secretion against pH gradients is a function of the active component of H^+ transport. Since apical areas do not change during acute luminal pH changes, the J_H vs Δ pH relation reflects the intrinsic properties of the H^+ pump (or of a given population of H^+ pumps). Transport stops at an opposing Δ pH of 3 U or a PD of 180 mV. At favorable gradients the transport rate reaches a maximal value. Andersen et al. [15] were able to simulate the observed J_H vs Δ pH relation by means of a set of assumptions about kinetic factors and a two component model of the H^+ pump complex. As shown in Fig. 6, their working model consisted of a catalytic unit where translocation of H^+ was coupled to ATP hydrolysis and a passive transmembrane channel linked to the catalytic unit through a buffer compartment (antechamber). Over the last few years, the biochemical studies of Gluck and Caldwell [11] and Stone and coworkers [16] have provided important new information about the subunit structure of vacuolar H^+-ATPase. The immunopurification studies of Gluck and coworkers have characterized the vacuolar ATPase of kidney medulla as a large protein of about 580 kD. There appear to be 3 subunits of 70 kD where ATP is bound during its hydrolysis and where NEM may inhibit. A smaller subunit of 56 kD is part of the catalytic unit and the structure of this unit has been highly conserved all the way from the archaebacteria to the mammalian kidney. The transmembrane channel appears to be formed by 6 copies of a 15 kD subunit which binds DCCD. On the whole, the subunit structure is consistent with the two component model of the physiologists [15].

Organization of α Cell:Basolateral Membrane

The basolateral cell membrane of the α cell contains a Cl-HCO_3 exchanger that is closely related to the band 3 protein of red cell. Messenger RNA studies of the kidney anion exchanger indicate that this exchanger is close to the red cell exchanger, except for a series of amino acids at the aminoterminal end. In any event, the α cells of turtle bladder, OMCD, and CCD contain a band 3-like exchanger in their basolateral membrane, as judged from immunocytochemical studies by Drenckhahn et al. [9], Schuster [17], and Verlander et al. [18], and as judged from the traditional response to stilbenes and Cl-removal. It is of interest that the turnover rate of the anion exchanger is much higher than that of the H^+ pump, so that a cell with 5 million H^+ pumps may only require some 50000 exchangers. Recent studies of cell attached patches have revealed the existence of high conductance Cl^- channels with possible transport rates well over a million/s. For the sake of comparison, that α cell would require only a small number, less than 50, of Cl channels in its basolateral membrane to accommodate the recycling of Cl^-. I have mentioned the intrinsic regulation of the H^+ pump rate by $\Delta \tilde{\mu}H$ and the regulation of the pump number by CO_2. At the basolateral membrane, the activity of Cl channels would directly affect the transfer of negative charge and, thereby, $\Delta \tilde{\mu}H$ across the apical membrane. In some α cells, the basolateral membrane may also contain Na/H antiporters. These antiporters are in the wrong position for vectorial H^+ secretion, but may play a role when the cell is acid loaded.

β Cell Function of HCO_3 Secretion

The next major transport function is HCO_3^- secretion by β cells. Renal tubular secretion of HCO_3 was first described in the 1950s, in the alligator. In the early 1970s, when Leslie, Schwartz, and I [19] found an electroneutral transport system for HCO_3^- secretion in turtle bladder, we were afraid that the system might be a reptilian peculiarity that would complicate the model. Subsequently, McKinney and Burg [20] and others showed a similar transport system in rabbit CCD. Following the discovery of two subtypes of carbonic anhydrase cells [5,21] with opposite functional polarities, this system has received considerable attention. Figure 7 shows a double membrane model for the β cell of turtle bladder operating under ordinary conditions, that is, without stimulation by cAMP. The net rate of HCO_3^- secretion equals the net rate of Cl-absorption and both rates are independent of sodium transport. H^+ pumps are located at the basolateral cell membrane, along with parallel Cl^- channels. For each H^+ ion extruded, a HCO_3^- ion is generated and subsequently secreted into the urine via a neutral Cl-HCO_3 exchanger. The Cl entering across the apical membrane exits through conductive basolateral channels, so that the overall exchange operation remains neutral. The ultrastructural and immunocytochemical evidence for baso-

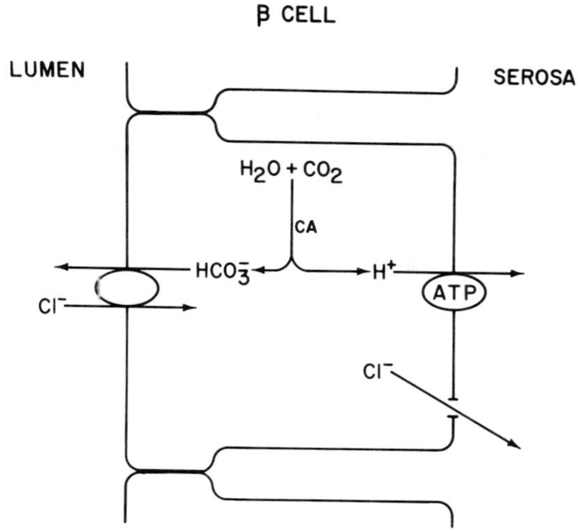

Fig. 7. Cellular organization of electroneutral HCO_3 secretion in β carbonic anhydrase (*CA*) cell

lateral H^+ pumps is compelling, but the nature of the apical Cl-HCO_3 exchanger remains to be clarified. The apical exchanger differs from the basolateral one in that antibodies to various parts of the band 3 protein have failed to react with it [9,17] and in that it is relatively resistant to inhibitors, as shown by Kohn et al. [22]. As you can see, the β cell is not a simple mirror reversal of the α cell. In turtle bladder, the electroneutral model for HCO_3^- secretion is modified and HCO_3^- secretion is stimulated by maneuvers that increase cAMP, such as phosphodiesterase inhibitors and certain peptides.

Cyclic AMP introduces an apical anion conductance for Cl^- and, to some extent, for HCO_3^- (Fig. 8). Total HCO_3^- secretion is increased as an electrogenic component of HCO_3^- secretion is added. A Cl ion entering the cell on the exchanger has two options. It can recycle across the apical membrane or it can exit across the basolateral membrane. In turtle bladder, the basolateral exit rate and therefore the neutral component, is decreased. Studies by Stetson [23] suggest that cAMP may cause selective addition of Cl^- channels to the apical membrane. Activation or insertion of Cl channels by cAMP is also a mechanism for anion secretion in other epithelia, such as tracheal and intestinal epithelia. In turtle bladder, cAMP increases HCO_3 secretion and has little effect on H^+ secretion, so that the combined effect is usually one of reducing net acid secretion. In the rabbit CCD, it appears that electroneutral rather than the electrogenic HCO_3 secretion is increased [17], an effect somewhat different from that in turtle bladder. Furthermore, there appear to be species differences among the mammalian CCDs studied. It should not be surprising that the overall effects of cAMP vary among tissues. Not only are there different cell types and different prevalences of α or β cells, but also, within a single cell type, cAMP may cause activation of Cl channels in different cell membranes. In this example, apical activation decreases transcellular Cl absorption, whereas

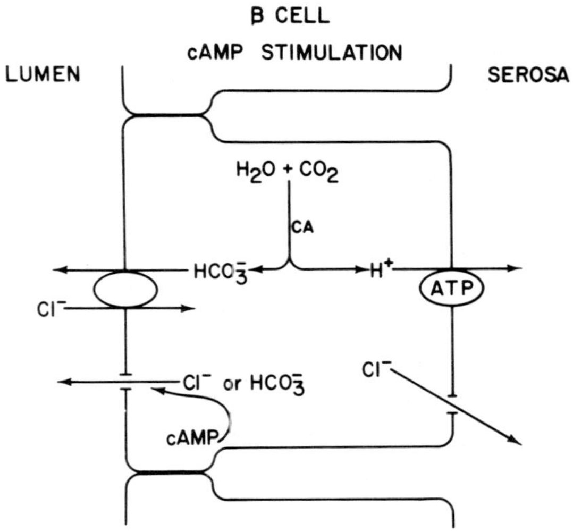

Fig. 8. Stimulation of electrogenic HCO_3^- secretion by cAMP in β carbonic anhydrase (*CA*) cell

basolateral activation might increase Cl absorption, depending on the initial conditions. It is clear that activation (used as an operational term) of Cl channels may have potent effects on the transport rate and on the electrogenicity of acid-base transport, but it is also clear that such effects depend very much on the precise membrane sites being activated.

In terms of β cell function, it is well to remember that this cell is found in very limited regions of the collecting duct system. β cells are confined to the cortical segments of the collecting duct. Their numbers, furthermore, depend on the acid-base condition of the animal. In rabbits on an alkaline ash diet, the majority of intercalated cells (IC) have a functional polarity of β cells. Schwartz, Barasch, and Al-Awqati [24] showed that acid loading would reverse the functional polarity of these intercalated cells to the H^+ secreting αform, as judged from their pH response to basolateral Cl removal. In turtle bladder, β cells make up about a third of the intercalated cells and the α and β forms appear to maintain a relatively stable polarity. For example, turtle α or β cells are clearly unipolar, as judged from their ultrastructure, i.e., cytoplasmic studs and rod-shaped intramembrane particles are either on one or the other pole, i.e., more than 95% are on the apical side in α cells and more than 95% are on the basolateral side in β cells. However, in rabbit CCD, one finds these elements on both poles, with one pole having a greater abundance than the other. The rabbit IC may be described as bipolar. It is likely that the adoptive response of the IC of rabbit CCD does not involve a complete reversal of all transporters between the two poles, but rather some remodelling that shifts the bulk of the H^+-ATPase molecules to the other cell membrane by some means of vesicular traffic. According to current models, the basolateral Cl^- conductance stays in place; the fate of the Cl-HCO_3 exchanger in this reversal remains poorly understood.

Acid-Base Function of Sodium-Transporting Cells

The third topic deals with acid-base transport in Na transporting cells. The granular cells transport Na and their O_2 consumption is not affected by carbonic anhydrase inhibition, as shown by Schwartz and coworkers in turtle bladder [25]. Conversely, the carbonic anhydrase rich cells are not affected by ouabain, in terms of either O_2 consumption or transport. Hence, vectorial acid-base transport and sodium transport appear to be separated into different cells in turtle bladder. In the CD the separation of function is less clear and varies with the segments.

In general, the intercalated cells of the CD contain both carbonic anhydrase and Na, K-ATPase, as shown by Ridderstrale et al. [26] in the rabbit. Electrophysiologic studies, however, by Koeppen [14] have shown that the OMCD intercalated and inner stripe cells behave like H^+ secreting cells. They have extremely high apical membrane resistances without detectable Na conductances and their basolateral membranes have Cl conductances, instead of the usual K conductances of principal cells. The separations between H^+ transport and Na transport become unclear in other segments of the CD. For example, in the initial segment of the IMCD, α cell function and Na reabsorption may well coexist in the same cells. Brown et al. [13] demonstrated H^+-ATPase in the apical regions of the cells of this segment. Since the vacuolar H^+-ATPase dates back to the primitive archaebacteria, it appears that H^+ pumps preceded the development of Na^+ pumps by a long period. In some instances, the H^+-ATPases continued to serve as the primary plasma membrane pumps, in other instances they became incorporated in Na^+ transporting cells.

Aside from incorporating H^+ pumps for vectorial transport, Na^+ transporting cells have acid-base transporters for housekeeping functions. These transporters have been defined, to an important extent, by means of fluorescence techniques for intracellular pH. For example, all Na-transporting cells that have been studied in the collecting duct appear to contain basolateral Na/H antiporters which play a role in the recovery from an acid load, but are in the wrong position to contribute to H^+ secretion into the urine. In some more proximal segments, like the thick ascending limb of Henle's loop and the distal convoluted tubule, there appear to be apical Na/H antiporters which resemble the antiporters of the proximal tubule and do contribute to H^+ secretion. The principal cells of the CCD may also contain a basolateral Cl/HCO_3 exchanger, as described by Weiner and Hamm [27]. The basolateral Cl/HCO_3 exchanger and Na/H antiporter are involved primarily in intracellular pH regulation.

Overall Function of Distal Urinary Acidification

How is distal urinary acidification integrated? Asking the question, we tend to assume that the processes are part of a system that is completely determined. This assumption goes back to Laplace, who believed in a universe that operates like clockwork. If you know all components and their initial conditions and all laws, you can predict all events. The problem for urinary acidification is that the components interact with each other and rarely can be measured simultaneously under identical conditions. Also, the rules underlying these interactions are not precisely known. Hence, we end up with a lot of isolated systems that can't be simply added up to get the whole

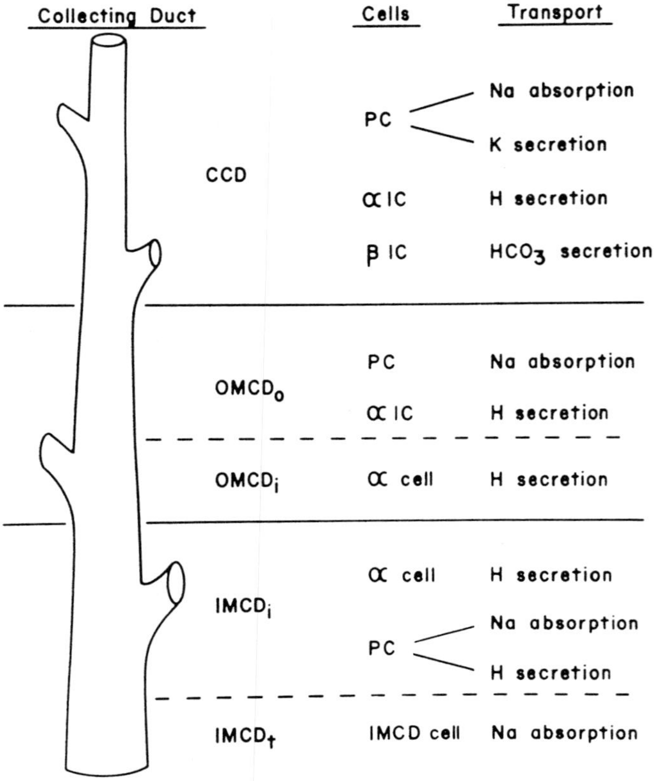

Fig. 9. Major transepithelial transport processes in collecting duct (*CD*). CCD, cortical CD; $OMCD_o$, outer stripe of outer medullary CD; $OMCD_i$, inner stripe of OMCD; $IMCD_i$ and $IMCD_t$, initial and terminal segments of inner medullary CD; PC, principal cell; IC, intercalated cell

system in vivo. Often, subsystems have their own evolutionary history, which bears little relation to acid-base transport. The best thing to do is to characterize each system (as we have always done) and to recognize the common, as well as the local, features, and to determine the context in which they should be taken within the overall system. Now that we work at the cellular and molecular level we need fewer black boxes, but we need more storage boxes to place the numerous local data and bits of incomplete knowledge into. Each student of urinary acidification must find the best simplification for his or her vantage point.

Figure 9 provides such a simplication of the collecting duct system. The fluid enters the cortical collecting duct (CCD) through connecting tubules, which are similar to the CCD. Much of the filtered HCO_3 has been reabsorbed in the proximal tubule (PT). In the thick ascending limb of Henle's loop and in the distal convoluted tubule this reabsorption is continued by transporters similar to those of the PT, namely an apical Na/H antiporter and, probably, a basolateral $Na3(HCO_3)$ cotransporter. The filtered HCO_3 is nearly reabsorbed by the time the CD begins contributing to net acid excretion.

The CCD is extremely versatile. The principal cells reabsorb Na and secrete K, at rates regulated by aldosterone. The intercalated cells secrete H^+ in cells with predominant α polarity and HCO_3^- in cells with predominant β polarity. This is the only segment where HCO_3^- secretion has been observed. None has been found beyond the cortical segment. The cortical segments also respond to K^+ depletion with increased K-ATPase activity of an ouabain resistant variety. Whether this ATPase is a H^+/K^+ ATPase or a Na^+/K^+ ATPase in a storage or ouabain resistant form, remains to be further explored. The regulation of acid-base transport is also versatile. Acute increases in peritubular HCO_3^- increase HCO_3^- secretion. Slower HCO_3^- loading increases the β polarity of IC cells and, thereby, the IC capacity to secrete HCO_3^-. Increases in CO_2 tension stimulate H^+ secretion under some, but not all, conditions. Aldosterone increases H^+ secretion via the voltage effect of stimulated Na^+ transport, as well as directly by some unspecified increase in H^+ pumps. Maneuvers increasing cellular cAMP tend to increase HCO_3^- secretion and, thereby, reduce any net H^+ secretion. Several peptide hormones such as VIP, glucagon, and, in some species, isoproterenol, stimulate HCO_3^- secretion. The catecholamines may stimulate both α and β cells, with the net outcome depending on the initial conditions. Paillard and Bishara [28] and Schuster and [17] have recently reviewed this field.

The OMCD is less versatile, but may serve as a better prototype for the study of H^+ secretion and α cell function. All intercalated cells of this segment are cells with a clearly unipolar organization. It has not been possible to bring about a polarity reversal by alkali loading. Na^+-transporting cells dominate in the outer stripe. In the less aerobic inner stripe, most cells behave as α cells secreting H^+. Their electrophysiology is one of H^+ secretion, with the typical basolateral Cl conductance and almost no apical ion conductance. H^+ secretion in this segment is stimulated directly by aldosterone. It is also regulated by CO_2 and HCO_3 in the expected directions.

The IMCD has been studied in vivo by microcatherization and perfusion, as well as in vitro, in culture preparations. The initial IMCD contains an apical membrane H^+-ATPase, as shown by Brown et al. [13]. Carbonic anhydrase is also present in the initial, but *not* in the terminal segments. The initial segment contributes to urinary acidification through H^+ secretion by apical H^+ pumps, a function comparable to α cell function. This segment, as well as the terminal segment, also contains Na/H antiporters. Their cellular distribution is not well characterized. In principle, an apical antiporter might contribute to urine acidification when concentration gradients are favorable, i.e., when the urine concentration of Na^+ is high and that of H^+ is low.

These are the main segments and functions along the CD system. In the overall system, the bulk of distal H^+ secretion is performed by α cells or α-like cells. As we have discussed, the regulation of H^+ secretion is a function, first, of the size of the H^+ pump population facing the lumen, and second, of the electrochemical potential difference for protons, $\Delta \tilde{\mu}H$, across the apical membrane. The intrinsic properties of the H^+ pumps are such that the pumps stop pumping as the pH gradient or the $\Delta \tilde{\mu}H$ approaches 3 pH units. The importance of the negative feedback inhibition of H^+ secretion cannot be overestimated. Significant net acid excretion can be achieved only if H^+ acceptors are available in the lumen. In the CD, ammonia and ammonium are the major buffer pair. Recent studies by Good and Knepper [29] have clarified the ways by which NH_3 and NH_4 ion accumulate within the medullary interstitium. They have shown how the transport of NH_4 ion is an important component of total ammonium transport in the proximal tubule and the thick ascending limb of Henle's loop. Once the NH_4^+ and NH_3 have accumulated within the interstitium, however, the diffusible NH_3 continues to play an old-fashioned role as a major proton acceptor within the lumen. This H^+ acceptor allows the H^+ pumps to secrete H^+ ions without self inhibition. Impaired H^+ secretion or impaired availability of ammonia can lead to a renal tubular acidosis.

Much less is known about the pathophysiology of HCO_3^- secretion. In principle, the β cells could play a role in preventing a dietary alkalosis. Since the apical exchanger is regulated by the luminal Cl^- concentration, reduced HCO_3^- secretion could contribute to Cl depletion alkalosis.

To conclude, despite the remarkable heterogeneity observed within distal urinary epithelia, we can recognize distinct cellular and molecular mechanisms that are central to acid-base transport and we can understand many of the principles by which they are regulated. Over the next few years, our knowledge of the major transport proteins—the H^+-ATPase, the kidney-related anion exchangers, and the Cl channels—is likely to expand. We shall learn more about the way these proteins are targeted to their membrane sites and the way they are expressed and regulated.

Acknowledgment. This work was supported by NIH research grant DK-30693.

References

1. Steinmetz PR, Husted A, Mueller A, Beauwens R (1981) Coupling between H^+ transport and anaerobic glycolysis in turtle urinary bladder: effects of inhibitors of H^+ ATPase. J Membr Biol 59:27–34
2. Beauwens R, Al-Awqati Q (1976) Active H^+ transport in the turtle urinary bladder:coupling of transport to glucose oxidation. J Gen Physiol 68:421–439
3. Rosen S (1972) Localization of carbonic anhydrase activity in turtle and toad urinary bladder mucosa. J Histochem Cytochem 20:696–702
4. Husted RF, Mueller AL, Kessel RG, Steinmetz PR (1981) Surface characteristics of carbonic-anhydrase rich cells in turtle urinary bladder. Kidney Int 19:491–502
5. Stetson DL, Steinmetz PR (1985) α- and β-types of carbonic anhydrase-rich cells in turtle bladder. Am J Physiol 249 (Renal Fluid Electrolyte Physiol 18):F553–F565
6. Stetson DL, Steinmetz PR (1986) Correlation between apical intramembrane particles and H^+ secretion rates during CO_2 stimulation in turtle bladder. Pflugers Arch 407(Suppl 2):S80–S84
7. Gluck S, Cannon C, Al Awqati Q (1982) Exocytosis regulates urinary acidification in turtle bladder by rapid insertion of H^+ pumps into the luminal membrane. Proc Natl Acad Sci USA 79:4327–4331
8. Steinmetz PR (1986) Cellular organization of urinary acidification. Am J Physiol 251 (Renal Fluid Electrolyte Physiol 20):F173–F187
9. Drenckhahn D, Oelmann M, Schaaf P, Wagner M, Wagner S (1987) Band 3 is the basolateral anion exchanger of dark epithelial cells of turtle urinary bladder. Am J Physiol 252 (Cell Physiol 21):C570–C574
10. Dixon TE, Al-Awqati A (1979) Urinary acidification in turtle bladder is due to a reversible proton-translocating ATPase. Proc Natl Acad Sci USA 76:3135–3138

11. Gluck S, Caldwell J (1988) Proton-translocating ATPase from bovine kidney medulla:partial purification and reconstitution. Am J Physiol 254:F71–F79
12. Brown D, Gluck S, Hartwig J (1987) Structure of the novel membrane-coating material in proton-secreting epithelial cells and identification as an H^+-ATPase. J Cell Biol 105:1637–1648
13. Brown D, Hirsch S, Gluck S (1988) Localization of a proton pumping ATPase in rat kidney. J Clin Invest 82:2114–2126
14. Koeppen BM (1985) Conductive properties of the rabbit outer medullary collecting duct:inner stripe. Am J Physiol 248 (Renal Fluid Electrolyte Physiol 17):F500–F506
15. Andersen OS, Silveira JEN, Steinmetz PR (1985) Intrinsic characteristics of the proton pump in the luminal membrane of a tight urinary epithelium. The relation between transport rate and $\Delta \tilde{\mu}$H. J Gen Physiol 86:215–234
16. Stone DK, Crider BP, Xie XS (1990) Structure of vacuolar proton pumps. Semin Nephrol 10:159–165
17. Schuster VL (1990) Bicarbonate reabsorption and secretion in the cortical and outer medullary collecting tubule. Semin Nephrol 10:139–147
18. Verlander JW, Madsen KM, Low PS, Allen DP, Tisher CC (1988) Immunocytochemical localization of band 3 protein in the rat collecting duct. Am J Physiol 255 (Renal Fluid Electrolyte Physiol 24):F115–F125
19. Leslie BR, Schwartz JH, Steinmetz PR (1973) Coupling between Cl^- absorption and HCO_3 secretion in turtle urinary bladder. Am J Physiol 255:610–617
20. McKinney TD, Burg MB (1978) Bicarbonate secretion by rabbit cortical collecting tubules in vitro. J Clin Invest 61:1421–1427
21. Stetson DL, Beauwens R, Palmisano J, Mitchell PP, Steinmetz PR (1985) A double-membrane model for urinary bicarbonate secretion. Am J Physiol 249 (Renal Fluid Electrolyte Physiol 18):F546–F552
22. Kohn OF, Mitchell PP, Steinmetz PR (1990) Characteristics of apical Cl-HCO_3 exchanger of bicarbonate-secreting cells in turtle bladder. Am J Physiol 258:F9–F14
23. Stetson DL (1989) Turtle urinary bladder:regulation of ion transport by dynamic changes in plasma membrane area. Am J Physiol 257:R973–R981
24. Schwartz GJ, Barasch J, Al-Awqati Q (1985) Plasticity of functional epithelial polarity. Nature 318:368–371
25. Schwartz JH, Bethencourt D, Rosen S (1982) Specialized function of carbonic anhydrase-rich and granular cells of turtle bladder. Am J Physiol 242 (Renal Fluid Electrolyte Physiol 11):F627–F633
26. Ridderstrale Y, Kashgarian M, Koeppen B, Giebisch G, Stetson D, Ardito T, Stanton B (1988) Morphological heterogeneity of the rabbit collecting duct. Kidney Int 34:655–670
27. Weiner ID, Hamm LL (1990) Regulation of intracellular pH in the rabbit cortical collecting tubule. J Clin Invest 85:274–281
28. Paillard M, Bichara M (1989) Peptide hormone effects on urinary acidification and acid-base balance: PTH, ADH, and glucagon. Am J Physiol 256:F973–F985
29. Good DW, Knepper MA (1990) Mechanisms of ammonium excretion:role of the renal medulla. Semin Nephrol 10:166–173

Osmolytes and Cell Osmoregulation in the Kidney

F.X. Beck, K. Thurau, M. Schmolke, and W.G. Guder

Chair: Tadao Niijima

Osmolytes and Cell Osmoregulation in the Kidney

F.X. BECK, K. THURAU[1], M. SCHMOLKE, and W.G. GUDER[2]

SUMMARY. The cells of the renal papilla are subject to widely varying extracellular osmolalities. In antidiuresis these cells are surrounded by hypertonic fluids, while in diuresis interstitial solute concentrations decline to levels comparable to those of the renal cortex. Papillary cells adapt to these extreme variations in extracellular tonicity by modulating the intracellular concentrations of small organic osmoeffectors (osmolytes), such as trimethylamines (glycerophosphorylcholine, betaine) and polyols (sorbitol, inositol). Variations in the intracellular concentrations of these osmolytes are accomplished by transmembrane net movement of water (cell swelling or shrinkage), by regulation of release and/or uptake of osmoeffectors via specific transmembrane transport pathways, and by changes in the intracellular synthesis of these organic compounds. These adaptive mechanisms allow intracellular electrolyte concentrations to remain relatively constant, despite extreme fluctuations in extracellular salinities. Accumulation of nonperturbing, organic osmolytes rather than inorganic electrolytes at high extracellular tonicities avoids the deleterious effects of elevated electrolyte concentrations on intracellular macromolecules. In addition, some of these osmolytes (trimethylamines) are assumed to counteract the adverse effects of high urea concentrations on the structure and function of cell proteins.

Introduction

The osmolality of the body fluids is maintained within narrow limits by the adequate response of the kidney to alterations in the organism's water balance. When water intake exceeds non-renal water loss and dilution of the body fluids develops, the kidney excretes the excess water, without major changes in solute excretion, by forming a hypoosmotic urine. On the other hand, during water shortage, the solutes to be

[1]Physiologisches Institut der Universität und [2]Institut für Klinische Chemie, Städtisches Krankenhaus München-Bogenhausen, 8000 Munich, Federal Republic of Germany

eliminated by the kidney are excreted in as small a volume of water as possible—hyperosmotic urine is produced.

The stability of the body fluids' osmolality contrasts sharply with the extreme variability of the renal medulla's solute concentrations. In antidiuresis, osmolalities many times higher than plasma osmolality prevail in the papilla, while in a state of diuresis papillary solute concentrations are decreased almost to isotonicity [1]. The cells of the renal medulla are thus subject to extreme changes in extracellular osmolality. In addition to this osmotic challenge, these cells are endangered by high urea concentrations in antidiuresis. This solute, which in the presence of antidiuretic hormone readily equilibrates across inner medullary cell membranes, may adversely affect the structure and function of cell proteins at these very high concentrations [2]. During the past few years concepts have emerged which allow us to explain how medullary cells are able not only to cope with extreme water stress, but also how they may escape the deleterious effects of high intracellular urea concentrations.

The study of intracellular electrolyte concentrations; in the rat renal papilla in antidiuresis, provided one of the first clues for the dominant role that organic osmolytes play in medullary cell osmoadaptation [3,4]. Using electron microprobe analysis on freeze-dried cryosections of the papillary tip, intracellular electrolyte concentrations were obtained which did not differ fundamentally from those of cells surrounded by isotonic fluids, such as proximal tubule cells [3,4]. These observations contrasted with earlier studies in which high sodium chloride concentrations, measured in medullary cells in antidiuresis, were assumed to balance the high extracellular salt concentrations (for review see [1]). Since, in antidiuresis, urea can be assumed to distribute freely across cell membranes, it is virtually certain that this substance does not impose any major osmotic stress on medullary cells. The finding of low cell sodium and chloride concentrations [3,4] implied that the high interstitial salt concentrations had to be balanced osmotically by equivalent concentrations of osmotically active substances, not directly detectable by electron microprobe analysis. For this phenomenon the term "osmotic gap" was coined (Fig. 1) [4]. Already at that time, it was clear that at least part of this gap could be filled by some organic osmoeffector, the so-called organic osmolytes.

Three classes of organic compounds must be considered as potential intracellular osmolytes: amino acids and their derivatives, methylamines, such as glycerophosphorylcholine and betaine, and polyols, such as sorbitol and inositol.

Although substantial amounts of amino acids and their derivatives (often assessed as ninhydrin-positive substances) have been demonstrated in the renal papilla, it is uncertain whether this group of osmolytes contributes significantly to cellular osmoadaptation, because high concentrations of amino acids have also been measured in extracellular compartments of the papilla [5]. In addition, information on the effect of alterations in the diuretic state on papillary amino acid contents is conflicting. While Law and Turner observed the concentrations of ninhydrin-positive substances to increase in papillary cells on exposure to hypertonic bathing solutions [6], Gullans and coworkers were unable to demonstrate any effect of water deprivation on papillary levels of ninhydrin-positive substances in vivo [7].

Analyses of the intrarenal distribution of glycerophosphorylcholine, betaine, sorbitol, and inositol have shown that substantial amounts of these osmolytes are present in the papillary tip in antidiuresis [8–12]. Since it is reasonable to assume that these compounds are located mainly in the intracellular compartment (see

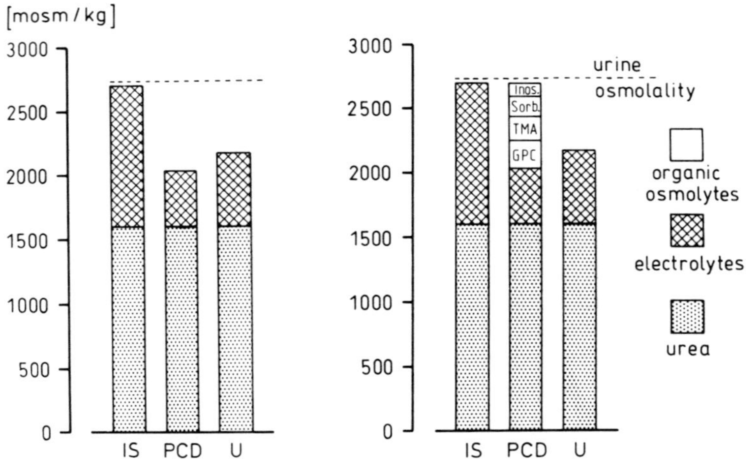

Fig. 1. Contribution of different osmoeffectors to total solute concentrations in the interstitium (*IS*), papillary collecting duct cells (*PCD*) and urine (*U*) in antidiuresis. The urea concentration and osmolality measured in the urine are assumed to exist in all tissue compartments. The contribution of inorganic electrolytes to total osmolality is assumed to be twice the sum of the sodium and potassium concentrations in a given compartment. The intracellular concentrations of glycerophosphorylcholine (*GPC*), other trimethylamines (*TMA*, mainly betaine), sorbitol (*sorb.*), and inositol (*inos.*) were calculated from total tissue contents of organic osmolytes, assuming the intracellular compartment to comprise 40% of papillary volume. (Adapted from [13])

below), and since the intracellular compartment comprises about 40% of total papillary tissue volume, estimates of intracellular concentrations of these organic osmolytes can be obtained [1,13]. These calculations suggest that most of the intracellular osmotic gap can be accounted for by trimethylamines and polyols (Fig. 1) [1,13].

Electron microprobe studies have also shown that the electrolyte concentrations of tubule cells in the inner stripe of the outer medulla are very similar to those of cortical tubule cells [14]. These results were taken to indicate that these cells achieve osmotic equilibrium with their hypertonic environment by accumulating organic osmolytes [1,14], as do inner papillary cells. Since the predominant osmolytes in the outer medulla are inositol and betaine (see below), it seems reasonable to assume that these osmoeffectors play a dominant role in the osmoadaptation of renal tubule cells located in the outer medulla.

Intrarenal Distribution of Organic Osmolytes During Different States of Diuresis

Methylamines

Glycerophosphoryl Choline (Fig. 2)

An analysis, by Ullrich and Pehling in the mid-fifties, of the spatial distribution of phosphorus-containing substances in the kidney showed the tissue content of an acid

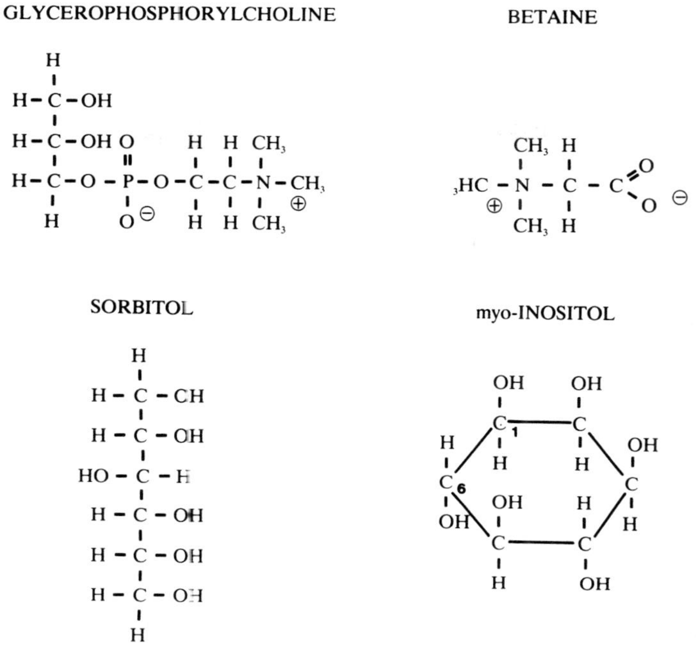

Fig. 2. Structural formulae of four types of organic osmolytes

soluble phosphorus compound to increase steeply between the outer medulla and the papillary tip in antidiuresis [15]. The remarkable concentration gradient of this substance was greatly attenuated during water diuresis [15]. Three years later this substance was identified by Schimassek, Kohl, and Bücher as glycerophosphorylcholine [8]. An important role in the osmotic adaptation of papillary cells was ascribed to glycerophosphorylcholine by these authors [8]. Several studies conducted on different species have, since then, confirmed these early observations of steeply increasing concentrations of glycerophosphorylcholine along the cortico-papillary axis in antidiuresis [8–12,16–17]. This gradient is markedly attenuated during states associated with low urine osmolalities [9,11,15–17]. Hence, glycerophosphorylcholine meets two requirements of an intracellular osmolyte, namely, that tissue glycerophosphorylcholine contents rise in parallel with tissue osmolality between cortex and papillary tip and that they are changed appropriately by the diuretic state.

Several lines of evidence suggest that glycerophosphorylcholine is restricted to the intracellular compartment. Urine concentrations of glycerophosphorylcholine are very low, as are the phosphorus concentrations of both the interstitial and intravascular compartments of the papilla [3,4,9]. These extracellular spaces are thus excluded from containing substantial amounts of glycerophosphorylcholine. In addition, intracellular phosphorus concentrations are high and are closely related to interstitial sodium concentration [3]. Finally, in isolated papillary collecting ducts, glycerophosphorylcholine has been found in concentrations similar to those of tissue homogenates of total papillae [9,10,12].

Betaine (Fig. 2)

Using ^{14}N nuclear magnetic resonance, high concentrations of trimethylamines, other than glycerophosphorylcholine, were detected by Balaban and Knepper in the inner medulla of antidiuretic rabbits [18]. Subsequent studies by Bagnasco and coworkers directly demonstrated that, in addition to glycerophosphorylcholine, betaine was abundant in the inner medulla of antidiuretic rabbits and that these high tissue contents of betaine were sharply reduced by diuresis [19]. Similar results in various species have been obtained since then by several laboratories [11,17,20–22]. In addition, tissue levels of betaine have been shown to increase between the outer medulla and the papillary tip [11,23]. Hence, this substance also meets the basic requirements of an intracellular osmoeffector, both with respect to its intrarenal distribution pattern and in its response to alterations in the diuretic state.

Polyols

Sorbitol (Fig. 2)

The tissue concentrations of sorbitol, a polyhydric alcohol, in several species have been shown to rise steeply between papillary base and tip in antidiuresis (Fig. 3) [10–12,21]. In the outer medulla, tissue levels are low; in the renal cortex, sorbitol frequently even escapes detection [10–12,17,19,21]. When inner medullary osmolality is diminished by diuresis, sorbitol levels in this zone are sharply reduced [10–12,19–22]. A preferential intracellular localization of sorbitol can be inferred from the observation that papillary collecting ducts isolated from hydropenic rats contain high concentrations of sorbitol [10,12,24].

Inositol (Fig. 2)

The intrarenal distribution of inositol, a cyclic polyol, contrasts markedly to that of the trimethylamines and sorbitol, since the highest tissue contents of inositol are found in the outer, rather than in the inner medulla [11,12,17,25]. In fact, inositol levels tend to decrease between papillary base and tip. In most species investigated, though not in all [17], inositol levels in the papilla are significantly reduced by diuresis [11,12,20,22,25].

Metabolism and Transmembrane Transport of Organic Osmolytes

Trimethylamines

Glycerophosphorylcholine

Glycerophosphorylcholine is thought to be liberated from phosphatidylcholine (lecithin) via the sequential action of phospholipase(s) A [13,26]. A second, direct metabolic pathway, in which choline is transferred from cytidinediphosphocholine to glycerophosphate [13] is less likely, since isolated rat papillary collecting duct cells incorporate inorganic phosphate into phosphatidylcholine before the label appears in the glycerophosphorylcholine pool [27]. In addition, while biosynthesis of glycerophosphorylcholine is slow and exhibits a considerable time lag after addition of its

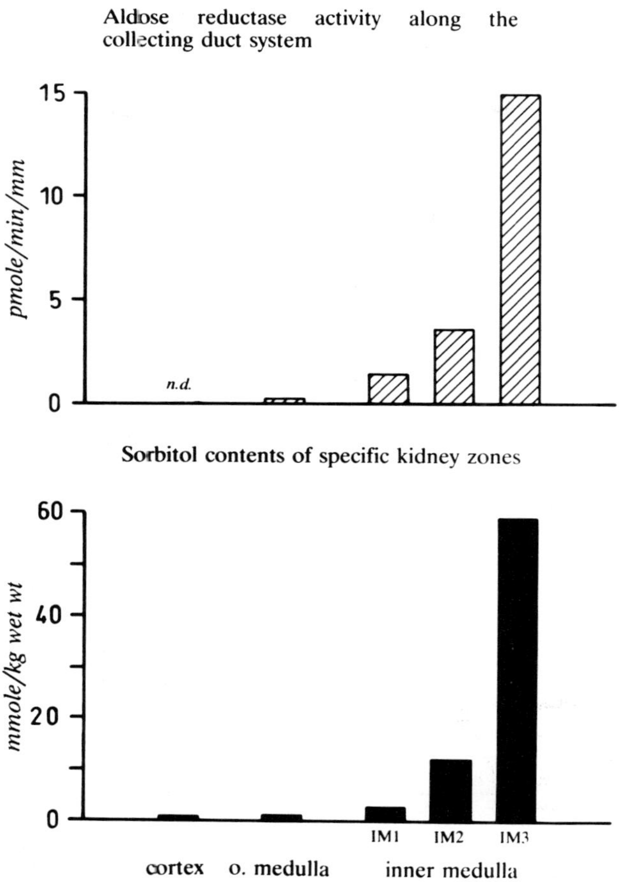

Fig. 3. Distribution of aldose reductase activity along the rat collecting duct system (*upper panel*). Sorbitol contents of different kidney zones (rat, antidiuresis) are shown *below*. (Adapted from [10,35])

precursors, the precursor choline is rapidly incorporated into tubular phospholipids [27]. The glycerophosphorylcholine degrading activity of papillary tissue has been shown to be low and not to be activated by diuresis [9]. On the other hand, isolated papillary collecting duct cells rapidly release glycerophosphorylcholine, without signs of osmotic cell rupture, when extracellular tonicity is reduced (Fig. 4) [12]. Available evidence thus suggests that the fall of the intracellular contents of glycerophosphorylcholine induced by diuresis is not due to enhanced intracellular degradation, but rather to activation of efflux into the extracellular compartment. At present, it is unclear whether uptake of glycerophosphorylcholine from the extracellular compartment into papillary cells contributes to the intracellular glycerophosphorylcholine pool. Likewise, information on the mechanisms mediating

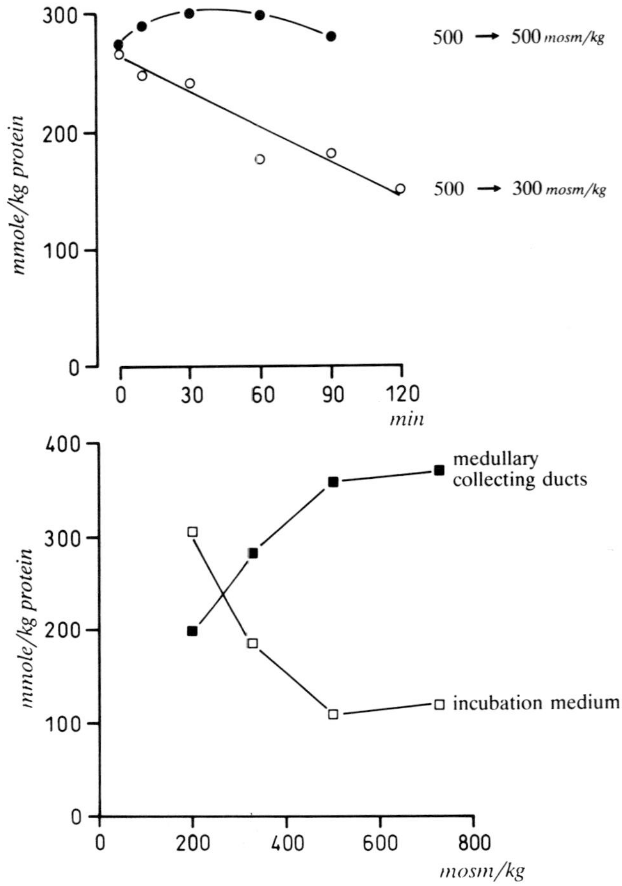

Fig. 4. Glycerophosphorylcholine contents of isolated papillary collecting ducts after transfer from hypertonic (500 mosm/kg) to isotonic (300 mosm/kg) incubation media (*upper panel*). Glycerophosphorylcholine contents of isolated collecting ducts and of the incubation media, measured after incubation (90 minutes) at different osmolalities, are shown in the *lower panel*. (Adapted from [12])

intracellular accumulation of glycerophosphorylcholine during the transition from diuresis to antidiuresis (reduced efflux enhanced uptake, enhanced liberation from phosphatidylcholine) is also scarce.

Betaine

Betaine is synthesized from choline via betaine aldehyde, a reaction which proceeds in mitochondria and is catalyzed by choline dehydrogenase and by betaine aldehyde dehydrogenase [26,28]. In the rabbit nephron, betaine synthesis has been found in proximal (S_3) and inner medullary tubules, but not in the thick ascending limb or in cortical and outer medullary collecting tubules. In accordance with these observations, betaine formed in vivo from labeled choline is rapidly accumulated in inner medulla and cortex in antidiuresis [29]. Grossmann and Hebert have shown choline dehydrogenase to be present in the inner medulla [28]. During chronic hypernatremia this enzyme was moderately stimulated in the medulla, but much more so in the cortex [28]. The uptake of the precursor choline into isolated papillary collecting ducts proceeds via a specific, sodium-independent transmembrane transport pathway [30]. This entry step is not stimulated by incubation in hypertonic bathing media [30], suggesting that modulation of choline uptake does not play a major role in regulating intracellular betaine levels, at least during acute changes of papillary osmolality. On the other hand, transport systems have been described which mediate uptake of betaine into renal tubule cells against steep transmembrane concentration gradients. This specific betaine transport has been shown in cortical tubule cells and in Madin-Darby canine kidney (MDCK) cells, a permanent line of renal tubule cells. Nakanishi and coworkers were able to demonstrate that a major portion of betaine uptake in MDCK cells is sodium-dependent and activated by chronic incubation in hypertonic media [31]. This raises the possibility that betaine synthesized in cortical tubules is taken up into medullary cells during hypertonic stress.

The response of intracellular betaine to decreasing extracellular concentrations of poorly permeable solutes has, as yet, not been studied directly in cells of the renal papilla. Investigations addressing this problem have, however, been performed on MDCK cells kept chronically in media of high tonicity. After switching the incubation medium from hypertonic to isotonic, betaine efflux from these cells rose significantly, while betaine uptake into the cells gradually declined [32].

Polyols

Sorbitol

Sorbitol is synthesized from glucose by the action of aldose reductase, and further metabolized to fructose by sorbitol dehydrogenase [13,26,33]. Glucose is taken up by papillary collecting duct cells via a sodium-independent mechanism, similar to that found in the basolateral membranes of proximal tubule cells [34]. Both enzymes of the sorbitol pathway, aldose reductase and sorbitol dehydrogenase, have been found in the renal inner medulla. Aldose reductase is present in all nephron segments of the renal medulla, as well as in the epithelium lining the papilla [33,35]. Studies on single nephron segments by Sands and coworkers have shown the activity of aldose reductase to increase steeply toward the tip of the papilla along both the collecting duct system (Fig. 3) and the thin descending and ascending limbs [35]. On the other hand, sorbitol dehydrogenase activity is much lower in the terminal papillary collecting duct than in proximal tubules [35]. These observations suggest that cell sorbitol contents may be regulated by changing aldose reductase, rather than sorbitol dehydrogenase, activity.

The sharp fall of tissue sorbitol contents in the inner medulla, seen after the transition from an antidiuretic to a diuretic state, is most likely due to rapid efflux of sorbitol out of medullary cells. Evidence for this has been obtained from in vitro experiments on isolated papillary collecting ducts, which demonstrate that sorbitol is rapidly released from the collecting duct cells when transferred from hypertonic to isotonic media [12,24]. Since the release of intracellular marker molecules, such as lactate dehydrogenase or ATP, was not increased by this experimental maneuver [12,24], this enhanced exit of sorbitol is not due to osmotic rupture of the cell membrane. The adaptation of intracellular sorbitol levels to acute alterations in extracellular tonicity is thus mainly achieved by alteration in sorbitol permeability of these cells. Changes in sorbitol efflux were not seen when urea was used to vary the osmolality of the incubation media [12].

The production of sorbitol, however, was not affected by acute reduction of extracellular solute concentration. Similarly, furosemide diuresis for 2 hours also failed to change aldose reductase activity [22]. The amount of aldose reductase mRNA in the papilla of the diuretic rats in this study, was, however, significantly reduced [22]. In agreement with these results, aldose reductase activities are diminished in the papilla of diabetes insipidus rats, in which interstitial tonicities are chronically low compared with normal rats [22]. The concept that cells in the renal medulla adjust their intracellular sorbitol levels to altered extracellular solute concentrations by rapid changes in cell sorbitol permeability and slow modulation of sorbitol synthesis is supported by observations on papillary cells in culture. In these cells, reduction of extracellular tonicity from 500 to 300 mosm/kg leads to rapid sorbitol efflux within a few minutes and to a slow fall of aldose reductase activity during the next few days [36].

One of the variables determining the production of sorbitol by inner medullary collecting duct cells is the glucose concentration of the incubation fluid [10,12]. It is, thus, not surprising that very high sorbitol levels are observed in the inner medulla of diabetic rats [23,37]. Grunewald and Kinne have shown that these high sorbitol contents are not due only to increased glucose availability, but are due also to enhanced aldose reductase activity in the inner medulla of diabetic rats [37]. Despite augmented capacity for sorbitol production, sorbitol permeability is not increased in these cells. This imbalance of sorbitol production and sorbitol release may contribute to necrosis of the inner medulla, which is a late complication in diabetes.

Inositol

The cyclic polyol, inositol, is an essential precursor of inositol-containing phospholipids and of inositolpolyphosphates which act as second messengers in a variety of cells. Inositol derives from D-glucose via three consecutive enzymatic steps: Myo-inositol 1-phosphate synthase acts on glucose-6-phosphate to form L-myo-inositol 1-phosphate. This is utilized subsequently by myo-inositol 1-phosphate phosphatase to produce myo-inositol [13,26]. Inositol can also be liberated from phosphatidylinositol via D-inositol 1-phosphate [26]. Up to now, it is, however, not completely clear whether intracellular accumulation of inositol in the outer and inner medulla occurs via these pathways. There is evidence that inositol can be catabolized to CO_2 via the glucuronate-xylulose pathway in the cortex and medulla, but not in the papilla [13].

On the other hand, specific uptake mechanisms for inositol have been demonstrated in MDCK cells. These transport pathways are activated by chronic incubation in hypertonic or inositol-free media, and they accomplish sodium-dependent inositol uptake against steep transmembrane inositol gradients [38]. If a similar transport system is also responsible for inositol uptake in renal medullary cells in vivo, the increase in extracellular sodium concentration during the transition from a diuretic to an antidiuretic state may help to achieve steep transmembrane inositol gradients.

Inositol is rapidly released from isolated papillary collecting duct cells on transfer from hypertonic incubation medium to a medium of lower tonicity [12]. Inositol efflux appears to proceed via specific pathways and appears not to be caused by osmotic rupture of cell membranes, since the release of marker molecules for cellular integrity, such as ATP or lactate dehydrogenase, was not increased by reducing extracellular tonicity [12]. Similar observations have been made in MDCK cells [32].

The major regulatory mechanisms responsible for the adjustment of intracellular inositol levels appear to be the appropriate modulation of inositol efflux and uptake. While changes in inositol permeability appear to constitute the short-term response to altered extracellular tonicity, alterations in inositol uptake become effective only after long-term perturbation of extracellular tonicity.

Information on the signals which trigger the increase or decrease of intracellular levels of organic osmolytes is scanty. Antidiuretic hormone, an obvious candidate, is probably not involved directly in the regulation of intracellular osmolytes, since studies on Brattleboro rats have shown that there is a considerable delay between the rise in urine osmolality and the increase of osmolytes in the papillary tissue [39]. In addition, accumulation of osmolytes in MDCK cells, in response to elevated extracellular tonicity, is partially inhibited by antidiuretic hormone [40]. The induction of aldose reductase has been studied in greater detail in a line of renal cells derived from the papillary surface epithelium. In these cells, expression of aldose reductase correlated with an increase in cell potassium concentration, but even better with an increase in the sum of intracellular sodium plus potassium concentrations [41]. This observation suggests that a rise in intracellular ionic strength may play an important role in the regulation of sorbitol production. Another variable influencing intracellular accumulation of sorbitol is the concentration of glucose in the extracellular compartment. In several studies, a clear correlation between extracellular glucose concentration and cell sorbitol levels was demonstrated [12,37]. Recent evidence suggests that increased intracellular calcium activities may contribute to the release of sorbitol from papillary collecting duct cells after hypotonic stress [42].

Even less is known about the factor which regulate intracellular levels of inositol and methylamines. Uptake of sorbitol, betaine, and inositol is modulated by the intracellular concentration of the respective osmolyte. When high intracellular concentrations of these osmolytes are reached, the uptake (inositol, betaine) or the production (sorbitol) slows [23,31,38,43]. It is conceivable, that, as for aldose reductase, the uptake of osmolytes or their precursors depends in some way on intracellular ionic strength. Such a betaine uptake system is well characterized in bacteria. This transporter contributes significantly to the osmotic adaptation of these cells to hypertonicity. The expression of a gene (proU) which codes for this betaine transporter is greatly stimulated by increased cell potassium concentrations [44].

Response of Inner Medullary Cells to Hyper- and Hypotonic Stress

Changes in intracellular concentrations of organic osmolytes may, however, be caused not only by changing the amount of intracellular organic osmoeffectors, but also by changing the amount of cell water. Electron microprobe studies on freeze-dried cryosections show the volume of papillary cells to increase when interstitial tonicity decreases [4]. Water shifts across the cell membranes, which are associated with dilution or passive concentration of intracellular osmoeffectors, may thus contribute to the osmotic adaptation of medullary cells. Moreover, these cell volume changes seem to persist in vivo for prolonged periods, because they could still be observed several hours after the onset of diuresis [4]. Complete volume regulation was, however, seen in isolated perfused papillary collecting ducts [45]. In these studies, elevation of extracellular tonicity induced cell shrinkage and subsequent restoration of cell volume by uptake of sodium and chloride via parallel Na-H-and Cl-HCO_3-exchangers [45]. The volume regulatory decrease was dependent on the presence of ADH in the peritubular bathing solution. On the other hand, complete volume regulation after hyperosmotic stress was not observed in a cell line derived from the papillary surface epithelium [41] and in the renal papillary surface epithelium in vitro [46].

The response of medullary cells to environmental hypertonic stress may thus comprise three phases. First, osmometric water efflux into the extracellular compartment produces cell shrinkage, with passive concentration of intracellular inorganic and organic osmoeffectors. Second, the subsequent activation of sodium and chloride uptake mechanisms favors restoration of cell volume. Enhanced entry of sodium can be assumed to stimulate active pump-mediated Na-K-exchange, so that in this phase increased amounts of intracellular potassium chloride primarily mediate cell osmoadaptation. Cell volume recovery in vivo is probably incomplete, so that cell concentrations of organic osmolytes may already be elevated at this stage, due to persistent moderate cell shrinkage. In the third phase, transport or/and metabolic pathways of organic osmolytes are modulated so as to attain increased cell levels of these osmoeffectors. This allows reduction of monovalent electrolyte concentrations to steady state values—thereby achieving full osmotic adaptation.

Lowering extracellular tonicity is associated with cell swelling and concomitant dilution of intracellular osmoeffectors. Subsequent stimulation of potassium chloride efflux may accomplish partial volume recovery. Even at this stage, exit of organic osmolytes may participate in the adaptive response. The final osmotic adjustments are achieved by appropriate modulation of those transport and metabolic pathways responsible for setting the intracellular levels of organic osmolytes.

Functional Advantages of Organic Osmolytes

For the cells of the renal medulla, the strategy of accumulating organic osmolytes, rather than inorganic electrolytes, in antidiuresis is advantageous in several respects [1,2].

First, high concentrations of inorganic electrolytes are known to perturb the structure and function of proteins [2]. This is well known from in vitro experiments, in which specific functional properties of enzymes, such as affinities and maximal turnover rates, are greatly diminished by increasing salt concentrations in the incubation medium. These adverse effects on enzyme function can be avoided if the solute concentration is increased by the addition of organic osmolytes, such as betaine, glycine, or trimethylamine oxide, rather than inorganic electrolytes.

Due to these non-perturbing properties, these osmoeffectors have been termed "compatible" osmolytes.

The second advantage concerns the role of urea. In antidiuresis, a major portion of total intracellular osmolality in the papilla is made up by urea. In the rat, for instance, urea concentrations of 1500 mmole/l or more are observed at the tip of the papilla [1]. These urea concentrations are high enough to destabilize protein structure and severely impair protein function. Trimethylamines have been shown to counteract this destabilizing effect of urea [2]. Trimethylamines, thus, may serve not only as *compatible* osmoeffectors, but also as *counteracting* osmoeffectors. Although the underlying mechanism is not completely understood, the most popular view is that these trimethylamines stabilize hydrogen bonds and are thus able to impair the weakening of these intramolecular bonds by urea. The native state of proteins is thus conserved and the unfolding of proteins is impeded.

Finally, the ability of renal papillary cells to respond to increased extracellular salt concentrations, with accumulation of organic osmolytes, allows the retention of low cell sodium concentrations. This is important because many transmembrane transport pathways, such as Na-H- and Na-Ca-exchange, rely on steep transmembrane sodium gradients. It is thus likely that high intracellular sodium concentrations would compromise cell proton and cell calcium homeostasis. In addition, intracellular accumulation of certain organic osmolytes themselves, such as betaine and inositol, is sodium-dependent and thus relies on steep transmembrane sodium gradients (see above).

Finally, it should be remembered that, in vivo, the alterations of extracellular tonicity during the transition from diuresis to antidiuresis, and vice versa, are gradual, rather than abrupt. This implies that the different phases of cell osmoadaptation in the papilla, enumerated above, are most likely not strictly separated, but may represent a continuum of states, in which activation and/or suppression of transport pathways for inorganic electrolytes and organic osmolytes, as well as metabolism of organic osmolytes, occurs in a coordinate and well balanced manner.

Acknowledgments. Studies carried out in the authors' laboratories were supported by grants from the Deutsche Forschungsgemeinschaft (Be 963/2-2, 2-3; Gu 82/3-2, 3-3).

References

1. Beck FX, Dörge A, Thurau K (1988) Cellular osmoregulation in renal medulla. Renal Physiol Biochem 11:174–186
2. Yancey PH, Clark ME, Hand SC, Bowlus RD, Somero GN (1982) Living with water stress: evolution of osmolyte systems. Science 217:1214–1222
3. Beck F, Dörge A, Rick R, Thurau K (1984) Intra- and extracellular element concentrations of rat renal papilla in antidiuresis. Kidney Int 25:397–403
4. Beck F, Dörge A, Rick R, Thurau K (1985) Osmoregulation of renal papillary cells. Pflügers Arch 405:S28–S32
5. Dantzler WH, Silbernagl S (1988) Amino acid transport by juxtamedullary nephrons: distal reabsorption and recycling. Am J Physiol 255:F397–F407
6. Law RO, Turner DPJ (1987) Are ninhydrin-positive substances volume-regulatory osmolytes in rat renal papillary cells? J Physiol 386:45–61

7. Gullans SR, Blumenfeld JD, Balschi JA, Kaleta M, Brenner RM, Heilig CW, Hebert SC (1988) Accumulation of major organic osmolytes in rat renal inner medulla in dehydration. Am J Physiol 255:F626–F634
8. Schimassek H, Kohl D, Bücher T (1959) Glycerylphosphorylcholine, die Nierensubstanz "Ma-Mark" von Ullrich. Biochem Z 331:87–97
9. Wirthensohn G, Beck FX, Guder WG (1987) Role and regulation of glycerophosphorylcholine in rat renal papilla. Pflügers Arch 409:411–415
10. Wirthensohn G, Lefrank S, Guder WG, Beck FX (1987) Studies on the role of glycerophosphorylcholine and sorbitol in renal osmoregulation. In: Kovacevic Z, Guder WG (eds) Molecular nephrology: biochemical aspects of kidney function. Walter de Gruyter, Berlin, pp 321–327
11. Yancey PH, Burg MB (1989) Distribution of major organic osmolytes in rabbit kidneys in diuresis and antidiuresis. Am J Physiol 257:F602–F607
12. Wirthensohn G, Lefrank S, Schmolke M, Guder WG (1989) Regulation of organic osmolyte concentrations in tubules from rat renal inner medulla. Am J Physiol 256: F128–F135
13. Beck FX, Dörge A, Thurau K, Guder WG (1990) Cell osmoregulation in the countercurrent system of the renal medulla: The role of organic osmolytes. In: Beyenbach KW (ed) Cell volume regulation, comp physiol. Karger, Basel, pp 132–158
14. Beck FX, Dörge A, Ring T, Sauer M (1989) Element composition of tubule cells in the inner stripe of the renal outer medulla. Miner Electrolyte Metab 15:144–149
15. Ullrich KJ, Pehling G (1956) Über das Vorkommen von Phosphorverbindungen in verschiedenen Nierenabschnitten und Änderungen ihrer Konzentration in Abhängigkeit vom Diuresezustand. Pflügers Arch 262:551–561
16. Philippson C (1964) Der Gehalt an Glycerylphosphorylcholin und Glycerylphosphoryläthanolamin von Nierenmark und Nierenrinde hochreiner Wistarratten während forcierter Wasserdiurese und extrem langer Durst-Antidiurese. Pflügers Arch 280:30–37
17. Yancey PH (1988) Osmotic effectors in kidneys of xeric and mesic rodents: corticomedullary distributions and changes with water availability. J Comp Physiol 158:369–380
18. Balaban RS, Knepper MA (1983) Nitrogen-14 nuclear magnetic resonance spectroscopy of mammalian tissues. Am J Physiol 245:C439–C444
19. Bagnasco S, Balaban R, Fales HM, Yang YM, Burg M (1986) Predominant osmotically active organic solutes in rat and rabbit renal medullas. J Biol Chem 261:5872–5877
20. Wolff SD, Stanton TS, James SL, Balaban RS (1989) Acute regulation of the predominant organic solutes of the rabbit renal inner medulla. Am J Physiol 257:F676–F681
21. Chambers ST, Kunin CM (1987) Osmoprotective activity for Escherichia coli in mammalian renal inner medulla and urine. Correlation of glycine and proline betaines and sorbitol with response to osmotic loads. J Clin Invest 80:1255–1260
22. Cowley BD, Ferraris JD, Carper D, Burg M (1990) In vivo osmoregulation of aldose reductase mRNA, protein, and sorbitol in renal medulla. Am J Physiol 258:F154–F161
23. Guder WG, Beck FX, Schmolke M (1991) Organic compounds in renal volume regulation. Proceedings of the XIth Congress of nephrology, July 15–20 1990. Springer, Tokyo Berlin Heidelberg.
24. Grunewald RW, Kinne RKH (1989) Intracellular sorbitol content in isolated rat inner medullary collecting duct. Pflügers Arch 414:178–184
25. Cohen MA, Hruska KA, Daughaday WH (1982) Free myo-inositol in canine kidneys: selective concentration in the renal medulla. Proc Soc Exp Biol Med 169:380–385
26. Wolff SD, Balaban RS (1990) Regulation of the predominant renal medullary organic solutes in vivo. Annu Rev Physiol 52:727–746
27. Schmolke M, Bornemann A, Guder WG (to be published) Distribution and regulation of organic osmolytes along the nephron. In: Koide H, Endou H, Kurokawa K (eds) Cell biology of nephron heterogeneity: fine structure and functions. Karger, Basel

28. Grossman EB, Hebert SC (1989) Renal inner medullary choline dehydrogenase activity: characterization and modulation. Am J Physiol 256:F107–F112
29. Eng J, Berkowitz BA, Balaban RS (to be published) Renal distribution and metabolism of [$^2H_9$]choline. A^{2}H NMR and MRI study. NMR Biomed
30. Bevan C, Kinne RKH (1990) Choline transport in collecting duct cells isolated from the rat renal inner medulla. Pflügers Arch 417:324–328
31. Nakanishi T, Turner RJ, Burg MB (1990) Osmoregulation of betaine transport in mammalian renal medullary cells. Am J Physiol 258:F1061–F1067
32. Nakanishi T, Burg MB (1989) Osmoregulatory fluxes of myo-inositol and betaine in renal cells. Am J Physiol 257:C964–C970
33. Terubayashi H, Sato S, Nishimura C, Kador PF, Kinoshita JH (1989) Localization of aldose and aldehyde reductase in the kidney. Kidney Int 36:843–851
34. Grunewald RW, Kinne RKH (1988) Sugar transport in isolated rat kidney papillary collecting duct cells. Pflügers Arch 413:32–37
35. Sands JM, Terada Y, Bernard LM, Knepper MA (1989) Aldose reductase activities in microdissected rat renal tubule segments. Am J Physiol 256:F563–F569
36. Bagnasco S, Murphy HR, Bedford JJ, Burg MB (1988) Osmoregulation by slow changes in aldose reductase and rapid changes in sorbitol flux. Am J Physiol 254:C788–C792
37. Grunewald RW, Kinne RKH (1989) Sorbitol metabolism in inner medullary collecting duct cells of diabetic rats. Pflugers Arch 414:346–350
38. Nakanishi T, Turner RJ, Burg MB (1989) Osmoregulatory changes in myoinositol transport by renal cells. Proc Natl Acad Sci USA 86:6002–6006
39. Schmolke M, Beck FX, Guder WG (1989) Effect of antidiuretic hormone on renal organic osmolytes in Brattleboro rats. Am J Physiol 257:F732–F737
40. Heilig CW, Brenner BM, Yu ASL, Kone BC, Gullans SR (1990) Modulation of osmolytes in MDCK cells by solutes, inhibitors, and vasopressin. Am J Physiol 259:F653–F659
41. Uchida S, Garcia-Perez A, Murphy HR, Burg M (1989) Signal for induction of aldose reductase in renal medullary cells by high external NaCl. Am J Physiol 256:C614–C620
42. Bevan C, Theiss C, Kinne RKH (1990) Role of Ca^{2+} in sorbitol release from rat inner medullary collecting duct (IMCD) cells under hypoosmotic stress. Biochem Biophys Res Comm 170:563–568
43. Moriyama T, Garcia-Perez A, Burg MB (1989) Osmotic regulation of aldose reductase protein synthesis in renal medullary cells. J Biol Chem 264:16810–16814
44. Epstein W (1986) Osmoregulation by potassium transport in Escherichia coli. FEMS Microbiol Rev 39:73–78
45. Sun A, Hebert SC (1989) Rapid hypertonic cell volume regulation in perfused inner medullary collecting duct. Kidney Int 36:831–842
46. Sands JM, Knepper MA, Spring KR (1986) Na-K-Cl cotransport in apical membrane of rabbit renal papillary surface epithelium. Am J Physiol 251:F475–F484

The Pathogenesis of Tubulointerstitial Nephritis

PETER S. HEEGER, GUNTER WOLF
and ERIC G. NEILSON

Chair: Priscilla Kincaid-Smith

The Pathogenesis of Tubulointerstitial Nephritis

Peter S. Heeger, Gunter Wolf, and Eric G. Neilson[1]

Summary. Tubulointerstitial nephritis is a common form of both acute and chronic renal disease in humans. Over the last 12 years we have been studying the pathogenic mechanisms involved in tubulointerstitial nephritis, using several animal models which are similar to distinct forms of human interstitial injury. The immunopathogenesis of tubulointerstitial nephritis can be arbitrarily divided into three phases. The afferent, or antigen recognition phase, involves expression of the nephritogenic antigen, recognition and presentation of the nephritogenic antigen in the context of appropriate MHC determinants, and circumvention of the usual mechanisms of tolerance. The immunoregulatory phase consists of multiple counter-regulatory events, both humoral and cell-mediated, that influence the amplitude and qualitative nature of the immune response. The final, effector, phase includes the various mechanisms directly responsible for tubulointerstitial injury and subsequent fibrosis. Additionally, once the immune response has been initiated, a number of factors can influence the progression of tubulointerstitial injury toward end stage renal disease.

Introduction

Tubulointerstitial nephritis accounts for up to 15% of cases of acute renal failure, and as many as 25% of cases of chronic renal failure have been ascribed to the long term sequelae of this disease [1,2]. Additionally, interstitial inflammation and subsequent fibrosis occur in most forms of renal failure resulting in end stage renal disease, regardless of the primary etiology. The significance of this form of renal disease is underscored by morphometric correlations suggesting that changes in tubular function and glomerular filtration rate correlate more strongly with histologic deteriora-

[1]Renal-Electrolyte Section of the Department of Medicine, and the Cell Biology and Immunology Graduate Groups, University of Pennsylvania, Philadelphia, PA 19104–6144, USA

Table 1. Immune mechanisms of tubulointerstitial nephritis

Immune mechanism	Animal model	Human disease
Immune deposit disease	NZB/W mouse or immunization with Tamm-Horsefall protein	Systemic lupus erythematosis Sjögren's syndrome Planted antigens Drugs Infections
Anti-TBM disease	Anti-TBM models in rats, mice, and guinea pigs	Drugs Idiopathic Renal transplantation Anti-GBM disease
Primarily cell-mediated disease	Spontaneous TIN in kdkd mice	Infections Drugs Pyelonephritis Medullary cystic disease Idiopathic

tion of interstitial architecture than with changes in glomerular structure. Our laboratory has long been interested in elucidating the pathogenic mechanisms involved in the initiation, regulation, expression, and progression of tubulointerstitial nephritis, and it is the purpose of this report to summarize some of our views. Due to space limitations, many of the references cited herein are recent, fully referenced review articles.

Although virtually all forms of human tubulointerstitial nephritis probably have an immune basis regardless of etiology, most of the information on pathogenesis of this disease comes from animal models [1–3]. There are three distinct immunohistological forms that can be recognized (Table 1). First, immune deposits, usually formed in situ through the reaction of antibodies with planted antigen, can mediate the inflammatory response. Preformed circulating immune complexes preferentially deposit in the glomerulus, and are not commonly implicated as causative in tubulointerstitial nephritis. Subsequent to immune complex deposition, activation of complement, and infiltration by polymorphonuclear leukocytes and lymphocytes eventually result in interstitial fibrosis. Animal models providing insight into this form of tubulointerstitial nephritis include the NZB/W mouse, as well as mice immunized with Tamm-Horsfall protein [3]. In humans, tubulointerstitial nephritis associated with immune deposits has been observed with lupus erythematosus and Sjögren's syndrome, and accompanies various forms of glomerulonephritis [2,3].

Secondly, anti-tubular basement membrane (anti-TBM) antibodies can promote tubulointerstitial nephritis. Anti-TBM disease can be induced in mice, rats, and guinea pigs following immunization with heterologous renal tubular antigens [3,4]. After 2 weeks, circulating antibodies and a linear deposition of IgG along the TBM can be observed by immunofluorescence. Later, mononuclear cells infiltrate the tubulointerstitium and progressive interstitial fibrosis ensues. Although both the humoral and cell-mediated arms of the immune system are activated in all forms of anti-TBM disease, the relative contribution of these arms toward disease expression varies between the different models studied [1–3]. Anti-TBM disease may occur in humans as a complication of drug therapy, infection, after renal transplantation, following Goodpasture's syndrome, or in an idiopathic form [2].

Finally, polymorphonuclear and mononuclear cell infiltration can occur in the absence of antibody deposition. Spontaneous tubulointerstitial nephritis in the kdkd mouse is an experimental model of this cell-mediated injury [5]. Similar lesions are found in human tubulointerstitial disease after chronic obstructive pyelonephritis and hydronephrosis, and in medullary cystic disease [2].

The pathogenesis of tubulointerstitial nephritis can be arbitrarily divided into three general phases [1,6]. Antigen recognition, the afferent phase, begins with the loss of tolerance to self-antigens, and loss of the genetically determined ability to respond to foreign antigens. The second immunoregulatory phase comprises protective processes that influence the amplitude and qualitative nature of the immune response. The final efferent, or effector, phase includes the mechanisms directly responsible for producing interstitial damage. These processes, as well as factors influencing disease progression once established, will be discussed in the ensuing sections.

Antigen Recognition Phase

Initiation of an autoimmune response requires the overcoming of protective mechanisms that result in tolerance to self-antigens. Tolerance to one's own parenchymal tissues can occur through failure of antigen to properly associate with MHC molecules on the surface of antigen presenting cells, through clonal deletion in the thymus or peripheral clonal anergy of self-reactive T cells, or through the action of specific suppressor cells [1].

Target antigen

The first and foremost factor in overcoming tolerance is that the inciting antigen must be present, and must be accessible to the immune system. The antigen may be endogenous, or may result from exposure to exogenous agents. Infectious agents (particularly viruses), can provide appropriate target antigens through molecular mimicry, or may damage interstitial tissues through toxic mechanisms and thereby expose novel immunogenic antigens [7]. Drugs can also act as hapten bridges to the tubulointerstitium, and can target the immune response towards previously unrecognized self-antigens [1].

The target antigen of murine anti-TBM disease is called 3M-1 [8]. It was recently identified as a glycoprotein with a molecular weight of 30–48 Kd, and can be localized to the lateral site of proximal tubular basement membrane. This nephritogenic antigen is expressed in an autosomal dominant pattern and is controlled by a single group of genes which are independent of the MHC, but closely linked to the gene for albinism on the first linkage group [9]. Using a monoclonal anti-3M-1 antibody, a closely related antigen with a similar molecular weight was isolated from the kidney of a human patient, suggesting significant evolutionary conservation [10]. Not all mammals tested have an accessible form of this antigen, however. Lewis rats, a strain not susceptible to anti-TBM disease following immunization with heterologous renal tubular antigen, do not bind anti-TBM antibodies in a linear pattern [3]. These animals develop circulating serum anti-TBM antibodies, however, and in vitro collagenase solubilization of the TBM preparations uncovers anti-TBM binding, implying that the reactive epitopes are normally sequestered from the immune system.

Additionally, 3M-1 may be absent in certain humans, explaining the development of anti-TBM disease after kidney transplantation (the recipient does not express the antigen but is given a graft that does, resulting in an immune response) [2]. Recently, screening of a cDNA expression library from murine proximal tubule cells has resulted in the isolation of a unique family of isoforms with transcripts of 1.7–1.9 kb, encoding the 3M-1 antigen [11]. These genes, and their transcripts, can be localized to tubular epithelium by in situ hybridization (E.G. Neilson unpublished observations). A synthetic peptide deduced from the cDNA framework region binds anti-3M-1 monoclonal antibodies and can function as specific antigen for a 3M-1 reactive helper T cell line (E.G. Neilson unpublished observations).

MHC Determinants

Effector T-cells recognize their target antigen in the context of specific MHC-determinants, thus defining genetic restriction. Murine anti-TBM disease, for example, is genetically restricted, and maps, in an autosomal dominant fashion, to H-$2K^s$ [12]. The induction of anti-TBM disease, or its aberrant expression in normally non-susceptible animals, also depends on the visibility of MHC class II determinants. These have traditionally been localized to the surface of macrophages, dendritic cells, or B lymphocytes. More recently, however, it has been appreciated that epithelial cells (including renal tubular cells) can act as antigen-secreting, as well as antigen-presenting, cells, and may express class II MHC molecules under certain conditions. We have shown in an in vitro system that a proximal tubular cell line secreting the 3M-1 target antigen (MCT cells) can present this self-antigen to syngeneic T helper cells in the context of class II MHC determinants [13,14]. Furthermore, treatment of MCT cells with γ-interferon increases the expression of class II molecules on the cell surface [14]. Interestingly, exogenous interferon treatment of a mouse strain that is normally not susceptible to anti-TBM disease converts this mouse to a susceptible strain. On the other hand, anti-tubular basement membrane antibodies, which bind to tubular epithelium, protectively down regulate the transcription and subsequent surface expression of class II MHC determinants on tubular cells [14]. The regulation of MHC class II determinants in the kidney is closely modulated by the immune repertoires expressing interstitial disease.

Other Factors

Despite the presence and accessibility of a target antigen and its association with the appropriate MHC molecule, other factors may lead to tolerance, and inhibit the expression of disease. Clonal deletion of specific reactive T cells during ontogeny could theoretically prevent the autoimmune response. There are, however, no major detectable differences yet, other than genetic restriction and selected cell phenotype, in the recognition properties of the T cell repertoires in mice that are susceptible or nonsusceptible to anti-TBM disease [1]. In addition, there is no evidence that clonal anergy, the inability of a T cell clone to react to an appropriately recognized antigen-MHC complex, plays a role in the susceptibility to anti-TBM disease.

Tolerance, of course, can also be overcome through the effects of regulatory T lymphocytes. Suppressor T cells can actively inhibit the activation of specific helper or effector T cells, despite their appropriate recognition of the antigen-MHC complex.

Since suppression is also an important immunoregulatory mediator, relevant examples will be discussed in the next section.

Immune Regulatory Phase

Activation of the nephritogenic T and B cell repertoires is normally self-limited by specific down regulatory events. These regulatory events are controlled either by complementary interactions in the immune repertoire, or by the immunologic visibility of the target antigen. In anti-TBM disease, helper T cells responding to tubulointerstitial antigens (after circumventing the above mentioned mechanisms of tolerance) induce the differentiation of nephritogenic effector T cells and anti-TBM antibody secreting B cells, and are thus central participants in these immunoregulatory events [1].

In Brown Norway rats, anti-TBM antibody production and cell-mediated events are quantitatively and temporally related to the expression of disease [1,3]. It has been demonstrated in our laboratory that an anti-idiotypic humoral immune response can modulate the idiotypic humoral and cell-mediated responses in this model [3,15]. Exogenous anti-idiotypic antibodies decrease the delayed-type hypersensitivity (DTH) response to renal tubular antigen, as well as limit disease progression, even if administered two weeks after initial immunization. Rats that are not susceptible to anti-TBM disease develop their own anti-idiotypic network upon immunization, which prevents disease [3]. The Brown Norway rat, however, does not normally develop an anti-idiotype response. This is due to the emergence of a specific suppressor cell that inhibits clonal expansion of these T and B cells. Idiotypically marked humoral and cell-mediated (anti-renal tubular antigen) responses thus go unchecked, leading to disease expression [1,3,15]. Additionally, a suppressor network can be induced in Brown Norway rats through immunization with renal tubular antigen and incomplete Freund's adjuvant. The induced suppressor cells have a cross-reactive idiotype to anti-TBM antibodies, and are able to specifically decrease production of anti-TBM antibodies, as well as abrogate disease progression [3].

The regulatory events involved in murine anti-TBM disease are somewhat analogous (Fig. 1). Antibody quality and quantity, however, do not differ between susceptible and nonsusceptible strains of mice. As discussed in the previous section, however, anti-TBM antibodies can down regulate the transcription of MHC class II molecules, and therefore decrease the immunologic visibility of available antigen. The important role of cell-mediated immune responses operating in anti-TBM disease was largely worked out in mice [1]. An antigen-specific, I-A restricted, CD4+ helper T cell (Th) emerges first, and is an essential mediator of subsequent events [16]. This helper cell induces both a CD4+ and a CD8+ effector cell (Te) early in the immune response of both susceptible and nonsusceptible mice [1]. The CD4+ effector cells recognize antigen in vitro, are class II restricted, but have difficulty normally recognizing relevant tubular antigen locally within the kidney. These cells preferentially emerge in nonsusceptible mouse strains [1]. The nephritogenic class I restricted CD8+ effector cell emerges in susceptible strains and directly causes disease. Nonsusceptible mice have such CD8+ effector cells, but their clonal expansion is inhibited by other regulatory T cells residing in the immune system [1]. These CD8+, I-J+ suppressor cells (Ts) prevent the emergence of the CD8+ effector cells.

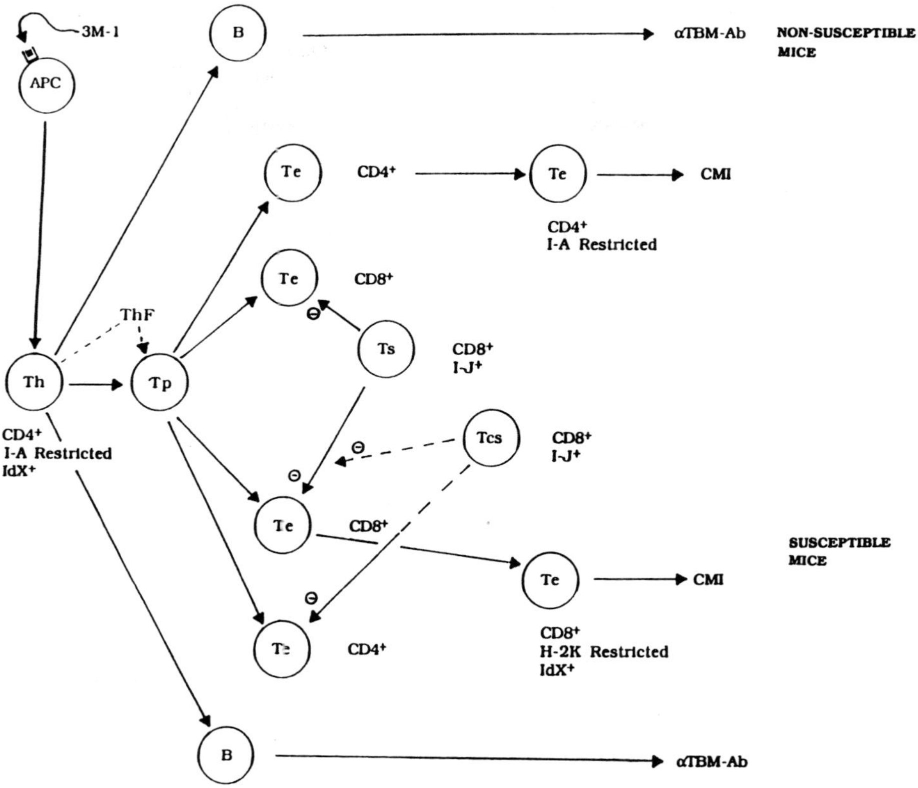

Fig. 1. Development of the immune response in murine anti-TBM disease. See text for explanation. APC, antigen presenting cell; B, B lymphocyte; Th, helper T lymphocyte; ThF, helper factor; Tp, undifferentiated precursor T lymphocyte; Te, effector T lymphocyte; Ts, suppressor T lymphocyte; Tcs, contrasuppressor T lymphocyte; CMI, cell mediated immune response; IdX+, idiotype +

In susceptible mice, the disease-protective suppressor cells are subverted, in turn, by CD8+, class I restricted contrasuppressor cells (Tcs), allowing immune injury to occur [17]. Immune regulation of effector T cell preference thus critically determines susceptibility to the development of anti-TBM disease [1,17].

Suppression is also an important influence on the expression of disease in the kdkd mouse model of tubulointerstitial nephritis. The kdkd mouse is a congenic subline of the CBA/Ca mouse, and is uniquely susceptible to a spontaneous, CD8+ T cell-mediated, autosomally dominant tubulointerstitial nephritis [1]. The nonsusceptible wild-type CBA/Ca mouse contains, in its immune system, a specific suppressor T cell that inhibits activation of the CD8+ effector cell, and thus prevents the expression of disease [1,18]. In the kdkd mouse, this suppressor cell, in turn, is inhibited by a specific contrasuppressor cell, thus facilitating clonal expansion of the CD8+ effector cell, and allowing expression of disease [17,18].

Another potentially important regulatory aspect of murine anti-TBM disease is that the central CD4+ helper T cell (Th) secretes an antigen-specific, class II restricted cytokine, T helper factor (ThF), that can specifically induce the CD8+ effector cell population to cause disease [19]. Molecular cloning of the antigen binding chain of ThF has yielded a family of cDNA that is currently being further characterized. Antisense oligonucleotides to this cDNA specifically inhibited the production of ThF, validating the relevance of this novel cDNA family [20]. Future work will focus on the factors controlling synthesis of this unique cytokine, in an effort to understand another regulatory mechanism for disease expression.

Effector Phase

A variety of potential effector mechanisms can lead to tubulointerstitial injury during the nephritogenic immune response (Fig. 2). Antibodies to interstitial structures may directly produce inflammation by activating the terminal membrane attack complex of complement, inducing chemotaxis of granulocytes and macrophages (with subsequent superoxide, protease, prostaglandin, and thromboxane release), invoking tubular injury through direct cytotoxicity of tubular cells, or by acting as an informational bridge targeting natural killer cells to the tubular epithelium [1,2]. An IgE humoral immune response may be preferentially produced when the inciting antigen derives from certain parasites, bacterial antigens, drug hapten-carrier molecules, or allergens. The produced IgE can then bind to special receptors on eosinophils, basophils, and primed mast cells, and a coordinated hypersensitivity response ensues [1].

Complement proteins have been observed to a varying degree in interstitial lesions. Complement activation can be seen in association with immune deposits, but it has also been occasionally observed when the nephritogenic process does not involve a humoral response. Exact mechanisms of activation under these circumstances are not fully worked out, but there is evidence that increased renal ammoniagenesis can activate complement [21]. Interstitial injury is not dependent on complement activation, however, in that C4 and C5 deficient animals can develop interstitial nephritis [1].

The hallmark of interstitial nephritis is the presence of mononuclear cells, mostly T cells, macrophages, and occasionally, eosinophils [1]. Effector T cells can induce delayed-type hypersensitivity responses with the release of inflammatory lymphokines, or they can directly produce cell-mediated cytotoxicity. Recently, a class I restricted CD8+ effector T cell line has been established in culture, and future work will further elucidate this cell's mechanism of cytotoxicity [22]. Additionally, T cells release a variety of lymphokines (including epidermal growth factor, transforming growth factor β, platelet derived growth factor, interleukins 1–6 (IL1–6), tumor necrosis factor, and others), that modulate the growth and biosynthesis of extracellular matrix in tubular epithelium and fibroblasts, as well as mediate the regenerative and hypertrophic responses of remnant epithelial tissue [23]. All of these factors can modulate procollagen deposition in the tubulointerstitial microenvironment, either through an increase in de novo procollagen biosynthesis, or through a decrease in proteolytic degradation. In addition, supernatants derived from cultured class II restricted T helper cells can influence the secretion of various

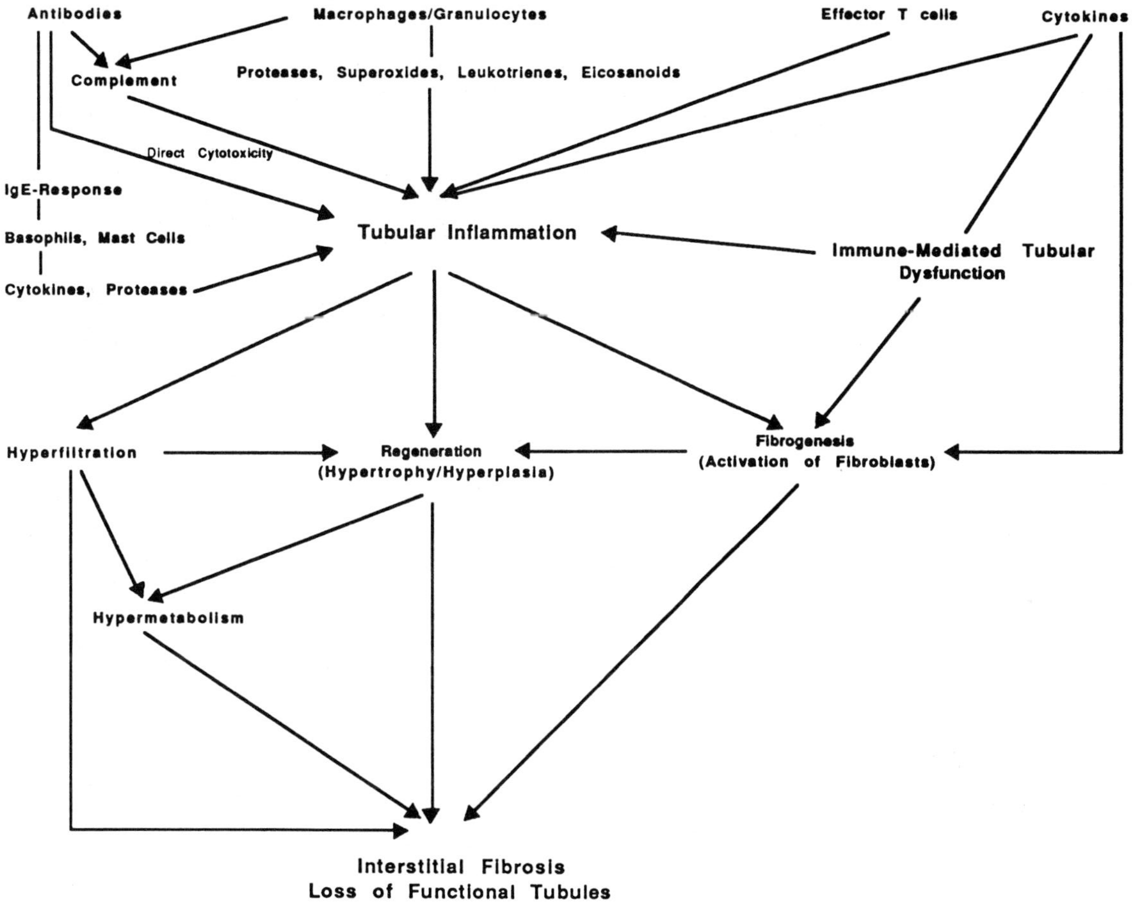

Fig. 2. Overview of the different effector mechanisms causing tubular injury, with interstitial fibrosis culminating in permanent loss of functional tubules

procollagens from tubular cells and interstitial fibroblasts [24]. More recent studies suggest that this effect is mediated through the aforementioned T helper factor (E.G. Neilson unpublished observations). The growth response itself may also lead to hypermetabolism of tubular cells, ultimately resulting in oxygen deprivation and the transformation of functional tubules into scar tissue. The importance of fibrogenesis and scar formation cannot be overstated. Irreversibility of the disease process correlates with the amount of fibrous tissue deposited, and can occur to a significant degree in as short a time as 7–10 days after the initial injury.

Tubulointerstitial nephritis is often accompanied by abnormalities of renal function, including sodium retention and a decrease in the glomerular filtration rate. Although altered renal plasma flow might be responsible for changes in tubular transport, there is increasing evidence that cytokines can directly influence these processes. IL-1 can significantly enhance sodium-dependent solute transport in proximal tubular cells, through steps requiring RNA and protein synthesis [25]. Similarly, tumor necrosis factor can stimulate sodium-dependent fluid transport in cultured proximal tubule cells. IL-1 has also been shown to mediate a decrease in glomerular filtration rate in some models of autoimmune renal injury. One can reasonably speculate, therefore, that the lymphocyte and macrophage infiltration found in tubulointerstitial nephritis could result in cytokine release that contributes to subsequent abnormalities in renal function.

Mediators of Disease Progression

Once a nephritogenic immunologic process has established itself in the kidney of an otherwise untreated animal, tubulointerstitial nephritis can ensue, and often progresses inexorably toward end-stage renal failure. A huge amount of literature has appeared in recent years concerning glomerular hypertension and hyperfiltration of remaining nephron units as causes of glomerulosclerosis, interstitial scarring, and progression of renal disease. It is also becoming clear that correction of these abnormalities can potentially slow down the progressive process. A full discussion of this topic is beyond the scope of this review, and the reader is referred elsewhere for details [26]. Our laboratory, among others, however, has noted several additional factors that can ameliorate the progressive process in immune-mediated tubulointerstitial nephritis.

Reduced caloric intake, without a change in total protein intake, has been shown to inhibit the development of renal disease and to prolong the lifespan of kdkd mice with spontaneous tubulointerstitial nephritis [27]. Prompt development of renal disease and death occurred after returning these mice to a higher calorie diet. A similar effect of calorie, but not protein, restriction decreasing the severity of disease has been noted in other models of immunologic renal injury. NZB/W mice spontaneously develop a lupus-like immune complex nephritis with interstitial immune deposits. Low calorie feeding reduces anti-DNA binding, improves T cell mitogenesis, and leads to less severe renal disease in these mice [6]. The precise mechanisms responsible for the preservation of renal function through calorie restriction are still under investigation.

A low protein diet, independent of caloric intake, can also favorably influence the outcome of immune-mediated renal disease. A low protein diet (3% versus 27%) at the time of immunization prevented the development of anti-TBM disease in rats, and stabilized histology and renal function in animals with already established disease [28]. This effect was most likely caused by nonspecific inhibition of T cell function, because DTH reactions to antigen were blunted in the 3% group. Other potential mechanisms for the protective effect of low protein diet include a decrease in glomerular hypertension, an alteration of mitochondrial oxygen consumption, and a modulation of tubular cell metabolism, all resulting in preservation of injured tubuloepithelial cells.

Furthermore, it has been shown that primary nonimmunological lesions, such as an acute reduction in renal mass, can lead to the stimulation of tubular ammoniagenesis by remnant nephrons, subsequent complement activation, and the production of chronic tubulointerstitial nephritis [21]. A protein restricted diet would, therefore, reduce the dietary acid load, decrease ammoniagenesis, and inhibit the nonspecific activation and deposition of complement in the renal tubulointerstitium.

Hyperlipidemia and hypercholesterolemia have been shown to contribute to the progression of glomerular renal disease in several animal models, but such a role in immune-mediated tubulointerstitial nephritis has yet to be proven [29]. Animals fed a high-cholesterol diet frequently do develop foam cells in the tubulointerstitium. Although the origin of foam cells is unknown, they appear to have characteristics of monocytes and macrophages, and can produce reactive oxygen intermediates which may be directly toxic to the tubular epithelium. The occurrence of foam cells has also been described in human tubulointerstitial nephritis, but the relevance of these cells in the pathogenesis of disease is presently unknown [2].

Our laboratory has also been interested in the disease abrogating effect of prostaglandin E_1 (PGE_1) treatment on tubulointerstitial nephritis. Administration of PGE_1 at the time of immunization delayed development of murine anti-TBM disease and diminished the DTH response in SJL mice. When begun on day 7 after immunization, however, this effect was not seen, suggesting that the immunosuppressive effect of PGE_1 occurs during the period of CD8+ nephritogenic effector T cell induction [30]. Further in vitro analysis revealed that PGE_1 led to the release of a nonspecific suppressor factor from T cells. Murine IL-1 was then shown to inhibit this PGE_1 suppressive effect [30]. When started during the first week after immunization, PGE_1 treatment also inhibited the development of acute and chronic inflammation in Brown Norway anti-TBM disease [3].

Conclusions and Future Directions

The immunopathogenesis of tubulointerstitial nephritis involves a complex interaction of genetic, immunologic, and environmental factors that determine initiation, development, and progression of disease in a given individual. The disease process proceeds through the expression and recognition of the nephritogenic antigen, the selection of an appropriate helper, effector, and regulatory T cell repertoire, the production of anti-TBM antibody, and finally, the various effector mechanisms responsible for tubular injury, fibrosis, and scarring. The next step in furthering our understanding of the pathogenesis of tubulointerstitial nephritis will be the molecular characterization of the various events in the disease process, with the ultimate goal of modifying these molecular interactions so as to prevent or attenuate the disease.

Acknowledgments. Original work in the authors' laboratory was supported by grants from the National Institute of Health (AR-20553, DK-30280, and DK-41110). Dr. Heeger is a recipient of a National Research Service Award (DK-08446) from the National Institutes of Health. Dr. Wolf is a recipient of a fellowship from the Boehringer Ingelheim Funds, Stuttgart, Federal Republic of Germany. Dr. Neilson is the recipient of an Established Investigator Award (85-108) from the American Heart Association and its Pennsylvania affiliates.

References

1. Neilson EG (1989) Pathogenesis and therapy of interstitial nephritis. Kidney Int 35:1257–1270
2. Neilson EG, Clayman MD, Kelly CJ (1989) The immunopathogenesis of interstitial nephritis. In: Massry S, Glassock R (eds) Textbook of nephrology, 2nd edn. Williams and Wilkins, Baltimore, pp 578–584
3. Wilson CB (1989) Study of the immunopathogenesis of tubulointerstitial nephritis using model systems. Kidney Int 35:938–953
4. Neilson EG, Phillips SM (1979) Cell-mediated immunity in interstitial nephritis. I. T lymphocyte systems in nephritic guinea pigs: the natural history and diversity of the immune response. J Immunol 123:2373–2380
5. Neilson EG, McCafferty E, Feldman A, Clayman MD, Zakheim B, Korngold R (1984) Spontaneous interstitial nephritis in kdkd mice. I. An experimental model of autoimmune renal disease. J Immunol 133:2560–2565
6. Kelly CJ, Haverty T, Neilson EG (1989) Control of the nephritogenic immune response. In: Wilson CB, Brenner BM, Stein JH (eds) Contemporary issues in nephrology. Churchill Livingstone, New York, pp 35–57 (Immunopathology of renal disease, vol 18)
7. Cameron JS (1989) Immunologically mediated interstitial nephritis: primary and secondary. Adv Nephrol 18:207–248
8. Clayman MD, Martinez-Hernandez A, Michaud L, Alper R, Mann R, Kefalides NA, Neilson EG (1985) Isolation and characterization of the nephritogenic antigen of anti-tubular basement membrane disease. J Exp Med 161:290–305
9. Neilson EG, Gasser DL, McCafferty E, Zakheim B, Phillips SM (1983) Polymorphism of genes involved in anti-tubular basement membrane disease in rats. Immunogenetics 17:55–65
10. Claymann MD, Michaud L, Brentjens J, Andres GA, Kefalides NA, Neilson EG (1986) Isolation of the target antigen of human anti-tubular basement membrane antibody-associated interstitial nephritis. J Clin Invest 77:1143–1147
11. Neilson EG, Sun MJ, Emergy J, Kelly C, Haverty T, Clayman M, Cooke NE (1989) Molecular cloning of the 3M-1 nephritogenic antigen. Kidney Int 35:358
12. Neilson EG, Phillips SM (1982) Murine interstitial nephritis. I. Analysis of disease susceptibility and its relationship to pleiomorphic gene products defining both immune response genes and a restrictive requirement for cytotoxic T cells at $H\text{-}2^K$. J Exp Med 155:1075–1085
13. Haverty TP, Kelly CJ, Hines WH, Amenta PS, Watanabe M, Harper RA, Kefalides NA, Neilson EG (1988) Characterization of a renal tubular epithelial cell line which secretes the autologous target antigen of autoimmune experimental interstitial nephritis. J Cell Biol 107:1359–1368
14. Haverty TP, Watanabe M, Neilson EG, Kelly CJ (1989) Protective modulation of class II MHC gene expression in tubular epithelium by target antigen-specific antibodies. Cell-surface directed down-regulation of transcription can influence susceptibility to murine tubulointerstitial nephritis. J Immunol 143:1133–1141

15. Neilson EG, Zakheim B (1983) T cell regulation, anti-idiotypic immunity, and the nephritogenic immune response. Kidney Int 24:289–302
16. Neilson EG, McCafferty E, Mann R, Michaud L, Clayman M (1985) Murine interstitial nephritis. III. The selection of phenotypic (Lyt and L3T4) and idiotypic T cell preferences by genes in Igh-1 and H-2^k characterizes the cell-mediated potential for disease expression: susceptible mice provide a unique T cell repertoire in response to tubular antigen. J Immunol 134:2375–2382
17. Kelly CJ, Neilson EG (1988) Contrasuppression in autoimmunity. Immunol Res 7:56–66
18. Kelly CJ, Neilson EG (1987) Contrasuppression in autoimmunity. Abnormal contrasuppression facilitates expression of nephritogenic effector T cells and interstitial nephritis in kdkd mice. J Exp Med 165:107–123
19. Hines WH, Mann RA, Kelly CJ, Neilson EG (1990) Murine interstitial nephritis IX. Induction of the nephritogenic effector T cell repertoire with an antigen-specific T cell cytokine. J Immunol 144:75–83
20. Saad T, Mandelbrot D, Sun MJ, Kelly CJ, Hines WH, Neilson EG (1990) Isolation of the cDNA for the antigen binding chain of a helper T cell factor in murine interstitial nephritis. Kidney Int 37:430
21. Nath KA, Hostetter MK, Hostetter TH (1985) Pathophysiology of chronic tubulo-interstitial disease in rats. Interactions of dietary acid load, ammonia, and complement component C3. J Clin Invest 76:667–675
22. Meyers CM, Kelly CJ (1990) An antigen specific CTL line transfers interstitial nephritis and is cytotoxic to antigen expressing tubular epithelial cells. Kidney Int 37:423
23. Wolf G, Neilson EG (to be published) Molecular mechanisms of tubulointerstitial hypertrophy and hyperplasia. Kidney Int
24. Neilson EG, Jimenez SA, Phillips SM (1980) Cell-mediated immunity in interstitial nephritis. II: T lymphocytes-mediated fibroblast proliferation and collagen synthesis: An immune mechanism for renal fibrogenesis. J Immunol 125:1708–1714
25. Schreiner GF, Kohan DE (1990) Regulation of renal transport processes and hemodynamics by macrophages and lymphocytes. Am J Physiol 258:F761–F767
26. Klahr S, Schreiner G, Ichikawa I (1988) The progression of renal disease. N Engl J Med 318:1657–1666
27. Fernandes G, Yunis EJ, Miranda M, Smith J, Good RA (1978) Nutritional inhibition of genetically determined renal disease and autoimmunity with prolongation of life in kdkd mice. Proc Natl Acad Sci USA 75:2888–2892
28. Agus D, Mann R, Cohn D, Michaud L, Kelly C, Clayman M, Neilson EG (1985) Inhibitory role of dietary protein restriction on the development and expression of immune-mediated antitubular basement membrane-induced tubulointerstitial nephritis in rats. J Clin Invest 76:930–936
29. Keane WF, Kasiske BL, O'Donnell MP (1988) Hyperlipidemia and the progression of renal disease. Am J Clin Nutr 47:157–160
30. Kelly CJ, Zurier RB, Krakauer KA, Blanchard N, Neilson EG (1987) Prostaglandin E_1 inhibits effector T cell induction and tissue damage in experimental murine interstitial nephritis. J Clin Invest 79:782–789

Lipids and the Pathogenesis of Kidney Disease

John F. Moorhead

Chair: Roscoe R. Robinson

Lipids and the Pathogenesis of Kidney Disease

JOHN F. MOORHEAD[1]

SUMMARY. The nephrotic syndrome presents clinically with a pattern of proteinuria, edema, albuminuria, hypoalbuminemia, and hyperlipidemia. Despite, or perhaps because of, familiarity with the syndrome, its possible implications for the progression of renal disease have been neglected. However, a large amount of information has been accumulated from animal models in the last decade, which, in aggregate, strongly suggests an important role for abnormalities of lipid metabolism in progressive renal disease. This review considers the metabolic background against which some of the pathological changes in animal models of nephrotic syndrome take place. Analogies between glomerular disease and atherosclerosis are discussed in the context of cellular pathology, the cardiovascular complications of nephrosis, and the relative protection of females from atherosclerosis. The role of lipid lowering drugs is discussed in relation to disease prevention in animal models. Reference is made to the role of excess eicosanoid synthesis in glomerular disease. Lack of information on the value or otherwise of long term lipid lowering therapy in patients with proteinuria, hyperlipidemia, and progressive renal disease emphasizes the need for long term studies of lipid lowering therapy in these patients.

Introduction

The clinicopathological components of the nephrotic syndrome are very familiar. An initial glomerular injury, usually unrecognized, leads to proteinuria, edema, hypoproteinemia, hyperlipidemia, and lipoproteinuria. These are the cardinal clinicopathological features of the nephrotic syndrome, however initiated. This review will explore the mechanisms by which hyperlipidemic glomerular injury may take place, and will examine some of the difficulties which are likely to occur in the interpretation and prevention of lipoprotein induced disease in man.

[1]Department of Nephrology, The Royal Free Hospital, Hampstead, London, NW3 2QG, UK

In 1982 we proposed that lipoproteins could be a cause of progressive kidney disease [1]. This hypothesis suggested that any (possibly self-limiting) condition which resulted in albuminuria and hyperlipidemia could establish secondary self perpetuating renal damage, with further loss of protein in the urine and continued inappropriate liver synthesis of lipoprotein. The excess circulating lipoprotein would then both cause and maintain further glomerular injury, so perpetuating the cycle. Other risk factors, such as continued activity of immune processes, increased glomerular pressure, and dietary factors, would continue to contribute to glomerular disease unless independently controlled. It is not yet certain how all these factors combine to produce irreversible glomerular damage. However, much experimental evidence has accumulated since 1982 which implicates lipids in the pathogenesis of progressive renal disease, and a review of this complex process is therefore timely.

Historical Evidence

Nephrotic hyperlipidemia has, until recently, been regarded as an epiphenomenon having little relevance to the pathogenesis of the underlying kidney disease. There has, however, been considerable interest in hyperlipidemia, both as a secondary metabolic phenomenon and for the abundant deposits of lipid in renal tissue in patients with nephrotic syndrome. Virchow [2] characterized lipid deposition in the kidney as "fatty metamorphosis" and Munk first described the plasma lipid abnormalities of the nephrotic syndrome in 1913 [3]. In their study of diabetic kidneys, Kimmelstiel and Wilson noted the presence of fat in some glomeruli [4], and subsequently Wilens et al. [5] reported that in diabetics glomerular lipidosis occurred only with glomerular sclerosis. The presence of glomerular lipid in 75% of sclerotic diabetic kidneys was reported by Hartroft [6] who, interestingly, also suggested for the first time that elevated intraglomerular pressure might contribute to glomerular lesions. French et al. [7] showed that feeding a 1% cholesterol diet to guinea pigs caused severe glomerular disease with cholesterol crystals in glomerular capillaries and intraglomerular proliferation of monocytes, a finding confirmed by Al-Shebeb in guinea pigs and New Zealand rabbits [8]. The first observation that abnormalities of lipid metabolism might be linked to glomerular disease in man was made by Gjone [9] in a report of the rare familial condition of lecithin:cholesterol acyl transferase (L:CAT) deficiency. Charlesworth and Edwards [10] suggested that hypertriglyceridemia was a risk factor in the outcome of renal transplantation in man. This concept was later supported in animal work by Edwards [11], who showed that pre-existing hyperlipidemia inhibited normal healing in female Sprague-Dawley rats with aminonucleoside nephrotic syndrome. In this study, high fat diets accelerated glomerular disease and lipid lowering drugs reduced proteinuria and glomerulosclerosis. Pavlovic et al. [12] observed that increased dietary fat prolonged proteinuria in the acute phase of puromycin aminonucleoside (PAN) nephrosis. An interesting animal model of hyperlipidemic renal disease is the obese Zucker rat, which is insulin resistant, hyperphagic, and hyperlipidemic, and develops heavy proteinuria and glomerular sclerosis [13]. Its lean litter mates do not develop hyperlipidemia and renal disease. Kasiske et al. [14], using clofibrate in these animals, confirmed Edwards' observation that lipid lowering effectively reduced proteinuria [15].

Pathological and Metabolic Background

The nephrotic syndrome is characterized by a striking increase in plasma lipoproteins. The liver cell secretes excess very low density lipoprotein (VLDL) which is carried in the circulation by apo-B100. Removal of fatty acids and trialglycerol from this particle gives rise to low density lipoprotein (LDL), which carries apo-B100 throughout its normal 36-hour life cycle. In the nephrotic syndrome, increased concentrations of apo-B are partly due to increased secretion of VLDL, the stimulus for which is low plasma albumin concentration. Despite this clear clinical correlation, the precise signal at a cellular level which causes lipoprotein secretion, rather than albumin synthesis alone, has not been elucidated. In vitro, relative increases in the viscosity of the culture medium, obtained by the addition of compounds of widely differing mass concentration and osmolarity, have been shown to inhibit VLDL secretion from rat hepatocytes [16]. It has also been shown that apo-B secretion by HepG2 cells is influenced in a dose-dependent manner by albumin in the culture medium, although no change in the level of apo-B mRNA occurred when apo-B output was modulated [17]. In man, plasma oncotic pressure, but not plasma viscosity, has been shown to influence total plasma cholesterol concentration.

The excess synthesis of lipoprotein is accompanied by slower than normal metabolism in the peripheral circulation [18]. The turnover rate of VLDL and LDL is prolonged for several reasons, which include decreased activity of two enzymes, lipoprotein lipase (LPL) and lecithin: cholesterol acyl transferase (L:CAT). Reduction in LPL activity may be due to a combination of inhibition and urinary loss of cofactors. L:CAT activity is reduced both as a result of urinary losses of co-factors associated with high density lipoprotein (HDL), and as a result of product inhibition caused by reduction in plasma albumin concentration, since albumin is responsible for removing the reaction product, lysolecithin, thus allowing the reaction to continue.

Since the glomerulus may be damaged by immunological, toxic, hemodynamic, and other insults, it seems, a priori, unlikely that it should be always protected from high concentrations of lipoproteins. However, glomerular disease does not occur (as far as is known) in primary hyperlipidemia. This may reflect a need for a combination of two predisposing conditions, prior glomerular vascular injury and a hyperlipidemic response to proteinuria. However, the absence of data on renal function in primary hyperlipidemias could also reflect failure to investigate. It is not known, for example, whether microproteinuria exists in hyperlipidemias, or whether such patients have an increased risk of developing renal diseases. The characteristics of the glomerular microcirculation may also have a role. For example, the mesangium is focused at the glomerular stalk and the small area it presents to the circulating plasma may reduce its susceptibility to circulating lipoproteins.

Comparisons with atheromatous disease in other parts of the vascular system have given rise to useful speculation that some glomerular diseases have much in common with atherosclerosis.

Analogies with Atherosclerosis

The fact that glomerulosclerosis and atherosclerosis occur in widely different anatomical sites need not preclude or deter interpretation along similar lines. Many of the requirements for atherosclerosis are satisfied by the cellular and metabolic conditions found in hyperlipidemic renal disease. Although elevated LDL is not regularly accompanied by renal disease, it is not known whether the normal glomerulus is ever susceptible to LDL damage. It is more likely that damage is initiated by some other agent, commonly immunological, and then sustained by the resulting hyperlipidemia. In fact, the details of the pathogenesis of progressive disease, as proposed [1], coincided to some extent with those proposed at that time for atherosclerosis [19]. The proposed pathogenesis of atherosclerosis in blood vessels bears similarities to that suggested for glomerulosclerosis. Thus endothelial injury, and lipid infiltration, are basic requirements. LDL is proposed as the endothelial damaging agent, with monocytes being attached to endothelium and infiltrating the subendothelial tissue. Leary [20] was the first to suggest that monocytes were implicated in the pathogenesis of the atherosclerotic lesion, and Ross [19], more recently, observed that monocytes interact with altered endothelium, penetrating subendothelial areas and accumulating lipid to form the foam cells which constitute part of the atherosclerotic plaque. Smooth muscle cells may also cause free radical damage to LDL and then internalize the altered lipoprotein, becoming foam cells.

The Role of the Macrophage

The macrophage is important in the pathogenesis of atherosclerosis, and may have a similar role in glomerular disease. The combination of endothelial injury by glomerular inflammatory processes, followed by neutrophil and macrophage influx, is probably a common event in certain forms of glomerulonephritis. The transformation of bone marrow derived monocytes into lipid laden macrophages (foam cells) takes place in vivo by the internalization of cholesterol ester from plasma lipoproteins. This occurs via the scavenger receptors, of which there are three, one of which prefers acetyl LDL, one oxidized LDL, the third binding both. As in atheromatous plaques, there are probably several glomerular mechanisms for the modification of LDL which allow its uptake by the macrophage. Acetylation, which increases the net negative charge of the lipoprotein, is mimicked by oxidation of unsaturated fatty acids into oxides and aldehydes which then attach to lysines of apoB-100, increasing its negative charge. A second method, oxidation of LDL by macrophages, occurs in response to several stimuli, including IgG and IgA immunoglobulins, and can be prevented by the antioxidant probucol. Finally, oxidized LDL can combine in vitro with proteoglycan [21] and collagen, forming a complex which may independently promote foam cell formation. The charge and conformational changes in LDL induced by these reactions preclude normal LDL receptor-mediated clearance. Since the macrophage is unable to clear cholesterol, it accumulates as droplets in the cytoplasm, forming the foam cell. The uptake of oxidized LDL by the macrophage may stimulate it to produce growth factors, cytokines, and other mediators capable of stimulating collagen synthesis and proliferation of mesangial cells. The combined effect of these changes would eventually produce irreversible scarring in the glomerular tuft.

Does evidence exist that these processes might take part in progressive glomerular disease? Monocytes are involved in the pathogenesis of several renal diseases in man, including focal glomerulosclerosis. Cotran [22] drew attention to the presence of monocytes in glomerular proliferative lesions. In studies of rabbit nephrotoxic serum nephritis, Thomson et al. [23] reported that macrophages accumulated in damaged glomeruli and infiltrated Bowman's space.

It would be surprising if the activity of infiltrating glomerular monocytes exposed to trapped LDL differed substantially from their behavior in the more familiar atherosclerotic plaque. In fact, experimental evidence now supports a link between the presence of glomerular monocytes, hyperlipidemia and glomerulosclerosis. Early experiments in guinea pigs fed a 1% cholesterol diet showed striking glomerular monocyte infiltration, associated with glomerular sclerosis, glomerular fat droplets, an increase in mesangial cells and fiber, and macrophage-like cells [7]. On the other hand, Grond et al. [24] found no excess of monocytes in male Wistar rats with chronic puromycin aminonucleoside (PAN) nephrosis after 20 weeks of weekly injections of PAN. This negative result may have been due to the late stage of the examination, since others have reported that, in rabbit nephrotoxic serum nephritis, macrophages have disappeared by 40 days [23]. The removal of macrophages from the glomeruli of rabbits with acute serum sickness by anti macrophage serum resulted in both a profound reduction in proteinuria and only mild histological lesions. It has recently been shown that essential fatty acid deficiency (EFAD) depletes Sprague-Dawley rat glomeruli of resident macrophages [25]. Using this information in hyperlipidemic PAN nephrosis, Diamond [26] showed that glomerular macrophages, glomerular sclerosis, and proteinuria are all reduced, and that the late chronic phase of PAN is ameliorated. In experiments in which 17β-ethinylestradiol was given to uninephrectomized obese Zucker rats, it was observed that improvement in glomerular disease was accompanied by significant reductions in plasma cholesterol, glomerular macrophages, and in vitro glomerular eicosanoid synthesis (J.F. Moorhead, submitted for publication).

The Role of the Mesangial Cell

The principal sites in which lipoprotein trapping may occur in injured glomeruli are the mesangium and the basement membrane. In physiological conditions in vitro, apo-B basic residues enable receptor binding to mesangial cells in culture, so promoting internalization. But the mesangial cell is also susceptible to lipoprotein damage. Thus, it was found that rat mesangial cells were killed in vitro by LDL in a concentration-dependent fashion [27]. Others have shown that this toxicity is mediated more efficiently by oxidized LDL, which may be present under conditions of local inflammation and monocyte ingress. In addition, mesangial cells, like the smooth muscle cells with which they share some characteristics, proliferate in vitro when stimulated appropriately by LDL [27]. Furthermore, infiltrating macrophages produce mediators which stimulate mesangial cell proliferation. Together, these observations may explain why mesangial hypercellularity and scarring is found in several models of nephritis. Lipoproteins may be captured by charge affinity in basement membrane glycosaminoglycans. ApoB binds, in vivo and in vitro, to collagen, and in vitro to heparan sulfate glycosaminoglycans (HSGAG) [21], a major constituent of the glomerular basement membrane (GBM). This binding may be enhanced by the reported presence in the GBM of a 130Kd residue with sequence homology to the LDL receptor [28]. Thus, apo-B alone may exert its pathological effects by neutralizing glomerular charge, added to which the combination of LDL-GAG, referred to previously, may permit internalization by macrophages.

Cardiovascular Complications

Since the postulated lesions of lipoprotein-mediated glomerular disease and atherosclerosis have a similar pathological basis it would be expected that extrarenal atherosclerosis would be recognized frequently in persistent proteinuria. The few studies which have examined ischemic heart disease and nephrotic syndrome have, in general, supported an association. Elevation of plasma lipids has been claimed as a risk factor in nephrotics [29], and has been reported to have caused premature atherosclerosis in a five-year-old child [30]. Mallick and Short [31] concluded that patients with persisting heavy proteinuria appear to be at substantial risk of developing ischemic heart disease. Wass et al. [32], in a study of 159 patients of whom more than 25% had minimal change disease, were less confident of a connection, but their paper was difficult to interpret. The report of the European Dialysis and Transplant Association (EDTA) for 1978 revealed a dramatically higher death rate from cerebrovascular accident (CVA) for patients on regular dialysis programs, suggesting, perhaps, that a substantial number of dialysis patients acquire their vascular disease while their renal function is declining and before dialysis starts.

Gender

Females are relatively protected from atherosclerosis, and it follows that any consideration of hyperlipidemia and progression of renal disease should include the contribution of gender. It is noteworthy that animal models of glomerular disease often make the distinction clear For example, male Munich-Wistar rats develop heavy proteinuria and nephrotic syndrome while females do not [33], and in an immune complex model of nephritis, proteinuria is more severe in males [34]. Further, glomerulosclerosis after subtotal nephrectomy is less severe in female rats [35]. One possible non-hormonal, cholesterol related, explanation for these sex differences may be the operation of the mevalonate 'shunt.' Mevalonate, a precursor of cholesterol, is metabolized by normal rat kidney, but to a lesser extent in females than in males. More mevalonate is therefore available for cholesterol metabolism in males than in females with significant renal disease. This may result in more lipoprotein being available to damage the glomeruli of male rats.

In man, two studies of patients with renal impairment, one of mixed pathogenesis [36] and the other in membranous nephropathy [37], reported a male-female ratio of 2:1. In a follow-up study of 139 patients with idiopathic membranous glomerulonephritis, Murphy et al. [38] reported that the patients whose renal function deteriorated were mainly nephrotic males. Hopper et al. [37], in a study of 100 patients with membranous nephropathy, found that this form of nephropathy was less frequent and more benign in women. On the other hand, immune reactivity is greater in females than in males, possibly due to down regulation of T-cell function and stimulation of B-cell function by estrogens [39].

This decreased susceptibility may account for the fact that renal failure programs care for fewer females than males. Carlsten and coworkers' study [39] cited polycystic kidney disease, but similar observations have been made in IgA nephropathy [40], although sex distribution in this group of conditions is not uniform worldwide [41]. Also, there are gender-dependent differences in age-specific changes of renal function, so that while renal function declines in males continuously [42], in the female it begins to decline gradually after the menopause. There is some evidence that renal disease in general is more common in men than in premenopausal women, and that this difference is not present before the menarche.

Could some of this difference be accounted for by protection from abnormalities of lipid metabolism in females with proteinuria and hyperlipidemia? Perhaps the protection of normal premenopausal women from atherosclerosis extends to lipid abnormalities in women with the nephrotic syndrome. Females with renal failure seem to be relatively immune from the cardiovascular complications of renal failure. For example, The 1987 European Dialysis and Transplant Association study of cardiovascular complications of renal failure found that the myocardial death rate was twice as high in males than in females. Whether this effect could have been influenced by estrogens in women or by androgens in men is unknown: we are ignorant of the effects of physiological concentrations of estrogens in human renal diseases. In comparing male and female disease, it should be remembered that the combination of relatively small effects in amelioration of disease in females and aggravation in males would combine to accentuate differences, necessitating caution in the interpretation of results.

Proteinuria and Hyperlipidemia: a Neglected Association

Proteinuria is recognized as an important feature of progressive disease, often being used as a direct measure of the effect of treatment or experiment. There are strong relationships between proteinuria and serum albumin, and between serum albumin and plasma cholesterol concentrations (Figs. 1,2). Warwick et al. [43] confirmed an association between proteinuria, LDL cholesterol, and plasma triglyceride, and in their study the absolute synthetic rate of LDL was also strongly correlated with proteinuria. Proteinuria correlates closely with deterioration of renal function, and reduction of proteinuria by administration of low protein diets may be associated with slowing of the rate of progression [44]. In IgA nephropathy, reputedly the most common worldwide form of glomerular disease, four independent indicators of poor outcome include proteinuria and glomerulosclerosis [41]. By inference, deterioration or improvement in renal function could have been caused by changes in plasma lipoproteins. Unfortunately, no large studies of proteinuria have related glomerular disease to changes in plasma lipids. Gross obesity has been reported to cause the nephrotic syndrome [45] and has been associated with focal segmental glomerular sclerosis. Recently, a number of cases of apo-E associated proteinuric lipoprotein glomerulopathy have been reported from Japan, and further developments of this work are awaited with great interest. Aside from these special cases, there is a consensus that most glomerular diseases which are accompanied by proteinuria have a worse prognosis than non-proteinuric renal

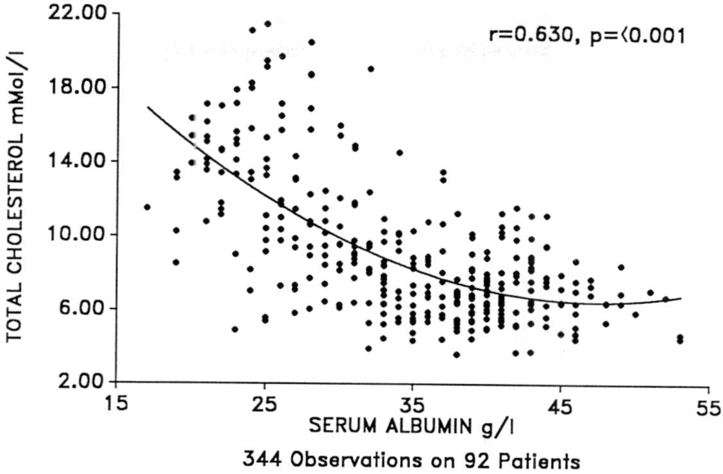

Fig. 1. The relationship between plasma cholesterol and serum albumin in nephrotic patients

diseases; it is likely that lipoprotein-mediated damage contributes to progression in some or all of these conditions.

Lipid Lowering

The few clinical studies of lipid lowering in the progression of renal disease have been short term and uncontrolled. Existing long term studies have concentrated on factors such as hypertension and the role of dietary protein, and have usually begun

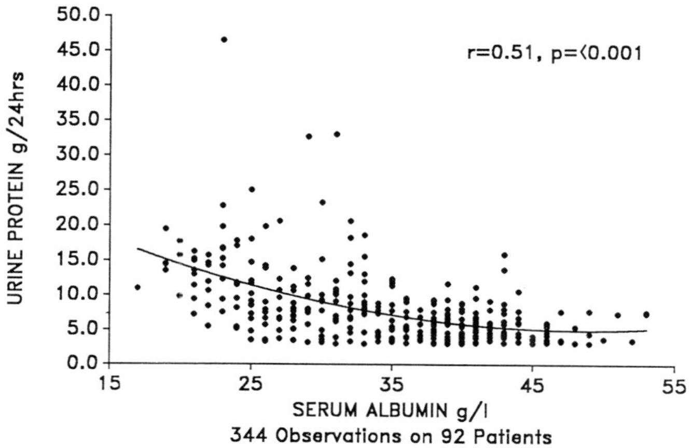

Fig. 2. The relationship between proteinuria and serum albumin in nephrotic patients

at a late stage in the decline of function. There is, therefore, no reliable evidence from controlled clinical trials that progressive renal disease can be slowed by drugs or diets designed to reduce plasma lipids. However, probucol has been shown to be effective in reducing plasma cholesterol in the nephrotic syndrome [46]. Recently, synvinolin, in short term administration, has also been shown to be an effective lipid lowering agent in nephrotics [47], but no reduction in proteinuria was reported in this uncontrolled study. Dietary treatment has been shown to be effective in lowering lipids in transplant patients, but patient compliance is likely to cause difficulties. In a controlled trial of fish oil in the treatment of chronic vascular rejection in man, Sweny et al. [48] showed that intervention preserved renal function by significantly reducing its rate of decline. Prospective drug treatment in man would need to be accompanied by dietary assessment and control in patients with nephrosis, as well as a decision on the plasma concentration of cholesterol to aim for. Raising plasma cholesterol by diet aggravates renal disease in puromycin-treated rats [12], while dietary reduction of plasma cholesterol in five-sixths nephrectomized rats [49] or in uninephrectomized obese Zucker rats [13] reduces renal damage. Dietary enrichment with eicosapentaenoic acid reduces renal disease, proteinuria, and mortality in murine lupus nephritis.

An important question relates to the timing of intervention. At present, there is little evidence favoring any particular time for diet or drug intervention and such questions will be resolved only by well designed clinical trials. In animals, evidence from many studies suggests that prevention or very early intervention is effective.

Renal Eicosanoids

Renal eicosanoid synthesis may have an important role in the mediation of some of the phenomena discussed here. Eicosanoid synthesis requires the presence of C_{20} unsaturated fatty acids in unesterified form before prostaglandin synthesis can take place. The source of free acids may be cholesterol esters, triglycerides, or phospholipids, from which they are freed by the actions of phospholipases. Perfusion of organs with arachidonic acid results in prostaglandin synthesis, which can be blocked pharmacologically, suggesting that conversion to prostaglandins take place as soon as substrate is available [50]. In hyperlipidemic nephrotics, substrate supply is presumably virtually unlimited. If the normal supply is substituted by fish oil, eicosanoid synthesis shifts to less vasoactive and less phlogistic metabolites, with decreased proteinuria and less glomerular scarring [51].

The dependency of eicosanoid synthesis on substrate supply offers a simple explanation for the fact that cholesterol-lowering drugs prevent renal disease in some animal models of nephrotic syndrome. HMG CoA reductase inhibitors and clofibrate [52] both reduce total plasma cholesterol, proteinuria, and glomerular scarring in a Zucker rat model. Fish oil (MaxEPA) administration also resulted in significant lowering of glomerular eicosanoid synthesis, which paralleled reduction in glomerular sclerosis [51]. We obtained similar data for clofibrate in the uninephrectomized (UNx) Zucker rat [13]. Recently we found that 17β-ethinyl-estradiol (17-EE), dramatically reduced plasma cholesterol and glomerular eicosanoids in the same model. These findings offer encouragement for the argument that therapeutic lowering of plasma cholesterol in man may also be beneficial to the kidney.

Conclusions

Clinical and experimental evidence available to date permits the following broad conclusions. In experimental animal models of non immune mediated nephrotic syndrome, treatment which lowers plasma lipoprotein cholesterol, diverts eicosanoid synthesis to less active metabolites, or deprives the animal of essential fatty acids, ameliorates renal disease. On the other hand, feeding saturated fat either delays recovery, in the case of PAN nephrosis, aggravates disease. In immune mediated systems, e.g., murine systemic lupus erythematosus (SLE), the renal disease is largely prevented by unsaturated fatty acid feeding.

To summarize the evidence to date, the glomerular structures susceptible to lipoprotein mediated injury are the mesangium, the basement membrane, and the resident and infiltrating glomerular monocytes. Lipoprotein (apoB-100) may damage the glomerular basement membrane directly or may damage it after peroxidation by activated macrophages. Lipid peroxidation results in foam cell formation via the macrophage scavenger receptors, with further glomerular and interstitial damage resulting from activated macrophages. The glomerular injury is perpetuated by continued exposure to lipoproteins. Comparisons with systemic atherosclerosis have helped to explain many of the glomerular abnormalities found in glomerulosclerosis.

References

1. Moorhead JF, Chan MK, El-Nahas M, Varghese Z (1982) Lipid nephrotoxicity in chronic progressive glomerular and tubulo-interstitial disease. Lancet II:1309–1312
2. Virchow R (1860) A more precise account of fatty metamorphosis. London, Churchill, pp 342–366
3. Munk F (1913) Klinische diagnostik der degenerativen nierenerkrankungen. Z Clin Med 78:1–52
4. Kimmelstiel P, Wilson C (1936) Intercapillary lesions in the glomeruli of the kidney. Am J Pathol 12:83–98
5. Wilens SL, Elster SK, Baker JP (1951) Glomerular lipidosis in intercapillary glomerulosclerosis. Ann Intern Med 24:592–607
6. Hartroft WS (1955) Fat emboli in glomerular capillaries of choline deficient rats and of patients with diabetic glomerulosclerosis. Am J Pathol 31:381–391
7. French SW, Yamanaka W, Ostwald R (1967) Dietary induced glomerulosclerosis in the guinea pig. Arch Pathol Lab Med 83:204–210
8. Al-Shebeb T, Frohlich J, Magil AB (1988) Glomerular disease in hypercholesterolemic guinea pigs: A pathogenetic study. Kidney Int 33:498–507
9. Gjone E, Blomhoff JP, Skarbovik AJ (1974) Possible association between an abnormal low density lipoprotein and nephropathy in lecithin cholesterol acyltransferase deficiency. Clin Chim Acta 54:11–18
10. Charlesworth JA, Edwards KDG (1974) Relation of hypertriglyceridemia to kidney transplant dysfunction and rejection, and response to antilymphocyte globulin therapy. Prog Biochem Pharmacol 9:107–120
11. Edwards KDG (1981) Controversies in nephrology. New York, Masson, pp 3–15
12. Pavlovic NM, Malik S, Chan MK, Z Varghese, Persaud JW, Moorhead JF (1984) The influence of high fat diet on the proteinuria in puromycin induced nephrotic syndrome in rats. Clin Sci 66:26P

13. Wheeler DC, Nair DR, Singh GS, Persaud J, Sweny P, Varghese Z, Moorhead JF (1988) Lipid-lowering therapy reduces proteinuria in the uninephrectomised obese Zucker rat. Nephrol Dial Transplant 3:533
14. Kasiske BL, O'Donnell, Keane WF (1986) The lipid lowering agent clofibric acid reduces glomerular injury in obese Zucker rats. Clin Res 34:600A
15. Zucker LM (1965) Hereditary obesity in the rat associated with hyperlipemia. Ann NY Acad Sci 131:447–458
16. Yedgar S, Weinstein DB, Patsch W, Schonfeld G, Casanada FE, Steinberg D (1982) Viscosity of culture medium as a regulator of synthesis and secretion of very low density lipoproteins by cultured hepatocytes. J Biol Chem 257(5):2188–2192
17. Pullinger CR, North JD, Teng BB, Rifici VA, De Brito AER, Scott J (1989) The apolipoprotein B gene is constitutively expressed in HepG2 cells:regulation of secretion by oleic acid, albumin, and insulin, and measurement of the mRNA half-life. J Lipid Res 30:1065–1077
18. Moorhead JF, Wheeler DC, Varghese Z (1989) Glomerular structures and lipids in progressive renal disease. Am J Med 87:12N–20N
19. Ross R (1986) The pathogenesis of atherosclerosis – an update. N Engl J Med 314:488–500
20. Leary T (1941) The genesis of atherosclerosis. Arch Pathol Lab Med 32(4):507–555
21. Iverius PH (1972) The interaction between human plasma lipoproteins and connective tissue glycosaminoglycans. J Biol Chem 247(8):2607–2613
22. Cotran RS (1978) Monocytes, proliferation, and glomerulonephritis. J Lab Clin Med 92:837–840
23. Thomson NM, Holdsworth SR, Glasgow EF, Atkins RC (1979) The macrophage in the development of experimental crescentic glomerulonephritis. Am J Pathol 94:223–240
24. Grond J, Van Goor H, Erkelens DW, Elema JD (1986) Glomerular sclerotic lesions in the rat. Virchows Arch [Cell Pathol] 51:521–534
25. Lefkowith JB, Schreiner G (1987) Essential fatty acid deficiency depletes rat glomeruli of resident macrophages and inhibits angiotensin II - induced eicosanoid synthesis. J Clin Invest 30:947–956
26. Diamond JR (1990) Effects of dietary interventions on glomerular pathophysiology. Am J Physiol 27:F1–F8
27. Wheeler DC, Persaud J, Kingstone D, Sweny P, Varghese Z, Moorhead JF (1989) Receptor mediated binding of human low density lipoprotein (LDL) to rat mesangial cells in vitro (abstract) Kidney Int 35:439
28. Pietromonaco SF, Farquhar MG (1989) Identification and characterization of a cDNA encoding the core protein of heparin sulfate proteoglycans from the rat glomerular basement membrane (abstract). Kidney Int 35:163
29. Alexander JH, Schapel GJ, Edwards KDG (1974) Increased incidence of coronary heart disease associated with combined elevation of serum triglyceride and cholesterol concentrations in the nephrotic syndrome in man. Med J Aust 2:119–122
30. Kallen RJ, Brynes, Aronson AJ, Lichtig C, Spargo BH (1977) Premature coronary atherosclerosis in a 5-year-old with corticosteroid-refractory nephrotic syndrome. Am J Dis Child 131:976–980
31. Mallick NP, Short CD (1981) The nephrotic syndrome and ischemic heart disease. Nephron 27:54–57
32. Wass VJ, Chilvers C, Jarrett RJ, Cameron JS (1979) Does the nephrotic syndrome increase the risk of cardiovascular disease? Lancet II:664–667
33. Remuzzi A, Puntorieri S, Mazzoleni A, Remuzzi G (1988) Sex related differences in glomerular ultrafiltration and proteinuria in Munich-Wistar rats. Kidney Int 34:481–486
34. Gretz N, Zeier M, Geberth S, Strauch M, Ritz E (1989) Is gender a determinant for evolution of renal failure? A study in autosomal dominant polycystic kidney disease. Am J Kidney Dis 14:178–183

35. Lombet JR, Adler SJ, Anderson PS, Nast CC, Olsen D, Glassock RJ (1988) Sex vulnerability in the subtotal nephrectomy (Nx) model of glomerulosclerosis (abstract). Kidney Int 33:378
36. Hunt LP, Short D, Mallick NP (1988) Prognostic indicators in patients presenting with the nephrotic syndrome. Kidney Int 34:382–388
37. Hopper JJR, Trew PA, Biava CG (1981) Membranous nephropathy:its relative benignity in women. Nephron 29:18–24
38. Murphy BF, Fairley KF, Kincaid-Smith PS (1988) Idiopathic membranous glomerulonephritis:long term follow up in 139 cases. Clin Nephrol 30:175–181
39. Carlsten H, Holmdahl R, Tarkowski A, Nilsson LA (1989) Oestradiol- and testosterone-mediated effects on the immune system in normal and autoimmune mice are genetically linked and inherited as dominant traits. Immunology 68:209–214
40. D'Amico G, Imbasciati E, Belgioioso GB, Bertoli S, Fogazzi G, Ferrario F, Fellini G, Ragni A, Colasanti G, Minetti L, Ponticell C (1985) Idiopathic IgA mesangial nephropathy. Medicine 64(1):49–60
41. D'Amico G (1987) The commonest glomerulonephritis in the world. IgA nephropathy. Q J Med 64:709–727
42. Lindeman RD, Tobin J, Shock W (1985) Longitudinal studies on the rate of decline in renal function with age. J Am Geriatr Soc 33:278–285
43. Warwick GL, Caslake MJ, Boulton-Jones JM, Dagen M, Packard CJ, Shepherd J (1990) Low-density lipoprotein metabolism in the nephrotic syndrome. Metabolism 39:187–192
44. El Nahas AM, Masters-Thomas A, Brady SA, Farrington K, Wilkinson V, Hilson AJW, Varghese Z, Moorhead JF (1984) Selective effect of low protein diets in chronic renal diseases. Br Med J [Clin Res] 289:1337–1342
45. Weisinger JR, Kempson RL, Eldridge FL, Swenson RS (1974) The nephrotic syndrome: a complication of massive obesity. Ann Intern Med 81:440–447
46. Appel G, Gelfand J, Kunis C, Blum C (1985) Treatment of hyperlipidemia of the nephrotic syndrome: a controlled trial (abstract). Kidney Int 270:131
47. Rabelink AJ, Erkelens DW, Hene RJ, Joles JA (1988) Effects of simvastatin and cholestyramine on lipoprotein profile in hyperlipidaemia of nephrotic syndrome. Lancet II:1335–1337
48. Sweny P, Wheeler DC, Lui SF, Amin NS, Moorhead JF, Jeremy JY, Mikhailidis DP, Varghese Z, Fernando ON, et al. (1989) Dietary fish oil supplements preserve renal function in renal transplant recipients with chronic vascular rejection. Nephrol Dial Transplant 4:1070–1075
49. Kasiske BL, O'Donnell MP, Daniels F, Keane WF (1985) The lipid lowering agent clofibric acid ameliorates renal injury in the 5/6 nephrectomy model of chronic renal failure. Clin Res 33:488A
50. Walker LA, Frolich JC (1987) Renal prostaglandins and leukotrienes. Rev Physiol Biochem Pharmacol 107:1–72
51. Wheeler DC, Nair DR, Persaud JW, Varghese Z, Moorhead JF (1990) Dietary fatty acid intake influences progression of glomerulosclerosis in the obese Zucker rat (abstract). Kidney Int 37:524
52. Kasiske BL, O'Donnell MP, Cleary MP, Keane WF (1988) Treatment of hyperlipidemia reduces glomerular injury in obese Zucker rats. Kidney Int 33:667–672

Symposia

Immunological and Cellular Mechanisms of Glomerulonephritis

Chair: William G. Couser (USA)
Leishi Li (China)

Glomerular Injury Induced by the C5b-9 Membrane Attack Complex of Complement

William G. Couser[1]

Summary. Strong evidence implicates the assembly and glomerular epithelial cell membrane insertion of C5b-9 in mediating proteinuria in experimental membranous nephropathy. The cellular basis for this effect may involve cell activation by sublytic concentrations of C5b-9, resulting in release at the epithelial cell interface of inflammatory mediators. Potential mediators released by the epithelial cell may include oxidants, proteases or prostaglandins. Epithelial cell detachment from underlying basement membrane may also be involved. Further studies to define the cellular basis of the C5b-9 effect are required.

The intracellular processing and excretion of C5b-9 into the urinary space by glomerular epithelial cells under antibody and C5b-9 attack has led to studies showing that elevated urinary C5b-9 is a sensitive marker of on-going deposition of antibody to epithelial cell membrane antigens in the rat. The presence of elevated urinary C5b-9 in a subset of human patients with membranous nephropathy suggest that a similar mechanism may be operative in this disease.

Introduction

Considerable progress has been made in recent years in clarifying the mechanisms by which glomerular immune deposits induce tissue injury [1]. This has included recognition that the role of complement in the mediation of glomerular disease, which was clearly established in the 1960s [2], includes not only generation of chemotactic factors such as C5a which lead to neutrophil localization, but also the formation of the C5b-9 membrane attack complex of complement which inserts into the lipid bilayer of glomerular cell membranes and leads to a non-inflammatory type of renal lesion [3]. In this paper, I will present briefly the evidence in support of a role for the C5b-9

[1]Division of Nephrology, University of Washington, Seattle, WA 98195, USA

complex in glomerular disease and review what little is currently known of the cellular mechanism for this effect. This subject has been reviewed in more detail elsewhere [4, 5].

The human glomerular disease in which this mechanism is most likely operative is membranous nephropathy, but a role is probable in other lesions as well, particularly if subepithelial immune deposits are present [5].

Evidence for C5b-9 Mediated Proteinuria in Experimental Membranous Nephropathy

The first evidence for C5b-9 induced glomerular injury derived from studies of the mediation of proteinuria in the passive Heymann nephritis (PHN) model of MN in rats. PHN is induced by injection of a heterologous antibody to a proximal tubular brush border fraction termed FxlA. Studies by several laboratories over the past decade have demonstrated that the subepithelial immune complex deposits which develop in PHN form in situ [6,7] due to IgG antibody reacting with antigens on the membrane of the GEC. The best characterized of these at the present time is GP330 [8]. These antigen-antibody complexes activate complement producing glomerular deposits of the C5b-9 membrane attack complex, but the antigen-antibody complexes themselves are patched, capped, and shed from the cell surface by mechanisms requiring an intact GEC cytoskeleton to form the discontinuous subepithelial immune complex deposits characteristic of MN [9,10]. In PHN, proteinuria develops four to five days after antibody injection, when sufficient IgG has deposited to induce injury; it is morphologically indistinguishable from MN in man, in that no circulating effector cells or other inflammatory changes are present [11,12]. Despite the lack of inflammatory changes, however, studies in which rats were depleted of complement with cobra venom factor during the five days required for proteinuria to develop, demonstrated that complement-depletion totally abolished proteinuria in PHN without altering antibody deposition [12]. We speculated that this lesion involved a glomerular effect of C5b-9 rather than generation of chemotactic or opsonic factors such as C5a, the only complement-mediated mechanism previously implicated in glomerular injury.

A macromolecular complex, C5b-9 results from proteolytic cleavage of C5 to generate C5b, which then combines with C6 and C7 to form the C5b6,7 complex, an amphophilic molecule which has binding sites for the lipid bilayer of cell membranes (reviewed in 13). With binding of C8 and multiple C9 molecules, the C5b-9 complex inserts into the lipid bilayer of cell membranes [13]. A protective mechanism for C5b-9 injury may be afforded by plasma S-protein (vitronectin), which results in formation of SC5b-7 complexes which can bind C8 and C9 but cannot insert into cell membranes and are therefore considered inactive [14]. Membrane insertion of C5b-9 results in rapid lysis of non-nucleated cells such as erythrocytes, but lysis of nucleated cells is much more difficult to achieve.

Confirmation that C5b-9 assembly is critical in the mediation of proteinuria in PHN has been provided now by studies in the intact animal, in the isolated perfused kidney, and in isolated glomeruli. In intact rats, selective depletion of C6 to prevent assembly of C5b-9 can be maintained throughout the four to five day period required for proteinuria to develop following antibody injection [15]. Selective C6 depletion prevents glomerular assembly of C5b-9 complexes, as detected by staining for C5b-9 neoantigens, and abolishes the development of proteinuria without altering glomerular deposition of antibody or C3. In the isolated perfused rat kidney, proteinuria does not develop when antibody deposition occurs in the presence of serum deficient in C6 or C8, but appears immediately following addition of normal serum containing all complement components [16]. In collaboration with Dr. Virginia Savin, we have recently shown, in the isolated rat glomerulus, that glomerular permeability to albumin, reflected by changes in the reflection coefficient for albumin (which is calculated from the volumetric response in isolated glomeruli to changes in oncotic pressure gradient), is increased within 10 minutes in normal glomeruli exposed to anti Fx1A antibody IgG and normal serum as a complement source *in vitro* [17]. No change in permeability is induced by antibody in the presence of C6 or C7 deficient serum [17]. Since the principal biologic function of C6, C7, and C8 is the assembly of the C5b-9 membrane attack complex, these studies provide convincing evidence that proteinuria in experimental MN induced by antibody to GEC antigen is mediated by C5b-9 in the intact animal, the isolated perfused kidney, and the isolated glomerulus.

A role for C5b-9 has also been established in mediating injury in MN induced by other mechanisms. In the autologous phase of PHN where injury results from antibody reacting with previously deposited but sub-nephritogenic quantities of antibody to GEC, injury also appears to be C5b-9 mediated in the intact animal [18,19] and in the isolated perfused kidney [20]. Similar results are obtained when subepithelial deposits form in situ, due to localization of cationic antigens and antibodies to them. Thus the onset of proteinuria is delayed in genetically C6 deficient rabbits with cationic BSA induced serum sickness, compared to normal controls, despite comparable amounts of glomerular immune complex deposits [21]. Rats selectively depleted of C6 develop significantly less proteinuria in response to a nephritogenic quantity of cationic IgG containing immune complexes, compared to controls [22]. Evidence for a nephritogenic role for C5b-9 has also been obtained in models of anti-GBM nephritis in rabbits [23,24].

Cellular Basis for C5b-9 Effect

The cellular basis for the C5b-9 effect has not been defined. To better understand this process we developed a monoclonal antibody directed against a C9 neoantigen present only in the assembled rat C5b-9 complex [25]. This antibody stains PHN glomeruli in a pattern similar to staining for IgG and similar to that reported in human MN and other diseases by Falk and others [26]. Immunoultrastructural studies in PHN, utilizing this reagent, demonstrate early C5b-9 localization in subepithelial deposits and along the surfaces of the GEC membrane, particularly in regions of clathrin coated pits where the putative GP330 antigen is expressed [27]. The cell bound C5b-9 then undergoes endocytosis and is transported through the GEC in large multivesicular bodies before being exocytosed into the urinary space [27]. This is in contrast to the cellular handling of antigen-antibody complexes which are primarily patched and capped and then shed from the cell surface where they form granular deposits that become non-covalently bound to the GBM (Reviewed in

[10]). Several authors have demonstrated S protein in subepithelial immune deposits in MN [28]. This finding has prompted comment that the glomerular C5b-9 deposits are inactivated, cannot insert into cell membranes, and are therefore not likely to be pathogenic. We believe this is probably the case with SC5b-9 deposits, which remain extracellularly with the immune complex and may represent most of the glomerular C5b-9. However, freeze-fracture studies in early PHN reveal clusters of large 200–250 A intramembrane particles, which compare in size and appearance to membrane inserted C5b-9 [27]. Although these active, membrane-inserted complexes may represent a small fraction of the total glomerular C5b-9 deposits, they appear to be sufficient to cause disease.

Despite these advances in understanding the role of C5b-9 in the mediation of MN, the cellular consequences of C5b-9 attack on the GEC remain poorly understood. There appear to be both structural and functional consequences of GEC C5b-9 attack. The structural changes are predominantly an increase in thickness of the GBM, due primarily to an accumulation of laminin along the outer surface and in the characteristic spikes projecting from the subepithelial surface [29,30]. This process progresses to glomerulosclerosis resulting from an accumulation of normal extracellular matrix components, predominantly type IV collagen [31]. Functional changes in the barrier to protein filtration consist of the development of large pore defects [32] which appear to represent areas of GEC detachment from underlying basement membrane [33]. At present it is unclear what the relationship is, if any, between the structural and functional changes in the basement membrane.

One possibility for the C5b-9 effect might be that C5b-9 induces an abnormality in GEC production of laminin or other constituents of the basement membrane, resulting over time in a persistent remodeling of the basement membrane structure, with altered barrier function. Hansch et al. have reported a several-fold increase in production of type IV collagen by rat GEC following C5b-9 attack [34], but no studies of laminin production have appeared. However, the alteration which occurs in glomerular permeability in experimental MN induced by C5b-9 can develop in minutes in the isolated kidney and glomerulus and therefore seems unlikely to result from an alteration in matrix component metabolism.

As in non-inflammatory lesions induced by antibody alone, GEC detachment appears to underlie the permeability defect in MN as well [33]. Thus, a C5b-9 induced alteration in expression or function of integrins, or the matrix components to which they bind, might lead to epithelial cell detachment and proteinuria. One study showed no alteration in expression or distribution of a beta one integrin in human MN [35]. However, other integrins and cell membrane receptors have not been explored.

A third mechanism by which C5b-9 might be pathogenic at the cellular level may involve cell activation, with release of potentially toxic inflammatory mediators by the GEC itself. Although membrane insertion of C5b-9 leads to lysis of non-nucleated cells such as erythrocytes, nucleated cells are relatively resistant to C5b-9 attack and may actually be stimulated by this [14]. With respect to GEC, Quigg et al. have shown that antibody to GEC membrane, in the presence of sublytic concentrations of complement, induces non-cytolytic injury, as evidenced by the release of low molecular weight intracellular markers and formation of membrane vesicles similar to those excreted in the urine in PHN [36]. Sublytic C5b-9 attack also results in increased intracellular calcium, activation of phospholipase C, increased levels of

IP2, IP3, diacyl glycerol, and phosphatidic acid, with release of arachidonic acid, $PGF_2\alpha$, and thromboxane [37,38]. Enhanced prostaglandin production by GEC following sublytic C5b-9 attack has also been reported by Hansch [39]. Similar changes occur in mesangial cells in response to C5b-9 [40]. This phenomenon of C5b-9 induced cell activation could result in release, at the GBM-GEC interface, of several cell-derived substances. Three potential inflammatory mediators warrant consideration: prostaglandins, oxidants, and proteinases.

With respect to prostaglandins, Cybulsky et al. reported a reduction in C5b-9 mediated proteinuria in the isolated perfused kidney when a thromboxane synthesis inhibitor was employed [41]. Two groups have demonstrated a reduction in proteinuria with indomethacin in models of MN [42,43], although these results may in part reflect a reduction in glomerular filtration rate [43]. We have demonstrated, in PHN rats, a marked increase in glomerular PGE_2 and thromboxane production by glomeruli that was complement dependent and may have derived from the GEC [44]. However, administration of a thromboxane synthesis inhibitor, which reduced glomerular thromboxane production by over 80%, had no effect on C5b-9 induced proteinuria in PHN [44] or in another model of MN induced with cationized IgG which is believed to be C5b-9 mediated [22,45]. Thus it seems unlikely that alterations in GEC prostaglandin metabolism account directly for the altered permeability to protein induced by C5b-9.

A second possible GEC-derived mediator would be reactive oxygen species. Oxidants including H_2O_2, superoxide anion, and hydroxyl radical have all been implicated in various forms of inflammatory renal injury [46]. Adler et al. have shown that C5b-9 can directly stimulate cultured mesangial cells to produce H_2O_2 and superoxide anion [14]. Although oxidant production by the GEC is relatively low, three studies have described a beneficial effect of administration of the hydroxyl radical scavengers DMSO and dimethylthiourea (DMTU) on proteinuria in PHN [47–49]. Moreover, a beneficial effect of the iron chelating agent deferoxamine suggests participation of the Haber-Weiss reaction to form hydroxyl radical [49]. However, a direct effect of C5b-9 on GEC oxidant production remains to be documented.

A final potential candidate for a GEC derived mediator would be a GBM-degrading proteinase. From our laboratory, preliminary evidence exists for the production of a proteinase with type IV collagenase activity by GEC. A stimulation of proteinase production by sublytic C5b-9 attack could lead to an immediate and non-inflammatory type of glomerular lesion such as that seen in early MN.

Urinary C5b-9 Excretion as an Index of Disease Activity in Membranous Nephropathy

The observation that membrane inserted C5b-9 is transported intracellularly and exocytosed into the urinary space prompted us to develop a sensitive ELISA assay for both rat and human C5b-9 in urine. In the rat, urinary C5b-9 excretion is elevated only when subepithelial deposits result from antibody to the GEC membrane, and C5b-9 excretion in urine is not seen in a variety of other experimental immune glomerular diseases with comparable glomerular C5b-9 deposits, or in non-immune proteinuric glomerular lesions [3,50]. In the rat, urinary C5b-9 excretion closely parallels disease activity (on-going glomerular immune deposit formation). Within hours of the onset of antibody deposits C5b-9 excretion is increased in both the heterologous and autologous phases of PHN and before proteinuria appears; C5b-9 excretion ceases promptly when antibody deposition is halted by transplanting a nephritic kidney to a normal host [19,50]. Of interest, glomerular C3 deposition follows a very similar course and may also serve as a marker of disease activity [19,51]. Similar results have been obtained in the autologous immune complex nephritis (active Heymann nephritis) model [51].

We have attempted to extend these observations in the experimental animal to study MN in man with some success. In studies of 148 patients with proteinuric glomerular diseases, elevated urinary C5b-9 (analyzed as differences from expected values based on urinary C5 excretion) was found in only nine (of 40) patients with idiopathic MN and in four (of six) patients with lupus MN, and not in a variety of other diseases with comparable levels of proteinuria, or in controls [52]. These findings have now been confirmed by Coupes et al. [53]. Patients with elevated urinary C5b-9 values were generally studied earlier in the course of disease and had higher levels of urine protein excretion than MN patients with normal urinary C5b-9 values, findings consistent with a greater likelihood of disease activity in high C5b-9 excretors [52]. These results imply that, in at least one subset of patients with idiopathic and lupus MN, the disease mechanism is analogous to the autoimmune process involving antibody to the GEC defined in the Heymann models in rats and that GEC membrane insertion of C5b-9 also takes place in man. Urinary C5b-9 excretion may serve as a useful marker of immune disease activity in MN in the absence of an assay for the pathogenic antibody.

References

1. Couser WG (1985) Mechanisms of glomerular injury in immune-complex disease (nephrology forum). Kidney Int 28:569–583
2. Cochrane CG, Unanue E, Dixon FJ (1965) A role of polymorphonuclear leukocytes and complement in nephrotoxic nephritis. J Exp Med 122:99–110
3. Couser WG, Baker PJ, Adler S (1985) Complement and the direct mediation of immune glomerular injury: A new perspective (editorial review). Kidney Int 28:879–890
4. Cybulsky AV, Quigg RJ, Salant DJ (1988) Role of the complement membrane attack complex in glomerular injury. In: Wilson CB, Brenner BM, Stein J (eds) *Contemporary issues in nephrol*, vol 18. Churchill Livingston, New York, pp 57–86
5. Couser WG, Abrass CK (1988) Pathogenesis of membranous nephropathy. Annu Rev Med 39:517–530
6. Van Damme BJC, Fleuren GJ, Bakker WW, Vernier RL, Hoedemaeker Ph.J (1978) Experimental glomerulonephritis in the rat induced by antibodies directed against tubular antigens. V. Fixed glomerular antigens in the pathogenesis of heterologous immune complex glomerulonephritis. Lab Invest 38:502
7. Couser WG, Steinmuller DR, Stilmant MM, Salant DJ, Lowenstein LM (1978) Experimental glomerulonephritis in the isolated perfused rat kidney. J Clin Invest 62:1275
8. Kerjaschki D, Farquhar MG (1982) The pathogenic antigen of Heymann nephritis is a membrane glycoprotein of the renal proximal tubular brush border. Proc Natl Acad Sci USA 79:5557–5561
9. Camussi G, Brentjens JR, Noble B, Kerjaschki D, Malavasi F, Roholt OA, Farquhar MG, Andres G (1985) Antibody-induced redistribution of Heymann's antigen on the surface of

cultured glomerular visceral epithelial cells: Possible role in the pathogenesis of Heymann glomerulonephritis. J Immunol 135:2409
10. Brentjens JR, Andres GA (1989) Interaction of antibodies with renal cell surface antigens. Kidney Int 35:954–968
11. Salant DJ, Darby C, Couser WG (1980) Experimental membranous glomerulonephritis in rats. Quantitative studies of glomerular immune deposit formation in isolated glomeruli and whole animals. J Clin Invest 66:71–81
12. Salant DJ, Belok S, Madaio MP, Couser WG (1980) A new role for complement in experimental membranous nephropathy in rats. J Clin Invest 66:1339–1350
13. Muller-Eberhard HJ (1988) Molecular organization and function of the complement system. Annu Rev Biochem 57:321–347
14. Adler S, Baker PJ, Johnson RJ, Ochi RF, Pritzl P, Couser WG (1986) Complement membrane attack complex stimulates production of reactive oxygen metabolites by cultured rat mesangial cells. J Clin Invest 77:762–767
15. Baker PJ, Ochi RF, Schulze M, Johnson RJ, Campbell C, Couser WG (1989) Depletion of C6 prevents development of proteinuria in experimental membranous nephropathy in rats. Am J Pathol 135:185–194
16. Cybulsky AV, Quigg RJ, Salant DJ (1986) The membrane attack complex in complement-mediated glomerular epithelial cell injury: Formation and stability of C5b-9 and C5b-7 in rat membranous nephropathy. J Immunol 137:1511–1516
17. Savin VJ, Johnson RJ, Couser WG (1990) Antibody induced complement activation increases albumin permeability of isolated rat glomeruli (abstract). Kidney Int 37: 430
18. Adler S, Salant DJ, Dittmer JE, Rennke HG, Madaio MP, Couser WG (1983) Mediation of proteinuria in membranous nephropathy due to a planted glomerular antigen. Kidney Int 23:807–815
19. Pruchno CJ, Burns MW, Schulze M, Johnson RJ, Baker PJ, Couser WG (1989) Urinary excretion of C5b-9 reflects disease activity in passive Heymann nephritis. Kidney Int 36:65–71
20. Cybulsky AV, Rennke HG, Feintzeig ID, Salant DJ (1986) Complement-induced glomerular epithelial cell injury. Role of the membrane attack complex in rat membranous nephropathy. J Clin Invest 77:1096–1107
21. Groggel GC, Adler S, Rennke HG, Couser WG, Salant DG (1983) Role of the terminal complement pathway in experimental membranous nephropathy in the rabbit. J Clin Invest 72:1948–1957
22. Ochi RF, Johnson RJ, Baker PJ, Adler S, Couser WG (1986) C6 depletion diminishes proteinuria in experimental membranous nephropathy induced by an exogenous antigen (abstract). Kidney Int 29:287
23. Groggel GC, Salant DJ, Darby C, Rennke HG, Couser WG (1985) Role of the terminal complement pathway in the heterologous phase of anti-glomerular basement membrane nephritis in the rabbit. Kidney Int 27:643–651
24. Tipping PG, Boyce NW, Holdsworth SR (1989) Relative contributions of chemo-attractant and terminal components of complement to anti-glomerular basement membrane (GBM) glomerulonephritis. Clin Exp Immunol 78:444–448
25. Perkinson DT, Baker PJ, Couser WG, Johnson RJ, Adler S (1985) Membrane attack complex deposition in experimental glomerular injury. Am J Pathol 120:121–128
26. Falk RJ, Dalmasso AP, Kim Y, Tsai CH, Scheinman JI, Gewurz H, Michael AF (1983) Neoantigen of the polymerized ninth component of complement. Characterization of a monoclonal antibody and immunohistochemical localization in renal disease. J Clin Invest 72:560–573
27. Kerjaschki D, Schulze M, Binder S, Kain R, Ojha PP, Susani M, Horvat R, Baker PJ, Couser WG (1989) Transcellular transport and membrane insertion of the C5b-9 membrane attack complex of complement by glomerular epithelial cells in experimental membranous nephropathy. J Immunol 143:546–552

28. Bariety J, Hinglais N, Bhakdi S, Mandet C, Rouchon M, Kazatchkine MD (1989) Immunohistochemical study of complement S protein (Vitronectin) in normal and diseased human kidneys: relationship to neoantigens of the C5b-9 terminal complex. Clin Exp Immunol 75:76–81
29. Fukatsu A, Matsuo S, Killen PD, Martin GR, Andres GA, Brentjens JR (1988) The glomerular distribution of type IV collagen and laminin in human membranous glomerulonephritis. Hum Pathol 19:64–68
30. Matsuo S, Brentjens JR, Andres G, Foidart J-M, Martin GR, Martinez-Hernandez A (1986) Distribution of basement membrane antigens in glomeruli of mice with autoimmune glomerulo-nephritis. Am J Pathol 122:36–49
31. Adler S, Striker LJ, Striker LJ, Striker GE, Perkinson DT, Hibbert J, Couser WG (1986) Studies of progressive glomerular sclerosis in the rat. Am J Pathol 123:553–562
32. Shemesh O, Ross JC, Deen WM, Grant GW, Myers BD (1986) Nature of the glomerular capillary injury in human membranous glomerulopathy. J Clin Invest 77:868–877
33. Schneeberger EE, O'Brien A, Grupe WE (1979) Altered glomerular permeability in Munich-Wistar rats with autologous immune complex nephritis. Lab Invest 40:227–235
34. Torbohm I, Schonermark M, Wingen A-M, Berger B, Rother K, Hansch GM (1990) C5b-8 and C5b-9 modulate the collagen release of human glomerular epithelial cells. Kidney Int 37:1098–1104
35. Kerjaschki D, Ojha PP, Susani M, Horvat R, Binder S, Hovorka A, Hillemanns P, Pytela R (1989) A β_1-integrin receptor for fibronectin in human kidney glomeruli. Am J Pathol 134:481–489
36. Quigg RJ, Cybulsky AV, Jacobs JB, Salant DJ (1988) Anti-Fx1A produces complement-dependent cytotoxicity of glomerular epithelial cells. Kidney Int 34:43–52
37. Cybulsky AV, Salant DJ, Quigg RJ, Badalamenti J, Bonventre JV (1989) Complement C5b-9 complex activates phospholipases in glomerular epithelial cells. Am J Physiol 257:F826–F836
38. Cybulsky AV, Bonventre JV, Quigg RJ, Lieberthal W, Salant DJ (1990) Cytosolic calcium and protein kinase C reduce complement-mediated glomerular epithelial cell injury. Kidney Int 38:803–811
39. Hansch GM, Betz M, Gunther J, Rother KO, Sterzel B (1988) The complement membrane attack complex stimulates the prostanoid production of cultured glomerular epithelial cells. Int Arch Allergy Appl Immunol 85:87–93
40. Lovett DH, Hansch G-M, Goppelt M, Resch K, Gemsa D (1987) Activation of glomerular mesangial cells by the terminal membrane attack complex of complement. J Immunol 138:2473–2480
41. Cybulsky AV, Lieberthal W, Quigg RJ, Rennke HG, Salant DJ (1987) A role for thromboxane in complement-mediated glomerular injury. Am J Pathol 128:45–51
42. Zoja C, Benigni A, Verroust P, Ronco R, Bertane T, Remuzzi G (1987) Indomethacin reduces proteinuria in passive Heymann nephritis in rats. Kidney Int 31:1335–1343
43. Kirschenbaum MA, Liebross BA, Serros ER (1985) Effect of indomethacin on proteinuria in rats with autologous immune complex nephropathy. Prostaglandins 30:295–303
44. Stahl RAK, Adler S, Baker PJ, Chen Y-P, Pritzl PM, Couser WG (1987) Enhanced glomerular prostaglandin formation in experimental membranous nephropathy. Kidney Int 31:1126–1131
45. Thaiss F, Germann PJ, Kahf S, Schoeppe W, Helmchen U, Stahl RAK (1989) Effect of thromboxane synthesis inhibition in a model of membranous nephropathy. Kidney Int 35:76–83
46. Johnson RJ, Klebanoff SJ, Couser WG (1988) Oxidants in glomerular injury. In: Wilson CB, Brenner BM, Stein J (eds) *Contemporary issues in nephrology*, vol 18. Churchill Livingston, New York, pp 87–110

47. Lotan D, Kaplan BS, Fong JSC, Goodyer PR, DeChadarevian J-P (1984) Reduction of protein excretion by dimethyl sulfoxide in rats with passive Heymann nephritis. Kidney Int 25:778–788
48. Kaplan BS, Milner LS, Lotan D, Mills M, Goodyer PR, Fong JSC (1986) Interaction of dimethyl sulfoxide and nonsteroidal anti-inflammatory agents in passive Heymann's nephritis. J Lab Clin Med 107:425–430
49. Shah SV (1988) Evidence suggesting a role for hydroxyl radical in passive Heymann nephritis in rats. Am J Physiol 254:F337–F344
50. Schulze M, Baker PJ, Perkinson DT, Johnson RJ, Ochi RF, Stahl RA, Couser WG (1989) Increased urinary excretion of C5b-9 distinguishes passive Heymann nephritis in the rat. Kidney Int 35:60–68
51. Pruchno CJ, Burns MW, Schulze M, et al. (to be published) Urinary excretion of the C5b-9 membrane attack complex of complement is a marker of immune disease activity in autologous immune complex nephritis. Am J Pathol
52. Schulze M, Donadio JV, Pruchno CJ, et al. (to be published) Elevated urinary excretion of the complement C5b-9 complex in a subset of patients with membranous nephropathy. N Engl J Med

Platelets in Immune Mediated Glomerular Disease

Richard J. Johnson[1]

Summary. Platelets are recognized for their role in hemostasis, but may also act as proinflammatory cells capable of releasing vasoactive, chemotactic, proliferative, and proteolytic factors or enzymes. Platelet activation and localization to glomeruli can be demonstrated in numerous experimental and human glomerular diseases, especially in diseases associated with endothelial cell or mesangial cell injury. Proposed roles for platelets in glomerular injury include initiating glomerular thrombosis, facilitating immune complex deposition, modulating hemodynamic changes and mediating glomerulosclerosis. We have recently demonstrated a critical requirement for platelets in neutrophil-mediated glomerulonephritis. The mechanism may involve an augmentation of neutrophil injury by the platelet or platelet products. Platelets also mediate mesangial cell proliferation in immune complex nephritis. The effect involves a platelet-mediated induction of platelet-derived growth factor (PDGF) and PDGF-receptor synthesis by the mesangial cell, and is also associated with the acquisition by the mesangial cell of a smooth muscle phenotype. Thus, the platelet has important and diverse roles in glomerular inflammation. Platelets can mediate direct effects, such as in the formation of platelet-fibrin thrombi, but may effect glomerular inflammation indirectly via their ability to interact with neutrophils and glomerular mesangial cells.

Platelets as Inflammatory Effector Cells

The blood platelet is well-recognized for having a major role in hemostasis and thrombosis. It is becoming increasingly evident that the platelet, like the neutrophil and monocyte, may also function as an inflammatory effector cell independent of its role in coagulation. Platelets contain numerous inflammatory mediators within their alpha, and dense granules, as well as within lysosomes, and can release their contents

[1]Division of Nephrology, Department of Medicine, University of Washington, Seattle, WA 98195, USA

Table 1. Platelet products important in inflammation

Adhesive proteins: Fibrinogen, fibronectin, von-Willebrand factor, thrombospondin, GMP140
Lipid mediators: Thromboxane A_2, lipoxygenase products, platelet activating factor (PAF)
Cationic proteins: β-thromboglobulin, platelet factor 4, platelet basic protein, connective tissue activating peptide III
Degrading enzymes: Heparanase, neutral proteinases, acid hydrolases
Vasoactive amines: Histamine, serotonin
Adenine nucleotides: ADP, ATP
Growth factors: Platelet derived growth factor (PDGF), transforming growth factor-β (TGF-β), epidermal growth factor/TGF-α, hepatocyte growth factor, endothelial cell growth factor, and interleukin I (IL-1)
Oxidants: Superoxide anion (O_2^-), H_2O_2
Anti-inflammatory products: α-1 antiproteinase, α-2 macroglobulin, superoxide dismutase, catalase, glutathione peroxidase, adenosine

following stimulation. Platelet releasates contain vasoactive, thrombogenic, chemotactic, proliferative, and proteolytic factors/enzymes (Table 1) [1]. Platelets, like leukocytes, can undergo chemotaxis, phagocytosis, degranulation, and generate cytotoxicity. Platelets do not contain an NADPH oxidase (which is present in neutrophils), but nevertheless are capable of generating small quantities of oxidants via both the cycloxygenase and lipoxygenase pathways [2]. Platelet generation of oxidants may mediate killing of various parasites as well as cultured endothelial cells [3,4]. Platelets can generate C5a (via platelet chemotactic factor) and can release terminal complement components that participate in additional C5b-9 formation [1,5]. Finally, platelets and megakaryocyte can endocytose plasma components, including IgG, and can subsequently release these components at sites of inflammation [6].

Platelet Participation in Glomerular Diseases

Platelets and platelet antigens have been described in glomeruli in numerous experimental glomerular diseases, particularly diseases associated with endothelial [7,8] or mesangial cell [9,10] injury. Platelets and platelet antigens can also be documented in glomeruli in a wide variety of human glomerular diseases, including IgA nephropathy, diffuse proliferative lupus nephritis, hemolytic uremic syndrome, and membranoproliferative glomerulonephritis (GN) [11]. In many of these diseases evidence for systemic platelet activation is often present, and is manifested by decreased platelet survival, the presence of platelet release products in plasma, and occasionally, thrombocytopenia [12,13].

Mechanisms for Platelet Localization and Activation in GN

The mechanisms responsible for the platelet localization are probably the consequence of the cellular injury and subsequent exposure of the subendothelium and basement membrane. It is known that *collagen fragments* can act as a strong chemotactic stimulus for platelets [14]. Another chemoattractant for platelets may be *platelet activating factor (PAF)*. Ito, Andres, and colleages have reported that the influx of platelets and neutrophils in glomeruli of rabbits with hyperacute transplant rejection may be due to the release by damaged glomerular cells of PAF, which can be detected in high levels in the renal veins of these animals [15]. In addition, activated neutrophils may cause intraglomerular platelet aggregation and activation by releasing oxidants that inactivate local ADPase within the glomerular capillary wall, resulting in increased concentrations of ADP [16]. This is consistent with our observation that glomerular endothelial cell and mesangial cell injury secondary to neutrophil oxidants produced by the myeloperoxidase-hydrogen peroxide reaction results in a marked influx of platelets [7].

Recently we have also reported an important *role for complement* in platelet localization in a model of subendothelial immune complex nephritis (the con A model) [8], and in the model of mesangial proliferative GN induced by anti-Thy 1 antibody [10]. Using ^{111}In-labeled platelets, we were able to demonstrate significant platelet accumulation in glomeruli, which in the con A model peaked with over 5000 platelets per glomerulus 10 minutes after disease induction [8]. Rats with con A GN that were depleted of complement with cobra venom factor had minimal glomerular platelet localization [8]. It is possible that the complement-dependent platelet localization results from tissue injury by the terminal membrane attack complex of complement [17]. It is also possible that the platelets are responding to complement activation products. It is known, for example, that guinea pig platelets can be activated by C3a and C5a [18]. The mechanism does not appear to be due to complement-mediated neutrophil localization. At least for the con A model, the initial platelet influx precedes the neutrophil localization and occurs despite profound leukocyte depletion [8].

Once localized, platelet activation ensues, with a change in shape from discoid to round, the formation of filopodia, and the centralization of granules. Platelet aggregation occurs secondary to a conformational change in the cell surface glycoprotein GPIIb-GPIIIa, allowing the platelet to bind fibrinogen which acts as an interconnecting link between platelets. Platelets also adhere to exposed areas of basement membrane and subendothelium, by utilizing the GPIb receptor to bind to von Willebrand factor. Immune adherence mechanisms may also be operative, resulting in the direct binding of the platelet to immune complexes by the platelet Fc receptor (primarily in primates) or by the CR1 receptor (as in rabbits and rats) [1]. Human platelets also have CR2, CR3, and CR4 receptors, but their functional significance remains to be established. Platelet activation is also associated with a "release" reaction in which the platelets discharge numerous mediators from alpha, dense, and lysosomal granules into the extracellular space.

Roles for the Platelet in Immune Mediated Glomerular Injury

The platelet has been proposed to have several important roles in immune mediated glomerular injury. The first major role ascribed to the platelet was to *facilitate immune complex deposition* in glomeruli in acute serum sickness [19]. The proposed mechanism involves antigen binding to IgE-sensitized basophils, followed by release from the basophil of PAF [20,21]. PAF causes platelet activation with the release of vasoactive amines and cationic proteins that subsequently mediate an increase in glomerular permeability, thus facilitating immune complex deposition [20,21]. Platelets may also mediate *glomerular thrombosis* [22]. Platelets, when activated, expose phospholipids on their cell surfaces which act as a matrix for coagulation reactions, providing binding sites for activated coagulation factors and generating prothrombinase activity that accelerates the formation of thrombin [23]. Platelets can also potentiate tissue factor production by monocytes and endothelial cells [24,25]. This latter observation is important, as recent experimental data strongly suggests that monocyte-macrophage release of tissue factor may be responsible for fibrin deposition in several glomerular diseases [26]. We have also reported that platelet depletion markedly reduces fibrin deposition in the con A model of subendothelial immune complex nephritis [27]. Platelets may also *modulate glomerular hemodynamics*, particularly by the release of vasoactive substances, such as thromboxane, that can mediate a significant reduction in the glomerular filtration rate (GFR). Other platelet products can also mediate mesangial cell contraction, and thus potentially modulate GFR; these include PDGF, PAF, and histamine [28]. Platelets have also been proposed to have a role in *glomerulosclerosis*. Platelet infiltration and thrombosis may precede glomerulosclerosis both in experimentally mediated glomerular injury [29,30] and in lupus nephritis in man [31]. Anti-platelet agents have also been reported to inhibit the glomerulosclerosis that develops following renal ablation [32,33]. A potential mechanism may involve release by the platelet of transforming growth factor (TGF)-β, which can induce mesangial cells to produce collagen, fibronectin, and heparan sulfate proteoglycans [34,35].

Recently we have performed studies on two additional roles for the platelet in glomerular injury; specifically, that of *augmenting neutrophil-mediated injury*, and that of *mediating mesangial cell proliferation and activation*. These studies are summarized below.

Platelets are Required for Neutrophil-Mediated Glomerular Injury

Early in our studies we were impressed by the frequent coexistence of platelets and neutrophils in glomeruli of both human and experimentally-induced glomerular diseases [8]. Platelets and neutrophils have been noted to co-localize in numerous inflammatory conditions, including the Arthus reaction, the Shwartzman reaction, hyperacute transplant rejection, and in various inflammatory skin lesions. Studies by Henson in the late 1960s demonstrated that in passive cutaneous anaphylaxis in rabbits both platelets and neutrophils were required for injury to occur [36]. The importance of platelets in neutrophil-mediated injury was further demonstrated by Ward et al. who reported that platelet depletion could prevent neutrophil-mediated injury in a rat model of the adult respiratory distress syndrome [37].

To investigate a potential interaction of the platelet and neutrophil in immune glomerular injury, we performed platelet depletion studies in the neutrophil and complement-dependent model of immune complex nephritis induced with concanavalin A (con A) and anti-con A antibody [27]. Platelet depletion completely prevented proteinuria in this model. The decrease in albuminuria could not be attributed to differences in blood or glomerular neutrophil counts, complement, or glomerular antibody binding.

It is possible that the mechanism involves an additive effect of platelets and neutrophils in mediating glomerular injury. As shown in Table 1, platelets can release a variety of mediators that could, theoretically, mediate changes in glomerular permeability. For example, the release of platelet cationic proteins, which could bind to anionic sites present in the glomerular basement membrane (GBM) could thus neutralize the charge barrier [20,21]. PAF can also induce direct changes in vascular permeability [20]. Platelets can contain the endoglycosidase, heparanase, which can degrade glycosaminoglycans such as the heparan sulfate component of heparan sulfate proteoglycan [38]. Kanwar and colleagues have reported that intrarenal perfusion of heparanase will lead to increased glomerular permeability to protein [39]. Platelets can also release oxidants and proteases, although the quantities are small relative to the neutrophil or monocyte [1,3,4].

Although it is possible that the platelet and neutrophil mediated effects are additive, we believe that a more likely mechanism involves an interaction of these two cell types within the glomerulus. Platelets and/or platelet products can, under certain conditions, augment neutrophil adherence, aggregation, CR3 expression, phagocytosis, degranulation, oxidant release, and cytotoxicity [1]. Platelets can also interact with neutrophils to potentiate PAF production, augment leukotriene B_4 formation, and generate new eicosanoids [1]. However, platelets or platelet products have also been reported to inhibit certain neutrophil functions, due to the presence within the platelet of anti-proteinases, adenosine, glutathione peroxidase, and other anti-inflammatory substances (Table 1). The complexity of the platelet-neutrophil interaction can be appreciated when one considers the multiple proinflammatory (as well as anti-inflammatory) mediators/substances that both cells can release. Nevertheless, the observation that both platelets and neutrophils are required for proteinuria to develop in the con A model of nephritis suggests an important synergy of these two cells in glomerular inflammation.

Role of Platelets in Glomerular Cell Proliferation

Studies in several experimental models of glomerular disease, including "Arthus"-type nephritis [30,40] and the glomerular injury induced by the myeloperoxidase system [7] have shown that these diseases are characterized by an initial platelet infiltration followed by endothelial cell or mesangial cell proliferation. Whereas these studies suggest an important association of platelets with glomerular cell proliferation, the first demonstration that platelets actually mediated the cell proliferation was reported by Cattell, who noted that platelet-depleted rats with Habu snake venom-induced glomerular injury had significantly less glomerular hypercellularity [9].

We examined the role of platelets in a rat model of GN induced with antibody to the Thy 1 antigen present on the mesangial cell membrane [41]. This model results in acute complement-dependent mesangiolysis (i.e., mesangial cell loss with dissolution of mesangial matrix) followed by marked hypercellularity in mesangial areas [17]. Because the hypercellularity represents both endogenous glomerular cell proliferation and leukocyte infiltration, we identified proliferating cells by immunostaining tissue sections for the proliferating cell nuclear antigen (PCNA) [41]. PCNA is an auxiliary protein to DNA polymerase δ that is expressed during the cell cycle from late G1 until the M phase (peaking during the S phase) [42]. In addition, double immuno-labeling was performed in which tissue sections were stained for both PCNA and the common leukocyte antigen (CD45). This was performed because some leukocytes may have recently proliferated in the marrow prior to localizing in the glomerulus, and also because certain leukocyte populations, such as monocytes and lymphocytes, can proliferate at sites of inflammation. Thus, double immunolabeling allowed us to distinguish proliferating glomerular cells (i.e., PCNA+, CD45-) from proliferating cells of bone marrow origin (PCNA+, CD45+). Utilizing these special methods, we were able to demonstrate that platelet depletion significantly reduced *glomerular cell proliferation*, independent of effects on glomerular antibody binding or complement levels.

There are several potential mechanisms by which the platelet could mediate glomerular cell proliferation. First, proliferation could be mediated by the direct release of platelet growth factors such as PDGF. Activated platelets have also been reported to express interleukin (IL)-1 on their cell surfaces [43]. It is also possible that the platelet mechanism is indirect, and involves a platelet-mediated induction of monocyte-macrophages or glomerular cells to release their own growth factors. Alternatively, the platelet mechanism could involve induction of the mesangial cell to upregulate growth factor receptors that would increase responsiveness of the mesangial cell to growth factor action.

In this regard an important growth factor is PDGF. Not only is it a major growth factor present in platelets, but it is capable of inducing mesangial cell proliferation [44]. Mesangial cells will also produce their own PDGF when they are exposed to a variety of growth factors (including PDGF), thus providing for a potential autocrine-mediated amplification of the proliferative stimulus [45].

Role of PDGF in Mesangial Proliferative GN

Gesualdo et al. recently reported that PDGF A-chain and B-chain mRNA were markedly elevated in whole kidney RNA from mice with an experimental IgA nephropathy [46]. However, studies using whole kidney RNA do not distinguish between PDGF mRNA of tubular or glomerular origin. Kidney epithelial cells in culture can express PDGF B-chain mRNA [47].

Recent studies by H. Iida and others in our laboratory have provided evidence that mesangial cell proliferation in anti-Thy 1 GN is associated with markedly increased gene expression for PDGF A and B chain in *glomerular RNA* extracts [48]. *In situ* hybridization has allowed us to identify individual cells that are expressing PDGF B chain mRNA in mesangial regions of glomeruli of these diseased rats (unpublished work).

The identification of the cells expressing PDGF B-chain protein in the rat model of anti-Thy 1 GN has been further studied by immunostaining. Double-immunostaining with a monoclonal antibody to the PDGF B-chain and to α-smooth muscle actin suggests that the majority of cells expressing PDGF are also α-smooth muscle actin positive [48]. This suggests that the majority of cells expressing PDGF B-chain are mesangial cells (see below).

An increase in gene and protein expression for PDGF β receptor in glomeruli also occurs in the anti-Thy 1 model of mesangial proliferative GN [48]. Immunostaining with a polyclonal antibody to the PDGF receptor β-subunit strongly suggests that the PDGF-R is expressed by mesangial cells. A similar upregulation of the PDGF-R β protein has also been reported in various types of mesangial proliferative nephritis in man [49].

Rats with anti-Thy 1 GN that were platelet depleted had significantly reduced PDGF and PDGF receptor gene and protein expression [48]. This suggests that one mechanism for platelet-mediated proliferation may be to induce mesangial cells to produce their own PDGF and PDGF receptors. This would allow for an autocrine-mediated amplification of the initial proliferative stimulus.

Platelet-Mediated Mesangial Cell Activation

We also have recent data that the platelet-mediated mesangial cell proliferation in anti-Thy 1 GN is associated with a phenotypic change of the mesangial cell to assume smooth muscle-like features. Specifically, there appears to be de novo expression of α-smooth muscle actin, by proliferating mesangial cells, that is mediated by platelets and complement [50]. Thus, platelets not only mediate mesangial cell proliferation, but they may also modulate changes in mesangial cell phenotype that may be potentially significant in active GN.

Conclusion

The platelet is a diverse cell that may play a major role in many forms of glomerular injury. One of the major roles may be to augment neutrophil-mediated injury of the glomerular capillary wall. Also important is the role of the platelet in inducing mesangial cell proliferation and activation. This mechanism may involve a platelet mediated stimulation of mesangial cells to produce PDGF that can act as an autocrine growth factor. Further studies are needed to determine the potential benefits of therapy designed to inhibit platelet activation in glomerulonephritis.

Acknowledgments. The author would like to acknowledge Dr. H. Iida, Dr. A. Yoshimura, and Dr. D.F. Bowen-Pope for their important contributions on the PDGF studies, and also Dr. W.G. Couser and Dr. C.E. Alpers for their valuable advice and suggestions.

Support for these studies was provided by U.S. Public Health Service grants DK-39068, DK-40802, and by research grants from the Northwest Kidney Foundation and the Jules and Gwen Knapp Charitable Foundation.

References

1. Weksler BB (1988) Roles for human platelets in inflammation. Prog Clin Biol Res 283: 611–638
2. Worner P (1981) Arachidonic acid-induced chemiluminescence of human platelets: contribution of the prostaglandin and lipoxygenase pathways. Thromb Haemost 46:584–589
3. Joseph M, Capron A, Ameisen J-C, Capron M, Vorng H, Pancre V, Kusnierz J-P, Auriault C (1986) The receptor for IgE on blood platelets. Eur J Immunol 16:306–312
4. Larsen T, Sorensen MB, Olsen R, Jorgensen L (1989) Effect of scavengers of active oxygen species and pretreatment with acetyl-salicylic acid on the injury to cultured endothelial cells by thrombin-stimulated platelets. In Vitro Cell Devel Biol 25:276–282
5. Houle JJ, Leddy JP, Rosenfeld SI (1989) Secretion of the terminal complement proteins, C5-C9, by human platelets. Clin Immunol Immunopath 50:385–393

6. George JN, Saucerman S, Levine SP, Knieriem LK, Bainton DF (1985) Immunoglobulin G is a platelet alpha granule-secreted protein. J Clin Invest 76:2020–2025
7. Johnson RJ, Guggenheim SJ, Klebanoff SJ, Ochi RF, Wass A, Baker P, Schulze M, Couser WG (1988) Morphologic correlates of glomerular oxidant injury induced by the myeloperoxidase-hydrogen peroxide-halide system of the neutrophil. Lab Invest 58:294–301
8. Johnson RJ, Alpers CE, Pruchno C, Schulze M, Baker PJ, Pritzl P, Couser WG (1989) Mechanisms and kinetics for platelet and neutrophil localization in immune complex nephritis. Kidney Int 36:780–789
9. Cattell V (1979) Focal mesangial proliferative glomerulonephritis in the rat caused by habu snake venom: the role of platelets. Br J Exp Pathol 60:201–208
10. Johnson RJ, Pritzl P, Iida H, Alpers CE. Platelet-complement interactions in mesangial proliferative nephritis in the rat. Amer J Path (in press)
11. Duffus P, Parbtani A, Frampton G, Cameron JS (1982) Intraglomerular localization of platelet related antigens, platelet factor 4 and β-thromboglobulin in glomerulonephritis. Clin Nephrol 17:288–297
12. George CRP, Slichter SJ, Quadracci LJ, Striker GE, Harker L (1974) A kinetic evaluation of hemostasis in renal disease. N Engl J Med 29:1111–1115
13. Parbtania A, Frampton G, Cameron JS (1980) Platelet and plasma serotonin concentrations in glomerulonephritis, II. Clin Nephrol 14:112–123
14. Lowenhaupt RW (1982) Human platelet chemotaxis can be induced by low molecular substance(s) derived from the interaction of plasma and collagen. In: Jamieson GA, Scipio AR (eds) Interaction of platelets and tumor cells. Alan R. Liss, New York, pp 269–280
15. Ito S, Camussi G, Tetta C, Milgrom F, Andres G (1984) Hyperacute renal allograft rejection in the rabbit. Lab Invest 51:148–161
16. Poelstra K, Hardonk MJ, Koudstaal J, Bakker WW (1990) Intraglomerular platelet aggregation and experimental glomerulonephritis. Kidney Int 37:1500–1508
17. Yamamoto T, Wilson CB (1987) Complement dependence of antibody-induced mesangial cell injury in the rat. J Immunol 138:3758–3765
18. Meuer S, Ecker U, Hadding U, Bitter-Suermann D (1981) Platelet-serotonin release by C3a and C5a: Two independent pathways of activation. J Immunol 126:1506–1509
19. Kniker WT, Cochrane CG (1968) The localization of circulating immune complexes in experimental serum sickness. J Exp Med 127:119–135
20. Camussi G (1986) Potential role of platelet-activating factor in renal pathophysiology (editorial review). Kidney Int 29:469–477
21. Barnes JL, Venkatachalam MA (1985) The role of platelets and polycationic mediators in glomerular vascular injury. Semin Nephrol 5:57–68
22. Kincaid-Smith P (1972) Coagulation and renal disease. Kidney Int 2:183–190
23. Walsh PN (1985) Platelet-mediated coagulant protein interactions in hemostasis. Semin Hematol 22:178–186
24. Johnsen ULH, Lyberg T, Galdal KS, Prydz H (1983) Platelets stimulate thromboplastin synthesis in human endothelial cells. Thromb Haemost 49:69–72
25. Niemetz J, Marcus AJ (1974) The stimulatory effect of platelets and platelet membranes on the procoagulant activity of leukocytes. J Clin Invest 54:1437–1443
26. Tipping PG, Worthington LA, Holdsworth SR (1987) Quantitation and characterization of glomerular procoagulant activity in experimental glomerulonephritis. Lab Invest 56: 155–159
27. Johnson RJ, Alpers CE, Pritzl P, Schulze M, Baker P, Pruchno C, Couser WG (1988) Platelets mediate neutrophil-dependent immune complex nephritis in the rat. J Clin Invest 82:1225–1235
28. Schlondorff D (1987) The glomerular mesangial cell: an expanding role for a specialized pericyte. FASEB J 1:272–281

29. Jorgensen L, Glynn MF, Hovig T, Murphy EA, Buchanan MR, Mustard JF (1970) Renal lesions and rise in blood pressure caused by adenosine diphosphate-induced platelet aggregations in rabbits. Lab Invest 23:347–357
30. Gabbiani G, Badonnel M-C, Vassalli P (1975) Experimental focal glomerular lesions elicited by insoluble immune complexes. Lab Invest 32:33–45
31. Kant KS, Pollak VE, Weiss MA, Glueck HI, Miller MA, Hess EV (1981) Glomerular thrombosis in systemic lupus erythematosus: Prevalence and significance. Medicine (Baltimore) 60:71–86
32. Purkerson ML, Heinrich-Joist J, Yates J, Valdes A, Morrison A, Klahr S (1985) Inhibition of thromboxane synthesis ameliorates the progressive kidney disease of rats with subtotal renal ablation. Proc Natl Acad Sci USA 82:193–197
33. Zoja C, Perico N, Bergamelli A, Pasini M, Morigi M, Dadan J, Belloni A, Bertani T, Remuzzi G (1990) Ticlopidine prevents renal disease progression in rats with reduced renal mass. Kidney Int 37:934–942
34. MacKay K, Striker LJ, Stauffer JW, Doi T, Agodoa LY, Striker GE (1989) Transforming growth factor-β. Murine glomerular receptors and responses of isolated glomerular cells. J Clin Invest 83:1160–1167
35. Border WA, Okuda S, Languino LR, Ruoslahti E (1990) Transforming growth factor-β regulates production of proteoglycans by mesangial cells. Kidney Int 37:689–695
36. Henson PM, Cochrane CG (1969) Immunological induction of increased vascular permeability. I. A rabbit passive cutaneous anaphylactic reaction requiring complement, platelets, and neutrophils. J Exp Med 129:153–164
37. Ward PA, Macconi D, Sulavik MC, Till GO, Warren JS, Johnson KJ, Powell J (1988) Rat neutrophil-platelet interactions in oxygen radical-mediated lung injury. UCLA symposium on molecular and cellular biology, new series, 82:83–98
38. Yahalom J, Eldor A, Fuks Z, Vlodavsky I (1984) Degradation of sulfated proteoglycans in the subendothelial extracellular matrix by human platelet heparitinase. J Clin Invest 74:1842–1849
39. Kanwar YS, Linker A, Farquhar MG (1980) Increased permeability of the glomerular basement membrane to ferritin after removal of glycosaminoglycans (heparan sulfate) by enzyme digestion. J Cell Biol 86:688–693
40. Shigematsu H, Niwa Y, Takizawa J, Akikusa B (1979) Arthus-type nephritis I. Characterization of glomerular lesions induced by insoluble and poorly soluble immune complexes. Lab Invest 40:492–502
41. Johnson RJ, Garcia RL, Pritzl P, Alpers CE (1990) Platelets mediate glomerular cell proliferation in immune complex nephritis induced by anti-mesangial cell antibodies in the rat. Am J Pathol 136:369–374
42. Kurki P, Vanderlaan M, Dolbeare F, Gray J, Tan EM (1986) Expression of proliferating cell nuclear antigen (PCNA)/cyclin during the cell cycle. Exp Cell Res 166:209–219
43. Hawrylowicz CM, Santoro SA, Platt FM, Unanue ER (1989) Activated platelets express IL-1 activity. J Immunol 143:4015–4018
44. Shultz PJ, Dicorleto PE, Silver BJ, Abboud HE (1988) Mesangial cells express PDGF mRNAs and proliferate in response to PDGF. Am J Physiol 255:F674–F684
45. Silver BJ, Jaffer FE, Abboud HE (1989) Platelet-derived growth factor synthesis in mesangial cells: Induction by multiple peptide mitogens. Proc Natl Acad Sci USA 86:1056–1060
46. Gesualdo L, Abboud HE, Pinzani M, Floriano J, Lamm ME, Emancipator SN (1990) Platelet-derived growth factor (PDGF) expression in increased in murine IgA nephropathy (IgAN). Kidney Int 37:414
47. Kartha S, Bradham DM, Grotendorst GR, Toback FFG (1988) Kidney epithelial cells express c-sis protooncogene and secrete PDGF-like protein. Am J Physiol 255:F800–F806
48. Iida H, Alpers CE, Seifert R, Gown A, Ross R, Bowen-Pope D, Johnson R. (1990) Platelet-derived growth factor (PDGF) and PDGF receptor (PDGF-R) expression in mesangial

proliferative nephritis. J Amer Soc Neph 1:526 (abstr)
49. Fellstrom B, Klareskog L, Heldin CH, Larsson E, Ronnstrand L, Terracio L, Tufveson G, Wahlberg J, Rubin K (1989) Platelet-derived growth factor receptors in the kidney—upregulated expression in inflammation. Kidney Int 36:1099–1102
50. Johnson RJ, Iida H, Alpers CE, Majesky MW, Schwartz SM, Pritzl P, Gordon K, Gown AM (1991) Expression of smooth muscle cell phenotype by rat mesangial cells in immune complex nephritis. J Clin Invest (in press)

The Role of Eicosanoids in Glomerular Immune Injury

ROLF A.K. STAHL[1]

Introduction

The characteristic features of several models of experimental glomerular immune injuries are reduction of the glomerular filtration rate and loss of the permselectivity of the glomerular filtration barrier, with the appearance of proteinuria [1]. These alterations are, in most cases, the consequence of glomerular antibody binding, immune complex formation, activation of mediator systems, and the glomerular infiltration of inflammatory cells (polymorphonuclear neutrophils (PMNs), monocytes, and platelets) [2]. In this initial process of experimental glomerular injuries, formation of eicosanoids in whole isolated glomeruli is enhanced [3–6].

Eicosanoids are oxygenic products of 20 carbon polyunsaturated fatty acids. In the enzymatic pathway of arachidonic acid the cyclooxygenase forms prostanoids (prostaglandins (PGE_2, PGI_2, $PGF_{2\alpha}$) and thromboxane A_2, the lipoxygenase converts polyunsaturated fatty acids in hydroxyeicosatetraenoic acids (HETEs) and leukotrienes ($LTBC_4$, LTB_4) (see Fig. 1). Eicosanoids exert their functional effects as local hormones and represent a group of autacoids.

Recent studies have addressed the question of which mechanisms lead to increased glomerular eicosanoid formation in experimental glomerular injury and which cellular components in whole nephritic glomeruli are the sources of increased eicosanoid formation. There is good evidence that prostanoids and thromboxane A_2 (TxA_2) are produced by resident glomerular cells and infiltrating monocytes [5–7], whereas HETE and leukotrienes derive from glomerular resident cells and PMNs [8,9]. It has also become clear that the intraglomerular activation of the complement system plays an important role in the release of eicosanoids in glomerular immune injury [6,7,9]. Even though the mechanisms of the release, and the cellular sources of eicosanoids

[1]University of Frankfurt, Department of Medicine, Division of Nephrology, Theodor-Stern-Kai 7, 6000 Frankfurt 70, Federal Republic of Germany

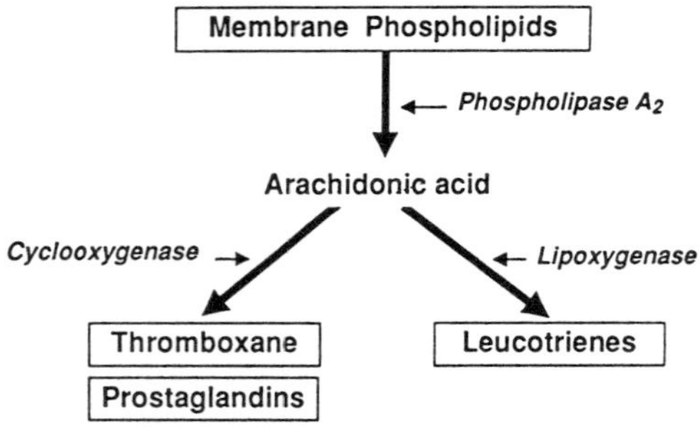

Fig. 1. Eicosanoids are products of arachidonic acid, which is converted by cyclooxygenase to thromboxane and prostaglandins and by lipoxygenase to leukotrienes

in nephritic glomeruli have been reasonably well characterized, their possible role in experimental glomerular injury is still being debated. There is now sufficient evidence to support the view that eicosanoids participate in the regulation of renal hemodynamics in glomerular disease. In most animal models studied, the reduction of glomerular filtration rate can be ameliorated by inhibition of the synthesis of TxA_2 or by its blockade [3,10]. On the other hand, increased formation of PGE_2 and PGI_2 in glomerular injury maintains impaired hemodynamic renal function [4,11]. Besides these hemodynamic functions, which are at least partially attributable to changes in the contractility of mesangial cells [12], there is still little information on whether eicosanoids are actively involved in other processes which appear in glomerular diseases, i.e., the attraction of inflammatory cells, growth of resident glomerular cells, formation of matrix components, or effects on the permselectivity of the glomerular filtration barrier.

This short review will therefore focus on information which deals with the role of eicosanoids, other than their vasoactive effects on the glomerulus. This review includes data from animal experiments; however, the majority of the information is derived from cell culture studies.

The Effect of Prostaglandins of the E Series on Experimental Glomerular Immune Injuries

The first evidence that prostaglandins of the E series might effect glomerular immune injury is derived from Zurier et al. [13]. NZB/NZW mice treated with prostaglandin E_1 had a decrease of immune complexes deposited in the glomeruli and a reduction of glomerular hypercellularity. PGE treatment also increased survival of these animals.

Similar data on different animal models of glomerular immune injury were collected by other investigators [14–17].

Most investigators observed beneficial effects on glomerular morphology and function. The beneficial effects, however, were attributed to different mechanisms by different investigators. These included influences of PGE_1 on immune complex formation [14], antibody synthesis [15], recruitment of PMNs [16], or recruitment of monocytes [17,18].

These experiments demonstrate that exogenous prostaglandins of the E series uniformly improve morphology and function of different models of glomerular immune diseases. The mechanisms by which PGs of the E series exert their beneficial effects, however, seem to be different and might involve immune complex formation, antibody synthesis, inflammatory cell recruitment, and more or less undefined effects. The influences of exogenous PGs might thus be systemic or could also appear on the glomerular level. The question therefore arises, whether prostaglandins formed locally, either by glomerular resident cells or by blood borne inflammatory cells during glomerular injury, participate in disease mechanisms.

There is currently no evidence from animal experiments, besides the hemodynamic function, which would clearly demonstrate that endogenous PGE_2 has such effects. There is, however, some information, obtained from recent studies in cell cultures of glomerular mesangial cells, which suggests that PGs can be involved in the growth of resident glomerular cells, and that PGs might be involved in the release of cytokines and in the formation of matrix components.

Prostanoids and Mesangial Cell Function

The mesangial cell, due to its ability to regulate perfusion, produce matrix components, express antigens of the MHC II class, proliferate and release several inflammatory mediators, has a central role in the pathophysiology of glomerular disease [19]. The mesangial cell is also a source of prostanoid formation in the glomerulus, $PGF_{2\alpha}$, PGE_2, and PGI_2 being the major products. In inflammatory processes, several mediators, including cytokines and growth factors, complement components, free oxygen radicals, bacterial toxins, and antibody binding stimulate mesangial cell prostanoid formation (for review see [20]).

Since increased formation of prostanoids and enhanced mesangial cell proliferation are characteristic features of several entities of glomerular immune injury, we addressed the question whether endogenous prostanoids formed by mesangial cells might be involved in the growth of mesangial cells. For this purpose rat mesangial cells were exposed to the cytokines interleukin-1β (IL-1β), tumor necrosis factor (TNF), and granulocyte macrophage colony stimulating factor (GMCSF), all inflammatory mediators which are supposed to be released during the process of inflammation on the glomerular level [19].

Without exception, all cytokines increased mesangial cell PGE_2 formation (see Fig. 2). On a molar basis TNF was the most potent stimulator of mesangial cell PGE_2 formation, whereas the effect of IL-1β was comparatively mild.

With regard to the effects on mesangial cell DNA synthesis there were, however, differences between the cytokines studied (see Fig. 3). IL-1β induced a small but significant increase of mesangial cell growth (evaluated by ^{3}H-thymidine uptake), whereas TNF and GMCSF reduced ^{3}H-thymidine incorporation in mesangial cells (see Fig. 3). The decrease in mesangial cell growth with TNF and GMCSF was paralleled by an increase in mesangial cell PGE_2 formation. The growth promoting activity of IL-1β was not dose-dependent, but rather showed a decrease when the concentration of the cytokine was increased.

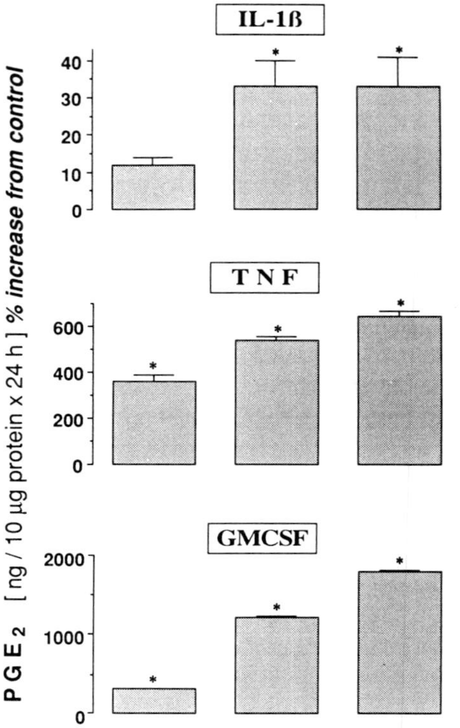

Fig. 2

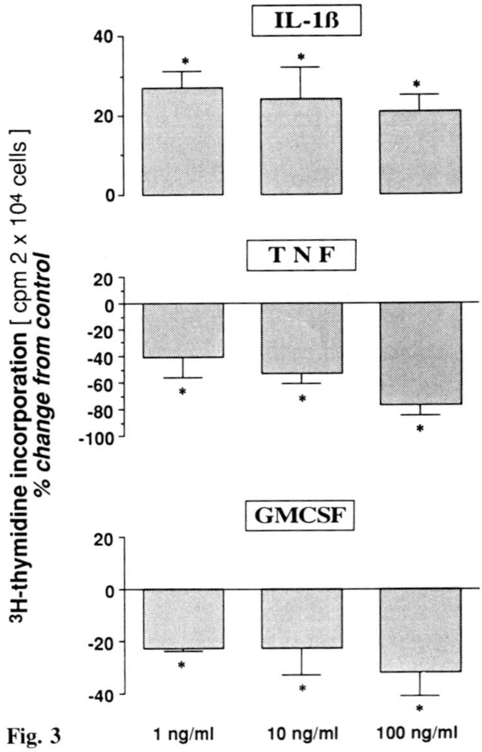

Fig. 3

Fig. 2. To study the effect of recombinant Interleukin-1β (IL-1β) (rat), Tumor Necrosis Factor (*TNF*) (human), and Granulocyte Macrophage Colony Stimulating Factor (*GMCSF*) (murine) on proliferating mesangial cell prostaglandin E_2 production, rat mesangial cells (2nd subculture) were grown in 24 well dishes in 5% fetal calf serum (*FCS*) and were incubated for 24 hours with increasing concentrations (1,10,100 ng/ml) of the cytokines. Prostaglandin E_2 (*PGE_2*) formation was analyzed in the supernatants by radioimmunoassay. Compared to control levels (5% FCS alone) all cytokines significantly increased PGE_2 production. The relative responses, however, were different. The most potent stimulator on a molar basis was TNF, whereas the stimulatory influence of IL-1β was relatively mild. The data (n=6, each variable) are given as means ± S.E. in % change from control. *P values < 0.05 were considered significant

Fig. 3. To assess the influence of IL-1β, TNF, and GMCSF (see Fig. 2 for definitions) on cell growth, mesangial cells (2nd subculture) were incubated in 96 well dishes (2×10^4 cells) either with 5% FCS or with 5% FCS and increasing concentrations of the cytokines (1,10,100 ng/ml). Prior to the experiments, cells were kept for 48 h on 0.5% FCS. Growth effects were evaluated over 48 h. ^{3}H-thymidine incorporation (last 6 h of the experimental period) and cell counts were applied to study growth.
Interleukin-1β induced a small, but significant increase of ^{3}H-thymidine uptake which was independent of the increasing concentration of the cytokine. TNF and GMCSF, however, significantly inhibited mesangial cell growth with increasing concentrations. The data (n=12, each variable) are given in % changes from control (5% FCS alone). *P values < 0.05 were considered significant

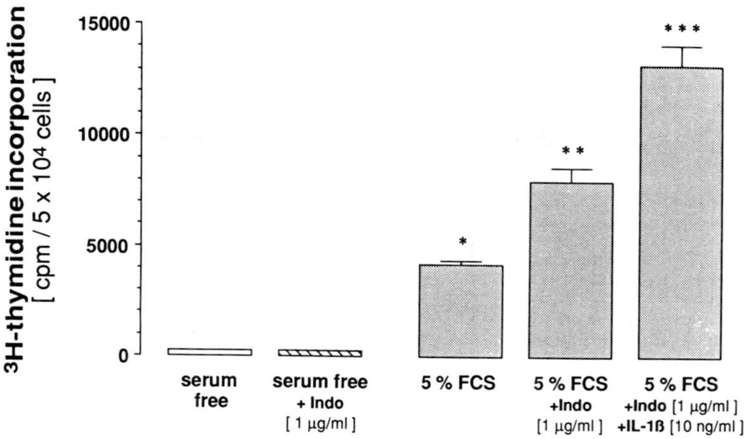

Fig. 4. To study the role of endogenous cyclooxygenase products of mesangial cells on growth, cells were incubated with endomethacin (*Indo*) in the presence and absence of serum. Indomethacin significantly increased ^{3}H-thymidine uptake by mesangial cells, however, only when serum was present. When IL-1β was added to the cyclooxygenase inhibitor, the growth promoting activity of FCS and indomethacin was further enhanced. Data (n=12, each variable) are given as means ± S.E. P values < 0.05 were considered significant.[a] FCS vs serum free; [b]FCS + Indo vs FCS; [c]FCS + Indo + IL-1β vs FCS + Indo

To study the possible role which endogenous cyclooxygenase products have in this growth promoting activity of IL-1β and fetal calf serum (FCS), mesangial cells were incubated with the cyclooxygenase inhibitor indomethacin (see Fig. 4).

Incubation with indomethacin significantly enhanced the ^{3}H-thymidine uptake in rat mesangial cells; however, the effect required the presence of FCS. In the absence of serum the cyclooxygenase inhibitor did not influence DNA synthesis.

The growth stimulatory effect of IL-1β increased with the degree of the reduction of mesangial cell PGE_2 formation, which appeared in a dose-dependent manner with increasing indomethacin concentrations (see Fig. 5).

These data demonstrate that endogenous formation of cyclooxygenase products might inhibit serum or cytokine (IL-1β) stimulated mesangial cell growth in culture. This growth inhibitory effect is unmasked when cyclooxygenase is inhibited. It appears from our experiment that TNF and GMCSF significantly stimulate mesangial cell prostaglandin formation and thereby might enhance growth inhibitory effects. These cytokines, however, do not further stimulate mesangial cell growth in mesangial cells incubated with a cyclooxygenase inhibitor (data not shown). It is unclear which cyclooxygenase metabolite derived from mesangial cells is responsible for the antiproliferative effect. When exogenous eicosanoids (PGE_2, $PGF_{2\alpha}$, AA), however, are added to mesangial cells in the presence of cyclooxygenase, only PGE_2 exerts antiproliferative effects [20]. It might therefore be possible that PGE_2 produced on the glomerular level, either by resident glomerular cells or by infiltrating inflammatory cells (i.e., monocytes), might inhibit mesangial cell growth in glomerular diseases.

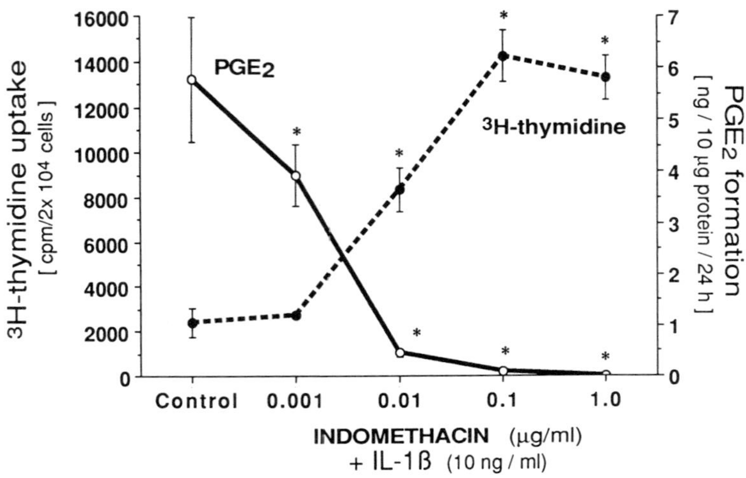

Fig. 5. Rat mesangial cells were incubated with increasing concentrations of indomethacin in the presence of interleukin 1-β and FCS 5% in order to evaluate the effect of endogenous cyclooxygenase products on mesangial cell growth. With the stepwise increase of indomethacin (0.001 to 1.0 μg/ml) PGE_2 formation decreased and was almost completely inhibited with 0.1 μg/ml indomethacin. Corresponding with the reduction of mesangial cell PGE_2 formation, ^{3}H-thymidine uptake increased significantly and reached a maximum at an indomethacin concentration of 0.1 μ/ml, when PGE_2 formation was completely inhibited. PGE_2, Prostaglandin E_2. The data (n=12, each variable) are given as means ± S.E. *P values < 0.05 were considered significant

There is also evidence, however, that endogenously added cyclooxygenase products can enhance mesangial cell growth in culture. Mene and Dunn [22] found that prostaglandin $F_{2\alpha}$, a compound which is present in significant amounts in isolated glomeruli, can induce rat mesangial cell proliferation in culture and, further, this compound enhances growth factor-induced proliferation. In a way similar to the stimulatory effect of the cyclooxygenase inhibitors (as mentioned), $PGF_{2\alpha}$ did not exert its effect without additional cofactors or serum.

In addition to the effects of eicosanoids on mesangial cell proliferation, endogenous cyclooxygenase products are probably involved in the release of cytokines and matrix components of resident glomerular cells.

Baud et al. [23] studied the mechanism of lipopolysaccharide (LPS)-induced release of TNF by rat mesangial cells in culture. In their studies LPS caused an increase in TNF secretion which was paralleled by stimulated mesangial cell PGE_2 formation. Treatment of mesangial cells with indomethacin promoted an increase in TNF synthesis, an effect which could be suppressed by the addition of PGE_2 and a cyclic AMP analogue. These observations strongly suggest that PGE_2 might regulate the release of TNF on a feedback mechanism.

There is also some evidence that cyclooxygenase products might be involved in the formation of basement membrane proteins and matrix components of the glomerulus.

In diabetic mice with progression of the disease, Ledbetter et al. [24] found an increase in mRNA expression of the α-1 chain of type IV collagen in the kidneys, which was paralleled by an increase in albuminuria. When the diabetic mice were treated with an inhibitor of thromboxane synthesis over a period of 1 month, albuminuria was reduced and mRNA expression of type IV collagen was not different from that of non-diabetic control mice. The authors conclude from their studies that thromboxane might play a role in progressive renal disease in diabetic mice and that thromboxane might be a mediator of increased collagen type IV production in diabetic mice.

Preliminary evidence, derived from studies by Ardaillou et al. [25], suggests that prostaglandin E_2 inhibits mesangial cell uptake of proline, probably due to the activation of cAMP, and that prostaglandin E_2 might be of significance in the production of matrix components, suggestions which have also been made earlier by others [26].

In summary, these recently obtained data suggest that endogenous eicosanoids are involved in the process of glomerular resident cell growth, cytokine release, and possibly, in glomerular matrix formation. Prostaglandin E_2 in this context might exert a "protective" effect by inhibiting cell growth, cytokine release, and matrix component formation. On the other hand $PGF_{2\alpha}$ and TxA_2 seem to exert effects which might be interpreted as "propagating" glomerular disease. One has to consider, however, that most of this information is obtained from tissue culture experiments and has yet to be confirmed in disease states.

References

1. Wilson CB, Blantz RC (1985) Nephroimmunopathology and pathophysiology (editorial review). Am J Physiol 248:F319–327
2. Couser WG, Baker PJ, Adler S (1985) Complement and the direct mediation of immune glomerular injury: A new perspective. Kidney Int 28:879–886
3. Lianos EA, Andres GA, Dunn MJ (1983) Glomerular prostaglandin and thromboxane synthesis in rat nephrotoxic nephritis. J Clin Invest 72:1439–1448
4. Stork JE, Dunn MJ (1985) Hemodynamic roles of thromboxane A_2 and prostaglandin E_2 in glomerulonephritis. J Pharmacol Exp Ther 233:672–678
5. Kelley VE, Sneve S (1986) Increased renal thromboxane production in murine lupus nephritis. J Clin Invest 77:252–259
6. Stahl RAK, Adler S, Baker PJ, Chen YP, Pritzl PM, Couser WG (1987) Enhanced glomerular prostaglandin formation in experimental membranous nephropathy. Kidney Int 31:1126–1131
7. Stahl RAK, Thaiss F, Kahf S, Schoeppe W, Helmchen UM (to be published) Immune mediated mesangial cell injury: biosynthesis and function of prostanoids. Kidney Int
8. Lianos EA (1988) Synthesis of hydroxyeicosatetraenoic acids and leukotrienes in rat nephrotoxic serum glomerulonephritis. J Clin Invest 82:427–435
9. Lianos EA, Noble B, Hucke B (1989) Glomerular leukotriene synthesis in Heymann nephritis. Kidney Int 36:998–1002
10. Thaiss F, Germann PJ, Kahf S, Schoeppe W, Helmchen U, Stahl RAK (1989) Effect of thromboxane synthesis inhibition in a model of membranous nephropathy. Kidney Int 35:76–83
11. Stahl RAK, Kudelka S, Paravicini M, Schollmeyer P (1986) Prostaglandin and thromboxane formation in glomeruli from rats with reduced renal mass. Nephron 42:252–257

12. Mene P, Dunn MJ (1988) Eicosanoids and control of mesangial cell contraction. Circ Res 62:916–925
13. Zurier RB, Damjanov I, Syadoff M, Rothfield NF (1977) Prostaglandin E_1 treatment of NZB/NZW F_1 hybrid mice. II. Prevention of glomerulonephritis. Arthritis Rheum 20:1449–1456
14. McLeish KR, Gohara AF, Gunning III WT, Senitzer D (1980) Prostaglandin E_1 therapy of murine chronic serum sickness. J Lab Clin Med 96:470–479
15. McLeish KR, Gohara AF, Gunning III WT (1982) Suppression of antibody synthesis by prostaglandin E as a mechanism for preventing murine immune complex glomerulonephritis. Lab Invest 47:147–152
16. Kunkel SL, Thrall RS, Kunkel RG, McCormick JR, Ward PA, Zurier RB (1979) Suppression of immune complex vasculitis in rats by prostaglandin. J Clin Invest 64:1525–1529
17. Kelley VE, Winkelstein A, Izui S (1979) Effect of prostaglandin E on immune complex nephritis in NZB/W mice. Lab Invest 41:531–537
18. Cattell V, Smith J, Cook HT (1990) Prostaglandin E_1 suppresses macrophage infiltration and ameliorates injury in an experimental model of macrophage-dependent glomerulonephritis. Clin Exp Immunol 79:260–265
19. Sterzel RB, Lovett DH (1988) Interactions of inflammatory and glomerular cells in the response to glomerular injury. In: Brenner BM, Stein JH (eds) Immunopathology of renal disease. Churchill Livingstone, pp 18:137–173
20. Stahl RAK, Thaiss F: Eicosanoids (1987) biosynthesis and function in the glomerulus. Renal Physiol 10:1–13
21. Stahl RAK, Thaiss F, Haberstroh U, Kahf S, Shaw A, Schoeppe W (to be published) Cyclooxygenase inhibition enhances rat Il-1β induced proliferation of mesangial cells. Am J Physiol
22. Mene P, Dunn MJ (1990) Prostaglandins and rat glomerular mesangial cell proliferation. Kidney Int 37:1256–1262
23. Baud L, Oudinet J-P, Bens M, Noe L, Peraldi M-N, Rondeau E, Etienne J, Ardaillou R (1989) production of tumor necrosis factor by rat mesangial cells in response to bacterial lipopolysaccharide. Kidney Int 35:1111–1118
24. Ledbetter S, Copeland EJ, Noonan D, Vogeli G, Hassell JR (1990) Altered steady state mRNA levels of basement membrane proteins in diabetic mouse kidneys and thromboxane synthase inhibition. Diabetics 39:196–203
25. Ardaillou N, Nivez PM, Ardaillou R (1990) Effect of prostaglandin E2 on proline uptake and collagen synthesis by cultured human mesangial cells (abstract). Kidney Int 37:344
26. Homma T, Ichikawa I, Hoover RL (1988) Prostaglandins of mesangium origin inhibit mesangial cell (MC) proliferation and matrix synthesis (abstract). Kidney Int 33:268

Mechanisms of Glomerular Fibrin Deposition in Glomerulonephritis

S. R. Holdsworth and P. G. Tipping[1]

Summary. Evidence points to glomerular fibrin deposition (GFD) as an important mediator of renal injury and crescent formation. GFD appears to be initiated by intraglomerular stimuli related to local immune inflammatory events. Macrophages expressing augmented procoagulant activity (PCA) are likely to be important initiators of GFD. Antibody Fc direction or delayed type hypersensitivity (DTH) mechanisms may be the primary initiating event. Other factors, including contact activation of coagulation and inhibition of fibrinolytic clearance, may act in concert to exacerbate fibrin accumulation, especially in Bowman's space. The importance of GFD in human GN is highlighted by evidence that it may be prevented or reversed by therapeutic intervention, thereby offering the potential for limiting the progression of injury in these forms of GN.

Introduction

Glomerular deposition of fibrin is observed in the most severe forms of glomerulonephritis (GN), in which the outcome for renal function is often poor. Paradoxically however, it is these forms of GN which offer the greatest potential for treatment. Defibrination studies in experimental GN demonstrate that prevention of fibrin deposition preserves renal function and abrogates crescent formation. Fibrin deposition in GN is restricted to the glomerulus, and is deposited in response to local immunologically initiated inflammatory events.

Fibrin Deposition in GN

Glomerular fibrin deposition (GFD) is observed in many histological types of GN but is most prominent in association with proliferative GN, and particularly with crescent formation [1,2]. Similar observations have been made in experimental GN. It is

[1]Department of Medicine, Prince Henry's Hospital, St. Kilda Road, Melbourne 3004, Australia

those forms of injury which are associated with severe proliferation, renal failure, and crescent formation where GFD is also most abundant. This occurs regardless of the nature of the immune initiating events. GFD occurs in GN initiated by anti-glomerular basement membrane (GBM) antibodies, immune complexes, and planted antigens and is common to a variety of species, including rabbit, mouse, rat, and sheep. Recent studies also suggest a close association between GFD and macrophage accumulation in human and experimental GN.

Pathological Effects of Glomerular Fibrin Deposition

Observations of human GN confirm the association of prominent GFD with loss of glomerular filtration, crescent formation, and a poor prognosis. In experimental GN, specific depletion of fibrin can be induced without altering other immune initiating events, allowing studies of the specific consequences of GFD. Ancrod is a component of cobra venom which converts fibrinogen to soluble fibrin monomer which cannot crosslink and is rapidly cleared from the circulation, resulting in severe hypofibrinogenemia. When employed in models of experimental GN with prominent GFD, immunofluorescence studies demonstrate complete abrogation of GFD with the use of this agent [3–5]. Similar results can be obtained with the fibrinolytic agent streptokinase [6,7]. Blocking GFD maintains urine output and preserves glomerular filtration, suggesting that fibrin deposition may result in a physical barrier limiting filtration. The second striking consequence of preventing GFD is the reduction in crescent formation. Early in experimental GN, fibrin collects in Bowman's space, forming an acellular proteinaceous crescent. Accumulation of monocytes and proliferation of epithelial cells leads to cellular crescent formation. Prevention of crescent formation by defibrination suggests a pivotal role for fibrin in the pathogenesis of these events. Fibrin is chemotactic for macrophages [8] and may induce macrophage localization in Bowman's space, but is also likely to act as an extracellular substratum facilitating cellular proliferation and organization. Studies in vitro demonstrate that fibrin degradation products may be toxic to mesangial cells [9], however, the observation of prominent mesangial proliferation in fibrin related GN in man clearly demonstrates that this potential toxicity is not a limiting feature in vivo.

Systemic Coagulation Changes in GN

A variety of alterations in systemic coagulation have been reported in patients with GN. These are largely due to the consequences of the nephrotic syndrome or the effects of systemic inflammation in diseases where GN is secondary to disease processes such as sepsis, vasculitis, or connective tissues diseases (principally SLE). In these inflammatory diseases, disturbance of coagulation may include thrombocytosis, hyperfibrinogenemia, and increased levels of acute phase proteins with anti-fibrinolytic activity [10–12], including C4 binding protein and α2 antiplasmin. Reduction in levels of anti-thrombin III may occur as a result of the nephrotic syndrome [13,14]. All of these changes in circulating coagulation factors shift the balance of procoagulant and anti-coagulant pathways in favor of clotting. Increased

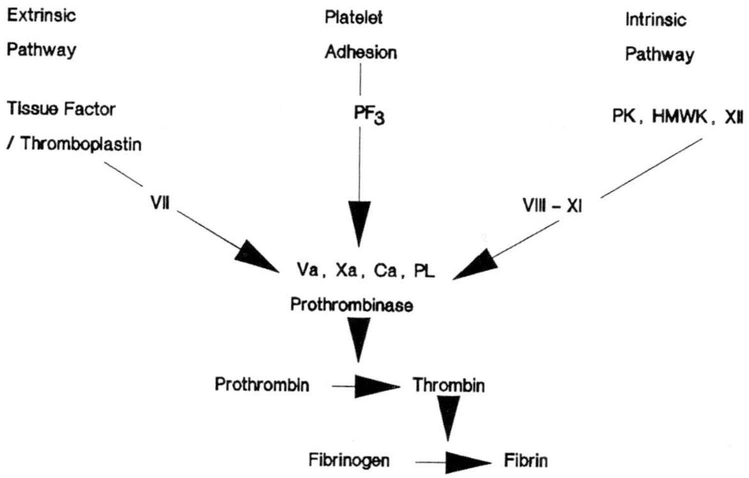

Fig. 1. Potential pathways for initiation of fibrin deposition in GN

levels of activated Factor VIII have been reported in some patients with GN [10,11]. Despite these reports, the majority of patients with GFD in association with GN have no systemic disturbance in coagulation. Similarly, experimental animal studies strongly support the view that GFD occurs as the result of local procoagulant stimuli rather than systemic coagulation changes.

Local Events Initiating Coagulation

The occurrence of GFD in glomeruli with evidence of capillary wall injury (manifested by histological changes and proteinuria) naturally led to the view that GFD was initiated by contact coagulation activation. Fibrin deposition is not a universal feature of all histological types of GN. In human GN, it is usually associated with proliferative and crescentic disease. However, in some types of GN associated with significant GBM injury, significant glomerular fibrin deposition is absent. These observations suggest that GFD is not a consequence of GBM injury alone.

Support for this hypothesis is provided by studies of experimental models of anti-GBM antibody initiated GN in rabbits [15]. Comparing the heterologous and autologous phases of this disease, similar levels of proteinuria and histological evidence of glomerular injury were observed. However, significant GFD was seen only in the autologous phase, indicating that capillary wall damage per se was not sufficient to initiate GFD. The mechanisms responsible for GFD have recently been explored in some detail.

Coagulation may be initiated by a number of different mechanisms, as demonstrated in Fig. 1.

Intrinsic Pathway Activation

Activation of the intrinsic coagulation pathway by contact with negatively charged molecules such as collagen, exposed as a result of endothelial injury, is clearly a potential trigger for GFD. A number of observations, however, suggest that this is not a significant initiating factor for fibrin deposition in GN. Hoyer et al. [16] observed that GFD in human GN was not associated with demonstrable glomerular factor VIII related antigen, suggesting lack of participation of intrinsic pathway coagulation factors. In contrast, in hemolytic-uremic syndrome, hyperacute homograft rejection, and post partum renal failure, factor VIII related antigen was prominent in association with GFD. Rats congenitally deficient in high molecular weight kininogen show no impairment of GFD in experimental crescentic GN [17], further indicating the lack of participation of the intrinsic coagulation pathway.

Hageman Factor (factor XII), similarly, is not deposited with fibrin in the glomerular tufts in rabbits developing crescentic GN, [18] although late passive accumulation in Bowman's space, along with other serum proteins, was noted. Factor VIII related antigen deposition also occurs well after the initiation of glomerular fibrin deposition and is restricted to Bowman's space in crescentic GN in rabbits [19]. These studies together provide consistent evidence for the lack of participation of intrinsic coagulation pathway factors in glomerular fibrin deposition.

Platelets and GFD

Platelets are a major component of intravascular thrombus although they are not essential for coagulation in vitro. Platelet phospholipid membrane provides an important co-factor for activation of coagulation proteins, and platelets themselves are a source of coagulation factors, including thrombin. Therefore it would seem difficult to entirely discount a role for platelets in GFD. However, available evidence does not suggest an important role for platelets in GFD associated with GN. Platelets are infrequently observed in proliferative forms of human GN [20], although they have been identified in experimental anti-GBM GN [21] and immune complex GN [22]. Induction of profound thrombocytopenia or use of anti-platelet drugs in experimental GN, however, did not reduce GFD [23,24].

Extrinsic Pathway Activation

The lack of involvement of intrinsic pathway factors and platelets in GFD in GN, raises the potential of a pivotal role for extrinsic pathway activation. The extrinsic pathway is triggered by activation of factor VII by tissue thromboplastin (tissue factor). Tissue factor is a membrane bound phospholipid expressed constitutively by many cells and may be upregulated in inflammation. Monocytes and macrophages in particular are an abundant source of tissue factor. The recognition of the close association between macrophages and GFD, both in human [25–28] and in experimental GN [1,5,7,15], suggested that monocytes may be responsible for glomerular fibrin deposition via tissue factor induced activation of the extrinsic coagulation pathway. We assessed the capacity of monocytes to induce glomerular fibrin deposition by studying the effects of monocyte depletion and selective repletion in a model of anti-GBM GN with prominent fibrin deposition in rabbits [15] (Fig. 2). These studies

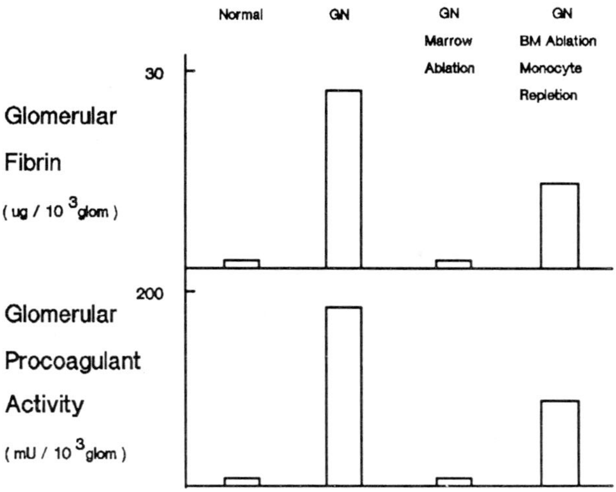

Fig. 2. The effect of macrophage depletion and repletion on glomerular fibrin deposition and procoagulant activity in anti-GBM GN

clearly indicated that GFD was dependent on monocyte infiltration in this model. Fibrin deposition was associated with monocyte induced GN, but not with neutrophil induced glomerular injury, indicating that the capacity of these leukocytes to induce glomerular injury was unrelated to their capacity to initiate GFD. Although both neutrophils and monocytes have the capacity to induce glomerular injury, only macrophages express procoagulant activity enabling them to initiate fibrin deposition by activation of the extrinsic pathway. To assess extrinsic pathway activation during development of GN, expression of procoagulant activity by nephritic glomeruli was measured. When compared to normal glomeruli and glomeruli from rabbits with heterologous phase injury, monocyte infiltrated nephritic glomeruli had greatly augmented levels of PCA. Depletion and repletion studies confirmed that glomerular monocyte influx accounted for the augmented expression of PCA [15] (Fig. 2).

The functional characteristics of glomerular PCA indicate it activates the extrinsic pathway and is tissue factor. Its activity is dependent on coagulation factors VIII and V and independent of factors VIII and XII. It is inhibited by phospholipase C and concanavalin A and by antibodies to tissue factor [29] (Fig. 3). Expression of PCA by macrophages isolated from nephritic glomeruli was compared with PCA expression by blood monocytes and pulmonary alveolar macrophages in the same animals. These studies indicated that infiltrating glomerular macrophages express vastly augmented levels of procoagulant activity (PCA) compared to other macrophage populations during the development of GN, indicating that they are locally activated, further suggesting a pivotal role for macrophages in the initiation of fibrin deposition in GN [30].

Macrophage Mechanisms for Promoting Coagulation (Fig. 4)

Activated monocytes are capable of influencing coagulation directly, by their expression of procoagulant and anti-coagulant molecules and indirectly, by their production

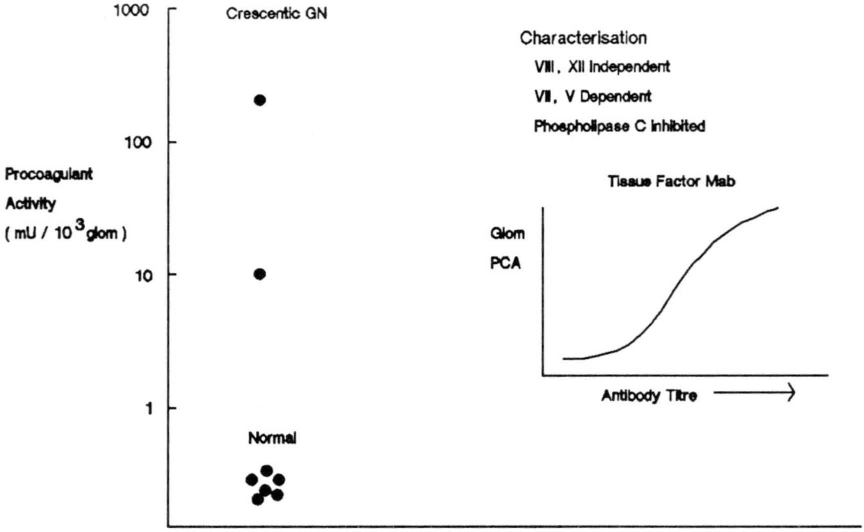

Fig. 3. Procoagulant activity in glomeruli from 2 patients with crescentic GN, and in normal glomeruli. Functional characteristics of glomerular procoagulant activity and its inhibition by a monoclonal anti-tissue factor antibody

of proinflammatory cytokines, principally interleukin 1 (IL1) and tumor necrosis factor (TNF), which alter the expression of procoagulant and anti-coagulant molecules by endothelial cells [31–33]. Endothelial cells normally exhibit a number of functions which result in a net anti-coagulant effect [12]. These include thrombomodulin, heparin-like proteoglycans that facilitate anti-thrombin III activity, plasminogen activator, and PGI_2 (prostacycline) which inhibits platelet aggregation. Macrophage cytokines have been shown both to downregulate these functions and to upregulate procoagulant endothelial function including plasminogen activator inhibitor, procoagulant activity, and Von Willebrand factor activity [31] (Fig. 4).

Mechanisms of Activation of Macrophage Procoagulant Functions

There are a number of mechanisms, of potential relevance to GN, by which macrophages may be stimulated to augment their PCA expression and thereby initiate GFD.

Complement

Glomerular complement deposition is prominent in many types of human and experimental GN and is often present in association with GFD. In experimental GN, depletion studies have demonstrated that complement is a pivotal chemoattractant

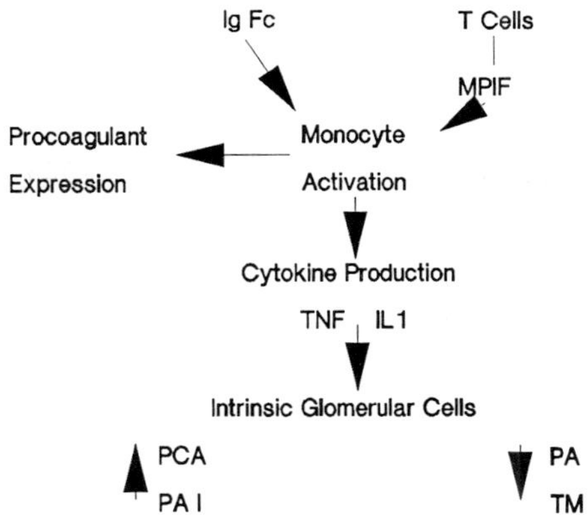

Fig. 4. Potential mechanisms for macrophage initiation of fibrin deposition. MPIF, macrophage procoagulant inducing factor; PA, plasminogen activator; PA1, plasminogen activator inhibitor; TM, thrombomodulin.

for neutrophils, but is not essential for glomerular monocyte accumulation. Complement fragments can activate macrophages and then augment monocyte PCA expression [33], however, in experimental GN, complement depletion does not alter glomerular PCA expression. (Lowe, Tipping and Holdsworth, unpublished observations)

Immunoglobulin

Immunoglobulin Fc is an important stimulus for macrophage localization in GN. Immunoglobulin and immune complexes are potent stimuli for augmentation of macrophage PCA expression [34–35], however the contribution of these to the augmented glomerular PCA in GN is unknown.

T Lymphocytes

T lymphocytes have recently been demonstrated in proliferative forms of human and experimental GN. They are particularly abundant in human GN, with prominent glomerular fibrin deposition macrophage accumulation and tissue factor expression. T lymphocytes are potent activators of macrophages [26–28], and have the capacity to augment macrophage PCA expression via release of the lymphokine macrophage procoagulant inducing factor (MPIF). T cell directed macrophage induced fibrin deposition is a characteristic feature of delayed type hypersensitivity (DTH) reactions occurring in the skin in response to a locally represented antigen. In both human and experimental GN there is now good evidence for the participation of these same mediators of injury, T cells [39–41], macrophages expressing tissue factor, and fibrin deposition [42], suggesting the potential for T cell augmentation of glomerular fibrin deposition via mechanisms akin to DTH.

The Role of Intrinsic Glomerular Cells in Glomerular Fibrin Deposition

Epithelial, endothelial, and mesangial cells all have the potential to interact in the coagulation process. However, there is a scarcity of studies addressing their contribution to GFD in GN. Indirect evidence comes from demonstration of the potential of intrinsic glomerular cells to release products which interact with various elements of the coagulation cascade, particularly via effects on endothelial cell procoagulant and anti-coagulant molecules. Isolated glomeruli can produce both thromboxane and PGI_2 in response to oxygen radicals [43]. Isolated glomeruli and mesangial cells can synthesize platelet aggregation factor (PAF) [43] and mesangial cells have the potential to express augmented PCA activity following TNF stimulation [44]. Mesangial cells have the potential to produce proinflammatory cytokines [45] which may modulate endothelial cell functions.

Both endothelial and mesangial cells synthesize tissue type plasminogen activator (t-PA) [46] and glomerular endothelial cells express thrombomodulin, and important anticoagulant molecule expressed by endothelial cells elsewhere [47]. Human glomeruli contain t-PA and a minor component of urokinase type plasminogen activator (u-PA). It is reported that mesangial cells release t-PA and plasminogen activator (PA) inhibitor type 1 while epithelial cells release an inactive form of u-PA [48].

Macrophage Modulation of Intrinsic Glomerular Cell Coagulant Functions

Endothelial cell expression of PCA is augmented by soluble products released from monocyte infiltrated isolated nephritic glomeruli [30]. This effect is not observed with culture supernatants of normal glomeruli or with nephritic glomeruli from macrophage depleted animals, suggesting that macrophage products (possibly proinflammatory cytokines) are responsible for this endothelial cell PCA augmentation. Monocytes in experimental models of GN with prominent GFD have been shown to express augmented levels of IL-1 and TNF [49] and these cytokines have the capacity to augment endothelial cell PCA in vitro. While these data confirm the potential for intrinsic cells to contribute to the augmented PCA in GN there is no direct evidence of a significant contribution to glomerular PCA by this mechanism in vivo, as nephritic glomerular supernatants capable of enhancing endothelial cell PCA failed to measurably enhance the PCA of intact glomeruli in vitro. Intrinsic glomerular cells and cytokine activated endothelial cells express 100–1000-fold less PCA than glomerular macrophages. This suggests that the contribution of intrinsic cells to the augmented PCA in GN with prominent macrophage infiltration may be insignificant, and that macrophages themselves are likely to account for most of the augmented procoagulant activity observed in nephritic glomeruli with prominent GFD.

Alterations in other coagulant functions of intrinsic cells may be relevant to GFD in GN. Glomerular fibrinolytic activity and t-PA activity has been assessed in models of GN with prominent fibrin depositions. In rabbits with chronic serum sickness, glomerular fibrinolytic activity was reduced in association with glomerular deposition of fibrin [50]. In anti-GBM antibody induced GN in rats, glomerular fibrinolytic activity and t-PA expression were enhanced [51] while procoagulant activity was reduced [52]. This is consistent with the observation that rats appear resistant to the development of crescentic GN and develop only sparse GFD. Blockade of fibrinolytic activity enhances crescent formation [53] in this model. In mercuric chloride induced GN in rats, enhanced glomerular PCA is associated with prominent GFD [54].

Mechanisms of Fibrin Deposition in Human Glomerulonephritis

In human GN, fibrin deposition is associated with the severe proliferative crescentic forms of GN. This has been demonstrated by immunohistochemical staining for fibrin in renal biopsies [1,2] and measurement of urinary fibrin degradation products [55,56]. The cellular mechanisms of GFD in human GN can only be studied indirectly, however there are now a number of histological studies of the participation of coagulation factors in renal tissue of patients with GN.

Absence of Factor VIII in glomeruli of patients with prominent GFD mitigates against a major role for intrinsic pathway initiation of fibrin deposition in human GN. Aggregation of platelets in glomeruli is not a prominent feature in human GN [20].

Recent evidence suggests that mechanisms similar to those observed in experimental GN may be operative in man. Glomerular macrophage influx is observed in forms of GN accompanied by prominent GFD [25–28]. Studies of the expression of procoagulant activity in human GN have recently been performed. Two patients who died with acute crescentic GN with prominent fibrin deposition and without substantial immunosuppression therapy provided renal tissue soon after death [57]. Isolated glomeruli from these patients showed vast augmentation of procoagulant activity when compared to levels expressed by non-nephritic human glomeruli. The procoagulant had the functional characteristics of tissue factor, being factor VII and V dependent and factor VIII and XII independent, and being inhibitable by phospholipase C and by a monoclonal antibody specific for human tissue factor. Nonspecific esterase staining demonstrated a significant macrophage presence in these glomeruli, indicating the potential for macrophages to be responsible for the augmented glomerular PCA in these patients.

The recent demonstration of the participation of T lymphocytes, particularly in proliferative forms of GN where fibrin deposition is associated with prominent macrophage infiltration, raises the possible involvement of delayed type hypersensitivity mechanisms in GFD. In a study of 62 renal biopsies, all those showing GN with fibrin deposition and random biopsies showing fibrin negative GN were studied for the presence of the essential elements of DTH; T lymphocytes, macrophages, and tissue factor [42]. Fibrin negative biopsies did not have substantial lymphocyte, monocyte, or tissue factor presence and, in general, exhibited features of less aggressive forms of GN. Fibrin positive biopsies, however, had marked tissue factor expression together with evidence of lymphocyte and macrophage accumulation, indicating the simultaneous deposition of the essential components of DTH in association with fibrin in human GN (Table 1).

Glomerular fibrin deposition occurs in experimental anti-GBM GN in association with macrophages and augmented PCA when injury is induced passively by antibody, without involvement of sensitized T lymphocytes. In this passive model of anti-

Table 1. The association of mediators of delayed type hypersensitivity, (*DTH*) and fibrin deposition in human GN

DTH Reactant	Fibrin negative biopsies $n = 19$	Fibrin positive biopsies $n = 10$
Macrophages	0.6 ± 0.02	18.9 ± 6.2
T Cells	0.2 ± 0.002	9.9 ± 0.6
Tissue Factor	–	++/+++

GBM GN, GFD, assessed quantitatively by ^{125}I fibrinogen accumulation, was substantially less than in the active form of this disease which is associated with glomerular T lymphocyte accumulation. A greater augmentation of glomerular PCA is also seen in the active model in association with T cells. Thus, in experimental GN, although T lymphocytes may have an important role in augmenting GFD, glomerular injury, initiated by immunoglobulin and mediated by macrophages in the absence of T cells, has the capacity to induce GFD.

On the other hand, GFD in human GN has been observed in the absence of any immunoglobulin deposition. In these patients with so called "immune negative" GN, fibrin deposition occurs in the presence of T cells and macrophages [42], providing strong evidence for the capacity of DTH, in the absence of antibody induced mechanisms, to induce GFD.

Alterations in the glomerular fibrinolytic system have been assessed in human GN. In the large study of human biopsies by Bergstein and Michael [56] no overall change in glomerular fibrinolytic or t-PA activity was observed. Recent studies have reported increased expression of PA inhibitor in crescentic GN with fibrin deposition [59]. Increased expression of PA inhibitor, synthesized by glomerular epithelial cells, may represent a further mechanism for preventing the clearance of deposited fibrin [48].

References

1. Kincaid-Smith P (1972) Coagulation and renal disease. Kidney Int 2:183–190
2. McCluskey RT, Vassalli P, Gallo G, Baldwin DS (1966) An immunofluorescent study of pathogenic mechanisms in glomerular diseases. N Engl J Med 274:695–701
3. Naish P, Penn GB, Evans DJ, Peters, DK (1972). The effect of defibrination on nephrotoxic serum nephritis in rabbits. Clin Sci 42:643–646
4. Naish PF, Evans DJ, Peters DK (1975) The effects of defibrination with ancrod in experimental allergic glomerular injuries. Clin Exp Immunol 20:303–309
5. Thomson NM, Simpson IJ, Evans DJ, Peters, DK (1975) Defibrination with ancrod in experimental chronic immune complex nephritis. Clin Exp Immunol 20:527–535
6. Tipping PG, Holdsworth SR (1986) Fibrinolytic therapy with streptokinase in established experimental glomerulonephritis. Nephron 43:258–264
7. Tipping PG, Thomson NM, Holdsworth SR (1986) A comparison of fibrinolytic and defibrinating agents in established experimental glomerulonephritis. Brit J Exp Pathol 67:481–491
8. Humair L, Kwann HC, Potter E (1969) The role of fibrinogen in renal disease II. Effects of anticoagulants and urokinase on experimental lesions in mice. J Lab Clin Med 74:72–78
9. Tsumagari T, Tanaka K (1984) Effects of fibrinogen degradation products on glomerular mesangial cells in culture. Kidney Int 26:712–718

10. Salem HH, Whitworth JA, Koutts J (1981) Hypercoagulation in glomerulonephritis. Br Med J 282:2083–2086
11. Adhikari M, Coovadia HM, Greig HBW, Christensen S (1978) Factor VIII procoagulant activity in children with nephrotic syndrome and post-streptococcal glomerulonephritis. Nephron 22:301–305
12. Esmon CT (1987) The regulations of natural anticoagulant pathways. Science 235: 1348–1352
13. Kendall AG, Lohmann RC, Dossetor JB Nephrotic syndrome a hypercoagulable state. Ann Intern Med 127:1021–1031
14. Vaziri ND (1983) Nephrotic syndrome and coagulation and fibrinolytic abnormalities. Am J Nephrol 3:1
15. Holdsworth SR, Tipping PG (1985) Macrophage induced fibrin deposition in experimental glomerulonephritis in the rabbit. J Clin Invest 76:1367–1374
16. Hoyer JR, Michael AF, Hoyer LW (1974) Immunofluorescent localization of antihemophiliac factor antigen and fibrinogen in human renal disease. J Clin Invest 53:1375–1384
17. Villaro J, Errasti P, Goni M, Monzo A, Purroy A, Sanchez-Ibarrola A (1984) Pathogenesis of glomerular fibrin deposition: Role of the contact system (abstract). Kidney Int 26:219
18. Wiggins RG (1985) Hageman factor in experimental nephrotoxic nephritis in the rabbit. Lab Invest 53:335–348
19. Tipping PG, Holdsworth SR (1986) The participation of macrophages, glomerular procoagulant activity and factor VIII in glomerular fibrin deposition. Studies in anti-glomerulonephritis basement membrane antibody induced glomerulonephritis in rabbits. Am J Pathol 124:10–17
20. George CPR, Clark WF, Cameron JS (1975) The role of platelets in glomerulonephritis. Adv Nephrol 5:19–65
21. Vassali P, McCluskey RT (1964) The pathogenic role of the coagulation process in rabbit Masugi nephritis. Am J Path 45:653–677
22. Gabbiani G, Boadonnel MC, Vassoli P (1975) Experimental focal glomerular lesion elicited by insoluble immune complexes: ultrastructural and immunofluorescent studies. Lab Invest 32:33–45
23. Ogawa S, Naruse T (1982) Effects of various antiplatelet drugs and a defibrinating agent on experimental glomerulonephritis in rats. J Lab Clin Med 99:428–435
24. Sindrey M, Marshall TI, Naish P (1979) Quantitative assessment of the effects of platelet depletion in the autologous phase of nephrotoxic serum nephritis. Clin Exp Immunol 36:90–96
25. Atkins RC, Holdsworth SR, Glasgow EF, Matthews FE (1976) The macrophage in human rapidly progressive glomerulonephritis. Lancet I:830–832
26. Monga G, Mazzucco G, Barbiano di Belgiojoso GB, Busnach G (1979) The presence and possible role of monocyte infiltration in human chronic proliferative glomerulonephritides. Light microscopic, immunofluorescence and histochemical correlation. Am J Pathol 94:271–284
27. Ferrario F, Castiglione A, Colasanti G, Barbiano di Belgiojoso G, Bertoli S, D'Amico G (1985) The detection of monocytes in human glomerulonephritis. Kidney Int 28:513–519
28. Magil AB, Wadsworth AB (1981) Monocytes in human glomerulonephritis. An electromicroscopic study. Lab Invest 34:77–81
29. Tipping PG, Worthington LA, Holdsworth SR (1987) The quantitation and characterization of glomerular procoagulant activity in experimental glomerulonephritis. Lab Invest 56:155–159
30. Tipping PG, Lowe MG, Holdsworth SR (1988) Glomerular macrophages express augmented procoagulant activity in experimental glomerulonephritis in rabbits. J Clin Invest 82:1253–1259
31. Cotran RS (1987) New roles for the endothelium in inflammation and immunity. Am J Pathol 129:407–413

32. Bevilacqua MP, Schleef RR, Gimbrone MA, Loskutoff DJ (1986) Regulation of the fibrinolytic system of cultured human vascular endothelium by interleukin 1. J Clin Invest 78:581–591
33. Mulfelder TW, Niemetz J, Kreutzer D, Beebe D, Ward PA, Rosenfeld SI (1979) C5 chemotactic fragment induces leukocyte production of tissue factor activity: A link between complement and coagulation. J Clin Invest 63:147–150
34. Rothberger H, Zimmerman TS, Spiegleberg HL, Vaughan JH (1977) Leukocyte procoagulant activity. Enhancement of production "in vitro" by IgG and antigen-antibody complexes. J Clin Invest 59:549–557
35. Schwartz BS, Edgington TS (1981) Immune complex-induced human monocyte procoagulant activity. I. A rapid unidirectional lymphocyte instructed pathway. J Exp Med 154:892–906
36. Edwards RL, Rickles FR, Bolorove AM (1979) Mononuclear cell tissue factor. Cell of origin and requirements for activation. Blood 54:359–370
37. Helin H, Edgington TS (1983) Allogenic induction of the human T cell instructed monocyte procoagulant response is rapid and is elicited by HLA-DR. J Exp Med 58:962–975
38. Gregory SM, Edgington TS (1985) Tissue factor induction in human monocytes. Two distinct mechanisms displayed by different alloantigen-responsive T cell clones. J Clin Invest 76:2440–2445
39. Tipping PG, Neale TJ, Holdsworth SR (1985) T-lymphocyte participation in antibody induced experimental glomerulonephritis. Kidney Int 27:530–537
40. Stachura I, Si L, Whiteside TL (1984) Mononuclear cell subsets in human idiopathic crescentic glomerulonephritis: Analysis in tissue sections with monoclonal antibodies. J Clin Immunol 4:203–208
41. Nolasco FEB, Cameron JS, Hartley B, Coelho A, Hildreth G, Reuben R (1987) Intraglomerular T cells and monocytes in nephritis: Study with monoclonal antibodies. Kidney Int 31:1160–1166
42. Neale TJ, Tipping PG, Carson S, Holdsworth SR (1988) Evidence for the participation of cell mediated immunity in the deposition of fibrin in glomerulonephritis. Lancet II:421–424
43. Baud L, Sraer J, Delarue F, Bens M, Balavoine F, Schlondorff D, Ardaillou R, Sraer JD (1985) Lipoxygenase products mediate the attachment of rat macrophages to glomeruli in vitro. Kidney Int 27:855–863
44. Wiggins RC, Njoku N, Sedor JR (1990) Tissue factor production by cultured rat mesangial cells. Stimulation by TNFα and lipopolysaccharide. Kidney Int 37:1281–1285
45. Boswell JM, Tui MA, Burt DW, Kelly VE (1988) Increased tumor necrosis factor and IL1-β gene expression in the kidneys of mice with lupus nephritis. J Immunol 141:3052–3054
46. Angles Cano E, Balaton A, Le Bonniec B, Genot E, Elion J, Sultan Y (1985) Production and immunolocalization of monoclonal antibodies to the high fibrin affinity tissue type plasminogen activator of human plasma: Demonstration of its endothelial origin by immunolocalization. Blood. 66:913–920
47. Hancock WW (1990) IL1 and TNF depress glomerular endothelial thrombomodulin expression in vitro and in vivo (abstract). Kidney Int 38:557.
48. Sraer JD, Kanfer A, Rondeau E, Lacaux R (1988) Glomerular hemostasis in normal and pathologic conditions. Adv Nephrol 17:27–56
49. Tipping PG, Lowe MG, Holdsworth SR (1991) Glomerular interleukin 1 production is dependent on macrophage infiltration in anti-GBM glomerulonephritis. Kidney Int (in press)
50. Stark H, Miller K, Michael AF (1979) Renal cortical fibrinolytic activity in rabbits with chronic immune complex nephritis. Isr J Med Sci 14:610–612
51. Giroux L, Verroust P, Morel-Maroger L, Delarue F, Delauche M, Sraer JD (1979) Glomerular fibrinolytic activity during nephrotoxic nephritis. Lab Invest 40:415–422

52. Kanfer A, De Prost D, Le Floch V (1985) Procoagulant activity in isolated glomeruli from normal and glomerulonephritic rats (abstract). Eur J Clin Invest 15:A43.
53. Clark BE, Ham KN, Tange JD, Ryan GB (1983) Macrophages and glomerular crescent formation: Studies with rat nephrotoxic nephritis. Pathology 15:75–81
54. Kanfer A, de Prost D, Guettier C, Nochy D, Le Floch V, Hinglais N, Druet P (1987) Enhanced glomerular procoagulant activity and fibrin deposition in rats with mercuric chloride-induced autoimmune nephritis. Lab Invest 57:138–143
55. Ekberg M, Pandolli M (1975) Origin of urinary fibrin fibrinogen degradation products in glomerulonephritis. Br Med J [Clin Res] 2:17–21
56. Clarkson AR, McDonald MK, Petrie JJB, Cash JD, Robson JS (1971) Serum and urine fibrin/fibrinogen degradation products in glomerulonephritis. Br Med J [Clin Res] 3:447–451
57. Tipping PG, Dowling JP, Holdsworth SR (1988) Glomerular procoagulant activity in human proliferative glomerulonephritis. J Clin Invest 81:119–125
58. Bergstein JM, Michael AF (1972) Cortical fibrinolytic activity in normal and diseased human kidneys. J Lab Clin Med 79:701–709
59. Mougenot B, Rondeau E, Kruithof B, Sraer JD (1988) Presence of type 1 plasminogen activator inhibitor (PA1-1) in renal fibrin deposits in human pathological conditions (abstract) Kidney Int 33:330

Hapten-Specific Cellular Immune Response Producing Glomerular Injury

TAKASHI OITE[1]

SUMMARY. A new model of experimental glomerulonephritis (GN), in which a cell-mediated reaction predominated, was established. Attachment of the haptens trinitrophenol (TNP) and fluorescein isothiocyanate (FITC) to a cationic carrier protein (bovine serum albumin:BSA) enabled their plantation in the glomerular capillary wall. Epicutaneous sensitization of the TNP without carrier protein induced a TNP-specific cell-mediated immunity. When we perfused the left kidneys of these sensitized rats with cationized TNP-BSA, proliferative glomerulonephritis with proteinuria could be induced without deposition of any autologous immunoglobulins and complement. Here, we will focus on the involvement of the cellular immune response in this experimental glomerulonephritis (GN) model.

Materials and Methods

Rats

All experiments were performed on male Wistar rats of body weight 160–180 g (Doken Japan).

Preparation of Hapten-Carrier Proteins and Their Cationization

2,4,6-trinitrobenzene-1-sulfonic acid sodium salt (TNBS), and fluorescein isothiocyanate (FITC) were conjugated to bovine serum albumin (BSA) by the method previously described [1]. Then TNP-BSA and FITC-BSA preparations were cationized as described previously [2]. Isoelectric points of the antigenic materials

[1]Department of Immunology, Institute of Nephrology, Niigata University School of Medicine, Asahimachi-dori 1, Niigata, 951 Japan

used in this study were determined by isoelectric focusing. The average degree of conjugation of haptens to BSA was determined spectrophotometrically.

Estimation of Serum Anti-TNP Antibody

Rat anti-TNP antibody was determined by enzyme-linked immunosorbent assay (ELISA), described previously [3].

Contact Hypersensitivity to the Haptenic Groups

Wistar rats were sensitized by applying 0.1 ml of 4% TNP or 4% FITC in absolute ethanol intradermally to the abdominal wall. Seven days later, 0.02 ml of 1% TNP or 1% FITC in olive oil was supplied to each side of the ear from a 25 gauge needle. Ear thickness was measured using a Peacock G1 dial thickness gauge (Ozaki Co., Tokyo). The results were expressed as the mean increment of ear thickness (10^{-2} mm).

Glomerular Labeling

Isolated glomeruli were incubated with monoclonal antibodies according to a modification of the method described by Schreiner et al. [4]. After washing, each preparation was incubated with FITC-conjugated rabbit anti-mouse immunoglobulins. The number of labeled cells per glomerulus was determined by focusing through whole glomerulus and counting.

Histological Examination

For light microscopy, renal tissue was fixed in buffered formalin and embedded in paraffin; 4 μm sections were stained with hematoxylin-eosin, periodic acid-Schiff, or periodic acid silver hematoxylin. For immunofluorescence, the material was snap-frozen in hexane cooled to −70 C.

Experimental Schedule

Unilateral renal perfusion was carried out to examine the nephritogenic potential of the test materials. Four groups of experiments were performed according to Table 1 in the Result section.

Results and Discussion

Characterization of Antigen Preparation

Table 1 shows the experimental schedule and characterization of the hapten-carrier protein used in each group. Native or cationized hapten-carrier protein, 500 μg, was injected intrarenally.

Table 1. Experimental design

Group	Sensitization	Renal perfusion
Group A	TNP	TNP.cat-BSA (P I≥9.3)
Group B	TNP	FITC.cat-BSA (P I=6.5–7.5)
Group C	FITC	TNP.cat-BSA (P I≥9.3)
Group D	–	TNP.nat-BSA (P I=4.6)

TNP, trinitrophenol; BSA, bovine serum albumin; FITC, fluorescein isothiocyanate

Contact Hypersensitivity to the TNP Haptenic Group

In TNP-sensitized group A, the standard ear-reaction when challenged with TNP showed an enhancement significantly greater than that of the FITC-sensitized group (Table 2).

Histological Changes

Light microscopically, there were no significant abnormalities in the right, unperfused kidneys from rats in TNP-sensitized group A and in bilateral kidneys from control groups B, C, and D. In the perfused kidneys from group A, there were prominent histological changes, such as endocapillary cell proliferation and adhesion of the glomerular capillary wall to Bowman's capsule, as described previously [1]. Figure 1 shows localization of immune reactants in the left kidney from group A. Hapten-specific binding to the glomerular capillary was found, as shown in Fig. 1a (1 hour after injection). The TNP bound to the glomerular capillary wall decreased rapidly with time, leading to moderate staining in a focal pattern within the first 24 hours (Fig. 1b). An interesting finding was that there was no deposition of rat IgG and C3, even in the TNP-sensitized group A, during the examination period (Fig. 1c and d). Immunofluorescent examination revealed a similar distribution and disappearance of TNP in both groups A and C. This finding is consistent with similar disappearance kinetics of ^{125}I-labeled cationized TNP-BSA from the perfused, left kidneys in both groups A and B, as described previously [1]. We have already reported that the presence of cationized antigen in the glomeruli, especially in the glomerular capillary walls, is markedly prolonged when complexed with antibody [2,5]. Since the elimination of the cationized TNP-BSA was not prolonged in sensitized animals, it is unlikely that, in group A, enough antibody was present to produce abnormal lesions with proteinuria.

Table 2. Contact hypersensitivity to TNP

			Increment of ear thickness (10^{-2} mm)		
Group	Sensitization	Challenge	Day 1	Day 2	Day 3
A	TNP	TNP	0.68±0.07	0.85±0.15	0.59±0.14
B	FITC	TNP	0.30±0.03	0.30±0.14	0.18±0.005

TNP, trinitrophenol; FITC, fluorescein isothiocyanate

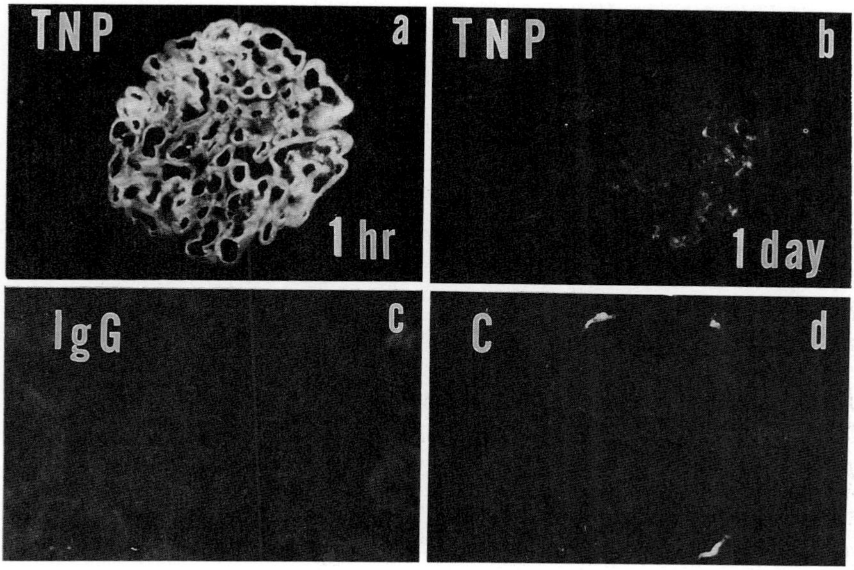

Fig. 1a-c. Cryostat sections of rat glomeruli from group A rats, **a** staining with FITC-anti-TNP-human IgG. At 1 h after renal perfusion with cationized TNP-BSA, **b** Staining with FITC-anti-TNP-human IgG. At 24 h after renal perfusion with cationized TNP-BSA, **c** and **d** Staining for rat IgG (Fig. 2c), and for rat C3 (Fig. 2d), at 1 h. FITC, fluorescein isothiocyanate; TNP, trinitrophenol; BSA, bovine serum albumin

Urinary Protein Analysis

Abnormal urinary protein excretion was seen on day 1 in all rats of the TNP-sensitized group A. The mean was 95 mg per day, but the level varied individually from rat to rat within a range of 35–170 mg per day. The amount of urinary protein in group A decreased rapidly to the point when, by day 2, it was already 13 mg per day. In groups B, C, and D there was no abnormal urinary protein excretion.

Labeled Cells Present in Isolated Glomeruli in this Experimental Glomerulonephritis

We quantified the number of cells bearing the rat leukocyte common antigen, and the Ia antigen, detected by mouse monoclonal antibodies. Many cells were significantly positive for leukocyte common antigen and Ia antigen in the glomerulus from the diseased left kidney (Fig. 2a). In contrast, fewer cells with these markers could be seen in the unperfused right kidney (Fig. 2b). As a control, the monoclonal antibody, RVG1, of the same subclass, IgG1, was substituted for the primary antibody (Fig. 2c).

In general, exudates induced by inflammatory, nonimmunological stimuli, such as thioglycollate broth or mineral oil were enriched for Ia-negative cells. Only 1%–4% of circulating monocyte-macrophages were Ia-positive. On the other hand, it is well

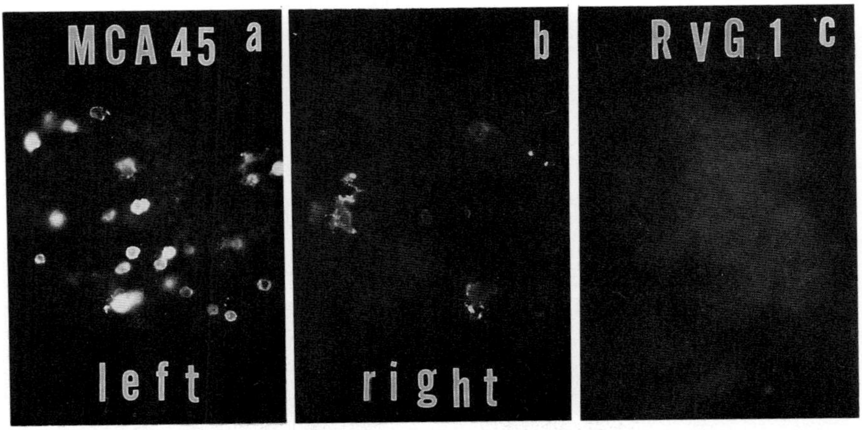

Fig. 2a-c. Fluorescent micrographs of isolated glomeruli on day 1, stained for cells bearing the rat Ia antigen, **a** A glomerulus from the perfused left kidney, **b** A glomerulus from the unperfused right kidney, **c** A glomerulus from the perfused left kidney, reacted with the control monoclonal antibody RVG1, instead of MCA 45, as a primary antibody

known that Ia-positive macrophages predominate in the exudates induced by the interaction of antigen-stimulated T cells and macrophages.

We have reported here that the development of proliferative glomerulonephritis with transient, but significant, proteinuria resulted from sensitization with a hapten, TNP. A cellular influx, including Ia-positive cells, was seen without deposition of any autologous antibody. We believe that the glomerular injury produced in this model is induced solely by cell-mediated immune reaction.

Acknowledgment. This work was supported by research grants (59570145, 60570153, 63570155) from The Ministry of Education, Science and Culture, Japan.

References

1. Oite T, Shimizu F, Kagami S, Morioka T (1989) Hapten-specific cellular immune response producing glomerular injury. Clin Exp Immunol 76:463–468
2. Oite T, Batsford SR, Mihatsch MJ, Takamiya H, Vogt A (1982) Quantitative studies of in situ immune complex glomerulonephritis in the rat induced by planted, cationized antigen. J Exp Med 155:460–474
3. Kagami S, Miyao M, Shimizu F, Oite T (1988) An active in situ immune complex glomerulonephritis using the hapten-carrier system: role of epitope density in cationic antigens. Clin Exp Immunol 74:121–125
4. Schreiner GF, Kiely J-M, Cotran RS, Unanue ER (1981) Characterization of resident glomerular cells in the rat expressing Ia determinants and manifesting genetically restricted interactions with lymphocytes. J Clin Invest 68:920–931
5. Oite T, Shimizu F, Kihara I, Batsford SR, Vogt A (1983) An active model of immune complex glomerulonephritis in the rat employing cationized antigen. Am J Pathol 112:185–194

Role of Potassium in Acid-Base Disturbances

Chair: F. John Gennari (USA)
Yasushi Asano (Japan)

Acid-Base Implications of the K-NH_4 Interactions

RICHARD L. TANNEN[1]

SUMMARY. Observations in animals and humans in vivo, as well as direct investigation of kidney tissue in vitro, indicate that alterations in potassium have a profound effect on renal ammonia production. Potassium depletion results in an adaptive increase in ammonia production by the kidney similar to the changes produced by chronic metabolic acidosis, suggesting that altered ammoniagenesis in both conditions may be initiated by a decrease in proximal tubular intracellular pH. Hyperkalemia inhibits ammonia production directly, but does not appear to induce an adaptive down regulation in the renal capacity to produce ammonia. The direct effects of a low potassium concentration on ammonia production are not definitively resolved.

Potassium-induced alterations in ammonia homeostasis appear to play an important role in the pathogenesis of metabolic alkalosis induced by potassium depletion and in the hyperchloremic metabolic acidosis found in patients with Type IV renal tubular acidosis (RTA).

Introduction

Ammonia production and excretion are crucial components of the kidney's capacity to excrete acid. It is now well established that potassium as well as on acid-base status can exert profound effects on ammonia metabolism. This review will address the physiologic observations relevant to this relationship in animals and humans, the biochemical studies focused on the impact of potassium on the regulation of ammonia production, and the role played by the interaction between potassium and ammonia in the production of the acid-base abnormalities which accompany states of potassium depletion and excess.

[1]LA County/USC Medical Center, 2025 Zonal Ave., Rm. 7900, Los Angeles, CA 90033, USA

Physiologic Observations

Studies, dating back to the 1950s, of potassium depletion induced experimentally or produced clinically by several conditions, including laxative abuse, primary hyperaldosteronism, and fasting, have suggested that urinary pH and ammonium excretion were perturbed. Increased ammonium excretion, a high urine pH with normal ammonium excretion, and a high rate of ammonium excretion relative to urine pH, were all described (See [1] for a listing of these publications).

In order to investigate the relationship between potassium depletion and ammonia in more detail, I carried out a study of urine acidification in normal men, who were subjected to mild, experimentally-induced potassium depletion [2]. After ingestion of a standard acute ammonium chloride load, urine pH was found to be higher in the potassium depleted state in comparison with paired observations obtained under conditions of normal potassium balance. The increase in urine pH was accompanied by an increase in ammonium and net acid excretion; calculated urinary free ammonia concentration was also higher during potassium depletion. These changes were demonstrable with deficits of potassium as modest as approximately 200 mEq.

This combination of findings, i.e., a concurrent increase in both urine pH and ammonium excretion, seemed to be best explained by an enhanced rate of ammonia diffusion into the urine as a result of a primary increase in renal ammonia production. Alternatively, a decrease in renal blood flow could, theoretically, result in urinary elimination of a higher percentage of the ammonia produced by the kidney, with a concurrent reduction of ammonia release into the renal venous effluent.

Similar studies of urine acidification were also performed in normal men who had had a high potassium intake (3.0 − 6.0 mmoles/kg per day) for five days [3]. As found in studies of potassium depletion, chronic potassium loading produced no detectable effects on blood acid-base parameters, on urinary flow rate, or on nonvolatile buffer excretion (i.e., phosphate, creatinine, and organic acids). Urine pH in the potassium loaded state was lower than during control conditions by a mean of 0.21 U. Furthermore, the largest decrements in urine pH were accompanied by decreased excretion rates of both ammonium and net acid.

These findings suggested that a potassium surfeit diminished renal ammonia production. However, the possibility that an increase in renal blood flow accounted for the primary decrease in ammonia diffusion into the urine could not be excluded [4].

In the aggregate, these studies with potassium depletion and loading indicated that an important relationship existed between potassium homeostasis and renal ammonia production. Furthermore, the ability to detect alterations in ammonia metabolism with a modest potassium depletion of only 200 mmoles (i.e., approximately 5% of total body stores) and an equally modest potassium retention, which approximated 219 mmoles, suggested that this relationship might be a physiologic, rather than a pathologic, phenomenon. A variety of experimental approaches have been utilized to more precisely delineate the biochemical mechanisms underlying the influence of potassium on ammonia metabolism.

Biochemical Studies

The impact of potassium depletion on ammoniagenesis has been subjected to intense scrutiny. Increased renal ammonia production, with potassium depletion, has been documented in intact humans and rats by the simultaneous measurement of urinary and renal venous ammonia content [5–8]. Furthermore, studies utilizing renal cortical tissue and isolated mitochondria from both rats and dogs have shown that an adaptive increase in the capacity to produce ammonia is induced by potassium depletion [9–14].

The adaptive alterations produced by potassium depletion in the rat are virtually identical, for the most part, with those manifested during the adaptation of ammoniagenesis to chronic metabolic acidosis (see [1]). Both these conditions increase the activity of the cytosolic enzymes of the glutaminase II pathway and purine nucleotide cycle, and decrease the conversion of glutamate to glutamine, suggesting an inhibition of glutamine synthetase activity. They also similarly affect the intramitochondrial ammoniagenic pathway, which is currently believed to be the primary regulator of renal ammoniagenesis. The activity of phosphate dependent glutaminase (PDG) is increased with specific localization to the proximal tubule [15]; mitochondrial entry of glutamine is enhanced; ammonia production by rotenone-inhibited mitochondria is increased, providing a functional correlate of increased glutamine transport and/or PDG activity; flux through glutamate dehydrogenase is accelerated; the activity of phosphoenolpyruvate carboxykinase (PEPCK) and the production of glucose is increased; the generation of 14 CO_2 from U-14C glutamine is modified, suggesting alterations in metabolism of the glutamine carbon skeleton by the tricarboxylic acid (TCA) cycle; and the rate of citrate decarboxylation is increased.

The controversy regarding which metabolic alteration is primarily responsible for the increase in ammoniagenesis in potassium depletion is as equally unresolved as the controversy over metabolic acidosis. The data suggest that alterations, in either the mitochondrial glutamine transporter and/or the activity of PDG, are essential components of the adaptive response, but the precise importance of alterations in flux through glutamate dehydrogenase and through PEPCK to glucose are still unclear.

In view of the similarities, it is tempting to suggest that a similar mechanism might account for the development of an adaptive increase in the capacity to produce ammonia with both potassium depletion and chronic metabolic acidosis. Supporting this view, the production of metabolic alkalosis by the ingestion of sodium bicarbonate suppresses renal ammonia production in rats with potassium deficiency [7]. The most attractive unifying hypothesis is that both conditions are accompanied by a similar decrease in intracellular pH of the proximal tubular cells. This concept is supported, indirectly, by the changes in citrate metabolism produced by both conditions [16]. Direct measurements of renal intracellular pH using nuclear magnetic resonance (NMR) are also consistent with this hypothesis [17].

The direct effect of a low potassium concentration, per se, on renal ammonia production is not resolved definitively. Studies employing renal cortical slices bathed in a potassium free medium have reported an increase in ammonia production [18]. However, experiments in our laboratory did not detect increased ammoniagenesis by isolated renal cortical mitochondria exposed to a low potassium concentration; nor did we detect increased ammoniagenesis by either isolated cortical tubules or the isolated perfused rat kidney subjected to a reduction of ambient potassium concentration to 2.0 mM [13,19]. A recent preliminary report, in which isolated microperfused proximal tubules from the mouse were used, found that when the bath potassium was reduced to 2.0 mM there was a 20% increase in ammonia production [20].

There has been considerably less investigation of the effects of a potassium surfeit, as compared with a deficit, on ammonia production. To date, despite a variety of observations in humans, rats, and dogs, that a high potassium diet decreases urine pH and ammonium excretion, no direct measurements of the effects of high potassium on renal ammoniagenesis in vivo have been reported.

Furthermore, studies of isolated tissues in vitro have not yielded any convincing evidence that a potassium surfeit results in an adaptive down regulation of the ammoniagenic capacity of the kidney. Ingestion of a high potassium diet had no discernible effect on ammonia production by either isolated renal cortical mitochondria or by the isolated perfused kidney [13,19]. An earlier report from our laboratory found that ingestion of a high potassium diet produced a 5% decline in ammoniagenesis, seen in slices from the renal cortex, and a more impressive 36% decline, seen in slices from the outer medulla, but the implications of this finding are currently unclear [14]. However, it is important to emphasize that all these studies examined only the effects of a high potassium diet and not the potential effects of sustained hyperkalemia on adaptive changes in ammoniagenesis.

The direct effect of a high potassium concentration on renal ammonia production has also not undergone extensive investigation; but the results reported are quite uniform. Studies utilizing the isolated perfused kidney, renal cortical tubules, renal cortical slices, and isolated microperfused mouse proximal tubules, all indicate that a high potassium concentration directly inhibits ammonia production [18–20]. The suppressive effect has been demonstrated with potassium concentrations in the range of 7.5–10.4 mM. While it is tempting to speculate that this direct effect of potassium concentration accounts for the apparent inhibition of ammonia production by a potassium surfeit in vivo, it is important to recognize that some studies have reported urinary changes consistent with diminished ammoniagenesis in the absence of detectable changes in plasma potassium concentration [3,21].

The precise metabolic step at which hyperkalemia influences ammoniagenesis is also unresolved. Some data point to inhibition of glutamate deamination, while other information suggests an inhibition of glutamine deamidation [18,19]. More direct methods of investigating the pathways of ammoniagenesis are required to resolve this issue.

In addition to its effects on ammonia production, hyperkalemia may also directly inhibit the excretion of ammonium into the urine. Recent studies have shown that an increase in bath potassium concentration reduces ammonium absorption by isolated perfused thick ascending limbs of Henle [22,23]. Since ultimate elimination of the ammonium produced and secreted by the proximal tubule is dependent upon reabsorption by the ascending limb, hyperkalemia might directly impair urinary secretion, as well as production, of ammonium.

Acid-Base Abnormalities

As discussed in detail in another contribution to this symposium, (see List of Contents) there is now convincing evidence that potassium depletion can play a role in the development and maintenance of metabolic alkalosis. It seems highly likely that, when an increase in acid excretion is a central part of the pathophysiology, the potassium depletion-induced increase in ammonia production contributes to the generation of alkalosis. Furthermore, potassium depletion-induced increase in ammonia production may also play an important role in the maintenance of metabolic alkalosis by sustaining ammonium, and thereby acid excretion, in the face of the suppressive effects of metabolic alkalosis.

Although ingestion of a high potassium diet in normal humans appears to have no effect on systemic acid-base homeostasis [3], the hyperkalemic effect on ammonia production appears to play a crucial role in the metabolic acidosis associated with two important clinical hyperkalemic syndromes. It is now widely recognized that hyperkalemia, often in association with hyperchloremic metabolic acidosis, is a manifestation of the renal disease which is associated with either hyporeninemic hypoaldosteronism or with aldosterone independent defects in tubular potassium secretion.

The seminal study in humans, done by Szylman and co-workers [24], and subsequent detailed investigations by Sebastian, Schambelan, and their co-workers [25,26], demonstrated that correction of hyperkalemia by the use of cation exchange resins, mineralocorticoids, or dietary potassium restriction, produced a concomitant correction of metabolic acidosis. Furthermore, the improvement in acid-base status was accompanied by changes in urinary pH and ammonium excretion consistent with an increase in renal ammonia production.

In contrast to the findings in humans, correction of hyperkalemia in mineralocorticoid-deficient dogs does not improve metabolic acidosis, despite the anticipated changes in urine pH and ammonium excretion [27]. However, additional studies from this same laboratory have elegantly shown that adrenalectomized, steroid-replaced dogs maintained on a phosphate restricted diet develop hyperkalemia and metabolic acidosis when challenged with a high KCl intake [28]. In response to KCl, these animals exhibited a reduction in urinary net acid excretion, accompanied by a decrease in urine pH and ammonium excretion, which was consistent with a reduction in ammonia production. Thus, it seems clear that in certain circumstances in animals, as well as in humans, hyperkalemia can result in metabolic acidosis. Furthermore, the acid-base abnormality appears to result, at least in part, from an effect of potassium on ammonia metabolism.

References

1. Tannen RL (1977) Relationship of renal production and potassium homeostasis. Kidney Int 11:453–465
2. Tannen RL (1970) The effect of uncomplicated potassium depletion on urine acidification. J Clin Invest 49:813–827
3. Tannen RL, Wedell E, Moore R (1973) Renal adaptation to a high potassium intake: The role of hydrogen ion. J Clin Invest 52:2089–2101
4. Hollenberg NK, Williams G, Burger B, Hooshmand I (1975) The influence of potassium on the renal vasculature and the adrenal gland, and their responsiveness to angiotensin II in normal man. Clin Sci 48:527–534
5. Baertl JM, Sancetta SM, Gabuzda GH (1963) Relation of acute potassium depletion to renal ammonium metabolism in patients with cirrhosis. J Clin Invest 42:696–706
6. Gabuzda GJ, Hall PW III (1966) Relation of potassium depletion to renal ammonium metabolism and hepatic coma. Medicine (Baltimore) 45:481–490

7. Tollins JP, Hostetter MK, Hostetter MK, Hostetter TH (1987) Hypokalemic nephropathy in the rat: The role of ammonia in chronic tubular injury. J Clin Invest 79:1447–1458
8. Yablon S, Relman AS (1977) Excretion and total renal production of ammonia in K^+-depleted rats. Clin Res 25:452A
9. Adam WR, Simpson DP (1975) Renal mitochondrial glutamine metabolism and dietary potassium and protein content. Kidney 7:325–330
10. Kamm DE, Strope GL (1973) Glutamine and glutamate metabolism in renal cortex from potassium-depleted rats. Am J Physiol 224:1241–1248
11. Pagliara AS, Goodman AD (1970) Relation of renal cortical gluconeogenesis, glutamate content, and production of ammonia. J Clin Invest 49:1967–1974
12. Sastrasinh S, Sastrasinh M (1986) Renal mitochondrial glutamine metabolism during K^+ depletion. Am J Physiol 250:F667–F673
13. Tannen RL, Kunin AS (1976) Effect of potassium on ammoniagenesis by renal mitochondria. Am J Physiol 231:44–51
14. Tannen RL, McGill J (1976) The influence of potassium on renal ammonia production. Am J Physiol 231:1178–1184
15. Nonoguchi H, Takehara Y, Endou H (1986) Intra- and inter-nephron heterogeneity of ammoniagenesis in rats: effects of chronic metabolic acidosis and potassium depletion. Pflugers Arch 407:245–251
16. Adler S, Zett B, Anderson B (1974) Renal citrate in the potassium deficient rat: Role of potassium and chloride ions. J Lab Clin Med 84:307–316
17. Adam WR, Koretsky AP, Weiner MW (1986) ^{31}P-NMR in vivo measurement of renal intracellular pH: Effects of acidosis and K^+ depletion in rats. Am J Physiol 251:F904–F910
18. Sleeper RS, Belanger P, Lemieux G, Preuss HG (1982) Effects of in vitro potassium on ammoniagenesis in rat and canine kidney tissue. Kidney Int 21:345–353
19. Sastrasinh S, Tannen RL (1983) Effect of potassium on renal NH_3 production. Am J Physiol 244:F383–F391
20. Nagami GT, Lee P (1987) Ammonia production by isolated perfused mouse proximal tubules. Effect of bath and luminal potassium concentration. Abstr Am Soc Nephrol 20:258A
21. Kamm DE (1971) Dissociation of urine pH and NH_3 excretion during KCl and NaCl loading. Abstr Am Soc Nephrol 5:36
22. Good DW (Nov 1987) Effects of potassium on ammonia transport by medullary thick ascending limb of the rat. J Clin Invest 80:1358–1365
23. Good DW (1988) Active absorption of NH^+_4 by rat medullary thick ascending limb: inhibition by potassium. Am J Physiol 255 (Renal Fluid Electrolyte Physiol 24):F78–F87
24. Szylman P, Better OS, Chaimowitz C, Rosler A (1976) Role of hyperkalemia in the metabolic acidosis of isolated hypoaldosteronism. New Engl J Med 294:361–365
25. Sabastian A, Schambelan M, Lindenfeld S, Morris RC Jr (1977) Amelioration of metabolic acidosis with fluorocortisone therapy in hyporeninemic hypoaldosteronism. New Engl J Med 297:576–583
26. Maher T, Schambelan M, Kurtz I, Hulter HN, Jones JW, Sebastian A (1984) Amelioration of metabolic acidosis by dietary potassium restriction in hyperkalemic patients with chronic renal insufficiency. J Lab Clin Med 103:432–445
27. Hulter HN, Licht JH, Glynn RD, Sebastian A (1979) Renal acidosis in mineralocorticoid deficiency is not dependent on NaCl depletion or hyperkalemia. Am J Physiol 236:F283–F294
28. Hulter HN, Toto RD, Iinicki LP, Sebastian A (1983) Chronic hyperkalemic renal tubular acidosis induced by KCl loading. Am J Physiol 244:F255–F264

Reabsorption of Bicarbonate Along the Nephron: Importance of Potassium

GIOVAMBATTISTA CAPASSO[1], ROBERT UNWIN[2], and GERHARD GIEBISCH[3]

SUMMARY. In order to assess the relationship between potassium and renal bicarbonate transport, micropuncture studies were carried out on superficial rat nephrons. The microcalorimetric method was used to quantitate bicarbonate reabsorption ($JHCO_3$). Two segments were studied: 1) the loop of Henle and 2) the distal tubule. In the first set of experiments, superficial loops of Henle were microperfused in vivo from late proximal to early distal tubule. Three groups of rats were investigated: 1) control rats 2) rats maintained either on 2) low or 3) high potassium diets. The loops were perfused with solutions containing 2 or 4 mM K^+. In control conditions $JHCO_3$ was 150.3 ± 5.0 pmol/min. This value was not affected by low or high potassium diet. In the second set of experiments free-flow micropuncture studies were carried out on superficial rat distal tubules. Experiments were performed in a) control conditions and b) during dietary potassium withdrawal. In normal conditions we observed highly significant, load dependent, net $JHCO_3$. Distal bicarbonate reabsorption persisted in hypokalemic alkalosis and, at comparable early distal loads, hypokalemia exerted a powerful stimulation on distal $JHCO_3$. These data demonstrate that along the loop of Henle, $JHCO_3$ is unaffected by changes in potassium intake, while in the distal tubule $JHCO_3$ is stimulated by potassium depletion.

Introduction

It is well established that, between potassium and hydrogen ions, there is a very close interaction at the cellular level that can lead to a mutual interplay of acid-base and potassium regulation. For example, changes in whole acid-base balance have been shown to influence the level of intracellular potassium activity [1], while alterations

[1]Chair of Nephrology, University of Naples, 80100 Naples, Italy

[2]Department of Cellular and Molecular Physiology, Yale Medical School, USA

[3]Department of Clinical Pharmacology, Hammersmith Hospital, London, UK

in potassium balance exert important effects on intracellular pH [2]. With respect to the kidney function it has been found that acidosis inhibits K^+ secretion in the distal tubule [2], while changes in body potassium distribution may influence acid-base transport along the nephron [3].

Although the proximal tubule is thought to be the major site of renal acidification [4], recent studies have shown that the distal nephron can make a significant contribution to the final urine pH. Our interest has been focused on two nephron segments: the loop of Henle and the cortical distal tubule. As opposed to the so-called proximal nephron, these segments have a much more pronounced heterogeneity, both from a morphological and from a functional point of view [5]. The loop of Henle comprises: a part of the late proximal convoluted tubule and the straight portion of the proximal tubule, the thin descending and ascending limbs, the thick ascending limb, and a small portion of the early distal tubule. The distal tubule is considered to be the segment starting at the macula densa and ending at the first junction with another distal tubule to form the collecting duct. It is certainly the most heterogeneous segment of the nephron; it contains at least three distinct sub-segments. The first of these is the distal convoluted tubule; the following segment is the connecting tubule which is lined by connecting tubule cells and by intercalated cells in relatively low density. The last segment is the initial cortical collecting duct, composed of a majority of principal cells and containing, in addition, intercalated cells (alfa and beta forms).

In the present study we have pursued two objectives: first, to assess the contribution and to elucidate the mechanisms involved in acid-base transport along these two heterogeneous segments. Second, to evaluate, in the same segments, the relationship between serum potassium level and bicarbonate transport. This last issue was studied by modulating the potassium intake through diets of different potassium content.

Methods

Preparation of Animals

Male rats were anesthetized with Inactin (Promonta, West Germany) using a dose of 120 mg/kg body weight, intraperitoneally; they were then tracheostomized and placed on a thermoregulated table designed to hold body temperature at 37°C. The right carotid artery was catheterized for blood pressure monitoring and periodic blood sampling for measurements of hematocrit, radioactive inulin, pH and total CO_2 concentration. The left jugular vein was cannulated with PE-50 tubing and used for infusion via a syringe pump. The left kidney was exposed through a flank incision, made free of perirenal fat, decapsulated and immobilized in a lucite chamber. The left ureter was catheterized for collection of urine. Three groups of rats were studied: (1) control rats maintained on a diet of standard Purina laboratory chow; (2) low potassium rats, maintained on a low potassium diet for at least three weeks; and (3) rats maintained on 10% potassium diet (potassium adapted animals).

Microperfusion of the loop of Henle

A perfusion pipette was inserted in the last surface loop of the proximal tubule and a castor oil block was placed upstream of the perfusion pipette. Microperfusion was

Table 1. Summary of baseline data (mean ± SEM) of rats fed with diet at different K content (*$p<0.005$ vs control)

Rats	Blood K^+ (nEq/lt)	Blood pH	Blood HCO_3 (mM)
Control	4.1 ± 0.1	7.348 ± 0.04	29.3 ± 0.3
Low K	2.5 ± 0.1*	7.532 ± 0.1*	36.0 ± 1.3*
K adapted	4.0 ± 0.2	7.372 ± 0.05	29.1 ± 0.7

started at 20 nl/min with a thermally shielded microperfusion pump. The perfusion solution was an end-proximal solution containing, in addition, 0.07% FD&C blue dye and ^{14}C-insulin.

Free-flow collections

After completion of surgery, methoxy-^3H-inulin (110 μCi/h following a priming injection of 90 μCi) was infused i.v. Collections of tubule fluid samples were begun after a 1 h equilibration period. Early and late distal segments were identified by the i.v. injection of 20 μl FDC solution. Puncture sites were recognized by filling the tubule with a microfil silicone rubber compound. The kidneys were then macerated overnight in 25% NaOH and the puncture sites determined by microdissection.

Analytical methods

Tubule fluid total CO_2 concentration was determined by microcalorimetry. The blood acid-base status of each animal was measured with a blood-gas analyzer. Radioactivity was measured by a liquid scintillation counter and plasma electrolytes were measured by flame photometry.

Results

Table 1 summarizes data on blood electrolytes and systemic acid-base parameters in control, potassium depleted, and potassium adapted animals. As expected, plasma potassium was markedly depressed in group (2), whereas blood pH and bicarbonate were significantly increased. In potassium adapted rats (group 3) no changes were detected.

Loop of Henle

Figure 1 shows the effects of various inhibitors on fractional bicarbonate transport ($FRHCO_3$) along the loop of Henle. In the presence of the carbonic anhydrase inhibitor methazolamide (2.10^{-4} M) $FRHCO_3$ was reduced by 73% ($P<0.01$); the Na^+-H^+ exchange inhibitor ethylisopropylamiloride (2.10^{-4} M) reduced $FRHCO_3$ by 39% ($P<0.01$); and the H^+-ATPase inhibitor bafilomycin A_1 reduced $FRHCO_3$ by 26% ($P<0.01$). The Cl^- channel blocker NPPB (5-nitro-2′-(3-phenylpropylamino)-benzoate) (2.10^{-4} M) and the anion exchange inhibitor DIDS (diidothiocyanato-2,2′-stilbenedisulfonate) (5.10^{-5} M) had no effect on $FRHCO_3$.

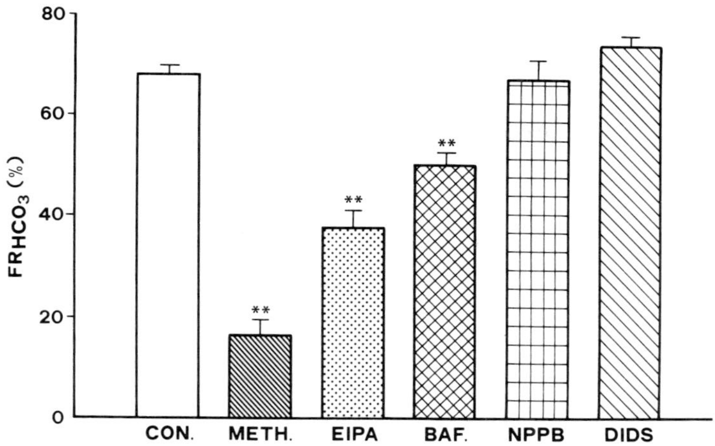

Fig. 1. Effect of several transport inhibitors on fractional bicarbonate reabsorption (*FRHCO$_3$*) along the loop of Henle ($^{**}P<0.01$ vs CON). CON, control; METH, methazolamide; EIPA, ethylisopropylamiloride; BAF, bafilomycin A_1; NPPB, 5-nitro-(-3-phenylpropylamino) benzoate; DIDS, diisothiocyanato-2-2′-stilben edisulfonate

In hypokalemic rats, $JHCO_3$ in the loop was 150.9±8.6 pmol/min (n=19); this value was not different from that obtained in control rats perfused with the same solution containing 2 mM K^+ (152.3±11.2 pmol/min, n=17).

In potassium adapted animals, loop $JHCO_3$ was 152.1 ± 6.3; this value was similar to that found in control animals.

Distal tubule

Figure 2 shows fractional bicarbonate delivery in the control group plotted as function of distal tubular length. Between 20% and 95% distal tubular length, a mean of some 6% of the filtered bicarbonate was reabsorbed. Accordingly, significant bicarbonate reabsorption takes place along the superficial distal tubule.

Figure 3 shows the data on the fractional reabsorption of bicarbonate along the distal tubule during hypokalemia. The figure clearly indicates that significant net bicarbonate reabsorption was uniformly observed along the distal tubule in hypokalemic rats.

Figure 4 provides a schematic overview of absolute bicarbonate reabsorption rates along the distal tubule, with and without bicarbonate loading, in control and hypokalemic conditions. It is important to note that in the presence of closely similar early distal bicarbonate loads in control and in K depletion, distal $JHCO_3$ was significantly higher in low-K rats compared with control rats. Moreover, both values are severalfold higher than corresponding values for bicarbonate reabsorption in the non-bicarbonate-loaded conditions. Thus, distal $JHCO_3$ in bicarbonate loaded control rats was 3.6 times higher than in non loaded rats, whereas in low-K rats, bicarbonate loading resulted in 5.4-fold stimulation of $JHCO_3$.

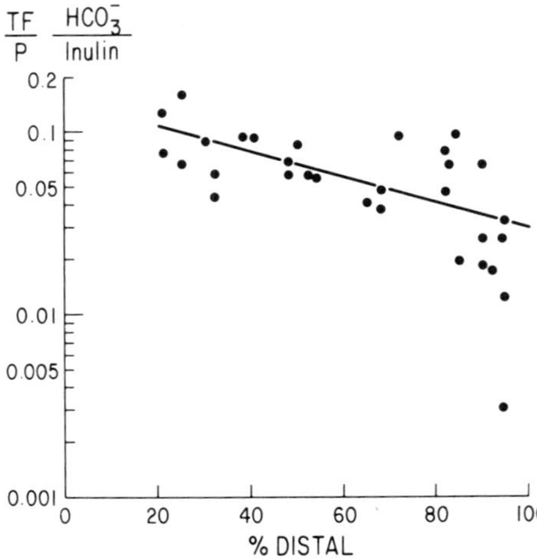

Fig. 2. Summary of fractional bicarbonate concentration ratios as function of distal tubular length of control rats. (From [10] with permission)

Discussion

Bicarbonate transport along the loop of Henle

The data presented show that about 15% of filtered bicarbonate is reabsorbed along the loop of Henle. Such transport is sensitive to inhibition by carbonic anhydrase, but there appears to be a carbonic anhydrase insensitive component. There was no major

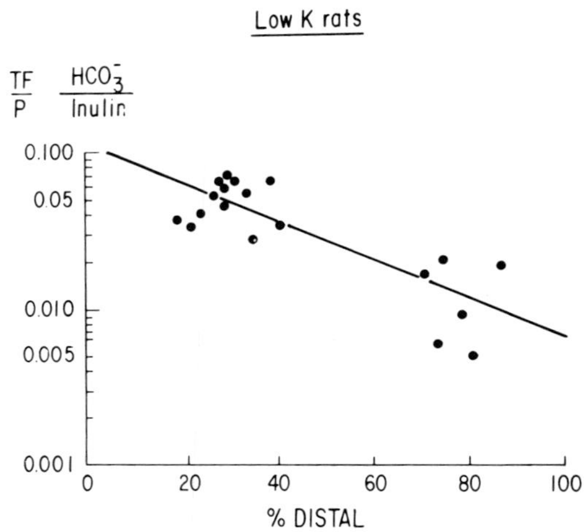

Fig. 3. Summary of fractional bicarbonate concentration ratios as function of distal tubular length of hypokalemic rats. (From [10] with permission)

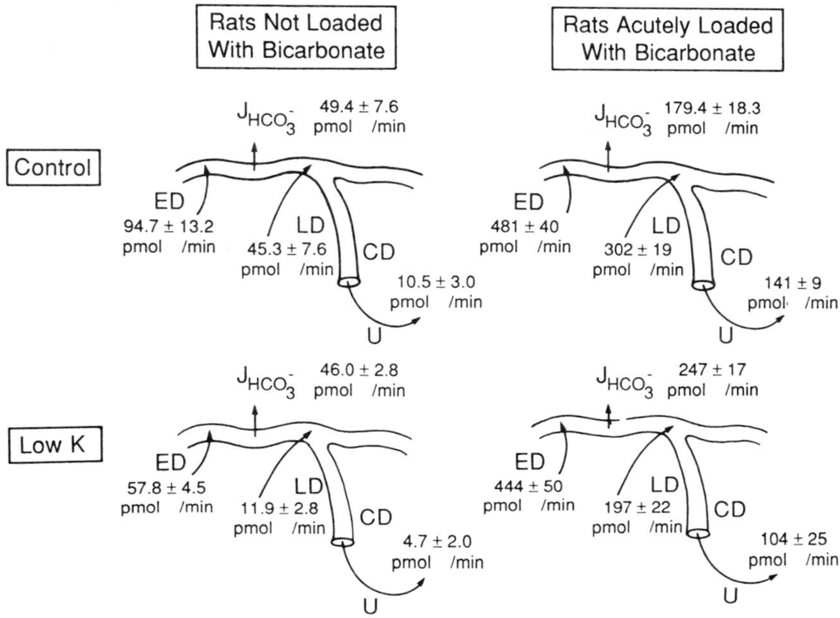

Fig. 4. Schematic summary of bicarbonate reabsorption along the superficial distal tubule of the rat. (From [14] with permission).

contribution to net bicarbonate transport by the Cl-HCO_3 exchanger. The bulk of loop of Henle bicarbonate transport is dependent on the presence of Na^+-H^+ exchanger and the proton pump. The data on the effect of potassium depletion on $JHCO_3$ are interesting. In contrast with the distal tubule, where in low K rats we found an increase in $JHCO_3$, we measured no difference in $JHCO_3$ between control and low K rats, when the loops were perfused with the same potassium concentration. One possible explanation could be related to the higher back-flux of bicarbonate. This effect would be facilitated by the steeper bicarbonate gradient and the relatively high bicarbonate permeability of the various segments that make up the loop of Henle. Such an interpretation is consistent with the data of Byers et al. [6], who found an accumulation of 6 mM bicarbonate in loops of Henle perfused with bicarbonate free solutions; and consistent with our observations that even in the presence of a potent carbonic anhydrase inhibitor, like methazolamide, we did not measure a bicarbonate concentration of less than 4 mM in collected fluid. Therefore it is entirely possible that in low potassium rats there could be an increase in bicarbonate transport, but this is offset by the larger bicarbonate back flux. With respect to $JHCO_3$ along the loop in potassium adapted animals the data presented seem to indicate that such a maneuver has no significant influence on loop bicarbonate handling.

Bicarbonate transport in the distal tubule

Studies in which luminal pH was used to estimate bicarbonate concentrations showed that bicarbonate remained approximately constant along the distal tubule. Distal bicarbonate reabsorption calculated from these values, and from inulin concentration ratios, yields an overall reabsorption rate of 5–8% of the filtered load along the distal tubule [7]. Pump-perfusion experiments in distal tubules have cast doubts on the capacity of these segments to acidify the urine. Lucci et al. [8] perfused these tubules with bicarbonate containing solutions and found that only in chronic metabolic acidosis was significant reabsorption of bicarbonate observed. These studies were more recently confirmed by Levine [9]. In our free-flow micropuncture study [10] the results obtained did not differ from the experiments in which bicarbonate concentrations were evaluated by measuring the pH of tubule fluid [7]. The fact that the bicarbonate concentration along the distal tubule was maintained at low levels, despite significant fluid reabsorption, demonstrates significant net bicarbonate reabsorption along the distal tubule in conditions of normal acid-base balance. Very recently, Levine et al. found that overnight fasting induced significant, load dependent distal bicarbonate reabsorption, whereas when normally fed rats were studied no net bicarbonate reabsorption was found [11].

In K-depleted rats, a distal reabsorption rate of 46 pmol/min was measured at a distal load of 58 pmol/min, that is, about 80% of the segmental load was reabsorbed. In control rats a similar net amount of bicarbonate was reabsorbed at a distal load of 95 pmol/min, corresponding to a reabsorption of only 52% of the segmental load. When low K rats were compared with control rats subject to acute bicarbonate loading, both groups having a similar distal bicarbonate load, significantly more bicarbonate was reabsorbed along the distal tubule in low K rats. Although direct cell pH measurements have not yet been done in cells of the distal tubule, it is possible that cell acidification, postulated to occur in tubule cells during hypokalemia, may be responsible for enhanced bicarbonate transport. Furthermore, the observation that during potassium depletion there is an activation along the distal tubule of a K/H-ATPase [12], would be consistent with our findings. Such an interpretation would be strengthened by the observation that the intercalated cells of the rat medullary collecting duct exhibit an increase in luminal membrane surface area under conditions of K^+ depletion [13]. Finally we would like to emphasize that the changes in bicarbonate transport could not have been due to alteration in circulating aldosterone, since hypokalemia depressed aldosterone secretion.

References

1. Kubota TK, Biagi BA, Giebisch G (1983) Effects of acid base disturbances on basolateral membrane potential and intracellular potassium activity in the proximal tubule of Necturus. J Membr Biol 73:61–68
2. Stanton BA, Giebisch G (1982) Effects of pH on K^+ transport by renal distal tubule. Am J Physiol 241:F544–F551
3. Chan YL, Biagi B, Giebisch G (1982) Control mechanisms of bicarbonate transport across the rat proximal convoluted tubule. Am J Physiol 242:F532–F543
4. Cogan MG, Alpern RJ (1984) Regulation of proximal bicarbonate reabsorption. Am J Physiol 247:F387–F395
5. Madsen KM, Tisher CC (1986) Structural-functional relationship along the distal nephron. Am J Physiol 250:F1–F15
6. Byers MK, Levine DZ, McLeod RA, Luisello JA (1979) Loop of Henle bicarbonate accumulation in vivo in the rat. J Clin Invest 63:59–66

7. Malnic G, De Mello, Aires M, Giebisch G (1972) Micropuncture study of renal tubular hydrogen ion transport in the rat. Am J Physiol 222:147–158
8. Lucci MS, Pucacco LR, Carter NW, Dubose TD (1982) Evaluation of bicarbonate transport in rat distal tubule: effects of acid-base status. Am J Physiol 243:F335–F341
9. Levine DZ (1985) An in vivo microperfusion study of distal tubule bicarbonate absorption in normal and ammonium chloride rats. J Clin Invest 75:588–595
10. Capasso G, Kinne R, Malnic G, Giebisch G (1986) Renal bicarbonate reabsorption in the rat. I, Effects of hypokalemia and carbonic anhydrase. J Clin Invest 78:1558–1567
11. Levine DZ, Iacovitti M, Nash L, Vandorpe D (1988) Secretion of bicarbonate by rat distal tubules in vivo. J Clin Invest 81:1873–1878
12. Doucet A, Marsy S (1987) Characterization of K-ATPase activity in distal nephron: stimulation by potassium depletion. Am J Physiol 253:F418–F423
13. Stetson DL, Wade JB, Giebisch G (1980) Morphologic alteration in the rat medullary collecting duct following potassium depletion. Kidney Int 17:4556
14. Capasso G et al. (1987) Renal bicarbonate reabsorption in the rat -II. Distal tubule load dependence and the effect of hypokalemia. J Clin Invest 80:409–414

Role of Acid-Base Disturbance on Potassium Transport Along the Nephron

Kaoru Tabei, Shigeaki Muto, Hiroaki Furuya, Yasunori Sakairi, Yasuhiro Ando, and Yasushi Asano[1]

Summary. We evaluated the role of acidosis on the regulation of transepithelial potassium transport in rabbit early proximal convoluted tubules (PCT) and cortical collecting ducts (CCD) by using in vitro microperfusion and conventional microelectrode methods. In PCT, when the bath medium pH declined from 7.4 to 6.8, transepithelial voltage (Vt) and net potassium flux (JK) increased; however, in CCD, Vt and JK decreased significantly without changing net Na flux. In CCD, basolateral acidosis decreased basolateral membrane voltage and increased transepithelial resistance, with an increment of calculated fractional resistance of apical membrane in principal cells. Inhibition of JK by basolateral acidosis remained significant in the presence of 2mM luminal $BaCl_2$. Elimination of ambient bicarbonate (Hepes buffer solution) did not affect the inhibitory effect of basolateral acidosis on JK. Basolateral 1 mM amiloride diminished the inhibitory effect of basolateral acidosis on JK. The ^{86}Rb and ^{22}Na efflux coefficients were not significantly affected by basolateral acidosis.

In conclusion, the present study demonstrates that basolateral acidosis affects JK in both PCT and CCD, but it does so in opposite directions. In CCD, basolateral pH is indeed an important modulator of epithelial K transport. Mechanistically, basolateral acidosis appears to inhibit apical K conductance independently of Na conductance or ambient bicarbonate in rabbit CCD.

Introduction

The maintenance of potassium balance is vital in several respects; in particular, a high intracellular potassium concentration is essential for operating cell functions and for keeping the normal electrical gradients across the cell membranes, which is essential for various forms of electrolyte transport. Since the maintenance of potas-

[1]Div. of Nephrology, Dept. of Medicine, Jichi Medical School, 3311-1 Minamikawachi-machi, Kawachi-gun, Tochigi, 329-04 Japan

sium balance is critical for the maintenance of cellular metabolism, potassium homeostasis should be efficiently regulated in a narrow range by several mechanisms. The acid-base balance is also critical for cell viability, therefore, several buffering systems should be necessary. It has long been known that changes in acid-base balance have significant effects on both renal and extrarenal potassium homeostasis [1]. It has been generally accepted that acidosis increases, while alkalosis decreases, plasma potassium concentration [2]. A common rule of thumb states that for every 0.1 unit change in blood pH the potassium concentration will change in the opposite direction by approximately 0.1–1.2 mEq/l [3,4]. Whether the acidosis is respiratory or metabolic in origin has an important effect on the magnitude of the hyperkalemic response. Respiratory acidosis causes little increase in the plasma potassium concentration; for every 0.1 unit change in blood pH the plasma potassium concentration increases by only 0.1–0.3 mEq/l [5]. Recent studies have indicated that the relationship between changes of blood pH and plasma potassium concentration is quite complex, and is influenced by several factors, including the origin of the acid-base disturbance, the nature of the anion accompanying the increase in hydrogen ion, change in plasma bicarbonate concentration, per se, duration of acidosis, and extent of intracellular buffering. Extrarenal potassium homeostasis is very important in keeping plasma potassium levels within a narrow range, especially in a rapid potassium loaded condition such as occurs just after meals. Several factors, such as insulin, catecholamines, aldosterone, and maybe other peptides, by controlling renal and/or extrarenal potassium regulatory systems, may contribute to keeping plasma potassium levels constant [1].

We have examined the relationship between acid-base disturbance and potassium transport in hemodialyzed patients [6]. In hemodialyzed patients, erythrocyte potassium concentration increased in patients with severe metabolic acidosis, and the amount of potassium removed into the dialysate was significantly smaller than that in patients without metabolic acidosis. These findings clearly showed the shift of potassium into the cells when metabolic acidosis was corrected by hemodialysis. To confirm this finding, in vitro ^{86}Rb uptake was examined in erythrocytes of control subjects and uremic patients. ^{86}Rb uptake was performed by incubation of cell suspensions of erythrocytes for 60 min with Hepes buffer. Acidification of the incubation medium, from 7.4 to 6.8, diminished Rb uptake significantly, by 15% [7]. In the presence of 10^{-5}M ouabain, Rb uptake was markedly inhibited, and the pH-dependent suppression of Rb uptake was also abolished. In the presence of 10^{-5} M amiloride and furosemide, acidification of the incubation medium failed to suppress Rb uptake in control subjects; however, in uremic patients, furosemide did not affect the pH-dependent suppression of Rb uptake. These data suggested that 1) in extrarenal potassium regulatory mechanisms, erythrocytes also play an important role in regulating plasma potassium level, 2) metabolic acidosis depletes erythrocyte potassium contents, and rapid correction of metabolic acidosis during hemodialysis shifts potassium into erythrocytes, and 3) metabolic acidosis, directly or indirectly suppresses ouabain-sensitive Na-K ATPase activity. In renal potassium homeostasis, a number of clearance studies have demonstrated that both metabolic and respiratory acidosis decrease urinary potassium excretion; in contrast, both metabolic and respiratory alkalosis increase urinary potassium excretion [8–11]. In renal potassium regulatory mechanisms, increased plasma potassium concentration, itself, stimulates urinary potassium secretion [12,13]; however, both metabolic and respiratory acidosis depress urinary potassium excretion independent of changes in plasma potassium concentration [14].

The role of acidosis in potassium transport along the nephron has been examined only in distal tubules. In the proximal tubules, several microelectrode and patch clamp studies suggest the possibility that metabolic acidosis affects potassium transport in these segments [15–20]; however, up to the present, no direct data is available. Nephron segments responsible for the alteration of potassium secretion in acid-base disturbance have been examined by the use of the free flow micropuncture method. Malnic et al. [21] and Stanton et al. [22] demonstrated that both metabolic and respiratory acidosis decreased potassium secretion in distal tubules. They also demonstrated that both metabolic and respiratory alkalosis stimulated potassium secretion in distal tubules. However, by using the micropuncture method, the nephron segments really responsible were not identified, because the distal tubules included distal convoluted tubules, connecting tubules, and cortical collecting ducts. So far, the nephron segments most responsible for final urinary potassium excretion have not yet been determined. Using isolated tubular microperfusion, Boudry et al. [23] reported the effect of luminal acidosis on potassium secretion in rabbit cortical collecting ducts. They demonstrated that luminal acidification, from 7.4 to 6.8, depolarized transepithelial voltage and decreased bath to lumen ^{86}Rb flux, without changing lumen to bath ^{22}Na flux. O'Neil et al. [24] demonstrated that luminal acidification, from 7.4 to 4.0, markedly inhibited luminal potassium conductance, by 70%, in rabbit cortical collecting ducts with microelectrode techniques. However, the effect of basolateral acidosis on potassium transport has not been examined. Using the in vitro microperfusion method, we examined the effect of metabolic acidosis on potassium transport in rabbit proximal convoluted tubules and cortical collecting ducts.

Methods

Protocol 1. The Effect of Metabolic Acidosis on Potassium Transport in Rabbit Proximal Convoluted Tubules

Proximal convoluted tubules, dissected from New Zealand white rabbits anesthetized with pentobarbital (50 mg/kg body weight), were placed in Euro Collins solution (mM): $NaHCO_3$ 10, K_2HPO_4 42.5, KH_2PO_4 15.0, KCl 15.0, and Glucose 3.5 g/dl; osmolarity was adjusted to 375 mOsm/kg.H_2O, at 4°C. Isolated tubular microperfusion was performed by the method of Burg et al. [25] with minor modifications [26]. Artificial solution was used as perfusate; the composition was (mM): NaCl 105, $NaHCO_3$ 25, KCl 5, NaH_2PO_4 1.6, Na_2HPO_4 0.4, $CaCl_2$ 1.8, Na acetate 10, d-glucose 8.3, and l-alanine 5.0; pH was adjusted to 7.4 after bubbling with 95% O_2/5% CO_2 gas mixture; osmolarity was adjusted to 298 mOsm/kg H_2O. For the bathing medium, bovine serum albumin 6.0 g/dl was added instead of d-glucose and l-alanine. The pH and osmolarity were identical with those of the perfusate. Metabolic acidosis was carried out by reducing the $NaHCO_3$ concentration from 25 to 5 mM/l and replacing the amount removed with 20 mmol Na cyclamate. pH was adjusted to 6.8, and osmolarity was identical with the control solution. The perfusate contained methoxy ^3H Inulin for a volume marker, and FD and C Green dye was used for the detection of damaged cells. Potassium transport was examined as a net flux by measuring the potassium concentration of the perfusate and collected fluid. Potassium concentration was measured with an ultramicroflamephotometer (Apel Co. Japan). Sample collections were performed, one by one, for measurement of water flux and potassium flux. After dissection, PCT were transferred to a Lucite bath chamber and were perfused in vitro. After a 20 min equilibrium period, control collections were performed: three for measuring water flux and three for measuring potassium flux. The bathing medium was then changed to an acidic solution, and the same samplings were performed, followed by consecutive changes of perfusate to acidic solution, change of bathing medium to 7.4 solution and, lastly, perfusate and bathing medium were returned to 7.4 solution.

Protocol 2. The Effect of Metabolic Acidosis on Potassium Transport in Rabbit Cortical Collecting Ducts

Rabbit cortical collecting ducts were perfused by the in vitro microperfusion method, as described above. In addition to measuring the net potassium flux under various conditions, ^{86}Rb flux and ^{22}Na flux were also examined. Either ^{86}Rb or ^{22}Na was added to the perfusate for measuring the unidirectional efflux coefficient. The isotope count was measured by the Chelencof method in ^{86}Rb and by gamma counter in ^{22}Na. In order to clarify the detailed mechanisms of the effect of acid-base disturbance on potassium transport, several maneuvers were performed: 2 mM $BaCl_2$ was added to the perfusate; 1 mM amiloride was added to the bathing medium. In order to examine the effect of bicarbonate on K transport, Hepes buffer was used instead of $NaHCO_3$ in both the 7.4 solution and the 6.8 solution. Conventional microelectrodes were used to impale the principal cells of rabbit cortical collecting ducts, in order to measure the basolateral membrane voltage by the method reported previously [27]. The electrolyte composition of the perfusate and the bath solution was identical to that used in the in vitro microperfusion experiments, except that the perfusate did not contain d-glucose and l-alanine, and the bath solution did not contain bovine serum albumin. Also, a constant current was passed through the perfusate and the bath solution, so that the transepithelial and fractional apical membrane resistances could be calculated.

Statistical analysis was performed by Student's *t*-test. A P value less than 5% was considered as significant.

Results

Protocol 1. The Effect of Metabolic Acidosis on K Transport in Rabbit Proximal Convoluted Tubules

Basolateral acidosis achieved by changing the bathing medium pH from 7.4 to 6.8 solution decreased transepithelial voltage by -2.36 ± 1.4 to -1.48 ± 0.85 mV ($P<0.05$); however, water transport did not significantly change. On the other hand, basolateral acidosis enhanced potassium secretion from -5.08 ± 1.76 to -11.97 ± 2.14 pmol/min per mm ($P<0.05$) without any change of sodium flux. Additional luminal acidosis depressed potassium secretion to -2.84 ± 3.04 pmol/min

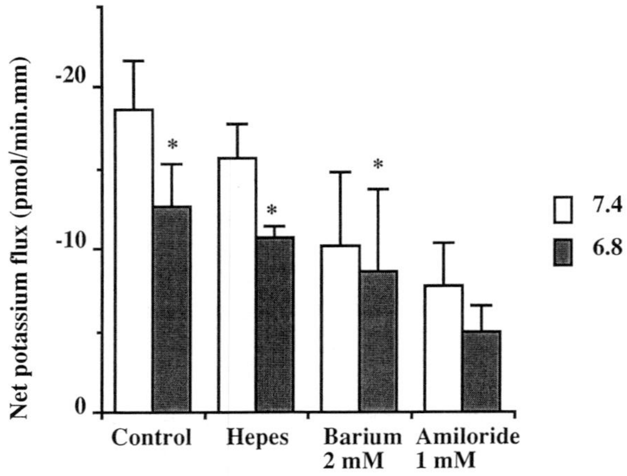

Fig. 1. Basolateral acidosis suppressed potassium secretion in rabbit cortical collecting duct. This effect was studied in isolated microperfused tubules in vitro. The inhibitory effect of basolateral acidosis on potassium transport was not affected by the elimination of bicarbonate, but was diminished in the presence of either luminal 2 mM barium or basolateral 1 mM amiloride

per mm; however, transepithelial voltage did not change. The change of bath solution to pH 7.4 did not affect potassium transport, water transport, and transepithelial voltage.

Protocol 2. The Effect of Metabolic Acidosis on Potassium Transport in Rabbit Cortical Collecting Ducts

When the pH of the bathing medium was changed from 7.4 to 6.8, transepithelial voltage was depolarized from -9.62 ± 2.18 to -3.84 ± 2.70 mV ($P < 0.005$), without significant recovery. Net potassium flux also decreased from -18.69 ± 3.00 to -10.98 ± 2.16 pmol/min per mm ($P < 0.025$), however, net sodium flux did not significantly change. In the presence of 2 mM barium chloride, a potent potassium channel blocker in the perfusate, the inhibitory effect of basolateral acidosis on potassium secretion and transepithelial voltage was diminished, but still remained significant (Fig. 1). Basolaterally, a high dose of amiloride, (1 mM), which is thought to inhibit both sodium channel and sodium-proton exchanger, diminished the inhibitory effect of basolateral acidosis on potassium flux and transepithelial voltage. When Hepes buffer solution was used as perfusate and bathing medium instead of bicarbonate, the inhibitory effect of basolateral acidosis remained unchanged. Neither the ^{86}Rb efflux coefficient nor the ^{22}Na efflux coefficient was significantly affected by the basolateral acidosis. Electrophysiological studies also revealed that basolateral acidosis depolarized transepithelial voltage and a simultaneous record of basolateral membrane voltage also showed deporalization in the principal cells, from -83.5 ± 2.3 to -74.75 ± 3.07 mV ($P < 0.001$). Basolateral acidosis also significantly increased transepithelial resistance, from 81.7 ± 7.08 to 93.4 ± 9.7 ohm.cm^2

(P<0.001), and significantly increased the calculated fractional resistance of apical membrane, from 0.47 ± 0.07 to 0.57 ± 0.08 ($P<0.001$).

Discussion

A high intracellular potassium concentration, essential for operating cell functions, is kept by sodium-potassium ATPase on the various epithelial membranes. Potassium ions can be shifted out of the extracellular space and taken up by body cells so that only a small fraction of any potassium added remains in the extracellular fluid compartment. Conversely, extracellular losses can be mitigated by transfer of potassium ions from the cell pool to the extracellular fluid. Since potassium imbalance, whether manifested as hypokalemia or hyperkalemia, leads to lethal disorders, plasma potassium levels should be regulated within a strictly narrow range. Clinically, it is a well-known phenomenon that acidosis induces hyperkalemia and that alkalosis induces hypokalemia. The real mechanisms of these interactions between acid-base disturbance and potassium homeostasis has remained uncertain [1].

Both metabolic and respiratory acidosis decrease urinary potassium excretion and, in contrast, both metabolic and respiratory alkalosis increase urinary potassium excretion, independently of extrarenal potassium regulatory systems [14]. In the renal potassium regulatory mechanisms, increased plasma potassium concentration, itself, stimulates urinary potassium secretion [12,13]; however, both metabolic and respiratory acidosis depress urinary potassium excretion, independently of changes in plasma potassium concentration.

Bulk reabsorption of electrolytes and water in the kidney occurs mainly in the proximal tubules and in Henle's loop, but the site of the final regulation of renal water and electrolyte excretion is the distal nephron segment, particularly the collecting duct system.

In the proximal tubules, there are no data available which would allow us to assume the effect of metabolic acidosis on net potassium transport. We demonstrated previously that potassium was secreted in rabbit proximal convoluted tubules in vitro when studied by isolated tubular microperfusion [28]; however, micropuncture studies have found that potassium is reabsorbed in the proximal tubules, to the extent of about 50%–80% of the filtered load. Similar findings were reported from Wasserstein [29] and Work [30] in proximal straight tubules. We further examined the effect of basolateral barium on potassium secretion in proximal convoluted tubules. Basolateral barium stimulated potassium secretion, perhaps due to the inhibition of basolateral barium-sensitive potassium channel [28], resulting in reduced potassium leaking out from basolateral membrane and an increment of luminal potassium extrusion. Intracellular recordings with conventional microelectrodes have demonstrated that changes in extracellular pH greatly affect the basolateral membrane potential in renal proximal tubules [15–18]. This fact may suggest that the basolateral potassium conductance is sensitive to external pH. As a change in extracellular pH is known to give rise to a change in intracellular pH [19], the potassium conductance might be regulated by intracellular pH [20]. Recent patch clamp studies in opossum kidney proximal tubular cells revealed that apical membrane potassium channel was calcium sensitive and basolateral membrane potassium channel was barium sensitive [20]. As we have shown in this paper, in the proximal convoluted tubules, basolateral acidosis enhanced potassium channels, contrary to our expectations. Although the detailed mechanisms have not yet been clarified, it is suggested that basolateral acidosis may enhance potassium secretion by the inhibition of basolateral barium sensitive potassium channel. Unless sodium and water reabsorption is reduced, proximal potassium transport is thought to be less important in the regulation of final urinary potassium excretion. However, the fact should be mentioned that basolateral acidosis stimulates potassium secretion in proximal convoluted tubules, although the physiological significance of this phenomenon has not yet been clarified.

In the loop nephron, the interaction of metabolic acidosis and potassium transport has not been examined; however, the upper portion of long-loop nephron segments is highly cation selective [31] and potassium permeability is very much higher here than that in other nephron segments [32]. A mathematical model of the transport profiles along the descending loop clearly demonstrated that potassium loading from the proximal tubules does not affect potassium transport in the long-loop nephron [33].

Thus, the cortical collecting duct has been identified as a major site of potassium secretion; it is also at this nephron site that hormones exert their typical sodium and potassium effects. The original potassium secretion model in cortical collecting ducts consists of a two-step process. The first step includes active, ATP-dependent sodium extrusion and active potassium uptake across the basolateral membrane, resulting in a high cell potassium concentration and an appropriate potassium gradient. The second step consists of potassium extrusion from cell to lumen, via potassium conductance of apical membrane [34].

Segments responsible for the interaction of acid-base disturbance and potassium transport along the nephron were examined by in vivo micropuncture and microperfusion [21,22] and in vitro microperfusion [23]. Luminal acidification depolarized transepithelial voltage and depressed bath to lumen ^{86}Rb flux, without changing lumen to bath ^{22}Na flux. However, the detailed mechanisms of the relationship between acid-base disturbance and potassium secretion in distal tubules remained unclear. We examined the effect of basolateral acidosis on potassium transport in the rabbit cortical collecting ducts. Our data clearly showed the inhibitory effect of basolateral acidosis on potassium secretion. Basolateral acidosis suppressed potassium secretion and depolarized transepithelial voltage, as seen in the luminal acidosis reported previously [23]. However, sodium flux did not change as a result of the acidification of the bathing medium.

It is well established that two distinct cell types constitute the cortical collecting duct; principal cells and intercalated cells. Several kinds of evidence suggest that principal cells are involved in sodium reabsorption and potassium secretion. As mentioned before, sodium is extruded and potassium is taken up by sodium-potassium ATPase pump in the basolateral membrane of the principal cell, and potassium diffuses and sodium enters across the apical membrane. These transporters of the apical membrane are mediated by amiloride-sensitive sodium channels and barium-sensitive potassium channels [35]. However, recent patch clamp studies clearly demonstrated the existence of at least three types of potassium channels; a so-called Maxi K channel, a small conductance channel, and a calcium-activated K channel [35–38]. The Maxi K channel is identified in the apical membrane of rat cortical collecting duct; this channel has a high conductance, is barium sensitive, and may be involved in potassium secretion; the pH sensitive conductance change is still controversial. The small conductance K channel is located in both apical and basolateral membranes; however, its role in potassium secretion is much different. The apical small conductance K channel is involved in potassium secretion in cortical collecting duct; this channel is pH-sensitive, barium-insensitive, and voltage independent. The calcium-activated K channel exists in basolateral membrane, although the physiological role of this channel is limited to that of cell volume regulation, and it has almost no significant role in the potassium secretory mechanism. That is, in hypotonic shock, membrane stretch activates this calcium-sensitive K channel.

Regarding the inhibitory effect of basolateral acidosis on potassium secretion, we showed that in the presence of luminal barium, the inhibitory effect of basolateral acidosis diminished, but still remained significant. However, the question remains whether 2 mM barium is enough to block luminal potassium channel, since recent microelectrode studies have suggested that more than 5 mM barium is required to completely block the potassium channel [24]. Thus, although it is indirect evidence, intracellular acidosis might inhibit barium-sensitive and, probably, barium-insensitive, pH-dependent K channels in the apical membrane, the so-called small K conductance channels.

However, problems remained in the interpretation of our data. We showed that basolateral acidosis inhibited potassium secretion via barium-sensitive and -insensitive pathways and that basolateral acidosis also deporalized transepithelial voltage. If pH-sensitive potassium channel blockade is the primary event in the inhibitory effect in cortical collecting ducts, the decrement of potassium secretion should result primarily in transepithelial voltage hyperporalization, because basolateral acidosis did not affect either net sodium reabsorption or unidirectional sodium efflux. This means that neither the change of sodium channel activity nor the change of sodium-proton ATPase activity might be involved in the effect of basolateral acidosis. How basolateral acidosis depolarizes transepithelial voltage remained to be resolved. There are two possibilities. One is that basolateral acidosis affects conductances other than sodium or potassium, such as sodium-proton exchanger, potassium-chloride cotransporter, and chloride-bicarbonate exchanger, in depolarizing transepithelial voltage. Another possibility is that basolateral acidosis affected intercalated cells, in which proton secretion might be stimulated in basolateral acidosis, resulting in deporalization of transepithelial voltage, independent of changes in sodium and potassium conductance. Indirect evidence suggested that this latter thesis better explained the facts. The addition of ouabain to the bathing medium induced marked depolarization, from negative transepithelial voltage to markedly positive voltage. This finding suggests that the complete block of principal cell function by ouabain revealed the voltage generation of intercalated cells. That is, the stimulation of proton secretion in the intercalated cells can deporalize transcellular voltage, resulting in the reduction of voltage-dependent potassium secretion. However, our electrophysiological data suggested that principal cells are the cells responsible, at least in part, for the inhibitory effect of basolateral acidosis on potassium secretion. The fact that addition of high dose amiloride from the basolateral side diminished the inhibitory effect of basolateral acidosis also suggested an effect of the sodium-proton exchanger system on the basolateral membrane of either principal cells or intercalated cells.

We summarized the data as follows: 1) Basolateral acidosis inhibited potassium secretion without changing sodium reabsorption in rabbit cortical collecting ducts, 2) basolateral amiloride diminished the effect of basolateral acidosis on potassium secretion, 3) luminal barium diminished the inhibitory effect of basolateral acidosis on potassium secretion, 4) ambient bicarbonate ion was not essential for the inhibitory effect of basolateral acidosis on potassium secretion, and 5) basolateral acidosis depolarized both transepithelial voltage and basolateral membrane voltage by increasing relative luminal resistance.

The present study further confirmed the previous assumption, based on clearance studies and in vivo micropuncture data, that the cortical collecting duct is involved in an reduced renal potassium secretion in acidosis. The mechanism of basolateral acidosis-induced inhibition of potassium secretion appears to involve: the inhibition of luminal barium-sensitive and barium-insensitive potassium channels and the basolateral amiloride-sensitive Na-H exchanger system, but not bicarbonate ion on either side of the epithelium in the principal cells.

References

1. De Fronzo RA, Bia M (1985) Extrarenal potassium homeostasis. In: Seldin DW, Giebisch G (eds) The kidney; physiology and pathophysiology. Raven, New York, pp 1179–1206
2. Simmons DH, Avedon M (1959) Acid base alterations and plasma potassium concentration. Am J Physiol 197:319–326
3. Burnell JM, Villamil MF, Uyeno BT, Scribner BH (1956) Effect in humans of extracellular pH change in relationship betwen serum potassium concentration and intracellular potassium. J Clin Invest 35:935–939
4. Adrogue HJ, Madias NE (1981) Changes in plasma potassium concentration during acute acid-base disturbances. Am J Med 71:456–467
5. Schwartz WB, Brackett N, Cohen JJ (1965) The response of extracellular hydrogen ion concentration to graded degrees of chronic hypercapnia. The physiologic limits of the defense of pH. J Clin Invest 44:291–301
6. Tabei K, Furuya H, Shimanaka K, Shindo Y, Hosoi H, Asano (1986) Changes of erythrocyte K concentration and K removal by hemodialysis. J Japn Soc Dial Ther 19:793–802
7. Sakairi Y, Tabei K, Furuya H, Ando H, Asano Y (1990) Regulation of extrarenal potassium (K) homeostasis in chronically hemodialyzed patients (pts) (abstract). Proceedings of the XIth international congress of nephrology, July 15–20, 1990. Tokyo, Japan
8. Berliner RW, Kennedy TJ, Orloff J (1951) Relationship between acidification of the urine and potassium metabolism. Am J Med 11:274
9. Berliner RW (1952) Renal secretion of potassium and hydrogen ions. Fed Proc 11:695
10. Schwartz WB, Cohen JJ (1978) The nature of the renal response to disorders of acid-base equilibrium. Am J Med 64:417
11. Seldin DW, Rector FC Jr (1972) The generation and maintenance of metabolic alkalosis. Kidney Int 1:306
12. Khuri RN, Windderholt M, Strieder N, Giebisch G (1975) Effects of flow rate and potassium intake on distal tubular potassium transfer. Am J Physiol 228:1249
13. Muto S, Giebisch G, Sanson S (1988) An acute increase of peritubular K stimulates K transport through cell pathways of CCT. Am J Physiol 255:F108–F114
14. Toussaint C, Vereerstraeten P (1962) Effect of blood pH changes on potassium excretion in the dog. Am J Physiol 202:768
15. Biagi B, Kubota T, Sohtell M, Giebsch G (1981) Intracellular potentials in rabbit proximal tubules perfused in vitro. Am J Physiol 240:F200–F210
16. Boron WF, Boulpaep EL (1983) Intracellular pH regulation in the renal proximal tubules of the salamander. J Gen Physiol 81:53–94

17. Kubota T, Biagi BA, Giebisch G (1983) Effects of acid base disturbances on basolateral membrane potential and intracellular potassium activity in the proximal tubule of Necturus. J Membr Biol 73:61–68
18. Steels PS, Boulpaep EL (1987) pH-dependent electrical properties and buffer permeability of the Necturus renal proximal tubule cell. J Membr Biol 100:165–182
19. Burckhardt BC, Fromter E (1987) Evidence for OH^-/H^+ permeation across the peritubular cell membrane of rat renal proximal tubule in HCO_3^--free solution. Pflügers Arch 409:132–137
20. Ohno-Shosaku T, Kubota T, Yamaguchi J, Fujimoto M (1990) Regulation of inwardly rectifying K^+ channels by intracellular pH in opossum kidney cells. Pflügers Arch 416:138–143
21. Malnic G, deMello-Aires M, Giebisch G (1971) Potassium transport across renal tubules during acid-base disturbance. Am J Physiol 211:1192
22. Stanton BA, Giebisch G (1982) Effect of pH on potassium transport by renal distal tubules. Am J Physiol 242:F544
23. Boudry JF, Stoner LC, Burg MB (1976) The effect of luminal pH on potassium transport in renal cortical collecting tubules. Am J Physiol 230:239
24. O'Neil RG, Sansom SC (1984) Characterization of apical cell membrane Na^+ and K^+ conductances of cortical collecting duct using microelectrode techniques. Am J Physiol 247:F14–F24
25. Burg MB, Grantham J, Abramow M, Orloff J (1966) Preparation and study of fragments of rabbit nephron. Am J Physiol 210:1293–1298
26. Ando Y, Tabei K, Furuya H, Asano Y (1989) Glucagon stimulates chloride transport independently of cyclic AMP in the rat medullary TAL. Kidney Int 31:760–767
27. Muto S, Sansom S, Giebisch G (1988) Effects of a high potassium diet on electrical properties of cortical collecting ducts from adrenalectomized rabbits. J Clin Invest 81:376–380
28. Tabei K, Furuya H, Muto S, Asano, Y (1988) Potassium (K) is secreted in rabbit proximal convoluted tubules (PCT) in vitro. Kidney Int 35:489
29. Wasserstein AG, Agus ZS (1983) Potassium secretion in the rabbit proximal straight tubule. Am J Physiol 245:F167–F174
30. Work J, Troutman L, Schafer JA (1982) Transport of potassium in the rabbit pars recta. Am J Physiol 242:F226–F237
31. Tabei K, Imai M (1986) Permselectivity for cations over anions in the upper portion of the descending limb of the long-loop nephron (LDLu) of hamsters. Pflügers Arch 406:279–284
32. Tabei K, Imai M (1987) K transport in upper portion of descending limb of long-loop nephron from hamsters. Am J Physiol 252:F387–F392
33. Taniguchi J, Tabei K, Imai M (1987) Profile of water and solute transport along long-loop descending limb: analysis by a mathematical model. Am J Physiol 252:F393–F402
34. Giebisch G, Malnic G, Berliner RW (1986) Renal transport and control of potassium excretion. In: Brenner BM, Rector FC Jr (eds) The kidney. Saunders, Philadelphia, pp 177–205
35. Giebel J, Zweifach A, White S, Wang W, Giebisch G (1990) K^+ channels of the mammalian collecting duct. Renal Physiol Biochem 13:5969
36. Koeppen B, Biagi BA, Giebisch G (1983) Electrophysiology of mammalian renal tubule: influences from intracellular microelectrode studies, Annu Rev Physiol 45:497–517
37. Wang W, Giebisch G (1989) The regulation of the small conductance K^+ channel in the apical membrane of rat cortical collecting tubule (abstract). Proc Am Soc Nephrol 21:386A
38. Frint G, Palmer IG (1987) Ca-activated K channels in apical membrane of mammalian CCT, and their role in K secretion. Am J Physiol 252:F458–F467

Mechanisms of Transcellular Potassium Shifts in Acid-Base Disorders

Horacio J. Adrogué[1]

Introduction

A substantial improvement in our understanding of the determinants of internal potassium balance, the regulation of acidity within body fluids, and the relationship between potassium transport and pH levels has been accomplished in the last forty years [1–4]. Yet, a number of fundamental questions on the linkage between acid-base and potassium transport at the cellular level remain unanswered. I will attempt to summarize our view of this puzzling relationship with the understanding that alternative explanations have been or might be offered at this time. Our analysis of the internal K^+ exchanges in acid-base disorders will be performed considering the existence of basic determinants of the K^+-H^+ relationship as well as modulators of this relationship. The wide range of Δ $[K^+]/\Delta$ pH values in the extracellular fluid observed among the various acid-base disorders [5] may be largely explained by the differential effects of the basic determinants of the K^+-H^+ relationship on each disorder. The modulators of the K^+-H^+ relationship might either ameliorate or exaggerate the translocation of potassium under a variety of pathophysiological conditions.

A. Basic Determinants

All cells contain a cytosolic fluid rich in proteins and phosphate compounds, which are polyvalent macromolecules essential for normal cell function. These macromolecules have, at normal cell pH, a net negative charge that accounts for more than two thirds of the anionic equivalency of the intracellular fluid. Furthermore, these cell-restricted anions are responsible for the peculiar distribution of the diffusable anions and cations on both sides of the cell membrane, as dictated by the physical

[1]Chief, Renal Section (151-B), Veterans Affairs Medical Center, 2002 Holcombe Blvd., Houston, TX 77030, USA

chemical principles of equilibrium in aqueous solutions, theoretically conceived by Gibbs and experimentally verified by Donnan. In most cells potassium and chloride are the dominant conductive species across the cell membrane and, in accordance with Gibbs-Donnan postulates, these permeant ions must be in electrochemical equilibrium. The negative charge of the cell-restricted anions is predominantly carried by the amino-acid residues of proteins, by ATP, and by other organic phosphate compounds. This charge is balanced by the positive charge of potassium, the exclusively permeant cation. Although sodium is not strictly impermeant, its rapid extrusion upon entering the cell makes this cation effectively impermeant. As a consequence a K^+-rich cytosolic fluid is created; the cell-restricted anions produce a much higher concentration of this diffusable cation within the cell compared to the extracellular fluid. In addition, the cell-restricted anions force an unequal distribution of chloride, the permeant anion, which largely accumulates in the extracellular fluid. Obviously, another cation must balance the negative charge of chloride outside the cells; the cation that fills this function is sodium.

The cellular accumulation of K^+ and exclusion of Cl^- generates an electrical potential across the membrane where the cytosol is negative with respect to the extracellular fluid. The polarized cell membrane, which repels anions and attracts cations, develops an electrical potential difference that satisfies the electrochemical equilibrium of the permeant ions potassium and chloride. The experimental verification of these assumptions required the measurement of ion permeabilities, intracellular voltage, and the chemical composition of the cytosolic fluid. Since several ions are permeant under steady-state conditions in most cells (i.e., K^+, Cl^- and to some extent Na^+) the membrane potential may be estimated by the Goldman-Hodgkin-Katz (GHK) constant field equation, that is a modification of the Nernst equation:

$$E_m = \frac{RT}{F} \ln \frac{P_K[K]_e + P_{Na}[Na]_e + P_{Cl}[Cl]_i}{P_K[K]_i + P_{Na}[Na]_i + P_{Cl}[Cl]_e}$$

which takes into account the main permeant (P = permeability) ions at rest which are Na^+, K^+ and Cl^-. Most cells have resting cell membrane potentials of −60 mV to −90 mV and these values are close to E_K (equilibrium potential for potassium) since their highest permeability at rest is to potassium ions. The cell membrane also has a relatively high resting permeability to Cl^- and low permeability to Na^+ which accounts for the proximity of the resting cell membrane potential to the equilibrium potential for potassium and chloride ions, but not to sodium. An examination of the Nernst potentials at 37°C, calculated according to the extracellular and intracellular concentrations of the different ions in mammalian cells, depicted below, helps to better recognize these phenomena.

Nernst Equilibrium Potential (mV)		Concentration (mmol/l)
Na^+	+71	(i = 10; e = 142)
Ca^{2+}	+150	(i = <0.0001; e = 2.5)
K^+	−98	(i = 155; e = 4)
Cl^-	−29 to −90	(i = 5-30; e = 101)

The application of the Gibbs-Donnan rules to the cellular membrane satisfactorily explains a large fraction of the available data on the peculiar distribution of electro-

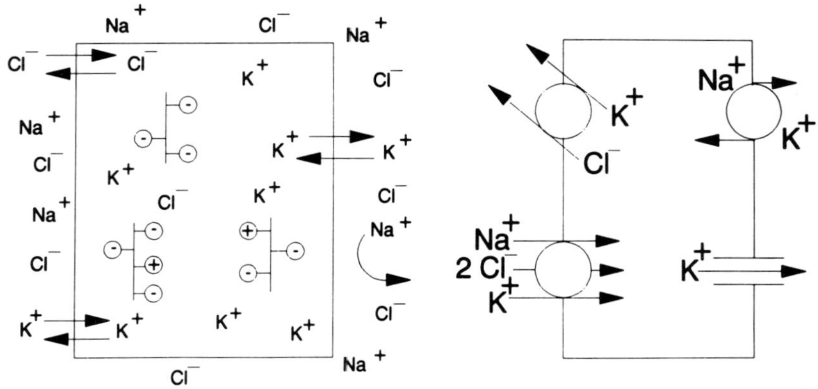

Fig. 1. The Gibbs-Donnan theory (*left panel*) and Pump/Leak hypothesis (*right panel*) properly account for the distribution of major electrolytes across the cell membrane (Modified from [6])

lytes in the cytosolic and extracellular fluids [6]. We believe that additional information, collectively described as the Pump/Leak hypothesis, completes the Gibbs-Donnan rules, resulting in a coherent overall account of the distribution of electrolytes in cells and extracellular fluid (Fig. 1). The exclusion of Na^+ from cells, for example, is not simply the result of a nonpermeant condition of this ion but is best explained by active pumping of sodium from cells by the Na^+, K^+ ATPase. Since this pump moves 3 Na^+ out in association with 2 K^+ into the cell, it generates an electrical potential. The Na^+-K^+ pump maintains the steady-state intracellular levels of high potassium and low sodium by creating a flux of ions that counterbalance the passive cellular loss of potassium and the influx of sodium. The action of the pump also accounts for the presence in some cells of K^+ levels that are above its electrochemical equilibrium.

The combination of ionic gradients of K^+, Cl^-, and Na^+ across the cell membrane, the permeability of the membrane to these ions, and the contribution from electrogenic pumping (i.e., Na^+-K^+ pump) determine the resting membrane potential. In most cells the resting membrane potential is largely generated by the potassium diffusion potential.

Effect of Cell pH on the Interaction Between Intracellular Proteins and Potassium

Intracellular proteins interact with potassium almost exclusively by electrostatic binding, that is in a salt-type manner, and the approximately 55 mEq/l of anionic proteins within skeletal muscle are balanced by equal amounts of potassium ions. Since proteins in an electrolyte solution contribute to both the anionic and the cationic properties of the solution, the 55 mEq/l of anionic proteins referred to above, are also known as the *net cationic equivalency* or *net negative charge* of the proteins. It has been estimated that the minimum acid/base buffer value of cell proteins in muscle is about 15 mmol/l per unit pH change (slyke), and this value agrees with data obtained in vivo in muscle from intact animals [7]. The ion-binding sites of proteins appear to

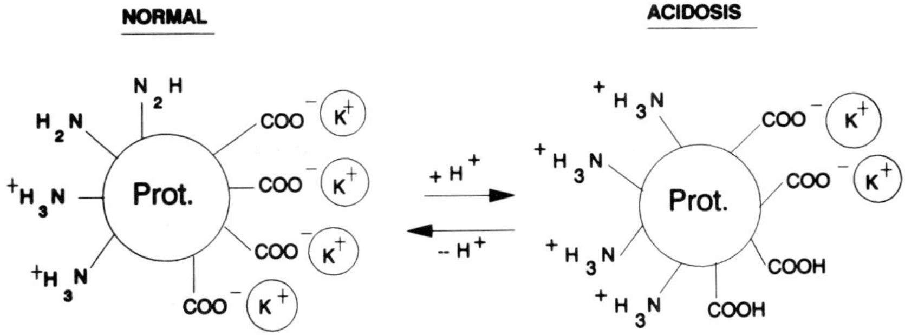

Fig. 2. Schematic representation of the decreased potassium-binding capacity of intracellular proteins in acidosis (Modified from [1])

have preference for H^+ ions so that other cations can compete only if their concentration is considerably higher than that of the H^+-ions [8]. This requisite is amply satisfied in the cytosolic fluid by K^+-ions because their concentration is six orders of magnitude higher than that of H^+-ions ($[K^+] = 10^{-1}M$; $[H^+] = 10^{-7}M$). Thus, as cell pH falls, the electrostatic binding of K^+-ions to cytosolic proteins decreases and H^+ ions displace K^+ ions from the proteins (Fig. 2); the opposite process occurs when pH increases. The magnitude of the change in K^+-binding capability is similar to the change in the net cation equivalency of intracellular proteins, which is a function of the deviation in cell pH multiplied by the buffer value of the proteins. The nature of the phenomenon that takes place in the cytosolic fluid is similar to the pH-related effect on plasma proteins, which partially accounts for the alteration in the plasma anion gap in the course of acid-base disturbances [9].

The diminished binding of K^+ by proteins within the cell in acidosis will alter the electrochemical equilibrium for this ion, favoring the cellular exit of potassium. By contrast, an increased intracellular pH will have the opposite effect which will favor the uptake of potassium by cells.

Intracellular Concentration of Bicarbonate

The intracellular level of bicarbonate of about 12 mEq/l in skeletal muscle balances an equal concentration of cations, most of which are potassium ions. Thus, increases and decreases in cytosolic bicarbonate concentration should be accompanied by parallel alterations in the levels of potassium bound to this anion within the cell. Respiratory acidosis and metabolic alkalosis are characterized by elevated levels of intracellular bicarbonate and consequently they have increased levels of anionic sites for K^+-binding. The opposite occurs in respiratory alkalosis and metabolic acidosis. The magnitude of the alteration in the concentration of bicarbonate is dependent on the severity of the acid-base disorder.

Increases and decreases of about 4 mEq/l in the cellular bicarbonate concentration have been described in skeletal muscle in moderately severe respiratory acidosis and respiratory alkalosis, respectively [10]. Yet, the changes in K^+-binding by cytosolic bicarbonate in each respiratory acid-base disorder occur in association with an opposite change in the K^+-binding properties of intracellular proteins. In fact, the titration of carbonic acid by non-bicarbonate buffers (mostly proteins) in respiratory acidosis and alkalosis fully accounts for the above mentioned changes in bicarbonate concentration.

In contrast to respiratory acid-base disorders, in metabolic acid-base disturbances there exists an additive change in the K^+-binding properties of intracellular anions, proteins and bicarbonate. Thus, a substantial decrease in K^+ bound to cellular anions occurs in metabolic acidosis and the opposite takes place in metabolic alkalosis.

Intracellular Concentration of Phosphate and Organic Acids

The concentration of organic and inorganic phosphate in skeletal muscle is high, with levels between 40 and 70 millimols per liter. The pK′ of all these phosphate compounds is about 6.5 and the resulting aggregate buffer value amounts to approximately 18 slykes [7]. By contrast, creatine phosphate has a very low pK′ of about 4.5, so that its buffer value is negligible.

The substantial acid/base buffer value of cell phosphates should result in a significant decrement in potassium-binding capability in acidosis and the opposite effect in alkalosis. However, changes in the levels of organic and inorganic phosphates in the cytosol, due to alterations in energy requirements, metabolic pathways, or other processes may substantially alter the predicted change in K^+-binding by phosphate moieties in acidosis and alkalosis.

Organic acid acidosis results in abnormally high cellular levels of protons and organic anions. Proton accumulation will displace potassium ions that were electrostatically bound to proteins, phosphate, and bicarbonate. Yet the organic anion may act as a sink for the displaced potassium ions, counterbalancing the effects of the protons released by the organic acid. The effect of changes in cell pH on organic acid production and disposal further complicates the basic interaction just mentioned.

In contrast to organic acid-acidosis, the cellular retention of protons, due to an impairment in renal acid excretion or to infusion of mineral acids, will not only diminish the K^+ binding by proteins, phosphate, and bicarbonate but also fails to offer a cellular anion to help with the disposal of the displaced potassium ions.

B. Modulators of the K^+-H^+ Relationship

The effect of changes in the cytosolic levels of hydrogen ions and sodium, and the role of insulin will be summarized below, since these are the dominant modulators of the K^+-H^+ relationship. Other influences of less importance [11], that include the effects of catecholamines, mineralocorticoids, and osmolality, will not be reviewed due to space limitation. A brief overview of the transport pathways of H^+ and K^+ will precede our evaluation of the interplay of these ions at the cell membrane.

A lipid bilayer that prevents the translocation of most ions is a basic component of the cell membrane. Yet, the exchange of potassium and other ions between cells and the interstitial fluid is allowed to occur through proteins that span the lipid bilayer of the cell membrane. Four distinct pathways are involved in the traffic of potassium.

Potassium may exit the cytosol satisfying the electrochemical gradient, either through K^+-channels or by a K^+/Cl^- cotransport, given that chloride is also accumulated above its electrochemical equilibrium in at least some cells.

The most important and best studied potassium influx mechanism occurs via the Na^+-K^+ pump, also known as Na^+-K^+ ATPase. This pump, which is present in all animal cells, is an ATP-dependent enzyme that catalyzes the movement of both Na^+ and K^+ in opposite directions. ATP hydrolysis acts as the energy source. A second K^+-influx pathway has been described in several cell types and involves the obligatory cotransport of one K^+, one Na^+ and two Cl^- ions across the cell membrane. This pathway is electroneutral and from an energetic point of view is a secondary active transport process. The uphill movement of K^+ and Cl^- into the cell is driven by the downhill movement of Na^+ toward the cells. The sodium gradient is in turn established by the Na^+-K^+ pump, which is the primary active transport mechanism.

The development of accurate measurements of intracellular pH and voltage has demonstrated that H^+ activity inside cells is lower than would be predicted if protons were simply distributed to satisfy electrochemical equilibrium. Thus, the cells are faced with a passive influx of protons which must be counterbalanced by active pumping of H^+ toward the extracellular fluid. An exception to this rule occurs in red cells and possibly hepatocytes, where H^+ effux is passive. Since cell metabolism is also a significant source of intracellular acidification, cells have developed effective acid-extruding mechanisms. The Na^+/H^+ exchange system is the most important mechanism that protects cells against intracellular acidosis by the countertransport of external Na^+ for internal H^+. This system extrudes H^+ from the cells because the net thermodynamic driving force on the Na^+-H^+ exchangers in the plasma membrane favors this process. The higher ratio of $[Na^+]e/[Na^+]_i$ in comparison with the $[H^+]e/[H^+]_i$ accounts for the direction of the ion fluxes mentioned above. This countertransport process is not directly dependent upon ATP hydrolysis, but the energy for the uphill extrusion of H^+ derives from the downhill inwardly directed Na^+ gradient. The primary active extrusion of Na^+ mediated by the Na^+-K^+ ATPase is responsible for the sodium gradient between interstitial and cytosolic fluid.

The Na^+/H^+ countertransport mechanism appears to play an important role in the control of cell pH, protecting cells against intracellular acidosis. A second system involved in cell pH regulation is an electroneutral Cl^-/HCO_3-exchanger that, under physiological conditions, protects cells against intracellular alkalosis. The latter mechanism exchanges external Cl^- for internal HCO_3. The pH-dependence of the two systems is quite different. The Na^+/H^+ exchanger predominates at acidic cell pH values and the defense of cell acidosis takes place at the expense of the transmembrane sodium gradient. By contrast, at alkaline cell pH levels the Cl^-/HCO_3 exchanger is activated, extruding cytosolic bicarbonate, which is driven by the transmembrane chloride gradient in the opposite direction.

Changes in cell and extracellular acidity alter the acid-loading and/or the acid-extruding mechanisms previously described, which in turn regulate the absolute values of pH in all the body compartments. In addition, the interdependence of intracellular and extracellular pH results from passive fluxes of H^+, HCO_3 and other weak acids and bases.

Intracellular Ion Levels

Changes in intracellular pH may alter K^+ transport across the cell membrane, acting on the Na^+-K^+ pump and on the conductance of K^+ channels [4,6]. Cell acidosis has been shown to depress both the activity of the pump and K^+-conductance through the cell membrane in some cell-types. Conversely, an alkaline cell pH stimulates the Na^+/K^+ pump and activates K^+ channels. The magnitude of this effect as well as the significance in overall extrarenal K^+ homeostasis is yet undefined.

The cytosolic concentration of sodium may also modulate the activity of the Na^+-K^+ pump as well as the activity of some K^+ channels. The effects of $[Na^+]_i$ on the pump have been previously discussed. The physiologic importance of the effects of intracellular sodium levels on the conductance of cell membrane K^+ channels remains unknown.

Insulin

Insulin is a major modulator of extrarenal potassium homeostasis and promotes potassium uptake in many cell types, including those from skeletal muscle and liver. The hypokalemic action occurs at very low concentrations of insulin and is independent from the effect of insulin on glucose uptake. The precise mechanism of action remains to be defined but appears to involve the activation of several transport proteins. Stimulation of Na^+-H^+ countertransport, resulting in cytosolic alkalinization, has been demonstrated in response to insulin in the skeletal muscle. The rise of cell pH caused by insulin is inhibited by lowering the extracellular Na^+ level and by amiloride. The insulin-induced cell alkalosis increases the K^+-binding capacity of intracellular anions and also stimulates the Na^+-K^+ pump, therefore favoring cellular K^+-loading. The increased cellular Na^+ concentration secondary to enhanced Na^+ entry via Na^+-H^+ exchange is also a stimulus for the action of the Na^+-K^+ pump to enhance potassium influx. This is the case because the Na^+ concentration for half-maximal activity of this pump is between 10 and 50 mM and the cellular concentration of sodium in most cells is 10–20 mM.

A direct stimulatory effect of insulin on the Na^+, K^+-ATPase in skeletal muscle and adipose tissue has been described. This stimulatory action is blocked by ouabain, a specific inhibitor of the pump. The mechanisms involved are an increase in the turnover rate of the pump or an unmasking of latent pump sites. In contrast with the action of thyroid hormones and adrenal steroids on the Na^+-K^+ pump, insulin does not appear to promote the synthesis of new pump units. The extent to which the activation by insulin of other transport mechanisms, including the Na^+-H^+ exchange, is important in the K^+ uptake by the pump remains undefined.

The hypokalemic action of insulin might also involve a direct effect on potassium channels [12]. One type of K^+ channel of significant relevance in the skeletal muscle is the inward rectifier channel, which accounts for most of the K^+ conductance in the resting state. This channel allows potassium to flow into cells much more easily than to exit cells. Thus, when the cell membrane is hyperpolarized the high inward conductance facilitates K^+ entry to cells. When the cell membrane is depolarized the low outward conductance reduces potassium exit from cells. The effect of insulin on the conductance of the inward rectifying potassium channels of skeletal muscle has been examined in potassium-depleted rats. Under these conditions a large K^+ conductance, defined by the presence of a steep slope in the current-voltage relationship, was found when the membrane was hyperpolarized. Insulin had no effects on this K^+ conductance. Preservation of the high conductance coupled to the hyperpolarization of the cell membrane due to stimulation of the Na^+-K^+ pump by insulin, would enhance cell potassium stores. By contrast to the lack of effect of insulin on K^+ conductance when

Table 1. Insulin-mediated cellular K^+ loading mechanisms

Primary action	Immediate result	Secondary effect
Stimulation of Na^+-H^+ exchanger	Cytosolic alkalinization	Increased K^+ binding capacity Stimulation of Na^+-K^+ ATPase
	Increased cell [Na^+]	Stimulation of Na^+-K^+ ATPase
Stimulation of Na^+-K^+ ATPase	Hyperpolarization of cell membrane	New electrical gradient favors K^+ entry Deactivation of K^+ channels turned on by depolarization prevents K^+ exit
K^+ Channels (inward rectifier)	Depressed K^+ conductance when membrane is depolarized	Exaggeration of the inward rectifying properties

the cell was hyperpolarized, a major depression of K^+ conductance occurred when the cell membrane was depolarized. This latter effect of insulin is in fact an exaggeration of the inward rectifying properties of this class of potassium channels. Thus insulin action on the inward rectifier K^+ channels may facilitate the accumulation of potassium by a dual effect of stimulation of K^+ entry and depression of K^+ exit.

Insulin produces hyperpolarization of the cell membrane in a number of tissues, including the skeletal muscle. The hyperpolarization might result from stimulation of the sodium-potassium pump or, less likely, might be the result of an increased K^+ conductance. Since the effect on membrane potential precedes cellular potassium accumulation, a primary effect on the pump is presumed. Yet the specific inhibitor of the Na^+-K^+ pump, ouabain, does not consistently block this insulin action.

The effect of insulin on the cell membrane potential might be of great relevance to the hypokalemic effect by a different mechanism that involves the modulation of K^+ currents in voltage-gated K^+ channels. Many potassium channels are activated by depolarization of the membrane (i.e., Ca^{2+}-activated K^+ channels, classic Hodgkin-Huxley/delayed rectifier K^+ channels) which increases the fraction of time that the channel is in the open state. In this circumstance K^+ is lost from the cell into the extracellular fluid. An example of this situation occurs in uremia, in which the depressed skeletal muscle potential may facilitate the cellular exit of potassium. The administration of insulin will hyperpolarize the cell membrane, which will in turn deactivate K^+ channels preventing the exit of cellular potassium. In some cells, such as those in the renal proximal tubule, gating of K^+ channels has the opposite voltage dependence so that when the membrane is hyperpolarized more channels are open. Thus, insulin action will enhance the potassium stores in these and other cells which have channels activated at hyperpolarized potentials.

Insulin action on glucose metabolism is pH-dependent and known to be impaired in acidosis [13]. Whether changes in pH have a similar effect on the kalemic effect of insulin remains unknown. It should be also recognized that increased insulin levels in the course of an acid-base disorder, as in the case of exogenous ketoacidosis, might substantially alter the K^+-H^+ relationship [14,15]. Table 1 summarizes the various insulin-mediated potassium loading mechanisms.

In summary, we envision the existence of basic determinants, as well as modulators, of the K^+-H^+ relationship. The action of the basic determinants is the result of changes in the anionic binding sites for K^+ in the cytosol, which in turn alter the electrochemical equilibrium for this ion, favoring either the cellular exit or the uptake of potassium. Intracellular proteins and phosphate interact with K^+ by electrostatic binding and their net anionic change is balanced with K^+ ions. As cell pH falls, H^+ ions displace K^+ ions from these compounds, while the opposite process occurs when cell pH increases. The intracellular level of bicarbonate also balances an equal concentration of cations, most of which are potassium ions. Thus, elevated levels of intracellular bicarbonate (respiratory acidosis and metabolic alkalosis) should be accompanied by parallel alterations in the levels of potassium bound to this anion within the cell. The opposite occurs in respiratory alkalosis and metabolic acidosis. Consequently, the changes in K^+ binding by cytosolic bicarbonate in each respiratory acid-base disorder occur in association with an opposite change in the K^+-binding properties of intracellular proteins. In contrast to the respiratory type, in metabolic acid-base disturbances there exists an additive change in the K^+-binding properties of intracellular anions, proteins and bicarbonate. The net result is the development of a substantial decrease in K^+ bound to cellular anions in metabolic acidosis; the opposite occurs in metabolic alkalosis. Organic acid acidosis is a special situation which results in abnormally high cellular levels of protons and anions of organic acids; the latter act as a sink for the displaced K^+, counterbalancing the effects of cell acidosis on the K^+-H^+ relationship. The most significant modulators of the K^+-H^+ relationship include the effects of cell pH and cytosolic [Na^+] on K^+ pathways and the action of insulin on the transport of H^+ and K^+ across the cell membrane. The importance of the modulators is modest in comparison to that of the basic determinants with respect to the Δ [K^+] Δ pH in the various acid-base disorders.

Acknowledgments. I am indebted to Debby S. Verrett for skillful assistance in preparing the manuscript. This study was supported in part by the Medical Research Service of the Veterans Affairs Medical Center in Houston and by the American Heart Association, Texas Affiliate.

References

1. Davenport HW (1974) The ABC of acid-base chemistry. The University of Chicago Press, Chicago, pp 3–53
2. Pitts RF (1976) Volume and composition of the body fluids. In: Pitts RF (ed) Physiology of the Kidney and Body Fluids. Year Book Medical Publishers, Chicago, pp 11–35
3. Boron WF (1989) Cellular buffering and intracellular pH. In: Seldin DW, Giebisch G (eds) The regulation of acid-base balance. Raven, New York, pp 33–56
4. Williams ME, Epstein FH (1989) Internal exchanges of potassium. In: Seldin DW, Giebisch G (eds) The regulation of potassium balance. Raven, New York, pp 3–29
5. Adrogué HJ, Madias NE (1981) Changes in plasma potassium concentration during acute acid-base disturbances. Am J Med 71:456–467
6. Palmer LG (1989) The regulation of intracellular potassium. In: Seldin DW, Giebisch G (eds) The regulation of potassium balance. Raven, New York, pp 89–119
7. Woodbury JW (1974) Regulation of pH. In: Ruch TC, Patton HD (eds) Physiology and Biophysics. WB Saunders, Philadelphia, pp 901–933

8. Van Leeuwen AM (1964) Net cation equivalency ("base binding power") of the plasma proteins. Acta Med Scand [Suppl] 422:1–212
9. Adrogué HJ, Brensilver J, Madias NE (1978) Changes in the plasma anion gap during chronic metabolic acid-base disturbances. Am J Physiol 235:F291–F297
10. Brown EB Jr (1965) Blood and tissue buffers. Arch Intern Med 116:665–669
11. Susuki H, Hishida A, Ohishi K, Kimura M, Honda N (1990) Role of hormonal factors in plasma K alterations in acute respiratory and metabolic alkalosis in dogs. Am J Physiol 258:F305–F310
12. Ruff RL (1989) Periodic paralysis. In: Seldin DW, Giebisch G (eds) The regulation of potassium balance. Raven, New York, pp 303–323
13. Adrogué HJ, Chap Z, Okuda Y, Michael L, Hartley C, Entman M, Field JB (1988) Acidosis-induced glucose intolerance is not prevented by adrenergic blockade. Am J Physiol 255:E812–E823
14. Adrogué HJ, Chap Z, Ishida T, Field JB (1985) Role of the endocrine pancreas in the kalemic response to acute metabolic acidosis in conscious dogs. J Clin Invest 75:798–808
15. Adrogué HJ, Lederer ED, Suki WN, Eknoyan G (1986) Determinants of plasma potassium levels in diabetic ketoacidosis. Medicine Baltimore 65:163–172

Hypokalemia in Metabolic Alkalosis: A New Look at an Old Controversy

F. John Gennari[1]

Summary. Metabolic alkalosis can be induced in humans either by potassium, or by chloride depletion, but the selective removal of one of these ions is almost invariably associated with losses of the other. As a result, a controversy persists concerning which of these ions is critical for the development of this common acid-base disorder. In the last decade, epithelial membrane ion transporters, identified in the loop and distal nephron, have provided new insights into the close linkage between K^+ and Cl^- transport in this part of the nephron. These transporters can also explain how each of these ions influences H^+ and HCO_3^- transport. Results from membrane transport studies provide the basis for explaining the effect of K^+ depletion on stimulating NH_4^+ excretion, impeding Cl^- reabsorption, and on stimulating H^+ secretion. The membrane transport studies also show how Cl^- depletion promotes K^+ excretion and inhibits HCO_3^- excretion. Review of human and animal studies reveals a coherent story, which indicates that both K^+ and Cl^- depletion contribute to the pathogenesis and maintenance of metabolic alkalosis.

Introduction

Metabolic alkalosis is invariably associated with potassium depletion and hypokalemia. However, the role of potassium depletion, per se, in the pathogenesis and maintenance of this acid-base disturbance has been a matter of controversy for over 30 years. The extreme positions in this controversy are: 1) potassium depletion is an essential feature, causing the changes in renal bicarbonate reabsorption and acid excretion responsible for maintaining metabolic alkalosis, and 2) potassium depletion is simply an epiphenomenon, playing no role whatever in maintaining the disorder in the most common forms of metabolic alkalosis. The latter position maintains that chloride depletion, rather than K^+ depletion, is the responsible factor for induc-

[1]University of Vermont, Burlington, VT 05405, USA

ing and maintaining the most common form of sustained metabolic alkalosis. The controversy has persisted, because in whole animal studies, it is difficult to separate K^+ depletion from Cl^- depletion. Despite this experimental problem, it is now clear that both Cl^- and K^+ depletion can play contributory roles in maintaining metabolic alkalosis, and that their respective roles vary depending on the pathogenetic mechanism involved. Most exciting has been the identification of apical membrane transport proteins which specifically link K^+, Cl^-, HCO_3^-, H^+ and NH_4^+ transport in the loop of Henle and distal nephron. From our new knowledge of these membrane transporters, a logical story is emerging which can explain the pathogenesis and maintenance of metabolic alkalosis. This story illustrates the interdependence of K^+ and Cl^- transport in the renal response to metabolic alkalosis.

Discussion

Metabolic alkalosis can be induced in a variety of ways (Table 1). To undertake a discussion of the role of K^+ and Cl^- in the pathogenesis of this disorder, one first needs to define what type or types of metabolic alkalosis one is discussing. Although metabolic alkalosis can be induced by acute bicarbonate loading, this model has little relevance to the clinical disorder. From a clinical perspective, two types of metabolic alkalosis are of interest. The first type is initiated primarily by selective loss of chloride from either the gastrointestinal tract (vomiting, nasogastric drainage) or kidney (after administration of certain diuretics). This type accounts for over 90% of the metabolic alkalosis seen in clinical settings and is termed "chloride-responsive." The second type is initiated by a primary increase in distal nephron hydrogen ion secretion, in most cases induced by increased mineralocorticoid activity (due either to endogenous secretion or exogenous administration). This type is termed "chloride-resistant."

The first issue to be addressed is whether the maintenance of the alkalosis in these two subtypes is due to different factors. In both types, K^+ depletion and hypokalemia occur. In both types, in addition, chloride loss occurs, although the loss may be

Table 1. Experimental models of metabolic alkalosis

1. Acute alkali administration
2. Chloride depletion
   - gastric drainage
   - peritoneal dialysis with $NaHCO_3$
   - hemofiltration and replacement with $NaHCO_3$
   - Furosemide
   - Furosemide + $NaHCO_3$
   - recovery from respiratory acidosis
3. Potassium depletion
   - low K^+ diet
   - low K^+ diet + $NaHCO_3$
   - low K^+ diet + DOCA
   - Aldosterone administration
   - DOCA + $NaHCO_3$

DOCA, desoxycorticosterone acetate

minimal in some models of chloride-resistant alkalosis. In clinical medicine, management of the two types of metabolic alkalosis differs, and thus it is useful to subdivide them. From a pathophysiologic perspective, however, it is less clear that a major difference exists. This point is illustrated below in reviewing the experimental studies directed at gaining insight into the pathophysiology of this disorder.

Role of Potassium Depletion

The best experiment to determine whether K^+ depletion plays a specific role in the production and maintenance of metabolic alkalosis is to induce negative K^+ balance by means of dietary K^+ restriction. This type of experiment has been carried out in rats [1–8], dogs [2,9,10], and humans [11,12]. Although at first glance, the results appear to differ in all three species, on further analysis it appears that the rat and human are quite similar in their response to this maneuver.

In the rat, dietary K^+ restriction for 3 weeks or longer leads to marked and sustained metabolic alkalosis ($HCO_3^- > 35$mEq/l) [2,3]. Shorter term K^+ restriction, which presumably produces less severe K^+ depletion, fails to produce alkalosis [4,5]. The increase in bicarbonate concentration that occurs with K^+ depletion in the rat is modulated by the concurrent Cl^- intake [2,6]. In rats given NaCl in their drinking water, the increase in bicarbonate concentration is less than one-third as great as that in animals drinking tap water [2]. In addition, renal Cl^- wasting and Cl^- depletion occur in severely K^+ depleted rats, in association with metabolic alkalosis [7,8]. These same features are found in human K^+ depletion. In humans fed a normal salt intake (1.8mEq/kg body weight), dietary K^+ restriction produces a small but significant increase in serum bicarbonate concentration (2mEq/l) [11]. When chloride as well as K^+ is restricted, the accompanying K^+ depletion induces an increment in bicarbonate concentration that is nearly four times as great as that in the K^+ only restricted cases [12]. Although the increase in bicarbonate in humans is smaller in magnitude than that in the rat, it should be noted that the K^+ depletion is much less severe in these human studies than in the rat. In severely K^+ depleted humans, the alkalosis is quite severe, and in addition, renal Cl^- wasting has been documented to occur, just as it does in the rat [13].

The response in the dog to dietary K^+ restriction is strikingly different. In this species, K^+ depletion produces a mild metabolic acidosis rather than metabolic alkalosis [2,9,10]. Thus, K^+ depletion stimulates renal H^+ secretion in the human and rat kidney, but inhibits it in the dog. The reason for this striking species difference is unclear, but suggests that the dog may not be a useful model for studying this type of metabolic alkalosis. In contrast to its response to dietary K^+ depletion, the dog responds in the same fashion as do humans and rats to mineralocorticoid administration. In all 3 species, mineralocorticoids induce metabolic alkalosis, if sufficient sodium is present in the diet [1,7,14–19]. The effect is enhanced, moreover, if mineralocorticoids are given together with sodium bicarbonate [1,15,18]. In addition, prior K^+ depletion, or concomitant K^+ restriction, worsens the resultant alkalosis [1,16]. In humans, there is no direct experimental evidence for this last observation, but a clear correlation exists between the severity of the hypokalemia and the steady-state bicarbonate concentration in primary hyperaldosteronism [19].

Although the response in humans and animals to mineralocorticoid administration clearly indicates that K^+ depletion is a contributory factor in the development and maintenance of metabolic alkalosis, it should be pointed out that mineralocorticoids also produce chloride depletion by increasing renal chloride excretion [15]. Moreover, to the extent that chloride losses exceed dietary intake, chloride administration is required for full correlation of the alkalosis [15]. To summarize, K^+ depletion produces alkalosis in humans and rats, but not in dogs. In all species tested, chloride is a modulating factor and is necessary for full repair of the acid-base disorder when chloride depletion is also present.

Role of Chloride Depletion

Experiments designed to isolate a specific role for chloride depletion in the generation and maintenance of metabolic alkalosis have been carried out in rats [20,21], dogs [15,22], and humans [23] as well. In all 3 species, chloride depletion produces metabolic alkalosis. Unfortunately, it is virtually impossible to avoid producing simultaneous K^+ depletion in experimental Cl^- depletion alkalosis. To get around this problem, Kassirer and Schwartz tested whether the alkalosis induced by chloride depletion could be fully corrected by Cl^- administration without repair of the accompanying K^+ deficit [23]. They induced metabolic alkalosis by gastric drainage in subjects on a low electrolyte diet. After stable metabolic alkalosis was present (and K^+ stores were depleted by some 300mEq), they administered 120mEq/day of NaCl and demonstrated full correction of the alkalosis with no change in body K^+ stores [23]. This experiment has often been cited as evidence that K^+ depletion is not a contributory factor in maintaining chloride-depletion metabolic alkalosis in man. However, correction of metabolic alkalosis in these K^+ depleted subjects did not occur until 400–500 mEq of chloride was retained above and beyond the chloride originally lost during induction of the alkalosis [23]. An alternative explanation of Kassirer and Schwartz's experiment is that chloride retention and extracellular fluid (ECF) volume expansion markedly increased distal Cl^- delivery, overcoming the effect of K^+ depletion on distal nephron acid and bicarbonate transport (see later for proposed mechanism) [12].

Galla and co-workers produced chloride depletion alkalosis in the rat by a single peritoneal dialysis against 150mM $NaHCO_3$ [20]. This maneuver results in selective chloride loss and alkalosis which is sustained by dietary chloride restriction. In this model, as in other forms of chloride-depletion alkalosis, significant K^+ depletion develops over time [20,21]. These investigators showed that chloride-depletion alkalosis in the rat could be corrected by chloride administration, without repleting K^+ losses, or indeed, without even administering Na^+ (using choline chloride) [20,21]. This experiment provides evidence for a specific role for chloride in the maintenance of this type of metabolic alkalosis. Even in this experiment, however, some K^+ retention occurred during the correction phase. Thus, a contributing role for potassium cannot be excluded.

The most striking experiment constructed to try and separate K^+ depletion from metabolic alkalosis was carried out in the dog by Bleich and co-workers [22]. They induced metabolic alkalosis by gastric drainage in animals fed a low electrolyte diet, and then completely corrected the alkalosis by HCl administration. After a new steady-state was achieved, they administered either potassium sulfate or potassium phosphate to these K^+ depleted, sodium-avid animals. This maneuver produced a dramatic increase in serum bicarbonate concentration (metabolic alkalosis) while at

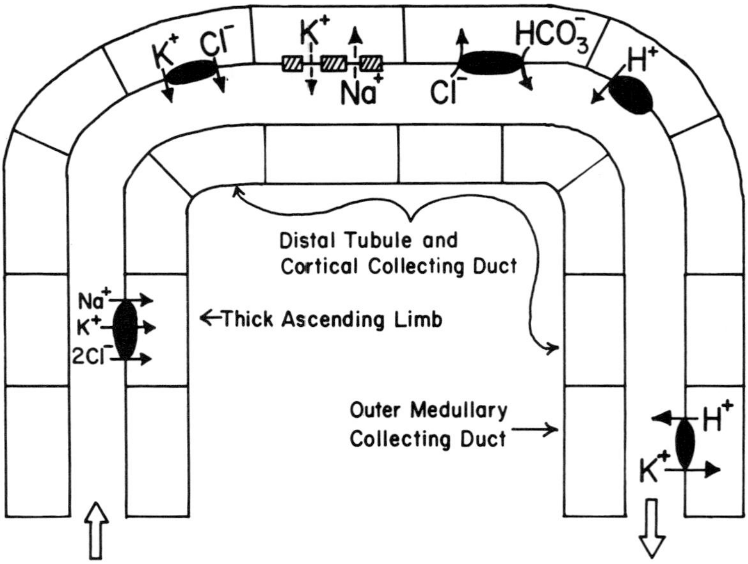

Fig. 1. Membrane ion transporters and channels linking potassium and chloride with hydrogen and bicarbonate secretion in the loop of Henle and the distal nephron

the same time completely replacing the K^+ lost as a result of the original gastric alkalosis. Bleich and co-workers concluded that as K^+ was retained, sodium was released from cells and delivered to the distal nephron with phosphate or sulfate rather than with chloride. Delivery of sodium without chloride to this site in the nephron in these sodium-avid animals stimulated hydrogen ion secretion, inducing metabolic alkalosis again. Although these ingenious experimental manipulations would seem to exclude a causal role for K^+ depletion in metabolic alkalosis, one must be cautious in extrapolating these findings to metabolic alkalosis in man. Firstly, as noted earlier, K^+ depletion in dogs does not produce metabolic alkalosis as it does in man. Secondly, it is possible that HCl administration conditioned the nephron to respond to sodium delivery by secreting hydrogen ions. These chloride-depletion studies in dogs, rats, and humans demonstrate a key role for chloride in the pathogenesis and maintenance of metabolic alkalosis, but they do not exclude a contributory role for K^+ depletion.

Linkage Between K^+, Cl^-, and H^+ Transport

The difficulty of separating the roles of K^+ and Cl^- in producing and maintaining metabolic alkalosis may well be due to the linked transport pathways of these two ions along the nephron. Potassium and chloride reabsorption and secretion are not only linked with one another by specific transporters, but also are linked with H^+, HCO_3^- and NH_4^+ transport in the loop and distal nephron [24–28]. Figure 1 illustrates the apical transporters where such interaction occurs. The primary cation reabsorptive site in the thick ascending limb of Henle's loop requires 2 Cl^- ions and one K^+ ion for each Na^+ ion which enters the apical membrane of the epithelial cell. Thus, severe K^+ depletion could impair Na^+ and Cl^- reabsorption in the loop. In fact, early distal Cl^- concentration is increased significantly in rats with K^+ depletion [29]. On this transporter, NH_4^+ can substitute for K^+ [28], and thus K^+ depletion could also enhance NH_4^+ entry, leading to more delivery of NH_4^+ to the papillary interstitium. This effect probably accounts for the stimulation of NH_4^+ excretion by K^+ depletion [30]. In the distal tubule and cortical collecting duct, a K^+/Cl^- cotransporter has been identified [31,32]. A low chloride concentration in the tubular fluid in this segment of the nephron promotes K^+ secretion by this mechanism, and a high chloride concentration inhibits it [31,32]. This could be one mechanism whereby chloride depletion promotes K^+ loss. A K^+ conductive channel is also present, and Cl^- depletion coupled with a driving force for Na^+ reabsorption creates a favorable electrochemical gradient for K^+ secretion via this channel [24]. The same luminal factors also create a favorable environment for H^+ secretion via the apical H^+-ATPase transporter.

Two additional transporters link K^+ and Cl^- directly with acid and alkali secretion. A K^+/H^+ exchanger, which reabsorbs K^+ in exchange for H^+ by an ATP driven mechanism, has been identified in the outer medullary collecting duct [25]. In K^+ depletion this transporter could be activated, promoting H^+ secretion (and thereby, bicarbonate reabsorption). Luminal chloride concentration is independently linked to bicarbonate transport through an apical transporter, the Cl^-/HCO_3^- exchanger, in the cortical collecting duct. The presence of chloride in the lumen promotes HCO_3 secretion (and excretion); the absence of chloride inhibits this process [26,27]. Microperfusion studies in the rat distal tubule have shown that the addition of chloride to the perfusate can convert a bicarbonate reabsorptive epithelium into a bicarbonate secreting epithelium [27]. This transporter could be the mechanism by which chloride ions modulate the alkalosis induced by K^+ depletion; it could also be the mechanism by which chloride depletion prevents recovery from alkalosis.

Conclusions

Thus, the presence of these newly identified membrane ion transporters can, in theory, account for 1) the effect of K^+ depletion to stimulate NH_4^+ excretion and to enhance distal H^+ secretion, 2) the effect of chloride intake to modulate the alkalosis-producing potential of K^+ depletion, 3) the effect of severe K^+ depletion to produce renal chloride wasting, 4) the effect of chloride depletion to promote renal K^+ excretion, and 5) the effect of chloride depletion to sustain alkalosis by inhibiting distal nephron bicarbonate secretion. The relative roles of each of these transporters in producing and maintaining metabolic alkalosis remains to be determined. Nonetheless, they provide a logical framework for understanding how K^+ and Cl^- interact to regulate bicarbonate reabsorption and NH_4^+ excretion by the kidney. Given this new information, further studies aimed at determining which ion is the "critical" one for maintaining metabolic alkalosis are not likely to be useful. It is clear that loss of either potassium or chloride can lead to a loss of the other ion, and that relatively normal stores of each of these ions are necessary for the kidney to regulate acid-base homeostasis in a normal fashion.

References

1. Seldin DW, Welt LG, Cort JH (1956) The role of sodium salts and adrenal steroids in the production of hypokalemic alkalosis. Yale J Biol Med 29:229–247
2. Garella S, Chang B, Kahn SI (1979) Alterations of hydrogen ion homeostasis in pure potassium depletion: Studies in rats and dogs during the recovery phase. J Lab Clin Med 93:321–331
3. Capasso G, Kinne R, Malnic G, Giebisch G (1986) Renal bicarbonate reabsorption in the rat. I. Effects of hypokalemia and carbonic anhydrase. J Clin Invest 78:1558–1567
4. Levine DZ, Walker T, Nash LA (1973) Effects of KCl infusions on proximal tubular function in normal and potassium-depleted rats. Kidney Int 4:318–325
5. Adam WR, Simpson DP (1975) Renal mitochondrial glutamine metabolism and dietary potassium and protein content. Kidney Int 7:325–330
6. Cooke RE, Segar WE, Reed C, Etzwiler DD, Vita M, Brusilow S, Darrow DC (1954) The role of potassium in the prevention of alkalosis. Am J Med 17:180–195
7. Luke RG, Levitin H (1967) Impaired renal conservation of chloride and the acid-base changes associated with potassium depletion in the rat. Clin Sci 32:511–526
8. Luke RG, Wright FS, Fowler N, Kashgarian M, Giebisch GH (1978) Effects of potassium depletion on renal tubular chloride transport in the rat. Kidney Int 14:414–427
9. Burnell JM, Teubner EJ, Simpson DP (1974) Metabolic acidosis accompanying potassium depletion. Am J Physiol 227:329–333
10. Hulter HN, Sebastian A, Sigala JF, Licht JH, Glynn RD, Schambelan M, Biglieri EG (1980) Pathogenesis of renal hyperchloremic acidosis resulting from dietary potassium restriction in the dog: Role of aldosterone. Am J Physiol 238:F79–F91
11. Jones JW, Sebastian A, Hulter HN, Schambelan M, Sutton JM, Biglieri EG (1982) Systemic and renal acid-base effects of chronic dietary potassium depletion in humans. Kidney Int 21:402–410
12. Hernandez RE, Schambelan M, Cogan MG, Colman J, Morris RC Jr, Sebastian A (1987) Dietary NaCl determines severity of potassium depletion-induced metabolic alkalosis. Kidney Int 31:1356–1367
13. Garella S, Chazan JA, Cohen JJ (1970) Saline-resistant metabolic alkalosis or "chloride-wasting nephropathy." Ann Intern Med 73:31–38
14. Orloff J, Kennedy TJ Jr, Berliner RW (1953) The effect of potassium in nephrectomized rats with hypokalemic alkalosis. J Clin Invest 32:538–542
15. Atkins EL, Schwartz WB (1962) Factors governing correction of the alkalosis associated with potassium deficiency; the critical role of chloride in the recovery process. J Clin Invest 41:218–229
16. Hulter HN, Sigala JF, Sebastian A (1978) K^+ deprivation potentiates the renal alkalosis-producing effect of mineralocorticoid. Am J Physiol 235:F298–F309
17. Relman AS, Schwartz WB (1952) The effect of DOCA on electrolyte balance in normal man and its relation to sodium chloride intake. Yale J Biol Med 24:540–558
18. Kassirer JP, Appleton FM, Chazan JA, Schwartz WB (1967) Aldosterone in metabolic alkalosis. J Clin Invest 46:1558–1571
19. Kassirer JP, London AM, Goldman DM, Schwartz WB (1970) On the pathogenesis of metabolic alkalosis in hyperaldosteronism. Am J Med 49:306–315
20. Galla JH, Bonduris DN, Luke RG (1983) Correction of acute chloride-depletion alkalosis in the rat without volume expansion. Am J Physiol 244:F217–F221
21. Wall BM, Byrum GV, Galla JH, Luke RG (1987) Importance of chloride for the correction of chronic metabolic alkalosis in the rat. Am J Physiol 253:F1031–F1039
22. Bleich HL, Tannen RL, Schwartz WB (1966) The induction of metabolic alkalosis by correction of potassium deficiency. J Clin Invest 45:573–579
23. Kassirer JP, Schwartz WB (1966) Correction of metabolic alkalosis in man without

repair of potassium deficiency. A reevaluation of the role of potassium. Am J Med 40:19–26
24. Field MJ, Giebisch G (1989) Mechanisms of segmental potassium reabsorption and secretion. In: Seldin DW, Giebisch G (eds) The regulation of potassium balance. Raven, New York, pp 139–155
25. Wingo CS (1989) Active proton secretion and potassium absorption in the rabbit outer medullary collecting duct. J Clin Invest 84:361–365
26. Star RA, Burg MB, Knepper MA (1985) Bicarbonate secretion and chloride absorption by rabbit cortical collecting ducts. Role of chloride/bicarbonate exchange. J Clin Invest 76:1123–1130
27. Levine DZ, Vandorpe D, Iacovitti M (1990) Luminal chloride modulates rat distal tubule bidirectional bicarbonate flux in vivo. J Clin Invest 85:1793–1798
28. Knepper MA, Packer R, Good DW (1989) Ammonium transport in the kidney. Physiol Rev 69:179–249
29. Luke RG, Booker BB, Galla JH (1985) Effect of potassium depletion on chloride transport in the loop of Henle in the rat. Am J Physiol 248:F682–F687
30. Tannen RL (1987) Effect of potassium on renal acidification and acid-base homeostasis. Semin Nephrol 7:263–273
31. Ellison DH, Velazquez H, Wright FS (1986) Unidirectional potassium fluxes in renal distal tubule: Effects of chloride and barium. Am J Physiol 250:F885–F894
32. Wingo CS (1989) Reversible chloride-dependent potassium flux across the rabbit cortical collecting tubule. Am J Physiol 256:F697–F704

Role of Kidney in the Pathogenesis of Hypertension

Chair: Maarten ADH Schalekamp (The Netherlands)
Takao Saruto (Japan)

The Renin Angiotensin System, the Kidney, and the Pathogenesis of Hypertension

NORMAN K. HOLLENBERG[1] and GORDON H. WILLIAMS[2]

SUMMARY. Some individuals enjoy a high salt diet with impunity: others, on the other hand, raise their blood pressure and suffer the consequences. Multiple observations suggest that familial, probably genetic, factors are involved and that the abnormality resides in the kidney. We have identified a group of patients, called "non-modulators," in whom impaired responsiveness of the kidney and adrenal to Angiotension II (AII) with shifts in salt intake, is associated with failure of renal blood flow to change as salt intake changes, impaired ability to handle a salt load, and sodium-sensitive hypertension. The abnormality is familial and probably inherited. Angiotensin converting enzyme (ACE) inhibition corrects many of the associated abnormalities, increases renal blood flow, and enhances the ability of the kidney to handle a salt load—an important contribution, we believe, to the antihypertensive effect. The renal abnormality may also predispose to progressive renal injury if an additional abnormality, such as diabetes mellitus, is superimposed.

Introduction

Recognition of a crucial contribution of genetics to the pathogenesis of hypertension is longstanding, but precisely what is inherited as the predisposing abnormality has remained remarkably elusive. Interest in the kidney has recently been renewed by recognition of the fact that hypertension follows the kidney after transplantation in animals and in humans [1–5]. A series of abnormalities, potentially involving the kidney and sodium homeostasis, has been recognized over the years, including familial factors in renal sodium handling [6] and in the control of the renal circulation [7,8]. Relevant abnormalities in angiotensin-mediated control of the renal circulation and adrenal aldosterone release have been documented worldwide, in the relatively homogeneous populations of Japan [8] and Switzerland [9], and the relatively heterogeneous population of the United States [10].

[1]Departments of Medicine[1] and Radiology[2], Harvard Medical School and Brigham and Women's Hospital, Boston, MA 02115, USA

The thrust of this essay will be to organize a growing body of evidence which indicates that an abnormality of the kidney, and the adrenal, involving disordered regulation through the renin-angiotensin system, is responsible for the pathogenesis in about 45% of patients – a discrete subgroup that may be the most common cause of hypertension. That fundamental abnormality leads to disordered renal sodium handling and sodium-sensitive hypertension, abnormalities in the renal vascular response to changes in sodium intake and to angiotensin II, blunted decrements of renin release in response to saline or angiotensin II, and an accentuated renal vasodilator response to angiotensin converting enzyme (ACE) inhibition. ACE inhibition increases renal blood flow substantially more in these patients than it does in normal subjects or other essential hypertensives. ACE inhibition also restores to normal the renal vascular and adrenal response to angiotensin II, renin release in response to angiotensin II, renal sodium handling, and, ultimately, blood pressure. Finally, and perhaps most intriguing, similar abnormalities have been found in 50% of the normotensive offspring of patients with essential hypertension; evidence is accruing to indicate that the abnormality is inherited, perhaps via a major gene.

Sodium and Renal Vascular Responses to Angiotensin II

Dahl, in a 1963 review of metabolism in hypertension, was puzzled by five then recent publications, which described a paradoxical, natriuretic response to angiotensin II associated with a blunted or absent renal vascular response in some patients with essential hypertension [11]. He noted the parallel with hepatic cirrhosis. Since then, the mechanism in cirrhosis has become clear [12]. The paradoxical natriuresis reflects the effects on renal sodium handling of the pressor response, when the renal vascular bed can no longer respond to angiotensin II because of angiotensin-mediated renal vasoconstriction.

During the time since Dahl's review, two separate lines of investigation on disordered control of the renal blood supply [13] and the adrenal [14] with shifts in state of sodium balance led to the recognition that both abnormalities occur in the same patient [15]. This followed recognition of a highly predictable shift in renal vascular and adrenal responses to angiotensin II with changes in sodium intake: the renal vasculature is more sensitive to angiotensin II on a high salt diet, and adrenal aldosterone release is more sensitive with restriction of sodium intake [16]. Because the term "modulation" had been employed to describe such shifts in responsiveness in other endocrine systems, the inability of these individuals to change renal vascular and adrenal responsiveness to angiotensin II [17] was called "non-modulation" [10,18].

Several lines of evidence indicate that "non-modulation" is not part of a continuum, but rather represents a discrete subgroup present in about 45% of patients with normal renin and high renin essential hypertension [10,18].

Sodium Sensitive Hypertension

The frequent sensitivity of hypertension to sodium intake has long been recognized. In 1904, within a few years of the first recognition that hypertension represents a clinical disorder, Ambard and Baujard proposed that the increase in blood pressure reflected a failure to adapt to an excess of salt in the diet [19]. Not long thereafter, Allen, in the United States, demonstrated that a severe reduction of salt in the diet was effective in reducing blood pressure in about 60% of patients with hypertension [20]. Both the French group and Allen believed that hypertension reflected an unknown renal defect that limited the individual's ability to handle salt. Since that time, confirmation of the frequency of sodium sensitive hypertension has come from estimates based on sodium intake as therapy [21], the frequency of response to diuretics [22], and from careful metabolic balance studies [23,24], which have confirmed a frequency of about 50%–60%. The metabolic balance studies failed to identify a mechanism responsible for the blood pressure rise, but did demonstrate that individuals with salt-sensitive hypertension showed more positive sodium balance and gained more weight as their blood pressure rose [23,24].

An abnormality involving the renal blood supply and adrenal aldosterone release, both crucial for sodium handling, raised the possibility, intriguing to us, that the unidentified patients in the metabolic balance studies were the non-modulators. Indeed, that has turned out to be the case. Whether the pattern by which external sodium balance is achieved when sodium intake is restricted [25] or the acute response to a saline load [26] is employed as the index, non-modulators show a clear inability to handle sodium. When the earlier metabolic balance study was replicated in a study in which external balance was first achieved on a restricted and then on a high salt intake, the non-modulators showed more positive sodium balance, as they gained more weight [25]; all of the sodium-sensitive hypertension that was identified occurred in that group [27].

Control of the Renal Circulation

In addition to blunted renal vascular responses to angiotensin II, two other abnormalities in the control of the renal circulation, that are germane both to renal vascular responses to angiotensin II and to renal sodium handling, occur in non-modulators. Normal individuals display parallel changes in renal blood flow as they change salt intake: in a shift from a high sodium to a low sodium intake renal blood flow falls, and rises with an increase in salt intake [10,13,17]. Patients with essential hypertension who have intact modulation show similar changes, but renal blood flow is fixed with shifts in sodium intake in non-modulators [10,13,17,15–17]. Again, this abnormality is not part of a continuum, but rather reflects a discrete limitation reflected in a bimodal distribution [25]. To the extent that intrarenal physical forces and filtration fraction contribute to the ability of the kidney to handle sodium, the limited renal vascular response to changes in sodium intake could account for the limited capacity of the kidney to handle sodium (described above).

A fixed renal blood supply in response to a physiological stimulus could reflect fixed, organic disease so common as a byproduct of hypertension. On the other hand, multiple lines of evidence suggest that in some patients there is a functional abnormality of the renal blood supply, vasoconstriction, that contributes to the reduced renal blood flow [10]. ACE inhibition, long recognized as inducing a potentiated renal vasodilatation in essential hypertension [28,29], is now recognized as producing preferential renal vasodilatation in the non-modulator. Indeed, only non-modulators display renal vasodilatation when an ACE inhibitor is administered on a high salt diet, when the renin system is suppressed [27].

ACE inhibition also restores renal vascular responsiveness to angiotensin II [27] and restores the capacity of the kidney to handle a sodium load [26]. We believe that the restoration of the ability of the kidney to handle a sodium load represents a major factor by which ACE inhibitors are effective at achieving goal blood pressure in patients with essential hypertension who enjoy a typical high salt diet, and thus have a suppressed circulating renin-angiotensin system.

The restoration of the renal vascular response to angiotensin II following ACE inhibition also provides insight into mechanisms. If the renal vasodilatation reflected the accumulation of bradykinin because of reduced degradation, or because of prostaglandin release, the renal vasodilator response to ACE inhibition should have been associated with further blunting of renal vascular responsiveness to angiotensin II, since both prostaglandins and kinins share this characteristic [30].

Renin Release and Non-Modulation

Patients with non-modulation at the steady state have either a normal or increased level of plasma renin activity [10,15–17], but two abnormalities of renin release have been identified in non-modulators. In normal subjects on a low salt diet, intravenous infusion of saline rapidly reduces plasma renin activity and plasma aldosterone concentration, but only about 50% of the patients with essential hypertension show this rapid fall [31]. The same patients that had a blunted renin response also had a reduced rate of sodium excretion, and a transient pressor response to the saline infusion. These observations suggested the possibility that non-modulation was involved. Indeed, subsequent studies showed that it was the non-modulator that showed the delayed response to saline [32].

Saline induced suppression of the renin-angiotensin system in the normal subjects did not involve simple plasma volume expansion, since the infusion of dextran in a volume to produce similar or more plasma volume expansion aldosterone concentration [31]. This observation made it possible to divide the stimulus into "sodium sensitive" and "volume sensitive" elements. The rate of fall of plasma renin activity in response to saline in non-modulators is identical to the normal response to dextran, the volume-sensitive signal. One attractive, but speculative, interpretation of these data is that non-modulators have a normal volume-sensing system, but lack the ability to respond to the specific signal emitted by sodium.

A second evidence of disregulation of renin release involves the so-called "short feedback loop," by which angiotensin II reduces renin release. The response occurs within minutes, as opposed to the "long feedback loop," which involves aldosterone release and sodium retention. Patients with essential hypertension frequently do not show renin suppression with angiotensin II infusion [33], an abnormality once again corrected by converting enzyme inhibition [34]. Again, after identification of the non-modulating group, this abnormality was found to occur only in the non-modulator [35].

Genetic Factors

A contribution of heredity to hypertension in many patients has long been recognized, but the precise factors inherited have been remarkably elusive. Information from renal transplantation, both in inbred animal models [1–3] and in man [4,5], has suggested that the genetic information, at least some of the time, is coded in the kidney. Four lines of investigation have suggested that non-modulation is inherited.

The first clue came from the frequency of a family history of hypertension in the parents of non-modulators [25]. In the neighborhood of 90% of the non-modulators in two studies have a parent with hypertension, where the family history could be evaluated, as opposed to a rate of about 30% in essential hypertensives in whom modulation was intact. The second line of investigation involves the identification of features identical to non-modulation, involving both the adrenal gland and the kidney, in the offspring of hypertensives. In the adrenal, plasma aldosterone concentration in the offspring of hypertensives studied on a low salt diet was substantially lower than the concentration in the offspring of normotensive parents, despite a similar level of plasma renin activity and plasma angiotensin II concentration [7]. In an elegant study on aldosterone release in response to angiotensin II infusion, performed by Beretta-Piccoli and his co-workers, aldosterone release was shown to be blunted in the offspring of hypertensives [9], but not normotensive, parents. In Japan, ACE inhibition increased renal blood flow, not only in essential hypertensives with a family history of hypertension, but also in their normotensive offspring [8]. This study was especially impressive because it was performed in Japan, where an ad libitum intake is especially rich in sodium chloride. We have confirmed that observation retrospectively in data for our earlier studies, and prospectively, the calcium channel blocking agent, diltiazem, increased renal blood flow, preferentially in 50% of the offspring of hypertensives, but not in the control group made up of the normotensive offspring of normotensive parents [37]. Diltiazem blocked the action of angiotensin II on the renal blood supply in that study. The specificity of that response was confirmed by the observation that no difference could be identified, in the renal vascular response to the vasodilator acetylcholine, as a function of family history.

A third line of evidence involves red blood cell sodium:lithium countertransport. Lithium countertransport is increased not only in many hypertensives, but also in their normotensive offspring [36–38]. There is a striking increase in the frequency with which increased lithium countertransport occurs in non-modulation [39]. Unfortunately, because of the number of confounding variables that influence lithium countertransport, that determination will be useful in identifying non-modulators only at the extremes of countertransport.

In a study still in progress, involving multiple family members, renal plasma flow and its response to angiotensin have been found in aggregate significantly in the non-modulator [40,41]. There is evidence that sodium handling also is influenced by heredity, and is modified by a family history of hypertension [6]. It will be intriguing to ascertain whether that genetic influence reflects non-modulation and its influence on the renal circulation and aldosterone, or abnormalities in other systems identified in these patients [39,40].

Equally speculative, and equally intriguing, is the possibility that non-modulation has implications for the pathogenesis of renal disease. About one-third of patients with type I diabetes mellitus will develop nephropathy, and two thirds will not, despite an apparently identical severity and duration of disease. Studies in animal models have suggested a powerful role for renal hemodynamic factors, but have not provided an explanation for the fact that 100% of rats but only 33% of people will progress to nephropathy. The information to indicate that the control of the renal circulation is altered not only in non-modulators, but also in their normotensive offspring, may be relevant. Patients with diabetes mellitus at risk of nephropathy display elevated red blood cell sodium: lithium countertransport and a striking family history of hypertension [41,42], features that they share with non-modulators. To the extent that non-modulators and their normotensive offspring act as though they have elevated intrarenal angiotensin II concentration – reflected in a blunted renal vascular response to angiotensin II, blunted renin release in response to saline and angiotensin II, and a potentiated renal vascular response to converting enzyme inhibition – the metabolic disarray of diabetes mellitus superimposed on a disordered control of the renal circulation could lead to glomerular hypertension and its consequences.

That speculation is most sweet when it leads to a testable hypothesis. The speculation that we have indulged in passes that test.

References

1. Bianchi G, Fox U, DiFrancesco GF, et al (1974) Blood pressure changes produced by kidney cross transplantation between spontaneously hypertensive rats (SHR) and normotensive rats (NR). Clin Sci 47:435–448
2. Dahl LK, Heine M (1975) Primary role of renal hemografts in setting blood pressure levels in rats. Circ Res 36:692–696
3. Kawabe K, Watanabe TX, Shiono K, et al (1978) Influence of blood pressure of renal isografts between spontaneously hypertensive and normotensive rats utilizing the F1 hybrids. Jpn Heart J 19:886–894
4. Guidi E, Bianchi G, Dallosia V, et al (1982) Influence of familial hypertension of the donor on the blood pressure and antihypertensive therapy of kidney grafat recipients. Nephron 30:318–323
5. Curtiss JJ, Luke RG, Dustan HP, et al (1983) Remission of essential hypertension after renal transplantation. N Engl J Med 309:1009–1015
6. Luft FC, Rankin LI, Bkloch R, et al (1979) Cardiovascular and humoral responses to extremes of sodium intake in normal black and white men. Circulation 60:697–703
7. Blackshear JL, TGarnic D, Williams GH, et al (1987) Exaggerated renal vascular response to calcium entry blockade in first degree relatives of essential hypertensives: Possible role of intrarenal angiotensin II. Hypertension 9:384–389
8. Uneda S, Fukishima S, Fujika Y, et al (1986) Renal hemodynamics and renin angiotensin system in adolescents genetically predisposed to essential hypertension. J Hypertens 2(Suppl 3):437–439
9. Beretta-Picolli C, Pusterla C, Stadler P, et al (1988) Blunted aldosterone responsiveness to AII in normotensive subjects with familial predisposition to essential hypertension. J Hypertens 61:57–61
10. Hollenberg NK, Williams GH (1986) Sensitivity to sodium and nonmodulation of renal and adrenal responsiveness to angiotensin II. Implications for the pathogenesis of hypertension. In: Zanchetti A, Tarazi RC (eds) Handbook of hypertension, vol 8. Elsevier, New York, pp 520–522
11. Dahl LK (1963) Metabolic aspects of hypertension. Annu Rev Med 14:69–98
12. Gutman RA, Forrey AW, Flet WP, et al (1973) Vasopressor-induced natriuresis and altered intrarenal hemodynamics in cirrhotic man. Clin Sci 45:19–34
13. Hollenberg NK, Merrill JP (1970) Intrarenal perfusion in the young essential hypertensive: A subpopulation resistant to sodium restriction. Trans Assoc Am Physicians 83:93–101
14. Williams GH, Rose LI, Dluhy RG, et al (1970) Abnormal responsiveness of the renin aldosterone system to acute stimulation in patients with essential hypertension. Ann Intern Med 72:317–326

15. Williams GH, Tuck ML, Sullivan JM, et al (1982) Parallel adrenal and renal abnormalities in the young patient with essential hypertension. Am J Med 72:907–914
16. Hollenberg NK, Chenitz WR, Adams DF, et al (1974) Reciprocal influence of salt intake on adrenal glomerulosa and renal vascular responses to angiotensin II in normal man. J Clin Invest 54:34–42
17. Shoback DM, Williams GH, Hollenberg NK, et al (1983) Endogenous angiotensin II as a determinant of sodium modulated changes in tissue responsiveness to angiotensin II in normal man. J Clin Endocrinol Metab 57:764–770
18. Williams GH, Hollenberg NK (1985) Abnormal adrenal and renal responses to angiotensin II in essential hypertension: Implications for pathogenesis. In: Carey RM (ed) Clinical endocrinology: is essential hypertension an endocrine disease?, vol 7. Butterworth, London, pp 184–211
19. Ambard L, Beaujard E (1904) Causes de l'hypertension arterielle. Arch Intern Med 1:520–533
20. Allen FM (1925) Treatment of kidney disease and high blood pressure. The Psychiatric Institute, Morristown, p 206
21. Chapman B (1951) Some effects of the rice-fruit diet in patients with essential hypertension. In: Bell ET (ed) Hypertension: A symposium. Minneapolis, pp 504–516
22. Freis E (1979) Comparative effects of tierynafen and hydrochlorothiazide in the treatment of hypertension (Veterans Administration Cooperative Study Group on Antihypertensive Agents). N Engl J Med 301:293–297
23. Kawasaki T, Delea CS, Bartter FC, et al (1978) The effect of high sodium and low sodium intakes on blood pressure and other related variables in human subjects with idiopathic hypertension. Am J Med 64:193–198
24. Fujita T, Henry WL, Bartter FC, et al (1980) Factors influencing blood pressure in salt sensitive patients with hypertension. Am J Med 69:334–344
25. Hollenberg NK, Williams GH (1986) Abnormal renal sodium handling in essential hypertension: Relation to failure to renal and adrenal modulation of responses to angiotensin II. Am J Med 81:412–418
26. Rystedt LL, Williams GH, Hollenberg NK (1986) The renal and endocrine response to saline infusion in essential hypertension. Hypertension 8:217–222
27. Redgrave JE, Rabinowe SL, Hollenberg NK, et al (1985) Correction of abnormal renal blood flow response to angiotensin II by converting enzyme inhibition in essential hypertensives. J Clin Invest 75:1285–1290
28. Williams GH, Hollenberg NK (1977) Accentuated vascular and endocrine responses to SQ 20881 in hypertension. N Engl J Med 297:184–188
29. Hollenberg NK, Meggs LG, Williams GH, et al (1981) Sodium intake and renal responses to captopril in normal man and in essential hypertension. Kidney 20:240–245
30. Meggs LG, Katzberg RW, DeLeeuw P, et al (1985) Specific desensitization of the canine renal vasculature to angiotensin II despite cycloxygenase inhibition. Yale J Biol Med 58:453–458
31. Tuck ML, Williams GH, Dluhy RG, et al (1976) A delayed suppression of the renin aldosterone axis following saline infusion in human hypertension. Circ Res 39:711–716
32. Rabinowe SL, Redgrave JE, Rysedt LL, et al (1987) Renin-suppression by saline is blunted in non-modulating essential hypertension. Hypertension 10:404–408
33. Dluhy RG, Bavli SZ, Leung FK, et al (1979) Abnormal adrenal responsiveness and angiotensin II dependency in high renin essential hypertension. J Clin Invest 64:1270–1276
34. LeBoff MS, Dluhy RG, Hollenberg NK, et al (1982) Abnormal renin short feedback loop in essential hypertension is reversible with converting enzyme inhibition. J Clin Invest 70:335–341
35. Seely EW, Moore TJ, Rogacz S, Gordon M, Gleason RE, Hollenberg NK, Williams GH

(1989) Angiotensin-mediated renin suppression is alterd in non-modulating hypertension. Hypertension 13:31–37
36. Redgrave JE, Canessa M, Gleason R, Hollenberg NK, Williams GH (1989) Red blood cell Na-Li countertransport in non-modulating essential hypertensives. Hypertension 13:721–726
37. Dluhy RG, Hopkins P, Hollenberg NK, Williams GH, Williams RR (1988) Heritable abnormalities of the renin-angiotensin-aldosterone system in essential hypertension. J Cardiovasc Pharmacol 12(3):149–154
38. Lifton RP, Hopkins PN, Williams RR, Hollenberg NK, Williams GH, Dluhy RG (1989) Evidence for heritability of non-modulating essential hypertension. Hypertension 13: 884–889
39. Gordon MS, Steunkel CA, Conlin PR, Hollenberg NK, Williams GH (1989) The role of dopamine in nonmodulating hypertension. J Clin Endocrinol Metab 69(2):426–432
40. Conlin PR, Gleason RE, Hollenberg NK, Williams GH (1989) Altered aldosterone and norepinephrine responses to upright posture in nonmodulating hypertension (abstract No. 61). Hypertension 14:346
41. Krolewski AS, Canessa M, Warram JH, et al (1988) Predisposition to hypertension and susceptibility to renal disease in insulin-dependent diabetes mellitus. N Engl J Med 318: 140–145
42. Mangill R, Bending JJ, Scott G, et al. Increased sodium-lithium countertransport activity in red cells of patients with insulin-dependent diabetes and nephropathy. N Engl J Med 318:146–150

Renal Microcirculation in Essential Hypertension

Koichi Hayashi, Murray Epstein[1,2], and Rodger D. Loutzenhiser[1,2]

Summary. The past several years have witnessed important advances in characterizing the renal microvascular response to pressure as a determinant of renal autoregulation. Utilizing diverse in vitro models, including the juxtamedullary nephron preparation and the isolated perfused hydronephrotic kidney, several investigators have demonstrated that pressure-dependent alterations of the renal microvessels are mediated, in part, independent of signals from the macula densa. Furthermore, recent evidence indicates that the afferent arterioles of normotensive and genetically hypertensive animals respond differently to changes of renal arterial pressure (RAP). Thus, hypertension is associated with a compensatory shift in the pressure response of the afferent arteriole, such that higher RAPs are required to elicit vasoconstriction in this vessel. Calcium antagonists attenuate pressure-induced afferent arteriolar vasoconstriction, suggesting the participation of dihydropyridine-sensitive calcium channels in mediating pressure-induced vasoconstriction of this microvessel.

Introduction

The rediscovery, by Goldblatt and his co-workers [1], that partial ligation of the renal artery induces hypertension raised the possibility that essential hypertension could be renal in origin due to abnormalities of renal perfusion. Subsequently, a large body of evidence has accumulated, recognizing the important role of structural and functional changes in the renal microcirculation in the initiation and maintenance of hypertension in animals, as well as in humans [2–4]. In this brief survey, we review recent studies which further characterize the renal microvascular response to pressure elevation utilizing diverse in vitro models.

[1]Nephrology Section, Veterans Administration Medical Center, Miami, FL 33125, USA
[2]Nephrology Division, Department of Medicine, University of Miami School of Medicine, Miami, FL 33125, USA
(Address correspondence to: Dr. Murray Epstein, at above address.)

Sustained hypertension markedly alters the renal response to elevations in renal perfusion pressure; shifting the threshold pressure of autoregulation of renal blood flow [5] and pressure-induced natriuresis [6,7] to higher pressures. This resetting of the renal response to pressure represents a renal adaptation to hypertension. Pressure-induced vasoconstriction of renal microvessels constitutes an important determinant of renal autoregulation [8,9]. It is extremely difficult, however, to assess directly the renal microvascular response to pressure in situ. The ability to directly observe microvascular responses would obviously facilitate the characterization of the determinants of the autoregulatory response. Unfortunately, the vascular pole of the glomerulus is not accessible to direct intravital microscopic observation. An early attempt to circumvent this problem involved transplantation of glomeruli into the hamster cheek pouch and subsequent observation following revascularization [10]. Using this approach, Click et al. demonstrated differences in the responsiveness of renal microvessels to various hormones in normotensive and hypertensive animals [10]. The effects of hypertension on renal microvascular responsiveness during acute changes of perfusion pressure have, until recently, not been directly ascertained.

Finally, it is apparent that when arterial pressure is altered in vivo, concomitant changes in the neural and humoral determinants of renal microvascular tone tend to counter the induced changes, thereby confounding the interpretation of results [11,12]. Recently, a number of investigators have succeeded in characterizing the determinants of the renal autoregulatory response to pressure, utilizing diverse in vitro models.

Role of TGF and Myogenic Vasoconstriction in Autoregulation

Sanchez-Ferrer et al. [13] utilized the in vitro perfused juxtamedullary nephron preparation perfused with cell-free artificial media to directly assess the determinants of the microvascular response to elevated pressure. Their studies demonstrated an afferent arteriolar vasoconstriction in response to elevated renal arterial pressure (120–180 mm Hg). When the tubuloglomerular feedback mechanism was blocked, either with furosemide administration, or by removal of the renal papilla (by interrupting the delivery of fluid to the macula densa), pressure-induced afferent arteriolar vasoconstriction was eliminated. Based on these observations, the authors concluded that pressure-induced pre-glomerular vasoconstriction is mediated entirely by feedback signals from the macula densa without any remaining, i.e., myogenic, component.

In contrast, Moore [14] has advocated that an important tubuloglomerular feedback (TGF)-independent component contributes to the renal microvascular response to pressure. Carmines et al. [15] demonstrated myogenic pressure-dependent contractions of interlobular arteries in the blood-perfused juxtamedullary nephron preparation.

Recently our laboratory has investigated, in a quantitative manner, the role of preglomerular microvessels, i.e., the interlobular artery and the afferent arteriole, in mediating the vasoconstrictor response to changes in perfusion pressure [16]. We have utilized the isolated perfused hydronephrotic kidney model to delineate the renal microvascular response to changes in perfusion pressure. This model is uniquely

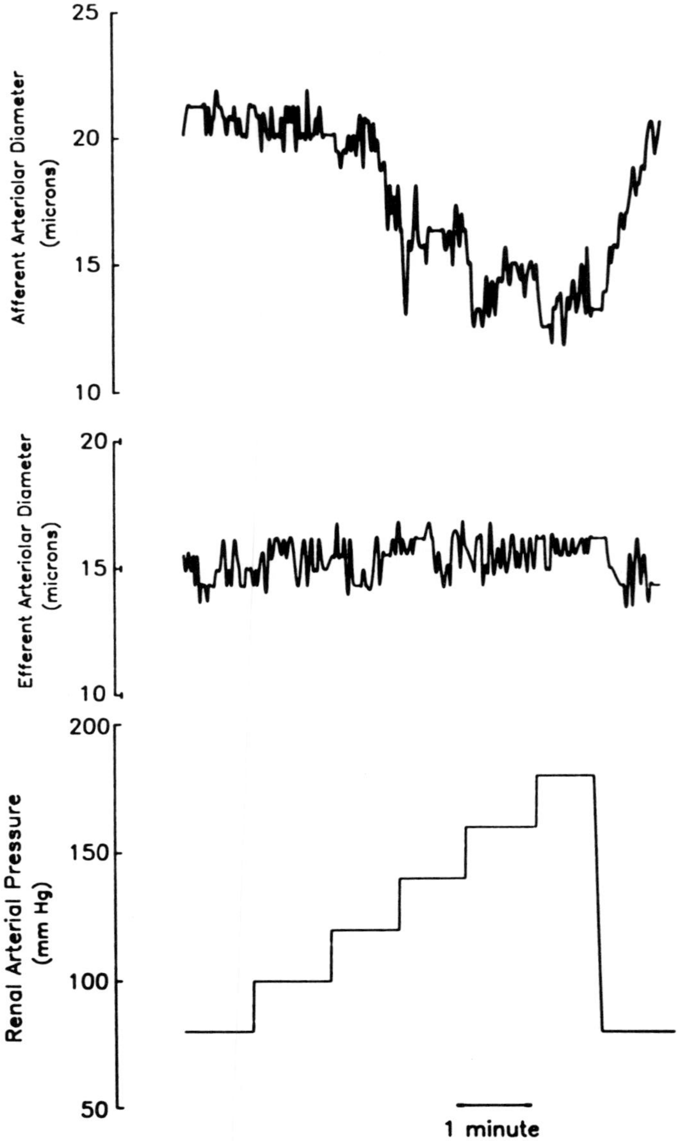

Fig. 1. Representative tracings depicting the response of afferent and efferent arterioles of an isolated perfused hydronephrotic kidney to alterations in renal arterial pressure. Increasing pressure in the renal artery (*bottom*) elicited a vasoconstriction of the afferent arteriole (*top*), but not of the efferent arteriole (*center*). (Reproduced from [11] with permission)

suited for the study of renal microvascular responsiveness to alterations in perfusion pressure [11]. The renal microvessels can be visualized in an intact in situ setting, but under in vitro conditions in which RAP is under direct experimental control. Extrarenal neural and humoral influences on renal vascular tone are eliminated. Furthermore, as detailed previously [11], because hydronephrosis induces tubular atrophy [17], tubulo-glomerular feedback is absent in this model. Thus, pressure-dependent alterations of the renal microvessels must occur independent of signals from the macula densa. As demonstrated by the original tracing in Fig. 1, the afferent arteriole constricted markedly as renal arterial pressure was elevated, whereas the efferent arteriole was unresponsive to this manipulation.

Recent studies by Hayashi et al. [16] utilizing the isolated perfused hydronephrotic kidney have delineated the marked segmental heterogeneity in the response of the afferent arteriole to pressure. These findings are summarized in Fig. 2. Both SHR and WKY manifested a blunted response to elevated perfusion pressure at the segment near the glomerulus. Thus, this segment of the afferent arteriole vasoconstricted only modestly in response to elevating RAP from 80 mm Hg to 180 mm Hg (i.e., 7.4±2.5% and 8.1±2.0% decreases in vessel diameters in WKY and SHR, respectively). In contrast, the same change in RAP resulted in marked decreases in the diameters of the segments of the afferent arteriole near the interlobular artery (−22.3±1.6% and −19.9±1.6% in WKY and SHR, respectively and at the mid-portion (−20.2±1.6% and −18.5±2.7% in WKY and SHR, respectively). These findings are in accord with the observation by Steinhausen et al. [18] that reducing renal arterial pressure in vivo causes less vasodilation in the afferent arteriolar segment near the glomerulus than in the more proximal portions of this vessel. In contrast to these observations in both in vivo and in vitro hydronephrotic kidneys, Carmines [19] reported that in the perfused juxtamedullary nephron preparation the portion of the afferent arteriole nearest the glomerulus manifests the major resistance adjustment to alterations in RAP. These divergent findings may be attributable to differences in the role of TGF in these two models. In the juxtamedullary nephron, TGF is intact, whereas the tubular atrophy associated with chronic hydronephrosis disrupts this mechanism [11,17]. In concert, these observations suggest that the portion of the afferent arteriole near the glomerulus may be under predominant control by TGF [20], whereas more proximal segments exhibit an intrinsic, e.g., myogenic, vasoconstrictor response to elevated pressure.

As discussed above, Sanchez-Ferrer et al. have recently reported that the pressure-induced decrement in arteriolar diameter and regulation of glomerular pressure in juxtamedullary nephrons were completely abolished by pharmacologic or surgical disruption of TGF [13]. Based on these findings, the authors concluded that TGF-induced vasoconstriction represented the sole mechanism whereby afferent arteriolar tone is modulated by elevated pressure. Our demonstration that the afferent arteriole of the hydronephrotic kidney constricts in response to pressure elevation, despite the absence of TGF mechanism, clearly indicates an important contribution of non-TGF mediated vasoconstriction in the pressure response of the renal microvasculature.

One possible explanation for these apparent discrepancies relates to the region of the afferent arteriole under observation. As detailed above, the segment of the affer-

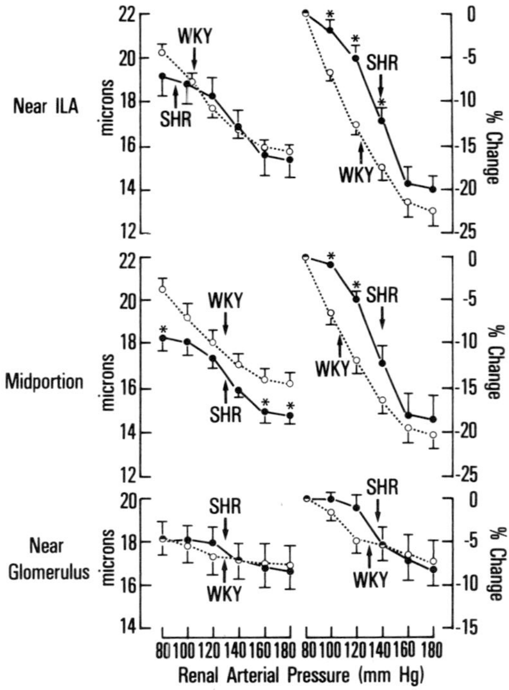

Fig. 2. Effects of renal arterial pressure on the diameters of afferent arterioles in kidneys from WKY (*open circle*) and SHR (*closed circle*). Regions of afferent arterioles observed were classified as segments near the interlobular artery (*ILA*, *top*), of midportion (*center*), and near the glomerulus (*bottom*). In the lower range of renal arterial pressure, pressure-induced afferent arteriolar vasoconstriction was blunted in SHR as compared with that in WKY (*left panel*). Plotting the data as the percent change in vessel diameter revealed a marked shift of the response of afferent arterioles in SHR kidneys (*right panel*). Note the diminished response of segments near the glomerulus to an increase in renal arterial pressure as compared with other segments. Results are mean±SE; *$P<0.05$ vs. WKY. (Reproduced from [16] by permission of the American Heart Association, Inc.)

ent arteriole near the glomerulus does not respond directly to elevated pressure (Fig. 2), whereas this site is the major region affected by TGF [20]. In contrast, more proximal portions of the afferent arteriole respond markedly to pressure, but are not likely to be influenced by the macula densa signal. Finally, it should be noted that we studied vessels arising from small caliber (ca. 30 μm) interlobular arteries, suggesting an origin in the superficial cortex. These afferent arterioles had a mean basal diameter of approximately 20 μm. In contrast, the afferent arterioles observed in the juxtamedullary nephron preparation arise primarily from the arcuate artery and have basal diameters of 32 μm. Thus, differences in myogenic responsiveness may be related to regional factors and may be influenced by vessel diameter.

Sites of Preglomerular Vasoconstriction

Although pre-glomerular vessels are thought to be primarily responsible for the autoregulatory response [21,22], controversy remains concerning the relative role of the afferent arteriole and the interlobular artery. Tønder et al. [23] demonstrated that the pressure within the interlobular artery in the outer cortex was substantially lower than that of the aorta. Furthermore, Källskog et al. [24] demonstrated that within the autoregulatory range, the pressure in the superficial interlobular artery was maintained relatively unchanged. These observations indicate that the interlobular artery contributes importantly to renal autoregulation. In contrast, Carmines and colleagues [15] reported that in juxtamedullary nephrons, afferent arteriolar pressure was variably regulated, whereas interlobular arterial pressure was not. Thus, these observations suggest a predominant contribution of the afferent arteriole to renal autoregulation, at least in the juxtamedullary portion of the renal microcirculation. Of interest, Carmines et al. demonstrated the presence of pressure-induced vasoconstriction in both afferent and interlobular artery [15]. Thus, the lack of pressure regulation within this segment of the interlobular artery may simply reflect the larger diameter of this vessel near the arcuate artery (ca. 50 μm).

We have recently demonstrated that the intralobular artery of the isolated perfused hydronephrotic kidney responds markedly to elevated pressure. More importantly, the responsiveness of this vessel to pressure is dependent on the basal diameter, with the smaller diameter, i.e., distal, segments demonstrating a much more marked response than the larger, i.e., proximal, segments [25]. Since vascular resistance is inversely related to the fourth power of the radius, it follows that a pressure-induced vasoconstriction of the smaller caliber segments of this vessel, i.e., in the outer cortex, may contribute more to autoregulation than the larger segments, i.e. in the juxtamedullary region. Taken together, these findings are consistent with the postulate that the segments of the interlobular artery in the superficial cortex contribute importantly to the regulation of renal hemodynamics.

Altered Autoregulation in Hypertension

Sustained hypertension influences several aspects of the renal response to elevated renal perfusion pressure. Autoregulation of renal blood flow and the pressure-natriuresis relationship are both reset toward higher pressure level in hypertensive animals [5–7]. In a recent study [16], we have demonstrated that the RAP at which a significant increase in total renal vascular resistance is attained is higher in kidneys isolated from SHR (180 mm Hg) than in those from WKY (140 mm Hg). This observation indicates a resetting of the relationship between RAP and total renal vascular resistance in our experimental model.

There is little information on the functional modification of the responsiveness of microvessels to changes of perfusion pressure in hypertensive animals. Previous investigations have demonstrated that arterioles from the gracilis muscle in SHR exhibited a higher threshold for pressure-induced vasoconstriction than in WKY, indicating the shift of pressure-diameter relationship at arteriolar levels in the microcirculatory bed of skeletal muscle [26].

We recently characterized for the first time, in a controlled in vitro setting, the responsiveness of the renal microvessels to changes of RAP in kidneys from normotensive and hypertensive rats. Direct assessment of the microvascular response to elevated RAP suggests that the renal hemodynamic adaptation in hypertension involves an alteration in the responsiveness of the afferent arteriole. Thus, we observed a shift to the right in the pressure response curves of afferent arterioles in kidneys from SHR (Fig. 2). The threshold RAP that elicited a significant afferent arteriolar vasoconstriction was 20 mm Hg higher in SHR than in WKY. Furthermore, the pressure at which half maximum vasoconstrictor response was elicited was also shifted to a higher pressure level in SHR at every segment of the afferent arteriole (Fig. 2). In contrast, interlobular arteries exhibited no shift of pressure-diameter relationship in kidneys from hypertensive animals. Thus, our study indicates that the adaptive changes in the responsiveness of renal microvessels to changes of RAP in hypertensive animals is restricted to the afferent arteriole. To our knowledge, this finding constitutes the first direct demonstration that renal arteriolar behavior adapts to a higher pressure level in hypertensive animals.

Although our recent study clearly demonstrates a shift in the relationship between RAP and pressure-induced afferent arteriolar tone, an influence of pre-afferent arteriolar resistance cannot be ruled out. Sustained hypertension causes structural changes which could decrease vessel diameters and thus increase passive resistance of larger vessels [27]. Thus, a greater pressure drop in pre-afferent arteries may be responsible for the observed shift in the relationship between RAP and afferent arteriolar vasoconstriction in kidneys from SHR. However, as detailed elsewhere in this volume [25], we observed that hypertension alters the responsiveness of the interlobular artery in an entirely different manner, potentiating the response of the intermediate segment. The distal portions of the interlobular arteries that we examined exhibited no shift in pressure-induced response. Furthermore, the basal (i.e., at 80 mm Hg) vessel diameters of the interlobular artery were identical (WKY; 28.4 ± 1.6 vs. SHR; 27.3 ± 2.0 μm, $P > 0.5$). This latter observation tends to militate against a difference in luminal pressure in WKY and SHR arterioles.

Effects of Calcium Antagonists

Calcium antagonists have been demonstrated to abolish autoregulation both in isolated kidney preparations [28,29] and in intact animals [30,31]. In isolated renal interlobular arteries from the dog, Harder et al. have demonstrated that verapamil abolishes pressure-induced vascular tone [32]. In an attempt to directly characterize the effects of calcium antagonists on the renal microvascular response to pressure, we have examined the actions of nifedipine on pressure-induced afferent arteriolar vasoconstriction in WKY and SHR in isolated perfused hydronephrotic kidneys.

The effects of nifedipine on pressure-induced afferent arteriolar vasoconstriction in kidneys from WKY and SHR are depicted in Figs. 3 and 4. As depicted in Fig. 3, before administration of nifedipine, the afferent arteriole constricted in response to graded increases in RAP. In the presence of nifedipine (10^{-6} M), the pressure-induced afferent arteriolar vasoconstriction was completely abolished.

Figures 4a and 4b depict the effects of nifedipine on pressure-induced afferent arteriolar vasoconstriction in WKY (n=7) and SHR kidneys (n=6). As detailed

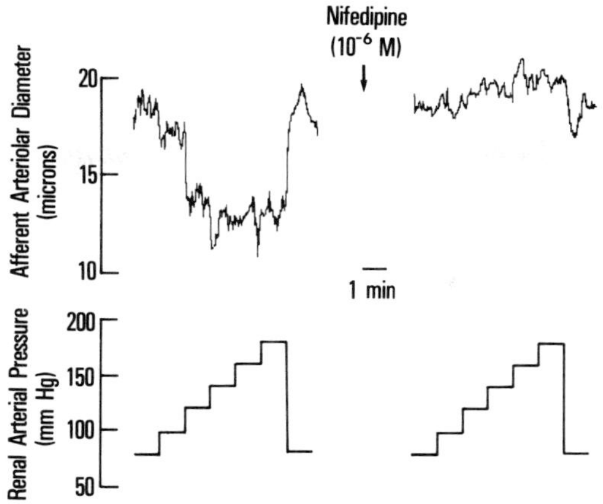

Fig. 3. Representative tracings depicting the effects of nifedipine on the pressure-induced vasoconstrictor response of an afferent arteriole in an isolated perfused kidney from SHR. In the absence of nifedipine, an increase in renal arterial pressure induced a pressure-dependent vasoconstriction (*left*). The addition of 10^{-6} M nifedipine to the perfusate abolished this response (*right*). (Reproduced from [16] by permission of the American Heart Association, Inc.)

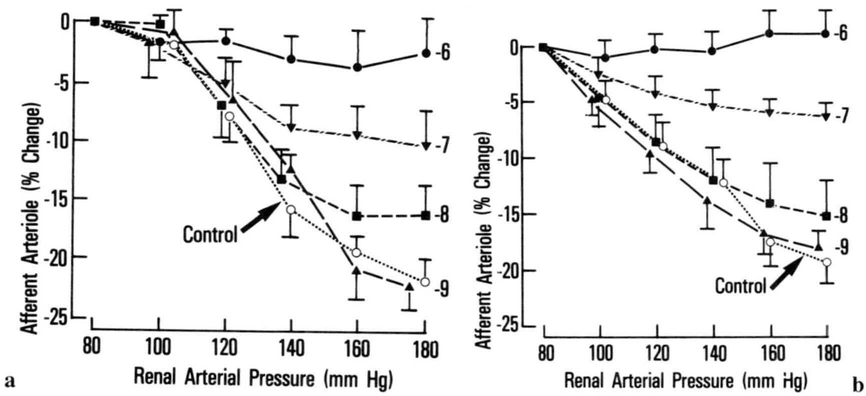

Fig. 4a,b. Effects of nifedipine on pressure-induced afferent arteriolar vasoconstriction in kidneys from Wistar Kyoto control (*WKY*) **a,** n=7 and Spontaneously hypertensive rat (*SHR*) **b,** n=6. In the absence of nifedipine (control, *open circle*), an increase in perfusion pressure induced a decrease in afferent arteriolar diameter. The addition of nifedipine to the perfusate inhibited the afferent arteriolar vasoconstriction in a dose-dependent manner (nifedipine concentrations depicted on *right* as log M). At 10^{-6} M, nifedipine completely abolished the response in both WKY ($P>0.5$) and SHR ($P>0.1$). Results are mean±SE. (Reproduced from [16] by permission of the American Heart Association Inc.)

above, in the absence of nifedipine, afferent arteriolar diameters decreased in both WKY and WHR as RAP was increased. The administration of 10^{-9} M–10^{6} M of nifedipine did not alter basal afferent arteriolar diameters in either strain. Nevertheless, nifedipine markedly inhibited pressure-induced afferent arteriolar vasoconstriction in a dose dependent manner in both WKY (Fig. 4a) and SHR (Fig. 4b). The concentrations at which half maximal inhibition was observed, i.e. IC_{50}, were identical (WKY; 63 ± 27 nM vs. SHR; 60 ± 32 nM, $P > 0.5$). At 10^{-6} M, nifedipine completely abolished the pressure-induced afferent arteriolar vasoconstriction in both strains. In concert, these observations suggest the participation of dihydropyridine-sensitive calcium channels in mediating pressure-induced vasoconstriction of this microvessel.

Conclusions

It is evident that major strides have been made in characterizing the renal microvascular response to pressure. Utilizing diverse in vitro models, including the juxtamedullary nephron preparation and the isolated perfused hydronephrotic kidney, investigators have demonstrated that elevated pressure elicits afferent arteriolar vasoconstriction directly by a pressure-dependent (i.e., myogenic) mechanism, and indirectly by signals originating from the macula densa (i.e., TGF). Therefore, the available evidence suggest that both TGF-induced and myogenic vasoconstriction act in concert to mediate renal autoregulation. Furthermore, recent evidence indicates that hypertension is associated with a compensatory shift in the pressure response of the afferent arteriole, such that higher RAPs are required to elicit vasoconstriction in this vessel. Finally, we have demonstrated in a direct and conclusive manner that calcium antagonists attenuate pressure-induced afferent arteriolar vasoconstriction, suggesting the participation of dihydropyridine-sensitive calcium channels.

Acknowledgments. We wish to thank Audrey M. Kincaid for expert preparation of this manuscript.

Portions of this review were adapted by permission of the American Heart Association, Inc. from our article "Pressure-induced vasoconstriction of renal microvessels in normotensive and hypertensive rats: Studies in the isolated perfused hydronephrotic kidney", Circulation Research 65:1475–1484, 1989.

References

1. Goldblatt H, Lynch J, Hanzal RF, Sommerville WW (1934) Studies in experimental hypertension. The production of a persistent elevation of systolic blood pressure by means of renal ischemia. J Exp Med 59:347–379
2. Folkow B, Hallback M, Lundgred Y, Sivertson R, Weiss L (1973) Importance of adaptive changes in vascular design for establishment of primary hypertension, studied in man and in spontaneously hypertensive rats. Circ Res 32:2–16
3. Mulvany MJ, Hansen PK, Aalkjaer C (1978) Direct evidence that the greater contractility of resistance vessels in spontaneously hypertensive rats is associated with a narrowed lumen, a thickened media, and an increased number of smooth muscle cell layers. Circ Res 43:854–864

4. MacKay A, Brown JJ, Lever AF (1983) Unilateral renal disease in hypertension. In: Roberson JIS (ed) Handbook of hypertension, vol 2: Clinical aspects of secondary hypertension. Elsevier, Amsterdam, pp 33–78
5. Iversen BM, Sekse I, Ofstad J (1987) Resetting of renal blood flow autoregulation in spontaneously hypertensive rats. Am J Physiol 252:F480–F486
6. Roman RJ, Cowley AW Jr (1985) Abnormal pressure-diuresis-natriuresis response in spontaneously hypertensive rats. Am J Physiol 248:F199–F205
7. Roman RJ (1987) Altered pressure-natriuresis relationship in young spontaneously hypertensive rats. Hypertension 9 (Suppl III):130–136
8. Aukland K, Øien AH (1987) Renal autoregulation:models combining tubuloglomerular feedback and myogenic response. Am J Physiol 252:F768–F783
9. Lush DJ, Fray JCS (1984) Steady-state autoregulation of renal blood flow: a myogenic model. Am J Physiol 247:R89–R99
10. Click RL, Joyner WL, Gilmore JP (1979) Reactivity of glomerular afferent and efferent arterioles in renal hypertension. Kidney Int 15:109–115
11. Loutzenhiser R, Epstein M (1990) Renal hemodynamic effects of calcium antagonists. In: Epstein M, Loutzenhiser R (eds) Calcium antagonists and the kidney. Hanley and Belfus, Philadelphia, pp 33–75
12. Epstein M, Flamenbaum W, Loutzenhiser R (1980) Characterization of the renin-angiotensin system in the isolated perfused rat kidney. Renal Physiol 2:244–256
13. Sanchez-Ferrer CF, Roman RJ, Harder DR (1989) Pressure-dependent contraction of rat juxtamedullary afferent arterioles. Circ Res 64:790–798
14. Moore LC (1984) Tubuloglomerular feedback and SNGFR autoregulation in the rat. Am J Physiol 247:F267–F276
15. Carmines PK, Inscho EW, Gensure RC (1990) Arterial pressure effects on preglomerular microvasculature of juxtamedullary nephrons. Am J Physiol 258:F94–F102
16. Hayashi K, Epstein M, Loutzenhiser R (1989) Pressure-induced vasoconstriction of renal microvessels in normotensive and hypertensive rats: Studies in the isolated perfused hydronephrotic kidney. Circ Res 65:1475–1484
17. Fleming JT, Garthoff B, Mayer D, Rosen B, Steinhausen M (1987) Comparison of the effects of antihypertensive drugs on pre- and postglomerular vessels of the hydronephrotic kidney. J Cardiovasc Pharmacol 10(Suppl 10):S149–S153
18. Steinhausen M, Fleming JT, Holz FG, Parekh N (1987) Nitrendipine and the pressure-dependent vasodilation of vessels in the hydronephrotic kidney. J Cardiovasc Pharmacol 9(Suppl 1):S39–S43
19. Carmines PK (1989) Responses of the renal microvasculature to changes in renal arterial pressure (abstract). FASEB J M19:A1381
20. Schnermann J, Briggs J (1985) Function of the juxtaglomerular apparatus; local control of glomerular hemodynamics. In: Seldin DW, Giebisch G (eds) The kidney: physiology and pathology, vol 1. Raven, New York, pp 669–697
21. Navar LG, Marsh DL, Blantz RC, Hall J, Ploth DW, Nasjletti A (1982) Intrinsic control of renal hemodynamics. Fed Proc 41:3022–3030
22. Øien AH, Aukland K (1983) A mathematical analysis of the myogenic hypothesis with special reference to autoregulation of renal blood flow. Circ Res 52:241–252
23. Tønder KJH, Aukland K (1979) Interlobular arterial pressure in the rat kidney. Renal Physiol 80;2:214–221
24. Källskog Ö, Lindbom LO, Ulfendahl HR, Wolgast M (1976) Hydrostatic pressure within the vascular structures of the rat kidney. Pflügers Arch 363:205–210
25. Hayashi K, Epstein M, Loutzenhiser R (1991) Role of the interlobular (ILA) in protection against glomerular barotrauma in hypertension (abstract). Proceedings of the XIth International Congress of Nephrology, July 15–20 1990. Tokyo, Japan
26. Alson RL, Dusseau JW, Hutchins PM (1985) Arteriolar and systemic autoregulatory

responses during the development of hypertension in the spontaneously hypertensive rats. Proc Soc Exp Biol Med 180:62–71
27. Heptinstall RH (1983) Pathology of the kidney, vol 1, 3rd edn. Little, Brown, Boston, pp 181–246
28. Ono H, Kokubun H, Hashimoto K (1974) Abolition by calcium antagonists of the autoregulation of renal blood flow. Naunyn Schmiedebergs Arch Pharmacol 285:201–207
29. Cohen AJ, Fray JCS (1982) Calcium ion dependence of myogenic renal plasma flow autoregulation: evidence from the isolated perfused rat kidney. J Physiol 330:449–460
30. Lin H, Young DB (1988) Verapamil alters the relationship between renal perfusion pressure and glomerular filtration rate and renin release: The mechanism of the antihypertensive effect. J Cardiovasc Pharmacacol 12(Suppl 6):S57–S59
31. Navar LG, Champion WJ, Thomas CE (1986) Effects of calcium channel blockade on renal vascular resistance responses to changes in perfusion pressure and angiotensin-converting enzyme inhibition in dogs. Circ Res 58:874–881
32. Harder DR, Gilbert R, Lombard JH (1987) Vascular muscle cell depolarization and activation in renal arteries on elevation of transmural pressure. Am J Physiol 253:F778–F781

The Pathogenesis of Salt-Sensitive Hypertension

TOSHIRO FUJITA[1]

SUMMARY. Patients with normal plasma renin and essential hypertension can be divided into two groups according to blood pressure response to salt loading; salt-sensitive (SS) and non-salt-sensitive (NSS). With a high-sodium diet SS patients retained more sodium, and had a greater increase in cardiac output, as compared to NSS patients. Despite the markedly increased cardiac output, systemic vascular resistance did not change with sodium loads in the SS patients, suggesting inappropriately elevated systemic vascular resistance. The greater increase in blood pressure with sodium loads seems to be characterized by a very inhomogeneous distribution of local flow and resistance in SS patients; renal and hepatic blood flow remains essentially unchanged and skeletal muscle blood flow receives almost all of the increase in cardiac output. Moreover, systemic vascular resistance changes did not reflect the resistance of individual beds because vasoconstriction appeared in the kidney and in the splanchnic area but was masked by prominent vasodilation in the skeletal muscle. Because this hemodynamic pattern is similar to the pattern evoked during defense reaction, it is suggested that sympathetic overactivity on a selective basis might be involved in the impaired renal function for sodium excretion and the increase in blood pressure with sodium loads in SS patients.

Introduction

It is widely believed that excessive sodium intake plays a role in the development of hypertension in man. Epidemiological studies have shown that the prevalence of hypertension in a population increases with the usual sodium intake of that population. Even in populations habitually consuming large amounts of sodium, however, 60% of the population remains free of hypertension, suggesting that some individuals are susceptible to the pressor effects of sodium while others are resistant.

[1]The Fourth Department of Internal Medicine, University of Tokyo School of Medicine, 3-28-6 Mejirodai, Bunkyo-ku, Tokyo, 112 Japan

In our previous studies [1–6], we found that patients with essential hypertension could be divided into two groups according to the blood-pressure response to salt load; salt-sensitive (SS) and non-salt-sensitive (NSS). On a high-salt diet, the salt-sensitive hypertensive patients retained more sodium and gained more weight, with greater increase in blood pressure, as compared to the non-salt-sensitive patients [1]. It seems that human hypertensive subjects show heterogeneous responses to sodium loading.

Systemic Hemodynamics in Patients with Salt-Sensitive Hypertension

In partially nephrectomized dogs, salt loading increases blood pressure, possibly by causing sodium retention. During the early period of salt loading, cardiac output increases, but later, systemic vascular resistance increases in association with the restoration of cardiac output. Although the precise mechanism for the increased vascular resistance with salt loading is still unknown, Guyton et al. [7] postulated that total body autoregulation might contribute to an increase in vascular resistance during exposure to salt and water in excess.

Cardiac output increased with salt loading in all patients, but the extent of the increase was significantly greater in the salt-sensitive patients than in the non-salt-sensitive ones. The elevation of blood pressure with salt loading in the salt-sensitive patients may be partly due to the increased cardiac output, possibly caused by sodium retention [1,6].

With increased cardiac output, the non-salt-sensitive patients had significantly decreased systemic vascular resistance with salt loading. In contrast, systemic vascular resistance remained unchanged with salt loading in the salt-sensitive patients, in spite of the pronounced increase in cardiac output. In the salt-sensitive patients, the fall in peripheral resistance was not adequate to maintain pressure hemeostasis when the magnitude of the increase in cardiac output with salt loading was relatively greater than in the non-salt-sensitive patients.

In another study [5], we investigated sodium susceptibility and hemeodynamics in young patients with borderline hypertension, since young borderline hypertensives are at least three times more likely to develop established essential hypertension than are age-matched normotensive subjects. After a period of sodium depletion with a diuretic, short-term sodium loading caused blood pressure to increase significantly in a group of young subjects with borderline hypertension but not in a group of normal subjects of comparable age, sex, and body weight.

Hemodynamic responses of borderline hypertensives to sodium loads after sodium depletion showed increased cardiac output, while in the normal subjects cardiac output did not change significantly. Calculated systemic vascular resistance did not change in either group. The blood pressure of borderline hypertensives was associated with an apparent increase in cardiac output and with inappropriately elevated systemic vascular resistance. Further, we divided thirty-four borderline hypertensives into two groups, according to blood-pressure responses to salt loads. Of the 34 borderline hypertensives 14 salt-sensitive patients had greater increases in cardiac output with salt loading than did the 20 non-salt-sensitive patients. With increased cardiac output, the non-salt-sensitive patients had significantly decreased

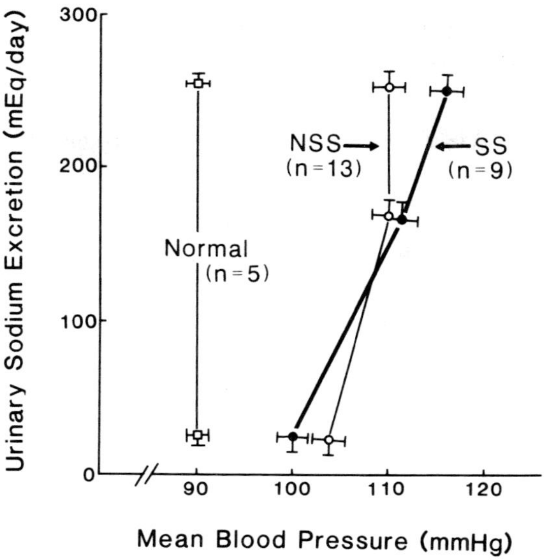

Fig. 1. Renal function curve in salt-sensitive (*SS*) and non-salt-sensitive (*NSS*) patients

systemic vascular resistance with salt loading. In contrast, systemic vascular resistance remained unchanged with salt loading in the salt-sensitive patients, which is consistent with the hemodynamic pattern in salt-sensitive essential hypertensive patients. Salt-induced elevation of blood pressure in the salt-sensitive patients with both borderline and established hypertension might be due to a disproportionate increase in cardiac output and inadequate fall in systemic vascular resistance.

Impaired Renal Function in Patients with Salt-Sensitive Hypertension

During salt loading, the salt-sensitive patients excreted less sodium in the urine than did the non-salt-sensitive patients. The salt-sensitive patients retained more sodium than did the other patients. In fact, the extent of the increases in plasma volume and body weight was significantly greater in the salt-sensitive patients than in the non-salt-sensitive patients [1,6].

Guyton et al. postulated that the blood pressure/urinary sodium excretion curve for the kidney of hypertensive subjects is shifted to the right, with a decreased slope [7]. Renal function curves of both salt-sensitive and non-salt-sensitive patients were shifted to the right, as compared to those of normotensive subjects (Fig. 1). However, the slope of the renal function curve for the kidney of salt-sensitive patients apparently decreased as compared with that of the non-salt-sensitive patients.

There was no significant difference in blood pressure, nor in creatinine clearance, between the two groups. Salt-sensitive patients have impaired renal function for sodium excretion, despite having normal glomerular filtration rates.

Regional Hemodynamics in Patients with Salt-Sensitive Hypertension

Although calculated systemic vascular resistance did not differ between the groups, the salt-sensitive patients had significantly higher renal vascular resistance than did the non-salt-sensitive patients. This suggests that vasoconstriction appeared specifically in the kidneys of salt-sensitive patients [6].

Salt-sensitive patients had significantly lower renal blood flow than did the non-salt-sensitive patients, but there was no significant difference between the two groups in hepatic nor in forearm blood flow. Impaired renal function for sodium excretion might be involved in the abnormality of renal hemodynamics in salt-sensitive patients.

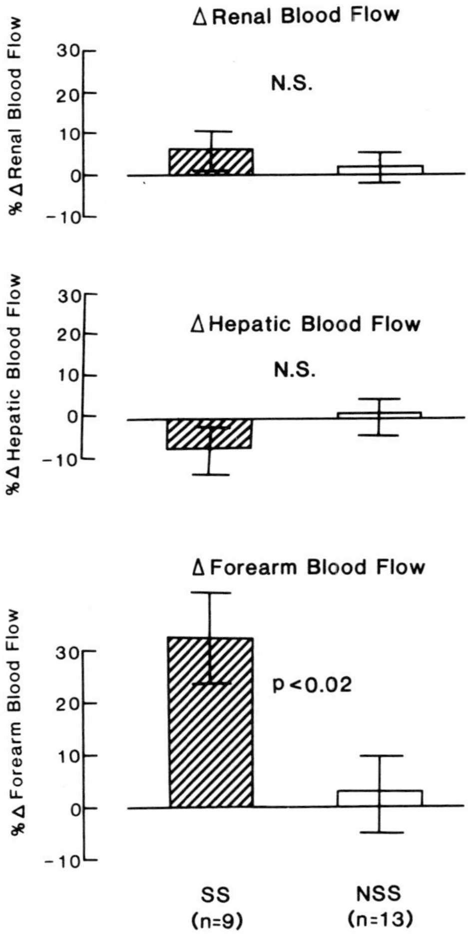

Fig. 2. Changes in renal, hepatic, and forearm blood flow with sodium loads in salt-sensitive (*SS*) and non-salt-sensitive (*NSS*) patients with hypertension. N.S., not significant

Although many extrarenal factors regulate renal vascular tone and change renal function in sodium excretion, neural mechanisms may play an important role in the control of renal sodium handling.

In our first study [1], we demonstrated that patients with salt-sensitive hypertension had inappropriately high levels of plasma norepinephrine during sodium loading, compared with the non-salt-sensitive hypertensive patients, thus suggesting that the persistence of autonomic "drive" in the sodium-loaded patients with salt-sensitive hypertension contributed to the relative sodium retention with sodium loads and to the increase in blood pressure.

In general, autonomic activation in essential hypertension is regional rather general, so that the measurement of total plasma norepinephrine and tests for generalized activation are inadequate. In our recent study [6], therefore, we measured regional blood flows in order to further assess changes in sympathetic nerve activity with salt loading in individual vascular beds.

We measured changes in renal, hepatic, and forearm blood flows with salt loading in the two groups [6]. Renal and hepatic blood flows remained essentially unchanged in both groups. In contrast, skeletal muscle blood flow increased profoundly in the salt-sensitive patients, and it received almost all of the increase in cardiac output (Fig. 2). Therefore, the greater increase in blood pressure with sodium loads seems to be characterized by a very inhomogeneous distribution of local flow and resistance in salt-sensitive patients.

Despite unchanged systemic vascular resistance, a high salt intake in salt-sensitive patients was associated with increases in hepatic and renal vascular resistances but with a decrease in forearm vascular resistance. This result suggests that analysis of systemic vascular resistance alone is inadequate for understanding the vascular changes that take place during elevation of blood pressure with sodium loading.

In this hemodynamic study, vasoconstriction appeared in the kidney and in the splanchnic area but, in salt-sensitive patients, vasoconstriction was masked by prominent vasodilation in skeletal muscle. Since this hemodynamic pattern is similar to the pattern evoked during defense reaction, in which sympathetic activity is selectively increased in the kidney and splanchnic area, this hemodynamic pattern might be involved in the impaired renal function for sodium excretion and blood pressure elevation which occurs with sodium loading in salt-sensitive patients [6].

The Antihypertensive Effect of Potassium in Salt-Sensitive Rats

A dietary potassium supplement is antihypertensive in animals and in humans, and protects against the hypertensinogenic effects of excessive dietary sodium. In our previous study [8], a high sodium diet for 4 weeks significantly increased blood pressure in salt-sensitive young spontaneously hypertensive rats (SHR). However, although potassium supplementation attenuated the elevation of blood pressure with the sodium loading, potassium had little effect on blood pressure in normal sodium-SHR.

The blood pressure/urinary sodium excretion curve for the kidneys of young SHR was shifted to the right and its slope apparently decreased as compared with that of Wistar Kyoto (WKY) control rats (Fig. 3). However, potassium supplements restored the slope toward normal, suggesting that potassium could normalize the increased salt-sensitivity of blood pressure in young SHR.

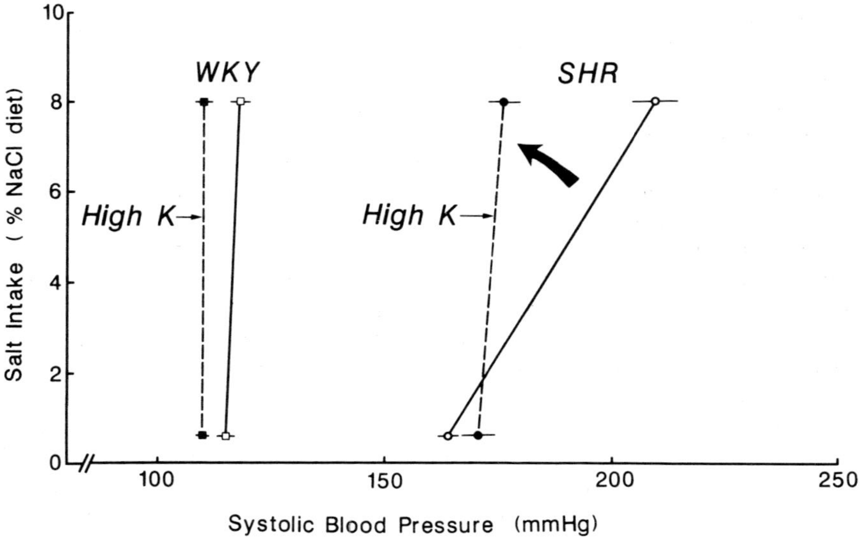

Fig. 3. Effects of potassium supplements on pressure-renal sodium excretion relationship in 5-week spontaneously hypertensive rats (*SHR*) and age-matched control Wistar-Kyoto rats (*WKY*) [8]

In the study of renal hemodynamics, sodium loads significantly increased renal vascular resistance in SHR, as was observed in salt-loaded patients with salt-sensitive hypertension. However, potassium supplementation attenuated the increased renal vascular resistance of salt-loaded SHR, although it did not affect renal vascular resistance in normal sodium-SHR. The salt-induced increase in renal vascular resistance, which might be intimately related to the impaired renal sodium handling, appears to be involved in the increased salt-sensitivity in young SHR.

Similar findings for potassium effects were observed in rats with desoxycorticosterone acetate (DOCA)-salt hypertension, another salt-sensitive model [9–11]. Salt loading increased blood pressure in DOCA-treated rats. However, the supplementation of potassium attenuated the development of hypertension in DOCA-salt rats.

From the data for cumulative sodium retention, it was found that potassium supplementation, as a result of natriuresis, attenuated the increase in the amount of sodium retained throughout the experimental period in DOCA-salt rats. We evaluated the effect of potassium supplementation on the blood pressure/urinary sodium excretion curve for the kidney of DOCA-salt rats. The slope of the renal function curve for DOCA-salt rats apparently decreased, with shifting, but potassium restored it toward normal (Fig. 4).

To further evaluate the role of renal sympathetic activity in the impaired sodium-excreting ability of the kidneys of DOCA-salt rats [11] and salt-sensitive SHR [12], the tissue norepinephrine turnover rate was measured in vivo by using alpha-methyl-p-tyrosine, an inhibitor of catecholamine synthesis. Norepinephrine turnover in the kidneys of DOCA-salt rats was significantly accelerated compared to that in control rats, but potassium supplement normalized this turnover [11,12]. According to

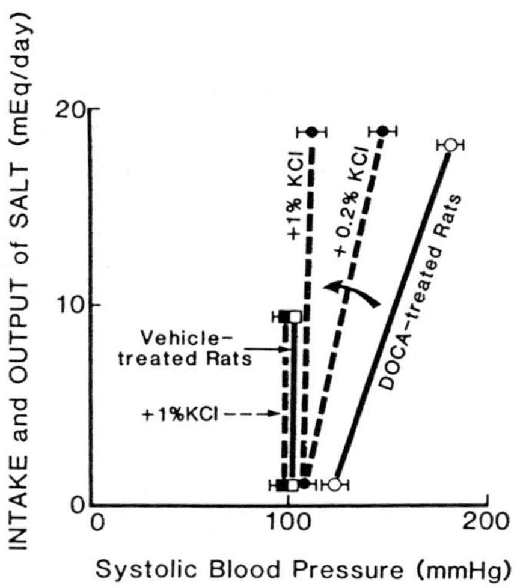

Fig. 4. Effects of potassium supplements on pressure-renal sodium excretion relationship in DOCA-salt treated rats. Potassium restored the decreased slope of the renal function curve toward normal but did not affect the curve in control vehicle-treated rats. DOCA, desoxycorticosterone acetate

changes in renal norepinephrine turnover, moreover, hypothalamic norepinephrine turnover, on exposure to cold, was markedly accelerated in salt-sensitive hypertensive animals, but the potassium supplement normalized this turnover [12]. The normalization of increased renal sympathetic activity, which is intimately related to central noradrenergic mechanisms, may be involved in the natriuretic and antihypertensive actions of potassium in salt-sensitive hypertensive animals [11,12].

Effects of Air Stress on Urinary Sodium Excretion in Salt-Sensitive Hypertensive Rats

Recently, Anderson reported that the combination of avoidance-conditioning tasks and saline infusion for 2 weeks could increase blood pressure in intact dogs, but blood pressure remained unchanged on an avoidance schedule or on saline infusion alone, indicating a significant interaction between environmental stress and dietary sodium in renal sodium handling and the development of hypertension [13]. We then studied the interaction of mental stress and dietary sodium and potassium in salt-sensitive hypertension.

To clarify the neural mechanisms for the antihypertensive and natriuretic actions of potassium in salt-sensitive hypertension, we studied the effects of potassium supplementation on urinary sodium excretion and renal function responses to a stressful environmental stimulus, air stress, in DOCA-salt rats (Y. Sato et al., manuscript in preparation).

In conscious DOCA-salt rats, air stress decreased urine flow rate and urinary sodium excretion, but in normotensive sham-operated rats air stress had no effects on these parameters. Renal denervation abolished the antidiuretic and antinatriuretic responses to air stress in DOCA-salt rats, suggesting that air stress decreased urinary sodium excretion, possibly by causing increased renal sympathetic activity. Correspondingly, potassium supplementation in DOCA-salt rats attenuated the antidiuretic and antinatriuretic responses to air stress, as in the renal-denervated DOCA-salt rats. This suggests that the attenuation achieved by potassium supplementation of the air stress-induced decrease in urinary sodium excretion in DOCA-salt rats might be attributable to normalization of the increased sympathetic activity in the kidney, possibly through changes in the central nervous system. This hypothesis is supported by the results of norepinephrine turnover studies [11,12].

The Antihypertensive Effects of Potassium Supplementation in Patients with Salt-Sensitive Hypertension

Salt loading after low sodium diets increased blood pressure in patients with essential hypertension. However, potassium supplementation during a high sodium diet period showed a lesser elevation of blood pressure with sodium loading than in the potassium-untreated group [14]. Potassium may counteract the pressor actions of dietary sodium in patients with salt-sensitive hypertension. In our previous studies [1,6], salt-sensitive patients had decreased urinary sodium excretion during high sodium diets, as compared to the non-salt-sensitive patients, but potassium supplementation promoted urinary sodium excretion in these hypertensive subjects with impaired renal sodium handling. Sodium retained during salt loading was attenuated by potassium supplementation. Correspondingly, potassium supplementation inhibited the increase in plasma volume with sodium loads. Moreover, potassium attenuated the salt-induced increase in cardiac output.

Further, we measured plasma norepinephrine in order to estimate sympathetic activity, since the sympathetic nervous system is known to control urinary sodium excretion. From the low sodium diet to Day 3 of the high sodium diet, plasma norepinephrine decreased significantly in the potassium-supplemented patients, but it remained unchanged in the non-potassium-supplemented patients. Concurrently, the heart rate of the potassium-supplemented patients decreased significantly in the early period of salt loading.

Concomitantly, in the potassium-supplemented group, as compared to the other group, urinary sodium excretion was significantly greater in the early period of salt loading. Moreover, there was a significant negative correlation between the degree of the decrease in plasma norepinephrine concentration from the end of the low sodium diet to the 3rd day of the high sodium diet and the amount of urinary sodium excretion in the early period of salt loading.

Taken together, these data suggest that potassium supplementation could shift the renal function curve toward normal, partly by inducing decreased sympathetic nerve activity in the kidney, which would result in natriuresis (Fig. 5).

Finally, we evaluated the antihypertensive effects of potassium when the potassium-supplemented patients were divided into two groups. The antihypertensive effect of potassium was greater in five salt-sensitive patients than in six non-salt-

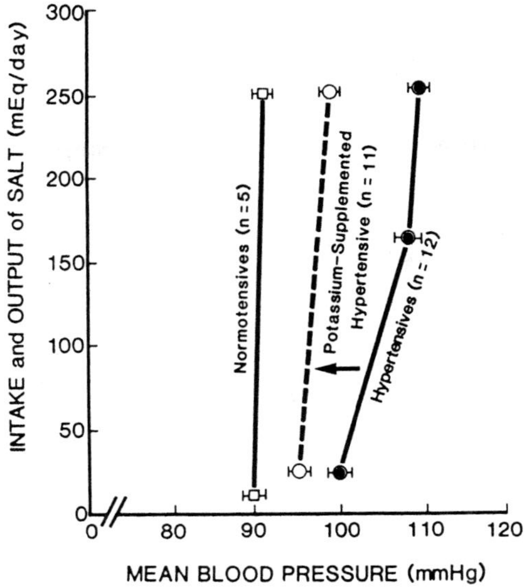

Fig. 5. Effects of potassium supplements on pressure-renal sodium excretion relationship in hypertensives

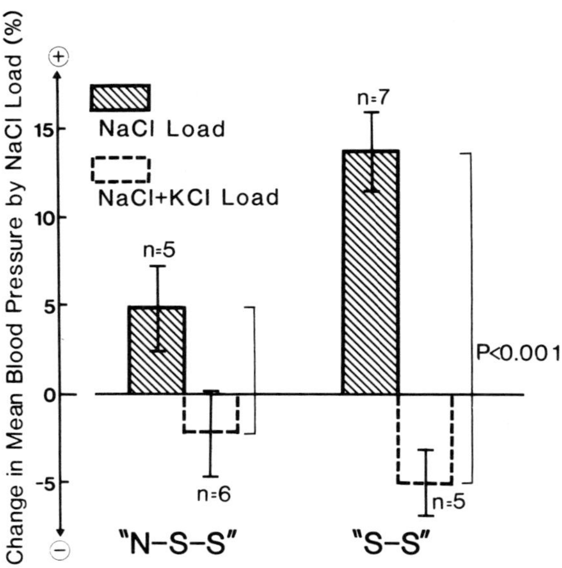

Fig. 6. Effects of potassium supplements on salt-loaded blood pressure increase in salt-sensitive (*SS*) and non-salt-sensitive (*NSS*) patients

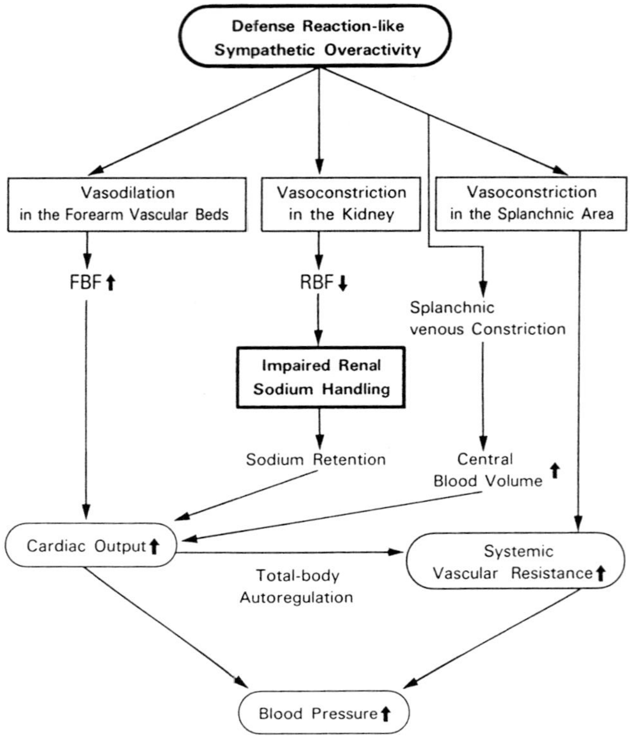

Fig. 7. The mechanism for blood-pressure rise with salt loads in patients with salt-sensitive hypertension

sensitive patients (Fig. 6). Potassium supplementation can prevent the increase in blood pressure induced with sodium loading in salt-sensitive hypertensive subjects.

Conclusion

Figure 7 shows our hypothesis regarding the mechanism of blood pressure elevation with sodium loading in salt-sensitive hypertensive subjects. With sodium loading, the salt-sensitive patients had markedly increased cardiac output and inappropriately elevated systemic vascular resistance, in which sympathetic overactivity on a selective basis, similar to that of the defense reaction, might be involved. Selective vasoconstriction in the kidney during salt loading, caused by increased renal sympathetic activity, may produce sodium retention, through the decreased slope of the renal function curve for sodium excretion, leading to increased cardiac output. In contrast, sympathetic nerve activity, which can readily be lowered by salt loading in the non-salt-sensitive patients, causes natriuresis through renal vasodilation. Vasoconstriction in the splanchnic bed during salt loading may contribute to the rise in blood pressure, not only by increased vascular resistance but also by increased cardiac output, through increased central blood volume via splanchnic venous constriction. In contrast to the renal and hepatic vasoconstriction, prominent vasodilation occurred in muscle blood flow in salt-loaded SS patients; this might contribute to the profound increase in cardiac output through a faster average venous return to the heart by means of the shorter time constant pathway, suggesting that, with sodium loading in the SS patients, skeletal muscle blood flow maintains high cardiac output. Not only this selective sympathetic overactivity, but also autoregulation in the setting might represent a response to the inappropriately high blood flow produced by increases in blood volume and cardiac output, resulting in increased vascular resistance during exposure to salt and water in excess. Because our study was a short-term one that did not include serial measurements of hemodynamic parameters, we could not examine the possibility of total body autoregulation as postulated by Guyton and his group [7].

Finally, an altered dietary sodium to potassium ratio may have possible significance in the development of hypertension. The high sodium-low potassium environment of civilized people, operating on a genetic substrate of susceptibility, is the cardinal factor in the genesis and perpetuation of 'essential hypertension'. Moreover, there is significant interaction between environmental stress and dietary sodium and potassium in renal sodium handling and the development of hypertension.

References

1. Fujita T, Henry WL, Bartter FC, Lake CR, Delea CS (1980) Factors influencing blood pressure in salt-sensitive patients with hypertension. Am J Med 69:334–344
2. Fujita T, Ando K, Noda H, Sato Y, Yamashita N, Yamashita K (1982) Hemodynamic and endocrine changes associated with captopril in diuretic-resistant hypertensive patients. Am J Med 73:341–347
3. Fujita T, Sato Y, Ando K (1983) Role of sympathetic nerve activity and natriuresis in the antihypertensive actions of potassium in NaCl hypertension. Jpn Circ J 47:1227–1231
4. Ando K, Fujita T, Ito Y, Noda H, Yamashita K (1986) The role of renal hemodynamics in the antihypertensive effects of captopril. Am Heart J 111:347–352
5. Fujita T, Noda H, Ando K (1984) Sodium susceptibility and potassium effects in young patients with borderline hypertension. Circulation 69:468–476
6. Fujita T, Ando K, Ogata E (1990) Systemic and regional hemodynamics in patients with salt-sensitive hypertension. Hypertension 16:235–244
7. Guyton AC, Coleman TG, Cowley AE, Scheeel KW, Manning RD, Norman RA (1972) Arterial pressure regulation: Overriding dominance of the kidneys in long-term regulation and in hypertension. 52:584–594
8. Sato Y, Ando K, Ogata E, Fujita T (to be published) High potassium diet attenuates salt-induced acceleration of hypertension in SHR. Am J Physiol
9. Fujita T, Sato Y (1983) Natriuretic and antihypertensive effects of potassium in DOCA-salt hypertensive rats. 24:731–739
10. Fujita T, Sato Y (1984) Changes in renal and central noradrenergic activity with potassium in DOCA-salt rats. 246:F670–F675
11. Sato Y, Fujita T (1984) Suppression of renal sympathetic activity with potassium supplement in DOCA-salt rats. Jpn Heart J 25:253–261
12. Sato Y, Ogata E, Fujita T (to be published) High potassium diet attenuates salt-induced acceleration of renal and hypothalamic norepinephrine turnover in young SHR. Hypertension

13. Anderson DE, Murphy P, Kearns WD (1983) Progressive hypertension via avoidance conditioning and saline infusion in the dog. Hypertension 5:286–293
14. Fujita T, Ando K (1984) Hemodynamic and endocrine changes associated with potassium supplementation in sodium-loaded hypertensives. Hypertension 6:184–192

Ion Transport Abnormalities in the Development of Hypertension

GIUSEPPE BIANCHI, DANIELE CUSI[1], PATRIZIA FERRARI, MARIA GRAZIA TRIPODI, and BARRY BARBER[2]

During the last decade mechanisms of ion transport across the cell membrane have been studied by many investigators interested in arterial hypertension [1–4], because ion transport is fundamental in the regulation of body fluids, renal function, hormone secretion and activity, nerve activity, etc. So far, many abnormalities of various ion transport systems have been described in hypertensive rats and in men with "hereditary" forms of hypertension. Such abnormalities regarding Na-K cotransport [5–7], Na/Li countertransport [6,8–10], Na/H countertransport [11,12], Na-K pump [13], passive permeability or leak [14], Ca pump [15], Ca channels [16] etc. have been reported in the literature. Therefore, theoretically, an abnormality of ion transport might be involved in the pathogenesis of "hereditary" or "primary" forms of hypertension.

Instead of discussing all the experimental data so far collected on this issue, we would prefer to discuss in detail one of these ion transport abnormalities, namely the Na-K cotransport, in order to evaluate the problems to be solved before we can say whether or not a given ion transport abnormality is useful in the detection of the genes responsible for hereditary forms of hypertension. The reasons for this choice should be clear. In fact, in our present state of knowledge, we do not know whether abnormalities in ion transport are directly linked to the genetic causes of hereditary forms of hypertension, or whether they are just epiphenomena with no relevance to the genetic mechanisms of hypertension. This distinction is obviously crucial in establishing the role and the importance of these transport systems, which will lead toward understanding the pathogenesis of hypertension. The problems to be considered include:

1) Differences in the methodological approaches used to measure ion transport systems. For instance, some workers have measured outward ion transport and others

[1]University of Milan, Nephrology and Hypertension Unit, Department of Science and Biomedical Technology, Ospedale San Raffaele, Via Olgettina 60, Milan, Italy

[2]Prassis, Research Institute, Via Forlanini 1/3, Settimo Milanese, Milan, Italy

have measured inward ion transport, without considering that the same molecular mechanism may be involved, differently, in both modes of transport [17].

2) A variety of environmental or physiological variables can, per se, affect these ion transport systems; the influence of such variables has been considered in only very few publications [18,19].

3) In many of these studies, ion transport systems were measured in erythrocytes, on the assumption that the functional pattern is similar to that in the plasma membrane of the cells (renal, vascular, nervous) more directly involved in blood pressure regulation. However, for most of the ion transport systems, there is no real experimental basis for this assumption.

4) Differences may be found in opposite directions among different individual patients and different rat strains. For instance, the rate of Na-K cotransport in hypertensive patients or rat strains may be either similar to, lower than, or higher than that in their normotensive controls [6,20,21].

5) It is not clear whether the differences in ion transport are directly linked to the primary molecular genetic mechanisms, or whether these differences are just the expression of secondary efforts to re-establish a cellular ion homeostasis after cellular dysfunction that has been caused by another genetic-molecular mechanism far from those directly involved in the ion transport systems. Even though both possibilities may occur in nature, this distinction is crucial for establishing the usefulness of these ion transport system abnormalities for the detection of gene or gene product candidates for genetic forms of hypertension.

6) Even though there is general agreement about the multifactorial nature of human primary hypertension, there are no precise and accepted clinical or biochemical criteria for sub-classification of the overall population of patients into distinct clinical entities with distinct and specific pathogenetic mechanisms. Therefore, we do not know whether the variability of the different patients mentioned in point 4 is due to our inability to classify them correctly or whether it is just an expression of epiphenomena not closely related to the primary pathogenetic mechanisms.

All of this suggests to us that the most productive way to find a clear answer to these problems is to use animal models of primary hypertension in which the genetic and environmental backgrounds can be properly evaluated, in order to understand how abnormal cotransport is linked to both the primary genetic molecular mechanisms and to the other cellular or organic dysfunctions which we believe to be the cause of hypertension. Since the ion transport systems of the MHS and SHR strains of rats are the most widely studied, we shall consider these two strains first.

Na-K cotransport measured in washed MHS erythrocytes is faster than in MNS erythrocytes [21]. This has been confirmed by another group of investigators [22] using slightly different methods, but with rats supplied from our breeding colony. Kinetic studies showed that the Km for internal Na is lower for MHS than for MNS, while the Vmax is similar for both strains [23,24]. The MHS erythrocyte is smaller than the MNS erythrocyte [21]. In renal vesicles prepared from the luminal membrane of the ascending limb [25], or in cultured vascular smooth muscle cells [26], Na-K cotransport is faster in MHS than MNS. Therefore, the assumption that there is widespread abnormality of the same ion transport system in erythrocytes and in the cells more directly involved in blood pressure regulation may be considered as proven, at least for the MHS strain.

When the Na-K cotransport of SHR was compared with that of WKY, conflicting results were obtained. Rosati et al. [20] found decreased cotransport affinity for internal Na in the erythrocytes of SHR, with a consequent decrease in Na-K cotransport, measured as bumetanide sensitive sodium efflux within the physiological ranges of intracellular sodium. On the other hand, Orlov et al. [22] found increased Na-K cotransport, measured as furosemide-sensitive ^{86}Rb influx, in SHR erythrocytes. Others have also found more active Na-K cotransport in the erythrocytes of SHR than in those of WKY [27,28]. It is not possible to say whether these discrepancies are due to differences in the methodology or to the genetic heterogeneity of the WKY strains, which would affect comparisons of WKY and SHR rats carried out in different Institutions using different commercial rat suppliers [29]. Conflicting results were also obtained for cultured vascular smooth muscle cell Na-K cotransport from SHR and from WKY rats [30,31]. Therefore, at this time, it is not possible to know whether the abnormality of Na-K cotransport is the same in erythrocytes and in vascular or renal tubular cells of SHR, even though a more uniform picture seems to be demonstrable for other cell membrane abnormalities in Ca or Na handling [1]. However, the question of the genetic heterogeneity of the different WKY substrains casts serious doubt on the validity of comparing the results obtained in different Institutions [29]. For these reasons, we shall not consider the results in SHR and WKY rats in the present discussion, which is aimed at comparing abnormalities in different types of cells. In fact, to our knowledge, there are no published results generated in the same Institution, with the same WKY substrain, in which different ion transports across different cell types are compared. This is a rather sad conclusion, in view of the tremendous amount of work that has so far been published on the variety of biochemical abnormalities in SHR.

For man there have been studies aimed at correlating abnormal transport rates across erythrocyte cell membranes with renal functional abnormalities [32,33] and some correspondences have been found, although at a much lower degree of precision than for rats. We shall discuss the Na-K cotransport in the last paragraph.

How Can a Faster Rate of Na-K Cotransport be Linked to the Organ Dysfunctions Involved in the Pathogenesis of Hypertension?

We have tried to answer this question as follows: in MHS, hypertension can be transplanted with the kidney [34–36], therefore the genetic message responsible for it may be transmitted through modification of renal function. When studied in vitro, isolated kidneys of MHS showed faster Na reabsorption and greater O_2 consumption than MNS kidneys [37,38]. Na transport across the luminal membrane was also faster in vesicles from proximal [39,40] or ascending portions of the tubules [25]. For the luminal membrane of the proximal tubules, faster Na transport seems to be mediated, at least in part, by the Na-H exchange pathway, while in the luminal membrane of the ascending limb, it is Na-K cotransport that is responsible for faster sodium transport [25]. This last conclusion is also supported by the results of comparisons of the diuretic effects of bumetanide, hydrochlorothiazide and amiloride in kidneys isolated from MHS and MNS. Na excretion after bumetanide is higher in MHS than in

MNS kidneys or in MHS kidneys given the other two diuretics [41]. The key role of Na-K cotransport in the transmission of the signal into the macula densa cells for generation of the tubulo-glomerular feedback mechanism is supported by much experimental data [42]. When measured in MHS and MNS, the tubulo-glomerular feedback mechanism in MHS is depressed at the pre-hypertensive stage although it is more active during the development of hypertension [43,44]. This depression at the pre-hypertensive stage in MHS is very likely due to increased renal interstitial pressure, which disappears during the development of hypertension, thus unmasking the underlying greater sensitivity of the feedback in MHS. The Na-K ATPase activity of isolated proximal tubules is also higher in MHS than in MNS [45]. Taken together, these findings are consistent with the notion that faster Na transport across the tubular epithelial cells is an important cause of hypertension in MHS and that an abnormality of Na-K cotransport may well be linked to the primary defect responsible for renal dysfunction.

The Possible Link Between Faster Na-K Cotransport and the Primary Genetic Mechanisms of Hypertension

This is certainly most relevant to today's discussion. A biochemical abnormality on a plasma membrane may be due to three different causes: 1) genetic, 2) environmental, 3) secondary readjustment through extracellular mechanisms (for instance, hormonal or other humoral changes) or intracellular ones. In order to differentiate between some of these mechanisms we transplanted bone marrow from MHS or MNS into (MHS × MNS) F_1 hybrids that had been previously irradiated to destroy their own bone marrow [46]. Erythrocyte volume was measured three months after transplantation and was found to be smaller in recipients of MHS bone marrow than in those that received MNS bone marrow. Also, the rate of Na-K cotransport was faster in MHS recipients. This clearly demonstrates that the genetic message responsible for faster Na-K cotransport and for the smaller volume of MHS erythrocytes was present in the stem cells, and that environmental factors or secondary readjustments through extracellular mechanisms are not responsible for these differences between MHS and MNS. Moreover, in F_2 hybrids, obtained by crossing the (MHS × MNS) F_1 hybrids, the rate of erythrocyte Na-K cotransport and the erythrocyte cell volume were correlated with the level of blood pressure, suggesting a genetic association between these traits [46]. However, these experiments do not exclude the possibility that faster Na-K cotransport might result from a readjustment of the cellular biochemical machinery. This readjustment would be aimed at re-establishing a cell homeostasis compatible with life, after a given mutation of a gene whose product is quite distant from the proteins directly involved in controlling Na-K cotransport. To evaluate this possibility we carried out a series of experiments which we shall summarize as follows: first of all, we wanted to see whether Na-K cotransport was still faster in inside out vesicles (IOV) prepared from MHS erythrocytes [47]. In these vesicles the transmembrane proteins responsible for ion translocation across the cell membrane should remain, while all the cytoplasm and the membrane skeleton proteins are removed. Na-K cotransport was similar for IOV prepared from MHS and MNS, and the Km for the internal site of Na on the Na-K cotransport system became similar for the two strains, excluding the possibility that transmembrane protein, by itself, was a possible cause of the differences between the intact erythrocytes [24]. Moreover, for resealed ghosts, in which the membrane skeleton is still present without the cytoplasmic component of the cell, the difference in cell volume between MHS and MNS remained [48]. This suggests that the membrane skeleton component may be involved in causing the overall cell dysfunction of MHS. With the aim of discovering possible differences in structural protein between MHS and MNS, we then injected extracts of erythrocyte membranes or membrane skeletons from MNS into MHS and vice-versa. After two immunizations, MNS recipients treated with MHS extract selectively produced an antibody against 105 KDa membrane skeleton protein. This protein was subsequently characterized as adducin [49].

Using this antibody, a cDNA library was screened and a clone was isolated. The study of the structure of the adducin gene is still in progress. However, we know almost ⅓ of the nucleotide sequence; the determination of such sequences in the MHS and MNS genes revealed a point mutation which was responsible for the coding of a glutamine (GLN) in place of an arginine (ARG) [50]. We had already noticed some degree of polymorphism in the MNS strain, but not in the MHS, in the antibody responses of the two strains to injection of antigen [49]. Evaluation of the genotypes also confirmed this phenomenon. Namely, all the MHS rats studied were ARG/ARG, while there were three MNS genotypes, ARG/ARG, ARG/GLN and GLN/GLN, suggesting that, in spite of close inbreeding for more than 50 generations, something had prevented achievement of homozygosis for the adducin locus in the normotensive strain. It should be noted that 11 other loci of MNS were homozygotic (Barber BR, personal communication). Theoretically there are four possible reasons for this selective heterozygosis at the adducin locus in the MNS inbred strain of animals:

1) homozygosis is lethal
2) homozygosis reduces biological fitness
3) mutation
4) selection for lower pressure favours heterozygosis

The first two reasons are not likely because we have animals homozygotic at the adducin locus and they show no differences from heterozygotic animals in body growth. Possibility No. 3 is also unlikely, because the difference in the antibody response was detected for the first time 4 years ago, and since then more than 10 generations have been obtained, with the maintenance of heterozygosis throughout these generations. Therefore, if a point mutation occurred without any relationship to the process of selection, we would expect its disappearance in the following generations. We are left with possibility No. 4 as the most likely one; first, by exclusion of the other three, second, because the blood pressure of rats with the genotype ARG/GLN is significantly lower than that of the rats of genotype ARG/ARG (Tripodi G, Piscone A, Ferrari P, Torielli L, Baralle T, Bianchi G, 1990, unpublished work). Also, the GLN/GLN genotype has slightly lower BP than the ARG/GLN genotype, even though the difference is not statistically significant (Tripodi G et al., 1990, unpublished work). There are major differences in ion transport systems and in BP between MHS and MNS. The mutation within the adducin gene, detected in MNS, may account for only minor differences in BP within this strain, and we do not yet know whether it may also account for minor differences in ion transport systems. However, we do not know whether or not other differences between MHS and MNS in the adducin gene might generate other adducin alleles that could be responsible for differences in blood pressure and ion transport much greater than those caused by the mutation studied so far.

This series of experiments was one attempt to establish a cause/effect relationship between a given alteration of a gene, membrane ion transport, and renal dysfunction responsible for increase in blood pressure. In our opinion, this body of knowledge can be used to approach our stated problem No. 4, that is, the meaning of ion transport system abnormalities in human essential hypertension. In fact, we have already shown that a subgroup of patients with essential hypertension had increased erythrocytic outward Na-K cotransport, increased renal Na excretion after furosemide, increased proximal reabsorption of urate (an index of proximal tubular reabsorption) [33], and lower plasma renin, with a greater blood pressure fall with diuretic compared to ACE inhibitors or β blockers, than other hypertensive patients or normal controls [51]. This overall clinical picture may well delineate a new nosologic entity with its own pathogenetic mechanisms. However, to prove the existence of this new clinical entity, we need to demonstrate that such biochemical, cell or organ dysfunctions are accompanied by precise genetic-molecular abnormalities which might explain such dysfunctions. Only by measuring all these factors (or the most important of them), in individual patients or subjects within a family tree, can we evaluate the genetic mode of transmission of a given ion transport system abnormality and its relevance to the determination of the blood pressure level. Indeed, the complexity of the interaction between the variety of genetic and environmental factors that may determine the level of blood pressure hampers attempts to study the mode of genetic transmission of this variable in an individual member of a family tree [52]. We might reduce the complexity of these factors by studying the genetics of ion transport systems as an intermediate phenotype. A better understanding of such an intermediate phenotype might help to dissect such complexity into relatively simpler systems [52]. The recent studies, by mixture analysis, of erythrocyte Li-Na countertransport [9] and blood pressure, or recent studies of the differences in Li-Na countertransport between "modulators" and "non-modulators" [53] are very helpful for drawing our attention to the importance of a particular ion transport system abnormality, in understanding the genetic and physiological mechanisms of hypertension. However, we must recognize that we are only at the start of a new avenue of research. This will give us meaningful results only if we take into consideration all the requirements for the approaching clarification of the role of genetic-molecular mechanisms in understanding the pathogenesis of complex diseases like arterial hypertension. In our opinion, the most important of these requirements is genetic homogeneity of the strain of animals used for these experiments. Only when the sequence of events from a given genetic abnormality to arterial hypertension has been clarified in animal models of primary hypertension, will we have the theoretical background to approach the enormous complexity of the relationship, in man, between the ion transport system and both the primary genetic-molecular abnormality and the cell dysfunction responsible for arterial hypertension.

Acknowledgments. The studies reported in this paper were supported in part by grants from the Ministry of Public Institutions, 1985–1989, (2-GB+DC), and by Research Grant on Hypertension from the Cassa di Risparmio delle Province Lombarde, Milano.

References

1. Postnov YV (1990) An approach to the explanation of cell membrane alteration in primary hypertension. Hypertension 15:332–337
2. Ives HE (1989) Ion transport defects and hypertension: Where is the link? Hypertension 14:590–597
3. Aviv A, Lasker N (1990) Proposed defects in membrane transport and intracellular ions as pathogenic factors in essential hypertension. In: Laragh, Brenner (eds) Hypertension: Pathophysiology, Diagnosis, and Management, vol 1. Raven, pp 923–937
4. Bianchi G (1986) Ion transport across blood cell membrane in essential hypertension. Curr Opin Cardiol 1:634–639
5. Garay RP, Dagher G, Pernolett MG, Dewynck MA, Meyer P (1980) Inherited defect in Na^+,K^+-cotransport system in erythrocyte from essential hypertensive patients. Nature 284:281–283
6. Cusi D, Barlassina C, Ferrandi M, Lupi GP, Ferrari P, Bianchi (1981) Familial aggregation of cation transport abnormalities and essential hypertension. Clin Exp Hypertens [A] 3:871–884
7. Canessa M, Spalvins A, Adragna N, Falkner B (1984) Red cell sodium countertransport and cotransport in normotensive and hypertensive blacks. Hypertension 6:344–351
8. Canessa M, Adragna N, Solomon HS, Connolly TM, Torteson D (1980) Increased sodium-lithium countertransport in red cells of patients with essential hypertension. N Engl J Med 302:772–776
9. Weder AB, Schork NJ (1989) Mixture analysis of erythrocyte lithium-sodium countertransport and blood pressure. Hypertension 2:145–150
10. Woods JW, Falk RJ, Pittman AW, Klemmer PJ, Watson BS, Namboodiri K (1982) Increased red cell sodium-lithium counter-transport in normotensive sons of hypertensive patients. N Engl J Med 306:593–595
11. Livne A, Balfe JW, Veitch R, Marquez-Julio A, Grinstein S, Rothstein A (1987) Increased platelet Na^+-H^+ exchange rates in essential hypertension: Application of a novel test. Lancet I:533–536
12. Semplicini A, Canessa M, Mozzato MG, Ceolotto G, Marzola M, Buzzaccarini F, Casolino P, Pessina AC (1989) Red blood cell Na^+/H^+ and Li^+/Na^+ exchange in patients with essential hypertension. Am J Hypertens 2:903–908
13. Diez J, Hannaert P, Garay R (1987) Kinetic study of Na^+-K^+ pump in erythrocytes from essential hypertensive patients. Am J Physiol 252:H1–H6
14. Garay RP, Nazaret C (1985) Na^+ leak in erythrocytes from essential hypertensive patients. Clin Sci 69:613–624
15. de la Sierra A, Hannaert P, Ollivier JP, Senn N, Garay R (1990) Kinetic study of the Ca^{2+} pump in erythrocytes from essential hypertensive patients. J Hypertens 3:285–293
16. Hermsmeyer K, Rusch N (1989): Calcium channel alterations in genetic hypertension. Hypertension 4:453–456
17. Canessa M, Brugnara C, Tosteson DC, Cusi D (1986) Modes of operation and variable stoichiometry of furosemide-sensitive Na and K fluxes in human red cells. J Gen Physiol 87:113–147
18. Canessa M, Brugnara C, Escobales N (1987) The Li^+-Na^+ exchange and Na^+-K^+-Cl^- cotransport systems in essential hypertension. Hypertension 10:4–10
19. Adragna NC, Chang JL, Morey MC, Williams R (1985) Effect of exercise on cation transport in human red cells. Hypertension 7:132–139
20. Rosati C, Meyer P, Garay R (1988) Sodium transport kinetics in erythrocytes from spontaneously hypertensive rats. Hypertension 1:41–48
21. Ferrari P, Ferrandi M, Torielli L, Canessa M, Bianchi G (1987) Relationship between erythrocyte volume and sodium transport in the Milan hypertensive rat and age-dependent changes. J Hypertens 5:199–206

22. Orlov SN, Postnov IY, Pokudin NI, Kukharenko VY, Postnov YV (1989) Na^+-H^+ exchange and other ion-transport systems in erythrocytes of essential hypertensives and spontaneously hypertensive rats: a comparative analysis. J Hypertens 7:781–788
23. Ferrari P, Torielli M, Ferrandi M, Bianchi G (1988) The role of membrane skeleton in the alteration of Na-K cotransport (CO) in Milan hypertensive rats (MHS) (abstract) 12th scientific meeting of the International Society of Hypertension, May 22–26 1988. Kyoto, Japan
24. Ferrari P, Torielli L, Cirillo M, Salardi S, Bianchi G (to be published) Sodium transport kinetics in erythrocytes and inside-out vesicles from Milan rats.
25. Ferrandi M, Salardi S, Parenti P, Ferrari P, Bianchi G, Braw R, Karlish SJD (1990) $Na^+/K^+/Cl^-$-cotransporter mediated Rb^+ fluxes in membrane vesicles from kidneys of normotensive and hypertensive rats. BBA Biomembranes 1021:13–20
26. Socorro L, Vallega G, Nunn A, Moore TJ, Canessa M (1990) Vascular smooth muscle cells from the Milan hypertensive rat exhibit decreased functional angiotensin II receptors. Hypertension 15(part 1)
27. Feig PU, Mitchel PP, Boylan JW (1985) Erythrocyte membrane transport in hypertensive humans and rats: Effect of sodium depletion and excess. Hypertension 7:423–429
28. Duhm J, Göbel BO, Beck FX (1983) Sodium potassium ion transport accelerations in erythrocytes of DOC, DOC-salt, two kidney, one clip, and spontaneously hypertensive rats: Role of hypokalemia and cell volume. Hypertension 5:642–652
29. Kurtz TW, Montano M, Chan L, Kabra P (1989) Molecular evidence of genetic heterogeneity in Wistar-Kyoto rats: Implications for research with spontaneously hypertensive rat. Hypertension 13:188–192
30. Tokushige A, Kino M, Tamura H, Hopp L, Searle BM, Aviv A (1986) Bumetide-sensitive sodium-22 transport in vascular smooth muscle cell of the spontaneously hypertensive rat. Hypertension 8:379–385
31. O'Donnel ME, Owen NE (1988) Reduced Na-K-Cl cotransport in vascular smooth muscle cells from spontaneously hypertensive rats. Am J Physiol 255 (Cell Physiol 24):C169–C180
32. Weder AB (1986) Red-cell lithium-sodium countertransport and renal lithium clearance in hypertension. N Engl J Med 314:198–201
33. Cusi D, Barlassina C, Tripodi G, Alberghini E, Pozzoli E, Stella P, Bianchi G (to be published) Mixture analysis of erythrocyte Na-K cotransport and Li-Na countertransport in essential hypertension. Am J Hypertens
34. Bianchi G, Fox U, Di Francesco G.F, Bardi U, Radice M (1973) The hypertensive role of the kidney in spontaneously hypertensive rats. Clin Sci Mol Med, 45(Suppl I):135S–139S
35. Bianchi G, Fox U, Di Francesco G.F, Giovanetti AM, Pagetti D (1974) Blood pressure changes produced by kidney cross-transplantation between spontaneously hypertensive rats and normotensive rats. Clin Sci Mol Med 47:435–448
36. Fox U, Bianchi G (1976) The primary role of the kidney in causing the blood pressure difference between the Milan Hypertensive strain (MHS) and the normotensive rats (MNS). Proceedings of the symposium on spontaneous genetic hypertension in rats, Dunedin, New Zealand, 4–6 March 1976. Clin Exp Pharmacol Physiol (Suppl 3):71–74
37. Salvati P, Pinciroli G.P, Bianchi G (1984) Renal function of isolated perfused kidneys from hypertensive (MHS) and normotensive (MNS) rats of the Milan strain at different ages. J Hypertens 2 (Suppl 3):351–353
38. Salvati P, Ferrario R.G, Parenti P, Bianchi G (1987) Renal function of isolated perfused kidneys from hypertensive (MHS) and normotensive (MNS) rats of the Milan strain: role of calcium. J Hypertens 5:31–38
39. Parenti P, Hanozet G, Bianchi G (1986) Sodium and glucose transport across renal brush-border membranes of Milan hypertensive rats. Hypertension 8:932–939

40. Hanozet GM, Parenti P, Salvati P (1985) Presence of potential-sensitive Na^+ transport across renal brush-border membrane vesicles from rats of the Milan hypertensive strain. BBA 819:179–186
41. Salvati P, Ferrario RG, Bianchi G (1990) Diuretic effect of bumetanide in isolated perfused kidneys of Milan hypertensive rats. Kidney Int 37:1084–1089
42. Lapointe JY, Bell PD, Cardinal J (1990) Direct evidence for apical Na^+:$2Cl^-$:K^+ cotransport in macula densa cells. Am J Physiol 258(Renal Fluid Electrolyte Physiol 27):F1466–F1469
43. Persson A.E, Bianchi G, Boberg U (1984) Evidence of defective tubuloglomerular feed-back control in rats of the Milan hypertensive strain (MHS). Acta Physiol Scand 122: 215–217
44. Persson AE, Bianchi G, Boberg U (1985) Tubuloglomerular feedback in hypertensive rats of the Milan strain. Acta Physiol Scand 123:139–146
45. Melzi ML, Bertorello A, Fukuda Y, Muldin I, Sereni F, Aperia A (1989) Na, K-ATPase activity in renal tubule cells from Milan hypertensive rats. Am J Hypertens 2:563–566
46. Bianchi G, Ferrari P, Trizio D, Ferrandi M, Torielli L, Barber B.R, and Polli E (1985) Red blood cell abnormalities and spontaneous hypertension in the rat: A genetically determined link. Hypertension 7:319–325
47. Ferrari P, Torielli L, Ferrandi M, Cirillo M, Bianchi G (1986) Volumes and Na transports in intact red blood cells, resealed ghosts and inside-out vesicles of Milan hypertensive rats J Hypertens, 4(Suppl 6):S379–S381
48. Ferrari P, Torielli L, Ferrandi M, Bianchi G (1986) Volumes and Na transports in intact red blood cells, resealed ghosts and inside out vesicles of Milan hypertensive rats. In: Bianchi G, Carafoli E, Scarpa A (eds) Ann NY Acad Sci 488:561–563
49. Salardi S, Saccardo, Borsani, Modica, Ferrandi M, Tripodi G, Soria, Ferrari P, Barralle, Sidoli I, Bianchi G (1989) Erythrocyte Adducin Differential Properties in Normotensive and Hypertensive rats of the Milan Strain: Characterization of Spleen Adducin m-RNA. Am J Hypertens 2:229–237
50. Tripodi G, Borsani G, Piscone A, Tisminetzky S, Salardi S, Sidoli A, Baralle FE, Bianchi G (1990) Difference between MNS and MHS rats in the cDNA coding for adducin (abstract). 13th scientific meeting of the International Society of Hypertension, 24–29 June 1990. Montreal, Canada
51. Niutta E, Cusi D, Colombo R, Tripodi G, Pellizzoni M, Pati P, Cesana B, Alberghini E, Barlassina C, and Bianchi G (1988) Antihypertensive Effect of Captopril, Canreonate Potassium, and Atenolol; Relations with Red Blood Cell Sodium Transport and Renin. Am J Hypertens 1:364–371
52. Camussi A, Bianchi G (1988) Genetics of Essential Hypertension From the Unimodal-Bimodal Controversy to Molecular Technology. Hypertension 12:620–628
53. Redgrave J, Canessa M, Gleason R, Hollenberg NK, Williams GH (1989) Red blood cell lithium-sodium countertransport in non-modulating essential hypertension. Hypertension 13:721–726

Cellular and Integrative Functions of the Juxtaglomerular Apparatus

Chair: Jurgen B. Schnermann (USA)
Toshikazu Takabatake (Japan)

Cell Volume Regulation and Transport Characteristics of Macula Densa Cells

A. Erik G. Persson, Max Salomonsson, Per Westerlund[1], Rainer Greger, Eberhard Schlatter[2], and Ernesto Gonzalez[3]

SUMMARY. To study the sensing step of the juxtaglomerular apparatus, we have performed studies using isolated perfused ascending limb of the loop of Henle with attached glomeruli and macula densa segments (c-TAL-MD). Both from measurement of macula densa cell volume and from measurements of the electrical potential of MD cells it can be proposed that a Na-K-2Cl cotransport mechanism is involved in the sensing step of the juxtaglomerular apparatus. To study this question further, measurements of MD cell chloride concentration have been made, using the fluorophore SPQ and a digital imaging system. A chloride concentration of 47 mM was found in the MD cells with 150 mM NaCl in both lumen and bath. The MD cell concentration was reduced to 6 mM when furosemide was added to the lumen solution and to 35 mM when lumen NaCl concentration was reduced to 30 mM. These results strongly support the view of a Na-K-2Cl cotransport mechanism in the entry step of the sensing mechanism. To study whether MD cell calcium concentration changes were involved in the activation of the MD cells, intracellular calcium was measured when changes in luminal NaCl were induced. NaCl was reduced from 150 to 30 mM and then there was an increase in macula densa cell calcium from 90 nM to 110 nM. However, we feel that this small change is not sufficient to explain activation of the cells. Other routes of activation could be involved and for the time being the exact mechanism for this activation is not clear.

Introduction

One way by which the kidney controls glomerular filtration is through the action of the tubuloglomerular feedback (TGF) control mechanism [1]. For the operation of this mechanism, the load to the distal nephron is sensed at the macula densa site,

[1]Department of Physiology and Biophysics, Sölvegatan 19, 223 62 Lund, Sweden
[2]Department of Physiology, University of Freiburg, Federal Republic of Germany
[3]Department of Physiology, University Central, Caracas, Venezuela

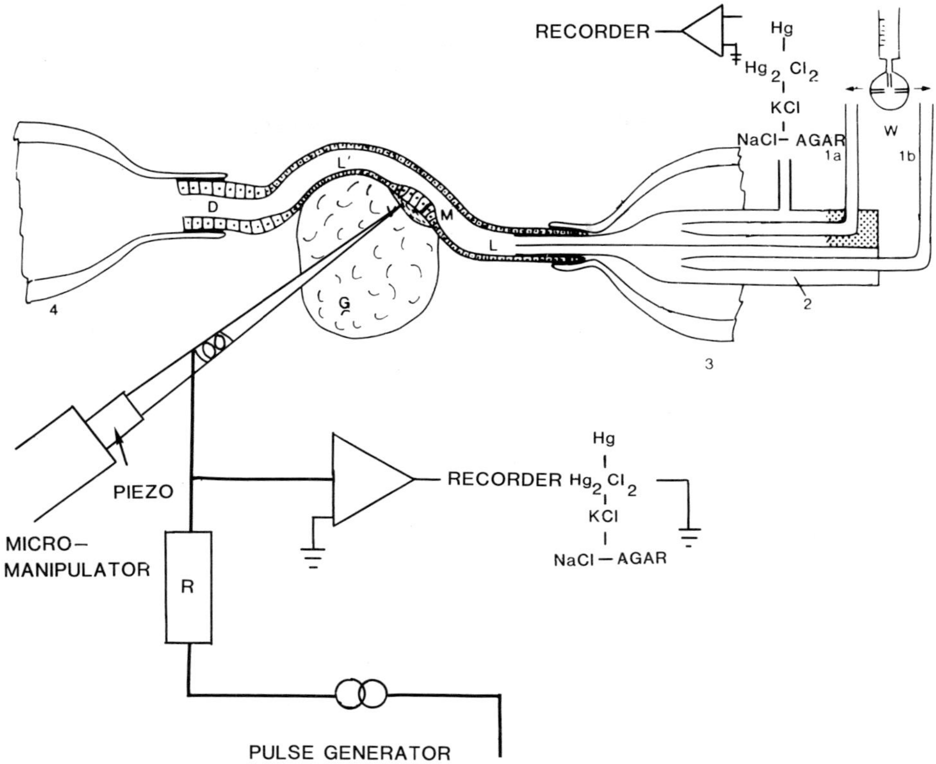

Fig. 1. Schematic view of the arrangement of the pipettes and the c-TAL and MD preparations. The tubular segment is perfused from right to left through a dual channel perfussion pipette. *2*. The active channel is determined by the position of a pneumatic three-way valve *W*. The composition of the perfusate in the two channels of the perfusion pipette can be varied through two fluid exchange pipettes *la* and *lb*. Two polyethylene catheters inserted through a lateral hole and sealed with epoxy resin serve as a fluid exchange pipette, *la*. The tubular segment is held by the perfusion holding pipette *3* and by the collection holding pipette *4*, the latter coated with solid and liquid Sylgard 184. Note the cellular heterogeneity in the perfused tubular segment: the transition from the cortical ascending limb in front of (*L*) and behind (*L'*) and the macula densa (*M*) to the beginning of the distal convoluted tubule (*D*). The macula densa cells are interposed in the cortical ascending limb-macula densa (CAL-MD) only on the side that is in contact with the vascular pole of the juxtaglomerular apparatus (*V*). *G*, glomerulus. With another micromanipulator a microelectrode connected to a piezo stepper was used to puncture macula densa cells. A pulse generator was connected to the microelectrode to be able to continuously monitor electrical resistance

probably by the macula densa cells. Information about the load is then transferred to the effector site, the arterioles, via cells in the juxtaglomerular apparatus. The signal may become modulated during its transmission, possibly by the extraglomerular mesangial cells located between the sensing and effector sites.

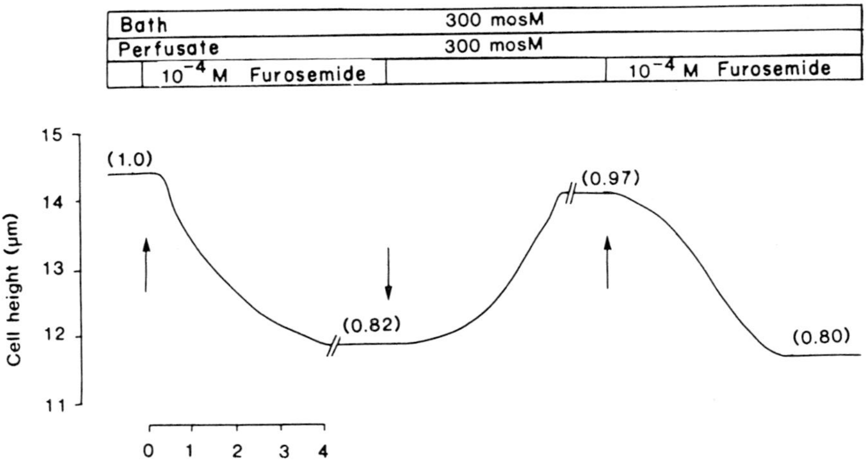

Fig. 2. Actual trace from an experiment illustrating the time course of the cell volume on exposure of the MD plaque to 10^{-4} M furosemide on the apical side. The numbers in parentheses are the relative cell volumes at different times during the experiment. (From [3] with permission)

Macula Densa Cell Volume Measurements

To study the sensing step, we performed the following sets of experiments [2–3]. The methods used were essentially the same as those described by Greger and Schlatter [4]. New Zealand white rabbits were used, and segments of cortical thick ascending limbs (c-TAL), 300–600 μm long, with attached glomeruli were isolated by manual dissection. Figure 1 shows how the tubules were mounted. The perfusion was carried out through a dual channel perfusion pipette which was put into the tubule and inserted into a holding pipette which kept the tubule in place. The tubule was mounted so that the macula densa (MD) cells were observed from the side. Experimental volume challenges caused no changes in the measured length or width of the MD cell plaque, but resulted in a change in its height [2]. The dimensions of these cells were measured with an image-splitting eyepiece to increase the resolution of the system. In the c-TAL segment the outer diameter was 25.2 μm, the inner tubular diameter was 7.1 μm, and the cell height was 4.8 μm. The height of the MD cell plaque was 13.3 μm, its length was 50 μm, and its width was 21.8 μm. Perfusion of furosemide rapidly reduced the cell volume to 0.82 compared with the control volume (see Fig. 2). This change was reversed on removal of the furosemide. When the luminal solution was modified by replacing most of the NaCl by mannitol, the cell volume decreased in the same way as with furosemide, resulting in an average cell volume of 0.83 compared with the control value. On calculation of the rate of cell volume decrease in the initial phase after removal of Na from the luminal fluid, a sodium flux of 0.28 nmol s^{-1} cm^{-2} was found. Since it is known from the work of Dr. Greger [5] that c-TAL segments reabsorb 5–10 nmol s^{-1} cm^{-2}, and from the work of Schnerman and Marver (in [1]) who found that the amount of Na-K-ATPase activity in MD cells was 1/37 of that in c-TAL cells, a sodium transport rate in MD cells of 0.14 – 0.27 nmol s^{-1} cm^{-2} may be predicted. The measured value is in the same range as the calculated value. Thus, it seems clear that the rate of transport of the Na-K pump is only about 1/40 of that in the c-TAL cells, and that this rate is in good accordance with other data. The reduction in cell volume strongly suggested that furosemide inhibitable Na-K-2Cl co-transport was involved in the transport of Na and K into the MD cells.

We have also determined the osmotic water permeability of the basolateral and apical MD cell membranes [3]. Either the luminal or the basal side of tubules was perfused with oil, and an osmotic change of 150 mOsm was induced on the other side. The hydraulic conductance could then be calculated from the initial slope of the volume change curves. It was found that the water permeability of the apical cell membrane was much lower than on the basolateral side, and it was therefore concluded that the apical cell membrane constituted the primary barrier to water flow. The water permeability in c-TAL constituted about 10% of that in the MD cells. A greater membrane, due to a larger number of villi in the MD cells, might explain the higher water permeability in the MD cells, might explain the higher water permeability in the MD cells compared with the cells of the c-TAL. Nevertheless, the water permeability of the apical cell membrane was quite low. The high water permeability of the basolateral side, together with the low permeability of the luminal membrane, would mean that osmotic changes in the tubular lumen would give rise to only minor changes in cell volume, because of the rapid water movement across the basolateral cell membrane. When the luminal osmolarity was changed while the osmolarity of the outside bath was kept constant, only 10% of the expected volume change occurred, because of basolateral water flow. It was also found that when the luminal NaCl concentration was decreased from 60 mM to 15 mM without any compensation for a change in osmolarity, the steady state cell volume remained unaltered after the initial osmotic swelling and compensatory volume regulation. From these results it seems less likely to us that the lumen osmolarity, per se, is the factor involved in the sensing step.

Electrical Potential Measurements in Macula Densa Cell

The basolateral cell membrane potential in the macula densa cells has been measured [6]. The cortical thick ascending limbs were cannulated and perfused in vitro as described by Greger and Schlatter [4]. Both the transepithelial and the basolateral membrane voltages were measured with microelectrodes. The electrode tip was positioned next to macula densa cells by visual observation and was then advanced with the piezo stepper. Electrode resistances were constantly measured by injection of current pulses of 5 nA, 500 ms, and 1 Hz to detect any clogging of the pipette that might build up tip potentials in the order of −20 mV or more.

A concentration of 150 mM NaCl was usually used on both sides of the tubule. During the experiments of Schlatter et al. [6] on 166 perfused segments, some 3000 cell penetrations were attempted, and of these, eight impaled tubule cells showed stable recordings for up to 47 minutes. The mean PD_{bl} was −56 mV, and when furosemide was present in the lumen, PD_{bl} hyperpolarized by 27 mV, suggesting the

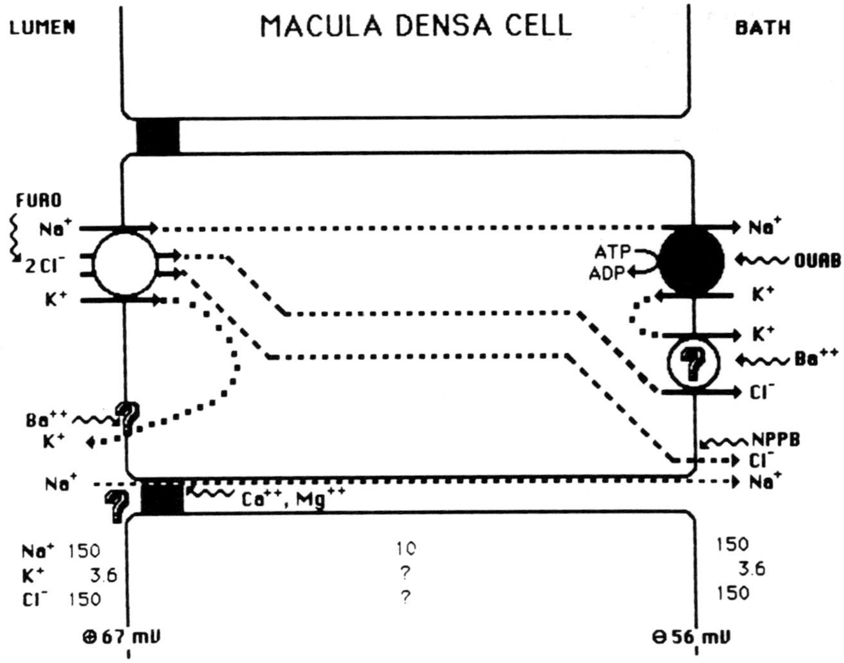

Fig. 3. Schematic diagram of ionic transport mechanisms in macula densa cells. Ouab, ouabain; Furo, furosemide. (From [16] with permission)

presence of a Na-K-2Cl co-transport system in the luminal cell membrane of the MD cells. This hyperpolarization dissipated when the furosemide was removed. It is possible that inhibition of Cl^- uptake hyperpolarized the cells, as the basolateral cell membrane was also Cl^- conductive. The Cl conductance of the basolateral cell membrane was also responsible for the increased depolarization of PD_{bl} when the bath Cl^- concentration was reduced from 150 to 30 mM.

The above results in the macula densa cells are compatible with the findings by Dr. Greger concerning the properties of c-TAL cells [5] (see Fig. 3). In the luminal membrane there is a Na-K-2Cl co-transport mechanism. When furosemide is added, the co-transport is blocked, the intracellular Cl concentration decreases, and the Cl conductance across the basolateral cell membrane is reduced, so that hyperpolarization of the basolateral cell membrane is reduced, so that hyperpolarization of the basolateral cell membrane takes place. The membrane potential then approaches the potassium equilibrium potential. Potassium recycling may also be suggested. The chloride conductance of the basolateral cell membrane is also supported by the finding of PD_{bl} depolarization when the bath concentration of Cl was reduced from 150 to 30 mM, as would be predicted for a Cl^- permeable membrane. In addition, the Cl channel blocker NPPB in the bath hyperpolarized PD_{bl}. Ouabain depolarized PD_{bl} from −68 to 12 mV, indicating the presence of Na-K pump activity.

Table 1.

Luminal perfusate	Macula densa cell (mM)	Thick ascending limb cell (mM)
150 mM NaCl	47	54
30 mM NaCl	35*	–
150 mM NaCl + 10^{-6} M furosemide	6*	5*

*$P < 0.06$

Macula Densa Cell Chloride Concentration

Recently, to test the hypothesis of Na-K-2Cl co-transport, we have performed direct measurements of chloride concentrations in cells of the cortical thick ascending limb and macula densa by use of the fluorophore SPQ, with a digital imaging system [7]. Chloride was measured in the macula densa and in the cortical thick ascending limb cells in the control states and after blockade with furosemide, or at a low sodium chloride concentration in the lumen perfusate. SPQ is quenched by a collisional mechanism without any change in the shape of its excitation or emission spectra [8]. SPQ follows a Stern-Volmer equation, and with knowledge of the Stern-Volmer constant K_{Cl^-}, the chloride concentration can be calculated;

$$F_o/F = 1 + K_{Cl}[Cl]$$

where F_o/F is the total fluorescence measured in the abscence of Cl divided by the fluorescence in the presence of Cl and K_{Cl} is the Stern-Volmer constant. The leakage of SPQ in the macula densa cells had a half-time of 197 minutes, which allowed sufficient time to perform the experimental protocol without losing too much SPQ. The chloride constant in the Stern-Volmer equation has to be determined for the macula densa cells, but it has been measured for proximal tubular cells [9] and for several types of fibroblasts [8] and does not seem to vary very much between the different cells. On the basis of the value for the proximal tubule, the concentration in the macula densa cells can be calculated. With this assumption the absolute value has to be considered with some caution. In the macula densa cells, as can be seen in Table 1, we found a chloride concentration of 47 mM at an NaCl concentration of 150 mM, both in the bath and in the lumen [7]. When furosemide was added to the luminal perfusion solution, the chloride concentration was reduced by 85% to 6 mM. The corresponding value in the cortical thick ascending limb cells was 54 mM, with a 90% reduction to 5 mM in the presence of furosemide. At a low NaCl of 30 mM in the tubular lumen, the chloride concentration in the macula densa cells was significantly reduced to 35 mM. The present results provide strong evidence that a Na-K-2Cl co-transport mechanism exists at the luminal cell membrane and that this mechanism allows NaCl to enter the macula densa cells and the cells of the cortical thick ascending limb at a fast rate, so that the chloride concentration is higher than that expected for passive distribution of chloride. When furosemide inhibits the Na-K-2Cl co-transport, the intracellular chloride concentration decreases to values close to the passive distribution of some 5 mM, calculated on theoretical grounds. On conversion of our furosemide values from ascending limb cells, the intracellular chloride activities were found not to be different from those obtained in rabbit cortical thick ascending limb cells by Dr. Greger and co-workers, using chloride selective microelectrodes [10].

Macula Densa Cell Calcium Concentration

It has been suggested that activation of macula densa cells may involve changes in the intracellular calcium concentration as one link in the chain of events leading to activation of TGF and release of renin. We therefore investigated the intracellular calcium concentration with fura-2, using a digital imaging system in macula densa cells, and compared it with the corresponding concentrations in the cells of the ascending limb of the loop of Henle. We found that our technique could be used to determine intracellular calcium. We found that the calibration curve for calcium and the K_d value of 228 nM was not different from that obtained by Grynkiewicz and co-workers [11]. An intracellular calcium concentration of about 90 nM was found both in the macula densa and in the cortical thick ascending limb cells, and the calcium concentration in the macula densa cells increased by about 20 nM when the tubular lumen was perfused with low Na and Cl concentrations. Addition of furosemide did not significantly increase the intracellular calcium concentration. We consider it less likely that this small change in the calcium concentration could be responsible for the full activation of renin release or the full inactivation of the TGF control mechanism. It would seem that the signal transmission from the macula densa cells could take routes other than through activation of intracellular calcium.

Sensing Step

Now, how can we envision the sensing step? Is it Na, Cl, NaCl, or osmolarity that is the flow dependent signal? On the basis of the present studies, it appears likely that MD cells have a Na-K-2Cl co-transport that carries Na-K and Cl into the cells. This can be concluded both from cell volume measurements and from the electrical measurements. An increase in the luminal NaCl concentration will increase the transport rate in the co-transport system, and a higher MD chloride will result, in association with a small increase in cell volume. The increase in conductive chloride flux across the basolateral cell membrane will depolarize the cell membrane potential. Since the Na-K-2Cl co-transport system has a higher affinity for Na than for Cl, as found in studies of the c-TAL segment [5], it is likely that the luminal Cl concentration is the most critical signal. The Na concentration will probably never fall so low as to limit the transport rate of the co-transporter.

Now, how is the signal from increased NaCl transport mediated across the macula densa cells to the effector site? For the time being there are several possibilities, of which we will briefly mention two. The first one is a metabolic control in which the intracellular formation of adenosine, and its leakage out of the cell, could transmit the response [12]. The formation of adenosine would increase on increased breakdown of ATP. These results are also particularly interesting in view of the findings of Bleich et al. [13], who demonstrated the existence of a luminal cell membrane K channel in the c-TAL cells that is inhibited by ATP. Thus, if a similar channel existed in the macula densa cells, increased NaCl transport through the macula densa cells would cause ATP breakdown. This would give rise to less inhibition of the K channel used for K recycling, thereby promoting this K recycling. At the same time more adenosine could leak out of the cell and mediate the response to the rest of the juxtaglomerular apparatus. One other possible explanation is that the NaCl concentration within the interstitial space of the extraglomerular mesangium is very high, and that this concentration is dependent on the NaCl transport in the macula densa. Dr. Bo Erik Persson and Dr. Marsh found that the Cl concentration within the renal interstitial space in the Amphiuma, as measured by chloride electrodes, was very high and was also flow-dependent [13]. It is possible that this high flow-dependent interstitial Cl concentration elicits the response from the arterioles or from the mesangial cells, as suggested by Dr. Kurokawa [14].

References

1. Schnermann J, Briggs J (1985) Function of the juxtaglomerular apparatus: local control of glomerular hemodynamics. In: Seldin DW, Giebisch G (eds) The kidney: physiology and pathophysiology. Raven, New York, pp 669–697
2. Gonzalez E, Salomonsson M, Müller-Suur C, Persson AEG (1988) Measurements of macula densa cell volume changes in isolated and perfused rabbit cortical thick ascending limb. I. Isosmotic and anisosmotic cell volume changes. Acta Physiol Scand 133: 149–157
3. Gonzalez E, Salomonsson M, Müller-Suur C, Persson AEG (1988) Measurements of macula densa cell volume changes in isolated and perfused rabbit cortical thick ascending limb. II. Apical and basolateral cell osmotic water permeabilities. Acta Physiol Scand 113:159–166
4. Greger R, Schlatter E (1983) Properties of the lumen membrane of the cortical thick ascending limb of Henle's loop of rabbit kidney. Pflugers Arch 396:315–324
5. Greger R (1985) Ion transport mechanisms in thick ascending limb of Henle's loop of mammalian nephron. Physiol Rev 65:760–797
6. Schlatter E, Salomonsson M, Persson AEG, Greger R (1989) Macula densa cells sense luminal NaCl concentration in furosemide sensitive Na^+-$2Cl^-$-K^+ cotransport. Pflugers Arch 414:286–290
7. Salomonsson M, Gonzalez E, Westerlund P, Persson AEG (to be published) The effect of furosemide on chloride concentration in macula densa and in cortical thick ascending limb cells. Acta Physiol Scand
8. Chao AC, Dix JA, Sellers MC, Verkman AS (1989) Fluorescence measurement of chloride transport in nonlayer cultured cells. Biophys J 56:1071–1081
9. Krapf R, Berry CH, Verkman AS (1988) Estimation of intracellular chloride activity in isolated perfused rabbit proximal convoluted tubules using a fluorescent indicator. Biophys J 53:955–962
10. Greger R, Oberleitner H, Schlatter E, Cassola A, Weidtke C (1983) Chloride activity in cells of isolated perfused thick ascending limb of rabbit kidney. Pflugers Arch 399:29–34
11. Grynkiewicz G, Poenie M, Tsien RY (1985) A new generation of Ca^{2+} indicators with greatly improved fluorescence properties. J Biol Chem 260:3440–3450
12. Osswald H (1988) Metabolic control of organ function—does it apply to the kidney. In: Persson AEG, Boberg U (eds) The juxtaglomerular apparatus. Elsevier, Amsterdam, pp 155–166
13. Persson B-E, Marsh D (1988) The flow sensor of tubuloglomerular feedback in the early distal tubule of Amphiuma. In: Persson AEG, Boberg U (eds) The juxtaglomerular apparatus. Elsevier, Amsterdam, pp 121-128

14. Kurokawa K (1989) Biology of glomerular mesangial cells (abstract). Int Eup Physiol Sci Proc Int Union Physiol Sci XVII. Helsinki, p 130
15. Schnermann J, Ploth DW, Hermle M (1976) Activation of tubuloglomerular feedback by chloride transport. Pflugers Arch 362:229–240
16. Persson AEG, Salomonsson M, Westerlund P, Greger R, Schlatter R, Gonzalez E. Macula densa cell function. Kidney Int in press

Intracellular and Membrane Events in the Activation of Afferent Arteriolar and Granular Cells

ARMIN KURTZ[1]

SUMMARY. There is accumulating information about the existence of membrane-bound signal transduction systems in renal afferent arteriolar and granular cells. The second messenger generating systems, which include phospholipases, nucleotide cyclases, and ion channels, become activated upon ligand binding to cell surface receptors. Subsequently they exert influence on the cellular functions, which predominantly are contraction and renin secretion, in these cells.

It is the aim of this contribution to summarize what we know at present about the existence of signal transduction systems, about their way of activation, and about their possible intracellular effects in renal arteriolar and granular cells.

Introduction

The renal afferent arterioles fulfill two important physiological functions. Firstly, they regulate the rate of glomerular filtration by determining preglomerular resistance. Secondly, they secrete renin into the circulation and thus determine the activity of the systemic renin-angiotensin-aldosterone system. Regulation of renin secretion and regulation of afferent vascular tone share a number of similarities. Both functions are elaborated by the same cell type, namely vascular smooth muscle cells (VSMC), because renin producing granular juxtaglomerular (JG) cells develop from the neighboring VSMC by a reversible metaplastic transformation [1,2]. There exists moreover, a small but significant degree of electrical coupling between the VSMC and JG cells in the afferent arterioles [3]. In most instances, both functions are influenced by the same parameters. Those parameters, for instance, comprise blood pressure, a signal generated by the macula densa, sympathetic transmitters that are released from sympathetic nerve endings in the juxtaglomerular region, and a

[1]Physiologisches Institut der Universität Zürich, Winterthurerstrasse 190, CH-8057 Zürich, Switzerland

number of circulating or locally generated hormones. A superior principle in the regulation of preglomerular vascular tone and renin secretion even appears to exist. Factors causing a contraction of afferent arterioles usually lead to an inhibition of renin secretion, while stimulators of renin secretion most often cause a relaxation of afferent vessels. For instance, a rise of blood pressure, activation of the macula densa, and vasoconstrictive hormones such as angiotensin II cause a contraction of the VSMC in the afferent arterioles and inhibit renin secretion, cf [4]. A fall of blood pressure, β-adrenergic agonists, and other vasodilating hormones, on the other hand, lead to relaxation of VSMC and enhancement of renin secretion, cf [4]. From a physiological point of view, such a kind of interrelation between VSMC contraction and renin secretion appears ingenious. By its action renin generates the vasoconstrictor hormone angiotensin II (ANG II), which itself is an important determinant of blood pressure. Inhibition of renin secretion during states of contraction of the afferent arteriole therefore reflects a very powerful negative feedback control of renin release in particular, and of blood pressure in general.

The mechanism by which VSMC contraction and renin secretion are interrelated is still speculative. It is also not well understood how the blood pressure, the macula densa, and a number of hormones exert their effects on VSMC and JG cells located in afferent arterioles. A common feature of the parameters affecting afferent arteriolar function as alluded to above is that they exert their effects on cell contraction and exocytosis of renin via specific signal transduction systems.

The identification of such signal transduction systems in afferent arteriolar VSMC and in JG cells was hampered by the fact that these cells lie buried within the renal cortex and are not accessible for direct investigation. The development of new techniques, such as the split hydronephrotic kidney [5], isolation techniques for juxtaglomerular apparatuses [6] and JG cells [7], and the application of sophisticated techniques on these preparations have enabled investigators to get some first-hand insight into the intracellular and membrane events in VSMC and JG cells in afferent arterioles. In this contribution I shall summarize the knowledge which is presently available on those processes occurring in afferent vessels. In this context I will focus my considerations on classic signal transduction systems such as phospholipases, nucleotide cyclases, and ion channels as they occur in a variety of tissues.

Phospholipases

Phospholipase C

A phospholipase C (PLC) is a phosphodiesterase that splits a phospholipid into diacylglycerol and a phosphorester compound. As long as several decades ago it was recognized that phospholipases C and their substrates played a role in transmembrane signalling [8,9]. The hydrolysis of phosphatidylinositolbisphosphate (PIP_2) in particular, has attracted interest, because it provides two second messengers that cause release of calcium from intracellular stores (via inositoltrisphosphate) and that activate protein kinase C (via diacylglycerol) [10]. Today we know that this important reaction takes place in almost every eukaryotic cell, provided that the essential enzyme (PLC) is present in the cell membrane and is subject to regulated activation. The physiological relevance of PLC as a signal transduction system is made clear by the fact that PLC is coupled to cell surface receptors via coupling proteins that have been characterized as heterotrimer guanosine triphosphate GTP-binding proteins, cf. [11].

The first evidence that an activatable PLC also existed in JG cells was obtained in primary cultures of rat juxtaglomerular cells. Addition of angiotensin II (ANG II), arginine-vasopressin (AVP) and norepinephrine (NE) to those cells led to a significant breakdown of PIP_2 and simultaneous increase of diacylglycerol (DAG) [12]. Although a rise in IP_3 level was not demonstrated in that study it was considered likely that a receptor coupled PLC exists in JG cells and can be activated by ANG II, AVP, and to a lesser extent, by NE. This conclusion was recently supported by the observation that ANG II also causes the mobilization of calcium from intracellular stores in JG cells [3], an effect that is considered to be dependent on the generation of IP_3 [13]. Moreover, it was found that the calcium mobilizing effect of ANG II was dependent on the presence of intracellular GTP and could be mimicked by a stable GTP analogue, suggesting that the activation of PLC by ANG II in JG cells is also mediated by G-proteins [3]. Indirect evidence that the effect of ANG II on JG cells could be mediated by G proteins had already been provided by the findings that pertussis toxin, which functionally inactivates a number of GTP-binding proteins, attenuated the effect of ANG II on renin secretion from isolated kidneys and also attenuated the effect of ANG II on renal vascular resistance [14]. This was also the first indication that the signal transduction mechanisms for ANG II in renal VSMC and in JG are not principally different, a consideration that has been corroborated by two previous studies [3,15].

Summing up, there is good evidence for the existence of functional receptor -G-protein-PLC complexes in the membranes of VSMC and JG cells in afferent arterioles.

As already mentioned, activation of PLC, for instance by ANG II, leads to a rise of diacylglycerol (DAG) and subsequently to an activation of protein kinase C [16]. The subcellular effects of protein kinase C activation in afferent arteriolar and granular cells have so far been assessed in experiments with tumor promoting phorbol esters that are considered as artificial activators of C-kinase, as well as by the use of putative C-kinase inhibitors. It appears as if C-kinase activation is important for the contraction of renal VSMC induced by ANG II [17]. Phorbol esters in high concentrations were also found to enhance transmembrane calcium influx and to attenuate renin secretion from isolated JG cells [12]. Whether the latter effects are really due to C-kinase activation or to side effects of phorbol esters needs to be clarified. Recent findings, moreover, suggest that phorbol esters at concentrations typical for C-kinase activation cause an electrical decoupling of VSMC and JG cells in the afferent arterioles (A. Kurtz and R. Penner, unpublished work). Other effects of C-kinase activation that occur in cells and might be important in the future, but have so far not been proven for JG cells, are enhancement of phospholipase A_2 activity [18] and activation of sodium/proton exchange, cf [19]).

The partner messenger molecular arising simultaneously with DAG is inositol-trisphosphate (IP_3). The outstanding role of IP_3 as a second messenger causing intracellular calcium release is well established [10]. Recent evidence, moreover, suggests that IP_3 or its derivatives have—at least in some cell types—an important role in the regulation of transmembrane calcium influx [20]. The changes which take place in the intracellular concentration of calcium in JG cells and VSMC in afferent

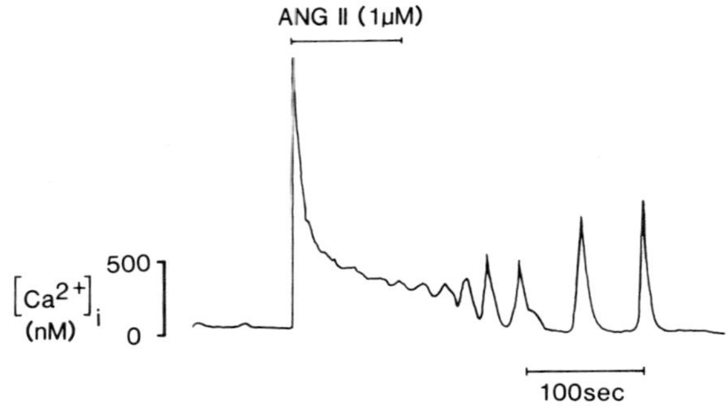

Fig. 1. Intracellular calcium concentration ([Ca]$_i$) in a juxtaglomerular cell from mouse kidney after addition of angiotensin II

arterioles upon activation of PLC by ANG II or by stable GTP-analogues are impressive (Fig. 1). Within a few seconds, cytosolic calcium rises transiently, as a result of calcium release from intracellular stores. This initial calcium transient, during which calcium levels rise from 90nM to 1µM or even higher, is then followed by an interval lasting 1–4 minutes, during which intracellular calcium stays constantly elevated at a level of about 200nM. When $[Ca^{2+}]_i$ declines to near resting levels, the cytosolic calcium concentration starts to oscillate. Such calcium oscillations after PLC-stimulation have already been observed in a number of cells, cf [21]. However, the pattern and the characteristics of the oscillations vary markedly between the cells. In JG cells the oscillations are very regular, with an average duration of 10 seconds and an average frequency of about 2 min^{-1} during continuous stimulation of PLC by stable GTP analogues [3]. The oscillatory calcium spikes result from intracellular calcium release. Their frequency, however, is strongly coupled to the extracellular concentration of calcium [3]. How extracellular calcium influences calcium release from internal stores in JG cells is not yet understood. Possible explanations could be that external calcium modulates PLC in a stimulatory fashion and/or that external calcium influences the refilling of internal calcium stores.

Another link between extra- and intracellular calcium concentrations is shown by the existence of calcium influx mechanisms, the activation of which causes the stable elevation of intracellular calcium after the initial calcium transient [3,12]. The mechanism activating the calcium influx in JG cells and in VSMC is not yet known. In analogy with other cell types, both receptor-operated or second messenger-operated calcium channels could be candidates. From the observation that not only ANG II, but also stable GTP analogues, can activate calcium influx in JG cells one could speculate that second messenger-operated channels rather than receptor-operated channels exist there. Whether IP_3 or one of its derivatives is the key activator of those channels still remains to be clarified.

What are the cellular events which follow a rise of calcium in renal afferent arteriolar VSMC and JG cells?

Doubtless, a rise of intracellular calcium is the key signal which activates myosin light chain kinase and it is thus the crucial event for the contraction of VSMC, the essential function of this cell type [22].

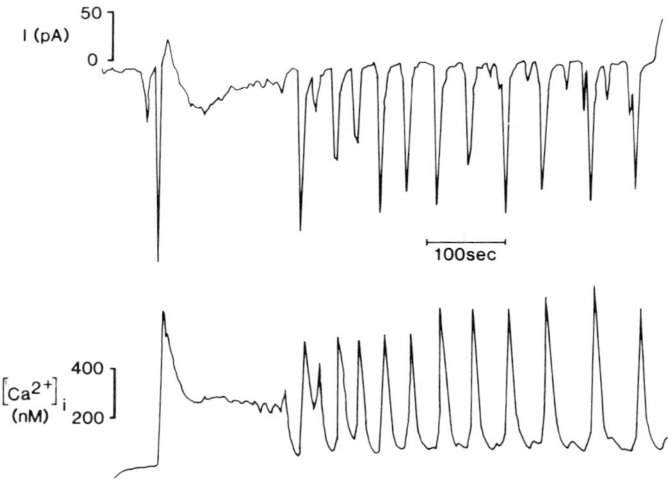

Fig. 2. Simultaneous recordings of membrane current and intracellular calcium concentration in a mouse JG cell during stimulation with GTP-γ-S (100μM). Voltage clamp potential was −60 mV

It is more difficult to find a clearcut answer for JG cells. Although it is generally assumed that a rise of calcium blocks the exocytosis of renin we still await unequivocal experimental proof of this hypothesis [23]. Therefore we should concentrate here on the cellular effects of calcium that have been measured in JG cells. In fact, so far, there is only one effect of calcium that has clearly been demonstrated in JG cells: the activation of calcium-dependent chloride channels (Fig. 2) that have been found to exist in high numbers in JG cells [3]. From the existence of these channels, a calcium-regulated cell volume control can be predicted for JG and VSMC cells in afferent arterioles [24]. A rise in internal calcium will lower the cell volume and, conversely, a drop in internal calcium will raise the cell volume. As outlined elsewhere, such a calcium-dependent volume control could, in fact, explain an inhibitory control function of calcium on renin secretion from JG cells [24].

Phospholipase A_2

Phospholipase A_2 (PLA_2) is a monoesterase that liberates fatty acids which are esterified in the 2 position of phospholipids. Since the bulk of arachidonic acid is bound in this position, activation of PLA_2 leads to a rise of the cytosolic level of arachidonic acid [25]. Arachidonic acid (AA) is the reaction limiting substrate for the AA-cascade leading to prostaglandins, thromboxanes, lipoxygenase products, and leukotriens. PLA_2-activity is highly calcium sensitive and it is not so surprising that it was at first thought that hormones activating PLC, and in consequence calcium release also led to an activation of PLA_2 [26,27]. This simpler view is now being expanded by recent findings that hormones can directly activate PLA_2, probably via GTP-binding proteins [28]. Regardless of the exact mechanisms of PLA_2 activation, it can be assumed that most hormones which stimulate PLC in JG cells and afferent arteriolar VSMC also lead to liberation of arachidonic acid and thus start the AA-cascade. By the action of cyclooxygenase AA is then converted into endoperoxides and subsequently into prostaglandins and thromboxanes. Lipoxygenases convert AA into hydroxyperoxide derivatives and also into leukotrienes. It is of some interest in this context that in canine renal afferent arterioles, prostaglandin formation is not stimulated by ANG II in a concentration range up to 100 nM [29]. Only at very high concentrations, such as 1 μM, did ANG II stimulate prostacyclin formation in superficial, but not in juxtamedullary afferent arterioles. If this observation holds also for renal afferent arterioles of other species, one would infer that receptor activation of PLA_2 or cyclooxygenase activity is relatively poorly expressed in afferent arteriolar VSMC and JG cells. If the latter is true then free arachidonic acid would be predominantly converted into lipoxygenase products and perhaps into leukotrienes.

Evidence exists to indicate that lipoxygenase products can inhibit renin secretion in vitro [30]. From indirect evidence it has been, moreover, speculated that ANG II inhibits renin secretion from JG cells via the lipoxygenase pathway [31]. Whether leukotrienes also affect renin secretion is not yet known. First evidence also suggests that lipoxygenase and epoxygenase products also affect the function of renal blood vessels [32].

Nucleotide Cyclases

Adenylate Cyclase

The adenylate cyclase (AC) generating cyclic AMP from ATP was the first among the, today, classic signal transduction systems whose existence was postulated for juxtaglomerular cells. Based on the observations that β-adrenergic agonists, as well as forskolin, exert profound stimulatory effects on renin secretion it was logical to assume first, the existence of AC and, secondly, the existence of a receptor coupling of AC in the membrane of JG cells, cf [4]. In experiments with isolated JG cells it has been confirmed that forskolin, isoproterenol, and also calcitonin gene related peptide (CGRP), increase the intracellular level of cAMP, cf [4]. The increase of cAMP caused by these agents is amplified when cAMP degradation is inhibited, thus suggesting strongly that they act, via cAMP formation, by stimulating adenylate cyclase. Forskolin causes receptor independent activation of AC, whereas, in contrast, receptor operated activation of AC, for instance, that caused by isoproterenol or by CGRP, only leads to a transient stimulation of AC (Fig. 3). This suggests that in JG cells, as in other cells, receptor mediated activation of AC is subject to desensitization, most likely to receptor downregulation. Irrespective of that fact, the effects of cAMP in JG cells appear to be longer lasting than the actual rise in cAMP (Fig. 3). This phenomenon is most likely due to phosphorylation processes that are performed by cAMP-dependent A-kinase and that last longer than the measurable rise of cAMP. It is generally agreed upon that a rise of cAMP enhances the exocytosis of renin from JG cells, cf [4]. The cellular mechanisms for this effect have not yet been identified. Recently it has been observed that the calcium mobilization induced by PLC activation is inhibited in JG cells if cAMP levels are elevated [3].

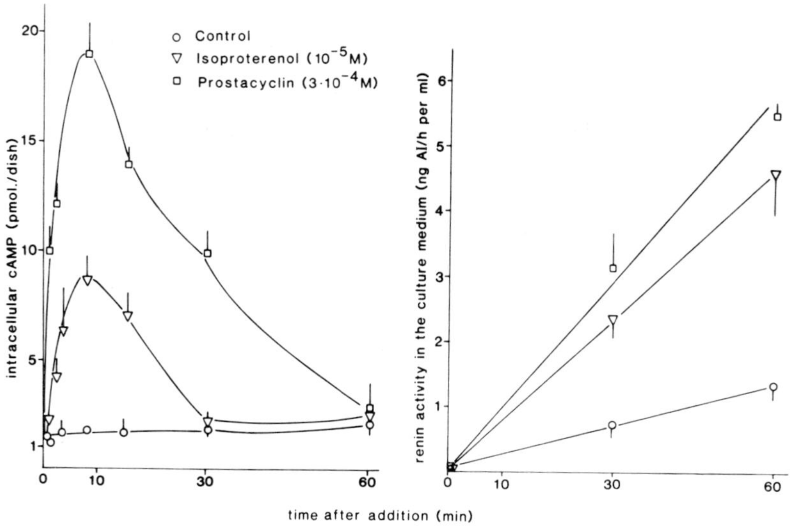

Fig. 3. Temporal change of intracellular cAMP levels (*left*) and renin secretion rates (*right*) from cultured rat juxtaglomerular cells after addition of prostacyclin and isoproterenol. (From [4])

Under the assumption that calcium is an inhibitory signal for renin secretion, the inhibition of calcium mobilization by cAMP could help us to understand, at least in part, the stimulatory effect of cAMP on renin secretion.

Cyclic AMP-dependent phosphorylation of the myosin light chain kinase has been recognized as a powerful negative regulatory element in the contraction of vascular smooth muscle cells [22]. If one assumes that receptor linked AC also exists in VSMC in afferent arterioles, then two potent vasorelaxant events can be postulated for these cells. First, inhibition of calcium mobilization, thus removing the key signal for smooth muscle cell contraction, and secondly, inhibition of myosin light chain kinase (MLCK), which is the key enzyme for the induction of smooth muscle cell contraction.

The juxtaglomerular region is well innervated with sympathetic nerve endings [1] and equipped with membrane bound β-adreno-receptors. Assuming continuous nerve activity, one can infer a steady activation of AC in VSMC and JG cells in the juxtaglomerular region.

This constellation provides a possible basis for another signal transduction system, namely for receptor mediated inhibition of cAMP formation. So far only a few hormones have been found to inhibit AC. Among these adenosine and α-adrenergic agonists are the best characterized ones, cf [33]. In several tissues, adenosine has been found to inhibit AC activity via A_1-subtype receptors, cf [33], while α-adrenergic agonists have been found to inhibit AC via α_2-subtype receptors, cf [33]. While the existence of α_2-receptors in afferent vessels is so far only speculative [34], there exists good evidence for the existence of adenosine A_1-receptors [35,36]. If they would negatively interfere with the steady state activation of AC in the juxtaglomerular region, then they should lower cellular cAMP levels. As a result, afferent arteriolar constriction and inhibition of renin secretion should arise from A_1-receptor activation, due to disinhibition of both MLCK and calcium mobilization. These effects have indeed been observed in a number of studies, cf [37]. Since, in this concept, adenosine appears only as a facilitator of calcium effects, one would expect that adenosine requires an additional agent that should directly stimulate PLC, and in consequence, calcium mobilization. Indeed, it has been found that the apparent "vasoconstrictory" effect of A1-receptor activation in vivo requires the presence of ANG II [38]; but not so the inhibitory effect on renin secretion that can also be observed in isolated glomeruli [39] and in isolated JG cells [40]. A possible explanation for these different effects of adenosine on the function of VSMC and JG cells could be provided by the observation that adenosine also causes small, but significant, elevations of cGMP in JG cells [40]. While guanosine monophosphate (cGMP) acts as a vasorelaxant in VSMC it most likely is an inhibitory signal for renin secretion [4]. The cellular mechanisms by which adenosine acts on afferent arteriolar and granular cells will attract increasing interest, because recent studies suggest that adenosine is a likely candidate for the macula densa signal [41,42].

Guanylate Cyclase

With the exception of the retina, a second messenger role of cyclic GMP in tissues has been speculated on for a long time. The discovery of atrial natriuretic peptide (ANP) as a physiologically important hormone has supported an important second messenger function of cGMP. The ANP-receptor that is anchored in the cell membrane has been identified as an intrinsic guanylate cyclase (GC), generating cyclic GMP from GTP [43].

Meanwhile several cGMP-mediated reactions have been characterized, cf [44], the most outstanding of which are, apart from light transduction, vasorelaxation and inhibition of renal sodium reabsorption.

The functional existence of ANP receptors has been shown for juxtaglomerular cells [7]. From that we may infer that JG cells and presumably also VSMC in the afferent arteriole are equipped with a membrane-bound guanylate cyclase.

There is good evidence that cGMP causes relaxation of VSMC in the afferent arterioles [45,46]. The precise mechanism leading to this effect is not yet known. It could be due to an increased calcium clearing from the cytosol, or could be due to a direct inhibitory action on myosin light chain kinase, cf [44].

The effect of ANP or cGMP on renin secretion from JG cells is less unequivocal. While the majority of the studies suggest an inhibitory effect of ANP and of cGMP on renin secretion, cf [4], there are also studies reporting no effect [47] and, in a single case, even a stimulatory effect of ANP/cGMP on renin secretion [48]. In my opinion these divergent results with ANP/cGMP result from the fact that cGMP has no direct effect on renin secretion, as cAMP has. In independent experiments, we have obtained evidence that ANP/cGMP requires calcium for its inhibitory effect on renin secretion [49] and that cGMP enhances the calcium sensitivity of the calcium-activated chloride channels in JG cells [3]. In consequence, ANP/cGMP requires at least normal calcium concentrations for its inhibitory effect on renin secretion. Given normal, or even elevated, calcium concentrations in JG cells an inhibitory effect of ANP/cGMP could be predicted for most experimental situations. Nevertheless, in some instances calcium levels could also drop below normal levels, and in these situations the inhibitory effect of ANP will be absent. An inhibitory effect of cGMP on renin secretion could gain importance in view of the fact that the recently discovered endothelial derived relaxing factor (EDRF) stimulates soluble guanylate cyclase activity and thus stimulates cGMP formation, cf [44]. Since there is evidence that JG cells contain a soluble guanylate cyclase [7], it is tempting to speculate about a possible endothelial control of renin secretion from JG cells via EDRF. First evidence in fact indicates that EDRF inhibits renin release in vitro [50]. Among the parameters stimulating EDRF formation by endothelial cells, the shear stress on the endothelial surface could play an important role, cf [51]. It will be interesting therefore, in future experiments, to test whether these mechanisms are involved in the process by which the blood pressure controls renin secretion from JG cells.

Ion Channels

Ion channels play an important role in signal transduction in excitable tissues. Since, in principle, vascular smooth muscle cells belong to the group of excitable cells it is obvious to question electrical events in JG cells upon activation and to consider the role of the membrane potential in the function of JG cells and VSMC in the afferent arterioles.

The first evidence for the occurrence of electrical events in JG cells was provided by microelectrode studies showing that the membrane potential of JG cells slightly hyperpolarized in response to β-adrenergic agonists [52]. More prominent, however, are changes of the membrane potential in response to vasoconstrictors. In elegant microelectrode investigations it was demonstrated that JG cells and VSMC in the afferent arterioles respond to ANG II and to other vasoconstrictors with a strong depolarization, with an amplitude ranging from 10 to 50mV [15]. In these studies no clear evidence for changes of electrical membrane resistance was found. Therefore it was not possible to attribute the observed depolarization to the opening or to the closing of certain types of ion channels. The resting membrane potential of VSMC and JG cells in afferent arterioles ranges between −70 to −80mV [3,15,52] and is thus close to the potassium equilibrium potential, suggesting that potassium conductances play a major role in the electrical properties of JG cells. In fact, a recent study has identified two types of potassium channels in JG cells and VSMC in afferent arterioles [3]. Both types are voltage activated but their activation potential differs markedly. One type of K^+-channel becomes activated upon depolarization of the cells to −10mV or more positive potentials. This type of K^+-channel is known in a variety of tissues; the sum current produced by these channels is named delayed (outward) rectifier for potassium. The second type of voltage gated K^+-channel present is inwardly rectifying and the channels become activated, upon hyperpolarization of the cells, to potential values lower than the resting membrane potential. This type of current, which also occurs in several other cell types, is named anomalous inward rectifier for potassium. So far no positive evidence has been produced for the existence of other potential activated ion channels, in particular sodium or calcium channels, in JG cells.

On the other hand there is good evidence for the existence of calcium-permeable channels which are activated by ANG II or by stable GTP analogues [3,53]. The question of whether these channels are directly coupled to receptors via GTP-binding proteins or whether they are activated by second messengers that result from G-protein mediated reactions, still has to be clarified.

Another type of second messenger operated ion channels has also been identified in JG cells and VSMC in afferent arterioles. These are calcium activated chloride channels, which have a small single channel conductance and which exist in high numbers in JG cells (Fig. 2) [3]. Together with the voltage gated K^+-channels the calcium activated chloride channels could manage an effective cell volume control, which in turn could govern renin secretion [24].

Having now considered the equipment of JG cells with ion channels we should recall the question of the mechanism by which ANG II leads to a depolarization of JG cells and VSMC in afferent arterioles.

As mentioned before, ANG II does cause calcium mobilization and calcium influx into JG cells. In parallel with the changes of calcium the chloride conductance of the cells will change and will therefore produce an electrical driving force toward the chloride equilibrium potential. The chloride equilibrium potential for JG cells has, so far, not been measured. If it is similar to that found in other smooth muscle cells it should be in the range of −20 to −30mV [54], a value that is far more positive than the resting membrane potential of −70 to −80mV in JG cells. In consequence, JG cells should depolarize upon a rise of intracellular calcium, and since the chloride conductance mirrors the intracellular calcium concentration, the time course of the membrane potential should mirror the time course of the intracellular calcium after stimulation of the cells by ANG II. In fact, the changes of membrane potential measured in microelectrode studies resemble the pattern of calcium changes in response to ANG II [15]. However, the depolarization usually lasts longer than the rise of calcium, suggesting that an additional depolarizing force is evoked by ANG II. This additional depolarizing force is most likely produced by a reversible inhibition of the anomalous inward rectifier for potassium caused by ANG II (Fig. 4), an event that removes a strong hyperpolarizing force. Interestingly, the inhibition of the inward rectifier can also be produced by stable GTP-analogues (Fig. 4), suggesting that it is mediated by a G-protein, or caused by a second messenger that is generated by G-protein mediated reaction. A third depolarizing force that is produced by the action of ANG II and also by stable GMP analogues is the increase of the calcium conductance of the cell membrane, which manifests itself as an increase of calcium influx [3,12,53]. Until recently, the depolarizing effect of ANG II in renal JG cells has been attributed mainly to the activation of potential operated calcium channels (POCC) [15]. However, a recent study failed to detect such channels in JG cells [53].

Summing up, the depolarization produced by ANG II in JG cells and VSMC in the afferent arterioles is probably a multifactorial event involving calcium activation of chloride conductance, increase of calcium conductance, and inhibition of potassium conductance.

Apart from the ion channels, ion exchange mechanisms could also gain importance for the regulation of function of JG cells. It has been observed that ANG II either directly, or indirectly via activation of protein kinase C, causes a stimulation of the sodium/proton exchange, cf [19]. This event leads to a transient alkalinization of the cytosol in response to ANG II. This effect could be of particular importance for JG cells, because recent studies on isolated JG cells have shown that inhibition of Na/H exchange leads to a marked stimulation of renin secretion (A. Kurtz et al., unpub-

Fig. 4. Block of inwardly rectifying potassium current in mouse JG cells by angiotensin II (*top*) and GTP-γ-S (*lower*). *Arrow* indicates establishment of whole cell configuration. Note that outward current is not blocked by GTP-γ-S

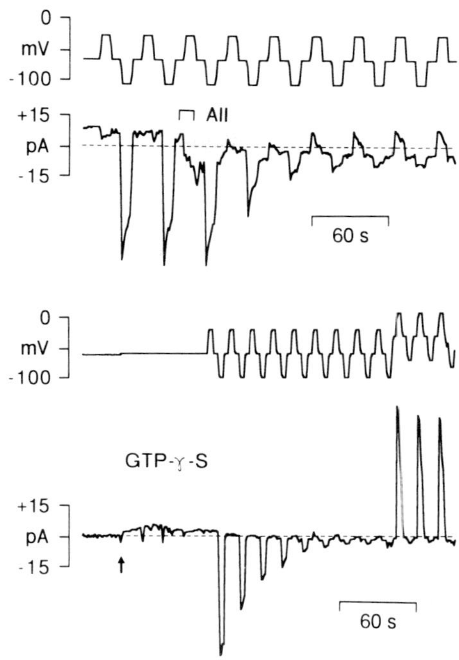

lished). If ANG II would activate Na/H exchange in JG cells also, then this action could causally contribute to the inhibitory effect of ANG II on renin secretion.

Cross-Talk Between Signal Transduction Systems

The accumulation of knowledge of intracellular events in JG cells has also revealed that the different signal transduction systems are not isolated units that produce specific cellular effects, but that the signal transduction systems communicate with each other (summarized in Fig. 5).

Receptor operated stimulation of PLC, for instance, causes activation of protein kinase C and the mobilization of calcium via IP_3 formation. C-kinase activation itself interferes with other second messenger systems in JG cells. First, it causes a negative feedback on PLC activation [55]. Secondly, presumably it activates Na/H exchange, cf [19], and could, as in neighboring mesangial cells, increase PLA_2 activity [18]. Calcium mobilization by IP_3 alters electrical behavior by influencing chloride channels [3]. Membrane depolarization, produced by calcium activation of chloride channels and by inhibition of potassium channels, has an inhibitory effect on the oscillatory calcium release [3].

A rise of cAMP produced by activation of adenylate cyclase impairs calcium mobilization in JG cells [3]. A rise of cGMP produced by activation of guanylate cyclase probably increases the calcium sensitivity of the chloride channels (A. Kurtz and R. Penner, unpublished work).

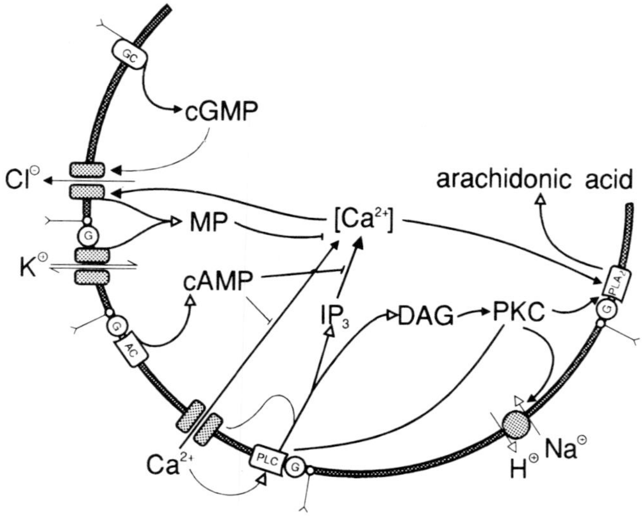

Fig. 5. Interaction of second messenger systems in afferent arteriolar and granular cells. PLC, phospholipase C; PLA_2, phospholipase A_2, DAG, diacyglycerol; IP_3, inositoltrisphosphate; PKC, protein kinase C; AC, adenylate cyclase; GC, guanylate cyclase; G, GTP-binding protein; MP, membrane potential

Acknowledgments. The author wishes to thank O. Stoupa for secretarial help and C. Gasser for doing the artwork. This work was financially supported by a grant from the Swiss National Science Foundation (31-26381.89)

References

1. Barajas L (1979) Anatomy of the juxtaglomerular apparatus. Am J Physiol 236:F333–F343
2. Taugner R, Bührle CP, Hackenthal E, Mannek E, Nobiling R (1984) Morphology of the juxtaglomerular apparatus and secretory mechanisms. In: Berlyne GM, Giovanetti S (eds) Contributions to nephrology, vol 43. Karger, Basel, pp 76–101
3. Kurtz A, Penner R (1989) Angiotensin II induces oscillations of intracellular calcium and inhibits anomalous inward rectifying potassium current in renal juxtaglomerular cells. Proc Natl Acad Sci USA 86:3423–3427
4. Kurtz A (1989) Cellular control of renin secretion. Rev Physiol Biochem Pharmacol 113:1–40
5. Steinhausen M, Snoei H, Parekh N, Baker R, Johnson PC (1983) Hydronephrosis: a new method to visualize vas afferens, efferens, and glomerular network. Kidney Int 23:794–806
6. Skott O, Briggs JP (1987) Direct demonstration of macula densa mediated renin release. Science 237:1618–1620
7. Kurtz A, Della Bruna R, Pfeilschifter J, Taugner R, Bauer C (1986) Atrial natriuretic peptide inhibits renin release from isolated renal juxtaglomerular cells by cGMP-mediated process. Proc Natl Acad Sci USA 83:4769–4773

8. Hokin MR, Hokin LE (1953) Enzyme secretion and the incorporation of ^{32}P into phospholipids of pancreas slices. J Biol Chem 203:967–977
9. Michell RH (1975) Inositol phospholipids and cell surface receptor function. Biochim Biophys Acta 415:81–147
10. Berridge MJ (1987) Inositoltriphosphate and diacylglycerol; two interactive second messengers. Annu Rev Biochem 56:159–193
11. Cockcroft S, Stutchfield (1988) G-proteins, the inositol lipid signalling pathway, and secretion. Philos Trans R Soc Lond [Biol] B320:247–265
12. Kurtz A, Pfeilschifter J, Hutter A, Bührle CP, Nobiling R, Taugner R, Hackenthal E, Bauer C (1986a) Role of protein kinase C in vasoconstrictor caused inhibition of renin release from isolated juxtaglomerular cells. Am J Physiol 250:C563–C571
13. Streb H, Irvine RF, Berridge MJ, Schulz I (1983) Release of Ca^{2+} from a nonmitochondrial store in pancreas acinar cells by inositol-1,4,5-triphosphate. Nature 306:67–68
14. Hackenthal E, Aktories K, Jakobs KH (1985) Pertussis toxin attenuates angiotensin II-induced vasoconstriction and inhibition of renin release. Mol Cell Endocrinol 42: 113–117
15. Bührle CP, Nobiling R, Taugner R (1985) Intracellular recordings from renin-positive cells of the afferent glomerular arteriole. Am J Physiol 249:F272–F281
16. Nishizuka Y (1984) Turnover of inositol phospholipids and signal transduction. Science 225:1365–1369
17. Scholz H, Kurtz A (1990) Role of protein kinase C in renal vasoconstriction caused by angiotensin II. Am J Physiol 259:C421–C426
18. Pfeilschifter J, Kurtz A, Bauer C (1986) Role of phospholipase C and protein kinase C in vasoconstrictor-induced prostaglandin synthesis in cultured rat renal mesangial cells. Biochem J 234:125–130
19. Smith JB (1986) Angiotensin receptor signalling in cultured vascular smooth muscle cells. Am J Physiol 250:F759–F769
20. Penner R, Matthews G, Neher E (1988) Second messenger control of calcium influx in rat peritoneal mast cells. Nature 334:499–504
21. Jacob R (1990) Calcium oscillations in electrically non-excitable cells. Biochim Biophys Acta 1052:427–438
22. Adelstein RS (1983) Regulation of contractile proteins by phosphorylation. J Clin Invest 72:1863–1866
23. Fray JCS (1990) Control of renin secretion by extracellular calcium. Cell Calcium 11:339–341
24. Kurtz A (1990) Do calcium-activated chloride channels control renin secretion? News Physiol Sci 5:43–46
25. Irvine RF (1982) How is the level of free arachidonic acid controlled in mammalian cells? Biochem J 204:3–16
26. Van den Bosch H (1980) Intracellular phospholipases A. Biochim Biophys Acta 604:191–246
27. Lapetina EG (1982) Regulation of arachidonic acid production: role of phospholipase C and A_2. Trends Pharmacol Sci 3:115–118
28. Axelrod J, Burch RM, Jelsema CL (1988) Receptor-mediated activation of phospholipase A_2 via GTP-binding proteins: arachidonic acid and its metabolites as second messengers. Trends Neurosci 11:117–123
29. Hura CE, Kunau RT (1988) Angiotensin II-stimulated prostaglandin production by canine renal afferent arterioles. Am J Physiol 254:F734–F738
30. Antonipillai I, Nadler JL, Robon EC, Horton R (1987) The inhibitory role of 12- and 15-lipoxygenase products on renin release. Hypertension 10:61–66
31. Antonipillai I, Nadler J, Horton R (1988) Angiotensin feedback inhibition on renin is expressed via the lipoxygenase pathway. Endocrinology 122:1277–1281

32. Takahashi K, Capdevila J, Karara A, Falck JR, Jacobson HR, Badr KF (1990) Cytochrome P-450 arachidonate metabolites in rat kidney: characterization and hemodynamic responses. Am J Physiol 258:F781–F789
33. Limbird LE (1988) Receptors linked to inhibition of adenylate cyclase: additional signalling mechanisms. FASEB J 2:2686–2695
34. Pettinger WA, Umemura S, Smyth DD, Jeffries WB (1987) Renal α_2-adrenoreceptors and the adenylate cyclase-cAMP system: biochemical and physiological interactions. Am J Physiol 252:F199–F208
35. Churchill PC, Churchill MC (1985) A1 and A2 adenosine receptor activation inhibits and stimulates renin secretion of rat renal cortical slices. J Pharmacol Exp Ther 232: 589–594
36. Holz FG, Steinhausen M (1987) Renovascular effects of adenosine receptor agonists. Renal Physiol 10:272–282
37. Spielman WS, Thompson CJ (1982) A proposed role for adenosine in the regulation of renal hemodynamics and renin release. Am J Physiol 242:F423–F435
38. Hall JE, Granger JP (1986) Adenosine alters glomerular filtration control by angiotensin II. Am J Physiol 250:F917–F923
39. Skott O, Baumbach L (1985) Effects of adenosine on renin release from isolated glomeruli and kidney slices. Pflugers Arch 404:232–237
40. Kurtz A, Della Bruna R, Pfeilschifter J, Bauer C (1988b) Role of cGMP as second messenger of adenosine in the inhibition of renin release. Kidney Int 33:798–803
41. Schnermann J, Weihprecht H, Briggs JP (1990) Inhibition of tubuloglomerular feedback during adenosine1 receptor blockade. Am J Physiol 258:F553–F561
42. Weihprecht H, Lorenz JN, Schnermann J, Skott O, Briggs JP (1990) Effect of adenosine 1-receptor blockade on renin release from rabbit isolated perfused juxtaglomerular apparatus. J Clin Invest 85:1622–1628
43. Chinkers M, Garbers DL, Chang MS, Lowe DG, Chin H, Goeddel DV, Schulz S (1989) A membrane form of guanylate cyclase is an atrial natriuretic peptide receptor. Nature 338:78–83
44. Walter U (1989) Physiological role of cGMP and cGMP-dependent protein kinase in the cardiovascular system. Rev Physiol Biochem Pharmacol 113:41–88
45. Marin-Grez M, Fleming JT, Steinhausen M (1986) Atrial natriuretic peptide causes preglomerular vasodilatation and post-glomerular vasoconstriction in rat kidney. Nature 324:473–476
46. Ohishi K, Hishida A, Honda N (1988) Direct vasodilatory action of atrial natriuretic factor on canine glomerular afferent arterioles. Am J Physiol 255:F415–F420
47. Takagi M, Franco-Saenz R, Mulrow PJ (1988) Effect of atrial natriuretic peptide on renin release in a superfusion system of kidney slices and dispersed juxtaglomerular cells. Endocrinology 122:1437–1442
48. Hiruma M, Ikemoto F, Yamamoto K (1986) Rat atrial natriuretic factor stimulates renin release from renal cortical slices. Eur J Pharmacol 125:151–153
49. Kurtz A, Della Bruna R, Pfeilschifter J, Bauer C (1986c) Effect of synthetic atrial natriuretic peptide on rat renal juxtaglomerular cells. J Hypertens 4:S57–S60
50. Vidal MJ, Romero JC, Vanhoutte PM (1988) Endothelium-derived relaxing factor inhibits renin release. Eur J Pharmacol 149:401–402
51. Daniel TO, Ives HE (1989) Endothelial control of vascular function. News Physiol Sci 4:139–142
52. Fishman MC (1976) Membrane potential of juxtaglomerular cells. Nature 260:542–544
53. Kurtz A, Skott O, Chegini S, Penner R (1990) Lack of direct evidence for a functional role of voltage gated calcium channels in renal juxtaglomerular cells. Pflugers Arch 416:281–287

54. Aickin CC, Brading AF (1985) Advances in the understanding of transmembrane ionic gradients and permeabilities in smooth muscle obtained by using ion-selective microelectrodes. Experientia 41:879–887
55. Kurtz A, Penner R (1990) Effects of angiotensin II on intracellular calcium and electrical function of mouse renal juxtaglomerular cells. Kidney Int 38:S-51–S-54

Macula Densa Control of Renin Secretion

Josie P. Briggs, John N. Lorenz, Horst Weihprecht, and Jürgen Schnermann[1]

Summary. Macula densa (MD) controls on renin secretion have recently been studied by examining the renin secretory response of the isolated perfused rabbit juxtaglomerular apparatus (JGA). Single JGAs, consisting of a segment of distal tubule including the macula densa, with adherent glomerulus and short vascular fragments, are dissected from rabbit kidney, and the tubule is perfused. Renin secretion from this preparation shows an inverse dependency on NaCl concentration in the tubular lumen. When perfused with a low NaCl solution, renin secretion is inhibited by addition of NaCl, choline Cl, and RbCl, but not by addition of Na acetate or Na isethionate. Renin secretion is stimulated by addition of 10^{-6}M bumetanide to the tubular perfusate but not to the bathing solution. It is concluded that renin secretion is inversely related to the rate of tubular transport, and that the pattern of ion specificity is consistent with participation of the Na-K-2Cl co-transporter. Other studies examined possible stimulus-response coupling mechanisms. Renin secretion was found to be stimulated by the adenosine1 analog CHA (N^6-cyclohexyladenosine), an effect that was blocked by the specific adenosine 1 blocker, CPX(8-cyclopentyl-1,3-dipropylxanthine). The inhibitory effect of a high luminal NaCl solution at the MD was markedly blunted in the presence of the A1 blocker CPX, but CPX did not significantly affect renin secretion when luminal NaCl was low, suggesting that adenosine formation is dependent upon luminal NaCl concentration, and supporting the hypothesis that variation in the local levels of adenosine may be at least partially responsible for macula densa signal transmission.

Introduction

The terminal end of the thick ascending limb of Henle, the site of the macula densa (MD), is a position uniquely suited for monitoring flow dependent changes of NaCl

[1]The University of Michigan, Department of Internal Medicine, Division of Nephrology, 1150 W. Medical Center Drive, 1560 MSRBII, Ann Arbor, MI 48109-0676, USA

concentration. Along the proximal tubule, flow is not a major determinant of salt concentration. In more distal nephron segments, Na and Cl concentrations are largely determined by the actions of aldosterone and vasopressin. At the macula densa, however, NaCl concentration is primarily dictated by tubular flow rate. The transport properties of the thick ascending limb of Henle (TALH), and active NaCl transport by a water impermeable epithelium, result in the transformation of a flow signal into a change in salt concentration.

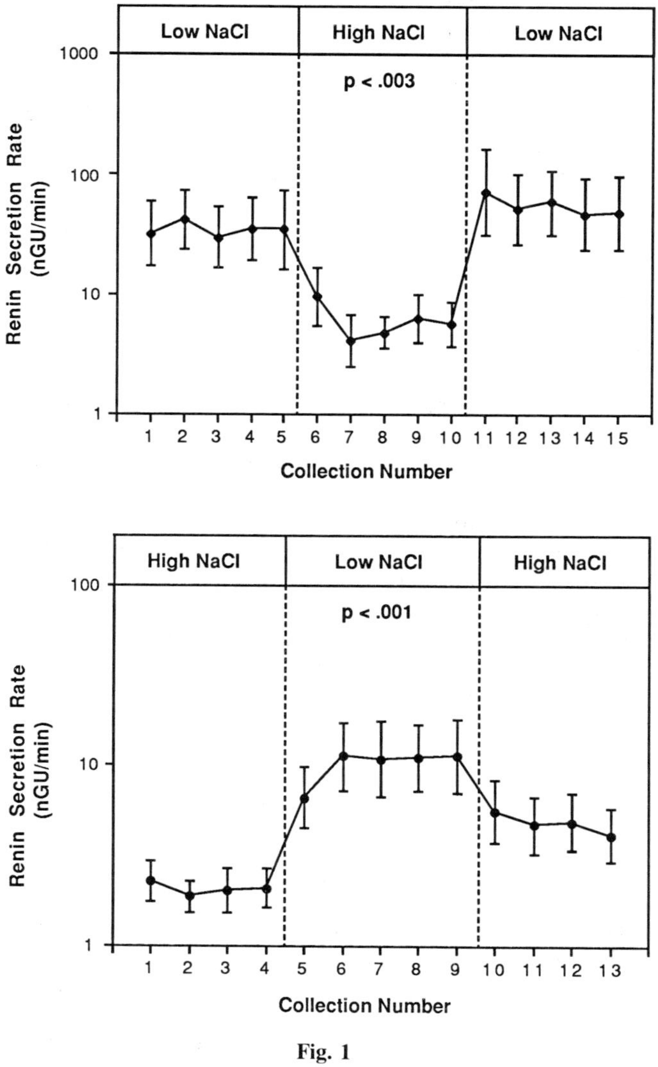

Fig. 1

An influence of tubular fluid composition on renin release was first proposed by Goormaghtigh [1]. In 1965 Vander summarized a substantial body of experimental evidence and concluded that a change in distal NaCl delivery induced inverse changes of renin secretion and that the input from the MD was the major control mechanism of renin secretion in states of salt depletion and excess [2]. Nevertheless, as judged from the continued controversy over existence and mechanisms of MD control of renin secretion, the experimental work in intact kidneys has remained remarkably inconclusive. Several problems have made limited progress in this area. First, the signal arriving at the MD often cannot be determined precisely, because the MD is located below the surface of the kidney. Secondly, renin secretion is also influenced by sympathetic tone, the baroreceptor mechanism [3], and the local levels of a number of hormones and autocoids [4]. Attempts to draw definitive conclusions from complex in vivo models, such as the non-filtering kidney, in which the MD influence is assumed to be eliminated, or the denervated, β-blocked, papaverine treated dog, in which sympathetic and baroreceptor influences are considered to be excluded [5,6], have been somewhat helpful, but in general these techniques have not been able to yield unequivocal answers. Finally, renin secreted from a single JGA cannot be sampled quantitatively in vivo, since it is secreted to a sizable extent into the renal interstitium. This limitation has prevented assessment of the response of MD secretion to single nephron perturbations in a manner comparable to that used for the evaluation of the tubuloglomerular feedback (TGF) response.

Two attempts have been made to evaluate the effect of changes in MD NaCl concentration at the single nephron level in vivo, but these studies have yielded contradictory results. Renin concentration was found to decrease in surface venules draining a group of oil-blocked nephrons in the cat, suggesting that a reduction in MD NaCl concentration inhibits renin release [7]. In contrast, tubular and postglomerular renin concentration varied inversely with changes in distal NaCl in micropuncture studies in the rat [8].

Isolated explants of juxtaglomerular cells have been a useful tool for in vitro evaluation of mechanisms of renin release [9,10] but this preparation has a disrupted JGA morphology and can therefore not be used for studying MD influences on renin secretion. Several laboratories have recently applied the isolated perfused tubule technique to studying various aspects of MD function [11–14]. Using this approach it has been possible, for the first time, to investigate MD control of renin secretion in the absence of baroreceptor and adrenergic inputs and during precise control of tubular fluid composition [14].

Evidence for MD Control of Renin Secretion

Effect of Changes in Luminal NaCl Concentration

Using the isolated perfused JGA it has been demonstrated that increasing NaCl concentration at the MD produces a suppression of renin secretion and that a reduction of NaCl concentration produces stimulation [14,15,16,17] (see Fig. 1). These results yield clear evidence for an inverse relationship between renin secretion and MD NaCl concentration. MD-dependent renin secretion is characterized by a rapid onset and offset following step changes in NaCl concentration and by reversibility of the induced changes [15,16]. Renin responses were independent of whether the tubule was perfused in an orthograde fashion from the TALH or in a retrograde fashion from the distal convoluted tubule [16]. Renin secretion was not altered when NaCl concentration was reduced from isotonicity to about 80 mM, but the full renin response was seen when NaCl concentrations were varied between 7 and 61 mM (Cl) and between 26 and 80 mM (Na)[17], that is, within the range that seems to be physiologically relevant. It is of note that this is the same concentration range in which the tubuloglomerular feedback response occurs.

These studies yield a quantitative estimate of the effect of MD NaCl concentration on renin secretion [16]. Assuming a linear relationship between the changes in NaCl concentration and renin release, the in vitro results predict that single JGA renin secretion increases by about 0.5 nGU/min per mM decrement of NaCl concentration. Using this approximation, one can estimate that plasma renin activity could increase approximately fivefold if NaCl concentration at the MD fell by 10 mM for ten minutes. Nonetheless, extrapolation from this in vitro system to the in vivo response must be made with caution. The assumption of a linear response of renin release over the concentration range studied may not be valid. Furthermore, in vitro, renin secretory responses are assessed in the absence of stabilizing feedback loops that may be important in vivo. For example, stimulation of renin secretion in vivo will increase angiotensin II levels and thereby depress steady-state renin secretion below that predicted for the prevailing MD NaCl concentration. Since renin is effectively removed in the in vitro preparation this negative feedback is eliminated. The TGF mechanism is another feedback system which would tend to minimize deviations in NaCl concentration at the MD and thereby dampen the signal for renin release.

NaCl Concentration vs NaCl Delivery

It has been an unresolved issue whether renin secretion responds to a reduction in NaCl concentration or in NaCl delivery (concentration times flow rate). When luminal NaCl load was reduced by 80% by decreasing perfusate flow at constant NaCl concentration, a small, approximately twofold increase in the rate of renin secretion was noted. In contrast, when NaCl load was reduced to a similar degree by decreasing perfusate NaCl concentration, renin secretion increased nearly eightfold [16]. These studies show clearly that, at least in the isolated perfused JGA, NaCl concentration is a more important determinant of renin release than NaCl delivery. The notion that NaCl load is of primary importance in MD-dependent renin secretion was derived from two observations. Stimulation of renin secretion by dietary Na restriction was associated with an increased distal NaCl concentration, but a reduced NaCl load [18], suggesting an inverse relationship between renin secretion and Na load, but not Na concentration. However, there is substantial evidence that NaCl measurements in the early distal tubule significantly overestimate NaCl concentrations at the MD when tubular flow rates are low, such as those observed in Na restricted animals [19,20]. It is therefore likely that NaCl at the level of the MD is in fact reduced during Na restriction. Another finding supporting load dependency of renin secretion was the observation that an osmotic diuresis produced by hypertonic mannitol infusions was associated with an inhibition of renin release, even though distal NaCl concentration was reduced [21–23]. A possible explanation is that the stimulatory signal exerted through the MD was overcome by other inputs. For example, the increase in plasma osmolality produced by mannitol may have suppressed renin release [24]. Studies with isolated superperfused glomeruli reveal marked sensitivity of renin release to the ambient osmolarity [25]. In contrast to the direct effects of osmolality on granular cells, stimulation of renin secretion by a reduction in luminal NaCl at the MD was also seen when perfusate osmolality was kept constant by the addition of mannitol [14]. Thus, changes in tubular fluid osmolality independent of NaCl variations do not seem to exert control over renin secretion. These findings attest to the specificity of compositional changes within the tubular compartment.

The Sensing Mechanism for MD-Mediated Renin Secretion

The Tubular Sensor

An important aspect of the use of the isolated JGA preparation is that it limits the possible sites of tubulo-vascular information transfer to cells present in the area of contact. Since only MD cells, and possibly a small number of surrounding TAL cells, are found in the area of contact, it is the cellular response of these cell types to luminal NaCl concentration which is probably the critical event in MD-regulated renin release.

It was suggested earlier that inhibition of MD Na transport is an early step in the stimulation of renin secretion [2,26]. This supposition was in part based on observations showing that increasing the delivery of NaCl to the MD prevented or reversed the stimulation of renin secretion produced by a fall in arterial pressure [26]. The subsequent finding that loop diuretics consistently stimulate renin secretion appeared to confirm transport dependency of MD-mediated renin secretion [4], but the in vivo effects of diuretics are complex, and alterations in the baroreceptor signal or in adrenergic input could also explain these effects. The first direct evidence for a MD mediated effect of furosemide on renin secretion came from experiments in which renin secretion from non-perfused afferent arterioles was measured; it was found to be lower when the MD segment was included in the dissected specimen, and higher in specimens which lacked a MD [27]. Addition of furosemide increased renin release in the presence of the MD, but not in its absence [27]. In the isolated perfused JGA preparation, luminal application of bumetanide in a concentration of 10^{-6} M stimulated renin secretion, while bath application had no effect [17]. Since bumetanide did not affect renin secretion when added to the bath it seems unlikely that it interacts directly with granular cells. In view of the low concentration required to observe this effect it seems likely that bumetanide interferes with the operation of the Na,K,2Cl-cotransporter and that the subsequent reduction in the rate of NaCl transport stimulates renin secretion. This proposal is consistent with the recent evidence in support of the presence of this transporter on MD cells [11,13,28].

Ion Specificity of Renin Secretory Responses

Renin secretion in intact animals has been shown to be suppressed by oral or intravenous administration of various Cl or Br salts, but not by Na salts including Na acetate [29,30]. An acute selective depletion of chloride by peritoneal dialysis increased plasma renin activity [31]. In addition, substitution of chloride by nitrate or thiocyanate in the perfusate of isolated kidneys has been shown to stimulate renin secretion [32]. In isolated perfused JGAs, ion selectivity has been examined by measuring the inhibitory effect of addition of various Na and Cl salts to a low NaCl perfusate. The inhibitory response was unchanged when most of the luminal Na was replaced by choline or rubidium. On the other hand, substituting chloride by isethionate or acetate virtually eliminated the response to increased Na concentration [17]. These results are similar to the pattern of ion specificity shown for TGF responses, and are compatible with the hypothesis that both mechanisms share a common sensing step. It has been outlined previously that the known binding affinities of the Na K 2Cl-cotransporter permit some predictions as to the efficacy of Na and Cl to affect MD-dependent processes. The expectation would be that changes in Cl concentration should have a more pronounced effect on renin secretion than changes in Na concentration, above a concentration of about 10 mM where Na binding sites are virtually saturated [33]. In summary, there is now good evidence in support of the hypothesis that the initiating signal for MD control of renin secretion is a change in NaCl transport rate, via a luminal Na K 2Cl-cotransporter whose physiological activity is determined by a change in luminal Cl concentration.

The Stimulus-Response Coupling Mechanism

Adenosine

In intact animals (rats or dogs) exogenous adenosine usually inhibits renin release [34–36]. Theophylline blocks the inhibitory effect of adenosine on renin secretion in dogs [37–40], and itself stimulates renin release [38]. Effects of adenosine analogs are generally dose dependent. At low concentrations, the adenosine1 analogs such as CHA (N^6-cyclohexyl adenosine) produce inhibition of release from intact kidneys [40,41], isolated cortical slices [42], and isolated perfused JGAs [43], but at higher concentrations these analogs may lose their specificity and stimulate renin secretion by interaction with adenosine 2 receptors [44].

In the isolated perfused JGA, addition of the adenosine1 analog CHA resulted in significant inhibition of renin release stimulated by low MD NaCl [43]. The selective adenosine$_1$-receptor blocker 8-cyclopentyl-1,3-dipropylxanthine (CPX) was noted to reverse the inhibiting effect of CHA [43]. Adenosine itself did not significantly inhibit renin secretion unless the adenosine deaminase inhibitor pentostatin (deoxycoformycin) was present in the bath (J. Briggs, H. Weihprecht, unpublished observations). These findings support the conclusion that receptors of the adenosine$_1$-subclass are present on renin-secreting cells at the glomerular vascular pole, and that their activation can initiate inhibition of renin secretion independent of changes in renal hemodynamics or sympathetic nerve activity.

Support for the hypothesis that transport-dependent alterations in local generation of adenosine serve as a paracrine mediator for renin release within the JGA comes from studies using agents which block adenosine receptors. Theophylline has been shown to stimulate renin secretion in isolated non-perfused arterioles that include a MD, but not in specimens lacking a MD [44]. Further evidence comes from experiments with perfused JGAs in which the MD signal was directly manipulated. The inhibitory effect of a high luminal NaCl solution at the MD was markedly blunted in the presence of the A1 blocker CPX, but CPX did not significantly affect renin secretion when luminal NaCl was low, suggesting that adenosine formation is dependent upon luminal NaCl concentration [43].

Prostaglandins

Alterations in renal prostaglandins are known to alter renin secretory responses to a variety of stimuli. For example, cyclooxygenase inhibition has been shown to reduce the stimulation of renin release by salt depletion [4], converting enzyme inhibitors [4], and adrenalectomy [45]. Infusion of arachidonic acid stimulates renin release from intact animals and isolated perfused kidneys; in most preparations administration of PGE_2 or PGI_2 is also stimulatory [4]. Indirect evidence supports PG participation in MD mediated effects on renin secretion. The acute stimulation of renin release produced by furosemide [4,46] and theophylline [38] is blunted by administration of indomethacin. Stimulation of renin secretion by supra-aortic constriction in denervated kidney of dogs treated with papaverine, a model of MD responses, is also blocked by indomethacin and meclofenamate [47].

Histochemical studies have provided evidence that cyclo-oxygenase, although abundant in renal endothelial cells, is low or absent in the MD [48]. This finding suggests that it is unlikely that a cyclo-oxygenase metabolite functions as a paracrine mediator transmitting a signal from the macula densa to the granular cell. However, cyclo-oxygenase products, particularly PGE_2 and PGI_2, appear to be produced by mesangial cells and isolated glomeruli [49,50]; a local autacoid or paracrine function of PGs within the JGA is possible. In cultured mesangial cells, medium Cl concentration has been shown to modify PGE_2 production, with reductions in Cl stimulating the formation of the measured prostaglandin [51].

Renin Secretion and Tubuloglomerular Feedback

Changes in NaCl concentration in the tubular fluid in the region of the MD exert two effects on cells of the afferent arteriole. They induce direct changes of the tone of contractile smooth muscle cells (the tubuloglomerular feedback response) and they inversely affect renin secretion from granular cells. Both responses have a number of similarities and it is possible that they are mediated through the same extracellular and intracellular mediators. One aspect of the MD-mediated control mechanisms which deserves some consideration is that they have the potential of influencing each other. Angiotensin has been shown to markedly enhance the contractile response of afferent arterioles to the MD signal [52,53]. An increase in NaCl at the MD will lead to an increase in afferent tone, which will tend to lower distal NaCl through its effect on GFR and proximal absorption. But since this compensation is likely to be incomplete, there will be a decrease in renin secretion simultaneously. The resulting change in plasma angiotensin concentration will decrease the sensitivity of the vascular response to NaCl and attenuate the dependency of GFR on the MD signal. These changes will relax control of NaCl at the MD and permit salt excretion to rise. The opposite sequence of events will occur when MD NaCl decreases.

This dual effect of MD NaCl may contribute to the adjustments in TGF responsiveness which are seen during alterations in extracellular volume. The reduction in TGF sensitivity, caused by volume expansion, is to a large extent explicable by reductions in angiotensin levels [52], suggesting that depression of renin secretion plays an important role in the adjustment of GFR during volume expansion, is predicted to uncouple GFR from MD control, because the simultaneous inhibition of renin secretion will, after a time, reduce TGF sensitivity. Since the resulting increase in GFR will further inhibit renin secretion, a positive feedback cycle is initiated which will allow filtrate formation to become independent of MD control. However, the fall in angiotensin levels will induce an increasing release of renin secretion from the inhibiting effects of angiotensin. Thus, resulting from a balance of these interconnected feedback loops, a new steady-state in salt excretion and in renin secretion will occur.

Acknowledgments. L.N. Lorenz is the recipient of an Individual National Research Service Award, DK-08411. H. Weihprecht is supported by a Fellowship from the Michigan Affiliate of the American Heart Association. Work performed in this laboratory is funded by the National Institutes of Health Grants DK-37448, DK-39255, and DK40042.

References

1. Goormaghtigh N (1939) Une glande endocrine dans la paroi des arterioles renales. Bruxelles-Med 19:1541–1549
2. Vander AJ (1967) Control of renin release. Physiol Rev 47:359–382
3. Bock HA, Hermle M, Fiallo A, Osgood RW, Fried TA (1990) Measurement of renin secretion in single perfused rabbit glomeruli. Am J Physiol 258:F1460–F1465
4. Keeton TK, Campbell WB (1980) The pharmacologic alteration of renin release. Pharmacol Rev 32:81–227
5. Blaine EH, Davis JO, Witty RT (1970) Renin release after hemorrhage and after suprarenal aortic constriction in dogs without sodium delivery to the macula densa. Circ Res 27:1081–1089
6. Witty RT, Davis JO, Johnson JA, Prewitt RL (1971) Effects of papaverine and hemorrhage on renin secretion in the non-filtering kidney. Am J Physiol 221:1666–1671
7. Morgan T, Gillies A (1977) Factors controlling the release of renin. A micropuncture study in the cat. Pflügers Arch 368:13–18
8. Leyssac PP (1986) Changes in single nephron renin release are mediated by tubular fluid flow rate. Kidney Int 30:332–339
9. Kurtz A (1989) Cellular control of renin secretion. Rev Physiol Biochem Pharmacol 113: 1–40
10. Carey RM, Geary KM, Hunt MK, Ramos SP, Forbes MS, Inagami T, Peach MJ, Leong DA (1990) Identification of individual renocortical cells that secrete renin. Am J Physiol 258:F649–F659
11. Bell PD, Lapointe JY, Cardinal J (1989) Direct measurement of basolateral potentials from cells of the macula densa. Am J Physiol 257:F463–F468
12. Kirk KL, Bell PD, Barfuss D, Ribadeneira M (1985) Direct visualization of the isolated and perfused macula densa. Am J Physiol 248:F890–F894
13. Schlatter E, Salomonsson M, Persson AEG, Greger R (1989) Macula densa cells sense luminal NaCl concentration via furosemide sensitive $Na^{+}2Cl^{-}K^{+}$ cotransport. Pflügers Arch 414:286–290

14. Skøtt O, Briggs JP (1988) A method for superfusion of the isolated perfused tubule. Kidney Int 33:1009–1012
15. Skøtt O, Briggs JP (1987) Direct demonstration of macula densa-mediated renin secretion. Science 237:1618–1620
16. Lorenz JN, Weihprecht H, Schnermann J, Skøtt O, Briggs JP (to be published) Characterization of the macula densa stimulus for renin secretion. Am J Physiol
17. Lorenz JN, Weihprecht H, Schnermann J, Skøtt O, Briggs JP (to be published) Renin release from the isolated juxtaglomerular apparatus depends on macula densa chloride transport. Am J Physiol
18. Churchill PC, Churchill MC, McDonald FD (1978) Renin secretion and distal tubule Na+ in rats. Am J Physiol 235:F611–F616
19. Schnermann J, Schubert G, Briggs JP (1982) In situ studies of the distal convoluted tubule in the rat. I. Evidence for NaCl secetion. Am J Physiol 243:F160–F166
20. Baines AD, Basmadjian D, Wang BC (1979) Computer simulation of flow-dependent absorption in microperfused short Henle's loop of rats. Biophys J 27:21–38
21. Churchill PC, Churchill MC, McDonald FD (1979) Effects of saline and mannitol on renin and distal tubule Na in rats. Circ Res 45:786–792
22. Di Bona GF (1971) Effect of mannitol diuresis and uretal occlusion on distal tubular reabsorption. Am J Physiol 221:511–514
23. Vander AJ (1968) Renin secretion during mannitol diuresis and ureteral occlusion. Proc Soc Exp Biol Med 128:518–520
24. Skøtt O (1988) Do osmotic forces play a role in renin secretion? Am J Physiol 255:F1–F10
25. Frederiksen O, Leyssac PP, Skinner SL (1975) Sensitive osmometer function of juxtaglomerular cells in vitro. J Physiol 252:669–679
26. Vander AJ, Miller R (1964) Control of renin secretion in the anaesthetized dog. Am J Physiol 207:537–546
27. Itoh S Carretero OA (1985) Role of the macula densa in renin release. Hypertension 7 (Suppl. 1):49–54
28. Gonzales E, Salomonsson M, Müller-Suur C, Persson AEG (1988) Measurements of macula densa cell volume changes in isolated and perfused rabbit cortical thick ascending limb. I. Isosmotic and anisosmotic cell volume changes. Acta Physiol Scand 133: 149–157
29. Kirchner KA, Kotchen TA, Galla JH, Luke RG (1978) Importance of chloride for acute inhibition of renin by sodium chloride. Am J Physiol 235:F444–F450
30. Kotchen TA, Welch WJ, Ott CE (1984) The renal tubular signal for renin release. J Hypertension 2(suppl 1):35–42
31. Abboud HE, Luke RG, Galla JH, Kotchen TA (1979) Stimulation of renin by acute selective chloride depletion in the rat. Circ Res 44:815–821
32. Rostand SG, Work J, Luke RG (1985) Effect of reduced chloride reabsorption on renin release in the isolated rat kidney. Pflugers Arch 405:46–51
33. Greger R (1985) Ion transport mechanisms in thick ascending limb of Henle's loop of mammalian nephron. Physiol Rev 65:760–797
34. Arend LJ, Haramati A, Thompson CL, Spielman WS (1984) Adenosine-induced decreases in renin release: dissociation from hemodynamic effects. Am J Physiol 247:F447–F452
35. Osswald H, Schmitz H-J, Heidenreich O (1975) Adenosine response of the rat kidney after saline loading, sodium restriction and hemorrhagia. Pflugers Arch 357:323–333
36. Tagawa A, Vander AJ (1970) Effects of adenosine compounds on renal function and renin secretion in dogs. Circ Res 26:327–338
37. Johns EJ, Singer B (1973) Effect of propranolol and theophylline on renin release caused by furosemide in the cat. Eur J Pharmacol 23:67–73
38. Oliw E, Anggard E, Fredholm BB (1977) Effect of indomethacin on the renal actions of theophylline. Eur J Pharmacol 43:9–16

39. Spielman WS (1984) Antagonistic effect of theophylline on the adenosine-induced decrease in renin release. Am J Physiol 247:F246–F251
40. Churchill PC, Bidani AK (1990) Adenosine and Renal Function. In: Adenosine and Adenosine Receptors, Williams M (ed), Humana, Clifton, pp 335–380
41. Cook CB, Churchill PC (1984) Effects of renal denervation on the renal responses of anesthetized rats to cyclohexyladenosine. Can J Physiol Pharmacol 62:934–938
42. Churchill PC, Churchill MC (1985) A_1 and A_2 adenosine receptor activation inhibits and stimulates renin secretion of rat renal cortical slices. J Pharmacol Exp Ther 232:589–594
43. Weihprecht H, Lorenz JN, Schnermann J, Skøtt O, Briggs JP (1990) Effect of adenosine$_1$-receptor blockade on renin release from rabbit isolated perfused juxtaglomerular apparatus. J Clin Invest apparatus. J Clin Invest 85:1622–1628
44. Itoh S, Carretero OA, Murray RD (1985) Possible role of adenosine in the macula densa mechanism of renin release in rabbits. J Clin Invest 76:1412–1417
45. Meyer DK, Benzing A (1979) Studies on the inhibitory effect of indomethacin and meclofenamate on the adrenalectomy-induced increase in plasma renin concentration. Naunyn Schmiedebergs Arch Pharmacol 309:25–27
46. Bailie MD, Crosslan K, Hook JB (1976) Natriuretic effect of furosemide after inhibition of prostaglandin synthetase. J Pharmacol Exp Ther 199:459–476
47. Olson RD, Skoglund ML, Nies AS, Gerber JG (1980) Prostaglandins mediate the macula densa stimulated renin release. Adv Prostaglandin Thromboxane Res 7:1135–1137
48. Smith WL, Bell YG (1978) Immunohistochemical localization of the prostaglandin-forming cyclooxygenase in renal cortex. Am J Physiol 235:F451–F457
49. Schlöndorff D, Ardaillou R (1986) Prostaglandins and other arachidonic acid metabolites in the kidney. Kidney Int 29:108–119
50. Mene P, Simonson MS, Dunn, MJ (1989) Physiology of the mesangial cell. Physiol Rev 69:1347–1424
51. Okuda T, Kojima I, Ogata E, Kurokawa K (1989) Ambient Cl^- ions modify rat mesangial cell contraction by modulating cell inositol trisphosphate and Ca^{2+} via enhanced prostaglandin E_2. J Clin Invest 84:1866–1872
52. Schnermann J, Briggs JP (to be published) Restoration of tubuloglomerular feedback in volume expanded rats by angiotensin II. Am J Physiol
53. Mitchell K, Navar LG (1988) Enhanced tubuloglomerular feedback during peritubular perfusions of angiotensins I and II. Am J Physiol 255:F383–F390

Macula Densa Control of Renin Secretion and Proximal Tubular Pressure

Paul P. Leyssac[1]

Summary. Early studies suggested that the proximal tubular pressure was regulated by a negative feedback mechanism operating via the juxtaglomerular (JG) apparatus, involving changes in renin secretion. Subsequent and recent studies have confirmed this hypothesis. The tubuloglomerular feedback (TGF) response oscillates with a frequency of about 30 mHz, and is sensitive to changes in late proximal flow of less than 3 $nl.min^{-1}$. It is specifically abolished by loop diuretics. Micropuncture studies have shown that single nephron renin release is increased when Henle loop flow is decreased and conversely, that single nephron renin release is decreased when Henle loop flow is increased. Studies on isolated JG-apparatuses have shown that this is due to the flow-dependent changes in luminal sodium chloride concentration at the level of the macula densa (M.D.). Thus, both the TGF-mediated afferent vasoconstriction and the M.D.-mediated renin secretion share the same luminal signal. The intracellular (i.c.) signal is probably also the same, since an increase in i.c. calcium causes vasoconstriction and inhibition of renin release from the JG cells. Both responses may therefore be considered as part of the TGF-mechanism.

Introduction

Present knowledge of glomerular and tubular pressures and flow rates through the different nephron segments indicates that the flow resistance across the glomerular membrane is 30–40 times less than the total resistance downstream from the proximal tubule. One could therefore predict that a primary change in the filtration pressure (P_{UF}) initially results in a nearly parallel increase in proximal tubular pressure (P_{prox}), thus leaving glomerular filtration rate (GFR) largely unchanged. However, the proximal hydrostatic pressure is very well regulated by tubuloglomerular feed-

[1]Institute of Experimental Medicine, University of Copenhagen, DK-2200 Copenhagen, Denmark

back mechanisms, and therefore rapidly returns to its control value [1]. In the steady state after such a change, at least after a moderate change of a few (e.g., 5) mm Hg, proximal intratubular pressure is always equal to its control value.

We have tested the concept that an increase in filtration pressure does in fact result in a parallel increase in proximal pressure, and that this pressure is regulated back to its stable steady state level by the TGF mechanism. We have also tested the postulate that the renin-angiotensin system (RAS) is involved in this regulation, and we conclude that it does participate, mainly by its effect on the efferent arteriolar resistance (R_e).

Results and Discussion

My first attempt dates back to 1969 [2], when tubular pressures were measured by the old-fashioned Landis technique, which only gives point-measurements. This is shown in Fig. 1, where pressure is followed as a function of time after an intravenous infusion of 2.5 ml of Ringer solution (equal to 1% of body weight), as shown by closed squares, or of rat plasma (circles), which gave the same plasma volume expan-

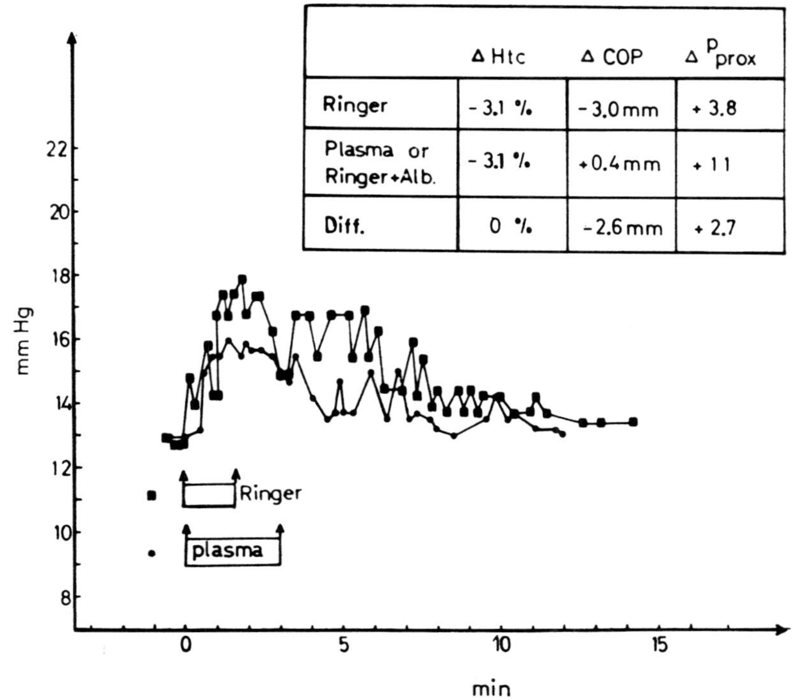

	Δ Htc	Δ COP	Δ P_{prox}
Ringer	- 3.1 %	- 3.0 mm	+ 3.8
Plasma or Ringer+Alb.	- 3.1 %	+0.4 mm	+ 11
Diff.	0 %	- 2.6 mm	+ 2.7

Fig. 1. Changes in proximal intratubular pressure following extracellular volume expansion with 2.5 ml of Ringers and of rat plasma, respectively. Htc, hematocrit; COP, oncotic pressure (mm Hg); P_{prox}, proximal intratubular pressure (mm Hg)

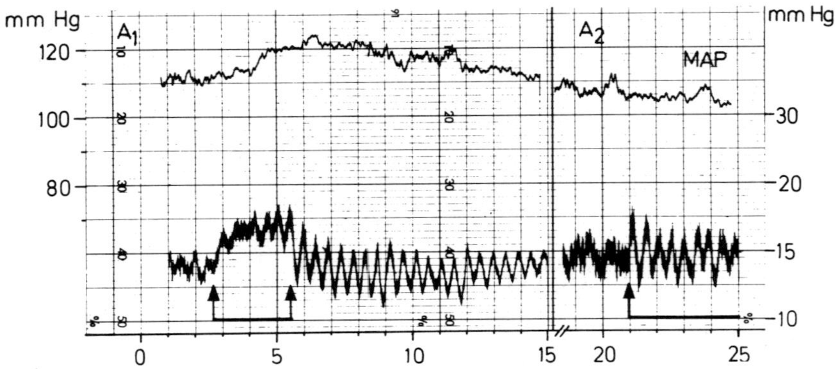

Fig. 2. Mean arterial pressure (*MAP*) and proximal tubular pressure recordings. **a_1** 2.5 ml of isotonic saline was given *between the arrows*. **a_2** After stabilization of the proximal pressure a micropertusion pipette was impaled into the last proximal convolution of the same nephron while leaving the pressure pipette in situ. The pump was started at 5 nl·min^{-1} *at the arrow*. (From [3] with permission)

sion, as seen from the change in hematocrit. The proximal tubular pressure increased and then returned to its control value. The difference in proximal peak pressure between Ringer and plasma equals the difference in filtration pressure caused by the drop in plasma oncotic pressure after Ringer infusion. It could therefore be concluded that the initial change in proximal tubular pressure quantitatively paralleled the change in filtration pressure. Now, when we look back on these recordings, it is possible to distinguish an oscillating character of the response, but this was not recognized until measurements could be made with the servo-nulling system for pressure recordings, as shown in Fig 2 a_1. The decrease in oncotic pressure following infusion of 2.5 ml of saline results in an increase in filtration pressure and thereby in the initial increase in proximal tubular pressure, which then begins to oscillate with a regular rhythm of 2 cycles per minute (30 mHz) while it returns to control pressure.

It was intuitively apparent that this oscillatory response looked like a physiological response and had the appearance of a high-gain negative feedback mechanism with a certain delay. Then, when the same nephron was microperfused into the last proximal convolution (Fig. 2 a_2), the same oscillation appeared with a similar amplitude, indicating that this response could be elicited in the single individual nephron.

This rhythmic response is extremely sensitive to changes in late proximal flow rate. A difference of less than 3 nl/min causes a significant change in the amplitude [4].

The individual character of the oscillatory response is also apparent from the observation that neighboring nephrons usually oscillate in different phase [4]. However, this is not always so. Holstein-Rathlou has shown that nephrons originating from the same interlobular artery may interact so that they become phase-locked, i.e., synchronized, and so that a change in Henle loop flow in one nephron also results in a response in its neighbor [5].

Further evidence that these oscillations represent a TGF-mediated response transmitted by the macula densa were obtained from experiments with loop diuretics. Figure 3 shows the effect of late proximal microperfusion with furosemide on the

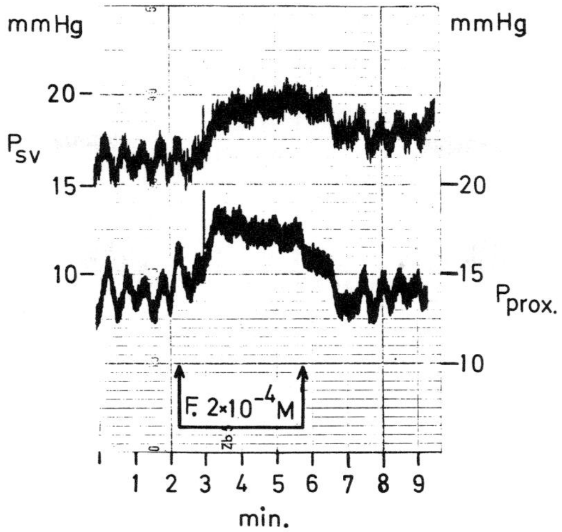

Fig. 3. Simultaneous recordings of pressures in the proximal tubule (P_{prox}) and in the star vessel of the same nephron (P_{SV}). Furosemide (*F.*) was microperfused into the last proximal convolution at 7.1 nl·min^{-1} *between the arrows*. (From [4] with permission)

proximal tubular and star vessel pressures. The oscillations disappear, and the increase in pressure indicates that the nephron is no longer able to regulate its pressure, probably due to the afferent arteriolar vasodilation, as suggested also by the increase in efferent arteriolar pressure. This effect is specific for loop diuretics, since it is not seen after microperfusion with acetazolamide or amiloride [6].

Thus, it seems safe to conclude that the pressure oscillations reflect a TGF response transmitted by the reabsorptive function of the macula densa.

If this oscillatory phenomenon was simply the result of the operation of the TGF system, it should be possible to design a dynamic mathematical model by combining previous steady state models of all the individual steps. Holstein-Rathlou elegantly solved this task, and with this first dynamic model of the nephron we could now follow the changes in all parameter values with time, in response to a change in one of them, e.g., in the Henle loop flow rate [7].

The first version of the model consisted of a glomerular model, a tubular model, and a model of the afferent arteriolar feedback. Figure 4 shows various model simulations of effects after changes in Henle loop flow compared with direct experimental recordings of the same changes. It is seen how well the model simulates the in vivo responses, both regarding frequency and amplitude, and that the mean proximal free flow pressure is stabilized by the feedback.

However, there are significant differences, which indicate that the model is incomplete in this version. Firstly, increasing Henle loop flow, e.g., by i.v. isotonic saline infusion causes renal blood flow (RBF) to increase, whereas the model predicts that RBF is depressed. Secondly, the proximal tubular pressure is more accurately regulated in vivo than in the model simulations, as seen in Fig. 4. Thus, something is missing in the model. This could be the renin-angiotensin system.

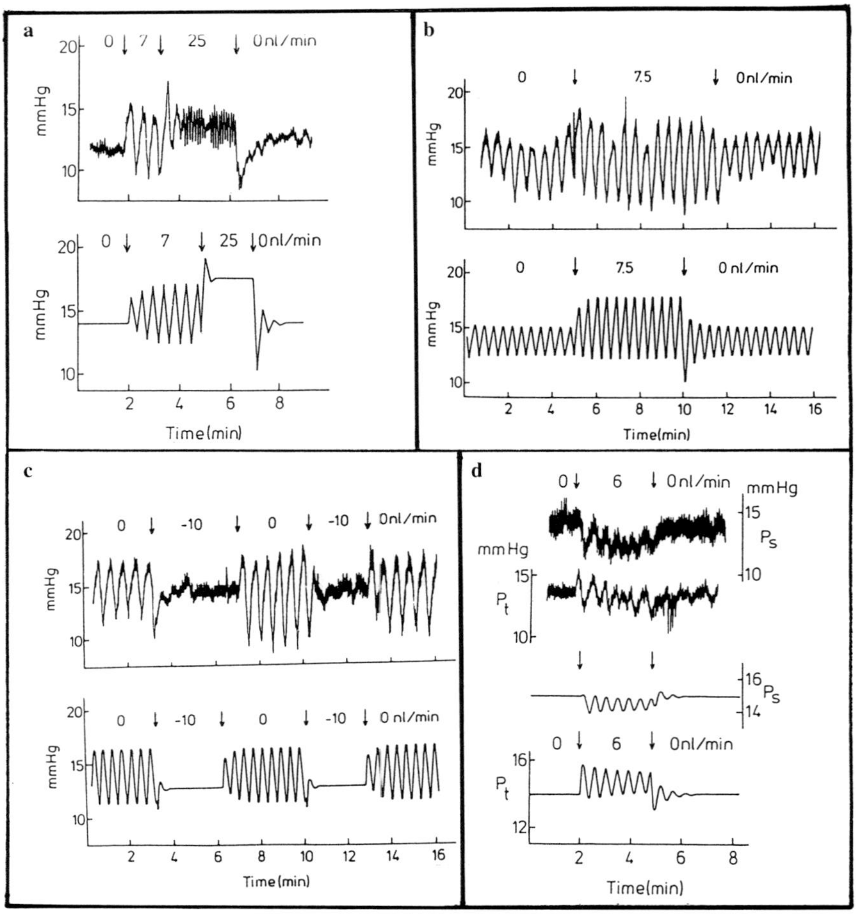

Fig. 4a-d. Effects of changing late proximal flow rate by microperfusion/suction. *Upper traces* experimental recordings of proximal intratubular pressures (**a**,**b**,**c**) and star vessel pressure (P_s) (**d**). *Lower traces* corresponding model simulations P_t. (From [7] with permission)

Since 1964 I have hypothesized that the renin-angiotensin system is directly involved in the control of tubular pressure and flow by the effects of angiotensin-II on the efferent arteriole and on proximal tubular reabsorption [8]. For this regulation it was postulated that macula densa-mediated renin release is depressed by an increase in proximal pressure and Henle loop flow.

When a sufficiently sensitive radio-immunoassay (RIA) had been developed, we tested this hypothesis directly in vivo in two series of microperfusion experiments.

In one series, early proximal tubular fluid was collected before and after changing late proximal microperfusion rate. Tubular fluid renin concentration was measured by RIA, corrected for water reabsorption, and normalized with respect to the systemic plasma renin concentration. Increasing the late proximal flow rate from 12 to

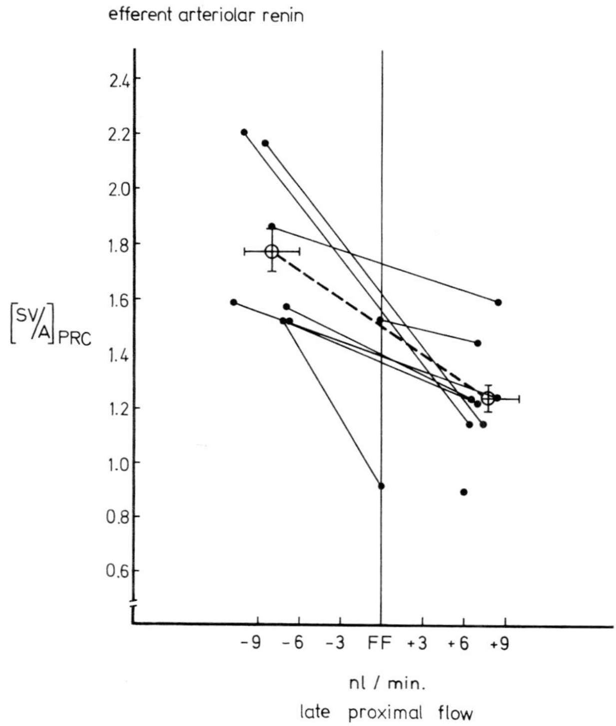

Fig. 5. Efferent arteriolar (*SV*) plasma renin concentration (*PRC*) versus changes in late proximal fluid flow. (From [9] with permission)

18 nl/min reduced tubular fluid renin concentration, while reducing the flow from 12 to 6 nl/min caused an increase in concentration [9]. In the other series, in order to ascertain that these changes in ultrafiltrate renin concentration represented changes in renin release rather than changes in glomerular membrane permeability to renin, blood was also collected at the end of the efferent arteriole, from the so-called star vessel [9].

The results are shown in Fig. 5, in which star vessel plasma renin concentration is normalized with respect to the systemic plasma renin concentration (PRC). Again, a reduction in late proximal flow caused an increase, while an increase in flow caused a decrease, in efferent arteriolar PRC. We conclude that an increase in Henle loop flow depresses macula densa-mediated renin release, and, conversely, that a decrease in Henle loop flow stimulates macula densa-mediated renin release. These results are in perfect agreement with those subsequently obtained by Skøtt and Briggs in their elegant in vitro studies with isolated, microperfused, and superfused juxtaglomerular apparatuses [10].

Thus, within recent years it has been firmly established that not only afferent arteriolar TGF, but also single nephron renin release responds to flow-dependent changes in sodium chloride concentration at the level of the macula densa.

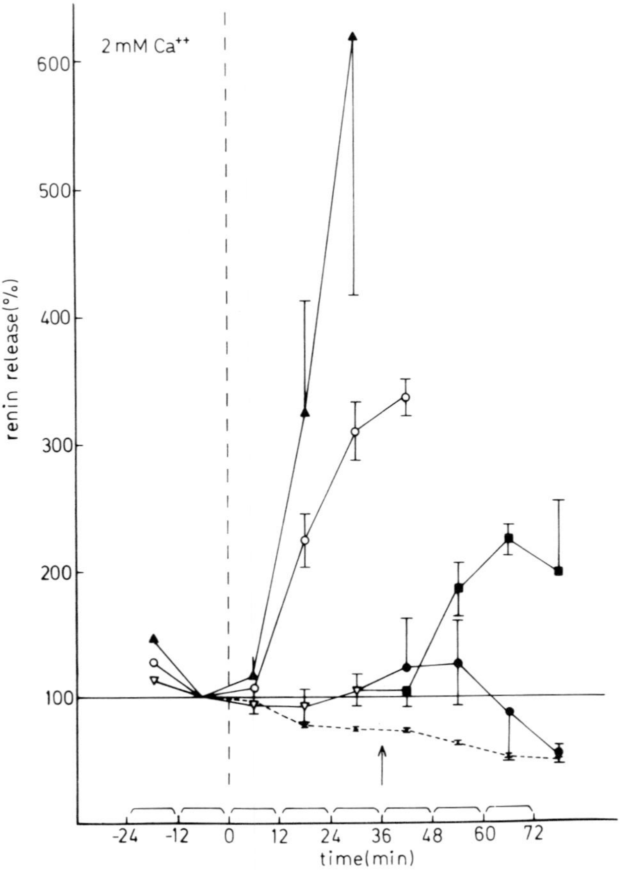

Fig. 6. Changes in renin release from isolated superfused glomeruli. Effect of changing superfusate calcium in the presence or absence of the calcium ionophore A_{23187}. In the control period superfusate was bicarbonate-Ringer containing 2 mM calcium. At time zero superfusate composition was changed: to Ca-free Ringer with A_{23187} (*open triangles*) and subsequently back to Ca-free Ringer without A_{23187} (*closed squares*) or back to control Ringer (*closed circles*); or to Ca-free Ringer containing 0.5 mM EGTA without A_{23187} (*open circles*) to be compared with Ca-free Ringer with A_{23187} (*closed triangles*). The *dashed line* indicates basal renin release with time in control Ringer. Means $\pm$ SEM

These two responses from the afferent arteriole therefore share the same luminal signal. As for the intracellular signal in the afferent arteriole there is also an intriguing parallelism between the signal leading to vasoconstriction and the inhibition of renin release. The arterioles constrict when intracellular calcium increases. But much to our surprise we found 13 years ago that renin release was inhibited when calcium was increased [11]. Figure 6 shows these old data from isolated, superfused rat glomeruli. The data indicate that lowering intracellular calcium concentration stimulates renin release. This finding has been confirmed and extended by my collaborators Lars Baumbach and Ole Skøtt and by many others, and suggests that intracellular calcium may serve as a common trigger for the afferent vasoconstriction and the inhibition of renin release. The demonstration by Kurtz and Penner [12] that intracellular calcium concentration in the JG cells also oscillates with a frequency similar to that of the pressure, and the observation by Skøtt [13] that renin is released in pulses, fits together, and opens the possibility that a stimulus to renin release from the individual nephron may vary as a function of the amplitude of the pressure oscillation, in spite of a stable mean pressure and flow to the macula densa.

Viewed together, I think that it would be reasonable to consider both responses as part of the TGF mechanism. Both responses cooperate in changing glomerular capillary pressure and in counteracting any acute primary change in the filtration pressure and/or in the Henle loop flow rate, since an increase in Henle loop flow causes afferent vasoconstriction, and the accompanying decrease in renin release and local angiotensin concentration will cause relaxation mainly of the efferent arteriole, both of which will reduce glomerular capillary pressure.

References

1. Leyssac PP, Holstein-Rathlou N-H (1988) Dynamics of TGF mediated regulation of proximal tubular pressure. Role of the renin system. In: Persson AEG, Boberg U (eds) The juxtaglomerular apparatus, Fernström Foundation Series vol 11. Elsevier Scientific, Amsterdam, pp 237–247
2. Leyssac PP (1969) New aspects of the mechanisms of renal sodium excretion. Proc R Soc Med 62:1111–1116
3. Leyssac PP, Baumbach L (1983) An oscillating intratubular pressure response to alterations in Henle loop flow in the rat kidney. Acta Physiol Scand 117:415–419
4. Leyssac PP (1986) Further studies on oscillating tubulo-glomerular feedback responses in the rat kidney. Acta Physiol Scand 126:271–277
5. Holstein-Rathlou N-H (1987) Synchronization of proximal intratubular pressure oscillations: evidence for interaction between nephrons. Pflugers Arch 408:438–443
6. Leyssac PP, Holstein-Rathlou N-H (1986) Effects of various transport inhibitors on oscillating TGF pressure responses in the rat. Pflugers Arch 407:285–291
7. Holstein-Rathlou N-H, Leyssac PP (1987) Oscillations in the proximal intratubular pressure: a mathematical model. Am J Physiol 252:F560–F572
8. Leyssac PP (1964) The effect of partial clamping of the renal artery on pressures in the proximal and distal tubules and peritubular capillaries of the rat kidney. Acta Physiol Scand 62:449–456
9. Leyssac PP (1986) Changes in single nephron renin release are mediated by tubular fluid flow rate. Kidney Int 30:332–339
10. Skøtt O, Briggs JP (1987) Direct demonstration of macula densa-mediated renin secretion. Science 237:1618–1620
11. Baumbach L, Leyssac PP (1977) Studies on the mechanism of renin release from isolated superfused rat glomeruli: effects of calcium, calcium ionophore and lanthanum. J Physiol 273:745–764
12. Kurtz A, Penner R (1989) Angiotensin II induces oscillations of intracellular calcium and blocks anomalous inward rectifying potassium current in mouse renal juxtaglomerular cells. Proc Natl Acad Sci USA 86:3423–3427
13. Skøtt O (1986) Episodic release of renin from single isolated superfused rat afferent arterioles. Pflügers Arch 407:41–45

The Afferent Arteriole in Tubuloglomerular Feedback and Autoregulation

LEON C. MOORE[1] and DANIEL CASELLAS[2]

Introduction

The preglomerular vasculature of the kidney has long been known to be the principal site of autoregulatory adjustments in vascular resistance and the major effector site of the tubuloglomerular feedback (TGF) mechanism [1]. This paper will review some recent studies from our laboratories that have provided new evidence about the function of the renal preglomerular microvasculature and, in particular, the role of the afferent arteriole in autoregulation and TGF [2,3]. These results have helped to resolve several important issues regarding the regulation of renal hemodynamics.

Role of the Afferent Arteriole in Autoregulation

Although the afferent arteriole (AA), as a whole, is known to be an important site of nephron blood flow and filtration regulation [1,4–6], it has been proposed that the terminal, juxtaglomerular segment of the AA (jAA) is incapable of active vasoconstriction, owing to the low myosin content of the renin-positive granulated cells in this segment [7] and the lack of significant autoregulatory vasoconstriction in the terminal AA found in rat hydronephrotic kidneys [6]. Further, the descending myogenic hypothesis forwarded by Øien and Aukland [8] suggests that the autoregulatory responses of the terminal AA should only be manifested near the limits of the autoregulatory pressure range, after saturation of the autoregulatory responses of all upstream vascular segments.

We have recently succeeded in obtaining high resolution video images of the entire afferent arteriole and juxtaglomerular apparatus of blood-perfused juxtamedullary

[1]Department of Physiology and Biophysics, State University of New York, Stony Brook, NY 11794, USA
[2]Groupe Rein et Hypertension, St. Charles Hospital, Montpellier, France

(JM) nephrons in vitro. This has provided us with the ability to specifically examine the hemodynamic function of the juxtaglomerular and mid-afferent (mAA) segments of the afferent arteriole. The studies were conducted in vitro in the blood-perfused, JM nephron preparation [9]. This preparation is unique in that all preglomerular vascular segments and the macula densa (MD) are visible. The nephrons in this preparation retain basic vascular, glomerular, and tubular function [2–5,9,10]. Detailed descriptions of the in vitro perfused JM nephron preparation are available elsewhere [2,9,10]. Briefly, a rat kidney is removed and extensively dissected to expose an area of juxtamedullary cortex that lies under the pelvic mucosa. The major arteries supplying the rest of the kidney are ligated. During dissection, the kidney is perfused with a gassed Krebs-bicarbonate-Ringer (KBR) solution containing 4% albumin. During measurements, the kidney is perfused with a blood solution prepared from fresh rat blood. The red cells are separated, washed, and resuspended in KBR-6%-albumin solution (pH 7.4) to a hematocrit of 30%. The preparation is superfused with a warm (37°C) KBR solution with 1% albumin. In this region, AA length varies from around 200 to 1400 μm. Where possible, responses were measured at two sites in each AA, the terminal, juxtaglomerular segment (jAA) consisting of the final approximately 50 μm of the AA, and a mid-afferent site (mAA) located around 130–150 μm upstream from the vascular pole. In most JM nephrons, the jAA lumen also narrows by about 33% and the vessel wall thickens as it approaches the vascular pole. These jAA segments have been shown to contain renin [11].

Autoregulatory Responses of the AA

Figure 1 illustrates a typical autoregulatory response in the jAA segment of a JM AA, while Fig. 2 summarizes the results obtained for the mAA and the jAA. Significant perfusion-pressure-dependent vasoconstriction was found in both segments. In response to increasing perfusion pressure from 60 to 140 mmHg, mAA luminal diameter decreased by 23% $\pm$ 4%, while jAA diameter decreased by 40% $\pm$ 4%. In contrast, the diameter of the efferent arteriole was unaffected by perfusion pressure. The autoregulatory responses were calcium-dependent, as superperfusion with 1 μM nimodipine resulted in pressure-dependent dilation rather than constriction. These results are consistent with earlier measurements by others in mid afferent segments and with the results of micropressure measurements in JM vessels [4–6]. However, they extend previous findings by clearly demonstrating that the terminal, renin-containing segment of the AA is also capable of strong autoregulatory adjustments in resistance. These results also contrast sharply with studies of isolated rabbit AA in vitro, where only weak autoregulatory vasoconstriction was found in the distal region [12].

Another noteworthy feature of the autoregulatory responses of the distal AA and jAA is that they were distributed approximately uniformly over the pressure range of 60–140 mmHg, which exceeds the autoregulatory range in rat JM nephrons [13]. The monotonic, almost linear responses are basically inconsistent with the descending myogenic hypothesis (DMH) of renal blood flow autoregulation [8]. The DMH predicts little or no autoregulatory compensation by the distal AA at arterial pressures around the normotensive level, where all autoregulatory compensation is predicted to occur in the proximal preglomerular vascular segments. In contrast, our results show

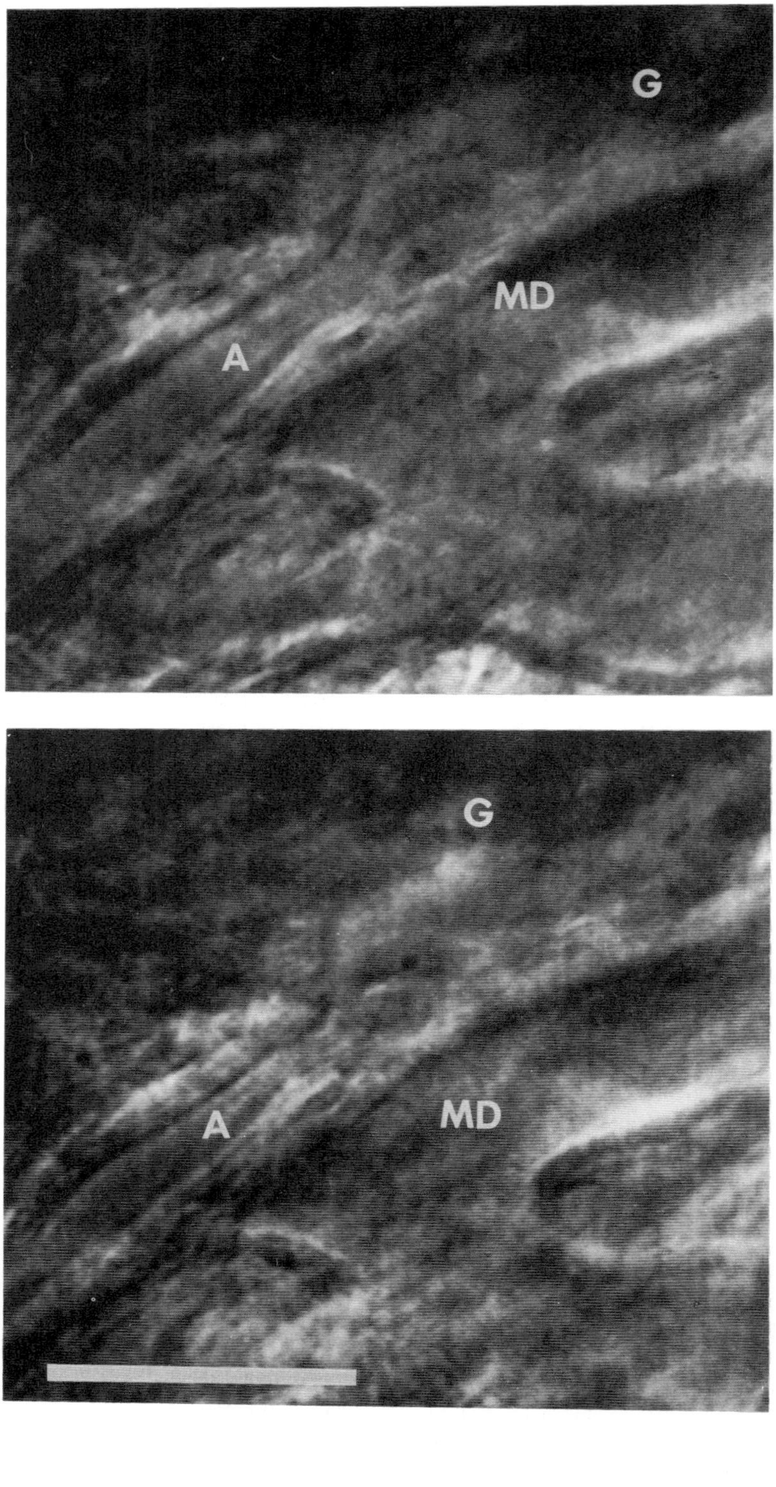
G
MD
A
G
A
MD

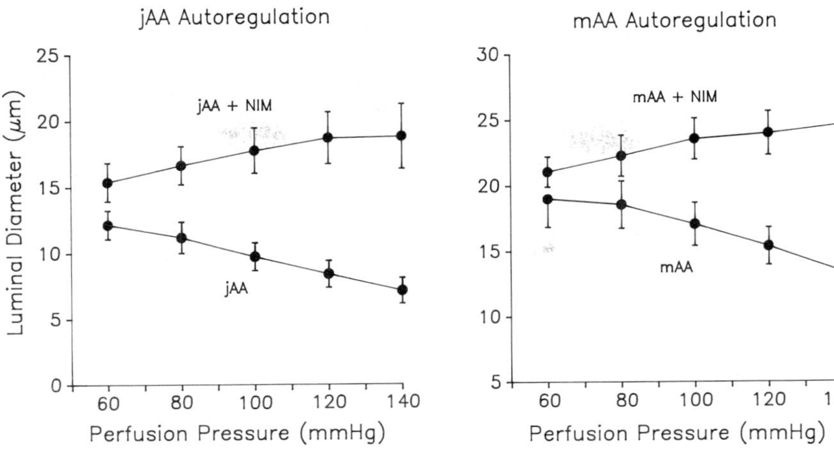

Fig. 2. Autoregulatory responses of the juxtoglomerular afferent arteriole (*jAA*), (*left*) and the mid-afferent arteriole (*mAA*), (*right*). Mean$\pm$SE, n=8 for jAA, n=7 for mAA. Responses are shown before and after calcium channel blockade with 1 µM nimodipine (*NIM*). The mAA and jAA responses and the inhibition by nimodipine were statistically significant in all cases. (Data from [2])

that the autoregulatory responses of the mid- and jAA are at least as strong in the region around 100 mmHg as they are at 60 and 140 mmHg. Hence, our results in JM vessels are inconsistent with the pattern of strong, sequential, descending responses predicted by the DMH. A similar conclusion was reached by Carmines et al. [4] on the basis of measurements of intravascular pressure in JM vessels. However, the DMH may be much more important in superficial cortical nephrons, where the cortical radial arteries are longer and show substantial autoregulatory ability [14].

TGF Responses in the Terminal Segment of the AA

It has long been known that the effector site of the TGF system was in the preglomerular vasculature, as TGF stimulation reduces glomerular capillary pressure and nephron glomerular filtration rate (GFR) in parallel [1]. However, the exact

Fig. 1. Micrograph illustrating typical autoregulatory vasoconstriction in a juxtaglomerular afferent arteriole (*jAA*). *Upper* Control measurement of jAA lumen diameter at 60 mmHg perfusion pressure. *Lower* The same vessel at a perfusion pressure of 120 mmHg. The *bar* is 50 µm. A, jAA lumen; G, glomerular tuft; MD, macula densa. Vessels were visualized through a compound microscope (Leitz 12-FS) with a 25X long-working distance objective (Leitz Fluorotar). Illumination was provided by low-angle incident light from a fiber optic guide. Video images were obtained with a CCD camera, edge-enhanced on-line, and recorded. Vessel dimensions were measured with a video-caliper system

site at which TGF-mediated vasoconstriction occurs, and the strength and speed of the TGF response have never been directly measured. We characterized TGF system in JM nephrons in vitro by directly observing changes in jAA luminal diameter elicited by direct microinjection of isotonic Ringers solution into an unblocked cortical thick ascending limb (cTAL) near the MD. The cTAL is readily identified in these nephrons, owing to marked differences in appearance between it and the surrounding proximal convoluted tubules, and the fact that it makes contact with jAA. Macula densa NaCl concentration was raised from its steady state level by the direct injection, with a micropipette, of 30–80 nl/min of stained (0.1% FD and C green) Ringers solution into the cTAL near the MD. The nephrons were unblocked and tubular fluid flow was verified by observing the washout of stained fluid from the cTAL after cessation of the microinjection. These experiments were conducted at 60 mmHg perfusion pressure to relax the TGF system which, in JM nephrons, is almost fully excited at normotensive pressure levels [15].

The observed TGF responses are shown in Fig. 3. TGF stimulation reduced jAA diameter by 34% $\pm$ 4% (n=8) from a control value of 12.0 $\pm$ 1.0 μm. These measurements were made at sites averaging 22 $\pm$ 3 μm from the end of the AA. We also demonstrated that the response is rapid, requiring around 5 s to develop fully [2]. In the same nephrons, the addition of 0.1 mM furosemide to the injected fluid completely inhibited the TGF response, as observed in many earlier studies [1].

These are the first direct observations of TGF-mediated vasoconstriction, and the results demonstrate that the terminal portion of the AA is a major effector site of the TGF mechanism. Further, the magnitude and location of the TGF responses are similar to earlier conclusions reached by Schnermann and Kriz [16], who measured afferent arteriolar dimensions in sections of flash-frozen kidneys and found smaller diameters in nephrons subjected to maximal TGF stimulation.

Physiological Significance of AA Responses

An interesting feature of these results is the magnitude of TGF-mediated and autoregulatory jAA vasoconstriction. To explore the functional significance of the observed responses, we estimated the relative increments in segmental structural resistance elicted by TGF stimulation, and increased perfusion pressure. These values were calculated from the measured changes in vessel caliber, assuming an inverse 4th power relationship between vessel radius and resistance. The results of this analysis are shown in Fig. 4. For maximal TGF stimulation, the 34% $\pm$ 4% reduction in lumen diameter corresponds to an increase of about 5-fold in segmental vascular resistance. In response to a doubling of perfusion pressure, jAA segmental resistance increased approximately 4-fold, while mAA segmental resistance increased in proportion to perfusion pressure. At first glance, the degree of jAA autoregulatory and TGF-mediated vasoconstriction appears to be excessive. Similar large TGF-mediated increments in structural resistance were observed by Schnermann and Kriz in superficial rat nephrons [16]. However, in vessels of this size, the increment in the structural component of vessel resistance may substantially overestimate the true hemodynamic resistance, owing to the fact that the hematocrit and the apparent viscosity of blood in small vessels is an inverse function of vessel diameter [17]. The observations that glomerular capillary pressure is well autoregulated in JM nephrons

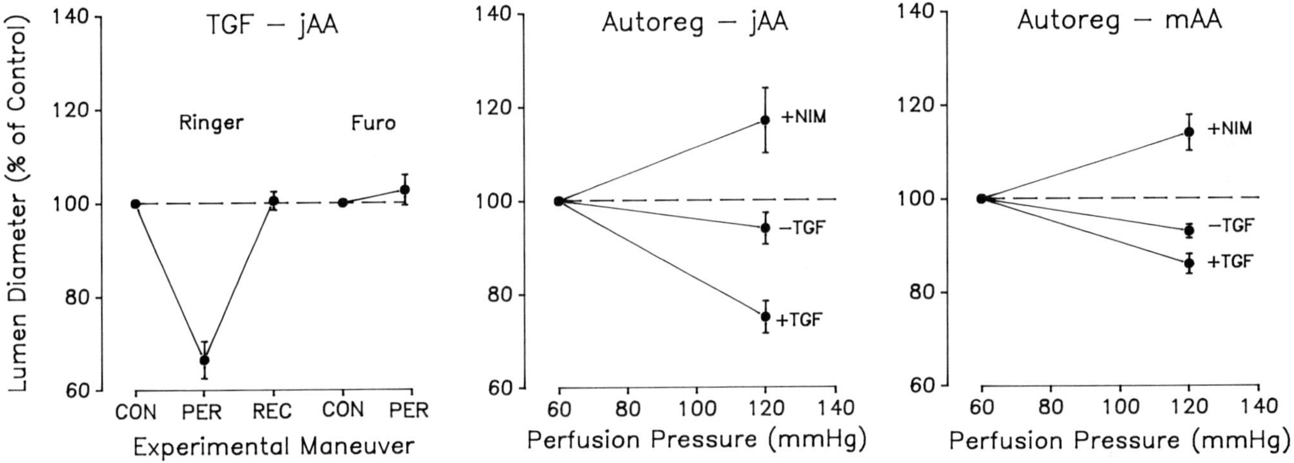

Fig. 3. TGF responses (*left*) ($n=8$) are shown before (*CON*), during (*PER*) and after (*REC*) the injection of Ringer solution into the macula densa region. Also shown are TGF responses in the juxtaglomerular afferent arteriole (*jAA*) ($n=7$) before (*Con*) and during microinjection of Ringer with 0.1 mM furosemide (*Furo*). The TGF response and the inhibition by furosemide were both statistically significant ($P<0.05$, paired t-test). Autoregulatory responses of the jAA (*middle*) and the mid-afferent arteriole (*mAA*) (*right*). Mean (±SE, $n=8$) responses are shown before (*+TGF*) and after TGF inhibition (*−TGF*), and after calcium channel blockade with 1 μM nimodipine (*NIM*). The inhibition of mAA and jAA responses by TGF inhibition and nimodipine were statistically significant in all cases, and the responses after TGF inhibition remained significant for both segments ($P<0.05$, paired t-test). The jAA and mAA measuring sites were 19 ± 3 and 130 ± 9 μm from the vascular pole. (Data from [3])

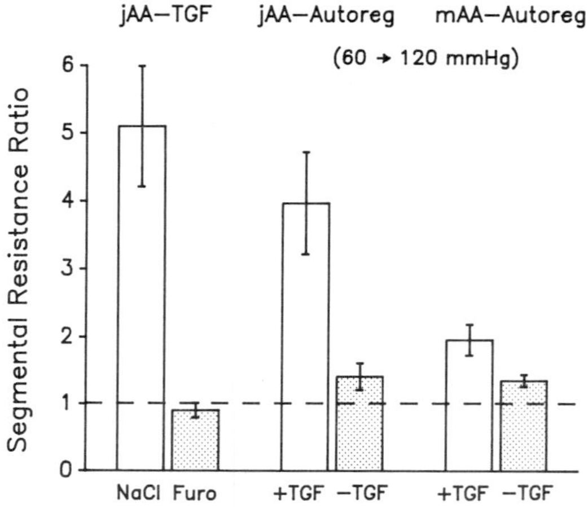

Fig. 4. Comparison of calculated increases in juxtaglomerular afferent arteriole (*jAA*) segmental structural resistance in response to maximal TGF stimulation with and without furosemide (*Furo*), and in response to a doubling of perfusion pressure before (*+TGF*) and after (*−TGF*) TGF inhibition. The responses of the mAA are also shown. The resistance ratios were calculated from measured decreases in luminal diameter assuming an inverse fourth-power relationship between segmental resistance and vessel radius. The *dashed line* at unity indicates no change in resistance. Data are given in Fig. 3

in vitro [4,5] suggest that such large reductions in vessel diameter may be necessary to counteract the decline in blood viscosity that will occur when the vessel constricts. This effect should be most apparent in the jAA, the narrowest preglomerular vascular segment.

Myogenic and TGF Components of AA Autoregulatory Responses

In a third investigation, we examined the extent to which the autoregulatory responses of the AA are dependent upon TGF, and whether the AA possesses TGF-independent, myogenic autoregulatory capability. In this study, a control measurement of jAA and mAA autoregulation was obtained, and nephron flow was verified by injecting a small bolus of stained Ringers solution into the cTAL and observing its washout. The TGF system was then inhibited by filling the MD region with castor oil, and the autoregulatory measurements were repeated. Finally, autoregulation was measured again after calcium-channel inhibition with 1 μM nimodipine added to the superfusate. The results, illustrated in Figs. 3 and 4, show strong calcium-dependent autoregulatory responses in the entire AA, with the strongest responses in the jAA. Mean fractional decreases in jAA and mAA lumen diameter were 25% ± 3% and 15% ± 2% from baseline (60 mmHg) diameters of 15.3 ± 1.8 and 24.0 ± 0.8 μm, respectively. Inhibition of TGF markedly attenuated the autoregulatory response of the jAA segment, reducing the mean fractional diameter decrease from 25% ± 3%

to 6% ± 3%. In the mAA, as in the jAA, the autoregulatory responses were also significantly attentuated by TGF inhibition, with the mean fractional reduction in mAA diameter reduced to 7% ± 2%. In both segments, however, there was also a significant degree of TGF-independent myogenic autoregulation that was most prominent in the mAA.

The dependence of afferent arteriolar autoregulation on TGF is consistent with micropuncture studies of single nephron GFR (SNGFR) autoregulation and with studies of isolated JM nephrons [1,5,16,18]. The results also explain the absence of substantial autoregulatory responses in late AA in hydronephrotic kidneys [6] and in AA segments in vitro [12], where the renal tubular system and, hence, TGF are absent. The results also clearly show a substantial TGF-independent myogenic autoregulatory component in both mAA and jAA segments, again in agreement with micropuncture and isolated nephron studies [1,4,18–20]. However, there is substantial evidence that relative contributions of the myogenic and TGF autoregulatory mechanisms may differ between species and may be altered by changes in physiological state. For example, autoregulation in the dog appears to be more dependent upon TGF than is autoregulation in the rat [21]. Further, two micropuncture studies have shown significantly enhanced myogenic autoregulation under conditions where the normal ability of TGF to participate in the autoregulatory process is inhibited by maintaining TGF under constant, maximal stimulation [19,20]. Although the mechanisms that underlie these intriguing observations of TGF-independent autoregulation are as yet unclear, they do suggest that renal autoregulation is a robust process, in that both TGF and myogenic mechanisms appear to be able to, at least partially, compensate when the other mechanism is impaired.

Communication Between Preglomerular Vascular Segments

Several recent studies have suggested that TGF responses that originate in the jAA can influence vascular reactivity in upstream AA segments and in neighboring nephrons. In our studies, we found substantial TGF-depencency of mAA autoregulation, where TGF inhibition attenuated the mAA autoregulatory increment in mAA segmental resistance by around 60%. This observation suggests that the effect of TGF stimulation can be seen over 100 μm upstream from the jAA segment. Further, the early studies by Schnermann and Kriz [16] in superficial cortical AA found that TGF stimulation resulted in a variable degree of vasoconstriction in the mid and early AA, with some vessels constricting along their entire length. Perhaps the most dramatic evidence that TGF has significant effects on upstream vessels is provided by a recent study by Källskog and Marsh [22]. They demonstrated that nephron stop-flow pressure, a variable that changes in parallel with glomerular capillary pressure, is reduced significantly when TGF in an adjacent nephron is subjected to maximal stimulation. As this response was seen only when both nephrons arose from a common feed vessel, the clear implication is that there is some communication pathway between afferent arterioles branching from the same cortical radial artery. The underlying mechanism has yet to be clearly identified. One possibility is electrotonic conduction of the local TGF signal for vasoconstriction along the arteriole. Although there are numerous gap junctions between endothelial cells in the AA, they are less prevalent between smooth muscle cells [23]. One investigation has failed to show extensive electrotonic conduction in the late AA in hydronephrotic kidneys [24], but it is unclear at present if results from this pathophysiological model can be extrapolated to normal renal vessels. A second possible mechanism is that a strong TGF response, localized in the jAA, enhances the degree of mAA myogenic vasconstriction indirectly by increasing upstream intravascular pressure. Such a mechanism was first proposed by Johnson [25], and would operate in parallel with any electrotonic coupling mechanism that might operate along the arteriole. As yet, no direct evidence has been obtained concerning intravascular-pressure-mediated spread of the TGF response, although two mathematical models suggest that it might have a significant impact on renal autoregulation [20,26]. Much of our current understanding of the regulation of renal hemodynamics is based on single nephron and single vessel studies, yet overall kidney function is determined by the ensemble action of all individual nephrons. Hence, elucidating how TGF and autoregulatory responses are propagated along the afferent arteriole and, perhaps, to the large renal arterial vessels, is likely to be of critical importance in understanding renal autoregulation and how it is altered in disease.

Acknowledgments. These studies were supported by grants from INSERM (CRE 875003) and NIK (DK 26341). During these studies, L.C. Moore was the recipient of a Poste Orange Fellowship from INSERM. Expert technical assistance was provided by Aija Birzgalis and Annie Artuso.

References

1. Schnermann J, Briggs J (1985) Function of the juxtaglomerular apparatus: local control of glomerular hemodynamics. In: Seldin DW, Giebisch G (eds) The kidney: physiology and pathophysiology. Raven, New York, Ch 28
2. Casellas D, Moore LC (1990) Autoregulation and tubuloglomerular feedback in juxtamedullary glomerular arterioles. Am J Physiol 258:F660–F669
3. Moore LC, Casellas D (1990) Tubuloglomerular feedback dependency of autoregulation in rat juxtamedullary afferent arterioles. Kidney Int 37:1402–1408
4. Carmines PK, Inscho EW, Gensure RC (1990) Arterial pressure effects on preglomerular microvasculature of juxtamedullary nephrons. Am J Physiol 258:F94–F102
5. Sanchez-Ferrer CF, Roman RJ, Harder DR (1989) Pressure-dependent contraction of rat juxtamedullary afferent arterioles. Circ Res 64:790–798
6. Steinhausen M, Blum B, Fleming JT, Holz FG, Parekh N, Wiegman DL, Dussel R (1989) Visualization of renal autoregulation in the split hydronephrotic kidney of rats. Kidney Int 35:1151–1160
7. Taugner R, Rosivall L, Bührle CP, Gorschel-Steward U (1987) Myosin content and vasoconstrictive ability of the proximal juxtaglomerular (renin-positive) segments of the afferent arteriole. Cell Tissue Res 248:579–588
8. Øien AH, Aukland K (1983) A mathematical analysis of the myogenic hypothesis with special reference to autoregulation of renal blood flow. Circ Res 52:241–252
9. Casellas D, Navar LG (1984) In vitro perfusion of juxtamedullary nephrons in rats. Am J Physiol 246:F349–F358
10. Casellas D, Carmines PK, Navar LG (1985) Microvascular reactivity of in vitro blood perfused juxtamedullary nephrons from rats. Kidney Int 28:752–759

11. Casellas D, Taugner R (1987) Renin status of the afferent arteriole and ultrastructure of the juxtaglomerular apparatus in superficial juxtamedullary nephrons from rats. Renal Physiol 9:348–356
12. Edwards RM (1983) Segmental effects of norepinephrine and angiotensin II on isolated renal microvessels. Am J Physiol 244:F526–F534
13. Cohen HJ, Marsh DJ, Kayser B (1983) Autoregulation in the vasa recta of the rat kidney. Am J Physiol 245:F32–F40
14. Källskog O, Lindbom LO, Ulfendahl HR, Wolgast M (1976) Hydrostatic pressures within the vascular structures of the rat kidney. Pflugers Arch 363:205–210
15. Müller-Suur R, Ulfendahl HR, Persson AEG (1982) Evidence for tubuloglomerular feedback in juxtamedullary nephrons of young rats. Am J Physiol 244:F425–F431
16. Schnermann J, Briggs J, Kriz W, Moore LC, Wright FS (1980) Control of glomerular vascular resistance by the tubuloglomerular feedback mechanism. In: Leaf A, Giebisch G (eds) Renal pathophysiology. Raven, New York, pp 165–182
17. Fung YC (1984) Biodynamics Circulation. Springer, New York, pp 238–249
18. Moore LC (1984) Tubuloglomerular feedback and SNGFR autoregulation in the rat. Am J Physiol 247:F267–F276
19. Schnermann J, Briggs JP (1989) Interaction between loop of Henle flow and arterial pressure as determinants of glomerular pressure. Am J Physiol 256:F421–F429
20. Davis JM, Kawata T, Häberle D (1988) The influence of renal autoregulation on TGF control of glomerular filtration rate. In: Persson AEG, Boberg U (eds) The juxtaglomerular apparatus. Elsevier, Amsterdam, ch 34
21. Navar LG, Bell PD, Burke TJ (1982) Role of a macula densa feedback mechanism as a mediator of renal autoregulation. Kidney Int 22(Suppl 12):S157–S164
22. Kallskog O, Marsh DJ (to be published) TGF-initiated vascular interactions between adjacent nephrons in the rat kidney. Am J Physiol
23. Taugner R, Hackenthal E (1989) The Juxtaglomerular Apparatus. Springer, Berlin, pp 33–40
24. Nobiling R, Bührle CP (1989) Cell to cell coupling at the afferent arteriole: A combined electrophysiological and morphological study (abstract). Kidney Int 36:307
25. Johnson PC (1986) Autoregulation of blood flow. Circ Res 59:483–495
26. Moore LC, Rich A (1988) Mathematical model of ascending myogenic responses to tubuloglomerular feedback induced changes in afferent vascular resistance (abstract). Kidney Int 33:412

Systemic Dysfunctions in Renal Failure and Their Management

Chair: August Heidland (FRG)
Tsan-Shin Yen (Taipei, China)

Neutrophil Function in Uremia: Inhibition by Endogenous Plasma Inhibitor(s)

WALTER H. HÖRL[1]

Introduction

Infectious complications in patients with end-stage renal disease result in significant morbidity and mortality. Uremia is an immunocompromised state which is due to the direct effects of uremic toxins and to indirect factors, e.g., malnutrition, dialysis membranes with their effects on complement system and white blood cells, or vascular access for dialysis providing a portal of entry for microorganisms [1]. Dysfunction of polymorphonuclear cells (PMN) in uremia includes adherence, the first step in neutrophil migration, chemotaxis, phagocytotic capacity, generation of reactive oxygen intermediates, or intracellular killing of bacteria [2].

Chemotaxis and Phagocytotic Activity of PMN

A reduction in generation of chemotactic activity in experimentally induced acute renal failure has been reported by Clark et al. [3]. This reduction was proportional to the degree of azotemia. Baum et al. [4] demonstrated that chemotaxis of PMN was impaired in the presence of undialyzed uremic sera, but that hemodialysis seemed to correct the defect. A chemotactic inhibitor found in sera of uremic patients acted directly on leukotactic factors (C_3 and C_5 chemotactic fragment and bacterial factor) to render them irreversibly inactive [5]. Pedersen et al. [6] studied the ability of serum to attract PMN in uremic patients before and after hemodialysis. The chemotactic response toward serum from uremic patients were significantly decreased prior to hemodialysis and were normalized thereafter.

Phagocytosis in uremic patients is either normal or slightly diminished. Hirabayashi et al. [7] observed decreased phagocytic uptake of IgG-coated particles in

[1]Department of Medicine, Division of Nephrology, University of Saarland, D-6650 Homburg, Federal Republic of Germany

patients before hemodialysis therapy, which was restored by hemodialysis. The phagocytotic responsiveness of PMN increased after exposure to cuprophane filter, although exposure to polyacrylonitrile and polysulfone hemodialyzers did not affect phagocytotic activity [8]. A dramatic fall was observed in phagocytotic activity after 15 minutes of hemodialysis with cuprophane membranes. Reused cuprophane caused a minor decrease in phagocytotic activity, whereas hemodialysis with polyacrylonitrile and polysulfone produced no significant change in phagocyte populations at this time [8].

Kinetic measurements of the serum-independent uptake of IgG-coated polyvinyl toluene latex particles by isolated PMN cells have been performed in patients undergoing hemodialysis or peritoneal dialysis [9]. The mean phagocytic rate for the patient group was significantly reduced when compared to the reference group of apparently healthy individuals. After 4 months of adequate dialysis, the phagocytic uptake was significantly higher than the uptake shortly after the beginning of dialysis. It was suggested that elevated serum phosphate levels may, in part, be responsible for the impaired phagocytic activity of uremic patients [9].

Oxidative Metabolism and Glucose Metabolism

Ritchey et al. [10] studied superoxide anion production and luminol-amplified chemiluminescence in PMN from chronic hemodialysis patients and in age-matched controls in the resting state; he also studied response to phorbol myristate acetate (PMA). Studies in autologous serum showed higher chemiluminescence resting values in PMN from hemodialysis patients, with a significant reduction after dialysis. Cross-incubation studies indicated that this was a result of factor(s) in the patients' serum. In response to PMA, neutrophils from chronic hemodialysis patients in autologous serum had a significantly smaller increase in chemiluminescence compared with controls, suggesting that there was a defect intrinsic to the patient PMN [10]. Hirabayashi et al. [7] also found that impaired hydrogen peroxide production by PMA-stimulated PMN before dialysis was restored to the control level by hemodialysis.

Different changes in oxidative metabolism have been observed in PMN when exposed to a cuprophane filter, but not with a polyacrylonitrile filter membrane [11]. Reduced PMN activity of both chemiluminescence and H_2O_2 occurred as a consequence of hemodialysis when a cuprophane dialyzer was employed; however, the diminished activity was no longer detectable after the filter had been hemophane modified [12].

Markert et al. [13] found an increase, compared to the control cells, of lucigenin-amplified chemiluminescence, stimulated by phorbol myristate, acetate in PMN isolated after 5 and 60 minutes during hemodialysis with cuprophane, cellulose acetate, and polyacrylonitrile during the first and/or second use. Luminol increased chemiluminescence during the initial use of three filters: cuprophane, polycarbonate, and polysulfone.

Although numerous studies have affirmed changes of PMN metabolism and function in uremia, most of the evidence has come from data obtained before and during hemodialysis. However, information comparing PMN function after hemodialysis treatment with that prior to treatment is lacking. Studies on glucose metabolism have revealed that glucose intolerance and impaired utilization of glucose are improved

Table 1. Biological activity of granulocyte inhibiting protein (GIP)

Test condition	GIP concentration which inhibits 50% of maximal stimulation (IC_{50})
^{3}H d-glucose uptake[a]	5.2 ± 1.2 μg/ml (n=5)
Chemotaxis[a]	7.2 ± 1.7 μg/ml (n=6)
Oxidative metabolism[a]	8.1 ± 1.4 μg/ml (n=5)
Intracellular killing[b]	7.9 ± 1.7 μg/ml (n=6)

[a]stimulation with FMLP
[b]stimulation with *S. aureus* 502

significantly after uremic patients have undergone hemodialysis treatment. This suggests that a circulating plasma factor is responsible for inducing insulin resistance [14–16]. A variety of normal tissues obtained from animals have inhibited basal uptake of glucose following incubation with whole or partially purified sera obtained from uremic patients [17–19]. The insulin stimulation of glucose uptake and the metabolism of rat adipocytes were also reduced following preincubation with serum from uremic patients [20]. This irregularity occurred without affecting either insulin binding or the antilipolytic action of insulin [15].

Cellular activation of PMN by microbial antigens and certain toxins is achieved by the stimulation of phosphoinositol (PI) turnover and activation of protein kinase C. For example, the stimulus-response coupling in PMN is induced by a chemotactic peptide. Concanavalin A, immune complexes, and PMA showed an increase of calcium uptake preceding the onset of degranulation and of O_2-generation [21]. The stimulation of hexose transport by PMNs is associated with the activation of protein kinase C [22]. Furthermore, pertussis toxin, which is known to involve the activation of G proteins, effectively stimulates PI turnover with regard to increased formation of IP_3 and an increased elevation of intracellular calcium [23].

We have observed that PMN from uremic patients have diminished responsiveness to chemotactic peptide FMLP-induced hexose uptake, enzyme release, and chemotaxis [24]. This lack of responsiveness is improved after the patients have undergone hemodialysis. Moreover, when normal PMN were exposed to various concentrations of ultrafiltrates from uremic patients, there was an increased loss of responsiveness of these cells with regard to hexose uptake [25] and enzyme release. In addition, washing the PMN with buffered saline restored their function to normal, which suggests that a plasma-derived constituent is responsible for these effects. There is further evidence for the existence of such a putative entity, from initial experiments that have employed one species with a molecular weight (MW) of 8-30 Kda that was partly purified by column chromatography (Sephadex G-100) from the ultrafiltrate of uremic patients. The factor greater than 10 Kda MW appears to be heat labile, which suggests that it can be further purified, characterized, and its biochemical and immunochemical properties further elucidated.

Physiochemical Characterization of a Novel Polypeptide

Recently, a novel protein (molecular weight 28 Kda) was isolated and characterized from uremic serum of patients undergoing regular hemodialysis therapy. This polypeptide inhibits chemotaxis, oxidative metabolism, the uptake of glucose, and intracellular bacterial killing by polymorphonuclear leukocytes [26]. The IC_{50} of the granulocyte inhibiting protein required to inhibit both the biochemical and the functional changes is in the nanomolar range. Therefore, the efficacy of the protein is well within the range of physiological effector substances (Table 1). A specific rabbit polyclonal antibody raised against the protein nullified these inhibitory changes [26]. In summary, a granulocyte inhibitory protein was isolated from ultrafiltrates of patients on regular hemodialysis treatment. A polysulfone membrane (Fresenius, Oberursel, FRG) was used. The protein is capable of inhibiting four fundamental PMN cell functions. Its exact role remains to be elucidated.

References

1. Tolkoff NE, Rubin RH (1990) Uremia and host defenses. N Engl J Med 322:770–772
2. Haag-Weber M, Hable M, Schollmeyer P, Hörl WH (1989) Metabolic response of neutrophils to uremia and dialysis. Kidney Int 36(Suppl 27):S293–S298
3. Clark RA, Hamony BH, Ford G, Kimball HR (1972) Chemotaxis in acute renal failure. J Infect Dis 126:460–463
4. Baum J, Cestero RVM, Freeman RB (1975) Chemotaxis of polymorphonuclear leukocytes and delayed hypersensitivity in uremia. Kidney Int 7(Suppl 2):S147–S153
5. Siriwatratananonta P, Sinsakul V, Stern K, Slavin RG (1978) Defective chemotaxis in uremia. J Lab Clin Med 92:402–407
6. Pedersen JO, Knudsen F, Nielsen AH, Grunnet N (1987) The ability of uremic serum to induce neutrophil chemotaxis in relation to hemodialysis Blood Purif 5:24–28
7. Hirabayashi Y, Kobayashi T, Nishikawa A, Aoki T, Takaya J, Kobayashi Y (1988) Oxidative metabolism and phagocytosis of polymorphonuclear leukocytes in patients with chronic renal failure. Nephron 49:305–312
8. Vanholder RC, Dhondt A, Ringoir SMG (1988) Challenge of phagocyte metabolism by extracorporeal test. Trans Am Soc Artif Intern Organs 34:214–218
9. Hällgren R, Fjellström KE, Venge P (1979) Kinetic studies of phagocytosis. II. The serum-independent uptake of IgG-coated particles by polymorphonuclear leukocytes from uremic patients on regular dialysis treatment. J Lab Clin Med 94:277–284
10. Ritchey EE, Wallin JD, Shah SV (1981) Chemiluminescence and superoxide anion production by leukocytes from chronic hemodialysis patients. Kidney Int 19:349–358
11. Nguyen AT, Lethias C, Zingraff J, Herbelin A, Naret C, Descamps-Latscha B (1985) Hemodialysis membrane-induced activation of phagocyte oxidative metabolism detected in vivo and in vitro within microamounts of whole blood. Kidney Int 28:158–167
12. Kolb G, Schönemann H, Fischer W, Bittner K, Lange H, Höffken H, Damann V, Joseph K, Havemann K (1988) Hemodialysis with cuprophane membranes leads to alteration of granulocyte oxidative metabolism and leukocyte sequestion in the lung. In: Hörl WH, Heidland A (eds) Proteases: Potential role in health and disease II. Plenum, New York, pp 377–384
13. Markert M, Heierli C, Kuwahara T, Frei J, Wauters JP (1988) Dialyzed polymorphonuclear neutrophil oxidative metabolism during dialysis: a comparative study with 5 new and reused membranes. Clin Nephrol 29:129–136
14. McCaleb ML, Izzo MS, Lockwood DH (1985) Characterization and partial purification of a factor from uremic human serum that induces insulin resistance. J Clin Invest 75:391–396
15. DeFronzo RA, Tobin JD, Rowe JW, Andres R (1978) Glucose intolerance in uremia. J Clin Invest 62:425–435

16. Hampers CL, Soeldner JS, Doak PB, Merrill JP (1966) Effect of chronic renal failure and hemodialysis on carbohydrate metabolism. J Clin Invest 45:1719–1731
17. Balesteri P, Rindi P, Biagini M, Giovaneti S (1972) Effects of uremic serum, urea, creatinine and methylguanidine on glucose metabolism. Clin Sci 42:395–404
18. Morgan JM, Morgan RE (1964) Study of the effect of uremic metabolites on erythrocyte glycosis. Metabolism 13:629–635
19. Dzurik R (1980) Metabolic alterations caused by uremia. Proc Eur Dial Transplant Assoc 17:577–586
20. McCaleb ML, Mevorach R, Freeman RB, Izzo MS, Lockwood DH (1984) Induction of insulin resistance in normal adipose tissue by uremic human serum. Kidney Int 25:416–421
21. Korchak HM, Rutherford LE, Weissman G (1984) Stimulus response coupling in the human neutrophiles. I. Kinetic analysis of changes in calcium permeability. J Biol Chem 259:4070
22. McCall C, Schmitt J, Cousart S, O'Flaherty J, Bass D, Wykle R (1985) Stimulation of hexose transport by human polymorphonuclear leucocytes: a possible role of protein kinase C. Biochem Biophys Res Commun 126:450–456
23. Krause KH, Schlegel W, Wollheim CB, Andersson T, Waldvogel FA, Lew PD (1985) Chemotactic peptide activation of human neutrophils and HL-60 cells. Pertussis toxin reveals correlation between inositol triophate generation, calcium ion transients, and cellular activation. J Clin Invest 76:1348–1354
24. Haag-Weber M, Hable M, Schollmeyer P, Hörl WH (1989) Hemodialysis improves carbohydrate metabolism in polymorphonuclear neutrophils (PMN) (abstract). Kidney Int 35:248
25. Haag-Weber M, Schollmeyer P, Hörl WH (1989) Neutrophil activation during hemodialysis. In: Hörl WH, Schollmeyer P (eds) New perspectives in hemodialysis, peritoneal dialysis, arteriovenous hemofiltration, and plasmapheresis. Plenum, New York, pp 27–37
26. Hörl WH, Haag-Weber M, Georgopoulos A, Block LH (1990) The physicochemical characterization of a polypeptide present in uremic serum that inhibits the biological activity of polymorphonuclear cells. Proc Natl Acad Sci USA 87:6353–6357

The Impact of Anemia in the Pathogenesis of Endocrine Abnormalities in Chronic Renal Failure

Franciszek Kokot, Andrzej Więcek, Mariusz Klin[1], and Jolanta Klepacka[2]

Summary. Endocrine abnormalities are well characterized in uremic patients. On the other hand it is known that erythropoietin (EPO) treatment in patients with chronic uremia is accompanied by several beneficial, as well as by adverse effects, which suggest the participation of endocrine organs in the pathogenesis of this disease. In this paper we report the effects of three months EPO treatment on the function of several endocrine organs in hemodialyzed patients. Endocrine parameters were assessed before and after 3 months on EPO treatment, as well as 3 months after EPO administration was discontinued. Results obtained in these patients were compared with those established in appropriately selected healthy subjects, as well as with those found in hemodialyzed uremic patients (not receiving EPO) with a hematocrit value of the same magnitude as that determined in patients after EPO treatment. Treatment with EPO was followed by suppression of basal plasma levels of somatotropin, prolactin, follitropin, lutropin, adrenocorticotropic hormone (ACTH), cortisol, and aldosterone and by a moderate increase of plasma parathyroid hormone (PTH) and testosterone. Treatment with EPO did not significantly influence plasma calcitonin and 25-OH-D levels or the function of the pituitary-thyroid feedback. After 3 months of EPO treatment we found a suppression of plasma renin activity, but an increase of plasma atrial natriuretic peptide level. Treatment with EPO increased insulin, but suppressed plasma levels of glucagon, gastrin, and to a lesser degree, those of the pancreatic polypeptide. Some EPO-induced endocrine alterations were still present three months after the discontinuation of EPO therapy. From data presented in this study, it follows that EPO treatment is accompanied by profound endocrine alterations and that these alterations do not seem to be related only to the improvement of anemia.

[1]Department of Nephrology, Silesian School of Medicine, ul. Francuska 20, Katowice, Poland
[2]Institute of Transplantology, Medical Academy, Warsaw, Poland

Introduction

Erythropoietin (EPO) is a factor which undoubedly participates in the pathogenesis of anemia in patients with chronic renal failure. Several lines of evidence suggest that additional factors are also involved in the pathogenesis and maintenance of such anemia. Among these factors we refer to endocrine abnormalities [1]. On the other hand, some hormones (corticoids, thyroid, and gonadal hormones) are proven modulators of erythropoiesis, even under physiological conditions. Finally, from data obtained in the last 3–4 years, it seems that some clinical signs and symptoms, such as increased well-being, increased libido and potency, increased appetite, exacerbation of preexisting elevated blood pressure, and improvement of physical and mental activity, as well as some side effects of EPO treatment (hyperkalemia, hypocalcemia, periarticular inflammation due to calcified deposits) are not related only to the amelioration of anemia (for review see references in [1]).

In this paper we summarize our extensive studies on the influence of EPO treatment on the function of endocrine organs in hemodialyzed patients. Results of some of these studies are already published [2–5] while others are to be published [7–9]. In these studies we aimed to answer the following questions:

1) Does EPO treatment influence the function of endocrine organs in hemodialyzed patients with chronic renal failure? and
2) What is the impact of anemia in the pathogenesis of endocrine abnormalities in chronic renal failure?

Material and Methods

Three groups of patients were examined. The first one consisted of hemodialyzed patients treated with EPO (EPO group). The second one comprised hemodialyzed patients not treated with EPO (no EPO group), but who showed hematocrit values similar to those of patients in the first group after those patients had completed EPO therapy. The third group consisted of healthy control subjects. In the EPO group, baseline plasma levels of hormones were assessed before EPO treatment, after three months on EPO treatment, and three months after the discontinuation of EPO therapy, while in the other two groups baseline plasma concentrations of the individual hormonal parameters were estimated only once. The number of subjects examined is listed in Table 1. The mean age of the three groups was of similar magnitude. In hemodialyzed patients, blood samples for the assessment of the individual hormones were withdrawn from fasting subjects immediately before the dialysis session. EPO (EPREX from Cilag) was administered intravenously as a bolus injection at the end of the dialysis session three times per week. The mean dose of EPO was 75 U/kg b.w. In all blood samples, in addition to assessing parameters, hemoglobin concentration (Hb), hematocrit value (Hct), and plasma levels of calcium, phosphorus (inorganic), sodium, potassium, and creatinine were also assessed. All hormones were assessed by radioimmunoassay (for reference see [2]). Statistical evaluation of results was performed using Student's "*t*" test for paired and unpaired variables, respectively.

Table 1. Baseline plasma levels of hormones in patients of the NO-EPO group (*D*), in healthy subjects (*controls*) and in hemodialyzed patients before (*B*) and after (*A*) three months of EPO therapy, and 3 months after discontinuation of EPO therapy (*C*). Means ± SEM. The number of patients examined is shown in parentheses. The degree of statistical significance in EPO-treated patients concerns the difference B-A and B-C respectively, while in patients of the NO-EPO group the difference concerns D-A. CRF, chronic renal failure
$^{x}P < 0.05$ $^{y}P < 0.01$ $^{z}P < 0.001$

	Patients with CRF on EPO				
	Before EPO	After EPO	3 Months after discontinued EPO	NO-EPO group	
	B	A	C	D	Controls
Somatotropin (STH) ng/ml	9.5±1.1 (11)	4.8 ±0.7^{z} (11)	4.6±1.1^{z} (11)	7.0±1.7 (7)	3.5±0.5
ACTH pg/ml	58.8±4.4 (5)	13.2 ±2.2^{z} (5)	65.6±9.5 (5)	82.9±21.2^{y} (7)	23.6±1.9 (15)
Prolactin ng/ml	36.8±4.7 (11)	12.9 ±2.6^{z} (11)	48.2±14.2 (11	11.6±2.9 (7)	12.1±1.6 (12)
Follitropin (FSH) mU/ml	46.8±11.7 (5)	13.6 ±5.3^{y} (5)	16.4±9.0^{x} (5)	28.4±3.3^{x} (7)	5.7±0.4 (15)
Lutropin (LH) mU/ml	17.5±1.5 (5)	7.9 ±1.1^{z} (5)	5.4±1.7^{z} (5)	18.0±1.0^{z} (7)	8.2±0.5 (15)
Thyrotropin (TSH) mU/ml	2.2±0.3 (5)	2.2 ±0.4 (5)	2.1±0.3 (5)	2.0±0.2 (7)	2.6±0.3 (12)
Thyroxin (T_4) μmol/l	80.0±11.4 (5)	86.3 ±4.2 (5)	103.0±10.9 (5)	103.1±9.3 (7)	120.0±5.6 (12)
Triiodothyronine (T_3) mmol/l	1.2±0.2 (5)	1.3 ±0.2 (5)	1.7±0.1 (5)	2.0±0.2 (7)	2.1±0.2 (12)
Parathyroid hormone (PTH) ng/ml	1.6±0.3 (5)	2.08±0.31 (5)	1.7±0.3 (5)	1.3±0.4 (7)	0.6±0.05 (12)
Calcitonin (CT) pg/ml	109±20 (5)	149±11 (5)	133±9 (5)	194±31 (7)	23±14 (12)
25-OH-D ng/ml	17.4±2.4 (5)	19.7 ±1.6 (5)	12.5±0.8 (5)	14.0±0.8^{y} (7)	16.2±0.8 (12)
Plasma renin activity (PRA) ng/ml per h	5.4±0.8 (11)	3.3 ±0.6^{y} (11)	3.9±1.4 (11)	2.9±0.9 (7)	2.8±0.2 (10)
Aldosterone (Ald) ng/dl	14.8±1.4 (5)	11.3 ±1.3^{x} (5)	16.3±2.9 (5)	15.3±1.4^{x} (7)	9.8±0.7 (10)
Cortisol μg/dl	13.2±2.1 (5)	7.9 ±1.2^{y} (5)	18.7±4.7 (5)	19.2±1.3^{z} (7)	12.4±1.8 (12)
Atrial natriuretic peptide (ANP) pg/ml	159±13 (5)	255±38^{x} (5)	117±14 (5)	149±7^{y} (7)	74±1 (10)
Vasopressin pg/ml	6.4±1.7 (5)	6.2 ±1.3 (5)	9.8±1.6 (5)	9.3±1.5 (7)	2.1±0.2 (10)
Glucagon pg/ml	256±61 (5)	114±42^{y} (5)	275±28 (5)	174±43 (7)	115±17 (15)
Gastrin pg/ml	125±19 (5)	53±9^{y} (5)	120±9 (5)	265±16^{z} (7)	38±6 (15)
Pancreatic polypeptide (PP) pg/ml	735±92 (5)	526±93^{x} (5)	250±34^{z} (5)	682±32 (7)	80±12 (15)
Insulin μU/ml	19.8±3.6 (11)	29.2 ±3.4^{x} (11)	40.8±7.3^{y} (11)	27.9±6.2 (7)	8.6±1.2 (15)
Testosterone ng/ml	1.9±0.8 (5)	3.0 ±0.7^{x} (5)	1.9±0.3 (5)	4.2±0.5 (7)	8.2±0.3 (15)

Results

Influence of EPO Therapy on Blood Hemoglobin Concentration, Hematocrit Value, and Plasma Levels of Creatinine and Electrolytes

Treatment with EPO did not significantly influence plasma levels of creatinine (1208 ± 47 μmol/l before EPO vs 1236 ± 62 μmol/l after EPO treatment).

Treatment with EPO was accompanied by a significant increase of hemoglobin, from 4.47 ± 0.14 to 6.67 ± 0.15 mmol/l, and by a significant increase of the Hct value, from 23 ± 0.89 to 34.8 ± 0.75% ($P < 0.001$). Three months after EPO therapy was discontinued both Hb (=5.3 ± 0.15 mmol/l) and Hct (=27.6 ± 0.97%) values were found to have declined, although these values were still significantly ($P < 0.05$) higher than pre-EPO values.

Treatment with EPO did not influence plasma sodium levels, but was accompanied by a slight increase of plasma potassium (from 5.06 ± 0.09 to 5.38 ± 0.06 mmol/l) and inorganic phosphorus (from 1.68 ± 0.18 to 1.94 ± 0.2 mmol/l), and by a significant ($P < 0.05$) decline of plasma total calcium (from 2.44 ± 0.07 to 2.25 ± 0.08). Three months after EPO therapy was discontinued the respective plasma levels of K, Ca, and P did not differ from pretreatment values.

Endocrine Alterations Induced by EPO Therapy

As can be seen in Table 1, pretreatment baseline plasma levels of most hormones (cortisol, thyrotropin, T_3, T_4, 25-OH-D, and testosterone excepted) were significantly higher than the respective values in the control group. After three months of EPO therapy a significant decline or even normalization, of plasma levels of somatotropin (STH), ACTH, follitropin (FSH), lutropin (LH), prolactin, glucagon, gastrin, cortisol, and of plasma renin activity was noticed. In contrast EPO did not significantly influence plasma concentrations of thyrotropin (TSH), triiodothyronine (T_3), thyroxine (T_4), arginine vasopressin (AVP), parathyroid hormone (PTH), calcitonin (CT), and 25-OH-D, while a marked increase of atrial natriuretic peptide (ANP), insulin, and testosterone was observed. Three months after EPO therapy was discontinued, baseline plasma renin activity (PRA) and plasma levels of ACTH, prolactin, PTH, CT, aldosterone, vasopressin, cortisol, glucagon, gastrin and testosterone were similar to pretreatment values, while plasma levels of STH, FSH, LH and pancreatic polypeptide (PP) were still significantly lower than pretreatment values; in contrast, the plasma level of insulin was significantly higher, while ANP levels were significantly lower than their respective pretreatment concentrations.

Discussion

From the data presented in these studies it follows that EPO treatment markedly influences the function of many endocrine organs. Although the pathophysiology of most of these hormonal alterations has not been clarified, it seems that at least some of these alterations are of clinical relevance. For example, it seems likely that the observed suppression by EPO treatment of PRA and aldosterone, as well as the increase of plasma ANP levels, are purposeful compensatory mechanisms which counteract hypervolemia (induced by increased erythropoiesis), as recently suggested by Kühn et al. [10]. As is well known, hypervolemia suppresses the activity of the renin-angiotensin-aldosterone system, but stimulates ANP release. Based on this reasoning, a reduction of plasma AVP level should also be expected. As this was not the case (EPO did not change plasma AVP level), it seems that factors other than hypervolemia are involved in the pathogenesis of reduced PRA and aldosterone, and of increased ANP levels in EPO treated patients, and/or that EPO therapy does not normalize the normal volumetric regulation of AVP secretion in uremic patients.

As shown in Table 1, EPO treatment was followed by a significant decrease in the plasma levels of STH, ACTH, cortisol, prolactin, PP, glucagon, and gastrin. It remains to be clarified whether these endocrine alterations are caused by direct effects of EPO on the respective endocrine organs, or whether these alterations are a consequence of the improvement of anemia.

As recently reported by Schäfer et al. [4,5] EPO treatment significantly suppresses plasma prolactin levels in uremic patients. This EPO effect could be involved in the causation of the improved sexual activity of these patients. As already reported by Bommer et al. [11], suppression of prolactin secretion by α-bromcriptin is accompanied by improvement of sexual activity in patients with endstage renal failure. As EPO treatment was also followed by a significant increase in plasma testosterone levels, it seems likely that improved function of the Leydig's cells may be involved in the causation of improved sexual activity in these patients. Very recently, an increase of plasma testosterone level in EPO treated patients was also reported by other authors [12].

The importance of the observed increase of immunoreactive insulin (IRI) and decrease of plasma levels of STH, ACTH, cortisol, and glucagon in EPO treated patients has been insufficiently elucidated. It seems likely that these EPO induced alterations may be involved in the pathogenesis of improved carbohydrate tolerance in uremic patients [8].

As already mentioned, EPO treatment was accompanied by a mild increase of PTH plasma levels, probably induced by an enhanced ingestion of food (as a consequence of increased appetite). Short term EPO treatment did not significantly influence thyroid function in uremic patients.

As shown in Table 1, in patients of the No-EPO group (with a Hct values similar to the posttreatment values in the EPO group) plasma levels of several hormones differed significantly from the respective posttreatment values of the EPO group. This fact suggests the participation of factors other than anemia in the pathogenesis of endocrine alterations induced by EPO therapy.

The results presented in this paper suggest that, in patients with endstage renal failure, elevated levels of some hormones are not caused only by the reduced degradation or excretion of these hormones by the failing kidneys. Thus, reconsideration of the pathogenesis of endocrine abnormalities in patients with endstage renal failure seems to be mandatory. It remains to be clarified as to what extent endocrine alterations in EPO-treated patients are due to improvement of erythropoiesis and oxygen supply to different organs or whether they are specific EPO effects.

References

1. Kokot F, Więcek A (1989) Endocrine changes in chronic dialysis patients. In: Maher JF (ed) Replacement of renal function by dialysis. Kluwer, Dordrecht, pp 953–971
2. Kokot F, Więcek A, Grzeszczak W, Klepacka J, Klin M (1989) Influence of erythropoietin treatment on endocrine abnormalities in haemodialyzed patients. In: Baldamus CA, Scigalla P, Wieczorek L, Koch KM (eds) Erythropoietin: from molecular structure to clinical application. Contrib Nephrol, Karger, Basel, pp 257–272
3. Kokot F, Więcek A, Grzeszczak K, Klin M (1990) Influence of erythropoietin treatment on function of the pituitary adrenal axis and somatotropin secretion in hemodialyzed patients. Clin Nephrol 33:241–246
4. Schaefer RM, Kokot F, Heidland A (1989) Impact of recombinant erythropoietin on sexual function in hemodialysis patients. In: Baldamus CA, Scigalla P, Wieczorek al, Koch KM (eds) Erythropoietin: from molecular structure to clinical application. Contrib Nephrol, Karger, Basel, pp 273–282
5. Schaefer RM, Kokot F, Kürner B, Zech M, Heidland A (1988) Normalization of elevated prolactin levels in hemodialysis patients on erythropoietin. Nephron 50:400–401
6. Kokot F, Więcek A, Grzeszczak W, Klin M (1990) Influence of erythropoietin treatment on plasma renin activity, aldosterone, vasopressin and atrial natriuretic peptide in haemodialyzed patients. Min Electrol Metab 16:25–29
7. Kokot F, Więcek A, Grzeszczak W, Klin M (to be published) Influence of erythropoietin treatment on follitropin and lutropin response to luliberin and plasma testosterone levels in haemodialyzed patients. Nephron
8. Kokot F, Więcek A, Grzeszczak W, Klin M, Żukowska-Szczechowska E (to be published) Influence of erythropoietin treatment on glucose tolerance, insulin, glucagon, gastrin and pancreatic polypeptide secretion in haemodialyzed patients with endstage renal failure. Contrib Nephrol, Karger, Basel
9. Kokot F, Więcek A, Grzeszczak W, Klin M (to be published) Der Einfluss von Erythropoietin auf die Funktion der Schilddrüse und Nebenschildrüsen bei dialysierten Patienten mit chronischer Niereninsuffizienz. Z Klin Med
10. Kühn K, Talarschik H, Koch KM, Eisenhauer T, Nonast-Daniel B, Scheler F, Brunkhorst R, Reimers E (1988) Plasma atrial natriuretic peptide after partial correction of renal anaemia by recombinant human erythropoietin. Nephrol Dial Transplant 3:497–498
11. Bommer J, DelPozo E, Ritz E, Bommer G (1979) Improved sexual function in male haemodialysis patients on bromocriptin. Lancet II:496–497
12. Haley NR, Matsumoto AM, Eschbach JW, Adamson JW (1988) Low testosterone levels increase in male hemodialysis patients treated with recombinant human erythropoietin (abstract). 21st annual meeting of the American Society of Nephrology, December 11–12, 1988. San Antonio, USA

Growth Hormone Treatment for Patients with Renal Failure

JOEL D. KOPPLE, GIULIANO BRUNORI, MARC LEISEROWITZ, CRYSTAL MATTIMORE, and RAIMUND HIRSCHBERG[1]

Growth Hormone (GH), so called for its ability to induce an increase in linear growth, is secreted by the somatotrophes of the anterior pituitary gland. It is a single-chain polypeptide with a molecular weight of 22000 and contains 191 amino acid residues. Its configuration is determined by two intrachain disulfide bridges. The factors controlling the secretion and plasma levels of GH have been reviewed elsewhere [1].

GH exerts many metabolic and anabolic effects on skeletal and soft tissues. Some of these actions appear to be mediated directly by GH. Others GH effects are dependent on the synthesis and release of two polypeptide growth factors. These compounds are called, for their structural homology to proinsulin and similar activity to insulin, IGF-I and IGF-II [2]. Growth hormone stimulates IGF-I production in many cells including those in liver, kidney, cartilage, and the pituitary gland. Nutritional status also plays an important role in IGF-I production. During conditions associated with negative calorie balance or negative nitrogen balance, the circulating levels of IGF-I are reduced [3], even though plasma GH levels are elevated. IGF-II production is less GH-dependent; like IGF-I, it is produced in many tissues.

The most important metabolic effects of GH include increased cellular DNA, RNA, protein synthesis, and sulfate incorporation, positive nitrogen balance, enhanced lipolysis and release of free fatty acids. Growth hormone decreases urinary excretion of phosphorus, sodium, potassium and chloride. Acutely, GH may exert an insulin-like effect on carbohydrates; later it may cause insulin antagonism, carbohydrate intolerance and diabetes mellitus [1]. Thus, GH can be considered an anabolic hormone that stimulates postnatal growth and positive protein balance, antagonizes the glucose-lowering action of insulin, and possesses lipolytic activity.

The kidneys play an important role in the turnover of circulating GH. Johnson and Maack reported that in rats about 70% of the total turnover of GH occurs in the kid-

[1]Division of Nephrology and Hypertension, Harbor UCLA Medical Center and Schools of Medicine and Public Health, UCLA Torrance, CA 90509, USA

neys [4]. This may account for the increased plasma levels and decreased plasma turnover of GH in anephric animals and in humans with chronic renal failure.

Almost all studies of the nutritional status of patients with advanced chronic renal failure, including patients undergoing maintenance hemodialysis or peritoneal dialysis, indicate that they often demonstrate wasting or protein calorie malnutrition [5,6]. In many individuals, malnutrition is mild or moderate. There are a number of causes for wasting and malnutrition in renal failure. Probably the most important cause is poor dietary intake. Other causes include intercurrent illnesses, blood loss, the hemodialysis procedure itself, which may both stimulate protein breakdown and also engender losses of amino acids and proteins, and the altered metabolic and hormonal environment of renal failure. Malnutrition has been shown to be an important risk factor for high morbidity and mortality in patients with chronic renal failure [7,8]. It is not established whether low protein and calorie intake and malnutrition cause the adverse effects or whether underlying illnesses are responsible for both the inadequate intake and the increased morbidity and mortality. There is the sense among many nephrologists that poor nutritional intake negatively affects the course of patients with chronic renal failure.

Many studies have suggested that the uremic environment itself is antianabolic or catabolic. Indeed, inhibitors to protein synthesis, glucose uptake by muscle, and the effects of insulin-like growth factor-I (IGF-I, somatomedin C) have been described in uremic sera [9–11]. In both children and adults with chronic renal failure, serum GH levels are generally increased [4,12] and serum somatomedin C concentrations are normal or slightly elevated [11,13]. However, in children [14] and adults [11] with kidney failure, the biological activity of somatomedin C is reported to be reduced. Bioactivity of serum somatomedin C increases after a hemodialysis treatment [11].

Several investigators have attempted to use anabolic steroids to promote anabolism in acutely or chronically uremic patients [15,16]. These agents, which usually are similar in structure to androgens, could induce anabolic effects; but the results appear to be transient [15]. Because of the evidence for an inhibiting effect of uremia on IGF-1 activity [11] and the fact that GH has been shown to both increase IGF-1 levels and to promote anabolism, several researchers have began to investigate whether GH injections may improve the nutritional status and body composition of patients with chronic renal failure.

At present, most research on the effects of GH in renal failure has focused on children. Growth retardation is a prominent manifestation in children with advanced chronic renal failure. The heights and weights of children undergoing maintenance dialysis are frequently in the lower 3 percentile as compared to normal children of the same sex and chronological age [17]. With conventional treatment, children with advanced renal failure may grow normally, but catch-up growth is rare. Fortunately, bone epiphyses often close late and, hence, uremic children may continue to grow at a chronological age where height gain usually has ceased in normal individuals [17]. Nonetheless, children with advanced renal failure usually have short stature when they become adults. Children who have a renal transplant often continue to demonstrate low growth rates and short stature. Glucocorticoid therapy and the persistence of some degree of renal insufficiency in the transplanted kidney may contribute to this phenomenon. It should be emphasized that in children with end stage renal disease, body weight and most other anthropometric parameters, when adjusted for height age rather than chronological age, tend to be normal; on the other hand, their serum albumin is often low [18].

The pathogenesis of impaired growth in renal failure probably involves many factors including inadequate calorie and protein intake, the uremic environment, renal osteodystrophy, aluminum toxicity, 1,25-dihydroxycholecalciferol deficiency, acidemia, glucocorticoid therapy and superimposed illnesses [5,17]. As in adults, serum IGF-1 measured by bioassay is low, suggesting an inhibitory effect of the uremic environment on IGF-1 and, hence, GH activity.

Since the early 1960s GH, initially obtained by extraction from human pituitary glands, has been used to treat humans with catabolic stress [19]. The data suggested that GH promoted anabolism in these patients. As a result of the relative scarcity, cost and, more recently, the recognized potential hazards of human GH, its use was largely limited to growth retarded patients with GH deficiency [20]. With the development of recombinant human GH (rhGH), the potential for synthesizing large amounts of GH was now at hand, and its greater purity reduced the hazards of treatment. Several investigators have begun to explore the use of rhGH to promote growth and anabolism in patients with chronic renal failure. Initially, chronically azotemic rats were studied. Growth hormone extracted from human pituitary glands and injected intraperitoneally, 0.5 IU/day, was stated to be unsuccessful at increasing growth in azotemic or normal rats [21]. However, rhGH was successful at promoting growth and anabolism in these animals [21]. Subsequently, the growth promoting and anabolic effects of this hormone were tested, first in children and then in adults with chronic renal failure. The following paragraphs briefly review these studies.

Mehls et al. examined the effects of rhGH on the growth rate, the food conversion ratio and the rate of longitudinal growth at the proximal tibia level in female rats with subtotal nephrectomy or sham operation [21]. The rats received rhGH or vehicle either by continuous subcutaneous infusion using osmotic minipumps or by intraperitoneal injection for 14 days. Azotemic rats infused with GH, as compared to the pairfed azotemic rats given the vehicle, demonstrated significantly improved gain in body length ($P<0.01$), and weight ($P<0.01$) and an increased food utilization ratio ($P<0.01$). The sham operated control rats infused with GH, as compared to pairfed sham animals given vehicle, also displayed a greater increase in growth and food utilization ratios. The growth velocity and weight gain in the azotemic rats given GH tended to be lower than the normal values of the sham-operated control rats treated with GH. These observations are consistent with the thesis that there is resistance to the actions of GH in chronic renal failure. The findings are also consistent with a lower ^{3}H-thymidine incorporation in cartilage chondrocytes in GH retarded chronically azotemic vs GH treated controls [22]. Curiously, serum IGF-1 levels did not rise in the GH treated rats.

Nakano and colleagues studied the effects of daily subcutaneous injections of rat GH in rats with mild to moderate renal insufficiency that were fed a low 8% protein diet [23]. The low protein diet was selected in order to reduce the potential hazards of higher protein diets on the survival of the remnant kidneys. Rats underwent 75% nephrectomy or sham surgery. The azotemic rats were randomly assigned to receive rat GH or vehicle; sham rats received only vehicle. Animals were studied for 20 days while they ate ad libitum. The azotemic rats treated with GH, as compared to azotemic animals given vehicle, demonstrated significantly greater body weight, length, head size, food efficiency ratios, and serum albumin. There were no apparent differences in these parameters between the azotemic GH treated rats and vehicle treated sham controls. In this experimental model of mild to moderate renal failure, GH was growth-enhancing, despite the low 8% protein diet.

Koch, Lippe, and associates studied the effects of rhGH in five children with chronic renal failure who were not receiving dialysis treatment and who had growth retardation [13]. All five patients were treated for one year with 0.125 mg/kg of rhGH (methionyl human GH [Protropin],Genentech Inc.) three times per week. Before treatment, the children had a mean annual growth velocity of 4.9±1.4 (SD) cm/year, with a mean standard deviation score for height (height SDS) of less than −2.0. After one year of rhGH treatment, the mean growth rate increased to 8.9±1.2 cm/year, and the mean height SDS rose from −2.98±0.73 to −2.36±0.83 ($P<0.02$). In one patient, the rhGH dosage was increased after 6 months to 0.250 mg/kg three times per week, because the height gain with rhGH was only 20% greater than his baseline growth rate; there was no further increase in his growth velocity with the higher rhGH dose. For the five patients, the mean weight gain during the year before the therapy was 1.5±0.5 kg/year; this increased to 2.8± 0.8 kg/year by the end of the rhGH treatment. The creatinine clearances remained stable during the period of the study in all five patients. This was an issue of some concern because of the possibility that the hyperfiltration induced by GH might accelerate the rate of progression of the renal failure [24]. The glucose tolerance test was not significantly different in the pre- vs the post-treatment period. Antibodies to GH did not develop in any patient. The mean acid-chromatographed serum IGF-1 levels were normal in all the children at the start of the study and increased during rhGH treatment.

Tonshoff and coworkers gave rhGH to nine prepubertal children, eight of whom were undergoing continuous ambulatory peritoneal dialysis (CAPD, $n=7$), or maintenance hemodialysis (HD, $n=1$) and one of whom had advanced chronic renal failure not treated with dialysis [25]. Patients received growth hormone, 4U/m^2 (Genotropin, KabiVitrum), in daily subcutaneous injections for six months. During the six months of treatment, the mean annualized height velocity increased from −2.77±1.69 (SD) to +2.5±2.43 (i.e., from 4.5±2.47 cm to 8.3±1.77 cm) ($P<0.01$). Serum IGF-1 and IGF-II, measured by radioimmunoassay and expressed as percent of normal mean values, increased from 91±60 to 308±215 ($P<0.01$), and from 155±26 to 202±23 ($P<0.01$), respectively. Serum IGF-1 bioactivity, expressed as percent of normal, also rose from 40±7 to 119±35 ($P<0.01$). Bone age increased by an average of only 0.4 years during the six months of treatment, suggesting that rhGH treatment will not accelerate bone aging and closure of the epiphyses. There was no change in glucose tolerance or in serum insulin levels.

Two studies with rhGH have been carried out in adult patients undergoing maintenance hemodialysis. Ziegler and colleagues performed six studies in four men and one woman undergoing maintenance hemodialysis as outpatients [26]. Patients received rhGH, 5 or 10 mg, subcutaneously, postdialysis, three times weekly for two weeks. Net urea generation fell from 6.2±0.7 g/day during the week prior to treatment to 4.8±0.6 and 4.5±0.6 during the first and second weeks after therapy. Net protein catabolic rate also fell from 1.1±0.1 g/kg per day before treatment to 0.9±0.1 and 0.8±0.1 ($P<0.05$) during the first two weeks of treatment. Similarly, the mean weekly serum urea nitrogen (SUN) and the time averaged SUN fell during the two weeks of rhGH therapy. The authors reported that the dietary protein and energy intake did not change during treatment.

Table 1. Response of serum urea nitrogen (*SUN*) to daily growth hormone injections in a malnourished maintenance hemodialysis patient

Day of study	SUN (mg/dl) pre/post	Day of study	SUN (mg/dl) pre/post
5	90/32	21	93/35
7	91/37	22	Start GH, 0.05 mg/kg per day
12	97/43	23	82/33
14	92/40	26	75/33
19	96/44	28	56/26

GH, growth hormone

We have commenced a series of studies to evaluate the role of rhGH in malnourished maintenance hemodialysis patients. Criteria for acceptance into the study included evidence for protein-calorie malnutrition, as indicated by a body weight of 90% or less of desirable, determined from the Metropolitan Life Insurance Tables [27], or a serum albumin of 3.4 g/dl or less. Patients were studied for five weeks in the Clinical Research Center at Harbor UCLA Medical Center, where they ingested a constant diet that provided, each day, the patients' usual protein and energy intake. All diets were supplemented with calcium, at least 800 mg/day, and multivitamins, including folic acid. After the first 14 days of baseline study, rhGH (Somotrem [Genentech Inc.]) was administered at 0.05 mg/kg per day for 21 days. The key outcome measures included SUN, nitrogen balance, serum albumin and anthropometry.

At present two men and one women have been studied. All showed substantial evidence for malnutrition or protein calorie wasting. Edema-free relative body weights at the onset of study in the three patients were 70%, 74%, and 71%, respectively. The prestudy bone-free upper arm muscle areas in the three patients were in the <5, 7, and <5 percentiles, respectively, for normal adults of similar sex, height, and frame sizes and roughly similar age range. Patient 1 developed an unrelated illness and was removed from the study after 8 days of rhGH injections. Patients 2 and 3 left the study after 19 and 21 days of rhGH treatment.

After commencing the rhGH therapy, the predialysis SUN levels fell, even though the daily protein and energy intake and the hemodialysis regimen did not change. In Patient 1, the decrease in predialysis SUN appeared to begin within 24 hours of starting GH therapy (Table 1). Predialysis SUN also fell in Patients 2 and 3 within one day after starting daily growth hormone injections. However, the fall in SUN in Patient 3 was substantially less and transient, possibly because she developed pancreatitis during the course of the study. Analyses of the nitrogen balance data to date have been completed only in Patient 1. The results indicate that this patient went into markedly positive nitrogen balance.

These initial data suggest that rhGH may markedly improve protein balance in at least some malnourished maintenance hemodialysis patients. It must be emphasized that these GH studies are both very preliminary and of short duration. It has not yet been demonstrated that the chronic use of GH will improve body composition, clinical status, and quality of life, or that its chronic use will reduce symptoms, or reduce morbidity or mortality. Longterm studies of GH treatment in more maintenance hemodialysis patients will be necessary to examine these questions.

Another potential use of GH is for the treatment of patients with renal disease or acute or chronic renal failure who have a superimposed catabolic illness. It has been suggested that GH may reduce the degree of catabolism in these patients, and that this might improve host resistance, reduce morbidity and mortality, and facilitate recovery and convalescence. If these hypotheses can be proven, it could be particularly beneficial for the severely ill patient with acute renal failure. The mortality rate for acute renal failure patients remains very high. This is especially true for those acute renal failure patients who have surgical problems, have multiple complications, or require hemodialysis. Patients who have shock or sepsis as the cause of acute renal failure, and are not able to be nourished enterally because of a poorly functioning gastrointestinal tract, also have a marked morbidity and mortality rate; their overall mortality is about 85% [28–30].

These individuals may be severely catabolic, with a net rate of protein degradation that may rise to 150 g per day or greater [29,30]. Provision of intravenous nutrition to these individuals often has little effect on their degree of negative nitrogen balance. This is due to their metabolic status, which is programmed toward degrading fuel substrates, including protein and amino acids. It has been speculated that administration of anabolic agents, including growth factors, may alter the metabolic status of these patients and facilitate their ability to utilize both exogenous and endogenous nutrients more effectively. An hypothesis that underpins this approach is that if hypercatabolic individuals can be induced to improve their utilization of nutrients and to reduce their marked degree of wasting, they will demonstrate improved morbidity and mortality.

At present, growth hormone treatment has not been specifically studied in catabolic patients with renal failure. However, such studies have been performed in acutely catabolic or malnourished surgical patients who usually did not have renal failure. The results of these studies will be briefly reviewed, since the results may be pertinent to the use of GH for stressed patients with renal failure.

Okamura and associates studied the effects of rhGH on protein metabolism in rats with sepsis induced by cecal ligation [31]. Ten rats underwent sham-operation. All rats were nourished with total parenteral nutrition. Cumulative nitrogen balance was significantly more positive in the septic rats given TPN and 200 mU/day of rhGH as compared with the septic animals given TPN without rhGH. In the former rats, as compared to the sham-operated controls, cumulative nitrogen balance was not statistically different, although it tended to be less positive; serum albumin was slightly lower ($P<0.05$), and urinary N^T-methylhistidine (3-methylhistidine), a marker of myofibrillar protein breakdown, was slightly greater ($P<0.01$).

Several studies indicate that in postoperative patients, GH in pharmacological doses may promote an anabolic response [32–34]. Zhu-Ming et al. investigated the effects of hypocaloric feedings with or without injections of rhGH in 18 patients who underwent gastrointestinal surgery [32]. This was a placebo-controlled double blind randomized trial. Starting on the third day before surgery and continuing throughout the postoperative period of study, patients were given intravenous infusions of nutrient solutions providing 20 kcal/kg body weight per day and 1 g amino acids/kg per day. Commencing with the first day after the day of surgery, nine patients received daily subcutaneous injections of placebo (control group) and nine patients received intramuscular injections of 0.15 IU rhGH/kg per day. This rhGH regimen was continued for seven postoperative days. In the control group, the subjects were consistently in negative nitrogen balance (-32.6 ± 4.2 g/8 days). The urinary excretion of N^T-methylhistidine rose from preoperative values of 4.4 ± 0.7 to

7.26±1.01 umol/kg per day. In the GH treated group, the nitrogen balance was less negative, −7.1±3.12 g/8 days ($P<0.001$ vs controls), and the N^{T}-methylhistidine excretion was 3.6±0.3 and 4.4±0.3 umol/kg per day, respectively, before surgery and on postoperative day 7 (postoperative N^{T}-methylhistidine excretion in GH treated vs controls, $P<0.05$). The patients receiving rhGH lost, on average, 1.7% of their body weight, whereas the control group lost a mean of 6% of their body weight. Analysis of body composition revealed that the patients receiving GH maintained their lean body mass. The authors concluded that the postoperative catabolic response in patients receiving hypocaloric nutrients can be significantly ameliorated with the use of GH.

Ziegler et al. studied the metabolic effects of rhGH in nine clinically stable malnourished patients receiving hypocaloric parenteral nutrition [33]. Patients were studied for two consecutive 7-day periods while they received a hypocaloric intake that provided approximately 1100 kcal/day and 1.3 g amino acids/kg per day. During the 7 day control period, patients received a daily subcutaneous injection of saline; during the treatment period, the rhGH was given subcutaneously at a dose of 10 mg/day. In seven studies rhGH was given in the second week and in two studies it was given during the first week. Nitrogen balance was +0.5±0.9 (SEM) g/day during the control period and +3.4±0.5 g/day during the treatment period ($P<0.001$). Phosphorus balance was 0±29 mg/day during the control period and +218±32 mg/day during the GH period ($P<0.001$).

Six patients of Ziegler et al. received rhGH for 13–25 days [33]. Significantly positive nitrogen balance was observed for the entire period of rhGH administration. No side effects were observed. Serum IGF-1 increased markedly during rhGH treatment.

Manson and coworkers studied four healthy men who underwent eight paired studies in which they were given a constant amount of parenteral nutrition for two 7-day periods separated by at least two weeks [34]. The energy intake in the paired studies was calculated to provide 100% (2 studies), 50% (4 studies), or 30% (2 studies) of the subjects' calculated energy needs. During the first 7-day period, the individuals received GH, 10 mg/day, subcutaneously. In the second 7-day period, they received a daily injection of saline. With the GH as compared to the saline injections, the subjects demonstrated significantly more positive nitrogen balance and protein synthesis and increased serum insulin and plasma IGF-1 concentrations. After an oral glucose load, the GH-treated individuals appeared to show higher blood glucose values and attenuated muscle uptake of glucose and release of amino acids.

In contrast to these studies, Dahn et al. gave rhGH (methionyl human GH) 1 mg intramuscularly every six hours for 48 hours to acutely ill septic patients [35]. During the 48-hour period, the septic patients displayed no increase in plasma IGF-1 or in urinary urea nitrogen, and manifested a fall in splanchnic amino acid uptake. The normal control subjects, who were similarly treated with GH, showed a rise in plasma IGF-1, a fall in urinary urea nitrogen and no change in the splanchnic amino acid uptake. These findings suggest that GH may not be effective at promoting anabolism in acutely and severely stressed patients, at least when given over short periods of time. Since plasma IGF-1 also did not rise in response to the GH injections in these patients, it is possible that an injection of IGF-1 might be more effective at promoting anabolism in acutely and severely ill patients. It is pertinent in this regard that Mehls et al. found no increase in ^{3}H-thymidine incorporation into growing cartilage chondrocytes in rats with acute uremia that were given GH vs those given the solvent [22].

In summary, rhGH shows great promise for promoting longterm (i.e., at least one year) increased growth in children with chronic renal failure. In malnourished adults with chronic renal failure, preliminary studies indicate that rhGH increases nitrogen balance. Whether increased protein balance will enhance nutritional or clinical status or improve morbidity and mortality in these patients is not yet known. In nonuremic catabolic patients, GH may improve protein balance. However, in severely ill septic patients, GH may not exert these effects, at least during the first two days of treatment. It is possible that most, or all, of these effects of GH are mediated by IGF-1; whether giving IGF-1 will improve nutritional status in these patients is not known. The role of GH for growth enhancement in nondialyzed children with renal disease needs to be clarified; whether this therapy will accelerate the rate of progression of renal failure must be examined. Further studies are necessary to define more precisely the role for GH in the treatment of growth retarded, malnourished, or catabolic patients with acute or chronic renal disease and renal failure.

References

1. Felig P, Baxter JD, Broadus AE, Frohman LA (eds) (1987) Endocrinology and metabolism. McGraw-Hill, pp 264–269, 1584–1589
2. Daughday WH, Hall K, Salmon WD (1987) On the nomenclature of the somatomedins and insulin like growth factors. Endocrinology 121:1911–1912
3. Ronge H, Blum J (1989) Insulin-like growth factor I responses to recombinant bovine growth hormone during feed restriction in heifers. Acta Endocrinol (Copenh) 120:735–744
4. Johnson V and Maack T (1977) Renal extraction, filtration, absorption and catabolism of growth hormone. Am J Physiol 233 (3):F185–F196
5. Kopple JD (1978) Abnormal amino acid and protein metabolism in uremia. Kidney Int 14:340–348
6. Blumenkrantz MJ, Kopple JD, Gutman RA, Chan YK et al (1980) Methods for assessing nutritional status of patients with renal failure. Am J Clin Nutr 33:1567–1585
7. Acchiardo SR, Moore LW, Latour PA (1983) Malnutrition as the main factor in morbidity and mortality of hemodialysis patients. Kidney Int 24 (Suppl 16):S199–S203
8. Lowrie EG, Lew NC (1990) Death risk in hemodialysis patients: the predictive value of commonly measured variables and an evaluation of death rate differences between facilities. Am J Kidney Dis 15:458–482
9. Delaporte C, Gros F, Anagnostopoulos T (1980) Inhibitory effects of plasma dialysate on protein synthesis in vitro: influence of dialysis and transplantation. Am J Clin Nutr 33:1407–1410
10. Dzurik R, Hupkova V, Cernaceck P, Valovicova E, Niederland TR (1973) The isolation of an inhibitor of glucose utilization from the serum of uremic subjects. Clin Chim Acta 46:77–83
11. Phillips LS, Kopple JD (1981) Circulating somatomedin activity and sulfate levels in adults with normal and impaired kidney function. Metabolism 30:1091–1095
12. El-Bishti M, Counahan R, Bloom S (1978) Hormonal and metabolic responses to intravenous glucose in children on regular hemodialysis. Am J Clin Nutr 31:1865–1869
13. Koch VH, Lippe BM, Nelson PA, Boechat MI, Sherman BM, Fine RN (1989) Accelerated growth after recombinant human growth hormone treatment of children with chronic renal failure. J Pediatr 115:365–371

14. Mehls O, Fine RN (1989) The use of human recombinant growth hormone for treatment of growth failure in uremia. Semin Nephrol 9:43–48
15. Linder A, Tenckhoff H (1972) Influence of anabolic steroids on nitrogen balance in chronic peritoneal dialysis. Nephron 9:77–83
16. Gjorup S, Thaysen JH (1960) The effect of anabolic steroid (Durabolin [R]) in the conservative management of acute renal failure. Acta Med Scand 167:227
17. Fine RN (1984) Growth in children with renal insufficiency. In: Nissensen AR, Fine RN, Gentile DE (eds) Clinical Dialysis. Appleton-Century-Crofts, Norwalk, pp 661–669
18. Salusky IB, Fine RN, Nelson P, Blumenkrantz MJ, Kopple JD (1983) Nutritional status of children undergoing continuous ambulatory peritoneal dialysis. Am J Clin Nutr 38:595–611
19. Wilmore DW, Moylan JA, Bristow BF, Masom AD, Pruitt BA (1974) Anabolic effects of human growth hormone and high caloric feedings following thermal injury. Surg Gynecol Obstet 138:875–884
20. Brown P, Gajdusek DC, Gibbs CJ, Asher DM (1985) Potential epidemic of Creutzfeldt-Jakobs disease from human growth hormone therapy. N Engl J Med 313:728–731
21. Mehls O, Ritz E, Hunziker E-B, Eggli P, Heinrich U, Zapf J (1988) Improvement of growth and food utilization by human recombinant growth hormone in uremia. Kidney Int 33:45–52
22. Mehls O, Ritz E, Hunziker E-B, Tonshoff B, Heinrich U (1988) Role of growth hormone in growth failure of uremia. Perspective for application of recombinant growth hormone. Acta Paediatr Scand [Suppl] 343:118–126
23. Nakano M, Kainer G, Foreman JW, Ko D, Chan JCM (1989) The effects of exogenous rat growth hormone therapy on growth of uremic rats fed an 8% protein diet. Pediatr Res 26:204–207
24. Doi T, Striker LJ, Quaife C, Conti FG, Palmiter R, Behringer R, Brinster R, Striker GE (1988) Progressive glomerulosclerosis develops in transgenic mice chronically expressing growth hormone releasing factor but not in those expressing insulin like growth factor-1. Am J Pathol 131:398–403
25. Tonshoff B, Mehls O, Schauer A, Henrich U, Blum W, Ranke M (1989) Improvement of uremic growth failure by recombinant human growth hormone. Kidney Int 36 (Suppl 27):S201–S204
26. Ziegler TR, Lazarus JM, Young LS, Hakim R, Wilmore DW (1990) Growth hormone administration decreases urea generation in patients undergoing chronic hemodialysis. Clin Res 38:355A
27. Metropolitan Life Insurance Co (1983) Metropolitan height and weight tables. Stat Bull Metrop Life Found 64:1
28. Kopple JD (1988) Dietary considerations in patients with advanced chronic renal failure, acute renal failure and transplantation. In: Schrier RW, Gottschalk CW (eds) Diseases of the kidney. Little Brown, Boston, pp 3387–3436
29. Feinstein EI, Blumenkrantz MJ, Healy M, Koffler A, Silberman H, Massry SG, Kopple JD (1981) Clinical and metabolic responses to parenteral nutrition in acute renal failure. Medicine (Baltimore) 60:124–137
30. Feinstein EI, Kopple JD, Silberman H, Massry SG (1983) Total parenteral nutrition with high or low nitrogen intakes in patients with acute renal failure. Kidney Int 26 (Suppl. 16):S319–S323
31. Okamura K, Toshitada O, Tabira Y, Miyauchi Y (1989) Effect of administered human growth hormone on protein metabolism in septic rats. Journal Parenteral and Enteral Nutrition (Baltimore) 13:450–454
32. Zhu-Ming J, Gui-Zhen H, Si-Yuan Z, Xiu-Rong W, Nai-Fai Y, Yu Z, Wilmore DW (1989) Low-dose growth hormone and hypocaloric nutrition attenuate the protein catabolic response after major operation. Ann Surg 210:513–524

33. Ziegler TR, Lorraine SY, Manson JM, Wilmore DW (1988) Metabolic effects of recombinant human growth hormone in patients receiving parenteral nutrition. Ann Surg 208:6–16
34. Manson JM, Smith RJ, Wilmore DW (1988) Growth hormone stimulates protein synthesis during hypocaloric parenteral nutrition. Ann Surg 208:136–142
35. Dahn MS, Lange P, Jacobs LA (1988) Insulin like growth factor 1 production is inhibited in human sepsis. Arch Surg 123:1409–1414

Myocardial Function in Hemodialysis Patients

D.C. Schohn, P.A. Petitjean, and H.A. Jahn[1]

Summary. Myocardial impairment in hemodialysis patients is mainly due to the alterations induced by the predialytic uremic stage. Hemodialysis treatment may improve some of these disturbances: by maintaining a normal salt and fluid balance, by clearing uremic toxins, and by ameliorating nutritional status. But hemodialysis treatment may also have deleterious effects: due to A.V. fistula, to hypotension related to ultrafiltration or acetate dialysate, or due to bioincompatibility and β^2 accumulation with amyloid deposition.

Treatment of hypertension, anemia and hyperparathyroidism needs particular attention and care.

Introduction

Cardiovascular complications take a prominent place in the statistical evaluation of morbidity and mortality in hemodialysis patients and promoting the prevention of these complications remains a constant endeavor. Awareness of the fundamental alterations of the myocardium needs efficient diagnostic investigations of the cardiovascular status. These are most often based on pressure measurements, on ejection fraction and circumferential fiber shortening determinations, and on morphologic evaluations of ventricular wall thickening.

The tremendous work accomplished to elucidate the role of pathogenetic factors, such as ventricular pre and afterload modifications, metabolic, endocrine, toxic and nutritional disturbances may provide helpful hints for management strategies. In recent years great progress, which appears very promising, has been made in the control of hypertension, nutritional prevention of uremic toxemia and in the correction of anemia both in predialytic uremics and in hemodialysis patients.

[1]Nephrology Department, Louis Pasteur University, 67092 Strasbourg Cedex, France

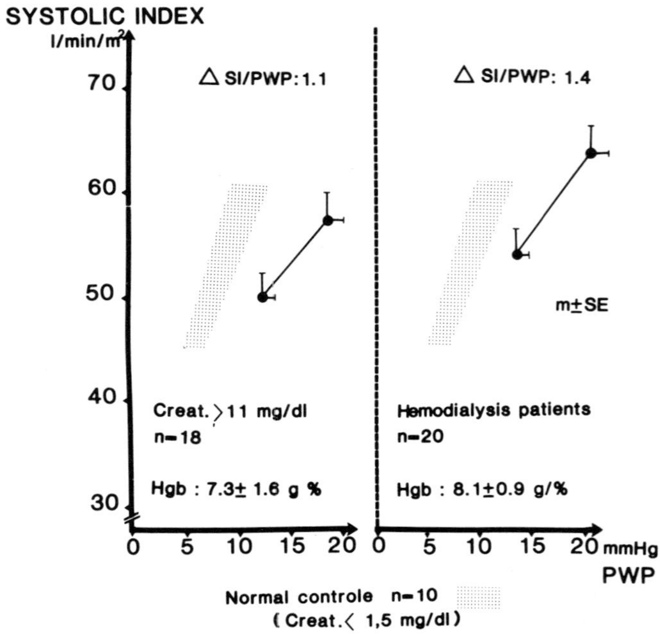

Fig. 1. Cardiac function curves (according to Frank and Starling) in chronic renal failure patients (creatinine > 11 mg/dl) and in hemodialysis patients compared with the area of normal function curves. PWP, pulmonary wedge pressure; SI, systolic index

The place of myocardial dysfunction in cardiovascular mortality statistics is difficult to evaluate. The European Dialysis and Transplant Association (EDTA) report of 1983 [1] mentions that cardiovascular disease represents 52.6% of all causes of death in hemodialysis patients, with the following origins: 14.1% cardiac failure, 12.9% cardiac arrest, 12.3% coronary disease, and 10.9% cerebrovascular lesions. Echocardiographic studies show that a high percentage of hemodialysis patients present with myocardial disturbances. Ejection fraction of left ventricle is reduced [2,3]. Left ventricular hypertrophy has been found in up to 66% of patients [4]. Invasive investigations have shown that cardiac function curves display reduced ventricular performance (Fig. 1).

Pressure Measurements and Myocardial Performance

Intracardiac pressures determine the cardiac output and reflect the adequacy of myocardial performance. In renal failure with disturbed volume homeostasis, pressure elevations are correlated to increased blood volume due to fluid overload. Pressure measurements are therefore an important clue for correction of volume disturbances. They represent the earliest sign of increased preload related to fluid overload and high fistula blood flows [5].

Table 1. Hemodynamic parameters in hemodialysis patients versus normal subjects and end stage renal failure patients

	$\overline{AP}$ (mm Hg)	HR (bpm)	$\overline{RAP}$ (mm Hg)	$\overline{PWP}$ (mm Hg)	CI (1/min per m^2)	SI (ml/b per m^2)	SVR (dyn/sec per cm^{-5})
* Normal subjects	103 ± 17	72 ± 8	0 ± 2	9 ± 3	3.08 ± 0.06	43.82 ± 6.11	1420 ± 210
n=29	(88 → 121)	(60 → 82)	(−3 → 3)	(5 → 13)	(2.91 → 3.36)	(36.12 → 53.11)	(799 → 1715)
* End stage renal failure	117 ± 15[a]	84 ± 13	4 ± 3[a]	12 ± 4[a]	4.11 ± 0.22[b]	50.17 ± 9.15[a]	1546 ± 329
n=51	(92 → 141)	(68 → 106)	(0 → 8)	(7 → 16)	(3.53 → 4.66)	(40.76 → 64.13)	1022 → 2113
* Hemodialysis patients	115 ± 14[a]	76 ± 8	5 ± 2[a]	13 ± 3[a]	3.97 ± 0.41[a]	54.25 ± 7.28[b]	1609 ± 281[a]
n=113	(88 → 136)	(64 → 91)	(1 → 10)	(8 → 18)	(3.01 → 4.42)	(37.16 → 71.81)	(713 → 2088)

m±sd
[a]$P<0.05$
[b]$P<0.01$ versus normal subject extreme values in brackets ( )
AP, arterial pressure; HR, heart rate; RAP, right atrial pressure; PWP, pulmonary wedge pressure; CI, cardiac index; SI, saturation index; SVR, systemic vascular resistance

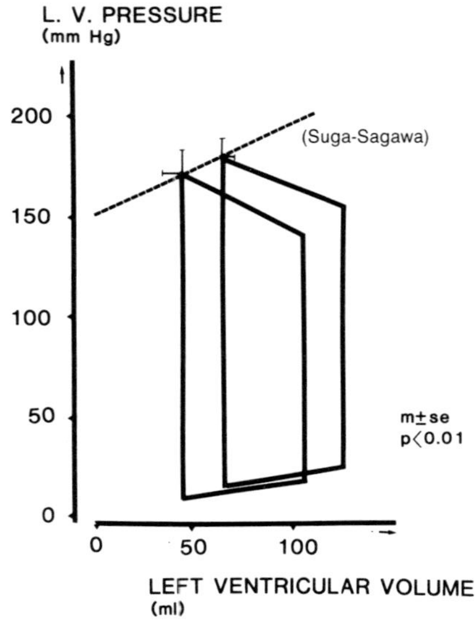

Fig. 2. Left ventricular pressure/volume relation before and after 0.9% saline infusion in dialysis patients (n=7) (plasma creat.: 10.6±3.1 mg/dl). Suga-Sagawa line less steep than normal indicates reduced inotropic state

Usually, right atrial pressure and pulmonary wedge pressure are slightly higher in chronic hemodialysis patients than in normal subjects (Table 1). It is not clearly established whether these values indicate inadequacy of myocardial performance or a slight increase of volume. When distinctly elevated they usually indicate myocardial failure with more or less fluid overload [5].

In Table 1 we show the hemodynamic parameters obtained in normal subjects in chronic renal failure and in hemodialysis patients. The cardiac output and systolic index are increased and are related to the degree of anemia [5,6]. The cardiac function curves, following Frank Starling, obtained by volume expansion with saline [7] are shifted to the right and are less steep in comparison to normal curves. These curves display a diminished contractile state and impaired myocardial performance and may also imply a diminished myocardial compliance (Fig. 1).

The left ventricular systolo-diastolic pressure/volume loop permits a load independent evaluation of left ventricular performance. In hemodialyzed patients it is shifted to the right and the Suga-Sagawa curve is less steep, indicating reduced inotropy [5,7,8] (Fig. 2).

The echocardiographic established ejection fraction and circumferential fiber shortening of the left ventricle produce similar results when confirmed myocardial impairment exists; they are less efficient in early states characterized only by abnormal pressures.

Ventricular function seems, therefore, to be impaired in hemodialysis patients. The degree of impairment is different from patient to patient, extending from near normal to profound disturbance. Hyperdynamic circulatory states were observed due

Table 2. Echocardiographic studies

	51 CHD patients[a]	14 out of 51 CHD patients with L.V. hypertrophy
Age (years)	50.14 ± 17.35	52.5 ± 19.1
Duration of dialysis (months)	34.96 ± 47.49	48.6 ± 70.49
Systolic AP (mmHg)	145.55 ± 32.6	155 ± 29.2
Diastolic AP (mmHg)	85.39 ± 13.78	87.76 ± 16.8
$\overline{\text{AP}}$ (mm Hg)	105.33 ± 17.31	104.9 ± 23
IST (mm)		
Systolic	13.87 ± 2.97	16.61 ± 2.47
Diastolic	10.46 ± 2.72	13.85 ± 1.75
LVPW (mm)		
Systolic	11.6 ± 2.55	13.33 ± 2.26
Diastolic	8.5 ± 2.0	9.9 ± 1.85
LVD (mm)		
Systolic	37.3 ± 8.8	40.1 ± 9.2
Diastolic	52.2 ± 7.6	54.1 ± 7.6
L.V. mass (gr)	243.7 ± 108	342.6 ± 140.8
EF (%)	63.4 ± 11.7	59 ± 14.5
Vcf (%)	29.3 ± 8.3	27.9 ± 9.8

CHD, chronic hemodialysis; AP, arterial pressure; IST, interventricular septum thickness; LVPW, left ventricular posterior wall; LVD, left ventricular dimension; EF, left ventricular ejection fraction; Vcf, circumferential fiber shortening of left ventricle
[a]mean values ± standard deviation

to anemia and to inotropic stimulation of parathyroidhormone. Associated heart disease contributes, in many situations, to the alterations of cardiac performance [9].

Immediate dialysate and ultrafiltration effects have been studied extensively: acetate dialysate enhances the peripheral contractile state due to vasodilatation and has a direct inotropic effect on the myocardium. During ultrafiltration, acetate vasodilatation mainly imprints the cardiovascular function and may induce severe hypotension [10,11]. Bicarbonate dialysate, per se, has no direct effect on myocardial performance; during ultrafiltration, peripheral vasoconstriction occurs and cardiac output diminishes.

Echomorphologic Changes of the Myocardium

Echocardiographic studies provide reliable information on the morphologic status of the myocardium; these studies comprise analysis of the interventricular septum, the left ventricular posterior wall, and the left ventricular mass and diameter.

The occurrence of the changes is diversely evaluated from 30% (Table 2)–66% [3,4]. The modifications consist of:

1) an increase in the diameter of the left and right atrium and left ventricle,
2) an increase in ventricular posterior wall thickness,
3) an asymmetric increase of interventricular septum,
4) an augmentation of left ventricular mass.

These modifications may all be found in the predialytic state.

Table 3. Risk involved in the genesis of arrhythmias in chronic hemodialysis patients

Myocardiopathy
Hypertrophy and/or dilatation
Pericardial disease
Electrolyte disturbances:
K^+, Ca^{2+}, Mg, Acidosis
Hypoxemia
Hypocapnia
Autonomous nervous system disturbances
Renin angiotensin system activation
Dialysis technique
rapid ultrafiltration
inadequate dialysate
Drugs: cardiac glycosides

A few observations provide some evidence of the role of hemodialysis in patients with uncontrollable weight gain. It is common to observe that fluid removal by ultrafiltration modifies the X ray silhouette and the echocardiographic images of the heart. In two observations we observed hypokinetic wall motion. In one patient it was located mainly in the right ventricle and was due to amyloid infiltration, perhaps related to bioincompatibility.

Severe morphologic abnormalities aggravate functional performance, conceivably both by impairment of myocardial compliance and contractility, but moderate modifications do not correlate with the results of functional investigations.

Clinical Manifestations

Slight impairments of myocardial performance remain asymptomatic or induce various intensities of exercise intolerance which are involved with the effects of anemia on oxygen supply.

In hemodialysis patients the degree of weight gain inducing dyspnea, may be a hint of the degree of myocardial impairment. Such weight gains are accompanied by elevations of pulmonary wedge pressure. Conversely, fluid removal by ultrafiltration may also be the expression of myocardial impairment: in such cases hypotension occurs as a consequence of inadaptation of cardiac output to removal of even a small volume of fluid.

Overt heart failure is rarely due to an impaired myocardial performance alone, usually other causes are added, such as salt and fluid overload; high A.V. fistula flows; hypertension; valvulopathy; coronary heart disease; and arrhythmias.

Myocardial intolerance may be expressed by dysrhythmias, tachycardia, and arrhythmia, which usually occur during dialysis treatment. Their pathogenesis is not yet clear (Table 3).

Factors Influencing Myocardial Function

Related to Renal Failure

Most of the disturbances of myocardial function and morphology may be present in the uremic state before dialysis treatment. Uremic myocardiopathy results from the

Table 4. Factors influencing myocardial function in chronic hemodialysis patients

Preload and/or afterload
Weight gain and fluid overload
Hypertension
Hypotension
Pericardial involvements
Myocardial cell function
K^+, Ca^{2+}, acidosis
Oxygen supply:
anemia
coronary atherosclerosis
Nutritional supply:
amino acids, fatty acids, carnitine, insulin sensitivity
Toxic influences:
biocompatibility
uremic toxins
Disturbed control systems
Autonomic nervous system
Catecholamines, receptors
Hyperparathyroidism
Hypocalcitriolemia
Renin angiotensin

consequences of renal failure and the associated organic metabolic and endocrine disorder. (enumerated in Table 4).

Hypertension, with its increase of afterload, has the most deleterious effects on the heart. It is one of the main factors of left ventricular hypertrophy. Its effects on coronary arteries enhance development of atherosclerosis [12].

Anemia reduces oxygen supply. It is one of the factors which induces increased cardiac output and acceleration of heart rate [5].

Hyperparathyroidism may enhance cardiac contractility [13] but its ionophore effects determine myocytic calcinosis [14]. Its effects on mitochondrial energy production make excess parathyroid hormone a dangerous uremic toxin [15]. It has been shown to be responsible for myocardial hypertrophy [16].

Hypocalcitriolemia has been experimentally shown to be responsible for hypertrophy of myocardial interstitium at the expense of myofibrills [17]. Angiotensin may also contribute to the hypertrophy of myofibrills.

Autonomic nervous system disturbances comprise high levels of catecholamines and alteration of receptor activity. They therefore diminish the capacity of the myocardium to adapt to the necessity of the organism and to induce regulation which interferes with load problems. The sensitivity of the beta-adrenergic receptors is decreased in renal failure and is reduced much more in hemodialysis patients, as shown by the response of the heart rate to injection of increasing doses of isoproterenol. The dose response curve (injected dose of isoproterenol versus delta heart rate increase) is shifted to the right, compared with the curve obtained in normal subjects. The chronotropic dose 25 is significantly increased [18].

The negativity of nitrogen balance in uremia denotes profound effects on striated muscle cells. These problems with disturbed aminograms of uremia and altered carnitine metabolism have been implicated in the genesis of uremic myocardiopathy [19].

Dialysis Related Effects

Fistula flow has been compared to the effects of arterio-venous aneurysm on heart function. High blood flow may induce modifications of preload. Heart failure has been reported. Shunt effects may also produce blood steeling effects on coronary flow.

Dialysis hypotension has deleterious effects on coronary circulation and must be avoided. The causes of hypotension are related to ultrafiltration rate, acetate dialysis, and bioincompatibility. These factors need therefore to be strictly monitored. Other factors which have to be taken into account are: antihypertensive drugs, autonomic neuropathy, and myocardiopathy itself.

Electrolyte disturbances and acidosis interfere with myocardial function and need to be monitored.

Beta 2 microglobulin which is retained in renal failure and is elevated in hemodialysis patients may be a factor in the genesis of amyloidosis.

Prevention of Myocardial Dysfunction

Prevention of myocardial dysfunction has to begin during the predialytic uremic state. Four main fields of progress seem to be promising:

1) The nutritional management of uremia, with drastic protein restriction and reduced accumulation of uremic toxins [20], usually supplemented with essential amino acids or keto acids of essential amino acids which ameliorate calcium phosphate metabolism and diminish hyperparathyroidism.
2) Administration of calcitriol may have protective effects per se on the myocardium [17] and may diminish hyperparathyroidism [21].
3) Administration of erythropoietin for correction of anemia maintains normal oxygen supply and avoids increased cardiac work. Data on beneficial effects have been reported [22,23].
4) The improved treatment of hypertension. Direct influences of medications on the myocardium have been suggested and need confirmation. Beta-blockers seem to prevent hypertrophy. Ca-channel blockers have been reported to influence coronary atherosclerosis. Converting enzyme inhibition prevents the hypertrophic effects of angiotensin II on myocardial cells.

Several improvements of hemodialysis techniques may reduce the influence of hemodialysis on the myocardial function.

It is most important to maintain the patient near his/her dry weight with normal pulmonary wedge pressure, to avoid the effects of increased preload.

Bicarbonate dialysate seems to ease fluid removal. Both hemofiltration and hemodiafiltration have, in this respect, advantages over conventional hemodialysis. More biocompatible membranes and better extractions of β^2 microglobulin will perhaps bring further ameliorations.

References

1. Geerling W, Tufveson G, Broyer M, Brunner FP, Brynger H, Fassbinder W (1983) Combined report on regular dialysis and transplantation in Europe. Proc Eur Dial Transplant Assoc 17:52–54
2. MacDonald IL, Uldall R, Buda AJ (1981) The effect of hemodialysis on cardiac rhythm and performance. Clin Nephrol 6:321–327
3. Lai KN, Whitford J, Buttfield I, Fasset RG, Mathew TH (1985) Left ventricular function in uremia: echocardiographic and radionuclide assessment in patients on maintenance hemodialysis. Clin Nephrol 23:125–133
4. London GM, Marchais SJ, Guérin AP, Fabiani F, Métivier F (1990) Fonction cardiovasculaire du sujet Hémodialysé. In: Hamburger J (ed) Actualités Néphrologiques. Flammarion, Paris, pp 283–302
5. Jahn HA, Schohn DC, Schmitt RL (1986) The heart in renal disease. In: Cheng Tsung O (ed) The international textbook of cardiology. Perga, New York, 988–1009
6. Jahn HA (1988) The cardiovascular system in uremia. Report of the Xth International Congress of Nephrology, London, pp 1026–1037
7. Jahn H, Schmitt R, Schohn D, Olier P (1984) Aspects of myocardial function in chronic renal failure. Contrib Nephrol 41:240–250
8. Kramer W, Wizemann V, Lämmlein G, Thormann J, Kindler M, Schlepper M, Schütter G (1986) Cardiac dysfunction in patients on maintenance hemodialysis. Contrib Nephrol 52:110–124
9. Kramer W, Wizemann V, Thormann J, Kindler M, Mueller K, Schlepper M (1986) Cardiac dysfunction in patients on maintenance hemodialysis. I) The importance of associated heat diseases in determining alterations of cardiac performance. Contrib Nephrol 52:97–109
10. Schohn D, Schmitt R, Jahn H (1986) Myocardial impairment in chronic hemodialysis patients. Effect of acetate hemodialysis. Contrib Nephrol 52:69–85
11. Jahn H, Schohn D, Schmitt R (1983) Hemodynamic modifications induced by fluid removal and treatment modalities in chronic hemodialysis patients. Blood Purif (1)80: 80–89
12. Rostand SG, Kirk KA, Rutsky EA (1982) Relationship of coronary risk factors to dialysis-associated ischemic heart disease. Kidney Int 22:304–308
13. Jahn H, Schohn D, Schmitt R Plasma parathormone levels (PTH) and heart function in end stage renal failure patients (abstract). IXth International Congress of Nephrology, June 11–16 1984. Los Angeles, USA, 51A
14. Massry SG (1987) Cardiovascular complications in chronic renal failure. Contrib Nephrol 54:177–189
15. Bogin E, Massry SG, Harray I (1981) Effects of parathyroid hormone on rat heart cells. J Clin Invest 67:1215–1227
16. London GM, Vernejoul De MC, Fabiani F, Marchais SJ, Guérin AP, Métivier F, London AM, Llach F (1987) Secondary hyperparathyroidism and cardiac hypertrophy in hemodialysis patients. Kidney Int 32:900–907
17. Weishaar RE, Sang-Nam K, Dwit ES, Robert US (1990) Involvement of vitamin D3 with cardiovascular function. III. Effects of physical and morphological properties. Am J Physiol 258:E134–E142
18. Schohn DC, Weidmann P, Jahn HA, Beretta-Piccoli C (1985) Norepinephrine-related mechanism in hypertension accompanying renal failure. Kidney Int 28:814–822
19. Drüeke T, Le Pailleur C (1981) Cardiomyopathy in uremia: hemodynamic and metabolic aspects. Nephrologie 2:63
20. Kopple JD (1988) Dietary considerations in patients with advanced chronic renal failure, acute renal failure and transplantation. In: Schrier RW, Gottschaltk CW (eds) Diseases of the kidney, vol 3, 4th edn. Little, Brown, New York pp 3387–3436

21. Mc Gonigle C, Fowler MB, Timmis AB, Weston MJ, Parsons Y (1984) Uremic cardiomyopathy: potential role of vitamin D and parathyroid hormone. Nephron 36:94–100
22. Tsutsui M, Suzuki M, Hirasawa Y (1989) Renewed cardiovascular dynamics induced by recombinant erythropoietin administration. Nephrol Dial Transplant 4:146–150
23. London GM, Zins B, Pannier B, Naret C, Berthelot JM, Jacquot C, Safar M, Drüeke TB (1989) Vascular changes in hemodialysis patients in response to recombinant human erythropoietin. Kidney Int 36:878–882

Electrophysiological and Biofunctional Abnormalities in Uremic Neuropathy

Alberto Albertazzi, Mario Bonomini, and Bruno Di Paolo[1]

SUMMARY. The pathophysiology of central and peripheral nervous system dysfunctions in uremia has been extensively evaluated by neurophysiological studies and biofunctional techniques during the last few years. In order to investigate uremia-related nervous alterations in our cohort of patients clinical research was supported by electrophysiology and experimental work in synaptosomes drawn from uremic rats.

During a thirteen-year period, a cohort of 408 patients, subdivided into eight groups, was examined: 100 controls; 88 patients on a conventional low nitrogen diet (CLND); 25 on a very low nitrogen diet supplemented with a mixture of essential aminoacids and ketoanalogues (SD); 105 on Regular dialysis treatment (RDT); 10 on high-efficiency dialysis strategies with different membranes and techniques, 25 on continuous ambulatory peritoneal dialysis (CAPD); 23 treated with erythropoietin; the final group of 32 were transplanted. Data on electrogenesis of Evoked Potentials were drawn by: Electroencephalogram (EEG) with Berg's analysis, Visual (VEP), Brainstem (BAER), Somatosensory Evoked Potentials (SEP), electromyogram (EMG), and motor and sensory nerve conduction velocities (MNCV-SNCV). The synaptosomes were isolated from the cortices of normal and uremic rats (Blood urea nitrogen (BUN) $\simeq$ 250 mg%).

A good correlation was found between EEG activity, VEP, BAER, SEP wave modification and the decline of renal function and/or the quantitative estimates of dialysis treatments (RDT + CAPD). The nerve conduction velocity was lowered earlier in peroneal than in median nerve and the sensory conduction was implicated to a greater extent than the motor one. In the uremic synaptosomes, normal and stimulated Na^+ uptake was significantly increased when compared to the controls; the same behavior was seen for Ca^{++} uptake. Spontaneous evoked potentials and biochemical research appear to be promising methods for investigating uremic neuropathy. It is to be hoped that bio-functional abnormalities in the modifications

[1]Institute of Nephrology and Dialysis, S. Camillo De Lellis Hospital, Via C. Forlanini, 66100 Chieti, Italy

of energy reserves will yield an explanation for the intrinsic and functional defects of nervous structures.

Introduction

Neurologic abnormalities specifically related to uremia occur constantly in chronic renal failure, although they do not become clinically well defined until late in the course of the uremic syndrome [1]. The presence of clinical features of uremic encephalopathy and neuropathy seems to correlate with the severity of the renal failure [2]. The symptomatology, the electrophysiology, and the biochemistry of uremic encephalopathy are incompletely relieved by dialysis and are generally ameliorated after successful renal transplantation [3–5]. It has not been established whether uremic encephalopathy is due to "uremic intoxication" per se, to the unphysiological nature of different dialysis treatments, or whether it is due to more strictly technical factors such as the type of membrane employed, the dialysis schedule, the composition of the dialysate or trace elements in it, or to concomitant therapy [6]. The pathogenesis of neurologic abnormalities is still speculative and is the subject of continuing investigation. It is desirable to utilize noninvasive methods for the early detection of neurological impairments. The reproducibility of modern electrophysiological tests, which we have utilized for many years, has allowed even early alterations of the nervous system to be revealed while clinical symptomatology was completely silent.

In order to exemplify a very complicated issue – in one word, the pathophysiology of uremic encephalopathy – clinical research has attempted to evaluate the effects of uremia on the central and peripheral nervous systems by using the sophisticated techniques of electrophysiology and of subcellular analysis. Many studies are now beginning to appear; they utilize additional techniques for assessing the relationships between electrocortical activity and uremia [7]. The present study deals with the evaluation of the effects of chronic renal failure, of uremia and of metabolic derangements related to the central and peripheral nervous systems. In order to determine the possible causes of electrophysiological abnormalities we designed functional and biochemical assessments of pathways and of nervous cells whose alterations are associated with the uremic state.

Material and Methods

During a thirteen-year period, 408 subjects, subdivided into various groups, were examined: 100 were healthy subjects; 88 were patients with chronic renal failure (creatinine clearance 15.5 ± 8.20 ml/min), treated with a conventionally low nitrogen diet (0.6 g/kg bw/daily of proteins, CLND); 25 patients (creatinine clearance 6.83 ± 3.31 ml/min) whose very low nitrogen diet (0.3 g/kg bw/daily of unselected proteins) was supplemented with a mixture of essential aminoacids and ketoanalogues (SD); 105 patients who underwent regular dialysis treatment (RDT) for 12 to 15 hours/weekly for 70.5 ± 13.4 months, and 10 patients who were on high-efficiency dialysis strategies with different membranes (polysulphon, polymethylmethacrylate, polyacrylonitrile) and different techniques (hemofiltration, hemodiafiltration, biofiltration) using such replacement only fluids as lactate and bicarbonate. Twenty-five patients were on CAPD from 34.5 $\pm$ 10.7 months, essentially with commercially available 2000 ml bags which were changed four times a day. The CAPD was performed in accordance with internationally recommended guidelines [8]. Twenty-three dialysis patients were treated with r-HuEPO given as an i.v. bolus 50-100 UI/kg thrice weekly, for at least 6 months. Thirty-two patients underwent cadaver-donor renal transplantation (T) from 13.4 $\pm$ 7.5 months, and were treated with methyl-prednisolone plus cyclosporine A, azathioprine or both. Patients with diabetes mellitus and/or systemic diseases which can involve the nervous system were excluded. Medications, antihypertensives in particular, that influence the nervous system, were not given to any of the patients, or were stopped two weeks before the examination.

The following electrophysiological parameters were studied: Electroencephalogram with Berg's analysis (EEG), Visual Evoked Potentials (VEP), Brainstem Auditory Evoked Potentials (BAER), Somatosensory Evoked Potentials (SEP), Electromyogram with Motor and Sensitive Nerve Conduction Velocities (EMG, MNCV, SNCV). All the tests were recorded in accordance with our previous papers [9] and checked at least once per year in the same patient during the span of the study period. Particular attention was paid to the modifications induced by conservative dietary treatment, by different dialysis techniques at various degrees of efficiency, and after renal transplantation.

Since numerous attempts have been made to elucidate the mechanisms by which uremia interferes with brain electrocortical activity, we performed biochemical and functional studies to ascertain the biochemical basis of dysfunctions of the central nervous system. These were done in vitro models such as the vesicles of synaptic junctions, called synaptosomes. Basically, the synaptosomes showed abnormalities both in enzyme activity and in certain transport phenomena. When brain tissue is homogenized in isoosmotic solution, the bulblike presynaptic nerve endings are sheared off and resealed to form intact vesicles. The synaptosomes function morphologically and biochemically as intact nerve endings [10]. Similarly to nerve terminals, the synaptosomes contain synaptic vesicles, mitochondria, and cytoplasmic volume and are metabolically active. Synaptosomes have been used for the investigation of the synthesis, storage and release of neurotransmitters; because of their unique properties, they appear to be appropriate models for the investigation of the effects of uremia on the central nervous system.

The synaptosomes were isolated from 200 g male Sprague-Dawley rats; the isolation was carried out in paired groups of normal and uremic rats. The rats were made acutely uremic (blood urea nitrogen $\simeq$ 250 mg%) by performing bilateral ureteral ligation under intramuscularly administered general anesthesia. At 45 h the rats were killed by decapitation; their forebrains were removed and immediately placed in 10 ml of ice-cold isolation medium at 0–4°C. The normal and uremic brains were processed simultaneously, but kept separately in distinctly marked containers.

In the synaptosomes we carried out protein determination; we calculated the total intern synaptosomal volume, ATP, Na^+-uptake, K^+-uptake, ATP-stimulated Na^+-uptake, oxygen consumption, and investigated enzymes. We measured Na^+ uptake using $^{22}Na^+$ under controlled conditions and under treatment with veratridine or tetrodotoxin. These studies were carried out in pH- and temperature-controlled conditions. Furthermore, our study was designed to investigate the role that the calcium transport may play in the abnormalities of synaptosomes taken from uremic rat brain cerebral cortex.

Results

The neurological manifestations of uremia are quite numerous. EEG changes include disorganization, slowing down and loss of alpha frequency, slow background activity together with an excess of theta and delta waves, linked with a decreased metabolic rate typical of all metabolic encephalopathies. There is a good correlation between the percentage of EEG frequencies and power below 7 Hz and the decline of renal function as estimated by serum creatinine [11]. The measurement of Central Nervous System function might yield quantitative estimates of relevant impairment in uremic patients, as well as their responses to treatment. That is why we employed some electrophysiological and biochemical dynamic measures which reflect the activity of central and peripheral neurons.

The VEPs represent a useful method of studying and following the cerebral alterations of the uremic cerebral cortex. In our experience P_{100} wave latency increased in the uremic population (115.7 $\pm$ 8.4 msec vs 106.4 $\pm$ 7.7 msec, $P < .01$) and correlated directly with serum creatinine concentration ($P < .01$). The uremic patients exhibited an increase in latency of BAER waves I, III, and V and an increase in interpeaks I-III, I-V, and III-V compared to normal subjects. The BAER were abnormal in 32/88 patients (36.3%) on CLND, in 44/105 (41.9%) on RDT, and in 13/25 (52%) on CAPD. The peak latencies for spinal and cortex SEP from median and peroneal nerves are summarized in Figs. 1 and 2. During median nerve stimulation the peaks were delayed in 43 out of 88 (48.8%) CLND patients and in 43/130 (33.0%) dialyzed patients (RDT + CAPD). During peroneal nerve stimulation the lumbar compound action potential was polyphasic in 17 out of 88 (19.3%) CLND patients and in 20 out of 130 dialyzed (RDT + CAPD) patients (15.3%). Latencies and morphologies of peroneal SEP were quite different in CLND and RDT patients.

Even though the whole EMG is extremely useful in the evaluation of uremic myopathy, the Fast Fourier Transform is fundamental in analyzing the sinusoidal components of a given waveform. In the uremic patients we found different populations of motor unit potentials. A normal one with a spectral distribution around 150–200 Hz was found in 25% of CLND patients, in 19% of RDT patients, and in all the transplanted patients; a high frequency-low voltage wave group around 500 Hz was found in 44% of CLND patients and in 35% of the RDT group, and a polymorphic pattern with a multiple spectral distribution at low and high frequencies was found in 24% of CLND and in 43% of RDT patients. Figs. 3 and 4 compare MNCV and SNCV in the control, CLND, RDT, and T groups. Decreased MNCV was found in 37% from the lower limb and in 32% from the upper limb of CLND patients, while RDT patients had slowed MNCV in 45% and 40% respectively. The SNCV was compromised more frequently than the MNCV in 44% and 35%, respectively, of CLND patients and in 52% and 45%, respectively, of RDT patients. In the first 6 months after transplantation the conduction velocity and the distal latency in median and peroneal nerves improved somewhat in all patients; a few achieved normal values. By 12 months most values were normal; the others were only slightly prolonged.

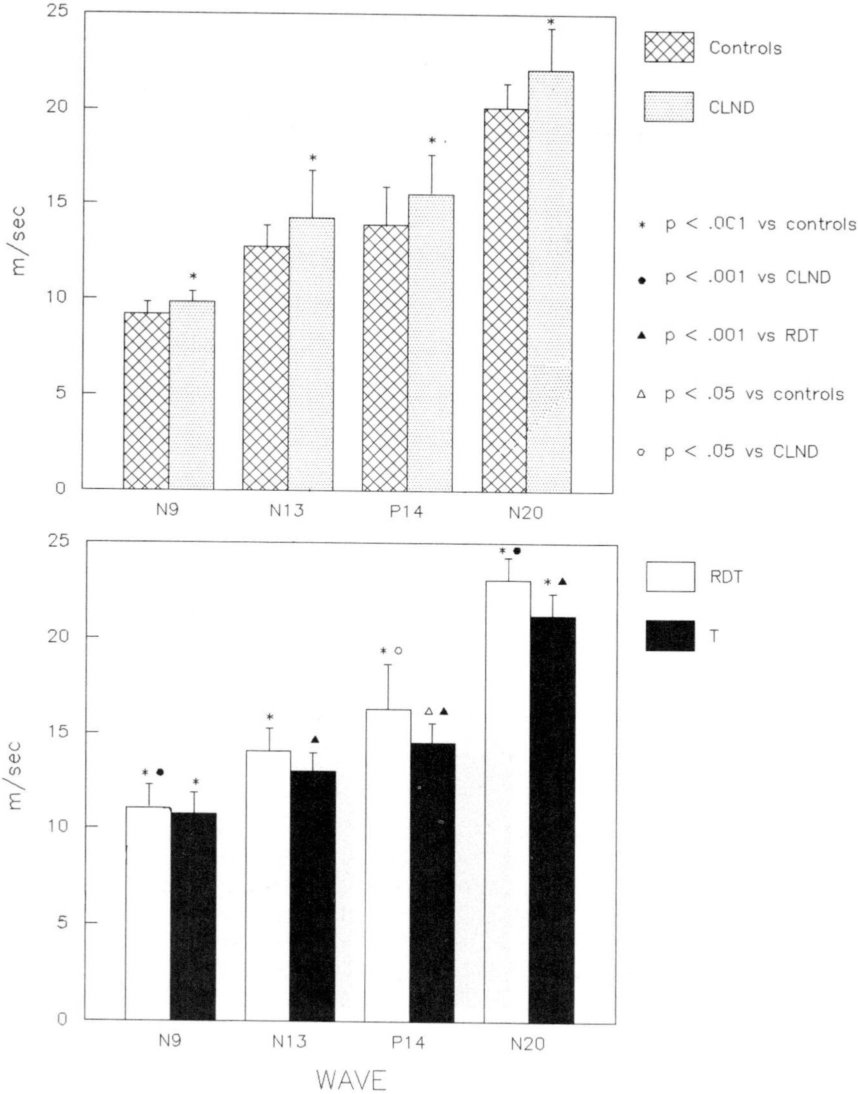

Fig. 1. Somatosensory evoked potentials (*SEP*) from median nerve in controls, diet (*CLND*), dialysis (*RDT*), and transplanted (*T*) patients. Latencies of main waves registered in posterior roots ganglia (*N9*), cervical medulla (*N13*), and pre-rolandic area (*P14* and *N20*)

Paradoxically, during the first year after transplantation, the improvement was greater in those patients affected most severely prior to transplantation. The synaptosomes function morphologically, biochemically, and from an electrophysiological point of view, as intact nerve endings do. To assess the ability of uremic synaptosomes to transport sodium, we first evaluated Na^+ uptake in normal synaptosomes.

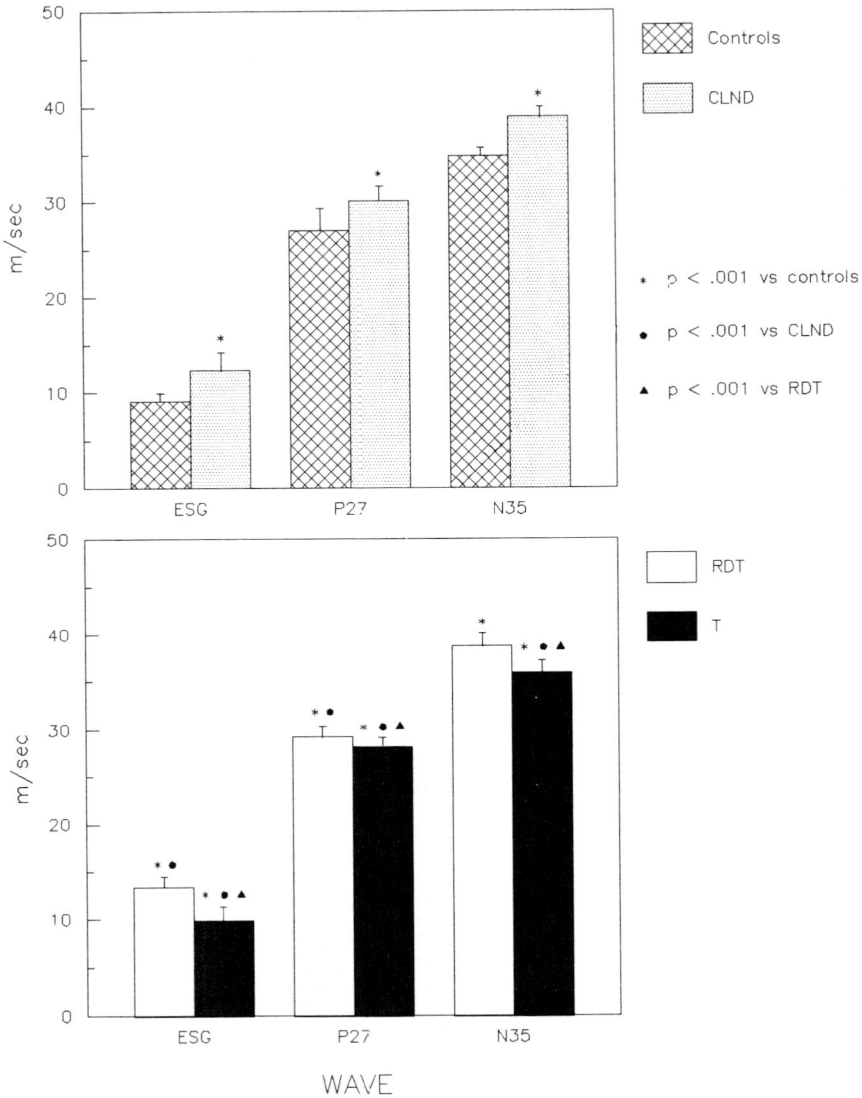

Fig. 2. Somatosensory evoked potentials (*SEP*) from peroneal nerve in controls, diet (*CLND*), dialysis (*RDT*), and transplanted (*T*) patients. Latencies of main waves registered from third lumbar vertebra (*ESG*) and cortical post-rolandic area (*P27* and *N35*)

Using synaptosomes from uremic rats, stimulated Na^+ uptake was increased significantly when compared with normal (4.12 nmol/mg vs 5.53 nmol/mg of protein, $P < .001$ respectively). Potassium uptake in uremic synaptosomes was only 78% of normal (6.0 nmol/mg vs 7.7 nmol/mg of protein) and was significantly less than normal ($P < .005$).

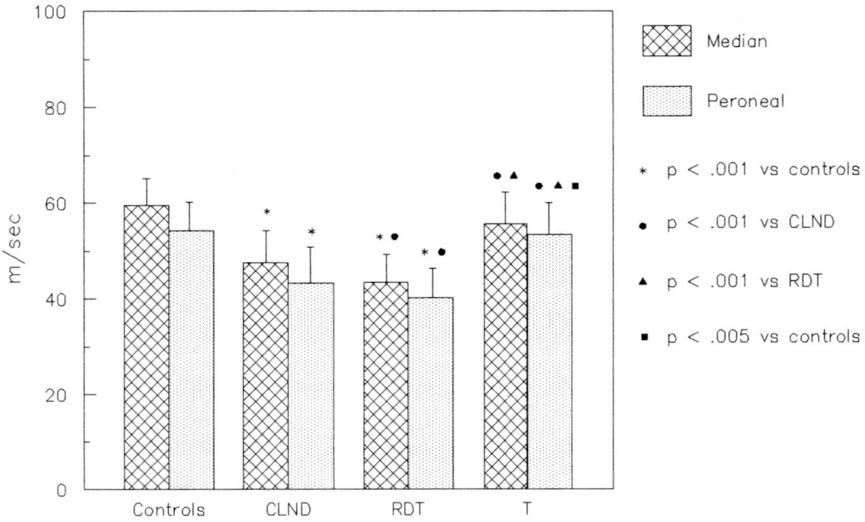

Fig. 3. Motor nerve conduction velocities (*MNCV*) from median and peroneal nerves comparing controls, diet (*CLND*), dialysis (*RDT*), and transplanted (*T*) patients

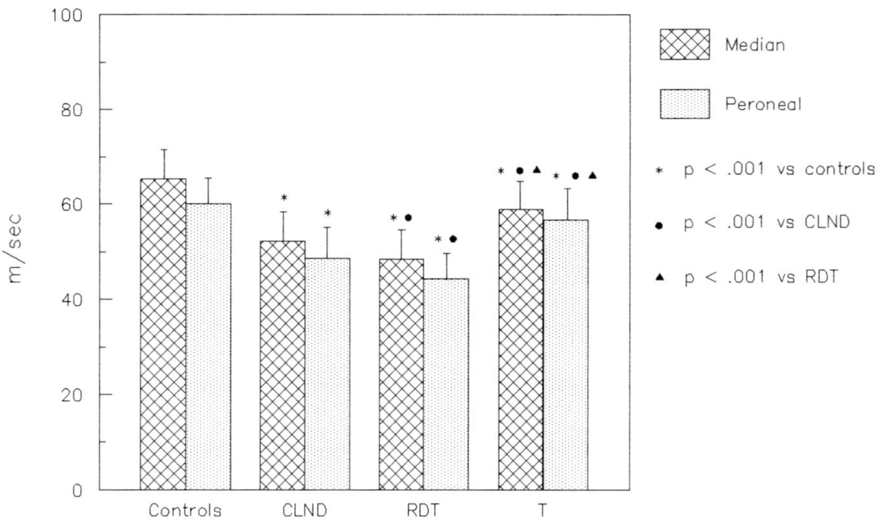

Fig. 4. Sensory nerve conduction velocities (*SNCV*) from median and peroneal nerves comparing controls, diet (*CLND*), dialysis (*RDT*), and transplanted (*T*) patients

The decreased K^+ accumulation in uremic synaptosomes may be due to a decreased amount of available intravesicular ATP and therefore to a dysfunction of the Na^+-K^+ ATPase pump. The Ca^{2+}-uptake was greater in uremic than in normal synaptosomes (13.0 nmol/mg vs 10.3 nmol/mg protein, $P < .005$). Both Na^+-Ca^{2+} exchange and ATP-dependent Ca^{2+} transport processes appear to be increased in uremia.

Two likely mechanisms may explain the differences between the normal synaptosome and the uremic synaptosome with its correlated electrophysiological abnormalities: firstly, increased synaptosomal membrane permeability to sodium in the uremic synaptosomes allows more sodium to enter the vesicles. This produces an increase in the size and/or the number of opened sodium channels which induces an enhancement of membrane permeability. Secondly, this could be the cause of electrical modifications which we examined by evoked potentials. The inability of the accumulated sodium to leave the synaptosomes suggests a decrease in the activity of the Na^+-K^+ ATPase pump. Since, in vivo, both the Na^+-Ca^{2+} exchange and the ATP-dependent Ca^{2+} transport processes function to extrude Ca^{2+} from within the cells, both abnormalities would thus tend to favor delayed latencies in evoked potentials, modification of amplitudes in wavelets, and in any event, all the modifications documented by electrophysiological examinations.

Discussion

Electrophysiological evaluation of the central and peripheral nervous systems and use of evoked potentials appear to be promising methods for investigating the cortical and sub-cortical functions of the uremic brain. The analysis of multimodal evoked potentials which was used to evaluate patients treated by CLND, RDT, or transplantation indicated diffuse structural and/or functional abnormalities, depending on the variety of alterations observed. More relevant was the fact that in uremic brains, electrical activity, with Berg's analysis, was usually accompanied by high voltage and slow wave forms. The VEPs were sensitive in detecting abnormalities that correlated with the concentrations of uremic toxins. Further studies are needed to disclose the underlying mechanisms which produce, in uremic patients, a prolongation of the interval between the latencies of the cerebral responses elicited by VEP. The alterations of BAER observed in uremic patients might be ascribed to defective impulse propagation along brainstem auditory relays secondary to structural and/or functional abnormalities, which are induced by an unfavorable perineuronal environment. The SEP technique has opened new dimensions for the study of "uremic nervous disease". In the end stage renal disease (ESRD) patients, median nerve SEP was involved to a lesser degree than peroneal SEP. Since the central conduction time during upper and lower limb stimulation was seldom impaired, most of the problems should be focused along the spinal afferents connected to lower limb receptors.

It was therefore suggested that most of the latency delay of the scalp SEP to peroneal nerve stimulation was secondary to defective propagation in the most distal axons. This is the mechanism proposed to explain uremic neuropathy; it implies that circulating agents might primarily affect the large diameter bipolar dorsal root ganglion cells, decreasing the axoplasmic flow in the most distal areas of their central and peripheral prolongations, which have the longest trajectories. A slowed lumbar-to-vertex central velocity could be due partly to a synaptic malfunction. However, this does not satisfactorily explain why, within the same anatomical structures, synapses interrupting ascending pathways from lower limbs should be more affected than those interposed between long sensory fibers from upper limbs. Slowing of the velocities of SEP, BAER, and VEP could be due partially to a synaptic malfunction, even though within the same anatomical loci, some synapses would be more affected than others.

Thus, it appears that the effects of uremia on both central and peripheral nervous systems are generated by intrinsic functional defects in various membranes. This could be the general meaning of uremic neuropathy and that is why we decided to study, in the synaptosomes, the biofunctional abnormalities induced by uremia. Our findings of increased Na^+ concentration and of decreased Na^+-K^+ ATPase pump activity may be significant factors in the observed central nervous system manifestations of uremia. The calcium transport in uremic synaptosomes is altered and this alteration results in increased Ca^{2+} uptake by both Na^+-Ca^{2+} exchange mechanisms and by the ATP-dependent calcium transport system [12]. The demonstrated in vitro abnormalities of intracellular Na^+ and Ca^{2+} flux in the uremic central nervous system may in fact lead to alterations in vivo in any of these electrophysiological processes mentioned. All these defects do not appear to be due to "uremic toxins" per se, but rather to an effect of uremia that alters synaptosomial function. In uremia, central nervous system function is impaired and is only partially corrected by dialysis, which corrects the abnormalities found in the uremic milieu (elevated BUN, creatinine, metabolic acidosis, etc.).

Further research into the role of brain energy metabolism in uremia should probably be addressed toward metabolic rates and electrophysiological implications rather than toward static levels of uremic metabolites. It is quite possible that the demonstration of a more than strict correlation between the electrophysiology of the nervous system and energy-using-producing reactions may not be a useful concept for investigating the pathophysiology of uremic encephalopathy. From a clinical point of view, the "neutralization" of uremic neurotoxicity, as achieved by a functioning transplant seems to be quite important [13]. Modern guidelines in the treatment of uremic neuropathy are leading towards the control of hypertension, towards counteracting anemia and aluminum intoxication, towards the employment of more biocompatible membranes in dialysis, and towards taking all those measures that modern research can foster.

References

1. Albertazzi A, Di Paolo B (1989) Neurologic abnormalities of uremia. In: Bonomini V, Scolari MP, Stefoni S, Vangelista A (eds) Biotechnology in renal replacement therapy. Contrib Nephrol, Karger, Basel, pp 188–193
2. Albertazzi A, Di Paolo B, Cappelli P, Spisni C, Del Rosso G (1985) Evoked potentials in uremia. In: D'Amico G, Colasanti G (eds) Advances in nephrology and dialysis. Contrib Nephrol, Karger, Basel, pp 60–68
3. Raskin NH, Fishman RA (1976) Neurologic disorders in renal failure. N Engl J Med 294:143–148, 204–210
4. Teschan PE, Arieff AI (1985) Uremic and dialysis encephalopathies. In: McCandless DW (ed) Cerebral energy metabolism and metabolic encephalopathy. Plenum, New York, pp 263–286

5. Arieff Al (1985) Effects of water, electrolyte and acid base disorders on the central nervous system. In: Arieff Al, DeFronzo RA (eds) Fluid, electrolyte and acid base disorders. Churchill Livingstone, New York, pp 969–1040
6. Savazzi GM (1988) Pathogenesis of cerebral atrophy in uremia. Nephron 49: 94–103
7. Di Paolo B, Arieff Al, Del Rosso G, Di Mizio GF, Campanella M, Muscianese P, Colacelli R, Bonomini M, Albertazzi A (1989) Alterazioni del trasporto di Na^+ e Ca^{2+} in sinaptosomi de encefalo di ratto uremico: vi è correlazione con la trasmissione sinaptica? In: Saporiti E, Bazzato G (eds) Atti del XXX Congresso Nazionale della Società Italiana di Nefrologia. Acta Medica Roma 835–836
8. Clayton S, Quinton C, Oreopoulos D (1981) Training technique for continuous ambulatory peritoneal dialysis (with discussion). Perit Dial Bull 1: S23–S28
9. Di Paolo B, Di Marco T, Cappelli P, Spisni C, Del Rosso G, Palmieri PF, Evangelista M, Albertazzi A (1988) Electrophysiological aspects of nervous conduction in uremia. Clin Nephrol 29: 253–260
10. Booth RFG and Clark JB (1978) A rapid method for the preparation of relatively pure metabolically competent synaptosomes from rat brain. Biochem J 176: 365–370
11. Albertazzi A, Di Paolo B, Del Rosso G, Gambi D, Rossini PM (1981) Neurophysiological abnormalities in uraemic encephalopathy. In: Robinson BHB, Hawkins JB, Davison AM (eds) Proc XVIII EDTA. Pitman, London, pp 652–656
12. Rasmussen H, Goodman DBP (1977) Relationships between calcium and cyclic nucleotides in cell activation: cellular calcium metabolism and calcium-mediated cellular processes. Physiol Rev 57: 428–441
13. Albertazzi A, Di Paolo B, Cappelli P, Evangelista M, Di Marco T, Varanese L (1985) Uremic polyneuropathy: electrophysiologic findings after renal transplantation. In: Najarian JF, Bach FH, Sutherland DER (eds) Transplantation proceedings, Grune and Stratton, New York, p 127

ATPases of the Kidney

Chair: Peter Leth Jørgensen (Denmark)
Stephen L. Gluck (USA)

Localization of Transport ATPases in the Mammalian Nephron

Adrian I. Katz[1]

Summary. Tubule microdissection and enzymatic microassays have allowed measurement of transport adenosine triphosphatases (ATPases) in individual nephron segments. Such studies have mapped the distribution of ATPases involved in the active transport of Na^+,K^+,Ca^{2+}, and H^+ along the nephron of several mammalian species, and have enabled investigators to correlate the activity of these enzymes with transport events mediated by them in the same tubule segment. This brief survey summarizes current knowledge of the nephron localization and function of Na-K-ATPase, the most abundant and best studied transport ATPase in the kidney, as well as of low- and high affinity Ca-ATPases, proton translocating ATPases, and K-activated ATPase—which have been examined in isolated tubules only in the last decade. In view of the remarkable functional heterogeneity of the nephron, information obtained about transport ATPases in its component units has contributed to an improved understanding of kidney function.

Introduction

In the preceding two decades, studies utilizing tubule microdissection and microperfusion techniques have revealed the remarkable biochemical diversity of the nephron and the heterogeneity of transport processes along its longitudinal axis [1–4]. By examining metabolic and transport functions in discrete tubule segments, such studies have greatly expanded previous knowledge obtained with classical biochemical methods in tissue slices or homogenates, or with clearance measurements which provided information about the kidney as a whole rather than about its component units. Given the functional specialization of different regions of the nephron, it is easy to appreciate why understanding kidney function requires its examination in the

[1]Department of Medicine, The University of Chicago Pritzker School of Medicine, Chicago, IL 60637, USA

individual segment(s) of interest. This is particularly true for epithelial transport and the various ATPases which are responsible for the active translocation of electrolytes across the renal tubule, as physiologic alterations, hormones, and dietary manipulations that affect transport do so in certain regions of the nephron and not in others. Equally important, determination of ATPase in specific nephron segments allows quantitative correlations between its activity and transport events measured in the corresponding segment with micropuncture or isolated tubule microperfusion techniques.

Localization of ATPases in the nephron has been attempted principally with two techniques: immunohistochemistry, lately utilizing monoclonal antibodies to the purified enzyme or its subunits [5–7] and, more often, tubule microdissection and enzymatic microassay (see below). The latter offers the advantage of quantitative measurements in nephron segments of unequivocal origin which, in addition, have preserved their linear architecture and cell orientation. Despite the technical difficulty and low tissue yield of this technique, its use has generated a large body of information on the location and function of transport ATPases in the nephron [8–10].

Na-K-ATPase

Na-K-ATPase, the biochemical equivalent of the Na:K pump, mediates the active reabsorption of Na from lumen to blood and secretion of potassium in the opposite direction by effecting the coupled countertransport of these ions at the basolateral membrane of renal tubule cells. In addition, Na-K-ATPase participates indirectly in the translocation of numerous other solutes ("secondary-active transport") via the sodium gradient that it generates. Because of its central role in epithelial transport in general, and kidney function in particular, this enzyme was the first and most extensively studied of renal transport ATPases.

Na-K-ATPase is not distributed evenly in the kidney, its activity being highest in the outer medulla, intermediate in the cortex, and lowest in the inner medulla-papilla. Because the concentration of Na:K pumps varies along the nephron, these differences reflect the relative abundance of the different nephron segments in each of the 3 zones of the kidney. For example, the renal outer medulla is rich in Na-K-ATPase because it contains chiefly thick ascending limbs of Henle's loops, one of the segments with the highest density of Na:K pumps in the nephron.

The first measurements of Na-K-ATPase in discrete nephron segments were reported by Schmidt and Dubach, who examined lyophilized tubules and used an enzymatic cycling method based on the fluorometric measurement of generated NADPH [11,12]. Because the use of freeze-dried tissue has certain limitations and because the method in general was too cumbersome for routine application, my colleagues and I developed an alternative technique that utilizes freshly microdissected tubules and measures directly radiolabeled P_i liberated from the hydrolysis of [γ-^{32}P]ATP [13,14]. This method is simple enough to allow simultaneous measurement of Na-K-ATPase in large numbers of tubules, and sufficiently sensitive to determine the enzyme activity in tubule segments 100–200 μm in length. Alternative techniques that combine certain features of those listed above have been introduced more recently [15,16].

Na-K-ATPase activity has been determined in individual nephron segments of several species, including the rabbit, rat, and mouse (see Table 1). Not surprisingly,

Table 1. Distribution of Transport ATPases in the Mammalian Nephron

ATPase	Species	Segment with highest activity	pmol·mm^{-1}·h^{-1}	PCT	PST	tDL	tAL	MAL	CAL	DCT	CNT	CCT	OMCT	IMCT	Ref.
				(% of segment with highest activity)											
Na^+-K^+-ATPase	Rabbit	MAL	3080[a]	33[b] 75[c]	–[d]	–	–	100	41	–	–	37	29	–	17
	Rabbit	DCT	3091	75	21	(3.5)[e]	–	80	32	100	–	27	17	–	14
	Mouse	DCT	5171	34	9	5	–	71	71	100	–	21	5	–	14
	Rat	DCT	6679	36	8	4	(2)	68	74	100	–	12	11	–	14
	Rabbit	DCT	9120	69	15	(3)	(2)	82	20	100	83	15	13	–	15
Ca^{2+}-ATPase (low-affinity)	Rabbit	DCT	1200	36	32	11	–	92	23	100	–	79	65	–	19
Ca^{2+}-Mg^{2+}-ATPase (high-affinity)	Rabbit	DCT	243	58	40	–	–	56	21	100	–	86	21	–	20
H^+-ATPase (NEM-sensitive)	Rat	PCT	550	100	64	–	–	66	78	–	–	64	45	–	21
	Rat	DCT	1980	–	–	–	–	44	49	100	–	39	38	32	23
	Rabbit[f]	CNT	1810	–	–	–	–	–	28	76	100	29	30	25	22
	Rat	PCT	450	100	9	0	0	51	80	82	–	61	48	72/17[g]	24
HCO_3^--ATPase	Rabbit	PST	330	64	100	–	–	(7)	(2)	55	91[h]	50	39	–	26
K^+-ATPase	Rabbit	CNT[h]	328	0	0	–	–	0	0	(3)	100[h]	55	20	–	27
	Rabbit	CNT	1000	(11)	(9)	–	–	(3)	(2)	(20)	100	40	54	–	28

[a]calculated from authors' data; [b]cortical nephron; [c]juxtamedullary nephron; [d]not measured; [e]values in parentheses are not significantly different from zero; [f]adrenalectomized rabbits receiving aldosterone replacement (1.5 μg/100g per day × 7); [g]before/after entry into the ducts of Bellini; [h]granular (terminal) portion of DCT

PCT, proximal convoluted tubule; PST, proximal straight tubule; tDL,tAL, thin descending and ascending limb of Henle's loop; MAL,CAL, medullary and cortical thick ascending limb of Henle's loop; DCT, distal convoluted tubule; CNT, connecting tubule; CCT, cortical collecting tubule; OMCT, IMCT, outer and inner medullary (papillary) collecting tubule

the absolute levels of enzyme activity measured by different investigators using diverse methods corresponded only for some segments and differed for others. In contrast, however, the enzyme distribution profile along the nephron was remarkably similar regardless of species studied or methods used, the greatest activity being always measured in the distal convoluted tubule (DCT) and thick ascending limb. Considerable activity is also found in proximal convoluted tubules (PCT), but the enzyme is present in lesser amounts in the collecting tubule and pars recta (PST), and is barely detectable in the thin limbs of Henle's loops [14,15,17]. When measured with the same technique, Na-K-ATPase activity was, in general, comparable in the three species studied, being greater in the rat, lesser in the rabbit, and intermediate in the mouse [14]. It should be noted, however, that even in the same nephron segment the enzyme is not distributed homogeneously. In the collecting tubule of the rat, for example, it is found in principal, but not in intercalated cells [5]. Finally, examination of Table 1 reveals that Na-K-ATPase is by far the most abundant transport ATPase in the nephron.

The nonuniform distribution of Na-K-ATPase activity along the nephron poses the question whether the enzyme has the same characteristics in all its subdivisions. Earlier studies which showed that cortical and outer medullary Na-K-ATPase have the same affinity (K_m) for ATP and sodium appear to support this view, as did observations that pump density ([^{3}H] ouabain binding) varies along the nephron exactly in parallel with Na-K-ATPase hydrolytic activity, so that the turnover rate of the pump is the same in all nephron segments. In contrast, a more recent report describing increased sensitivity to ouabain of the cortical collecting tubule (CCT) compared with the thick ascending limb and PCT [18] raised speculations that Na-K-ATPase may vary in different nephron segments, for example because it may contain different isoforms of its catalytic (α) subunit. As of the time of this writing, however, there is no convincing evidence for the presence of other isoforms of the enzyme besides α_1 in the kidney, and therefore its different affinity for ouabain probably reflects the local influence of factors extrinsic to the pump itself, as originally suggested by the authors.

Ca-ATPases

The bulk of filtered Ca is reabsorbed in the proximal convoluted tubule, but substantial reabsorption also occurs in the pars recta, thick ascending limb, distal convoluted tubule, and early cortical collecting tubule; indeed, the final regulation of Ca excretion takes place in the distal segments of the nephron.

The mechanisms responsible for tubular Ca reabsorption are incompletely understood, as both active and passive modes of transport have been proposed, sometimes for the same nephron segment. Cytoplasmic free Ca concentrations are several orders of magnitude lower than in plasma, and this gradient is maintained both by ATP-dependent Ca pumps and Ca:Na and Ca:H exchange mechanisms located in the plasma membrane as well as in cell organelles. When located in the membrane of transporting epithelia these systems participate in the vectorial transport of Ca, besides maintaining cell Ca homeostasis.

Ca-activated ATPases have been demonstrated in kidney cortex homogenates, suspensions of cortical tubules, and microsomes or membrane vesicles from several species. Supporting a physiologic role of these enzymes is their location in the basolateral membrane, across which the large Ca concentration gradient is maintained, and observations that they operate optimally in the presence of ATP concentrations found in kidney cells' cytosol.

Low-Affinity Ca-ATPase

A calcium-stimulated ATPase that could be activated by either Ca *or* Mg in millimolar amounts has been described in basolateral membranes of kidney cortex. We determined the distribution of this enzyme along the rabbit nephron with the microassay previously used for measuring Na-K-ATPase in individual nephron segments [13]. The enzyme was found along the entire nephron, and was activated by millimolar concentrations of Ca or Mg, neither of which was necessary for activation by the other cation [19]. This Ca-ATPase originated both in the mitochondria and in the plasma membrane, as it was inhibited to a substantial extent by oligomycin and azide; its activity in the combined presence of these inhibitors ranged between 200 and 400 pmols $Pi.mm^{-1} \cdot h^{-1}$ in most segments examined, being lower in the cortical thick ascending limb.

The physiologic role of this enzyme in transmembrane Ca transport (i.e., whether it behaves like a Ca pump) is not clear, because it is activated by Ca in millimolar concentrations, whereas cytosolic free Ca in kidney cells is orders of magnitude lower. Although its function remains obscure, it is of interest that such an enzyme was also found in red blood cell ghosts, brain synaptosomes, and eel gills. Perhaps its high capacity compensates for its low affinity, or it may act at the outer surface of the membrane.

High-Affinity Ca-Mg-ATPase

A more attractive hypothesis is that calcium extrusion from renal tubule cells is mediated, in part, by a high-affinity calcium-stimulated ATPase, activated by Ca in concentrations normally present in the cytosol. Supporting this view is the identification of such an enzyme exclusively in basolateral membrane vesicles, and the correspondence between the K_m for calcium of this Ca-Mg-ATPase and that of the ATP-dependent Ca uptake in this preparation. It is also recalled that cytosolic free Ca in kidney cells averages 0.1–0.45 μM. For these reasons we sought to determine whether a high-affinity calcium-ATPase could be detected in isolated rabbit tubules and to measure its activity in individual nephron segments [20].

A Mg-dependent ATPase, maximally activated by Ca concentrations between 1.1 and 2.3 μM and with an apparent K_m of 0.3 to 0.4 μM (hence Ca-Mg ATPase), was found in all the nephron segments examined: Its activity was greatest ($\geq$200 $pmols.mm^{-1}.h^{-1}$) in distal convoluted and cortical collecting tubules, intermediate in the proximal convoluted tubule and medullary thick ascending limb, and least in the pars recta, cortical thick ascending limb, and medullary collecting tubule [20]. Because we measured Ca-Mg-ATPase in intact tubules, the cellular component where it originates is uncertain. However, sodium azide, an inhibitor of mitochondrial ATPase, did not affect the enzyme, so that enzyme location in the plasma membrane (or in the endoplasmic reticulum) seems likely. This enzyme differed from the

Ca-ATPase described above in its absolute requirement for magnesium, high affinity for calcium, and lack of inhibition by azide.

To our knowledge Ca-Mg-ATPase has not been determined in microdissected nephron segments by other investigators. Borke et al. [6] have demonstrated this enzyme in basolateral membranes of the human DCT with an immunohistochemical method, using monoclonal antibodies against Ca-Mg-ATPase purified from red cell ghosts.

H-ATPase

ATPases in general are classified into two broad categories: Those of the F_0-F_1 type, characterized by a complex structure with several subunits, lack of a phosphorylated intermediate, and resistance to vanadate; and those of the E_1-E_2 type, which have a simpler subunit structure, undergo phosphorylation in the catalytic cycle, and are inhibited by vanadate. In recent years much attention has been devoted to a proton-translocating ATPase (H-ATPase) not strictly belonging to either type. This enzyme is associated with cell organelles such as clathrin-coated vesicles and lysosomes, and is not affected by ouabain, vanadate, oligomycin or azide, but is inhibited by dicyclohexylcarbodiimide (DCCD) and N-ethylmaleimide (NEM), which helps define it operationally. This vacuolar H-ATPase, thought to be the biochemical expression of proton pumps involved in ATP-dependent H secretion, has been characterized in the turtle urinary bladder and purified from bovine renal medulla, where it is found in the intercalated cells of collecting ducts. Its activity is regulated by insertion of vesicles into the membrane, e.g., in response to respiratory acidosis or increased ambient CO_2 in vitro.

Active H secretion in the kidney occurs primarily in the proximal tubule, where it brings about the reclamation of filtered bicarbonate, and in the collecting tubule, where it regenerates bicarbonate consumed in metabolism. Proton secretion in the proximal tubule is largely sodium-dependent and electroneutral, whereas in the collecting tubule it has the opposite characteristics. Proximal acidification is thus accomplished mainly via luminal Na:H exchange, but recent studies also suggest a role for a proton pump in the proximal tubule, as well as in the other segments besides the collecting tubule (reviewed in [7]). Distal acidification, on the other hand, is mediated by the electrogenic proton pump found in the intercalated cells of the collecting tubule, especially in its medullary portion.

Several studies have attempted to localize the vacuolar proton pump in the nephron, taking advantage of its inhibition by N-ethylmaleimide. Ait-Mohamed et al. [21] were the first to describe the distribution of a NEM-sensitive ATPase along the nephron. Interestingly, the highest activity was found in proximal convoluted tubules, whereas the activity in medullary collecting tubules, although substantial, was lowest among the segments tested. More recently, Garg and Narang have measured NEM-sensitive ATPase in the distal segments of the rat and rabbit nephron [22,23], where it was highest in the DCT and connecting tubule (CNT), respectively; the activity of this enzyme in outer and inner medullary collecting tubules was about one third that in the DCT and CNT (see Table 1). Finally, in a study that included the proximal nephron, Sabatini et al. [24] found a distribution of NEM-sensitive ATPase in the rat nephron similar to that originally reported in this species [21].

The distribution of vacuolar H-ATPase in the kidney has also been examined by immunocytochemistry, using affinity-purified antibodies to several subunits of the proton pump from bovine kidney medulla [7]. This study also revealed a widespread occurrence of the enzyme, which was found in most nephron segments. In the PCT it was present in the apical plasma membrane, where it would be expected to reside if it contributed to H transport. In the collecting duct only intercalated cells showed staining, which was located to the apical membrane in cells of the medullary portion, but to either side of the cell membrane in cells of the cortical collecting duct. The latter observation reflects the presence of different populations of intercalated cells (α and β subtypes) involved in proton – or bicarbonate secretion, respectively.

Besides being stimulated by respiratory acidosis, NEM-sensitive ATPase in distal segments is also stimulated by aldosterone [22], metabolic acidosis [24,25], and K-depletion [23,25]. Although abundant in PCT, the enzyme therein (to the extent that it has been tested) is not increased by these stimuli, and its precise role in urine acidification remains unclear.

HCO_3-ATPase

Another enzyme putatively involved in H secretion is an ATPase stimulated by intracellular HCO_3 (HCO_3-ATPase). However, the nature of this enzyme, and specifically whether it is of mitochondrial or extramitochondrial origin, has been the subject of intense controversy that continues to the present. Advocates of a plasma membrane location of HCO_3-ATPase postulate that by stimulating H secretion via this mechanism, reabsorbed HCO_3 may act as a positive promoter of additional HCO_3 reabsorption from the tubular lumen, but the role of this enzyme is far from being settled.

Perhaps because of the controversy surrounding its cellular location and physiologic function, HCO_3-ATPase in isolated tubules has been studied less extensively than other transport ATPases. In a thorough study describing an extramitochondrial HCO_3-ATPase in discrete rabbit nephron segments [26], the highest activity was found in proximal straight tubules and in the late ("granular") DCT, although substantial activity was also found in all other segments examined except in the thick ascending limb of Henle's loop (see Table 1). In distal portions of the nephron the enzyme was stimulated by chronic desoxycorticosterone acetate (DOCA) treatment [26].

K-ATPase

An enzyme stimulated by potassium and inhibited by vanadate (but not by ouabain) has been recently reported by two groups of investigators [27,28]. Unlike all the other ATPases described in this review, this enzyme is present only in distal portions of the nephron, where its activity is highest in the late ("granular") DCT [27] or connecting tubule [28], and decreases in the cortical and medullary collecting duct. Distribution of the enzyme is proportional to the number of intercalated cells in these segments, and its activity is stimulated by K depletion. For these reasons it has been postulated that K-ATPase is located in intercalated cells where it participates in active K reabsorption, although it should be mentioned that enzyme activity is highest at nephron sites proximal to the outer medullary collecting duct where most of the K reabsorption is thought to occur.

Because of certain shared characteristics with the gastric H-K-ATPase, including inhibition by vanadate, omeprazole, and Sch 28080, it has also been proposed that the K-ATPase found in distal nephron segments might be similar to or identical with the gastric enzyme. This intriguing hypothesis depends, first, on the demonstration that H-K-ATPase is present in the kidney. While this has not yet been established with certainty, preliminary studies suggest that the rat kidney expresses a mRNA encoding for a molecule closely related to (albeit not identical with) gastric H-K-ATPase [29]. Madin-Darby canine kidney (MDCK) cells, derived from a distal tubular epithelium, may have a H-K-pump, but this appears to be immunologically distinct from the gastric pump [30].

Acknowledgment. This paper was supported by National Institutes of Health Grant DK 13601 and by the American Heart Association.

References

1. Jacobson HR (1981) Functional segmentation of the mammalian nephron. Am J Physiol 241:F203–F218
2. Ross BD, Guder WG (1982) Heterogeneity and compartmentation in the kidney. In: Sies H (ed) Metabolic Compartmentation. Academic, New York, pp 363–409
3. Berry CA (1982) Heterogeneity of tubular transport processes in the nephron. Annu Rev Physiol 44:181–201
4. Schlondorff D (1986) Isolation and use of specific nephron segments and their cells in biochemical studies. Kidney Int 30:201–207
5. Kashgarian M, Biemesderfer D, Caplan M, Forbush B (1985) Monoclonal antibody to Na, K-ATPase: immunocytochemical localization along nephron segments. Kidney Int 28: 899–913
6. Borke JL, Minami J, Verma A, Penniston JT, Kumar R (1987) Monoclonal antibodies to human erythrocyte membrane $Ca^{2+}Mg^{2+}$ adenosine triphosphatase pump recognize an epitope in the basolateral membrane of human kidney distal tubule cells. J Clin Invest 80: 1225–1231
7. Brown D, Hirsh S, Gluck S (1988) Localization of a proton-pumping ATPase in rat kidney. J Clin Invest 82:2114–2126
8. Katz AI (1986) Distribution and function of classes of ATPases along the nephron. Kidney Int 29:21–31
9. Doucet A (1988) Function and control of Na-K-ATPase in single nephron segments of the mammalian kidney. Kidney Int 34:749–760
10. Katz AI (1988) Role of Na-K-ATPase in kidney function. In: Skou JC, Norby JG, Maunsbach AB, Esmann M (eds) The Na^+,K^+-Pump, Part B: Cellular Aspects. Alan R Liss, New York, pp 207–232
11. Schmidt U, Dubach U (1969) Activity of (Na^+K^+)-stimulated adenosintriphosphatase in the rat nephron. Pflugers Arch 306:219–226
12. Schmidt U, Dubach U (1974) Induction of Na K ATPase in the proximal and distal convolution of the rat nephron after uninephrectomy. Pflugers Arch 346:39–48
13. Doucet A, Katz AI, Morel F (1979) Determination of Na,K-ATPase activity in single segments of the mammalian nephron. Am J Physiol 237:F105–F113
14. Katz AI, Doucet A, Morel F (1979) Na,K-ATPase activity along the rabbit, rat and mouse nephron. Am J Physiol 237:F114–F120

15. Garg LC, Knepper MA, Burg MB (1981) Mineralocorticoid effects on Na,K-ATPase in individual nephron segments. Am J Physiol 240:F536–F544
16. O'Neil RG, Dubinsky WP (1984) Micromethodology for measuring ATPase activity in renal tubules: Mineralocorticoid influence. Am J Physiol 247:C314–C320
17. Schmidt U, Horster M (1977) Na-K-activated ATPase: activity maturation in rabbit nephron segments dissected in vitro. Am J Physiol 233:F55–F60
18. Doucet A, Barlet C (1986) Evidence for differences in the sensitivity to ouabain of Na-K-ATPase along the nephron of rabbit kidney. J Biol Chem 261:993–995
19. Katz AI, Doucet A (1980) Calcium-activated adenosine triphosphatase along the rabbit nephron. Int J Biochem 12:125–129
20. Doucet A, Katz AI (1982) High-affinity Ca-Mg-ATPase along the rabbit nephron. Am J Physiol 242:F346–F352
21. Ait-Mohamed AK, Marsy S, Barlet C, Khadouri C, Doucet A (1986) Characterization of N-ethylmaleimide-sensitive proton pump in the rat kidney. Localization along the nephron. J Biol Chem 261:12526–12533
22. Garg LC, Narang N (1988) Effects of aldosterone on NEM-sensitive ATPase in rabbit nephron segments. Kidney Int 34:13–17
23. Garg LC, Narang N (1990) Effects of low-potassium diet on N-ethylmaleimide-sensitive ATPase in the distal nephron segments. Renal Physiol Biochem 13:129–136
24. Sabatini S, Laski ME, Kurtzman NA (1990) NEM-sensitive ATPase activity in rat nephron: effect of metabolic acidosis and alkalosis. Am J Physiol 258:F297–F304
25. Hayashi M, Chekal MA, Katz AI (1986) Proton ATPase in isolated rat medullary collecting tubules: effects of systemic acidosis, K depletion and aldosterone. Kidney Int 29:368
26. Ben Abdelkhalek M, Barlet C, Doucet A (1986) Presence of an extramitochondrial anion-stimulated ATPase in the rabbit kidney: localization along the nephron and effect of corticosteroids. J Membr Biol 89:225–240
27. Doucet A, Marsy S (1987) Characterization of K-ATPase activity in distal nephron: stimulation by potassium depletion. Am J Physiol 253:F418–F423
28. Garg LC, Narang N (1988) Ouabain-insensitive K-adenosine triphosphatase in distal nephron segments of the rabbit. J Clin Invest 81:1204–1208
29. Okusa MD, Unwin R, Wright FS, Giebisch G, Caplan MJ (1990) H^+,K^+-ATPase mRNA expression in rat kidney. Kidney Int 37:568
30. Eisen TD, Caplan MJ, Boron WF (1990) Intracellular pH regulation in MDCK cells. Kidney Int 37:535

Regulation of Tubular Na-K-ATPase

C. Barlet-Bas, L. Cheval, E. Feraille, S. Marsy, and A. Doucet[1]

Summary. This review summarizes some studies from our laboratory which illustrate the wide variety of mechanisms through which renal Na-K-ATPase activity is controlled by hormones. A special emphasis is given to those regulation processes which alter Na-K-ATPase activity and renal Na handling with similar time-courses. Analysis of Na-K-ATPase was carried out at the level of single nephron segments obtained by microdissection of collagenase-treated kidneys.

Introduction

The functional polarization of renal epithelial cells results from the presence of segregated permeability and transport properties in apical and basolateral membranes (Fig. 1). In fact most uphill transepithelial transport processes in tubular cells are coupled to cell metabolism through Na-K-ATPase, either directly or undirectly. This enzyme, which is located in basolateral cell membranes [1,2], converts the energy-rich P_i bond of ATP into electrochemical gradients of Na and K. The low intracellular Na concentration generated thereby can drive Na entry across the luminal cell membrane, and thus creates a net transepithelial, transcellular Na reabsorption flux. Despite the marked axial heterogeneity of the nephron, this general scheme applies to the successive nephron segments, which differ from one another mainly by the nature of transport systems which allow luminal sodium entry.

In renal cells, transcellular Na flux is intense, since it accounts for 1–10 times the intracellular Na content per minute, according to the cell type. Furthermore, in a given nephron segment this flux may vary within a wide range according to the metabolic and/or hormonal status of the organism. Confronted which such large variations of the transcellular sodium flux, maintaining cellular homeostasia requires the

[1]Laboratoire de Physiologie Cellulaire, URA 219 CNRS, Collège de France, 11 Place M. Berthelot, 75231 Paris Cedex 05, France

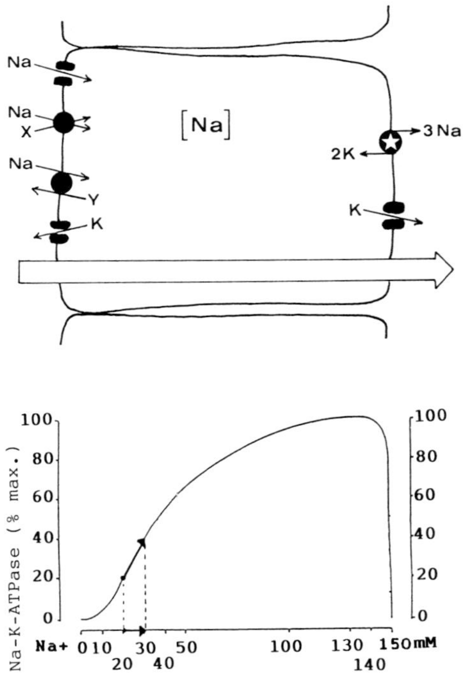

Fig. 1. *Top*, schematic representation of the segregation of Na transport systems in apical and basolateral membrane which leads to Na-K-ATPase generated transcellular Na transport. *Bottom*, activation of Na-K-ATPase activity by increasing Na concentration. Na-K-ATPase, expressed as percent of its V_{max}, was determined in the presence of varying Na concentrations, the sum of Na and K concentrations being maintained equal to 150mM. The *left part of the curve* corresponds to what occurs at the intracellular site (low Na, high K). It indicates that increasing Na concentration activates Na-K-ATPase which will extrude more Na out of the cell and, thereby, decrease Na concentration

existence of a tight coupling between the Na-transporting systems which operate at both cell borders. Thus, Na flux through Na-K-ATPase must exactly balance luminal Na entry, whatever the changes of the latter might be.

It has long been admitted that the adaptation of Na-K-ATPase pumping rate to alterations of luminal Na entry was accounted for by changes in intracellular Na concentration. Indeed, since intracellular Na is rate limiting for Na-K-ATPase, any increase in luminal Na entry will increase intracellular Na concentration, and thereby activate Na-K-ATPase. In turn, the pump will extrude more Na out of the cell, thus contributing to restore basal conditions (Fig. 1). Conversely, decreased luminal Na entry will inhibit basolateral Na exit through the pump. Although efficient, this automatic control process does require transient changes in Na (and K) concentration, which may be prejudicial to cell survival, even in the short term. The purpose of this work is to present evidence that, besides its control by intracellular Na concentration, the activity of renal Na-K-ATPase can be controlled by metabolic and/or hormonal parameters through other mechanisms, although within short latency.

As long as the cellular heterogeneity of the nephron can be overcome, the renal tubule reveals itself as a highly suitable model for the study of Na-K-ATPase regulation because: 1) it is the target for a great number of hormones, 2) some of these hormones induce very large changes in the Na transport capacity of target cells, and 3) within the same organ, some cells are sensitive to a given hormone whereas others are not, which proves useful for assuming the specificity of the responses. Our approach to circumvent the renal heterogeneity has consisted in measuring Na-K-ATPase in single nephron segments obtained by microdissection of collagenase-treated kidney [3]. This allowed us to obtain large numbers of well-characterized nephron segments which, although not suitable for in vitro microperfusion, could be used for biochemical studies since they displayed a cellular polarity, they responded to hormones, and they could be maintained in vitro for several hours while keeping their transport and regulatory properties.

On such samples, the hydrolytic activity of Na-K-ATPase can be measured by the rate of ouabain-sensitive production of $^{32}P_i$ from $[\gamma^{-32}P]ATP$ [4]. Although it has been fruitful, this methodological approach suffers several limitations. First, it permits the measurement of Na-K-ATPase activity mainly under V_{max} conditions, which may mask regulatory phenomena which do not alter V_{max}. Secondly, it requires the previous permeabilization of cell membranes to allow the entrance of exogenous ATP, and this leads to the loss of transmembrane gradients, and possibly of intracellular regulatory components. To palliate these limitations we recently developed another microassay which permits the quantitation of Na-K-ATPase-mediated ionic flux in intact tubular cells, i.e., transport generated through the cellular metabolism and against the transmembrane gradients prevailing under physiological conditions. This assay is based on the determination of the initial rate of ouabain-sensitive ^{86}Rb influx in single nephron segments [5].

To elucidate the molecular mechanisms underlying changes in Na-K-ATPase activity, in particular to determine whether such changes are due to activation of preexisting pump units or to induction of new ones, it has been necessary to quantitate the number of active Na-K-ATPase units. This is feasible by measuring specific ^{3}H-ouabain binding under saturating conditions in intact tubules [6]. Unfortunately, this method is hardly applicable to the rat nephron, because of the very low affinity for ouabain of this species. Therefore, we are presently developing a substitutive method, utilizable in all species, which consists in quantifying the phosphointermediate of the Na-K-ATPase cycle. The simultaneous application of these methods, which are not further discussed in this article, allowed the characterization of some regulatory processes of tubular Na-K-ATPase which are summarized below. A special emphasis will be given to those processes which do not involve long term, secondary adaptations of tubular cells.

Activation of Na-K-ATPase Activity by Intracellular Na

As discussed above, intracellular Na is the main rate limiting factor of Na-K-ATPase activity. Thus, changes in its concentration modify the pump activity in a way which tends to restore basal Na level. In addition, it should also be noted that Na-K-ATPase sensitivity to Na is modulated by intracellular K, since the two cations compete for the occupancy of intracellular Na sites [7,8]. Thus the apparent $K_{0.5}$ for Na deter-

Table 1. Kinetic properties of Na-K-ATPase along the rabbit nephron

	App $K_{0.5}$ for Na (mM)		App K_i for ouabain (μM)	App K_D for ouabain (μM)
	[K]=5mM	[Na]+[K]=150mM		
Proximal tubule	9.5	65.0	1.8	4.0
Thick ascending limb	10.2	48.0	0.5	0.6
Collecting tubule	3.1	25.0	0.06	0.1

Apparent $K_{0.5}$ for Na was measured either at low K concentration ([K]=5mM) or at high K concentration, under conditions in which the sum of the Na and K concentrations remained constant and equal to 150mM([Na]+[K]=150mM). The apparent $K_{0.5}$ for K was 0.4 mM for all nephron segments. (Data from [9] and [10])

mined at low K concentration ([K] = 5mM) is five–eightfold lower than that measured at high K concentration ([Na] + [K] = 150mM) (Table 1). In other words, at a constant Na concentration, Na-K-ATPase activity increases when intracellular K concentration decreases, and this is particularly marked when the latter varies within the 120–100mM range [9], i.e., within the physiological range of variation of cell K concentration. If one assumes that the sum of Na and K concentrations within the cell remains constant under all conditions, this property enhances the self regulatory ability of Na-K-ATPase. Indeed, in response to increased intracellular Na concentration, Na-K-ATPase will be stimulated through: 1) the enhancement of the concentration of its rate limiting substrate, i.e., Na, and 2) the enhancement of its affinity for Na (due to decreased K concentration).

A specific feature of kidney cells is that the sensitivity of Na-K-ATPase for Na varies along the nephron: The collecting tubule is two-threefold more sensitive to Na than more proximal segments, whether this sensitivity is determined at low or high K concentration (Table 1). Therefore, the collecting tubule is more sensitive to physiological changes of intracellular Na concentration, a property likely related to the role of this nephron segment in the ultimate control of Na/K excretion.

Again it should be emphasized that these auto-regulation processes of Na-K-ATPase activity require changes in intracellular Na concentration, which often are not observed, and which may be unsuitable for the maintenance of cellular homeostasia.

Can Endogenous Ouabain-Like Factor Control Renal Na-K-ATPase?

It is beyond the scope of this review to analyze the pieces of evidence which suggest that the specific ouabain-binding site present on the catalytic subunit (α) of Na-K-ATPase may be the receptor for a circulating modulator (hormone?) of this enzyme. If one admits that such a modulator(s) exists, which is most likely, even though it proves difficult to purify, the problem in question here is whether the kidney may or may not be a target for its action. Indeed, there was a paradox in the findings that kidney has a low affinity for ouabain on the one hand [10], and that ouabain-like factors are natriuretic on the other [11].

However, analysis of renal ouabain-sensitivity at the level of single nephron segments instead of whole kidney homogenates or membrane fractions thereof revealed that, conversely to most nephron segments, the collecting tubule is highly sensitive to ouabain [12]. Indeed, apparent K_i as well as apparent K_D for ouabain are 10–30-fold lower in the rabbit collecting tubule (either in its cortical or medullary portions) than in more proximal nephron segments (Table 1). A posteriori, it appears obvious that such a property could not be observed on whole kidney preparations because Na-K-ATPase activity originating in the collecting tubule represents only a minute fraction of the whole kidney enzyme's activity since: 1) this nephron segment represents a small fraction (<5%) of total kidney mass, and 2) the collecting tubule has among the lowest Na-K-ATPase activities, when expressed per millimeter of tubule length (or per unit of mass). These results suggest that ouabain-like factors may act on the kidney, and that the collecting tubule likely represents their target site.

Together with the higher affinity for Na described above (Table 1), the higher affinity of the collecting tubule for ouabain may suggest that this nephron segment expresses the α_3 isoform of the catalytic subunit of Na-K-ATPase rather than the α_1 isoform, which is admittedly found in kidney [13]. However, confirmation of this hypothesis will require different experimental approaches at the level of isolated segments of collecting tubule. In any case, whether α_3 is present in the collecting tubule or not, this does not change the conclusion that this nephron segment is the major renal target of ouabain-like factors. In contrast, this has functional implications regarding the regulation of the synthesis of Na-K-ATPase, since the genes encoding for the α_1 and α_3 subunits are likely not controlled by the same parameters.

Control of Na-K-ATPase Synthesis by Aldosterone in the Collecting Tubule

Among the numerous hormones which control renal Na-K-ATPase, mineralocorticoids play a central role because the kidney is their major target. The antinatriuretic action of mineralocorticoids results from the induction of specific genes encoding for aldosterone-induced proteins (AIP) which are responsible for the hormonal action. Since adrenalectomy decreases Na-K-ATPase activity in the collecting tubule [14,15] and since in vivo administration of aldosterone to adrenalectomized rats [14] or rabbits [15] restores it within 3 h, the question arises, whether or not Na-K-ATPase is an AIP.

In vitro experiments [16] demonstrated that incubation, for 2.5 h at 37° C, of cortical collecting tubules of 7-day-adrenalectomized rats resulted in a marked stimulation of Na-K-ATPase activity and specific binding of ^3H-ouabain (Fig. 2). This stimulation was totally abolished in the presence of actinomycin D or of cycloheximide (Fig. 2), suggesting that aldosterone induced the synthesis of Na-K-ATPase. Alternatively, however, these results could suggest that aldosterone induces the synthesis of a protein which, in turn, would activate preexisting units of Na-K-ATPase. The demonstration that aldosterone indeed induces Na-K-ATPase synthesis was provided by the work of Verrey et al. who showed that in A_6 cells, aldosterone enhances the number of mRNAs encoding for the α and β subunits of the enzyme [17].

Although it is usually admitted that Na-K-ATPase has a long half-life (7–15 h), it is noteworthy that the time-course of aldosterone action on the pump synthesis is fast (30 min latency, maximal stimulation within 2.5–3 h) and coincides with the

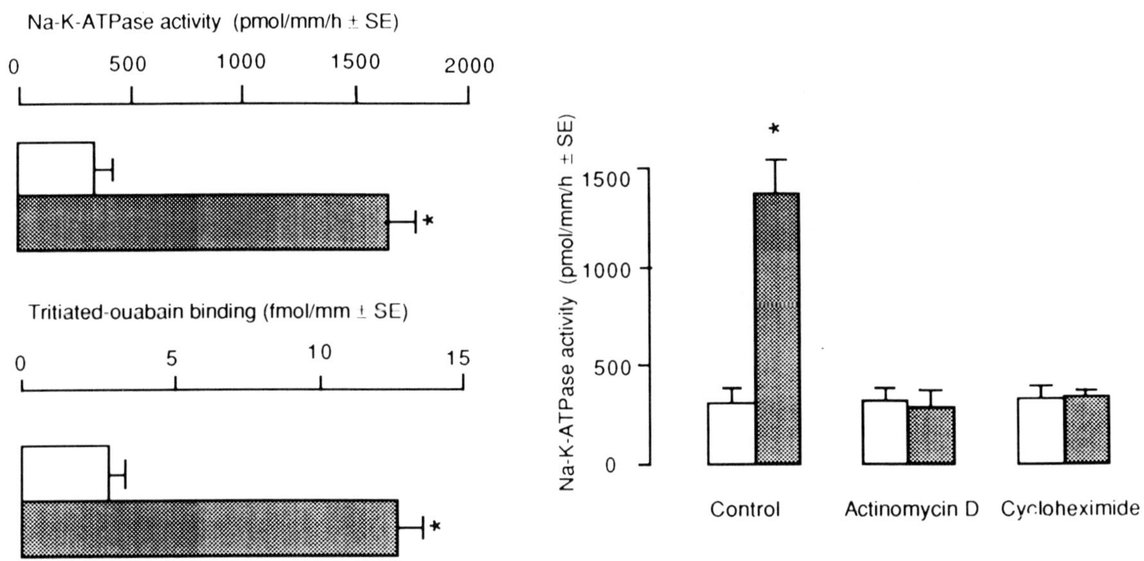

Fig. 2. Effect of aldosterone on Na-K-ATPase in the cortical collecting tubule (*CCT*) of 7-day-adrenalectomized rats. *Left*, Na-K-ATPase activity and specific binding of ^{3}H-ouabain were measured in CCT incubated for 2.5h at 37°C in the absence (*open bars*) or in the presence of $10^{-8}M$ aldosterone (*dark bars*). *Right*, CCT were incubated without (*open bars*) or with aldosterone (*dark bars*) in same conditions as above, and in the presence of 5µM actinomycin D, 20µM cycloheximide or in the absence of drug (control). Statistical significance according to Student's t-test:*, $P<0.005$. (Redrawn from [16])

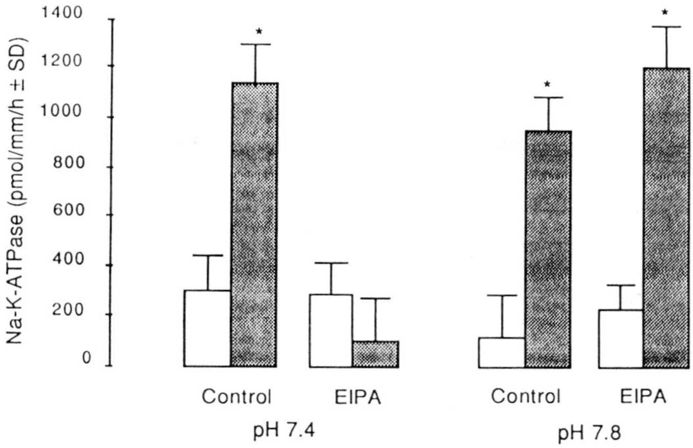

Fig. 3. Effect of ethylisopropyl amiloride (*EIPA*) and pH on aldosterone action in the cortical collecting tubule (*CCT*) of adrenalectomized rats. Na-K-ATPase activity was measured in CCT incubated for 2.5h at 37°C in the absence (*open bars*) or in the presence of 10^{-8}M aldosterone (*dark bars*), under normal conditions (control) or in the presence of 25μM EIPA. The pH of the medium was adjusted to either 7.4 or 7.8, which corresponds to intracellular pH of 7.3 and 7.6, respectively. Statistical significance according to Student's t-test:*,$P<0.001$

antinatriuretic response to aldosterone [14]. Despite this synchronization between the actions of aldosterone on Na-K-ATPase activity and on urinary Na excretion, it has been postulated that induction of Na-K-ATPase synthesis could be a secondary action of aldosterone due to enhanced intracellular Na concentration, itself brought about by the primary stimulation by aldosterone of luminal Na channels. This hypothesis was based on the finding that in vivo administration of the Na channel blocker amiloride prior to aldosterone abolished the stimulation of collecting tubule Na-K-ATPase [18]. However, such inhibitory action of amiloride could result from unspecific effects of this drug which, depending on its concentration, can also inhibit the Na/H exchanger [19], Na-K-ATPase [20], and even protein synthesis [21]. And indeed, low concentrations of amiloride sufficient to inhibit Na channels, but with no action on other systems had no effect on the in vitro induction of Na-K-ATPase by aldosterone, whereas higher concentrations known to inhibit the Na/H exchanger totally abolished Na-K-ATPase stimulation [16]. That induction of Na-K-ATPase synthesis by aldosterone requires the integrity of the Na/H exchanger is confirmed by experiments showing that ethylisopropylamiloride (EIPA), a specific inhibitor of the Na/H exchanger [19], totally abolished aldosterone action (Fig. 3). Thus, induction of ATPase synthesis by aldosterone may require the preliminary stimulation of the Na/H exchanger which has previously been observed by Oberleithner et al. [22]. In fact, it seems to require an intracellular alkalinization, brought about by stimulation of Na/H exchanger, since the inhibitory action of EIPA can be curtailed when artificial intracellular alkalinization is produced by incubating the samples at pH 7.8 (which corresponds to a pH_i of 7.6) instead of 7.4 (which corresponds to a pH_i of 7.3) (Fig. 3).

In conclusion, Na-K-ATPase of the collecting tubule is likely an AIP. However, its induction requires other factors, which include intracellular alkalinization as well as the presence of triiodothyronine [16]. The time-course of Na-K-ATPase stimulation correlates with that of the antinatriuretic action of aldosterone.

Sodium-Induced Recruitment of Latent Na-K-ATPase Units in the Collecting Tubule

Besides its stimulatory role as a substrate of Na-K-ATPase (see above) intracellular Na also controls the number of pump units in several cell types [23]. However, this regulation displays specific features in kidney cells, in particular as regards its time-course and mechanism.

Thus, incubation of rat cortical collecting tubules in the presence of extracellular Na and of Na ionophores such as nystatin or amphotericin B results, within 2–3 h, in a marked stimulation of Na-K-ATPase activity, and, to a similar extent, of the specific ^{3}H-ouabain binding (Fig. 4). However, this induction of new pump units by increased intracellular Na concentration does not involve de novo synthesis of the enzyme, since it is not altered by either actinomycin D or cycloheximide (Fig. 4). Rather, these observations suggest the existence of a pool of latent Na-K-ATPase units which can be recruited in response to a transient increment of intracellular Na concentration [24]. The localization of this pool and its mode of recruitment are not, as yet, known.

Another feature of this regulatory process is that the latent pool of Na-K-ATPase does not exist (or is not recruitable) in collecting tubules of adrenalectomized rats [24], suggesting that its synthesis is controlled by corticosteroids. In fact, during the first 24 h following adrenalectomy, the pool of latent Na-K-ATPase is progressively recruited so as to maintain constant the pool of active Na-K-ATPase; this latter decreasing because of the decline in its rate of synthesis (see above). Thus, following adrenalectomy, a decreased rate of Na-K-ATPase synthesis may generate an increase in intracellular Na concentration, which triggers the recruitment of the latent pool of ATPase, until its total disappearance.

Besides the nature and the intracellular localization of this latent pool of Na-K-ATPase, several other questions have to be solved. Among them, it will be important to know whether or not this reserve of Na-K-ATPase is a special feature of the collecting tubule.

Control of Na-K-ATPase Activity by Locally Generated Mediators

Another mechanism of rapid regulation of Na-K-ATPase involves metabolites of arachidonic acid which can be produced in the medullary thick ascending limb (MTAL) in response to vasopressin (AVP).

Thus, we observed [25] that incubation of MTAL, microdissected from normal rats, in the presence of AVP 10^{-7} M for 15 min induced a marked inhibition of Na-K-ATPase

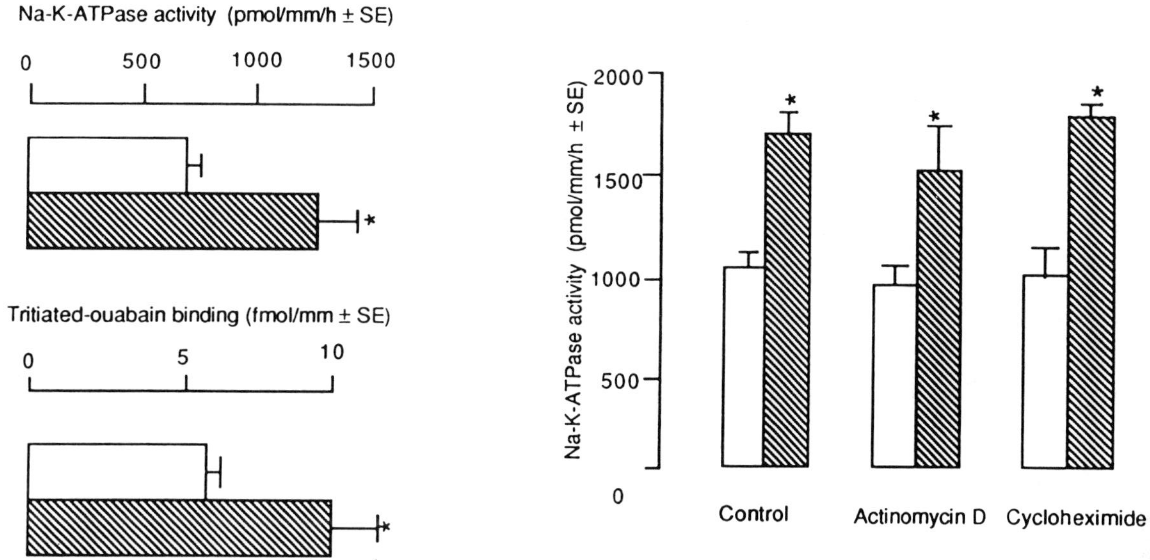

Fig. 4. Effect of increasing intracellular Na concentration on Na-K-ATPase in rat cortical collecting tubule (*CCT*). *Left*, Na-K-ATPase activity and specific binding of ^{3}H ouabain were measured in CCT incubated for 2.5h at 37°C in the absence (*open bars*) or in the presence of 0.1U/μl of the sodium ionophore nystatin (*hatched bars*). *Right*, Before incubation without (*open bars*) or with nystatin (*hatched bars*) for 2h in same conditions as above, CCT were preincubated for 1 h with 5μM actinomycin D, 20μM cycloheximide, or in the absence of drug (control). Statistical significance according to Student's t-test:*,$P<0.001$. (Redrawn from [24])

activity (control: 3740±210 pmol/mm per h ±SE; AVP: 2280±110 pmol/mm per h ± SE; n=5, $P<0.001$ by Student's t-test). This inhibition was dose-dependent (app $K_{0.5} \sim 2.10^{-8}$M) and reached its maximum within 5 min. Inhibition of Na-K-ATPase activity by AVP was accompanied by a similar inhibition of ouabain-sensitive ^{86}Rb uptake (Control: 42.8±2.8 pEq/mm per min ±SE; AVP: 29.9±1.9 pEq/mm min ±SE, n=6, $P<0.005$). Inhibition of ATPase activity and Rb uptake was mediated by cyclic AMP since it was mimicked by cAMP generating hormones (calcitonin and glucagon), by forskolin, and by dibutyryl cAMP.

Earlier, Schwartzman and colleagues reported that cells from rabbit MTAL displayed a cytochrome P450-dependent monoxygenase pathway which metabolized arachidonic acid into two biologically active compounds, one of which was a potent inhibitor of purified Na-K-ATPase [26]. Thus, we investigated whether this metabolite could be responsible for AVP-induced inhibition of Na-K-ATPase in rat MTAL.

Results indicated that: 1—preincubation of MTAL with 10^{-4}M arachidonic acid mimicked the action of AVP; 2—the inhibitory actions of AVP and arachidonic acid were not additive; 3—addition of 10^{-5}M of the phospholipase A_2 inhibitor, quinacrine, abolished the inhibitory action of AVP, and 4—addition of 5.10^{-5}M of the monoxygenase inhibitor SKF525A curtailed the actions of both AVP and arachidonic acid. These findings confirmed that AVP promotes its inhibitory action on Na-K-ATPase by inducing the monoxygenase-dependent synthesis of an arachidonate-derived inhibitor of Na-K-ATPase.

From a physiological point of view, this inhibitory action of AVP on Na-K-ATPase is paradoxical, since this hormone is known to increase Na reabsorption in the thick ascending limb [27]. It is possible, however, that the inhibitory action, which requires higher concentrations of hormone, may represent a regulatory feedback mechanism preventing excessive dilution of the tubular fluid.

Other local mediators have been shown to control Na-K-ATPase activity. Thus, prostaglandins, which were reported to inhibit Na-K-ATPase in the gastric mucosa [28], liver [29], and brain [30], also inhibit the renal enzyme. Indeed, Cordova et al. have shown that Na-K-ATPase activity was increased in the cortical collecting tubule of rabbits chronically treated with the prostaglandin synthesis inhibitor indomethacin [31]. Similar results were observed by Wald et al. [32] on rat MTAL. Furthermore, these authors reported that in vitro addition of 10^{-4}M PGE_2 inhibited Na-K-ATPase activity in rat MTAL within 15 min [32]. It is interesting to note that this regulatory pathway could also be triggered by AVP in vivo, since this hormone stimulates prostaglandin synthesis in the collecting tubule [33,34], from where it can be expected to act on both collecting tubule and thick ascending limb.

Control of Na-K-ATPase Mediated Ion Flux by Insulin in the Collecting Tubule

Besides its metabolic effects, insulin controls urinary sodium excretion directly at the tubular level. Thus, insulin reduces natriuresis in isolated kidneys perfused at constant GFR [35]. Since, in several tissues, insulin was shown to stimulate Na-K-ATPase activity [36–38], we investigated whether the antinatriuretic action of insulin could be mediated by stimulation of the pump activity. A likely target for this

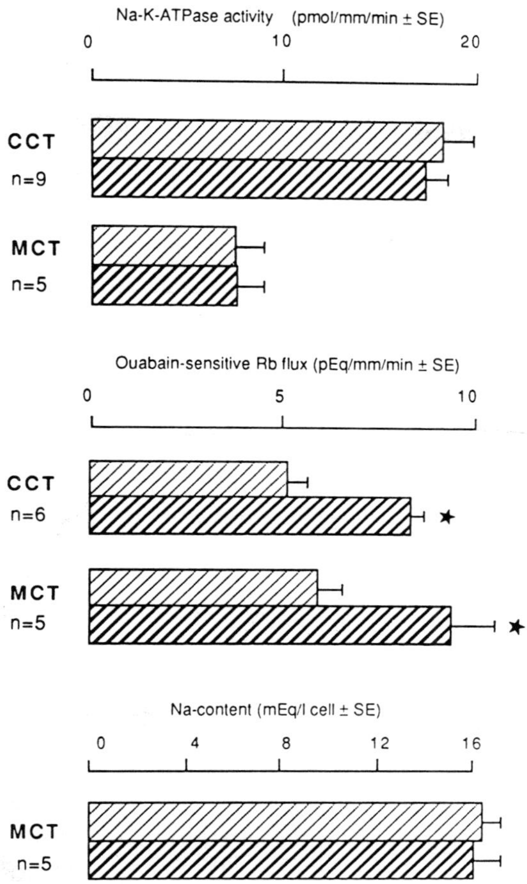

Fig. 5. Effect of insulin on Na-K-ATPase and Na concentration in rat cortical (*CCT*) and medullary collecting tubule (*MCT*). Na-K-ATPase activity, ouabain sensitive Rb uptake and intracellular Na concentration were measured in CCT and MCT incubated for 15–120 min at 37°C in the *absence* ( ) or in the *presence* of 10^{-8}M insulin ( ). Statistical significance according to Student's t-test:*,$P<0.05$

action is the collecting tubule, since it has been reported previously that insulin increased active transepithelial Na transport in amphibian bladder and in cultured A_6 cells [39,40].

In vitro preincubation of rat collecting tubules at 37°C for 15–120 min in the presence of 10^{-8}M insulin did not modify the V_{max} of the ATP hydrolytic activity of Na-K-ATPase (Fig. 5). However, under the same conditions, insulin markedly increased (+60%) the ouabain-sensitive influx of Rb (Fig. 5). This stimulation was dose-dependent (app $K_{0.5}$ ~ 10^{-9}M) and reached its maximum within the first 5 min of incubation with insulin (E. Feraille et al., unpublished work).

Such a discrepancy between the absence of insulin action on Na-K-ATPase activity on the one hand, and the stimulation of Rb influx on the other, may have several origins. First, it may be secondary to the tubule permeabilization necessary to measure Na-K-ATPase activity, which may result in the loss of some insulin-sensitive intracellular factor controlling the V_{max} of the enzyme. Alternatively, it may indicate that insulin does not alter the V_{max} of Na-K-ATPase (the number of pump units), but rather alters the pumping rate of preexisting units. This last hypothesis seems more likely, since in several other cell types insulin was reported to stimulate the pump activity by increasing either intracellular Na concentration [37,41] or the pump affinity for Na [42]. In the collecting tubule, however, we did not observe any change in intracellular Na concentration in response to insulin, under conditions in which this hormone increased Rb influx (Fig. 5). Thus, it is likely that insulin stimulates Na-K-ATPase in the collecting tubule by increasing its affinity for Na. This hypothesis is presently being tested in this laboratory.

If this hypothesis is confirmed, it will be interesting, since the collecting tubule is likely to contain the α_3 isoform of Na-K-ATPase catalytic subunit (see above) and, in adipocytes, Lytton has reported that insulin increased the affinity for Na of the α_3 isoform exclusively [42]. Thus, besides the existence of specific processes of regulation of their genomic expression, the α_1 and α_3 isoforms may also display different regulation properties at the protein level.

Conclusions

This review briefly describes some mechanisms through which a hormone may control the activity of basolateral Na-K-ATPase. As summarized in Fig. 6 (from top to bottom), a hormone may: 1) through induction of genomic expression, increase the rate of synthesis of Na-K-ATPase; 2) alter some intracellular metabolic pathway leading to the production of an inhibitor (or an activator) of the pump; 3) directly inhibit Na-K-ATPase via its binding to the extracellular ouabain site; or 4) increase intracellular Na concentration through activation of luminal Na entry, and thereby either activate preexisting pump units (substrate effect) or induce the recruitment of latent pump units (possibly through exocytosis). Other possible mechanisms which have been described in the literature include alterations of the basolateral membrane potential (which might alter the pump activity because of its electrogenicity) or alterations of the basolateral K conductance associated with the recycling of K [43,44). Finally, it has also been proposed that, in the proximal tubule, Na-K-ATPase could be controlled through a G protein [45].

The two main conclusions which can be drawn are the following: Firstly, in many circumstances, control of Na-K-ATPase activity in kidney cells is fast and is concomitant with the hormone action on Na transport. Thus, changes in Na-K-ATPase primarily participate in the hormonal response, rather than being, as considered hitherto, secondary adaptations to this response. Secondly, there is a wide heterogeneity of hormone actions on Na-K-ATPase along the nephron (even though the collecting tubule appears as a major site of control). This heterogeneity may be due either to the distinct nature of regulatory proteins present in each cell type (hormone receptors, transduction mechanisms, intracellular metabolic pathways, . . .) or to the very nature of Na-K-ATPase itself, i.e., the presence of α_1 versus α_3 isoforms of the pump.

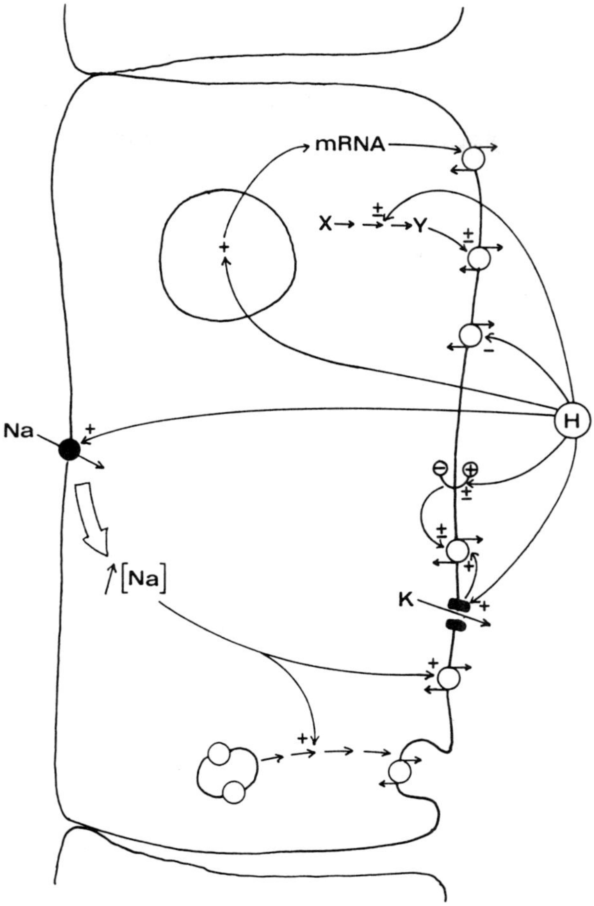

Fig. 6. Schematic summary of the different modes of control of Na-K-ATPase by a hormone (*H*)

Acknowledgments. The authors are grateful to L. Bonnet-Lericque for her secretarial assistance during the preparation of this manuscript. Work from our laboratory was supported in part by grants from the Centre National de la Recherche Scientifique to the Unité de Recherche Associée 219. L. Cheval and E. Feraille were assisted by grants from the Ministère de la Recherche et de la Technologie and from the Fondation pour la Recherche Médicale, respectively.

References

1. Kyte J (1976) Immunoferritin determination of the distribution of Na, K-ATPase over the plasma membranes of renal convoluted tubules. I. Distal segment. J Cell Biol 68:287–303

2. Kyte J (1976) Immunoferritin determination of the distribution of Na, K-ATPase over the plasma membranes of renal convoluted tubules. II. Proximal segment. J Cell Biol 68:304–318
3. Morel F, Chabardes D, Imbert-Teboul M (1978) Methodology for enzymatic studies of isolated tubular segments: Adenylate cyclase. In: Martinez-Maldonado M (ed) Methods in Pharmacology, vol 4B. Plenum, New York, pp 297–323
4. Doucet A, Katz AI, Morel F (1979) Determination of Na-K-ATPase activity in single segments of the mammalian nephron. Am J Physiol 237 (Renal Fluid Electrolyte Physiol 6):F105–F113
5. Cheval L, Doucet A (1990) Measurement of Na-K-ATPase-mediated rubidium influx in single segments of rat nephron. Am J Physiol 259 (Renal Fluid Electrolyte Physiol 28):F111–F121
6. El Mernissi G, Doucet A (1984) Quantitation of [^{3}H] ouabain binding and turnover of Na-K-ATPase along the rabbit nephron. Am J Physiol 247 (Renal Fluid Electrolyte Physiol 16):F158–F167
7. Knight AB, Welt LG (1974) Intracellular K. A determinant of Na:K pump rate. J Gen Physiol 63:351–373
8. Skou JC (1960) Further investigations of a Mg^{2+} and Na^+-activated adenosine triphosphatase possibly related to the active, linked transport of Na^+ and K^+ across the nerve membrane. Biochim Biophys Acta 42:6–23
9. Barlet-Bas C, Cheval L, Khadouri C, Marsy S, Doucet A (1990) Difference in the Na affinity of Na-K-ATPase along the rabbit nephron:modulation by K. Am J Physiol 259 (Renal Fluid Electrolyte Physiol 28):F246–F250
10. Jorgensen PL (1980) Sodium and potassium ion pump in kidney tubules. Physiol Rev 60:864–917
11. De Wardener HE, Mills IH, Clapham WF, Hayter CJ (1961) Studies on the efferent mechanism of the sodium diuresis which follows the administration of intravenous saline in the dog. Clin Sci 21:249–263
12. Doucet A, Barlet C (1986) Evidence for differences in the sensitivity to ouabain of Na-K-ATPase along the nephrons of rabbit kidney. J Biol Chem 261:993–995
13. Sweadner KJ (1989) Isozymes of the Na^+/K^+-ATPase. Biochim Biophys Acta 988:185–220
14. El Mernissi G, Doucet A (1983) Short-term effect of aldosterone on renal sodium transport and tubular Na-K-ATPase in the rat. Pflugers Arch 399:139–146
15. El Mernissi G, Doucet A (1983) Short term effects of aldosterone and dexamethasone on Na-K-ATPase along the rabbit nephron. Pflugers Arch 399:147–151
16. Barlet-Bas C, Khadouri C, Marsy S, Doucet A (1988) Sodium-independent in vitro induction of Na-K-ATPase by aldosterone in renal target cells: permissive effect of triiodothyronine. Proc Natl Acad Sci USA 85:1707–1711
17. Verrey F, Schaerer E, Zoerkler P, Paccolat MP, Geering K, Kraehenbuhl JP, Rossier BC (1987) Regulation by aldosterone of Na^+, K^+-ATPase mRNAs, protein synthesis, and sodium transport in cultured kidney cells. J Cell Biol 104:1231–1237
18. Petty KJ, Kokko JP, Marver D (1981) Secondary effect of aldosterone on Na-K-ATPase activity in the rabbit cortical collecting tubule. J Clin Invest 68:1514–1521
19. Frelin C, Vigne P, Barbry P, Lazdunski M (1987) Molecular properties of amiloride action and of its Na^+ transporting targets. Kidney Int 32:785–793
20. Soltoff SP, Mandel LJ (1983) Amiloride directly inhibits the Na, K-ATPase activity of rabbit kidney proximal tubules. Science 20:957–959
21. Leffert HL, Koch KS, Fehlmann M, Heiser W, Lad PJ, Skelly H (1982) Amiloride blocks cell-free protein synthesis at levels attained inside cultured rat hepatocytes. Biochem Biophys Res Commun 108:738–745
22. Oberleithner H, Weigt M, Westphale HJ, Wang W (1987) Aldosterone activates Na^+/H^+ exchange and raises cytoplasmic pH in target cells of the amphibian kidney. Proc Natl Acad Sci USA 84:1464–1468

23. Fambrough DM, Wolitzky BA, Tamkun MM, Takeyasu K (1987) Regulation of the sodium pump in excitable cells. Kidney Int 32:S97–S112
24. Barlet-Bas C, Khadouri C, Marsy S, Doucet A (1990) Enhanced intracellular sodium concentration in kidney cells recruits a latent pool of Na-K-ATPase whose size is modulated by corticosteroids. J Biol Chem 265:7799–7803
25. Doucet A (1988) Multiple hormonal control of the Na/K-ATPase activity in the thick ascending limb. In: Davison AM (ed) Nephrology, vol 1. Baillière Tindall, London, pp 247–254
26. Schwartzman M, Ferreri NR, Carroll MA, Songu-Mize E, McGiff JC (1985) Renal cytochrome P450-related arachidonate metabolite inhibits (Na^+ + K^+) ATPase. Nature 314: 620–622
27. Greger R (1985) Ion transport mechanisms in thick ascending limb of Henle's loop of mammalian nephron. Physiol Rev 65:760–797
28. Mazsik G, Kutas J, Nagy L, Nameth G (1974) Inhibition of Mg^{2+}, Na^+-K^+-dependent ATPase system in human gastric mucosa by prostaglandin E_1 and E_2. Eur J Pharmacol 29:133–137
29. Verna R (1984) Effects of prostaglandins on rat liver plasma membrane-bound Na^+-K^+-ATPase. In: Braquet P, et al (eds) Prostaglandins and membrane ion transport. Raven, New York, pp 227–233
30. Yasuko S, Hideramro O, Masarori S, Yasahiko S, Hisashi T (1982) Inhibitory effect of PGA_2 on Na-K-ATPase in synoptic plasma membrane of rat brain in vitro. Int J Biochem 14:347–350
31. Cordova HR, Kokko JP, Marver D (1989) Chronic indomethacin increases rabbit cortical collecting tubule Na^+-K^+-ATPase activity. Am J Physiol 256 (Renal Fluid Electrolyte Physiol 25)F570–F576
32. Wald H, Scherzer P, Rubinger D, Popovtzer MM (1990) Effect of indomethacin in vivo and PGE_2 in vitro on MTAL Na-K-ATPase of the rat kidney. Pflugers Arch 415:648–650
33. Kirschenbaum MA, Lowe AG, Trizna W, Fine LG (1982) Regulation of vasopressin action by prostaglandins. Evidence for prostaglandin synthesis in the rabbit cortical collecting tubule. J Clin Invest 70:1193–1204
34. Schlondorff D, Satriano JA, Schwartz GJ (1985) Synthesis of prostaglandin E_2 in different segments of isolated collecting tubules from adult and neonatal rabbits. Am J Physiol 248 (Renal Fluid Electrolyte Physiol 17):F134–F144
35. Nizet A, Lefèbvre P, Crabbé J (1971) Control by insulin of sodium potassium and water excretion by the isolated dog kidney. Pflugers Arch 323:11–20
36. Clausen T, Flatman JA (1987) Effects of insulin and epinephrine on Na^+-K^+ and glucose transport in soleus muscle. Am J Physiol 252 (Endocrinol Metab 15)E492–E499
37. Gelehrter TD, Shreve PD, Dilworth VM (1984) Insulin regulation of Na/K pump activity in rat hepatoma cells. Diabetes 33:428–434
38. Rosic NK, Standaert ML, Pollet RJ (1985) The mechanism of insulin stimulation of (Na^+-K^+)-ATPase transport activity in muscle. J Biol Chem 260:6206–6212
39. Cobb MH, Yang CPH, Brown JA, Scott WN (1986) Insulin stimulated sodium transport in toad urinary bladder. Biochim Biophys Acta 856:123–129
40. Fidelman ML, May JM, Biber TVL, Watlington CO (1982) Insulin stimulation of Na^+ transport and glucose metabolism in cultured kidney cells. Am J Physiol 242 (Cell Physiol 11):C121–C123
41. Resh MD, Nemenoff RA, Guidotti G (1980) Insulin stimulation of (Na^+,K^+)–adenosine triphosphatase dependent $^{86}Rb^+$ uptake in rat adipocytes. J Biol Chem 255:10938–10945
42. Lytton J (1985) Insulin affects the sodium affinity of the rat adipocyte (Na^+,K^+)-ATPase. J Biol Chem 260:10075–10080

43. Capasso G, Lin JT, DeSanto NG, Kinne R (1985) Short term effect of low doses of triiodothyronine on proximal tubular membrane Na-K-ATPase and potassium permeability in thyroidectomized rats. Pflugers Arch 403:90–96
44. Schultz SG (1981) Homocellular regulatory mechanisms in sodium-transporting epithelia: Avoidance of extinction by "flush-through." Am J Physiol 241 (Renal Fluid Electrolyte Physiol 10):F579–F590
45. Bertorello A, Aperia A (1989) Regulation of Na^{+}-K^{+}-ATPase activity in kidney proximal tubules: involvement of GTP binding proteins. Am J Physiol 256 (Renal Fluid Electrolyte Physiol 25):F57–F62

Properties and Function of the Kidney Vacuolar H^+ ATPase: a Versatile Proton Pump Responsible for Urinary Acidification

STEPHEN GLUCK, BAHAR BASTANI, RAOUL NELSON, HENRY PURCELL, ZHI-QIANG WANG, KUN ZHANG, MICHAEL MARUSHACK, BETH LEE, XIAO-LI GUO, KHALID MASOOD, and PHILIP HEMKEN[1]

Introduction

Approximately 30%–40% of hydrogen ion transport in the proximal tubule, and most or all of proton transport in the distal nephron, is generated by proton pumps belonging to the vacuolar class of H^+ATPases. This ubiquitous type of proton pump is found in all eukaryotic cells, where it serves to acidify intracellular compartments, such as endosomes, lysosomes, and secretory vesicles, in the endocytic and secretory pathways. Certain renal tubular epithelial cells have amplified the expression of the enzyme, and are able to direct it in a polarized manner to specific domains of the plasma membrane, where it carries out transepithelial proton secretion. How amplified expression and polarized localization are achieved, how the enzyme is regulated, and the abnormalities in these processes that underlie disease processes, remain among the most important unanswered questions in this field.

Structure of the Vacuolar H^+ ATPases

Progress in understanding the structure and function of the vacuolar class of H^+ATPases has come from studies in several systems, including the fungal and plant enzymes, and the kidney, coated vesicle, and chromaffin granule enzymes from mammalian sources. The vacuolar H^+ATPases were first identified as electrogenic proton pumps that were resistant to azide and oligomycin, inhibitors of the mitochondrial proton pump, and resistant to vanadate, an inhibitor of the gastric electroneutral H^+/K ATPase. The plant, fungal, and mammalian enzymes were all purified independently from different sources, but showed remarkably similar structures. The vacuolar H^+ATPases are all 500–600000 molecular weight (*M*r) proteins with, generally, at

[1]Depts. of Medicine and Cell Biology and Physiology, Washington University School of Medicine, and The Renal Division, Jewish Hospital, St. Louis, MO 63178, USA

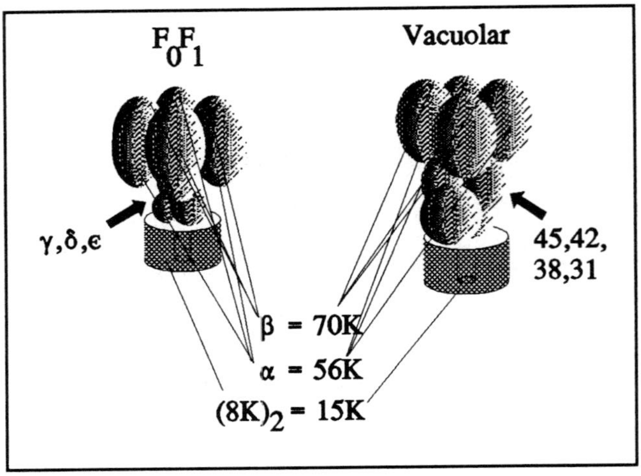

Fig. 1

least 8 different component subunits. All have subunits of approximately 70 kD, 56 kD, several subunits between 30 and 50 kD, and at least one low molecular weight subunit of 17 kD. In all of the enzymes, most of the large molecular weight proteins are peripheral membrane proteins that do not have any membrane spanning portions, and the small molecular weight proteins are intrinsic membrane proteins that span the lipid bilayer. Purification of the bovine kidney H^+ATPase by two different methods yielded an identical pattern of composite polypeptides with relative molecular weights of 70, 56 (a cluster), 45, 42, 38, 33, 31, 15, 14, and 12 kD.

Advance in understanding the basic structure of the enzyme and the function of the subunits has been relatively rapid because of the remarkable similarity of these enzymes to the F0F1 class of H^+ATPases, whose structure and function have been investigated extensively. The known structure of the F0F1 H^+ATPases has provided a conceptual framework for most of the experiments probing the structure of the vacuolar enzymes (Fig. 1). The α and β subunits which form the major structural part of the catalytic domain of the F0F1 ATPases share significant sequence homology with the 56 kD and 70 kD subunits of the vacuolar enzymes. Recent sequence analysis shows that the sequences of the 70 kD and 56 kD subunits are also highly similar to the two largest subunits of the archaebacterial H^+ATPases. Thus, it is likely that the vacuolar and F0F1 classes of H^+ATPases share a common ancestral proton pump, from which both diverged, dating back to the earliest life forms.

The vacuolar H^+ATPases have two major domains, the cytoplasmic domain and the transmembrane domain, each of which is composed of a multitude of subunits. The cytoplasmic domain is the locus of the catalytic and probably regulatory sites of the enzyme, and is composed of peripheral membrane proteins. The transmembrane domain forms the channel through which protons cross the lipid bilayer, and is composed of intrinsic membrane proteins which span the cytoplasmic domain and anchor it on the membrane (Fig. 2).

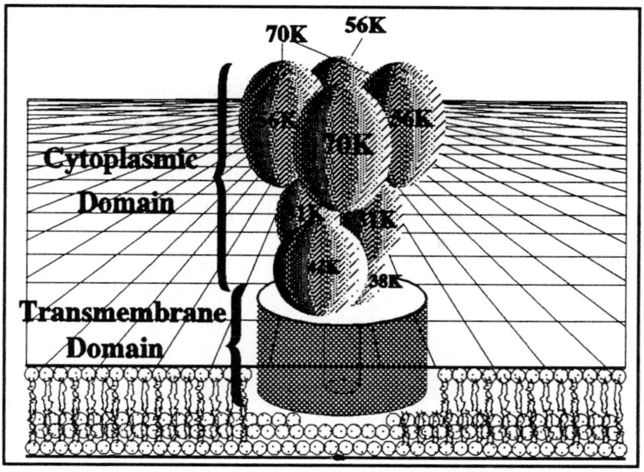

Fig. 2

The Cytoplasmic Domain

The 70 kD molecular weight of the vacuolar H$^+$ATPases appears to be the site where ATP is hydrolyzed during proton transport. Thee are three duplicates of the subunit in each complete proton pump. The evidence available at present suggests that there is only one gene for the 70 kD subunit. The sequences of the 70 kD subunit and its homolog have a highly conserved domain in the mid coding region, which probably comprises the nucleotide binding and catalytic site. The sequence of the bovine kidney subunit, compared with the subunits of plant and fungal enzymes, shows wide divergence at the amino-terminal and carboxyl-terminal domains, with no sequence conservation. It is possible that these regions have a regulatory or non-catalytic role.

There are three duplicates of this subunit per H$^+$ATPase as well. The function of the 56 kD subunit is uncertain. The subunit is homologous to the α subunit of the F0F1 H$^+$ATPases. The α subunit does not have a catalytic ATP binding site, but is required for catalytic activity. It has a high affinity nucleotide binding site, which is though to be involved either in regulation of the enzyme, or as a non-hydrolytic part of the reaction mechanism. The function of the 56 kD subunit of the vacuolar H$^+$ATPases is unknown, although evidence from the plant enzyme suggests that it may have an ATP binding site. In kidney H$^+$ATPase, isolated by affinity chromatography on a monoclonal antibody column, several 56 kD subunits were observed which differed slightly in *M*r. cDNA cloning of the subunit has revealed that there are at least two different isoforms of the 56 kD subunit in the kidney, and that these are encoded by different genes. The isoforms have 93% sequence identity in the mid coding region, but are completely different at the amino and carboxyl terminal domains. H$^+$ATPase affinity purified from a bovine kidney cortex microsomal fraction had different enzymatic properties from H$^+$ATPase isolated from bovine kidney brush border. The microsomal enzyme also exhibited a pattern of 56 kD polypeptides that differed from

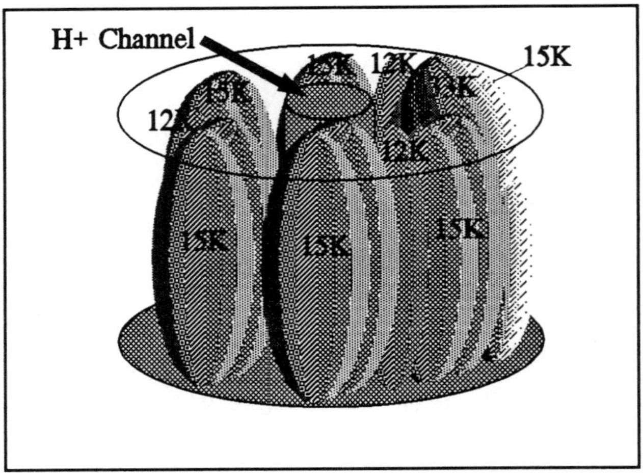

Fig. 3

the 56 kD subunit pattern in the H⁺ATPase isolated from brush border. The 56 kD subunit may therefore have an important role in determining the enzymatic properties or compartmentation of the vacuolar H⁺ATPase.

There are from one to three duplicates of the 31 kD subunit per H⁺ATPase; the exact composition is unresolved. Results to date indicate only one gene for this subunit in mammalian cells. The amino acid sequence of the subunit is 98% identical in different mammalian species, far higher than for the 70 and 56 kD subunits. The function of the 31 kD subunit is unknown. Experiments on the biosynthesis of the enzyme suggest a possible role in nucleating its extramembranous catalytic head. Free 70 and 56 kD subunits could be immunoprecipitated from the cytosol of 35-S methionine-labeled cultured renal cells, but free 31 kD subunit could not, although this subunit could be immunoprecipitated associated with the other two subunits.

The function of the other subunits of the cytosolic domain is not established, but they may constitute a "stalk" domain connecting the catalytic portion to the intrinsic membrane domain, a construction similar to that of the F0F1 enzymes.

The Transmembrane Domain

The transmembrane domain forms a proton conducting channel that spans the lipid bilayer. Although the entire composition of this portion of the enzyme remains in dispute, all of the vacuolar H⁺ATPases have an approximately 17 kD (or 15 kD in the kidney) polypeptide that reacts readily with the hydrophobic carboxyl reagent DCCD. The F0F1 H⁺ATPases all have a DCCD binding protein which is approximately 8 kD, and is present in 9 or more duplicates per enzyme. The 17 kD subunit of the mammalian and fungal H⁺ATPases has been cloned, and the vacuolar subunit appears to have arisen from a duplication and fusion of the F0F1 gene.

This suggests that this subunit forms at least part of the proton conducting channel spanning the membrane. The function of the other subunits is unclear. Evidence from other vacuolar H^+ATPases suggests that the 33 kD subunit may be part of the transmembrane domain. By functional analogy with the F0F1 H^+ATPases, it may serve as a binding and regulatory subunit for anchoring the cytosolic domain on the membrane.

Specialized Use of the Vacuolar H^+ATPase in Renal Hydrogen Ion Excretion

As indicated above, most eukaryotic cells have the vacuolar H^+ATPase primarily, or exclusively, on the plasma membrane. This is true even in cultured renal epithelial cells such as the LLC-PK1 and MDCK lines. However, some specialized cells, such as certain proton-transporting renal epithelial cells, are able to direct the enzyme to the plasma membrane and employ it to engender hydrogen ion or bicarbonate secretion. To do so, proton transporting renal epithelial cells impart four specialized functions to the vacuolar H^+ATPase, functions not observed in other cells: 1) Amplified expression of the H^+ATPase, 2) appearance of the enzyme in abundance on the plasma membrane, 3) polarization to different plasma membrane or cellular domains, and 4) physiologic regulation geared to maintain extracellular fluid homeostasis. How the kidney uses the enzyme to accomplish these tasks, while still employing vacuolar H^+ATPases to acidify and energize transport in intracellular compartments, remains a central question.

Several lines of evidence indicate that the vacuolar H^+ATPase in mammalian kidney is actually composed of a mixture of several different enzymes with subtle differences in structure. We postulate that these structural variations impart different physiologic properties to the enzyme, enabling renal cells to establish the differentiated functions outlined above. The first evidence for different forms of the H^+ATPase was obtained from the SDS gels of fractions from a high performance liquid chromatography (HPLC) ion exchange column originally used to purify the bovine kidney enzyme (Fig. 4). Two partially resolved peaks of ATPase activity were observed eluting off the column. Gels of these revealed the complicated polypeptide composition described above. However, the first peak of ATPase activity had a polypeptide at *M*r 58 kD, whereas the second peak of activity had a peak at 56 kD. This suggested that different forms of the ATPase might exist, which differed in the composition of the 56 kD subunit. Recent experiments have continued to provide support for this view. As discussed above, at least two different genes for the 56 kD subunit are expressed in mammalian kidney, and these differ in composition prominently at the amino and carboxyl termini, while the central portion, which contains the domain thought to participate in catalysis, is highly conserved.

A second approach to this question has been to compare the properties of vacuolar H^+ATPase isolated from different kidney membrane compartments, such as microsomes (which likely includes plasma membrane from intercalated cells), and brush border microvilli. H^+ATPase, purified from kidney microsomes and brush border on a monoclonal antibody affinity column and analyzed on 2D gels, revealed a different composition of polypeptides in the 56 kD *M*r range. H^+ATPase purified from brush

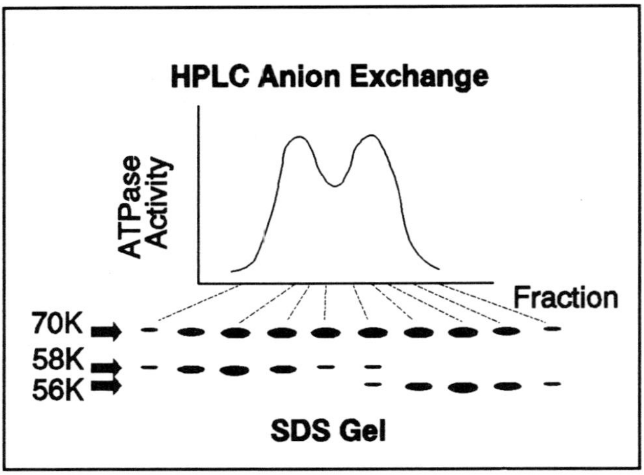

Fig. 4

border had different enzymatic properties from H⁺ATPase purified from renal microsomes, with different pH optima, ATP:GTP substrate preference, and response to the addition of various divalent cations. We have subsequently isolated H⁺ATPase from bovine kidney cortex lysosomes, and found that its properties differ from both the microsomal and brush border enzymes.

The 31 kD subunit may also be a site for variations in structure between different forms of the H⁺ATPase (Fig. 5). Two monoclonal antibodies, E11 and H8, were

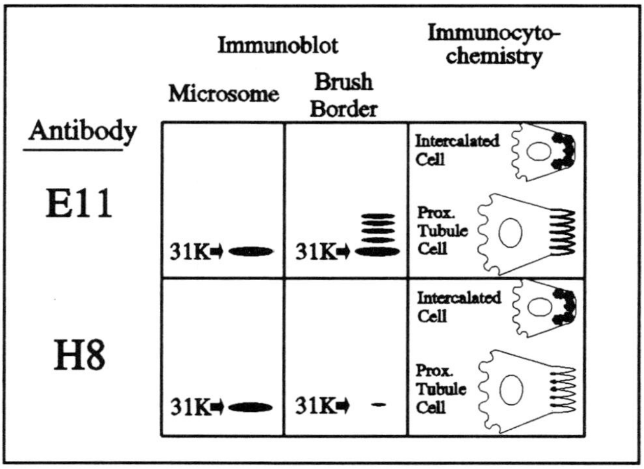

Fig. 5

generated to the 31 kD subunit. The patterns of reactivity of the two antibodies on immunoblots of the isolated brush border and microsomal H^+ATPase, and the distribution of immunocytochemical staining with the two antibodies differed greatly. E11 reacted strongly with both the microsomal and brush border enzymes, but the brush border immunoblot showed several additional immunoreactive bands at apparent molecular weights slightly higher than 31 kD. H8 reacted strongly with the microsomal H^+ATPase, but showed only faint immunoreactivity against the brush border enzyme. On immunocytochemistry, both E11 and H8 stained the intercalated cells strongly. E11 also stained both the brush border and the invaginations at the base of the brush border in the proximal tubule. H8 stained only the invaginations, and did not stain the brush border. These observations suggest that structural differences in the 31 kD subunit exist between the brush border and microsomal H^+ATPase, and that the differences may have a role in directing the enzyme to the brush border. The higher molecular weight forms of the 31 kD subunit were visible on two dimensional silver stained gels of the purified brush border H^+ATPase, but were not seen in the microsomal H^+ATPase.

These observations show that enzymatic differences exist between vacuolar H^+ATPase isolated from different kidney membrane fractions, and that structural differences can be detected in at least two of the subunits of the enzyme. It remains to be determined whether these differences in structure underlie the specialized functions of the vacuolar H^+ATPase in epithelial cells, discussed above.

Mechanisms for Regulating Renal Hydrogen Ion Secretion

Hydrogen ion transport could be regulated, in principle, by three different mechanisms, illustrated in Fig. 6. Regulation could involve a redistribution of the enzyme,

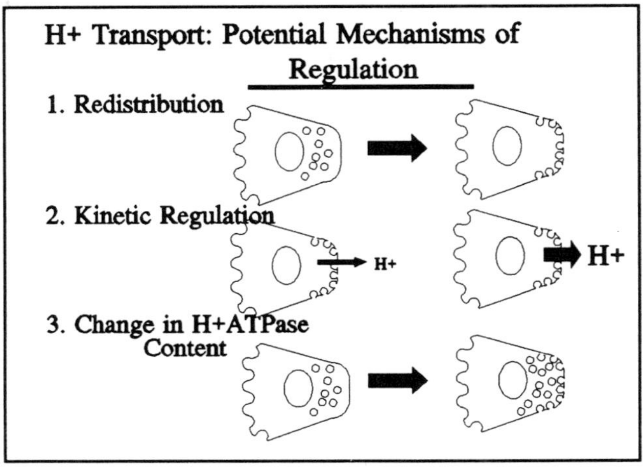

Fig. 6

kinetic regulation of the enzyme, or a change in the quantity of enzyme. Acute redistribution of the enzyme is known to occur in the kidney in response to a change in pCO_2. Increases in the pCO_2 stimulate the recruitment of H^+ATPase from intracellular membrane vesicles, and its insertion in the plasma membrane. This response is prevented by the microtubule destabilizing agent, colchicine. Recent micropuncture studies have shown that in the outer stripe of the outer medulla, only half of the increase in hydrogen ion secretion in response to CO_2 is inhibited by colchicine, suggesting that mechanisms other than insertion operate to regulate hydrogen ion transport.

Our laboratory recently discovered that kidney cytosol contains proteins that both inhibit and stimulate the purified H^+ATPase, and that these proteins appear to do so by binding to the enzyme. The binding of the activator is enhanced at low pH, implying that the protein could activate the H^+ATPase, were cytosolic pH to fall. The binding of the inhibitor protein is prevented at low pH. The partially purified inhibitor suppresses both purified H^+ATPase and proton transport in vesicles by up to 80%, but has no activity against Na-K, Ca^{2+}, or F0F1 ATPases. Though additional studies are needed to establish the cellular distribution and physiologic role of these proteins, they appear to be candidates as kinetic regulators.

Renal hydrogen ion excretion increases in response to acid loading, which has prompted the speculation that the response is, in part, due to an increase in the H^+ATPase content of the intercalated cells. We examined this directly by using monoclonal antibodies and a cDNA clone probe for the 31 kD subunit to measure quantities of H^+ATPase protein, 31 kD subunit transcript, and the distribution of the H^+ATPase by immunocytochemistry in rats subjected to acid and alkali loading over a 14-day period. No change in 31 kD subunit protein or in mRNA levels was detected during the 2-week period, either in the cortex or in the medulla. In contrast, there was a striking change in the distribution of the enzyme. In both the inner and outer stripe of the outer medulla, acid loading produced a progressive shift of H^+ATPase from intracellular vesicles to the plasma membrane. Similar changes were seen in a major subpopulation of intercalated cells in the cortex. Changes in the distribution of the H^+ATPase also appear to have a role in the adaptive response of the remnant kidney, and in the acidification defect which follows relief of acute ureteral obstruction.

SUMMARY. Proton transporting renal epithelial cells employ a vacuolar H^+ATPase to produce the final acidification of urine. Vacuolar H^+ATPases normally reside in intracellular membrane compartments at low abundance levels. Their specialized use in renal cells may be the result of different structural isoforms of the enzyme that serve unique functions in the kidney. Acute regulation of acidification occurs through changes both in the distribution, and, probably, in the kinetics of the enzyme, and kinetic regulation may be controlled by cytosolic inhibitor and activator proteins. Chronic regulation also occurs through shifts in the distribution of the enzyme between intracellular vesicles and the plasma membrane, without major changes in abundance.

References

1. Forgac M (1989) Structure and function of vacuolar class of ATP-driven proton pumps. Physiol Rev 69:765–796
2. Steinmetz PR (1974) Cellular mechanisms of urinary acidification. Physiol Rev 54:890

3. Gluck S, Caldwell J (1988) Proton-translocating ATPase from bovine kidney medulla: partial purification and reconstitution. Am J Physiol (Renal Fluid Electrolyte Physiol 23)254:F71–F79
4. Gluck S, Caldwell J (1987) Immunoaffinity purification and characterization of vacuolar H^+ATPase from bovine kidney. J Biol Chem 262:15 780–15 789
5. Yurko M, Gluck S (1987) Production and characterization of a monoclonal antibody to vacuolar H^+ATPase of renal epithelia. J Biol Chem 262:15 770–15 779
6. Brown D, Gluck S, Hartwig J (1987) Structure of the novel membrane-coating material in proton-secreting cells and identification as an H^+ATPase. J Cell Biol 105:1637–1648
7. Brown D, Hirsch S, Gluck S (1988) An H^+ATPase in opposite plasma membrane domains in kidney epithelial cell subpopulations. Nature 331:622–624
8. Brown D, Hirsch S, Gluck S (1988) Localization of a proton-pumping ATPase in rat kidney. J Clin Invest 82:2114–2126
9. Madsen KM, Tisher CC (1984) Response of intercalated cells of rat outer medullary collecting duct to chronic metabolic acidosis. Lab Invest 51:268–276
10. Hirsch S, Strauss A, Masood K, Lee S, Sukhatme V, Gluck S (1988) Isolation and sequence of a cDNA clone encoding the 31-kDa subunit of bovine kidney vacuolar H^+ATPase. Proc Natl Acad Sci USA 85:3004–3008
11. Alper S, Natale J, Gluck S, Lodish H, Brown D (1989) Intercalated cell subtypes in rat kidney collecting duct defined using antibodies against erythrocyte band 3 and renal vacuolar H^+ATPase. Proc Natl Acad Sci USA 86:5429–5433
12. Gluck S, Cannon C, Al-Awqati Q (1982) Exocytosis regulates urinary acidification in turtle bladder by rapid insertion of H^+ pumps into the luminal membrane. Proc Natl Acad Sci USA 79:4327–4331
13. Wang Z-Q, Gluck S (to be published) Isolation and properties of bovine kidney brush border vacuolar H^+ATPase. A proton pump with enzymatic and structural differences from kidney microsomal H^+ATPase. J Biol Chem
14. Wang Z-Q, Hemken P, Gluck S (1989) Role of the vacuolar H^+ATPase 31K subunit in targeting to renal brush border. J Cell Biol 109:297a
15. Hemken P, Wang Z-Q, Gluck S (1990) Role of 31k subunit in targeting renal H^+ATPase to brush border. Kidney Int 37:225a
16. Schwartz GJ, Al-Awqati Q (1985) Carbon dioxide causes exocytosis of vesicles containing H^+ pumps in isolated perfused proximal and collecting tubules. J Clin Invest 75:1638–1644

Role of Ca^{2+} ATPase and Plasma Membrane Ca^{2+} Pump in Ca^{2+} Transport by the Mammalian Kidney

JOHN T. PENNISTON[1]

SUMMARY. Current evidence suggests that Ca^{2+} transport in the distal nephron involves transit of Ca^{2+} through the epithelial cells and movement out of these cells on the basolateral side via the ATP-powered plasma membrane Ca^{2+} pump.

Introduction

In its role of reclaiming the Ca^{2+} from the filtrate, the kidney faces very different problems in the proximal and distal portions of the nephron. In the proximal nephron the freshly formed ultrafiltrate has nearly the same Ca^{2+} concentration as does the blood, so that the Ca^{2+} needs to be moved up only a very shallow concentration gradient as it moves into the blood. In the distal nephron, the Ca^{2+} concentration in the ultrafiltrate is very low and the remaining Ca^{2+} must be moved up a steep concentration gradient in order to reclaim it. Since plasma membrane Ca^{2+} pumps are ubiquitous in mammalian cells [1], it is natural to suppose that an asymmetrical distribution of the Ca^{2+} pumps in the epithelial cells of the nephron might be responsible for Ca^{2+} transport. In order for this to work, Ca^{2+} would have to enter the epithelial cells from the villous side and then be extruded by Ca^{2+} pumps located only on the basolateral side. This supposition has been supported by studies on plasma membranes isolated from whole kidney homogenates; when basolateral kidney membranes were isolated, they contained Ca^{2+} pump, consistent with the suggestion that Ca^{2+} pumps were present in these membranes, but not ruling out their presence in the villous membranes on the other side of the epithelium [2,3]. The studies on isolated plasma membranes also did not address the question of whether the amount and location of Ca^{2+} pump differed in the proximal and distal nephrons.

[1]Department of Biochemistry and Molecular Biology, Mayo Clinic, Rochester, MN 55905, USA

Table 1. Ca^{2+} pump and Na^+/Ca^{2+} exchange in Ca^{2+} efflux

	V_{max} nmol/(mg,min)	
	Ca^{2+} pump	Na^+/Ca^{2+} exchange
Kidney	80	10
Heart	90	1200

Additional information on localization was provided by the use of monoclonal antibody 5F10, raised against the human erythrocyte Ca^{2+} pump. This antibody cross-reacted with tissues other than erythrocyte and with species other than human. When applied to the kidney, this antibody stained specifically the basolateral side of epithelial cells only in the distal nephron (not in the proximal). This was observed in both human and rat kidneys [4,5]. This results suggests that the proximal and distal portions of the nephron employ different strategies to move Ca^{2+} across the epithelium. The lack of an obvious asymmetric staining in the proximal nephron may mean that transcellular Ca^{2+} transport is not highly important here, but that paracellular Ca^{2+} transport mechanisms are in operation. In paracellular transport, the Ca^{2+} does not pass into an epithelial cell, but rather passes through a channel between epithelial cells. This Ca^{2+} transport may be driven by the potential difference across the epithelial layer. On the other hand, the distal nephron must put more energy into the Ca^{2+} transport process in order to move Ca^{2+} up the steep concentration gradient between the filtrate and the blood. This can be done by allowing Ca^{2+} to diffuse passively into the cell. Although the Ca^{2+} concentration in the ultrafiltrate is much lower than that in the blood, it is high compared with that inside the cell, so that no energy input is needed for this phase of the Ca^{2+} movement. By allowing Ca^{2+} to enter the cell, the epithelium can employ the cell's highly developed mechanisms for controlling Ca^{2+}. In other types of cells, these same mechanisms are used to manage the intracellular Ca^{2+} signal, which controls contraction, secretion, etc. Once the Ca^{2+} has entered the cell, it must be exported through the basolateral membrane, up a 10000-fold concentration gradient. The necessity of moving Ca^{2+} up such a steep gradient is not unique to epithelial cells; in mammals all types of cells must extrude Ca^{2+} against such a gradient. The plasma membrane Ca^{2+} pump exists in all kinds of mammalian cells and is specialized for moving Ca^{2+} up this gradient. Thus, it appears likely that the specific staining for Ca^{2+} pump in the distal nephron reflects a special role for this pump in Ca^{2+} transport by the epithelial cells of the distal nephron.

In considering the ejection of Ca^{2+} from cells, the Na^+/Ca^{2+} exchanger must also be taken into account. This exchanger performs a specific exchange of Na^+ for Ca^{2+} in such a way that the gradient of Na^+ ions across the plasma membrane drives the ejection of Ca^{2+}. Table 1 is a brief summary of data accumulated by Van Os [6], showing the relative capacities of the Na^+/Ca^{2+} exchanger and the plasma membrane Ca^{2+} pump in kidney and in heart. As Table 1 shows, the Na^+/Ca^{2+} exchanger is extremely active in heart muscle (and also in nervous tissue and skeletal muscle). In these tissues, the exchanger probably moves most of the Ca^{2+} out of the cell. However, in kidney, the situation is very different; the Na^+/Ca^{2+} exchanger is present only in rather low concentrations and is probably not capable of moving very much Ca^{2+} out of the cell. This indicates that the Ca^{2+} pump is probably a primary mechanism of transepithelial Ca^{2+} transport.

We still do not know whether the packaging of Ca^{2+} into vesicles [7] is an important part of transcellular Ca^{2+} movements in any tissue. The formation of vesicles packed with Ca^{2+} at one side of the cell, followed by the movement of the vesicle through the cell and the dumping of this Ca^{2+} on the other side of the cell is still a possible mechanism for transcellular Ca^{2+} transport. However, no conclusive evidence in favor of the existence of such a mechanism has yet been introduced.

A feature of plasma membranes which complicates the study of the Ca^{2+} pump is the presence of non-pump Ca^{2+} ATPases. Plasma membranes in many kinds of cells have very active ATPases which are stimulated by the presence of Ca^{2+}. These ATPases are entirely separate from the Ca^{2+} pump and frequently are so high in activity as to mask the Ca^{2+} ATPase activity of the pump. Several different kinds of enzymes can give such ATPase activity, so that the use of ATPase to measure pump activity requires great care and definitive proof that the ATPase activity observed is due to the Ca^{2+} pump. In kidney plasma membranes, an ATPase activity stimulated by either Mg^{2+} or Ca^{2+} is present at an activity of about 700 nmol/(mg,min) [2,3,8]. This ATPase is not specific for ATP, but hydrolyzes other nucleotides equally well [2]. Compared to the ATPase activity of this enzyme, the ATPase due to the Ca^{2+} pump is relatively low in activity, being between 10 and 50 nmol/(mg,min). By taking special care, it is possible to demonstrate the presence of the Ca^{2+} ATPase due to the pump, but routine measurements of Ca^{2+} ATPase will measure primarily the other activity. Thus, in order to measure with certainty the activity of the Ca^{2+} pump in various parts of the kidney or along the nephron, it is necessary to measure Ca^{2+} uptake by inside-out plasma membrane vesicles or to measure Ca^{2+} ATPase with special precautions such as were used in the references cited above.

Four different genes which code for the plasma membrane Ca^{2+} pump in mammals are now known [9–12]. Northern blots performed on messenger RNA (mRNA) from rats shows that, of the first three isozymes, only the mRNA of isozyme 1 is present to a significant degree in rat kidney [11]. The mRNA for this isozyme was present in all tissues tested, so that kidney is not unusual in having it. The functions of the isozymes are not known, and much remains to be done in determining the details of the role of the plasma membrane Ca^{2+} pump in Ca^{2+} transport by the kidney.

References

1. Penniston JT (1983) Plasma membrane Ca^{2+}-ATPases as active Ca^{2+} pumps. In: Cheung WY (ed) Calcium and cell function, vol 4. Academic, New York, pp 99–149
2. Ghijsen W, Gmaj P, Murer H (1984) Ca^{2+}-stimulated Mg^{2+}-independent ATP hydrolysis and the high affinity Ca^{2+}-pumping ATPase. Two different activities in rat kidney basolateral membranes. Biochim Biophys Acta 778:481–488
3. van Heeswijk MPE, Geertsen JAM, van Os CH (1984) Kinetic properties of the ATP-dependent Ca^{2+} pump and the Na^+/Ca^{2+} exchange system in basolateral membranes from rat kidney cortex. J Membr Biol 79:19–31
4. Borke JL, Minami J, Verma A, Penniston JT, Kumar R (1987) Monoclonal antibodies to human erythrocyte membrane Ca^{2+}-Mg^{2+} adenosinetriphosphatase pump recognize an epitope in the basolateral membrane of human kidney distal tubule cells. J Clin Invest 80:1225–1231

5. Borke JL, Minami J, Verma AK, Penniston JT, Kumar R (1988) Co-localization of erythrocyte Ca^{2+}-Mg^{2+} ATPase and vitamin D-dependent 28-kilodalton calcium binding protein in the cells of human kidney distal tubules. Kidney Int 34:262–267
6. van Os CH (1987) Transcellular calcium transport in intestinal and renal epithelial cells. Biochim Biophys Acta 906:195–222
7. Terepka AR, Coleman JR, Armbrecht HJ, Gunter TE (1976) Transcellular transport of calcium. Symposia of the Society for Experimental Biology, No. XXX, Calcium in biological systems. Cambridge University Press, Cambridge, pp 117–140
8. Gmaj P, Murer H, Carafoli E (1982) Localization and properties of a high-affinity Ca^{2+} + Mg^{2+} ATPase in isolated kidney cortex plasma membranes. FEBS Lett 144:226–230
9. Verma AK, Filoteo AG, Stanford DR, Wieben ED, Penniston JT, Strehler EE, Fischer R, Heim R, Vogel G, Matthews S, Strehler-Page MA, James P, Vorherr T, Krebs J, Carafoli E (1988) Complete primary structure of a human plasma membrane Ca^{2+} pump. J Biol Chem 263:14152–14159
10. Strehler EE, James P, Fischer R, Heim R, Vorherr T, Filoteo AG, Penniston JT, Carafoli E (1990) Peptide sequence analysis and molecular cloning reveal two calcium pump isoforms in the human erythrocyte membrane. J Biol Chem 265:2835–2842
11. Greeb J, Shull GE (1989) Molecular cloning of a third isoform of the calmodulin-sensitive plasma membrane Ca^{2+}-transporting ATPase that is expressed predominantly in brain and skeletal muscle. J Biol Chem 264:18569–18576
12. Shull GE, Greeb J (1988) Molecular cloning of two isoforms of the plasma membrane Ca^{2+}-transporting ATPase from rat brain. Structural and functional domains exhibit similarity to Na^+, K^+- and other cation transport ATPases. J Biol Chem 263:8646–8657

Vitamin D and Uremic Bone Disease

Chair: Francisco Llach (USA)
Shozo Koshikawa (Japan)

Vitamin D_3 and Uremic Bone Disease

Harmut H. Malluche and Marie-Claude Faugere[1]

Summary. The failure of patients with renal insufficiency to produce vitamin D_3 plays a major role in the initiation and progression of uremic bone disease. The longevity that dialysis affords patients is accompanied by severe clinical symptoms which reduce the quality of life of chronically dialyzed patients.

Relative or absolute D_3 deficiency results in secondary hyperparathyroidism [1]. Research is under way to determine the mechanisms which link the diminished endocrine function of the kidneys and increased synthesis and secretion of parathyroid hormone (PTH) seen in patients with early renal failure [2–4].

The uremic bone disease seen in end-stage renal failure and in chronically dialyzed patients is caused by a variety of independent and interrelated factors. These factors include altered set point for calcium-regulated PTH secretion, phosphate retention, hypocalcemia, aluminum intoxication, metabolic acidosis, putative abnormalities in calcitonin secretion, primary kidney disease and dialytic therapies [5]. This explains the heterogeneity of the syndrome.

Histological Abnormalities of Uremic Bone Disease

Mild to Moderate Renal Failure

Uremic bone disease develops in the early stages of loss of kidney excretory function. Half of those patients with a glomerular filtration rate (GFR) equal to or less than 50% of normal exhibit abnormal bone histology. Bone biopsies indicate increased PTH activity, increased volume and surface of osteoid bone, and increased number of osteoclasts and osteoblasts. Mineralization status, as measured by tetracycline uptake, is usually normal until the GFR reaches 40 ml/min. Below 40 ml/min, woven

[1]Department of Medicine, Division of Nephrology, Bone and Mineral Metabolism, University of Kentucky Medical Center, Lexington, KY 40536-0084, USA

osteoid is present and some individuals exhibit impaired mineralization at the osteoid surface [6].

Advanced Renal Failure

When end-stage renal failure ensues, necessitating chronic dialysis, nearly all patients have abnormal bone histology and approximately 5% have stainable aluminum at the mineralization front [7].

Advanced renal bone disease can be divided into three primary histological groups: predominant hyperparathyroid bone disease, low turnover osteomalacia and adynamic bone disease, and mixed uremic osteodystrophy [8]. These groups do not represent fully separate entities and transformation from one form to another can occur. However, characterization is useful because therapy can be tailored according to the predominant histological finding.

Predominant Hyperparathyroid Bone Disease

This disease is seen in 5%–30% of dialyzed patients and is characterized by a marked increase in bone turnover due to longstanding, excessive PTH secretion. The morphological cellular abnormalities present are accompanied by profound perturbation of cell function. Excessive production of collagen fibers results in an increase in osteoid surface and volume. Osteoid is primarily of the woven, irregular type. Although mineralization sites and apposition rate are increased, as documented by tetracycline labelling, mineralization of woven osteoid is deficient and haphazard.

Cortical bone volume is reduced due to increased bone turnover, while cancellous bone volume depends upon calcium balance. However, bone mass cannot be equated with bone strength in predominant hyperparathyroid bone disease, because of the prevalence of mechanically deficient woven bone.

Low Turnover Osteomalacia and Adynamic Bone Disease

This disease is seen in 5%–35% of individuals on chronic maintenance dialysis and is characterized by a profound decrease in the number of active remodelling sites. In addition to aluminum overload, pathogenetic factors include parathyroidectomy, medications, and underlying disease.

The dramatic reduction in the number of bone forming and resorbing cells is associated with greatly diminished bone formation and mineralization. Osteoblasts in particular are reduced in number and/or activity.

Two subgroups may be characterized: adynamic bone disease, where few osteoid seams are present, and low turnover osteomalacia, where an accumulation of unmineralized matrix prevails.

Bone volume is usually reduced in adynamic uremic bone disease. Although total bone volume may vary in low turnover osteomalacia, mineralized bone volume is invariably low. This, in addition to increased osteoid, renders osteomalacic bone soft and subject to deformity and fractures.

Mixed Uremic Osteodystrophy

This disease is seen in 45%–80% of patients on chronic dialysis, and in most individuals in end-stage renal failure. Hyperparathyroidism and defective mineralization, with or without decreased bone formation, are pathogenetic factors in mixed uremic osteodystrophy.

Woven osteoid may be found adjacent to lamellar sites. Mineralization surfaces and apposition rates are increased in woven bone, whereas in lamellar bone the obverse is true.

Bone volume is variable within this group and is relative to the predominant pathogenetic factor.

Aluminum-Related Bone Disease

Aluminum-related bone disease may be found superimposed upon any of the three groups previously described.

Aluminum deposition at the bone-osteoid interface and within trabecules is seen in approximately 90% of patients with low turnover uremic bone disease, in 50% of patients with mixed uremic bone disease and in 10%–15% of those individuals with predominant hyperparathyroid osteodystrophy [7] for whom aluminum deposition should not be regarded as an epiphenomenon [9].

The influence of parathyroid hormone on aluminum-related bone disease is controversial. On the one hand, the occurrence of stainable aluminum in patients with predominent hyperparathyroid bone disease is less frequent than in the other types of uremic bone disease [7,10]. On the other hand, high serum PTH levels seem to augment aluminum uptake [11]. Indeed, clinicians point out that patients with severe hyperparathyroid bone disease may have higher total bone aluminum content than patients with aluminum-related osteomalacic.

Prophylaxis and Therapy of Uremic Bone Disease Using Vitamin D_3

Supplementation of the renal hormone vitamin D_3 has been in use since 1972 for the prevention of uremic bone disease. Reversal of secondary hyperparathyroidism and increased growth velocity in children have been observed.

Effects of Vitamin D_3 on Bone in Mild to Moderate Renal Failure

Widespread prophylactic use of the active vitamin D metabolite by $1{,}25D_3$ has been hampered by its cost, concern regarding a deleterious effect on renal function, and by the metabolite's tendency to suppress bone turnover. Recent trials using low dose therapy (not exceeding 0.50 μg/day) and careful monitoring of serum and urinary calcium failed to demonstrate impaired renal function [12]. Suppression of bone turnover can be avoided by intermittent therapy.

Effects of Vitamin D_3 on Bone in Advanced Uremic Bone Disease

Most studies indicate that vitamin D_3 has a beneficial effect on the biochemical and histological abnormalities seen in hyperparathyroid bone disease. The drug's effect on osteomalacic abnormalities must be re-evaluated in the light of aluminum's pathogenetic influence on uremic bone disease. Moreover, studies indicate that the presence or absence of aluminum may influence the efficacy of vitamin D_3 therapy.

Recently, 1,25$(OH)_2D_3$ became available for intravenous injection. Daily injections of vitamin D_3 may induce hypercalcemia, a situation further aggravated by use of calcium salts to bind aluminum. Alternative approaches such as "pulse therapy," with high doses of the metabolite given twice weekly at the end of dialysis, or modulation of calcium supplement, dialysate calcium, and oral vitamin D_3 dosage have been shown to decrease hyperparathyroidism while reducing the incidence of hypercalcemia [13–15].

The efficacy and safety of intravenous vitamin D_3 administration needs further study.

New Avenues for Research

Recent studies report the mechanisms involved in the effects of vitamin D_3 on bone histology [16].

Vitamin D_3 exerts an antiproliferative effect on bone cells and promotes their activity, whereas parathyroid hormone stimulates increased numbers of cells. This explains how vitamin D_3 suppresses the accelerated bone turnover characteristic of hyperparathyroid osteodystrophy (by decreasing parathyroid hormone secretion), but is able to promote normal lamellar bone growth. In contrast, vitamin D_3 is of little value in low turnover states characterized by a paucity of bone cells.

Parathyroid hormone had long been thought to be influenced solely by abnormalities in plasma calcium. Current studies in our laboratory indicate that during early renal failure serum phosphorus and calcium concentrations increase as 1,25 vitamin D_3 levels decline. This is followed by increased PTH levels, while calcium remains elevated and serum phosphorus decreases toward normal. After normalization of serum phosphorus, serum calcium remains high and serum 1,25 Vit D_3 rises. Consequently, we have advanced the hypothesis that PTH secretion (secondary hyperparathyroidism) functions as a compensatory mechanism used to correct low levels of circulating vitamin D_3 occurring during the earliest stages of loss of kidney function.

References

1. Oldham SB, Smith R, Hartenbower DL (1979) The acute effects of 1,25-dihydroxycholecalciferol on serum immunoreactive parathyroid hormone in the dog. Endocrinology 104:248–254
2. Silver J, Russell J, Serwood LM (1985) Regulation by vitamin D metabolites of messenger ribonucleic acid for preproparathyroid hormone in isolated bovine parathyroid cells. Proc Natl Acad Sci USA 82:4270–4273

3. Lopez-Hilker S, Galceran T, Chan U-L, Rapp N, Martin KJ, Slatopolsky E (1986) Hypocalcemia may not be essential for the development of secondary hyperparathyroidism in chronic renal failure. J Clin Invest 78:1097–1102
4. Faugere M-C, Friedler RM, Fanti P, Malluche HH (1988) Lack of histologic signs of Vit D deficiency in early development of renal osteodystrophy. J Bone Mineral Res 3(Suppl 1):S95
5. Malluche HH, Faugere M-C (1990) Renal bone disease 1990: An unmet challenge for the nephrologist. Kidney Int 38:193–211
6. Maluche HH, Ritz E, Lange HP, Lutschere K, Hodgson M, Seiffert U, Schoeppe W (1976) Bone histology in incipient and advanced renal failure. Kidney Int 9:355–362
7. Smith AJ, Faugere M-C, Abreo K, Fanti P, Julian B, Malluche HH (1986) Aluminum related bone disease in mild and advanced renal failure. Evidence for high prevalence and morbidity, and studies on etiology and diagnosis in 197 patients. Am J Nephrol 6:275–283
8. Malluche HH, Faugere M-C (1986) Atlas of Mineralized Bone Histology. S. Karger, New York
9. Malluche HH, Faugere M-C, Smith AJ, Friedler RM (1986) Aluminum intoxication of bone in renal failure: Fact or fiction? Kidney Int 29(Suppl 18):70–73
10. Ott SM, Maloney NA, Coburn JW, Alfrey AC, Sherrard DJ (1982) The prevalence of bone aluminum deposition in renal osteodystrophy and its relation to the response to calcitriol therapy. N Engl J Med 307:709–713
11. Alfrey AC, Sedman A, Chan Y-L (1985) The compartmentalization and metabolism of aluminum in uremic rats. J Lab Clin Med 105:227–233
12. Baker LRI, Abrams SML, Roe CJ, Faugere M-C, Fanti P, Subayti Y, Malluche HH (1989) $1,25(OH)_2D_3$ administration in moderate renal failure: A prospective double-blind trial. Kidney Int 35:661–669
13. Slatopolsky E, Weerts C, Thielan J, Horst R, Harter H, Martin KJ (1984) Marked suppression of secondary hyperparathyroidism by intravenous administration of 1,25-dihydroxycholecalciferol in uremic patients. J Clin Invest 74:2136–2143
14. Salusky IB, Goodman WC, Norris KC, Horst R, Fine RN, Coburn JW (1988) Bioavailability of calcitriol: comparison of oral, intravenous and intraperitoneal routes of administration in CAPD patients (abstract). Kidney Int 33:250
15. Andress DL, Norris KC, Coburn JW, Slatopolsky EA, Sherrard DJ (1989) Intravenous calcitriol in refractory osteitis fibrosa of chronic renal failure. N Engl J Med 321:274–279
16. Malluche HH, Matthews CM, Faugere M-C, Fanti P, Friedler RM (1986) 1,25 dihydroxyvitamin D maintains bone cell activity and parathyroid hormone modulates bone cell number in dogs. Endocrinology 119:1298–1304

The Therapeutic Role of 24,25 Dihydroxycholecalciferol in Dialysis Patients with Secondary Hyperparathyroidism

Mordecai M. Popovtzer[1]

Summary. In early renal insufficiency, secondary hyperparathyroidism can be controlled with calcium/vitamin D and low-phosphate intake. In advanced disease, secondary hyperparathyroidism becomes refractory, displaying variable suppression with high levels of $1,25(OH)_2D_3$. However, $1,25(OH)_2D_3$ directly blocks bone formation and induces resorption, the latter being undesirable.

As shown in experimental and clinical studies, $24,25(OH)_2D_3$ administration (1) lowers parathyroid hormone (PTH) mRNA, (2) directly blocks PTH action on the bone, (3) reduces osteoclast number, suppresses resorption, and normalizes mineralizing surface, when combined with 1 alpha$(OH)D_3$ analogues. These findings demonstrate that $24,25(OH)_2D_3$, combined with 1 alpha$(OH)D_3$, reverses the osseous abnormalities of secondary hyperparathyroidism and proves to be an effective therapy for uremic osteodystrophy in patients on chronic dialysis.

Introduction

Secondary hyperparathyroidism is evident in the majority of patients with chronic renal disease, even in those with minimal functional impairment [1–4]. The pathogenesis of this abnormality is still unknown. In the early phase of renal disease there is already a decrease in the urinary excretion and an increase in the fractional reabsorption of calcium and an increase in the fractional excretion of phosphate, both factors reflecting secondary hyperparathyroidism [3,4]. Serum levels of calcium and phosphate are not significantly altered, whereas $1,25(OH)_2D_3$ levels are variable, but still in the normal range [5,6]. At this early stage the parathyroid hyperactivity is amenable to suppression by intravenous calcium [1,4] and can be normalized with dietary phosphate restriction and oral physiological doses of $1,25(OH)_2D_3$ [7]. As

[1]Nephrology and Hypertension Services, Hadassah University Hospital, 91120 Jerusalem, Israel

renal failure progresses the parathyroid glands become less suppressible [1,4] and eventually become refractory to most medical treatments. The end-organ damage that is caused by secondary hyperparathyroidism consists of an incapacitating bone disease, osteitis fibrosa cystica [8], metastatic calcifications, and presumed damage to many other systems, including the central nervous system, the bone marrow, and the heart muscle.

The deleterious consequences of secondary hyperparathyroidism have led to clinical trials in which attempts have been made to optimize the management of this complication. Attempts to reduce PTH levels by calcium supplementation have met with variable success [9]. In patients with end-stage renal disease the parathyroid glands exhibit a reduced sensitivity to calcium suppression. This abnormality can be quantitated by the assessment of the "set point," which is defined as the calcium level that produces 50% of the maximum decrement in PTH level. In patients on dialysis there is a shift in that "set point," i.e., to achieve a 50% of maximum suppression of PTH, "supraphysiological" degrees of hypercalcemia are necessary [10]. Yamamoto et al. [11] have recently shown that in rats with normal kidney function, sustained moderate hypercalcemia can elicit a significant decrease in the steady state levels of PTH messenger RNA in the parathyroid tissue. This finding implied that hypercalcemia not only suppresses the secretion, but also inhibits the synthesis of PTH. The effect of sustained hypercalcemia on messenger RNA levels in rats with chronic renal failure has not been studied in detail. Hypercalcemia induced by the intravenous infusion of calcium in patients on dialysis fails to produce a substantial decrease in PTH level [10].

Vitamin D Treatment of Secondary Hyperparathyroidism

In vivo experiments have demonstrated that physiological or nearly physiological amounts of $1,25(OH)_2D_3$ inhibit the levels of messenger RNA, independent of serum calcium levels [12,13]. These findings, reported in rats with both normal and reduced renal effects of $1,25(OH)_2D_3$ on PTH-gene transcription, suggested that this active metabolite of vitamin D directly regulates PTH synthesis. Furthermore, it has been shown that the suppression of PTH mRNA by $1,25(OH)_2D_3$ is dose-dependent [12,13].

In patients undergoing chronic dialysis, the oral administration of 1 alpha-hydroxylated analogues of vitamin D, in many instances, failed to elicit a therapeutically effective suppression of PTH [15,16]. Two major disadvantages are inherent in the oral route of administration. First, the direct action on the gut absorption of minerals may result in prohibitively high concentrations of calcium and phosphate that limit continuation of therapy. Second, the enhanced intestinal break-down of orally administered $1,25(OH)_2D_3$ [17] precludes achievement of high serum levels of this metabolite, which are essential for a direct suppression of PTH synthesis in uremic patients.

In view of the above limitations of oral therapy with 1 alpha-hydroxylated analogues of vitamin D, the intravenous route of administration has emerged. In clinical studies, intravenous administration of $1,25(OH)_2D_3$ was associated with a striking increase in serum levels that led to a fall in PTH levels, an effect which could not be accomplished with equal oral doses of $1,25(OH)_2D_3$ [15]. The suppression of PTH levels in uremic patients receiving the intravenous $1,25(OH)_2D_3$ was apparent before measurable changes in serum calcium were evident [15]. Furthermore, the intravenous administration of 1,25$(OH)_2D_3$ was associated with a shift toward normal in the set point for PTH suppression [10]. In a recent clinical trial it was shown that long term treatment with intravenous 1,25$(OH)_2D_3$, in patients with secondary hyperparathyroidism undergoing chronic dialysis, was associated with significant changes in bone histology [16]. These changes consisted of a striking and significant decrease in bone formation without significant changes in the osteoclast number [16]. The authors commented that these changes in bone histology could not be fully explained by the suppression of PTH, and a possible direct effect of 1,25$(OH)_2D_3$ on the bone was implied. High levels of 1,25$(OH)_2D_3$ are known to exert a direct effect on the bone which is independent of the inhibitory effect on PTH secretion. This direct effect on the bone consists of: 1] An induction of osteoclast differentiation from proliferating and from post-mitotic precursors, 2] an enhanced formation of multinucleated cells bearing the characteristics of osteoclasts including an augmented osteoclastic resorption [18–22], 3] a decrease in the rate of bone matrix apposition and a decrease in the rate of osteoblast proliferation, 4] a suppression of collagen synthesis [18–25], and 5] an impairment of bone mineralization [22]. It is felt that the anabolic effects of 1,25$(OH)_2D_3$ on bone growth are mediated by its intestinal actions through an increased supply of calcium and phosphate to the bone [22]. Popovtzer et al. [27] were the first to demonstrate a complete clinical and histological healing of vitamin D deficiency osteomalacia in man, without vitamin D therapy, solely with the intravenous administration of calcium and phosphate.

The net effect of high levels of 1,25$(OH)_2D_3$ on bone metabolism will be determined by the balance of the two main processes triggered by this active metabolite:

1) Suppression of PTH secretion.
2) Direct action on the bone.

Suppression of PTH will remove the major stimulus for the increased bone turnover rate which is the main feature of secondary hyperparathyroidism. This will reduce equally both the bone formation and the bone resorption. In clinical studies, the intravenous administration of 1,25$(OH)_2D_3$ was associated with a reduction in PTH [16]; however, even after a prolonged treatment the PTH level was still very high. Through its direct action 1,25$(OH)_2D_3$ will reduce bone formation, yet will increase bone resorption. Thus, the interaction between declining PTH levels and high 1,25$(OH)_2D_3$ will result in a synergism with respect to bone formation, but will result in an antagonism with respect to bone resorption (see Table 1). This interaction will invariably result in reduced bone formation, whereas the effect on resorption will vary.

In a recent report we described the effects of high doses of 1,25$(OH)_2D_3$ in rats with 5/6 nephrectomy [28]. The elevated PTH in these animals declined to a normal level and bone formation decreased markedly; however, the osteoclast number did not change significantly. Similar results were recorded in a recent clinical study employing long-term intravenous therapy with 1,25$(OH)_2D_3$ in uremic patients with secondary hyperparathyroidism [16]. There was a significant fall in PTH levels, normalization of bone formation rate, and a non-significant change in the osteoclast count.

The above clinical and experimental studies suggest that high circulating concentrations of 1,25$(OH)_2D_3$ may suppress PTH hyperactivity, however, their direct resorptive actions on the bone may be therapeutically counterproductive (Table 1).

Table 1. Effects of the interaction of $1,25(OH)_2D_3$ with suppressed PTH on bone metabolism

	Bone formation	Bone resorption
1. Direct effect of $1,25(OH)_2D_3$ on the bone	↓	↑
2. Effect of suppressed PTH on the bone[a]	↓	↓
3. Net result of the combined effects of 1. and 2. on the bone	↓↓	0

[a]Suppressed by high levels of $1,25(OH)_2D_3$. ↓, Decreased; ↑, Increased

In this regard, the administration of $24,25(OH)_2D_3$ in combination with 1 alpha hydroxylated metabolites of vitamin D, as will be further elaborated, may be the optimal formulation of vitamin D therapy for uremic patients.

Treatment with $24,25(OH)_2D_3$ in Combination with 1 Alphahydroxylated Analogues of Vitamin D

Experimental Studies

The exact physiological function of $24,25(OH)_2D_3$ has not yet been fully elucidated. There is, however, an accumulation of experimental and clinical data suggesting a biological role for $24,25(OH)_2D_3$ in bone metabolism. Galus et al. [29] showed, in vitamin D deficient dogs, that the administration of $24,25(OH)_2D_3$ increased bone formation and mineralization, but decreased bone resorption, while 1 alpha$(OH)D_3$ increased both bone mineralization and bone resorption. Thus, the difference in the action of these two metabolites was with respect to bone resorption; $24,25(OH)_2D_3$ effected a decrease while 1 alpha$(OH)D_3$ caused an increase in this parameter.

In a dose-dependent manner, $24,25(OH)_2D_3$ blocked PTH-activated adenylate cyclase in rat calvaria and in osteoblastic cells [30,31], but enhanced calcitonin-stimulated adenylate cyclase. Long-term administration of $24,25(OH)_2D_3$ to vitamin D replete rats obliterated PTH-sensitive adenylate cyclase activity in crude calvarial membrane fractions [31]. Activation of adenylate cyclase is believed to be the mechanism of the skeletal action of PTH. Specific inhibition of this activity by $24,25(OH)_2D_3$ both in vivo and in in vitro experiments, suggests that $24,25(OH)_2D_3$ interferes directly with the skeletal action of PTH [30–32].

We have shown that $24,25(OH)_2D_3$ suppresses the hypercalcemic effect of $1,25(OH)_2D_3$ in rats with reduced renal mass (5/6 nephrectomy), a model of chronic renal failure with secondary hyperparathyroidism [33]. Furthermore, our histomorphometric bone studies demonstrated that the effect of $24,25(OH)_2D_3$ in blunting the hypercalcemic effect of $1,25(OH)_2D_3$ was associated with striking decrease in osteoclastic activity [34]. In this experimental model, even though $1,25(OH)_2D_3$ lowered the elevated PTH to normal levels, it reduced osteoclastic bone resorption only modestly [28]. The combined administration of $24,25(OH)_2D_3$ with $1,25(OH)_2D_3$ elicited the most profound suppression of osteoclastic resorption, even though it did not reduce the PTH to a level below that achieved with $1,25(OH)_2D_3$

alone. These findings implied that $24,25(OH)_2D_3$ acts to reverse osteoclastic bone resorption in rats with chronic renal failure, independent of PTH suppression. The synergism with $1,25(OH)_2D_3$, however, is probably related to calcitriol's inhibitory action on PTH secretion.

In rats with intact kidney function, $24,25(OH)_2D_3$ similarly to $1,25(OH)_2D_3$, suppresses the levels of prepro PTH mRNA. It is, however, less potent than $1,25(OH)_2D_3$ in this regard. At a dose of 100 pmol, $24,25(OH)_2D_3$ elicits a 52% decrease in prepro PTH mRNA in 24 hours, compared with an 82% reduction with an equimolar dose of $1,25(OH)_2D_3$ [12,13]. Fukagawa et al. [14] have recently shown, in rats 4 weeks after 5/6 nephrectomy, a steady state elevation of PTH mRNA. They were able to suppress the elevated PTH mRNA with either 100 pmol of $1,25(OH)_2D_3$ or 500 pmol of $24,25(OH)_2D_3$. Fukagawa et al. suggested that the diminished levels of these 2 metabolites of vitamin D in chronic renal failure may play a critical role in the pathogenesis of secondary hyperparathyroidism. These results suggest that $24,25(OH)_2D_3$ directly suppresses PTH synthesis. This effect, however, is by far smaller when compared with that of $1,25(OH)_2D_3$.

Clinical Studies

Brickman et al. [35] and Piraino et al. [36] demonstrated a calcium lowering effect of $24,25(OH)_2D_3$, both in normocalcemic and in hypercalcemic patients undergoing chronic hemodialysis. It has been pointed out that when $24,25(OH)_2D_3$ is added to 1 alpha-hydroxylated analogues of vitamin D it lowers the risk of hypercalcemia and increases the tolerance to these agents.

Long-term administration of $24,25(OH)_2D_3$, in combination with dehydrotachysterol, to children undergoing chronic hemodialysis brought about a 70% reduction in bone surface covered with osteoclasts [37].

Mortensen et al. [31,32] showed that serum levels of $24,25(OH)_2D_3$ in normals and in patients with chronic renal failure were inversely correlated with PTH-stimulated adenylate cyclase from iliac crest biopsies. The adenylate cyclase activity correlated directly with bone resorption. This finding was interpreted to indicate that $24,25(OH)_2D_3$ serves as an important physiological modulator of PTH-induced bone resorption. Mortensen et al. [32] extended their observations by investigating 3 groups of uremic patients: (1) Patients treated with $1,25(OH)_2D_3$ alone, (2) patients treated with a high dose of $24,25(OH)_2D_3$, and (3) patients treated with a combination of both $1,25(OH)_2D_3$ and $24,25(OH)_2D_3$. Net bone PTH-activated adenylate cyclase was completely abolished after 2 months of treatment with $24,25(OH)_2D_3$ or with the combination, while $1,25(OH)_2D_3$ alone yielded a minor decrease in the enzyme activity. The authors concluded that the effect of $24,25(OH)_2D_3$ might be to restore normal bone turnover in uremia in concert with $1,25(OH)_2D_3$.

We have conducted the first controlled trial evaluating the effect of $24,25(OH)_2D_3$ combined with 1 alpha$(OH)D_3$, as compared with the effect of 1 alpha$(OH)D_3$ alone on renal osteodystrophy in patients undergoing chronic hemodialysis [38].

Fifty eight patients were randomly divided into: (1) a control group receiving 1 alpha$(OH)_2D_3$ alone and (2) a combined treatment group receiving both $24,25(OH)_2D_3$ and 1 alpha$(OH)D_3$. In 41 patients two bone biopsies, the first pretrial and the second at the end of the trial, about 12 months apart, were suitable for histomorphometric analysis. Nineteen patients were in the control and 22 in the

Table 2. Effects of the interaction of 1,25$(OH)_2D_3$ and 24,25$(OH)_2D_3$ with suppressed PTH on bone metabolism

	Bone formation	Bone resorption
1. Direct effect of 1,25$(OH)_2D_3$ on the bone	↓	↑
2. Direct effect of 24,25$(OH)_2D_3$ on the bone	↑	↓↓
3. Effect of suppressed PTH on the bone[a]	↓	↓
4. Net result of the combined effects of 1., 2., and 3. on the bone	↓	↓↓

[a]Suppressed both by high levels of 1,25$(OH)_2D_3$ and by 24,25$(OH)_2D_3$.
↓, Decreased; ↑, Increased

combined treatment group. No differences between the control and the combined treatment group were recorded in 25$(OH)D_3$ and 1,25$(OH)_2D_3$ levels in the serum; 24,24$(OH)_2D_3$ levels remained below normal in the control, but increased markedly in the combined treatment groups. Changes from the first to the second biopsy in the control were compared with those in the combined treatment group. A striking decrease (−10.5%) in the eroded surface was observed in the combined treatment, but not in the control group, leading to a significant difference in this change between the two groups ($P<0.01$). A significant decrease ($-0.22 mm^{-1}$) in the osteoclast number was observed in the combined treatment, but not in the control group, resulting in a significant difference in this change between the two groups ($P<0.05$). Likewise, a significant decrease (−15.8%) in mineralizing surface was recorded in the combined treatment, but not in the control group, leading to a significant difference in this change between the 2 groups ($P<0.01$). An increase (+5.6%) in bone volume was recorded in the control, but not in the combined treatment group, resulting in a significant difference in this change between the 2 groups ($P<0.01$).

The above results clearly demonstrated that the combined administration of 24,25$(OH)_2D_3$ with 1 alpha$(OH)D_3$ produced a striking improvement in the hyperparathyroid bone disease [38]. This was highlighted by a substantial fall in osteoclast number and a reduction in mineralizing surface. As summarized in Table 2, the combined administration of 24,25$(OH)_2D_3$ with 1 alphahydroxylated vitamin D_3 features an optimal integrated treatment with vitamin D. Not only does 24,25$(OH)_2D_3$ attenuate the effects of bone-resorbing factors, including those of PTH, but it also facilitates the effects of 1 alphahydroxylated vitamin D analogues in suppressing PTH secretion. Furthermore, 24,25$(OH)_2D_3$ has no significant side-effects. These unique attributes make 24,25$(OH)_2D_3$ an important therapeutic agent in the treatment of uremic osteodystrophy when given in combination with 1 alphahydroxylated vitamin D analogues.

References

1. Reiss E, Canterbury JH, Canter A (1969) Circulating PTH in chronic renal failure. Arch Intern Med 124:417–420

2. Popovtzer MM, Massry SG, Coburn JW, Kleeman CR (1969) The interrelationship between sodium, calcium and magnesium excretion in advanced renal failure. J Lab Clin Med 73:763–771
3. Popovtzer MM, Schainuck LI, Massry SG, Kleeman CR (1970) Divalent ion excretion in chronic kidney disease. Relation to degree of renal insufficiency. Clin Sci 38:297–307
4. Popovtzer MM, Massry SG, Coburn JW, Koppel M, Drinkard JH, Kleeman CR (1970) Calcium infusion test in chronic renal failure. Nephron 7:400–412
5. Llach F, Massry SG (1985) On the mechanism of secondary hyperparathyroidism in moderate renal insufficiency. J Clin Endocrinol Metab 61:601–606
6. Wilson L, Felsenfeld A, Drezner MK (1985) Altered divalent ion metabolism in early renal failure: role of $1,25(OH)_2D_3$. Kidney Int 27:565–573
7. Portale AA, Booth BE, Halloran BP, Morris RC (1984) The effect of dietary phosphorus on circulating concentrations of $1,25(OH)_2D_3$ and immunoreactive parathyroid hormone in children with moderate renal insufficiency. J Clin Invest 73:1580–1589
8. Huffer WE, Kuzela D, Popovtzer MM (1975) Metabolic bone disease in chronic renal failure. I. Dialyzed uremics. Am J Pathol 78:365–385
9. Popovtzer MM, Pinggera WF, Hutt MH, Robinette J, Halgrimson CG, Starzl TE (1972) The effect of sustained normocalcemia on serum levels of parathyroid hormone and renal handling of phosphorus in patients with chronic renal disease. J Clin Endocrinol Metab 35:213–218
10. Delmez JA, Tindira C, Grooms P, Dusso A, Windus DW, Slatopolsky E (1989) Parathyroid hormone suppression by intravenous 1,25-dihydroxyvitamin D. J Clin Invest 83:1349–1355
11. Yamamato M, Igarashi T, Muramatsu M, Fukagawa M, Motokra T, Ogata E (1989) Hypocalcemia increases and hypercalcemia decreases the steady-state level of parathyroid hormone messenger RNA in the rat. J Clin Invest 83:1053–1056
12. Silver J, Naveh-Many T, Mayer H, Schmelzer HJ, Popovtzer MM (1986) Regulation by vitamin D metabolites of parathyroid hormone gene transcription in vivo in the rat. J Clin Invest 78:1296–1301
13. Silver J, Naveh-Many T, Schmelzer H, Mayer H, Popovtzer MM (1987) Vitamin D metabolites regulate PTH gene transcription in vivo in the rat. In: DV Cohn, TJ Martin, PJ Meunier (eds) Calcium regulation and bone metabolism. Basic and clinical aspects, vol 9. Excerpta Medica, Amsterdam, pp 782–784
14. Fukagawa M, Kaname S, Igarashi T, Kurokawa K (1989) Regulation of PTH messenger RNA levels in parathyroid glands of chronic renal failure in rats. Kidney Int 35:392A.
15. Slatopolsky E, Weerts C, Thielan J, Horst R, Harter H, Martin KJ (1984) Marked suppression of secondary hyperparathyroidism by intravenous administration of 1,25-dihydroxycholecalciferol in uremic patients. J Clin Invest 74:2136–2143
16. Andress DL, Norris KC, Coburn JW, Slatopolsky E, Sherrard DJ (1989) Intravenous calcitriol in the treatment of refractory osteitis fibrosa of chronic renal failure. N Engl J Med 321:274–279
17. Napoli JL, Premanik BC, Royal PM, Reinhardt TA, Horst RL (1983) Intestinal synthesis of 24-keto 1,25-dihydroxyD_3. J Biol Chem 258:2100–2107
18. Raisz LG, Trummel CL, Holick MF, DeLuca HF (1972) 1Alpha,25-dihydroxycholecalciferol, a potent stimulator of bone resorption in tissue culture. Science 175:768–769
19. Bar-Shavit Z, Teitelbaum SL, Rietsma P, Hall A, Peg LE, Trail J, Kahn AJ (1983) Induction of monocytic differentiation and bone resorption by 1,25-dihydroxyvitamin D_3. Proc Natl Acad Sci USA 80:5907–5911
20. Pharaoh M, Heersche JNM (1985) 1,25-dihydroxyvitamin D_3 causes an increase in the number of osteoclast-like in cat bone marrow cultures. Calcif Tissue Int 37:276–281

21. McSeehy PMJ, Chambers TJ (1987) 1,25-Dihydroxyvitamin D_3 stimulates rat osteoblastic cells to release a soluble factor that increases osteoclastic bone resorption. J Clin Invest 80:425–428
22. Raisz LG (1990) Recent advances in bone cell biology: interactions of vitamin D with other local and systemic factors. Bone Min 9:191–197
23. Hock JM, Kream BE, Raisz LG (1982) Autoradiographic study of the effect of 1,25-dihydroxyvitamin D_3 on bone matrix synthesis in vitamin D replete rats. Calcif Tissue Int 34:347–351
24. Raisz LG, Kream BE, Smith MD, Simmons HA (1980) Comparison of the effects of vitamin D metabolites on collagen synthesis and resorption of fetal rat bone in organ culture. Calcif Tissue Int 32:135–138
25. Rowe DW, Kream BE (1982) Regulation of collagen synthesis in fetal rat calvaria by 1,25-dihydroxyvitamin D_3. J Biol Chem 257:8009–8015
26. Skjodt H, Gallagher JA, Beresford JN, Couch M, Poser JW, Russell RG (1985) Vitamin D metabolites regulate osteocalcin synthesis and proliferation of human bone cells in vitro. J Endocrinol 105:391–396
27. Popovtzer MM, Matthay R, Alfrey A, Block M, Beck P, Reeve EB (1973) Vitamin D deficiency osteomalacia: Healing of the bone disease in the absence of vitamin D with intravenous calcium and phosphorus infusion. In: Frame B, Parfitt AM, Duncan H (eds) Clinical aspects of metabolic bone disease. International Congress Series No. 270. Excerpta Medica, Amsterdam, pp 382–387
28. Rubinger D, Moscovitz A, Popovtzer MM, Bernheim J, Bab I, Gazit D (1990) $24,25(OH)_2D_3$ in combination with calcitriol reverses osteoclastic hyperactivity in chronic renal failure (CRF): evidence for a direct effect on the bone. Kidney Int 37:451A
29. Galus K (1980) Effects of 1alpha-hydroxyvitamin D_3 and 24,25-dihydroxyvitamin D_3 on bone remodeling. Calcif Tissue Int 31:209–213
30. Gordeladze JO, Gautvik KM (1986) Hydroxycholecalciferols modulate parathyroid hormone and calcitonin sensitive adenylyl cyclase in bone and kidney of rats. A possible physiological role for 24,25-dihydroxyvitamin D_3. Biochem Pharmacol 35:899–902
31. Mortensen B, Gordeladze JO, Aksnes L, Gautvik KM (1990) Long term administration of vitamin D_3 metabolites alters PTH-responsive osteoblastic adenylate cyclase in rats. Calcif Tissue Int 46:339–345
32. Mortensen B, Klem KH, Jablonski G, Haug E, Aarseth HP, Gautvik KM, Gordeladze JO (1990) The permissive role of $24,25(OH)_2D_3$ in treatment of renal osteodystrophy. Calcif Tissue Int 46:A56
33. Rubinger D, Cojocaru T, Popovtzer MM (1987) $24,25(OH)_2D_3$ attenuates the calcemic effect of $1,25(OH)_2D_3$ in rats with reduced renal mass. Proc Soc Exp Biol Med 186:64–69
34. Rubinger D, Moscovitz A, Popovtzer MM, Bab I, Gazit D (1989) $24,25(OH)_2D_3$ in combination with $1,25(OH)_2D_3$ ameliorates renal osteodystrophy in rats. Kidney Int 35:379(A)
35. Brickman AS, Llach FL, Coburn JW (1979) Preliminary report of biological actions of $24,25(OH)_2D_3$ in normal man and in patients with advanced renal failure. In: Norman, Schaefer, Herrath, Grigsleit, Coburn, DeLuca, Mawer, Suda (eds) Vitamin D, basic research and its clinical applications. Walter de Gruyter, Berlin, pp 1085–1090
36. Piraino BM, Rault R, Greenberg A, Dominguez JH, Wallia R, Houck P, Segre GV, Chent T, Foti FM, Puschett JB (1986) Spontaneous hypercalcemia in patients undergoing dialysis. Etiologic and therapeutic considerations. Am J Med 80:607–615
37. Van Diemen-Steenvoorde R, Donckerwolcke RA, Visser WJ, Raymakers JA, Duursma SA (1985) Treatment of renal osteodystrophy in children with dihydrotachysterol and 24,25-dihydroxyvitamin D_3. Clin Nephrol 24:292–299
38. Popovtzer MM (1989) $24,25(OH)_2D_3$ (OSTEO-D) combined with $1alpha(OH)D_3$ is an effective therapy for uremic bone disease. Report of the Collaborative Israeli Multicenter trial. Calcif Tissue Int 44:S-86

The Future of New Vitamin D Analogs in Uremic Bone Disease

Alex Brown, Jane Finch, Silvia Lopez-Hilker, Adriana Dusso, Jeremiah Morrissey, Junko Abe, Takashi Mori, Yasuho Nishii[2], and Eduardo Slatopolsky[1]

Summary. The spectrum of activities promoted by calcitriol has been found to extend far beyond a role in calcium homeostasis. Calcitriol has been shown to have important immunomodulating properties. The major limitation of calcitriol therapy is its accompanying calcemic activity. The recent development of analogs of vitamin D, that retain the properties of calcitriol with less calcemic activity, may offer a potential therapeutic tool in the treatment of uremic bone disease and other clinical conditions such as psoriasis and leukemia. Among these analogs 22-oxacalcitriol (OCT), 1,25-$(OH)_2$-24-homo-D_3, 1,25-$(OH)_2$-22-ene-24-homo-D_3, formerly MC 903 (now Calcipotriol), and 1,25-$(OH)_2$-16-ene-23-yne-D_3 have been shown to have important biological effects.

In studies in rats and dogs OCT has a low calcemic activity both in vitro and in vivo. In primary culture of bovine parathyroid cells, OCT is as active as calcitriol in suppressing parathyroid hormone (PTH) release. In studies in normal and uremic rats, OCT produced a significant decrease in pre-pro PTH mRNA. In addition, OCT decreased PTH secretion in dogs with chronic renal failure. This analog may provide a unique therapeutic tool for the treatment of secondary hyperparathyroidism in patients with chronic renal failure.

Introduction

In the past 10 years the biological functions induced by 1,25-$(OH)_2D_3$ (calcitriol) have been found to extend far beyond a role in calcium homeostasis. Calcitriol has been shown to have important cell differentiating activities and immunomodulating properties. Because hypercalcemia may preclude the administration of large

[1]The Renal Division, Department of Medicine, Washington University School of Medicine, St. Louis, MO 63110, USA
[2]Chugai Pharmaceutical Company Limited, 2-1-9 Kyobashi, Chuo-ku, Tokyo, 104 Japan

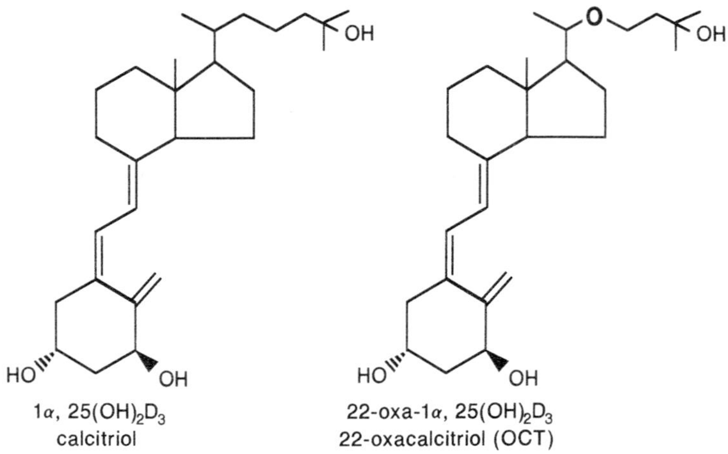

Fig. 1. Structure of 1,25-$(OH)_2D_3$ and 22-oxa-1,25-$(OH)_2D_3$[22-oxa-calcitriol (OCT). (Modified from [2])

doses of vitamin D in certain clinical disorders, the recent development of analogs of vitamin D that retain the properties of calcitriol with less calcemic activity may offer a potential therapeutic tool for the treatment of secondary hyperparathyroidism and renal osteodystrophy.

New Analogs of Vitamin D with Low Calcemic Activity

In 1986, Murayama et al. [1] studied the effects of a new analog with selective activity. This compound, 22-oxacalcitriol (OCT), developed by Chugai Pharmaceutical Co. in Japan, differs from 1,25-$(OH)_2D_3$ solely by the substitution of an oxygen atom for the methylene group at carbon 22 (Fig. 1). Abe et al. [2] demonstrated that OCT is more effective than 1,25-$(OH)_2D_3$ in suppressing cell growth and in inducing phagocytic activity in a mouse myelomonocytic leukemia cell line, WEHI-3. In addition, OCT is 10 times more effective than 1,25-$(OH)_2D_3$ in suppressing cell growth and in inducing phagocytic activity in a human leukemia cell line, HL-60. Despite this higher activity, OCT was found to bind 14 times less avidly to chicken intestinal receptor [1]. Calcemic activity was tested in vitro by measuring release of ^{45}Ca from prelabelled fetal mouse calvaria. OCT appeared to be 50–100 times less effective than 1,25-$(OH)_2D_3$ [2]. This low calcemic activity of OCT has been confirmed in vivo in both mice [2] and rats [3]. This analog is 100 times less effective than 1,25$(OH)_2D_3$ in mobilizing bone calcium and 1000 times less effective in stimulating intestinal calcium transport. Subsequently, Abe et al. [4] demonstrated that OCT markedly enhanced the immune response in mice. When mice were injected with a dose of antigen (10^7 sheep erythrocytes) that gave a submaximal antibody response, treatment with either OCT or 1,25-$(OH)_2D_3$ significantly increased the number of antibody-producing spleen cells. OCT was 50 times more potent than 1,25-$(OH)_2D_3$.

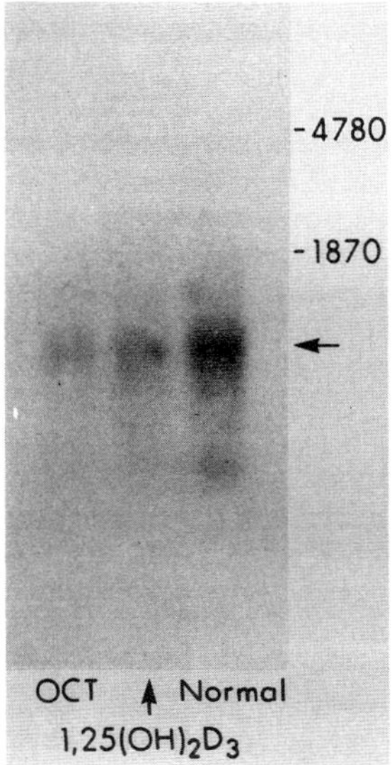

Fig. 2. Northern blot analysis of cytoplasmic RNA extracted from the parathyroid glands of normal, 1,25-$(OH)_2D_3$-treated and OCT-treated rats. The blot was hybridized with PTHm122cDNA. (Reproduced from the *Journal of Clinical Investigation* by copyright permission of the American Society for Clinical Investigation [3])

The doses of OCT that enhance the immune response are much lower than those capable of increasing serum calcium.

Further investigations of the activities of OCT by Brown et al. [3] have demonstrated that this analog can suppress the synthesis and secretion of PTH. The ability of OCT to suppress PTH secretion was assessed initially in primary cultures of parathyroid cells. Exposure of the cells to various doses of OCT and 1,25-$(OH)_2D_3$ for 48 hours revealed a similar dose-dependent inhibition of PTH secretion by these two compounds. The suppressive action of OCT in vivo was confirmed by measuring the pre-pro PTH mRNA levels in the parathyroid glands of normal rats 48 hours after a single 40 ng dose of 1,25-$(OH)_2D_3$ or OCT. Northern analysis and slot blot analysis showed that both 1,25-$(OH)_2D_3$ and OCT suppressed PTH mRNA levels by about 60%–80% (Fig. 2).

More recently in a preliminary study, we have confirmed that OCT effectively suppressed N-terminal PTH levels in dogs with chronic renal failure [5]. Administration of a single intravenous dose of 5 μg OCT decreased PTH by 80% toward normal levels in 24 hours. PTH levels were still suppressed at 69 hours. With this dose of OCT, no changes in serum calcium or phosphorus were observed (Fig. 3). Further studies indicate that even lower doses of OCT are capable of suppressing PTH to a similar degree. These data indicate that OCT may be effective for the treatment of secondary hyperparathyroidism.

In 1987, Ostrem et al. [6,7] demonstrated the effects of non-calcemic analogs that retained the ability of 1,25-$(OH)_2D_3$ to differentiate myeloid leukemia cells. Two of the analogs, 1,25-$(OH)_2$-24-homo-D_3 and 1,25-$(OH)_2$-22-ene-24-homo-D_3 had very low bone mobilizing activity. On the other hand, these analogs were about 10 times more potent than 1,25-$(OH)_2D_3$ in differentiating HL-60 cells, as assessed by the appearance of the macrophage-like activities, non-specific esterase and phagocytosis, after four days of exposure to the compounds. These analogs contain an extra carbon atom in the side chain; one also contains a double bond at the 22 position.

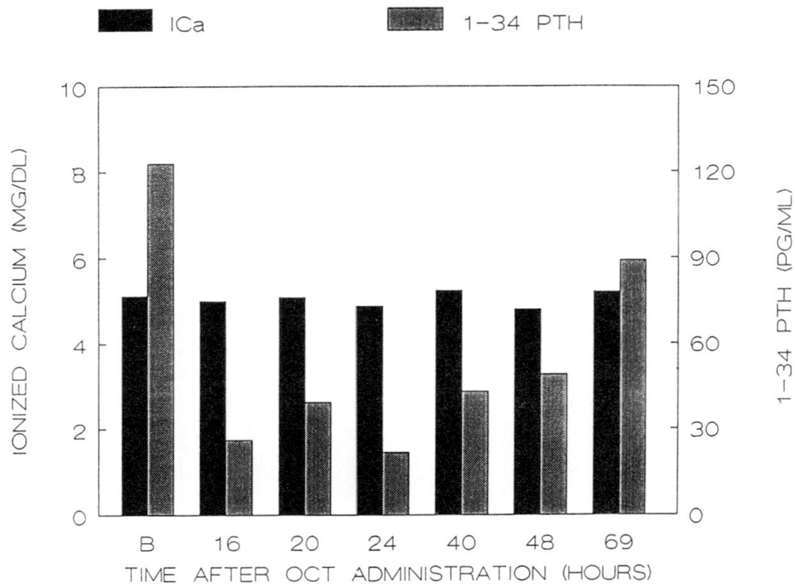

Fig. 3. The effects of a single dose of OCT (5 μg), given intravenously, on ionized calcium and amino-terminal PTH in a dog with chronic renal failure. (Reprinted from *Kidney International* with permission [5])

In 1988, Leo Pharmaceutical Products in Denmark [8] developed a new analog which was originally designated as MC 903 but is now referred to as calcipotriol. In this compound, the 26 and 27 carbons of the vitamin D side chain have been joined in a cyclopropyl ring, and the hydroxyl group is at the 24 position. Also, there is a double bond at the 22 position. This analog has twice the activity of 1,25-$(OH)_2D_3$ in blocking the proliferation of the histiocytic lymphoma cell line, U937. The calcemic response of MC 903 was assessed in normal rats on 1% calcium diet following daily intraperitoneal administration for one week. This analog was more than 200 times less potent than 1,25$(OH)_2D_3$ in its ability to increase urinary and serum calcium and decrease bone mass. Two clinical studies [9,10] have reported that topically-applied MC 903 is effective in the treatment of psoriasis, but has no effect on serum ionized calcium.

Recently Zhou et al. [11] tested eight analogs for their effects on hemopoietic cell growth and calcium metabolism. The most potent of these analogs in HL-60 cells is 1,25-$(OH)_2$-16-ene-23-yne-D_3. This compound is four times more effective than 1,25-$(OH)_2D_3$ in blocking HL-60 cell growth but is 33 times less active in stimulating intestinal calcium absorption and 50 times less active in bone calcium mobilization.

The general properties of these non-calcemic analogs can be summarized as follows: (1) All of these analogs are modified in the side chain, implicating this portion of the molecule in their selective action; (2) All of these analogs show selective activity on leukemia cells. They are more active than 1,25-$(OH)_2D_3$ in the differentiation of these malignant cells, but have much lower calcemic activity. (3) One analog,

OCT, is active in vivo in suppressing PTH synthesis and secretion and in enhancing the immune response, indicating that the lack of calcemic activity, at least for this analog, is not due to rapid clearance or inactivation in vivo.

The reason for the selective action of these analogs is not clear. Every analog tested had a relatively low affinity for the vitamin D binding protein (DBP) ranging from 50–500 times less than that of 1,25-$(OH)_2D_3$. The possible consequences of this low affinity for DBP are: (1) A higher proportion of the analog will be in the free, or active, form. This may explain why the analogs have a higher differentiating activity than expected based on the receptor-binding affinity. All leukemia cell cultures contained serum, usually 10%, during incubation with vitamin D compounds. Under these conditions, the greater proportion of the analogs will be unbound and more accessible to the cells. This hypothesis has not yet been tested. Bikle and Gee [12] indicate that in keratinocyte cell culture the free rather than the total 1,25-$(OH)_2D_3$ is responsible for the regulation of 25$(OH)D_3$ metabolism; (2) The analogs will be cleared more rapidly from the circulation which generally will decrease their effectiveness. Presumably, one of the important functions of DBP is to prolong the lifetime of 1,25-$(OH)_2D_3$ in the circulation. Despite the more rapid clearance, however, OCT is still active in vivo on the parathyroid glands and the immune system; (3) The low affinity for DBP suggests that these analogs may be carried by other serum proteins. Okano et al. [13] demonstrated that OCT is associated primarily with lipoproteins. A number of other possibilities also exist for the selective action of these analogs. Rapid degradation in the non-responsive target tissues, bone and intestine, may prevent the action of the analogs. Currently, little is known about the metabolism of any of these vitamin D analogs. Recently, Tanaka et al. [14] demonstrated that during differentiation of HL-60 cells, OCT differs from 1,25-$(OH)_2D_3$ in that it does not increase cytosolic calcium or prime the cells for oxidative burst. It is not known whether OCT is defective in stimulating cytosolic calcium in all target tissues or whether this phenomenon is related to its lack of calcemic activity. Although currently there is no clear explanation for the selective action of these analogs, their low calcemic activity may be useful for the treatment of a number of diseases that have been shown to respond to 1,25-$(OH)_2D_3$.

Therapeutic Potential of Non-Calcemic Analogs of Vitamin D

Suda and his co-workers demonstrated that 1,25-$(OH)_2D_3$ could differentiate myeloid leukemia cells from both mice and humans to non-proliferating monocyte/macrophage-like cells [15,16]. Smith et al. demonstrated an effect of 1,25-$(OH)_2D_3$ in the normal maturation of skin cells [17]. These newly discovered functions of 1,25-$(OH)_2D_3$ have also suggested new therapeutic uses of this hormone for the treatment of leukemia and psoriasis. The major limitation of 1,25-$(OH)_2D_3$ therapy is its accompanying calcemic activity. Thus, several investigators are currently determining the potential clinical application of these new vitamin D analogs. M C903 has been shown to be effective in the treatment of psoriasis [9,10]. Morimoto et al. demonstrated that OCT inhibited the growth of psoriatic fibroblasts more effectively than 1,25-$(OH)_2D_3$ [18]. We have found that OCT suppresses PTH synthesis and secretion. Studies in normal rats clearly demonstrated that OCT has a significant suppressive effect on pre-pro PTH mRNA. In addition, in preliminary studies on dogs with chronic renal failure, OCT greatly decreased the levels of circulating PTH, with no change in serum ionized calcium. This may be of utmost importance in the treatment of secondary hyperparathyroidism in patients with renal failure. The control of serum phosphorus is critical before calcitriol is administered to uremic patients. Since the long term administration of phosphate-binders containing aluminum is associated with a multitude of deleterious effects, calcium carbonate is currently the phosphate-binder of choice. However, the simultaneous administration of large doses of calcium carbonate, e.g., 6–10 gm daily, and calcitriol frequently induces severe hypercalcemia, precluding the administration of therapeutic doses of calcitriol. Thus, OCT, an analog of vitamin D which is without a calcemic effect, but which has properties similar to those of calcitriol in its action on PTH synthesis and release, may provide a unique therapeutic tool for the treatment of secondary hyperparathyroidism in patients with chronic renal failure.

References

1. Murayama E, Miyamoto K, Kubodera N, Mori T, Matsunaga I (1986) Synthetic studies of vitamin D_3 analogues. VIII. Synthesis of 22-oxavitamin D_3 analogues. Chem Pharm Bull (Tokyo) 34:4410–4413
2. Abe J, Morikawa M, Miyamoto K, Kaiho S-I, Fukushima M, Miyaura C, Abe E, Suda T, Nishii Y (1987) Synthetic analogues of vitamin D compounds with an oxygen atom in the side chain. FEBS Lett 226:58–62
3. Brown AJ, Ritter CS, Finch JL, Morrissey J, Martin KJ, Murayama E, Nishii Y, Slatopolsky E (1989) The noncalcemic analogue of vitamin D, 22-oxacalcitriol, suppresses parathyroid hormone synthesis and secretion. J Clin Invest 84:728–732
4. Abe J, Takita Y, Nakano T, Miyaura C, Suda T, Nishii Y (1989) A synthetic analogue of vitamin D_3, 22-oxa-1,25-dihydroxyvitamin D_3, is a potent modulator of in vivo immunoegulating activity without inducing hypercalcemia in mice. Endocrinology 124:2645–2647
5. Brown AJ, Finch JL, Lopez-Hilker S, Dusso A, Ritter C, Pernalete N, Morrissey J, Nishii Y, Slatopolsky E (1990) New active analogues of vitamin D with low calcemic activity. Kidney Int 38 S 29 22–27
6. Ostrem VK, Lau WF, Lee SH, Perlman K, Ikekawa N (1987) Induction of monocytic differentiation of HL-60 cells by 1,25-dihydroxyvitamin D analogues. J Biol Chem 262:14164–14171
7. Ostrem VK, Tanaka Y, Prahl J, DeLuca HF, Ikekawa N (1987) 24-and 26-homo-1,25-dihydroxyvitamin D_3: Preferential activity in inducing differentiation of human leukemia cells HL-60 in vitro. Proc Natl Acad Sci USA 84:2610–2614
8. Binderup L, Bramm E (1988) Effects of a novel vitamin D analogue MC903 on cell proliferation and differentiation in vitro and on calcium metabolism in vivo. Biochem Pharmacol 37:889–895
9. Staberg B, Roed-Petersen J, Menne T (1989) Efficacy of topical treatment in psoriasis with MC903, a new vitamin D analogue. Acta Derm Venereol (Stockh) 69:147–150
10. Kragballe K (1989) Treatment of psoriasis by the topical application of the novel cholecalciferol analogue calcipotriol (MC 903). Arch Dermatol 125:1647–1652
11. Zhou J-Y, Norman AW, Lubbert M, Collins ED, Uskokovic MR, Koeffler HP (1989) Novel vitamin D analogues that modulate leukemic cell growth and differentiation with little effect on either intestinal calcium absorption or bone calcium mobilization. Blood 74:82–93
12. Bikle DD, Gee E (1989) Free, and not total, 1,25-dihydroxyvitamin D regulates 25-hydroxyvitamin D metabolism by keratinocytes. Endocrinology 124:649–654

13. Okano T, Tsugawa N, Masuda S, Takeuchi A, Kobayashi T, Nishii Y (1989) Protein-binding properties of 22-Oxa-1α, 25-dihydroxyvitamin D_3, a synthetic analogue of 1α,25-dihydroxyvitamin D_3. J Nutr Sci Vitaminol (Tokyo) 35:529–533
14. Tanaka H, Hruska KA, Seino Y, Nishii Y, Teitelbaum SL (1989) Dissociation of the macrophage-maturational effects of vitamin D from respiratory burst priming. J Bone Mineral Res 4:S197
15. Abe E, Miyaura C, Sakagami H, Takeda M, Konno K, Yamazaki T, Yoshiki S, Suda T (1981) Differentiation of mouse myeloid leukemia cells induced by 1,25-dihydroxyvitamin D_3. Proc Natl Acad Sci USA 78:4990–4994
16. Tanaka H, Abe E, Miyaura C, Kuribayashi T, Konno K, Nishii Y, Suda T (1982) 1,25-Dihydroxycholecalciferol and a human myeloid leukemia cell line (HL-60). Biochem J 204:713–719
17. Smith EL, Walworth NC, Holick MF (1986) Effect of 1,25-dihydroxyvitamin D_3 on the morphologic and biochemical differentiation of cultured human epidermal keratinocytes grown in serum-free conditions. J Invest Dermatol 86:709–714
18. Morimoto S, Imanaka S, Koh E, Shiraishi T, Nabata T, Kitano S, Muyashita Y, Nishii Y, Ogihara T (1989) Comparison of the inhibitions of proliferation of normal and psoriatic fibroblasts by 1α,25-dihydroxyvitamin D_3 and synthetic analogues of vitamin D_3 with an oxygen atom in their side chain. Biochem Int 19:1143–1149

AIDS/AIDS-Nephropathy

Chair: Gerhard Treser (USA)
Filoteo A. Alano (Philippines)

Highlights of Major Differences Between Children and Adults with HIV-Associated Nephropathy

JOSE STRAUSS, GASTON ZILLERUELO, CAROLYN ABITBOL, BRENDA MONTANE, GWENDOLYN SCOTT, CHARLES MITCHELL, ANDREA GRECO,[1] and VICTORIANO PARDO[2]

SUMMARY. Major differences between human immunodeficiency virus (HIV) associated nephropathy (HIVN) in children and HIVN in adults include the following: HIVN occurs in both HIV-1+ and AIDS adults, but apparently only in AIDS children. In HIVN patients, the virus has been transmitted to adult males mostly by intravenous drug use, and to adult females mostly by intercourse with infected males, but the virus has been transmitted to male and female infants and children by the mother. Renal histology changes in HIVN adults are mostly of the focal and segmental sclerosis (FSS) type, but FSS type changes are found in only one-third–one-half of HIVN children. The onset of chronic renal failure in adults heralds a rapid (few weeks) course to death, but in children the course is much slower (several months). Acute renal failure is rarely diagnosed in HIVN children while it is commonly diagnosed in HIVN adults.

Introduction

The clinical and immunologic characteristics of patients with the human immunodeficiency virus (HIV) and the acquired immunodeficiency syndrome (AIDS) sparked our interest in 1981 and we began studying renal involvement in HIV and AIDS pediatric patients at the University of Miami/Jackson Memorial Medical Center. In 1984, urine and renal histology abnormalities in AIDS children were described by our group [1] and were described in AIDS adults by Pardo and Rao [2,3]. Subsequently, we published our updated data on HIV associated nephropathy (HIVN) in children [4]; also available are other investigators' data on children [5–13]

[1]Departments of Pediatrics and [2]Pathology, University of Miami School of Medicine, and Laboratory Services, Veterans Administration Medical Center (V.P.), Miami, FL 33101, USA

and on adults [9,10,12–29]. Based on these data, this paper presents and analyzes some of the differences between HIVN in children and in adults.

Occurrence of HIVN and Clinical Status of the HIV-1+ Patient

In 1984, the severity of renal histologic changes was found to be greater in AIDS adults than in AIDS pediatric patients, and it was concluded that AIDS children do not live long enough for severe changes to develop [1]. Now, however, with a greater number of children studied, more active search for urine changes, and availability of biopsy material, children have been found to have a broad range of renal abnormalities, including severe ones which lead to renal failure [4–13]. A major difference that seems to exist between adults as a group and children as a group is the occurrence of HIVN in HIV-1+ adult patients, without clinical manifestation of the infection. This has been well documented in numerous adults [13–29], while to date no such association has been found in children [4–13]. In adults, HIVN has been reported as being the first manifestation of the HIV-1 infection [21,22]. What could be the cause of this difference? Race can be excluded, since the great majority of children, as well as adult patients, who have HIVN are Black [1–29]. Possible causes are the manner in which the infection was acquired and the characteristics of the host.

Mode of Transmission of the Virus

Mode of transmission may play a role in determining the time of appearance of the nephropathy. Adult males who develop HIVN have acquired the infection almost exclusively through intravenous drug (IVD) use; children who develop HIVN seem to become infected only through their mothers, mostly in utero, but some in the perinatal period or even during lactation. Mothers may be IVD addicts, but most (about two-thirds) seem to have been infected through heterosexual intercourse with bisexual or IVD abuser men [30].

Characteristics of the Host

The difficulties the neonate has in fighting off infections are well known. Even so, only one-third–one-half of the babies born to HIV-1+ mothers are infected; most have maternal anti-HIV-1+ antibodies which have crossed the placenta [30]. What makes so many infants resistant to such a severe infection when for months all of their organs have been perfused by contaminated blood? Determinants may be the time at which the mother acquired the infection, the route by which the mother acquired the infection, and the stage of evolution of her disease. Another host difference is that HIVN children in our group were 2:1 male to female [4] while an overwhelming majority of HIVN adults are males [13–29]. In addition, since only a small percentage of patients infected with HIV-1 develop HIVN, the susceptibility of mesangial cells of glomeruli to the virus may be modified by predisposing agents or conditions [23].

Histologic Renal Changes

It has been amply documented that most adults with HIVN have focal and segmental sclerosis (FSS); this finding is regarded as the characteristic glomerular histologic change in an adult patient with suspected HIV-1 infection [13–29]. Mesangial hyperplasia has been reported in some adult patients [13]. From our data we concluded that a broader spectrum of disease seems to be present in younger patients: in our report five children had FSS, five had mesangial hyperplasia, one had segmental necrotizing glomerulonephritis, and one had minimal changes [4]. Even a rough estimate of the various reports on HIVN in children identified only 30 of 80 patients as evidencing FSS [24]. In addition, we have identified one patient with membranoproliferative changes and another with microangiopathic thromboses. Though an occasional adult patient also has been reported to have changes similar to those found in children, they occur much less frequently [25]. We also have identified the apparent conversion of mesangial hyperplasia (by biopsy) into FSS (by autopsy) in one child; this finding lends support to the belief that mesangial hyperplasia is an early stage of FSS in HIVN [23]. No differences have been identified between children and adults with HIVN in regard to the tubulointerstitial lesions or the tubuloreticular inclusions of glomerular endothelial cells [4,16,21].

HIVN Patients as Percentage of the HIV-1+/AIDS Population

As stated already, HIV-1+ patients with HIVN were found only among adults; HIVN has not been identified in any children who are HIV-1+ but who do not have AIDS [4]. This could be due to incomplete assessment of the population, since not all HIV-1+ children have been checked for urine changes; only those children admitted to our Medical Center for other AIDS-related problems have had their urines evaluated consistently. The only published data on adults have been almost equally biased; still, patients were seen by a nephrologist when a request for consultation was received [23] and a significant number of asymptomatic adults have had HIVN [23,24]. As already mentioned, renal involvement has even been reported as the first manifestation of the infection [21,22]. Requests for Nephrology consultations for patients with HIV-1 infection and with AIDS were received in 7%–12% of the total HIV-1+ and AIDS adult population [23]. In the pediatric AIDS population, a similar percentage of children was found to have HIVN [4]. The true incidence of HIVN in those populations can be identified only when *all* patients (those with only the infection and those with the syndrome) are assessed prospectively and at regular intervals. With the support of the National Institutes of Health, we are currently doing this in infants and children and hope to have meaningful data soon.

Impact of HIVN on Survival

AIDS adults who develop HIVN have a rapidly deteriorating course and die more rapidly than those without HIVN [23,24,27]; children with and without HIVN die at a similar age [4]. Some AIDS children under our care with biopsy-proven renal involvement have survived for up to one year after diagnosis of HIVN, while most AIDS adults who develop HIVN die within weeks [23].

Number of AIDS Children Who Develop HIVN

Between January 1981 and June 1987 (6.5 years) we identified 12 AIDS children who developed HIVN [4]. During the subsequent three years, we have identified 20 additional AIDS children with HIVN. Thus, we have gone from 12 HIVN patients out of 155 AIDS children (7.7%) in the first 6.5 years (1.85 patients/year), to 20 HIVN patients out of 195 AIDS children (10%) in 3.0 years (6.67 patients/year), or a total of 32 HIVN patients out of 350 AIDS patients in 9.5 years.

Other communities with endemic characteristics for HIV-1+ infection also have reported the identification of several children with HIVN. These communities include areas of Newark [7], New York [8,28], and Canada [6]. The reason for this increased occurrence or identification of new HIVN cases remains unknown.

Though in some patients the increase coincided with regular IV administration of gamma globulins [9], most of the patients from our Medical Center did not receive such medication. Increased awareness of the occurrence of proteinuria with or without hematuria among AIDS children may have led to early identification among patients who otherwise might have died before a nephrotic syndrome-like clinical picture was apparent.

Chronic/Renal Failure

As stated above, it was not uncommon for children who were diagnosed as having HIVN to live for a period which lasted several months from the time of diagnosis; this was true even (or particularly) in those who developed chronic renal failure [4]. Although children and adults with HIVN and FSS have in common the development of chronic renal failure, the latter was present in only 6 of 12 HIVN children, while sooner or later, it becomes a regular feature in HIVN adults [23].

Acute Renal Failure

This functional alteration has been diagnosed often in adults with the HIV infection or with AIDS [23,25]. For reasons not clearly understood, such a diagnosis has rarely, if ever, been made in the children admitted to our Medical Center. The difference may be due to a multiplicity of factors, among which repeated insults from allergenic medications, nephrotoxic drugs, x-ray contrast material, certain infections, etc., may play an important etiopathogenic role in adults. Ischemic renal injury also is more likely to occur in adults (often with other organ involvement through atherosclerosis, hypertension, etc.) than in children.

The possible delay in the increase of blood urea nitrogen and serum creatinine, because of severe malnutrition in children, may contribute to the lack of diagnosis of acute renal failure. Our use of radionuclides to assess glomerular filtration rate and renal blood flow prospectively should answer this question.

Summary and Conclusion

The differences between children and adults infected with HIV-1 or suffering from AIDS have been presented and briefly evaluated in terms of the reasons for those differences. It is hoped that in-depth prospective studies will help clarify these perplexing problems. The possibility is that careful follow-up of large numbers of children will eliminate some of the differences now seen between HIV infected or AIDS adults and children with renal involvement.

Acknowledgments. Supported in part by a grant (1R01 DK-40838-02) from the National Institute of Diabetes and Digestive and Kidney Diseases, a grant from Children's Medical Services, Florida Department of Health and Rehabilitative Services, and grants (5R01 AI-20736 and 5R37 AI-23524) from the National Institute of Allergy and Infectious Diseases.

We thank Pearl Seidler for study coordination, LaDemia Albury for typographical assistance, and Mozhe Jalali and Rhonda Davis for computer processing.

References

1. Strauss J, Montane B, Scott G, Freundlich M, Abitbol C, Zilleruelo G, Pardo V (1984) Urinary and renal histological changes in children with acquired immunodeficiency syndrome (AIDS). Pediatr Res 18(Suppl):371A
2. Pardo V, Aldana M, Colton RM, Fischl MA, Jaffe D, Moskowitz L, Hensley GT, Bourgoignie JJ (1984) Glomerular lesions in the acquired immunodeficiency syndrome. Ann Inter Med 101:429–434
3. Rao TK, Filippone EJ, Nicastri AD, Landesman SH, Frean E, Chen CK, Friedman EA (1984) Associated focal and segmental glomerulosclerosis in the acquired immunodeficiency syndrome. N Engl J Med 310:669–673
4. Gardenswartz MH, Lerner CW, Seligson GR, Zabetakis PM, Rotterdam H, Tapper ML, Michelis MF, Bruno MS (1984) Renal disease in patients with AIDS: a clinicopathologic study. Clin Nephrol 21:197–204
5. Strauss J, Abitbol C, Zilleruelo G, Scott G, Paredes A, Malaga S, Montane B, Mitchell C, Parks W, Pardo V (1989) A spectrum of renal disease in children with acquired immunodeficiency syndrome. N Engl J Med 321:625–630
6. Rousseau E, Russo P, Lapointe N, O'Reagan S (1988) Renal complications of acquired immunodeficiency syndrome in children. Am J Kidney Dis 11:48–50
7. Connor E, Gupta S, Joshi V, DiCarlo F, Offenberger J, Minnefor A, Uy C, Oleske J, Ende N (1988) Acquired immunodeficiency syndrome-associated renal disease in children. J Pediatr 113:39–44
8. Chander P, Sagel I, Weiss R, Pimentel C, Gupta A, Bamji M, Treser G (1989) Renal disease in human immunodeficiency virus infected children (abstract). Kidney Int 35:368
9. Ingulli E, Gonzalez R, Rajpoot D, Pomrantz A, Tejani A (1989) Demography, morphology, treatment and outcome of AIDs nephropathy. Pediatr Nephrol 3:C168
10. Kaplan MS, Wechsler M, Benson MC (1987) Urologic manifestations of AIDS. Urology 30:441–443
11. Cohen AH, Nast CC (1988) HIV-associated nephropathy: a unique combined glomerular, tubular, and interstitial lesion. Mod Pathol 1:87–97
12. Horowitz L, Greco MA, Feiner V (1988) Renal pathology in pediatric AIDS. Abstracts 4th international conference on AIDS. Stockholm pp 402

13. Rao TKS, Friedman EA, Nicastri AD (1987) The types of renal disease in the acquired immunodeficiency syndrome. N Engl J Med 316:1062–1068
14. Pardo V, Meneses R, Ossa L, Jaffe DJ, Strauss J, Roth D, Bourgoignie JJ (1987) Aids-related glomerulopathy: Occurrence in specific risk groups. Kidney Int 31:1167–1173
15. Vaziri ND, Barbari A, Licorish K, Cesario T, Gupta S (1985) Spectrum of renal abnormalities in acquired immune-deficiency syndrome. J Natl Med Assoc 77:369–375
16. D'Agati V, Suh JI, Carbone L, Cheng JT, Appel G (1989) Pathology of HIV-associated nephropathy: a detailed morphologic and comparative study. Kidney Int 35:1358–1370
17. Heredia JB, Angeles AA, Gutierrez ER, Correa-Rotter R, Saldiyar S, Pena JC (1987) Nephropatia associada al sindrome de inmunodeficiencia acquirida. Rev Invest Clin 39:105–115
18. Kim KK, Factor SM (1987) Membranoproliferative glomerulonephritis and plexogenic pulmonary arteriopathy in a homosexual man with acquired immunodeficiency syndrome. Hum Pathol 18:1293–1296
19. Cantor ES, Kimmel PK, Bosch JP (1989) Impact of race on renal disease in patients with AIDS (abstract). Kidney Int 35:222
20. Weiss MA, Daquioaq E, Margolin EG, Pollak VE (1986) Nephrotic syndrome, progressive irreversible renal failure, and glomerular "collapse:" A new clinicopathologic entity? Am J Kidney Dis 7:20–28
21. Chander P, Soni A, Suri A, Bhagwat R, Yoo J, Treser G (1987) Renal ultrastructural markers in AIDS-associated nephropathy. Am J Pathol 126:513–526
22. Alpers CE, Harawi S, Rennke HG (1988) Focal glomerulosclerosis with tubuloreticular inclusions: Possible predictive value for acquired immunodeficiency syndrome (AIDS). Am J Kidney Dis 12:240–242
23. Bourgoignie JJ (1990) Renal complications of human immunodeficiency virus type I. Kidney Int 37:1571–1584
24. Rao TKS, Fiedman EA (1989) AIDS (HIV)-associated nephropathy; Does it exist? Am J Nephrol 9:441–453
25. Rao TKS (1988) Renal complications in patients with AIDS. Kidney failure is potentially manageable and reversible. J Crit Illness 3:55–74
26. Chander P, Agarwal A, Soni A, Kim K, Treser G (1988) Renal cytomembranous inclusions in idiopathic renal disease as predictive markers for the acquired immunodeficiency syndrome. Hum Pathol 19:1060–1064
27. Humphreys MH, Schoenfeld PY (1987) Renal complications in patients with the acquired immune deficiency syndrome (AIDS). Am J Nephrol 7:1–7
28. Langs C, Gallo GR, Schacht RG, Sidhu G, Baldwin DS (1990) Rapid renal failure in AIDS-associated focal glomerulosclerosis. Arch Intern Med 150:287–292
29. Glassock RJ, Cohen AH, Danovitch G, Parsa KP (1990) Human immunodeficiency virus (HIV) infection and the kidney. Ann Intern Med 112:35–49
30. Scott GB, Hutto C, Makuch RW, Mastrucci MT, O'Connor T, Mitchell CD, Trapido EJ, Parks WP (1989) Survival in children with perinatally acquired human immunodeficiency virus type I infection. N Engl J Med 321:1791–1796

Human Immunodeficiency Virus Associated Nephropathy (HIVAN)

T.K. Sreepada Rao[1]

Summary. Although human immunodeficiency virus (the causative agent of acquired immunodeficiency syndrome) infection in man leads primarily to multiple infectious complications, it also results in multisystem disorders as well. While coincidental acute renal failure and fluid-electrolyte, acid-base disorders were commonly seen early in the AIDS epidemic, HIV associated nephropathy (HIVAN), an unusual disorder, was recognized only in 1984 in certain geographic areas in the United States. Approximately half the patients with HIVAN are intravenous drug abusers, and those remaining include recent immigrants from Haiti (mostly in Brooklyn and Miami) who deny drug use or homosexuality, gay men, sexual partners of HIV infected persons, contaminated blood/blood product recipients, and children born to infected women. HIVAN is typically a disease of young black men and is characterized by massive proteinuria, hypoalbuminemia, large echogenic kidneys, normotension, and a fulminant progression to end stage renal disease (ESRD) within a few months. The renal histopathology consists of focal and segmental glomerulosclerosis, with deposition of IgM, C3, C1q, and, rarely, other immune globulins. There is disproportionate tubular injury, manifested by microcystic dilatation of renal tubules, and sparse interstitial infiltrates and fibrosis. Ultrastructurally, tubulo-reticular structures and unusual cytoplasmic inclusions, along with peculiar nuclear chromatin changes, are present which suggests a possible viral etiology in the genesis of HIVAN. The pathogenesis of HIVAN is unknown, and no effective treatment exists at present. Patients with clinical AIDS and ESRD do poorly when supported by renal replacement therapy.

Introduction

Acquired immunodeficiency syndrome (AIDS), a disease identified in early 1980, is caused by human immunodeficiency virus (HIV), a retro virus which preferentially

[1]SUNY Health Science Center at Brooklyn, Brooklyn, NY 11203, USA

infects and depletes the T helper lymphocytes (CD4 cells), a key component of the immune system. Our understanding of HIV disease in man has evolved over the past decade, and we now recognize its clinical manifestations, which include various stages from an asymptomatic (HIV antibody seropositive) state, to non specific illnesses such as weight loss, persistent fever/diarrhea, lymphadenopathy (AIDS related complex (ARC)), and finally to the development of opportunistic infections and or unusual malignancies (clinical AIDS). In patients with HIV infection, the duration, and the factors which determine progression from an asymptomatic state to clinical AIDS are unclear. While HIV seropositive individuals survive for long periods, the mortality in patients with AIDS continues to be very high. Persons at risk for acquiring HIV infection include intravenous drug abusers (by needle sharing), homosexual and bisexual men, recipients of contaminated blood products, heterosexual partners of HIV infected persons, and children born to HIV infected mothers. In Miami and Brooklyn, the increased incidence of HIV infection in recent immigrants from Haiti, who deny homosexuality and intravenous drug use, remains unexplained. Although infectious complications dominate the clinical picture in AIDS, signs and symptoms referring to other organs, which contribute greatly to patients' morbidity and mortality, are increasingly being recognized. Renal syndromes encountered in patients with HIV infection include:

1. Coincidental diseases such as a spectrum of fluid-electrolyte, acid-base disorders, renal infections, infiltrations, and potentially reversible acute renal failure.
2. An unusual form of HIV associated nephropathy (HIVAN), possibly related to HIV infection, per se.
3. Various known forms of renal disease in patients already infected with HIV.
4. Patients with prior renal disease who subsequently acquire HIV infection through known modes of viral transmission.

Prior to the introduction of serological studies, such as enzyme-linked immunoadsorbent assay (ELISA) and Western Blot tests, which could detect HIV infection, clinicians followed the criteria established by the Center for Disease Control (CDC) to diagnose AIDS. Consequently, the initial descriptions in 1984 of a renal syndrome in AIDS patients was referred to as AIDS associated nephropathy (AAN). As the experience accumulated, it became evident that nephropathy could be an initial manifestation in asymptomatic HIV seropositive individuals. Hence, the terminology was changed to HIV associated nephropathy, a comprehensive name which included all HIV disease patients with the renal syndrome, irrespective of the clinical stage of their illness. This report will focus on clinical features of patients with HIVAN. The epidemiology and pathological features will be described in greater detail by other workers in this area.

Clinical Features of HIVAN

HIV associated nephropathy is not only a disease of clinically ill AIDS patients, as studies indicate that more than half the patients with nephrotic syndrome may be either asymptomatic seropositive carriers of the virus, or those with ARC. In our experience, about 15%–20% of patients with HIVAN at initial presentation do not have other signs and symptoms of ARC/AIDS. The commonest clinical manifestation is proteinuria, discovered either because of a routine urine examination during a clinic visit, or during investigation of patients with pedal edema. Proteinuria is usually massive and is a component of nephrotic syndrome (greater than 3.5 grams in 24 hour urine collections), along with hypoalbuminemia (serum albumin of less than 2.5 g/dl), and generalized edema. Hyperlipidemia may or may not be present. Nephrotic proteinuria is accompanied by normal glomerular filtration rate (Ccr), or varying degrees of azotemia. An analysis of the first 82 patients at our institutions revealed that 74 (90%) had nephrotic syndrome with normal to impaired Ccr, and only 8 (10%) presented with azotemia, hematuria, and proteinuria of less than 2 grams per day. The onset of edema with massive proteinuria and renal insufficiency can sometimes be abrupt. Many of our patients who have been followed in the HIV clinic, with no evidence of prior renal disease, have had explosive presentations with edema and or severe azotemia during routine follow-up visits. Investigations fail to reveal evidence for collagen vascular disease and other known causes of renal syndrome. The serum complement levels are not depressed, and polyclonal elevations of IgG and IgM levels in the blood are detectable. By definition, all nephropathy patients are HIV seropositive, and in our studies, absolute levels of circulating CD4 cells are low, along with a reversal in the ratio of T4:T8 cells (even in asymptomatic individuals with nephrotic syndrome). Ultrasound studies of the kidney reveal large echogenic kidneys in the nephrotic stage of the illness. When serially followed, despite progression to ESRD, renal size remains large; these findings have been repeatedly observed both in clinical and in autopsy studies. One major clinical finding in HIVAN is the notable absence of hypertension both in the early and in the late stages of the disease. The other distinctive feature in HIVAN is the malignant nature of the syndrome and the rapidity with which renal functional deterioration occurs in the absence of additional insult from anoxic injuries and nephrotoxic agents. In most large series, ESRD has developed in 4–6 months, although wide variations in renal progression have been observed. In our large experience, the mean duration from the discovery of proteinuria to irreversible renal failure was 16 weeks, as compared to several months to years in patients with heroin associated nephropathy (HAN). The reasons for the rapid renal failure in HIVAN are unclear. Some have speculated that HIV infection, per se, is responsible, and that HIVAN is a unique disease of combined glomerular, tubular, and interstitial lesions. The development of ESRD in HIVAN patients (those with clinical AIDS), also marks the beginning of a progressive clinical deterioration, ending in death in most patients in less than a year, despite maintenance dialysis. Some HIVAN patients, who do not manifest signs and symptoms of ARC/AIDS during renal replacement therapy, tolerate dialysis well and survival for prolonged periods has been reported.

The most frequently encountered renal pathology in HIVAN is focal and segmental glomerulosclerosis (FSGS). Other uncommonly reported renal histology in HIVAN includes minimal change disease, glomerular mesangial changes, and membranous and membrano proliferative glomerulonephritis. If the mesangial lesions represent an early change before evolution to focal sclerosis, then about 95% of all renal histological changes described in HIVAN will be comprised of FSGS. In the early stages of the disease, the visceral epithelial cells are enlarged, with coarse cytoplasmic vacuoles and with collapse of underlying capillary walls. In late stages, there is a pronounced obliteration of capillary lumen with increase in mesangial matrix and advanced sclerosis. The proximal renal tubular cells contain numerous protein absorption droplets. But the most striking feature is the dilatation of renal tubular lumen filled with pale staining casts, and hence the term "microcystic dilatation" to describe these changes. The dilated tubules are present throughout the cortex and medulla, although they may be more abundant at the cortico-medullary junction. Interstitial fibrosis, renal tubular atrophy, and vascular changes of arteriolosclerosis are minimally present, or strikingly absent, and there is sparse infiltration of interstitium by lymphocytes and other mononuclear cells. Immunofluorescent studies reveal intraglomerular deposition of IgM, C1q, and C3, and rarely, IgG, in the mesangium and sclerotic areas. The nature of these immune deposits is unknown. They may represent deposited immune complexes, or nonspecific trapping of immunoglobulins in the mesangium or sclerotic areas.

Ultrastructural renal changes consist of fusion of epithelial foot processes, increase in mesangial matrix, and detachment of epithelial cells from the basement membrane. Electron dense deposits may be found in the mesangium. But the most striking feature is the presence of abundant tubuloreticular structures in the endothelium of glomerular and peritubular capillaries, interstitial cells, and leukocytes. Multiple complex (Types III and IV) and budding forms of nuclear bodies are increasingly found in AIDS patients with proteinuria. Other ultrastructural changes, considered by some as distinctive in HIVAN, include peculiar nuclear cell bodies in the tubular and interstitial cells, a granulofibrillary transformation of tubular and interstitial cell chromatin, and the presence of intracytoplasmic and intranuclear inclusions of test tube and ring shaped forms in different cells. Based on these findings, a viral etiology for HIVAN has been strongly suggested. The recent in situ hybridization studies employing cDNA probes, and clearly demonstrating the localization of proviral HIV nucleic acid in the glomerular and renal tubular epithelium offer a strong support for the direct HIV infection theory in the initiation (causation) of HIVAN.

The clinical and pathological features of this renal syndrome, HIVAN, may be confused with those of heroin associated nephropathy (HAN), which is also a disease of young black addicts between the ages of 18 and 45 years. While in some patients this distinction may be impossible, the two diseases can be distinguished by some unusual characteristics, as described below. Although the light microscopic and immunofluorescence glomerular findings in HIV associated FSGS resemble those seen in heroin related, idiopathic variety, or other forms of focal sclerosis, the differentiating features in HIV include a larger percentage of "collapsed" glomeruli, a greater degree of tubular degeneration, and microcystic dilatation of renal tubules. Ultrastructurally, in HIVAN, there is an abundance of tubuloreticular inclusions in the glomerular endothelial cells; inclusions which are distinctively rare or absent in other forms of FSGS. Another major point of distinction between the two entities is that children, Haitian immigrants, and gay men constitute about 50% of patients with HIVAN, while HAN, by definition, includes only intravenous drug addicts. A fulminant clinical course of development of ESRD in 3–4 months, large kidney size, and persistent normotension, despite severe uremia in HIVAN patients contrasts clearly to the clinical course of patients with HAN, a disease marked by severe hypertension and shrunken kidneys, as azotemia progresses with the development of global glomerulosclerosis.

The pathogenesis of HIVAN is poorly understood. As is the case with idiopathic FSGS, in HIV associated glomerulosclerosis evidence is lacking which either supports or disputes the role of immune complexes in the development of the disease.

The significance of IgM, C3, and the occasional IgG, seen on immunofluorescent studies of the glomerulus, is unclear. These immune globulins may represent either localization of immune complexes, or merely a non specific trapping in the injured glomerulus. Attempts to localize HIV antigens in these presumed immune complexes have been uniformly unsuccessful. The electron microscopic features, and the in situ hybridization studies, on the other hand, lend a strong support for a direct role of HIV in the initiation and possibly in the progression of renal disease. An intriguing question, still unanswered, is the mechanism of HIV-induced renal injury, in the absence of CD4 receptors in various target cells in the kidney.

Other than symptomatic treatment of edema and hypoalbuminemia, consisting of salt restriction, diuretics, and protein supplementation, no specific treatment is available for HIV associated nephropathy. Neither short-term nor long-term use of corticosteroids or other immunosuppressive agents has been tested, because of fear of inducing infectious complications. Anecdotal data reportedly showing the efficacy of Zidovudine (AZT) in the treatment of patients with HIVAN needs confirmation by large prospective studies.

At present, the survival and rehabilitation of patients with chronic uremia and AIDS treated by maintenance dialysis can be summarized only as dismal and unsatisfactory. Despite renal replacement therapy, ESRD in AIDS is associated with a patient survival of under one year. During hemodialysis therapy, major problems contributing to a high mortality are unexplained malnutrition and a wasting phenomenon encountered in these patients, whether or not an underlying malignancy and/or opportunistic infection is present. During maintenance hemodialysis, AIDS patients manifest a “failure to thrive” syndrome, which fails to respond to nutritional support by hyperalimentation. Death usually results from a combination of cachexia and superimposed opportunistic and or other intercurrent infections.

References

1. Murray HW, Godbold JH, Jurica KB, Roberts RB (1989) Progression to AIDS in patients with lymphadenopathy or AIDS-related complex: reappraisal of risk and predictive factors. Am J Med 86:533–538
2. Rao TKS, Filippone EJ, Nicastri AD, Landesman SH, Frank E, Chen CK, Friedman EA (1984) Associated focal and segmental glomerulosclerosis in the acquired immunodeficiency syndrome. N Engl J Med 310:669–673
3. Rao TKS, Friedman EA, Nicastri AD (1987) The types of renal disease in the acquired immunodeficiency syndrome. N Engl J Med 316:1062–1068
4. Rao TKS, Friedman EA (1989) AIDS (HIV) associated nephropathy; does it exist?, an in-depth review. Am J Nephrol 9:441–453
5. Bourgoignie JJ, Meneses R, Pardo V (1988) The nephropathy related to acquired immunodeficiency syndrome. Adv Nephrol 17:113–126
6. Bourgoignie JJ, Meneses R, Ortiz C, Jaffe D, Pardo V (1988) The clinical spectrum of renal disease associated with human immunodeficiency virus. Am J Kidney Dis 12(2):131–137
7. Chander P, Soni A, Suri A, Bhagwat R, Yoo J, Treser G (1987) Renal ultrastructural markers in AIDS-associated nephropathy. Am J Pathol 126:513–526
8. Chander P, Agarwal A, Soni A, Kim K, Treser G (1988) Renal cytomembranous inclusions in idiopathic renal disease as predictive markers for the acquired immunodeficiency syndrome. Hum Pathol 19:1060–1064

9. D'Agati V, Suh JI, Carbone L, Cheng JT, Appel G (1989) Pathology of HIV-associated nephropathy: a detailed morphologic and comparative study. Kidney Int 35:1358–1370
10. Glassock RJ, Cohen AH, Danovitch G, Parsa P (1990) Human immunodeficiency virus (HIV) infection and the kidney. Ann Intern Med 112:35–49
11. Cohen AH, Nast CC (1988) HIV-associated nephropathy: a unique combined glomerular, tubular, and interstitial lesion. Mod Pathol 1:87–97
12. Cohen AH, Sun NCJ, Shapshak P, Imagawa DT (1989) Demonstration of human immunodeficiency virus in renal epithelium in HIV-associated nephropathy. Mode Pathol 2:125–128
13. Rao TKS (1988) Maintenance dialysis in patients with human immunodeficiency virus infection. Semin Dialysis 1(4):203–208
14. Ortiz C, Meneses R, Jaffe JA, Fernandez JA, Perez G, Bourgoignie JJ (1988) Outcome of patients with human immunodeficiency virus on maintenance hemodialysis. Kidney Int 34:248–253
15. Bowen II PA, Lobel SA, Caruana RJ, Leffell MS, House MA, Rissing PJ, Humphries AL (1988) Transmission of human immunodeficiency virus (HIV) by transplantation: clinical aspects and time course analysis of viral antigenemia and antibody production. Ann Intern Med 108:46–48

The Epidemiology of Human Immunodeficiency Virus-Associated Nephropathy

Jacques J. Bourgoignie, Carmen Ortiz-Interian, Dollie F. Green, David Jaffe, David Roth, and Victoriano Pardo[1]

Summary. The data from the literature and our own cumulative experience in Miami indicate differences in the occurrence of HIV-associated nephropathy among different groups at risk. HIV-associated glomerulosclerosis is observed almost exclusively among intravenous drug abusers and in blacks, often presenting with uremia or the nephrotic syndrome associated with rapidly progressive renal failure. In contrast, renal involvement in HIV-infected caucasians who do not use IV drugs is usually limited to diffuse mesangial hyperplasia with modest proteinuria and little progression of renal dysfunction. Socio-ethnic factors likely explain the variable occurrence of HIV-associated nephropathy reported from different geographic areas where HIV is widespread.

Introduction

In 1984, investigators in New York and Miami reported the clinical presentation of nephrotic syndrome accompanied by rapid progression into renal failure among patients with the acquired immunodeficiency syndrome (AIDS) [1–3]. Renal histology most often demonstrated an aggressive focal and segmental glomerulosclerosis (FSGS). These observations were later expanded upon by the original investigators and confirmed by others [4–11]. Since the nephropathy often occurred in asymptomatic carriers of the human immunodeficiency virus Type 1 (HIV) and in patients with AIDS-related complex before the opportunistic infections or the malignancies characteristic of AIDS developed, the syndrome was referred to as HIV- rather than AIDS-associated nephropathy.

These initial observations met with skepticism, largely because they were not confirmed in San Francisco, a center of AIDS [12]. Second, the nephropathy was not

[1]Departments of Medicine and Pathology, University of Miami School of Medicine, Miami, FL 33101, USA

Table 1. Glomerulosclerosis in AIDS patients at autopsy

		Non-Blacks %	IVDAs %
North America			
1983 Reichert (Bethesda) [13]	0/10	80	10
1984 Hui (Los Angeles) [14]	0/12	83	33
1984 Welch (San Francisco) [15]	0/34	97	0
1984 Guarda (Houston) [16]	0/13	NA	0
1985 Niedt (New York) [17]	0/56	89	7
1985 Mobley (New York) [18]	1/12	83	25
1986 Balow (Bethesda) [19]	0/50	100	4
1989 Pardo (Miami) [20]	24/240	+	+
1989 D'Agati (New York) [11]	1/30	53	13
1990 Mazbar (San Francisco) [21]	1/91	89	24
1990 Seney (Dallas) [22]	1/50	80	50
Central and South America			
1987 Heredia (Mexico [23]	16/21*	100	0
1990 Marques (Rio de Janeiro) [24]	7/77	NA	NA
Europe			
1988 Dratwa-De Meyer (Brussels)++	0/63	43	3
1989 van der Reijden (Amsterdam) [25]	0/47	95	0
1989 Burger (Zurich) [26]	3/210**	100	NA
1989 Giampalmo (Genoa) [27]	6/25	NA	80

IVDA, intravenous drug abuser; NA not available
+About 30% Non-Blacks and 40% IVDAs
*Clinically "silent" focal and segmental glomerulosclerosis
++Presentation, Societé de Néphrologie, Brussels, 1988
**All 3 with features of idiopathic FSGS

apparent in autopsy series even when it was specifically looked for [13–27] (Table 1). Finally, the same type of nephropathy was known to occur in intravenous drug abusers (IVDAs) irrespective of HIV infection [28]; IVDAs represented 30 to 50 percent of the patients with HIV-associated nephropathy described in New York and Miami.

By 1987, AIDS was recognized to occur in other risk groups besides homosexuals and IVDAs. From Miami, where the population of patients with AIDS is more heterogenous than that in New York or San Francisco, we published a large series of patients, including 8 children infected perinatally, with focal and segmental (or global) glomerulosclerosis or with diffuse mesangial hyperplasia [5]. We then called attention to the apparent preponderance of nephrotic proteinuria and glomerulosclerosis among IVDAs and Haitians, the latter a group in which IV drug use is rare and in which HIV is mostly transmitted heterosexually. In contrast, among homosexuals the incidence of heavy proteinuria and FSGS was low. This variable manifestation of renal disease among different groups at risk suggested the participation of co-factors in the expression of HIV-associated nephropathy. We found no statistically significant differences between the various groups at risk with regard to age, duration of disease, or the incidence and types of major opportunistic infections. Moreover, in many patients the nephrotic syndrome and FSGS preceded any opportunistic infection. The incidence of typical or atypical tuberculosis was greater in Haitians than in IVDAs or in homosexuals, a reflection of an increased exposure of the Haitian community in Miami to tuberculosis. It was not evident, however, whether race or the route of contamination was primarily responsible for the rare occurrence of the nephropathy among homosexuals. Three years later, it is timely to reexamine the epidemiology of HIV-associated nephropathy.

Epidemiology

Glomerulosclerosis is rarely found at autopsy of patients with AIDS, even in recent series aimed at evaluating HIV-associated nephropathy (Table I). In contrast, more than 200 cases of histologically proven (many by biopsy) HIV-associated glomerulosclerosis have been formally reported in adults. Half of the cases originated from New York [1,3,7,10,29–31] and 20% were from Miami [2,20], with the balance made up of small series or individual patients from within and outside the United States [6,21–24,26,33–38]. An additional 30 cases have been reported in infants and young children [8,39–43].

Social Factors: Role of IV Drug Use

The use of IV drugs certainly stands out as an important factor in the transmission of HIV. IVDAs represent a large group of patients with HIV-associated nephropathy, with a prevalence varying from 39–84% in the largest series reported [4,10,30,31, 44] from the United States. Of interest, Giampalmo et al [27] from Italy published the only autopsy series made up of a majority of IVDAs (presumably Caucasians) with HIV infection; in this series the prevalence of FSGS was 24% (Table I).

Overall, however, IVDAs represent a minority of patients with glomerulosclerosis and HIV infection. One hundred eighty-eight patients with HIV-associated glomerulosclerosis in whom IV drug use was specifically identified or excluded as a possible risk factor can be recognized in the literature; 50 (27%) were IVDAs and 138 (73%) were not. Thus, IV drug use does not fully explain the clustering of cases of HIV-associated nephropathy among groups living in metropolitan areas where IV drug use is prevalent.

Ethnic Factors

Table 2 is a census, from the literature, of patients with HIV-associated glomerulosclerosis for whom race and IV drug use were specifically identified. Whereas HIV-associated glomerulosclerosis was associated with IV drug use in 28% of the patients, the data identify the nephropathy in 113 Blacks (90%) but in only 14 Caucasians (10%). The 8:1 ratio of Blacks vs Caucasians with HIV-associated glomerulosclerosis increases to 11:1 after exclusion of IV drug users.

Worldwide Experience

In North America, HIV-associated nephropathy has been confined to metropolitan areas of the East Coast of the United States, such as New York, Miami, and Washington D.C. [1,3,4,7,10,29–31,33,44] Small series or individual patients have also

Table 2. Distribution of race and IV drug use in patients with HIV-associated glomerulosclerosis

	Blacks		Caucasians	
	IVDA*	No IVDA	IVDA	No IVDA
Rao (New York) [1]	5	5	–	–
Gardenswartz (New York) [3]	–	–	1	1
Pardo (Miami) [5]	11	16	3	1
Provenzano (Detroit) [6]	–	5	–	–
Cohen (Los Angeles) [8]	1	5	1	2
Alpers (Boston) [9]	1	1	1	–
Soni (New York) [10]	–	–	–	1
Mazbar (San Francisco) [21]	2	2	–	–
Carbone (New York) [30]	11	14	–	–
Weiss (Cincinnati) [32]	–	1	–	–
Cantor (Washington, DC) [33]	–	4	–	–
Patrick (Port of Spain) [34]	–	1	–	–
Dosquet (Paris) [35]	1	10	–	–
Hory (Besancon, France) [36]	–	1	–	–
Babut-Gay (Montfermeil, France) [37]	–	–	–	1
Baumelou (Paris) [38]	–	2	1	1
Connor (Newark) [39]	–	4	–	–
Rousseau (Montreal) [40]	–	4	–	–
Strauss (Miami) [41]	–	5	–	–
Burger (Zurich)**	–	1	–	–
Total	32	81	7	7

Numbers indicate number of patients
*IVDA, intravenous drug abuser
**Personal communication, 1990

been reported from Los Angeles, Dallas, Cincinnati, Boston, Detroit, and San Francisco [6,8,9,21,22,32]. Outside North America, isolated cases have been reported in black natives from the West Indies and Trinidad [34,35].

In Europe, HIV-associated nephropathy was identified in 2 white homosexuals in France (Table 2) and in IVDAs in Italy, but not in Caucasian homosexuals in the Netherlands or in Switzerland (Table I) [25–27,38]. In 1988, 13 cases of FSGS were reported from Brussels and Paris at the Meeting of the Societé de Néphrologie in Brussels in non-IVDAs (D. Kleinknecht, personal communication, 1990).

There are no data directly from Africa. However, several non-IVDA African patients with HIV infection and a nephrotic syndrome and glomerulosclerosis were identified in Belgium, France (Societé de Néphrologie, Brussels, 1988) [35], and Switzerland (HR Burger, German Society of Nephrology, Bern, 1989). These patients were from the Western part of Central Africa [Senegal, Zaire].

In Mexico, FSGS was identified at autopsy in 16 homo- or bisexual men; unlike all other patients reported elsewhere, however, clinically, these patients had minimal renal disease [23]. Seven patients with AIDS and FSGS and three with diffuse mesangial proliferation are reported from Brazil [24]. Cases of HIV-associated nephropathy have not been identified in Chile (A. Valdevieso, Santiago, personal communication, 1990) or in Venezuela (J. Weisinger, Caracas, personal communication, 1990).

There are no data from Asia.

Table 3. Clinical pathology of renal disease identified in Miami in HIV-infected adults who did not use IV drugs

		Clinical disease*	
		Severe	Minimal
Caribbean Blacks			
n=22 (9 ♀)	Glomerulosclerosis	12	2
	Diff. mes. hyperplasia	–	6
	Membranous GN	1	–
	Interstitial Nephritis	–	1
American Blacks			
n=11 (5 ♀)	Glomerulosclerosis	6	1
	Diff. mes. hyperplasia	–	3
	Membranous GN	–	1
Caucasians			
n=12 (1 ♀)	Glomerulosclerosis	–	2
	Diff. mes. hyperplasia	–	9
	Membranoproliferative GN	1	–

*Severe, proteinuria usually > 3.5 g/24 h and serum creatinine > 3 mg/dl; Minimal, proteinuria usually < 2g/24 h and serum creatinine < 2 mg/dl

In Miami

To examine the contribution of race per se, we reviewed our histologic and clinical experience in our adult population with HIV infection and renal disease, after exclusion of IVDAs.

Forty-five patients with abnormal renal biopsy or autopsy specimens were identified, for whom HIV infection was not associated with IV drug use. The patients were divided into Caribbean Blacks, American Blacks, and Caucasians (including Hispanics) (Table 3).

Half of the patients (22 of 45) were Caribbean Blacks (21 Haitians). All denied IV drug use or homosexuality and none had received prior blood transfusions. There were 13 men and 9 women. Fourteen had glomerulosclerosis, 6 had diffuse mesangial hyperplasia (DMH), one had a lupus membranous glomerulonephritis and one had an interstitial nephritis. Eleven American Blacks, 6 homosexual men and 5 women contaminated heterosexually, had a nephropathy characterized as glomerulosclerosis in 7, DMH in 3, and membranous glomerulonephritis in one. In contrast, the nephropathology in 12 Caucasians (11 homosexual men and 1 woman infected by blood transfusion) was limited to early FSGS in 2 patients and DMH in 9. The twelfth patient had a membranoproliferative glomerulonephritis associated with chronic active hepatitis B. Thus, we observed 21 Blacks, but only 2 Caucasians, with HIV infection and glomerulosclerosis in an HIV population where the racial distribution between Blacks and Caucasians was 3:1 [45].

The clinical presentation was also strikingly different, in that 18 Blacks but no Caucasians developed a severe nephropathy (Table 3). Typically, Blacks with advanced glomerulosclerosis presented with nephrotic-range proteinuria (> 3.5 g/24 h) and renal insufficiency (serum creatinine > 3 mg/dl); whereas Caucasians with DMH or FSGS had minimal renal involvement (proteinuria < 2 g/24 h and serum creatinine < 2 mg/dl), although a nephrotic syndrome was the reason for renal biopsy in one Caucasian HIV carrier with DMH.

Separately, we identified 11 additional Blacks (9 Caribbean, of whom 4 were women) and 3 Caucasians (all men) with HIV infection not associated with IV drug use, who developed nephrotic-range proteinuria and a progressive nephropathy. Renal tissue was not available for histologic examination in these patients.

Discussion

The literature and our experience in Miami indicate that factors other than IV drug use may be determinant in allowing the full expression of HIV-associated nephropathy. Race, more than IV drug use, seems to predispose Blacks to the development of progressive HIV-associated nephropathy. In contrast, uremia is rarely observed in Caucasian homosexuals in whom the nephropathology seems to be limited to DMH rather than FSGS. The increased expression of the nephropathy in Blacks infected with HIV may reflect a susceptibility of Blacks to develop FSGS. This is consistent with numerous studies reporting a higher incidence of chronic renal disease occurring in Blacks with hypertension, diabetes, or IV drug use without HIV infection when compared to a cohort of Caucasian patients (see references in [46,47]). In a large series mostly of IVDAs from New York, progression to endstage renal disease was also faster in Blacks than in Hispanics with HIV infection and equivalent proteinuria [10]. In the same context, infants and young children have been identified with HIV-associated glomerulosclerosis [8,39–43]. Of note, all children but one reported so far were Black.

Genetic factors may be involved in the expression of HIV-associated nephropathy. Specific immune response genes may be important in facilitating the expression of FSGS in Blacks or in repressing it in Caucasians. Alternatively, unrecognized environmental factors could be responsible for predisposing Blacks infected with HIV to progressive renal disease. The data indicate that HIV-associated glomerulosclerosis may afflict American Blacks and Caribbean Blacks; preliminary data suggest that West African Blacks may be affected as well. More epidemiologic and histologic data than those presently available are needed to determine whether progressive HIV-associated nephropathy is related to blacks in general or is limited to certain subsets of this population.

The finding of different renal manifestations in different groups at risk for HIV infection is intriguing, particularly since Cohen et al. ([8,48], and personal communication, 1990) have localized the HIV genome in renal glomerular and tubular epithelial cells from IVDAs as well as from Caucasians and Black homosexuals with HIV infection and glomerulosclerosis.

Whatever the reasons for the differences in the expression of HIV-associated nephropathy between Blacks and Caucasians who are not IV drug users, social and ethnic factors likely explain the discrepancies that exist in the literature regarding the occurrence of HIV-associated nephropathy reported from different geographic areas where HIV is widespread.

Acknowledgments. This work was supported by NIH Grant R01-DK 40836. The authors are grateful to Ms. Kim Schauers for expert secretarial assistance.

References

1. Rao TK, Filippone EJ, Nicastri AD, Landesman SH, Frean E, Chen CK, Friedman EA (1984) Associated focal and segmental glomerulosclerosis in the acquired immunodeficiency syndrome. N Engl J Med 310:669–673
2. Pardo V, Aldana M, Colton RM, Fischl MA, Jaffe D, Moskowitz L, Hensley GT, Bourgoignie JJ (1984) Glomerular lesions in the acquired immunodeficiency syndrome. Ann Intern Med 101:429–434
3. Gardenswartz MH, Lerner CW, Seligson GR, Zabetakis PM, Rotterdam H, Tapper ML, Michelis MF, Bruno MS (1984) Renal disease in patients with AIDS: A clinicopathologic study. Clin Nephrol 21:197–204
4. Rao TK, Friedman EA, Nicastri AD (1987) The types of renal disease in the acquired immunodeficiency syndrome. N Engl J Med 316:1062–1068
5. Pardo V, Meneses R, Ossa L, Jaffe DJ, Strauss J, Roth D, Bourgoignie JJ (1987) AIDS-related glomerulopathy: Occurrence in specific risk groups. Kidney Int 31:1167–1173
6. Provenzano R, Kupin W, Santiago GC (1987) Renal involvement in the acquired immunodeficiency syndrome: Presentation, clinical course and therapy. Henry Ford Hosp Med J 35:38–41
7. Kaplan MS, Wechsler M, Benson MC (1987) Urologic manifestations of AIDS. Urology 30:441–443
8. Cohen AH, Nast CC (1988) HIV-associated nephropathy: A unique combined glomerular, tubular and interstitial lesion. Mod Pathol 1:87–97
9. Alpers CE, Harawi S, Rennke (1988) Focal glomerulosclerosis with tubuloreticular inclusions: Possible predictive value for acquired immunodeficiency syndrome (AIDS). Am J Kidney Dis 12:240–242
10. Soni A, Agarwal A, Chander P, Yoo J, Singal D, Salomon N, Robinson B, Treser G (1989) Evidence for an HIV-related nephropathy: A clinicopathological study. Clin Nephrol 31:12–17
11. D'Agati V, Cheng JI, Carbone L, Cheng JT, Appel G (1989) The pathology of HIV-nephropathy: A detailed morphologic and comparative study. Kidney Int 35:1358–1370
12. Humphreys MH, Schoenfeld PY (1988) Renal complications in patients with the acquired immune deficiency syndrome. Am J Nephrol 7:1–7
13. Reichert CM, O'Leary TJ, Levens DL, Simrell CR, Macher A (1983) Autopsy pathology in the acquired immune deficiency syndrome. Am J Pathol 112:357–382
14. Hui AN, Koss MN, Meyer PR (1984) Necropsy findings in acquired immunodeficiency syndrome: A comparison of premortem diagnoses with postmortem findings. Hum Pathol 15:670–676
15. Welch K, Finkbeiner W, Alpers CE, Blumenfeld W, Davis RL, Smuckler EA, Beckstead JH (1984) Autopsy findings in the acquired immune deficiency syndrome. JAMA 252:1152–1159
16. Guarda LA, Luna MA, Smith JL Jr (1984) Acquired immune deficiency syndrome: postmortem findings. Am J Clin Pathol 81:549–557
17. Niedt GW, Schinella RA (1985) Acquired immunodeficiency syndrome. Arch Pathol Lab Med 109:727–734
18. Mobley K, Rotterdam HZ, Lerner CW, Tapper ML (1985) Autopsy findings in the acquired immune deficiency syndrome. Pathol Annu 20:45–65
19. Balow JE, Macher AM, Rook AH (1986) Paucity of glomerular disease in acquired immunodeficiency syndrome (AIDS) (abstract). Kidney Int 29:178
20. Pardo V, Bell M, Ortiz C, Strauss J, Bourgoignie JJ (1989) The spectrum of glomerular lesions in patients with HIV infection (abstract). Fed Proc 3:A1281
21. Mazbar SA, Schoenfeld PY, Humphreys MH (1990) Renal involvement in patients infected with HIV: Experience at San Francisco General Hospital. Kidney Int 37:1325–1332

22. Seney FD Jr, Burns DK, Silva FG (to be published) AIDS and the kidney. Am J Kidney Dis.
23. Heredia JB, Angeles AA, Gutierrez ER, Correa-Rotter R, Saldiyar S, Pena JC (1987) Nephropatia associada al sindrome di immunodeficiencia acquirida. Rev Invest Clin 39:105–115
24. Marques LPJ, Oliveira AV, Basilio de Oliviera CA, Riodja LS, Lopes GS, Santos OR (1990) Renal histologic alterations in AIDS. Abstracts 11th Int Congr Nephrology, 15–20 July, Tokyo, p. 174A
25. van der Reijden HJ, Schipper HE, Danner SA, Arisz L (1989) Glomerular lesions and opportunistic infections of the kidney in AIDS: an autopsy study of 47 cases. Adv Exp Med Biol 252:181–189
26. Burger HR, Kriemler S, Mihatsch M (1989) Gibt es eine AIDS-Nephropathie? Resultate von 210 Autopsiefällen (abstract). Nieren - und Hochdruck -Krankeiten 6:379
27. Giampalmo A, Ardoino S, Borghesi MR, Buffa D, Lapertosa G, Pagano S, Pesce C, Provaggi MA, Ravetti GL, Guaglia AC, Ravetti GL, Terragna A (1989) Anatomopathologic findings in 25 autopsy cases of AIDS. Pathologica 81:1–46
28. Rao TKS, Nicastri AD, Friedman EA (1977) Renal consequences of narcotic abuse. Adv Nephrol 7:261–290
29. Chander P, Agarwal A, Soni A, Kim K, Treser G (1988) Renal cytomembranous inclusions in idiopathic renal disease as predictive markers for the acquired immunodeficiency syndrome. Hum Pathol 19:1060–1064
30. Carbone L, D'Agati V, Cheng JT, Appel GB (1989) The course and prognosis of human immunodeficiency virus-associated nephropathy. Am J Med 87:389–395
31. Langs C, Gallo GR, Schacht RG, Sidhu G, Baldwin DF (1990) Rapid renal failure in AIDS-associated focal glomerulosclerosis. Arch Intern Med 150:287–292
32. Weiss MA, Daquioag E, Margolin EG, Pollak VE (1986) Nephrotic syndrome, progressive irreversible renal failure, and glomerular "collapse": A new clinicopathologic entity? Am J Kidney Dis 7:20–28
33. Cantor ES, Kimmel PL, Bosch JP (1989) Impact of race on renal disease in patients with AIDS (abstract). Kidney Int 35:222
34. Patrick AL, Roberts LA, Burton EN, Jankey N, Shah DH (1986) Focal and segmental glomerulosclerosis in the acquired immunodeficiency syndrome. West Indian Med J 35:200–202
35. Dosquet P, Michel C, Elyaszewicz M, Matheron S, Meychas MC, Ronco P, Mignon F (1990) Focal and segmental glomerulosclerosis (FSG) among HIV infected patients: possible favorable effect of treatment with azidothymidine (AZT). Abstracts 11th Int Congr Nephrology, 15–20 July, Tokyo, p 14A
36. Hory B, Bresson C, Lorge JF, Perol C (1988) Associated focal and segmental glomerulosclerosis in the acquired immunodeficiency syndrome. Am J Kidney Dis 12:169
37. Babut-Gay ML, Echard M, Kleinknecht D, Meyrier A (1989) Zidovudine and nephropathy with human immunodeficiency virus (HIV) infection. Ann Intern Med 111:856–857
38. Baumelou A, Assogba V, Beaufils H, Hinglais N, Ben Hmida M, Christin S, Eugene M, Deray G, Jacobs C (1989) Pathologie rénale associée à l'infection à virus VIH et au syndrôme d'immunodéficience acquise. In: Chatelain C, Jacobs C (eds) Séminaires d'Uro-Nephrologie. Masson, Paris, pp 42–49
39. Connor E, Gupta S, Joshi V, DiCarlo F, Offenberger J, Minnefor A, Uy C, Oleske J, Ende N (1988) Acquired immunodeficiency syndrome-associated renal disease in children. J Pediatr 113:39–44
40. Rousseau E, Russo P, Lapointe N, O'Regan S (1988) Renal complications of acquired immunodeficiency syndrome in children. Am J Kidney Dis 11:48–50
41. Strauss J, Abitbol C, Zilleruelo G, Scott G, Paredes A, Malaga S, Montane B, Mitchell C, Parks W, Pardo V (1989) A spectrum of renal disease in children with acquired immunodeficiency syndrome. New Engl J Med 321:625–630

42. Chandler P, Sagel I, Weiss R, Pimentel C, Gupta A, Bamji M, Treser G (1989) Renal disease in human immunodeficiency virus (HIV)-infected children (abstract). Kidney Int 35:368
43. Horowitz L, Greco MA, Feiner Y (1988) Renal pathology in pediatric AIDS. Abstracts 4th Int Conf on AIDS, Stockholm, I, 402
44. Bourgoignie JJ, Meneses R, Ortiz-Interian C, Jaffe D, Pardo V (1988) The clinical spectrum of renal disease associated with human immunodeficiency virus. Am J Kidney Dis 12:131–137
45. Bourgoignie JJ, Ortiz-Interian C, Green DF, Roth D (1989) Race, a co-factor in HIV-1 associated nephropathy. Transplant Proc 21:3899–3901
46. Rao TKS, Friedman EA (1989) AIDS (HIV)-associated nephropathy; Does it exist? An in-depth review. Am J Nephrol 9:441–453
47. Stephens GN, Gillaspy JA, Clyne D, Mejia A, Pollak VE (1990) Racial differences in the incidence of end-stage renal disease in types I and II diabetes mellitus. Am J Kidney Dis 15:562–567
48. Cohen AH, Sun NCJ, Shapshak P, Imagana DT (1989) Demonstration of human immunodeficiency virus in renal epithelium in HIV-associated nephropathy. Mod Pathol 2:125–128

Pathology of Human Immunodeficiency Virus (HIV) Associated Nephropathy in Adults and Children

PRAVEEN N. CHANDER[1], INGE SAGEL[2], and GERHARD TRESER[3]

SUMMARY. A variety of renal lesions are identified in patients infected with Human Immunodeficiency virus (HIV). A distinctive clinicopathologic entity, termed HIV-associated nephropathy (HIVAN) is noted in 7–10% of the unselected adult and pediatric hospital admissions for Acquired Immunodeficiency Syndrome (AIDS). Adult HIVAN is more common in Blacks and in intravenous (IV) drug users and is characterized clinically by acute onset of severe, often nephrotic range proteinuria with generally rapid and irreversible progression to renal failure. Histologically, focal segmental sclerosis (FGS) is frequently accompanied by a unique globally collapsing glomerulopathy with dilatation of Bowman's space, microcystic ectasia of tubules, scant interstitial cellular infiltrate and fibrosis in the well established lesions. A combination of these distinctive clinical features and histologic findings, along with abundant tubulo-reticular inclusions (TRI) in renal vascular endothelium on electronmicroscopy, distinguishes HIVAN from heroin-associated nephropathy (HAN). A constellation of these clinicopathological findings also allows one to make a presumptive diagnosis of HIV infection with a high degree of accuracy in an asymptomatic HIV carrier. Greater frequency of multiple, budding, and complex nuclear bodies, and various cytomembranous and intranuclear inclusions, presumed to be "viral footprints," suggest a viral etiology for HIVAN.

In children with HIV infection, the commonest lesion is proliferative glomerulonephritis, often present as mesangial hyperplasia, accompanied by a mild degree of focal segmental and global glomerulosclerosis, with clinically modest proteinuria and mild progression to renal insufficiency.

Introduction

A broad spectrum of renal lesions has been observed in patients infected with the Human Immunodeficiency Virus (HIV), ranging from renal infections and tumors to

[1]Departments of Pathology, Pediatrics[2], and Medicine[3], New York Medical College, Valhalla, NY 10595, USA

tubulointerstitial lesions and a variety of glomerular pathology [1–4]. The glomerular pathology includes focal segmental sclerosis (FGS), mesangial proliferation, membranoproliferative glomerulonephritis, minimal change disease, postinfectious glomerulonephritis, membranous nephropathy, amyloidosis, hemolytic uremic syndrome, infarcts, and cortical necrosis.

In spite of such a variety of observed "nonspecific" pathology, a more specific and characteristic clinical and pathological entity has been recognized and has been named HIV associated nephropathy (HIVAN). It was first described as a rapidly progressive renal disease accompanied by heavy proteinuria, with FGS as the glomerular lesion [5]. Subsequent investigations have broadened the clinical presentations and defined the structural lesions in the kidney [6–15]. In this report we have summarized our observations of the renal pathology of HIV infected adults and children and included a review of the literature, in an attempt to characterize the specific HIV associated nephropathy.

Renal Pathology in HIV-Associated Nephropathy in Adults

We compared the renal biopsy or autopsy tissues of patients with AIDS and severe proteinuria (> 2g/day) with the renal tissues of other AIDS patients with comparable clinical features, but without proteinuria, and with the renal tissues of patients with heroin associated nephropathy (HAN) [6]. The patients with HAN had a similar degree of proteinuria and were of comparable age. The HAN tissues were from our files and were taken prior to 1982 and the spread of the AIDS epidemic. The following account is a summary based on our cumulative experience and on the consensus of other published reports on this subject [2,6,7,12,15].

Histology

Histologically, nephropathy in patients with AIDS was characterized by segmental glomerulosclerosis which was quantitatively and qualitatively similar to HAN (Fig. 1). The FGS however, was often accompanied by a global collapse of capillary tufts with dilated Bowman Spaces, filled with bright eosinophilic proteinaceous material. Tubules were frequently enormously dilated, sometimes to microcystic proportions, and filled with large hyaline casts and often lined by degenerating and/or simplified flattened epithelium. Retracted glomerular capillary tufts were in general devoid of hyaline deposits, foam cells, and excessive accumulation of mesangial matrix and revealed mesangial hypocellularity in many of the autopsy specimens. Small shrunken capillary tufts retracted towards the vascular pole, giving the appearance of a rapidly progressive event, akin to the rapid progression of renal failure described clinically, due perhaps to the loss of axially supporting mesangial cells. Focal mesangial hyperplasia was observed in other areas of the same tissue. (Mesangial proliferation has also been reported in some patients with HIVAN. Many of these were non-IV-drug-user Caucasian men with mild to moderate proteinuria and slight progression to renal insufficiency.) In addition there was severe hypertrophy and focal hyperplasia of visceral epithelium, containing abundant and massive protein resorption droplets, overlying segmentally sclerotic areas of globally collapsing glomeruli. Interstitial infiltrate could be moderately dense, in the early lesions, particularly in

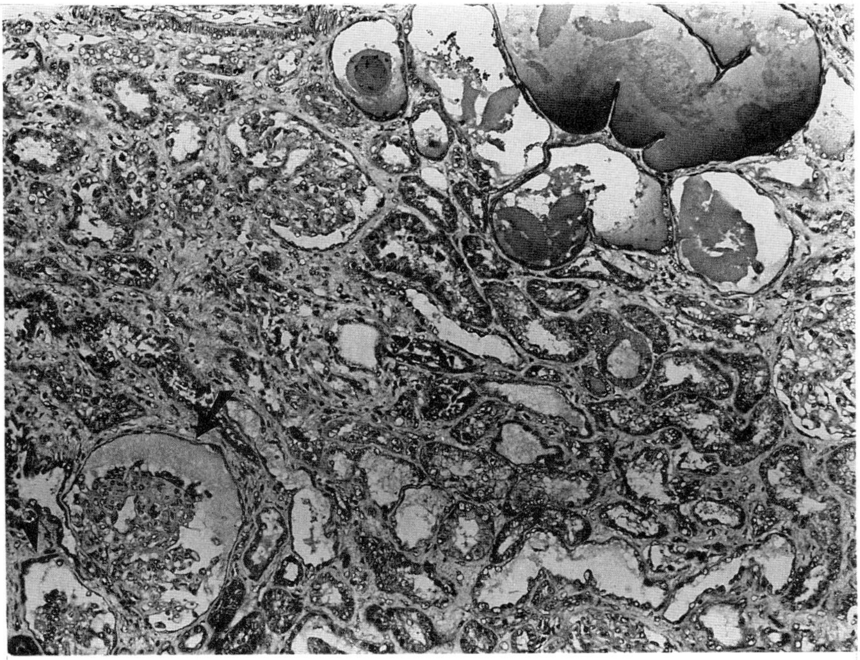

Fig. 1. Segmentally sclerotic glomerulus with global capillary tuft collapse and prominent visceral epithelial cells crowding the sclerotic tuft and dilated Bowman space (*arrow*). Another glomerulus with global capillary tuft retraction without deposits of hyaline, foam cells, or excessive mesangial matrix (*arrow head*). There is tubular degeneration, regeneration and microcystic ectasia. Interstitium is edematous with sparse inflammatory infiltrate. H&E, × 125

biopsy specimens (Chander, unpublished work), [14] but in the later stages, in the autopsy specimens, the infiltrate was invariably scanty in an interstitium that frequently appeared edematous and was sometimes replaced by a homogenous acidophilic substance [6,7]. The paucity of interstitial infiltrate in the autopsy specimens is perhaps related to leucopenia in patients dying of AIDS. Microscopic calcium deposits (nephrocalcinosis) were noted in tubules and interstitium.

In contrast, globally sclerosing glomeruli in HAN and idiopathic FGS appeared as solid mass consisting of excess accumulation of mesangial matrix and focal hyaline deposits. "Capping" by the hypertrophic and proliferated visceral epithelium, dilatation of Bowman's spaces, microcystic ectasia of tubules, and degenerative epithelial changes were not a prominent feature in either. Tubular atrophy and interstitial fibrosis were commensurate with the degree of glomerulosclerosis. The interstitium in HAN frequently contained marked infiltrates of lymphocytes and plasma cells in early, and in the well established late lesions.

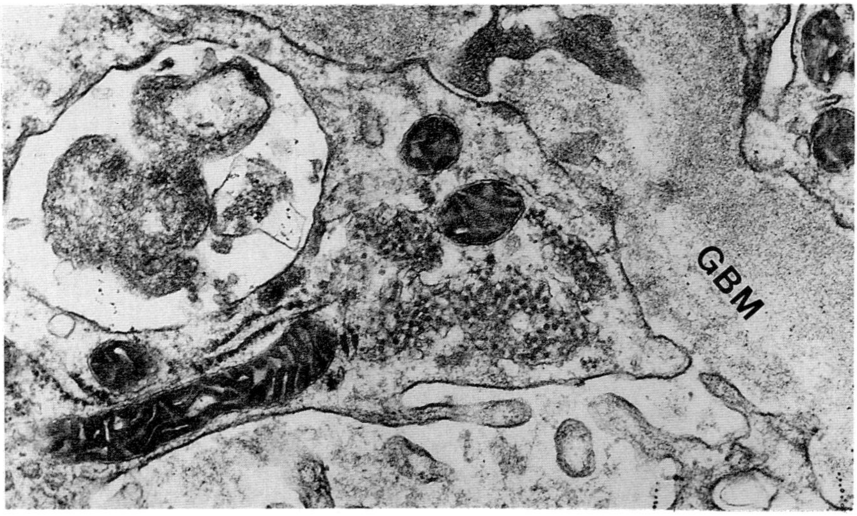

Fig. 2. Tubuloreticular inclusions in the endoplasmic cisternae of a swollen glomerular endothelial cell × 20,000. Glomerular basement membrane (GBM)

Immunofluorescent Findings

No distinctive pattern could be distinguished by immunofluorescence. Segmental coarsely granular deposits of IgM and C_3 were frequently seen in sclerosing glomeruli, similar to those seen in HAN and in idiopathic FGS. In addition, variable scattering of C_1, IgG, and IgA was also present. The same deposits however, could be identified in apparently normal glomeruli, in patients without the nephropathy who were dying of AIDS [2,6,7]. Deposits found by immunofluorescence and electron-microscopy correlated best with chronic infections such as hepatitis B virus infection [6].

Electronmicroscopy

On electron microscopy, in addition to scattered mesangial and, rarely, subendothelial and subepithelial deposits, GBM wrinkling and collapse was noted in the sclerosing glomeruli with, and often without, accumulation of mesangial matrix. Diffuse effacement and focal detachment of foot-processes were seen in such areas. Visceral epithelial cells were markedly swollen and hypertrophic and showed frequent villous transformation. The most notable finding on electron microscopy was the presence of numerous tubuloreticular inclusions (TRI) (Fig. 2) in the glomerular and peritubular capillary endothelium and interstitial leukocytes [6,9,12,15,17]. These TRI are reticular aggregates of apparently branching membranous tubules, measuring approximately 25 nm in diameter. The TRI have been described in association with a variety of different nephritides including HAN, SLE, and other collagen vascular, autoimmune, and viral diseases. Except for lupus nephritis, a persistent and diligent search is needed to document the presence of TRI in the renal parenchyma in most other nephritides. In contrast, in particular to HAN, TRI were in abundance in HIV associated nephropathy; with little experience they were detectable, at the low power scanning magnification, in the often swollen endothelial cells. Frequently, multiple aggregates of TRI were present in a single capillary loop as well as in different parts of the cytoplasm of the same endothelial cell. The clear abundance of TRI has also been documented by D'Agati et al. [15], who, by a semi-quantitative analysis of randomly taken electron-micrographs, arrived at the figure of 0.86 TRI on average per capillary loop in HIVAN. Cylindrical confronting cisternae (CCC), another ultrastructure marker of HIV infection described in peripheral leukocytes, were detected only rarely in the renal tissue, and required a more persistent and diligent search, than was needed for documenting TRI. Possibly derived from endoplasmic reticulum, CCC are parallel, cylindrical, or concentrically arranged cisternae with electron dense material interposed between the two membranous lamellae. They measure approximately 3.5 μm in length with a width of approximately 250 μm. In the kidney, CCC were found mostly in the glomerular endothelial cells, often in association with TRI [6,9,17]. These CCC have never been seen in HAN or in idiopathic FGS.

On comparative renal morphologic analysis of the HIV infected patients, with and without nephropathy, and the HAN patients, a variety of unusual ultrastructural findings were observed in HIVAN, and were observed with lesser frequency in AIDS without nephropathy. These are best described as viral "foot prints" and may suggest a viral etiology for HIVAN [6,17,18]. These findings are summarized as follows: Type I and II nuclear bodies are a ubiquitous feature of normal cells, but are induced in cells activated by viruses, amongst other stimuli. Nuclear bodies (NB) were seen in greater frequency, complexity, size, and budding configuration, and also in increased frequency of multiple NBs per cell, in HIV nephropathy, than in the cells without nephropathy and in the HAN cells.

A peculiar granulofibrillary change of the normal nuclear chromatin was seen with greater frequency in the interstitial and tubular cells in HIVAN. The nature of this transformation is unclear, but greater frequency and complexity of nuclear bodies in the nuclei thus affected, suggests "activated" rather than normally degenerating cells (Fig. 3). These findings were confirmed by D'Agati et al. [15]. In addition, we observed a great variety of other intranuclear inclusions in interstitial fibroblasts of HIV infected patients, with an even greater frequency in HIVAN. These included filamentous crystalline and fibrillary inclusions, membranous lamellae or profiles, vacuolar, lipid, and granular vesicles and, rarely, CCC. None were present in HAN. Some of these inclusions have been described in various human viral diseases. Except for CMV in 2 children with HIVAN, we have been unable, ultrastructurally, to detect other specific viral agents, including HIV-1, in spite of thorough search. A recent report of HIV nucleic acid and p-24 antigen in tubular and visceral epithelial cells, by in-situ hybridization and immunohistochemical techniques, respectively, deserves further study [19].

TRI as Predictive Markers for HIV Disease and HIVAN

In an effort to evaluate the value of TRI in the diagnosis of HIVAN we carefully studied the renal tissue available from 13 patients with risk factors for AIDS, who

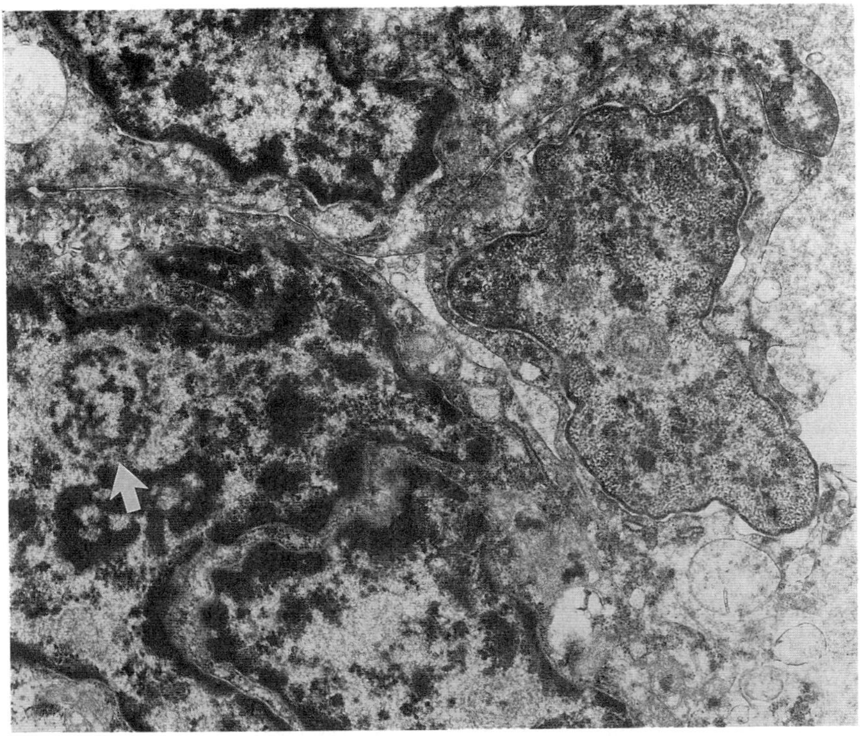

Fig. 3. Distal tubular cell nucleus with two type II nuclear bodies and partial granular fibrillary transformation (*right*). A type IV nuclear body is present in an adjacent cell nucleus (*arrow*) × 15,000

underwent renal biopsy for severe proteinuria. On the basis of the clinical presentation and follow up, these patients could be grouped into 4 categories: A. Two patients who had AIDS at the time of biopsy; B. four patients who had ARC; C. four patients who had risk factors for AIDS but no evidence of AIDS or ARC at the time of biopsy, but developed AIDS subsequently, and D. three patients who were similar to those in group C, except that AIDS did not manifest over a prolonged observation period (Table 1). Our findings and conclusions from this study [9] were: Renal pathology was similar in groups, A, B, and C; nephropathy with severe, often nephrotic range proteinuria, with or without rapid progression to endstage renal disease, can occur in patients with AIDS or with AIDS related complex, but most importantly, also in asymptomatic HIV carriers. Globally collapsing glomerulopathy was seen, frequently associated with focal and segmental glomerulosclerosis, dilated Bowman spaces and microcystic tubular ectasia.

Tubuloreticular inclusions were uniformly present in all biopsies of patients from groups, A, B, and C. They were not seen in the renal tissue of the 3 group D patients who subsequently never developed AIDS, in spite of the fact that one patient was documented to be HIV infected. Therefore, TRI are not uniformly present in

Table 1. Analysis of renal biopsies from patients with HIV risk factors and proteinuria

Groups	Risk factors	Follow-up average months (*n*)*	Histology FGS	GCG	PGN	TRI	Positive HIV Ab (*n* tested)
A AIDS(n−2)	IVDA-1 gay-1	14 (2)	1	2	0	2	1 (1)
B ARC(n−4)	IVDA-3 het-1	3 (1)	3	3	1	4	4 (4)
C Prturia to AIDS (n−4)	IVDA-1 gay-1 het -2	11 (4)	4	4	0	4	2 (2)
D Prturia No AIDS (n−3)	IVDA-2 gay-1**	16 (3)	1	0	2	0	1 (3)

FGS, focal and segmental glomerulosclerosis; GCG, globally collapsing glomerulopathy; het, heterosexual transmission in women; PGN, proliferative glomerulonephritis; Ab, antibody; Prturia, proteinuria; *number of patients available for follow-up; **died of lung cancer

glomerular lesions, other than in HIV associated nephropathy in HIV infected patients. We have confirmed these observations in some additional cases (Chander, unpublished work). Combination of the characteristic glomerulo-tubular findings described above and TRI on electron microscopic examination are almost pathognomonic and we suggested that a presumptive diagnosis of HIV infection and/or nephropathy can be made with a high degree of accuracy, in the appropriate clinical setting [9,17]. Similar observations have also been made by other investigators [15,20]. At present, however, it is not clear whether TRI in kidney are simply markers for systemic HIV disease or are specific for HIVAN in HIV infected patients.

Renal Pathology in Perinatally HIV Infected Children

In perinatally HIV-infected children, the occurrence of a nephropathy similar to that seen in adults, supports the existence of a specific HIV-associated nephropathy. Children with HIV infection were analyzed by us and by Strauss et al. [21,22]. Although mild proteinuria was very frequent, ranging from 40–50% of unselected admissions for AIDS, the incidence of heavy proteinuria, defined as >2+ on dipstick examination and/or > 1 g/day per square meter of body surface area, was between 8 and 9%, similar to that reported in adults. Altogether, 29 such cases are reported in the entire literature, all born to HIV infected mothers with IV drug use or heterosexual contact with an IV drug user as the risk factors [12,15,21–24]. Of these, 25 were Black and 4 were Hispanic children. Rapid progression to renal failure was rare and the nephropathy was generally milder than that seen in adults. The renal histology was variable, with several distinctive features different from the adult form of disease. Focal segmental sclerosis was not a dominant lesion, and was seen in only 9 of the 29 reported cases. An associated fulminant globally collapsing glomerulopathy with dilation of Bowman spaces and microcystic ectasia of tubules was infrequent and milder, when present. There were no distinctive histologic tubulo-interstitial findings. Proliferative glomerulonephritis was more prevalent, and was observed in 18 of the 29 reported cases. Mesangial proliferation or hyperplasia constituted the great majority. Although not an exclusive finding, greater than normal prevalence of segmental and often global glomerulosclerosis, (defined as >5% affected glomeruli), was observed frequently in association with proliferative glomerular disease. Deposits of the immune type were frequent on immunofluorescent and electron microscopic studies. These, along with abundant TRI in vascular endothelium and variable immunologic abnormalities suggested a superficial resemblance to lupus nephritis. Diagnosis of lupus nephritis was documented in 2 of the 29 cases in view of highly positive ANA and anti-double stranded DNA [15,22].

Since the children have milder renal disease and shorter survival, proliferative glomerulonephritis, frequently occurring with immune-deposits, may be considered an early mild form of HIV-associated nephropathy. However, a progression of mesangial proliferative lesion to segmentally sclerosing and globally collapsing glomerulopathy has not been documented. Only one case of minimal change disease (MCD) on biopsy that progressed to FGS has been reported [15] amongst several cases of MCD reported in the setting of HIV disease. It has been speculated that lymphokines liberated by T-cells are involved in the etiology of both MCD and HIV nephropathy. Alternatively, mesangial proliferation and FGS may be two separate independent lesions, with the former of post-infectious etiology.

Renal Pathology Other than HIVAN in HIV Infected Patients

The incidence of various renal lesions is different in large series reporting primarily on renal biopsy versus autopsy material [10,11,15]. There is a preponderance of tubulo-interstitial disease, such as acute tubular necrosis, allergic interstitial nephritis, colonization by opportunistic pathogens, nephrocalcinosis etc., in the autopsy series. These are often related to AIDS, its complications, and a variety of necessary therapeutic and diagnostic interventions. Table 2 lists the majority of non-glomerular renal lesions seen in patients with AIDS. Although focal segmental sclerosis was present in 28% and mesangial hyperplasia in 32% of the autopsy results

Table 2. Spectrum of non glomerular renal lesions in human immunodeficiency virus (HIV) infection

1. *Acute tubular necrosis*: toxic ischemic (e.g. sepsis, dehydration, amphotericin, pentamidine)
2. *Drug induced allergic interstitial nephritis* (e.g. trimethoprim-sulfamethoxazole, cephalosporines and other beta-lactam antibiotics)
3. *Renal infections*
   - CMV
   - Mycobacterium
   - Cryptococcus
   - Candida
4. *Tumors*
   - Kaposi's sarcoma
   - lymphomas
   - renal cell carcinoma
5. *Vascular* hemolytic uremic syndrome, renal cortical necrosis, vasculitis
6. *Nephrocalcinosis* amphotericin B

Table 3. Glomerular pathology in patients with human immunodeficiency virus (HIV) infection

1.	Focal and segmental glomerulosclerosis with epithelial "capping"
2.	Globally sclerosing (collapsing) glomerulopathy
3.	Mesangial Proliferation
4.	Membranoproliferative glomerulonephritis
5.	Acute postinfectious glomerulonephritis
6.	Membranous nephropathy
7.	Hepatitis B-Virus associated nephropathy
8.	Minimal change disease
9.	Heroin-associated nephropathy
10.	Amyloidosis
11.	Hemolytic-uremic syndrome with or without renal cortical necrosis
12.	Lupus nephritis
13.	? vasculitis
14.	End stage kidney

reported [3], the incidence of clinically evident glomerular disease was rather low [15]. In contrast, glomerular lesions predominate in renal biopsies obtained from HIV infected patients, including AIDS, ARC, and asymptomatic HIV carriers. This is undoubtedly related to selection bias, because renal biopsies were performed mostly in patients with unexplained proteinuria. Focal segmental sclerosis with globally collapsing glomerulopathy accounts for 83% biopsies reported in the literature, mesangial proliferation for 6%, minimal change disease for 3%, and other glomerulonephritides for 6%. The greater frequency of mesangial hyperplasia at autopsy, as compared to biopsy material, is also best explained by the lack of clinically significant proteinuria and progressive renal insufficiency in such cases [7]. Even though HIVAN is the most common lesion in those biopsied, present in 76% of cases in one series [15], not every HIV infected patient with proteinuria can be presumed to have HIVAN. Other glomerular lesions commonly seen in such patients include those associated with IV drug use (such as HAN, amyloidosis), and Hepatitis B Virus associated nephropathies, or perhaps nephropathies which are of post-infectious etiology (immune complex mediated proliferative glomerulonephritides) (Table 3). Rarely, vasculitis, hemolytic-uremic syndrome with or without renal cortical infarcts, and lupus nephritis are reported. These lesions are intriguing in view of the well known autoimmune abnormalities noted in patients with HIV infection [25].

References

1. Gardenswartz MH, Lerner CW, Seligson GR, Zabetakis PM, Rotterdam H, Tapper ML, Michelis MF, Bruno MS (1984) Renal disease in patients with AIDS – A clinicopathologic study. Clin Nephrol 21:197–204
2. Pardo V, Aldana M, Colton RM, Fischl MA, Jaffe D, Moskowitz L, Hensley GT, Bourgoignie JJ (1984) Glomerular lesions in the acquired immunodeficiency syndrome. Ann Intern Med 101:429–434
3. Bourgoignie JJ (1990) Renal complications of human immunodeficiency virus type 1. Kidney Int 37:1571–1584

4. Glassock RJ, Cohen AH, Danovitch G, Parsa P (1990) Human immunodeficiency virus (HIV) infection and the kidney. Ann Intern Med 112:35–49
5. Rao TKS, Filippone EJ, Nicastri AD, Landesman SH, Frank E, Chen CK, Friedman EA (1984) Associated focal and segmental glomerulosclerosis in the acquired immunodeficiency syndrome. N Engl J Med 310:669–673
6. Chander P, Soni A, Suri A, Bhagwat R, Yoo J, Treser G (1987) Renal ultrastructural markers in AIDS-Associated nephropathy. Am J Pathol 126:513–526
7. Pardo V, Meneses R, Ossa L, Jaffe DJ, Strauss J, Roth D, Bourgoignie JJ (1987) Aids-related glomerulopathy: Occurrence in specific risk groups. Kidney Int 31:1167–1173
8. Rao TKS, Friedman EA, Nicastri AD. The types of renal disease in the Acquired Immunodeficiency Syndrome (1987) N Engl J Med 316:1062–1068
9. Chander P, Agarwal A, Soni A, Kim K, Treser G (1988) Renal cytomembranous inclusions in idiopathic renal disease as predictive markers for the acquired immunodeficiency syndrome. Hum Pathol 19:1060–1064
10. Bourgoignie JJ, Meneses R, Pardo V (1988) The nephropathy related to acquired immunodeficiency syndrome. Adv Nephrol 17:113–126
11. Bourgoignie JJ, Meneses R, Ortiz C, Jaffe D, Pardo V (1988) The clinical spectrum of renal disease associated with human immunodeficiency virus. Am J Kidney Dis 12(2):131–137
12. Cohen AH, Nast CC (1988) HIV-associated nephropathy: a unique combined glomerular, tubular, and interstitial lesion. Mod Pathol 1:87–97
13. Soni A, Agarwal A, Chander P, Yoo J, Singal D, Salomon N, Robinson B, Tresser G (1989) Evidence for an HIV-related nephropathy: A clinicopathological study. Clin Nephrol 31:12–17
14. Carbone L, D'Agati V, Cheng JT, Appel GB (1989) The course and prognosis of human immunodeficiency virus-associated nephropathy. Am J Med 87:389–395
15. D'Agati V, Suh JI, Carbone L, Cheng JT, Appel G (1989) Pathology of HIV-associated nephropathy: a detailed morphologic and comparative study. Kidney Int 35:1358–1370
16. Langs C, Gallo GR, Schacht RG, Sidhu G, Baldwin DS (1990) Rapid renal failure in AIDS nephropathy. Arch Intern Med 150:287–292
17. Chander PN, Treser G (1987) Ultrastructural markers of "AIDS nephropathy." Kidney Int 31:335
18. Chander PN, Treser G (1987) Nuclear bodies and ultrastructural markers in "AIDS associated nephropathy." Lab Invest 56:39
19. Cohen AH, Sun NCJ, Shapshak P, Imagawa DT (1989) Demonstration of human immunodeficiency virus in renal epithelium in HIV-associated nephropathy. Mod Pathol 2:125–128
20. Alpers CE, Harawi S, Rennke HG (1988) Focal glomerulosclerosis with tubuloreticular inclusions: Possible predictive value for acquired immunodeficiency syndrome (AIDS). Am J Kidney Dis 12:240–242
21. Chander P, Sagel I, Weiss R, Pimentel C, Gupta A, Bamji M, Treser G (1989) Renal disease in human immunodeficiency virus infected children. Kidney Int 35:368
22. Strauss J, Abitbol C, Zilleruelo G, Scott G, Paredes A, Malaga S, Montane B, Mitchell C, Parks W, Pardo V (1989) A spectrum of renal disease in children with acquired immunodeficiency syndrome. N Engl J Med 321:625–630
23. Connor E, Gupta S, Joshi V, DiCarlo F, Offenberger J, Minnefor A, UyC, Oleske J, Ende N (1988) Acquired immunodeficiency syndrome-associated renal disease in children. J Pediatr 113:39–44
24. Rousseau E, Russo P, Lapointe N, O'Reagan S (1988) Renal complications of acquired immunodeficiency syndrome in children. Am J Kidney Dis 11:48–50
25. Kopelman RG, Zolla-Pazner S (1988) Association of human immunodeficiency virus infection and autoimmune phenomena. Am J Med 84:82–86

HIV-Associated Nephropathy in Children in Spain

SERAFÍN MÁLAGA*, FERNANDO SANTOS, CORSINO REY, and GONZALO OREJAS[1]

SUMMARY. Although it is well known that children who acquire HIV infection during the perinatal period may develop renal disease, the natural history of HIV-associated nephropathy (HIV-AN) remains to be determined. Although a variety of renal lesions may occur, both focal glomerulosclerosis (FGS) and mesangial hyperplasia are the most common. By the end of March 1990, 160 cases of pediatric AIDS and almost 1400 perinatally HIV-infected children had been reported in Spain, all of them Whites.

In order to identify the prevalence of HIV-AN in children in Spain, a survey of 20 Spanish hospital Divisions of Pediatric Nephrology was undertaken; 18 Divisions responded (90%). Three (3) HIV-infected children with renal disease were identified. Clinically, all three had proteinuria, two had hematuria and none had renal failure. One was found to have FGS. Only one is alive, free of proteinuria, after treatment with prednisone.

These findings provide evidence for the existence of renal disease in HIV-infected children in Spain, but the low incidence suggests that unrecognized co-factors, including race, may be important in the development of renal disease. Further studies are needed to determine the correlations between the clinical and the pathological features of HIV-AN in children.

Introduction

The acquired immunodeficiency syndrome (AIDS) is a lethal multisystemic disease that has become a major public health problem since its recognition in the USA in 1981. The syndrome, caused by the human immunodeficiency virus (HIV) has been described in children as well as in adults.

---

[1]Section of Pediatric Nephrology, Department of Pediatrics, Covadonga Hospital, University School of Medicine, 33006 Oviedo, Asturias, Spain

*Representing the Spanish Society of Pediatric Nephrology

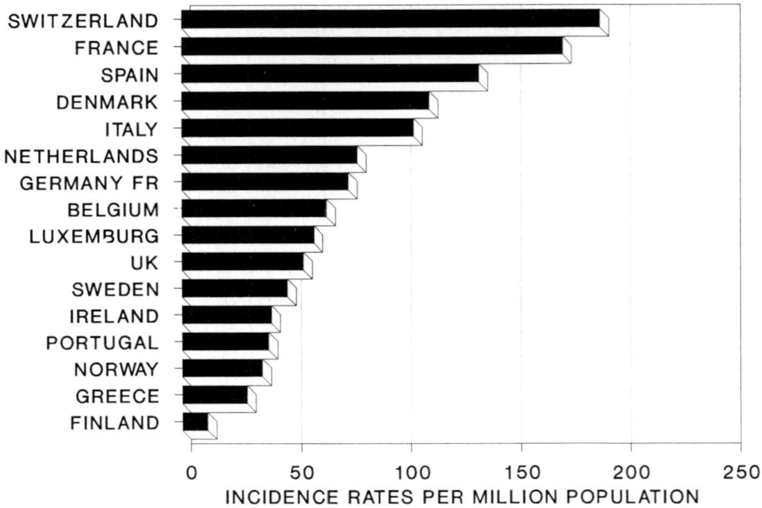

Fig. 1. AIDS cases in European countries. Reported by March 1990

The first cases suggestive of an AIDS-like illness in children were reported by the Center for Disease Control (CDC) in the United States in 1982. From then until June 1989, 1681 cases in patients under 13 years of age were registered [1]. These numbers represent only approximately 2% of all cases of AIDS reported to date in the United States.

Although the AIDS epidemic began in Europe in 1981, the first cases of pediatric AIDS were diagnosed in 1983. Since then the number, both of HIV infected children and of those with AIDS, has markedly increased [2].

According to the CDC definition, pediatric cases are limited to patients under 13 years of age. Thus, we shall discuss the problem only for this group of patients with AIDS. We shall use the current CDC definition of AIDS for this group [3] and we will also use the classification system developed by the CDC [4].

A positive HIV antibody test in a child over 15 months of age, born to an HIV infected mother, indicates that the child is also infected. In children younger than 15 months, HIV genome or HIV antigen has to be demonstrated before HIV infection is proven.

In Europe, the most comprehensive data are available from the World Health Organization Collaborating Center on AIDS, using the standard CDC definition [5].

By March 1990, sixteen participating European countries had reported 34047 cases of AIDS; 5295 (15.5%) of them are from Spain. Our country leads in those cases where intravenous drug abuse (IVDA) is the risk factor. Figure 1 summarizes the situation of AIDS in Europe by the end of March 1990.

Separate analysis of pediatric AIDS surveillance has revealed that until the end of December 1989 135 cases of pediatric AIDS were registered in Spain (Fig. 2) and at the end of March 1990 there were 165 cases [6]. This represents about 3.1% of all cases of AIDS, a percentage higher than the cumulative pediatric percentage observed in the United States and in the rest of Europe, where the incidence is

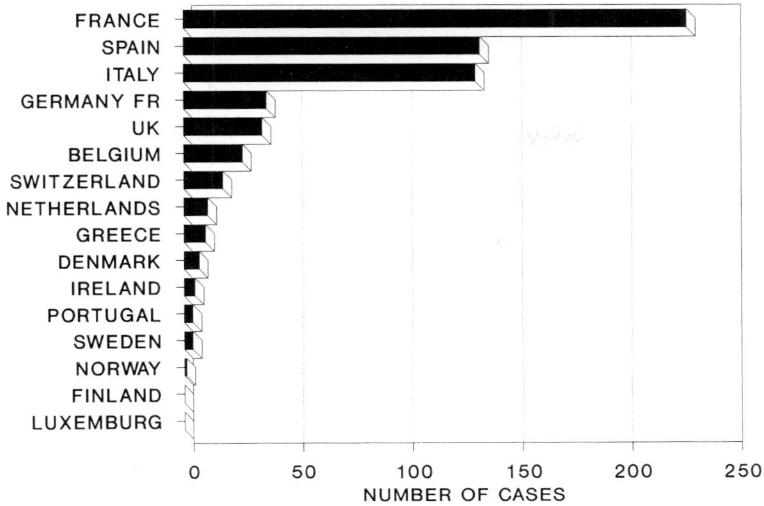

Fig. 2. Pediatric AIDS cases in Europe. Reported by December 1989

approximately 2%. The continuous increase in the relative percentage of these cases in Spain indicates rapid spread of the disease in this group. All cases of pediatric AIDS reported in Spain are in Whites and 60% of them are in males.

In Europe, pediatric AIDS is reported most frequently in France, followed by Spain and Italy. Most cases in Europe (77%) have been acquired vertically (Fig. 3).

Since the first reports of renal disease in patients with AIDS were published in 1984 [7,8], a variety of renal lesions have been described, although focal glomerulosclerosis (FGS) is the most common, and is thought by some authors, to be the true HIV-associated nephropathy (HIV-AN) [9,10].

Although renal disease is not considered a common clinical manifestation of AIDS, approximately 10% of adult and 7% of pediatric AIDS patients are affected (V. Pardo et al., manuscript in preparation). Children may represent a more appropriate

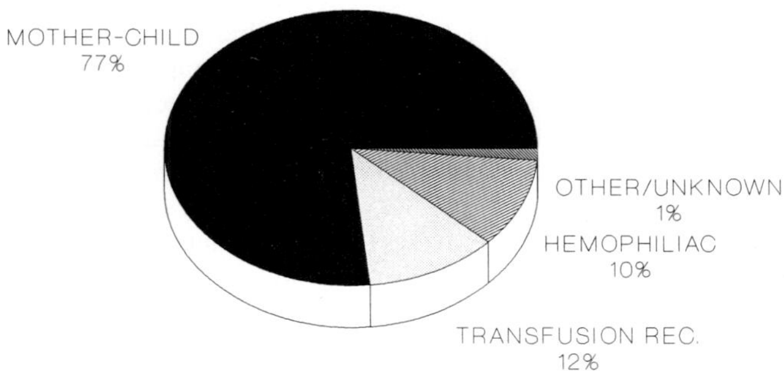

Fig. 3. Pediatric AIDS in Europe: Transmission groups. Reported by December 1989

group than adults for studying HIV-AN, because the onset of the infection may be accurately established, and complicating risk factors, frequently present in adults, such as homosexuality or IVDA, can be excluded.

There have been relatively few descriptions of HIV-AN in children; reports have been primarily from Miami (V. Pardo et al., manuscript in preparation [11]) and New York [12–15] on the East Coast of the United States, although recent reports attest to the presence of the disease in the West Coast [16] and in Canada [17]. Although at present HIV-AN has become a common problem in many hospitals, experience with appropriate diagnostic facilities is still limited to a few centers in the world.

To assess the situation of childhood HIV-AN in Spain, we would like to outline the present magnitude of the problem.

Design of the Study

In order to identify the prevalence of HIV-AN in the pediatric population in Spain, we performed a survey of all Spanish hospitals with Divisions of Pediatric Nephrology. During the period April–June 1990 a total of 20 centers were contacted.

The questionnaire included a retrospective analysis of their experience with HIV infected and HIV-AN infected children. Several aspects of clinical presentation were assessed.

HIV-AN was considered to be present when FGS or some degree of mesangial hyperplasia was confirmed by necropsy or biopsy. Clinical renal disease was considered when one or more of the following were present [11]:

– persistent urinary excretion (found on more than two occasions during a period of at least four weeks) of more than 0.1 g of protein per square meter of body surface area per day, an Albustix reading above 1+, or a urinary protein/creatinine ratio more than 0.1;

– heavy proteinuria, diagnosed when there was persistent excretion of more than 1 g of protein/m2 per 24 h, an Albustix reading above 2+, or a urinary protein/creatinine ratio more than 1.5.

Results

Eighteen centers (90%) responded to the questionnaire. Nine of them had screening programs to detect renal disease in HIV infected children. Of the responders 15 had not treated any patients with HIV-AN or HIV infected patients with clinical renal disease. Only 3 centers, 2 from Madrid and the other from Valencia, had had experience with HIV-AN or HIV infected patients with clinical renal disease. They reported 3 children with clinical manifestations of HIV infection and renal disease (one with FGS at autopsy).

All patients were followed prospectively. The clinical and pathological characteristics are shown in Table 1. There was a male predominance: (2/1), all were White, and all had perinatally acquired HIV infection. None of the children presented with peripheral edema or hypertension. Onset of the nephropathy was taken as the time of detection of persistent proteinuria or hematuria. Microscopic hematuria was seen in two of the children and proteinuria was seen in all of them, but was seen in

Table 1. Clinical and pathologic data of 3 children with HIV infection and renal manifestations

CDC Class	Sex Age[a] Race	Clinical finding Proteinuria (mg/dl)	Hematuria	Renal failure	Pathologic data	Outcome (months)
P_2	M/7/W	300	Not	Not	ND	Dead/8
P_2	F/21/W	300	++	Not	FGS	Dead/22
P_1	M/18/W	Heavy	+	Not	ND	Alive/42

FGS, focal glomerulosclerosis; ND, not done
[a]Age (months) at the time the nephropathy was detected

nephrotic range in only one child. None of the patients developed renal failure. The single child with nephrotic syndrome is alive after treatment with prednisone. The other two children died of infectious complications of AIDS.

Comments

At this time the natural history of HIV-infection in children remains to be determined. Children with HIV infection show both similarities to and differences from adults. The incubation period appears to be shorter in children who have acquired their infection perinatally than it is in adults with sexually or blood product acquired HIV. At the same time there is a spectrum for disease, because some children with perinatally acquired infection have not become symptomatic for 7–8 years, suggesting that genetic factors, virus strains, or cofactors might contribute to this heterogeneity [1].

Since multiorgan involvement, kidney included, is noteworthy in pediatric AIDS, it is possible that more widespread yet subtle deficits may become evident in the long term follow-up of congenitally infected infants who may be clinically free of AIDS in the first years of life.

The review of epidemiological aspects of pediatrics AIDS in Spain raises further questions. In Spain we have a high incidence of IVDA in women, nearly 79% of whom are of reproductive age (15–45 years). Perinatal infection in their infants may be anticipated. In a recent survey, performed in more than 70% of the hospitals in the country by The Spanish Pediatric Association [18], 1416 HIV-infected children were detected. In Spain the number of female HIV positive and AIDS cases is still increasing. Thus, for a significant number of years pediatricians have to expect a slowly increasing number of HIV positive children and children with AIDS.

By March 30, 1990, 165 cases of AIDS in children below 13 years of age had been reported to the *Centro Nacional de Epidemiologia* [16]. These represent 3.1% of all cases of AIDS reported in Spain until that time.

At least two factors account for the emerging impact of HIV as a serious disease among children. First, the criteria used to define AIDS in children have become less stringent and more concordant with the clinical profile of the disease in children. The revision of the CDC criteria [3] in September 1987 provided guidelines more consistent with the disease manifestations in children and offered the opportunity for more accurate reporting.

Most infants and children who have acquired HIV perinatally live in urban areas with a high frequency of IVDA. Among the most prominent of these high frequency IVDA areas are Madrid, Barcelona, Valencia, and Málaga.

Since the first reports of renal disease in patients with AIDS were published in 1984 [7,8], a variety of renal lesions have been described, although FGS is the most common [19–21]. It is characterized clinically by nephrotic range proteinuria and by rapidly advancing renal failure; it has been observed in about 10% of adult patients with AIDS [22].

Most of the cases of HIV-AN in adult patients have been observed in Blacks, with IVDA as the AIDS risk factor, suggesting that the HIV-AN could be a variant of heroin nephropathy, which is also characterized by FGS and is confined largely (90%) to black IVDA patients. However, only 53% of patients with HIV-AN are heroin addicts, so it is clear that IVDA plays a role in the development of renal disease [23].

On the other hand, again for unknown reasons, Blacks have increased risks for renal diseases of all types. While Blacks represent 12% of the United States population, they represent 28% of all end-stage renal disease (ESRD) cases. Adjusted for age and sex differences, Blacks had 3.8 times higher rates of new ESRD cases in 1987 than did Whites [24]. The predilection of HIV-AN for Black people is apparent in the unbalanced distribution of the disease according to race. In a review of the literature we found a 3:1 ration in the number of White vs Black people with AIDS, while HIV-AN has been reported ten times more frequently in Blacks (V. Pardo et al., manuscript in preparation). It seems evident that Black race is a major cofactor in the predisposition of patients with HIV infection to acquire the nephropathy. The reasons why HIV-AN occurs basically in Blacks and in IVDA patients are not well known. Although genetic factors may indeed play some role in the racial differences, both genetic and environmental theories have been proposed, suggesting higher susceptibility of the kidney to immunologic and vascular forms of injury in black people [25,26].

In recent reports, Rao et al. [9] and Mazbar et al. [26] recognize that Blacks with HIV infection are more likely, in general, to suffer from structural renal disease than are Whites. All adult HIV infected patients who develop renal disease share several features in common.

They are mostly young men, likely to be black, who have nephrotic syndrome, azotemia of varying degree, FGS, and IVDA as a risk factor; they have a low incidence of Kaposi's sarcoma.

Since, however, HIV-AN also develops in white homosexuals and in infants with AIDS, neither race nor IVDA is solely responsible.

The natural history of HIV-AN in children is, up to now, poorly understood, because there are only a few published cases (Table 2). In children, the predominant presenting symptoms include the nephrotic syndrome, and although the commonest renal lesions found are those of FGS, some degree of mesangial hyperplasia and the proliferative forms of glomerulonephritis are often observed [11,24]. Strauss et al. [11] found HIV-AN in 12 out of 155 children with perinatal HIV infection (7%). One additional series included 5 patients with FGS and mesangial hyperplasia [14]. A second additional series included two children with FGS and perinatal nephritis [13]. On the other hand, Rousseau et al. [17] studied 17 children with perinatal AIDS and described only one patient, a Haitian, with FGS and renal disease. Another study [15] showed proliferative glomerulonephritis as the predominant lesion.

Table 2. HIV-associated nephropathy in children

Ref.	Year	No. patients	Age (months)	FGS	MH
Kaplan et al. [13]	1987	5	3–36	NR	NR
Rao et al. [10]	1987	4	2–24	2	0
Connor et al. [15]	1988	5	6–108	2	3
Rousseau et al. [18]	1988	4	3–36	4	0
Cohen et al. [17]	1988	1	24	1	0
Horowitz et al. [14]	1988	3	3–60	2	0
Chandler et al. [16]	1989	38	NR	12	0
Strauss et al.[a] [12]	1989	12	7–95	5	5
Spanish serie	1990	3	7–21	1	0
Total		75		29	8

FGS, focal glomerulosclerosis; MH, Mesangial hyperplasia; NR, not reported
[a]Eight cases from Miami, reported previously by Pardo et al. [30] are included

Although various other parenchymal renal lesions have been described in HIV infection, including those of acute glomerulonephritis, membranous glomerulonephritis, etc., in these circumstances HIV infection is more coincidental than causative [27]. The HIV-AN in children has rarely been described in Europe.

Although the incidence of HIV-AN in children is similar to that in adults, the clinical criteria for defining renal disease are different, since only approximately 50% of pediatric patients exhibit FGS. This fact would explain that progression of HIV-AN in children is not as rapid as that in adults since renal failure occurred within a mean period of one year after recognition of the nephropathy (V. Pardo et al., manuscript in preparation). The rapid progression to ESRD which has previously been reported is not the universal outcome [26]. Some authors have recommended that the term HIV-AN should be reserved for those disorders with FGS, tubular and interstitial changes, ultrastructurally defined cytoplasmic and nuclear damage, heavy proteinuria, and renal impairment [9,27], in which mesangial changes represent an early form of the disease and are likely to progress to FGS with time.

Our report drew attention to the fact that the occurrence of HIV-AN in the pediatric population in Spain is extremely rare, but although many centers are only now beginning to detect this disease, we suggest that the occurrence of HIV-AN in children is, as of now, not a nationwide problem, but the problem will become serious if the epidemic continues. On the other hand, the fact that Zidovurine may slow the progression toward ESRD [28] may make early treatment with Zidovurine, as soon as proteinuria is detected in an HIV carrier, worthwhile.

At our present level of knowledge, we conclude that the occurrence of renal disease in children with HIV infection in Spain is not frequent. The reasons for the differences between our study and the experience reported by other centers from Miami or New York City may relate to our study having a lower proportion of black patients, as occurs in centers from the West coast of the United States [26,29]

Careful screening of proteinuria and microscopic hematuria in pediatric patients with HIV infection may lead to the discovery of further cases of HIV-AN. On the other hand, it is necessary to determine clinical criteria, which will be accepted by all centers for indications for renal biopsy only in children who exhibit evident symptoms suggesting HIV-AN.

Acknowledgments. The authors acknowledge the cooperation of the following Centers and physicians that kindly provided information about their patients: Barcelona: Hospital Infantil Vall d'Hebrón. L. Callís, M.D. Hospital Infantil San Juan de Dios. L. García, M.D. Hospital Clínico Universitario. C. Pérez Prado, M.D. Bilbao: Hospital Infantil Cruces. A. Vallo, M.D. Madrid: Hospital Infantil La Paz. M. Navarro, M.D. Hospital Infantil Niño Jesús. M. Vázquez, M.D. Hospital Infantil 12 de Octubre. R. Muley, M.D. Hospital Infantil Gregorio Marañón. A. Luque, M.D. Málaga: Hospital Infantil Carlos Haya. J.M. Millán, M.D. Murcia: Hospital Virgen de la Arritxaca. F. Rodrigo, M.D. Oviedo: Hospital Covadonga. L.M. Rodríguez, M.D. Hospital General de Asturias. M. Roza, M.D. Santander: Centro Médico Marqués de Valdecilla. M. García Fuentes, M.D. Sevilla: Hospital Infantil Virgen del Rocio. J. Martín Govantes, M.D. Valencia: Hospital Infantil La Fe. C. Canosa, M.D. and I. Zamora, M.D. Hospital General Universitario. A. Lurbe, M.D. Valladolid: Hospital Infantil Del Rio Ortega. F. de las Heras, M.D. Zaragoza: Hospital Infantil Miguel Servet. C. Loris, M.D. We also thank Jorge Román (Unidad de estadística e Informática. INSALUD-ASTURIAS), for his professional and technical assistance.

References

1. Pizzo Ph A (1990) Pediatric AIDS: Problems within problems. J Infect Dis 161:316–325
2. Wahn V, Tangermann R (1988) Pediatric AIDS in Europe. Pediatr Eur 2:16–21
3. Centers for Disease Control (1987) Revision of the CDC surveillance case definition for acquired immunodeficiency syndrome. Morb Mort Wkly Rep 36 (Suppl 15):3–15
4. Centers for Disease Control (1987) Classification system for human immunodeficiency virus (HIV) infection in children under 13 years of age. Morb Mort Wkly Rep 36:225–230
5. WHO Collaborating Centre on AIDS: AIDS surveillance in the European Community. (1990) Data reported by December 1989. Paris
6. Centro Nacional de Epidemiología: Registro Nacional del SIDA (1990) Ministerio de Sanidad y Consumo. marzo 1990. Madrid
7. Rao TKS, Filippone EJ, Nicastri AD, Landesman SH, Frank E, Chen CK, Friedman EA (1984) Associated focal and segmental glomerulosclerosis in the acquired immunodeficiency syndrome. N Engl J Med 310:669–673
8. Pardo V, Aldana M, Colton RM, Fischi NA, Jaffe D, Mokowitz L, Hensley GT, Bourgoignie JJ (1984) Glomerular lesions in the acquired immunodeficiency syndrome. Ann Intern Med 101:429–434
9. Rao TKS, Friedman EA (1989) AIDS (HIV)-Associated nephropathy. Does it exist? Am J Nephrol 9:441–453
10. Rao TKS, Friedman EA, Nicastri AD (1987) The types of renal disease in the acquired immunodeficiency syndrome. N Engl J Med 316:1062–1068
11. Strauss J, Abitbol C, Zilleruelo G, Scott G, Paredes A, Málaga S, Montané B, Mitchell C, Parks W, Pardo V (1989) Renal disease in children with the acquired immunodeficiency syndrome. N Engl J Med 321:625–630
12. Kaplan MS, Wechsler M, Benson MC (1987) Urologic manifestations of AIDS. Urology 30:441–443
13. Horowitz I, Greco MA, Feiner V, et al. (1988) Renal pathology in pediatric AIDS (abstract) Lab Invest 58:5
14. Connor E, Gupta S, Joshi V, DiCarlo F, Offenberg J, Minnefor A, Uy C, Oleske J, Ende N (1988) Acquired immunodeficiency syndrome-associated renal disease in children. J Pediatr 113:39–44

15. Chander P, Sagel I, Weis R, Pimentel C, Gupta A, Bamji M, Treser G (1989) Renal disease in human immunodeficiency virus (HIV)-infected children. Kidney Int 35:368
16. Cohen AH, Nast CC (1988) HIV-associated nephropathy: a unique combined glomerular, tubular, and interstitial lesion. Mod Pathol 1:87–97
17. Rousseau F, Russo P, Lapointe M, O'Regan S (1988) Renal complications of acquired immunodeficiency syndrome in children. Am J Kidney Dis 11:48–50
18. Asociación Española de Pediatría.: Registro español de la infección HIV en edad pediátrica. Noviembre 1989. Madrid
19. Soni A, Agarwal A, Chander P, Yoo J, Singal D, Salomon N, Robinson B, Treser G (1989) Evidence for an HIV-related nephropathy: a clinico-pathological study. Clin Nephrol 31:12–17
20. D'Agati V, Suh JI, Carbone L, Cheng JT, Appel (1989) Pathology of HIV-associated nephropathy: a detailed morphologic and comparative study. Kidney Int 35:1358–1370
21. Van der Reijden HJ, Schipper ME, Danner SA, Arisz LU (1989) Glomerular lesions and opportunistic infections of the kidney in AIDS: an autopsy study of 47 cases. Adv Exp Med Biol 252:181–188
22. Carbone L, D'Agati V, Cheng JT, Appel GB (1989) Course and prognosis of human immunodeficiency virus-associated nephropathy. Am J Med 87:389–95
23. Shemin D, Chazan JA (1989) A risk factor for AIDS nephropathy. Nephron 51:558
24. Gordon D (1990) Racial differences in ESRD. Dial Transplant 19:114–116
25. Bourgoignie JJ, Ortín-Interian C, Green DF, Roth D (1989) Race, a cofactor in HIV-1-associated nephropathy. Transplant Proc 21:3899–3901
26. Mazbar SA, Schoenfeld PY, Humphreys MH (1990) Renal involvement in patients infected with HIV: experience at San Francisco General Hospital. Kidney Int 37:1325–1332
27. Cohen AH (1990) Renal pathology of human immunodeficiency virus (HIV) infection. In: Glassock RJ (moderator) Human immunodeficiency virus infection and the kidney. Ann Intern Med 112:37–40
28. Kleinknecht D, Meyrier A, (1989) Zidovurine and nephropathy with human immunodeficiency virus (HIV) infection. Ann Intern Med 111:856–857
29. Humphreys MH (1990) Human immunodeficiency virus-associated nephropathy. East is East and West is West? Arch Intern Med 150:253–255
30. Pardo V, Menseses R, Ossa L (1987) AIDS-related glomerulopathy. Kidney Int 31:1167–1173

Considerations of Pathogenesis of HIV-Associated Nephropathy

ARTHUR H. COHEN[1]

SUMMARY. The structural abnormalities in HIV-associated nephropathy affect cells of all renal components and result in a combination of focal and segmental glomerulosclerosis and acute tubular necrosis. Ultrastructural features of the cellular injury are considered markers associated with viral infection, although not necessarily indicative of viral protein per se. The prominent abnormalities of glomerular visceral and tubular epithelium suggest that a single insult to these cells is responsible for the lesions. This led us to consider the role of HIV infection of renal epithelium; using in situ hybridization, we identified HIV genome in glomerular visceral and tubular epithelium in HIV-associated nephropathy. While these results are promising at elucidating the pathogenesis of this nephropathy, many unanswered questions remain. Are other infectious agents also necessary to produce the structural and functional abnormalities? How does the virus gain access to these cells which lack CD4 receptors? Why is the disorder so common in Blacks? Are other factors, such as heredity or drug use also necessary? What is the role of altered renal hemodynamics? At the present time, further studies, including a valid animal model, are needed to explain adequately these perplexing questions and other features of this renal disorder.

The structural abnormalities in HIV-associated nephropathy have been documented to be diverse and to affect cells of all renal components [1,2,3]. As emphasized in several series, focal and segmental glomerulosclerosis, often in an early stage of evolution, acute tubular cell injury with microcystically dilated tubules often containing precipitates of plasma proteins, and interstitial edema coexist to cause widespread renal structural and functional damage [1,3]. Glomerular visceral and tubular epithelial cells demonstrate a variety of degenerative features; vascular endothelium, among many cell types, contains large and numerous tubulo-reticular structures and cylindrical confronting cisternae, and nuclei from most cells have a

[1]Departments of Pathology and Medicine, Harbor-UCLA Medical Center, 1000 W. Carson Street, Torrance, CA 90509, USA

large variety of inclusion bodies and undergo peculiar granular and granulo-fibrillar transformations [4–6]. These and other alterations are considered morphological markers associated with viral infection, although they do not necessarily indicate viral protein per se [4].

Unlike many other glomerular disorders associated with infections, the glomerulopathy of HIV-associated nephropathy is not the result of accumulation of immune deposits. The positive immunofluorescence in HIV-associated nephropathy is on a non-immune basis; segmental IgM and complement deposits in focal and segmental glomerulosclerosis associated with other diseases or as a "primary" process are considered trapped in a nonimmune manner [7]. It is known that immune complex mediated glomerulonephritis occurs in some HIV infected individuals [1,3,8, 9,11,12]; however, it should be appreciated that that broad category of glomerular injury is not an integral part of the lesions of HIV-associated nephropathy [1]. Indeed, the pathological aspects of immune complex mediated glomerulonephritis do not bear any relationship to the types of renal injury encountered in HIV-associated nephropathy. While there is some question whether HIV antigen(s) may be a component of glomerular immune complexes, there is no evidence that HIV antigen is a part of the focal and segmental "deposits" in the glomerular lesion of HIV-associated nephropathy.

The pathogenesis of the lesion of segmental glomerulosclerosis is uncertain, although many theories exist. These include the effects of altered glomerular hemodynamics, glomerular hypertrophy, disordered lipid metabolism, other metabolic factors, persistent proteinuria, genetic factors, and aging, to cite but a few [13]. Regardless of which one or more of these "etiologic" considerations are favored, there is some debate as to the glomerular cell which is initially affected. Strong evidence exists to implicate visceral epithelial cells; perhaps equally compelling evidence favors primary mesangial cell injury. It is beyond the scope of this paper to cite all data favoring one or the other cell; however, persistent and pronounced morphological abnormalities are regularly evident in visceral epithelium early in the development of segmental glomerulosclerosis in all settings [7]. Hence, it seems appropriate to consider visceral epithelial cell injury to be important in the pathogenesis of this form of glomerular disease. The lesions manifested in visceral epithelium at the onset of development of focal and segmental glomerulosclerosis include localized hyperplasia and hypertrophy, coarse cytoplasmic vacuoles, protein reabsorption droplets, detachment of cells from basement membranes, and necrosis [1,2]. The stimulus(i) for these changes is unknown; direct cellular injury, e.g., by drugs such as puromycin of aminonucleoside has been suggested. Is it possible that viruses can infect glomerular visceral epithelium and result in similar cellular injury which may well lead to segmental glomerulosclerosis? Viral infection of glomerular cells has been documented in animal models of cytomegalovirus (CMV) and adenovirus infection [14]. With CMV, experimentally infected mice develop transient proteinuria; mesangial cell hyperplasia and intra-nuclear inclusions are found. Visceral epithelium is not regularly affected [15]. With adenovirus, glomeruli of infected dogs have cytopathic effect in and proliferation of mesangial and endothelial cells [14]. On the other hand, in disseminated human CMV infection, there may be viral inclusions in glomerular visceral epithelium as well as in tubular epithelial cells. Antigens of other viruses in humans, such as Coxsackie B, have also been demonstrated in glomerular and tubular epithelium [16]. It is uncertain whether glomerular epithelial localization of virus in these infections can cause the morphological and functional features of segmental glomerulosclerosis or other manifestations of glomerular injury. Nevertheless, it is important to appreciate that viruses can and do infect human glomerular visceral epithelium.

The other major components of the kidney with prominent cellular lesions are the tubules. It has been well established that tubular cell degeneration and necrosis are integral features of HIV-associated nephropathy; they occur in the absence of known eitologic or pathogenetic mechanisms such as renal ischemia and nephrotoxins [1,3]. Indeed, the tubular changes may be equally as prominent in patients who develop HIV-associated nephropathy prior to any other evidence of HIV infection as in those who already have fully developed acquired immunodeficiency syndrome. In a different setting, clinically relevant polyomavirus-induced tubular necrosis has been adequately documented in a child with immunodeficiency who presented with acute renal failure [17]. These and other data indicate that some viruses can and do directly infect tubular epithelium and, in some instances, produce renal functional impairment.

With the above background, we wondered if the major structural and functional components of the renal injury in HIV-associated nephropathy might well be the result of a single mechanism which simultaneously affected glomerular and tubular cells. It seemed appropriate, therefore, to consider the role of direct HIV infection of renal epithelium in its pathogenesis. We used two techniques – in situ hybridization using a cDNA probe for viral nucleic acid and a peroxidase labeled antibody to p24 core protein – to search for virus in renal tissue [18]. These procedures were performed on fixed paraffin-embedded specimens. We evaluated renal tissues (10 biopsies and one nephrectomy) from eleven patients with HIV-associated nephropathy and compared the results with kidney biopsy specimens from HIV infected patients with immune complex mediated glomerulonephritis, autopsy kidneys from AIDS patients without clinical or morphological evidence of renal disease, and biopsies or nephrectomies from patients with "idiopathic" focal and segmental glomerulosclerosis, heroin-associated nephropathy, and normal kidneys. Specimens from the last three groups were obtained prior to 1980. We found that in HIV-associated nephropathy, numerous tubular and glomerular visceral epithelial cells contained hybridization product (Fig. 1); in contrast, very few glomerular and tubular epithelial cells were positive in HIV-infected patients with glomerulonephritis, and rare tubular cell was positive in normal kidneys of patients with AIDS. In contrast, p24 antigen was localized to very few tubular cells and rare glomerular epithelial cells in HIV-associated nephropathy. We interpreted these findings to indicate that HIV infects renal epithelium and may be pathogenetically important in HIV-associated nephropathy. We also documented that in situ hybridization is a more sensitive technique than immunohistochemistry to detect HIV in cells. Two recent preliminary reports tend to support these conclusions. Cronin et al. [19] noted p24 antigen in some proximal tubular epithelial cells in AIDS patients without renal manifestations; they suggested that "silent" HIV infection of renal epithelium is possible. Genderini et al. were unable to demonstrate core (p18 and p25) and envelope (gp 45 and gp 100) antigens in glomerular and tubular epithelium in biopsies from patients with HIV-associated nephropathy [20]. However, they acknowledged that their results did not necessarily exclude direct viral infection of renal epithelium, because of the relative insensitivity of their methods.

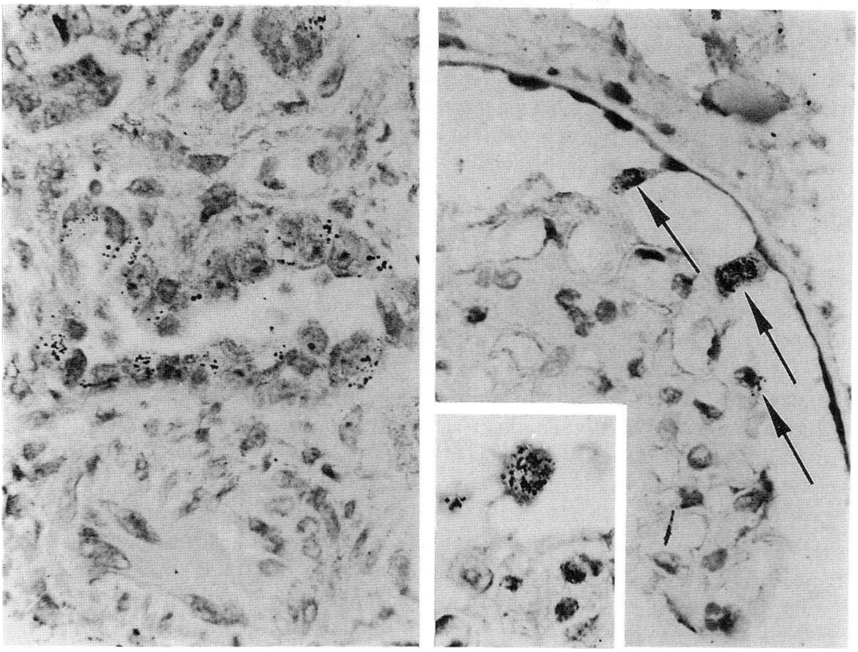

Fig. 1. HIV genome demonstrated in renal epithelium by in situ hybridization. **a** Virtually all cells of a single tubule are positive, ×400. **b** Portion of glomerulus with several positive visceral epithelial cells (*arrows*), ×350. *Inset*, enlarged positive visceral epithelial cell overlying a few patient capillaries, ×480. (Reprinted from [18] with permission]

Our observations actually raise more questions than they answer. How does the virus get to the kidneys? In the absence of CD4 receptors, how does the virus get into glomerular and tubular epithelium? Why is the virus not present in mesangial cells? Three to five percent of these cells are derived from bone marrow and possess CD4 receptors, as suggested by the work of Karlsson-Parra and colleagues [21]. Why has the virus not been identified in renal endothelial or interstitial cells? Is infection by HIV alone responsible for the morphological and functional features? Are other agents also necessary for producing damage? For example, is infection with CMV, hepatitis B, EB virus and/or herpes viruses important in the pathogenesis of HIV-associated nephropathy? What is the role, if any, of *Mycoplasma incognitus*? Why is HIV-associated nephropathy virtually limited to Blacks? What hereditary factors, such as HLA-BW53, influence the development of HIV-associated nephropathy? What is the relationship of HIV-associated nephropathy to heroin-associated nephropathy? What is the role of altered renal hemodynamics in the genesis of some features of the glomerular abnormalities and acute renal failure with tubular cell necrosis?

It is likely that HIV spreads to the kidneys in infected lymphocytes and monocytes [9]. Although the sequence of events following arrival in the kidneys has not been studied yet, certain suppositions are possible. The infected cells may infiltrate the interstitium; from this location, virus can migrate to and infect tubular cells. Either lymphocytes or monocytes can infiltrate into glomeruli; monocytes can extend into the mesangium. The exact route to visceral epithelium is clearly not known; however, passage of either free virus or infected cells across glomerular basement membrane is necessary to infect visceral epithelium. It is remotely possible that monocytes containing HIV can be partially responsible for mesangial hypercellularity observed in kidneys of some patients with proteinuria [9]. However, it should be noted that neither HIV genome, nor antigen, nor viral particles have been identified in cells in the glomerular mesangium. Furthermore, our study did not identify viral genome in interstitial mononuclear leukocytes [18].

Although most cells infected by HIV possess CD4 receptors and are, therefore, of hematopoietic origin, infection of brain cells (microglia, astrocytes, oligodendrocytes), brain endothelium, Langerhans' cells, perhaps myocardial cells, endothelium of endocervix, and other diverse cells has been well documented [22]. In addition, infection of bowel epithelium and enterochromaffin cells has been described in duodenal and rectal biopsies and in these cells in culture; the tissue specimens were from patients with chronic diarrhea with no other discernible cause [23]. This important observation indicates that HIV can infect epithelial cells and result in their functional derangement; it also indicates that the virus can and does infect cells which lack CD4 antigen expression. By direct analogy, it is possible that renal epithelium can be infected and that this can result in important functional consequences – proteinuria following infection of glomerular visceral epithelium and renal failure resulting from tubular cell injury.

No information is available on the possible role of other viral agents in the pathogenesis of HIV-associated nephropathy. However, because of the multiple infections which may be present in HIV infected individuals, other viruses may also infect renal epithelium and play a role in the pathogenesis. Some agents which should be considered include EB virus, hepatitis B virus, herpes virus and cytomegalovirus. We plan to search for these viruses using in situ hybridization and immunohistochemistry on renal specimens.

Although some investigators have postulated that simultaneous infection with HIV and a newly described microorganism, *Mycoplasma incognitus*, is necessary to produce the many and varied aspects of AIDS, there is little evidence that this combination is necessary to cause HIV-associated nephropathy. A single preliminary report has described immunohistochemical and ultrastructural localization of *Mycoplasma incognitus* in glomerular epithelium and endothelium, tubular epithelium and casts, interstitial mononuclear cells, and glomerular basement membrane in what was termed AIDS-associated nephropathy [24]. However, neither we nor others who have performed detailed ultrastructural studies of the kidneys have noted similar organisms. Clearly this observation needs confirmation.

There is some morphological similarity between heroin-associated nephropathy and HIV-associated nephropathy; this is mainly in the glomerular abnormalities, for both lesions are characterized by focal and segmental glomerulopathies; most investigators can distinguish one from the other [1,2,3,4]. However, both have epidemiological similarities in that they are disorders with an extraordinarily high prevalence in Blacks; in excess of 95% of reported cases of HIV-associated nephropathy are in Blacks, a disproportionate representation of HIV infected patients in the United States [25]. Furthermore, approximately 50% of reported patients with HIV-associated nephropathy are intravenous drug users [3,9]. A study by Haskell and colleagues [26] described an increased frequency of HLA-BW53 in patients with heroin-associated nephropathy, suggesting a genetic predisposition to this renal disorder. Similar studies have not yet been directed at patients with HIV-associated nephropathy. The close relationship between clinical and epidemiologic features of heroin-associated nephropathy and HIV-associated nephropathy has suggested to some investigators that HIV-infected patients who develop HIV-associated nephropathy are overt or covert intravenous drug abusers; hence, they consider the renal lesion to be heroin-associated nephropathy and, therefore, not related to HIV infection [27]. Unfortunately, this postulate does not explain the appearance of HIV-associated nephropathy in infants and children and in the many adults who clearly do not use intravenous drugs [1,3,10].

An alternative suggestion for an explanation for the rapidly developing renal failure which characterizes HIV-associated nephropathy was recently offered by Langs and coworkers [28]. They suggested that, rather than viral induced tubular necrosis, altered renal hemodynamics with profound renal ischemia would result in tubular necrosis and progressive renal failure and also in glomerular capillary collapse. No functional data were provided to support this thesis.

At the present time there are no adequate animal models of HIV-associated nephropathy. Focal and segmental glomerulosclerosis has been briefly described in a single rhesus monkey infected with simian AIDS virus [29]. Also briefly reported has been the development of focal and segmental glomerulosclerosis, heavy proteinuria, and renal failure with greatly diminished survival in transgenic mice bearing chromosomally integrated HIV-1 proviral DNA. The morphology of the renal damage is similar to human HIV-associated nephropathy. HIV-1 RNA expression has been documented in the kidneys; the study suggested that HIV-1 gene expression in glomerular epithelium may be responsible for the observed lesions [30]. This preliminary work serves to support our original thesis.

It is clear from the above that continued work on the role of infection, hereditary factors and race, renal hemodynamics, drugs and toxins, and other mechanisms of cell and tissue injury, is necessary before a better understanding of the pathogenesis of HIV-associated nephropathy is realized.

References

1. Cohen AH, Nast CC (1988) HIV-associated nephropathy: a unique combined glomerular, tubular and interstitial lesion. Mod Pathol 1:87–97
2. D'Agati V, Suh J-I, Carbone L, Cheng J-T, Appel G (1989) Pathology of HIV-associated nephropathy: a detailed morphologic and comparative study. Kidney Int 35:1358–1370
3. Glassock RJ, Cohen AH, Danovitch G, Parsa KP (1990) Human immunodeficiency virus (HIV) infection and the kidney. Ann Intern Med 112:35–49
4. Chander P, Soni A, Suri A, Bhagwat R, Yoo J, Treser G (1987) Renal ultrastructural markers in AIDS-associated nephropathy. Am J Pathol 126:513–526
5. Chander P, Agarwal A, Soni A, Kim K, Treser G (1988) Renal cytomembranous inclusions in idiopathic renal disease as predictive markers for the acquired immunodeficiency syndrome. Hum Pathol 19:1060–1064

6. Soni A, Agarwal A, Chander P, Yoo J, Singal D, Salomon N, Robinson B, Treser G (1989) Evidence for an HIV-related nephropathy: a clinico-pathological study. Clin Nephrol 31:12–17
7. Glassock RJ, Adler SG, Ward HJ, Cohen AH (1986) Primary glomerular disease. In: Brenner BM, Rector FC Jr (eds) The kidney. WB Saunders, Philadelphia, pp 929–1013
8. Cohen AH, Sun NCJ, Shapshak P, Imagawa D (1989) Immune complex (IC) glomerulonephritis (GN) in HIV infected patients: lack of HIV antigens in immune complexes (abstract). Lab Invest 60:18A
9. Bourgoignie JJ (1990) Renal complications of human immunodeficiency virus type I. Kidney Int 37:1571–1584
10. Strauss J, Abitbol C, Zilleruelo G, Scott G, Paredes A, Malaga S, Montane B, Mitchell C, Parks W, Pardo V (1989) Renal disease in children with the acquired immunodeficiency syndrome. N Engl J Med 321:625–630
11. Rao TKS, Friedman EA (1989) AIDS (HIV)-associated nephropathy: does it exist? Am J Nephrol 9:441–453
12. Mazbar SA, Schoenfeld PY, Humphreys MH (1990) Renal involvement in patients infected with HIV: experience at San Francisco General Hospital. Kidney Int 37:1325–1332
13. Silva FG, Hogg RJ (1989) Minimal change nephrotic syndrome – focal sclerosis complex (including IgM nephropathy and diffuse mesangial hypercellularity) In: Tisher CC, Brenner BM (eds) Renal pathology with clinical and functional correlations. JB Lippincott, Philadelphia, pp 265–339
14. Ronco P, Verroust P, Morel-Maroger L (1982) Viruses and glomerulonephritis. Nephron 31:97–102
15. Smith RD, Wehner RW (1983) Progressive cytomegalovirus glomerulonephritis: an experimental model. Am J Pathol 112:313–325
16. Burch GE, Chu KC, Colcolough HL, Sohal RS (1969) Immunofluorescent localization of Coxsackie B antigen in the kidney observed at routine autopsy. Am J Med 47:36–42
17. Rosen S, Harmon W, Krensky AM, Edelson PJ, Padgett BL, Grinnell BW, Rubino MJ, Walker DL (1983) Tubulointerstitial nephritis associated with polyomavirus (BK type) infection. N Engl J Med 308:1192–1196
18. Cohen AH, Sun NCJ, Shapshak P, Imagawa DT (1989) Demonstration of human immunodeficiency virus in renal epithelium in HIV-associated nephropathy. Mod Pathol 2:125–128
19. Cronin W, Sevchuck M, daSilva M, Bagchi S (1990) The prevalence of HIV positivity in kidneys of AIDS patients (abstract). Abstracts Sixth International Conference on AIDS 2:212
20. Genderini A, Vago L, Bertoli S, Scorza D, Barone MT, Landriani N, Milani S, Barbiano di Belgiojoso G (1990) HIV-associated-nephropathy: absence of HIV-antigens (abstract). Abstracts Sixth International Conference on AIDS 2:208
21. Karlsson-Parra A, Dimeny E, Fellstrom B, Klareskog L (1989) HIV receptors (CD4 antigen) in normal human glomerular cells. N Engl J Med 320:741
22. Levy JA (1989) The human immunodeficiency viruses. Detection and pathogenesis. In: Levy JA (ed) AIDS, pathogenesis and treatment. Marcel Decker, New York, pp 159–229
23. Nelson JA, Wiley CA, Reynolds-Kohler C, Reese CE, Margaretten W, Levy JA (1988) Human immunodeficiency virus detected in bowel epithelium from patients with gastrointestinal symptoms. Lancet I:259–262
24. Bauer FA, Wear DJ, Angritt P, Lo S-C (1990) *Mycoplasma incognitus* infection in kidneys of AIDS patients with AIDS-associated nephropathy (abstract). Abstracts Sixth International Conference on AIDS 1:255
25. Bourgoignie JJ, Ortiz-Interian C, Green DF, Roth D (1989) Race, a cofactor in HIV-1-associated nephropathy. Transplant Proc 21:3899–3901
26. Haskell LP, Glicklich D, Senitzer D (1988) HLA associations in heroin-associated nephropathy. Am J Kidney Dis 12:45–50

27. Balow JE, Macher AM, Rook AH (1986) Paucity of glomerular disease in acquired immunodeficiency syndrome (abstract). Kidney Int 29:178
28. Langs C, Gallo GR, Schacht RG, Sidhu G, Baldwin DS (1990) Rapid renal failure in AIDS-associated focal glomerulosclerosis. Arch Intern Med 150:287–292
29. Alpers CE, Baskin GB (1989) Sclerosing glomerulopathy in Rhesus monkeys with Simian AIDS (abstract). Kidney Int 35:339
30. Dickie P, Bryant J, Notkins AL, Silver J, Felser JM (1990) Glomerulosclerosis in transgenic mice expressing HIV-1 genes (abstract). Abstracts Sixth International Conference on AIDS 1:192

Cyclosporine Nephrotoxicity: From Experimental Animal to Clinical Practice

Chair: William M. Bennett (USA)
Michael J. Mihatsch (Switzerland)

Cellular Mechanisms of Cyclosporin Nephrotoxicity

ROBERT JAMES WALKER[1]

SUMMARY. Cyclosporin A (CsA) is a neutral lipophilic cyclic undecapeptide used extensively in transplantation. Cyclosporin A accumulates rapidly in renal tubular segments due to a partitioning process of the drug into the lipid components of the cellular membranes. Cyclosporin has been shown to inhibit protein kinase C and peptidyl-propyl *cis-trans* isomerase (identical to cyclophilin, an intracellular CsA-binding protein), as well as other intracellular enzymes. Inhibition of these intracellular regulatory enzymes, along with inhibition of intracellular Ca^{2+} flux, will significantly alter renal cellular function, including contractile activity, DNA and protein synthesis, and synthesis of prostaglandins. Inhibition of renal metabolic enzymes and alterations in renal glutathione content, in a hypoxic milieu, would enhance the toxic effects of cyclosporin.

Cellular toxicity probably has a multifactorial etiology which is related to alterations in renal vascular cells, modifying renal hemodynamics, and the relative ischemia induced by vasoconstriction potentiating sublethal changes in renal tubular epithelial cells. Histological evidence of cell damage will be apparent only if the toxic injury exceeds the capacity of the cellular mechanisms to respond to the toxic insult.

Introduction

Cyclosporin A (CsA) is a unique neutral lipophilic cyclical undecapeptide of fungal origin with potent immune-modulating properties, properties which have enabled dramatic improvements in solid organ transplantation to occur. However, the therapeutic window between immunosuppression and nephrotoxicity is very narrow with considerable overlap. Cyclosporin A-induced nephrotoxicity occurs in all forms of solid organ transplantation [1,2], as well as in bone marrow transplantation [3]. The

---

[1]Department of Medicine, Otago University Medical School, PO Box 913, Dunedin, New Zealand

clinical manifestations of cyclosporin A nephrotoxicity can be classified into two groups that are not necessarily exclusive. Cyclosporin A has been shown to modify renal tubular function with impaired distal tubular excretion of potassium and hydrogen ions, consistent with a voltage-dependent distal renal tubular acidosis [4,5], increased proximal tubular sodium reabsorption with decreased delivery of solute to the distal tubule [6], and impairment of urinary concentrating ability [6]. Cyclosporin A induces a marked increase in renal vascular resistance, associated with a fall in renal blood flow and a decrease in glomerular filtration rate. These changes are often associated with the development of de-novo hypertension [2,4,5].

Renal histological changes associated with CsA administration suggest injury to the proximal tubules, with foci of tubular dilatation, epithelial cell degeneration, fine reticulin deposition in the interstitium, and the presence of giant mitochondria [7,8]. Cyclosporin A may induce an arteriopathy with the development of constrictive intimal thickening together with mucoid thickening and arteriolar hyalinosis [7,8]. The development of diffuse interstitial fibrosis or striped interstitial fibrosis with tubular atrophy, an obliterative arteriolopathy and ischemic changes in some glomeruli are seen in chronic CsA nephrotoxicity [7–9].

It is difficult to correlate the histological changes and functional changes observed following the exposure to CsA [10,11]. Experimental studies have shown that there is considerable variation between species, strains, and sex of animals in their response to CsA and the development of nephrotoxicity [11]. Hence, there is no suitable experimental model that accurately reflects all the alterations seen in the human kidney.

Rats exposed to CsA will develop evidence of structural damage to the S_3 segment (straight segment) of the proximal tubule within four days [11]. Cellular damage includes vacuolation and dilatation of the endoplasmic reticulum (may also be a non-specific cellular response), tubular inclusion bodies, tubular microcalcification, tubular regeneration, and loss of brush border membranes [10–12]. Jackson and colleagues [13] found that cyclosporin induced focal areas of tubular atrophy and interstitial fibrosis in the outer cortex, and an increase in cell proliferation, the majority of which was located in the interstitium and not in the renal tubules. More recently, chronic CsA administration (12.5mg/kg per day for ten weeks) to rats was shown to produce histological injury to the inner stripe of the outer medulla and the medullary ray of the kidneys [14], similar to that seen in the striped interstitial fibrosis which is associated with chronic CsA administration in humans [8]. The features seen in the medullary ray included S_2-S_3 degenerative changes as well as tubulointerstitial fibrosis [14]. Of significance is that these morphological changes were demonstrated in nephron segments particularly sensitive to limited oxygen availability [14], thus, hypoxia secondary to vasoconstriction may further potentiate cellular injury.

Cyclosporin A has a high lipid solubility and is extensively distributed to extravascular tissues, with the highest concentrations found in fat, liver, and kidney. There is marked variation among individuals in its absorption, metabolism, and elimination [15]. Cyclosporin A has been shown to accumulate rapidly in renal segments in vitro; this accumulation being related to the lipid solubility of CsA and a partitioning process of the lipophilic drug into the lipid components of cellular membranes, which occurs in a saturable fashion. There is no evidence to suggest that CsA binds to a specific cell membrane receptor [16]. Metabolism of CsA is via the

Table 1. NADPH Cytochrome C reductase activity in renal cortical and hepatic microsomal enzymes from vehicle alone and CSA fed rats

	NADPH cytochrome C reductase enzyme activity		
	Specific activity[a]	Km[b]	Vmax[c]
	Hepatic microsomes		
Vehicle	237.2(6.4)	0.85(0.29)	300(29.5)
CSA	150.4(3.5)*	0.86(0.13)	204(8.45)
	Renal microsomes		
Vehicle	34.0(0.5)	1.78(0.08)	59.3(0.16)
CSA	31.1(0.9)*	1.51(0.24)	49.9(2.52)

[a]Specific enzyme activity expressed as nmol cytochrome C reduced/min per mg protein for cytochrome C [2mM] and NADPH [5mM]
[b]Km expressed in uM. (K^m, substrate concentration of half maximum velocity)
[c]Vmax expressed as nmol/min. (V_{max}, maximum enzyme velocity; substrate concentration not rate limiting)
Vehicle microsomes were obtained from pooled microsomes from 7 rats fed olive oil +0.1% ethanol for 4 days. CSA microsomes were obtained from pooled microsomes from 6 rats fed CSA 50mg/kg per day for 4 days. The microsomal protein concentration was kept constant for all reactions. Results are the mean±SE of 6 assays at each substrate concentrations. *$P<0.01$. (From [19] with permission)

cytochrome P-450-dependent mixed function oxidases, predominantly in the liver, with the generation of hydroxylated and N-demethylated metabolites [15].

Experimentally, CsA has been shown to significantly inhibit hepatic mixed function oxidases by uncompetitive inhibition [17,18]. The renal cortex contains similar cytochrome P-450-dependent mixed function oxidases located predominantly in the S_3 segment of the proximal tubules, a major site of histological injury produced by CsA, suggestive of a cause and effect relationship. Walker and colleagues [19] have demonstrated that CsA produces a significant uncompetitive inhibition of renal cortical NADPH cytochrome C reductase, an essential component of the mixed function oxidase enzyme complex (Table 1). Compared to the hepatic enzymes the specific activities of the renal enzymes were of a much lower order of magnitude. Despite similar tissue concentrations of cyclosporin A in the liver and kidney, the propensity for renal tubular damage is increased as compared to hepatic cellular damage. The combined effect of lower enzyme activity, together with a greater degree of uncompetitive inhibition and lower enzyme concentrations probably acting as a rate limiting step, may, in part, explain this propensity [19].

Ischemic damage to the kidney associated with transplantation, coupled with cyclosporin A-induced reduction in renal blood flow, would alter oxygen availability and metabolic requirements in the S_3 segment of the nephron. This reduced oxygen gradient would further limit the activity of the renal mixed function oxidases already compromised by the inhibitory effects of cyclosporin A.

In addition to alterations in metabolism, the hypoxic environment may also significantly impair cellular mechanisms essential for maintaining cell integrity. Cyclosporin A has been shown to reduce renal glutathione content [19] and to produce a small but significant increase in lipid peroxidation, in vitro, in renal cortical microsomes, mitochondria, and membrane fractions [19]. A reduced availability of glutathione (GSH) could impair the ability of glutathione peroxidases to metabolize fatty acid peroxides generated by lipid peroxidation. The net effect could be an increase in oxidant injury to renal tubular cells exposed to a hypoxic environment [19].

There is considerable debate over what influence CsA has on renal cell mitochondrial function and the subsequent development of nephrotoxicity. It has been suggested that decreased mitochondrial function in isolated renal cortical mitochondria following exposure to CsA in vivo and in vitro may contribute to renal tubulotoxicity [20]. Other workers have demonstrated that CsA administered to rats in nephrotoxic doses produced little or no change in mitochondrial function [21] and that these changes are probably in response to the renal hypoxia rather than a direct effect on mitochondrial function [21,22]. It is possible that the alterations in mitochondrial function may be due to alterations in the synthesis and activity of cellular protein components, including mitochondrial proteins, as discussed below [23].

Cyclosporin A has been demonstrated to alter cellular macromolecular synthesis in various cell lines [24]. Cyclosporin A and the immunologically inert cyclosporin, cyclosporin H (CsH), at concentrations comparable to those achieved in vivo, have been demonstrated to alter cellular DNA (^{3}H-thymidine incorporation) and protein synthesis (^{3}H-leucine incorporation) in renal tubular epithelial cells in culture, within two hours of exposure to cyclosporin, suggesting that cyclosporin might be altering the normal regulatory mechanisms that control the cellular enzyme systems [24]. Alterations in cellular synthesis were detected long before there were any substantial effects on cell growth or cell morphology [24]. Early sublethal damage, with altered membrane permeability, has been demonstrated in vascular endothelial cells after six hours exposure to CsA, measured by lactate dehydrogenase (LDH) and ^{51}Cr release [25]. Incubation at 4° prevented these changes, suggesting that CsA toxicity initially requires intact cellular metabolism [25].

Buss and colleagues [23] have demonstrated that a cyclosporin metabolite or a product induced by renal cells in response to CsA, directly interferes with renal microsomal protein translation or the regulation of translation. In vivo administration of CsA was required to produce inhibition of protein translocation. Renal cell sap from CsA-treated rats inhibited protein synthesis (^{3}H-leucine incorporation) in microsomes from control animals, demonstrating that a translocation inhibitor was present in the cell sap of CsA-treated rats (Fig. 1) [23]. Buss & colleagues postulate that this may be due to cyclosporin-induced inhibition of microsomal peptidyl-prolyl *cis-trans* isomerase [23], an enzyme that facilitates protein folding during synthesis and possibly may modulate some intracellular signal pathways [26]. Furthermore, CsA has been shown to inhibit peptidyl-prolyl *cis-trans* isomerase (PPI) activity in vitro [26,27], supporting the hypothesis that CsA may mediate some of its effects through alterations in protein synthesis and/or changes in protein configuration [26,27]. This enzyme has recently been demonstrated to be identical to cyclophilin (an intracellular cyclosporin binding protein, M_r 17000) [26,27], which is present in most cells and thought to be important in the intracellular transport of CsA. It has been suggested that CsA-induced inhibition of the Ca^{2+}-dependent Na^{+}/H^{+} antiport (in lymphocytes) might be mediated through CsA binding to cyclophilin [28]. Changes in protein confirmation and possible phosphorylation or dephosphorylation would alter enzyme activity. The exact role that CsA binding to and/or inhibition of cyclophilin (PPI) activity may play in renal toxicity requires further elucidation.

Ziegler and colleagues [29] have demonstrated selective binding of CsA to a M_r 75000 polypeptide component of the renal Na^{+}-D-glucose cotransporter, with a prob-

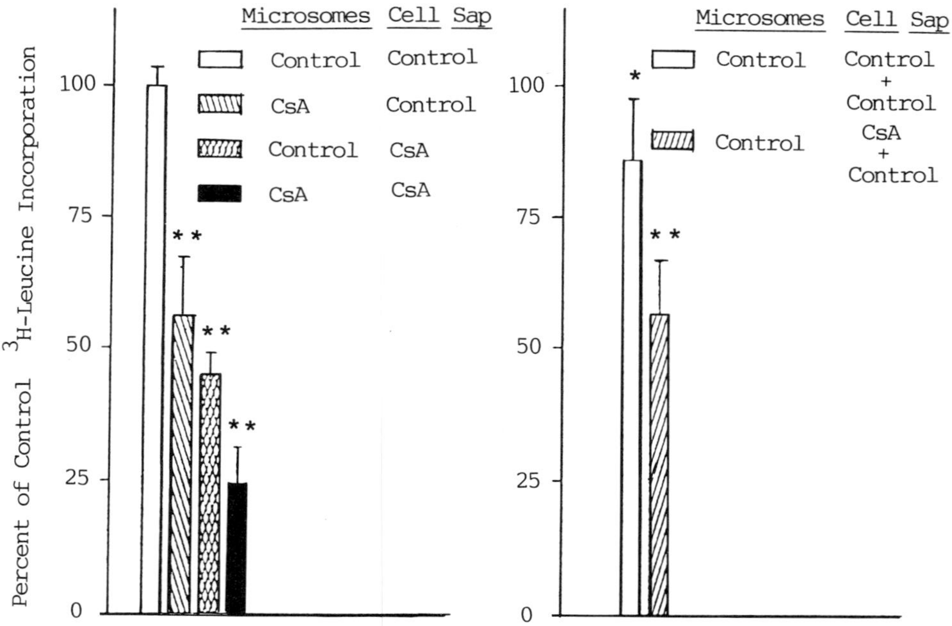

Fig. 1. Cyclosporin-induced inhibition of microsomal translocation in cross-over experiments using renal microsomes and cell saps. Microsomes and cell saps were prepared from CsA-fed (50mg/kg per day for 6 days) or vehicle-fed animals. Protein synthesis was measured as a percentage of control ^{3}H-leucine incorporation. $*P<0.02$; $**P<0.001$ compared to controls. (Reproduced with permission from Pergamon Press PLC 1989 [23])

able allosteric interaction between the binding sites for cyclosporin, D-glucose, and Na^+. Cyclosporin did not inhibit Na^+ D-glucose cotransport in isolated brush-border vesicles, suggesting that a direct effect of cyclosporin on Na^+ D-glucose cotransport across the brush-border membrane is not involved in nephrotoxicity. Rather, cyclosporin may modify the cellular turnover of the transporter protein [29]. Utilizing monoclonal antibodies directed against the cotransporter, increased localization of the antibody to the dilated endoplasmic reticulum following cyclosporin treatment was demonstrated. These authors postulate that cyclosporin, binding to a freshly synthesized component of the Na^+ D-glucose cotransporter, may inhibit the assembly of the intact transporter, with subsequent intracellular accumulation of the transport components [29]. The effect that this may have on renal tubular cellular function remains unknown, but it could play a significant role in mediating some of the cellular changes seen with cyclosporin.

Walker and colleagues [30], using partially purified protein kinase C extracts, have demonstrated that cyclosporin A significantly inhibits renal cellular protein kinase C activity both in vivo and in vitro (Fig. 2). Protein kinase C is a ubiquitous enzyme important in regulating a variety of intracellular functions by phosphorylating target proteins and enzymes [31]. It is interesting to speculate what regulatory mechanisms, such as protein phosphorylation, might be involved in regulating PPI (cyclophi-

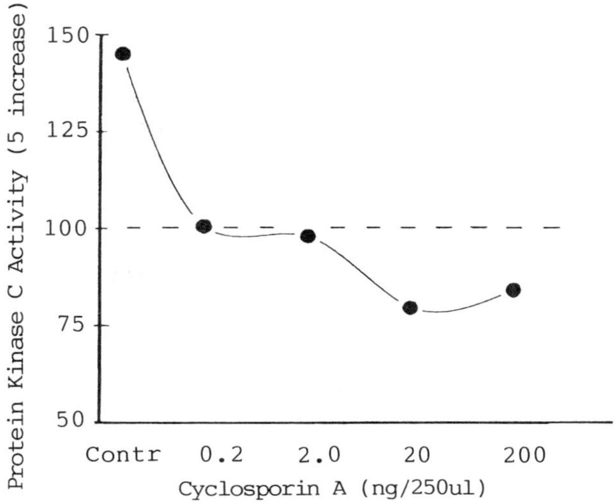

Fig. 2. Cyclosporin A inhibition of partially purified protein kinase C activity. Cytosolic protein kinase C was partially purified from pooled cytosol obtained from renal tubular epithelial cells in culture, using DEAE ion-exchange chromatography. Enzyme activity was measured as the increase in radioactivity (^{32}P) by the phosphorylation of histone. (From [30] with permission)

lin) activity and the synthesis of proteins related to the Na^+-D-glucose cotransporter. The net effect of the inhibition of various intracellular enzymes would be to impair the ability of renal cells to maintain their function and integrity in response to the toxic insult. Histological evidence of cell damage will be apparent only if the toxic injury exceeds the capacity of the cellular mechanisms to respond to the damage.

Within the literature there is controversy over the role of CsA as compared to the roles of cyclosporin metabolites or analogues in the generation of nephrotoxicity. Earlier studies, utilizing histological criteria for toxicity, suggested that it was the parent molecule of CsA, with its associated immunosuppressive properties, that was responsible for generating nephrotoxicity and that metabolites produced only minimal changes [10]. More recent studies (described below) suggest that toxicity, although variable in extent, is related to the unique cyclic ring structure of cyclosporin.

CsA has been shown to be rapidly metabolized by hepatocytes in culture, and, by 30 minutes, intracellular concentrations of metabolites were greater than the parent CsA [32]. Indirect evidence suggests that similar changes occur within renal tubular epithelial cells in culture, with an excess of metabolites present by two hours (RJ Walker, unpublished work). Renal clearance of CsA and metabolites is very low and it has been suggested that the high molecular weight of CsA and the metabolites would prevent the secretion of the drug. This would allow accumulation of both drug and metabolites in renal tubular cells which may then contribute to the development of nephrotoxicity [33,34].

As described above, CsH, an immunologically inert cyclosporin, produced changes similar to those induced by CsA in renal tubular cell DNA and protein synthesis [22].

Cyclosporin H (D N-MeVal [11]-cyclosporin) differs from CsA only by the substitution of the L-methyl valine at position 11 with its D-isomer. The primary and secondary structure of the molecule is preserved, with only a change in its tertiary structure rendering the molecule immunologically inert [35]. Cyclosporin H also has been demonstrated to inhibit glomerular mesangial cell prostaglandin synthesis to an extent similar to that seen with CsA [36]. Cyclosporin G (Nva^2-Cs) has been demonstrated to produce hemodynamic changes in vivo similar to those produced by CsA [37] (see subsequent sections). This would suggest that the mechanism by which renal cellular function is altered is common to all cyclosporins and is related to the basic molecular structure of cyclosporin.

Further supportive evidence is provided by Gschwendt and colleagues [38], who demonstrated that CsA, CsD, and CsH significantly inhibited phorbol ester-stimulated protein kinase C phosphorylation as well as Ca^{2+}/calmodulin-dependent phosphylation in vitro. This was associated with inhibition of protein and DNA synthesis, as well as with phorbol ester-induced tumor promotion in a mouse skin graft model. These actions were independent of the immunosuppressive actions of CsA [38].

The acute administration of cyclosporin A causes a dose-dependent increase in renal vascular resistance and a reduction in renal blood flow and glomerular filtration rate [39]. These early changes are functional, with no structural damage evident, and are reversible on withdrawal of the drug [39]. In the renal microcirculation similar reductions were observed. The reduction in single nephron glomerular filtration rate was associated with an increase in afferent and efferent arteriolar resistances and a fall in glomerular plasma flow. The mean glomerular capillary hydraulic pressure increased and the glomerular ultrafiltration coefficient decreased significantly [40].

The glomerular mesangial cells with their diverse roles of providing structural support for the capillary loops; modulation of the glomerular surface area and hence glomerular filtration by their smooth muscle activity, which is in turn regulated by vasoactive agents; and the ability of these mesangial cells to synthesize vasoconstrictor and vasodilatory hormones [41]; probably play a critical role in mediating the reductions in glomerular filtration rate produced by CsA administration.

Baxter and colleagues [42] have shown that cyclosporin A activates the renin angiotensin system in vivo and in vitro and that this is not accompanied by an appropriate release of the vasodilatory prostaglandins [42]. Similarly, cyclosporin A has been shown to stimulate and enhance the release of renin from juxtaglomerular cells in culture [43]. Cyclosporin A has been demonstrated to enhance arginine vasopressin stimulated mesangial cell and vascular smooth muscle cell contractility in vitro [44]. Stimulation of mesangial cells by cyclosporin A alone does not modify the release of the vasodilatory prostaglandin PGE_2, or produce an increase in the vasoconstricting prostaglandin thromboxane A_2 (TXA_2). However, CsA inhibited angiotensin II (AII)-stimulated prostaglandin release from mesangial cells (Fig. 3) [36], as well as in vascular smooth muscle cells in culture [45]. This was not associated with an increase in mesangial cell thromboxane A_2 release [36]. Alteration of mesangial cell phospholipid content, by substituting omega 3 fatty acids for omega 6 fatty acids, did not alter CsA-induced inhibition of AII-stimulated mesangial cell prostaglandin synthesis in vitro [46]. Cyclosporin H produced a similar degree of inhibition of AII-stimulated PGE_2 release [36]. Therefore, it would seem probable that cyclosporin-induced alterations in the concentrations of vasoactive hormones

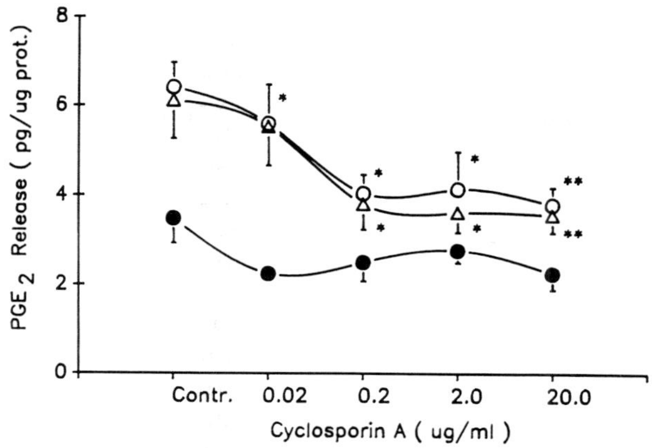

Fig. 3. Effects of CsA on Angiotensin II (*AII*)-stimulated PGE_2 release from rat mesangial cells. Following a 5 min pre-incubation with CsA, AII (0.1uM) was added to the culture media. PGE_2 release following 5 min and 15 min stimulation with AII was measured by radioimmunoassay (*RIA*). •–•, CsA alone; ∘–∘, CsA + AII 5min; ▲–▲, CsA + AII 15 min $^{*}P<0.01$; $^{**}P<0.001$ compared to control + AII. (From [36] with permission)

would allow mesangial cell contraction to predominate [36]. The net effect would be a reduction in the glomerular ultrafiltration coefficient, with an associated reduction in glomerular filtration rate, as seen both clinically and experimentally.

Exaggerated glomerular thromboxane synthesis has been suggested as a potential mechanism in producing the cyclosporin A-induced reductions in glomerular filtration rate. Perico and colleagues [47] have shown, in vivo, that glomerular synthesis and urinary excretion of thromboxane progressively increase with cyclosporin A therapy. Other studies have demonstrated that the increase in urinary thromboxane excretion is a consequence of intrarenal platelet and macrophage activation, probably triggered by cyclosporin-induced endothelial damage [48,49], rather than arising from glomerular mesangial cells [36,47]. The increased release of the vasoconstricting thromboxane from these non-renal sources could potentiate the reduction in glomerular filtration rate associated with cyclosporin A.

Cyclosporin A has been shown to enhance the transmembrane Ca^{2+} flux and to increase intracellular Ca^{2+} stores, which, in response to agonist stimulation, leads to enhanced contractility [44]. This effect on calcium flux appears to be dissociated from cyclosporin's immunosuppressive potential, as CsG and CsH, as well as CsA, have been demonstrated to significantly increase vasopressin-stimulated intracellular free calcium release from cultured rat mesangial cells [50]. Cyclosporin A inhibits protein kinase C activation [30] which also requires Ca^{2+} for its activity. Therefore, it is reasonable to assume that cyclosporin A is modulating the hormone receptor activated pathway, at several different points at least, with subsequent impairment of cellular function.

An alternative, but not necessarily opposing, hypothesis proposes that cyclosporin A nephrotoxicity, like its immunosuppressive action, is mediated by inhibition of gene transcription of critical humoral regulators of mesangial cell or vascular endothelial and/or vascular smooth muscle cell activity, particularly locally active vasodilatory agents [51]. As suggested above, this may be due to phosphorylation of critical regulatory cellular enzymes, including those responsible for transcription and translocation.

Cyclosporin has been shown to directly induce tension development in isolated rat aortic rings [52] and to augment the contractile response of arterial strips in vitro to endogenously released and exogenous norepinephrine [53]. It was suggested that CsA was acting at the level of the plasma membrane, decreasing the membrane potential, which would augment adrenergic neurotransmission and/or the response of the vascular smooth muscle cells to contractile stimuli [53]. One could speculate that the alterations in membrane potential could be mediated by CsA-induced changes in the membrane Na^+/ATPase pump [54], Na^+/H^+ antiport and intracellular pH [28], and intracellular Ca^{2+} flux [44].

Cyclosporin appears to affect many facets of renal function, from changes in whole kidney function in vivo, to alterations at a subcellular level demonstrated in cell culture models. Cyclosporin-induced changes in the renal vascular cells mediate changes in renal hemodynamics. As a consequence, the reduced oxygen availability must then influence the subsequent ability of the renal tubular epithelial cells to maintain their cellular integrity in response to cyclosporin-induced changes in cellular metabolism. The hypoxic milieu induced by CsA may be sufficient to allow potentially lethal changes in cellular function to occur, with the development of cell death and interstitial fibrosis as seen clinically. Despite the large number of studies investigating cyclosporin nephrotoxicity, there are still many unanswered questions as to how this unique agent produces the various changes that are manifested in the development of nephrotoxicity.

Acknowledgments. The expert technical assistance of Miss Vicki Lazzaro in all the studies carried out by the author is gratefully acknowledged. These studies were undertaken in, and with the valuable support of, the Department of Renal Medicine, Royal Prince Alfred Hospital, Sydney, Australia. Dr RJ Walker was the recipient of a National Health and Medical Research Council (Aust) Postgraduate Research Scholarship.

References

1. Klintmaln GBG, Iwatsuki S, Stazel TE (1981) Nephrotoxicity of cyclosporin A in liver and kidney transplantation patients. Lancet II:470–471
2. Hall BM, Tiller DJ, Duggin GG, Horvath JS, Farnsworth A, May J, Johnson JR, Shiel AGR (1985) Post-transplant acute renal failure in cadaver renal recipients treated with cyclosporine. Kidney Int 28:178–186
3. Atkinson K, Biggs JC, Hayes J, Ralston M, Dodds AJ, Concannon AJ, Naidoo D (1983) Cyclosporin associated nephrotoxicity in the first 100 days after allogenic bone marrow transplantation: 3 distinct syndromes. Br J Haematol 54:59–67
4. The Canadian Multicenter Transplantation Study Group (1986) A randomized clinical trial of cyclosporine in cadaveric renal transplantation: analysis at three years. N Engl J Med 314:1219–1225
5. Myers BD (1986) Cyclosporine nephrotoxicity. Kidney Int 30:964–974

6. Dieperink H, Leysacc PP, Kemp E, Starklint H, Frandsen NE, Tvede N, Moller J, Buchler Fredericksen P, Rossing N (1987) Nephrotoxicity of cyclosporine A in humans: effects on glomerular filtration and tubular reabsorption rates. Eur J Clin Invest 17:493–496
7. Fainsworth A, Hall BM, Ng ABP, Duggin GG, Horvath JS, Shiel AGR, Tiller DJ (1984) Renal biopsy morphology in renal transplantation: a comparative study of the light microscopic appearances of biopsies from patients treated with cyclosporine A or azathioprine prednisone and anti lymphocyte globulin. Am J Surg Pathol 8:243–252
8. Mihatsch MJ, Thiel G, Basler V, Ryffel B, Landmann J, van Overbeck J, Zollinger HU (1985) Morphological patterns in cyclosporine-treated renal transplant recipients. Transplant Proc 17(Suppl 1):101–116
9. Myers BD, Sibley R, Newton L, Tomlanovich SJ, Boshokos C, Stinson E, Luetscher JA, Whitney DJ, Kransey D, Coplaon NS, Perloth MG (1988) The long term course of cyclosporine-associated chronic nephropathy. Kidney Int 35:590–600
10. Ryffel B, Hiestand P, Foxwell B, Donatsch P, Boelsterli HJ, Maurer G, Mihatsch MJ (1986) Nephrotoxic and immunosuppressive potentials of cyclosporine metabolites in rats. Transplant Proc 18(Suppl 5):41–45
11. Duncan JI, Thomson AW, Aldridge RD, Simpson JG, Whiting PH (1986) Cyclosporine-induced renal structural damage: influence of dosage, strain, age and sex with reference to the rat and guinea pig. Clin Nephrol 25(Suppl 1):S14–S17
12. Bertani T, Perico N, Abbate M, Battaglia C, Remuzzi G (1987) Renal injury induced by long term administration of cyclosporin A to rats. Am J Pathol 127:569–579
13. Jackson NM, Hsu CH, Visccher E, Vankatachalam MA, Humes HD (1987) Alterations in renal structure and function in the rat model of cyclosporine nephrotoxicity. J Pharmacol Exp Ther 242:749–756
14. Rosen G, Greenfeld Z, Brezis M (1990) Chronic cyclosporine-induced nephropathy in the rat. Transplantation 49:445–452
15. Wood AJ, Lemaire M (1985) Pharmacologic aspects of cyclosporine therapy: pharmacokinetics. Transplant Proc 17(Suppl 1):27–32
16. Jackson NM, O'Conner RP, Humes HD (1988) Interactions of cyclosporine with renal proximal tubule cells and cellular membranes. Transplantation 46:109–114
17. Augustine JA, Zemaitis MA (1986) The effects of cyclosporin A on hepatic microsomal drug metabolism in the rat. Drug Metab Dispos 14:73–78
18. Cunningham C, Gavin MP, Whiting PH, Burke MD, MacIntyre F, Thomson AW, Simpson JG (1984) Serum cyclosporin levels, hepatic drug metabolism and renal tubulotoxicity. Biochem Pharmacol 33:2857–2861
19. Walker RJ, Lazzaro VA, Duggin GG, Horvath JS, Tiller DJ (1990) Cyclosporin-induced alterations in renal metabolism: The role of lipid peroxidation and enzyme inhibition in cyclosporin nephrotoxicity. Transplantation 50:487–492
20. Jung K, Reinholdt C, Scholz D (1987) Inhibited efficiency of kidney mitochondria isolated from rats treated with cyclosporin A. Nephron 45:43–45
21. Elzinga LW, Mela-Riker LM, Widener LL, Bennett WM (1989) Renal cortical mitochondrial integrity in experimental cyclosporine nephrotoxicity. Transplantation 48:102–106
22. Lemmi CAE, Pelikan PCD, Sikka SC, Hirschberg R, Geesaman B, Miller RL, Park KS, Liu SC, Koyle M, Rajfer J (1989) Cyclosporine augments renal mitochondrial function in vivo and reduces renal blood flow. Am J Physiol 257:F837–F841
23. Buss WC, Stepanek J, Bennett WM (1989) A new proposal for the mechanism of cyclosporine nephrotoxicity: Inhibition of renal microsomal protein chain elongation following in vivo cyclosporine A. Biochem Pharmacol 38:4085–4093
24. White DJG, Plumb AM, Pawlee G, Brons G (1979) Cyclosporin A: An immunosuppressive agent preferentially active against proliferating T cells. Transplantation 27:55–58
25. Zoja C, Furci, Ghilardi F, Zilio P, Benigni A, Remuzzi G (1986) Cyclosporin-induced endothelial cell injury. Lab Invest 55:455–462

26. Takahashi N, Hayano T, Suzuki M (1989) Peptidyl-prolyl *cis-trans* isomerase is the cyclosporin A-binding protein cyclophilin. Nature 337:473–475
27. Fischer G, Wittman-Liebold B, Lang K, Kiefhaber T, Schmid FX (1989) Cyclophilin and peptidyl-prolyl *cis-trans* isomerase are probably identical proteins. Nature 377:476–478
28. Rosoff PM, Terres G (1986) Cyclosporine A inhibits Ca^{2+} dependent stimulation of the Na^+/H^+ antiport in human T cells. J Cell Biol 103:457–463
29. Ziegler K, Frimmer M, Fritzsch G, Koepsell H (1990) Cyclosporin binding to a protein component of the renal Na^+-D-glucose cotransporter. J Biol Chem 265:3270–3277
30. Walker RJ, Lazzaro VA, Duggin GG, Horvath JS, Tiller DJ (1989) Cyclosporin A inhibits protein kinase C activity: A contributing mechanism in the development of nephrotoxicity? Biochem Biophys Res Commun 160:409–415
31. Nishizuka Y (1988) The molecular heterogeneity of protein kinase C and its implication for cellular regulation. Nature 334:661–665
32. Fabre G, Bertault-Peres P, Fabre I, Maurel P, Just S, Cano JP (1987) Metabolism of cyclosporin A. 1. A study in isolated fresh rabbit hepatocytes. Drug Metab Dispos 15:384–390
33. Caterson RJ, Duggin GG, Critchley L, Baxter C, Horvath JS, Hall BM, Tiller DJ (1986) Renal tubular transport of cyclosporin A and associated changes in renal function. Clin Nephrol 25(Suppl 1):S30–S35
34. Burke MD, Whiting PH (1986) The role of drug metabolism in cyclosporine A nephrotoxicity. Clin Nephrol 25(Suppl 1):S111–116
35. Walkinshaw MD, Weber HP, Widmir A (1986) Molecular recognition in biological systems: Models for rational drug design. Sandoz J Med 25:131–142
36. Walker RJ, Lazzaro VA, Duggin GG, Horvath JS, Tiller DJ (1990) Structure activity relationships of cyclosporins (II): Inhibition of angiotensin II stimulated prostaglandin release in rat mesangial cells. Transplantation 50:343–345
37. Pallor MS, Ferris TF (1987) Effects of Nva^2-cyclosporine on glomerular filtration rate and renal blood flow in rats. Transplantation 43:893–895
38. Gschwendt M, Kittstein W, Marks F (1988) The weak immunosuppressant cyclosporin D as well as the immunologically inert cyclosporin H are potent inhibitors in vivo of phorbol ester TPA-induced biological effect in mouse skin and of Ca^{2+}/calmodulin dependent EF-2 phosphorylation in vitro. Biochem Biophys Res Commun 150:545–551
39. Murray MS, Pallor MS (1985) Effect of cyclosporine administration on renal hemodynamics in conscious rats. Kidney Int 28:767–774
40. Barros ESG, Boim MA, Ajzen H, Ramos OL, Schor N (1985) Glomerular hemodynamics and hormonal participation in cyclosporine nephrotoxicity. Kidney Int 32:19–25
41. Schlondorff D (1987) The glomerular mesangial cell: an expanding role for a specialized pericyte. FASEB J 1:272–281
42. Baxter CR, Duggin GG, Hall BM, Horvath JS, Tiller DJ (1984) Cyclosporin A and renal prostaglandin biosynthesis. Res Commun Chem Pathol Pharmacol 45:69–80
43. Kurtz A, Bruna RB, Kuhn KW (1988) Cyclosporine A enhances renin secretion and production in isolated juxtaglomerular cells. Kidney Int 33:947–953
44. Meyer-Lehnert H, Schrier RW (1988) Cyclosporine A enhances vasopressin-induced Ca^{2+} mobilization and contraction in mesangial cells. Kidney Int 34:89–97
45. Kurtz A, Pfeilschifter J, Kuhn K, Koch KW (1987) Cyclosporin A inhibits PGE_2 release from vascular smooth muscle cells. Biochem Biophys Res Commun 147:542–549
46. Walker RJ, Lazzaro VA, Duggin GG, Horvath JS, Tiller DJ (1989) Dietary eicosapentaenoic acid does not modify cyclosporin-induced inhibition of angiotensin II stimulated prostaglandin synthesis in mesangial cells. Renal Failure 11:125–132
47. Perico N, Zoja C, Benigni A, Ghilardi F, Gualandris L, Remuzzi G (1986) Effect of short term cyclosporine administration in rats on renin-angiotensin and thromboxane A_2: possi-

ble relevance to the reduction in glomerular filtration rate. J Pharmacol Exp Ther 239:229–235

48. Benigni A, Chiabrandio C, Piccinelli A, Perico N, Gavinelli M, Furci L, Patino O, Abbate M, Bertani T, Remuzzi G (1988) Increased urinary excretion of thromboxane B_2 and 2,3-dinor TXB_2 in cyclosporin A nephrotoxicity. Kidney Int 34:164–174
49. Rogers TS, Elzinga L, Bennett WM, Kelley VE (1988) Selective enhancement of thromboxane in macrophages and kidneys in cyclosporine-induced nephrotoxicity. Transplantation 45:153–156
50. Goldberg HJ, Wong PY, Cole EH, Levey GA, Skorecki KL (1989) Dissociation between the immunosuppressive activity of cyclosporine derivatives and their effects on intracellular calcium signaling in mesangial cells. Transplantation 47:731–733
51. Kahan BD (1989) Cyclosporine. N Engl J Med 321:1725–1738
52. Xue H, Bukoski RD, McCarron DA, Bennett WM (1987) Induction of contraction in isolated rat aorta by cyclosporine. Transplantation 43:715–718
53. Lamb FS, Webb RC (1987) Cyclosporine augments reactivity of isolated blood vessels. Life Sci 40:2571–2578
54. Suzuki S, Oka T, Ohkuma S, Kuriyama K (1987) Biochemical mechanisms underlying cyclosporine A-induced nephrotoxicity. Effect of concurrent administration of prednisolone. Transplantation 44:363–368

Glomerular Hemodynamic Effects of Cyclosporine

Nestor Schor, Mirian A. Roim, Elvino J.G. Barros, and Oscar F.P. Santos[1]

Summary. We evaluated the effects of acute and chronic Cyclosporine (CsA) administration on renal microcirculation, as well as the role of hormonal systems in this nephrotoxicity. Studies were performed in euvolemic Munich-Wistar rats by using a micropuncture technique. Acute CsA infusion caused a decline in single nephron (SN) glomerular filtration rate (GFR) due to a decrease in glomerular plasma flow (Q_A) and a decrease in the glomerular ultrafiltration coefficient (K_f), despite an increase in transcapillary hydraulic pressure difference (ΔP). Both captopril and verapamil partially prevented the decrease in whole kidney function altered by acute CsA infusion. Conversely, indomethacin did not modify these parameters, suggesting that the renin-angiotensin system and calcium play a role in CsA nephrotoxicity, while the prostaglandin system participated in this event by a direct blocking of CsA. The platelet activating factor (PAF) antagonist, (BN 52 021), blunted CsA effects on superficial nephron function. Since dazmegrel, a thromboxane synthetase inhibitor, did not change the SNGFR already altered by CsA, the beneficial effects of BN 52 021 would appear to be related to a direct blocking of PAF actions. Acute CsA nephrotoxicity was not fully demonstrated in Brattleboro rats, who present a hereditary absence of antidiuretic hormone (ADH), thus suggesting that the absence of ADH can be a protective factor in CsA nephrotoxicity. Short-term chronic infusion of CsA provoked a decline in SNGFR due to a decrease in Q_A and ΔP, while K_f remained unaltered. Glomerular hemodynamic patterns in acute and chronic CsA administration were different, suggesting that distinct pathophysiological mechanisms were involved and that distinct pathophysiological approaches would be required to improve knowledge of CsA nephrotoxicity.

[1]Nephrology Division, Escola Paulista de Medicina, Rua Botucatu no. 740, 04023-Sao Paulo, SP-Brazil

Introduction

Cyclosporine A (CsA) is a potent immunosuppressor drug that has been successfully used to prevent rejection of kidney, heart, bone marrow, and other organ transplants [1]. However, a number of side effects are known, the most common and important one being its nephrotoxicity [2].

It has been suggested that hormonal factors might take part in this acute renal failure, since no significant glomerular lesions have been found by light, immunofluorescence, or electron microscopy [3]. Indeed, there is evidence of pronounced renal vasoconstriction after acute and chronic CsA administration [4].

In order to evaluate renal microcirculation and glomerular hemodynamics during acute or chronic CsA administration, as well as the role of some hormonal systems in these events, Munich-Wistar rats were submitted to micropuncture studies.

Material and Methods

Adult male euvolemic Munich-Wistar rats were submitted to a general protocol consisting of two study periods (Groups 1–7). In the first period, saline administration was followed by clearance and micropuncture evaluation, after that, CsA (50 mg/Kg BW, iv, in bolus) was infused and a second study was performed (Group 1, n=10). In Group 2 (n=7), indomethacin (INDO, 2 mg/Kg, iv, in bolus) was given in the first period and the same dose of CsA was infused. Group 3 (n=8) and Group 4 (n=7) were treated in the same way as Group 2, but captopril (CAPT, 2 mg/Kg per h, i.v.) and verapamil (VERA, 20 ug/Kg per min, i.v.), respectively, were infused throughout both periods; CsA was also simultaneously administered in the second study period. Group 5 (n=7), animals were treated with BN 52 021 (5 mg/Kg, i.v., in bolus), a platelet activating factor (PAF) antagonist, in the first period and with CsA in the second period. Group 6 (n=7) were given a thromboxane synthetase inhibitor, dazmegrel (DAZ, 5 mg/Kg, i.v., in bolus), in the first period and CsA in the second period. In order to evaluate the role of ADH in CsA nephrotoxicity, Brattleboro homozygote rats, with genetic diabetes insipidus, were studied before and after CsA administration (Group 8, Homo BB, n=9). Heterozygote rats (Group 9, Hetero BB, n=7) served as controls for Group 8. Finally, short-term CsA administration (Group 10, n=9, 25 mg/Kg, i.p., per day) during 9 days was also evaluated.

In all rats, glomerular filtration rate (GFR) and total renal plasma flow (RPF) were analyzed by inulin and p-amminohippuric acid clearance, respectively.

The total renal vascular resistance (TRVR) was calculated as the quotient between mean arterial pressure (MAP) and RPF. Groups 1, 5, 6, and 10 were submitted to micropuncture studies following the usual routine fashion [5]. Statistical analyses were performed by Student's paired and unpaired two-tailed t test, and by the Mann-Whitney test when appropriate. Statistical significance was defined as $P<0.05$. Data were presented as mean ($X \pm SEM$).

Results

Although not shown, when a CsA vehicle, cremophor, was acutely or chronically administered, no change in global or superficial renal function was observed.

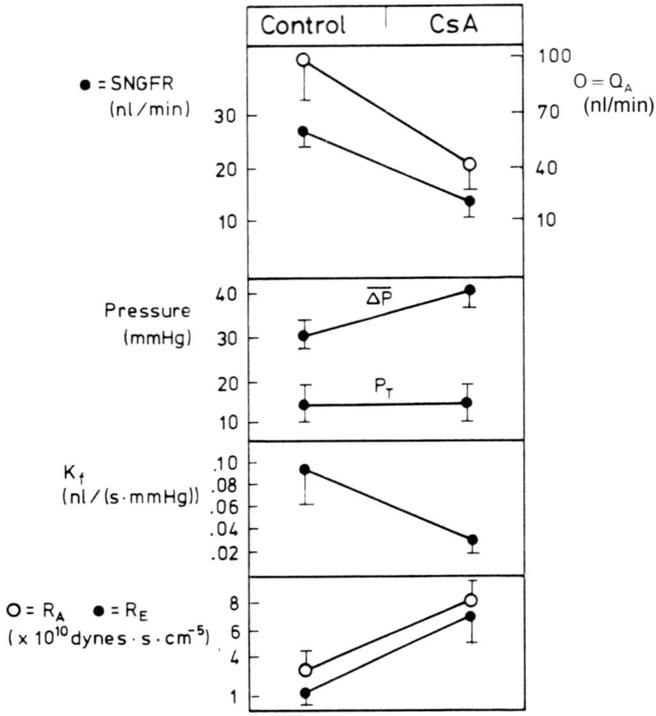

Fig. 1. Summary of CsA acute infusion.

Conversely, acute infusion of CsA induced an important decline in GFR and RPF, from 0.96±0.04 to 0.47±0.07 ml/min and from 2.91±0.19 to 1.30±0.23 ml/min ($P<0.05$), respectively. The TRVR was elevated three times (39±3 vs 129±40 mmHg/min per ml, $P<0.05$). As shown in Fig. 1, CsA, with results similar to those observed for global renal function, provoked a decline in single nephron GFR (SNGFR). A proportional decrease in glomerular plasma flow rate (Q_A) and in the glomerular ultrafiltration coefficient, K_f, were observed. The decline in Q_A was due to a great elevation in both afferent (R_A) and efferent (R_E) arteriolar resistances, mainly in R_E. Thus, this pattern of modification of arteriolar resistances provoked an increase in the mean transcapillary hydraulic pressure difference (ΔP). However, the increase in ΔP was not large enough to compensate for the decline in Q_A and K_f, and so, the SNGFR decreased.

Figure 2 shows the percentage changes from control values of GFR, first bar, renal plasma flow, second bar, and total renal vascular resistance, third bar. The decline of GFR and RPF and the increase in TRVR were not affected by indomethacin infusion when compared with the results for animals receiving CsA alone. On the other hand, both captopril and verapamil improved global renal function when CsA had been given previously. The decline in GFR and RPF, as well as the increase in TRVR, were partially prevented by these two drugs, suggesting that the renin angiotensin system and calcium participate in this model of nephrotoxicity.

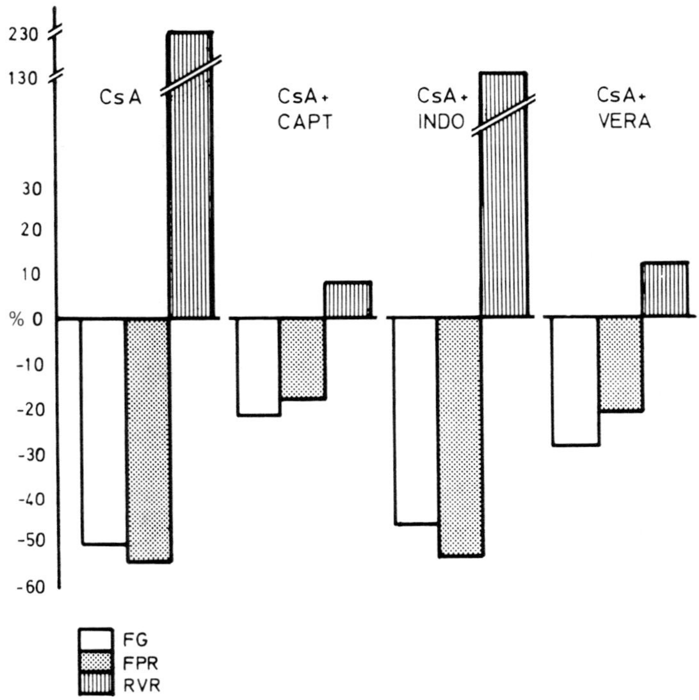

Fig. 2. Effects of CsA during captopril CAPT, Indomethacin (*INDO*), and Verapamil (*VERA*) administration

Simultaneous treatment with BN 52 021 and CsA provoked an improvement in SNGFR due to a normalization in glomerular plasma flow (Q_A) and glomerular capillary hydraulic pressure, P_{GC}. The K_f remained unchanged and the arteriolar resistances were not modified, suggesting that PAF could be one of the mediators involved in CsA nephrotoxicity (Fig. 3). In contrast, despite preventing the glomerular hypertension induced by CsA, DAZ did not modify the reduced SNGFR, Q_A and K_f, suggesting that thromboxane A_2 was not involved in the acute renal failure (ARF) induced by acute infusion of CsA.

As shown in Fig. 4, when renal function in Homo BB was compared with that in Hetero BB rats, it was observed that the declines in GFR and RPF were lower in rats without ADH than the declines in rats with ADH, and as well, the increase in TRVR was blunted in Homo BB rats. These data suggest that the absence of ADH appears to be a protective factor in the ARF induced by CsA.

In contrast to the results observed for acute CsA infusion, short-term CsA treatment provoked a decline in SNGFR with a decrease in Q_A. The reduction in Q_A occurred as a result of an elevation in both arteriolar resistances R_A and R_E, mainly in the afferent arteriolar resistance. This fact caused a decline in ΔP, while the K_f remained unaltered (Fig. 5).

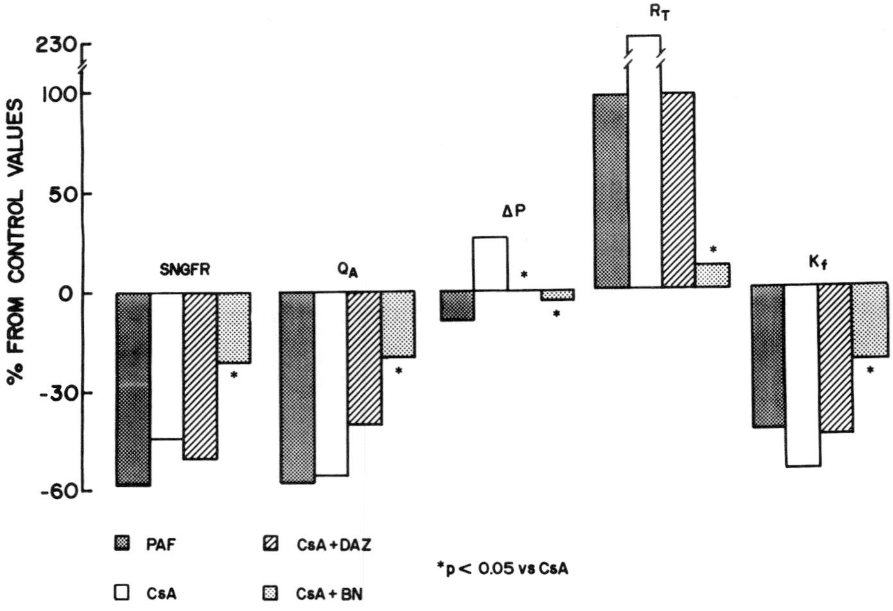

Fig. 3. Effects of PAF, CsA, CsA plus dazmegrel (*DAZ*), and CsA plus BN52 021 on glomerular hemodynamics

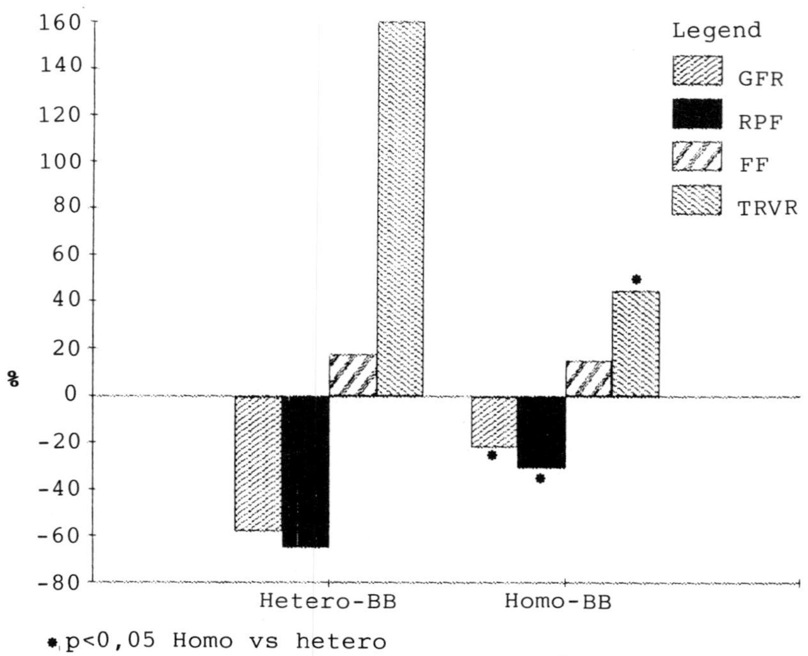

Fig. 4. Acute CsA administration in homozygote (*Homo-BB*) and heterozygote (*Hetero-BB*) Brattleboro rats

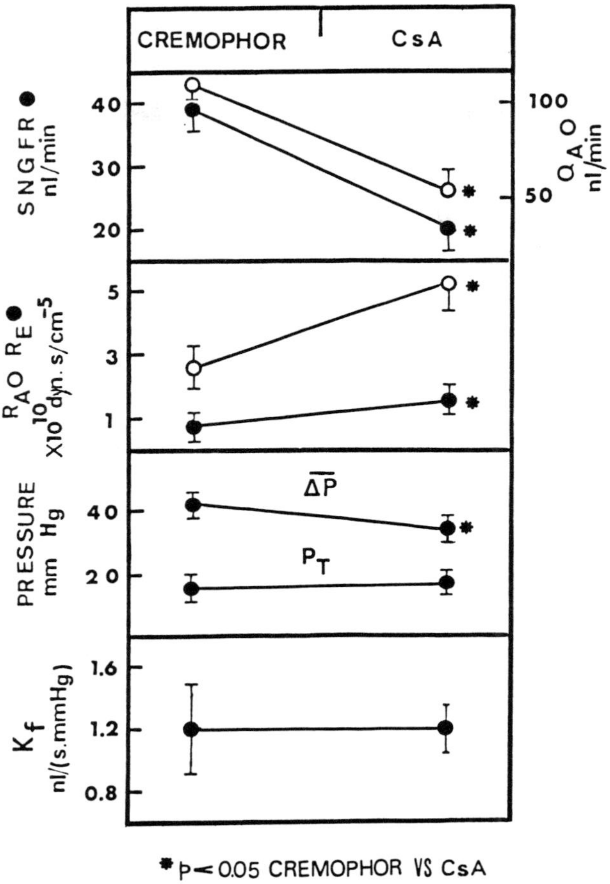

Fig. 5. Summary of CsA chronic treatment

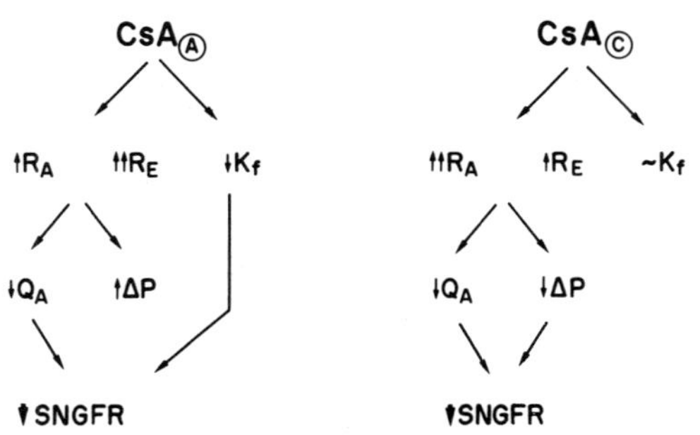

Fig. 6. Glomerular hemodynamic patterns after acute and chronic CsA administration

Thus, the glomerular hemodynamic patterns observed after acute and chronic administration of CsA were different. As presented in Fig. 6, acute CsA infusion caused a decline in SNGFR due to a decrease in Q_A and K_f, despite an increase in ΔP. On the other hand, chronic CsA nephrotoxicity showed decreases in SNGFR and Q_A, but with maintenance of K_f and decline in ΔP.

Discussion

Cyclosporine, an immunosuppressive agent used widely in organ transplantation and in several immune-mediated diseases presents potential nephrotoxicity. The acute renal failure (ARF) induced by CsA depends on its dosage and on the extent of treatment and is generally reversible after CsA reduction or discontinuation [2]. Since the toxicity of CsA has not been associated with glomerular lesions, this suggests that ARF might be mediated by hormonal factors [6]. Indeed, CsA produces activation of the renin angiotensin system (RAS) and platelet activating factor (PAF) and produces direct suppression of prostaglandin (PG) synthesis [6–8].

In this study (Fig. 1), acute CsA infusion provoked a great increase in both R_A and R_E, but the higher increment obtained in R_E determined a significant increase in ΔP. Despite the increase in ΔP, reduced values for SNGFR, due to an arteriolar vasoconstriction, were observed. The latter determined a fall in Q_A. Nevertheless, the fall in Q_A was not the only factor responsible for this. Our data indicate that SNGFR was also decreased by a significant fall in K_f [9]. Moreover, it was observed that CsA caused mesangial cell contraction in vitro [7], reducing glomerular surface available for filtration, thus leading to a lower K_f.

The data from micropuncture studies suggest that angiotensin II (AII), by increasing arteriolar resistance, has a role in the decline in Q_A and K_f [10]. In the animal group treated with captopril, it was observed that renal vasoconstriction induced by CsA was abolished. So, captopril partially prevented the fall in GFR and RPF (Fig. 2). This finding suggests that AII may play a role in the pathogenesis of renal vasoconstriction produced by CsA. Its participation could be mediated by a stimulation of the tubuloglomerular feedback mechanism or by a decrease in K_f [10,11].

Conversely, the use of indomethacin produced essentially the same results as those found with CsA alone (Fig. 2). This indicates that the PG system has a minor effect or that CsA directly decreases prostaglandin production [8].

Once CsA had caused an increase in total renal resistance, it became important to evaluate the observed Ca-channel blocker drug effect. Verapamil attenuated the CsA effects on TRVR and RPF, leading to an improvement in GFR (Fig. 2).

Antidiuretic hormone (ADH) is another vasoactive substance which is capable of influencing the process of glomerular ultrafiltration, mainly by reducing K_f [10]. In the present study, acute CsA administration in Homo BB rats produced only a slight decline in GFR and RPF when compared with both Hetero BB and Munich-Wistar rats (Fig. 4). Therefore, it can be postulated that the presence of ADH, in some way, is necessary for the full range of CsA nephrotoxic action which is observed in the rat kidney. It is possible that ADH participates in this pathophysiology either by its vasoconstrictor effects or by its known action of reducing K_f.

Continuous intravenous infusion of PAF provoked a decline in SNGFR due to a decrease in Q_A, K_f, and ΔP [12]. Thus, the pattern of glomerular hemodynamics induced by PAF and acute CsA was very similar. Moreover, it was observed that a PAF antagonist blunted the mesangial cell contraction induced by CsA [7]. Thus, PAF could be a mediator in this nephrotoxicity. Actually, acute treatment with BN 52 021, a PAF antagonist, before infusion of CsA prevented SNGFR, Q_A, ΔP, and K_f alterations. Thus, these protective actions could be due to an effect on mesangial cell contraction or an effect on minimizing the arteriolar vasoconstriction (Fig. 3). However, it has been shown that PAF can induce release of secondary mediators, including TxA_2, from various cell types and organs [13]. Indeed, increased production of renal thromboxane under chronic CsA treatment has been demonstrated [14]. Thus, the protective effects of BN 52 021 could be mediated by blunting the release of TxA_2 or by a direct action on PAF responses. In order to separate these two possible mechanisms, dazmegrel (DAZ), a thromboxane synthetase inhibitor, was employed. This inhibitor did not protect against the acute nephrotoxicity induced by CsA, since the SNGFR, Q_A, and K_f remained decreased, despite the decline in ΔP (Fig. 3). These data suggest that the improvement in SNGFR caused by BN 52 021 was mediated by a direct effect on PAF action and not by a blocker of TxA_2 release [15].

It was observed that the glomerular hemodynamic alterations induced by acute [9] or chronic [16] CsA administration were different. It is possible that the roles of vasoactive systems were modified during these two models of CsA nephrotoxicity. As chronic CsA toxicity is closer to clinical situations, we also decided to evaluate short-term CsA administration effects on renal function and glomerular hemodynamics in Munich-Wistar rats.

When CsA was given chronically, it was observed that great vasoconstriction, with increases in pre and post glomerular resistances occurred. However, the predominant rise in afferent arteriolar resistance produced a fall in Q_A and ΔP, both being responsible for the decrease in SNGFR.

In contrast with the results observed with acute CsA, K_f presented no significant change after chronic treatment (Fig. 5), despite multiple hormonal interactions.

In summary (Fig. 6), the glomerular hemodynamic patterns observed after acute and after chronic administration of CsA were different. As shown, acute CsA infusion caused a decline in SNGFR due to a decrease in Q_A and K_f, despite the increase in ΔP. On the other hand, chronic CsA nephrotoxicity showed decreases in SNGFR and Q_A, but with maintenance of mean K_f and decline of mean ΔP. These aspects of renal microcirculation, observed for both acute and chronic CsA administration, imply distinct pathophysiological mechanisms; in order to understand and, perhaps, to modify the nephrotoxicity of cyclosporine, distinct pathophysiological approaches will also be required. Also, the hormonal participation in chronic CsA treatment appears to be different from that in the acute model.

References

1. Kahan BD (1985) Cyclosporine: The agent and its actions. Transplant Proc 17:5–18
2. Flechner SM, Van Buren G, Herman RH, Kahan BD (1983) The nephrotoxicity of cyclosporine in renal transplant recipients. Transplant Proc 15:2689–2694
3. Mihatsch MJ, Ryffel B, Hermle M, Brunner FP, Thiel G (1986) Morphology of cyclosporine nephrotoxicity in the rat. Clin Nephrol 25:S2–S8

4. Murray BM, Paller MS, Ferris TF (1985) Effect of cyclosporine administration on renal hemodynamics in conscious rats. Kidney Int 28:767–774
5. Lugon JR, Boim MA, Ramos OL, Ajzen H, Schor N (1989) Renal function and glomerular hemodynamics in male endotoxemic rats. Kidney Int 36:570–575
6. Perilo N, Benigni C, Bosco E, Rossini M, Orisio S, Ghilardi E, Piccinilli A, Remuzzi G (1986) Acute cyclosporine A nephrotoxicity in rats: which role for renin-angiotensin system and glomerular prostaglandins? Clin Nephrol 25:583–588
7. Lama S, Oliveira A, Lopez-Novoa JM, Ortega G, Lopez-Forre A, Rodrigues-Puyol D (1988) El factor activador de las plaquetas (PAF) como mediador de la nefrotoxicidad inducida por ciclosporina A: estudios en glomerulos aislados humanos y de ratos. Nefrologia 7 (Suppl 1):24–29
8. Persan L, Kaskuel F, Barnett R, Wilson T, Moore L, Arbeit L, Schlondorff D (1989) Altered renal prostaglandin and thromboxane production in cyclosporine nephrotoxicity (abstract). Kidney Int 35:508
9. Barros EJG, Boim MA, Ajzen H, Ramos OL, Schor N (1987) Glomerular hemodynamics and hormonal participation in cyclosporine nephrotoxicity. Kidney Int 32:19–25
10. Schor N, Ichikawa I, Brenner BM (1981) Mechanisms of action of various hormones and vasoactive substances on glomerular ultrafiltration in the rat. Kidney Int 208:442–451
11. Siegl H, Ryffel B, Petric P, et al. (1983) Cyclosporine, the renin-angiotensin-aldosterone system, and renal adverse reactions. Transplant Proc 15:2719–2725
12. Badr KF, DeBoer DK, Takahashi K, Harris FC, Fogo A, Jacobson HR (1989) Glomerular responses to platelet-activating factor in the rat: role of thromboxane A_2. Am J Physiol 256:F35–F43
13. Weisman SM, Felsen D, Darracott Vaughan E Jr (1985) Platelet activating factor is a potent stimulus for renal prostaglandin synthesis: possible significance in unilateral ureteral obstruction. J Pharmacol Exp Ther 30:10–15
14. Perico N, Benigni A, Zoja C, Delaini F, Remuzzi G (1986) Functional significance of exaggerated renal thromboxane A_2 synthesis induced by cyclosporine A. Am J Physiol 251:F581–587
15. Santos OFP, Boim MA, Bregman R, Draibe SA, Barros EJG, Pirotzky E, Schor N, Braquet P (1989) Effect of platelet-activating factor on cyclosporine nephrotoxicity: glomerular hemodynamics evaluation. Transplantation 47:592–595
16. Thomson SC, Tucker BJ, Gabba F, Blantz RC (1989) Functional effects on glomerular hemodynamics of short-term chronic cyclosporine in male rats. J Clin Invest 83:960–969

Mechanisms and Mediators of Cyclosporine-Induced Renal Vascular Changes

NORBERTO PERICO and GIUSEPPE REMUZZI[1]

Cyclosporines are a family of structurally related endecapeptides isolated as metabolites during fermentation of the soil fungi *Trichoderma polysporum Rifae* and *Cylindrocarpon lucidum Booth* [1]. Cyclosporin A (CyA), the clinically active compound, is a hydrophobic cyclic peptide containing a unique, nine-carbon amino acid bearing an ethylene band, which is essential for its biological activity. In contrast with the conventional immunosuppressive drugs, azathioprine and adrenal corticosteroids, CyA selectively inhibits adaptive immune responses, primarily through the inhibition of interleukin-2 gene translocation to mRNA and reduction of interleukin-2 production at T-cell level, while other events of T-cell activation continue unabated [2]. By virtue of its peculiar and selective activity on the immune system, CyA has improved the management of patients with organ transplantation by increasing graft and patient survival rates [3,4]. Moreover, the use of CyA has recently been advocated for the prevention of graft-versus-host disease in bone marrow transplantation [5] and for the treatment of autoimmune diseases such as uveitis [6], systemic lupus erythematosus [7], rheumatoid arthritis [8], and various forms of glomerulonephritis [9]. However, the major concern regarding CyA therapy has focused upon its association with an array of side-effects, the most serious of which is nephrotoxicity [10,11]. Thus, acute reversible dose-related decreases in renal function have been observed in over 50% of cases in some series [12]. Persistent increase in serum creatinine has prompted discontinuation or reduction of the CyA dose in a large number of patients, with subsequent improvement in renal function [13]. In addition, the potential long-term nephrotoxicity of this drug has been suggested by the progressive decline in glomerular filtration rate associated with tubulo-interstitial scarring and the obliterative arteriolopathy and glomerular sclerosis seen in cardiac allograft recipients with excellent cardiac function [14] and in liver allograft recipients [15]. Despite the fact that the clinical and pathological features

[1]Mario Negri Institute for Pharmacological Research, Via Gavazzeni 11, 24100 Bergamo, Italy

of these syndromes differ, all these manifestations of nephrotoxicity are consistent with the changes induced by CyA in the renal vessels, in which elevation in renal vascular resistance is manifested. Extensive investigations have been performed in this area, but the cause of CyA-induced renal vascular damage and the reason for the peculiar susceptibility of renal vessels to CyA-induced injury remain ill defined.

Here we will describe the vascular effects of CyA, comparing the results of human data with experimental studies, and we will analyze the possible pathogenetic mechanism(s) underlying these lesions.

Acute Reversible Renal Vasoconstriction

The administration of CyA is complicated in most renal transplant recipients by the occurrence of one or more episodes of acute renal insufficiency [13,16], usually rapidly reversible after the daily dose of CyA is reduced [17]. Moreover, liver transplant recipients receiving intravenous CyA may develop a syndrome characterized by oliguria and low fractional excretion of sodium [18]. The acute effect of CyA on renal function in animal models varies with respect to species or strain of animal as well as dose, mode of administration, and duration of treatment with CyA [19]. Several investigators have reported elevated reno-vascular resistance, diminished renal blood flow, and functional renal impairment in the rat [19–21]. Because these studies were carried out in vivo, it is difficult to separate the direct acute effects of CyA on the kidney from the indirect effects caused by systemic CyA toxicity. This issue has been addressed, using an isolated perfused rat kidney model, a preparation in which systemic influences on renal function can be eliminated [22]. With this technique we have recently shown that CyA, but not vehicle, caused a dose-dependent fall in renal perfusate flow associated with a concomitant increase in renal vascular resistance [23]. These findings are in line with those of Rossi et al. [24] who found a concentration-dependent increase in perfusion pressure in isolated rat kidneys perfused at constant flow and exposed to CyA. Recently English and coworkers [25], in rat experiments, provided the morphological counterpart of CyA-induced vasoconstriction, showing by scanning electron microscopy a disproportionate and progressive narrowing of the diameter of afferent arterioles which paralleled the decrease in inulin clearance.

CyA-induced renal vasoconstriction has been studied extensively, yet the mechanism of the drug's renovascular activity is still not clearly understood. Because in several studies CyA administration was followed by activation of the renin-angiotensin system, it has been postulated that CyA-induced arteriolar vasoconstriction is mediated by angiotensin II. However, there is no definitive evidence of this. Thus, in animals, renin secretion and plasma renin are increased with CyA treatment, which suggests that angiotensin II might be a mediator [26–28]. In contrast, plasma renin is decreased significantly in some humans with CyA-induced renal failure [14]. Moreover, improvements in renal hemodynamics have not been uniformly observed following converting enzyme inhibition in rats given CyA [21,29–31]. The possible role of activation of the sympathetic nervous system as a cause of CyA-induced vasoconstriction has also been considered. The observation that denervated kidneys fail to constrict in response to CyA in vivo [21], together with findings that α-adrenergic inhibitors antagonize CyA-induced renal vasoconstriction in innervated kidneys [21] and findings that renal sympathetic nerve activity is augmented in CyA-treated rats [32], support the contention that the renal sympathetic nerves mediate CyA-induced renal vasoconstriction, at least in part. Regardless of the validity of these observations, such a mechanism cannot readily account for the acute decline in renal blood flow and glomerular filtration rate (GFR) seen early in transplanted, and therefore denervated, kidneys [33]. CyA has been reported to alter arachidonic acid metabolism in peripheral blood monocytes [34] and in smooth muscle cells in culture [35]. Since arachidonate metabolites generated via cyclooxygenase and lipoxygenase enzymes have been found to play an important role in regulating glomerular function [36,37], one would expect that these compounds may contribute to the renal vasoconstriction induced by acute CyA administration.

Among the arachidonate metabolites formed via cyclooxygenase enzyme, TxA_2, a potent vasoconstrictor, has been shown to reduce GFR in normal rats by increasing glomerular afferent and efferent arteriolar resistances [38] and it has been shown to contract cultured rat mesangial cells through an elevation of free cytosolic calcium [39], reducing the glomerular filtration surface area. To test the possibility that TxA_2 may participate in acute CyA nephrotoxicity we exposed bovine aortic endothelial cells in culture to different concentrations of CyA, and TxA_2 generation was evaluated. In contrast with vehicle only results, incubation of confluent monolayer endothelial cells with CyA caused a time- and concentration-dependent increase in TxA_2 production, measured as its stable breakdown product TxB_2 [40]. To further investigate, in more physiologic conditions, the potential role of TxA_2 in the renal function deterioration induced by CyA, we evaluated the effects of pharmacological inhibition of endogenous TxA_2 activity in an experimental model of acute CyA nephrotoxicity. A specific TxA_2 receptor antagonist, GR32191, but not its vehicle, partially prevented the decline in GFR and renal plasma flow induced by acute CyA administration [41], pointing out a major role for TxA_2 in mediating the acute renal vasoconstriction induced by CyA in the rat. The fact that after GR32191 administration, renal function increased, but did not reach control values suggests that in addition to TxA_2 other factor(s) might be involved in the reduction of GFR induced by CyA.

Sulfidopeptide leukotrienes LTC_4 and LTD_4, derived from the 5-lipoxygenase pathway of the oxidative metabolism of arachidonic acid [42], have recently received considerable attention as modulators of glomerular function, on the basis of the observation that they increase renal vascular resistance and reduce GFR when infused in the intact animal [37] as well as in the isolated perfused rat kidney [43]. That these eicosanoids may play an intermediary role in the renal functional impairment following CyA treatment has been recently documented by the demonstration that a specific LTC_4/D_4 receptor antagonist, L-649923, also partially prevented the fall in GFR and in renal plasma flow (RPF) caused by acute i.v. CyA administration to rats [41]. Of interest, the combined administration of the TxA_2 receptor antagonist, GR32191, and the LTC_4/D_4 receptor antagonist, L-649,923, completely abolished CyA-induced decline in GFR and RPF [41], indicating an additive contribution of TxA_2 and LTC_4/D_4 to the acute renal vasoconstriction caused by CyA, at least in rats. Whether the effect of TxA_2 and/or LTC_4/D_4 on renal vascular resistance is direct or is mediated, at least in part, by their capability of releasing other vasoactive substances from endothelial cells is a matter of debate. The recent isolation and identification of a novel constrictor peptide derived from vessel endothelial cells, termed endothelin [44], and the cloning and sequence analysis of the complementary DNA of its precursor, preproendothelin [44], has aroused interest in its potential physiologic/pathophysiologic significance. Thus in rats, endothelin infusion elicits a concentration-dependent increase in renal vascular resistance and reduction in GFR [45]. Similarly, in isolated perfused rat kidneys, proportional changes in GFR and RPF have been reported over a wide range of endothelin doses [46]. Preliminary experiments in our laboratories have shown that exposure of bovine aortic endothelial cells in culture to the TxA_2 analogue U-46619 increased the expression of preproendothelin mRNA associated with the synthesis and release of the corresponding peptide in the cell supernatant (C. Zoja, personal communication).

That TxA_2 may modulate endothelin gene expression and synthesis is further supported by the recent observation that the TxA_2 mimetic, U-46619, stimulates preproendothelin mRNA expression and endothelin production also in human glomerular mesangial cells in culture [47]. The demonstration that endothelin gene expression and production in endothelial and mesangial cells is regulated by molecules potentially released at glomerular level during CyA administration, may suggest that endothelin participates in the increased renal vascular resistance caused by the drug. This possibility also rests on the fact that if one compares the effect of endothelin on glomerular hemodynamics [48,49] with the effects reported for CyA [30], the two are very similar. We have recently addressed this issue.

In isolated perfused rat kidneys exposed to a specific anti-endothelin antibody, but not to a non-immunized rabbit serum, CyA-induced fall in renal perfusate flow and GFR were markedly prevented [23]. The role of endogenous endothelin in acute CyA nephrotoxicity has been documented in vivo by studies showing that the infusion of specific endothelin antiserum partially, but significantly, prevented the reduction of GFR and RPF induced by intravenous CyA administration [23]. The micropuncture studies of Kon and coworkers [50] also found that in glomeruli infused with anti-endothelin antibody the vasoconstriction induced by CyA was markedly attenuated. The same authors also reported that in rats serum levels of endothelin studied 20 minutes after the acute injection of CyA were elevated as compared to values in identically instrumented rats not given CyA [50]. Altogether, these data support the notion that increased levels of endothelin and intense microvascular constriction following CyA may reflect a perturbed endothelin synthesis and/or metabolism in the kidney. Since CyA nephrotoxicity encompasses a spectrum of renal damage, which also depends upon the length of treatment, it remains to be determined whether the mediator(s) potentially responsible for the acute vasoconstriction also play a role in the chronic form of renal damage associated with CyA.

Persistent Vasoconstriction as a Cause of Progressive Renal Damage in Chronic CyA Treatment

The chronic renal failure which develops after long-term exposure to the drug [14,51,52] is one of the main clinical problems associated with the administration of CyA to human beings. However, any attempt to define the nature and extent of CyA-associated chronic nephropathy in renal transplants is hampered by the contribution of concomitant chronic rejection. No such difficulties are encountered, however, in cardiac or liver transplant recipients who have healthy native kidneys and are also on long-term CyA treatment. Analysis of the available studies [14,15,51] clearly points to an impairment of renal function in patients chronically treated with CyA, which becomes manifest by the development of persistent azotemia and hypertension.

So far, no clear-cut evidence has been provided as to whether chronic exposure to CyA determines a progressive form of renal damage [53,54]. Heart transplant recipients on CyA for more than 1 year have renal vascular damage, the so-called CyA-associated arteriolopathy, associated segmental or global sclerosis of some glomeruli, and a patchy collagenization of the interstitial compartment [53]. Similar pathological changes except for the severe vascular lesions, have been reported in liver allograft recipients followed for up to 4 years [15]. That persistent renal vasoconstriction plays a central role in chronic CyA nephropathy has been suspected on the basis of elevated renal vascular resistance in cardiac transplant recipients treated with CyA for one year or more [53]. Moreover, since determination of renal arcuate vein occlusion pressure revealed an increasing renal artery-to-peritubular capillary pressure gradient occurring between 1 and 12 months of CyA therapy [53], a predilection for a preglomerular site of increased renovascular resistance in CyA-treated humans has been pointed out.

That the afferent arteriole is indeed the predominant site of increased renovascular resistance in CyA-treated heart transplant recipients was also suggested by the striking elevation of transglomerular dextran transport after both 1–4 weeks and 12 months of therapy [53]. However, in the absence of an experimental model, the precise cause of renal vasoconstriction associated with long-term CyA administration remains speculative. We have recently reported that rats given CyA for 5 months, at the dose of 40 mg/kg on alternate days, had a progressive decrease in GFR associated with pathological changes characterized by glomerular endothelial damage, intracapillary hypercellularity, increased mesangial matrix, diffuse isometric vacuolization in the proximal tubules, and interstitial fibrosis with tubular atrophy [55]. Similarly, other investigators have shown that CyA, at doses of 10 and 20 mg/kg [56] or 12.5 and 25 mg/kg [57], given daily to rats for a long-term period caused renal function deterioration with striped interstitial fibrosis. Of interest, the lack of correlation between the reduction in GFR and proximal tubule abnormalities that we found in our model [55] supports the notion that renal vasoconstriction, rather than tubular injury, is a major factor in chronic experimental CyA nephrotoxicity, as it is in humans.

In order to evaluate whether vasoactive substances previously recognized as participating in the acute form of CyA nephrotoxicity may also play a role in chronic renal vasoconstriction, we have recently measured the urinary excretion of endothelin, taken as a marker of intrarenal synthesis of the peptide [58], in rats chronically given CyA. In contrast to results obtained with vehicle, 30-day CyA administration resulted in significant increase in the urinary excretion of endothelin, measured by radioimmunoassay, as compared to pre-treatment values [59]. Since, in these animals, we found a significant correlation between the urinary excretion of endothelin and the serum creatinine concentration [59], a possible contribution of this vasoactive peptide, also, to chronic CyA nephrotoxicity has been postulated. In addition to being a vasoconstrictor, endothelin has been shown to stimulate 15-lipoxygenase activity leading to 15-hydroxyeicosatetraenoic acid (15-HETE) formation [60]. This compound, 15-HETE, is chemotactic for inflammatory cells [61], and may represent the signal for circulating inflammatory cells and platelets to accumulate within glomerular capillaries, such accumulation being a typical feature of rats chronically given CyA [55]. Activation of inflammatory cells and platelets entrapped within the glomerular tuft could explain the increased levels of urinary TxA_2 metabolites that negatively correlated with GFR values in our model [62].

Since a selective thromboxane synthase inhibitor ameliorated GFR in these animals [62] it has been suggested that TxA_2 plays a role in CyA associated chronic nephropathy. In order to discriminate between the relative contribution of extrarenal versus renal TxA_2 to the observed phenomenon we performed experiments with isolated perfused kidneys prepared from animals previously treated with CyA (30 days). The perfusion procedure removed virtually all the circulating inflammatory cells entrapped within glomerular capillaries [63]. In such conditions the ratio of 2,3-dinor-TxB_2/TxB_2 urinary excretion markedly decreased as compared to the values found in vivo [63]. Since urinary 2,3-dinor-TxB_2 is derived mainly from inflammatory cells and platelets, while urinary TxB_2 is a likely marker of renal TxA_2 synthesis [64], we concluded for an extrarenal source for urinary thromboxane in CyA-treated animals. The observation that chronic CyA administration to rats enhances urinary excretion of TxB_2 has been confirmed by Coffman et al. [65], who found, in a post-ischemic, denervated rat model, a decline in renal function associated with an increase in urinary excretion of 2,3-dinor-TxB_2 and TxB_2. Recently, Kuhn et al. [66], studying 40 patients with multiple sclerosis who received a two-year treatment with CyA (5 mg/kg per day), found an increased urinary excretion of 2,3-dinor-TxB_2 which was accompanied by a significant increase in serum creatinine. Of note, withdrawal of CyA was followed by return of renal function to normal and by a reduction in 2,3-dinor-TxB_2 excretion.

The persistent renal vasoconstriction caused by the increased generation of endothelin and TxA_2 may promote ischemic parenchymal injury associated with structural alteration and eventual obliteration of the renal vessels, which ultimately causes downstream, possibly irreversible, glomerular damage. This natural history of chronic CyA nephrotoxicity has been clearly defined by Myers and coworkers [53] in heart transplant recipients followed up for 48 months. Myers and coworkers found that, despite a stable GFR in the last 2 years, some glomeruli had collapsed and become sclerotic, probably as an effect of ischemia. Moreover, morphometric analysis showed that glomerular ischemic changes were associated with the appearance of small size glomeruli, together with a subset of remaining glomeruli larger than normal, probably compensating in this fashion for the loss of surface area in the damaged glomeruli [53] and contributing to the relative stability of the GFR. Similar findings have recently been reproduced in normal rats during long-term exposure to CyA [67]. Thus, CyA administration for 3 months resulted in a marked reduction of GFR and ischemic glomerular lesions. A complete reconstruction of the glomerular corpuscle, used to evaluate the consequences of CyA-induced renal ischemia on capillary tuft volume, showed that in these rats glomerular volume distribution was shifted toward small glomeruli. Prolongation of CyA administration for 5 months did not result in a further decrease in GFR, and was associated with the appearance of a subpopulation of glomeruli which became larger than normal.

Besides its potent vasoconstrictor activity, evidence now emerges for TxA_2 participation in the development of glomerulosclerosis. Thus, in differentiated teratocarcinoma (F9+) cells in culture, the TxA_2 analog, U46619, induced a dose-dependent increase in several components of the extracellular matrix, including laminin A, B1, and B2 chains [68]. Similarly, U46619 increased type IV collagen ($\alpha 1$ and $\alpha 2$) gene expression in mesangial cells in culture [69]. This is in line with the notion that spatial and temporal expression of specific proteins which constitute the glomerular basement membrane is altered in many forms of glomerular disease, as it can be in chronic CyA glomerulopathy. Indeed, in mice given CyA for 4 weeks, a dose-dependent increase in mRNA expression for protocollagens type I and IV has recently been reported in kidney fibroblasts [70]. In addition to increasing expression of basement membrane components, the TxA_2 mimetic, U-46619, stimulates [^3H]-thymidine uptake in quiescent human mesangial cells in culture [71], suggesting that TxA_2 could contribute to glomerulosclerosis, also inducing the proliferation of mesangial cells.

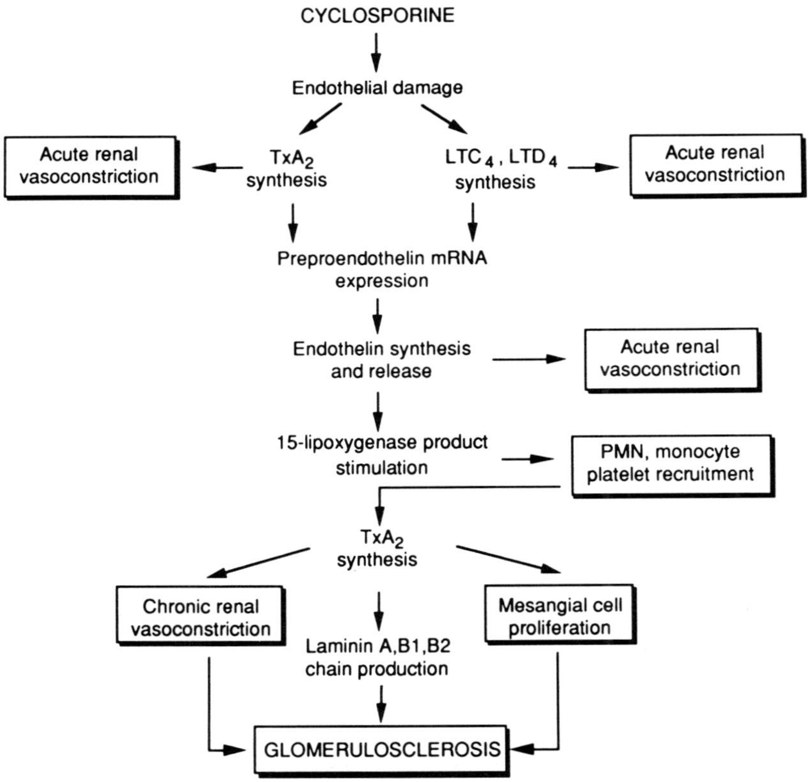

Fig. 1. Proposed mechanisms and mediators of cyclosporine A-induced renal vascular changes: possible link between clinical findings and experimental data. PMN, polymorphonuclear neutrophils

Conclusions

Because of its superior immunosuppressive properties, CyA has become the drug of choice for allograft rejection, and its use in suppressing immune inflammation associated with autoimmune diseases is rapidly increasing. Whereas bone marrow suppression or infections represent limitations to the use of conventional immunosuppressive agents, therapy with CyA is constrained chiefly by the development of protracted acute or progressive chronic renal insufficiency. The initiating event of CyA-induced decline in renal function is probably an intense vasoconstriction as documented by several recent studies that also tried to identify the responsible mechanisms(s) (Fig. 1). Among the potential vasoconstrictors, endothelin and TxA_2 have recently been shown to have pivotal roles in the pathophysiology of both acute and sustained renal vasoconstriction and glomerular dysfunction associated with CyA administration. Drugs that limit the functional consequences of excessive renal generation of endothelin and/or TxA_2 may become effective tools in the future treatment of CyA nephropathy.

Before a method of reducing CyA-induced renal vascular damage becomes available, the theoretical benefits of CyA should be weighed against its adverse effects on the kidney. While the risk of CyA nephropathy might be acceptable for patients with cardiac transplant, as long as no alternative immunosuppressive therapy is practicable, we argue against the use of this molecule in preventing rejection of isolated pancreas graft in non-uremic diabetics [72] and in autoimmune diseases [73] before control trials will convincingly document that the expected benefits overwhelm its toxicity.

References

1. Thomson AW, Whiting PH, Simpson JG (1984) Cyclosporine: immunology, toxicity and pharmacology in experimental animals. Agents and Actions 15:306–327
2. Kronke M, Leonard WJ, Depper JM Arya SK, Wong-Staal F, Gallo RC, Waldmann TA, Greene WC (1984) Cyclosporin A inhibits T-cell growth factor gene expression at level of m-RNA transcription. Proc Natl Acad Sci USA 81:5214–5218
3. Starzl TE, Hakala TR, Rosenthal JT, Arya SK, Wong-Stall F, Gallo RC, Waldmann TA, Greene WC (1983) The Colorado-Pittsburgh cadaveric renal transplantation study with cyclosporine. Transplant Proc 15:2463–2468
4. Oyer PE, Stinson EB, Jamieson SW (1983) Cyclosporine in cardiac transplantation: a 2½ year follow-up. Transplant Proc 15:2546–2549
5. Deeg HJ, Storb R, Thomas ED, Flournoy N, Kennedy MS, Banaji M, Appelbaum FR, Bensinger WI, Bunckner CD, Clift RA, Doney K, Fefer A, McGuffin R, Sanders JE, Singer J, Stewart P, Sullivan KM, Witherspoon RP (1985) Cyclosporine as prophylaxis for graft-versus-host disease: a randomized study in patients undergoing marrow transplantation for acute nonlymphoblastic leukemia. Blood 65:1325–1334
6. Nussenblatt RB, Palestine AG, Chan CC (1983) Cyclosporin A therapy in the treatment of intraocular inflammatory disease resistant to systemic corticosteroids and cytotoxic agents. Am J Ophthalmol 96:275–282
7. Feutren G, Querin S, Chatenoud L, Noel LH, Beaurain G, Tron F, Lesavre P, Bach JF (1985) The effects of cyclosporin in twelve patients with severe systemic lupus. In: Schindler R (ed) Cyclosporin in autoimmune diseases. Springer, New York, pp 366–372

8. Forre O, Bjerkhoel F, Salvesan CF, Berg KJ, Rugstad HE, Saelig G, Mellbye OJ, Kass E (1987) An open, controlled, randomized comparison of cyclosporine azathioprine in the treatment of rheumatoid arthritis: a preliminary report. Arthritis Rheum 30: 88–92
9. Lai KN, Mac-Moune Lai F, Vallance-Owen J (1988) A short-term controlled trial of cyclosporine A in IgA nephropathy. Transplant Proc 20 (Suppl 4):297–303
10. Myers BD (1986) Cyclosporine nephrotoxicity. Kidney Int 30:964–974
11. Kahan BD (1989) Cyclosporine. N Engl J Med 321:1725–1738
12. Salaman JR (1984) Cyclosporine in a renal transplantation: a guide to management. Lancet II:269–271
13. Cohen DJ, Loertscher R, Rubin MF, Tilney NL, Carpenter CB, Strom TB (1984) Cyclosporine: A new immunosuppressive agent for organ transplantation. Ann Intern Med 101:667–682
14. Myers BD, Ross J, Newton L, Leutscher J, Perloth M (1984) Cyclosporine-associated chronic nephropathy. N Engl J Med 311:699–705
15. Dische FE, Neuberger J, Keating J, Parsons V, Calne RY, Williams R (1988) Kidney pathology in liver allograft recipients after long-term treatment with cyclosporin A. Lab Invest 58:395–402
16. Calne RY, White DJG, Thiru S, Evans DB, McMaster P, Dunn DC, Craddock GN, Pentlow BD, Rolles K (1978) Cyclosporin A in patients receiving renal allografts from cadaver donors. Lancet II:1323–1327
17. Flechner SM, van Buren C, Kerman RH, Kahan DB (1983) The nephrotoxicity of cyclosporine in renal transplant recipients. Transplant Proc 15 (Suppl 1):2689–2694
18. Powell-Jackson PR, Young B, Calne RY, Williams R (1983) Nephrotoxicity of parenterally administered cyclosporine after orthotopic liver transplantation. Transplantation 36:505–508
19. Sullivan BA, Hak LJ, Finn WF (1985) Cyclosporine nephrotoxicity: studies in laboratory animals. Transplant Proc 17 (Suppl 1):145–154
20. Humes HD, Jackson NM, O'Connor RP, Hunt DA, White MD (1985) Pathogenetic mechanisms of nephrotoxicity: insights into cyclosporine nephrotoxicity. Transplant Proc 17 (Suppl 1):51–62
21. Murray BM, Paller MS, Ferris TF (1985) Effect of cyclosporine administration on renal hemodynamics in conscious rat. Kidney Int 28:767–774
22. Maack T (1980) Physiological evaluation of the isolated perfused rat kidney. Am J Physiol 238:F71–F78
23. Perico N, Dadan J, Remuzzi G (1990) Endothelin mediates the renal vasoconstriction induced by cyclosporine in the rat. JASN 1:76–83
24. Rossi NF, Churchill PC, McDonald FD, Ellis VR (1989) Mechanism of cyclosporine A-induced renal vasoconstriction in the rat. J Pharmacol Exp Ther 250:896–901
25. English J, Evan A, Houghton DC, Bennett WM (1987) Cyclosporine-induced acute renal dysfunction in the rat. Evidence of arteriolar vasoconstriction with preservation of tubular function. Transplantation 44:135–141
26. Siegl H, Ryffel B, Petric R, Shoemaker P, Muller A, Donatsch P, Mihatsch M (1983) Cyclosporine, the renin-angiotensin-aldosterone system, and renal adverse reactions. Transplant Proc 15 (Suppl 1):2719–2725
27. Baxter CR, Duggin GG, Hall BM, Horvath JS, Tiller DJ (1984) Stimulation of renin release from rat renal cortical slices by cyclosporin A. Res Commun Chem Pathol Pharmacol 43:417–423
28. Perico N, Zoja C, Benigni A, Ghilardi F, Gualandris L, Remuzzi G (1986) Effect of short-term cyclosporine administration in rats on renin-angiotensin and thromboxane A_2: Possible relevance to the reduction in glomerular filtration rate. J Pharmacol Exp Ther 239:229–235

29. Dieperink H, Leyssac PP, Kemp E, Steinbruchel D, Starklint H (1986) Glomerulotubular function in cyclosporine A treated rats. Clin Nephrol 25 (Suppl 1):S70–S74
30. Barros EJG, Boim MA, Ajzen H, Ramos OL, Schor N (1987) Glomerular hemodynamics and hormonal participation in cyclosporine nephrotoxicity. Kidney Int 3:219–225
31. Jao S, Waltzer W, Arbeit LA (1986) Acute cyclosporine induced decrease in GFR is mediated by changes in renal blood flow and renal vascular resistance. Kidney Int 29:431
32. Moss NG, Powell SL, Falk RJ (1985) Intravenous cyclosporine activates afferent and efferent renal nerves and causes sodium retention in innervated kidneys in rats. Proc Natl Acad Sci USA 82:8222–8226
33. Gazdar AF, Dammin GJ (1970) Neural degeneration and regeneration in human renal transplants. N Engl J Med 283:222–224
34. Whisler RL, Lindsey JA, Proctor KVM, Morisaki N, Cornwell DG (1984) Characteristics of cyclosporine induction of increased prostaglandin levels from human peripheral blood monocytes. Transplantation 38:377–381
35. Lindsey JA, Morisaki N, Stitts JM, Zager RA, Cornwell DG (1983) Fatty acid metabolism and cell proliferation. IV. Effect of prostanoid biosynthesis from endogenous fatty acid release with cyclosporin A. Lipids 18:566–569
36. Scharschmidt LA, Lianos E, Dunn MJ (1983) Arachidonate metabolites and the control of glomerular function. Fed Proc 42:3058–3063
37. Badr KF, Baylis C, Pfeffer JM, Pfeffer MA, Soberman RJ, Lewis RA, Austen KF, Corey EJ, Brenner BM (1984) Renal and systemic hemodynamic responses to intravenous infusion of leukotriene C_4 in the rat. Circ Res 54:492–499
38. Baylis C (1987) Effects of administered thromboxanes on the intact, normal rat kidney. Renal Physiol 10:110–121
39. Menè P, Dunn MJ (1986) Contractile effects of TxA_2 and endoperoxide analogues on cultured rat glomerular mesangial cells. Am J Physiol 251:F1029–F1035
40. Zoja C, Furci L, Ghilardi F, Zilio P, Benigni A, Remuzzi G (1986) Cyclosporin-induced endothelial cell injury. Lab Invest 55:455–462
41. Pasini M, Perico N, Remuzzi G (1990) Roles for thromboxane $(Tx)A_2$ and sulfidopeptide leukotrienes (LT) in cyclosporine (CsA)-induced acute renal failure. Kidney Int 37:350
42. Schlondorff D, Ardaillou R (1986) Prostaglandins and other arachidonic acid metabolites in the kidney. Kidney Int 29:108–119
43. Rosenthal A, Pace-Asciak CR (1983) Potent vasoconstriction of the isolated perfused rat kidney by leukotrienes C_4 and D_4. Can J Physiol Pharmacol 61:325–328
44. Yanagisawa M, Kurihara H, Kimura S, Tombe Y, Kobayashi M, Mitsui Y, Yazaki Y, Goto K, Masaki T (1988) A novel potent vasoconstrictor peptide produced by vascular endothelial cells. Nature 332:411–415
45. King AJ, Brenner BM, Anderson S (1989) Endothelin: a potent renal and systemic vasoconstrictor peptide. Am J Physiol 256:F1051–F1058
46. Perico N, Dadan J, Gabanelli M, Remuzzi G (1990) Cyclooxygenase products and atrial natriuretic peptide modulate renal response to endothelin. J Pharmacol Exp Ther 252:1213–1220
47. Zoja C, Orisio S, Perico N, Benigni A, Morigi M, Benatti L, Rambaldi A, Remuzzi G (to be published) Constitutive expression of endothelin gene in cultured human mesangial cells and its modulation by transforming growth factor β, thrombin and a thromboxane A_2 analogue. Lab Invest
48. Badr KF, Murray JJ, Breyer MD, Takahashi K, Inagami T, Harris RC (1989) Mesangial cell, glomerular and renal vascular responses to endothelin in the rat kidney. J Clin Invest 83:336–342
49. Kon V, Yoshioka T, Fogo A, Ichikawa I (1989) Glomerular actions of endothelin in vivo. J Clin Invest 83:1762–1767

50. Kon V, Sugiura M, Inagami T, Harvie R, Ichikawa I, Hoover RL (1990) Role of endothelin in cyclosporine-induced glomerular dysfunction. Kidney Int 37:1487–1491
51. Moran M, Tomlanovich S, Myers BD (1985) Cyclosporine-induced chronic nephropathy in human recipients of cardiac allografts. Transplant Proc 17 (Suppl 1):185–190
52. Remuzzi G, Bertani T (1989) Renal vascular and thrombotic effects of cyclosporine. Am J Kidney Dis 13:261–272
53. Myers BD, Newton L, Boshkos C, Macoviak JA, Frist WH, Derby GC, Perlroth MG, Sibley RK (1988) Chronic injury of human renal microvessels with low-dose cyclosporine therapy. Transplantation 46:694–703
54. Bantle JP, Paller MS, Boudreau RJ, Olivari MT, Ferris TF (1990) Long-term effects of cyclosporine on renal function in organ transplant recipients. J Lab Clin Med 115:233–240
55. Bertani T, Perico N, Abbate M, Battaglia C, Remuzzi G (1987) Renal injury induced by long-term administration of cyclosporin A to rats. Am J Pathol 127:569–579
56. Simpson JG, Saunders NJ, Thompson KJ, Whiting PH (1988) Chronic renal damage caused by cyclosporine. Transplant Proc 20 (Suppl 3):792–799
57. Dieperink H, Leyssac PP, Starklint H, Kemp E (1988) Long-term cyclosporin nephrotoxicity in the rat: Effect on renal function and morphology. Nephrol Dial Transpl 3:317–326
58. Benigni A, Perico N, Gaspari F, Zoja C, Bellizzi L, Gabanelli M, Remuzzi G (to be published) Increased renal endothelin production in rats with reduced renal mass. Am J Physiol
59. Perico N, Benigni A, Ladny R, Imberti O, Bellizzi L, Remuzzi G (1990) Chronic cyclosporine A (CyA) administration to rats increases urinary excretion of big-endothelin and endothelin. American Society of Nephrology Conference 1990
60. Nagase T, Fukuchi Y, Jo C, Teramoto S, Uejima Y, Ishida K, Shimizu T, Orimo H (1990) Endothelin-1 stimulates arachidonate 15-lipoxygenase activity and oxygen radical formation in the rat distal lung. Biochem Biophys Res Commun 168:485–489
61. Goetzl EJ, Pickett WC (1980) The human PMN leukocyte chemotactic activity of complex hydroxy-eicosatetraenoic acids (HETEs). J Immunol 125:1789–1791
62. Perico N, Benigni A, Zoja C, Delaini F, Remuzzi G (1986) Functional significance of exaggerated renal thromboxane A_2 synthesis induced by cyclosporin A. Am J Physiol 251: F581–F587
63. Benigni A, Chiabrando C, Piccinelli A, Perico N, Gavinelli M, Furci L, Patino O, Abbate M, Bertani T, Remuzzi G (1988) Increased urinary excretion of thromboxane B_2 in cyclosporin A nephrotoxicity. Kidney Int 34:164–174
64. FitzGerald GA, Pedersen AK, Patrono C (1983) Analysis of prostacyclin and thromboxane biosynthesis in cardiovascular disease. Circulation 67:1174–1177
65. Coffman TM, Carr DR, Varger WE, Klotman PE (1987) Evidence that renal prostaglandin and thromboxane production is stimulated in chronic cyclosporine nephrotoxicity. Transplantation 43:282–285
66. Kuhn K, Forstermann U, Frolich JC, Verterqvist O, Green K, Brunkhorst R, Koch KM, Haas J (1987) Effect of cyclosporine A (CyA) on blood pressure and prostacyclin and thromboxane A_2 production. Xth International congress of nephrology, July 26–31 1987. London, United Kingdom p 231
67. Perico N, Imberti O, Remuzzi A, Cavallotti D, Bertani T, Remuzzi G (1990) Distribution of glomerular capillary tuft volume in rats chronically treated with cyclosporine (CsA). Proceedings of the XIth international congress of nephrology, July 15–20 1990. Tokyo, Japan pp 438A
68. Klotmann P, Bruggeman L, Hassell J, Horigan E, Martin G, Yamada Y (1989) Regulation of extracellular matrix by thromboxane. Kidney Int 35:294
69. Bruggeman LA, Burbelo PD, Yamada Y, Klotman PE (1990) Regulation of renal transcriptional factors for type IV collagen gene expression by thromboxane. Proceedings of the XIth international congress of nephrology, July 15–20 1990. Tokyo, Japan pp 30A

70. Wolf G, Neilson EG (1990) Cyclosporine A (CyA) stimulates secretion of collagen IV in murine proximal tubular cells and of collagen I in kidney fibroblasts. Proceedings of the XIth international congress of nephrology, July 15–20 1990. Tokyo, Japan pp 50A
71. Menè P, Dubyak GR, Abboud HE, Scarpa A, Dunn MJ (1988) Mitogenic activity and intracellular signals for thromboxane A_2 in cultured human mesangial cells. Clin Res 36:627A
72. Sutherland DER, Kendall DM, Moudry KC (1988) Pancreas transplantation in non-uremic type I diabetic recipients. Surgery 104:453–464
73. Tegzess AM, Doornbos BM, Minderhound JM, Donker AJ (1988) Prospective serial function studies in patients with nonrenal disease treated with cyclosporine A. Transplant Proc 20 (Suppl 2):390–393

Animal Models of Cyclosporine Nephrotoxicity

Thomas M. Coffman[1]

Introduction

Cyclosporine nephrotoxicity is a significant clinical problem which has limited the therapeutic applications of this potent immunosuppressive agent. Most of the clinical experience defining cyclosporine nephrotoxicity has been in heart, liver and kidney transplant recipients. Since there are a number of factors which influence renal hemodynamics in these patients which are independent of cyclosporine, it has been difficult to isolate specific renal effects attributable to cyclosporine in these patient groups. Thus, much of what is known about the mechanisms of cyclosporine toxicity has been contributed through the development of animal models. The large number of potential cellular and molecular mechanisms of cyclosporine toxicity have been exhaustively reviewed recently [1,2]. In this paper, I will focus on animal models of cyclosporine nephrotoxicity and highlight similarities and differences between these animal models and cyclosporine toxicity in humans.

Clinical Syndromes of Cyclosporine A (CyA) Nephrotoxicity

The two most common clinical syndromes of cyclosporine nephrotoxicity can be broadly divided into acute reversible renal vasoconstriction and chronic irreversible nephropathy. Acute cyclosporine nephrotoxicity is most commonly observed within the first six to twelve months of initiating therapy and is characterized by acute or sub-acute reduction in renal function that is often dose dependent. Generally, this renal dysfunction is non-progressive and reverses with dose reduction or discontinuation of the drug. In renal allograft recipients, it is often difficult to differentiate acute cyclosporine nephrotoxicity from acute rejection. Renal biopsy can be helpful in this setting since aggressive inflammatory cell infiltrates are usually absent in

[1]RM. B3002-Nephrology (111I), VA Medical Center, Durham, NC 27705, USA

acute cyclosporine nephrotoxicity. Further, even stable allograft recipients who have been taking cyclosporine for periods exceeding twelve months will almost invariably manifest some reversible renal dysfunction which is apparent when cyclosporine is discontinued.

Chronic cyclosporine nephropathy is defined by the development of interstitial fibrosis and irreversible reduction in renal function. This form of nephrotoxicity is more ominous than the acute form and is most commonly observed after six to twelve months of therapy [3]. Morphologically, chronic cyclosporine nephropathy is characterized by focal or striped interstitial fibrosis with tubular atrophy [4a]. Often these changes are accompanied by obliterative arteriolar lesions. In more advanced cases, diffuse interstitial fibrosis accompanied by focal and segmental glomerular sclerosis may be seen. In some patients, renal fibrosis and loss of renal function may be progressive [5]. In renal allograft recipients, both the clinical presentation as well as histomorphologic findings in chronic cyclosporine nephropathy are similar to those of chronic rejection. These similarities have made it difficult to identify the role of cyclosporine in producing progressive renal injury in these patients.

While at the extremes these two clinical syndromes are distinct, there is significant overlap of features of both acute and chronic cyclosporine nephrotoxicity in individual patients. Furthermore, the causal relationship between the two syndromes is not clear. Although it has been suggested that chronic renal vasoconstriction and ischemia may produce fibrosis and irreversible renal injury in cyclosporine nephrotoxicity, this has not been proven and would be difficult to establish in clinical trials. Thus, animal models have been developed to attempt to uncover the mechanisms underlying cyclosporine's toxic effects in the kidney. Generally, it has been much easier to reproduce acute reversible renal vasoconstriction in animals than chronic nephropathy. However, several recent reports describe animal models which resemble chronic cyclosporine toxicity in humans [6–10].

Animal Models of Acute and Chronic Cyclosporine Nephrotoxicity

The effects of cyclosporine on the kidney have been evaluated in a number of species including rats, mice, dogs, goats, pigs, and sheep. However, the vast majority of published studies have used rat models and no other species studied present any particular advantage in terms of similarities to the human system. Although CyA pharmacokinetics are very similar in rats and humans [11], the doses of cyclosporine that are required to produce renal dysfunction in rats are generally much higher than those used in patients. The reasons for the rat's resistance to the nephrotoxic effects of CyA have been related to the increased ratio of kidney weight to body weight and increased GFR per kidney weight in rats compared to humans [11]. Despite the difference in dose required to produce nephrotoxicity, there are a number of qualitative similarities in cyclosporine's effects on renal hemodynamics in rats and humans.

As mentioned above, the acute effects of cyclosporine on renal function have been fairly easy to reproduce in animal models. For example, Murray and associates showed that intravenous infusion of cyclosporine to rats produced rapid reduction in renal blood flow and glomerular filtration rate associated with an increase in renal

Table 1. Rat models of chronic cyclosporine nephrotoxicity

Author	CyA dose	Description
Gillum et al.	25 mg/kg per day IP for 28 days	Focal interstitial fibrosis and tubular atrophy, interstitial inflammation and JG hypertrophy
Dieperink et al.	14 mg/kg per day PO for 26 weeks	40% of CyA treated rats developed striped IF
Simpson et al.	20 mg/kg per day for 28–84 days	Striped IF
Rosen et al.	12.5 mg/kg per day SQ for 3–10 weeks	Striped medullary fibrosis in salt depleted animals
Elzinga et al.	15 mg/kg per day SQ for 14–28 days	Tubulointerstitial nephropathy with striped IF in salt depleted animals; progression of IF after CyA withdrawn

vascular resistance [12]. A number of investigators subsequently showed that more prolonged oral or parenteral administration of cyclosporine to rats also caused renal dysfunction. Friedman and associates have shown that CyA has a similar effect on renal hemodynamics in sheep [13]. In studies by Perico et al., rats developed progressive deterioration in renal function over three months when cyclosporine was administered 40 mg/kg every other day [14]. After three months, the cyclosporine was discontinued and GFR rapidly returned to baseline levels. Thus, as in humans, the effects of CyA on renal hemodynamics in rats are reversible when the drug is discontinued.

Early studies of the effects of cyclosporine on the rat kidney focused on the observation of structural abnomalities in the proximal tubule, which included vacuolization and the development of giant mitochondria in proximal tubule cells [15]. Therefore, it was hypothesized that the primary effects of cyclosporine on renal function occurred as a result of this apparent tubular toxicity. However, English et al. subsequently showed that the effect of cyclosporine on renal function in rats was mediated primarily by hemodynamic factors [16]. These authors found that 50 mg/kg per day of cyclosporine caused a progressive fall in glomerular filtration rate without any change in fractional lithium excretion or development of enzymuria which might indicate ongoing tubular injury. In addition, casts made of the renal microvasculature showed a progressive reduction in the diameter of afferent arterioles to less than 50% of control after 14 days of treatment. Studies in humans have also failed to support a significant role for tubular toxicity in CyA associated renal dysfunction.

Although cyclosporine-induced renal vasoconstriction has been relatively easy to reproduce in animals, development of models of chronic cyclosporine nephropathy has been more difficult. Several groups have reported chronic treatment of rats with toxic doses of cyclosporine and have observed only minimal histomorphologic abnormalities [14,17,18]. More recently, several reports have appeared which describe the development of renal fibrosis in rats treated with cyclosporine [6–10]. These papers are summarized in Table 1. In several of these studies rats developed striped interstitial fibrosis which was similar to that described in patients with chronic cyclosporine nephropathy. While these papers have been largely descriptive, the existence of rat models of chronic cyclosporine injury may provide avenues for unravelling the mechanisms of this clinically devastating syndrome. Of particular interest are the

Table 2. Potential mediators of CyA-associated renal vasoconstriction

Sympathetic nervous system
Renin-angiotensin system
Reduced production of vasodilator prostanoids
Increased production of thromboxane A_2
Platelet activating factor
Sulfidopeptide leukotrienes
Endothelin

CyA, cyclosporine A

studies of Rosen et al. [9] and Elzinga et al. [10] which suggest that the development of fibrosis is accelerated by sodium depletion. Furthermore, in the model described by Elzinga, renal fibrosis did not remit when cyclosporine was discontinued. This phenomenon has also been observed in humans.

Mechanisms of Renal Vasoconstriction

Some of the proposed mechanisms of renal vasoconstriction caused by cyclosporine are shown in Table 2. A role for increased activity of the sympathetic nervous system was suggested by Moss et al. [19] who demonstrated increased activity of both efferent and afferent renal nerves in rats receiving intravenous infusions of cyclosporine. Murray and associates showed that renal denervation or treatment with the alpha sympathetic antagonists phenoxybenzamine and prazosin could lessen the degree of renal dysfunction caused by intravenous infusions of cyclosporine in rats [12,20]. Evidence for a role of the sympathetic nervous system in cyclosporine nephrotoxicity in humans is not as compelling. Clearly, cyclosporine nephrotoxicity can occur very soon after renal transplantation before re-innervation of the allograft would be expected to occur. In addition, clinical studies have failed to demonstrate beneficial effects of alpha sympathetic antagonists on renal function in cyclosporine treated renal allograft recipients [21].

There is evidence in both rat and human systems to support a role for altered arachidonic acid metabolism in cyclosporine toxicity. For example, in vitro studies have suggested that cyclosporine may inhibit prostaglandin production [22] and it was hypothesized that this reduced production of vasodilator prostanoids might lead to renal dysfunction. A physiologic role for vasodilator prostanoids was also suggested by the observation that cyclo-oxygenase inhibition exacerbated renal vasoconstriction caused by cyclosporine [12]. However, in vivo inhibition of vasodilator prostaglandins in rats treated with cyclosporine has not been observed [12,17]. Alternatively, pharmacologic doses of stable prostaglandin analogues ameliorate cyclosporine nephrotoxicity in rats [23,24]. For example, Paller showed that 100 μg/kg of the PGEl analogue misoprostol increased GFR and renal blood flow and reduced renal vascular resistance in cyclosporine treated rats [23]. Kobayashi et al. demonstrated a similar beneficial effect of a stable prostacyclin analogue in another rat model of cyclosporine nephrotoxicity [24]. Efficacy of prostaglandin analogues has also been demonstrated in human renal allograft recipients. Moran et al. showed that renal function in cyclosporine treated renal allograft recipients was improved significantly in patients who also received misoprostol 200 μg four times per day compared to patients who received placebo [25]. In this study, there were no differences in the number of "acute" episodes of cyclosporine nephrotoxicity between the groups. However, the observed differences in long term graft function may reflect a beneficial effect of misoprostol to lessen renal vasoconstriction.

In addition to the potential role of perturbations in the production of vasodilator prostanoids, a number of groups have demonstrated increased production of the vasoconstrictor eicosanoid thromboxane A2 in rats with cyclosporine toxicity [14,17,26,27]. Perico et al. first showed that this increase in thromboxane production is physiologically important by demonstrating an improvement in renal function in cyclosporine toxic rats treated with a thromboxane synthase inhibitor [14]. Several other groups have confirmed this finding. In addition, our group has shown that a thromboxane receptor antagonist had a similar beneficial effect [27]. In our study, intravenous administration of the thromboxane receptor antagonist GR32191 increased GFR and renal blood flow and reduced renal vascular resistance to control levels. We have recently completed a study which suggests that thromboxane may also be important in patients with cyclosporine nephrotoxicity [28]. In this study of cyclosporine-treated renal allograft recipients, we found that urinary excretion of the thromboxane metabolites TXB2 and 2,3 dinor TXB2 were significantly increased in cyclosporine treated patients compared to controls. Intravenous infusions of the thromboxane synthase inhibitor CGS 13080 increased renal plasma flow in eight of the ten patients.

Fish oil supplementation, a non-pharmacologic intervention which also alters arachidonic acid metabolism, has been similarly effective in ameliorating cyclosporine nephrotoxicity. Elzinga et al. have shown in a rat model that by using fish oil as the vehicle for cyclosporine, nephrotoxicity was dramatically reduced [29]. This improvement in renal function was associated with reduced renal cortical thromboxane production. A similar beneficial effect of fish oil in humans was shown by van der Heide [30]. This group found that dietary fish oil supplements improved GFR and renal plasma flow in cyclosporine treated renal allograft recipients. Corn oil supplements had no effect in these patients.

A role for the renin-angiotensin system in cyclosporine mediated renal vasoconstriction has also been postulated [1]. Several groups have reported increased plasma renin activity in rats treated with cyclosporine [12]. Cyclosporine has also been found to stimulate renin release from renal cortical slices [31] and isolated juxtaglomerular cells [32]. However, there have been conflicting reports regarding the efficacy of angiotensin converting enzyme inhibitors in rat models of cyclosporine nephrotoxicity. In addition, plasma renin activity is suppressed in cardiac and renal transplant patients treated with cyclosporine [33]. In renal allograft recipients, the renin-angiotensin system has also been shown to be relatively unresponsive to stimulatory maneuvers such as captopril and diuretics, or changes in posture [34]. Thus, support for a significant role of the renin-angiotensin system is uncertain.

Other isolated reports have suggested the potential involvement of other vasoactive compounds in cyclosporine nephrotoxicity. Santos et al. have demonstrated a beneficial effect of platelet activating factor antagonist on glomerular hemodynamics in rats given cyclosporine [35]. Pasini et al. have shown that a petidoleukotriene antagonist blunts the fall in GFR and renal blood flow caused by 50 mg/kg of cyclosporine given by IV injection [36]. Circulating levels of endothelin have been found to be elevated in rats treated with cyclosporine [37]. In addition, anti-endothelin antibodies given to rats in vivo or in isolated perfused rat kidneys prevent cyclosporine induced renal dysfunction [38]. The relevance of these observations to cyclosporine nephrotoxicity in humans remains to be explored.

Potential Role for Cyclophilin in Nephrotoxicity

Although the molecular mechanisms of cyclosporine's immunosuppressive properties have not been completely defined, recent studies have implicated a 17 kD cyclosporine binding protein as being important in this process [39]. This protein, which has been named cyclophilin, binds avidly and specifically to cyclosporine. It also has peptidyl-prolyl-cis-trans isomerase (PPIase) activity which is inhibited by cyclosporine binding [40]. This PPIase activity is thought to be important in the refolding of proteins. It has been suggested that inhibition of cyclophilin's PPIase activity by cyclosporine may be a mechanism of its immunosuppressive effects. For example, PPIase inhibition may interfere with the conformational assembly of DNA binding proteins which are involved in the transcriptional regulation of genes that are important in generating immune responses, such as interleukin-2.

A role for cyclophilin in animal models of cyclosporine nephrotoxicity has not been explored. However, there are at least three lines of indirect evidence that suggest that cyclophilin and inhibition of its PPIase activity might play a role in cyclosporine nephrotoxicity. Although cyclophilin is present in highest quantities in immune cells, kidney, brain, and liver all contain significant amounts of cyclophilin as well [41]. These organs also represent the three major targets for clinically important toxicities. In addition, the immunosuppressive properties of cyclosporine analogues correlate with cyclophilin binding and, thus far, the major immunosuppressive cyclosporine analogues also appear to be nephrotoxic. Finally, the activity of the new and very potent immunosuppressive agent FK506 also appears to depend on binding to its own specific binding protein which is also a PPIase [42]. The new agent FK506 also causes nephrotoxicity [43,44]. Studies in a rat model showed that renal dysfunction produced by the combination of low doses of cyclosporine and FK506 was greater than that produced by either agent alone [43]. Furthermore, this synergistic nephrotoxicity was also observed in liver transplant patients who were given FK506 as rescue therapy [44]. When FK506 and cyclosporine were being administered simultaneously, patients uniformly developed severe renal toxicities. While the information suggesting that inhibition of certain PPIase enzymes might produce renal toxicity is circumstantial, this area certainly deserves further consideration and study.

Conclusions

Animal models have been useful in defining the mechanisms of cyclosporine induced renal vasoconstriction. These studies suggest that there are similarities in renal hemodynamic responses to cyclosporine in rats compared to humans. Interventions such as treatment with prostaglandin analogues, thromboxane inhibition, and fish oil supplementation are effective in reversing renal hemodynamic abnormalities in both rats and humans treated with cyclosporine. Recent development of models of chronic cyclosporine nephropathy may allow for the definition of the events which lead to this most serious clinical manifestation of cyclosporine renal toxicity. The role of PPIase inhibition in cyclosporine nephrotoxicity is not known; however, there is indirect evidence suggesting its involvement in producing renal dysfunction in this setting.

References

1. Remuzzi G, Bertani T (1989) Renal vascular and thrombotic effects of cyclosporine. Am J Kidney Dis 13:261–272
2. Kopp JB, Klotman PE (1990) Cellular and molecular mechanisms of cyclosporin nephrotoxicity. JASN 1:162–179
3. Ruiz P, Kolbeck PC, Scroggs MW, Sanfilippo F (1988) Associations between cyclosporine therapy and interstitial fibrosis in renal allograft biopsies. Transplantation 45:91–95
4. Myers BD, Sibley R, Newton L, Tomlanovich SJ, Boshkos C, Stinson E, Luetscher JA, Whitney DJ, Krasny D, Coplon NS, Perlroth MG (1988) Kidney Int 33:590–600

4a. Mihatsch MJ, Thiel G, Ryffel B (1988) Histopathology of cyclosporine nephrotoxicity. Transplant Proc 20:759–771

5. Myers BD, Ross J, Newton L, Luetscher J, Perlroth M (1984) Cyclosporine-associated chronic nephropathy. N Engl J Med 311:699–705
6. Gillum DM, Truong L, Tasby J, Migliore P, Suki WN (1988) Chronic cyclosporine nephrotoxicity. Transplantation 46:285–292
7. Dieperink H, Kemp E, Starklint H (1988) Cyclosporine A in high dosages induces renal interstitial fibrosis in the rat. Transplant Proc 20:525–527
8. Simpson JG, Saunders NJ, Thompson KJ, Whiting PH (1988) Chronic renal damage caused by cyclosporine. Transplant Proc 20:792–799
9. Rosen S, Greenfeld Z, Brezis M (1990) Chronic cyclosporine-induced nephropathy in the rat. Transplantation 49:445–452
10. Elzinga LW, Rosen S, Porter GA, Bennett WM (1990) Progression of chronic cyclosporine tubulointerstitial nephropathy despite functional improvement by CSA withdrawal (abstract). Proc XIth Int Congress Nephrol, July 15–20 1990. Tokyo, Japan.
11. Sullivan BA, Hak LJ, Finn WF (1985) Cyclosporine nephrotoxicity: studies in laboratory animals. Transplant Proc 17:145–154
12. Murray BM, Paller MS, Ferris TF (1985) Effect of cyclosporine administration on renal hemodynamics in conscious rats. Kidney Int 28:767–774
13. Friedman AL, Kahng KU, Monaco DO, Rosen BD, Wait RB (1988) Cyclosporine nephrotoxicity in conscious sheep. Transplant Proc 20:595–602
14. Perico N, Benigni A, Zoja C, Delaini F, Remuzzi G (1986) Functional significance of exaggerated renal thromboxane A_2 synthesis induced by cyclosporin A. Am J Physiol 20:F581–F587
15. Thomson AW, Whiting PH, Simpson JG (1984) Cyclosporine: immunology, toxicity and pharmacology in experimental animals. Agents Actions 15:306–327
16. English J, Andrew E, Houghton DC, Bennett WM (1987) Cyclosporine-induced acute renal dysfunction in the rat. Transplantation 44:135–141
17. Coffman TM, Carr DR, Yarger WE, Klotman PE (1987) Evidence that renal prostaglandin and thromboxane production is stimulated in chronic cyclosporine nephrotoxicity. Transplantation 43:282–285
18. Jackson NM, Hsu C-H, Visscher GE, Venkatachalam MA, Humes HD (1987) Alterations in renal structure and function in a rat model of cyclosporine nephrotoxicity. J Pharmacol Exp Ther 242:749–756

19. Moss NG, Powell SL, Falk RJ (1985) Intravenous cyclosporine activates afferent and efferent renal nerves and causes sodium retention in innervated kidneys in rats. Proc Natl Acad Sci USA 82:8222–8226
20. Murray BM, Paller MS (1986) Beneficial effects of renal denervation and prazosin on GFR and renal blood flow after cyclosporine in rats. Clin Nephrol 25:S37–S39
22. Neild GH, Rocchi G, Imaberti L, Fumagalli F, Brown Z, Remuzzi G, Williams DG (1983) Effect of cyclosporine on prostacyclin synthesis by vascular tissue in rabbits. Transplant Proc 4:2398–2400
23. Paller MS (1988) Effects of the prostaglandin E_1 analog misoprostol on cyclosporine nephrotoxicity. Transplantation 45:1126–1131
24. Kobayashi M, Takaya S, Koie H (1988) Effect of a stable analogue of prostacyclin on cyclosporine A-induced nephrotoxicity: morphological qualitative and quantitative studies. Transplant Proc 20:183–186
25. Moran M, Mozes MF, Maddus MS, Veremis S, Bartkus C, Ketel B, Pollak R, Wallemark C, Jonasson O (1990) Prevention of acute graft rejection by the prostaglandin E_1 analogue misoprostol in renal-transplant recipients treated with cyclosporine and prednisone. N Engl J Med 322:1183–1188
25a. Pirotzky E, Colliez P, Guilmard C, Schaeverbeke J, Braquet P (1988) Cyclosporine-induced nephrotoxicity: preventive effect of a PAF-acether antagonist, BN52063. Transplant Proc 20:665–669
26. Petric R, Freeman D, Wallace C, McDonald J, Stiller C, Keown P (1988) Effect of cyclosporine on urinary prostanoid excretion, renal blood flow, and glomerulotubular function. Transplantation 45:883–889
27. Spurney RF, Mavros SD, Collins D, Ruiz P, Klotman PE, Coffman T (1990) Thromboxane receptor blockade improves cyclosporine nephrotoxicity in rats. Prostaglandins 39:135–146
28. Coffman TM, Smith SR, Creech EA, Schaffer AV, Martin LL, Rakhit A, Douglas FL, Klotman PE (1989) The thromboxane synthetase inhibitor CGS13080 improves renal allograft function in patients taking cyclosporine. Kidney Int 37:604A
29. Elzinga L, Kelley VE, Houghton DC, Bennett WM (1987) Modification of experimental nephrotoxicity with fish oil as the vehicle for cyclosporine. Transplantation 43:271–274
30. van der Heide JJH, Bilo HJG, Tegzess AM, Donker AJM (1990) The effects of dietary supplementation with fish oil on renal function in cyclosporine-treated renal transplant recipients. Transplantation 49:523–527
31. Baxter CR, Duggin GG, Hall BM, et al. (1984) Stimulation of renin release from rat renal cortical slices by cyclosporin A. Res Commun Chem Pathol Pharmacol 43:417–423
32. Kurtz A, Della Bruna R, Kuhn K (1988) Cyclosporine A enhances renin secretion and production in isolated juxtaglomerular cells. Kidney Int 33:947–953
33. Schuler S, Thomas D, Hetzer R (1987) Cyclosporine A-related nephrotoxicity after cardiac transplantation: the role of plasma renin activity. Transplant Proc 29:3998–4001
34. Curtis JJ, Luke RG, Jones P, et al. (1988) Hypertension in cyclosporine-treated renal transplant recipients is sodium dependent. Am J Med 85:134–138
35. Santos OFPD, Boim MA, Bregman R, Draibe SA, Barros EJG, Pirotzky E, Schor N, Braquet P (1998) Effect of platelet-activating factor antagonist on cyclosporine nephrotoxicity. Transplantation 47:592–595
36. Pasini M, Perico N, Remuzzi G (1989) Roles for thromboxane and sulfidopeptide leukotrienes in cyclosporine-induced acute renal failure. Kidney Int 37:350A
37. Dadan J, Perico N, Remuzzi G (1989) Role of endothelin in cyclosporine-induced renal vasoconstriction. Kidney Int 37:479A

38. Kon V, Sugiura M, Inagami T, Hoover RL, Fogo A, Harvie BR, Ichikawa I (1989) Cyclosporine causes endothelin-dependent acute renal failure. Kidney Int 37:486A
39. Harding MW, Handschumacher RE (1988) Cyclophilin, a primary molecular target for cyclosporine (1988) Transplantation 46:29S–35S
40. Takahashi N, Hyano T, Suzuki M (1989) Peptidyl-prolyl cis-trans isomerase is the cyclosporin A-binding protein cyclophilin. Nature 337:473–475
41. Koletsky AJ, Harding MW, Handschumacher RE (1986) Cyclophilin: distribution and variant properties in normal and neoplastic tissues. J Immunol 137:1054–1059
42. Harding MW, Galat A, Uehling DE, Schreiber SL (1989) A receptor for the immunosuppressant FK506 is a cis-trans peptidyl-prolyl isomerase. Nature 341:758–760
43. Nalesnik MA, Lai HS, Murase N, Todo S, Starzl TE (1990) The effect of FK 506 and CyA on the Lewis rat renal ischemia model. Transplant Proc 22:87–89
44. McCauley J, Fung J, Jain A, Todo S, Starzl TE (1990) The effects of FK 506 on renal function after liver transplantation. Transplant Proc 22:17–20

Clinical Aspects of Cyclosporine Nephrotoxicity

William M. Bennett[1]

Summary. Nephrotoxicity is the major adverse effect of the valuable immunosuppressive drug cyclosporine. The pharmacology and pharmacokinetic behavior of cyclosporine is complex; clinically relevant considerations, including drug interactions, are covered in this paper. In addition, the major clinical syndromes associated with cyclosporine nephrotoxicity are discussed. These include initial oligoanuria after renal transplant, acute reversible episodes of renal dysfunction, chronic nephrotoxicity with tubulointerstitial fibrosis, hemolytic-uremic syndrome, hypertension, and electrolyte disturbances. An algorithm for distinguishing renal dysfunction due to allograft rejection from acute cyclosporine nephrotoxicity is proposed, since this distinction continues to be a difficult problem for nephrologists. Although therapeutic drug monitoring using blood or plasma cyclosporine levels has not fulfilled its promise, practical guidelines for the use of these studies are presented.

Cyclosporine has emerged has emerged as the mainstay of most transplant immunosuppressive protocols over the past five years. This unique cyclic peptide, containing eleven amino acids, has become the primary immunosuppressive agent in recipients of heart, kidney, liver, heart-lung, and bone marrow allografts. In addition, there are expanding indications for cyclosporine in a wide variety of diseases thought to have an autoimmune or immunologic pathogenesis. This paper will review clinical aspects of cyclosporine nephrotoxicity, the most important adverse reaction observed with this valuable drug. The use of therapeutic drug monitoring as well as important drug interactions will be covered.

Clinically Relevant Pharmacology

Cyclosporine is a neutral hydrophobic compound which selectively inhibits activated lymphocyte function and interleukin-2 mediated events. It is a cyclic undecapeptide

[1]Division of Nephrology and Hypertension L463, Oregon Health Sciences University, 3181 S.W. Sam Jackson Park Road, Portland, OR 97201, USA

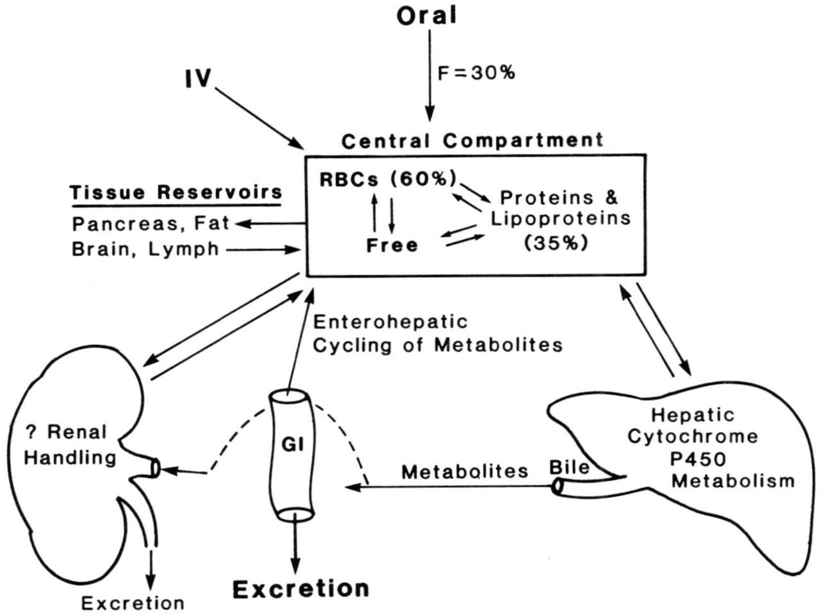

Fig. 1. Cyclosporine pharmacokinetics

produced in cultures as a metabolite of the fungal species *Tolypocladium inflatum gams*. Molecular weight is 1202 Daltons.

Cyclosporine pharmacokinetics are schematically shown in Fig. 1. The prescribing physician should realize that interindividual and intraindividual differences make average kinetic parameters of limited value in the individual complicated transplant recipient. Thus, in the clinical transplant setting, allowance for individual patient factors is necessary for the optimum use of cyclosporine [1].

Cyclosporine is poorly and variably absorbed from the upper part of the small intestine after oral administration. Peak blood concentrations are observed 1 to 8 hours after a given dose, and the extent of absorption varies from 20% to 60%. The extent of absorption and absorption half-life can vary in the same patient over time and differ widely between patients receiving identical doses of cyclosporine on a body weight basis. Time-dependent improvement of absorption is regularly seen in patients treated chronically with cyclosporine, who may increase absorption three- to five-fold over a few months.

Physiologic and pathologic conditions frequently present in transplant recipients may considerably modify cyclosporine absorption. Liver disease and cholestasis can markedly reduce cyclosporine absorption, particularly when there is impairment of bile delivery to the gastrointestinal tract. During the immediate postoperative period in liver transplant recipients, cyclosporine absorption may be less than 5 percent of an administered dose, due to external biliary drainage through a T-tube. When the external drainage of bile is discontinued, drug absorption may increase markedly [1]. Gastrointestinal mucosal disease resulting in diarrhea or poor gastric emptying, as in

Gastrointestinal mucosal disease resulting in diarrhea or poor gastric emptying, as in diabetes mellitus, may also decrease cyclosporine absorption. In liver and gastrointestinal diseases the use of intravenous cyclosporine may be needed in the early post-transplant period to provide consistent immunosuppression.

In whole blood, 55–60% of cyclosporine is bound to red cells, and an additional 30%–35% is bound to lipoproteins. Thus the distribution of cyclosporine in blood is dependent on the patient's hematocrit and lipoprotein concentration [2]. The blood cyclosporine increases linearly until whole blood concentrations reach 1000 ng/ml, after which red blood cells are substantially saturated. When cyclosporine blood concentrations drawn from patients are allowed to stand at room temperature, there is redistribution of cyclosporine from plasma into red cells, falsely lowering plasma concentrations. Thus, many centers prefer to monitor cyclosporine therapy with whole blood rather than plasma levels, particularly in situations where plasma and red cells cannot be separated immediately. The high-density lipoprotein, very low-density lipoprotein and low-density lipoprotein fractions bind virtually all of the cyclosporine in plasma [2]. In transplant patients with plasma lipid abnormalities, free and thus pharmacologically active cyclosporine concentrations may be altered. For example, serious neurotoxicity has been reported in liver transplant recipients with low total cholesterol concentrations and relatively increased concentrations of "free" cyclosporine [3].

Cyclosporine is extensively metabolized by hepatic P450 microsomal mixed function oxidase enzymes, with metabolites and unchanged parent compound appearing primarily in bile. Metabolites probably undergo enterohepatic recycling, resulting in small secondary and tertiary peak blood concentrations in some patients. The predominant metabolites result from demethylation and hydroxylation reactions, leaving the ring structure of the parent cyclosporine molecule intact. In normal volunteers, the elimination half-life of the parent compound is 6–8 h with a slightly longer value (8–9 h) for metabolites [1]. The metabolites of cyclosporine have less immunosuppressive effect than the parent cyclosporine molecule, although some metabolites demonstrate in vitro effects which decrease interleukin-2 production [4]. Since experimental nephrotoxicity can be reduced by hepatic microsomal enzyme inducers such as phenobarbital, it is presumed that the parent cyclosporine molecule, rather than a nephrotoxic metabolite, is the major cause of renal dysfunction. However, the activation of cyclosporine to a nephrotoxic metabolite, by renal tubular drug metabolizing enzymes, has been suggested by recent experimental data [5]. The presence of documented nephrotoxicity with "therapeutic" parent cyclosporine concentrations, as measured by HPLC, is consistent with a role for renally generated metabolites in cyclosporine nephrotoxicity.

Table 1. Clinical presentations of cyclosporine nephrotoxicity

1. Delayed initial function, oligoanuria and acute renal failure
2. Episodes of acute renal dysfunction
3. Chronic cyclosporine-associated nephropathy
   Reversible depression of glomerular filtration rate
   Progressive renal insufficiency
4. Hemolytic-uremic syndrome; thrombotic microangiopathy
5. Hypertension-*de novo* or aggravating pre-existing hypertension
6. Electrolyte disturbances: hyperkalemia, metabolic acidosis, Hypomagnesemia

Pediatric transplant recipients rapidly metabolize cyclosporine, necessitating larger doses on a weight basis to achieve any given cyclosporine blood concentration. Renal excretion plays a limited role in overall cyclosporine elimination, with small amounts of radiolabeled drug appearing in the urine within four days of drug administration. Thus the presence of renal failure does not influence cyclosporine pharmacokinetics, and no adjustment of dosage is required. Due to its high molecular weight and relatively avid binding to blood components, little cyclosporine is lost during hemodialysis or peritoneal dialysis, and no dosage adjustments are necessary.

Nephrotoxicity

Although the most frequent and potentially limiting consequence of cyclosporine immunosuppression is nephrotoxicity, the clinical presentations of these adverse effects are diverse [6] (Table 1). Each of these syndromes will be briefly summarized.

Oligoanuria and Acute Renal Failure

Lack of initial function of renal transplants, necessitating dialysis, is more frequent with cyclosporine immunosuppression than with azathioprine. This has been attributed to high initial cyclosporine doses ($>$ 15 mg/kg) or introduction of the drug prior to onset of urine flow. Ischemic injury to the kidney due to adverse procurement conditions potentiates this problem [7]. Cyclosporine-treated patients, even when function ultimately improves, have approximately twice as long a period of oligoanuria as azathioprine-treated patients [8]. There is evidence that cadaver kidneys experiencing prolonged oligoanuria have inferior one- and two-year survival despite the fact that serum creatinine often returns to normal following the oliguric period. There is an analogous period of acute renal failure following heart transplantation, presumably due to high initial cyclosporine doses interacting with the ischemic renal injury produced by heart bypass.

Reduction of initial cyclosporine doses to 5–8 mg/kg in renal transplantation and 8–10 mg/kg in cardiac transplantation has minimized the problem of poor initial renal function. Some centers prefer to withhold cyclosporine until serum creatinine falls below 2–3 mg/dl and urine output is well established. There is increasing use of induction immunosuppression with monoclonal antibodies or antilymphocyte globulin to prevent early rejection, prior to beginning cyclosporine.

Monitoring of cyclosporine blood levels and percutaneous allograft biopsy during the period of oligoanuria is crucial for minimization of this problem. In patients with non-function for more than 7–10 days, percutaneous biopsy of the allograft is very helpful in excluding clinically silent rejection so that anti-rejection treatment can be instituted.

Episodes of Acute Renal Dysfunction

Many renal transplant patients treated with cyclosporine develop episodes of acute renal insufficiency. Since these episodes improve rapidly within a few days if cyclosporine dosage is reduced, and since similar episodes are common in recipients of

Table 2. Renal histopathology in cyclosporine-treated allograft recipients[9]

Clinical condition	Finding	Comment
Acute renal dysfunction	Proximal tubular cell vacuolization Microcalcification in tubular cells	Nonspecific, probably a marker of cyclosporine treatment since tubular function preserved. Cell necrosis absent
	Glomerular capillary thrombi	Associated with a poor graft outcome; can be noted in grafts without cyclosporine and in grafts with stable function
	Obliterative arteriopathy of varying severity in interlobar and arcuate vessels; patchy cell necrosis	May produce microangiopathic hemolytic anemia and thrombocytopenia; results in graft loss; found in approximately 10 percent of cases
Initial oligoanuria with acute renal failure	Arteriolar wall hyalinosis	Present with prolonged renal failure; may be permanent; infrequently found
	Diffuse interstitial fibrosis	Renal failure may be partially reversible; seen primarily in nonbeating heart cadaver donors
	Normal post-transplant biopsy	Most frequent finding in first 3–4 post-transplant weeks
Chronic renal dysfunction	Striped pattern of tubulointerstitial fibrosis, glomerulosclerosis	Irreversible changes; frequently associated with hypertension
	Hyalinosis and sclerosis of arterioles and small arteries	May be observed in normotensive patients

non-renal allografts, they have been attributed to cyclosporine nephrotoxicity. In the renal transplant recipient these episodes are difficult to distinguish from rejection, particularly in the absence of fever, allograft tenderness, and oliguria. Both rejection and cyclosporine nephrotoxicity may be associated with decreased fractional sodium excretion and isosthenuria. Often the correct diagnosis of these episodes can be made only after observing the patient's response to a therapeutic maneuver such as antirejection therapy or cyclosporine dose reduction. Although trough cyclosporine levels may be high in patients subsequently proven to have acute cyclosporine nephrotoxicity, a normal or low level does not exclude the diagnosis. In some circumstances, cyclosporine can act synergistically with rejection to produce renal dysfunction.

Biopsy of the easily accessible renal allograft during episodes of acute renal dysfunction is often critical to exclude treatable rejection. The histopathologic features observed in patients treated with cyclosporine (summarized in Table 2) are largely markers of therapy with this agent, not necessarily indicative of toxicity.

The management of acute renal dysfunction can be difficult, particularly in renal transplant recipients, since rejection is often impossible to exclude confidently. Table 3 compares features of rejection to acute cyclosporine nephrotoxicity. Since rejection is still the most likely reason for renal dysfunction, especially in the first six months after transplant, this possibility needs to be actively excluded in order for the patient to receive appropriate therapy. An elevation of trough cyclosporine blood concentrations is helpful if present, but cyclosporine-induced renal dysfunction is frequently present despite "therapeutic" levels. Signs suggesting rejection include

Table 3. Comparison of acute rejection and cyclosporine-associated renal allograft dysfunction

Signs or symptoms	CSA	Rejection
Fever, graft tenderness	Absent	Present in 25%
Oliguria	Absent	Present in 50%
Graft swelling (clinical ultrasound, NMR, fine needle manometry)	Absent	Present in 50%
Hypertension	75%	50%
Blood CSA concentration	Normal or High	Normal
Renal perfusion by isotope scan	Decreased in 75%	Decreased in virtually all
Hyperkalemic metabolic acidosis with hyperchloremia	15%	5%
Factional excretion of sodium	Low	Low in first 2 days, then increased
Biopsy; fine needle aspirates	Subtle features; absence of rejection	Usually diagnostic

increase in graft size found by ultrasound, elevations of intra-renal hydrostatic pressure found by thin needle manometry, or tubular cell changes in fine needle aspirates. Most centers prefer to perform a core biopsy on the allograft to diagnose and treat subtle rejection, if present. If steroid or monoclonal antibody treatment for rejection is unsuccessful in effecting an improvement in renal function, reduction in cyclosporine dosage by 0.5–1.0 mg/kg every 5–7 days may be beneficial. Rejection can be diagnosed with confidence if a diffuse interstitial infiltrate or arteritis is present. Focal mononuclear infiltrates can be present with proven cyclosporine nephrotoxicity and thus are not specific for rejection. Arteriolar hyalinosis is more frequently observed in patients with cyclosporine nephrotoxicity [10]. If the transplant biopsy fails to show acute rejection, particularly if arteriolar hyalinosis is present, empiric dose reduction is indicated in an attempt to avoid chronic tubulointerstitial fibrosis, which has been noted in many patients with frequent episodes of reversible cyclosporine-induced creatinine rises. An algorithm which can be used for this differential diagnosis is shown in Table 4.

Chronic Cyclosporine-Associated Nephropathy

Progressive renal insufficiency is well documented in transplant recipients receiving cyclosporine for over 12 months. While this process can be attributed to chronic allograft rejection in renal transplant recipients, in non-renal recipients and in patients with autoimmune disease, it is most certainly due to a nephrotoxic effect of cyclosporine. Long-term cyclosporine treated recipients, as a group, have lower glomerular filtration rates than comparable patients immunosuppressed with azathioprine [11]. In a series of heart transplant recipients the decline in renal function could not be attributed to cardiac dysfunction since cardiac performance was normal and similar to that in azathioprine-treated heart recipients [12]. Similar chronic renal dysfunction has been described in long-term liver transplant recipients and patients receiving long-term cyclosporine therapy for autoimmune uveitis [13,14]. While excessive initial doses of cyclosporine may play a role in chronic nephrotoxicity, the condition may be progressive, despite dose reduction. In some patients, however, stopping cyclosporine altogether after a year of treatment results

Table 4. Algorithm for management of acute renal dysfunction in renal transplantation

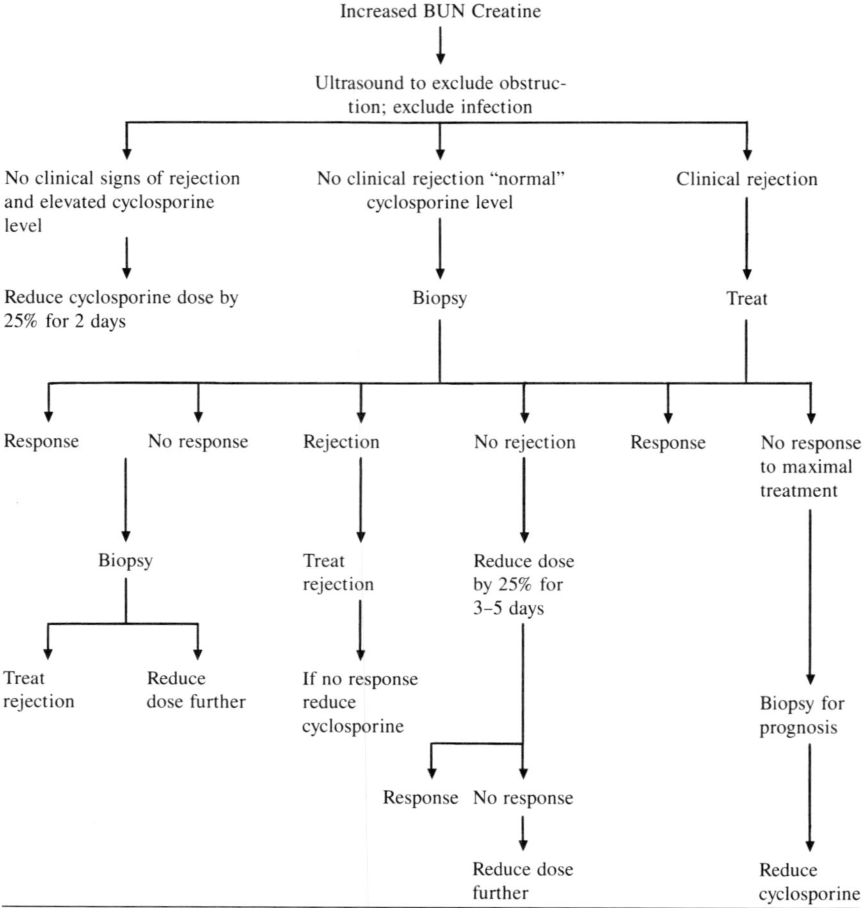

in rapid improvement in renal hemodynamics and function [15]. Whether permanent structural damage remains is unknown. Several patients have required dialysis for end-stage renal disease due to chronic cyclosporine nephrotoxicity [12]. Clinically, hypertension and proteinuria are noted even in non-renal recipients, excluding rejection as an explanation for the findings. Biopsy findings in renal and non-renal recipients show chronic tubulointerstitial fibrosis with focal and segmental glomerulosclerosis [12].

Patients treated with cyclosporine may have very subtle changes in renal function. In patients with autoimmune disease, for example, creatinine clearance commonly falls gradually. When the drug is withdrawn, renal function returns to baseline even after one year of treatment. Some, but not all, of these patients develop *de novo* hypertension, and most have rises in mean arterial pressure even though values remain less than 140/90. These patients generally have no other reason for the decline in renal function and maintain stable but elevated serum creatinine values during the entire treatment period. Reduction of dose and combination therapy with other immunosuppressive drugs may minimize the decline in creatinine clearance. The lack of sensitivity of the serum creatinine and creatinine clearance in discerning progressive tubulointerstitial renal disease make it difficult to dismiss this result of cyclosporine therapy as harmless and "reversible" until long-term follow-up is available. The number of cases of chronic nephrotoxicity evolving within the group thought to have stable but reversible renal dysfunction described above is unknown.

Gradual withdrawal of cyclosporine or triple-therapy regimens using low-dose cyclosporine with azathioprine and prednisone may reduce the severity and frequency of chronic cyclosporine nephrotoxicity [16,17].

Hemolytic-Uremic Syndrome: Thrombotic Microangiopathy

Rises in direct bilirubin without other liver function abnormalities have been reported with cyclosporine immunosuppression. In some patients this is associated with fulminant acute renal failure and thrombocytopenia [18]. This syndrome, reported primarily in bone marrow transplant recipients, also occurs *de novo* in renal transplantation [19]. In renal transplantation, this vasculopathy confers a poor prognosis on the allograft despite absence of pathologic changes of acute rejection. Histological examination of the kidneys reveals arteriolar lesions similar to the hemolytic-uremic syndrome, with thrombotic microangiopathy and occasionally afferent arteriolar thrombosis. Plasmapheresis has been used to induce hematological remission and renal recovery [20]. The causative role of the nodular hyalinotic vascular lesions, without obvious clinical rejection, seen in some renal transplant biopsies in this rare manifestation of cyclosporine nephrotoxicity is unclear, since a minority of patients develop clinical symptoms. However, thrombotic microangiopathy may occur in transplants not treated with cyclosporine, as recurrence of original disease or as a rare manifestation of allograft rejection.

During periods of renal dysfunction related to cyclosporine, high concentrations of factor VIII related antigen have been noted; these fall to normal as the dose of the drug is decreased [21]. This phenomenon has been interpreted as additional evidence that vascular injury is a major component of cyclosporine nephrotoxicity.

Hypertension

Increases of blood pressure, either *de novo* or from previously hypertensive levels, are frequently seen in cyclosporine treated patients [22]. In cardiac transplantation where renal rejection is not present, the majority of cyclosporine-treated patients are hypertensive, compared to historical data from azathioprine-treated patients [23]. Although renal function is usually also decreased, this is not uniformly true. Conventional approaches to antihypertensive therapy are often ineffective, necessitating multiple drug regimens. When measured, plasma volume is increased, plasma renin activity is low, and the renin-angiotensin axis is relatively unresponsive to stimulatory maneuvers such as upright posture and diuretics [24]. Increases in plasma renin activity in response to converting enzyme inhibition by captopril is blunted, compared to the usual hypertensive subject.

Despite this indirect evidence for volume expansion, diuretics may actually aggravate the pressure elevation. There is emerging evidence that calcium entry blockers are useful as monotherapy. Poor therapeutic results are often obtained with vasodilators, beta blockers, and converting enzyme inhibitors.

Electrolyte Disturbances

Hyperkalemia, with mild hyperchloremic metabolic acidosis, has been reported with cyclosporine therapy in patients with relatively well-preserved glomerular filtration rates [25]. Anion gaps are normal, and virtually all patients reported have urine pH values less than 6. Plasma renin activities are low or normal and plasma aldosterone levels are normal. When cyclosporine dosage is reduced, the electrolyte patterns return towards normal. Whether this is a primary renal effect of the drug or, more likely, the result of chronic tubulointerstitial fibrosis and hyporeninemic hypoaldosteronism is unclear. Detailed studies of the renin-angiotensin system correlated with renal histopathology are unavailable.

Hypomagnesemia is common during cyclosporine therapy, especially in bone marrow recipients. Accompanying tubular toxins such as aminoglycosides and amphotericin are often present. Occasionally serum magnesium concentrations fall to less than 1 mEq/l in conjunction with inappropriate urinary magnesium wasting [26]. Magnesium deficiency could partially explain some of the seizures which can occur in patients as an adverse effect of cyclosporine.

Drug Interactions

Drugs which influence hepatic drug metabolizing enzymes may cause clinically significant changes in cyclosporine pharmacokinetics. Drugs which interact with cyclosporine are listed in Table 5. Some of these interactions have been reported only in anecdotal case reports, and their clinical importance is unclear. Corticosteroids used in most transplant recipients have complex effects on cyclosporine metabolism. High doses of methylprednisolone used for treatment of rejection crises, as well as long-term steroid therapy, may increase cyclosporine biotransformation to inactive metabolites [27]. Any potential loss of immunosuppressive effect may be counterbalanced by an independent effect in which cyclosporine decreases prednisone metabolism [27,28].

Monitoring of Cyclosporine Blood Concentrations

Because of the multiple clinical and pharmacological variables present in any individual allograft recipient, therapeutic drug monitoring is practiced in some form by most transplant units. Whether such monitoring justifies its expense and inconvenience is still not clear after a decade of wide therapeutic use of cyclosporine. By monitoring blood concentrations, problems in patient compliance and/or drug absorption can be discovered. However, as a goal for therapy in individual patients, blood level monitoring may be disappointing. Rejection of an allograft frequently occurs with "therapeutic" blood levels, and reversible nephrotoxicity can be documented in patients when decreases in "nontoxic" blood concentrations result in

Table 5. Clinically relevant drug interactions with cyclosporine

Increased metabolism: Decreased blood levels, loss of immunosuppression
Anticonvulsants
Carbamazepine
Phenytoin
Phenobarbital
Antituberculous Drugs
Rifampicin
Isoniazid
Decreased metabolism: Increased blood levels, increased risk of nephrotoxicity
Antimicrobial Agents
Erythromycin
Fluconazole
Ketoconazole
Miscellaneous
Androgens, oral contraceptives[a]
Cimetidine
Calcium blockers—nicardipine, diltiazam, verapamil
Potentiated or Additive Nephrotoxicity
Aminoglycoside antibiotics
Amphotericin B
Cephalosporin antibiotics (cefotaxime, cefuroxime)[b]
Digoxin[d]
Etoposide[c]
Mannitol[b,7,5]
Furosemide[b]
Melphelan
Nonsteroidal anti-inflammatory drugs
Trimethoprim-sulfamethoxazole

[a]Hepatotoxicity reported
[b]Documented only in experimental animals
[c]Enhanced CNS and hepatotoxicity
[d]Reduced volume of distribution of digoxin

improved kidney function. Whenever a major change, such as a concomitant illness or a new therapeutic agent, occurs in the patient's condition it may be prudent to measure a cyclosporine level after two to three days to be assured that no major change in cyclosporine kinetics has occurred.

Because of the differences in absolute drug concentrations between individuals on given doses and the confounding effects of dose regimen (once versus twice daily dosing), food, age, meals, and even time of day, generalizations are difficult. These factors must constantly be considered before making changes in an effective therapeutic program simply because of a change in blood concentration. Most transplant programs monitor blood levels two to three times per week in the perioperative period, followed by a period of weekly surveillance for several months, and then checks at monthly or quarterly intervals. It should also be remembered that higher doses are required shortly after transplant and that target concentrations can be reduced at later time periods. Most transplant centers monitor the cyclosporine level prior to the next scheduled dose because of the marked variability in the time and height of peak concentrations.

References

1. Ptachcinski RJ, Venkataramanan R, Burckart GJ (1986) Clinical pharmacokinetics of cyclosporine. Clin Pharmacokinet 11:107–132
2. Sgoutas D, MacMahon W, Love A, Jerkunica I (1986) Interaction of cyclosporin A with human lipoproteins. J Pharm Pharmacol 38:583–588
3. de Groen PC, Aksamit AJ, Rakela J, Forbes GS, Krom RAF (1987) Central nervous system toxicity after liver transplantation: the role of cyclosporine and cholesterol. N Engl J Med 317:861–866
4. Freed BM, Rosano TG, Lempert N (1987) In vitro immunosuppressive properties of cyclosporine metabolites. Transplantation 43:123–127
5. Buss WC, Stepanek J, Bennett WM (1989) A new proposal for the mechanism of cyclosporine A nephrotoxicity: inhibition of renal microsomal chain elongation following *in vivo* cyclosporine A. Biochem Pharmacol 38:4085–4093
6. Von Graffenried B, Krupp P (1986) Side effects of cyclosporine (Sandimmun) in renal transplant recipients and in patients with autoimmune diseases. Transplant Proc 18:876–883
7. Canadian Multicentre Trial Group (1983) A randomized clinical trial of cyclosporine in cadaveric renal transplantation. N Engl J Med 309:809–815
8. Hall BM, Tiller DJ, Duggin GG, Horvath JS, Farnsworth A, May J, Johnson JR, Shiel AGR (1985) Post-transplant acute renal failure in cadaver renal recipients treated with cyclosporine. Kidney Int 28:178–186
9. Mihatsch MJ, Thiel G, Spichtin HP (1983) Morphological findings in kidney transplants after treatment with cyclosporine. Transplant Proc 15:2821–2835
10. Nield GH, Taube DH, Hartley RB, Bignardi L, Cameron JS, Williams DG, Ogg CS, Rudge CJ (1986) Morphological differentiation between rejection and cyclosporin nephrotoxicity in renal allografts. J Clin Pathol 39:152–159
11. Myers BD (1986) Cyclosporine nephrotoxicity. Kidney Int 30:964–974
12. Myers BD, Sibley R, Newton L, Tomlanovich SJ, Boshkos C, Stinson E, Luetscher JA, Whitney DJ, Krasney D, Coplon NS, and Perlroth M (1988) The long term course of cyclosporine-associated chronic nephropathy. Kidney Int 33:590–600
13. Dische FE, Neuberger J, Keating J, Parsons V, Calne RY, Williams R (1988) Kidney pathology in liver allograft recipients after long-term treatment with cyclosporin A. Lab Invest 58:395–402
14. Palestine AG, Austin HA, Balow JE, Antonovych TT, Sabnis SG, Preuss HG, Nussenblatt RB (1986) Renal histopathologic alterations in patients treated with cyclosporine for uveitis. N Engl J Med 314:1293–1298
15. Curtis JJ, Luke RG, Jones P, Dubovsky EV, Whelchel JD, Diethelm AG (1986) Cyclosporine in therapeutic doses increases renal allograft resistance. Lancet II:477–479
16. Kahan BD (1989) Cyclosporine. N Engl J Med 321:1725–1738
17. Bennett WM, Normal DJ (1986) Action and toxicity of cyclosporine. Ann Rev Med 37:215–224
18. Shulman H, Striker G, Deeg HJ, Kennedy M, Storb R, Thomas EG (1981) Nephrotoxicity of cyclosporin A after allogeneic marrow transplantation: Glomerular thromboses and tubular injury. N Engl J Med 305:1392–1395
19. Van Buren D, Van Buren CT, Flechner SM, Maddox AM, Verani R, Kahan BD (1985) *De novo* hemolytic uremic syndrome in renal transplant recipients immunosuppressed with cyclosporine. Surgery 98:54–62
20. Keusch G, Gmür J, Baumgartner D, Burger HR, Largiader F, Binswanger V (1986) *De novo* hemolytic uremic syndrome in two renal allograft recipients treated with cyclosporine: Successful therapy with plasmapheresis. Transplant Proc 18:1097–1098

21. Braun Z, Neild GH, Willougby JJ, Somia NV, Cameron SJ (1986) Increased Factor VIII as an index of vascular injury in cyclosporine nephrotoxicity. Transplantation 42:150–153
22. Luke RG (1987) Hypertension in renal transplant recipients. Kidney Int 31:1024–1037
23. Bellet M, Cabrol C, Sassano P, Leger P, Corvol P, Menard J (1985) Systemic hypertension after cardiac transplantation: Effect of cyclosporine on the renin-angiotensin-aldosterone system. Am J Cardiol 56:927–931
24. Bantle JP, Nath KA, Sutherland DE, Najarian JS, Ferris TF (1985) Effects of cyclosporine on the renin-angiotensin-aldosterone system and potassium excretion in renal transplant patients. Arch Intern Med 145:505–508
25. Stahl R, Kanz L, Maier B, Schollmeyer P (1986) Hyperchloremic metabolic acidosis with high serum potassium in renal transplant recipients: A cyclosporine A associated side effect. Clin Nephrol 25:245–248
26. June CH, Thompson CB, Kennedy MS, Nims J, Thomas ED (1985) Profound hypomagnesemia and renal magnesium wasting associated with the use of cyclosporine for marrow transplantation. Transplantation 39:620–624
27. Ost L, Klintmalm G, Ringden O (1985) Mutual interaction between prednisolone and cyclosporine in renal transplant patients. Transplant Proc 17:1252–1255
28. Burckart GJ, Canafax DM, Yee GC (1986) Cyclosporine monitoring. Drug Intell Clin Pharm 20:649–652

Evolution of Cyclosporin Nephrotoxicity

MICHAEL J. MIHATSCH and BERNHARD RYFFEL[1]

SUMMARY. Cyclosporine (CsA) nephrotoxicity is reviewed with special emphasis on the development of the morphological lesion. Renal lesions are essentially confined to the proximal tubules and arterioles. At both sites cellular degenerative changes develop, which consist of vacuolization, inclusion bodies, mitochondrial abnormalities, and single cell necroses. Similar morphological changes, which indicate a direct effect of the drug, are inducible in experimental animals and in cell culture.

In contrast to the occurrence of functional nephrotoxicity (reduction of glomerular filtration rate) the morphological changes essentially occur after high CsA exposure. Whereas tubular lesions are generally reversible, the arteriolar alterations may progress and cause irreversible ischemic tissue damage. From repeat biopsies in single patients the evolution, especially of the arteriolar lesions, was followed. Endothelial cell and myocyte degeneration with platelet deposition and protein extravasation was followed by tissue repair, resulting in luminal obliteration and downstream ischemic fibrosis.

Studies with radiolabelled CsA on cells from different sources revealed that CsA is concentrated intracellularly by the specific binding protein cyclophilin. Analyses of the radioligand data revealed two binding components: a saturable cytosolic binding and a non-saturable membrane binding. It is speculated that immunosuppression is mediated by cyclophilin, whereas morphological renal changes which occur at high drug levels are due to binding and probably disintegration of the cell membranes.

Introduction

Recently, there has been discussion of a variety of factors which may mediate Cyclosporin (CsA) toxicity [1,2], e.g., disturbed prostaglandin metabolism, release of endothelin, reduction of endothelium-derived relaxing factor, activation of the

[1]Institute of pathology, Schönbeinstrasse 40, CH-4003 Basel, Switzerland

renin-angiotensin system, and stimulation of the autonomous nervous system. However, changes of many of these factors are secondary rather than causative of CsA toxicity. This hypothesis is supported by experimental studies in rats in which glomerular filtration and prostaglandin metabolism was investigated. Whereas CsA caused immediate reduction in glomerular filtration rates, renal urinary prostaglandin excretion occurred at least 6 days after commencement of CsA treatment. Thus, alterations in prostaglandin metabolism are unlikely to be the cause of renal vasoconstriction. As a second example, the possible role of an activated renin-angiotensin system in CsA toxicity has been investigated. An immunohistochemical study of the juxtaglomerular apparatus was performed on kidney biopsies from patients before and after CsA therapy [3]. The CsA treatment group consisted of patients with kidney transplants, bone marrow transplants, heart transplants, and juvenile diabetes. The size of the juxtaglomerular apparatus did not differ in patients with either short or long term drug administration. This finding, however, does not invalidate the functional findings reported by Myers [4], who showed increased prorenin levels, but it does refute consistent hypertrophy of the juxtaglomerular apparatus. Without reviewing all the experimental evidence, the proposed pathogenic factors mentioned above cannot explain the morphologic lesions which possibly are the key to the understanding of CsA toxicity. The following overview, therefore, focuses on factors responsible for the development of morphologic lesions and addresses the question whether CsA has a direct toxic effect on target cells.

The concept of CsA nephrotoxicity was developed on the basis of morphological findings in man. Therefore, in the first part of this review, CsA toxicity found in man and duplicated in animal and cell culture is presented; with emphasis being placed on the development of the structural lesions. In the second part of this review, the role of cellular drug uptake, intracellular concentration, and binding to the cell membrane for the development of morphologic lesions is discussed.

Overview of CsA-Toxicity in Man

Based on morphological criteria, CsA toxicity can be divided into functional toxicity and morphological toxicity [1,2,5]. Functional and morphological toxicity occur in the renal tubule and in the vascular system, as shown in Fig. 1. Morphological lesions, which will be discussed here, may also be a key for understanding functional toxicity.

The morphological changes seen in *tubular toxicity* (Fig. 2) comprise inclusion bodies in tubular epithelial cells (corresponding to giant mitochrondria), isometric tubular vacuolization, and microcalcification. These different lesions of tubular toxicity are most often found in one and the same biopsy. They may occur, however, in any combination and even giant mitochondria or isometric vacuolization or microcalcification may be found alone. Vascular lesions (see below) may be present or absent. Tubular changes are found in kidney transplants as well as in bone marrow and heart transplant recipients and in patients with autoimmune diseases.

Giant mitochondria, usually one per cell, occur predominantly in the convoluted part (S 1,2 segment) of the proximal tubule. The morphology of giant mitochondria lacks any specificity. Isometric vacuolization is almost exclusively found in the straight part of the proximal tubule (S 3 segment) of a few nephrons. The light microscopic picture is identical to that of osmotic nephrosis. All or most of the

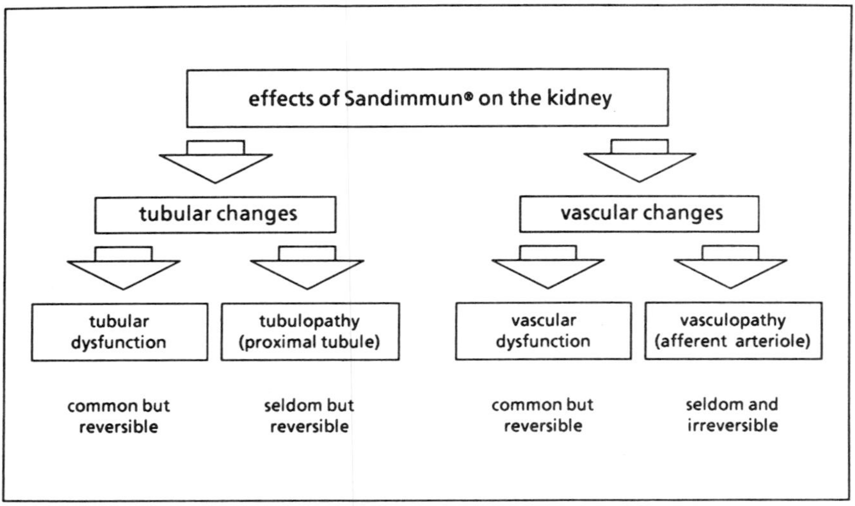

Fig. 1. Classification of CsA (Sandimmun)-toxicity

tubular cells in a cross-section contain densely packed empty vacuoles (free of lipids) of equal size. Vacuolization is at least partly due to a dilatation of the smooth endoplasmatic reticulum. Giant mitochondria and isometric vacuolization were never observed in one and the same cell. Sometimes the nuclei of the cells affected by isometric vacuolization are pycnotic, and the brush border of the cells may be missing. Single cell necroses are rare. Microcalcifications of a single cell or groups of tubular cells are found in various parts of the nephron. They are round, crescent,

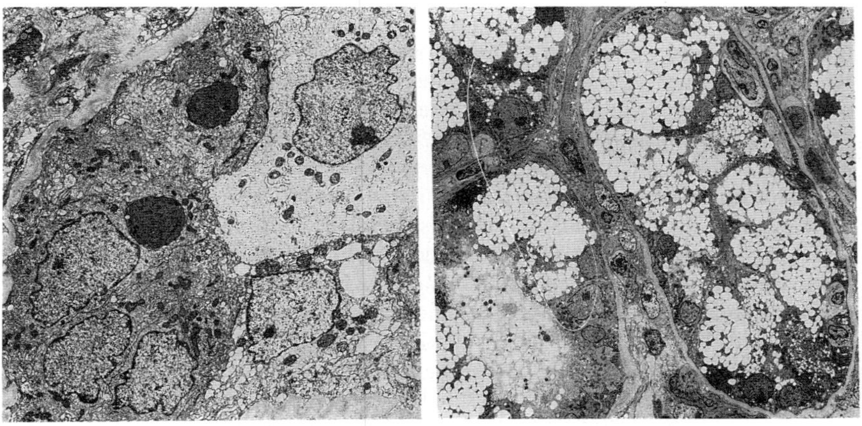

Fig. 2. Tubular toxicity: tubular cross-sections with inclusion bodies (giant mitochondria (*left*) or isometric vacuolization (*right*))

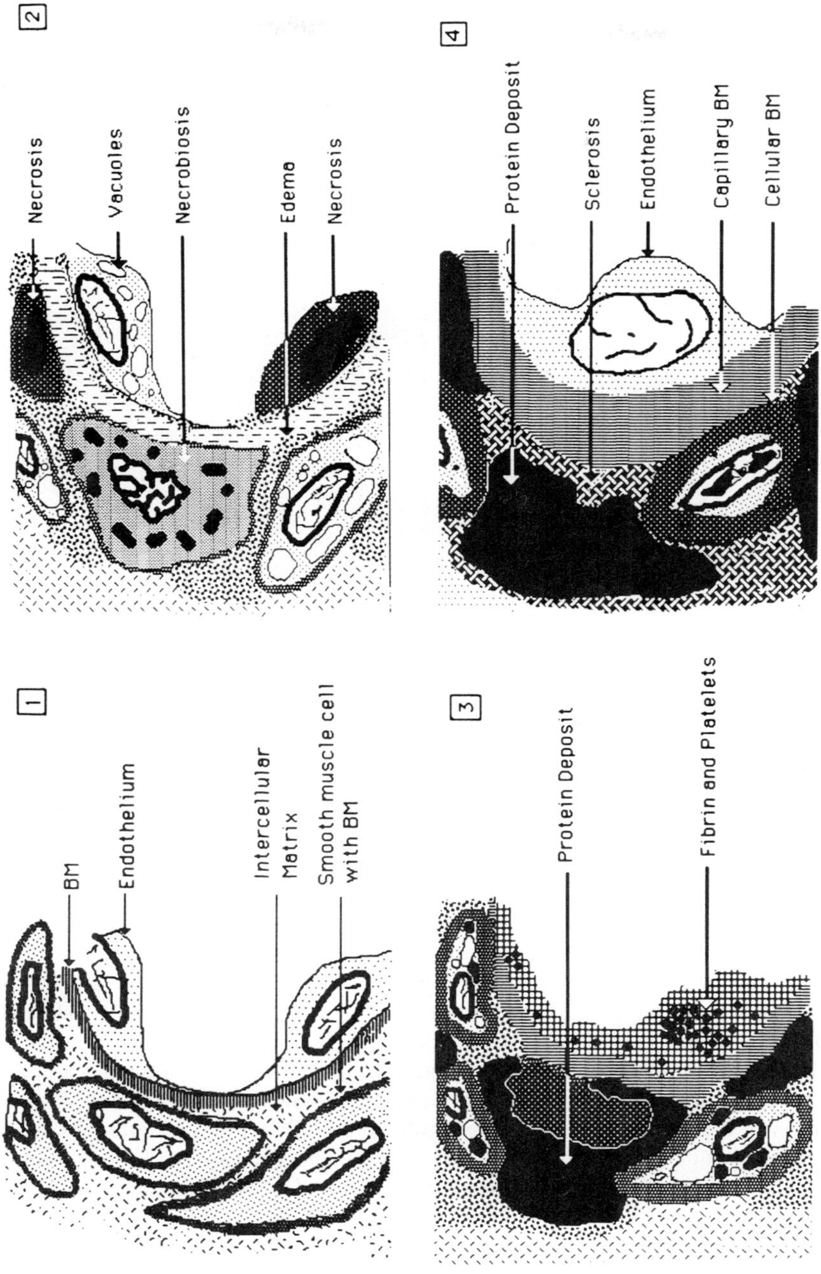

Fig. 3. Morphogenesis of CsA-associated arteriolopathy (see text)

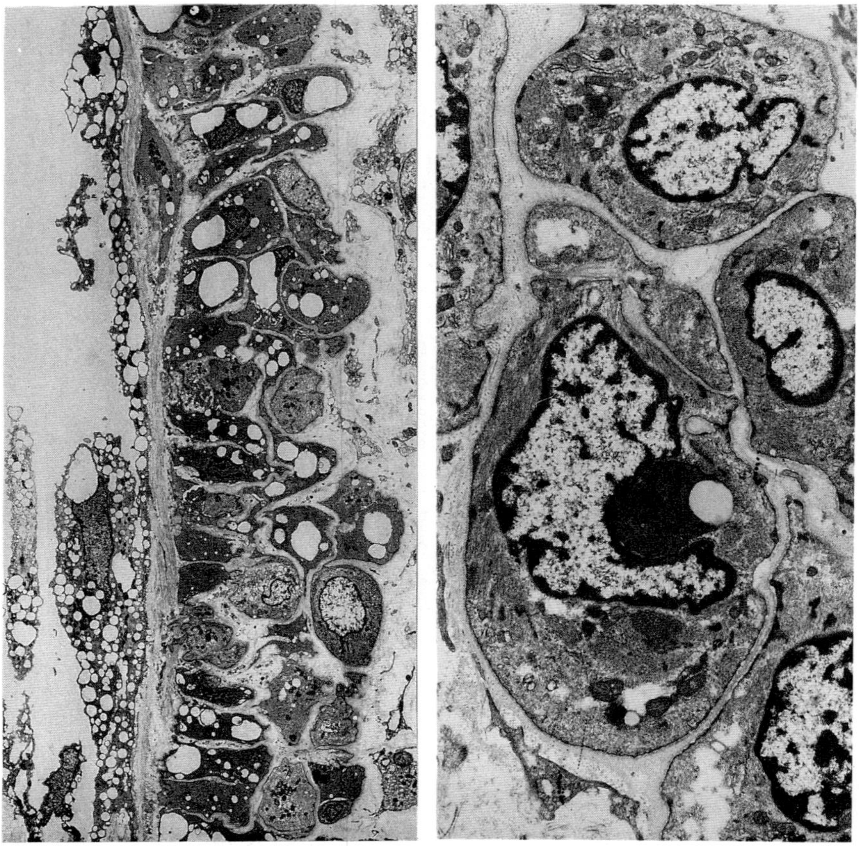

Fig. 4. Vascular toxicity: vacuolization of endothelial and smooth muscle cells of an arteriole (*left*) or inclusion body (*lysosome*) in a smooth muscle cell (*right*)

or polycyclic in shape. Microcalcification is the result of calcification of Tamm-Horsfall protein casts and possibly also of necrotic tubular cells.

By far the most frequent lesions and hallmarks of *vascular toxicity* are CsA-associated arteriolopathy and interstitial fibrosis of striped form with tubular atrophy. Vascular (interstitial) toxicity is found not only in kidney transplant recipients, but also in patients with bone marrow, liver, and heart transplants and in patients with autoimmune diseases. The vascular lesions are predominately in the periphery of the vascular tree. They are confined to the arterioles (afferent vessels) and arteries in up to two layers of smooth muscle cells. The vascular lesions sometimes extend to the vascular pole of the glomerulus and even into some glomerular segments and arteries close to the branching into arterioles.

The morphogenesis [6] is deduced from observations of the various stages occurring concurrently or in serial biopsies (Fig. 3). The earliest lesions visible by light microscopy, and seen even more clearly by electron microscopy, are endothelial or

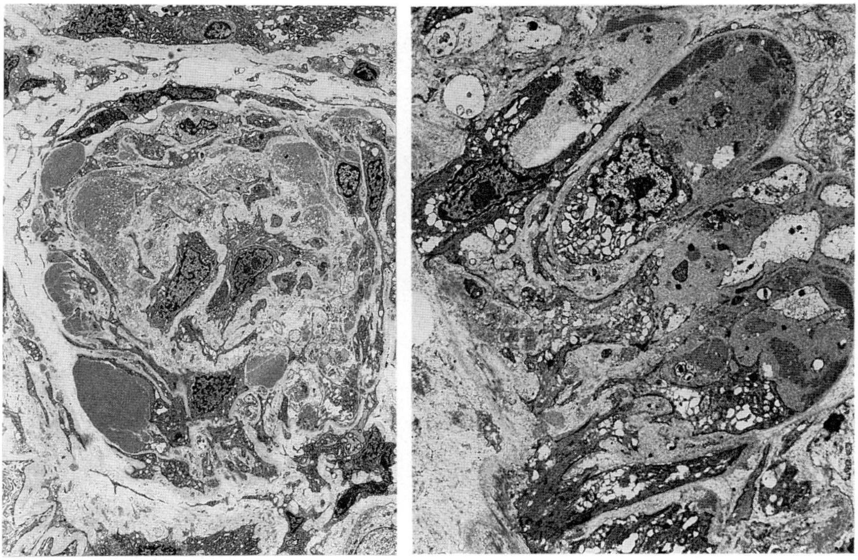

Fig. 5. Vascular toxicity: Nodular protein deposits in necrotic smooth muscle cells and complete occlusion of the arteriolar lumen (*left*). Higher magnification showing necrotic smooth muscle cells replaced by protein insudates (*right*)

myocyte damage with vacuolization, inclusion bodies (lysosomes), and single cell necrosis (Fig. 4). These lesions are followed by fibrin and platelet deposition in arterioles and/or in glomeruli. The full picture of CsA-associated arteriolopathy results from the insudation of plasma proteins into the damaged vessel wall giving rise to nodular and circular protein deposits, often at sites of necrotic myocytes (Fig. 5). The protein deposits give positive immunohistological reactions for complement components and also for IgM. If the arteriole is not completely occluded, the endothelium regenerates and rests upon a thickened basement membrane. In the arteriolar tunica media the nodular protein deposits persist and the remaining myocytes are surrounded by thickened basement membranes and embedded in a sclerotic matrix. If the arterioles are completely occluded, the glomeruli become obsolescent, but if the vascular lumen is only narrowed the glomerulus may collapse. Since the blood supply of the tubular-interstitial space depends on the integrity of the preglomerular vessels, narrowing of the arterioles results in the ischemic damage of these structures. Thus, tubular atrophy and interstitial fibrosis (Fig. 6) are the consequences of the arteriolar changes.

In summary, the primary morphological lesions seen in man are confined to the proximal tubules and the arterioles. They consist of mitochondrial abnormalities, vacuolization, and occasional single cell necrosis. All other lesions, e.g., fibrin or platelet thrombi, protein insudation in the vascular wall, and interstitial fibrosis with tubular atrophy—must be considered as sequelae of the primary lesions.

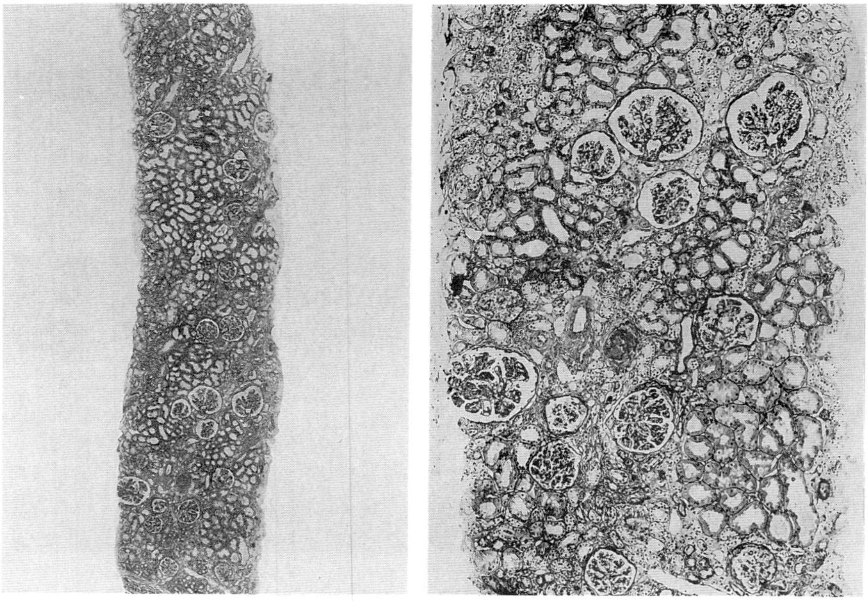

Fig. 6. Striped form of interstitial fibrosis and tubular atrophy as seen by lower and higher magnification

CsA-Toxicity in Animal Experiments and Cell Culture

To define the primary lesions described in man as specific for CsA toxicity and independent of species, animal experiments and cell culture studies were performed. Toxic tubulopathy (Fig. 7) can easily be reproduced in all commonly used animals and the morphology has been described identically by many investigators [7]. There are only minor differences in comparison with tubular toxicity in man. Tubular inclusion bodies in the rat correspond mainly to giant autophagolysosomes containing fragments of degenerate mitochondria; more rarely, typical giant mitochondria are present. Tubular vacuolization is more irregular in the rat than in man, i.e., the vacuoles are more variable in size and clearly due to dilatation of the endoplasmatic reticulum. After long-term treatment tubular microcalcifications are more widespread in the rat than in man and are found mainly along the cortical-medullary junction.

It is far more difficult to reproduce vascular toxicity in experimental animals. In normotensive animals single cell necrosis of vascular smooth muscle cells is seen rarely, but vacuolization of endothelial and smooth muscle cells is never observed [8]. In spontaneously hypertensive rats (SH), however, there is a significantly more pronounced vasculopathy than in the control animals, despite concomittant reduction of blood pressure, heart rate, and plasma renin activity [7] (Fig. 8). Electron microscopy shows the typical picture of necrotising hypertensive vasculopathy, similar to the spontaneously occurring vasculopathy seen in this rat strain without CsA treatment.

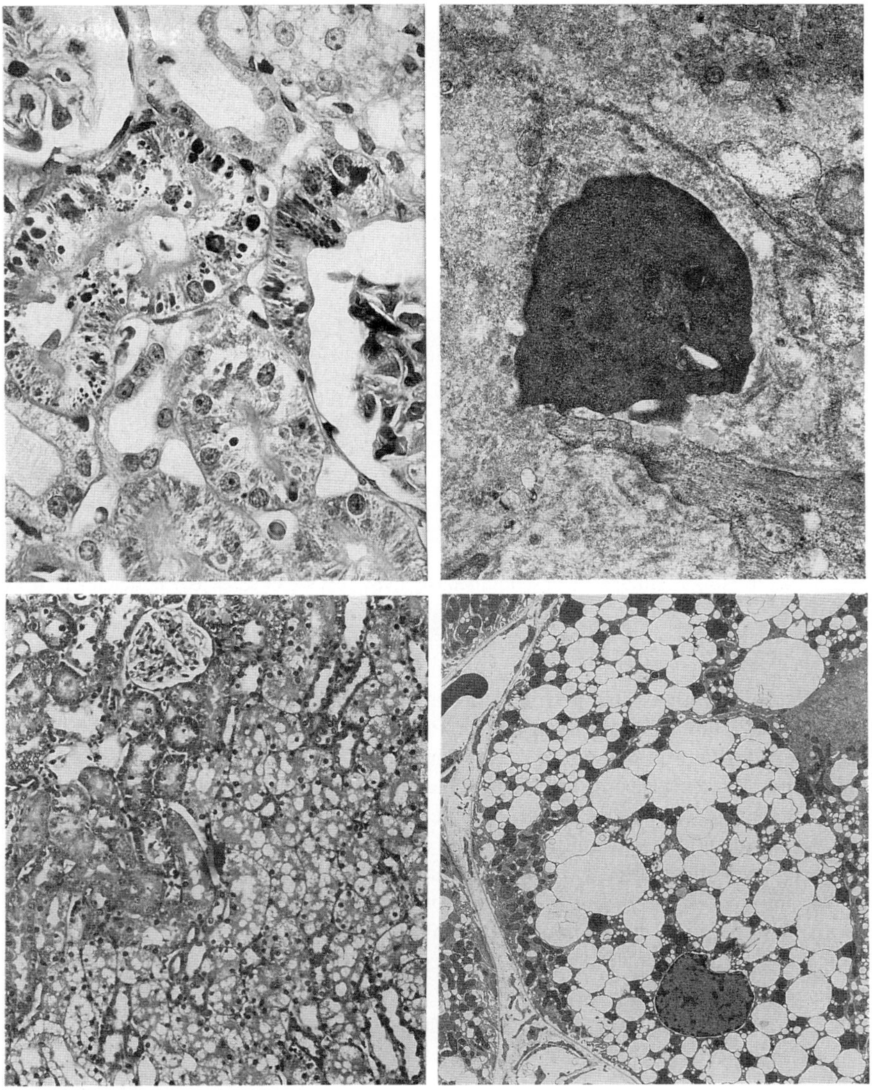

Fig. 7. Tubular toxicity in the rat: Cytoplasmatic inclusion bodies (*giant mitochondria*) in the convoluted part (*top*) and vacuolization (*dilatation of the endoplasmatic reticulum*) (*bottom*) in the straight part of the proximal tubule, by light and electron microscopy

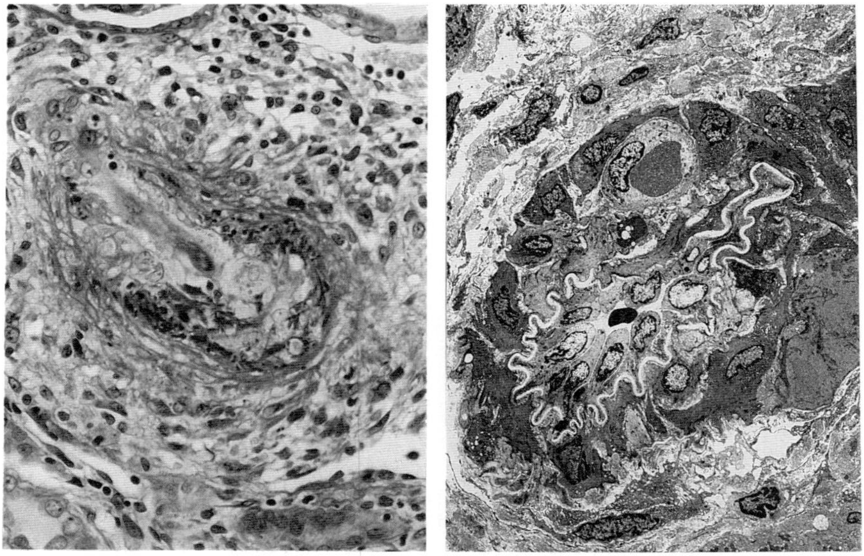

Fig. 8. Necrotising vasculopathy in spontaneously hypertensive rats, seen by light and electron microscopy

Cell culture studies using porcine and canine tubular cells (LICK-PK1 and MDCK, respectively), bovine endothelial cells (CPAE and FBHE), and human and gibbon T cell lines (Jurkat and MLA 144, respectively) exhibited, by light microscopy, cell enlargement, vacuolization, and lipid inclusions, as well as necrotic cells [9]. Electron microscopy showed dilatation of the endoplasmatic reticulum, giant mitochondria, lipid accumulation, and necrobiotic changes (Fig. 9).

In summary, morphological studies in man, animals, and cell culture show a group of lesions consisting of vacuolization (endoplasmatic reticulum), mitochondrial abnormalities (giant mitochondria, lysosomes), and cell necrosis.

CsA Uptake and Intracellular Accumulation

Cellular uptake was investigated by the use of radiolabelled CsA [10]. The cell membrane allows free permeability of CSA; there is no evidence of active or receptor mediated transport. It has recently been shown that the drug binds to specific membrane proteins, such as p-glycoprotein in liver and kidney apical membranes. Furthermore, binding to the Na^+-glucose co-transporter in the kidney and bile acid transporter in the liver were shown. The functional relevance of CsA binding to these proteins is not yet clear; however, these transporters are unlikely to be necessary for CsA transport.

Studies with radiolabelled CsA revealed intracellular accumulation of the drug, suggesting an intracellular binding protein. Two CsA binding proteins have been described, calmodulin and cyclophilin. Whereas the former's role in calcium-

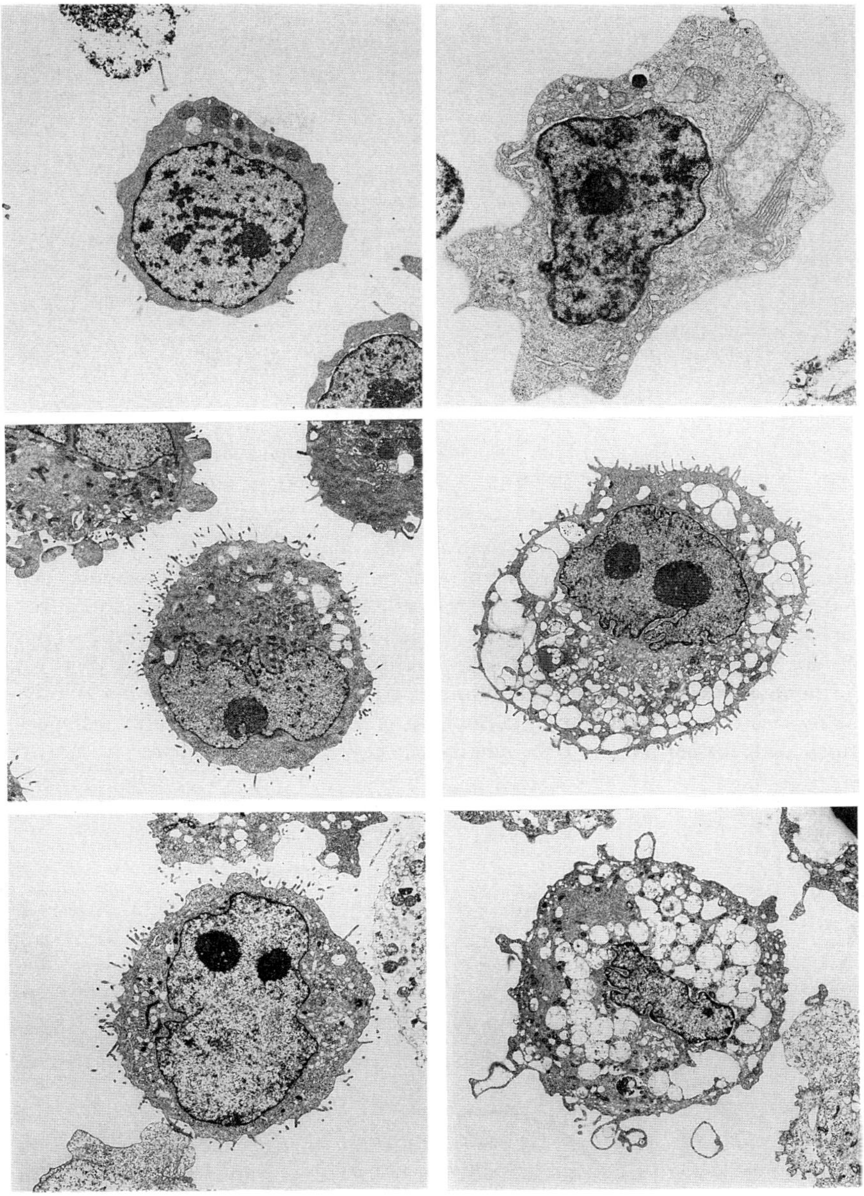

Fig. 9. Ultrastructural changes of Jurkat, FBHE, and PK1 cells after 24-h culture in the presence (*right*) or absence, of CsA (*left*). Cellular swelling and giant mitochondrion is noted in Jurkat cells (*top*), swelling and vacuolization are present in FBHE (*endothelial*) and PK1 (*tubular*) cells (*bottom*)

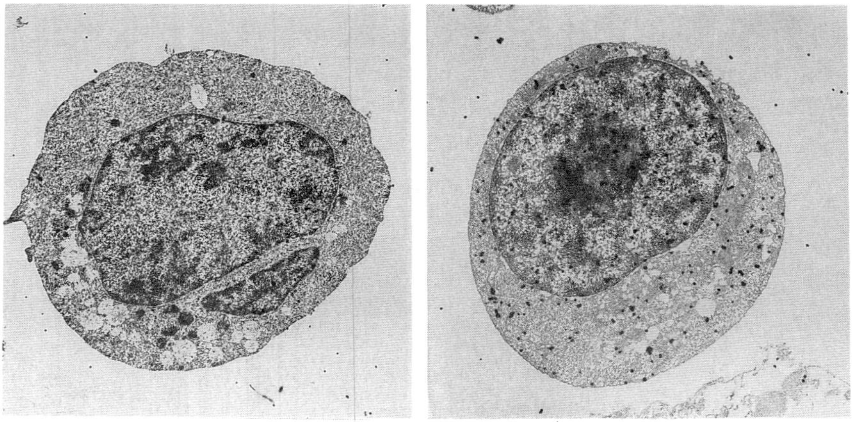

Fig. 10. Immunogold staining with anti-cyclophilin antiserum at the electron microscopic level. Control (*left*) with rabbit serum

dependent enzyme activation is well known, cyclophilin is another ubiquitous peptide which is present in all tissues at comparable concentrations. Investigations from our laboratory, as well as others, have suggested that calmodulin has little, if any, affinity for CsA. In contrast, cyclophilin has high affinity binding to CsA (Fig. 10). Furthermore, Quesniaux et al. [11] showed a good correlation between immunosuppressive activity and binding to cyclophilin of various CsA structural analogues, which lends further support to the relationship between immunosuppressive activity

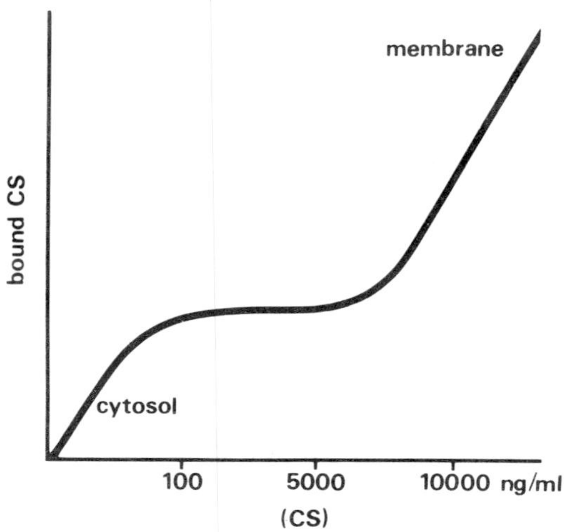

Fig. 11. CsA-binding characteristics: Cytosolic binding saturated below 1 μM, and non-saturable membrane binding

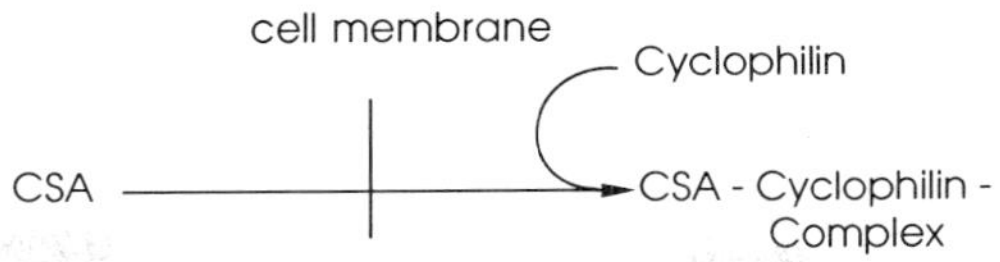

Low CSA - levels	High CSA- levels
Cyclophilin not saturated	Cyclophilin saturated CSA - binding to other cell constituents
Cell proliferation not inhibited	Cell proliferation arrested → toxic cellular damage
Functional Toxicity	Morphological Toxicity

Fig. 12. Hypothesis of cellular mechanisms responsible for CsA toxicity

and toxicity. Furthermore, the cloned protein has a cis-trans-isomerase activity, which may be necessary to the proper folding of regulatory proteins and which is inhibited by CsA. Based on present knowledge, it is assumed that binding to cyclophilin and inhibition of its enzymatic activity is in some way connected to immunosuppression. However, the specific substrate for this enzyme is presently unknown.

Analyzing the CsA binding properties of whole cells over a broad range of concentrations revealed two components: a] a saturable, cytosolic binding, which is most likely due to cyclophilin at concentrations below 1 μM and b] a non-saturable membrane associated binding (Fig. 11) [12]. Since CsA toxicity occurs only at concentrations above 1 μM, i.e., at concentrations which have already saturated cytosolic cyclophilin pools, we presently assume that its toxicity is related to non-specific insertion of the drug into cell membranes, disrupting their integrity. This accumulation of CsA occurs not only in the surface membrane but also intracellularly, e.g., in the endoplasmic reticulum, mitochondria, and Golgi apparatus.

Hypothesis for the Pathogenesis of CsA Toxicity

At pharmacological concentrations, i.e., below 1 μM, CsA binds to cyclophilin and inhibits specifically induced gene transcription in lymphoid cells (Fig. 12). At these concentrations there is no general inhibition of cell proliferation and protein synthesis. At higher concentrations CsA accumulates in the membranes and disrupts membrane functions. Concomitantly, cell proliferation and protein synthesis are inhibited and overt toxic changes are apparent. This may be the basis of the observed morphological toxicity which occurs in the tubular and vascular systems in man and animals as well as in cell culture. This hypothesis does not explain why the kidney is the main target of toxicity. Since CsA is not accumulated in renal tissue, other factors unique to the tubular, endothelial, and smooth muscle cells of the kidney must be involved.

References

1. Mihatsch MJ, Ryffel B, Gudat F, Thiel G (1988) Cyclosporin nephropathy. JB Lippincott, Philadelphia, 1555–1586
2. Mihatsch MJ, Thiel G, Ryffel B (1986) Morphology of Cyclosporin nephropathy. Prog Allergy 38:447–465
3. Nizze H, Mihatsch MJ (1989) Führt die diclosporintherapie zu Veränderungen des juxtaglomerulären Apparates? Nieren- Hochdruck. krankheiten 18:418
4. Myers B, Sibley R, Newton L, Tomlanovich S, Boshkos C, Stinson F, Leutscher J, Whitney D, Krasny D, Coplon N, Perlrothj M (1988) The long-term course of Cyclosporin-associated chronic nephropathy. Kidney Int 33:590–600
5. Bergstrand A, Bohmann S, Thiel G, Mihatsch MJ (1985) Renal histopathology in kidney transplant recipients immunosuppressed with Cyclosporin A: results from an international workshop. Clin Nephrol 24:107–119
6. Nizze H, Mihatsch MJ, Zollinger HU (1988) Cyclosporin-associated nephropathy in patients with heart and bone marrow transplants. Clin Nephrol 30:248–260
7. Thile G (1985) Experimental Cyclosporin A nephrotoxicity: a summary of the international workshop. Clin Nephrol 25:205–210
8. Fasel J, Kaissling B, Ludwig K, Ryffel B, Mihatsch MJ (1987) Light- and electron microscopic changes in the kidney of Wistar rats following treatment with Cyclosporine A. Ultrastruct Pathol 11:435–448
9. Ryffel B, Foxwell B, Gee A, Greiner B, Woerly G, Mihatsch MJ (1988) Cyclosporin-relationship of side effects to mode of action. Transplantation 46:90s–96s
10. Ryffel B (1989) Cellular activation: regulation of intracellular events by Cyclosporin. Pharmacol Rev 41:407–422
11. Quesniaux V, Schreier M, Wenger R, Hiestand PC, Haveling MW, van Regenmortel MHV (1987) Cyclophilin binds to the region of Cyclosporin involved in its immunosuppressive activity. Eur J Immunol 17:1359–1365
12. Foxwell B, Frazer G, Winters M, Hiestand PC, Wenger R, Ryffel B (1988) Identification of Cyclophilin as the erythrocyte Cyclosporin-binding-protein. Biochim Biophys Acta 938:447–455

Cell Volume Regulation in Health and Disease

Chair: Guillermo Whittembury (Venezuela)
Walter G. Guder (FRG)

Water Permeability, Reflection Coefficients, and Cell Volume Regulation

LARRY W. WELLING and DAN J. WELLING[1]

SUMMARY. Isolated, lumen collapsed, proximally and distally occluded segments of rabbit proximal tubule were equilibrated in isotonic medium and then exposed acutely to a medium identical to the first, except for the deletion or addition of a single test solute. The result was a water flux across the basolateral membrane and a swelling or shrinking of the tubule that could be measured within the first 0.1 s or less following a change from steady state. Tubule volume change was proportional to applied osmotic difference and differed consistently with the solute employed. By use of the impermeant solute raffinose, the membrane hydraulic conductivity was found to be 300 $\mu m \cdot s^{-1}$. By comparing their effects to that of raffinose, NaCl and KCl were found to have reflection coefficients of 0.56 and 0.70, respectively. Other considerations indicate that the reflection coefficients of Na^+, Cl^-, and K^+ are approximately 0.68, 0.50, and 0.94, respectively. The implications of these findings are considered in the context of cell volume maintenance and regulation.

Introduction

When challenged by an acute reduction in bathing osmolality, most tissues undergo a very rapid increase in volume and then, over a much longer period of time, recover toward their original volume. Dellesaga and Grantham observed these events in isolated renal tubules nearly 20 years ago [1]. They used the term "osmometric phase," to describe the very rapid initial increase in volume and the term "volume regulatory phase," to describe the subsequent volume decrease toward normal.

In this symposium, as in the recent literature, the main emphasis in this area of cell volume control is on the second, volume regulatory phase of the osmotic response,

[1]Research Service, Veterans Administration Medical Center, Kansas City, MO 64128, USA and Departments of Pathology and Physiology, University of Kansas Medical Center, Kansas City, KS 66103, USA

and on how cell membranes can accommodate the water and solute fluxes necessary to accomplish the regulatory task. However, since research in our laboratory touches more directly on the earlier events, the emphasis here will be on the osmometric phase and the information about cell membrane characteristics that can be gained from the study of such events. It will be assumed that membrane properties in the first instant after change from steady state will carry into and set a baseline for properties in the subsequent time periods. The membrane properties of principal interest will be hydraulic conductivity and solute reflection coefficients.

Experimental Method

The techniques we use are designed to evaluate rabbit, proximal renal tubule, basolateral cell membranes in the first instant after a change from steady state osmotic conditions, as close as possible to time $t = 0$ and before major fluxes of water or solutes dissipate the osmotic difference imposed by the anisotonic test medium [2–4].

Individual tubules are isolated, transferred to a long, narrow bathing chamber, and viewed through an inverted microscope. A 0.15 mm segment is then occluded at both ends by holding pipettes, oriented transverse to the long axis of the chamber, and positioned about 0.1 mm above a cover slip that forms the bottom of the chamber. All studies are performed at 37°C.

The volume of the bathing medium usually is 0.5 ml and is limited by the height of a suction drain. Immediately before a medium exchange, however, it is reduced to about 20 μl and to a hemispheric droplet covering only the tubule and pipette tips. Immediately thereafter, a large bolus of new medium is rapidly injected down the length of the bathing chamber. It is estimated that the original medium is displaced within 4 ms and that the unstirred layers at the tubule surface are less than 2.6 μm in thickness and 7 ms in duration [3,5].

The osmotic events are observed by video camera and recorder with 17 ms, field-by-field replay. Figure 1 shows a typical recorded image, along with an oscilloscopic display of the light intensity across a single raster line parallel to the tubule diameter. Diameter measurements are taken directly from the monitor screen and involve the eclipsing of the bright highlights at each tubule edge by the opaque jaws of a caliper. In our hands, a given tubule can be measured repeatedly with a standard deviation of ± 0.03 μm. These measurements are not limited by, nor are they closely related to, the Rayleigh criteria for estimating optical resolution.

The tubules are first equilibrated in an isotonic medium and then, to produce a rapid swelling or shrinkage, are exposed acutely to a medium identical to the first, except for the deletion or addition of a single test solute. The result is a water flow, into or out of the tubule, that can be described by the equation

$$J_{Vo} = (L_pA)\,(\sigma\Delta\pi)$$

in which J_{Vo} is the water flow per mm tubule length ($nl{\cdot}min^{-1}{\cdot}mm^{-1}$) at time $t = 0$, L_pA is the basolateral membrane hydraulic conductivity per mm tubule length ($nl{\cdot}min^{-1}{\cdot}mm^{-1}{\cdot}mOsm^{-1}$), σ is the reflection coefficient of the test solute used, and

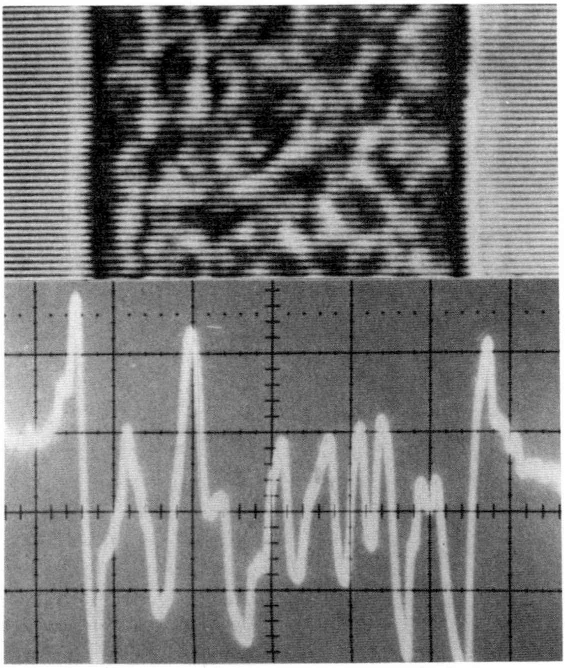

Fig. 1. *Top* Portion of typical S_2 segment as seen on monitor screen, diameter 38.20 μm. *Bottom* Light intensity pattern across single raster line in above tubule. (From [3] with permission)

$\Delta\pi$ is the mOsm difference between the equilibration medium and the test medium as measured by vapor pressure technique.

To approximate J_{Vo} at time $t = 0$, we use only those tubule diameters and changes in relative tubule volume recorded and measured to be linear during the first few 1/60 s time intervals following osmotic challenge and change from steady state dimensions. The slope of that linear fit divided by the change in medium osmolality then gives the reflection coefficient of the test solute times the membrane hydraulic conductivity. Thus, if the solute has a reflection coefficient of one, as is the case for raffinose, the result is the membrane hydraulic conductivity, L_PA. Similarly, if two different solutes of equal measured osmolality are used in the same or different tubules, the ratio of the results is equal to the ratio of the reflection coefficients for the two different solutes employed. If one of the two solutes is raffinose, the result is a measure of the reflection coefficient of the second solute.

Results

Figure 2 shows the changes that occur in S_1, S_2, and S_3 proximal tubule segments after challenge with 240 mOsm hypotonic or 320 mOsm hypertonic raffinose medium. Note that the time scale is in units of 1/60 s and that only the first few time

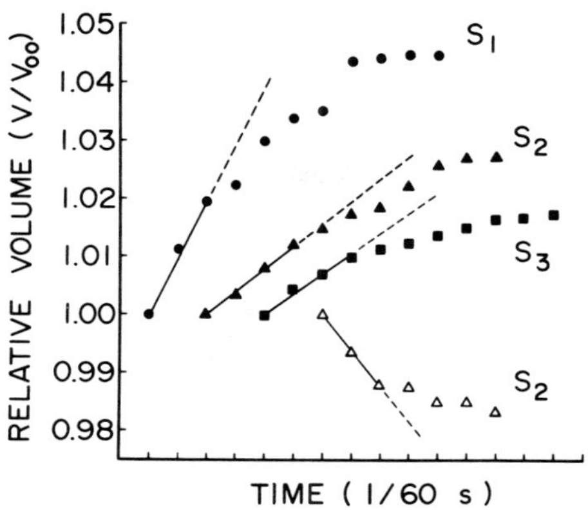

Fig. 2. Typical responses of S_1, S_2, and S_3 segments during first several 1/60 s time increments after hypotonic or hypertonic challenge of approximately 40 mOsm. (From [2] with permission)

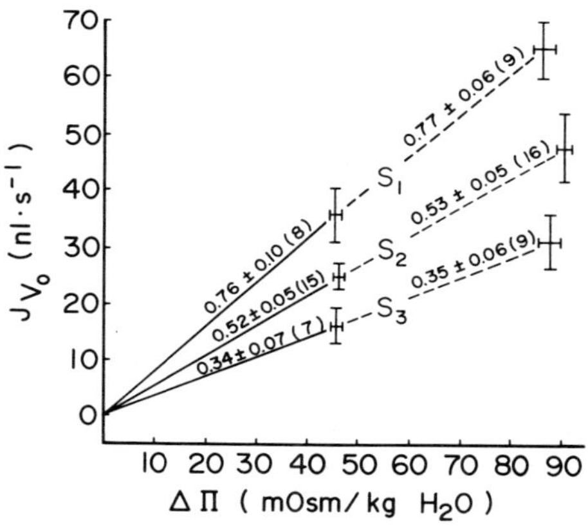

Fig. 3. Hydraulic conductivities of S_1, S_2, and S_3 segments given by the slopes of J_{V_o} vs magnitude of hypotonic challenge. (From [2] with permission)

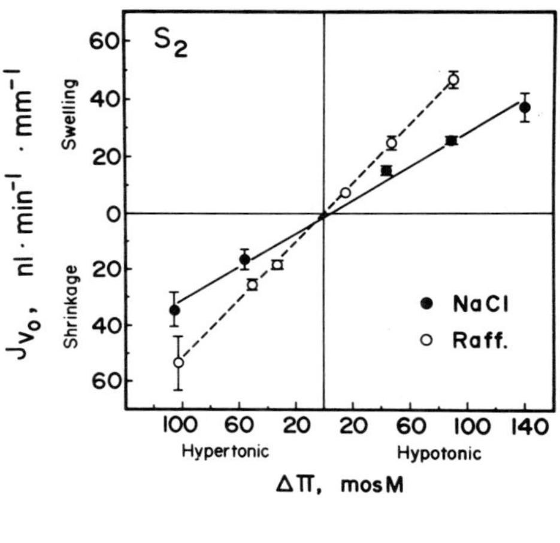

Fig. 4. Relationship in S_2 segments between J_{V_o} and magnitude of challenge produced by raffinose or NaCl. (From [3] with permission)

Table 1. Relative osmotic effectiveness of different solutes

	A		B		$\frac{\sigma_A}{\sigma_B}$
n	Solute	$\sigma L_P A$/mm	Solute	$\sigma L_P A$/mm	
		nl·min^{-1}·min^{-1}·mOsm^{-1}		nl·min^{-1}·min^{-1}·mOsm^{-1}	
54	KCl	0.36 ±0.02	Raffinose	0.51 ±0.03	0.70 ±0.02
13	NaCl	0.27 ±0.02	KCl	0.36 ±0.03	0.76 ±0.06
6	KCl	0.28 ±0.02	KCl + $BaCl_2$	0.29 ±0.02	0.97 ±0.06
9	Na gluconate	0.33 ±0.03	Raffinose	0.40 ±0.03	0.84 ±0.06
10	K gluconate	0.37 ±0.05	Raffinose	0.39 ±0.06	0.97 ±0.07
8	Choline Cl	0.34 ±0.04	Raffinose	0.45 ±0.04	0.75 ±0.06

n, number of S_2 segments studied; σ, reflection coefficient of test solute; L_PA, basolateral membrane hydraulic conductivity per mm tubule length. All data mean ± SE

increments following a change from steady state volume have been considered. Note also the break in the volume vs time data after the first three or four data points and recall that calculations are based only on the slopes of the volume vs time data collected before that break point.

In Fig. 3 the hydraulic conductivities are given by the slopes of J_{Vo} vs magnitude of osmotic challenge for the three segment types. Clearly, hydraulic conductivity is greater in S_1 segments than in S_2, and greater in S_2 than in S_3. It is important to recognize, however, that the calculated hydraulic conductivities are in units of L_PA, where L_P is an intrinsic property of the membrane and A is the area of the membrane across which water movement occurs. If one divides by the known areas of basolateral membrane per millimeter tubule length [6], the result for all three segments is found to be about 300 μm·s^{-1}, not statistically different among the three segments, and approximately that calculated for mammalian red blood cell membrane [2].

The conclusion from these studies, therefore, is that proximal tubule basolateral cell membranes are quite leaky to water and that, in terms of cell volume regulation, membrane hydraulic conductivity is unlikely to be a limiting factor.

Figure 4 shows a comparison between the effects of raffinose in 59 S_2 segments and the effects of NaCl in 44 other S_2 segments. Since raffinose has a reflection coefficient of one, the ratio of these two effects is a measure of the NaCl reflection coefficient. The result from those data is a σNaCl of 0.56 ± 0.07. A very similar result was found in S_1 segments [3].

Because the experiments just described required a statistical comparison between separate groups of tubules, the procedure subsequently was changed to allow comparisons in individual tubules, each exposed to two hypertonic test solutions in random sequence and with intervening periods of equilibration in isotonic medium. To date, that new technique has been used to study the relative effects of KCl vs NaCl and of raffinose vs KCL, Na gluconate, K gluconate, or choline chloride [4]. The results are summarized in Table 1.

The first horizontal line of Table 1 shows that the osmotic efficiency of KCl is quite different from that of raffinose, $P < 0.001$. The ratio of the effects, and thus the reflection coefficient of KCl, is calculated there to be 0.73. In the next line it is seen that the efficiency of NaCl is less than that of KCl by a factor of about 0.76. In other words, although KCl is 0.7 times as efficient as raffinose, it still is 1.3 times more efficient than NaCl across the basolateral cell membrane. This is completely consistent with the earlier finding of a NaCl reflection coefficient of 0.56.

Regarding the other data in Table 1, note that the use of Na gluconate and choline Cl, in which the gluconate and choline can be assumed to be impermeant ions, results in calculated reflection coefficients statistically different both from unity and from the 0.56 value for NaCl. The result with K gluconate, however, is not different from that with raffinose.

Discussion

The findings in these studies lend themselves to discussion in two broad areas, one dealing with steady state osmotic balance in renal tubules and another dealing with the nature of the water and ion channels in the basolateral cell membrane. The starting point for both discussions is the recognition that while raffinose is a single species in solution, the other solutes used here are electrolytes that completely dissociate into their respective ions. Their observed effects, therefore, are the net effects of their component parts.

Consider first the proposition that the reflection coefficient for an electrolyte is the simple average of the reflection coefficients of its component ions. For example, $\sigma KCl = (\sigma K^+ + \sigma Cl^-)/2$, $\sigma NaCl = (\sigma Na^+ + \sigma Cl^-)/2$, etc. Now, if one considered only the σKCl and $\sigma NaCl$ results and the fact that chloride is common to both, it would be possible to establish broad ranges for the individual ion reflection coefficients. However, the more valuable information comes from the Na gluconate, K gluconate, and choline Cl studies in which we have the advantage of knowing that gluconate and choline have reflection coefficients of one. Thus, if σ Na gluconate = 0.84, σNa^+ must be approximately 0.68; if σK gluconate = 0.97, σK^+ must be approximately 0.94; and if σ choline Cl = 0.75, σCl^- must be approximately 0.50. Each of these values is, in fact, quite consistent with what would have been expected from the KCl and NaCl studies alone. That is, calculating from $\sigma Na^+ = 0.68$ and $\sigma Cl^- = 0.50$, $\sigma NaCl$ should have a value of about 0.59. That result is in good agreement with the 0.56 value actually observed. Furthermore, using $\sigma KCl = 0.73$ and $\sigma Cl^- = 0.50$, σK^+ should have a value of approximately 0.96, a value also in good agreement with that calculated from the K gluconate studies.

Returning now to the question of steady state osmotic balance, it is of interest to point out a seeming paradox in the maintenance of cell volume, namely, that under normal circumstances the cells of proximal renal tubule contain approximately 140 mM K^+, 10 mM Na^+, and 30 mM Cl^- (a total of 180 mM), while the bathing medium contains approximately 5 mM K^+, 150 mM Na^+, and 120 mM Cl^- (a total of 275 mM). Thus there is a 95 mM discrepancy which, if the reflection coefficients of the principal solutes were taken to be unity, would represent an osmolality difference of 95 mOsm/kg that presumably would have to be made up by other intracellular solutes. The nature of those solutes, however, is not readily apparent. On the other hand, if one multiplies the intra- and extracellular potassium, sodium, and chloride concentrations by the reflection coefficients from the present studies, the missing osmoles are reduced dramatically to about 13 mOsm. Furthermore, of those remaining, perhaps 5 mOsm might be accounted for by large impermeant solutes [7], and a variety of other solutes could easily contribute the rest. In any case, the point to be made is that any consideration of cell volume maintenance or adjustment, be it in the osmometric phase or the recovery phase, cannot disregard the reflection coefficients of the solutes involved.

The second broad area of discussion to which our results contribute is the nature of the water and ion channels in the basolateral membranes. Several comments can be made.

First, since the reflection coefficients for sodium and for chloride are found to be less than unity, those solutes and water must have common pathways through the cell membrane. Since solute movement thus must accompany water movement, the cell cannot be viewed as a perfect osmometer.

Second, it might be seen to be inconsistent that we find σNa^+ to be considerably less than σK^+ in spite of the well-known fact that the diffusional permeability of potassium exceeds that of sodium. That could be explained, however, if potassium mostly employs a highly permeable channel from which water is excluded, while sodium shares a pathway with water, as would all other solutes with reflection coefficients less than unity. Since potassium channels in this membrane are known to be blocked by barium [8], the present finding that the osmotic effect of KCl is not affected by $BaCl_2$ supports both the finding of a potassium reflection coefficient near unity and the suggestion that K^+ and water do not share a common pathway.

The last point of discussion has to do with the earlier assumption that the reflection coefficient of an electrolyte can be considered to be the average of the reflection coefficients of its dissociated ions. In spite of the fact that calculations based on that assumption yield internally consistent results and predict individual ion values quite appropriate for the maintenance of steady-state cell volume, it still should be asked how this can be reconciled with the fact that, for reasons of transmembrane charge conservation, electrolyte reflection coefficients would be weighted toward the least permeant ionic species with the highest reflection coefficients [9]. In other words, if gluconate and choline are indeed impermeant, how could the reflection coefficients of sodium gluconate and choline chloride have been anything other than unity?

To this we have no answer except to point out the very acute nature of the studies and the possibility that, at the initial instant of osmotic change, the membrane is just penetrated to various degrees by the several ionic species that still behave as hydrated particles in the bathing solution. Subsequently, as the particles proceed through the membrane and the transient state is diminished, there presumably would have to occur either a change in the effective reflection coefficient or a change in the steady state charge condition near the membrane. In the latter case, the reflection coefficient might even become a function of the ambient environmental conditions and the recent past history of the cell.

References

1. Dellesega M, Grantham JJ (1973) Regulation of renal tubule cell volume in hypotonic media. Am J Physiol 224:1288–1294

2. Welling LW, Welling DJ, Ochs TJ (1983) Video measurement of basolateral membrane hydraulic conductivity in the proximal tubule. Am J Physiol 245 (Renal Fluid Electrolyte Physiol 14):F123–F129
3. Welling LW, Welling DJ, Ochs TJ (1987) Video measurement of basolateral NaCl reflection coefficient in proximal tubule. Am J Physiol 253 (Renal Fluid Electrolyte Physiol 22):F290–F298
4. Welling LW, Welling DJ, Ochs TJ (1990) Relative osmotic effects of raffinose, KCl, and NaCl across basolateral cell membrane. Am J Physiol (Renal Fluid Electrolyte Physiol 28):F594–F597
5. Pedley TJ (1983) Calculation of unstirred layer thickness in membrane transport experiments: a survey. Q Rev Biophys 16:115–150
6. Welling LW, Welling DJ (1988) Relationship between structure and function in renal proximal tubule. J Electron Microsc Tech 9:171–185
7. Linshaw MA, Stapleton FB, Cuppage FE, Grantham JJ (1977) Effect of basement membrane and colloid osmotic pressure on renal tubule cell volume. Am J Physiol 233 (Renal Fluid Electrolyte Physiol 2):F325–F332
8. Welling PA, Linshaw MA, Sullivan LP (1985) Effect of barium on cell volume regulation in rabbit proximal straight tubules. Am J Physiol 249 (Renal Fluid Electrolyte Physiol 18):F20–F27
9. Kedem O, Leaf A (1966) The relation between salt and ionic transport coefficients. J Gen Physiol 49:655–662

Fluid Transport by Leaky Epithelia and Cell Volume Regulation

KENNETH R. SPRING[1]

SUMMARY. The mechanism and pathways of fluid absorption by leaky epithelia are subjects of considerable investigation and controversy. Theories and models of fluid transporting epithelia are briefly reviewed and related to fluid absorption across renal proximal tubules. The relevance of cell volume regulation to transepithelial fluid absorption is also discussed.

The Movement of Water Through Membranes and Tight Junctions

The means by which water may cross cell membranes have been recently reviewed in detail [1]. The movement of water may be treated theoretically in the same manner as the flow of any substance: water is driven by the difference in its electrochemical potential. Flow always occurs as a result of the driving forces which comprise the electrochemical gradient for a substance. In the case of water, the primary factors are the relative concentration of water across a barrier (i.e., the solute concentration difference) and the hydrostatic pressure difference. Electro-osmotically driven flow does not appear to be a significant factor in the movement of water across cell membranes [1–3].

Inasmuch as the flow of water is dependent on its gradient, the issue of the mechanism of transepithelial water flow may be reduced to two considerations: (1) Determination of the site and magnitude of the differences in water activity, and (2) Measurement of the water permeability of the relevant pathways across the epithelium. Most attempts to directly determine the magnitude of the water activity differences have not been successful because of difficulties in sampling the relevant

[1]Laboratory of Kidney and Electrolyte Metabolism, National Heart, Lung, and Blood Institute, Building 10, Room 6N307, Bethesda, MD 20892, USA

compartments and of precisely analyzing collected samples. It should be clear from the above considerations that there must be, within or adjacent to the epithelium, a region in which water activity differs from that of the bulk solutions. Determination of the site of this region of altered osmolality, as well as the magnitude of the osmotic pressure difference, has occupied the interest of transport physiologists for over 30 years.

Osmolality of the Transported Fluid

The earliest investigators were impressed by the lack of measurable difference in the composition of the bulk solutions bathing small intestine studied in vitro [4,5]. A number of studies in intestine [6] and renal proximal tubule [7] supported these earlier workers, showing that the calculated osmolality of the transported fluid agreed, within experimental error, with that expected for isosmotic transport. The subject of the osmolality of the transported fluid was investigated again in both gallbladder [8–10] and renal proximal tubule [11,12]. No measurable transepithelial differences in macroscopic osmolality were detected in these studies, supporting the conclusion that transepithelial osmotic pressure differences did not exist. Differences in solute reflection coefficients, and therefore the effective osmotic pressure generated by the bathing solutions, have been proposed as important factors in the generation of transepithelial driving forces for fluid movement across renal proximal tubule [13,14]. Although cryoscopic osmolality may not differ, the effective osmolality of solutions depends on the relative reflection coefficients of the solutes across the epithelial layer.

As studies of fluid absorption by mammalian proximal tubule have progressed, the issue of the composition of the transported fluid has received a great deal of attention [15]. Evidence has been obtained that the fluid filling the lumen of the proximal tubule may become slightly hypotonic as transport of solutes and water progresses [13,14,16]. Collection of the proximal tubular absorbate showed it to be significantly hypertonic to the lumenal perfusate, with much of the preferentially absorbed solute being glucose and other organic solutes [17,18]. In tissues such as the intestine, the underlying connective tissue (submucosa) precludes the type of fluid collection experiments done in perfused renal tubules and the composition of the transported fluid may be determined only indirectly. However, estimates of the osmolality of the subepithelial layer in small intestine support the conclusion that the osmolality of the interstitial fluid may be altered as a result of fluid absorption [19].

Models of Epithelial Fluid Transport

Although it was generally agreed that transepithelial water movement must be the result of osmosis, workers were perplexed by the fact that no transepithelial osmotic gradients could be detected. In most epithelia the transepithelial potential was also near zero [2,9,10,20], ruling out simple electro-osmosis as a mechanism for fluid transport. The most widely accepted solution to these problems was put forward by Diamond and Bossert [21] in their “standing gradient” model for fluid transport. This model was an outgrowth of an earlier three compartment model for epithelial fluid transport developed by Curran and MacIntosh [22]. Curran and MacIntosh developed a three compartment model which resulted in vectorial fluid transport consequent to solute injection into the middle compartment. The membrane between the middle compartment and the outer bath was assumed to be similar to a cell membrane, while the membrane facing the inner bath was assumed to be similar to a basement membrane. The outer membrane was an effective semipermeable barrier, while the inner membrane was ineffective as an osmotic barrier. Thus, as solute was injected into the middle compartment by active transport, water was osmotically drawn into this compartment from the outer bath. Water was not drawn into the middle compartment from the inner bath because of the lack of solute reflection by the inner membrane, i.e., because the inner membrane was not semipermeable, but was freely permeable to both solutes and water. As water entered the middle compartment the pressure within it rose and forced fluid out across the leaky inner membrane. The pressure caused predominant flow across the inner membrane because of its high hydraulic conductivity (water permeability) compared to that of the outer membrane.

An analysis of models for fluid-transporting epithelial was done by Weinstein and Stephenson [23,24]; they characterized all epithelial models as variants of the original scheme of Curran and MacIntosh. The essential conclusion is that transepithelial water flow arises because there is, within the epithelium, a region of higher osmolality than the bulk solutions. The exact location of the middle compartment of the Curran and MacIntosh scheme was not defined by those investigators, although the characteristics of the limiting membranes were strictly delineated.

Whitlock and Wheeler [25] suggested, on the basis of morphological studies of the rabbit gallbladder, that the middle compartment of the Curran and MacIntosh model was the lateral intercellular space separating epithelial cells. Tormey and Diamond [26] confirmed and extended the work of Whitlock and Wheeler and provided the morphological basis for the mathematical model developed by Diamond and Bossert [27]. It is worthwhile recalling why Diamond and Bossert rejected the simple three compartment scheme for osmotic flow as the mechanism of transepithelial fluid transport. They reviewed the literature values for epithelial hydraulic water permeability and concluded that the water permeability of the cell membranes was too low to enable water and solute to move out of the cell with equal speed. In other words, they concluded that salt actively transported out of the cell would rapidly diffuse away before exerting significant osmotic effect across the basolateral membrane. They therefore proposed a region of restricted solute diffusion within the epithelium where water and solute could equilibrate and achieve isotonicity. The lateral intercellular space was the postulated site of solute-solvent coupling. The space geometry and the location of the solute pumps figured prominently in this model. The spaces had to be sufficiently narrow and tortuous to restrict solute diffusion; the pumps had to be located near the blind, tight junctional end of the channel. Alterations of interspace geometry, such as widening or shortening of the space, resulted in the formation of hypertonic absorbate. Thus, a model was developed and widely accepted which assigned critical importance to the morphology of the epithelium.

What has followed in the last 20 years is a large number of morphological and theoretical studies concerned with the geometric alterations associated with variations in the rate of transepithelial fluid transport. It became evident that several of the key assumptions of the standing gradient model were incorrect. It was convincingly demonstrated that the tight junction was leaky to solutes [28,15] and that solute pumps were uniformly distributed [29,30], rather than clustered at the apical end of the channel as required by the standing gradient model. Model calculations showed that it was theoretically impossible to achieve true isotonic transport with the standing gradient [15] and that all acceptable models reduced to the three compartment system of Curran and MacIntosh [23,24,59]. Although serious questions about the standing gradient model for transepithelial fluid transport were raised by Hill [20], Diamond [2] had already noted that difficulties with the model were primarily associated with uncertainties about the values for the hydraulic water permeability of the basolateral cell membrane. Diamond [2] pointed out the need for direct determination of cell membrane water permeability, as well as the need for better estimates of epithelial water permeability, free of the errors due to solute polarization in the unstirred layers. Finally Weinstein and Stephenson [24] pointed out that there was no need for a standing gradient to achieve solute-solvent coupling when cell membrane water permeability was in the range of experimentally determined values for nonepithelial cell membranes.

Water Permeability of Epithelia

Epithelial hydraulic water permeability (L_p) has been measured in a number of preparations by the imposition of transepithelial osmotic pressure gradients. As previously discussed, unstirred layers adjacent to or within the tissue cause substantial underestimates of L_p [2,31–34]. The extent of the unstirred layer dependent error in L_p has been extensively discussed and it has been generally concluded that the L_p of most epithelial has been underestimated by an order of magnitude or more [1,2,34]. The exception to this conclusion is the renal tubule which, because of its small size, is essentially free of unstirred layer related errors [16,35]. Even in renal proximal tubule there is a relatively wide range (approximately ten-fold) of estimated L_p values [35]. Knowledge of the L_p of the epithelium is essential both to determination of the route of transepithelial fluid flow as well as to estimation of the magnitude of the osmotic forces required to achieve that flow [36]. Finally, estimates of epithelial reflection coefficient for individual ions or solutes are dependent on the epithelial L_p value [36].

The most reliable estimates of L_p in leaky, flat epithelia have come from work on rabbit gallbladder done by Van Os et al. [37] using rapid stirring and a fast response flow measurement apparatus developed by Wiedner [7]. These investigators determined L_p by imposition of either osmotic or hydrostatic pressures and determined the resultant volume flows by a capacitance method. Hydrostatic pressures can be used to measure L_p without concern about unstirred layer related effects. It should be noted that the imposition of hydrostatic pressure differences across the epithelium results in alterations of cell geometry which have consequences on the rate of fluid transport. Naftalin and Tripathi [38] used high speed optical measurements combined with the capacitance probe technique to simultaneously measure the volume flows across rabbit ileum and estimate the flows across the individual cell membranes. They used both osmotic and hydrostatic pressures to drive fluid across the tissue and examined the magnitude of unstirred layer effects as well as possible electro-osmosis. They concluded that apical unstirred layer related effects were negligibly small in their system and that electro-osmosis was demonstrable, as evidenced by streaming potentials. Although their measurements are probably the most accurate estimate of intestinal water permeability made to date, I find their arguments concerning electro-osmosis to be unconvincing and conclude, as others have done [3,20], that electro-osmosis does not result in a significant transepithelial flow of water. It is clear that unstirred layers and the unfavorable tissue geometry of flat epithelia prevent a complete assessment of the fluid flows across these tissues.

Direct determination of cell membrane water permeability of an epithelium was first reported by Persson and Spring [39]. They used quantitative light microscopy to measure rapid changes in cell volume subsequent to alteration of the osmolality of the apical or basolateral solution bathing the Necturus gallbladder. Other investigators [21,40–43] estimated basolateral cell membrane L_p from the rate of swelling of collapsed renal proximal tubules suddenly exposed to hypotonic bathing solution. The accuracy, speed, and validity of these studies were questioned [35], and subsequent investigations [43,44] led to somewhat higher values for basolateral membrane L_p. Apical membrane L_p was measured in renal proximal tubules by Gonzalez et al. [21]. The first direct determinations of apical and basolateral cell membrane L_p in cortical collecting tubules of rabbit have also been made [33]. The inherent difficulties in making L_p measurements in cells with the high surface area and small volume of mammalian cells have been reviewed [45].

The reported values of cell membrane L_p for all epithelia fall into a relatively narrow range after correction for surface amplification. Unfortunately the units used to define water permeability values are confusing and inconsistent [1,39], making it difficult to directly compare results from different laboratories. The most commonly used units for hydraulic water permeability, L_p, are cm/s-atm; while water permeability, Posm, is usually expressed in μm/s. ($Posm = RTL_p/V_w$, where R is the gas constant, T is temperature, V_w is the partial molar volume of water). Rather than expose the reader to a plethora of values, it is more instructive to recognize that all epithelial cell membranes studied have L_p or Posm values that differ by no more than an order of magnitude. Most epithelial cell membranes have Posm values of 40–50 μm/s; the only exception being the "poorly permeable" membranes such as the apical membrane of toad urinary bladder [46] or cortical collecting duct [33] in the absence of antidiuretic hormone. These membranes have Posm values in the 5–25 μm/s range [1,33]; Posm increases 6–10-fold upon addition of the hormone. The high apparent L_p of epithelia such as the renal proximal tubule comes from the great area amplification created by the microvilli and extensive infoldings [24]. Necturus gallbladder apical area is increased 8-fold by microvilli and basolateral area is increased 26-fold [47]. In all absorptive tissues investigated to date, basolateral membrane area exceeded apical area, with the result that the effective basolateral membrane L_p was much larger than that of the entire apical membrane, even though the L_ps of the unit membranes were similar [33,39].

The most significant aspect of the L_p of epithelial cell membranes is the realization that water permeability is sufficiently large that water moves "freely" across these barriers. Once both apical and basolateral membrane water permeabilities are known, the driving forces and routes of transepithelial water movement may also be estimated.

Route of Transepithelial Fluid Flow

Transcellular movement of water may not be the sole pathway for transepithelial flow, because the tight junction is known to be leaky to ions. There is no reason to believe that the junctions are not also permeable to water and that some fraction of transepithelial fluid flow is paracellular [36,48]. Most conclusions about the routes taken by water and solutes across epithelia have come from model calculations based on the geometry and structure of the tight junction and shunt pathway. Disputes about these parameters have led to a wide range of estimates of the relative flows across the cellular and shunt pathways. General agreement does exist about the relative areas of the cell and tight junction at the mucosal surface. In most epithelia, the area of the apical cell membrane is approximately 10^4 times that of the cross sectional area of the tight junction [48–50]. Significant rates of transepithelial flow of water and solutes across the tight junction occur when the area-adjusted permeability of that pathway approaches or exceeds that of the cellular pathway. The driving force for transepithelial volume flow is the osmotic pressure difference between the basolateral space and the apical bathing solution. If the same osmotic pressure exists across the tight junction and the entire cell, the relative flow through each path depends on the area-adjusted water permeability of each. As mentioned above, the basolateral membrane of epithelia is far more water permeable than the apical membrane, and interspace hypertonicity must therefore lead to volume flow across that membrane, with resultant increase in cell osmolality. The primary cellular barrier to osmotic pressure gradients is, then, the apical membrane. In Necturus gallbladder, the area-adjusted apical membrane Posm is 550 μm/s [48]; to achieve equal flows across junctional and cellular routes a junctional water permeability 10^4 times greater is required. The required junctional Posm, 5 m/s, is physically unreasonable, leading me to conclude that transjunctional flow of water is not a significant factor in fluid absorption. Other investigators have made similar calculations and reached the same conclusion [2,32,35,51]. However, the issue of the magnitude of the transjunctional volume flow remains controversial, with several reports favoring substantial paracellular water flux [25,36,43]. The route taken by water as it crosses the epithelium determines the epithelial solute reflection coefficients, as well as the magnitude of solvent drag effects. Until this issue is resolved interpretation of experimental results will be clouded.

Osmotic Driving Force Required for Transepithelial Flow

The osmotic driving force required to achieve the observed rate of fluid absorption may be calculated directly from the L_p of the epithelium. Such calculations for renal proximal tubule indicate that the osmotic pressure difference required is between 2 and 25 mosmol [19]. A similar calculation for Necturus gallbladder led to the conclusion that only 3.5 mosmol driving force was needed to achieve the observed rates of fluid absorption [39,48]. Such small differences in osmotic pressure are not readily detectable by conventional means [35,48,52], even when attempts are made to magnify the differences [19,53]. Assuming such osmotic pressure differences exist within the lateral intercellular spaces, it is instructive to consider the consequences of a hypertonic interspace.

Transcellular Osmosis

On the basis of the preceding discussion, it is possible to estimate the transmembrane driving forces required to obtain the observed rates of fluid absorption by transcellular osmotic flow for tissues in which cell membrane water permeabilities have been determined. Extensive work on the mechanism of fluid flow across Necturus gallbladder [39,48,54] has provided the necessary permeability and fluid flow rate information for calculations for that leaky tissue.

Knowledge of the cell membrane water permeabilities permits calculations to be made of the osmotic driving forces required to transport water across each membrane. The rate of fluid transport across Necturus gallbladder is about 1.6×10^{-6} cm/s [54]. If virtually all of this fluid enters the cells across the apical membrane, the osmotic pressure difference required to achieve this rate of fluid flow is about 1.6 mosmol/kg. The cell osmolality must be 1.6 mosmol higher than that of the apical solution to result in this flow. Vectorial water flow across epithelia must be the result of a gradient in water activity across the epithelial cell layer. The water activity in the fluid surrounding the basolateral membrane of the cell must be lower than that in the cell for water movement across that membrane. The calculated osmotic gradient across the basolateral membrane, based on its water permeability and a volume flow of 1.6×10^{-6} cm/s, is about 0.7 mosmol/kg. In other words, the osmolality of the interstitial fluid must be 0.7 mosmol/kg greater than that of the cell for water to move out of the cell at the required rate. Thus, the basolateral interstitial space must be about 2.3 mosmol/kg hypertonic to the apical bathing solution to result in normal rates of fluid transport [48]. The hyperosmolality of the interstitial fluid will result in an absorbate which is hyperosmotic to the bathing solutions by 1.5%. As mentioned above, such a small difference in osmolality would be very difficult to detect by present techniques. It is clear, however, that the cells become slightly anisotonic as a result of water entry across the apical membrane. Conversely, water would not enter the cells if there were no gradient in its activity.

Mechanism of Fluid Exit from the Basolateral Spaces

As Curran and MacIntosh [22] showed in their model of fluid transport, hydrostatic pressure constitutes the driving force for fluid exit from the middle compartment (lateral intercellular spaces and basolateral interstitium). The basement membrane and underlying connective tissue are highly permeable structures with virtually no solute reflection capabilities [55]. As a result of the low reflection coefficient of connective tissue, osmotic pressures cannot develop across these tissues. Fluid will only move across the submucosa by hydrostatic or oncotic forces. As fluid leaves the epithelial cells, driven by the osmotic pressure difference across the basolateral membrane, the lateral intercellular spaces fill and become dilated [26,56,57]. From the pressure volume curves of the spaces [56], it is possible to calculate the hydrostatic pressure within the spaces. For Necturus gallbladder this pressure difference amounts to 3 cm of water or less at normal rates of fluid transport. The hydraulic properties of the underlying basement membrane and connective tissue determine the magnitude of the pressure rise in the spaces. The pressure will increase until it is sufficient to drive the transported fluid across the submucosa. The magnitude of the restriction of fluid movement offered by the submucosal structures is an important factor in determination of the rate of transepithelial fluid flow [5,15,19,23,24,48].

Another mechanism could account for some of the fluid exit from the lateral intercellular spaces during transepithelial fluid transport. McGlaughlin and Mathias [3] proposed that water could be driven out of the lateral spaces by electro-osmotic flow parallel to the plane of the lateral cell membrane. This type of electro-osmosis had not been previously proposed for biological systems; it is dependent on close approximation of the lateral membranes of adjacent cells. If the lateral membranes of the epithelial cells are separated by a distance of 0.2 μm or less, the electric field created by the current through the Na-K pump could constitute a driving force for electro-osmotic movement of fluid out of the interspace. Mammalian renal proximal tubule cells may have the correct geometry for such electro-osmosis to occur, and McGlaughlin and Mathias [3] suggested several experiments to test their hypothesis in this epithelium. This mechanism will not account for significant fluid flows in epithelia in which the lateral spaces are widely separated during fluid transport, but it represents a possible class of water transport that has been overlooked as a biologically relevant phenomenon.

Transjunctional Flows of Water and Ions

As discussed above, the tight junctions have been shown by many investigators to be leaky to solutes. It is unreasonable to assume that such an extracellular shunt pathway does not permit water to cross. The issue is not whether water will move across the junction, but the relative magnitude of the transjunctional fluid flux compared to the transcellular flow. Clearly, if one had accurate measurements of both epithelial and cell apical membrane L_p, the junctional contribution to transepithelial flow could be readily determined. Whittembury et al. [43] have attempted these measurements in renal proximal tubule and concluded that about one half of the transepithelial flow occurs across the tight junction. In other experiments Whittembury et al. [58] have attempted to demonstrate solvent drag of extracellular solutes across gallbladder. The demonstration of solvent drag is difficult, because the solutes employed diffuse across the junction into the interspace, while the fluid coming out of the cell across the lateral membranes is presumably free of these solutes. Thus the fluid within the spaces always has a lower concentration of the solute than does either bulk solution. Diffusion of solute from the apical bathing solution may then be mistaken for solvent drag [2,28].

In my opinion it is not possible to accurately estimate the magnitude of the transjunctional flow of water at present. Weinstein [36] has recently calculated that the permeability and solute reflection properties of the rat renal proximal tubule cannot be reproduced by a mathematical model which does not permit substantial (50% or greater) transjunctional water flow. These calculations do not agree with my conclusion that transjunctional flow is negligible in leaky epithelial [48]. Resolution of this issue awaits future experimental results.

The conflict over the magnitude of the transcellular versus transjunctional water flow does not extend to the area of ion movements across these pathways. Boulpaep [59] first showed that the paracellular pathway, constituted by the tight junction and lateral intercellular spaces, was the primary route for transepithelial ionic currents. This conclusion has been supported by innumerable observations in many tissues, notably those of Frizzell and Schultz [60] in intestine. In most tissues the apical cell membrane permeability to ions is about 10^{-5}–$[10]^{-7}$ cm/s. Equal diffusional flows through the cellular and junctional paths would occur when the junctional permeability is in the range of $[10]^{-1}$–10^{-3} cm/s. Transjunctional ion flows would predominate when the junctional permeability exceeds that of the cell membrane. The calculated maximum diffusional permeability of the tight junction of Necturus gallbladder [48] is about 1.5 cm/s. Thus, junctional ion permeability could be about 10–500 times that of the cellular pathway without any physically unrealistic assumptions. The difference in the paths taken by water and salt in response to transepithelial gradients arises not because the junctions are selectively permeable to salt, but because the cell membrane restricts the flow of salt markedly compared to that of water.

Fluid Transport and the Regulation of Cellular Volume

The large volumes of fluid which move across epithelial cell membranes would result in significant dilution or concentration of the cytoplasm if fluid entry and exit were not balanced. As an example, the rates of fluid movement across renal proximal tubule cells are sufficiently great that the entire cellular volume is replaced every 20 seconds (or every 40 seconds if only half of the fluid absorption is transcellular as discussed above). If entry or exit rates change as a result of altered solute movements, cell volume should change dramatically. Substantial experimental evidence has been obtained which shows that stimulating solute entry, for example by the addition of a sugar or amino acid to the apical bathing solution, leads to significant cell swelling [61,62]. Similarly, interfering with solute exit results in cell swelling because solute entry continues [54,63–65]. In these cases cell swelling did not result in the rapid volume regulatory decrease usually observed when bathing solution osmolality is decreased. Necturus gallbladder is an example of an epithelium which shows cell volume regulatory behavior as well as transport related volume alterations.

When solute entry into Necturus cells is blocked by the removal of Na or Cl from the apical bathing solution [39,54,57], shrinkage of the cell occurs. The shrinkage results from the continued operation of the solute exit mechanism, primarily the Na,K-ATPase [54,64,65]. No sign of volume regulatory increase is observed, although the shrinkage is large (17%) compared to the osmotic stimulus (6%) required to activate volume regulatory increase. Blockage of solute exit, by the addition of ouabain, a specific inhibitor of the Na,K-ATPase results in cell swelling at a constant rate of 4% per minute [54,64]. This swelling has been shown to result from the continued entry of NaCl from the apical bath into the cell across the apical membrane. After 10–30 minutes, cell volume reaches a maximum of about 1.4 times that of control and a slow shrinkage begins that persists for many minutes or hours [64]. If at any time during the swelling phase resulting from ouabain addition an osmotic perturbation is imposed, volume regulatory behavior is activated [39,65,66]. It is apparent that changes in osmolality trigger a specialized response in Necturus gallbladder cells that differs from the response to perturbations in solute entry or exit. I have speculated in the past on the physiologic basis for volume regulation [48,65], and have concluded that volume regulation may be a misnomer. Volume is really not regulated, per se, the intracellular concentration of some key solute may be what is being regulated.

The kind of volume regulatory behavior exhibited by Necturus gallbladder epithelial cells raises questions about the relevance of volume regulation to transepithelial fluid transport. The response to a sudden perturbation of the osmolality of the bathing solution is a very rapid (60–90 seconds) readjustment of cell volume to control size, despite the continued presence of the anisotonic bath [65]. Such a perturbation may not be an appropriate stimulus for the study of the control of cell volume or composition, as discussed by Lohr and Grantham [61]. These investigators reported that the response of collapsed renal proximal tubules to a change in solution osmolality depended on the rate at which the osmolality change occurred. Changes of bath osmolality between 167 and 361 mosmol/kg did not cause a change in tubule volume if the rate of osmolality alteration did not exceed 1 mosmol/kg per min. The response to a sudden osmolality change may be due to changes in cell pH or calcium secondary to the change in cell osmolality [65]. In addition, the role of organic solutes in the maintenance of epithelial cell volume is not well understood.

At present the relationship between transepithelial fluid transport and cell volume regulation is not clearly defined. Inasmuch as fluid transport involves osmotic gradients across the cell membranes, it is possible to regard the regulatory responses to external osmolality changes as a manifestation of the osmoregulation required for balanced fluid entry and exit. The intracellular indicator(s) which trigger volume regulatory responses have not been identified in epithelia; their role, if any, in the regulation of transepithelial fluid transport is also unknown. Clearly, there is a great deal yet to be learned about fluid transport by epithelia.

References

1. Finkelstein A (1987) Water movement through lipid bilayers, pores, and plasma membranes. J. Wiley, New York
2. Diamond JM (1979) Osmotic water flow in leaky epithelia. J Membr Biol 51:195–216
3. McGlaughlin S, Mathias RT (1985) Electro-osmosis and the reabsorption of fluid in renal proximal tubules. J Gen Physiol 85:699–728
4. Goldschmidt S (1921) On the mechanism of absorption from the intestine. Physiol Rev 1:421–453
5. Reid W (1902) Intestinal absorption of solutes. J Physiol 28:241–256
6. Curran PF, Solomon AK (1957) Ion and water fluxes in the ileum of rats. J Gen Physiol 41:143–168
7. Wiedner G (1976) Method to detect volume flows in the nanoliter range. Rev Sci Intrum 47:775–776
8. Diamond JM (1962) The reabsorptive function of the gallbladder. J Physiol 161:442–473
9. Diamond JM (1964) Transport of salt and water in rabbit and guinea pig gallbladder. J Gen Physiol 48:1–14
10. Diamond JM (1964) The mechanism of isotonic water transport. J Gen Physiol 48:15–42
11. Andreoli TE, Schafer JA, Troutman SL (1978) Perfusion rate-dependence of transepithelial osmosis in isolated proximal convoluted tubules: Estimation of the hydraulic conductance. Kidney Int 14:263–269
16. Schafer JA (1984) Mechanisms coupling the absorption of solutes and water in the proximal nephron. Kidney Int 25:708–716

17. Barfuss DW, Schafer JA (1981) Collection and analysis of absorbate from proximal straight tubules. Am J Physiol 241 (Renal Physiology 10):F597–F604
18. Williams JC, Barfuss DW, Schafer JA (1986) Transport of solute in proximal tubules is modified by changes in medium osmolality. Am J Physiol 250 (Renal Fluid Electrolyte Physiol 19):F246–F255
19. Hallback D-A, Jodal M, Lundgren O (1980) Villous tissue osmolality, water and electrolyte transport in the cat small intestine at varying luminal osmolalities. Acta Physiol Scand 110:95–100
20. Hill A (1980) Salt-water coupling in leaky epithelia. J Membr Biol 55:117–182
21. Gonzalez E, Carpi-Medina P, Linares H, Whittembury G (1984) Osmotic water permeability of the apical membrane of proximal straight tubular (PST) cells. Pflugers Arch 402:337–339
22. Curran PF, MacIntosh JR (1962) A model system for biological water transport. Nature 193:347–348
23. Weinstein AM, Stephenson JL (1981) Coupled water transport in standing gradient models of the lateral intercellular space. Biophys J 35:167–191
24. Weinstein AM, Stephenson JL (1981) Models of coupled salt and water transport across leaky epithelia. J Membr Biol 60:1–20
25. Whitlock RT, Wheeler HO (1964) Coupled transport of solute and water across rabbit gallbladder epithelium. J Clin Invest 48:2249–2265
26. Tormey JM, Diamond JM (1967) The ultrastructural route of fluid transport in rabbit gallbladder. J Gen Physiol 50:2031–2060
27. Diamond JM, Bossert WH (1967) Standing-gradient osmotic flow. A mechanism for coupling of water and solute transport in epithelia. J Gen Physiol 50:2061–2083
28. Berry CA, Boulpaep (1975) Nonelectrolyte permeability of the paracellular pathway in Necturus proximal tubule. Am J Physiol 228:581–595
29. DiBona DR, Mills JW (1979) Distribution of Na pump sites in transporting epithelia. Fed Proc 38:134–143
30. Kyte J Immunoferritin determination of distribution of [Na+K] ATPase over plasma membranes of renal convoluted tubules. I. Proximal segment. J Cell Biol 68:287–303
31. Pedley TJ (1983) Calculation of unstirred layer thickness in membrane transport experiments, a survey. Q Rev Biophys 16:115–150
32. Schafer JA, Patlak CS, Andreoli TE (1974) Osmosis in cortical collecting tubules. J Gen Physiol 64:201–227
33. Strange KB, Spring KR (1987) Cell membrane water permeability of rabbit cortical collecting duct. J Membr Biol 96:27–43
34. Weinstein AM, Stephenson JL, Spring KR (1981) The coupled transport of water. In: Bonting SL, de Pont JJHHM (eds) New comprehensive biochemistry. Membrane transport, vol 2. Elsevier, Amsterdam, pp 311–351
35. Berry CA (1983) Water permeability and pathways in the proximal tubule. Am J Physiol 245 (Renal Fluid Electrolyte Physiology 14):F279–F294
36. Weinstein AM (1987) Convective paracellular solute flux. J Gen Physiol 89:501–518
37. Van Os CH, Wiedner G, Wright EM (1979) Volume flows across gallbladder epithelium induced by small hydrostatic and osmotic gradients. J Membr Biol 49:1–20
38. Naftalin RJ, Tripathi S (1985) Passive water flows driven across isolated rabbit ileum by osmotic, hydrostatic and electrical gradients. J Physiol 360:27–50
39. Persson B-E, Spring KR (1982) Gallbladder epithelial cell hydraulic water permeability and volume regulation. J Gen Physiol 79:481–505
40. Carpi-Medina P, Lindemann B, Gonzales E, Whittembury G (1984) The continuous measurement of tubular volume changes in response to step changes in contraluminal osmolality. Pflugers Arch 400:343–348

41. Gonzalez E, Carpi-Medina P, Whittembury G (1982) Cell osmotic water permeability in isolated rabbit proximal straight tubules. Am J Physiol 242 (Renal Electrolyte Fluid Physiol 11):F331–F330
42. Welling LW, Welling DJ, Ochs TJ (1983) Video measurement of basolateral membrane conductivity in the proximal tubule. Am J Physiol 245 (Renal Fluid Electrolyte Physiol 14):F123–F129
43. Whittembury G, Paz-Aliaga A, Biondi A, Carpi-Medina P, Gonzalez E, Linares H (1985) Pathways for volume flow and volume regulation in leaky epithelia. Pflugers Arch 405(Suppl 1):S17–S22
44. Verkman AS, Ives HE (1986) Water permeability and fluidity of renal basolateral membranes. Am J Physiol 250 (Renal Fluid Electrolyte Physiol 19):F633–F643
45. Strange KB, Spring KR (1986) Methods for imaging renal tubule cells. Kidney Int 30:P192–200
46. Kachadorian WA, Sariban-Sohraby S, Spring KR (1985) Regulation of water permeability in toad bladder at two barriers. Am J Physiol 248 (Renal Fluid Electrolyte Physiol 17):F260–F265
47. Suzuki K, Kottra G, Kampmann L, Fromter E (1982) Square wave pulse analysis of cellular and paracellular conductance pathways in Necturus gallbladder epithelium. Pflugers Arch 394:302–312
48. Spring KR (1983) Fluid transport by gallbladder epithelium. J Exp Biol 106:181–194
49. Bentzel CJ, Parsa G, Hare DK (1969) Osmotic flow across proximal tubule of Necturus: correlation of physiologic and anatomic studies. Am J Physiol 217:570–580
50. Blom H, Helander HF (1977) Quantitative electron microscopical studies on in vitro incubated rabbit gallbladder epithelium. J Membr Biol 37:45–61
51. Preisig PA, Berry CA (1985) Evidence for transcellular osmotic flow in rat proximal tubules. Am J Physiol 249 (Renal Fluid Electrolyte Physiol 18):F124–F131
52. Ikonomov O, Simon M, Fromter E (1985) Electrophysiological studies on lateral intercellular spaces of Necturus gallbladder epithelium. Pflugers Arch 403:301–307
53. Zeuthen T (1983) Ion activities in the lateral intercellular spaces of gallbladder epithelium transporting at low external osmolalities. J Membr Biol 76:113–122
54. Larson M, Spring KR (1983) Bumetanide inhibition of NaCl transport by Necturus gallbladder. J Membr Biol 74:123–129
55. Persson B-E, Spring KR (1984) Permeability properties of the subepithelial tissues of Necturus gallbladder. Biochim Biophys Acta 772:135–139
56. Spring KR, Hope A (1978) The size and shape of the lateral intercellular spaces in a living epithelium. Science 200:54–58
57. Spring KR, Hope A (1979) Fluid transport and the dimensions of cells and interspaces of living Necturus gallbladder. J Gen Physiol 73:287–305
58. Whittembury G, Verde-Martinez C, Linares H, Paz-Aliaga A (1980) Solvent drag of large solutes indicates paracellular water flow in leaky epithelia. Proc R Soc Lond [Biol] 211:63–81
59. Boulpaep EL (1967) Ion permeability of the peritubular and luminal membrane of the renal tubule cell. In: Kruck F (ed) Transport und Funktion Intracellularer Elektrolyte. Urban and Schwarzenberg, Munich, pp 98–107
60. Frizzell R, Schultz SG (1972) Ionic conductances of extracellular shunt pathway in rabbit ileum. Influence of shunt on transmural sodium transport and electrical potential differences. J Gen Physiol 59:318–348
61. Lohr JW, Grantham JJ (1986) Isovolumetric regulation of isolated S_2 proximal tubules in anisotonic media. J Clin Invest 78:1165–1172
62. Tune BM, Burg MB (1971) Glucose transport by proximal renal tubules. Am J Physiol 221:580–585

63. Guggino WB (1986) Functional heterogeneity in early distal tubule of Amphiuma kidney: evidence for two modes of Cl and K transport across the basolateral cell membrane. Am J Physiol 250 (Renal Fluid Electrolyte Physiol 19):F430–F440
64. Jensen PK, Fisher RS, Spring KR (1984) Feedback inhibition of NaCl entry in Necturus gallbladder epithelial cells. J Membr Biol 82:95–104
65. Spring KR, Ericson A-C (1982) Epithelial cell volume modulation and regulation. J Membr Biol 69:167–176
66. Larson M, Spring KR (1984) Volume regulation by Necturus gallbladder: basolateral KCl exit. J Membr Biol 81:219–233

Organic Compounds in Renal Volume Regulation

WALTER G. GUDER, MICHAEL SCHMOLKE[1], and FRANZ X. BECK[2]

SUMMARY. Four small organic molecules belonging to the chemical groups of trimethylamines (betaine and glycerophosphorylcholine) and polyols (sorbitol and inositol) have been identified as acting as organic osmolytes in the kidney. When measured along the corticopapillary axis, each substance exhibits a specific distribution pattern, indicating a specific localization and function. Studying their behavior under vasopressin treatment in diabetes insipidus rats and after insulin treatment in diabetes mellitus rats confirmed this conclusion: arginine vasopressin (AVP) led to a steady increase of sorbitol and glycerophosphorylcholine over 7 days with no effect on inositol levels. Insulin treatment of diabetic rats, on the other hand, decreased sorbitol with a concomitant increase in glycerophosphorylcholine, again without any effect on tubular inositol concentrations. From this and in vitro studies it can be concluded that both hormones act by indirect mechanisms, which alter interstitial osmolality. This in turn leads to a change in tubular osmolyte synthesis, uptake, and release rates. In addition, the concentration of the respective precursors, glucose and choline, influences the formation rates of sorbitol and betaine.

Introduction

Extracellular osmolality in mammalian kidney exhibits a corticopapillary gradient, which changes with renal concentrating and diluting functions depending on water load, vasopressin activity, and other osmoregulatory factors [1]. Whereas the osmolality of interstitium and intracellular space of renal cortex changes only in a narrow range, in parallel with plasma osmolality, papillary osmolality of these compartments can vary from near-isotonicity during diuresis to some thousand mosmol/kg H_2O

[1]Institute of Clinical Chemistry, Bogenhausen Hospital, D 8000 Munich 81, Federal Republic of Germany
[2]Physiologisches Institut der Universität, D 8000 Munich 81, Federal Republic of Germany

during water deprivation [2]. Such dramatic changes impose a severe osmotic stress on all medullary cells, which would lead to cell damage if it were not accompanied by adequate osmoregulatory mechanisms. In various medullary cells, several mechanisms have been found which lead to intracellular osmotic equilibration during changing extracellular osmolalities while keeping intracellular electrolyte concentrations rather constant [2], with or without cell volume regulation [3,4].

Recently, four small organic molecules have been found in high concentrations intracellularly in renal medullary cells, where they form corticopapillary concentration gradients in parallel to the osmotic gradients [5,6]. These substances were identified as the polyols sorbitol and inositol and the trimethylamines betaine and glycerophosphorylcholine. Besides carrying out their role as osmotic effectors, methylamines have been shown to counteract the destabilizing effect of urea on enzymes (non-perturbing solutes) [7].

After reliable methods were developed to quantify individual organic osmolytes we were able to document their intracellular concentrations in inner and outer medullary tubules [6,8]. When polyols and methylamines were measured in more defined kidney and nephron segments, it turned out that each substance exhibited an individual concentration pattern (Fig. 1). This result implies that each osmolyte may have different functions in different osmotic states and may be regulated by specific mechanisms. This hypothesis was further substantiated in two diuretic models, the Brattleboro (diabetes insipidus centralis) and the streptozotocin treated (diabetes mellitus) rat.

Materials and Methods

Brattleboro rats, kindly provided by D. Ganten, Heidelberg, were treated with AVP (100 ng/day per 100 g b.w.) for up to 14 days, via intraperitoneal osmotic mini-pumps [9]. Diabetes mellitus rats, (diabetes mellitus induced by a single i.v. injection of 100 mg/kg b.w. streptozotocin) were obtained in collaboration with E. Schleicher, Institute for diabetes research, Munich. These rats were treated for 8 days with insulin or for 6 days with insulin followed by 2 days omitting the hormone [10]. As a control group, untreated Sprague-Dawley rats were run in parallel. Kidneys were excised and cut into five sections along the corticopapillary axis (Fig. 1); the organic osmolytes were quantitated by high performance liquid chromatography (HPLC) [11] and by enzymatic methods [6] described previously.

Results

Distribution of Organic Osmolytes Along the Corticopapillary Axis

When analyzed by HPLC [12] and by enzymatic methods [6] each organic osmolyte exhibited an individual distribution pattern along the corticopapillary axis in normal rat kidney (Fig. 1). Sorbitol was found nearly exclusively in the inner medulla, forming a steep gradient from inner/outer medullary border to papillary tip. In sharp contrast, inositol increased at the corticomedullary border (Fig. 1) [5,6,9], but seemed to have no gradient along the entire medulla. Glycerophosphorylcholine concentra-

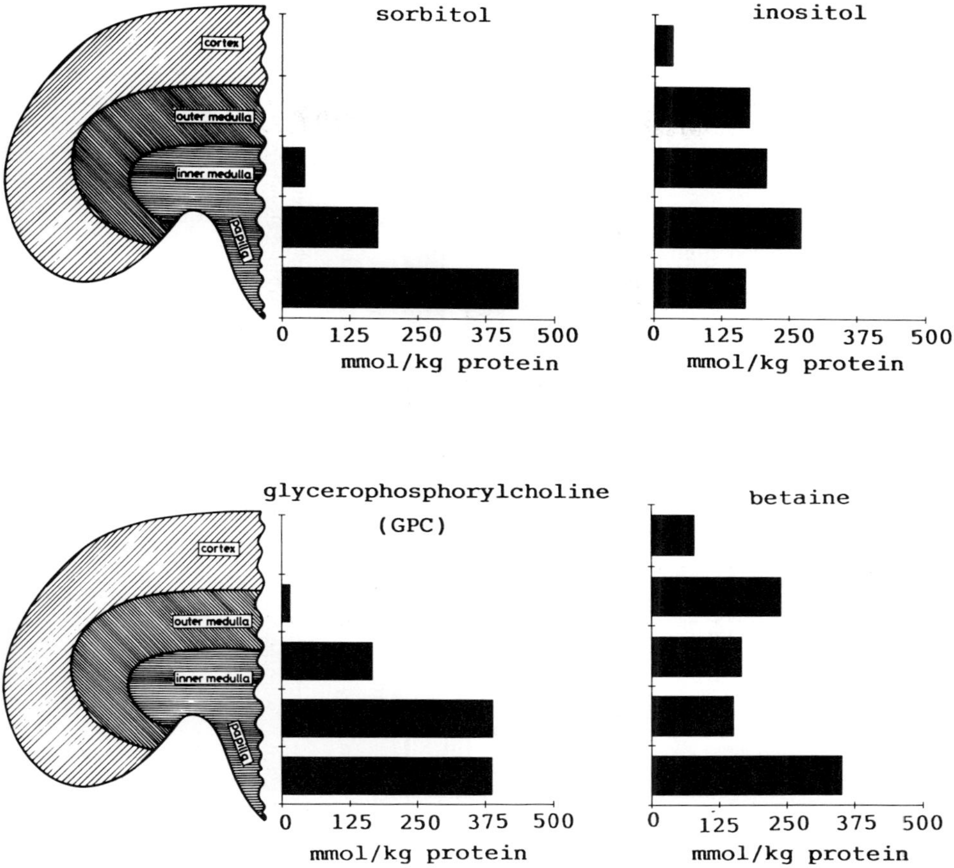

Fig. 1. Distribution of organic osmolytes in rat kidney. Sorbitol, inositol, glycerophosphorylcholine and betaine were quantitated in different sections of a normal rat kidney by the HPLC procedure described by Wolff et al. [11]. Results are given per tissue protein, measured by the biuret method in individual homogenates [6]

tion, on the other hand, increased from outer medullar to papilla, with negligible amounts in cortex. The betaine concentration increased in papillary tip, but in addition, it showed a unique gradient in the outer medulla decreasing to cortex. The latter finding has not been described before, whereas the other osmolyte patterns agree with those found in rabbit [12].

Changes in Diabetes Insipidus

Untreated Brattleboro rats were found to produce hypotonic urine (134 mosmol/kg, [9]). Under these conditions, sorbitol concentrations were reduced to 4–14% and glycerophosphorylcholine and betaine concentrations were reduced to 20–30%

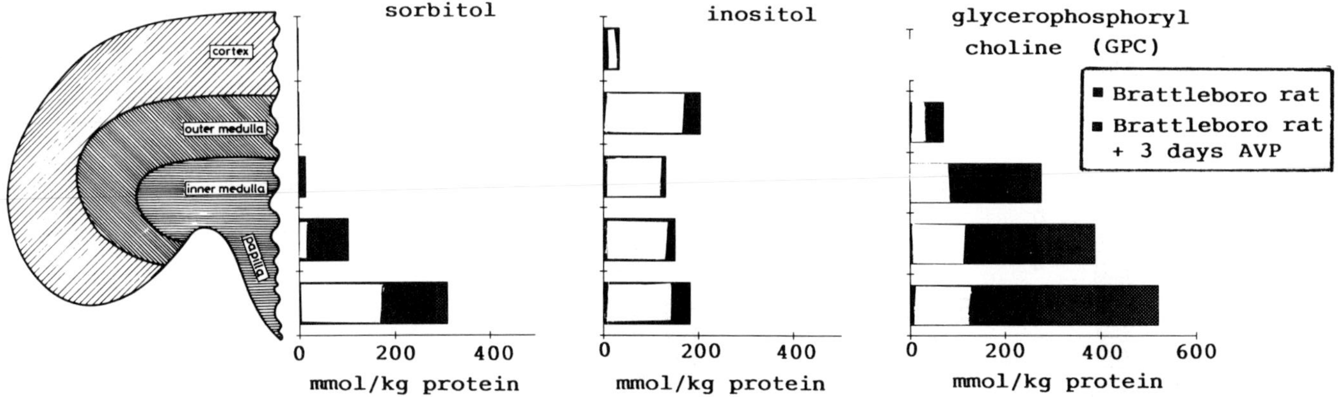

Fig. 2. Effect of arginine-vasopressin treatment on organic osmolyte concentrations in Brattleboro rat kidney sections. Brattleboro rats were treated with arginine vasopressin (*AVP*), 100 ng/100g bw per day, over 3 days, using osmotic mini-pumps; sorbitol, inositol, and glycerophosphorylcholine were quantitated by enzymatic methods as described elsewhere [9]. Results are means of four rats compared to those of three untreated Brattleboro rats

[9,13] of those found in control rats. In sharp contrast, inositol was little affected by diabetes insipidus, whereas furosemide, water and lithium diuresis decreased all four organic osmolytes [9,13,14,15,16].

Treatment with AVP led to normalization of organic osmolyte concentrations in 3 days (Fig. 2). Interestingly, urine osmolality increased before a significant effect of AVP on organic osmolyte content could be demonstrated. The conclusion that this finding indicates an indirect effect of AVP on organic osmolytes is confirmed by the lack of effect of this hormone on osmolyte content in isolated tubules (G Wirthensohn, unpublished work).

Osmolyte Content in Diabetes Mellitus

The sodium concentration of urine produced by insulin deficient diabetic rats was comparable to that in other diuretic states, but was of normal osmolality, due to high glucose concentration [10]. Therefore this model seemed to be suitable for the investigation of the possible role of sodium and glucose versus osmolality as possible triggers of organic osmolyte accumulation. In contrast to Brattleboro rats and furosemide diuresis, glycerophosphorylcholine was found to be only slightly decreased (Fig. 3) Inositol exhibited little change in diabetic animals. Sorbitol levels, on the other hand, increased 2–3-fold under these conditions, without significant changes in the distribution pattern (Fig. 3). Betaine was not measured in diabetic animals.

This glucose dependent increase in sorbitol, but not in inositol and glycerophosphorylcholine, was confirmed by in vitro experiments with inner medullary tubules: glucose increased sorbitol biosynthesis with a saturation above 10 mmol/l [6]. Distribution of newly synthesized sorbitol between cells and incubation medium was regulated by extracellular osmolality [6,8], pointing to a specific sorbitol export mechanism in papillary cells. In addition, diabetes mellitus was shown by Grunewald and Kinne [17] to increase the activity of the sorbitol forming enzyme, aldose reductase, known to be regulated at the gene level by extracellular osmolality in renal medullary cells [15].

Insulin treated diabetic rats showed a normalization of blood and urine glucose concentrations, urinary sodium, potassium, urea, and osmolality [10]. Accordingly, glycerophosphorylcholine increased slightly, inositol did not change, but sorbitol concentrations were reduced to levels between those of control and untreated diabetic rats. This decrease in cellular sorbitol was much less than expected from the normalization of glucose concentrations, indicating a time lag in adaptation of cellular osmolyte composition. Again the regional distribution pattern of organic osmolytes was not changed by insulin deficiency and insulin treatment.

Discussion

Why Four Different Organic Osmolytes?

The present findings and those of other investigators indicate that the four major substances found to be involved in renal medullary osmoregulation may have specific localization and specific regulation mechanisms, and may function under various physiological and pathophysiological conditions. This was confirmed by recent

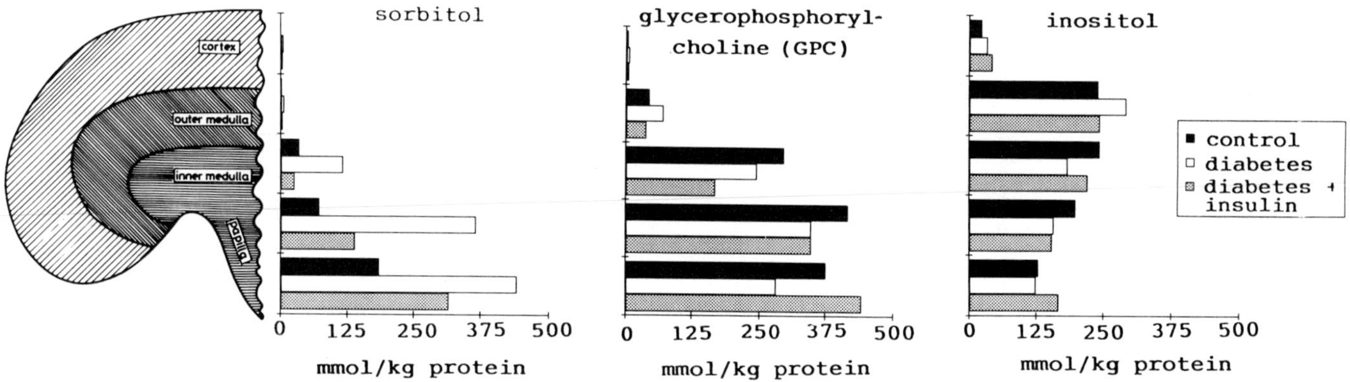

Fig. 3. Renal organic osmolytes in streptozotocin diabetic rats. Sorbitol, glycerophosphorylcholine, and inositol were measured by enzymatic methods in streptozotocin diabetic rats (100 mg/kg bw i.v.). *Black bars*: means of 3 untreated control rats run in the same series. *Open bars*: means of 9 diabetic animals, which were treated with insulin (2*5U per day) for 6 days after streptozotocin and analyzed on day 8, two days after insulin withdrawal. *Stippled bars*: means of 8 diabetic animals treated with insulin for 8 days

studies in microdissected nephron segments, showing a unique distribution of inositol in the segments of the thick ascending limb [18], whereas the enzymes for sorbitol synthesis [19] and sorbitol [18] were restricted to all tubular structures of the inner medulla. Choline oxidation to betaine, on the other hand, was shown to be highest in the S3 segment of the proximal tubule, but was also active in papillary tubules [20,21]. These findings point to a possible rôle of biosynthesis in regulating local osmolyte concentrations. On the other hand, cellular import and export mechanisms have been described as being involved in regulating tubular osmolyte concentrations [2].

Conclusions

From our present knowledge the following general conclusions may be drawn:

All four organic osmolytes described are present in papillary cells in concentrations which fill the osmotic gap between intracellular and extracellular salt concentration [2]. Moreover, betaine seems to play a specific role in cells at the corticomedullary border. Inositol forms high concentrations in loop cells of the thick ascending limb of Henle [20].

Betaine, glycerophosphorylcholine, and sorbitol are formed in tubular cells from their precursors choline [20,22] and glucose, [6,8,10] respectively; inositol and betaine, in addition, seem to be taken up by active transport from extracellular space [23]. All four osmolytes are highly concentrated in the cell, unless decreasing extracellular osmolality opens still undefined "gates" of cellular organic osmolyte export [6].

Besides their different locations along the nephron the presence of four different organic osmolytes in the renal papilla allows the kidney cell to adapt to various forms of changing osmolality in a flexible and specific way: Thus, vasopressin in vivo leads to an accumulation of all osmolytes [15], and water diuresis leads to rapid loss of all osmolytes [2] in the renal papilla, by changing interstitial osmolality. When sodium is replaced by glucose as extracellular osmolyte there is a specific increase in sorbitol [6,8,17].

Of all four organic osmolytes in the kidney, sorbitol is the best studied. The present study confirms that sorbitol is of special significance in diabetic states, where it seems to compensate for the high extracellular glucose concentrations [10,17,24]. Similar increases have been observed in diabetic eye lenses, nervous tissue, and blood cells [25]. The complications found in diabetes have partially been attributed to these changes. Consequently, aldose reductase inhibitors have been introduced to reduce tissue sorbitol levels. The present finding that, despite normoglycemia after two days of insulin treatment, sorbitol levels are still elevated, indicates slow adaptation of intracellular osmolality; this may help to explain osmoregulatory complications which appear during intensive treatment of hyperosmolar diabetic coma. On the other hand, aldose reductase inhibitors are expected to cause osmotic complications, if the missing sorbitol is not counterregulated by other osmolytes. The reciprocal changes in glycerophosphorylcholine and sorbitol concentrations in diabetic rats during treatment indicates that such mechanisms may exist in renal cells [10].

The lack of change in inositol concentration during AVP treatment in Brattleboro rats [9] and in diabetes mellitus [10] also contrasts with the behavior of the other polyols and suggests that the function of inositol in tubular osmoregulation differs from that of the other polyols.

In spite of our rapidly increasing knowledge of the mechanisms and sites of osmoregulation by organic osmolytes, major problems still remain to be investigated by future experiments: None of the transporters have been fully characterized, nor do we know the individual mediators that transfer the signal of changing extracellular osmolality to the intracellular sites. These unknown mediators seem to cause specific changes in the biosynthesis and transport of the individual osmolytes at the gene [15], protein [26], and membrane level [6,8,23]. Experiments in microorganisms, mammalian cell culture, and in vivo indicate that all kinds of mechanisms can be operative simultaneously, resulting in the specific osmolyte pattern observed in acute and chronic osmoregulation.

At present, little is known about the connection between cellular volume regulation and observed changes in organic osmolyte concentration. As extensively discussed in other contributions to these proceedings [2,4], cellular volume is expected to change upon rapid changes of intracellular osmolality. The rapidity and extent of volume regulatory changes may depend on the presence and velocity of changes in organic osmolyte concentrations. Thus, proximal tubule cells [27] and loop cells of the thick ascending limb of Henle [4] seem to be volume regulated, whereas in papillary collecting duct cells [2,3] this was not consistently observed.

Acknowledgment. The work reported herein was supported by the Deutsche Forschungsgemeinschaft (Gu 82/3-2 and Be 963/2-3).

References

1. Jamison RL, Kriz W (1982) Urinary concentrating mechanism. Oxford University Press, Oxford
2. Beck FX, Thurau K, Schmolke M, Guder WG (1991) Osmolytes and cell osmoregulation in the kidney. In: Proceedings of the XIth international congress of nephrology, July 15–20 1990. Tokyo, Japan
3. Law RO (1990) Adaptive volume responses of renal papillary cells exposed to hyperosmolal media. Renal Physiol Biochem 13:171–172
4. Hebert SC (1990) Rapid cell volume regulation. In: Proceedings of the XIth international congress of nephrology, July 15–20 1990. Tokyo, Japan
5. Bagnasco S, Balaban R, Fales H, Yang YM, Burg MB (1986) Predominant osmotically active organic solutes in rat and rabbit renal medullas. J Biol Chem 261:5872–5877
6. Wirthensohn G, Lefrank S, Schmolke M, Guder WG (1989) Regulation of organic osmolyte concentrations in tubules from rat renal inner medulla. Am J Physiol 256:F128–F135
7. Yancey P, Clark M, Hand S, Bowlus R, Somero G (1982) Living with water stress: evolution of osmolyte systems. Science 217:1214–1222
8. Schmolke M, Guder WG (1989) Metabolic regulation of organic osmolytes in tubules from rat renal inner and outer medulla. Renal Physiol Biochem 12:347–358
9. Schmolke M, Beck FX, Guder WG (1989) Effect of antidiuretic hormone on renal organic osmolytes in Brattleboro rats. Am J Physiol 257:F732–F737
10. Guder WG, Schleicher E, Schmolke M (to be published) Perturbation of renal polyols and glycerophosphorylcholine in streptozotocin diabetes and insulin treatment. Diabetologia
11. Wolff SD, Yancey PH, Stanton TS, Balaban RS (1989) A simple HPLC method for quantitating the major organic solutes of the renal medulla. Am J Physiol 256:F954–F956

12. Yancey PH, Burg MB (1989) Distribution of major organic osmolytes in rabbit kidneys in diuresis and antidiuresis. Am J Physiol 257:F602–F607
13. Blumenfeld J, Hebert S, Heilig C, Balschi J, Stromski M, Gullans S (1989) Organic osmolytes in inner medulla of the Brattleboro rat: effect of ADH and dehydration. Am J Physiol 256:F916–F922
14. Wirthensohn G, Lefrank S, Guder WG, Beck FX (1987) Studies of the role of glycerophosphorylcholine and sorbitol in renal osmoregulation. In: Kovacevic Z, Guder WG (eds) Molecular Nephrology: Biochemical aspects of kidney function. Walter de Gruyter, Berlin, pp 321–327
15. Cowley BD, Ferraris JD, Carper D, Burg MB (1990) In vivo osmoregulation of aldose reductase mRNA, protein, and sorbitol in renal medulla. Am J Physiol 258:F154–F161
16. Guder WG, Schmolke M, Lefrank S, Beck FX (1990) Specific changes of renal organic osmolyte pattern in different diuretic states (abstract). Renal Physiol Biochem 13:166–177
17. Grunewald W, Kinne RKH (1989) Sorbitol metabolism in inner medullary collecting duct cells of diabetic rats. Pflugers Arch 414:346–350
18. Schmolke M, Bornemann A, Guder WG (to be published) Polyol determination along the rat nephron. Biol Chem Hoppe Seyler
19. Sands JM, Terada Y, Bernard LM, Knepper MA (1989) Aldose reductase activities in microdissected rat renal tubule segments. Am J Physiol 256:F563–F569
20. Schmolke M, Bornemann A, Guder WG (to be published) Distribution and regulation of organic osmolytes along the nephron. In: Koide H, Endou H, Kurokawa H (eds) Cell Biology of Nephron Heterogeneity: Fine Structure and Functions. Karger Basel
21. Grossmann EB, Hebert SC (1989) Renal inner medullary choline dehydrogenase activity: characterization and modulation. Am J Physiol 256:F107–F112
22. Wirthensohn G, Guder WG (1982) Studies on renal choline metabolism and phosphatidylcholine synthesis. In: Morel F (ed) Biochemistry of kidney function. Elsevier, Amsterdam, pp 119–128
23. Nakanishi TR, Burg MB (1989) Osmoregulatory fluxes of myoinositol and betaine in renal cells. Am J Physiol 258:C964–C970
24. Burg MB (1988) Role of aldose reductase and sorbitol in maintaining the medullary intracellular milieu. Kidney Int 33:635–641
25. Burg MB, Kador PF (1988) Sorbitol, osmoregulation and the complications of diabetes: J Clin Invest 81:635–640
26. Bagnasco S, Uchida S, Balaban R, Kador P, Burg M (1987) Induction of aldose reductase and sorbitol in renal inner medullary cells by elevated extracellular NaCl. Proc Natl Acad Sci USA 84:1718–1720
27. Völkl H, Paulmichl M, Lang F (1988) Cell volume regulation in renal cortical cells. Renal Physiol Biochem 11:158–173

Volume Regulation in the Collecting Duct and Related Epithelia

KEVIN STRANGE[1]

SUMMARY. Under normal physiological conditions, cells of tight, Na^+-reabsorbing urinary epithelia, such as the collecting tubule, are exposed to both anisosmotic and isosmotic volume stress. A common but poorly understood response of these cells to volume perturbation is the activation of mechanisms that restore volume to its original resting value. The purpose of this article is to review briefly what is currently known about volume regulatory processes in the collecting tubule, amphibian and mammalian bladder, and frog skin. Specifically, the role of solute loss and accumulation pathways, transcellular cross-talk mechanisms, and volume sensor/transducer systems will be discussed. Key questions in need of future research will be emphasized.

Introduction

Under normal physiological conditions, cells of the renal collecting tubule are exposed to both anisosmotic and isosmotic volume stress. Anisosmotic volume changes are brought about by changes in extracellular osmolality, which fluctuates with the degree of diuresis or antidiuresis the animal is undergoing. In contrast, isosmotic volume perturbations occur when intracellular solute content changes. Variations in cell solute content take place during fluctuations in the activity of membrane transport processes.

In principle, it is teleologically desirable for cells to maintain a constant volume. Changes in cell volume can perturb flux through metabolic pathways, membrane transport processes, cellular signaling mechanisms, and the function of intracellular organelles. Excessive volume changes can result in cellular lysis. Many cell types, therefore, respond to volume perturbations by activating volume regulatory pathways. Cell volume regulation is brought about by the loss of, or accumulation of,

[1]The Children's Hospital, Division of Nephrology, Harvard Medical School, Boston, MA 02115, USA

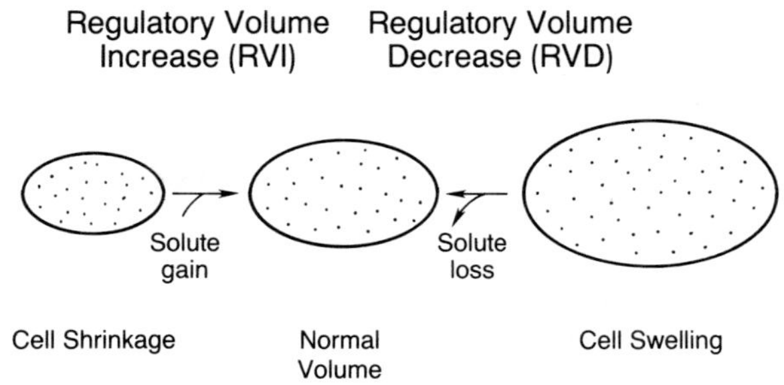

Fig. 1. Cells regulate their volume after swelling or shrinkage by the loss or gain of osmotically active solutes

inorganic ions and organic solutes, collectively referred to as osmolytes (Fig. 1). The purpose of this review is to discuss briefly the mechanisms and control of volume regulation in the renal collecting tubule and in three related epithelia, the amphibian bladder, the mammalian bladder, and frog skin. For additional discussions of cell volume regulation the reader should consult several articles published elsewhere in these proceedings (see List of Contents).

Volume Regulation Under Anisosmotic Conditions

One of the first studies of epithelial volume regulation was carried out by MacRobbie and Ussing in the frog skin [1]. These investigators demonstrated that dilution of the serosal bathing medium caused marked cell swelling, followed by a partial regulatory volume decrease (RVD) and significant loss of intracellular K^+. Ussing [2] demonstrated that RVD was inhibited by the Cl^- channel blocker, MK196, suggesting that parallel K^+ and Cl^- conductances mediate this process. Consistent with these observations are the recent microelectrode studies of Costa et al. [3], which suggest that cell swelling increases basolateral conductive K^+ permeability in this tissue.

MacRobbie and Ussing [1] also demonstrated that the frog skin was capable of undergoing regulatory volume increase (RVI). When volume-regulated skins were transferred from hypotonic to isosmotic medium, the cells shrank below their initial volume and then reswelled. Later studies by Ussing [4] demonstrated that this RVI process occurred only when Na^+, K^+, and Cl^- were present in the serosal bathing medium. In addition, the process was inhibited by furosemide and bumetanide, suggesting involvement of a basolateral Na/K/2Cl cotransport mechanism.

Optical studies carried out by Davis and Finn [5] have demonstrated that cells in the frog urinary bladder regulate their volume following exposure to serosal hypotonicity via a basolateral Ba^{2+}-sensitive K^+ channel. Interestingly, RVD is also blocked by luminal amiloride, which appears to decrease basolateral K^+ conductance via a transcellular cross-talk mechanism ([6]; discussed below). Studies by Lewis and coworkers [7–9] in both the toad and rabbit urinary bladders have indicated that cell shrinkage reduces basolateral K^+ conductance. Cell shrinkage also appears to inhibit the basolateral Cl^- conductance in rabbit bladder [8]. Downregulation of membrane ion permeability in these epithelia presumably reduces net cellular solute loss and aids in volume recovery. Donaldson and Lewis [9] have recently suggested that cell shrinkage in the rabbit bladder activates basolateral volume regulatory Na^+/H^+ and Cl^-/HCO_3^- exchangers.

Both principal and intercalated cells in the rabbit cortical collecting tubule (CCT) undergo nearly complete RVD following hypotonic cell swelling [10]. The mechanism by which this occurs, however, remains unknown. In this tissue RVD is not inhibited by bilateral addition of a variety of K^+ and Cl^- transport blockers (ouabain, bumetanide, Ba^{2+}, SITS, anthracene-9-carboxylic acid), bilateral HCO_3^- and CO_2 removal, bilateral elevation of K^+ concentration to 53 mM, or prolonged exposure of the tissue to K^+- or Cl^+-free media. These results suggest, very indirectly, that anisosmotic RVD may be mediated primarily by organic solute loss mechanisms such as occurs in medullary nephron segments and in cultured medullary cells [11].

The response of CCT cells to a volume decrease is variable. Principal cells show little or no capacity for RVI following 20–40 minutes of shrinkage [10,12]. In contrast, two populations of intercalated cell have been observed. One cell type shows no RVI capabilities, while the other undergoes a partial to complete volume recovery after shrinkage [10,12]. The mechanism of RVI and the relationship between volume regulation and the so-called type A and type B intercalated cell morphology is unknown.

Natke et al. [13] have reported that RVI can be activated in non-perfused rabbit CCT by exposure to low concentrations of butyrate. In perfused tubules, however, this organic acid has no effect on cell volume following hyperosmotic shrinkage (K. Strange, unpublished observations). It is interesting to speculate that the difference between the two preparations may be related to Na^+ transport. Sodium reabsorption in non-perfused tubules is blocked and, as such, it is likely that basolateral conductive pathways are downregulated (e.g., [6]; discussed below). Stimulation of solute influx pathways by butyrate (see [14]) may therefore allow net solute accumulation and RVI to occur.

Sun and Hebert [15] have examined volume regulation in the rat inner medullary collecting duct (IMCD). This nephron segment is normally exposed to variations in interstitial osmolality, which occur as part of the urinary concentrating mechanism. In the absence of antidiuretic hormone (ADH), the IMCD exhibits little or no RVI capabilities when exposed to a hypertonic medium. Peritubular addition of ADH or cAMP, however, stimulated a rapid RVI response following cell shrinkage. Volume regulation was inhibited by bilateral Na^+ or CO_2 and HCO_3^- removal and by peritubular addition of amiloride or DIDS, suggesting involvement of basolateral Na^+/H^+ and Cl^-/HCO_3^- exchangers. Luminal amiloride also inhibited RVI, suggesting that an apical cation channel or Na^+/H^+ exchanger may also mediate volume regulation.

The role of organic osmolyte transport and metabolism pathways in volume regulation has been examined in the intact renal medulla and in cultured renal medullary and Madin-Darby canine kidney (MDCK) cells (reviewed in [11]). Sands et al. [16] quantified aldose reductase activity in single, microdissected collecting tubule segments. The activity of this enzyme increased with depth into the medulla, suggesting that sorbitol is important for anisosmotic volume regulation in the medullary collecting duct. In suspensions of papillary tubules, Wirthensohn et al. [17] have observed high concentrations of inositol, sorbitol, and glycerophosphorylcholine. These organic compounds are transported out of the cell when extracellular osmolality is decreased, suggesting that they play an important role in RVD.

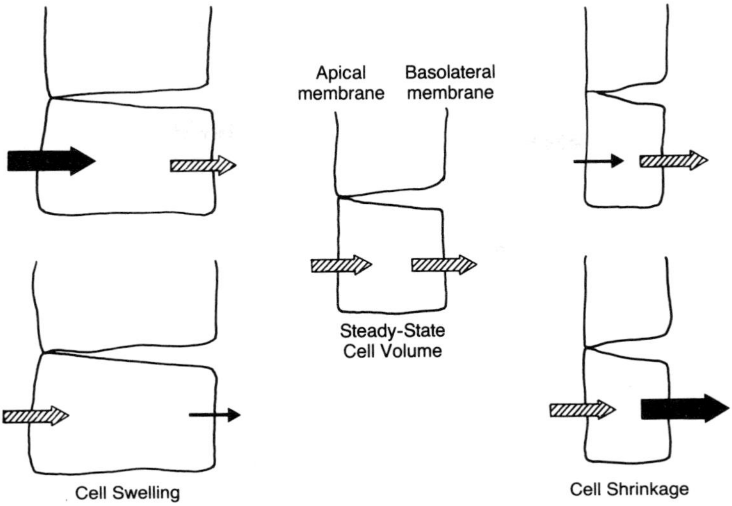

Fig. 2. Changes in the rates of apical and basolateral transport change epithelial cell volume. *Arrow size* reflects relative rate of solute influx or efflux (Modified from [30])

Volume Regulation Under Isosmotic Conditions

Under steady-state conditions, the rates of apical and basolateral membrane solute transport in epithelial cells are matched. These rates can, however, change independently of one another as the result of hormonal modulation of transport pathway activity and/or by variations in the concentration of transported solutes. This is particularly true in tight, Na^+-transporting, urinary epithelia. Tissues such as the collecting duct play a pivotal role in "fine tuning" whole animal salt and water balance. As such, transcellular transport rates can change rapidly and dramatically with changes in whole animal osmoregulatory demands. Figure 2 illustrates that independent changes in solute influx or efflux will alter intracellular solute content and cause cell swelling or shrinkage.

Regulation of epithelial cell volume during changes in transport is mediated by two distinct mechanisms. Transcellular cross-talk is a communication process that occurs between apical and basolateral cell membranes [18]. This communication allows epithelial cells to monitor rates of solute entry and exit and to adjust those rates so that they are matched. Return of epithelial cell volume to its original value following swelling or shrinkage is mediated by volume regulatory solute loss or accumulation pathways.

Transcellular Cross-Talk

The first observations of epithelial cross-talk were made by MacRobbie and Ussing in the frog skin [1]. These investigators noted that inhibition of basolateral Na^+ extrusion by ouabain caused an apparent reduction in apical Na^+, and basolateral K^+,

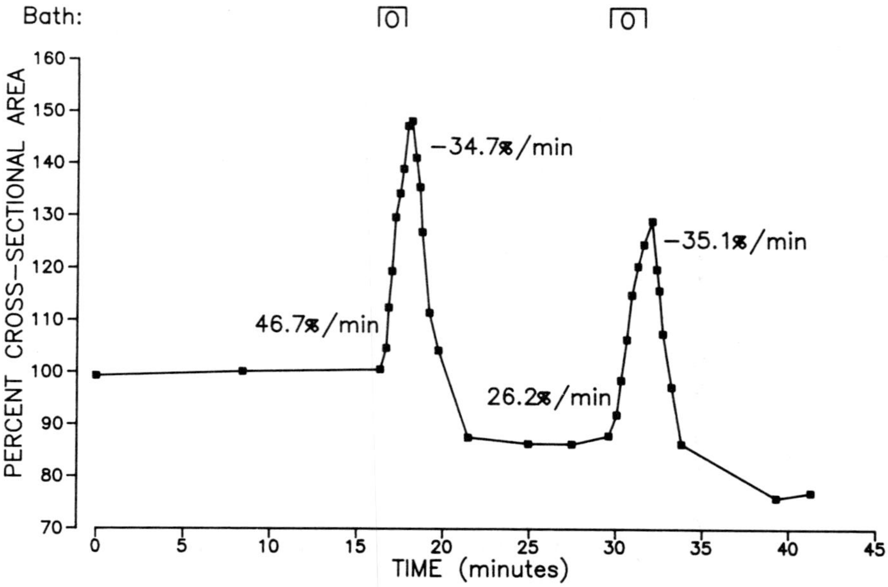

Fig. 3. Ouabain (O)-induced swelling in a principal cell of a CCT dissected from a mineralocorticoid-treated rabbit. The effects of ouabain on cell volume *per se* are readily reversible, but NaCl transport exhibits a long-term inhibition. Initial rates of cell swelling and shrinkage for the first and second periods of ouabain exposure and washout are shown. (See text and [20] for details)

permeability. Helman et al. [19] confirmed and extended these observations, using microelectrodes. Similar findings have also now been made in a variety of other Na^+ transporting epithelia [18].

In desoxycorticosterone acetate (DOCA)-treated rabbit CCT, ouabain causes principal cells to swell 50%–130% at rates of 25%–70%/min [20–21]. Cell swelling is due to net intracellular accumulation of NaCl and water during pump blockage. Sodium enters the cell primarily through an apical Na^+ channel. The mechanism and sidedness of Cl^- entry remains unclear at present.

As shown in Fig. 3, the effects of ouabain on principal cell volume are readily reversible. Removal of this inhibitor causes a rapid cell shrinkage as the pump is reactivated and NaCl is extruded from the cell. The effects of this compound on Na^+ reabsorption, measured as the rate of cell swelling, cannot be readily reversed, however. Brief, successive exposures to ouabain cause a rapid, concomitant reduction in the rate of Na^+ and/or Cl^- entry, while prolonged pump blockage results in a complete cessation of solute influx [20]. Reduction of apical solute entry during pump blockage prevents cell lysis and allows the cell to regulate its volume (discussed below).

Prolonged pump blockage also causes an apparent reduction of basolateral K^+ conductance in principal cells [21–22]. As discussed by Schultz [18], changes in basolateral K^+ permeability that occur with changes in Na^+ transport most likely reflect

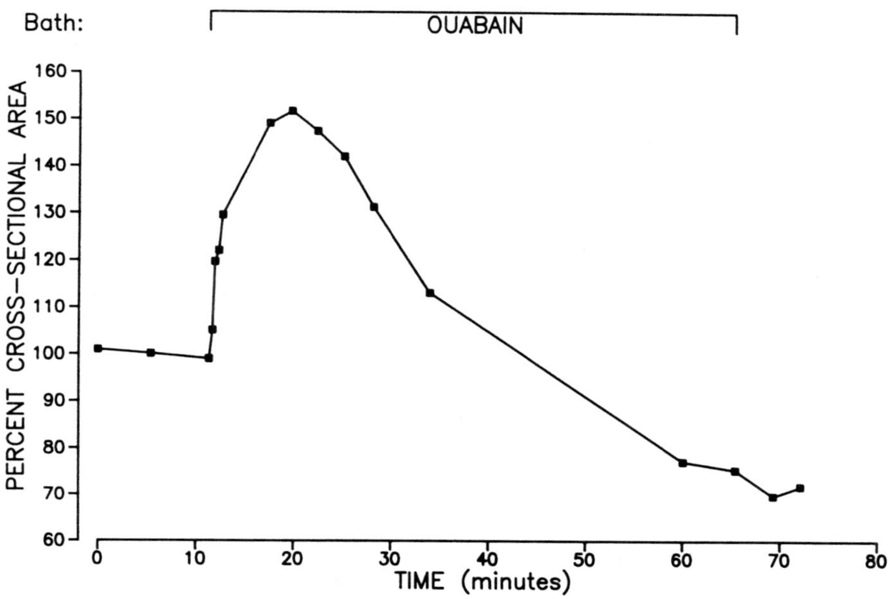

Fig. 4. Ouabain-induced swelling and RVD in a principal cell of a CCT dissected from a mineralocorticoid-treated rabbit

a close interaction between the Na^+/K^+ ATPase and K^+ channels. This pump-leak parallelism minimizes changes in cell K^+ when the activity of the Na^+ pump changes.

Primary changes in the rate of apical Na^+ entry also result in compensatory changes in rates of basolateral transport (see [18]). For example, in the amphibian urinary bladder, blockage of apical Na^+ channels with amiloride causes a rapid reduction in basolateral K^+ conductance [6].

Volume Regulatory Solute Loss and Accumulation

The mechanisms of isosmotic volume regulatory shrinkage or swelling are largely unknown. It is generally assumed that anisosmotic RVD and RVI pathways are the same as those activated following volume perturbations induced by changes in cell solute content. As discussed below, however, this may not be true in all cases.

The one tight epithelial cell type where isosmotic volume regulation has been examined in detail is the principal cell of the rabbit CCT. As discussed above, ouabain causes principal cells to swell rapidly. Attainment of the peak swelling volume is followed by volume regulatory shrinkage, which occurs at a rate of 4%–5%/min until a new volume 10%–15% below control is reached (Fig. 4). Bilateral addition of Ba^{2+} or tetraethylammonium $(TEA)^+$ inhibits [21] RVD 50%–60%. Bath addition of TEA^+ has no effect on RVD, but luminal perfusion with TEA^+ or quinidine inhibits the process by 50%–60% [21]. Since Ba^{2+}, TEA^+, and quinidine are blockers of K^+ channels, these results suggest that RVD is mediated in part by an apical K^+ conductance. Luminal K^+-induced cell swelling studies have indicated that the RVD channel is distinct from the resting apical K^+ conductance responsible for transepithelial K^+ secretion [21]. The RVD channel may be similar to the Ca^{2+}-activated high conductance channel described in patch clamp studies [23]. Ca^{2+}-sensitive, maxi K^+ channels mediate volume regulation in several cell types [24].

Volume regulatory K^+ loss must be accompanied by an equimolar loss of anion. The magnitude of the ouabain-induced volume increase requires that Cl^- accumulated in the cell be lost for RVD; no other intracellular anion is present in sufficient quantity to account for the magnitude of the observed volume regulatory shrinkage. Since K^+ efflux occurs via a conductive pathway, Cl^- loss should also occur by a channel mechanism. Recent studies from this laboratory have confirmed this prediction [22]. Reduction of peritubular Cl^- concentration transiently depolarizes the transepithelial potential by 35 mV and stimulates the rate of RVD 30-fold. Peritubular application of 0.5 mM DIDS inhibits RVD 74%. In contrast, luminal Cl^- reduction or application of DIDS has no effect on RVD.

Luminal K^+-induced swelling confirmed the presence of a Cl^- conductance in the basolateral membrane of volume-regulated principal cells [22]. The rate of K^+-swelling is unaffected by luminal Cl^- removal, but is inhibited 96%–99% by peritubular or bilateral replacement of Cl^- with isethionate. This unilateral inhibitory effect of Cl^- removal indicates clearly that the major pathway for KCl influx during luminal K^+-induced swelling is via K^+ and Cl^- channels located on opposing cell membranes.

K^+-swelling studies have demonstrated that the RVD Cl^- channel has a high selectivity for Cl^- over other anions [22]. Surprisingly, the channel has a very low NO_3^- permeability. Substitution of bath Cl^- for this anion inhibits the rate of K^+-swelling by 82%. The resting basolateral Cl^- channel also has a low NO_3^- permeability, suggesting, very indirectly, that it may be the predominant anion conductance responsible for RVD.

The volume regulatory response of principal cells to ouabain-induced swelling is likely to have a direct physiological correlate. Several endogenous substances have now been shown to inhibit the renal Na^+/K^+ ATPase, including prostaglandin E_2 (PGE_2), a potent natriuretic factor, and the vasoconstrictor substance, endothelin (reviewed in [21]). Rapidly accumulating evidence suggests that the hypothalamus produces a very high-affinity inhibitor of the Na^+/K^+ ATPase that functions in a manner similar to ouabain and may play a role in controlling renal salt and water excretion [25]. Doucet and Barlet [26] have suggested that the CCT may be a primary site of action of this so-called hypothalamic inhibitory factor (HIF).

An expected consequence of the action of endogenous pump blockers is cell swelling and volume regulation. In support of this prediction, Strange [21] has recently shown that micromolar concentrations of PGE_2 induce a pattern of swelling and RVD qualitatively identical to that seen with ouabain. Such results suggest strongly that the volume regulatory response to ouabain-induced swelling may occur with acute physiological downregulation of the Na^+ pump. Figure 5 illustrates a working model of isosmotic volume regulation in CCT principal cells.

It is interesting and important to note that anisosmotic and isosmotic volume regulation may not necessarily be carried out by the same transport pathways. As discussed above, hypotonic RVD in CCT principal cells does not appear to extensively involve passive KCl loss [10], whereas RVD following Na^+ pump blockage is clearly mediated by K^+ and Cl^- channels [21–22]. This suggests, indirectly, that the way in which cell volume is altered may influence the activity of volume regulatory path-

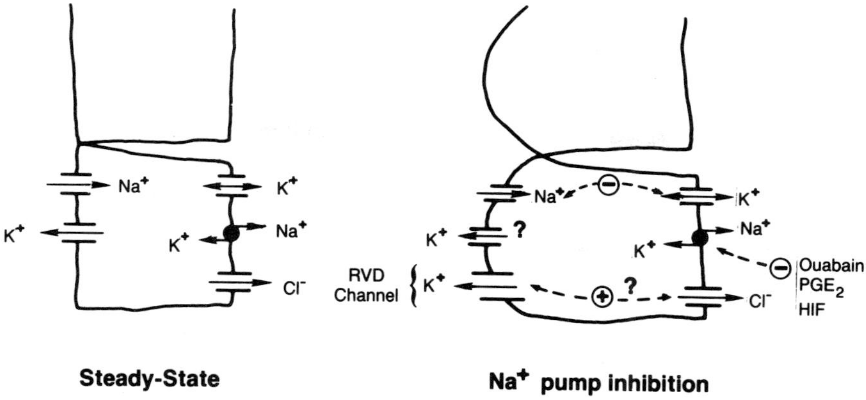

Fig. 5. Tentative cellular model of volume regulation in rabbit CCT principal cells following inhibition of the Na^+ pump. HIF, hypothalamic inhibitory factor. (See text and [20–22] for details)

ways. Such a possibility is supported strongly by recent studies of Rome et al. [14,27]. These investigators quantified volume regulatory electrolyte loss and uptake in rabbit proximal tubules by electron microprobe analysis. Their results demonstrate clearly that the mechanisms utilized by proximal tubule cells for RVD or RVI are influenced by the rate at which cell volume is changed. For example, during gradual exposure to hyperosmotic solutions, 52% of the observed RVI was due to uptake of inorganic ions. The remainder of the RVI was mediated by some unknown organic solute(s). When proximal tubules were abruptly exposed to hyperosmotic solutions, however, only 21% of the observed RVI was due to inorganic ion accumulation [14]. Similar findings were made during exposure of proximal tubules to rapid or gradual reductions in extracellular osmolality [27].

Control of Volume Regulatory Pathways

Control of volume regulation requires the involvement of two distinct processes. First, the cell must have a means to sense a change in volume and/or intracellular composition. Second, the cell must be able to transduce the volume or compositional change into a regulatory response. Very little is known about these processes in either epithelial or symmetrical cells.

Intracellular Ca^{2+} has been implicated extensively in the control of cross-talk during fluctuations in transcellular Na^+ transport [18]. Changes in cell Na^+ concentration are "sensed" by the basolateral Na^+/Ca^{2+} exchanger through changes in electrochemical driving forces. For example, increases in cell Na^+ lead to a reduction in the inward driving force for Na^+/Ca^{2+} exchange and lead to an elevation of cell Ca^{2+} concentration. Cell Ca^{2+}, in turn, transduces the primary change in cell Na^+ into a regulatory response by directly or indirectly inhibiting apical Na^+ channels.

Elevation of cell Ca^{2+} may also activate Ca^{2+}-sensitive, volume-regulatory solute loss mechanisms such as K^+ channels. For example, anisosmotic RVD in frog bladder is blocked when serosal Ca^{2+} is removed [5]. In toad bladder, Wong et al. [28] have demonstrated that hypotonic swelling induces large increases in cell Ca^{2+} levels. Furthermore, removal of extracellular Ca^{2+} or buffering of intracellular Ca^{2+} changes inhibits RVD in this tissue (reviewed in [28]). Other cellular messengers, such as inositol phosphates, leukotrienes, G proteins, protein kinase activity, etc., are also likely to be involved in the control of volume regulatory pathways [24].

Stretch activated and stretch inhibited [24,29] ion channels may play an important role in volume regulation in some cell types. Mechanosensitive transport pathways apparently sense membrane stretch, such as that induced by cell swelling or shrinking. This membrane stretch is then transduced directly into a change in transmembrane solute flux.

For long-term volume stress, changes in the synthesis of membrane transporters and metabolic enzymes are likely to play an important volume regulatory role (e.g., [11,24]). In this case, the genome senses cell structural or compositional changes directly and then transduces those changes into altered gene expression. Genetic sensor-transducer systems are important in bacterial volume regulation (reviewed in [24]).

Conclusions

From the above discussion it is clear that an understanding of anisosmotic and isosmotic volume regulation in "tight," Na^+-transporting epithelia is still very much in its infancy. Future research must provide a detailed description of the transport and metabolic pathways and driving forces responsible for RVD and RVI. The possibility that cells possess multiple volume regulatory mechanisms that are activated under different conditions needs to be examined. Changes in cell solute content accompanying volume regulation must be quantified and volume sensors and intracellular signaling pathways need to be elucidated. The technical challenges involved in investigating these important areas are formidable. An integrated use of electrophysiological, optical, biochemical, and molecular biological approaches is required.

References

1. MacRobbie EAC, Ussing HH (1961) Osmotic behaviour of the epithelial cells of frog skin. Acta Physiol Scand 53:348–365
2. Ussing HH (1986) Epithelial cell volume regulation illustrated by experiments in frog skin. Renal Physiol 9:38–46
3. Costa PMF, Fernandes PL, Ferreira HG, Ferreira KTG, Giraldez F (1987) Effects of cell volume changes on membrane ionic permeabilities and sodium transport in frog skin (*Rana ridibunda*) J Physiol 393:1–17
4. Ussing HH (1985) Volume regulation and basolateral co-transport of sodium, potassium and chloride ions in frog skin epithelium. Pflugers Arch 405:S2–S7
5. Davis CW, Finn AL (1987) Interactions of sodium transport, cell volume, and calcium in frog urinary bladder. J Gen Physiol 89:687–702
6. Davis CW, Finn AL (1982) Sodium transport inhibition by amiloride reduces basolateral membrane potassium conductance in tight epithelia. Science 216:525–527
7. Lewis SA, Butt AG, Bowler MJ, Leader JP, MacKnight ADC (1985) Effects of anions on cellular volume and transepithelial Na^+ transport across toad urinary bladder. J Membr Biol 83:119–137

8. Donaldson PJ, Chen LK, Lewis SA (1989) Effects of serosal anion composition on the permeability properties of rabbit urinary bladder. Am J Physiol 256:F1125–F1134
9. Donaldson PJ, Lewis SA (1990) Effect of hyperosmotic challenge on basolateral membrane potential in rabbit urinary bladder. Am J Physiol 258:C248–C257
10. Strange K (1988) RVD in principal and intercalated cells of rabbit cortical collecting tubule. Am J Physiol 255:C612–C621
11. Wolff SD, Balaban RS (1990) Regulation of the predominant renal medullary organic solutes in vivo. Annu Rev Physiol 52:727–746
12. Strange K, Spring KR (1987) Cell membrane water permeability of rabbit cortical collecting duct. J Membr Biol 96:27–43
13. Natke E, Terranova R, DiScala VA (1989) Importance of butyrate in hypertonic volume regulation of cortical collecting tubule (CCT). Kidney Int 35:500
14. Rome L, Grantham J, Savin V, Lohr J, Lechene C (1989) Proximal tubule volume regulation in hyperosmotic media: intracellular K^+, Na^+, and Cl^-. Am J Physiol 257:C1093–C1100
15. Sun A, Hebert SC (1989) Rapid hypertonic cell volume regulation in the perfused inner medullary collecting duct. Kidney Int 36:831–842
16. Sands JM, Terada Y, Bernard LM, Knepper MA (1989) Aldose reductase activities in microdissected rat renal tubule segments. Am J Physiol 256:F563–F569
17. Wirthensohn G, Lefrank S, Schmolke M, Guder WG (1989) Regulation of organic osmolyte concentrations in tubules from rat renal inner medulla. Am J Physiol 256:F128–F135
18. Schultz SG (1981) Homocellular regulatory mechanisms in sodium-transporting epithelia: avoidance of extinction by "flush-through." Am J Physiol 241:F579–F590
19. Helman SI, Nagel W, Fisher RS (1979) Ouabain on active transepithelial Na transport in frog skin: studies with microelectrodes. J Gen Physiol 74:105–127
20. Strange K (1989) Ouabain-induced cell swelling in rabbit cortical collecting tubule: NaCl transport by principal cells. J Membr Biol 107:249–261
21. Strange K (1990) Volume regulation following Na^+ pump inhibition in CCT principal cells: apical K^+ loss. Am J Physiol 258:F732–F740
22. Strange K Volume regulatory Cl^- loss following Na^+ pump inhibition in CCT principal cells. Am J Physiol, in press
23. Frindt G, Palmer LG (1987) Ca-activated K channels in apical membrane of mammalian CCT, and their role in K secretion. Am J Physiol 252:F458–F467
24. Chamberlin ME, Strange K (1989) Anisosmotic cell volume regulation: a comparative view. Am J Physiol 257:C159–C173
25. Haber E, Haupert GT (1987) The search for a hypothalamic Na^+-K^+ ATPase inhibitor. Hypertension 9:315–324
26. Doucet A, Barlet C (1986) Evidence for differences in the sensitivity to ouabain of NaK-ATPase along the nephrons of rabbit kidney. J Biol Chem 261:993–995
27. Rome L, Lechene C, Grantham JJ (1990) Proximal tubule volume regulation in hypoosmotic media: intracellular K^+, Na^+, and Cl^-. J Am Soc Nephrol 1:211–218
28. Wong SME, DeBell MC, Chase HS (1990) Cell swelling increases intracellular free [Ca] in cultured toad bladder cells. Am J Physiol 258:F292–F296
29. Morris CE (1990) Mechanosensitive ion channels. J Membr Biol 113:93–107
30. Reuss L (1988) Cell volume regulation in nonrenal epithelia. Renal Physiol Biochem 3-5:187–201

Rapid Cell Volume Regulation by the Mouse Medullary Thick Ascending Limb of Henle

Steven C. Hebert and Adam M. Sun[1]

Summary. In this paper, we summarize our current knowledge regarding cell volume regulation in mouse medullary thick ascending loop of Henle (MTAL) cells. It has become apparent that arginine vasopressin (ADH) plays a central role in this process (at least in certain species). During antidiuresis ADH increases the rate of NaCl absorption by the MTAL, thereby enhancing the single effect of countercurrent multiplication. In addition, ADH is required for MTAL cells to regulate their volume in the more hypertonic environment. ADH appears to activate normally quiescent basolateral Na^+:H^+ exchangers which mediate Na^+ uptake into MTAL cells during volume regulatory increase (VRI). This action of ADH may be mediated via an increase in cytosolic calcium. The trade off for this effect of ADH appears to be that the MTAL cells are no longer able to regulate their cell volume completely following reductions in interstitial osmolality. This is a direct result of an inverse relationship between the rates of salt absorption and volume regulatory decrease (VRD). This may not present a problem for the MTAL in vivo for two reasons. First, when interstitial osmolality is increased, NaCl absorption is reduced (see [1–3]). Second, when interstitial osmolality decreases during the transition from an antidiuretic to a water diuretic state the circulating level of ADH falls, and consequently, the rapid VRD response would be restored.

Introduction

Cell volume maintenance is one of the fundamental properties of renal epithelial cells. Over the last few years, much has been learned about how these cells maintain a constant, or nearly constant, cell volume under certain well-defined conditions. The medullary thick ascending limb of Henle (MTAL) has served as a valuable model

[1]Laboratory of Molecular Physiology and Biophysics, Renal Division, Department of Medicine, Brigham and Women's Hospital, Boston, MA 02115, USA

for the study of renal epithelial cell volume regulation. These studies have identified a new role for antidiuretic hormone (ADH, arginine vasopressin) in MTAL cells, that of activating normally quiescent, volume-responsive inorganic ion transporters.

Results and Discussion

Cell membranes are usually freely permeable to water, and thus, the distribution of water between cytosol and extracellular medium is in thermodynamic equilibrium. This is also true for "watertight" nephron segments such as the thick ascending limb of Henle (TAL). We have demonstrated in the isolated perfused MTAL that the apical cell membrane is the primary barrier that limits transcellular water movement and accounts for the very low hydraulic conductance of this nephron segment [4,5]. In contrast, the basolateral cell membrane of the MTAL is highly permeable to water, and differences in water activity between cell cytoplasm and the basolateral medium (interstitial fluid in vivo) provide the driving force for water movement into or out of these cells (i.e., changes cell volume).

Cell Volume Responses to Hypertonic Medium

Using quantitative morphological measurements of video images of cells obtained with differential interference contrast microscopy, we [4,6,7] have assessed the hypertonic Volume Regulatory Increase (VRI) responses of isolated perfused mouse CTAL and MTAL segments. The important observations are shown in Fig. 1. In the absence of ADH, MTAL cells behave as simple osmometers, showing no evidence of a rapid VRI response after cell shrinkage induced by a 50 mOsm increase in the osmolality of basolateral medium with mannitol (Fig. 1a). In contrast, following exposure of MTAL cells to physiological concentrations of ADH (25 μU/ml), a rapid VRI response is observed, with nearly complete recovery of cell volume in 2–5 minutes (Fig. 1b). The effect of vasopressin on the ability of mouse MTAL cells to express a VRI response is mimicked by the addition of dibutyryl cyclic AMP (Fig. 1c), and by direct activation of the catalytic subunit of adenylate cyclase with forskolin (Fig. 1d). These results indicate that the hypertonic VRI response of this medullary epithelial cell requires, at a minimum, an effect of ADH working through V_2 receptors. The increase in cell volume above baseline upon returning to the isotonic basolateral medium is consistent with net solute uptake into these cells during the VRI response. Since ADH has no effect on the negligible water permeability of the apical membrane [4], osmotic water uptake into these cells, which results from the increase in total cell osmoles, occurs exclusively across the basolateral membrane.

In contrast to the results in the MTAL, the mouse cortical thick ascending loop of Henle (CTAL) (Fig. 1e) shows no hypertonic VRI response even under conditions identical to those supporting VRI in the MTAL cells. The lack of a rapid hypertonic VRI response to a sudden increase in extracellular osmolality has also been observed in other renal cortical segments such as the proximal tubule [8] and cortical collecting duct. It should be noted, however, that Lohr and Grantham [9] have demonstrated that the rabbit proximal tubule is able to control cell volume when extracellular medium osmolality is increased slowly ($\cong$5 mosom/min).

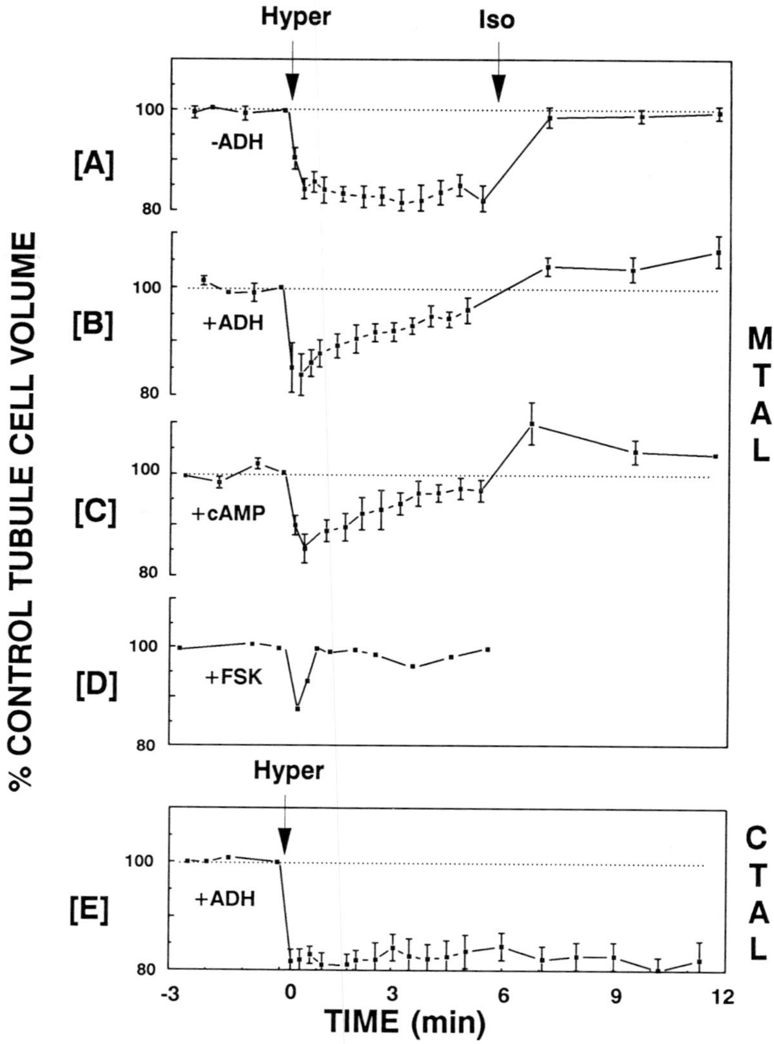

Fig. 1a-e. Hypertonic cell volume regulation in isolated perfused segments of mouse medullary (*MTAL*) or cortical (*CTAL*) thick ascending limbs of Henle. All studies were conducted at 37 °C in HCO_3^-/CO_2-buffered media. At the *first arrow, hyper,* peritubular osmolality was increased from 290 to 340 mosm/Kg H_2O with mannitol. At the *second arrow, Iso,* peritubular medium was changed back to the isotonic solution. In the MTAL studies were performed: in the absence of arginine vasopressin (*ADH*), (**a**) or in the presence of peritubular ADH (25 μU/ml), (**b**), one mM dibutyryl cyclic AMP, (**c**), or one μM forskolin (*FSK*), (**d**). In the CTAL, (**e**), 25 μU/ml ADH was present in the peritubular medium. (Data from [4])

The requirement for ADH in expressing a VRI response is also seen when MTAL cells are shrunken upon re-exposure to an isotonic medium after a Volume Regulatory Decrease (VRD) response. The role of ADH in this post-VRD VRI response is shown in Fig. 2 [7]. This requirement for ADH is an unusual feature of volume regulation by MTAL cells since most renal (and nonrenal) cells show a VRI response with pre-exposure to hypotonic media in the absence of vasopressin, even if they don't express a hypertonic VRI response [10]. Finally, a more general role for ADH (via cyclic AMP) in the VRI responses of renal medullary-papillary cells has been suggested by the recent observation that ADH is also required for hypertonic VRI in rat inner medullary collecting duct cells [11].

Cell Volume Responses to Hypotonic Media

VRD responses have been assessed in isolated perfused mouse MTAL segments under the different states of salt absorption shown in Fig. 2 [7]. In the absence of ADH (Fig. 2a), cells first swell and then rapidly decrease their volume toward the control isotonic value when exposed to a 50 mOsm reduction in the bath osmolality. Upon returning to the isotonic medium cells shrink, consistent with cell solute loss during the VRD response. When salt absorption is increased with ADH (Fig. 2b), the VRD response is markedly reduced (compare Figs. 2a and 2b). This hormone-associated impairment of VRD is in sharp contrast to the ADH requirement for either post-VRD VRI (compare Figs. 2a and 2b) or hypertonic VRI (compare 1a and 1b). The blunting of the VRD response in ADH-activated MTAL segments is due to the hormone-mediated increase in NaCl absorption on the hypotonic-induced solute efflux mechanism(s) rather than to a direct inhibitory effect of hormone, via cyclic AMP, on the signal transduction pathway leading to activation of volume-responsive solute efflux [7]. The relevant observation, shown in Fig. 2c, is that the rate of VRD is increased four-fold when the ADH mediated increase in salt absorption is abolished with luminal furosemide.

When the rates of VRD are plotted for the varying rates of NaCl absorption for the three different transport conditions shown in Fig. 2a-2c, a highly significant inverse relationship is observed, i.e., increasing the rate of NaCl absorption decreases the rate of the VRD response [7]. This inverse relationship suggests that both an increase in cell solute traffic and a decrease in extracellular osmolality activate similar mechanisms to enhance salt exit. The recent observations that both ADH [12,13] and hypotonicity [14] activate Ba^{2+}-sensitive K^+ channels in apical membranes of the TAL provide strong support for the latter suggestion. A large conductance, maxi-K^+ channel appears to be activated by cell swelling and likely mediates K^+ loss during VRD.

Coupled Basolateral Na^+:H^+ and Cl^-:HCO_3^- Exchangers and Apical Na^+:K^+:2Cl^- Cotransporters Mediate VRI

Two types of electroneutral NaCl transport mechanisms have been proposed to mediate rapid hypertonic VRI responses. One process requires CO_2/HCO_3^- and involves parallel Na^+:H^+ and Cl^-:HCO_3^- exchangers; the other process is independent of CO_2/HCO_3^- and involves a loop diuretic-sensitive Na^+:K^+:2Cl^- (or Na^+:Cl^-)

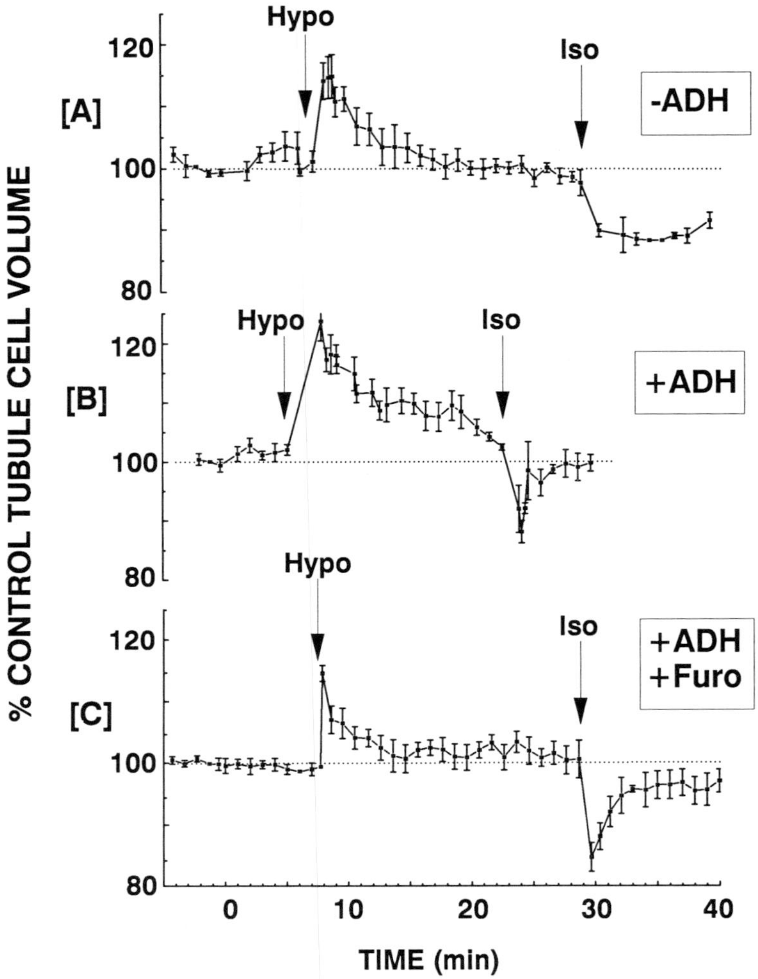

Fig. 2a-c. Hypotonic cell volume regulation in isolated perfused mouse medullary thick ascending loop of Henle (*MTAL*) segments. All studies were conducted at 37°C in HCO_3^-/CO_2-buffered media. At the *first arrow, hypo*, peritubular osmolality was decreased from 290 to 240 mosm/Kg H_2O by removal of 25 mM NaCl. At the *second arrow, Iso*, peritubular medium was changed back to the isotonic solution. Studies were performed: in the absence of arginine vasopressin (*ADH*), (**a**) or in the presence of peritubular ADH (10–25 μU/ml) (**b**), or in the presence of both ADH and 10^{-4} M luminal furosemide, (**c**). Cell volume changes following the return to isotonic basolateral media are referred to as post-volume regulatory decrease (*VRD*) VRI responses Furo, furosemide; VRI, volume regulatory increase. (Data from [7])

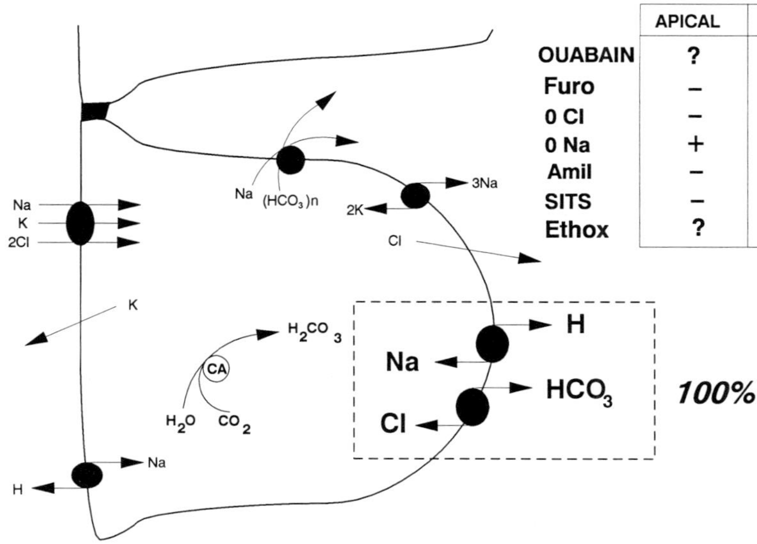

Inhibition of VRI	APICAL	BASAL
OUABAIN	?	+
Furo	–	?
0 Cl	–	+
0 Na	+	+
Amil	–	+
SITS	–	+
Ethox	?	+

Fig. 3. Mechanism of ion uptake mediating the arginine vasopressin (*ADH*)-dependent hypertonic volume regulatory increase (*VRI*) response of the mouse medullary thick ascending loop of Henle (*MTAL*). All of the NaCl uptake mediating the VRI response appears to be mediated by basolateral Na^+:H^+ and Cl^-:HCO_3^- exchangers. The *insert* lists the maneuvers utilized to deduce the VRI transport mechanism. Ouabain at 10^{-3} M, *Furo* is furosemide at 10^{-4} M, *Amil* is amiloride at 10^{-4} M, *SITS* is 4-acetamido-4′-isothiocyanostilbene-2,2′-disulfonic acid at 10^{-4} M, and *Ethox* is the carbonic anhydrase inhibitor, ethoxzolamide at 10^{-4} M. *CA* is carbonic anhydrase present in both the cytoplasm and along the basolateral membrane of mouse MTAL [30]

cotransporter [10,15–18]. Each of these transport mechanisms has been found to mediate NaCl uptake into mouse MTAL cells during the VRI response under certain conditions [4,6,7,19].

In both hypertonic and post-VRD VRI responses, NaCl uptake occurs via coupled Na^+:H^+ and Cl^-:HCO_3^- exchangers located in basolateral membranes (Figs. 3 and 4). The relevant observations are (see insert in Fig. 3; [4,6,7]): (i) both the hypertonic and post-VRD VRI responses are abolished either by symmetrical Na^+ deletion from extracellular media or by basolateral, but not luminal, Cl^- removal; (ii) since either addition of ouabain to the basolateral solution or cooling the tissue to 15°C reduces or abolishes the hypertonic VRI response, NaCl uptake during VRI is an active (i.e., secondary active) process ultimately dependent on basolateral Na^+:K^+-ATPase; (iii) both types of VRI responses can also be abolished by basolateral, but not by luminal, amiloride, by the isohydric replacement of CO_2/HCO_3^- with HEPES, or by basolateral addition of 4-acetamido-4′-isothiocyanostilbene-2,2′-disulfonic acid (SITS); and (iv) inhibition of carbonic anhydrase (CA) activity with ethoxzolamide inhibits hypertonic VRI (CA appears to be required in order to maintain an adequate supply of H^+ and HCO_3^- to the basolateral exchangers).

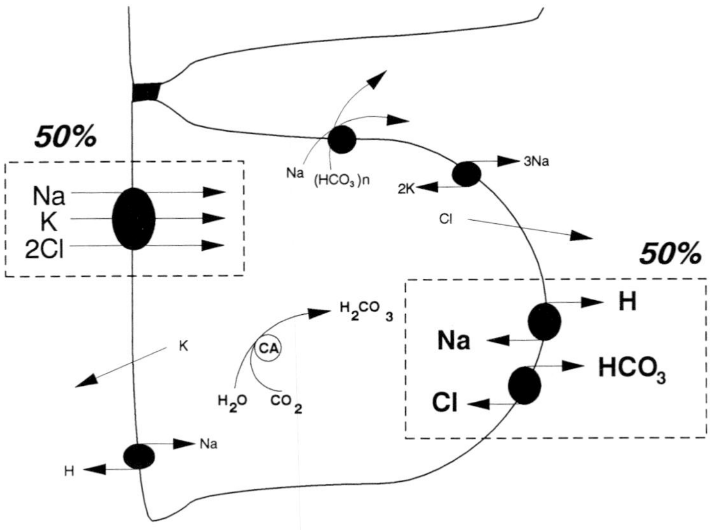

Fig. 4. Mechanism of ion uptake mediating the arginine vasopressin (*ADH*)-dependent post-volume regulatory decrease (*VRD*) VRI response of the mouse medullary thick ascending loop of Henle (*MTAL*). The apical Na^+:K^+:$2Cl^-$ cotransporter and the basolateral Na^+:H^+ and Cl^-:HCO_3^- exchangers each mediate about 50% of the net NaCl uptake during the VRI response. CA, carbonic anhydrase (see Fig. 3); VRI, volume regulatory increase

The contribution of the apical Na^+:K^+:$2Cl^-$ cotransporter to VRI depends explicitly on the method used to elicit the VRI response (see Table 1; Figs. 3 and 4). Inhibition of the apical Na^+:K^+:$2Cl^-$ cotransporter with furosemide (or the substitution of luminal Cl^- with isethionate) has no effect on the steady-state rate of VRI under hypertonic conditions (Fig. 3; [4,7]). On the other hand, the rate of post-VRD VRI is significantly reduced by this diuretic (Table 1; Figs. 2 and 4). The steady-state rate of post-VRD VRI is about three-fold higher than the rates of VRI under hypertonic conditions, with or without luminal furosemide, or the rate of post-VRD VRI in the presence of furosemide. Thus, the apical cotransporter provides a mechanism for enhancing ion uptake only during the post-VRD VRI response. In contrast, the contribution of the ADH-dependent, basolateral Na^+:H^+ and Cl^-:HCO_3^- exchangers to VRI does not appear to be altered by the method used to shrink MTAL cells.

ADH Activates Basolateral Na^+:H^+ Exchangers Mediating VRI

Our initial studies [4,6,7] suggested that the basolateral Na^+:H^+ and Cl^-:HCO_3^- exchangers involved in the VRI response of the mouse MTAL were either not functional, or not as active, during steady-state isotonic conditions. Using 2′,7′-bis(carboxyethyl)-5(6)carboxyfluorescein (BCECF) to measure pH_i in isolated perfused MTAL tubules and in suspensions of MTAL segments from mouse kidney, we have demonstrated that a Na^+:H^+ exchanger is present on basolateral membranes in the absence of ADH; we have confirmed that this exchanger has a very acid pH_i set

Table 1. Role of the apical $Na^+:K^+:2Cl^-$ cotransporter in the VRI responses of the mouse MTAL

	ADH	FURO	Rate of VRI (nl/min per cm)
Hypertonic			
	+	−	0.105 ± 0.032
	+	+	0.167 ± 0.032
Post-VRD VRI			
	+	−	0.310 ± 0.050[a]
	+	+	0.138 ± 0.096

[a]indicates significantly different from the rate of post-VRD VRI in the presence of furosemide.
VRI, volume regulatory increase; VRD, volume regulatory decrease; MTAL, medullary thick ascending loop of Henle; ADH, arginine vasopressin; FURO, furosemide. (Data from [4,6,7])

point of ≅6.7 so that it would be inactive at the resting pH_i (≅7.23 in the absence of CO_2/HCO_3^-) [19–22]. We also identified a $Na^+:H^+$ on apical membranes of the mouse MTAL. In contrast to the basolateral exchanger, this apical exchanger is active at the resting cell pH_i under isotonic conditions and in the absence of ADH ([19,20]; see Fig. 3) and functions importantly in pH regulation. The apical exchanger, however, appears to play no role in Na^+ uptake during VRI (luminal amiloride has no effect on the rate of cell volume recovery in either hypertonic VRI [6] or post-VRD VRI [7].

We have recently begun to assess the effects of ADH on both the apical and basolateral $Na^+:H^+$ exchangers in the isolated perfused mouse MTAL. The observation that VRI is supported by cyclic AMP (Fig. 1c) and forskolin (Fig. 1d) suggests that V_2 receptor-linked events may be involved in activation of the basolateral $Na^+:H^+$ exchanger by ADH. Interestingly, cyclic AMP, presumably working via activation of protein kinase A, inhibits $Na^+:H^+$ exchange activity in some cells [23–25], while this second messenger activates the exchanger in other cell types [26]. In fact, our recent preliminary studies in the mouse MTAL suggest that both effects of cyclic AMP may occur (see Table 2). The activity of the apical exchanger is reduced by ADH while the activity of the basolateral $Na^+:H^+$ exchanger is clearly enhanced by the hormone. We [21,22] have suggested that a hormone induced increase in cytosolic Ca^{2+} may be involved in the activation of the basolateral $Na^+:H^+$ exchanger by ADH. We found

Table 2. Effect of ADH on apical and basolateral $Na^+:H^+$ antiporters in mouse MTAL

	H^+ Efflux rate at pH_i = 6.48 (pmol/min per mm)	
ADH	Basolateral	Apical
−	3.40 ± 0.80	28.32 ± 1.81
+	8.41 ± 1.15[a]	14.61 ± 2.33[a]

[a]indicates P<0.05 compared to the -ADH condition.
MTAL, medullary thick ascending loop of Henle; ADH, arginine vasopressin

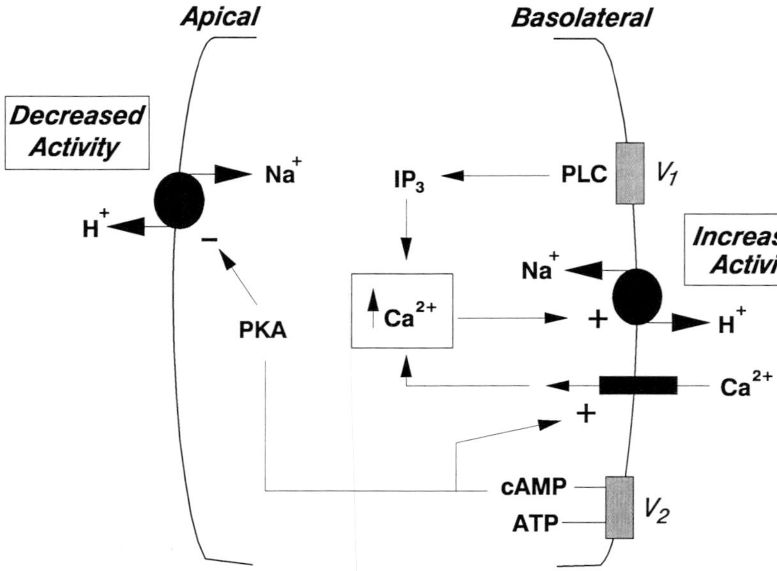

Fig. 5. Tentative model for the action of arginine vasopressin (*ADH*) on apical and basolateral Na^+:H^+ exchangers in the medullary thick ascending loop of Henle (*MTAL*)

that addition of one μM ionomycin to the basolateral solution in the absence of ADH markedly enhanced the activity of the basolateral Na^+:H^+ exchanger in isolated perfused mouse MTAL segments. A similar enhancement of Na^+:H^+ exchange activity by ionomycin-induced increases in cytosolic Ca^{2+} has previously been observed in lymphocytes by Grinstein and Cohen [27].

Although this effect of increased intracellular Ca^{2+} on exchanger activity might suggest that ADH-V_1 receptor-mediated events participate in the activation of the basolateral exchanger in the mouse MTAL, it is clear that cyclic AMP alone fully supports the VRI response. It is possible, however, that increased cytosolic Ca^{2+} may play a role in a further enhancement of the exchanger, mediated by cell shrinkage [27]. An alternative possibility is suggested by the recent preliminary studies of Hoffmann et al. [28] in the rabbit cortical collecting duct, which duct appears to possess both V_1 and V_2 receptors for ADH. These investigators found that a low concentration of ADH (100 μU/ml), working via V_2 receptor, increases the intracellular Ca^{2+} concentration of principal cells. This effect of hormone appears to be mediated virtually exclusively by an influx of Ca^{2+} from extracellular media, rather than by its release from intracellular Ca^{2+} stores.

A Tentative Model for the Action of ADH on Na^+:H^+ Exchangers

When taken together, our results suggested the tentative model for the action of ADH on apical and basolateral exchangers which is shown in Fig. 5. Activation of the basolateral exchanger is a two step process: an initial activation by ADH that prepares the cell for a second response induced by cell shrinkage. In the first step, ADH stimulates intracellular cyclic AMP production via activation of V_2 receptors. The increase in cyclic AMP, in turn, results in an enhanced activity of the basolateral Na^+:H^+ exchanger, possibly by induction of a Ca^{2+} influx, leading to an increase in cytosolic Ca^{2+} (how Ca^{2+} stimulates the exchanger is undetermined, but may also involve activation of a phosphorylation mechanism [27]). In the second step, cell shrinkage would further activate the exchanger, by as yet undetermined mechanisms. This latter activation step might lead to an additional alkaline shift in the pH_i dependence of the exchanger. Although it is possible that ADH-V_1 receptor-mediated events may play some role in augmenting the activation of the exchanger, we have not clearly identified this presence of the V_1 receptor on MTAL cells. Finally, the processes leading to activation of the basolateral Cl^-:HCO_3^- exchanger involved in the VRI response of the mouse MTAL are completely unknown at present. However, it seems reasonable to speculate that ADH (via cyclic AMP) may also activate this exchanger by a process similar to that depicted in Fig. 5. As discussed above, the coupling of the Na^+:H^+ and Cl^-:HCO_3^- exchangers appears to be critical to their function in volume regulation [29].

References

1. Hebert SC, Andreoli TE (1984) Control of NaCl transport in the thick ascending limb. Am J Physiol 246:F745–F75
2. Hebert SC, Culpepper RM, Andreoli TE (1981) NaCl transport in mouse medullary thick ascending limbs. III Modulation of the ADH effect by peritubular osmolality. Am J Physiol 241:F443–F45
3. Molony DA, Andreoli TE (1988) Diluting power of thick limbs of Henle: I. Peritubular hypertonicity blocks basolateral Cl channels. Am J Physiol 255:F1128–F1137
4. Hebert SC (1986) Hypertonic cell volume regulation in mouse thick limbs. I. ADH dependency and nephron heterogeneity. Am J Physiol 250:C907–C919
5. Hebert SC, Culpepper RM, Andreoli TE (1981) NaCl transport in mouse medullary thick ascending limbs. I Functional nephron heterogeneity and ADH-stimulated NaCl cotransport. Am J Physiol 241:F412–F431
6. Hebert SC (1986) Hypertonic cell volume regulation in mouse thick limbs. II. Na-H and Cl-HCO_3 exchange in basolateral membranes. Am J Physiol 250:C920–C931
7. Hebert SC, Sun A (1988) Hypotonic cell volume regulation in mouse medullary thick ascending limb: effects of ADH. Am J Physiol 255:F962–F969
8. Kirk KL, Schafer JA, DiBona DR (1987) Cell volume regulation in rabbit proximal straight tubule in vitro. Am J Physiol 252:F922–F932
9. Lohr J, Grantham JJ (1986) Isovolumetric regulation in anistonic media: A new approach to study compensated cell volume regulation in isolated proximal S2 segments. Kidney Int 29:419
10. Hoffmann EK, Simonsen LO (1989) Membrane mechanisms in volume and pH regulation in vertebrate cells. Physiol Rev 69:315–382
11. Sun A, Hebert SC (1989) Rapid hypertonic cell volume regulation in the perfused inner medullary collecting duct. Kidney Int 36:831–842
12. Hebert SC, Friedman PA, Andreoli TE (1984) Effects of antidiuretic hormone on cellular conductive pathways in mouse medullary thick ascending limbs of Henle: I. ADH increases transcellular conductive pathways. J Membr Biol 80:201–219
13. Reeves WB, McDonald GA, Mehta P, Andreoli TE (1989) Activation of K^+ channels in renal medullary vesicles by cAMP-dependent protein kinase. J Membr Biol 109:65–72

14. Taniguchi J, Guggino WB (1989) Membrane stretch: a physiological stimulator of Ca^{2+}-activated K^+ channels in thick ascending limb. Am J Physiol 257–26:F347–F352
15. Chamberlin ME, Strange K (1989) Anisotonic cell volume regulation: a comparative view. Am J Physiol 257(26):C159–C173
16. Hebert SC (1987) Volume regulation in renal epithelial cells. Semin Nephrol 7:48–60
17. Eveloff JL, Warnock DG (1987) Activation of ion transport systems during cell volume regulation. Am J Physiol 252:F1–F10
18. Blumenfeld JD, Grossman EB, Sun AM, Hebert SC (1989) Sodium-coupled ion cotransport and volume regulatory increase response. Kidney Int 36:434–440
19. Kikeri D, Azar S, Sun A, Zeidel ML, Hebert SC (1990) Na^+:H^+ antiporter and $Na^+(HCO_3^-)_n$ symporter regulate intracellular pH in mouse medullary thick limbs. Am J Physiol 258:F445–F456
20. Kikeri D, Sun A, Zeidel ML, Hebert SC (1989) Cell membranes impermeable to NH 3. Nature 339:478–480
21. Hebert SC, Sun A, Kikeri D (1990) Interrelationships among cell volume, pH and salt transport in thick ascending limb (TAL) and inner medullary collecting duct (IMCD) cells from mammalian kidney: Effects of vasopressin (abstract). Renal Physiol Biochem 13:168–169
22. Sun A, Hebert SC (1990) Antidiuretic hormone (ADH) and cytosolic Ca^{2+} regulate the basolateral (Bl) Na^+:H^+ antiporter involved in the rapid volume regulatory increase (VRI) response of mouse medullary thick limbs (MTAL) (abstract). Clin Res 38:313A
23. Grinstein S, Rothstein A (1986) Mechanism of regulation of the Na^+/H^+ exchanger. J Membr Biol 90:1–12
24. Ussing HH (1960) Active and passive transport of the alkali metal ions. In: Ussing HH, Kruhoffer P, Thaysen JH, Thorn NA (eds) The alkali metal ions in biology. Springer, Berlin, pp 45–143
25. Weinman EJ, Shenolikar S, Kahn AM (1987) cAMP-associated inhibition of Na^+-H^+ exchanger in rabbit brush-border membranes. Am J Physiol 252:F19–F25
26. Borgese F, Garcia-Romeu F, Motias R (1987) Control of cell volume and ion transport by β-adrenergic catecholamines in erythrocytes of rainbow trout, *Salmo gairdneri*. J Physiol (Lond) 382:123–144
27. Grinstein S, Cohen S (1987) Cytoplasmic [Ca^{2+}] and intracellular pH in lymphocytes. Role of membrane potential and volume-activated Na^+/H^+ exchange. J Gen Physiol 89:185–213
28. Hoffmann EK, Simonsen LO (1989) Membrane mechanisms in volume and pH regulation in vertebrate cells. Physiol Rev 69:315–382
29. Mason MJ, Smith JD, Garcia-Soto JD-J, Grinstein S (1989) Internal pH-sensitive site couples Cl^--HCO_3^- exchange to Na^+:H^+ antiport in lymphocytes. Am J Physiol 256-25: C428–C433
30. Dobyan DC, Magill LS, Friedman PA, Hebert SC, Bulger RE (1982) Carbonic anhydrase histochemistry in rabbit and mouse kidneys. Anat Rec 204:185–197

Mechanisms of Renal Cell Injury of Acute Renal Failure

Chair: Haskel E. Eliahou (Israel)
Robert W. Schrier (USA)

Evidence of Renal Cell Injury in Acute Renal Failure

H.E. Eliahou, C. Falconi, and L. Shulman[1]

The basis of the early irreversible stage of acute tubular necrosis (ATN), i.e., of established acute renal failure (ARF), is the cell injury and dysfunction which seem to be responsible for the lack of glomerular filtration. The loss of glomerular filtration occurs despite the fact that the initially raised plasma renin activity and the diminished renal blood flow (RBF) have returned to normal levels. Even at the onset of established acute renal failure in man, the RBF does not decrease to levels below 45% of normal [1], a rate which should allow some glomerular filtration. Thus, earlier conclusions that vasoconstriction is the factor responsible for the cessation of glomerular filtration seem inadequate to explain the phenomenon of renal failure following traumatic or hypovolemic shock.

It is well-known from experimental animal models of ARF that GFR remains negligible despite the return of renal blood flow to normal levels within 24 to 72 h after the injury. Renal failure persists in mercuric chloride-induced ARF, even though renal blood flow returns to normal by 24 h, after reaching 20% in the first 3–6 h after injection (Biber et al. [2]).

Similar findings of normal RBF after 1 or 2 days of mercuric chloride injection were described by Churchill et al. and Sherwood et al. [3,4]; findings after 3 days were described by Baehler et al. [5]. Renal blood flow was normal within 24 h in the glycerol model [6] and in the nor-epinephrine model [7] of ARF. Additional support for the dissociation between return to normal RBF and return to normal GFR has come from Blantz [8] who reported decreased glomerular permeability in the absence of detectable structural abnormalities in uranyl nitrate-induced ARF.

There is a similar dissociation between the RBF and GFR in man. For instance, Reubi [1] also showed adequate RBF in the presence of suppressed GFR in man in ARF after shock. Nevertheless, with the discovery of the extremely potent vasoconstrictor endothelin, and with the improvement in glomerular function obtained by the anti-endothelin antibodies in short term ischemic ARF, the question of continu-

[1]Department of Nephrology, Chaim Sheba Medical Center, S2621, Tel-Hashomer, Israel

ous sustained vasoconstriction has, once again, become important in understanding the pathogenesis of the renal failure in ARF.

Recently, Kon et al. [9] showed that continuous infusion of endothelin in a first-order branch of the left main renal artery was sufficient to induce ARF in Munich Wistar rats [9]. It was found by micropuncture that SNGFR was decreased by 35% in the glomeruli exposed to endothelin. Glomerular plasma flow was also reduced. This hypofiltration/hypoperfusion was associated with an increase in the afferent and efferent arteriolar resistance. The study of the effect of anti-endothelial antibodies on kidney function 48 hours after 25 min of renal artery clamping is even more interesting. The infusion of anti-endothelin antibody into one of the branches of the main renal artery ameliorated the characteristic post-ischemic vasoconstriction and significantly improved SNGFR. These findings tend to show that sustained vasoconstriction is important in the pathogenesis of ARF which results from 25 minutes of complete ischemia. However, the effect of deviation from the currently accepted 50–60 min period of ischemia required to produce ARF in the rat is not clear. The question is whether the anti-endothelin antibody would have acted to the same extent had the renal artery occlusion lasted 60 rather than 25 min, with the resultant, more definite, cell injury.

Conger et al. [10] produced ARF in uninephrectomized Sprague Dawley rats by the infusion of nor-epinephrine 0.6μg/kg per min for 90 min, using a micropipette directly into the renal artery. Seven days after this injury, the response to changes in renal perfusion pressure and renal nerve stimulation was measured.

Their investigation showed that, following nor-epinephrine induced ARF (NE-ARF), there was a marked sensitivity of the renal vessels to reductions in renal perfusion pressure (RPP) and to renal nerve stimulation. This was shown by a marked decrease in RBF with a decrease in RPP or renal nerve stimulation. Conger and colleagues were able to reverse this hypersensitivity with the calcium channel blockers verapamil or diltiazem. This seems to indicate that this hypersensitivity is dependent on intracellular calcium concentration. The use of endothelium-derived relaxing factor (EDRF) dependent agents, such as acetyl choline or bradykinin, was not successful in reversing this hypersensitivity. This would favor the possibility that endothelial injury results in a decrease in EDRF release, which allows sustained vasoconstriction. The authors claim that in such a condition, even subclinical reductions in blood pressure in the ARF patient could cause a great deal of vasoconstriction, which may result in ATN. Since this hypersensitivity is reversed by calcium channel blockers, it seems to be modulated by perturbations in cell calcium. Thus, endothelial cell injury resulting in the decreased release of EDRF, and therefore in vasoconstriction, may be the cause of the lack of filtration at the glomerulus. This vasoconstriction resulting from the high endothelin and the decreased release of EDRF is, in itself, a consequence of endothelial cell injury and dysfunction.

Calcium entry blockers were found to reverse the initial stages of ARF. In the renal artery clamping model in the rat, we found that orally administered verapamil was able to alleviate the functional damage of the involved kidney [11].

Verapamil also significantly improved renal function and was accompanied by less histologic damage in a rat model in which ARF was induced by cyclosporin treatment combined with mild renal ischemia of only 20 min. The authors concluded that transcellular calcium ion transport disturbances seemed to be important in the pathogenesis of ischemic as well as nephrotoxic ARF [12].

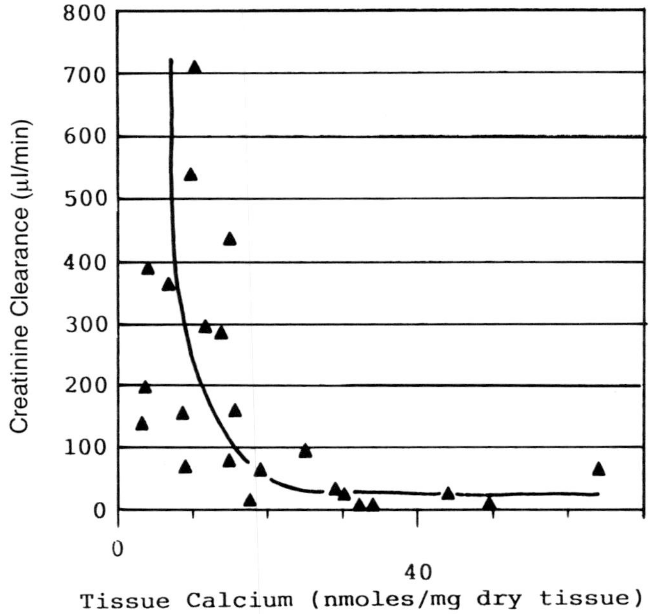

Fig. 1. Verapamil and mifedipine in rat ARF correlation of tissue Calcium and Ccr. Ccr, creatinine clearance; ARF, acute renal failure.

In our studies in rats, in which ARF was induced by uninephrectomy and contralateral clamping of the renal artery for one h, the tissue calcium content of the renal cortex correlated very well with creatinine clearance on the day following the operative procedure (Fig. 1).

Epithelial cell polarity is lost in ischemia [13]. The ARF produced in Sprague Dawley rats by 50 min clamping of the renal pedicle resulted in a loss of Na-K-ATPase polarity in the proximal tubular cells. This was demonstrated cytochemically and biochemically by the redistribution of Na-K-ATPase to apical membranes, where it should not be found. Furthermore, the relative percentage of sphingomyelin content at the apical membrane of the proximal tubular cell was considerably decreased allowing a decreased sphingomyelin/phosphatidyl choline ratio. This ratio is important in the determination of membrane fluidity [14] and therefore of transmembrane transport. The postulate is that one needs a re-establishment of lipid and protein polarity for the normalization of tubular cell function. An additional finding affecting another cell compartment was the significant decrease in the activity of sphingomyelinase in gentamicin-induced ARF in rats (50mg/kg per d for 4 days or 4 mg/kg per d for 8 days). This enzyme is responsible for the intra-lysosomal breakdown of sphingomyelin [15].

More evidence which demonstrates cell dysfunction in ARF is the finding, by microprobe analysis, of a marked increase in proximal tubule intracellular sodium and chloride concentrations. This seems to indicate that there is a marked disturbance in the sodium potassium pump [16].

What is the evidence for an effect of cell dysfunction on glomerular filtration? It has been claimed that when elevated arteriolar resistance in post-ischemic ARF is lowered by saline volume expansion, the rate of glomerular ultrafiltrate formation remains very depressed [17]. Thus, there is an intrinsic loss of normal ultrafiltration capacity at the glomerular capillary wall. This decrease in permeability is still undefined. A similar finding occurs in the tubule, where it has been shown that recovery from ARF coincided with the restoration of tubular impermeability to inulin [18].

Treatment of Wistar rats with either 4 or 40 mg gentamicin/kg per day for 10 days resulted in a marked decrease in the glomerular capillary ultrafiltration coefficient, Kf, in both gentamicin treatment groups. The ultrastructural changes in the proximal tubules (focal loss of brush border, myeloid bodies and cell vacuoles) were typical of gentamicin toxicity. Nevertheless, it seems surprising that there were no apparent ultrastructural differences between the control and experimental groups in the 3 different component layers of the glomerular capillary wall, i.e., the endothelium, GBM, and epithelial cell layer, despite the significant decrease in Kf [19].

Ultrastructural studies in the clamp model of ischemic ARF show that cell swelling, even in the glomeruli, is a predominant feature of this model. This feature occurred, together with a normal RBF measured with the Xenon-washout technique, 6 and 24 h after reflow [20]. In norepinephrine-induced acute renal failure in dogs, scanning electron microscopy revealed a marked abnormality in the epithelial structure of the glomerulus [17]. These studies indicate that ultrastructural changes may be an important aspect of the cell dysfunction which contributes considerably to lack of filtration.

In ischemic ARF the renal tissue calcium content is increased, as is the cytosolic Ca^{2+}. Calcium channel blockers improved experimental ischemic ARF. Observations on mitochondrial respiration, as assessed by state 4 and state 3 oxidative phosphorylation and by uncoupled respiration, show that the detrimental effects of ischemia on these various states of mitochondrial respiration are prevented by calcium channel blockers.

During ischemia, renal beta-ATP, as assessed by 31P-NMR in the renal cortex, fell rapidly to about 10% of control levels. During reflow and recovery, the tissue ATP returned slowly to near normal, but in rats given ATP-$MgCl_2$, the return of ATP levels to normal was accelerated [21].

Creatinine kinase determinations in freeze clamped kidney cortex in rats showed normal values in both control and experimental (60 min clamping of renal pedicle) kidneys, 24 h following the episode of ischemia (Shulman LM, Eliahou HE, unpublished work, 1990). This, together with the finding that cortex ATP returned to near normal within 24 h following the ischemia, seems to indicate that the energy system was functioning during this period, yet the glomerulus was not able to filter normally.

In 1974 Cox et al. [17] described nor-epinephrine-induced acute renal failure (NE-ARF) in a dog, induced by the intrarenal infusion of NE 0.75μg/kg per min for 2 h. In this model, the RBF decreased considerably (from 190ml/min to 116ml/min), 48 h after the NE infusion. The administration of 10% of body weight Ringer's solution resulted in a marked redistribution of flow to inner cortical nephrons in both control and experimental kidneys, with a marked increase in total RBF. In the experimental kidney, the increase was from 116 to 235 ml/min. Over 99% of the 15 μM spheres were extracted in one pass through the experimental kidney. However, despite the marked increase in RBF, there was essentially no urine flow.

Micropuncture showed that the surface tubules were collapsed with no evidence of tubular obstruction or leakage of filtrate. Scanning electron microscopy revealed a marked abnormality in the epithelial structure of the glomerulus. The authors suggest a decrease in the capillary permeability in this model of ARF. In this paper, the NE was infused for 2 h and therefore the damage was very severe, and probably of the irreversible type.

An interesting, somewhat similar, finding in the glomeruli was described by Kobayashi et al. [22]. They induced ARF, with uranyl acetate (2mg/Kg body weight IV), in rabbits. Five days later, scanning electron microscopy revealed a loss of epithelial foot processes and fattening and spreading of podocyte cell bodies. These changes were most pronounced in the maintenance stage of the ARF. In many areas the glomerular capillaries were covered by a continuous sheet of podocyte cytoplasm and the fine structure of the foot processes was not found. There was a decrease in the density of fenestrae in some areas. The authors found no correlation between the morphological findings and serum creatinine levels. Following ischemia, the mitochondria were severely affected. Immediately following 60 min of ischemia, the cells were seen to be swollen, but not necrotic, and the tubules were filled with eosinophilic debris. Six h after recovery from ARF, partial necrosis of tubular walls with some cell swelling was seen in the cytoplasm. At 12 h, severe necrosis of tubules was already seen. Electron microscopy showed large clear intracristal spaces, with swollen and distended microvilli and rounded swollen mitochondria [23].

In summary, there is much evidence to indicate that there is cellular injury and dysfunction in ARF. Such disturbances have been studied mainly in the tubule, apparently because the glomerulus does not lend itself to the study of the individual type of cell. Direct studies on the permeability at the glomerulus are needed to clarify the lack of filtration during ARF. Our present studies are being directed towards defining new molecules and biological response systems which can serve as markers of cell dysfunction in acute renal failure.

References

1. Reubi FC, Vorburger C (1976) Renal hemodynamics in acute renal failure after shock in man. Kidney Int 10:S137–S143
2. Biber TUL, Mylle M, Baines AD, Gottsschalk CW (1968) A study by micropuncture and microdissection of acute renal damage in rats. Am J Med 44:664–705
3. Churchill S, Zarlengo MD, Carvalho GF, Gottlieb MN, Oken D (1977) Normal renal cortical blood flow in experimental acute renal failure. Kidney Int 11:246–255
4. Sherwood T, Lavender JP, Russell SB (1974) Mercury induced renal vascular shutdown: Observations in experimental acute renal failure. Eur J Clin Invest 4:1–8
5. Baehler RW, Kotchen TA, Burke JA, Galla H, Bhathena D (1977) Considerations in the pathophysiology of mercuric chloride induced acute renal failure. J Lab Clin Med 90: 330–340
6. Kurtz TW, Maletz RM, Hsu CH (1976) Renal cortical blood flow in glycerol induced acute renal failure. Circ Res 38:30–35
7. Conger GD, Robinette JB, Guggenheim SJ (1981) Effect of acetyl choline on the early phase of reversible nor-epinephrine induced acute renal failure. Kidney Int 19:399–409
8. Blantz RC (1975) The mechanism of acute renal failure after uranyl nitrate. J Clin Invest 55:621–635

9. Kon V, Yoshioka T, Fogo A, Ichikawa I (1989) Glomerular actions of endothelin in vivo. J Clin Invest 83:1762–1767
10. Conger JD, Robinette JB, Schrier RW (1988) Smooth muscle calcium and endothelium-derived relaxing factor in the abnormal vascular responses of acute renal failure. J Clin Invest 82:532–537
11. Goldfarb D, Iaina A, Serban I, Gavendo S, Kapuler S, Eliahou HE (1983) Beneficial effect of verapamil in ischemic acute renal failure in rats. Proc Soc Exp Biol Med 172:389–392
12. Iaina A, Herzog D, Cohen D, Gavendo S, Kapular S, Schiby G, Eliahou HE (1986) Calcium entry blockade with verapamil in cyclosporin A plus ischemia induced acute renal failure in rats. Clin Nephrol 25(Suppl 1):S168–S170
13. Spiegel DM, Wilson PD, Molitoris BA (1989) Epithelial polarity following ischemia: A requirement for normal cell function. Am J Physiol 256 (Renal Fluid Electrolyte Physiol 25):F430–F436
14. Pottel H, VanDer Meer W, Herreman W (1983) Correlation between the order parameter and the steady state fluorescence anisotropy of 1,6 diphenyl-1,3,5 hexatriene and an evaluation of membrane fluidity. Biochim Biophys Acta 730:181–186
15. Morin JP, Viotte G, Vandewalle A, Van Hoof F, Tulkens P, Fillastre JP (1980) Gentamicin-induced nephrotoxicity: A cell biology approach. Kidney Int 18:583–590
16. Mason J, Beck F, Dorge A, Rick R, Thurau K (1981) Intracellular electrolyte composition following ischemia. Kidney Int 20:61–70
17. Cox JW, Baehler RW, Sharma H, O'Dorisio T, Osgood RW, Stein JH, Ferris TF (1974) Studies on the mechanism of oliguria in a model of unilateral acute renal failure. J Clin Invest 53:1546–1558
18. Finn WF, Chevalier RL (1979) Recovery from postischemic acute renal failure in the rat. Kidney Int 16:113–123
19. Baylis C, Rennke HR, Brenner BM (1977) Mechanisms of the defect in glomerular ultrafiltration associated with gentamicin administration. Kidney Int 12:344–353
20. Frega NS, DiBona DR, Guestler B, Leaf A (1976) Ischemic renal injury. Kidney Int 10:S17–S25
21. Siegel NJ, Avison MJ, Reilly HF, Alger JR, Shulman RG (1983) Enhanced recovery of renal ATP with postischemic infusion of ATP-$MgCl_2$ determined by 31P-NMR. Am J Physiol 245:F530–F534
22. Kobayashi S, Nagase M, Honda N, Hishida A (1984) Glomerular alterations in uranyl acetate acute renal failure in rabbits. Kidney Int 26:808–815
23. Glaumann B, Glaumann H, Trump BF (1977) Studies of cellular recovery from injury. Virchows Arch [Cell Pathol] 25:281–308

Pathogenetic Role of Calcium in Renal Cell Injury

ROBERT W. SCHRIER, JOHN D. CONGER, and THOMAS J. BURKE[1]

Introduction

In 1981 at the VIIIth International Congress of Nephrology in Athens, Greece, and subsequently at the Tel Aviv Satellite Symposium on Acute Renal Failure (ARF) in Israel, the first studies pointing to a pathogenetic role of Ca^{2+} in renal ischemic injury were reported by our group [1–3]. In those initial experiments it was shown that infusion of a calcium channel blocker (CCB) or mannitol prevented or greatly attenuated the severity of the functional defect in experimental, norepinephrine- (NE) induced ARF in dogs. Moreover, mitochondrial function assessed by mitochondrial Ca^{2+} content, respiration, and efflux rates was normal at 24 h after these treatments. Subsequent investigations in our laboratories have not only provided insight into the mechanism of Ca^{2+}-related tubular epithelial cell injury, but have also suggested that smooth muscle cell Ca^{2+} may contribute to the abnormal vascular reactivity that follows renal ischemia [4].

This report will first review evidence that CCBs, assumedly by attenuating increases in cell Ca^{2+}, are protective in the ischemic ARF. Next, experiments will be described that focus on the pivotal role of disordered Ca^{2+} metabolism in tubular epithelial cell ischemia and, finally, the potential mechanistic role of Ca^{2+} in the functional aberrations of the renal vasculature following transient interruption of renal blood flow (RBF) will be examined.

Effects of CCB in Ischemic ARF

In one of our early studies, verapamil or nifedipine was infused into the renal artery of dogs prior to the infusion into the renal artery of a dose of NE that resulted in total renal ischemia [5]. Dogs infused with these CCB did not develop ARF, as assessed

---

[1]Department of Medicine, University of Colorado School of Medicine, Denver, CO 80262, USA

by inulin clearance (C_{In}). Although we could find no evidence for an attentuation of the severe renal ischemia induced during the NE infusion, it was possible that the failure of ARF to develop was simply due to a small, continued level of RBF, undetected by flow meter methodology. However, improved C_{In} was also observed in dogs in which CCB were infused after, rather than before, NE. Since publication of our report, others have demonstrated protection against ischemic ARF in both rat and dog models when CCBs are infused while a totally occlusive clamp is in place on the renal artery. Such maneuvers should not be associated with a lessening of the ischemia during clamping induced by this mechanical obstruction to RBF.

The functional improvement we noted occurred as early as one hour after NE infusion was terminated and persisted at 24 h. In addition, the morphologic appearance of the kidney by light and electron microscopy was dramatically improved. The results of these experiments demonstrating an impressive protective effect of CCB in ischemic ARF suggested an important role of Ca^{2+} in cell injury. The pathogenesis of Ca^{2+}-mediated cell injury may relate to the dissipation of the very large gradient for Ca^{2+} ions between extracellular and intracellular fluid, since maintenance of this gradient requires expenditures of energy and, thus, O_2 dependent adenosine triphosphate (ATP) synthesis. In ischemia or anoxia where O_2 levels are very low or absent the mechanisms for the control of cytosolic-free Ca^{2+} ($[Ca^{2+}]_i$), such as Na^+/Ca^{2-} exchange, CaATPase, and mitochondrial buffering, fail, with the result that $[Ca^{2+}]_i$ increases and, in parallel, cell injury ensues.

Ca^{2+} in Tubular Epithelial Cell Ischemic Injury

Studies from our laboratories [6,7] and from those of other investigators [8] have demonstrated the critical contribution of tubular injury and obstruction to the acute deterioration in renal function following ischemia. Tubular obstruction from cellular debris and, to a varible extent, tubular fluid backleak as a result of disrupted tubular wall integrity are central factors in the reduction in glomerular filtration. Thus, an examination of Ca^{2+} kinetics in tubules or tubular epithelial cells was a logical first step in determining the mechanism of protection conveyed by CCB.

However, neither the mechanism of ischemic injury to tubules nor the site(s) at which CCB convey protection are precisely identified during in vivo studies. For example, it is difficult to argue against the suggestion that some of the improvement in glomerular filtration rate (GFR) or reduction in blood urea nitrogen (BUN) occurs as a direct result of the effects of improved renal hemodynamics which are induced by intrarenal or systemic CCB to cause improvement in O_2 and substrate delivery to the previously ischemic renal epithelial tissue. For this reason, we have turned to several in vitro models of tubular ischemic injury. Each model has, of course, its limitations and pitfalls, but use of the models in combination with the results of whole animal studies provides important data which help explain both the pathogenesis and prevention of ischemic injury.

One example of the in vitro model is that of the isolated perfused kidney (IPK) in which the vasculature is already maximally dilated (or nearly so) such that improved C_{In} is unlikely to be due solely to improved RBF. We have found that both low dose (2.5 and 5.0 μM) verapamil and high dose (100 μM) verapamil improved C_{In} after 40 min of warm ischemia in the rat IPK, and ATP regeneration was enhanced. Cold

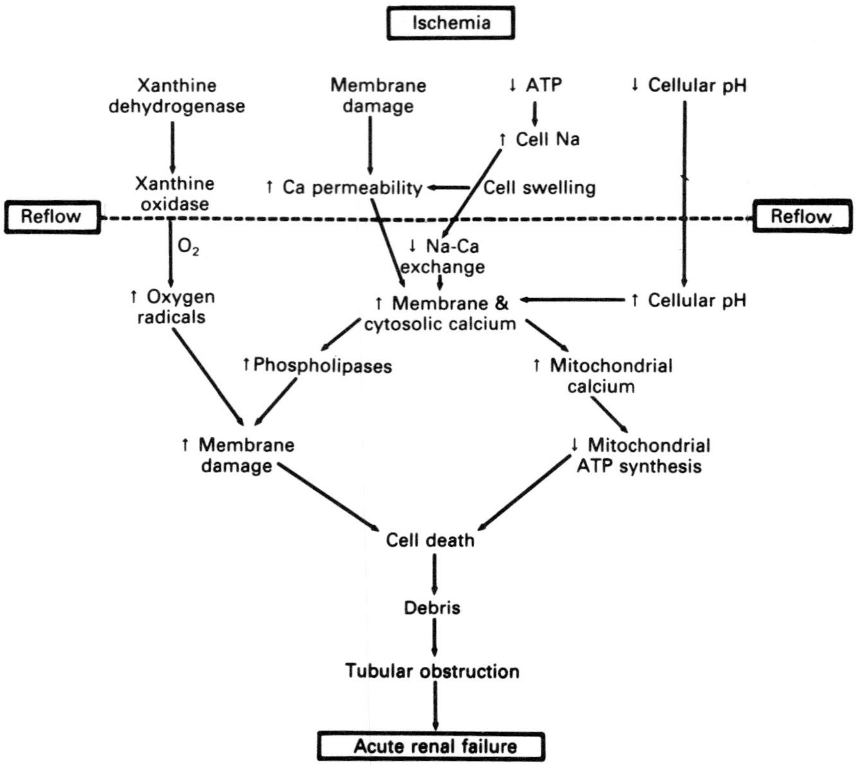

Fig. 1. Mechanisms of renal epithelial cell injury during ischemia and reflow. (From [20] with permission)

ischemia, a model of organ harvesting and storage prior to transplantation, also leads to renal injury and this can be attenuated, as assessed by better tubular Na^+ reabsorption (T_{Na}) when verapamil is added to the initial flush solution [9].

Together, the in vivo and in vitro demonstration of less renal tubular injury following ischemia when CCB are added led us to the hypothesis that ischemia is associated with an increased $[Ca^{2+}]_i$ burden, which may play a role in inducing epithelial (tubular) cell injury, thereby providing the source of tubular debris that causes nephron obstruction, as shown in Fig. 1. It is also likely that, at various times during reperfusion, the influx of Ca^{2+} into the mitochondria of tubular epithelial cells occurs at high but different rates, due in part to differences in the state of mitochondrial energization.

Mitochondrial respiration is impaired during ischemia (prior to reflow), subsequently improves during the first 3 h of reflow, and thereafter begins to deteriorate. The lowest values for basal respiration (S_4), adenosine diphosphate-stimulated (S_3), and uncoupled respiration are usually seen prior to reflow and after 24 h of reflow. Associated with reflow, mitochondrial Ca^{2+} content increases, reaching its highest level at 24 h post-ischemia [10].

To determine if the increase in renal mitochondrial Ca^{2+} noted at 24 h of reflow was simply a result of cell death, we measured the Ca^{2+} content of mitochondria harvested from renal cortical tissue of rat kidneys immediately after ischemia (prior to reflow) and after 1, 3, 6, 12, 18, and 24 h of reflow [11]. These data reveal that during the first 3 h of reflow, mitochondrial Ca^{2+} content increases only slightly, but that between 3 and 24 h, a progressive, significant, and further rise in mitochondrial Ca^{2+} content occurs. The 3 h time point appears to be a critical turning point, because during reflow, mitochondrial respiration steadily improves for the first 3 h and then becomes progressively impaired thereafter.

To determine if the mitochondria harvested from ischemic kidneys had been damaged in some way other than simply by the exposure to Ca^{2+} in vivo, we isolated normal rat kidney mitochondria in an isolation buffer that contained increasing concentrations of Ca^{2+}, much as might occur when calcified renal tissue is disrupted during the isolation of mitchondria. These mitochondria, exposed to a normal cytosolic-like fluid containing progressively higher Ca^{2+} concentrations, exhibited progressively more severe inhibition of mitochondrial respiration, even when all isolation and centrifugation steps were conducted at 4°C [11].

Since Ca^{2+} translocation across the mitochondrial inner membrane can be blocked by ruthenium red, we reexamined the interrelationship between mitochondrial Ca^{2+} overload and mitochondrial respiration during reperfusion when ruthenium red was present during isolation [11]. The magnitude of the rise in Ca^{2+} and the depression in respiration were reduced somewhat by this maneuver but the temporal changes were similar to those observed without ruthenium red. We conclude that tissue and mitochondrial Ca^{2+} overload occur after complete ischemia in vivo, primarily during reflow.

The uniqueness of mitochondrial injury was demonstrated by isolation of endoplasmic reticulum (ER) from ischemic kidneys [12]. This membrane preparation exhibited normal Ca^{2+} transport characteristics, unlike the decrement in mitochondrial respiration, 24 h after ischemia, for 50 or even 90 min duration. Thus, ischemic injury to renal cortical tissue, primarily epithelial tissue, may be manifested mainly by Ca^{2+}-mediated damage to mitochondria. The associated impairment in S_3 respiration limits the ability of the cells to reestablish normal structure and function. Provision of exogenous ATP to ER in vivo, 24 h after reflow, shows that this organelle's function of transporting Ca^{2+} is essentially intact. It is likely, however, that the reduction in S_3 respiration and the decreased mitochondrial ATP synthesis may impair Ca^{2+} uptake by the ER in vivo.

Ca^{2+} Handling by Injured Renal Tissue

As noted above, tissue and mitchondrial Ca^{2+} accumulation occur with reperfusion and, without ATP to extrude Ca^{2+}, could reflect the effect simply, of normal rates of Ca^{2+} uptake. Since it is possible that Ca^{2+} uptake rate from extracellular fluid (ECF) to tubules is increased following a period of O_2 deprivation, we have measured $^{45}Ca^{2+}$ uptake rates in isolated rat proximal tubules (RPT) [13]. Our data show that $^{45}Ca^{2+}$ uptake rate is increased in vitro during reoxygenation at a PH of 7.4 and that reduction in ECF pH to 6.9 normalizes $^{45}Ca^{2+}$ uptake. We have also shown that cellular death can be attenuated in primary cultures of rabbit tubule segments by removal of

Ca^{2+} from the media during the first 2 h of reoxygenation after anoxia; all tubule segments including S_1, S_2, and S_3 segments of the proximal tubule, as well as the cortical collecting duct and the medullary ascending limb were protected [14].

ATP and Cell Injury

As noted above, we have observed a decrease in mitchondrial respiration beginning about 3 h after reflow following ischemia. ATP is synthesized under normal conditions by substrates metabolized by mitchondria. In several glycolytic reactions, consumption of ATP is necessary and when ATP availability is reduced, as it is shortly after an ischemic insult, glycolytic processes, and thus mitchondrial respiration, are at risk.

We have attempted to increase ATP synthesis by addition of fructose 1,6-diphosphate to the perfusate in an isolated perfused kidney subjected to 40 min of warm ischemia. Both C_{In} and T_{Na} were markedly increased. Nuclear magnetic resonance spectroscopy of these kidneys showed that ATP concentrations had indeed improved quite substantially.

Together, data obtained in the experiments described above led to a tentative hypothesis as to how Ca^{2+} derangements occurring during ischemia and during reflow contribute to epithelial cell injury and manifest themselves as ARF (Fig. 1).

Mechanisms and Magnitude of Increased Ca^{2+} Uptake in O_2 Deprivation

We have begun to examine the cause(s) of incresed Ca^{2+} uptake which leads to time dependent, tissue Ca^{2+} overload during hypoxia. After determining that there was indeed a "window" of severe hypoxia (pO_2 range 40–60 mmHg) during which rat proximal tubule (RPT) Ca^{2+} content increased, as had been previously demonstrated by two groups in the rabbit proximal tubule, $^{45}Ca^{2+}$ uptake was measured in RPT during total anoxia (pO_2 = 0 mmHg). These results demonstrated that $^{45}Ca^{2+}$ uptake was indeed increased during anoxia, but only during the first 10 min; by 20 min of anoxia $^{45}Ca^{2+}$ uptake had returned to control levels. Verapamil reduced $^{45}Ca^{2+}$ uptake to near normal levels during the first 10 min of either anoxia or hypoxia, suggesting that at least one of the influx pathways for Ca^{2+} was via a potential operated channel (POC). Because one similarity between hypoxic or anoxic epithelial tissue and excitable tissues, which normally respond to CCB, is an altered transmembrane K^+ gradient, we have questioned whether K^+ loss from ischemic tissues and chronic membrane depolarization induced by O_2 deprivation may be related to the 1) opening of potential operated Ca^{2+} channels and to the 2) efficacy of CCB in preventing epithelial injury during O_2 deprivation.

The approach we have taken is to expose normoxic RPT to various drugs or incubation conditions which have the capacity to alter the transmembrane K^+ gradient (and therefore the membrane potential). We have used 3 and 30 μM valinomycine, 10 μM ouabain, 30 μM amphotericin, and 40 mM extracellular KCl. The Krebs Henseleit buffer (KHB) was modified by reducing NaCl, in order to keep extracellular osmol-

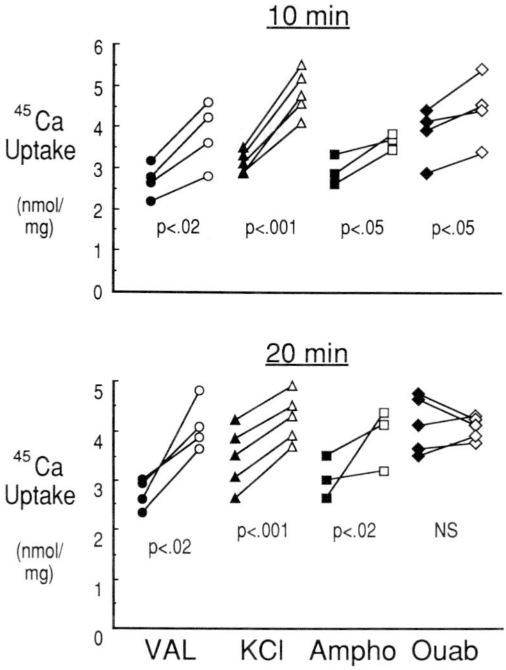

Fig. 2. $^{45}Ca^{2+}$ uptake, in freshly isolated rat proximal tubules incubated under normoxic conditions, is increased when the transcellular K^+ gradient is reduced. Studies were performed at 10 (*top panel*) and 20 min (*bottom panel*) after exposure to the experimental conditions. Val, valinomycin; Ampho, amphotericin; Ouab, ouabain; KCl, 40 mM extracellular potassium chloride

ality constant when KCl was increased from 4 to 40 mM and in other studies the independent effects of reducing NaCl by 40 mM and replacing it with choline chloride were also tested. The results of these studies demonstrate that each of the four different maneuvers increases $^{45}Ca^{2+}$ uptake rate (Fig. 2). This increase can be blocked by verapamil. Blockade of $^{45}Ca^{2+}$ uptake in depolarized, hypoxic tissue is not unique to verapamil because flunarizine, a non-specific CCB, also prevents $^{45}Ca^{2+}$ uptake and lessens lactate dehydrogenase (LDH) release.

Our final question concerned the mechanism for the abrupt cessation of Ca^{2+} uptake by anoxic RPT after an initial early increased rate. Takano and colleagues had suggested that the hypoxic rabbit proximal tubule accumulates Ca^{2+} in a time-dependent manner because the mitochondria remain partially energized, providing a site for sequestration of Ca^{2+} and therefore for sustained high Ca^{2+} uptake rates [15]. In anoxic tissue there would be no partially energized mitochondria, so that Ca^{2+} sequestration would not occur and any early increase in $^{45}Ca^{2+}$ uptake would simply increase the concentration of free Ca^{2+} in the cytosol. If this reasoning is correct then free Ca^{2+} ($[Ca^{2+}]_i$) measured by Fura2 should be similar in control and in hypoxic tissue but increased in anoxic tissue. Figure 3 demonstrates that this indeed is the case, since in anoxic RPT, $[Ca^{2+}]_i$ is 2- to 3-fold higher after 10 min of anoxia compared to normoxic RPT and there is virtually no difference in $[Ca^{2+}]_i$ between hypoxic and normal RPT. Furthermore, if hypoxic but not anoxic RPT accumulate Ca^{2+} in their mitochondria, then administration of FCCP, which collapses the mitochondrial membrane potential, should lead to release of Ca^{2+} from mitochondria of hypoxic RPT and to a much higher

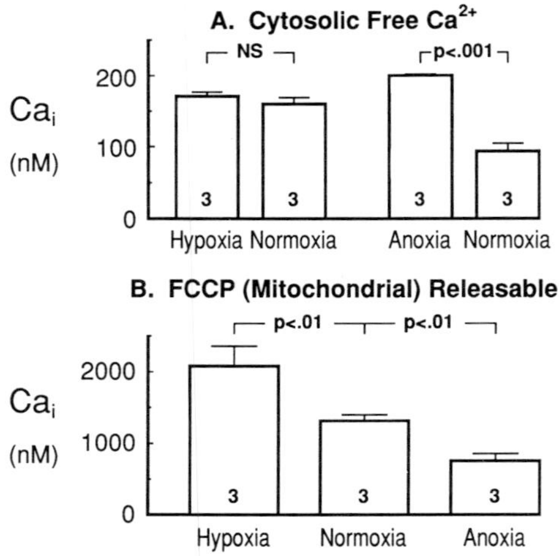

Fig. 3. Fura2 measurements of cytosolic free calcium ($[Ca^{2+}]_i$) in freshly isolated rat proximal tubules (*RPT*) under conditions of O_2 deprivation

Ca^{2+} signal (using Fura2) than in normoxic tissue, which in turn, should be higher than in anoxic tissue. Figure 3 also demonstrates that this is exactly what occurs.

Ca^{2+} in Vascular Ischemic Injury

While there has been considerable focus on post-ischemic tubular injury and the pathogenetic role of Ca^{2+}, there is a growing body of evidence indicating that renal ischemia results in specific abnormalities of the renal vasculature as well. There is also evidence that disordered smooth muscle cell Ca^{2+} metabolism may be a factor in the aberrations of vasoreactivity.

Following ischemic ARF induction, there are two recognized functional defects of the arterial system of the kidney: persistent focal pre-glomerular vasoconstriction and a loss of normal RBF autoregulation [7,16]. The former defect results in decreased driving forces for glomerular filtration and, in conjunction with tubular obstruction and tubular fluid backleak, is a significant pathogenetic mechanism in ischemic ARF. Persistent vasoconstriction is a focal rather than a diffuse process, as indicated by the heterogeneity of glomerular capillary pressure and glomerular plasma flow measurements by micropuncture and the near restoration of total kidney blood flow in established ARF [7]. Recently, we examined basal tone in afferent arterioles (AA) isolated from kidneys of rats that had undergone ARF induction with NE one week previously and had RBF and GFR that were 80% and 30% of control values, respectively. Mean lumen diameter of AA from ARF kidneys was less than that of sham-ARF control kidney over a physiologic pressure range (Fig. 4). These data indicate that there was an intrinsically greater arteriolar tone in AA from ARF kidneys. (It should be noted, however, that while there was a statistically lesser lumen diameter at physiologic pressures, there were occasional AA with diameters

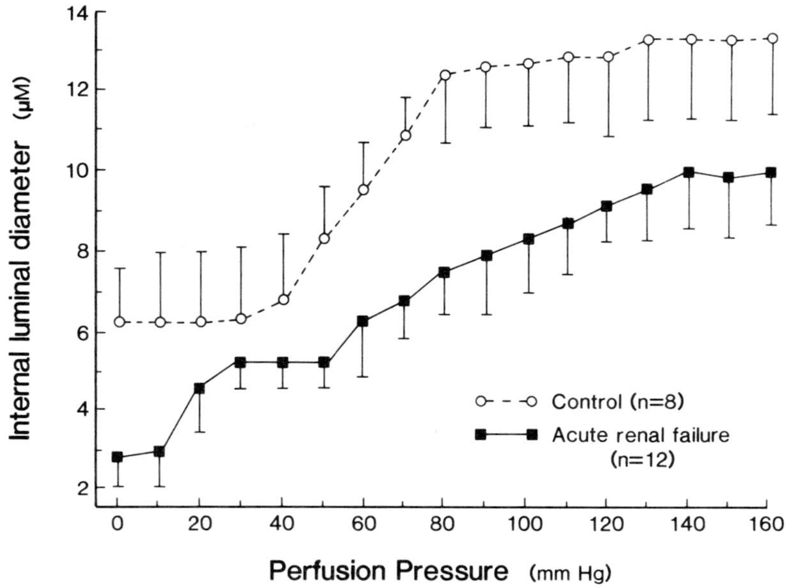

Fig. 4. Pressure-related changes in lumen diameter of afferent arterioles isolated from control and post-ischemic ARF rat kidneys. Over a physiologic range (60–100 mmHg) lumen diameter was less in the afferent arterioles from ARF kidneys ($P<.02$)

similar to sham-ARF controls, consistent with the heterogeneity of the vascular abnormality.) To assess the basis for differences in tone between AA from ARF and control kidneys, we examined smooth muscle $[Ca^{2+}]_i$ in these vessels at 80 mmHg pressure before and after the addition of the vasoconstrictor agonist angiotensin II by dual excitation fluorescence ratio imaging using Fura2. As can be seen from Fig. 5, the basal $[Ca^{2+}]_i$ was more than 2-fold higher in ARF vessels (equivalent to 200 vs 70 nM). There was an abrupt increase in $[Ca^{2+}]_i$ in response to angiotensin II in the control AA, but no detectable response in the AA from ARF kidneys. While one interpretation of these data is provided by the recent study of Kon et al. [17] indicating that persistent post-ischemic vasoconstriction is due to the paracrine action of endothelin, another explanation is possible. As in tubular epithelial cells, increases in smooth muscle Ca^{2+} may be a consequence of ischemia, per se, secondary to a loss of transmembrane potential difference. Although indirect evidence, the lack of receptor activation by angiotensin II in AA from ARF kidney suggests a loss of receptors from smooth muscle cells. If there was a similar loss of receptors to endothelin, then the latter explanation for increased $[Ca^{2+}]_i$ would be more tenable. In any case, the increase in post-ischemic smooth muscle cell Ca^{2+} is consistent with the demonstrated increase in basal tone in the majority of AA examined from ARF kidneys.

The second defect in post-ischemic vascular reactivity, loss of RBF autoregulation, is actually a paradoxical vasoconstriction to a reduction in renal perfusion pressure, when examined in the NE-induced ARF rat model [18]. The aberrant vasoconstriction in the autoregulatory pressure range, over which vasodilation is the normal

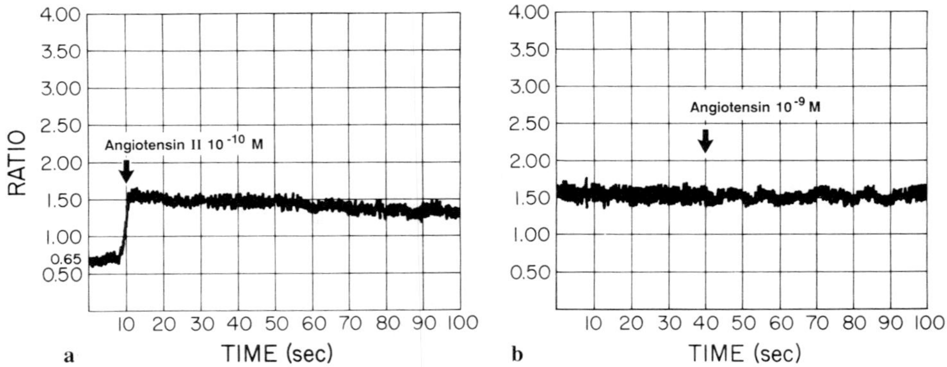

Fig. 5a-b. Real time cytosolic free calcium $[Ca^{2+}]_i$ transients in smooth muscle cells of afferent arterioles from normal (**a**) and post-ischemic ARF rats (**b**) in basal state and after addition of angiotensin II as determined by dual excitation fluorescence ratio imaging using Fura2. Note that basal state $[Ca^{2+}]_i$ was higher in afferent arterioles from ARF kidneys, but did not respond to angiotensin II despite the higher concentration used in comparison with AA from normal kidneys

response, is intimately related to a renovascular hypersensitivity to autonomic nerve activity. There is an increased vasoconstriction to renal nerve stimulation and a complete attenuation of the paradoxical vasoconstriction to renal perfusion pressure reduction if the kidney is denervated [18]. Interestingly, while renal denervation

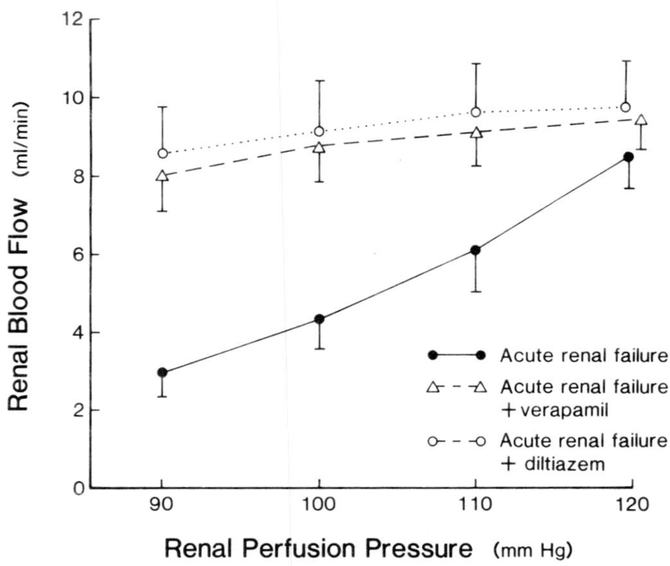

Fig. 6. Renal blood flow (*RBF*) response to reduction in renal perfusion pressure over the physiologic autoregulatory range in post-ischemic acute renal failure (*ARF*) kidneys without and with 90 min intrarenal infusion of calcium channel blockers

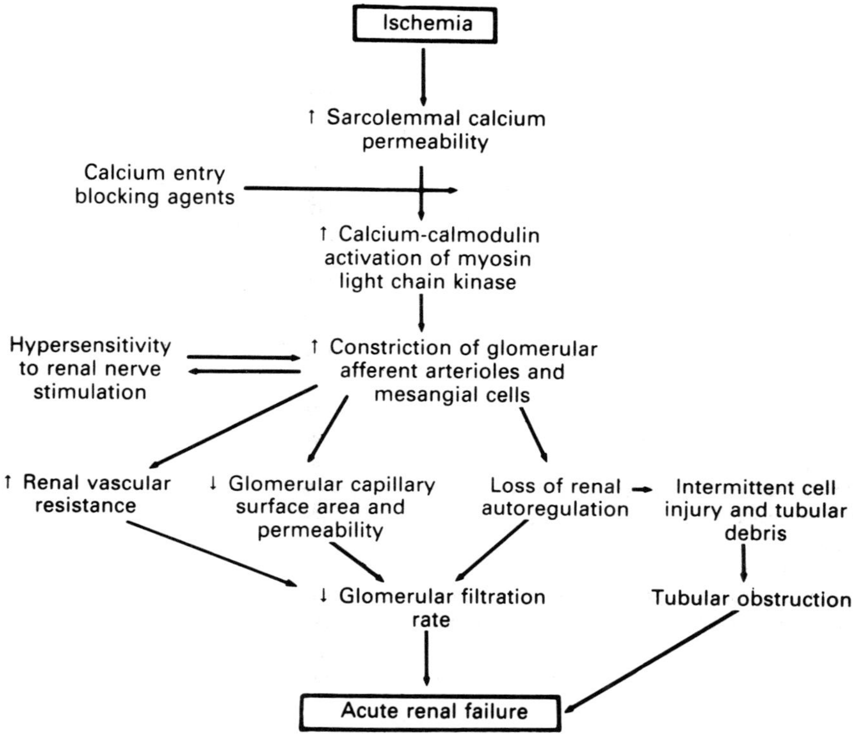

Fig. 7. Vascular and tubular contribution to ischemic acute renal failure (*ARF*). (From [20] with permission)

blocks the paradoxical vasoconstriction to renal perfusion pressure reduction, normal autoregulatory vasodilation is not restored. The abnormal vasoreactive response to renal perfusion pressure reduction following ischemic renal injury is complex and, likely, involves more than one mechanism, including an augmented release of neurotransmitter to autonomic nerve activity [19]. However, it is possible that abnormal smooth muscle cell Ca^{2+} also plays a role in this disordered autoregulatory response. We have found that 90 min, but not 30 min, intraarterial infusion of the CCB verapamil and diltiazem will completely block the renovascular hypersensitivity to renal nerve stimulation and renal perfusion pressure reduction [4]. In addition, the normal autoregulatory vasodilation is restored, as shown in Fig. 6. It is postulated that prolonged CCB infusion reduces smooth muscle cell Ca^{2+} (assuming continued Ca^{2+} extrusion and blocked Ca^{2+} entry) restoring a more nearly normal response to adrenergic neurotransmitters and appropriate vasodilation to renal perfusion pressure reduction. The inference derived from this postulate is that increased arteriolar $[Ca^{2+}]_i$, as demonstrated by Fura2 fluorescence of isolated AA, contributes both to exaggerated vasoconstriction to stimuli such as renal nerve stimulation, and to the failure to dilate appropriately to renal perfusion pressure reduction in the autoregulatory range (Fig. 7).

Conclusion

Our understanding of the pathogenesis and prevention of ARF has progressive dramatically over the last 20 years, from observations of whole animals in the 1970s to cells and organelles in the 1980s. Much of this information was recently synthesized in an editorial [20]. Nevertheless, even with present therapeutic approaches, the mortality in ARF is 35%–75% and thus there continues to be a dire need for interventional strategies. With the demonstration of altered Ca^{2+} kinetics in both vascular and epithelial tissue in ARF, further research into the mechanisms by which Ca^{2+} is mishandled by ischemic renal tissues may permit clinicians, in the near future, to reverse or eliminate this extraordinarily high mortality rate.

References

1. Schrier RW, Burke RJ, Conger JD, Arnold PE (1981) New aspects of acute renal failure. Proceedings of the 8th International Congress Nephrology, Athens. S Karger, pp 63–69
2. Schrier RW, Arnold PE, Burke TJ (1982) Alterations in mitchondrial respiration and calcium movements in norepinephrine-induced acute renal failure: modification by mannitol. In: Eliahou HE (ed) Acute renal failure. John Libbey, London, pp 21–22
3. Burke TJ, Arnold PE, Grossfeld PD, Schrier RW (1982) Effect of calcium membrane inhibition on norepinephrine-induced acute renal failure. In: Eliahou HE (ed) Acute renal failure. John Libbey, London, pp 239–240
4. Conger JD, Robinette JB, Schrier RW (1988) Smooth muscle calcium and endothelium-deprived relaxing factor in the abnormal vascular responses of acute renal failure. J Clin Invest 82:532–537
5. Burke TJ, Arnold PE, Gordon JA, Bulger RE, Dobyan DC, Schrier RW (1984) Protective effect of intrarenal calcium membrane blockers before or after renal ischemia. J Clin Invest 74:1830–1841
6. Burke TJ, Cronin RE, Duchin KL, Peterson LN, Schrier RW (1980) Ischemia and tubule obstruction during acute renal failure in dogs: Role of mannitol in protection. Am J Physiol 238:F305–F314
7. Conger JD, Robinette JB, Kelleher SP (1984) Nephron heterogeneity in ischemic acute renal failure. Kidney Int 26:422–429
8. Tannen GA, Sophasan S (1976) Kidney pressures after temporary renal artery occlusion in the rat. Am J Physiol 230:1173–1179
9. Shapiro JI, Cheung C, Itabashi A, Chan L, Schrier RW (1985) The effect of verapamil on renal function after warm and cold ischemia in the isolated perfused rat kidney. Transplantation 40:596–600
10. Wilson DR, Arnold PE, Burke TJ, Schrier RW (1984) Mitochondrial calcium accumulation and mitchondrial respiration in ischemic acute renal failure in the rat. Kidney Int 25:591–526
11. Arnold PE, Lumlertgul D, Burke TJ, Schrier RW (1985) In vitro versus in vivo mitchondrial calcium loading in ischemic acute renal failure. Am J Physiol 248:F845–F850
12. Schieppati A, Wilson PD, Burke TJ, Schrier RW (1985) Effect of renal ischemia on cortical microsomal calcium transport. Am J Physiol 249:C476–C483
13. Burnier M, Van Putten VJ, Schieppati A, Schrier RW (1988) Effect of extracellular acidosis on $^{45}Ca^{2+}$ uptake in isolated hypoxic proximal tubules. Am J Physiol 254:C839–C846
14. Wilson PD, Schrier RW (1986) Nephron segment and calcium as determinants of anoxic cell death in primary renal cell cultures. Kidney Int 29:1172–1179

15. Takano T, Soltolf SP, Murdaugh S, Mandel LJ (1985) Intracellular respiratory dysfunction and cell injury in short-term anoxia of rabbit renal proximal tubules. J Clin Invest 76:2377–2384
16. Conger JD (1983) The role of blood flow autoregulation in pathophysiology of acute renal failure. Circ Shock 11:235–244
17. Kon V, Yoshioka T, Fogo A, Ichikawa I (1989) Glomerular actions of endothelin in vivo. J Clin Invest 83:1762–1767
18. Kelleher SP, Robinette JB, Conger JD (1984) Sympathetic nervous system in the loss of autoregulation in acute renal failure. Am J Physiol 15:F379–F386
19. Robinette JB, Conger JD (1990) The roles of angiotensin II and thromboxanes in the hypersensitivity to renal nerve stimulation in acute renal failure. J Clin Invest 86:1532–1539
20. Schrier RW, Arnold PE, Van Putten VJ, Burke TJ (1987) Cellular calcium in ischemic acute renal failure: Role of calcium entry blockers. Kidney Int 32:313–321

Cyclosporine Nephrotoxicity in the 1990s

Kim Solez[1] and Lorraine C. Racusen[2]

Summary. As we approach the 18th year since the discovery of cyclosporine's immunosuppressive properties, the drug has now "come of age." Despite the advent of newer agents such as FK506, 15-deoxyspergualin, and rapamycin, cyclosporine is such a highly successful therapeutic agent that it is likely to remain in use for many years. Therefore, cyclosporine nephrotoxicity, the major side effect of the drug, will continue to be an important problem. Renal vasoconstriction appears to be the primary mechanism of toxicity, and thromboxane is likely to be the principal mediator of this effect. Thromboxane receptor blockade or inhibition of thromboxane synthesis may be a clinically effective means of lessening cyclosporine nephrotoxicity.

Introduction

It has now been 18 years since the discovery of the immunosuppressive properties of cyclosporine A by Borel et al., 12 years since the first clinical trials in kidney transplantation and graft-versus-host disease, 10 years since the total synthesis of the molecule, and 7 years since its approval and release for use as an immunosuppressive agent in the U.S. [1] Cyclosporine has moved from the status of a new drug to that of an established pharmaceutical agent which has had a major impact on medical practice.

Cyclosporine represents not only a major therapeutic and pharmacologic advance but also a major phenomenon in the medical literature. As depicted in Fig. 1, the number of articles per year devoted to cyclosporine, dubbed "the drug of the 1980s," has steadily risen from 3 in 1976 to nearly 1600 in 1988. The decline since 1988 has been more or less compensated for by a burgeoning literature on newer powerful and potentially clinically useful immunosuppressive agents, such as FK506, 15-deoxy-

[1]Department of Pathology, 5B4.02 Mackenzie Health Sciences Centre, University of Alberta, Edmonton, Alberta, T6G 2R7 Canada. Recipient of a Sandoz Travel Fellowship
[2]Department of Pathology, Johns Hopkins Hospital, Baltimore, Maryland 21205, USA

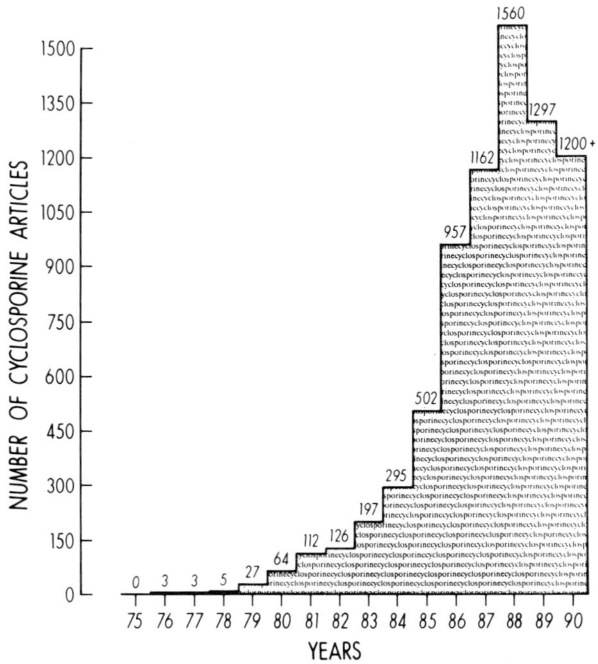

Fig. 1. Number of cyclosporine articles published per year, 1975–1990

spergualin, and rapamycin [2–14]. The best characterized of these three new agents, FK506, appears to have a mechanism of action similar to that of cyclosporine [15–20]. It has some potential for nephrotoxicity [21], but apparently lacks direct endothelial toxicity [22,23].

Much of the immense literature on cyclosporine deals with its nephrotoxicity, reflecting the fact that the renal toxicity of the drug, which manifests itself clinically in over half the patients who receive it, is the major side effect limiting its use [24] (Table 1). The 8000 articles on cyclosporine published between 1976 and 1990 could logically be expected to generate confusion. It is important in the nephrotoxicity area to try to provide some clarity and consensus out of the morass of conflicting studies. Clinical cyclosporine nephrotoxicity can be divided into six forms [24]:

1) Acute reversible renal functional impairment
2) Delayed renal allograft function
3) Acute vasculopathy (thrombotic microangiopathy)
4) Chronic nephropathy with interstitial fibrosis
5) Functional toxicity
6) Tubular toxicity

It is now clear that, clinically, the most important of these forms are 1, 4, and 5, and that these three clinical syndromes represent a spectrum of functional and morphologic abnormalities brought about in the kidney by cyclosporine-induced

Table 1. Reported adverse effects of cyclosporine-A in 3518 renal transplant recipients[a]

Adverse effect	Percentage
Renal dysfunction	54.3
Hypertension	42.4
Infections	
Bacterial	15.4
Viral	14.8
Fungal	3.3
Hypertrichosis	32.5
Tremor	22.1
Hepatic dysfunction	18.2
Gum hyperplasia	16.2
Nausea, vomiting	9.0
Paresthesia	5.2
Hyperuricemia	4.1
GI ulcer hemorrhage	3.2
Convulsions	1.8
Hyperkalemia	1.7
Malignancy (including 0.4% lymphoma)	1.3
Joint/muscle pain	1.1
Anemia	1.1

[a](Modified from [31])

vasoconstriction. Possible suggested mechanisms for this vasoconstriction have included:

1) A direct vasoconstrictive effect
2) Endothelin mediated vasoconstriction
3) Enhancement of local production of angiotensin in renal vessels
4) Decreased atrial natriuretic peptide
5) Increased production of thromboxane
6) Activation of the sympathetic nervous system

The renal vasoconstriction induced by cyclosporine is clearly not secondary to tubular injury, since it can be observed in the hydronephrotic rat model in which most tubular structures have been obliterated [25]. Enhanced thromboxane release is likely to be the most important mechanism of cyclosporine-induced renal vasoconstriction. Several studies document amelioration of cyclosporine nephrotoxicity after thromboxane receptor blockade or modulation of thromboxane metabolism in experimental animals [26–28]. Inhibition of thromboxane synthetase has recently been shown to improve renal allograft function in patients taking cyclosporine [29]. It is of interest that thromboxane synthetase inhibition has also been shown to be beneficial in another condition in which renal vasoconstriction plays an important role, acute renal failure accompanying systemic sepsis [30].

Concluding Remarks

Cyclosporine is such a successful drug that it is likely to remain in use for many years despite the discovery of other potent immunosuppressive agents. Elucidation of the mechanisms of cyclosporine-induced renal vasoconstriction will enable the development of better strategies to avoid this important side effect of the drug.

References

1. Borel JF (1982) The history of Cyclosporin A and its significance. In: White DJG (ed) Cyclosporin A. Elsevier Biochemical, Amsterdam, pp 5–17
2. Kino T, Hatanaka H, Miyata S, Inamura N, Nishiyama M, Yajima T, Goto T, Okuhara M, Kohsaka M, Aoki H, Ochiai T (1987) FK-506, a novel immunosuppressant isolated from *A Streptomyces*. II: Immunosuppressive effect of FK-506 *in vitro*. J Antibiot (Tokyo) 40(9):1256–1265
3. Goto T, Kino T, Hatanaka M, Nishiyama M, Okuhara M, Kohsaka M, Aoki H, Imanaka H (1987) Discovery of FK-506, a novel immunosuppressant isolated from *Streptomyces Tsukubaensis*. Transplant Proc 19(5):4–8
4. Starzl TE, Todo S, Fung J, Demetris AJ, Venkataramman R, Jain A (1989) FK 506 for liver, kidney and pancreas transplantation. Lancet II:1000–1004
5. Ochiai T, Sakamoto K, Gunji Y, Hamaguchi K, Isegawa N, Suzuki T, Shimada H, Hayashi H, Yasumoto A, Asano T, Isono K (1989) Effects of combination treatment with FK506 and cyclosporine on survival time and vascular changes in renal-allograft-recipient dogs. Transplantation 48:193–197
6. Hoffman AL, Makowka L, Banner B, Cai X, Cramer DV, Pascualone A, Todo S, Starzl TE (1990) The use of FK-506 for small intestine allotransplantation. Transplantation 49:483–490
7. Inagaki K, Fukuda Y, Sumimoto K, Matsuno K, Ito H, Takahashi M, Dohi K (1989) Effect of FK506 and 15-deoxyspergualin in rat orthotopic liver transplantation. Transplant Proc 21:1069–1071
8. Ishibashi M, Jiang S, Kokado Y, Takahara S, Sonoda T (1989) Immunopharmacologic effects of immunosuppressive agents explored by a new effector monocyte generation assay. Transplant Proc 21:1854–1858
9. Nakajima K, Sakamoto K, Ochiai T, Asano T, Isono K (1989) Effects of 15-deoxyspergualin and FK506 on the histology and survival of hamster-to-rat cardiac xenotransplantation. Transplant Proc 21:546–548
10. Ochiai T, Nakajima K, Sakamoto K, Nagata M, Gunji Y, Asano T, Isono K, Sakamaki T, Hamaguchi K (1989) Comparative studies on the immunosuppressive activity of FK506, 15-deoxyspergualin, and cyclosporine. Transplant Proc 21:829–832
11. Dumont FJ, Staruch MJ, Koprak SL, Melino MR, Sigal NH (1990) Distinct mechanisms of suppression of murine T cell activation by the related macrolides FK-506 and rapamycin. J Immunol 144:251–258
12. Dumont FJ, Melino MR, Staruch MJ, Koprak SL, Fischer PA, Sigal NH (1990) The immunosuppressive macrolides FK-506 and rapamycin act as reciprocal antagonists in murine T cells. J Immunol 144:1418–1424
13. Calne RY, Collier DStJ, Lim S, Pollared SG, Samaan A, White DJG (1989) Rapamycin for immunosuppressants in organ allografting. Lancet II:227
14. Thomson AW, Woo J (1989) Immunosuppressive properties of FK-506 and rapamycin. Lancet II:443–444
15. Harding MW, Galat A, Uehling DE, Schreiber SL (1989) A receptor for the immunosuppressant FK506 is a *cis-trans* peptidyl-prolyl isomerase. Nature 341:758–760
16. Siekierka JJ, Hung SHY, Poe M, Lin CS, Sigal NH A cytosolic binding protein for the immunosuppressant FK506 has peptidyl-prolyl isomerase activity but is distinct from cyclophilin. Nature 341:755–757
17. Freedman RB (1989) Convergence of drug action. Nature 341:692

18. Tocci MJ, Matkovich DA, Collier, Kwok P, Dumont F, Lin S, Degudicibus S, Siekierka JJ, Chin J, Hutchinson NI (1989) The immunosuppressive FK506 selectively inhibits expression of early T cell activation genes. J Immunol 143:718–726
19. Siekierka JJ, Staruch MJ, Hung SHY, Sigal NH (1989) FK-506, a potent novel immunosuppressive agent, binds to a cytosolic protein which is distinct from the cyclosporin A-binding protein, cyclophilin. J Immunol 143:1580–1583
20. Suzuki N, Sakane T, Tsunematsu T (1990) Effects of a novel immunosuppressive agent, FK506, on human B cell activation. Clin Exp Immunol 79:240–245
21. Stephen M, Woo J, Hasan NU, Whiting PH, Thomson AW (1989) Immunosuppressive activity, lymphocyte subset analysis, and acute toxicity of FK-506 in the rat. Transplantation 47:60–65
22. McCauley J, Bronsther O, Fung J, Todo S, Starzl TE (1989) Treatment of cyclosporin-induced haemolytic uraemic syndrome with FK506. Lancet II:1516
23. Brown Z, Neild GH (1990) FK-506 and haemolytic uraemic syndrome. Lancet I:412
24. Racusen LC, Solez K (1988) Cyclosporine nephrotoxicity. Int Rev Exp Pathol 30:107–157
25. Zimmerhackl LB, Fretschner M, Steinhausen M (1990) Cyclosporin reduces renal blood flow through vasoconstriction of arcuate arteries in the hydronephrotic rat model. Klin Wochenschr 68:166–174
26. Rossini M, Belloni A, Remuzzi G, Perico N (1990) Thromboxane receptor blockade attenuates the toxic effect of cyclosporine in experimental renal transplantation. Circulation 81:61–68
27. Spruney RF, Mayros SD, Collins D, Ruiz P, Klotman PE, Coffman T (1989) Thromboxane receptor blockade improves cyclosporine nephrotoxicity in rats. Prostaglandins 39:135–146
28. Teraoka S, Takahashi K, Tanabe K, Yamaguchi Y, Kawai T, Tojinbara T, Nakajima I, Nakagawa Y, Fujikawa H, Hayashi T, Oba S, Tagisama T, Honda H, Fuchinoue S, Toma H, Agishi T, Ota K (1989) Improvement in renal blood flow and kidney function by modulation of prostaglandin metabolism in cyclosporine-treated animals. Transplant Proc 21:937–940
29. Coffman TM, Smith SR, Creech EA, Schaffer AV, Martin LL, Rakhit A, Douglas FL, Klotman PE (1990) The thromboxane (TX) synthetase inhibitor CGS 13080 improves renal allograft function in patients taking cyclosporine (CYA). Kidney Int 37:604
30. Cumming AD, McDonald JW, Lindsay RM, Solez K, Linton AL (1989) The protective effect of thromboxane synthetase inhibition on renal function in systemic sepsis. Am J Kidney Dis 13:114–119
31. Krupp P, Gülich A, Timonen P (1986) Side effects and safety of Sandimmune in long-term treatment of renal transplant patients. Transplant Proc 18:991–992

Heterogeneity of Nephron Energy Metabolism: Implications for Response to Hypoxic Insult

Hitoshi Endou and Kyu Yong Jung[1]

SUMMARY. The mammalian kidney is known to consume ATP at high rates for various transporting processes. In order to evaluate energy metabolism and response to hypoxic insult along the nephron, we measured ATP content in each of the microdissected nephron segments from three animal species under various conditions using the luciferin/luciferase technique.

When proximal tubules from rats or mice were incubated at 37°C for 15 min without substrate, ATP content decreased rapidly in the following order; terminal (S_3) > middle (S_2) > early (S_1) segments, in rabbits, however, the order was reversed. This ATP decrease was restored with a sole preferred substrate at 2mM. ATP production from glucose was minimal in S_1 from three species, but was substantial in S_3. Glutamine or pyruvate was a preferred substrate in the proximal tubule. In lower nephron segments, although ATP was not reduced after 15 min incubation without substrate, a monovalent cationic ionophore, monensin, (10 μg/ml) decreased ATP, and this decrease was restored by 2mM glucose or pyruvate as preferred substrates.

In order to identify the portion within the proximal tubule most sensitive to hypoxic insult, each of three proximal segments was incubated with antimycin A, and ATP content was determined. In rats, antimycin A, at 5×10^{-7}M, decreased ATP content dramatically in S_3, moderately in S_2 and slightly in S_1, even in the presence of a preferred substrate.

These results suggest that energy metabolism differs from segment to segment, and that, in response to hypoxic insult, S_3 is the most fragile segment in rats.

Introduction

For active transporting systems, ATP is the major high-energy compound. To generate this energy source, the kidney metabolizes various substrates [1–3]. For each

[1]Department of Pharmacology, Faculty of Medicine, University of Tokyo, 113 Tokyo, Japan

defined nephron segment, however, with the exception of our recent reports [4,5], no clear-cut information is available about major substrates used for ATP synthesis along the nephron. We, therefore, report here that renal energy metabolism and its functions possess intranephron heterogeneity.

In addition, the kidney is very vulnerable to changes in metabolism and function caused by anoxia or by various chemicals such as drugs and hazardous xenobiotics. Since, in the field of renal toxicology, the relationship between ATP synthesis and consumption, as affected by exogenous materials in each nephron segment, has not yet been demonstrated, we also report here the effect of antimycin A, instead of anoxia, on cellular ATP within the rat proximal tubule.

Materials and Methods

Tissue preparation and tubule microdissection techniques used in this study have been previously described [6,7]. Incubation of microdissected nephron segments for ATP turnover determination and ATP assay were carried out as reported elsewhere [4,5]. Monensin and antimycin A were dissolved in ethanol, and the final concentration of vehicle was 0.2%. In preliminary experiments, this concentration of vehicle did not interfere with ATP biosynthesis.

Bovine serum albumin (BSA), collagenase (type 1, 240 U/mg), monensin, antimycin A, β-hydroxybutyrate, and DL-lactate were purchased from Sigma Chemical (St. Louis, Mo). Monitoring reagent for ATP was purchased from LKB-Wallac. All other compounds and reagents were of the highest grade available.

Values were expressed as means ± SE. Analysis of variance for multiple group comparisons and the Student's *t* test for unpaired data were used to determine statistical significance.

Results

Effect of Incubation Time on Cellular ATP Content in Individual Nephron Segments

When isolated nephron segments from kidneys of three animal species were incubated without any substrates, cellular ATP content was reduced dramatically in the proximal tubule, but not so conspicuously in the lower nephron segments (Table 1). In mice, the glomerulus also showed a decrease of ATP similar to that in the proximal tubule, where the straight portion (S_2 and S_3) showed a larger decrease than S_1. In rats, the most fragile segment was S_3, followed by S_2. In contrast, in rabbits, S_1 was the most sensitive suggesting a clear species difference in metabolic properties within the proximal tubule.

Substrate Specificities in the Maintenance of ATP Content in the Glomerulus and Proximal Tubule

When rat proximal tubules were incubated at 37°C for 15 min without exogenous substrate, cellular ATP content decreased significantly (Fig. 1). When glucose was

Table 1. Effect of incubation time on cellular ATP content in isolated nephron segments from three animal species

Species incubation	Mouse		Rat		Rabbit	
	0	30 min	0	[a]20 or 30 min	0	25 min
Glm	6.3±0.5	1.9±0.3	12.1±1.2	ND	14.3±1.9	11.1±1.5
S_1	12.2±1.2	2.2±0.4	17.4±2.2	[a]4.8±2.3	24.2±2.1	6.9±1.0
S_2	24.8±1.7	1.7±0.3	20.9±3.7	[a]4.9±1.4	29.8±2.8	12.4±3.0
S_3	25.2±2.8	2.7±0.3	20.0±1.7	[a]2.4±0.6	25.7±1.4	21.2±0.8
MAL	17.3±1.8	15.9±1.2	17.5±0.4	14.9±0.4	18.6±2.9	ND
CAL	12.8±1.2	10.3±1.3	9.9±0.4	ND	10.2±0.8	ND
DT	23.0±2.8	14.7±2.4	13.1±0.7	13.6±0.8	27.3±1.8	ND
CCT	20.8±2.8	15.2±1.5	13.9±0.7	ND	23.5±2.5	ND
MCT	14.0±1.2	10.0±1.3	17.6±1.1	16.0±0.6	29.2±2.2	ND

[a]S_1, S_2, and S_3 of rat were incubated for 20 min and MAL, DT, and OMCT were incubated for 30 min. Values ($\times 10^{-13}$ mol/glm or mm tubule) are means ± SE of 4–7 experiments. ND, not done; Glm, glomerulus; S_1 to S_3, first to third segments of the proximal tubule; MAL and CAL, medullary and cortical thick ascending limbs of Henle's loop; DT, distal tubule; CCT and MCT, cortical and outer medullary collecting tubules

added to the incubation medium as an exogenous substrate, ATP production by the proximal tubule cells was minimal (Fig. 1), whereas glutamine or pyruvate caused cellular ATP contents higher than those of other substrates used in this study. Figure 1 also shows that cellular ATP produced by lactic acid and β-hydroxybutyric acid was relatively high in the proximal tubule. In the glomerulus, however, no remarkable difference in ATP production was observed among these substrates. The order of preferred substrates for cellular ATP maintenance in the proximal tubule was pyruvate = glutamine > lactic acid > β-hydroxybutyric acid > glucose.

Substrate Specificities for Maintaining ATP in the Distally Located Nephron Segments

As shown in Table 1, a simple incubation of the distally located nephron segments does not change ATP content. Therefore, it is difficult to identify their preferred substrates by the same protocol as that used for the glomerulus or the proximal tubule. It should be possible to demonstrate that increasing the rate of active sodium transport by addition of a cationic ionophore, monensin, decreases cellular ATP content. Although the data are not shown, concentrations of monensin higher than 10μg/ml decreased ATP content significantly in the medullary thick ascending limb of Henle's loop (MAL), the distal tubule (DT), and the medullary collecting tubule (MCT).

In the presence of 10μg/ml monensin, cellular ATP content in distally located nephron segments decreased significantly without substrate (Fig. 2). When the ionophore was added to the incubation medium, the differences in each substrate's ability to maintain the ATP level also became clear in the distally located nephron segments. The pattern of substrate specificity in these segments (Fig. 2) was different from that in the proximal tubule (Fig. 1). The order of preferred substrates for cellular ATP maintenance in distally located nephron segments was glucose = pyruvate = lactate > β-hydroxybutyric acid > glutamine.

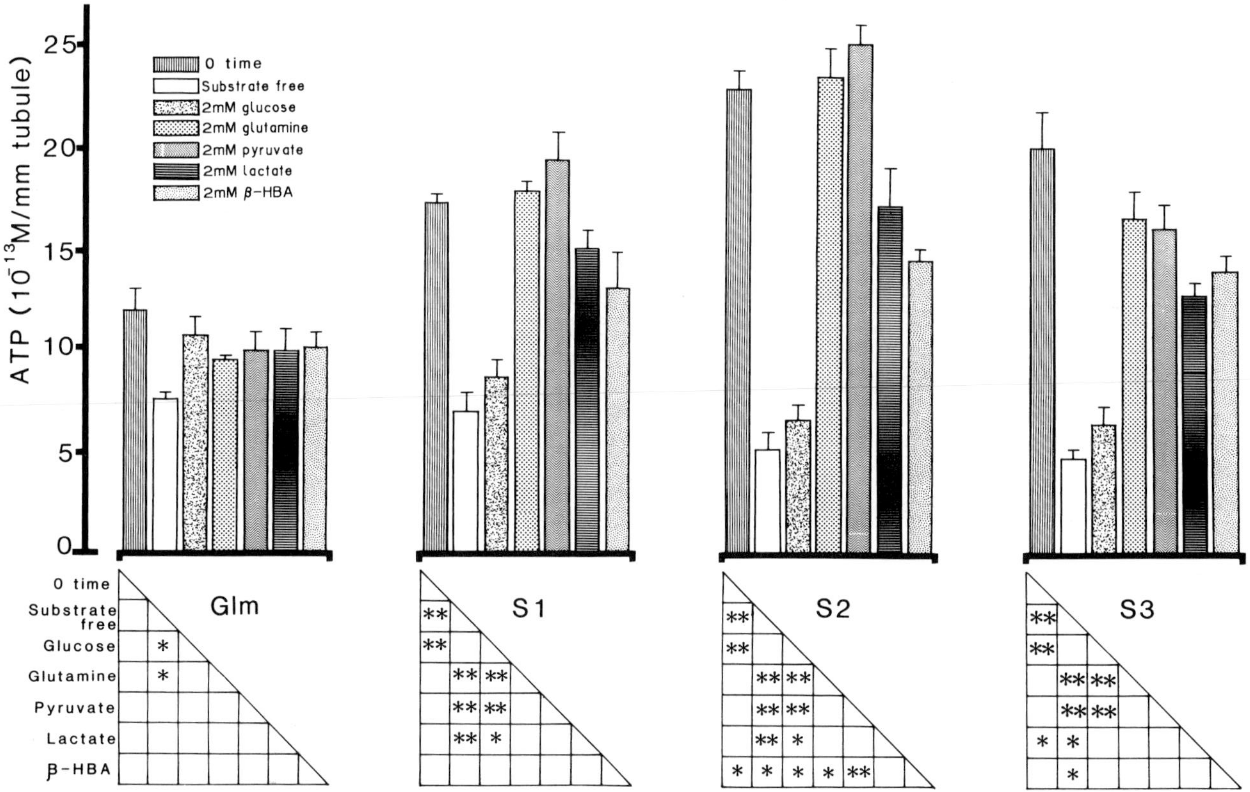

Fig. 1. Specificity of substrate utilization in maintaining cellular ATP content in the glomerulus and the proximal tubule. Immediately after microdissection, cellular ATP contents of the isolated glomerulus and proximal tubule were determined by microchemiluminescence (0 time). After 15 min of incubation at 37°C in Hanks' medium (oxygen saturated, pH 7.40) with each substrate (2 mM) cellular ATP was measured. β-HBA, β-hydroxybutyric acid. Statistical analysis was carried out by ANOVA (*$P < 0.05$, **$P < 0.01$). Values are means ± SE ($n = 5$) [5]

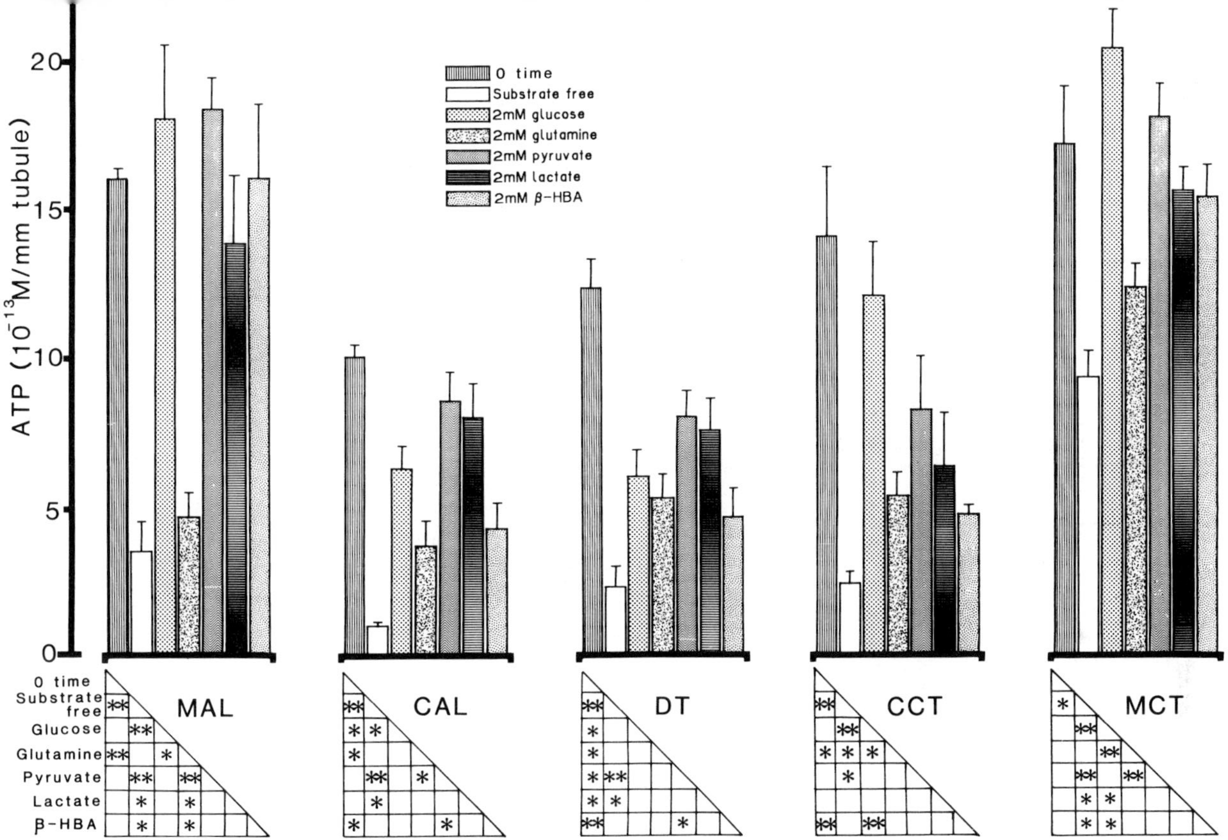

Fig. 2. Substrate specificity in the maintenance of cellular ATP content in distally located nephron segments. Assay protocol was the same as that described in Fig. 1, except that the incubation medium (pH 7.40) contained 10 μg/ml monensin to delete ATP by stimulating Na^+, K^+-ATPase activity. MAL and CAL, medullary and cortical thick ascending limbs of Henle's loop; DT, distal tubule; CCT and MCT, cortical and medullary collecting tubules; β-HBA, β-hydroxybutyric acid *Asterisks* denote significant differences among various substrates by ANOVA (*$P < 0.05$, **$P < 0.01$). Values are means ± SE ($n = 5$) [5]

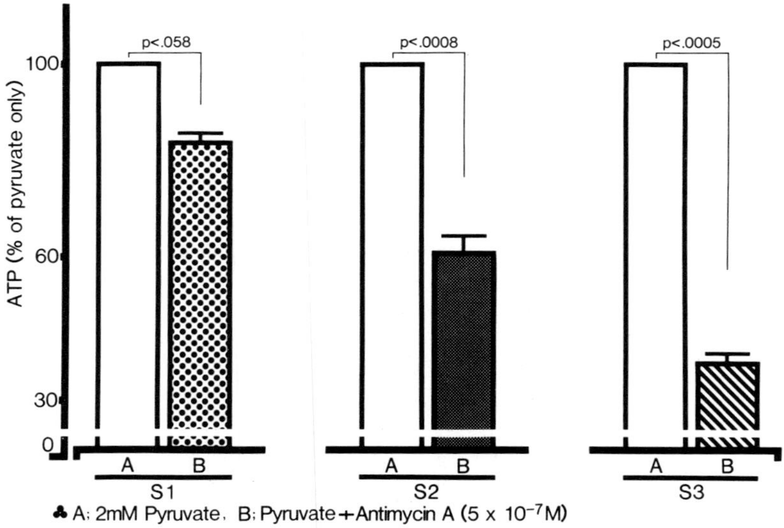

Fig. 3. Effect of antimycin A on cellular ATP content in rat proximal tubule. Each nephron segment isolated from male SD rat kidneys was incubated in the presence of 2mM pyruvate, with or without 5×10^{-7}M antimycin A, at 37°C for 15 min, and ATP content was assayed by the luciferin/luciferase method

Effect of Antimycin A on Cellular ATP Content in Rat Proximal Tubule

As illustrated in Fig. 3, antimycin A, at 5×10^{-7}M, significantly decreased ATP which had been restored by 2mM pyruvate in both S_2 and S_3; however, the decrease was insignificant in S_1. The decreased amount in S_3 was higher than that in S_2. This finding clearly suggests that, in rat kidneys, heterogeneity in response to hypoxic insult exists within the proximal tubule, where S_3 is most fragile. This result, shown in Fig. 3, is consistent with that shown in Table 1.

Although the data are not shown, the MAL and CAL (the cortical thick ascending limb of Henle's loop) of mouse kidneys are more sensitive to antimycin A than the CCT or MCT [4].

Discussion

The purpose of this study was to clarify the specificity of substrate utilization for ATP production along the single nephron and to identify the nephron segment(s) sensitive to hypoxic insult.

Since ATP is the most efficient high-energy compound used by the kidney to support its various functions, it is worthwhile to study nephron heterogeneity of ATP consumption and production. Levels of ATP in microdissected nephron segments have previously been reported [8]; however, information concerning the efficiency of ATP extraction from nephron segments was not provided. We found that the conventional ATP extracting agents, such as Extralight and Triton X-100, did not adequately extract ATP from the segments tested. Although there was no direct proof that TCA extraction used in this study was complete, the estimated ATP concentration, on the basis of the value obtained by TCA extraction, was calculated to be 3–6mM, using the available morphometry [9], values that are in accord with the physiological concentrations previously reported in in vivo freeze-clamp studies [10,11].

It became evident in this study that each nephron segment has its own distinct ability to utilize specific substrates. Studies on enzyme distribution in different nephron segments have also revealed distinct patterns, suggestive of specific substrate metabolism [12]. In glucose metabolism particularly, hexokinase, phosphofructokinase, pyruvate kinase, and pyruvate dehydrogenase are key enzymes [13]. Hexokinase activity was low in the proximal tubules, especially in S_1, but was slightly increased in S_3 [14]. Our results in Fig. 1 indicate that S_3, but not S_1 or S_2, could metabolize glucose to produce ATP. As predicted by hexokinase distribution [14], all distally located nephron segments tested readily utilized glucose to maintain cellular ATP.

We observed that a relatively low concentration of substrate (10^{-4}M) was sufficient to maintain cellular ATP in almost all segments (data not shown). Considering the physiological concentrations of these substrates, glomeruli and tubules would normally be surrounded by sufficient metabolic fuels in vivo. Endogenous substrates may also play a role in energy metabolism. The amount of glycogen stored in the kidney has been reported to be small [15], but Bastin et al. [10] showed that thick ascending limb and papilla had a tenfold larger glycogen content than did the proximal tubule. In our study, the decrease of ATP content after 30-min incubation without substrate (Table 1) was greater in proximal tubules than in distally located segments. Moreover, this conserved ATP content in MAL or CAL decreased remarkably when the MAL or CAL were incubated with antimycin A [4]. These observations suggest that the distally located nephron segments may contain more endogenous substrate(s) than do the proximal tubules, and that they might be more resistant to hypoxia. Indeed, S_3 is most vulnerable to ischemia [16], and this might be related to the observation that ATP content in proximal tubules, especially in S_3, decreased faster than that in distally located segments. In addition, we have recently found that the superoxide generating enzyme, xanthine oxidase, was densely distributed in the proximal tubule [17]. This factor may also be directly related to the vulnerability of that tubule.

In order to gain better understanding of unsolved species differences the remarkable difference between rats and rabbits, within the three portions of the proximal tubule, in ATP decrease after incubation without substrate (Table 1), should be further investigated.

Acknowledgments. This work was supported by grants from the Japanese Ministry of Education, Science, and Culture (Nos. 01480136 and 01870111), and by the Japanese Ministry of Health and Welfare, Hoansya and Shimabara Science Promotion Foundation.

References

1. Weidemann MJ, Krebs HA (1969) The fuel of respiration of rat kidney cortex. Biochem J 112:149–166

2. Pitts RF, Macleod MB (1975) Metabolism of blood glucose by the intact functioning kidney of the dog. Kidney Int 7:130–136
3. Wirthensohn G, Guder WG (1986) Renal substrate metabolism. Physiol Rev 66:469–497
4. Uchida S, Endou H (1988) Substrate specificity to maintain cellular ATP along the mouse nephron. Am J Physiol 255:F977–F983
5. Jung KY, Uchida S, Endou H (1989) Nephrotoxicity assessment by measuring cellular ATP content. Toxicol Appl Pharmacol 100:369–382
6. Morel F, Chabardes D, Imbert M (1976) Functional segmentation of the rabbit distal tubule by microdetermination of hormone-dependent adenylate cyclase activity. Kidney Int 9:264–277
7. Nonoguchi H, Uchida S, Shiigai T, Endou H (1985) Effect of chronic metabolic acidosis on ammonia production from L-glutamine in microdissected rat nephron segments. Pflügers Arch 403:229–235
8. Kiebzak GM, Yusufi ANK, Kusano E, Braun-Warness J, Dousa TP (1985) ATP and cAMP system in the in vitro response of microdissected cortical tubules in PTH. Am J Physiol 248:F152–F159
9. Pfaller W, Guder WG, Gstraunthaler G, Kotanko P, Jehart I, Purschel S (1984) Compartmentation of ATP within renal proximal tubular cells. Biochim Biophys Acta 805:152–157
10. Bastin J, Canbon N, Thompson M, Lowry OH (1987) Changes in energy reserves in different segments of nephron during brief ischemia. Kidney Int 31:1239–1247
11. Guder WG, Wagner S, Wirthensohn G (1986) Metabolic fuels along the nephron: pathways and intracellular mechanisms of interaction. Kidney Int 29:41–45
12. Guder WG, Ross B (1984) Enzyme distribution along the nephron. Kidney Int 26:101–110
13. Ross BD, Espinal J, Silva P (1986) Glucose metabolism in tubular function. Kidney Int 29:54–67
14. Vandewalle A, Wirthensohn G, Heidrich HG, Guder WG (1981) Distribution of hexokinase and phosphoenolpyruvatecarboxykinase along the rabbit nephron. Am J Physiol 240:F492–F500
15. Needleman P, Passonneau JV, Lowry OH (1968) Distribution of glucose and related metabolites in the kidney. Am J Physiol 215:655–659
16. Venkatachalam MA, Bernard DB, Donohoe JF, Levinsky NG (1978) Ischemic damage and repair in the rat proximal tubule; difference among S1, S2, and S3 segments. Kidney Int 14:31–49
17. Endou H, Yamada T, Takahashi T, Tamura K, Ito S (1987) Intranephron distribution and properties of xanthine oxidase, superoxide dismutase, and guanase activities in control and nephrotic rats. In: Kovacevic Z, Guder WG (eds) Molecular nephrology. Walter de Gruyter, Berlin, pp 347–352

Ischemia-Induced Loss of Epithelial Polarity

Bruce A. Molitoris[1]

Summary. Proximal tubular cells play a major role in the reabsorption of ions, water and solutes from the glomerular filtrate. This process is accomplished, in large part, by the cells having a polarized surface membrane with structurally, biochemically, and physiologically distinct apical and basolateral membranes separated by cellular junctional complexes. Establishment and maintenance of these unique membrane domains is essential for the normal functioning of proximal tubular cells. Ischemia results in the duration-dependent loss of apical and basolateral surface membrane lipid and protein polarity. This loss of surface membrane polarity is associated with disruption of the microfilament network and opening of cellular tight junctions. Surface membrane lipids and proteins are then free to diffuse laterally within the bilayer into the alternate membrane domain. Functionally, ischemia-induced loss of epithelial polarity is responsible for reduced sodium and glucose reabsorption and for the enhanced susceptibility of proximal tubular cells to aminoglycoside-induced nephrotoxicity. With recovery, proximal tubular cells undergo remodeling of the surface membrane, such that the unique apical and basolateral membrane domains are reestablished, allowing normal cellular function to return.

Introduction

Renal proximal tubular epithelial cells function to provide and regulate the unidirectional movement of ions, water, and macromolecules between the glomerular filtrate and the blood. This is accomplished, in large part, by having a surface membrane polarized into apical and basolateral components which are structurally, biochemically, and physiologically distinct membrane domains that contain different ion channels, transport proteins, enzymes, and lipids [1,2]. The establishment and maintenance of these unique surface membrane domains is dependent upon the polarized

[1]Denver VA Medical Center, Denver, CO 80220, USA

delivery of newly synthesized surface membrane components, cytoskeletal surface membrane interactions, and cell-cell junctional complexes which serve as a barrier between apical and basolateral domains [1,2]. The purpose of this review is to highlight the polar nature of proximal tubule cells, describe how ischemia disrupts the ability of proximal tubule cells to maintain polarity, and to discuss the cellular mechanisms involved and the functional consequences of loss of surface membrane polarity in proximal tubular cells.

Proximal Tubular Cells as a Polarized Epithelium

Renal proximal tubular cells possess highly polarized apical and basolateral membrane domains (Table 1). The apical membrane faces the urinary lumen (external compartment) and is composed of membrane proteins with specialized properties related to the reabsorption of water, electrolytes, and macromolecules. The basolateral membrane domain faces the internal milieu (blood compartment) and has a complement of intrinsic and extrincis membrane proteins which are involved in the maintenance of the normal physiologic state of the cell and also in signal recognition and transduction [1]. Extensive differences also exist between apical and basolateral membrane lipids, which are responsible for large physicochemical differences between the two different membrane domains [3–5]. Differences in membrane lipids also influence the function of numerous membrane proteins and the binding of certain macromolecules [6].

The functional necessity of the polarized distribution of surface membrane components into apical and basolateral domains is well illustrated by considering the

Table 1. Asymmetery of the surface of membrane of proximal tubular cells

Characteristics	Apical membrane	Basolateral membrane
Proteins		
Enzymes	Leucine aminopeptidase Maltase GPI-linked proteins (alkaline phosphatase)	Adenylate cyclase
Receptors		Insulin Parathyroid hormone Epidermal growth factor
ATPases	H^+-ATPase Mg^{2+}-ATPase	Na^+-K^+-ATPase Ca^{2+}-ATPase
Carriers	Na^+-dependent cotransporters Na^+-H^+ antiporter	Cl^-/HCO_3 exchanger Na^+-independent glucose carrier
Lipids		
Cholesterol/phospholipid	High	Low
Sphinogomyelin	High	Low
Phosphatidylcholine	Low	High
Phosphatidylinositol	Low	High
Physical properties		
Electrical resistance	High	Low
Membrane fluidity	Low	High

GPI, glycosyl-phosphatidylinositol

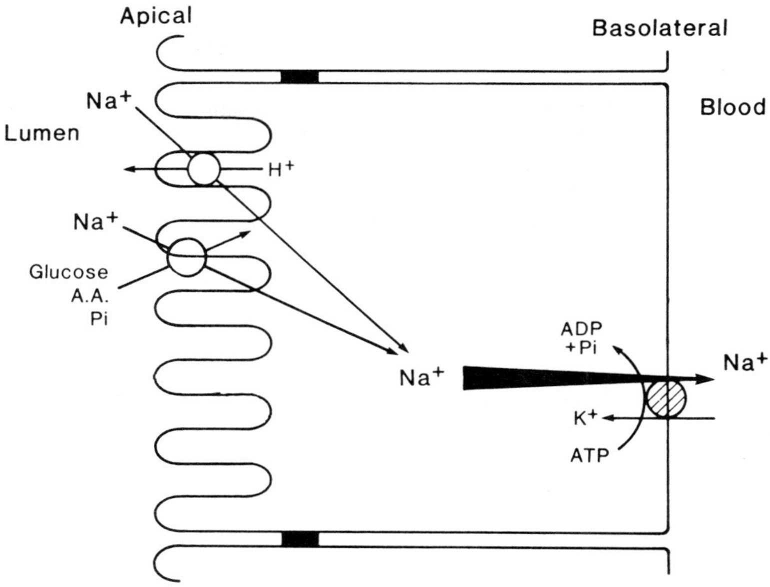

Fig. 1. Polarized proximal tubular cell. Sodium enters across the apical membrane down its electrochemical gradient providing the driving force for hydrogen ion secretion and the cellular uptake of glucose, amino acids, and phosphate, via co-transport processes. Sodium is then pumped up its electro-chemical gradient by NaK-ATPase, which is specifically localized to the basolateral membrane. This is an energy requiring process which also results in the inward movement of potassium

basolateral localization of NaK-ATPase (Fig. 1). NaK-ATPase is synthesized in the endoplasmic reticulum, transported to the Cis aspect of the golgi complex, buds off the Trans aspect of the golgi complex and is delivered in a polarized fashion to the basolateral membrane [7]. Upon arrival it associates with the actin cytoskeleton via a direct linkage of the alpha subunit to an ankryn-fodrin complex [2,8]. In this location the enzyme functions to bring about the ATP-dependent outward movement of sodium up its electro-chemical gradient, and the inward movement of potassium. This action, in conjunction with specialized apical membrane sodium-dependent carriers, results in the efficient reabsorption of sodium from the glomerular filtrate (Fig. 1).

Ischemia Alters Surface Membrane Protein and Lipid Polarity

That ischemia resulted in the loss of surface membrane protein and lipid polarity was suggested by our initial study, in which we were only able to isolate apical membrane fractions, following ischemia, that were markedly enriched for NaK-ATPase (our basolateral membrane marker) [9]. This redistribution of basolaterally associated NaK-ATPase into the apical membrane occurred rapidly during ischemia, with significant differences being documented following 10 minutes of ischemia [10,11].

Subsequent biochemical, histochemical, and immunocytochemical studies have now clearly demonstrated that ischemia induced a time-dependent loss of surface membrane lipid and protein polarity. Marked decreases in apical sphingomyelin and cholesterol content and increases in apical phosphatidylcholine and phosphatidylinositol content occurred within 5 minutes of generalized ischemia induced by renal pedicle clamping [10]. These lipid alterations occurred rapidly during the first 15 minutes of ischemia, and at a much slower rate thereafter [10,11]. Biochemical and immunocytochemical studies have also been used to demonstrate that apical lipids and proteins (leucine aminopeptidase) redistribute into the basolateral membrane during ischemic injury [11]. In summary, ischemia induced the rapid redistribution of apical and basolateral membrane domain specific proteins and lipids into the alternate surface membrane domain.

We have also documented that repolarization of surface membrane polarity occurred following the phase of cellular injury. The marked alterations in apical and basolateral lipids and the redistribution of leucine aminopeptidase and NaK-ATPase into the alternate surface membrane domain was corrected during reperfusion following reversible ischemic injury [11,12]. Since proximal tubule cells recover from ischemic injury by cellular repair and do not undergo cellular division [12], the changes observed represent actual remodeling of the surface membrane domains of recovering cells and are not due to cellular proliferation.

Functional Significance of Ischemia-Induced Loss of Epithelial Polarity

While loss of surface membrane polarity could lead to numerous alterations in the cell's ability to conduct its normal functions, my laboratory has concentrated on two specific areas known to be fundamentally important in proximal tubular function. The first area involved transcellular transport (reabsorption). Since ischemia led to the duration-dependent redistribution of NaK-ATPase into the apical membrane we reasoned that the redistributed enzyme could be functional and therefore able to carry out the transport of intracellular sodium to the nephron lumen (Fig. 2). This would lead to reduced effective Na^+ reabsorption and would also uncouple ATP and sodium reabsorption, resulting in inefficient utilization of an already limiting source of cellular energy (Fig. 2). Two approaches were used to test this hypothesis. Our first approach involved the use of in vivo micropuncture techniques to measure sodium reabsorption under control situations and then following 15 minutes of ischemia and two hours of reperfusion in the same nephron segment. Following two hours of reperfusion, cellular ATP, cellular morphology, and apical sodium permeability had all normalized. However, there was a marked reduction in both the reabsorption of sodium (37.4% vs 23.0%, $P < 0.01$) and water (48.6% vs 36.9%, $P < 0.01$) in these paired tubule studies [13]. In an additional in vivo study, following 50 minutes of ischemia, normalization of the transcellular transport sodium and lithium, a specific marker of proximal tubular reabsorption, was dependent upon the reestablishment of surface membrane NaK-ATPase polarity in proximal tubular cells. Normalization of glucose transport across proximal tubular cells following ischemic injury was also found to be dependent upon the reestablishment of surface

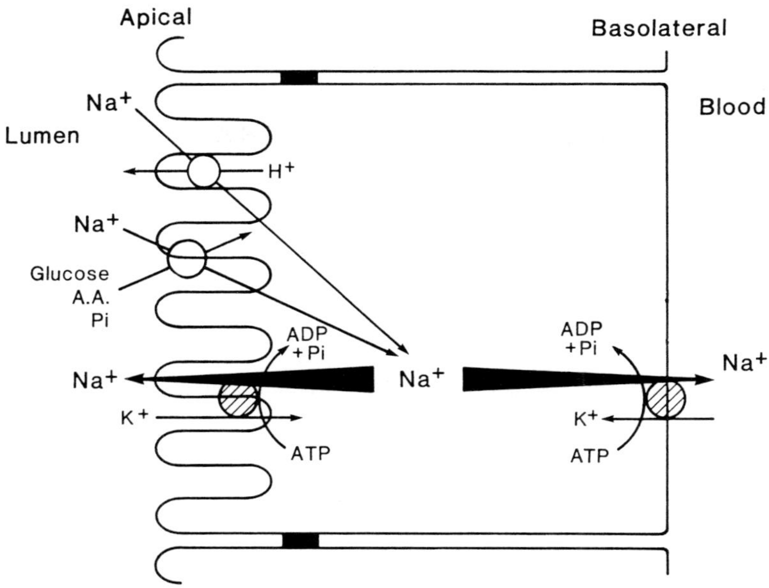

Fig. 2. Non-polarized renal proximal tubular cell following ischemic injury. Following ischemic injury NaK-ATPase is found in both the basolateral and the apical membrane domains. In the apical membrane NaK-ATPase maintains its functional activity and is, therefore, capable of competing for intracellular sodium ions. This markedly diminishes the efficiency of sodium transport and results in a high urinary excretion of sodium following ischemic injury. By pumping sodium back out of the lumen a futile cycle is also set up which uncouples ATP utilization and sodium transport

membrane apical lipid polarity [12]. In brush border membrane vesicle studies, alteration in the ability of the apical membrane to transport glucose was directly related to a decease in membrane fluidity and to the sphingomyelin/phosphatidylcholine ratio. These data suggest that the rapid ischemia-induced alteration in these lipids was responsible for reduced reabsorption of glucose following ischemic injury [14]. Furthermore, glucose transport increased to control levels concurrently with the reestablishment of the apical sphingomyelin/phosphatidylcholine ratio [12]. Taken together, these data indicate that the reabsorption of ions, water, and solutes by proximal tubular cells is dependent upon the establishment and maintenance of domain-specific lipid and protein polarity in apical and basolateral membranes. Furthermore, following ischemic injury, proximal tubular cells are unable to function properly until surface membrane polarity has been reestablished.

Recent evidence from our laboratory also indicates that alterations in the phospholipid content of the apical membrane may be of critical importance in determining the nephrotoxicity of aminoglycoside antibiotics. Aminoglycoside antibiotics are known to bind to phosphatidylinositol phospholipids with increased affinity [15] and are internalized via the endocytic process. Ischemia is known to rapidly increase the apical content of phosphatidylinositol [9–11]. We have now shown that mild, functionally insignificant, ischemia occurring prior to aminoglycoside administration, markedly enhanced the nephrotoxicity of gentamicin [16]. Additional preliminary evidence indicated that, following ischemic injury, gentamicin binding to the apical membrane increased markedly [17]. These data, when taken together, suggest the ischemia-induced increase in apical phosphatidylinositol content is directly responsible for enhanced gentamicin binding. This, in turn, may play a role in the ischemia-induced enhancement of aminoglycoside nephrotoxicity observed by our laboratory and others [16,18].

Mechanism of Ischemia-Induced Loss of Epithelial Polarity

Figure 3 indicates three potential avenues by which ischemia could induce loss of epithelial polarity in proximal tubular cells. First, the random (non-polar) delivery of newly synthesized membrane components to either the apical or the basolateral membrane could be responsible. This, however, seems unlikely because both the synthesis and intracellular translocation of these membrane components is ATP-dependent and during ischemia cellular ATP drops rapidly to non-detectable levels [13]. Second, abnormal migration and fusion of previously existent endocytic and

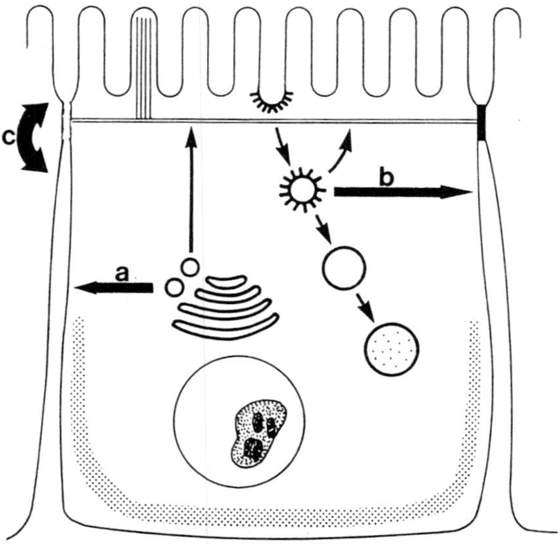

Fig. 3. Potential mechanisms for loss of epithelial polarity during ischemic injury. The first potential mechanism (*a*) involves the abnormal (random) translocation of newly synthesized membrane components from the trans golgi to the incorrect surface membrane domain. The second mechanism (*b*) involves the abnormal (random) intracellular movement of endocytic and exocytic vesicles and fusion with the alternate surface membrane domain. The final potential mechanism, resulting in loss of epithelial polarity (*c*) involves the opening of cellular tight junctions which then allows for the lateral diffusion of surface membrane lipids and proteins within the plane of the bilayer into the alternate surface membrane domain

exocytic vesicles to the alternate membrane domain could also lead to the loss of epithelial surface membrane polarity. Studies from our laboratory, published in preliminary form, indicate that this mechanism was also not involved in the loss of epithelial polarity [19]. We have, however, accumulated data which indicated that disruption of the tight junction is involved in the loss of surface membrane polarity during ischemic injury. In proximal tubular cells tight junctions between cells consist of one or two discontinuous strands. Proximal tubular cells are classified as "leaky" epithelia, as the electrical resistance across a monolayer of these cells is low. Since disruption of tight junctions by several mechanisms (calcium, chelation, monoclonal antibodies) results in loss of epithelial polarity, we investigated the effect of ischemia on tight junction functional integrity. In vivo microperfusion of early loops of proximal tubules with ruthenium red in glutaraldehyde was used to gain selective access to and outline the apical surface membrane and tight junctions. Ischemia resulted in a time-dependent stepwise increase in the number of tight junctions penetrated by ruthenium red, from less than 10% in control situations to 29%, 50%, and 62% after 5, 15, and 30 minutes of ischemia, respectively [10]. This was associated with the rapid duration-dependent redistribution of basolateral membrane domain specific lipids and NaK-ATPase into the apical membrane domain. We, therefore, believe that ischemia leads to rapid deterioration in the cells' ability to maintain the tight junction. Following the disassociation of the tight junction cellular barrier, apical and basolateral lipids and proteins are free to diffuse laterally within the plane of the bilayer and redistribute into the alternate membrane domain. That lipids moved more rapidly into the alternate membrane domain is consistent with their increased lateral mobility, as compared to proteins [20].

Since the tight junction is under the direct control of the microfilament cytoskeleton [21], we next undertook studies to determine the effect of ischemia on the proximal tubular cell microfilament network. Ischemia was associated with the rapid duration-dependent disruption of the apical microfilament network, with loss of the polarized distribution of microfilaments from the apical aspect of the cell into the entire cell cytoplasm. Disruption of the apical microfilament network was noticeable following only five minutes of ischemia and was present in all cells following 15 minutes of ischemia. To determine the functional significance of selective microfilament disruption, a microfilament selective dose of cytochalasin D (10 μM) was utilized in an isolated perfused kidney system. Structurally, cytochalasin D resulted in extensive disruption of the apical surface, with blebbing, vacuolization, fusion, and patchy loss of microvilli. Cytochalasin D also brought about a decrease in the reabsorption of sodium, from 97.1% ± 0.7% to 64.3% ± 7%, which occurred in a linear fashion throughout the duration of cytochalasin D exposure [22]. In control kidneys the reabsorption of Na^+ remained unchanged throughout the duration of the perfusion. Lithium reabsorption also decreased linearly and there was a high degree of correlation in individual kidneys between sodium and lithium reabsorption, indicating that the defect in Na^+ reabsorption induced by cytochalasin-mediated microfilament disruption was localized to proximal tubular cells. These data indicate that the selective disruption of microfilaments results in proximal tubular structural and functional alterations similar to those seen during ischemia. The data, therefore, imply that microfilament disruption may play an important role in the pathophysiology of ischemic injury.

In summary, ischemia leads to the duration-dependent loss of surface membrane polarity in proximal tubular cells. This appears to occur via loss of the cells' ability to maintain the actin cytoskeleton, and via the opening of cellular tight junctions. Following ischemic injury, proximal tubular cells function as non-polar cells until cellular remodeling occurs, allowing for the return of unique apical and basolateral membrane domains which can then function together in a coordinated fashion to bring out the vectorial transport ions, water, and macromolecules transcellularly. Further understanding of ischemia-induced loss of surface membrane polarity and cytoskeletal alterations will greatly enhance the understanding of the pathophysiology of ischemic injury and cellular recovery.

References

1. Molitoris BA, Nelson WJ (1990) Alterations in the establishment and maintenance of epithelial cell polarity as a basis for disease processes. J Clin Invest 85:3–9
2. Rodriquez-Boulan E, Nelson WJ (1989) Morphogenesis of the polarized epithelial cell phenotype. Science 245:718–725
3. Molitoris BA, Simon FR (1985) Renal cortical brush-border and basolateral membranes: cholesterol and phospholipid composition and relative turnover. J Membr Biol 3:207–215
4. Carmel G, Rodriquez F, Carriere S, LeGrimellec C (1985) Composition and physical properties of lipids from plasma membranes of dog kidney. Biochim Biophys Acta 818:149–157
5. Molitoris BA, Hoilien C (1987) Static and dynamic components of renal cortical brush border and basolateral membrane fluidity: role of cholesterol. J Membr Biol 99:165–172
6. Molitoris BA (1987) Membrane fluidity: measurement and relationship to solute transport. Semin Nephrol 7:61–67
7. Caplan MJ, Anderson HC, Palade GE, Jamieson JD (1986) Intracellular sorting and polarized cell surface delivery of Na^+, K^+-ATPase, an endogenous component of MDCK cell basolateral plasma membranes. Cell 46:623–631
8. Nelson WJ, Hammerton RW (1989) A membrane-cytoskeletal complex containing Na^+, K^+-ATPase ankyrin, and fodrin in Madin-Darby canine kidney (MDCK) cells. Implications for the biogenesis of epithelial cell polarity. J Cell Biol 108:893–902
9. Molitoris BA, Wilson PD, Schrier RW, Simon FR (1985) Ischemia induces partial loss of surface membrane polarity and accumulation of putative calcium ionophores. J Clin Invest 76:2097–2105
10. Molitoris BA, Dahl RH, Falk SA (1989) Ischemia-induced loss of epithelial polarity. Role of the tight junction. J Clin Invest 84:1334–1339
11. Molitoris BA, Hoilien CA, Dahl RH, Ahnen DJ, Wilson PD, Kim J (1988) Characterization of ischemia-induced loss of epithelial polarity. J Membr Biol 106:233–242
12. Spiegel DM, Wilson PD, Molitoris BA (1989) Epithelial polarity following ischemia: a requirement for normal cell function. Am J Physiol (Renal Fluid Electrolyte Physiol) 256:F430–F436
13. Molitoris BA, Chan LK, Shapiro JI, Conger JD, Falk SA (1989) Loss of epithelial polarity: A novel hypothesis for reduced proximal tubule Na^+ transport following ischemic injury. J Membr Biol 107:119–127
14. Molitoris BA, Kinne R (1987) Ischemia reduces surface membrane dysfunction. Mechanism of altered Na^+-dependent glucose transport. J Clin Invest 80:647–654
15. Hume HD (1988) Aminoglycoside nephrotoxicity. Kidney Int 33:900–911
16. Spiegel DM, Shanley PF, Molitoris BA (to be published) Mild ischemia predisposes the S_3 segment to gentamicin toxicity. Kidney Int
17. Molitoris BA, Geerdes A, Meyer C (1990) Ischemia enhanced gentamicin toxicity: Role of increased apical phosphatidylinositol. Clin Res 38:141A

18. Zager RA (1988) Gentamicin nephrotoxicity in the setting of acute renal hypoperfusion. Am J Physiol 254:F574–F581
19. Molitoris BA, Falk S, Dahl R (1989) Mechanism of ischemia-induced loss of epithelial polarity. Clin Res 37:497A
20. Salas PJI, Vega-Salas E, Hochman J, Rogriquez-Boulan E, Edidin M (1988) Selective anchoring in the specific plasma membrane domain. A role in epithelial cell polarity. J Cell Biol 107:2363–2376
21. Madara JL (1989) Loosening tight junctions. Lessons from the intestine. J Clin Invest 83:1089–1094
22. Kellerman PS, Clark PAF, Hoilien CA, Linas SL, Molitoris BA (to be published) Role of microfilament in maintenance of proximal tubule structural and functional integrity. Am J Physiol

Acquired Resistance to Rechallenge Injury to Acute Renal Failure

Akira Hishida, Hideo Yamada, Taisuke Isozaki, and Nishio Honda[1]

Summary. A smaller dose of uranyl acetate (0.8–0.9 mg/kg) lessened the severity of acute renal failure (ARF) following a rechallenge with a larger dose of the agent (2 mg/kg). This resistance to the rechallenge was not attributed largely to renal hemodynamic alterations, suppressed glomerular contractile response to vasoactive substances, smaller amount of uranium bound to regenerated tubular cells, and altered active oxygen scavenging enzyme and Na-K-ATPase activities in regenerated tubular cells.

Introduction

A number of studies have demonstrated that prior nephrotoxic acute renal failure (ARF) affords resistance to a rechallenge with the same or a different agent [1,2,3,4,5], though this is not a universal finding [5]. The mechanisms for acquired resistance to ARF are poorly understood, but possible mechanisms include renal hemodynamic alterations, suppressed glomerular response to vasoactive substances, altered glomerular capillary ultrafiltration coefficient (K_f), and the resistance of regenerated tubular epithelium to a rechallenge with renal failure insult [5]. In this paper, we summarize our data regarding the mechanisms for acquiring resistance to ARF.

Acquired Resistance to Uranyl Acetate(UA)-Induced ARF

Studies were performed on uranium-induced ARF rabbits. In this model, major determinants of ARF seem to be a decrease in glomerular filtration rate (GFR) due to reduced K_f, back-leakage of the filtrate across damaged tubular epithelia and, probably, tubular obstruction due to casts.

[1]The First Department of Medicine, Hamamatsu University School of Medicine, 3600 Handa-cho, Hamamatsu, 431-31 Japan

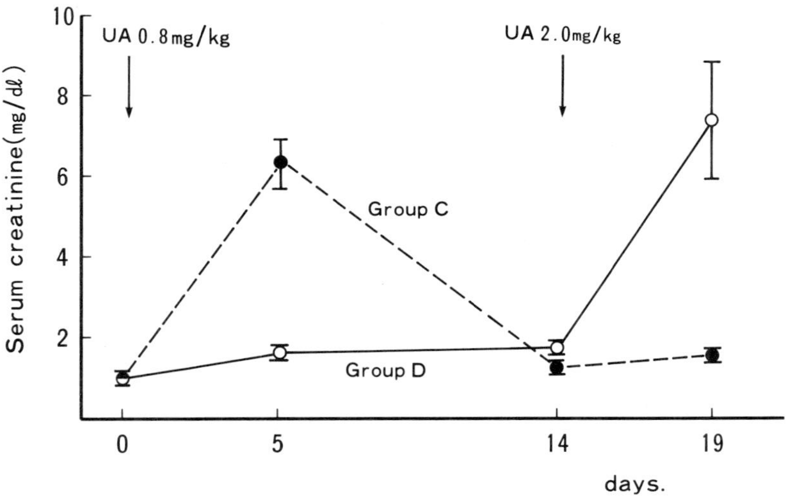

Fig. 1. Effects of a rechallenge with uranyl acetate (*UA*) on serum creatinine. *Group C*, rabbits which developed azotemia by UA (0.8 mg/kg) injection; *Group D*, rabbits which did not develop azotemia by UA (0.8 mg/kg) injection

In experiments, rabbits were classified into 4 groups: group A, normal controls; group B, in which a single dose of 2 mg/kg of UA was injected i.v.; groups C and D, in which a smaller dose of UA (0.8–0.9 mg/kg) was administered 14 days before a rechallenge with UA (2 mg/kg). In half of the rabbits examined (group C), 0.8–0.9 mg/kg of UA induced a decrease in GFR but in the remainder (group D), it did not induce a decrease. In groups B and D 2 mg/kg of UA induced a decrease in creatinine or inulin clearance and an increase in plasma creatinine, though these changes were much less in group D. In contrast, the animals recovering from ARF (group C) did not develop renal failure after the second UA injection [3] (Fig. 1). This resistance to ARF disappeared 4 weeks after the initial injection of UA [6].

Mechanisms for Resistance to a Rechallenge with UA

Vascular Factors

Renal blood flow (RBF) and intracortical blood flow distribution were estimated in all groups 5 days after the vehicle or UA (2mg/kg) injection. There was no significant difference in RBF or intracortical flow distribution between groups, except for redistribution of the regional flow toward the deep cortex in group B [3]. The data suggest that altered renal hemodynamics makes a minor contribution to resistance to ARF. Recent studies suggest that a decrease in K_f accounts for UA-induced reduction in GFR [7,8], and that this reduction in K_f is mediated by increased renin-angiotensin activity [8]. In our experiments, the plasma renin activity increased in both ARF-resistant (group C) and -less resistant (group D) rabbits following the rechallenge, as in animals subjected to a single UA injection. There was no significant difference in the plasma renin activity between groups [9].

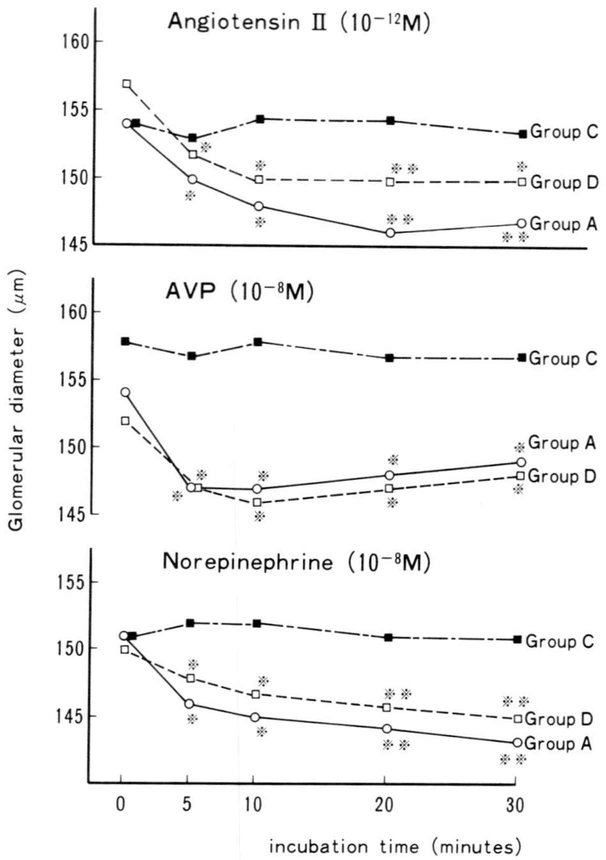

Fig. 2. Changes of glomerular diameter induced by angiotensin II, arginine vasopressin (*AVP*), and norepinephrine in rabbits. *Group A*, normal controls; *Group C*, ARF-resistant rabbits; *Group D*, ARF-less resistant rabbits

Unfortunately, K_f has not yet been estimated in ARF-resistant animals. Morphologic studies with scanning electron microscopy, including our study in UA-induced ARF, disclosed changes in the glomerular ultrastructure in various models of ARF [10,11,12,13]; this was characterized by a flattening and spreading of podocyte cell bodies associated with loss of epithelial foot processes, and reduction in the density of endothelial fenestrae, and suggested a causative role of these alterations in the diminution of K_f and thereby GFR [10,11,12]. To evaluate these glomerular changes semiquantitatively, we measured the percent fraction of the glomerular capillary surface covered only by processes narrower than 1 μm in width, percent fraction of the interpedicular space on the glomerular epithelial surface, and the density and diameter of the endothelial fenestrae in groups B, C, and D, 5 days after the UA (2 mg/kg) injection. No significant difference between groups, in changes of these parameters, was found [14].

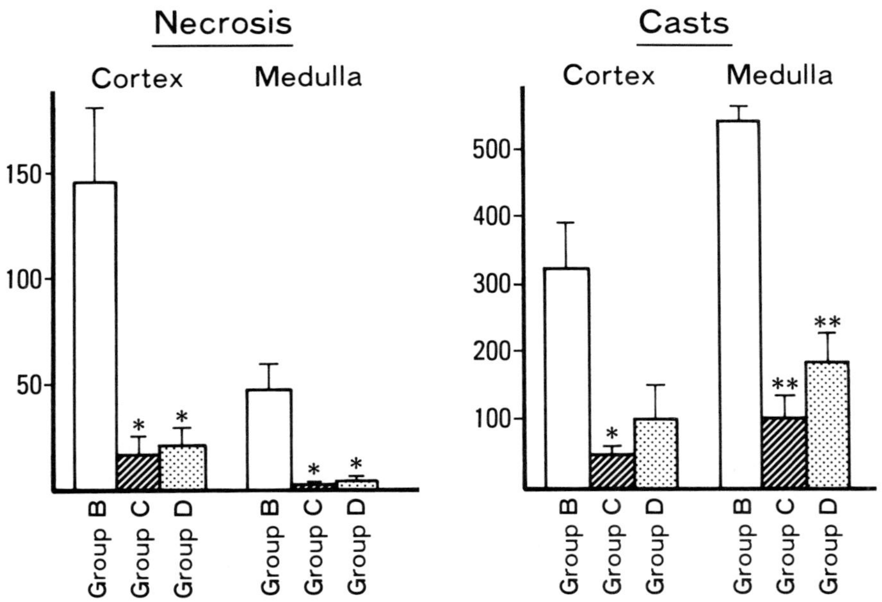

Fig. 3. The number of necrotic renal tubules (*necrosis*) and intratubular casts (*casts*) on day 5 after injection of uranyl acetate (2mg/kg). The number was counted in 50 fields at 400 magnification with a light microscope. *Group B*, UA (2mg/kg) single injection; *Groups C* and *D*, rechallenge with UA (2mg/kg) 14 days after 0.8mg/kg of UA injection; Group C developed azotemia and Group D did not. $*P<0.05$ and $**P<0.01$ compared with Group B

Wilkes et al. [15] demonstrated that the glomerular contractile response to angiotensin II(AII) was totally inhibited in rats recovering from glycerol-induced ARF; they suggested that loss of glomerular response to angiotensin contributed, at least in part, to the resistance to a subsequent renal failure challenge. We examined the glomerular response to AII, norepinephrine (NE), and arginine vasopressin (AVP) in controls (group A), ARF-resistant (group C), and ARF-less resistant (group D) rabbits, 14 days after the vehicle or the first UA injection. Angiotensin II, NE, and AVP significantly reduced the diameter of glomeruli derived from normal controls and ARF-less resistant animals. In contrast, these vasoactive substances did not provoke glomerular contraction in ARF-resistant rabbits [10] (Fig. 2). The suppressed glomerular response to the vasoactive substances was still observed 4 weeks after the initial UA injection, a time at which resistance to ARF disappeared. It is unlikely, therefore, that resistance to ARF is largely due to suppressed glomerular contractile response to vasoactive substances.

Tubular Factors

Previous studies suggested that tubular obstruction by casts [16] and back-leakage of the filtrate across damaged epithelia [7] also contributed to developing and maintaining UA-induced ARF. Following rechallenge with UA, intratubular cast formation and tubular necrosis lessened, in ARF-resistant (group C) than in ARF-less resis-

Table 1. Effects of uranyl acetate (*UA*) (0.9mg/kg) injection on kidney tissue enzyme activities

	n	SOD (U/mg)	GSH-Px (nmol/mg per min)	Catalase (U/mg)
Control	6	16.8 ± 0.6	330 ± 18	228 ± 22
UA 14 days	9	14.6 ± 0.5	351 ± 33	220 ± 26
		$P < 0.02$	NS	NS

SOD, superoxide dismutase; GSH-Px, glutathione peroxidase; NS, not significant

tant (group D) rabbits, though the difference was not statistically significant. When compared to group B subjected to a single UA injection, however, the severity of tubular damage was significantly less in groups C and D. This finding suggests that prior UA administration attenuates tubular damage caused by a rechallenge with a larger dose of the agent (Fig. 3).

A question arises as to why regenerated tubular cells are resistant to a nephrotoxic agent. There is a possibility that the resistance of regenerated tubular cells to the rechallenge is due to a smaller amount of uranium being bound to the cells. In our study, however, the kidney previously challenged by UA achieved tissue levels of uranium similar to those of the untreated kidney subjected to the second UA injection.

Some investigators have suggested that the peroxidative process contributes to heavy metal-mediated tubular damage [17,18]. An alternative possibility may be, therefore, that active oxygen scavenging enzymes might have been activated by the first UA injection, and thereby protect against the peroxidative action enhanced by the second UA injection. We measured the superoxide dismutase, glutathion-peroxidase, and catalase activities in the kidney tissue before, and 14 days after, the initial UA injection. There was no significant increase in the enzyme activities in the kidney tissues in previously UA-treated rabbits (Table 1).

Uranium and mercury have been found to inhibit Na-K-ATPase activity [19,20]. Kirschbaum and Oken [21] demonstrated that Mg-ATPase activity in the brush border membrane increases to 310% of the control value 10 days following $HgCl_2$-induced ARF. There is a possibility, therefore, that regenerated tubular cells are rich in Na-K-ATPase and resistant to the inhibition of Na-K-ATPase by uranium. In our experiment, however, no significant difference was found between normal controls and rabbits subjected to prior UA injection in Na-K-ATPase activity in tissue homogenates of whole kidney (control 30.8±6.9 vs. 14 days after UA 26.6±5.9 μmol Pi/mg prot per hr).

Acknowledgment. This work was supported by a research grant for Cardiovascular Diseases from the Ministry of Health and Welfare in Japan.

References

1. MacNider W deB (1929) The functional and pathological response of the kidney in dogs subjected to a second subcutaneous injection of uranium nitrate. J Exp Med 49:411–431
2. Elliott WC, Houghton DC, Gilbert DN, Baines-Hunter J, Bennett WM (1982) Gentamicin nephrotoxicity. II. Definition of conditions necessary to induce acquired insensitivity. J Lab Clin Med 100:513–525

3. Honda N, Sudo M (1982) Resistance to uranyl acetate-induced acute renal failure in rabbits: renal function and morphology. In: Eliahou HE (ed) Acute renal failure. John Libbey, London, pp 105–107
4. Yonemura K (1986) Acquired resistance to acute renal failure in ischemic and uranium-induced renal failure of rabbits. Nippon Jinzo Gakkai Shi 28:1221–1227
5. Honda N, Hishida A, Ikuma K, Yonemura K (1987) Acquired resistance to acute renal failure. Kidney Int 31:1233–1238
6. Ikuma K, Honda N, Yonemura K, Ohishi K, Hishida A, Nagase M (1988) Glomerular refractoriness to contractile stimuli in rabbits recovering from ischemic acute renal failure. Nephron 48:306–309
7. Blantz RC (1975) The mechanism of acute renal failure after uranyl nitrate. J Clin Invest 55:621–635
8. Blantz RC, Pelayo JC, Gushwa LC, Myers RR, Evan AP (1985) Functional basis for the glomerular alterations in uranyl nitrate acute renal failure. Kidney Int 28:733–743
9. Ikuma K, Honda N, Hishida A, Nagase M (1986) Loss of glomerular responses to vasoconstrictor agents in rabbits recovering from ARF. Kidney Int 30:836–841
10. Avasthi PS, Evan AP, Hay D (1980) Glomerular endothelial cells in uranyl nitrate-induced acute renal failure in rats. J Clin Invest 65:121–127
11. Avasthi PS, Evan AP, Huser JW, Luft FC (1981) Effect of gentamicin on glomerular ultrastructure. J Lab Clin Med 98:444–454
12. Solez K, Racusen LC, Whelton A (1981) Glomerular epithelial cell changes in early postischemic acute renal failure in rabbits and man. Am J Pathol 103:163–173
13. Kobayashi S, Nagase M, Honda N, Hishida A (1984) Glomerular alterations in uranyl acetate-induced acute renal failure in rabbits. Kidney Int 26:808–815
14. Kobayashi S, Yonemura K, Ikuma K, Hishida A, Nagase M, Honda N (1985) Glomerular alterations in acute renal failure-resistant rabbits (abstract). Nippon Jinzo Gakkai Shi 27:700
15. Wilkes BM, Caldicott WJH, Schulman G, Hollenberg NK (1981) Loss of the glomerular contractile response to angiotensin in rats following myohemoglobinuric acute renal failure. Circ Res 49:1190–1195
16. Hishida A, Yonemura K, Ohishi K, Yamada M, Honda N (1988) The effect of saline loading on uranium-induced acute renal failure in rats. Kidney Int 33:942–946
17. Gstraunthaler G, Pfaller W, Kotanko P (1983) Glutathione depletion and in vitro lipid peroxidation in mercury or maleate induced acute renal failure. Biochem Pharmacol 32:2969–2972
18. Shukla GS, Hussain T, Srivastava RS, Chandra SV (1989) Glutathione peroxidase and catalase in liver, kidney, testis and brain regions of rats following cadmium exposure and subsequent withdrawal. Ind Health 27:59–69
19. Nechay BR, Thompson JD, Saunders JP (1980) Inhibition by uranyl nitrate of adenosine triphosphatases derived from animal and human tissues. Toxicol Appl Pharmacol 53:410–419
20. Kramer HJ, Gonick HC, LU E (1986) In vitro inhibition of Na-K-ATPase by trace metals: relation to renal and cardiovascular damage. Nephron 44:329–336
21. Kirschbaum BB, Oken DE (1979) The effect of mercuric chloride on renal brush border membrane. Exp Mol Pathol 31:101–112

Cellular and Integrative Regulation of Renal Circulation

Chair: Hans R. Ulfendahl (Sweden)
Kenjiro Yamamoto (Japan)

Hormonal Control of Medullary Blood Flow

LOTHAR BERND ZIMMERHACKL[1]

SUMMARY. The medullary microcirculation is part of the countercurrent exchange system which is necessary for the regulation of salt and water homeostasis. To maintain mass balance, solute and fluid reabsorbed by tubular transport mechanisms are removed directly from the medullary tissue by the vasa recta. This role of the medullary microcirculation during the physiological changes of diuresis and water diuresis, regulated by the antidiuretic hormone, is firmly established.

Technical constraints still influence the investigation of medullary vascular regulation. New animal models – in-vitro perfusion of juxtamedullary nephrons and the split hydronephrotic rat kidney – stimulate the study of medullary blood flow regulation.

Besides its part in nephro-vascular coupling, the microvascular-tubular unit supports the tissue with energy. Oxygen delivery may be hampered by low medullary hematocrit. With regard to the high energy demand of active transport of solute in the thick ascending limb of Henle, the medullary blood flow has an important role under pathophysiological conditions of toxicity or ischemia.

The hormonal regulation of medullary blood flow differs from the regulation of cortical blood flow. Under physiological conditions, medullary blood flow is influenced by the renin-angiotensin system. Inhibition of angiotensin by converting enzyme antagonists significantly increase medullary blood flow. Infusion of angiotensin II decreases medullary blood flow. This action can be reversed by the activation of prostaglandins.

Cyclosporine reduces medullary blood flow after short term ischemia. This may reflect local activation of endothelin release.

[1]Department of Pediatrics, Albert-Ludwigs-University, Mathildenstr. 1, D-7800 Freiburg, Federal Republic of Germany

Introduction

Under physiologic conditions, the medullary microcirculation has three major tasks: (1) it plays an important role in nephro-vascular coupling; (2) it supports tissue energy supply and, (3) it participates passively in solute reabsorption from interacting tubules [1,2].

Under pathophysiologic conditions, in particular after renal ischemia, medullary congestion, with damage to the outer stripe of the medulla, is evident [3,4].

Medullary blood supply is distinct from renal cortical blood supply and may have different tasks [1,2,5]. The influence of vasoactive hormones under physiological and pathophysiological conditions may thus be important for the outcome of any renal disturbance.

New Animal Models for Studying Medullary Blood Flow

Technical constraints still hamper the investigation of medullary vascular regulation. New animal models – in-vitro perfusion of juxtamedullary nephrons [6,7] and the split hydronephrotic rat kidney [8] – stimulate the study of medullary blood flow regulation. These two new animal models may be important in the investigation of medullary blood flow in vitro and in vivo. In vitro perfusion of the excised medulla has been put forward by Casellas and co-workers [6,7]. With this animal model the influence of hormones, without the interaction of other systemically activated hormones, can be studied. With the hydronephrotic kidney model it is possible to investigate the influence of hormones on juxtamedullary glomerulus and the presumed vasa recta structures directly, without the interaction of tubular parameters. This model has no tubular structures remaining. According to Steinhausen et al. [7], sex difference may play an as yet neglected role in medullary flow regulation. In his preparation, female animals demonstrate medullary autoregulation, whereas male animals do not! This is in contrast to earlier observations in a different rat model [9]. However, both models allow the study of acute changes only. Long-term effects still cannot be studied with present techniques.

Fluid Reabsorption and Medullary Blood Flow: Effects of Furosemide and Adenosine

According to the mathematical concept of countercurrent exchange, medullary tonicity is inversely correlated to medullary blood flow [1,2,5]. During physiological changes in diuresis, total renal blood flow is unchanged. Medullary blood flow is diminished during diuresis, due to a direct vasoactive effect of vasopressin through its V_1-receptor [10]. The vasa recta are able to remove water from the medulla [5]. Under furosemide-induced diuresis (10 mg/kg/per h) vasa recta fluid flow was increased [11,12]. Red cell flux, an indicator of blood supply, was slightly elevated as well (Fig. 1; [11,12]). This situation of passive removal of fluid was already demonstrated in 1971 by Jamison and coworkers [13]. In several experimental protocols, the "passive" role of the medullary microcirculation as the route of fluid removal

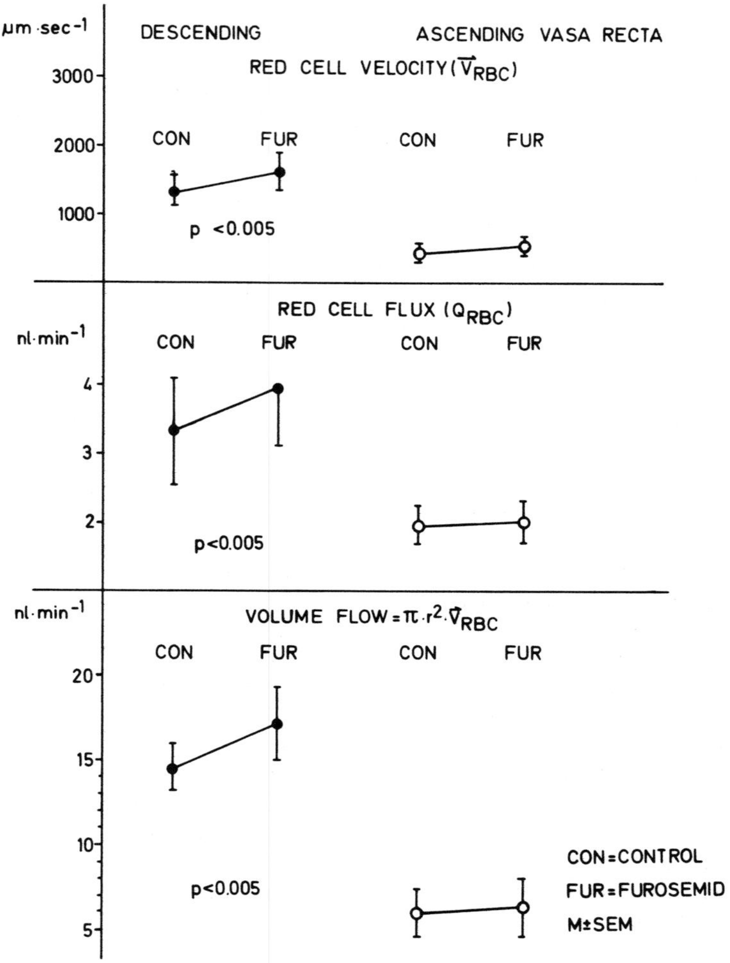

Fig. 1. Effect of furosemide on medullary erythrocyte velocity, red cell flux, and volume flow in rats, using videomicroscopy with fluorescent red cells and fluorescent plasma. After furosemide infusion significant increase occurred in volume flow, red cell velocity, and red cell flux. CON, control period; FUR, furosemide period (10 mg/kg i.v.); RBC, red blood cell

from the medulla, necessary for the maintenance of mass balance, could be confirmed [1,2].

Under experimental conditions, the "medullary washout" hypothesis was demonstrated by Thurau and collaborators in the dog [14]. Several studies in rats are in conflict with this thesis [1,2,15]. In a recent study by Miyamoto et al. [16] the influence of intrarenal adenosine on medullary blood flow was studied. Adenosine caused a dramatic natriuresis and diuresis with an infusion of as little as 2µg/min. In contrast, vasa

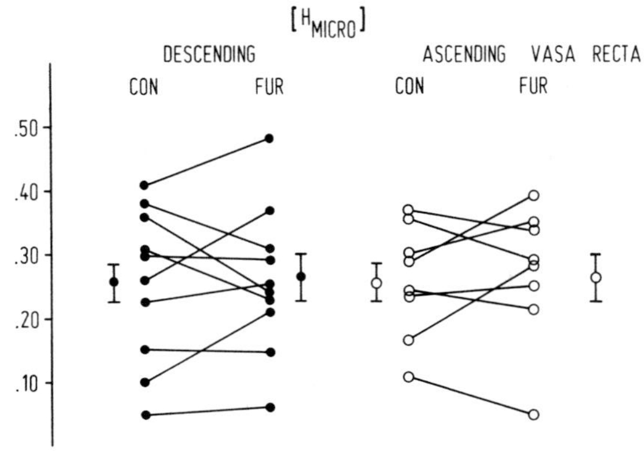

Fig. 2. Dynamic hematocrit in vasa recta in ascending and descending vessels of the rat. Hematocrit was calculated from flux of fluorescent red cells and volume flow was derived from diameter and red cell velocity (without correction for Fahräus effect). CON, control period; FUR, furosemide period

recta blood flow was increased at much higher infusion rates only. Although this study does not disprove the notion that medullary washout exists, it does not support it.

Medullary Congestion?

During pathophysiological situations, hormonal influence on medullary blood flow may be crucial in the maintenance of solute balance. Following the hypothesis of Epstein et al. [4] and Mason et al. [3], electrolyte transport of the thick ascending loop of Henle may be influenced by energy support from the vasa recta. Medullary hematocrit [1] is lower than cortical hematocrit (Fig. 2). In ischemic acute renal failure in particular, medullary congestion plays an important role. Recently Hellberg et al. [17] reported that neutrophils are involved in intravascular erythrocyte aggregation, particularly in the outer medulla. This finding supports the concept of a vulnerable region in the outer medulla, which is particularly prone to damage under conditions of high tubular transport activity and low medullary blood flow [3,4].

Influence of Angiotensin II

Under physiological conditions, medullary blood flow is influenced by the renin-angiotensin system. Exogenous infusion of angiotensin II in pharmacological concentrations reduces cortical and medullary blood flow by afferent and efferent arteriolar vasoconstriction [18]. Inhibition of angiotensin-mediated action by the angiotensin converting enzyme (ACE) antogonists captopril or enalapril significantly increases medullary blood flow without influence on water excretion [19–21]. Even under normal conditions blood flow is increased after saralasin or ACE-inhibition. Infusion of angiotensin II decreases medullary blood flow [18]. The effect of angiotensin on salt regulation is still not fully understood. In particular, understanding of the interaction between angiotensin, vasopressin, and prostaglandins [21] is incomplete. This is a situation of important clinical relevance, since the application of prostaglandin antagonists under conditions of hypovolemia (activation of angiotensin and vasopressin) can cause acute renal failure with medullary damage.[2]

Hormonal Influence After Renal Ischemia: Effects of Cyclosporin A

After short-term renal ischemia, medullary blood flow is maintained, or even enhanced. Using direct microscopic techniques, several authors were able to demonstrate early reflow with normal to increased blood flow [22,23], after 45–60 minutes of renal ischemia. However, ischemic endothelia may be prone to damage by nephrotoxic agents [24,25]. Acute infusion of Cyclosporine A (20 mg/kg i.v.) reduces cortical blood flow at the level of the arcuate arteries in the split hydronephrotic kidney model [26]. The same infusion rate in the intact kidney of the rat had no effect on medullary blood flow [27]. After ischemia, however, medullary blood flow was considerably reduced [27]. In addition, ischemia and cyclosporine can cause medullary tubular damage in humans as well [28]. Whether this is a direct action of cyclosporine or an indirect effect of local endothelin, as shown by Kon et al. [29] is under investigation.

Acknowledgment. This work was supported by the German Research Foundation.

References

1. Zimmerhackl B, Robertson CR, Jamison RL (1985) The microcirculation of the renal medulla. Circ Res 57:657–667
2. Chou S-Y, Porush JG, Faubert PF (1990) Renal medullary circulation: Hormonal control. Kidney Int 37:1–13
3. Brezis M, Seymour R, Silva P, Epstein FH (1984) Renal ischemia: a new perspective. Kidney Int 26:375–383
4. Mason J, Welsch J, Torhorst (1987) The contribution of vascular obstruction to the functional defect that follows renal ischemia. Kidney Int 31:65–71
5. Jamison RL, Kriz W (1982) Urinary concentrating mechanisms: structure and function. Oxford University Press, Oxford
6. Casellas D, Moore LC (1990) Autoregulation and tubuloglomerular feedback in juxtamedullary glomerular arterioles. Am J Physiol 258:F660–F669
7. Casellas D, Carmines PK, Navar LG (1985) Microvascular reactivity of in vitro blood perfused juxtamedullary nephrons from rats. Kidney Int 28:752–759
8. Steinhausen M, Ballantyne D, Fretschner M, Parekh N (1990) Sex differences in autoregulation of juxtamedullary glomerular blood flow in hydronephrotic rats. Am J Physiol 258:F863–F869

[2]This is, for example, the situation in preterm infants with open ductus arteriosus. These patients receive indomethacin for duct closure. Under hypovolemic and antidiuretic conditions these patients are prone to acute renal failure, which can be prevented by inducing water diuresis before the application of the prostaglandin antagonist.

9. Cohen HJ, Kayser B, Marsh DJ (1983) Autoregulation in vasa recta of the rat kidney. Am J Physiol 245:F32–F40
10. Zimmerhackl B, Jamison RL, Robertson CR (1985) Effect of arginine vasopressin on renal medullary blood flow. J Clin Invest 76:770–778
11. Zimmerhackl B, Dussel R, Steinhausen M (1986) Nieren Hochdruckkrankheiten 15:371
12. Spitalewitz S, Chou PF, Faubert PF, Porush JG (1982) Effects of diuretics on inner medullary hemodynamics in the dog. Circ Res 51:703–710
13. Jamison RL, Buerkert F, Lacy F (1971) A micropuncture study of collecting tubule function in rats with hereditary diabetes insipidus. J Clin Invest 50:2444–2452
14. Thurau K (1964) Renal hemodynamics. Am J Med 36:698–719
15. Sjöquist M, Görannson A, Hansell P, Ulfendahl HR (1985) Regulation of filtration rate and blood flow in juxtamedullary nephrons of the rat kidney. Acta Physiol Scand 123:4A
16. Miyamoto M, Yagil Y, Larson T, Robertson CR, Jamison RL (1988) Effect of intrarenal adenosine on renal function and medullary blood flow in the rat. Am J Physiol 255:F1230–F1234
17. Hellberg POA, Källskog ÖT, Öjteg G, Wolgast M (to be published) Peritubular permeability and intravascular RBC aggregation after ischemia: effects of neutrophils.
18. Zimmerhackl B, Parekh N, Kücherer H, Steinhausen M (1985) Influence of systemically applied angiotensin II on the microcirculation of glomerular capillaries in the rat. Kidney Int 27:17–24
19. Hansell P, Sjöquist M, Ulfendahl HR (1988) Effect of a converting-enzyme inhibitor on vasa recta blood flow in the rat kidney. Am J Physiol 254:F492–F499
20. Roman RJ, Kaldunski ML, Scicli AG, Carretero OA (1988) Influence of kinins and angiotensin II on the regulation of papillary blood flow. Am J Physiol 255:F690–F698
21. Cupples WA, Sakai T, Marsh DJ (1988) Angiotensin II and prostaglandins in control of vasa recta blood flow. Am J Physiol 254:F417–F424
22. Böttcher W, Steinhausen M (1976) Microcirculation of the renal papilla of rats under control conditions and after temporary ischemia. Kidney Int 10:S74–S80
23. Yagil Y, Miyamoto M, Jamison RL (1989) Inner medullary blood flow in postischemic acute renal failure in the rat. Am J Physiol 256:F456–F461
24. Brenner BM, Troy JL, Ballermann BJ (1989) Endothelium-dependent vascular responses. J Clin Invest 84:1373–1378
25. Devarakan P, Kaskel FJ, Arbeit LA, Moore LC (1989) Cyclosporine nephrotoxicity: blood volume, sodium conservation, and renal hemodynamics. Am J Physiol 256:F71–F78
26. Zimmerhackl LB, Fretschner M, Steinhausen M (1990) Cyclosporin reduces renal blood flow through vasoconstriction of arcuate arteries in the hydronephrotic rat model. Klin Wochenschr 68:166–174
27. Yagil Y (1990) Acute effect of cyclosporin on inner medullary blood flow in normal and postischemic rat kidney. Am J Physiol 258:F1139–F1144
28. Steidel K, Brandis M, Leititis JU, Kramer M, Zimmerhackl LB (1990) Cyclosporin causes hyperuricemia in renal transplants, not in children treated for nephrotic syndrome. Renal Failure 12:193–198
29. Kon V, Sugiura M, Inagami T, Harvie BR, Ichikawa I, Hoover RL (1990) Role of endothelin in cyclosporin-induced glomerular dysfunction. Kidney Int 37:1487–1491

On the Intrinsic Control of Capillary Permeability

M. Wolgast, Ö. Källskog, K. Nygren, and G. Öjteg[1]

Summary. The permeability of the renal capillary membranes is suggested to be controlled not only by external forces, but also by the prevailing Starling pressures, in the sense that a large net driving force is followed by a large hydraulic resistance, and vice versa. This means that, in spite of variations of the net driving force, the fluid transfer may remain fairly constant—in other words an *autoregulation* of the membrane permeability is suggested. The need for such a mechanism would seem obvious, i.e., since otherwise even small changes in glomerular filtration and/or peritubular capillary uptake might lead to drastic changes in the urinary output. The hypothesis has its basis in a new model, in which it is supposed that a *flexible* gel/fiber-matrix, rather than a rigid porous membrane, constitutes the membrane. The size, shape, and permeability characteristics of such a membrane will be the result of the balance between, on the one hand, the above mentioned physical forces and, on the other, the mechanics of the gel/fiber structure. Here, the tension of the fibers acts to restrict expansion, whereas membrane-fixed negative charges, via the resulting electroosmotic pressure and balancing hydrostatic pressure, act to resist compression. Regarding the intra-membranous net driving force, the hydrostatic pressure gradient valid in the Starling model will be replaced by an electroosmotic net driving force, i.e., where the magnitude and direction of the force is governed by the electric field. A gel/fiber-matrix membrane can furthermore be predicted to possess a self-rinsing ability, a feature typical of, e.g., the glomerular capillary membrane. Regarding external control of the membrane permeability, all factors which affect the isoelectric point of the structure carrying the charges can be predicted to govern the membrane characteristics.

[1]Department of Physiology and Medical Biophysics, University of Uppsala, S-75123 Uppsala, Sweden.

Introduction

The present paper aims to analyze whether the permeability of renal capillary membranes is governed not only by "external factors" (humoral factors, the action of contractile elements etc.), but also by physical factors such as the transmembranous Starling forces. More specifically, it is suggested that a high net driving force will induce a high hydraulic resistance, whereas a low net driving force will be concomitant with a reduced resistance such that the fluid transfer may remain largely unaltered – in other words, an autoregulation of the hydraulic permeability of the membrane is suggested.

The need for such a mechanism would seem obvious. Thus, if the permeability of the two renal capillary membranes would remain constant, even a minute increase in, e.g., the hydrostatic pressure would lead to a very large difference between fluid filtration and reabsorption and hence to a large urinary output.

The basis for the above hypothesis is a new model, in which it is suggested that flexible gel/fiber matrix, rather than a rigid porous membrane, constitutes the capillary membrane. From an anatomical point of view, this suggestion would not seem particularly provocative. Morphologists [1–6] have since long denied the existence of a rigid membrane penetrated by discrete cylindrical pores, but have claimed that capillary membranes are composed of highly specialized structural elements with a network of collagenous fibrils and, immobilized in this network, medium-sized polysaccharides known as glycosaminoglycans.

From a biophysical point of view, however, the assumption of a gel/fiber-matrix membrane does not merely imply a change of wording, but indeed a change of concept. The key point refers to the fact that, in the absence of rigid elements, other means of preserving membrane integrity have to be considered. Furthermore, since at least "dilute" gels do not allow for the development of hydrostatic pressure gradients, "new" forces accounting for the fluid transfer have to be considered. The ability of charged gel/fiber-matrix membranes to rinse themselves from entrapped proteins, a feature typical of biological membranes, will also be examined.

Model

Figure 1 depicts a capillary membrane with a network for fibers attached to each other by interconnecting filaments. If this membrane is exposed to a hydraulic pressure gradient, the pressure on the right hand side of each fiber will be higher than that on the left hand side. The fibers will then move in the left hand direction until eventually they will be packed one next to the other, with the formation of a very dense and tight capillary membrane. It is also evident that, on the plasma side, the plasma proteins will drag water out of the fiber-matrix, which again results in the formation of densely packed fibers.

In Fig. 2, this complete collapse of the membrane has been prevented by replacing the interconnecting fibers with strings able to resist both expansion and compression. Still, however, the fiber density will be dependent on the hydraulic pressure gradient, such that a low net driving force is followed by a low hydraulic resistance,

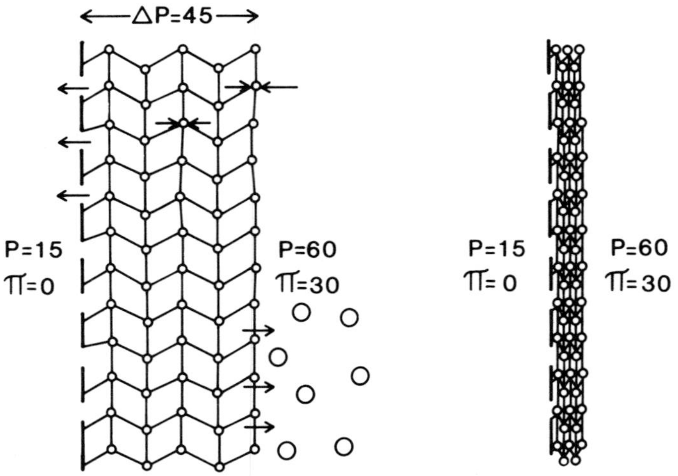

Fig. 1. Fiber-matrix of the glomerular capillary membrane. Since the pressure on the right hand side of the individual fibers is higher than that on the left hand side, the fibers will move in the right hand direction until they become packed, one next to the other, with the formation of a very dense tight matrix. At the plasma side of the membrane, the plasma proteins will drag water out of the membrane, which again results in a dense packing of the matrix fibers

whereas a high net driving force is followed by a high hydraulic resistance. As a result, fluid transfer may remain largely unaltered.

In order to test the expected dependency between net driving force and hydraulic resistance, the data on 1) the glomerular and 2) the peritubular capillary membranes, obtained in our previous investigation [7], were applied. The experimental condi-

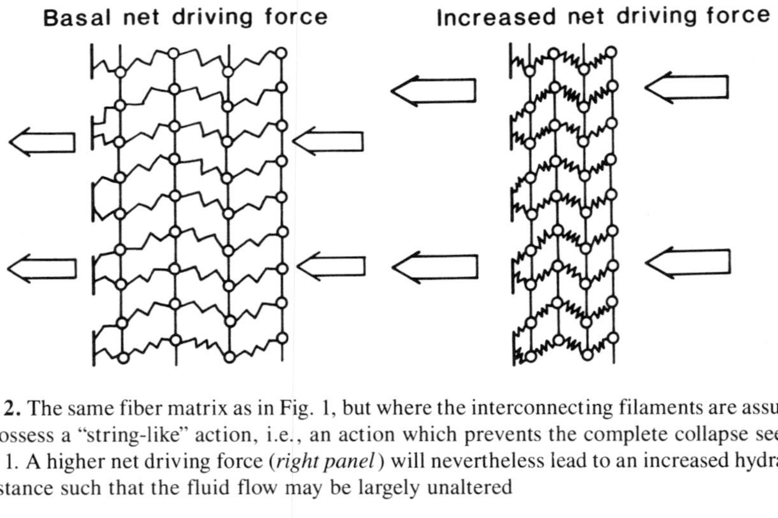

Fig. 2. The same fiber matrix as in Fig. 1, but where the interconnecting filaments are assumed to possess a "string-like" action, i.e., an action which prevents the complete collapse seen in Fig. 1. A higher net driving force (*right panel*) will nevertheless lead to an increased hydraulic resistance such that the fluid flow may be largely unaltered

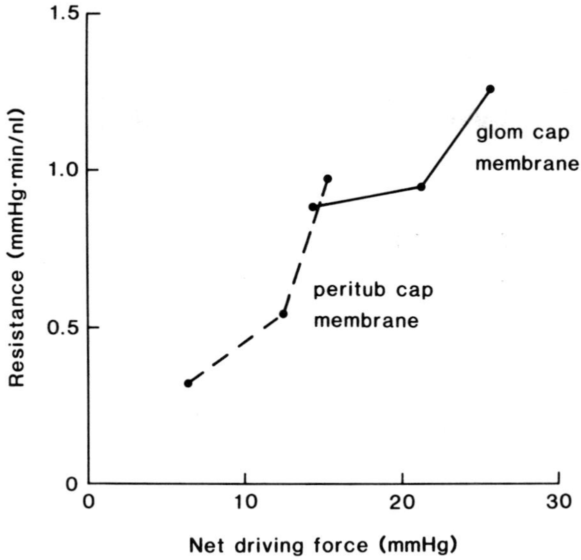

Fig. 3. Relation between the net driving force and hydraulic resistance in the glomerular and peritubular capillary membranes

tions were: a) control antidiuresis, b) 4% saline expansion, and c) 10% saline expansion. As shown from the two points in the middle of Fig. 3, the control net driving force and also the hydraulic resistance of the glomerular and peritubular capillary membrane would seem to be about the same. After saline expansion, however, the net driving force across the glomerular capillary membrane will increase, whereas in the peritubular capillaries, the same dilution leads to a reduction of the driving force. In both cases, however, a rise in the net driving force will be accompanied by an increased hydraulic resistance. The biological data thus supports the expected dependency between net driving force and hydraulic resistance.

Nature of the Elastic Forces

As regards the mechanical characteristics of a fiber matrix, it is easy to imagine that the collagenous fibers act to resist expansion of the gel/fiber-matrix. In contrast, however, they are probably less effective in restricting compression, i.e., unless the matrix is very dense.

A chemical osmotic force would also seem less likely, simply because the *molar concentration* of the structural elements is very small.

A third possibility arises from charged groups fixed to the matrix filaments [7–11]. Altough such charges, in themselves, do not induce an osmotic force, they will attract mobile ions of opposite charge, and it is these ions that induce the osmotic force. The consequent fluid entry and rise in the intramembranous hydrostatic pressure now enables the membrane to resist compression. Indeed, the charges will have a true

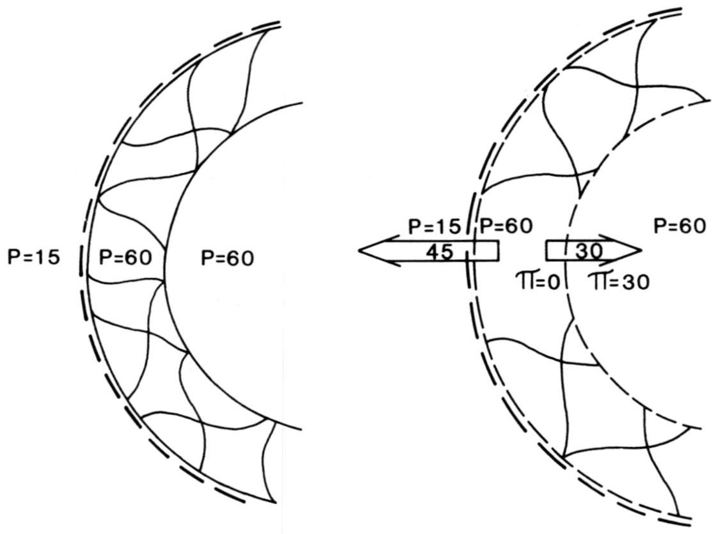

Fig. 4a,b. Structure of the glomerular capillary membrane consisting of a "loose" gel/fiber-matrix enclosed into two sheets; in **a** the two sheets are assumed to be watertight, in **b** they are permeable. In both cases the basement membrane offers mechanical support. Note that, since a gel (like water) is able to transmit pressures, the intra-membranous hydrostatic pressure must equal the glomerular capillary hydrostatic pressure of 60 mm Hg

"string-like" action in the sense that compression leads to a rise in the fixed charge density and hence to an increased electro-osmotic pressure, and vice versa.

It should be pointed out that the electro-osmotic pressure is independent of the sign of the charges. However, in most biological structures negatively charged groups seem to predominante.

Where the concentration of membrane-fixed charges is concerned, there are two alternatives, which both allow for the preservation of membrane integrity. In the first and simplest case, the charge density is so high that the resulting electoosmotic pressure and the balancing intramembranous hydrostatic pressure outrange the pressures in the free fluid phases surrounding the membrane. Since such an "overstretched" membrane thereby will be unaffected by the Starling forces in its surroundings, it will in fact behave as a rigid porous membrane.

In the second, and more probable, alternative the hydrostatic and osmotic pressures of the membrane are in balance with those in its surrounding free fluid phases. In the evaluation of this alternative, we may first assume (Fig. 4a) that the gel/fiber-matrix is enclosed between two flexible and *watertight* sheets, the sheet to the left faces the interstitium (or Bowman's space) and that to the right faces the capillary plasma. In order to prevent rupture of the structure, the membrane is supported by a relatively rigid (though still tensile) basement membrane (the heavy interrupted line in Fig. 4).

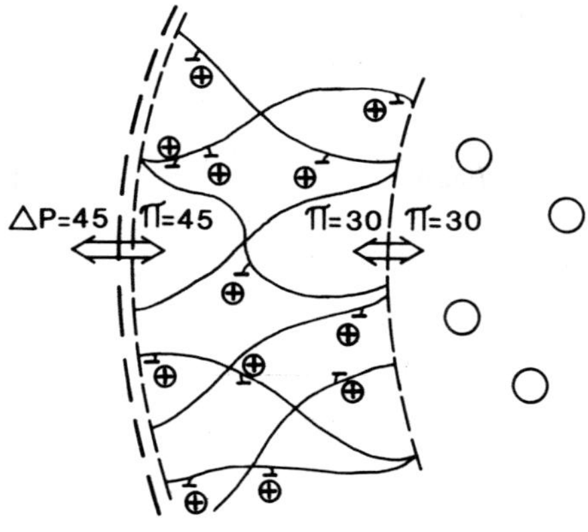

P (mmHg)	15	60	60	60
Π (mmHg)	0	45	30	30
X (mEq/l)	0	30.6	37.4	0
E (mV)	0	−3.33	−2.77	0
Na (mEq/l)	150	169.9	166.1	150
Cl (mEq/l)	150	132.4	135.5	150
Na+Cl (mEq/l)	300	302.4	301.6	300
Myo^{0} (mM)	0.67	0.67	1.07	1.07
Myo^{-6} (mM)	0.55	0.260	0.60	1.10

Fig. 5. Gel/fiber-matrix of the glomerular capillary membrane, where the electroosmotic force offered by positive mobile ions attracted to negative membrane-fixed charges enables fluid equilibria at the two interphases of the membrane

Since the membrane gel, like water, transmits hydrostatic pressures, exposure to a capillary hydrostatic pressure of 60 mm Hg (i.e., as in the glomerular capillaries) results in an intramembranous hydrostatic pressure of the same 60 mm Hg. However, since the two sheets enclosing the gel/fiber-matrix are watertight there will be no exchange of fluid. The integrity of the capillary membrane will thus be maintained.

Water-tightness is, however, not an obligatory prerequisite. We may also assume a fluid equilibrium across the two interphases. In this case, we have to balance a pressure difference of 45 mm Hg on the Bowman's space (interstitial) side and, on the plasma side, the glomerular plasma colloid osmotic pressure of 30 mm Hg (Fig. 4b).

This is accomplished (Fig. 5, upper panel) by introducing membrane-fixed negative charges such that the electroosmotic pressure becomes 45 mm Hg and 30 mm Hg, at the two sides of the membrane, respectively.

In order to calculate the fixed charge density producing the desired electroosmotic pressure, the distribution of the small mobile ions has first to be considered. Here,

Donnan equilibrium predicts that the concentrations of the mobile positive and negative ions (here denoted as Na and Cl) in the inside (index i) and outside (index o) solution are related to the electric potential, E, as:

$$E = z_{Na} \cdot F/RT \cdot \ln(Na_i/Na_o) = z_{Cl} \cdot F/RT \cdot \ln(Cl_i/Cl_o) \quad (1a)$$

where z_{Na} and z_{Cl} are the valences of Na and Cl, F is Faradays constant, R the gas constant, and T the absolute temperature.

The equality between the two expressions on the right hand side means that:

$$Na_i/Na_o = (Cl_i/Cl_o)^{-1} = Cl_o/Cl_i \quad (1b)$$

Utilizing the fact that in a negatively charged membrane with a charge density of X mEq/l, the intra-membranous concentration of chloride, $Cl_i = (Na_i - X)$, we obtain:

$$Na_i/Na_o = Cl_o/(Na_i - X) \quad (2)$$

Since Na_o and Cl_o in the outside solution are known, the intra-membranous concentrations of the ions can be obtained:

$$Na_i = X/2 + [(X/2)^2 + Na_o \cdot Cl_o]^{1/2} \quad (3a)$$

$$Cl_i = -X/2 + [(X/2)^2 + Na_o \cdot Cl_o]^{1/2} \quad (3b)$$

The sum of Na and Cl within the membrane is, accordingly:

$$Na_i + Cl_i = 2 \cdot [(X/2)^2 + Na_o \cdot Cl_o]^{1/2} \quad (4)$$

The osmotic force, II, generated by the intramembranous *excess* of Na and Cl, can now be obtained by van't Hoff's law, $\pi = RT \cdot \Delta C$, as:

$$\begin{aligned} \pi &= RT \cdot [(Na_i + Cl_i - (Na_o + Cl_o)] \\ &= RT \cdot \{2\,[(X/2)^2 + Na_o \cdot Cl_o]^{1/2} - (Na_o + Cl_o)\} \end{aligned} \quad (5)$$

Evidently, the electroosmotic force is dependent on both the fixed charge density, X, and the ionic strength (Na_o and Cl_o). If Na_o and Cl_o approach zero, the electroosmotic force will approach RT·X, i.e., it is directly proportional to the fixed charge density. For higher ionic strengths the electroosmotic presssure shows a progressive decrease; the figures at physiological ionic strength, where $Na_o = Cl_o = 150$ mEq/l, are shown in Fig. 6.

Utilizing this figure, we may obtain the fixed charge densities, X, for the sought electroosmotic pressures of 45 mm Hg and 30 mm Hg, respectively, valid for the glomerular capillary membrane discussed in Fig. 4. These figures, the electric potentials, the distributions of Na and Cl and sums, (Na+Cl), are given in the lower panel of Fig. 5. As expected from a negatively charged membrane, the intramembranous concentration of Na is higher than that of Cl.

Validification of the Hypothesis

As shown in Fig. 5, a low concentration of negative ions not only applies to Cl, but also to a negatively charged polyion such as Myoglobin:

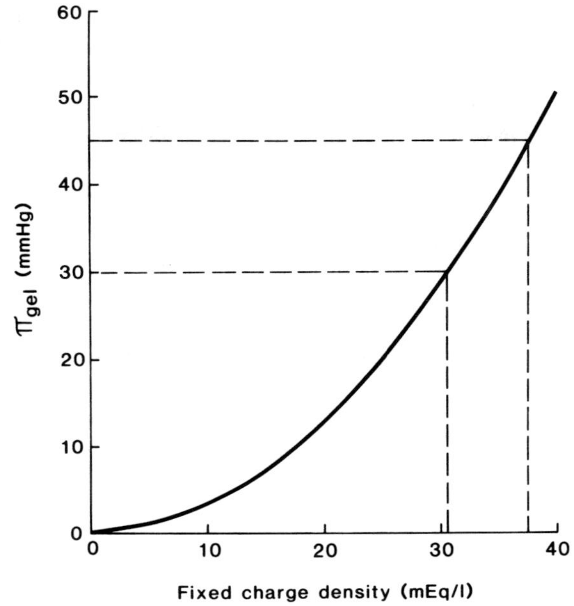

Fig. 6. Relation between fixed charge density and electroosmotic pressure at a physiological ionic strength

$$E = z_{Cl}\ F/RT \cdot \ln(Cl_i/Cl_o) = z_{Myo}\ F/RT \cdot \ln(Myo_i/Myo_o) \tag{6}$$

The transport, M, of myoglobin across the membrane is governed by Nernst's equation:

$$M = -A_P D'\ dC(x)/dx + V\ (1-\sigma)\ C(x) - A_P D'\ C(x) \cdot dE(x)/dx \tag{7}$$

where A_P is the pore area, D′ the coefficient for restricted diffusion, V the hydraulic fluid flow (in the glomerulus the glomerular filtration rate), σ the reflection coefficient and dE(x)/dx the electric field.

Assuming a constant electric field, i.e., $dE(x)/dx = \Delta E/\Delta x$, integration between $x=0$ (plasma side) and $x=\Delta x$ (Bowman's space side) gives:

$$M = [V\ (1-\sigma) - D'Ap/\Delta x\ (\Delta EzF/RT)]\cdot[C(\Delta x) - C(0)\ \exp K]/[1-\exp K],$$

where $K = [V\ (1-\sigma) - D'Ap/\Delta x\ (\Delta EzF/RT)]/[D'Ap/\Delta x]$

Details of analyses of pertinent parameters have been given elsewhere [11]. In brief, the terms $A_P/\Delta x$, D′ and σ are obtained (Table 1) from the transport of a series of neutral probes: inulin, myoglobin, horse radish peroxidase (HRP), and lactate dehydrogenase (LDH). Knowing the electric potential difference, ΔE (Fig. 5, lower panel), the transport, and hence also the interstitial (Bowman's space) concentration, of their negatively charged counterparts could be predicted. The latter figures, for both the glomerular and peritubular capillary membranes are shown in Table 1. As is evident from this table, the experimental data support the hypothesis.

Table 1. Experimental and predicted concentration of a series of neutral and charged molecular probes in Bowman's space (*upper panel*) and renal interstitium (*lower panel*). The concentration in systemic plasma is put at 1.0

Probe (plasma concentration)	Size	Valency	Experimental concentration	Predicted concentration
Bowman's space				
Inulin (1.01)	11 Å	0	0.94	0.94
Myoglobin (1.07)	17.5 Å	0	0.67	0.67
HRP (1.20)	32 Å	0	0.07	0.06
Myoglobin (1.10)	17.5 Å	−6	0.51	0.55
Myoglobin (1.05)	17.5 Å	+2	0.74	0.70
HRP (1.20)	32 Å	−14	0.01	0.01
Renal interstitial field				
HRP (1.13)	32 Å	0	0.32	0.32
LDH (1.13)	46 Å	0	0.12	0.12
HRP (1.13)	32 Å	−14	0.28	0.29
LDH (1.13)	46 Å	−19	0.08	0.07
LDH (1.13)	46 Å	+2	0.13	0.13
Myoglobin (1.13)	17.5 Å	−6	0.66	0.66

HRP, horseradish peroxidase; LDH, lactate dehydrogenase

Net Driving Force for Fluid Transfer

On inspecting the numbers in the lower panel of Fig. 5 one can see that gel osmotic pressures of 45 mm Hg and 30 mm Hg at the two sides of the membrane, respectively, are shown. The resulting net driving force will then be 15 mm Hg, i.e., the same as that calculated conventionally from the Starling forces in glomerular plasma and Bowman's space.

This force derives from the difference in osmolality on the two sides of the membrane; on the Bowman's space side (Na+Cl) = 302.4 mOsm/kg and at the plasma side (Na + Cl) = 301.6 mOsm/kg, i.e., a difference of 0.8 mOsm/kg. Utilizing van't Hoff's relation, $\pi = RT\Delta C$, the osmotic pressure difference would be the same − 15 mm Hg.

Such a calculation assumes, however, that the membrane is impermeable to the particles in question. Considering the small size of Na and Cl, this assumption most certainly is not valid. Instead, the required "impermeability" results from the electric potential difference (0.56 mV), which prevents a *net transport* of both Na and Cl. To be more precise, the momentum and hence the presssure generated by Na and Cl in the two directions will be the same. The only source of a difference in momentum or pressure is then that resulting from the difference in the water activity, i.e., from the difference of 0.8 mOsm/kg. Since this force is dependent on electric field, it should be denoted an electroosmotic force.

A second, and perhaps more adequate, mode of expressing the electroosmotic force π_{El}, is as:

$$\pi_{El} = -[Na(x) - Cl(x)] \cdot F \cdot dE(x)/dx = -X(x) \cdot F \cdot dE(x)/dx \qquad (8)$$

The advantage of this formulation is inherent in the fact that it more clearly demonstrates that the osmotic force is dependent on the magnitude and direction of the electric field. As regards the pressure in the direction perpendicular to the electric field, it remains the same (60 mm Hg, see Fig. 5) in all parts of the membrane. The membrane is thereby able to withstand the same pressure – 60 mm Hg – in glomerular capillary plasma.

So far, the analysis is based on the assumption of an equilibrium,i.e., no net transport of fluid, including its ions. This would, however, lead to the false conclusion that, since the intramembranous concentration of Na is higher than that of Cl, the bulk flow transport, $\dot{M} = \dot{V}\,(1-\sigma)\,C(x)$, for Na would exceed that of Cl, i.e., the prerequisite of electroneutrality would not be fulfilled. For this reason we have to adjust the electric potential difference, such that the transport of negative and positive ions becomes the same. However, since the adjustment needed is only of the order of 1%, this consideration does not alter the figures for the ion distribution outlined in Fig. 5.

Pore Structure of the Gel/Fiber Matrix

Figure 7a aims to illustrate the structure in a fenestra of the glomerular capillary membrane. It is assumed that the fibers (probably synthesized by the endothelial cells) carry specific binding sites able to form the regular network depicted in the figure. In order to prevent collapse of the meshes in the network, the fibers are also assumed to carry negatively charged groups, which, via the attraction of positive mobile ions, cause an inward transport of fluid and expansion of the meshes. This process will proceed until the "dilution" of the charges has resulted in an electroosmotic pressure equal to the colloid osmotic pressure of glomerular plasma (30 mm Hg).

At a given plasma colloid osmotic pressure, the size of the meshes is thus governed by the number of charges on each fiber. Many charges would thus lead to large meshes, and vice versa, i.e., providing that the fibers are tensile. Obviously, the density of the fiber network in the plasma-Bowman's space direction may also contribute to the resultant fixed charge density.

At the Bowman's space side of the membrane the electroosmotic pressure has to be somewhat higher (45 mm Hg). This might be accomplished either by 1) a larger number of charges on each fiber, or 2) by a slight narrowing of the meshes, or 3) by a compression of the matrix at this side of the membrane.

Rinsing of Entrapped Proteins from the Membrane

In Fig. 7b, a protein molecule has been trapped into one of the meshes of the membrane (the single mesh depicted above the fenestra). The space available for the positive mobile ions needed to neutralize the fixed negative charges is thereby reduced. Consequently, the *concentration* of the mobile ions, and hence the osmotic force, will increase. Fluid will then enter into the space between the protein molecule and the fibers, widen the mesh, which thence will allow the entrapped protein to move in the downstream direction until it will be expelled into the Bowman's space. A charged gel/fiber-matrix can thus be predicted to possess a self rinsing ability, an essential feature of membranes such as, e.g., the glomerular capillary membrane.

a

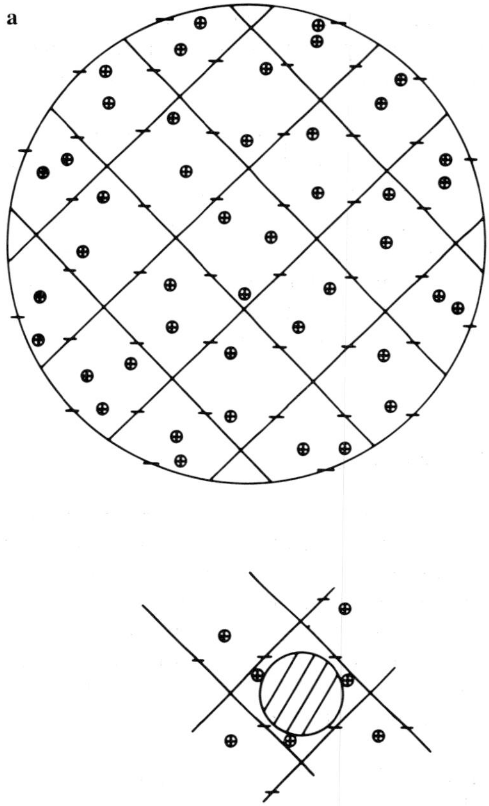

Fig. 7. a Capillary fenestra, where positive mobile ions attracted to membrane-fixed negative charges have induced an inward fluid flow and hence expansion of the meshes to the form depicted in the figure. **b** In this figure a relatively large protein molecule has been trapped into one of the meshes in the gel/fiber-matrix (the single mesh depicted above the fenestra). Since the space available for the positive mobile ions (needed to neutralize the membrane-fixed negative charges) is thereby reduced, the local concentration (not the number) of the mobile positive ions will be increased. The consequent fluid entry will then widen the mesh such that the protein molecule is free to move in the downstream direction

b

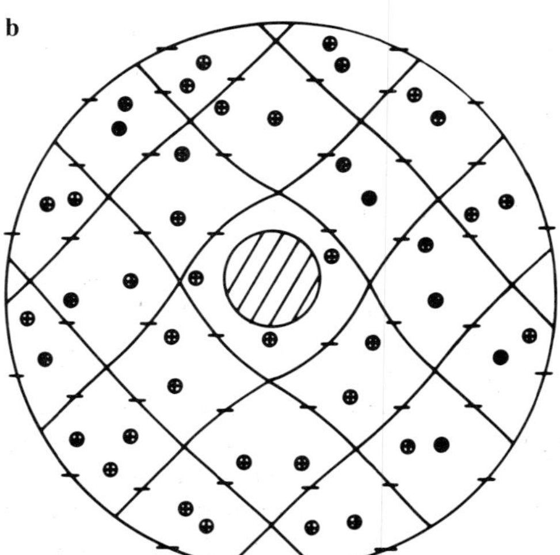

Discussion

The prediced dependency of the hydraulic resistance on the driving forces for fluid transfer will in fact constitute an "edema preventing mechanism." It will thereby add to the more classical mechanism, in which capillary fluid loss is prevented by a compensatory increase in the hydrostatic, and decrease in the colloid osmotic, pressure of the interstitial fluid.

In the kidney, the constancy of the glomerular filtration rate would be a result not only of autoregulation of the renal blood flow, but also of the mechanism discussed here. Where the peritubular capillaries are concerned, the above mentioned mechanism would seem even more essential. Thus, considering that, in man, the transcapillary fluid flow is about 150 l/day, a depression of the hydrostatic pressure in the two capillary beds of as little as 1.5 mm Hg (in both the capillary beds equal to 10% of the normal net driving force) would thus result in a urinary loss as excessive as 30 l/day!! Evidently, the delicate task of controlling extracellular volume cannot be attributed to such "unreliable" forces as the capillary Starling forces. If, on the other hand, the permeability of the peritubular capillary membrane adjusts itself such that, in all instances, the capillaries reabsorb all of the tubular reabsorbate, renal fluid handling will be regulated by the tubular epithelial cells, seemingly a more suitable target for systems aimed to control extracellular volume.

It should be noted, however, that although this reasoning speaks against a strict coupling between the capillary Starling forces and tubular reabsorption, it does not rule out the possibility of some sort of "peritubular control" of, e.g., proximal tubular fluid reabsorption. A further conclusion is that factors altering the fixed charge density might be powerful regulators of capillary permeability. A decline in the isoelectric point of the fibers carrying the charges, for instance, would thus increase the fixed charge density and hence increase capillary permeability.

References

1. Kritz W, Kaissling B (1985) Structural organization of the mammalian kidney. In: Seldin DW, Giebisch G (eds) The kidney: physiology and pathophysiology. Raven, New York, pp 265–306
2. Maul GG (1971) Structure and formation of pores in fenestrated capillaries. J Ultrastruct Res 36:768–782
3. Maunsbach AB, Olsen TS, Christensen EI (1980) Functional ultrastructure of the kidney. Academic, New York
4. Milici AJ, Lérnhault N, Palade GE (1985) Surface density of diaphragmed fenestrae and transendothelial channels in different murine capillary beds. Circ Res 56:709–717
5. Simioneski M, Simionescu N (1984) Ultrastructure of the microvascular wall: functional correlations. In: The Cardiovascular System. Microcirculation. American Physiology Society, Bethesda, pp 41–101 (Handbook of Physiology, sect 2, vol 4)
6. Levick JR, Smaje LH (1987) An analysis of the permeability of a fenestra. Microvasc Res 33:233–256
7. Larsson M, Nygren K, Sjöquist M, Wolgast M (1983) Functional characteristics of the peritubular capillary membrane in the rat kidney. Acta Physiol Scand 117:251–261
8. Deen WM, Satvat B, Jamieson JM (1980) Theoretical model for glomerular filtration of charged solutes. Am J Physiol 238:F126–F139

9. Deen WM, Bridges CR (1982) Molecular charge of horse radish peroxidase. Am J Physiol 242:F750–F762
10. Ötjeg G, Nygren K, Wolgast M (1987) Permeability of renal capillaries. II. Transport of neutral and charged protein molecular probes. Acta Physiol Scand 129:287–294
11. Öjteg G, Wolgast M (1988) Permeability of renal capillaries. III. Theoretical analysis of hydraulic conductivity, pore structure and electric properties. Acta Physiol Scand 133:459–468
12. Wolgast M, Öjteg G (1988) Electrophysiology of renal capillary membranes: gel concept applied and the Starling model challenged. Am J Physiol 254:F364–F373

Regulation of Renal Vascular Resistance: Studies Using Pharmacological Probes

Yasuharu Aki, Toshiaki Tamaki, Hideyasu Kiyomoto, Hiroshi Iwao, and Youichi Abe[1]

Introduction

The kidney has two resistance vessels, the afferent and the efferent arterioles, located in the pre- and post-glomerulus. Different reactions of each arteriole to endogenous and exogenous vasoactive agents regulate renal blood flow (RBF) and glomerular filtration rate (GFR). Functional and anatomical heterogeneity among nephrons has also been well recognized. Therefore, it might be expected that differences exist among nephrons in the relative tonus of afferent and efferent arterioles. However, there is no literature concerning these differences.

To understand the regulatory mechanisms of renal hemodynamics, we must have good pharmacological tools which act selectively either on the afferent arteriole or the efferent arteriole. For this purpose we have examined the effects of various renal vasodilators on renal hemodynamics and determined the intrarenal vascular action sites of these agents. Then, using these pharmacological tools, we clarified the vasodilatory characteristics of the afferent and efferent arterioles. In addition, the differences in the relative tonus of the afferent and efferent arterioles between the superficial and juxtamedullary nephron were also determined.

In the present study, we used glucagon, adenosine, dipyridamole, ATP, acetylcholine, forskolin and dibutyryl cyclic AMP as pharmacological tools. Adenosine has been noted to be one of the endogenous regulators of renal hemodynamics [1–3]. Osswald and colleagues [1] reported that adenosine is a mediator in the tubuloglomerular feedback mechanism. According to their hypothesis, increased GFR enhances sodium reabsorption and elevates renal oxygen consumption and energy utilization, thereby increasing ATP hydrolysis and adenosine production. Increased adenosine levels in renal tissue would then preferentially constrict the afferent arterioles, helping to return the GFR toward the control level. However, it has

[1]Department of Pharmacology, Kagawa Medical School, 1750-1 Ikenobe, Miki-cho, Kita-gun, Kagawa, 761-07 Japan

been reported that adenosine has both renal vasoconstrictive action, via the inhibition of adenylate cyclase and renal vasodilatory action, via the activation of adenylate cyclase [4,5]. In addition, the renal vasoconstrictive action of adenosine was found to be transient when it was infused into the renal artery [6,7]. Therefore, in this study we have focused on the renal vasodilatory action and have examined whether the vasodilation induced by adenosine might be induced via the activation of adenylate cyclase.

The vascular action sites of these agents were determined by an analysis of the renal arterial pressure (RAP)–RBF relationship. RBF remains relatively constant over a wide range of RAPs through adjustments in the resistance of the preglomular afferent arteriole [8–12]. Also, it is generally accepted that the resistance of the preglomerular vessels attains a minimum value at the RAP near the lower limit of the autoregulatory pressure range [11]. If a vasodilator such as adenosine impairs autoregulatory efficiency within an autoregulatory pressure range and has no potency to increase RBF at the lower limit of the autoregulatory pressure range, it should mainly dilate the afferent arterioles. In contrast, if a vasodilator maintains autoregulatory efficiency despite a higher RBF level, it should mainly dilate the efferent arterioles. Based on the above idea, RAP–RBF relationships were obtained during the infusion of adenosine, ATP and glucagon.

The vasodilatory capabilities of the superficial and the juxtamedullary nephrons were determined by flow measurements in the superficial and deep cortex zone, using the radioactive microsphere method. Based on the differences in the zonal flow responses to various agents, the relative tonus of the afferent and the efferent arterioles in each nephron was estimated.

Methods

Preparations

Experiments were performed on mongrel dogs of both sexes, weighing 12–19 kg, which were maintained on a standard sodium diet. Animals were anesthetized with sodium pentobarbital (30 mg/kg, i.v.), which was followed by a maintenance dose if necessary. A tracheotomy was performed, and the right brachial artery and vein were catheterized for the measurement of systemic blood pressure, sampling of arterial blood, and the infusion of saline and inulin. Another catheter was inserted into the left ventricle via the right carotid artery in order to inject the microspheres. The left kidney was exposed through a retroperitoneal flank incision. The kidney was denervated by a division of all visible periarterial nerve fibers and a sharp dissection of the tissue connected to the renal hilum cephalad to the renal artery. RAP was measured via a catheter inserted into the right femoral artery and advanced into the abdominal aorta just below the bifurcation of the left renal artery. An adjustable aortic clamp was placed on the aorta between the bifurcation of the right and left renal arteries. RAP was varied by means of that clamp. RBF was measured by an electromagnetic flowmeter (MPV-1200, Nihonkohden, Japan). RBF and RAP were continuously monitored and recorded on a polygraph (model No. 361, NEC San-ei, Japan). A curved 23-gauge needle was inserted into the left renal artery for the infusion of saline and drug solutions. The needle was maintained patent by a continuous infusion of saline at a rate of 0.19 ml/min. After the completion of surgery, an intravenous infusion of saline was initiated at the rate of 2 ml/min. For the measurement of GFR, a priming dose of inulin (100 mg/kg) was given intravenously, followed by a continuous infusion of inulin at a rate of 100 mg/kg per hr to maintain a constant plasma level. GFR was obtained by the renal clearance of inulin; inulin was determined by the method of Walser et al [13].

Protocols

The experiments were divided into the following groups: A; Effects of adenosine (20 μg/kg per min, n=12), ATP (40 μg/kg per min, n=5), glucagon (0.5 μg/kg per min, n=10), and acetylcholine (ACh, 4 μg/kg per min, n=8) on RAP–RBF relationships, B; Effects of glucagon, adenosine, and ACh on the intrarenal distribution of blood flow, C; Effects of dipyridamole (10 μg/kg per min) on RBF and GFR with and without a low dose of adenosine (1 μg/kg per min, n=5), D; Effects of forskolin (0.2 μg/kg per min, n=6), dibutyryl cyclic AMP (0.3 mg/kg per min, n=7) and a calcium channel blocker (nitrendipine, 0.5 μg/kg per min, n=7), and forskolin (0.2 μg/kg per min, n=7) on RBF and GFR. In group A, the RAP–RBF relationships were obtained during the infusion of each agent and also for control. RAP was sequentially altered in the 5 steps indicated in Fig. 1, i.e., normal pressure, 100, 75, 60 and 45 mmHg. Each pressure level was maintained for several minutes to allow for a complete autoregulatory response.

Analytical Procedures

The distribution of cortical blood flow was determined using the radioactive microsphere technique [14–16]. A suspension of microspheres labeled with different gamma emitters (85-Sr or 141-Ce), 15 μm in diameter and containing 0.5 mg of bead mass, was inserted into the left ventricle at control and 20 min after the start of the adenosine, glucagon, or ACh infusion. Then the kidney was excised and the renal cortex was cut, parallel to the surface, into four zones of equal thickness. These four cortex zones were analyzed for individual isotope counts, and the flow rate of each zone was calculated.

Data are presented as means ± SEM. The Student's t-test for paired comparisons was used for statistical analysis. Probability values of less than 0.05 were accepted as being statistically significant differences.

Results and Discussion

Intrarenal Vascular Sites of Action of Glucagon, Adenosine and ATP

The effects of glucagon, adenosine and ATP on RBF, GFR, and filtration fraction are shown in Table 1. The dose of each agent used was the respective submaximum dose on the basis of its renal vasodilatory action. In intrarenal infusion of adenosine caused a biphasic response in RBF. Following the initiation of the infusion, RBF decreased transiently and then increased to about 40% above the control level within 5 min, as reported previously [6,17]. This high level of RBF continued thereafter

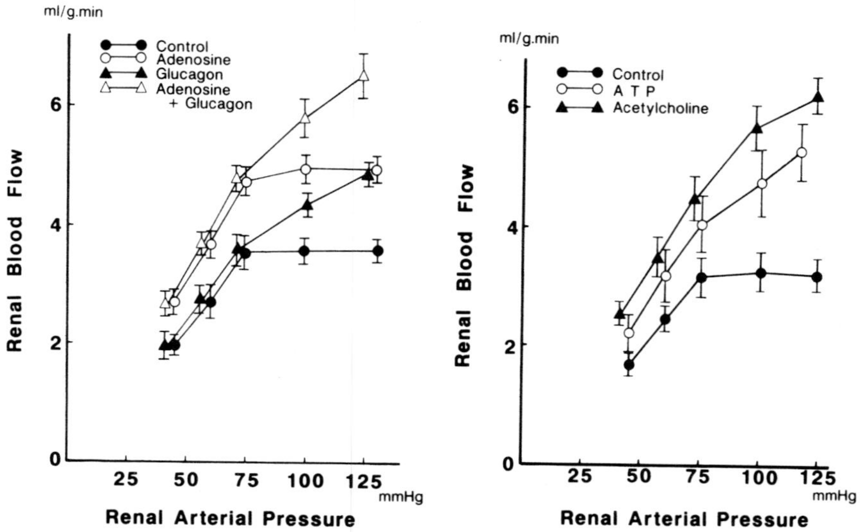

Fig. 1. The *left hand panel* shows the effects of adenosine alone, glucagon alone, and adenosine plus glucagon on the relationship between renal arterial pressure (RAP) and renal blood flow (RBF). Adenosine increased RBF at RAPs below, as well as within, the autoregulatory pressure range. In contrast, glucagon increased RBF at RAPs within the autoregulatory range. The superimposition of glucagon to adenosine infusion resulted in a further vasodilation which occurred at RAPs within the autoregulatory pressure range. The *right hand panel* shows the effects of ATP and acetylcholine (ACh) on the relationship between RAP and RBF. Both ATP and ACh increased RBF at RAPs below, as well as within, the autoregulatory pressure range and significantly impaired the autoregulation of RBF

during the infusion, but GFR was reduced significantly. As a result, the filtration fraction decreased significantly. Glucagon, which activates the adenylate cyclase [18,19], also increased RBF without the initial reduction seen during adenosine infusion. This renal vasodilation induced by glucagon was similar in magnitude to that produced by adenosine, however GFR increased significantly.

Fig. 1 compares the respective effects of adenosine, glucagon, and adenosine plus glucagon on RAP–RFB relationships. Although both adenosine and glucagon elicited vasodilation, the effects on the overall relationships were quite different. Adenosine increased RBF at RAPs below, as well as within, the autoregulatory pressure range. Although the autoregulatory capability was not perceptibly impaired by adenosine, the autoregulatory plateau was shifted upward. The responses obtained by the infusion of adenosine were consistent with the responses previously reported [6]. During the infusion of glucagon, RBF decreased in proportion to the reduction of RAP. At RAPs lower than the autoregulatory range, there were no significant differences between RBF in the absence of or in the presence of glucagon. That is, the vasodilation induced by glucagon was restricted to the RAPs within the autoregulatory pressure range. Glucagon completely abolished the autoregulation of RBF.

It is generally considered that autoregulation-induced resistance changes occur predominantly at the afferent arteriole and that the resistance of an afferent arteriole

Table 1. Effects of various vasodilators on renal hemodynamics in dogs

	Renal blood flow ml/g.min	Glomerular filtration rate ml/g.min	Filtration fraction
Control	3.67±0.18	0.75±0.03	0.32±0.02
glucagon (0.5 μg/kg/min)	5.08±0.23*	0.98±0.04*	0.32±0.02
Control	3.60±0.15	0.74±0.05	0.34±0.02
adenosine (20 μg/kg/min)	5.07±0.15*	0.55±0.04*	0.18±0.01*
adenosine + glucagon	6.63±0.33*+	0.73±0.02+	0.22±0.03+
Control	3.03±0.36	0.72±0.06	0.38±0.03
ATP (40 μg/kg/min)	5.03±0.44*	0.66±0.07	0.20±0.03*
Control	3.36±0.18	0.74±0.04	0.36±0.04
acetylcholine (4 μg/kg/min)	6.41±0.33*	0.74±0.04	0.20±0.02*
Control	3.40±0.20	0.72±0.05	0.35±0.05
forskolin (0.2 μg/kg/min)	4.15±0.30*	0.86±0.06*	0.34±0.05
Control	3.15±0.13	0.64±0.06	0.33±0.02
dibutyryl cyclic AMP (0.3 mg/kg/min)	5.10±0.38*	0.89±0.09*	0.30±0.03
Control	3.29±0.21	0.72±0.04	0.32±0.02
nitrendipine (0.5 μg/kg/min)	4.80±0.31*	0.96±0.04*	0.31±0.02

All values are means±S.E. * indicates significant difference from control ($P<0.05$); + indicates significant difference from adenosine alone ($P<0.05$)

attains a minimum value at the lower limit of the autoregulatory pressure range. Therefore, the observation that glucagon selectively interferes with the autoregulatory component suggests that glucagon dilates the afferent arteriole primarily. In contrast to the action of glucagon, adenosine increased RBF even at the RAP of 75 mmHg, having a minimum value of the afferent arteriolar resistance. This observation indicates that adenosine may dilate the postglomerular efferent arterioles preferentially. The RAP–RBF relationships obtained during the infusions of ACh, which dilates both afferent and efferent arterioles [10,20], and ATP are shown in the right hand panel of Fig. 1. During infusion of ATP or ACh RBF decreased in proportion to the reduction of RAP. But, unlike the effect of glucagon, during infusion of ACh or ATP RBF was significantly higher than the control at each pressure level. Thus, both ACh and ATP induced significant vasodilation characterized by a leftward shift in the RAP–RBF relationship. Thus, these findings show that both ATP and ACh dilate both arterioles. The superimposition of glucagon onto adenosine induced further vasodilation at RAPs within the autoregulatory pressure range. However, at RAPs lower than 75 mmHg there was no difference in RBF between the infusion of adenosine alone and the infusion of adenosine plus glucagon (Fig. 1). The superimposition of glucagon onto adenosine dilated the renal blood vessels such that there was a marked attenuation of the autoregulatory efficiency. Also, there were no significant differences between the RAP–RBF relationship obtained during the infusion of ACh and adenosine plus glucagon. These findings indicate the differences in the action sites of glucagon and adenosine, and support our conclusion.

Osswald et al. [21] reported that adenosine preferentially constricts the afferent arterioles in the superficial nephron of the canine kidney. It is well known that adenosine causes both vasoconstriction and dilation of renal blood vessels unlike that in other organ vascular beds [6,7,22]. The vasoconstriction may appear immediately after the start of infusion whereas the vasodilation appears gradually. Transient

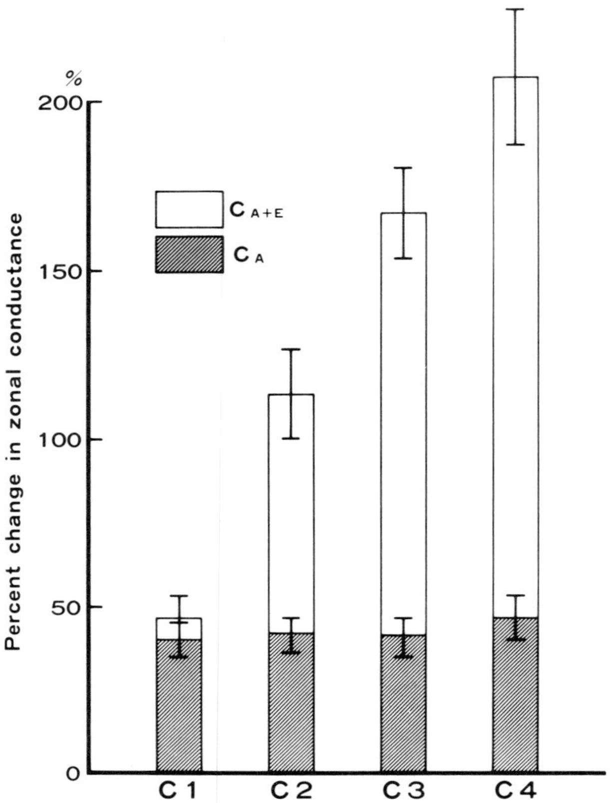

Fig. 2. Vasodilatory capabilities of the afferent and efferent arterioles in the renal cortex zone. The vasodilatory capability of the afferent arteriole (▨) was uniform among zones. That of the efferent arteriole (□) was not uniform and was characterized by a progressively proportional increase from the superficial to the deep cortex

reduction of RBF may be observed by the summation of both actions of adenosine. So, it could be considered that an abrupt change in adenosine concentration may induce transient vasoconstriction, but the gradual increase of adenosine concentration may not cause such transient vasoconstriction. To test the above hypothesis, the effect of dipyridamole, which inhibits the cellular uptake of adenosine [23] and the degradation of adenosine [24] on RBF, was examined. The intrarenal infusion of dipyridamole alone at a rate of 1 μg/kg per min did not affect RBF, but dipyridamole at a rate of 10 μg/kg per min increased RBF significantly, from 3.32 ± 0.15 to 3.75 ± 0.26 ml/g per min ($P<0.05$). The superimposition of dipyridamole at a rate of 1 μg/kg per min on adenosine infusion (0.05 μg/kg per min), which did not affect RBF, significantly increased RBF from 3.25 ± 0.20 to 3.81 ± 0.30 ml/g per min without any transient reduction of RBF ($P<0.05$). Thus, the moderate and gradual changes in adenosine concentration may not induce net vasoconstriction on a whole kidney basis. At present, the speed of changes of adenosine concentration in the renal tissue under various conditions is unknown. Nevertheless, it can be considered that the possible physiological action of adenosine may be preferential dilation of the efferent arterioles.

Differences Among Nephrons in the Vasodilatory Capacities and the Relative Tonus of the Afferent and Efferent Arterioles

In the previous section, the intrarenal action sites of adenosine and glucagon were determined. Glucagon preferentially dilates the afferent arteriole, while adenosine dilates the efferent arteriole. We examined the effects of both of these agents, and ACh, on the intrarenal distribution of blood flow. At basal condition, the flow rate of each cortex zone differed significantly from that of the other three. The inner zones were characterized by the lower perfusion rates. The response to glucagon (0.5 μg/kg per min) was characterized by an almost uniform increase in the flow rates in all four cortex zones. On the other hand, although adenosine induced a significant increase in flow rates in all zones, the zonal response pattern was not uniform. The response pattern was characterized by a progressively proportional increase in flow from the superficial to the deep cortex. Thus, glucagon, which dilates the afferent arterioles, increased the zonal flow rates by the same degree. Adenosine, which dilates the efferent arterioles, increased the inner cortical flow more than the outer cortical flow. These results indicate that the vasodilatory capability of the afferent arteriole is uniform among nephrons, whereas the vasodilatory capability of the efferent arteriole is not uniform and is highest in the juxtaglomerular nephron (Fig. 2). ACh, as well as adenosine, increased the deep cortical flow more than the superficial flow, but the flow response to ACh in each zone was higher than that to adenosine. Renal vasodilation induced by ACh reached a maximum at a dose of 4 μg/kg per min because other vasodilators such as bradykinin and prostaglandin E2 could not dilate the renal blood vessels more than ACh [15,25]. In addition, as shown in Table 1 and in Fig. 1, adenosine plus glucagon achieved almost the same degree of dilation as that achieved by ACh. Thus, it seems that glucagon and adenosine selectively dilate the afferent arteriole and the efferent arteriole, respectively, to the maximum extent.

Vasodilatory Mechanisms of Adenosine

Forskolin, which activates adenylate cyclase in various tissues, increased RBF and GFR concomitantly. Conversely, adenosine, which shows bi-directional action to adenylate cyclase, increased RBF and decreased GFR. If the efferent arteriolar dilation induced by adenosine is exerted exclusively by the activation of adenylate cyclase, it is unlikely that there are significant differences between GFR responses, even though adenosine dilates renal blood vessels in the same magnitude as forskolin. Thus, it is possible that the vasodilatory action of adenosine may not be induced via the activation of adenylate cyclase. The intrarenal infusion of dibutyryl cyclic AMP caused significant increases of both RBF and GFR, which were similar to those seen during the glucagon infusion.

We have previously reported that forskolin stimulated cyclic AMP production in the isolated canine afferent arteriole [26]. However, at present we do not have any data concerning the cyclic AMP production ability of the efferent arteriole. However, it seems likely that the efferent arteriole is also able to produce cyclic AMP. The present findings, that both forskolin and dibutryl cyclic AMP produced the same renal hemodynamic actions, suggest that differences between the intracellular signal-transduction systems of the afferent arteriole and the efferent arteriole may exist.

Conclusions

The present study clearly shows that glucagon and adenosine preferentially dilate the afferent arteriole and the efferent arteriole, respectively. Both agents can be considered to be useful pharmacological tools for clarifying the regulatory mechanisms of renal hemodynamics. The action of adenosine has demonstrated the importance of adenosine as a physiological controller of renal hemodynamics. The increase of adenosine production indicates the negative balance of oxygen supply. Adenosine reduced oxygen consumption in the kidney via the reduced GFR and increased the oxygen supply via the increased RBF. Thus, we suggest that adenosine plays an important role in linking the control of RBF and GFR with changes in renal metabolism. In addition, renal vasodilation by adenosine might not be mediated via the activation of adenylate cyclase. Both forskolin and dibutyryl cyclic AMP produced the same renal hemodynamic actions. These results substantiate the differences between the intracellular signal-transduction systems of the afferent arteriole and the efferent arteriole.

References

1. Osswald H, Hermes H, Nabakowski G (1982) Role of adenosine in signal transmission of tubuloglomerular feedback. Kidney Int 22: S136–S142
2. Osswald H, Nabakowski G, Hermes H (1980) Adenosine as a possible mediator of metabolic control of glomerular filtration rate. Int J Biochem 12: 263–267
3. Spielman WS, Thompson IC (1982) A proposed role for adenosine in the regulation of renal hemodynamics and renin release. Am J Physiol 242: F423–435
4. Van Calker D, Miller M, Hamprecht B (1978) Adenosine inhibits the accumulation of cyclic AMP in cultured brain cells. Nature 276: 839–841
5. Londos C, Cooper DMF, Wolff J (1980) Subclasses of external adenosine receptors. Proc Natl Acad Sci USA 77: 2551–2554
6. Premen AJ, Hall EJ, Mizelle LH, Cornell EJ (1985) Maintenance of renal autoregulation during infusion of aminophylline or adenosine. Am J Physiol 248 (Renal Fluid Electrolyte Physiol 17): F366–F373
7. Ueda J, Abe Y, Okahara T, Yamamoto K (1974) Adenine nucleotides and renal function: Special reference with intrarenal distribution of blood flow. Osaka City Med J 20: 33–50
8. Schmid HE, Garrett CR, Spencer PM (1964) Intrinsic hemodynamic adjustments to reduced renal pressure gradients. Circ Res 15(Suppl): 170–177
9. Selkurt EE, Hall WP, Spencer PM (1949) Influence of graded arterial pressure decrement of renal clearance of creatinine, p-aminohippurate and sodium. Am J Physiol 159: 359–378
10. Abe Y, Dixon F, McNay JL (1970) Dissociation between autoregulation of renal blood flow and glomerular filtration rate. Am J Physiol 219: 986–993
11. Navar LG (1970) Minimal preglomerular resistance and calculation of normal glomerular pressure. Am J Physiol 219: 1658–1664

12. Robertson CR, Deen MW, Troy LJ, Brenner MB (1972) Dynamics of glomerular ultrafiltration in the rat: III. Hemodynamics and autoregulation. Am J Physiol 223:1191–1200
13. Walser M, Davidson GD, Orloff J (1955) The renal clearance of alkali-stable inulin. J Clin Invest 34: 1520–1523
14. McNay JL, Abe Y (1970) Pressure dependent heterogeneity of renal cortical blood flow in dogs. Circ Res 27: 571–587
15. Abe Y, Okahara T, Kishimoto T, Yamamoto K, Ueda J (1973) Relationship between intrarenal distribution of blood flow and renin secretion. Am J Physiol 225: 319–323
16. Abe Y, Kishimoto T, Yamamoto K, Ueda J (1973) Intrarenal distribution of blood flow during ureteral and venous pressure elevation. Am J Physiol 224: 746–751
17. Ueda J (1972) Adenine nucleotides and renal function: Special reference with intrarenal distribution of blood flow (abstract). Jpn J Pharmacol 22: 5
18. Broadns AE, Kaminsky NI, Northcutt RC, Hardman JC, Sutherland EW, Liddle GW (1970) Effects of glucagon on adenosine 3′, 5′-monophosphate and guanosine 3′, 5′-monophosphate in human plasma and urine. J Clin Invest 49: 2237–2244
19. Mulvehill JB, Hui YS, Barnes LD, Palumbo PJ, Dousa TP (1976) Glucagon sensitive adenylcyclase in human renal medulla. J Clin Endocrinol Metab 42: 380–386
20. Abe Y (1971) Intrarenal blood flow distribution and autoregulation of blood flow and glomerular filtration rate. Jpn Circ J 35: 1163–1173
21. Osswald H, Spielman SW, Knox GF (1978) Mechanism of adenosine mediated decreases in glomerular filtration rate in dogs. Circ Res 43: 465–469
22. Murray RD, Churchill CP (1985) Concentration dependency of the renal vascular and renin secretory responses to adenosine receptor agonists. J Pharmacol Exp Ther 232: 189–193
23. Klabunde RE, Althouse DG (1981) Adenosine metabolism in dog whole blood: effects of dipyridamole. Life Sci 28: 2631–2641
24. Bunag RD, Douglas CR, Imai S, Berne RM (1964) Influence of a pyrimido-pyrimidine derivative on determination of adenosine by blood. Circ Res 15: 83–88
25. Imanishi M, Abe Y, Okahara T, Yukimura T, Yamamoto K (1980) Effects of prostaglandin I2, and E2 on renal hemodynamics and function and renin release. Jpn Circ J 44: 875–882
26. Tamaki T, Hura CE, Kunau RT (1989) Dopamine stimulates cAMP production in canine afferent arterioles via DA1 receptors. Am J Physiol 256: H626–H629

Role of Intracellular Calcium in the Regulation of Renal Hemodynamics

L. Gabriel Navar[1], Pamela K. Carmines[1], Kenneth D. Mitchell[1], and P. Darwin Bell[2]

SUMMARY. Intracellular calcium contributes to renal hemodynamic regulatory mechanisms in multiple ways. Calcium channel blockers elicit a selective vasodilation of preglomerular arterioles leading to increases in renal blood flow (RBF), glomerular filtration rate (GFR), and glomerular pressure, with marked attenuation of autoregulatory capability. The effects of these agents seem to be restricted to the component of renal vascular resistance responsible for autoregulation and contrast with other agents which vasodilate the kidney at arterial pressures below, as well as within, the autoregulatory range. This component of renal vascular resistance that is not influenced by calcium entry blockade can be altered by angiotensin converting enzyme inhibition. Studies at the microvascular level have demonstrated that the effects of angiotensin II on afferent arterioles are dependent upon calcium entry whereas the vasoconstrictor actions on efferent arterioles are not influenced by calcium channel blockade. The macula densa cells responsible for mediating tubular glomerular feedback (TGF) appears to utilize a different type of intracellular calcium mechanism for transmission of feedback signals. Increases in the intralumenal solute concentration at the macula densa elicit feedback signals to constrict the afferent arterioles and reduce glomerular pressure. These effects can be artificially induced by the intralumenal addition of calcium ionophores; however, intralumenal addition of calcium channel blockers or variation in intralumenal calcium concentration do not interfere with signal transmission. In contrast, agents that interfere with intracellular calcium mobilization can block TGF responses. Thus, intracellular mobilization of cytosolic calcium within the macula densa cells leads to transmission of TGF signals to the vascular cells. At the afferent arteriolar effector site, transmembrane calcium flux appears to serve as the dominant mechanism for regulating intracellular calcium, since TGF-mediated vasoconstrictor responses are abolished by calcium channel blockade. The efferent arterioles may be

[1]Department of Physiology, Tulane University School of Medicine, 1430 Tulane Ave., New Orleans, LA 70112, USA

[2]Department of Physiology, Nephrology Research and Training Center, University of Alabama at Birmingham, Birmingham, AL 35294, USA

less responsive to TGF signals because of their relative insensitivity to agents that alter transmembrane calcium flux.

Introduction

Although it is well recognized that activation of cytosolic calcium is a pivotal step in many intracellular processes, including vascular smooth muscle contraction, the mechanisms by which increases in cytosolic calcium can be achieved are varied [1–3]. Cytosolic calcium can be activated either by increasing calcium influx from the extracellular compartment through several mechanisms or by increased mobilization of intracellular calcium from sequestered sites. In many systems there is a complex coupling between intracellular mobilization mechanisms and calcium influx mechanisms [1–4]. For this presentation emphasis will be placed on the role of intracellular calcium in two specific aspects related to renal hemodynamic regulatory mechanisms. Initially, attention will be focused on the role of calcium entry mechanisms in regulating afferent arteriolar resistance in response to changes in perfusion pressure and in response to certain vasoactive peptides, such as angiotensin II. In the second part of this paper, consideration will be given to the role of intracellular calcium in the mediation of tubular glomerular feedback (TGF) signals from the macula densa cells to the afferent arterioles.

Vascular Control Mechanisms

The fact that transmembrane calcium flux is very important in mediating vascular contraction [2–4] should not be taken as evidence that fluctuations in the ionized calcium levels in the extracellular fluid environment within the physiologic range cause major effects. Indeed, because of the exquisite power which very small changes of cytosolic calcium have to cause major alterations in cellular function, the cell membrane has developed a high degree of impermeability to calcium ions. Calcium ions generally leak in very slowly from the extracellular fluid compartment and can be removed by a number of powerful transport mechanisms that return calcium to the extracellular fluid or compartmentalize it within the cell in an inactive form. Thus, although calcium concentration in the extracellular fluid is in the millimolar range, the intracellular concentration of free calcium is less than one micromolar [1–4]. In spite of this extremely large calcium gradient between the extracellular and the intracellular environments, the influx is considered to be rather limited and to be controlled primarily by mechanisms which activate calcium influx through specific calcium channels. Accordingly, previous studies have demonstrated that changes in plasma calcium concentration within the physiologic range elicit only subtle changes in renal vascular resistance and have rather negligible effects on renal autoregulatory capability [5].

Pharmacological agents which can directly alter transmembrane calcium influx have been shown to have powerful renal hemodynamic effects [6]. Systemic or intrarenal arterial infusion of calcium channel blockers increases RBF and GFR and causes a marked attenuation of the ability of the vasculature to respond to changes in arterial pressure with appropriate autoregulatory resistance adjustments [7,8].

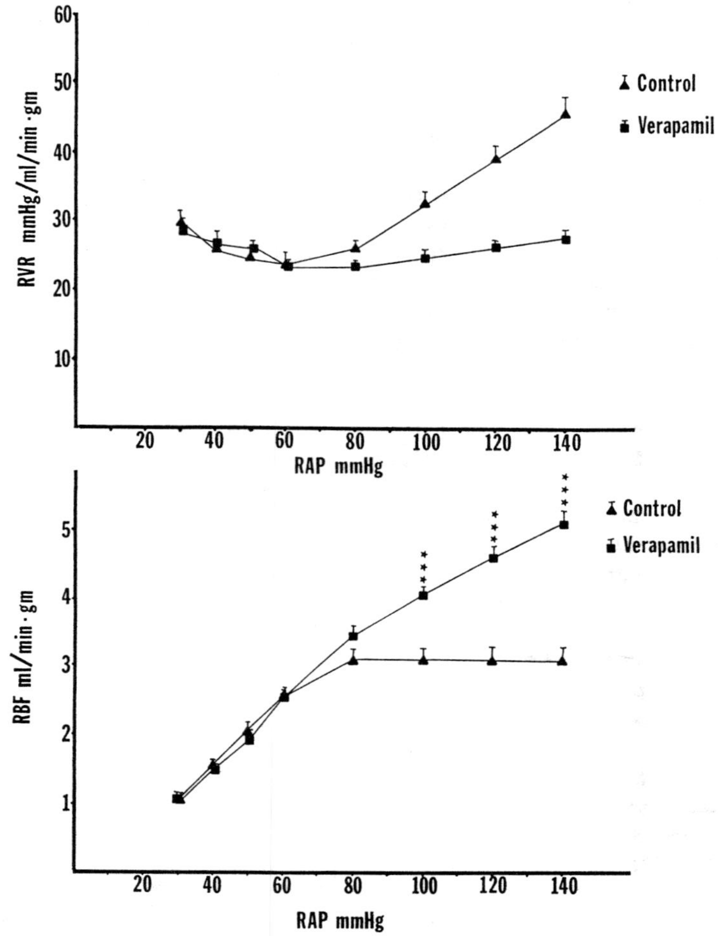

Fig. 1. Effects of verapamil on renal autoregulatory behavior. Data show the relationship between renal arterial pressure (*RAP*) and renal blood flow (*lower panel*) and between RAP and renal vascular resistance (*RVR*) (*upper panel*). (Data from [7])

Examples of such responses are shown in Fig. 1, which demonstrates the shift from a normal autoregulatory pattern to a near passive RBF response to decreases in renal arterial pressure which occurs during the intraarterial infusion of verapamil. Importantly, the verapamil-induced increase in RBF was restricted primarily to the range of arterial pressures associated with autoregulation. At these higher renal arterial pressures, the loss of autoregulatory capability resulted in the magnitude of the renal vasodilation being highly dependent on the level of renal arterial pressure. However, at arterial pressures below the autoregulatory range, there was little or no difference between RBF during control conditions and during calcium channel blockade. Coincident with the loss of RBF autoregulation, calcium channel blockers also attenuated

GFR autoregulation [7]. When these responses are assessed as changes in renal vascular resistance during reductions in arterial pressure, it can be observed that calcium channel blockers decrease renal vascular resistance only down to the minimal level achieved at the reduced levels of arterial pressure. Thus, calcium channel blockers appear to be unique in their ability to vasodilate the kidney. In contrast to other types of vasodilators, such as acetylcholine, which can vasodilate at renal arterial pressures below as well as within the autoregulatory range [9], or angiotensin converting enzyme (ACE) inhibitors, which increase RBF at all pressures but do not alter renal autoregulatory behavior [7,10], the calcium channel blockers seem to uniquely influence the autoregulatory portion of the curve with little or no effect on other components. Interestingly, pharmacological agents that interfere with intracellular mobilization of calcium are not as effective in blocking autoregulatory mediated changes in vascular resistance [11]. These observations suggest that one unique property of the renal vascular resistance segment responsible for autoregulation is its sensitivity to stimuli which alter transmembrane calcium flux.

In further studies it was demonstrated that infusion of an angiotensin converting enzyme inhibitor during calcium channel blockade caused additional dilation of the renal vascular bed [7]. The effect could be reversed by angiotensin II even though it was apparent that overall angiotensin II sensitivity was markedly reduced by calcium channel blockade. Thus, there is also an angiotensin sensitive vascular resistance component that is not susceptible to calcium channel blockers.

The whole kidney data suggest that calcium channel blockers predominately dilate the preglomerular resistance vessels responsible for mediating autoregulatory adjustments in renal vascular resistance. More recent micropuncture experiments using the peritubular capillary infusion technique have provided direct confirmation of this conclusion [12]. Peritubular capillary infusion is a particularly useful technique, because it allows infusion of high concentrations of hormones or pharmacological agents into the blood flow of a single large peritubular capillary welling point on the surface of the kidney. The infused agents diffuse out of the peritubular capillary network and infiltrate the surrounding interstitial spaces and can thus expose the adjoining microvasculature to high concentrations of vasoactive agents without affecting systemic arterial pressure. With this technique, the effects of maximally effective doses of calcium channel blockers on the superficial nephron vascular function can be assessed without the hypotensive effects elicited by intravenous or intraarterial infusion of these agents. One purpose of our study was to evaluate the effects of calcium entry blockers on glomerular pressure and glomerular pressure autoregulation, as assessed by proximal tubule stop flow pressure (SFP) measurements. As shown in Fig. 2, verapamil caused substantial increases in SFP and also increased the slope of the relationship between renal arterial pressure and SFP. Thus, even though the control SFP responses reflect only the residual autoregulatory capability occurring in the absence of the contribution of TGF influences from the nephron with interrupted distal flow [13], calcium entry blockade caused a further preglomerular dilation and a near passive relationship between arterial pressure and glomerular pressure.

Another important objective of this study was to evaluate the sensitivity of the effector component of the TGF mechanism to calcium channel blockers [12]. As shown in Fig. 3, SFP feedback responses were nearly abolished during peritubular capillary infusion with verapamil or nifedipine. These results provide further support for the

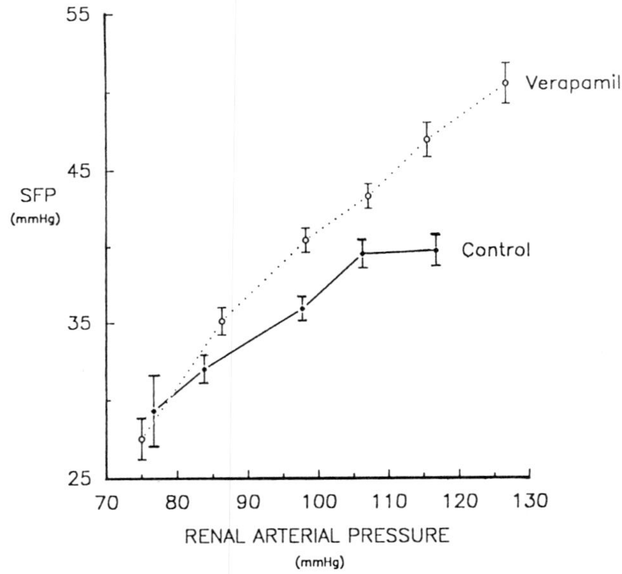

Fig. 2. Relationships between RAP and stop flow pressure (*SFP*) obtained during control conditions and during peritubular infusion of verapamil. (Data from [12])

contention that the preglomerular contractile elements responsible for autoregulatory capability, as well as for TGF responsiveness, can essentially be rendered passive by calcium entry blockers and suggest that transmembrane calcium flux through voltage-dependent channels serves as a common effector mechanism for both feedback-mediated and autoregulation-induced adjustments in preglomerular resistance.

Because of the evidence suggesting that complex intrarenal vascular control mechanisms are only partially dependent on transmembrane calcium movement through voltage-dependent channels, videomicroscopic measurements of vascular dimensions were performed on in vitro blood perfused juxtamedullary nephrons [14]. The effects of calcium channel blockers on control arteriolar diameters and on the vascular responsiveness to angiotensin II were evaluated. In particular, attention was focused on differences between afferent and efferent arterioles. The in vitro blood perfused juxtamedullary nephron technique is unique in that it provides accessibility to the preglomerular and postglomerular microvasculature, allowing videometric evaluation under well controlled in vitro conditions [14]. Kidney donors are heparinized and the right kidney is perfused through a double-barreled cannula with an oxygenated Tyrode's solution containing albumin. During continued perfusion, the kidney is removed and sectioned longitudinally to expose the pelvic cavity, leaving the papilla intact. Since the papilla normally overlies the tissue of interest, it is reflected back and the pelvic mucosa, adipose, and connective tissues which normally cover the inside cortical surface are removed and the veins are cut open. This procedure exposes the tubules and superficial microvasculature of juxtamedullary nephrons. The terminal portions of the vasculature giving rise to arterioles

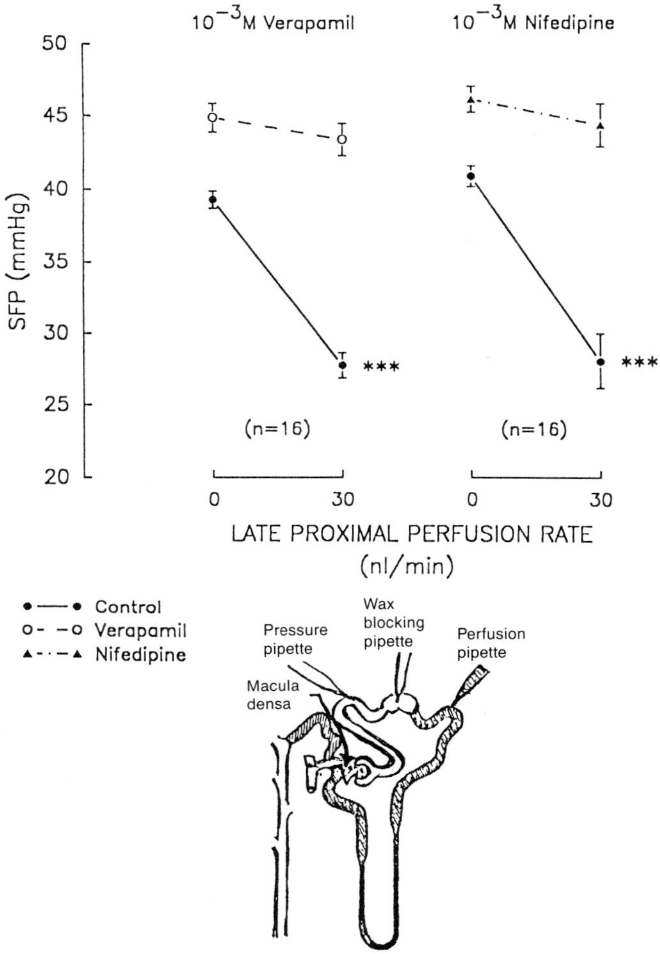

Fig. 3. Effects of calcium channel blockers on tubuloglomerular feedback responses. For these experiments, the normal TGF-mediated decrease in stop flow pressure (*SFP*) was assessed by increasing orthograde perfusion rate to 30 nl/min. After recovery, peritubular capillary infusion with either verapamil or nifedipine was started. After maximal response in SFP was achieved, the tubular perfusion rate was again increased to 30 nl/min. TGF-mediated vasoconstriction was nearly abolished during treatment with these agents. (Data from [12])

associated with these "superficial" juxtamedullary nephrons are isolated with tight ligatures [15]. It is important to emphasize that, although the technique for exposing these structures is extensive, the actual nephron segments and arterioles are not dissected and anatomical tubular-vascular relationships are not interrupted [15].

Videometric techniques were used to evaluate the afferent and efferent arteriolar responses to calcium channel blockade in this unique experimental setting. As shown in Fig. 4, these experiments provide direct confirmation of previous results showing

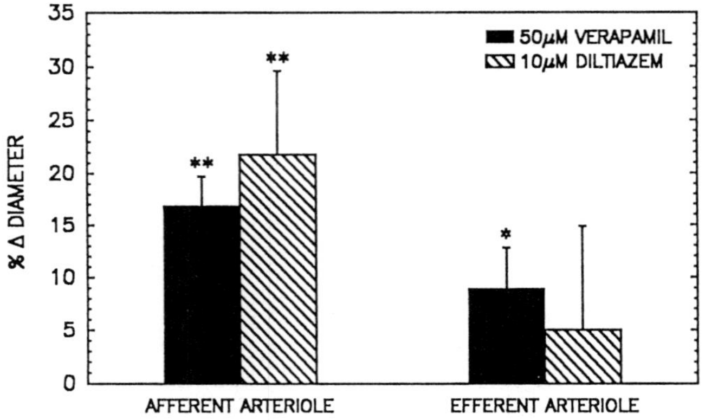

Fig. 4. Effects of calcium channel blockers on the afferent and efferent arteriolar diameters. Arteriolar inside diameters were measured utilizing videometric microscopy techniques. Control diameters averaged 23.0 ± 1.6 and 21.2 ± 2.2 μm for afferent and efferent arterioles, respectively. Verapamil and diltiazem were administered topically via the superfusing bathing solution. *, $P < 0.05$ vs control diameter; **, $P < 0.01$ vs control (Data from [14])

the ability of calcium channel blockers to dilate the afferent arterioles with maximal dilation of 17%–22% being observed. Interestingly, there was a mixed response of the efferent arteriole. Verapamil elicited a slight dilation of the efferent arterioles (9%), whereas diltiazem did not significantly influence efferent arteriolar caliber. Thus, these studies demonstrate further that calcium channel blockers predominantly dilate the afferent arterioles and provide further support to the interpretation based on whole kidney and micropuncture experiments. Other recent data have demonstrated that the calcium channel agonist, BAY K8644, constricts the preglomerular arterioles more than efferent arterioles [16]. Also, KCl-induced depolarization is a more effective constrictor of afferent than efferent arterioles [17]. In a recent micropuncture study, it was shown that manganese, which is capable of blocking transmembrane calcium flux through voltage gated as well as other entry pathways, exerted selective preglomerular vasodilation [18]. Collectively, these data support the premise that there is a fundamental difference between the intracellular calcium activation mechanisms in afferent and efferent arterioles, with voltage gated calcium channels being of predominant importance in afferent arterioles and intracellular mobilization mechanisms playing a greater role in efferent arterioles.

The influence of calcium channel blockers on the arteriolar responsiveness to angiotensin II was particularly intriguing. As shown in Fig. 5, both verapamil and diltiazem abolished the afferent arteriolar constrictor effect of angiotensin II at concentrations up to 10 nanomolar. In contrast to this effect, the responses of the efferent vessels were virtually unaffected by these calcium entry blockers. These results indicate that angiotensin II elicits its vasoconstrictor actions on afferent and efferent arterioles through different mechanisms of calcium entry, mobilization, or activation. At the afferent arterioles, essentially all of the contractile response can be explained on the basis of an increased transmembrane calcium influx. In contrast, the finding that angiotensin sensitivity persists in the presence of calcium channel block-

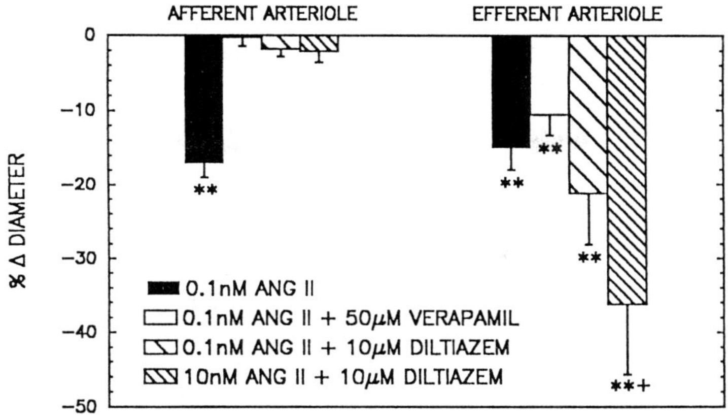

Fig. 5. Effects of calcium channel blockers on angiotensin-induced vasoconstriction of afferent and efferent arterioles. Arteriolar diameters were measured as described for Fig. 4. Responses to topical application of angiotensin II (ANG II) were assessed before and during exposure to either diltiazem or verapamil. **, $P < 0.01$ vs control diameter; +, $P < 0.05$ vs response to 0.1 nm ANG II plus 10 μm diltiazem. (Data from [14])

ade in efferent arterioles suggests a more complicated mechanism operating through receptor operated channels not sensitive to these blockers, or involving calcium mobilization from intracellular storage sites, as has been demonstrated for cultured vascular smooth muscle cells of aortic origin [19]. These results may have important implications that will help us to understand how, in certain pathophysiological states, the preglomerular vessels become unresponsive to angiotensin II. Such a selective loss of preglomerular sensitivity could have detrimental consequences due to altered glomerular pressure in conditions where the renin-angiotensin system is activated and only the efferent arterioles have retained their sensitivity to the elevated angiotensin II levels. Furthermore, such a setting may explain how the administration of ACE inhibitors could lead to the paradoxical reductions in glomerular function not infrequently observed in some patients [20]. These intriguing differential mechanisms of intracellular calcium activation of the afferent and efferent arterioles in response to angiotensin II emphasize the importance of studies on discrete segments of the renal microvasculature.

Macula Densa Intracellular Calcium Activating Mechanism

As already mentioned, the TGF mechanism serves as a communication link from the macula densa cells of the ascending limb of the loop of Henle to the afferent arterioles. Although signalling mechanisms remain uncertain, the effector responses at the level of the afferent arteriole appear to be dependent on voltage-dependent calcium entry mechanisms [12]. In contrast, the macula densa cells which are responsible for mediating TGF signals to the afferent arterioles appear to utilize a completely different intracellular calcium activating mechanism for the transmission of feedback

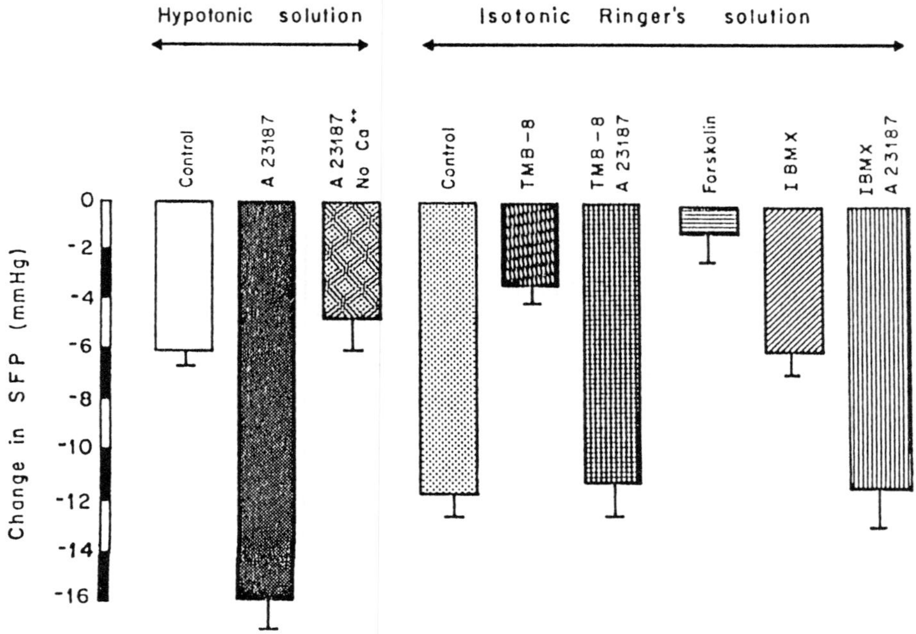

Fig. 6. Summary of the TGF responses during retrograde intralumenal perfusion with various agents that alter cytosolic calcium or cAMP. SFP, stop flow pressure. (Results taken from data in [23–25])

signals. Under normal conditions, tubular fluid osmolality at the level of the macula densa is in the range of 100 mOsm, but varies directly with flow [21]. The flow-dependent changes in solute concentration are sensed by the macula densa cells which initiate a sequence of events leading to the mediation of vasoactive signals to the afferent arteriole. Several studies have indicated that a critical intracellular event requisite for the transmission of these signals from the macula densa cells is activation of intracellular calcium [21,22].

Because of the frequent role of cytosolic calcium as a regulator of various cellular processes in other systems, we were prompted to consider how it may be involved in the mediation of TGF responses. This possibility was initially addressed by evaluating the consequences of increases in cytosolic calcium concentrations. TGF responses were assessed by the retrograde microperfusion technique, which involves perfusion of the macula densa segment with solutions of different solute concentrations. Previous studies have demonstrated that the magnitude of the TGF-mediated decrease in SFP depends on the total solute concentration of the perfusion solution, with maximum responses achieved with solutions of 120 mOsm/Kg [21]. A calcium ionophore (A23187) was utilized to artificially induce an increase in lumenal calcium permeability. As shown in Fig. 6, addition of the calcium ionophore to the perfusion solution (5–500 μM) elicited a marked augmentation of the TGF response during perfusion with a hypotonic solution (60 mOsm/Kg) which normally does not elicit substantive TGF-mediated decreases in SFP [23]. This effect of the calcium ionophore appeared to be due to calcium entry, as indicated by further studies in which calcium was eliminated from the tubular fluid perfusion solution. These results indicated that A23187 artificially increased macula densa cytosolic calcium concentration by allowing an entry of calcium from the tubular fluid into the cells. However, in further experiments in which the calcium ionophore was not used it was clear that changes in lumenal fluid calcium concentration normally had no significant effects. For example, total elimination of calcium from the perfusion solution or the addition of a calcium chelator to the perfusion solution did not inhibit normal TGF responses. Furthermore, the addition of verapamil in high concentrations to the perfusion solution did not interfere with the ability of increases in tubular fluid osmolality to induce feedback-mediated vasoconstriction [24].

These results support the hypothesis that an increase in intracellular calcium is a critical step in the mediation of TGF signals, but that under normal conditions, transmembrane calcium flux is probably not responsible for this increase in intracellular calcium. Additional experiments were conducted to evaluate the potential role of intracellular calcium mobilizing mechanisms in this phenomenon. TMB-8 (8-(N,N-diethylamino)-octyl-3,4,5-trimethoxybenzoate), an agent which binds to intracellular calcium and prevents the release of calcium from calcium sequestering sites, was utilized in this study. During perfusion with solutions containing TMB-8 in concentrations up to 500 micromolar, a normal feedback response was observed initially; however, the response slowly waned and was markedly attenuated after 3–5 minutes. Thus, it appeared that TMB-8 entered the macula densa cells and formed a stable complex with the intracellular calcium, thus preventing its release. Furthermore, it appeared that this inhibition of calcium release was a critical step necessary for normal mediation of feedback responses. In order to determine if the effects of TMB-8 were specifically related to alterations of intracellular calcium, we combined the calcium ionophore with the TMB-8. Under those conditions, the A23187 completely reversed the effects of TMB-8 and a maximal feedback response was restored [24]. These results provide further evidence that the effects of TMB-8 were not non-specific, and support the concept that activation of the TGF signaling pathway normally includes an intracellular calcium mobilizing event. It should also be noted that these effects were probably due to direct alterations in macula densa cell function, since it has been shown that systemic infusion of TMB-8 does not elicit renal vasodilator effects or interfere with renal autoregulatory behavior [11].

A number of other experiments have been conducted to probe the potential interactions between intracellular calcium mobilization and other signal transduction systems. Experiments using calmodulin inhibitors revealed little or no role for a calcium calmodulin-interaction in the mediation of feedback signals [25]. This is another important difference between the role of intracellular calcium in the macula densa signal mediating system compared to its role in vascular smooth muscle. Interestingly, calmodulin antagonists significantly prolonged the recovery response following cessation of perfusion, suggesting that one potential role of calmodulin in the TGF mechanism could be to promote calcium resequestration after termination of the stimulus.

Further experiments were conducted to evaluate the potential role of cAMP as a mediator of TGF signals. Various studies have previously suggested that cAMP might be involved, because treatment with agents capable of increasing cell cAMP levels led

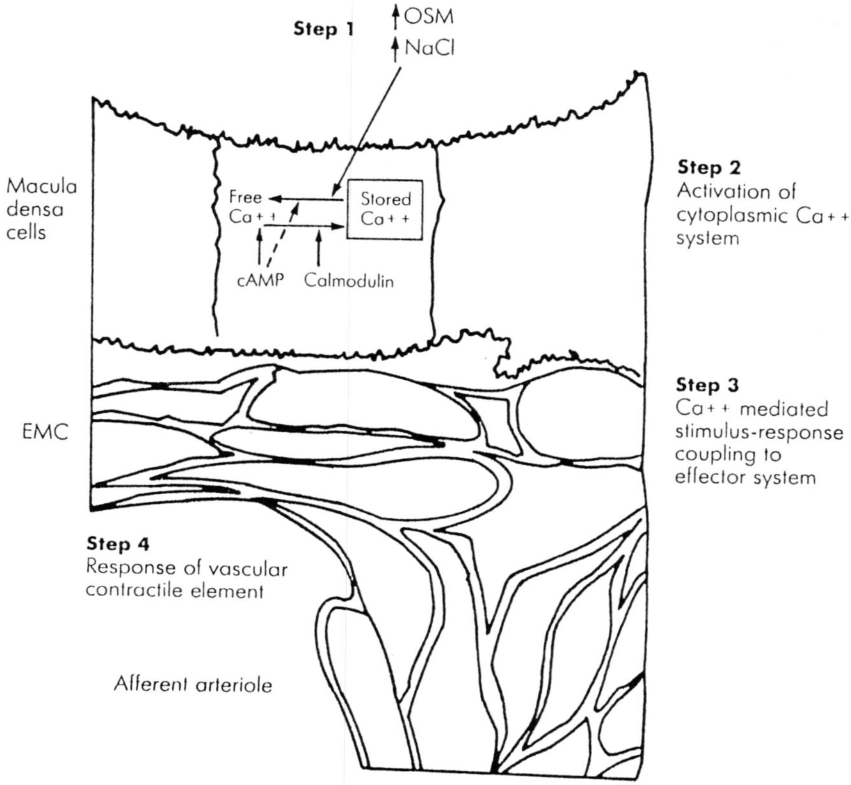

Fig. 7. Schematic presentation of macula densa signalling mechanism and the interaction of signal transduction mechanisms which regulate cytosolic calcium

to attenuation of TGF responses [26]. The inclusion of IBMX, a methylxanthine capable of increasing cAMP because of its action as a phosphodiesterose inhibitor, in the perfusion solution markedly attenuated the magnitude of the feedback response. This attenuation appeared to be primarily related to an increase in cell cAMP levels, because the increase in cellular cAMP levels elicited by treatment with dibutyryl cAMP in the presence of small concentrations of IBMX resulted in a similar attenuation of TGF vasoconstrictor responses [27]. Further experiments with forskolin, an activator of the catalytic subunit of adenylate cyclase, also caused a marked attenuation of the TGF response. Interestingly, the effects which increased cell cAMP had in attenuating TGF responses were completely abolished when we added A23187 to the perfusion solution [27]. Thus, the increase in intracellular calcium caused by the calcium ionophore reversed the inhibitory effects elicited by elevations in cAMP. These results suggest that the increases in cAMP are probably interacting with a cytosolic calcium system and may be causing TGF inhibition by reducing macula densa cytosolic calcium and preventing appropriate activation during intralumenal perfusion (Fig. 7). This conclusion, based on the results of micropuncture experiments, has received further support from recent studies on isolated perfused thick ascending limbs in which the cytosolic calcium level in the macula densa cells has been measured directly using fluorescence microscopy [28]. In response to increases in intratubular sodium chloride concentration, there was an increase in cytosolic calcium in the macula densa cells as assessed by changes in fura-2 fluorescence intensity.

Thus, one can conclude that the macula densa cells are capable of responding to increases in tubular fluid solute concentration by eliciting an increase in cell calcium that is primarily due to mobilization of calcium from intracellular sites. At present it is not clear how the increase in cell calcium may mediate feedback signals. It is possible that an increase in cytosolic calcium leads to the formation of a vasoactive agent which is secreted from the macula densa cells into the extraglomerular mesangial area and vascular cleft of the glomerulus. In turn, this agent may directly cause increase in calcium entry into afferent arteriolar smooth muscle cells by activating voltage-dependent calcium channels. It is likely that the relative insensitivity of the efferent arteriole to TGF signals is due to its lack of responsiveness to agents which influence voltage gated calcium channels and its ability to maintain vascular responsiveness to angiotensin II, even during exposure to calcium channel blockers. In terms of the TGF signal transmission pathway, some of the critical steps which remain uncertain relate to the membrane and transport events at macula densa cells which are actually responsible for detection of changes in lumenal fluid solute concentration and the ever elusive substance which is released by the macula densa cell and serves as the communication link with the smooth muscle cells of the afferent arteriole.

Acknowledgments. We would like to acknowledge the technical assistance of Anthony K. Cook and Lynn Debose and assistance from Agnes C. Buffone in preparing the manuscript. This work was supported by the National Institute of Health Grants HL18426, HL26371, and DK39202. P.K. Carmines and P.D. Bell are Established Investigators of the American Heart Association.

References

1. Exton JH (1985) Role of calcium and phosphoinositides in the action of certain hormones and neurotransmitters. J Clin Invest 75:1753–1757
2. Williamson JR, Monck JR (1989) Hormone effects on cellular calcium fluxes. Annu Rev Physiol 51:107–129
3. Cauvin C, Loutzenhiser R, Van Breemen C (1983) Mechanisms of calcium antagonist-induced vasodilation. Annu Rev Pharmacol Toxicol 23:373–396
4. Loutzenhiser R, Leyten P, Saida K, Van Breemen C (1985) Calcium compartments and mobilization during contraction of smooth muscle. In: Graver AK, Daniel EE (eds) Calcium and contractility. Humona, pp 61–92
5. Chomdej B, Bell PD, Navar LG (1977) Renal hemodynamic and autoregulatory responses to acute hypercalcemia. Am J Physiol (Renal Fluid Electrolyte Physiol 6) 232:F490–F496
6. Loutzenhiser R, Epstein M (1985) Effects of calcium channel antagonists on renal hemodynamics. Am J Physiol 249:F619–F629
7. Navar LG, Champion WJ, Thomas CE (1986) Effects of calcium channel blockade on renal vascular resistance responses to changes in perfusion pressure and angiotensin-converting enzyme inhibition in dogs. Circ Res 58:874–881

8. Ono H, Kokubun H, Hashimoto K (1974) Abolition by calcium antagonists of the autoregulation of renal blood flow. Naunyn Schmiedebergs Arch Pharmacol 285:201–207
9. Baer PG, Navar LG (1973) Renal vasodilation and uncoupling of blood flow and filtration rate autoregulation. Kidney Int 4:12–21
10. Rosivall L, Youngblood P, Navar LG (1986) Renal autoregulatory efficiency during angiotensin-converting enzyme inhibition in dogs on a low sodium diet. Renal Physiol 9:18–28
11. Ogawa N, Ono H (1988) Effect of 8-(N,N-diethylamino)octyl-3,4,5-trimethoxybenzoate (TMB-8), an inhibitor of intracellular Ca^{2+} release, on autoregulation of renal blood flow in the dog. Naunyn Schmiedebergs Arch Pharmacol 338:293–296
12. Mitchell KD, Navar LG (1990) Tubuloglomerular feedback responses during peritubular infusions of calcium channel blockers. Am J Physiol (Renal Fluid Electrolyte Physiol 27)258:F537–F544
13. Navar LG, Chomdej B, Bell PD (1975) Absence of estimated glomerular capillary pressure autoregulation during interrupted distal delivery. Am J Physiol 229:1596–1603
14. Carmines PK, Navar LG (1989) Disparate effects of Ca channel blockade on afferent and efferent arteriolar responses to ANG II. Am J Physiol (Renal Fluid Electrolyte Physiol 25)256:F1015–F1020
15. Casellas D, Navar LG (1984) In vitro perfusion of juxtamedullary nephrons in rats. Am J Physiol (Renal Fluid Electrolyte Physiol 15)246:F349–F358
16. Steinhausen M, Baehr M (1989) Vasomotion and vasoconstriction induced by a Ca^{2+}-antagonist in the split hydronephrotic kidney. Prog Appl Microcirc 14:25–39
17. Loutzenhiser R, Hayashi K, Epstein M (1989) Divergent effects of KCl-induced depolarization on afferent and efferent arterioles. Am J Physiol 257:F561–F564
18. Lafferty HM, Gunning M, Brady HR, Brenner BM, Anderson S (1990) Renal hemodynamic and natriuretic effects of manganese and interactions with atrial natriuretic peptide. Am J Physiol (Renal Fluid Electrolyte Physiol 27)258:F998–F1004
19. Smith JB (1986) Angiotensin-receptor signaling in cultured vascular smooth muscle cells. Am J Physiol (Renal Fluid Electrolyte Physiol 19)250:F759–F769
20. Curtis JJ, Luke RG, Welchel JD, Diethelm AG, Jones P, Dustan HP (1983) Angiotensin converting enzyme inhibition in renal transplant patients with hypertension. N Engl J Med 308:377–381
21. Bell PD, Navar LG (1982) Macula densa feedback control of glomerular filtration: Role of cytosolic calcium. Miner Electrolyte Metab 8:61–77
22. Bell PD, Franco M, Navar LG (1987) Calcium as a mediator of tubuloglomerular feedback. Annu Rev Physiol 49:275–293
23. Bell PD, Navar LG (1982) Cytoplasmic calcium in the mediation of macula densa tubuloglomerular feedback responses. Science 215:670–673
24. Bell PD, Reddington M (1983) Intracellular calcium in the transmission of tubuloglomerular feedback signals. Am J Physiol 245:F295–F302
25. Bell PD (1986) Tubuloglomerular feedback responses in the rat during calmodulin inhibition. Am J Physiol 250:F715–F719
26. Schnermann J, Osswald H, Hermle M (1977) Inhibitory effect of methylxanthines on feedback control of glomerular filtration in the rat kidney. Pflugers Arch 369:39–48
27. Bell PD (1985) Cyclic AMP-calcium interaction in the transmission of tubuloglomerular feedback signals. Kidney Int 28:728–732
28. Bell PD, Franco-Guevara M, Abrahamson DR, Lapointe JY, Cardinal J (1988) Cellular mechanism for tubuloglomerular feedback signalling. In: Persson AEG, Boberg U (eds) The juxtaglomerular apparatus. Elsevier, Amsterdam, pp 63–77

The Role of Angiotensin in the Control of Renal Vascular Resistance

László Rosivall[1]

Introduction

Not only does the kidney play an essential role in regulating the renin-angiotensin system by secreting renin in response to a variety of stimuli, but it also serves as an important target tissue for angiotensin II. The renal action of angiotensin II to conserve sodium and maintain appropriate extracellular fluid volume under the condition of volume and/or salt deprivation is evoked by the direct hemodynamic and also by the tubular effects of angiotensin II, and by the consequent indirect alterations in renal peritubular Starling forces. The details of these complex effects of angiotensin on kidney function have been widely studied for a long time, raising many different issues and utilizing many different approaches. Consequently, in the literature so much—in many cases conflicting—information has been gathered that the realistic aim of this review shouldn't be more than to select some topics and focus on issues that seem to be promising for future experimental and clinical research.

Effects of Angiotensin on Renal Hemodynamics

With the interesting exception of the large arteries of the kidney, the renal vasculature is highly sensitive to angiotensin II, although some heterogeneity of response has been noted within the renal vascular beds [1–6].

Angiotensin II elicits a dose-dependent decrease in renal blood flow and similar but more variable effects on glomerular filtration rate [2–4,7]. Also, infusions of moder-

[1]Department of Pathophysiology, Semmelweis University Medical School, Budapest P.O. Box 370, H-1445, Hungary

ate amounts of angiotensin do not prevent normal autoregulatory adjustment in vascular resistance following reductions in arterial pressure [8,9].

In micropuncture experiments it has been observed that angiotensin II infusions reduce single nephron glomerular filtration rate (SNGFR) and glomerular plasma flow, the latter reduction being proportionally greater [10,11]. Afferent and efferent arteriolar resistance increased and the glomerular filtration coefficient (K_f) was decreased [10–12]. These studies suggest that the changes in afferent arteriolar resistance are greater than could be attributed specifically to the autoregulatory mechanism. Uncertainty exists, however, as to whether angiotensin II normally has a direct vasoconstrictor effect on preglomerular vessels under physiological conditions. While in most of the cases it was found that either the infusion of angiotensin or the administration of converting enzyme inhibitor altered both pre-and post-glomerular resistances in anesthetized dog [3,11,13], it has been also demonstrated that angiotensin II infusions, in pharmacological concentrations, affected preglomerular resistance only when other autoregulatory mechanisms (tubuloglomerular feedback activating and myogenic mechanism) were intact, thereby negating direct constrictor effects of angiotensin II on preglomerular vessels [14]. Even the latter investigators, however, have reported that in the presence of high intrarenal levels of adenosine or under blockade of renal prostaglandin synthesis, angiotensin II appears to have a direct vasoconstrictor effect on the preglomerular vessels [15]. Also, protective effects of vascular prostaglandins, mainly on the afferent arteriole, against the vasoconstriction due to the circulating angiotensin II was recently suggested by others [16].

In another study, the pressure in the interlobular arteries was measured in anesthetized rats by micropuncture through conicotomy and the relative interlobular arterial resistance was calculated by utilizing the pressures and renal blood flow values [17]. It was demonstrated that angiotensin II infusion had a direct vasoconstrictor effect even in the interlobular arteriole as a preglomerular response, but the constriction of interlobular arteries elicited by intravenous angiotensin II reflected more autoregulatory response and less direct effect.

In normotensive rats there is a pressure drop along the interlobular arteries, resulting in different hemodynamic conditions in the outer and inner cortical nephrons [18]. The superficial afferent arterioles are almost maximally dilated, whereas the juxtamedullary ones are significantly constricted under the condition of normohydration [19]. Recently it was shown that inhibition of angiotensin converting enzyme in these deep nephrons markedly changed SNGFR [20], medullary plasma flow [21], and intratubular free-flow pressure [4], indicating that angiotensin II plays a role in the regulation of juxtamedullary vascular resistance. This conclusion is also supported by the recent demonstration of significant increase in red cell flux in the vasa recta in the exposed papilla during converting enzyme inhibition [22]. Earlier studies from the same laboratories have shown that captopril increased SNGFR to a lesser extent than it increased the inner medullary blood flow [4,20,21]. Thus the overall data suggest that both afferent and efferent arteriolar resistances are under the influence of angiotensin II in the juxtamedullary nephrons.

These data indicate that angiotensin II can serve to regulate both pre- and post-glomerular resistances. It is possible, however, that under some steady state conditions the influence of angiotensin on the preglomerular vessels is counteracted, either partially or completely, by other intrarenal humoral systems.

Direct Assessment of the Effects of Angiotensin II on Renal Segmental Vascular Diameter

The inaccessibility of renal vessels in vivo under normal experimental conditions has hindered assessment of the specific segmental vascular effects of angiotensin II. This holds true particularly for the intrarenal vasculature located in the juxtamedullary area. During the past few years this issue has benefitted from the development of a variety of in vivo or in vitro techniques which allow visualization of the vessels and direct approach to renal microcirculation [5].

Utilizing the technique of transplantation of renal tissue into hamster cheek pouch it was demonstrated that afferent and efferent arterioles responded to angiotensin II and that these responses were augmented in hypertension [23]. The effects appeared to be slightly greater on the efferent arteriole. Edwards [24], however, was able to document constriction of efferent, but not afferent arterioles during exposure of isolated microvessels to angiotensin II. More recently, in similarly isolated vessel segments, it was also demonstrated that the efferent arteriole was more sensitive than the afferent arteriole to angiotensin II, whereas the sensitivity of both arterioles to norepinephrine was similar [25].

In contrast to this, an extensive study using the split hydronephrotic kidney preparation demonstrated that 1] acute intravenous administration of angiotensin II produced a significant constriction of pre- and postglomerular vessels, 2] the constriction of the preglomerular vessels in response to acute angiotensin II infusion was greater than the postglomerular constriction, 3] the constriction of preglomerular vessels primarily resulted from a direct angiotensin II constrictor action mediated by angiotensin II receptors, and to much lesser extent, from a myogenic response due to elevation of blood pressure [6]. It is of interest that, in this preparation, these workers observed attenuated vascular responses to angiotensin II, following long-term exposure, similar to those which were earlier demonstrated in dog [7]. In these experiments several segments of the renal vasculature were studied by precise identification of proximal and distal parts of a. arcuata, vas afferens and vas efferens. The diameter of a. interlobularis was measured at the distal site, near the branching point of the terminal afferent arteriole. Approximate changes in vessel diameter at controlled blood pressure were as follows: a. arcuata, −15%, −20%; a. interlobularis, −25%; vas afferens, −18%, −20%; vas efferens, −16%, −8%. It is worth noting that the diameter of certain preglomerular vessels progressively increased following angiotensin II infusion, probably reflecting the action of vasodilator substances released by the peptide.

To gain further insight, both micropuncture and videometric technique have been used to elucidate the influence of angiotensin II on various segments of the in vitro blood perfused juxtamedullary nephrons. It was demonstrated that intravascular bolus injection of angiotensin II (12.5–20 ng) increased total vascular resistance, as revealed by a rise in perfusion pressure, and induced dose-dependent and reversible decreases in glomerular capillary pressure [26]. Such a change is indicative of predominantly preglomerular vasoconstriction which could not be attributed to an autoregulatory response. In subsequent studies on the same preparation, topical application of angiotensin II induced significant reductions in diameter of arcuate and interlobular arteries, as well as of afferent and efferent arterioles [27,28,9].

Table 1. Percent changes in vessel diameter during angiotensin II treatments

AII treatment	BP controlled	A. arcuata Early	A. arcuata Late	A. interlobularis	Afferent arteriole Early	Afferent arteriole Mid	Afferent arteriole Late	Efferent arteriole Early	Efferent arteriole Mid	Efferent arteriole Late	Doses	Ref. no	Preparation
Systemic	–	−17	−20	−30	−17		−11	−12		− 7	50mg/ min per kg	[6]	Hydronephrotic
	–	−18	−26	−35	−29		−22	−13		− 3	100mg/min per kg		split kidney
	±	−13	−20	−25	−19		−20	−17		− 7	100mg/min per kg		
Topical		− 4	− 5	− 5	− 2		− 9	− 9		− 5	10^{-9}M	[6]	Hydronephrotic
		−28	−22	−39	−35		−36	−33		− 9	10^{-7}M		split kidney
						− 5			− 9		10^{-13}M	[23]	Tissue transplant
						−24			−31		10^{-12}M		(cheek pouch)
				± 0		± 0			−10		10^{-12}M	[24]	Isolated vessel
				± 0		± 0			−60		10^{-8}M		
						± 0			− 5		10^{-12}M	[25]	Isolated vessel
						−20			−60		10^{-10}M		
						−80			−95		10^{-8}M		
				−18		−20	−14		−17		$10^{-12}-10^{-9}$M	[27]	Isolated nephron
						−17			−15		10^{-10}M	[28]	Isolated nephron

Taken together, these observations indicate that both circulating and extravascularly administered angiotensin II can, in most cases, induce major resistance effects at both preglomerular and efferent arteriolar sites (Table 1). The angiotensin-induced changes in the caliber of a. arcuata and a. interlobularis probably represent a relatively small overall effect on preglomerular resistance, due to the big size of these vessel segments and their minor contribution to the normal pressure drop along the renal vasculature. Nevertheless, it seems clear that angiotensin II is capable of influencing the renal microcirculation at all vascular levels. The reason why the isolated renal afferent arteriole is less responsive to angiotensin II than the efferent arteriole [24,25], which observation makes this preparation clearly distinct from others, is not obvious. This observation of efferent, but of no, or significantly fewer, preglomerular effects of angiotensin II was made under conditions of stop flow in the arteriole, when there were no tubular elements and there was no blood etc. It is important to emphasize that even under these conditions, angiotensin is able to constrict preglomerular arterioles, proving the presence of angiotensin receptors in this segment, but there is a decreased sensitivity [25]. This finding, however, may also indicate that angiotensin II-induced effects on pre- and postglomerular vessel segments operate through complex and/or disparate mechanisms [28,29].

Effects of Locally Formed Angiotensin II on Renal Hemodynamics

The significance of this issue depends on two basic problems: (1) Is there enough intrarenal angiotensin formation to substantially alter renal function? and (2) Is there any difference between the effects of angiotensin II formed intrarenally, versus delivered systemically, on renal hemodynamics?

Previous studies have demonstrated that a substantial amount of angiotensin II is formed within the kidney and that this formation shows a significant correlation with renin secretion [30]. In this study it was not possible to determine the source of angiotensin I (endogenously generated vs systemically delivered) utilized by the kidney to generate angiotensin II. It was suggested earlier, however, that 90% of angiotensin I is a result of an extravascular local production [31]. This is supported by recently published data, obtained in hypertensive patients, showing that there is a rapid metabolism of angiotensin in the kidney, while there is no difference between the arterial and venous angiotensin I concentrations [32]. It was calculated that less than 20%–30% of the de novo-produced angiotensin I could be accounted for by circulating renin, indicating that most of the intrarenally formed angiotensin II comes from locally produced angiotensin I. Whatever the source of angiotensin I in the kidney, it is important that at least 20% of the angiotensin I is converted to angiotensin II in a single passage through the kidney [33]. This conversion probably occurs not only intravascularly, but also extravascularly [34] and is induced not only by the angiotensin converting enzyme, but also by other enzymes [29,34,35]. Because the angiotensin I concentration in the blood may well be several-fold higher (10–15x) than the angiotensin II concentration, as was demonstrated in dog and in human [33,36], it is probable that most of the angiotensin effects on kidney function are due to the effect of intrarenally formed angiotensin II.

It cannot yet be determined what percentage of the angiotensin I formed in the kidney originates from circulating or from intrarenally produced angiotensinogen. Recent studies show that in the kidney angiotensinogen mRNA expression is altered by sodium intake and by various pathophysiological conditions such as hypertension and cardiac failure [37,38]. The change in angiotensinogen mRNA is not necessarily parallel with renal renin gene expression [39]. These findings support the theory that intrinsic renin-angiotensin may play a substantial role in the regulation of renal function under experimental and clinical conditions.

There are many—partly overlooked—examples of data in the literature that are indicative of differences in effects on renal hemodynamics induced by circulating or by locally formed angiotensin II. Intrarenally converted angiotensin II produced somewhat different intrarenal blood flow distribution than did circulating angiotensin II [40]. Topical administration of angiotensin II in the hydronephrotic kidney preparation produced concentration-dependent reductions in the diameter of all preglomerular vessels; results just like those achieved with intravenous infusion of angiotensin II. The constrictor response of afferent arteriole to local angiotensin II, however, was not followed by a dilation during the control period, as was the case with i.v. infusion [6].

In a recent series of experiments, where angiotensin I and angiotensin II infusion were studied concurrently, it was recognized that even equiconstrictor doses of these peptides might produce slightly different effects on renal hemodynamics, i.e., GFR was more consistently decreased during angiotensin I infusions [3]. According to the above-mentioned effects of topically administered angiotensin II, it is possible that locally formed angiotensin II causes less release of protective vasodilators than does the circulating peptide. These data also indicate that intrarenal conversion of circulating angiotensin I occurs at vascular sites early enough to allow the locally formed angiotensin to decrease glomerular function. Micropuncture data show that this augmented intrarenal conversion of circulating angiotensin I reduces GFR as a consequence of decreases in glomerular filtration coefficient as well as in glomerular plasma flow, the latter being due to concomitant increases in preglomerular and efferent arteriolar resistances in superficial nephrons [11]. The existence of the difference between the effects of circulating and locally formed angiotensin II is also supported by the observation that in the sodium restricted dog, intravenous angiotensin II infusion alone, even in doses sufficient to restore renal blood flow (RBF) to control during captopril treatment when both the circulating and local formation of angiotensin II is blocked, failed to restore the increase in GFR [41].

In a micropuncture study, angiotensin I or II was infused into peritubular capillary; the objective was to determine whether angiotensin I infusion could lead to sufficient de novo generation of angiotensin II, in the peritubular or interstitial environment, to elicit effects on glomerular function. It was found that angiotensin II formed beyond the glomerular circulation could reduce SNGFR and enhance proximal tubular reabsorption [42]. Presumably, angiotensin generated from interstitially formed angiotensin I due to the enhanced renin release into the interstitium would act in a similar manner.

In a subsequent study, peritubular infusion of both angiotensin I and II, in doses which did not effect base-line glomerular capillary pressure, increased the sensitivity of the tubuloglomerular feedback mechanism [43]. Angiotensin I or angiotensin II plus saralasin had no effects. These observations indicate that angiotensin II formed in the postglomerular capillary and/or interstitial environment can gain access to, and enhance the sensitivity of, the vascular elements that respond to signals from the macula densa cell. Considering recent morphological observations of the juxtaglomerular apparatus [44], it is also possible that the enhanced sensitivity of the tubuloglomerular feedback mechanism is due to the alteration of the interstitial fluid balance of the juxtaglomerular apparatus, caused by angiotensin II.

Thus, it can be concluded that the amount of angiotensin II formed intrarenally is enough to significantly contribute to the regulation of intrarenal hemodynamics and, indeed, it is probable that most of the effects of angiotensin on kidney function are due to the effects of intrarenally formed angiotensin II. According to experimental data, intrarenally formed angiotensin II may have effects on renal circulation which are basically similar to those of circulating angiotensin II; however, there are also some subtle, but significant, differences.

Conclusions

In this presentation, recent studies on (1) the effects of angiotensin on renal hemodynamics, (2) direct assessment of the effects of angiotensin II on renal vascular segmental diameter, and (3) the effects of locally formed angiotensin II on renal hemodynamics have been reviewed.

It has been demonstrated, in whole kidney and micropuncture studies, that angiotensin II, either delivered systematically or formed locally, has a crucial role in the regulation of both afferent and efferent arteriolar resistances throughout the cortex. Angiotensin-induced constriction of preglomerular arterioles has been further confirmed by direct assessment of segmental vascular responses during systemic or topical administration of the peptide. The preglomerular vasoconstrictor effects of the peptide are not restricted only to the afferent arteriole. Angiotensin II, formed even beyond the glomerular circulation in the postglomerular capillary and/or interstitial environment, can reduce glomerular and proximal tubular function. Recent findings on intrarenal angiotensin formation, e.g., the existence and response of angiotensinogen mRNA to different experimental and clinical conditions, the high intrarenal conversion of angiotensin I to II, the higher concentration of angiotensin I than angiotensin II in the blood, etc., all support the idea that the effects of angiotensin II on renal hemodynamics may be due mainly to the effects of the locally formed peptide. Therefore, it is especially important to emphasize that there are some observed differences between the effects of intrarenally formed angiotensin II versus systemically delivered angiotensin II on renal hemodynamics.

Acknowledgments. We are grateful to S. Adamkó for technical assistance. This study was supported by a Grant: OTKA/207 from the Hungarian Research Foundation.

References

1. Bohr DF (1974) Angiotensin on vascular smooth muscle. In: Page IH, Bumpus FM (eds) Angiotensin. Springer, New York, pp 424–440 (Handbook of experimental pharmacology, vol 37)

2. Fagard RH, Cowley AW, Navar LG, Langford HG, Guyton AC (1976) Renal responses to slight elevations of renal arterial plasma angiotensin II concentration in dogs. Clin Exp Pharmacol Physiol 3:531–538
3. Rosivall L, Navar LG (1983) Effects on renal hemodynamics of intrarenal infusions of angiotensins I and II. Am J Physiol 245:F181–F187
4. Göransson A, Sjöquist M, Ulfendahl HR (1986) Superficial and juxtamedullary nephron function during converting enzyme inhibition. Am J Physiol 251:F25–F33
5. Navar LG, Gilmore JP, Joyner WL, Steinhausen M, Edwards RM, Casellas D, Carmines PK, Zimmerhackl LB, Yokota SD (1986) Direct assessment of renal microcirculatory dynamics. Fed Proc 45:2851–2861
6. Steinhausen M, Sterzel RB, Fleming JT, Kühn R, Weis S (1987) Acute and chronic effects of angiotensin II on the vessels of the split hydronephrotic kidney. Kidney Int 31:S1–S10
7. Lohmeier TE, Cowley AW Jr (1979) Hypertensive and renal effects of chronic low level intrarenal angiotensin infusion in the dog. Circ Res 44:154–160
8. Kiil F, Kjekshus J, Loyning E (1969) Renal autoregulation during infusion of noradrenaline, angiotensin, and acetylcholine. Acta Physiol Scand 76:10–23
9. Casellas D, Carmines PK, Dupont M, Redon P, Moore LC (1990) Arteriolar renin and vascular effects of angiotensin II in juxtamedullary nephrons. Kidney Int 38:suppl 30:65–68
10. Blantz RC, Konnen KS, Tucker BJ (1976) Angiotensin II effects upon the glomerular microcirculation and ultrafiltration coefficient of the rat. J Clin Invest 57:419–434
11. Rosivall L, Carmines PK, Navar LG (1984) Effects of renal arterial angiotensin I infusion on glomerular dynamics in sodium replete dogs. Kidney Int 26:263–268
12. Schor N, Ichikawa I, Brenner BM (1980) Glomerular adaptations to chronic dietary salt restriction or excess. Am J Physiol 238:F428–F436
13. Navar LG, Jirakulsomchok D, Bell PD, Thomas CE, Huang WC (1982) Influence of converting enzyme inhibition on renal hemodynamics and glomerular dynamics in sodium-restricted dogs. Hypertension 4:56–68
14. Hall JE (1986) Regulation of glomerular filtration rate and sodium excretion by angiotensin II. Fed Proc 45:1431–1437
15. Olsen ME, Hall JE, Montani JP, Cornell JE (1987) Interaction between renal prostaglandins and angiotensin II in controlling glomerular filtration in the dog. Clin Sci 72:429–436
16. Heller J, Horácek V (1990) The effect of converting enzyme inhibitor, angiotensin II, and Saralasin on glomerular haemodynamics in the dog. Kidney Int 38:suppl 30:74–76
17. Keyeraas KJ, Aukland K (1987) Interlobular arterial resistance: influence of renal arterial pressure and angiotensin II. Kidney Int 31:1291–1298
18. Källskog Ö, Lindbom LO, Ulfendahl HR, Wolgast M (1976) Hydrostatic pressures within the vascular structures of the rat kidney. Pflugers Arch 363:205–210
19. Ericson A, Sjöquist M, Ulfendahl HR (1982) Single glomerular filtration rate in superficial and deep nephrons in rat kidneys. Acta Physiol Scand 114:201–209
20. Göransson A, Sjöquist M (1985) The effect of a converting enzyme inhibitor on autoregulation and intrarenal distribution of glomerular filtration in the rat. Acta Physiol Scand 124:515–523
21. Sjöquist M, Göransson A, Hansell P, Ulfendahl HR (1985) Regulation of filtration rate and blood flow in juxtamedullary nephrons of the rat kidney. Acta Physiol Scand 123:4A
22. Hansell P, Sjöquist M, Ulfendahl HR (1988) Effect of a converting-enzyme inhibitor on vasa recta blood flow in rat kidney. Am J Physiol 254:F492–F499
23. Click RL, Joyner WL, Gilmore JP (1979) Reactivity of glomerular afferent and efferent arterioles in renal hypertension. Kidney Int 15:109–115
24. Edwards RM (1983) Segmental effects of norepinephrine and angiotensin II on isolated renal microvessels. Am J Physiol 244:F526–534
25. Yuan BH, Robinette JB, Conger JD (1990) Effect of angiotensin II and norepinephrine on isolated rat afferent and efferent arterioles. Am J Physiol 258:F741–F750

26. Casellas D, Carmines PK, Navar LG (1985) Microvascular reactivity of in vitro blood perfused juxtamedullary nephrons from rats. Kidney Int 28:752–759
27. Carmines PK, Morrison TK, Navar LG (1986) Angiotensin II effects on microvascular diameters of in vitro blood-perfused juxtamedullary nephrons. Am J Physiol 251:F610–F618
28. Carmines PK, Navar LG (1989) Disparate effects of Ca channel blockade on afferent and efferent arteriolar responses to ANG II. Am J Physiol 256:F1015–1020
29. Okamura T, Okunishi H, Ayajiki K, Toda N (1990) Conversion of angiotensin I to angiotensin II in dog isolated renal artery: role of two different angiotensin II-generating enzymes. J Cardiovasc Pharmacol 15:353–359
30. Rosivall L, Narkates J, Oparil S (1987) De novo intrarenal formation of angiotensin II during control and enhanced renin secretion. Am J Physiol 252:F1118–F1123
31. Campbell DJ (1985) The site of angiotensin production. J Hypertens 3:199–207
32. Admiraal PJJ, Derkx FHM, Danser AHJ, Pieterman H, Schalekamp MADH (1990) Metabolism and production of angiotensin I in different vascular beds in subjects with hypertension. Hypertension 15:44–55
33. Rosivall L, Rinder DF, Champion J, Khosla MC, Navar LG, Oparil S (1983) Intrarenal angiotensin I conversion at normal and reduced renal blood flow in the dog. Am J Physiol 245:F408–F415
34. Bührle CP, Rosivall L, Taugner R (1987) Intrarenal generation of angiotensin II evaluated by an electrophysiological technique. Am J Physiol 252:F635–F644
35. Wintroub BU, Klickstein LB, Dzau VJ, Watt KWK (1984) Granulocyte-angiotensin system. Identification of angiotensinogen as the plasma protein substrate of leukocyte cathepsin G. Biochemistry 23:227–232
36. Kawamura M, Yoshida K, Akabane S, Matsushima Y, Kawano Y, Kojima S, Takahashi N, Shimamoto K, Ito K, Omae T (1987) A sensitive method for precise measurement of endogenous angiotensins I, II and III in human plasma. Clin Exp Theory Practice A9: 687–691
37. Ludwig G, Ganten D, Murakami K, Fasching U, Hackenthal E (1987) Relationship between renin mRNA and renin secretion in adrenalectomized, salt depleted, or converting enzyme inhibitor-treated rats. Mol Cell Endocrinol 50:223–229
38. Dzau VJ, Ingelfinger JR (1989) Molecular biology and pathophysiology of the intrarenal renin-angiotensin system. J Hypertens 7:S3–S8
39. Gomez RA, Lynch KR, Chevalier RL, Everett AD, Johns DW, Wilfong N, Peach MJ, Carey RM (1988) Renin and angiotensinogen gene expression and intrarenal renin distribution during ACE inhibition. Am J Physiol 254:F900–F906
40. Britton SL (1981) Intrarenal vascular effects of angiotensin I and angiotensin II. Am J Physiol 240:H914–H919
41. Carmines PK, Rosivall L, Till MF, Navar LG (1983) Renal hemodynamic effects of captopril in anesthetized sodium-restricted dogs. Renal Physiol 6:281–287
42. Mitchell KD, Navar LG (1987) Superficial nephron responses to peritubular capillary infusions of angiotensins I and II. Am J Physiol 252:F818–F824
43. Mitchell KD, Navar LG (1988) Enhanced tubuloglomerular feedback during peritubular infusions of angiotensins I and II. Am J Physiol 255:F383–F390
44. Rosivall L (1990) Morphology and function of distal part of the afferent arteriole. Kidney Int 38:suppl 30:10–15

Dietary Factors and Progression of Chronic Renal Failure

Chair: Giuseppe Maschio (Italy)
William E. Mitch (USA)

Effects of Lipid Manipulations in Chronic Renal Failure

William F. Keane, Bertram L. Kasiske, Michael P. O'Donnell, Paul G. Schmitz, and Youngki Kim[1]

Summary. Experimental results have demonstrated that a number of effects of hyperlipidemia are involved in the initiation and progression of glomerular injury. First, hyperlipidemia has been associated with the development of progressive mesangial expansion. This expanded mesangium is constituted, in part, by an accumulation of laminin, fibronectin and collagen. These changes in the mesangial region preceded the development of focal glomerulosclerosis (FGS). Similar changes in the mesangium have been observed in clinical and experimental studies, lending credence to the hypothesis that changes in mesangial matrix contribute to the development of FGS. The mechanisms whereby lipid-induced expansion of the mesangial region occur are poorly understood. A second effect of hyperlipidemia is to increase the number of glomerular Ia^+ macrophages. This influx of macrophages into glomeruli is reminiscent of the influence of hyperlipidemia on macrophage subendothelial localization seen in large vessels during the development of atherosclerosis. Macrophages have also been implicated in glomerular injury in a variety of experimental renal diseases. However, the role that the macrophage or macrophage derived products may play in the development of lipid-induced glomerular injury is at present unknown. Finally, lipid-induced glomerular injury may ultimately lead to altered glomerular hemodynamics, specifically glomerular hypertension, a factor that may contribute to glomerular injury. Indeed, experimental data suggest that an interaction between hypertension and hyperlipidemia may occur, resulting in additive glomerular damage. This interaction between risk factors for glomerular injury may be similar to the interaction between risk factors seen in patients with atherosclerosis.

Introduction

It has been established that once a critical number of functioning nephrons have been injured progressive loss of renal function may ensue, even though the original cause

[1]Department of Medicine, Division of Nephrology, Hennepin County Medical Center, and Division of Pediatric Nephrology, University of Minnesota Hospital, University of Minnesota Medical School, Minneapolis, MN 55415, USA

of injury is no longer present [1]. The mechanisms involved in progressive renal injury have been extensively investigated during the past decade, and it has been found that a number of physiologic and metabolic changes that occur in the course of progressive renal disease may contribute to glomerular destruction [2,3]. Based on pharmacological and dietary intervention studies, it has been postulated that hemodynamic factors, particularly glomerular hypertension, are important in the pathogenesis of progressive renal injury [1–4]. Additionally, experimental studies have demonstrated that genetic and metabolic factors, specifically abnormal lipid metabolism, may modulate glomerular damage [2,3,5–7]. The possibility that abnormal lipid metabolism could be important in the development and progression of renal injury has intrigued investigators for well over a hundred years. Support for the notion that lipids are involved in renal injury can be derived from three areas of experimental investigation. First, high cholesterol diets are associated with albuminuria and glomerular injury in different animal species. Second, pharmacological agents, including bile acid sequestrants, 3-hydroxy 3-methyl coenzyme A (HMG-CoA) reductase inhibitors, and fibrate derivatives have reduced circulating lipids and ameliorated glomerular injury in different experimental models of renal disease associated with hyperlipidemia. Third, the intake of large amounts of dietary polyunsaturated fatty acids of the omega-3 and omega-6 classes has also decreased circulating lipids and reduced glomerular injury in a variety of models of renal disease.

Dietary Induced Hypercholesterolemia

It is well established that feeding a high cholesterol diet to different animal species leads to focal glomerulosclerosis (FGS). Interestingly, the extent of glomerular injury has usually correlated with the circulating cholesterol level. The mechanism for these glomerular effects is, however, not completely understood. Glomerular hypercellularity and expansion of the mesangial matrix were demonstrated as early morphologic changes in animals fed a high cholesterol diet [8,9]. For example, in rats fed a diet of increased cholesterol content, significant albuminuria and, ultimately, FGS was observed [9]. Glomerular enlargement, mesangial expansion, and hypercellularity were evident after only one month of increased circulating cholesterol. These changes in the glomerular mesangium preceded the appearance of FGS. Immunocytochemical studies have demonstrated that glomerular hypercellularity was, in part, a result of an increase in Ia^+ macrophages [8]. A diet high in cholesterol has also led to an increased cortical content of cholesteryl esters [8,9]. In addition, a significant reduction in cortical arachidonic acid and an increased linoleic acid content were found in the cortical phospholipid fraction, suggesting an inhibitory effect of elevated cholesterol levels on desaturation and elongation of this essential fatty acid [9]. These changes in cholesteryl esters and fatty acids were also found to correlate significantly with the presence of glomerular injury [9]. Thus, high dietary cholesterol induced cellular, morphological, and biochemical changes in glomeruli similar to the changes, induced by hypercholesterolemia in large vessels, which were associated with the development of atherosclerosis. The precise role that these glomerular changes play in the development of FGS remains to be defined.

Recently, physiological studies in cholesterol fed rats have also been reported [9]. Micropuncture studies were performed after 6–8 weeks of a high cholesterol diet when albuminuria was minimal (>5mg/24h), and glomeruli demonstrated mesangial expansion but no FGS [9]. In these studies single nephron glomerular filtration rate and plasma flow were maintained. However, an increase in glomerular capillary pressure (P_{GC}) and an increase in the transcapillary hydraulic pressure were observed. This increment in hydraulic pressure occurred, in part, because of an increase in colloid osmotic pressure, and a trend toward an increase in efferent arteriolar resistance [9]. These changes in osmotic pressure are unique to this model of hypercholesterolemia. In addition to changes in osmotic pressure and arteriolar resistance, diet-induced hypercholesterolemia may alter blood rheologic properties and these effects could also contribute to changes in glomerular hemodynamic function. Thus, in this model of diet-induced hypercholesterolemia both hemodynamic and structural abnormalities have been described that could contribute to progressive glomerular injury. In addition, it has been demonstrated that unilateral nephrectomy, clip hypertension, chemically induced diabetes and the nephrotic syndrome exaggerated the degree of glomerular injury in cholesterol-fed animals [6,7,10]. Thus, it would appear that experimentally induced hemodynamic stresses, as well as direct glomerular injury, may also interact with hyperlipidemia to exaggerate nephron damage.

Although hypercholesterolemia is associated with glomerular injury, the mechanism whereby this occurs is unknown. Recent advances in our understanding of the metabolism of lipoproteins have suggested that modifications in the structure of lipoproteins may affect their potential for vascular injury. In this regard, probucol, an antilipemic agent with anti-oxidant activity, has been shown to modify diet-induced hypercholesterolemic glomerular injury independent of changes in circulating cholesterol levels [11]. These data suggested the possibility that the local glomerular deposition of lipoproteins and their oxidation might be important in lipid-induced glomerular injury. In support of this concept, mesangial cells have been shown to express receptors for low-density lipoproteins (LDL) [12]. In addition, LDL cholesterol induced a biphasic effect on mesangial cell proliferation. At lower concentrations (<200 μg/ml), LDL stimulated proliferation, while at higher concentrations of LDL (2000 μg/ml) inhibition of mesangial cell growth was observed and frank cytotoxicity was demonstrated [12–14]. The inhibition of mesangial cell growth at the higher LDL concentrations was associated with a tenfold increase in LDL malonaldehyde, a measure of lipid peroxidation [14]. Since mesangial cells are known to generate reactive oxygen molecules [15], we assessed whether scavengers of reactive oxygen molecules would be effective in preventing their peroxidation of lipoprotein and thus, their cytotoxicity. In these studies, both superoxide dismutase and butylated hydroxytoluene, scavengers of reactive oxygen molecules, decreased formation of malonaldehyde and abrogated the cytotoxic effects of oxidized LDL [14]. Thus, reactive oxygen molecules derived from mesangial cells might be important in altering lipids and rendering them cytotoxic. The possibility that mesangial cells can oxidize LDL is of more than passing interest. Oxidized LDL has recently been demonstrated to be present in atherosclerotic lesions in experimental models of atherosclerosis [16]. In addition, oxidized LDL is a chemo-attractant and is also endocytosed by macrophages and mesangial cells, through a scavenger receptor mechanism, at a more rapid rate than normal LDL [16]. This ultimately leads to increased formation of cholesteryl esters and foam cells. The biochemical demonstration of increased cholesteryl esters and the appearance of macrophages and foam cells in the glomerulus of cholesterol-fed rats [9] lends credence to the notion that oxidized LDL could participate in the glomerular injury seen in models of lipid-induced renal disease.

Pharmacological Treatment of Hyperlipidemia and the Pathogenesis of Glomerulosclerosis

In the obese Zucker rat, hyperlipidemia and microalbuminuria are present at 10–12 weeks of age [17,18]. Hypercholesterolemia becomes more pronounced as albuminuria increases. Mesangial matrix expansion and an increase in mesangial cellularity accompany the development of albuminuria. At 6 months of age, FGS is evident and subsequently progresses. Mild systemic hypertension and reduced renal function become manifest as glomerular and tubular interstitial injury evolve [17,18]. Immunohistochemical studies to define the changes which occurred in mesangial matrix in obese Zucker rats before the development of FGS have demonstrated that, at 24–28 weeks of age, obese rats have increased mesangial deposition of fibronectin, laminin, and type IV collagen, compared to lean Zucker rats. Glomerular staining for types I and III collagen was also increased in obese rats, but to a lesser extent. Thus, these studies indicated that the morphologic changes in the mesangial matrix by light microscopy are associated with an increase in accumulation of specific matrix proteins. In addition, we have demonstrated increased apolipoprotein (Apo) B deposits in glomerular sclerotic areas and in segmental areas of mesangial expansion. Since Apo B is the principal apolipoprotein of very low density lipoproteins in rats this observation may have important implications with respect to lipid-mesangial cell interactions. Characterization of the increased glomerular cellularity by immunocytochemical techniques demonstrated that obese rat glomeruli contain a three-fold increase in the number of Ia^+ macrophages in the mesangial region. These glomerular cellular changes were similar to those reported by us in dietary-induced hypercholesterolemic rats [9].

Micropuncture studies in obese and lean Zucker rats demonstrated normal glomerular function at 10–12 weeks of age, when only mild glomerular matrix expansion and minimal albuminuria (<5 mg/24h) were present [18]. We have recently studied older obese Zucker rats at 22–26 weeks of age when albuminura was increased (>50mg/24h), glomerular mesangial expansion was marked, but FGS was minimal [19]. In these studies, single nephron filtration rate was maintained by an increased P_{GC}. The mechanism responsible for the development of glomerular hypertension in older obese Zucker rats is unknown. Alterations in glomerular production of vasoactive substances or changes in blood rheology could have participated in the development of these hemodynamic changes. Thus, in this experimental model, glomerular hypertension developed late in the course of glomerular injury and may play a role in further amplifying renal injury.

Since hyperlipidemia was an early change in obese Zucker rats and preceded not only FGS, but also hemodynamic changes, we hypothesized that hyperlipidemia contributed to glomerular injury [20]. To test this thesis, we reduced circulating lipids with clofibric acid, the pharmacologically active form of clofibrate, or with lovastatin, an HMG-Co A reductase inhibitor. These therapies decreased serum lipids, reduced albuminuria, and prevented FGS [20]. In addition, with each of these therapies a decrease in mesangial cellularity and matrix expansion was observed. Micropuncture assessments performed after 4 weeks of antilipemic therapy failed to demonstrate alterations in glomerular hemodynamic function that could explain these beneficial effects [20].

The importance of systemic and glomerular hypertension in modulating progressive renal injury has been described [1–4]. In the remnant kidney model, for example, removal of 80%-90% of renal mass was accompanied by hypertension, proteinuria, uremia, and death. In addition, abnormal circulating lipids were found soon after ablative surgery, and secondary hypercholesterolemia developed as albuminuria worsened. We have shown that therapy with clofibrate or lovastatin effectively prevented secondary hypercholesterolemia in the remnant kidney model; this was associated with a reduction in proteinuria and decreased glomerular damage [21]. The effect of these agents appeared independent of effects on systemic or glomerular pressures [21].

The Dahl salt-sensitive rat is a model of systemic hypertension in which albuminuria and progressive glomerular damage are present [22]. Interestingly, hyperlipidemia was evident before many of the structural and functional changes developed in these rats [23]. Therapy with lovastatin has recently been shown to prevent the progressive increase in cholesterol levels and to have dramatically reduced albuminuria and FGS [24]. Thus, in two experimental models of systemic and glomerular hypertension associated with hypercholesterolemia, therapy with lipid lowering agents reduced the degree of proteinuria and the extent of glomerular injury. Finally, in studies of the nephrotic syndrome induced by the aminonucleoside of puromycin, a reduction in circulating lipids by cholestyramine or lovastatin has been shown to decrease glomerular injury and to preserve renal function [25,26]. Thus, in models of experimental disease in which hypercholesterolemia is a primary abnormality (obese Zucker rat), or in models in which abnormalities of lipids occur as a consequence of renal disease, pharmacologic modification of circulating lipids resulted in amelioration of glomerular injury and preservation of renal function.

The Effects of Polyunsaturated Fatty Acids in Glomerular Injury

The influence of dietary polyunsaturated fatty acid (PUFA) supplementation on the progression of glomerular injury has been evaluated in a number of immune and nonimmune models of renal disease [27]. In these studies, dietary supplementation with either the omega-3 or the omega-6 class of PUFAs has been evaluated and the results have shown that both PUFAs reduced proteinuria and decreased glomerular damage (Table 1). Recently, we have investigated the effects of PUFA supplementation in the obese Zucker rat. These studies were motivated by the observation that reduced cortical contents of omega-3 and omega-6 PUFAs were present in obese Zucker rats and that these changes correlated with glomerular injury [28]. We used diets containing sunflower and menhaden oils (diets enriched in omega-6 and omega-3 PUFA, respectively), and diets containing coconut oil or beef tallow (enriched in medium and long chain saturated fatty acids, respectively) and compared these to rats fed standard rodent chow. All rats were pair-fed and grew normally during the six-month study. Throughout the experiment, comparable blood pressures were measured in all groups. At the conclusion of the study, the PUFA diet rats demonstrated lower lipids

Table 1. Effects of polyunsaturated fatty acids on renal injury

Model	↑Linoleic acid (ω-6)	↑Eicosapentanoic acid (ω-3)
Murine lupus models	No change	↓
Murine immune-mediated models	↓	↓
5/6 Nephrectomy model	↓	↑/↓
Obese zucker model	↓	↓

↑, increase; ↓, decrease

and lower urine albumin excretion rates. In both the sunflower and menhaden oil supplemented groups of obese Zucker rats, there was a significant reduction in FGS and mesangial matrix expansion. Similar effects of a fish oil (Max EPA) supplemented diet in obese Zucker rats has also been recently reported [29]. The mechanisms whereby PUFA supplemented diets may ameliorate glomerular injury in obese Zucker rat are at present unknown. However, in addition to their lipid lowering effects, these fatty acids may influence renal hemodynamics, alter macrophage function, change eicosanoid production, and alter cell membrane biophysical properties [27]. Since many of these effects may modify renal injury, further investigations to define the role of these potential beneficial effects of PUFAs are necessary.

Acknowledgments. The authors acknowledge the assistance of Lee Schroeder and Ellen Davis in preparing this manuscript. Supported, in part, by grants received from the National Institutes of Health and the Baxter Extramural Grant Program.

References

1. Brenner BM (1985) Nephron adoption to renal injury. Am J Physiol 249:324–337
2. Keane WF, Anderson S, Aurell M, deZeeuw D, Narins RG, Povar G (1989) Angiotensin converting enzyme inhibitors and progressive renal insufficiency. Ann Intern Med 111:503–516
3. Klahr S, Schreiner G, Ishikawa I (1988) The progression of renal disease. N Engl J Med 318:1657–166
4. Anderson S, Rennke HG, Brenner BM (1986) Therapeutic advantage of converting enzyme inhibitors in arresting progressive renal disease associated with systemic hypertension in the rat. J Clin Invest 77:1993–2000
5. Moorhead JF, Chan MK, El-Nahas M, Varghese Z, et al. (1982) Lipid nephrotoxicity in chronic progressive glomerular and tubulointerstitial disease. Lancet I:1309–1311
6. Keane WF, Kasiske BL, O'Donnell MP (1988) Lipids and progressive glomerulosclerosis: A model analogous to atherosclerosis. Am J Nephrol 8:261–271
7. Diamond JR, Karnovsky MJ (1988) Focal and segmental glomerulosclerosis: Analogies to atherosclerosis. Kidney Int 33:917–924
8. Al-Shebeb T, Frohlich J, Magil AB (1988) Glomerular disease in hypercholesterolemic guinea pigs: a pathogenetic study. Kidney Int 33:498–507
9. Kasiske BL, O'Donnell MP, Schmitz PG, Kim Y, Keane WF (1990) Renal injury of diet induced hypercholesterolemia in rats. Kidney Int 37:880–891
10. Kasiske BL, O'Donnell MP, Cowardin W, Keane WF (1990) Lipids and the kidney. Hypertension 15:443–450

11. Kaplan R, Aynedjian HS, Bank N, Schlondorff D (1990) Cholesterol feeding causes renal vasoconstriction via oxidized lipoprotein activation of thromboxane. Kidney Int 37:371A.
12. Wasserman J, Santiago A, Rifici V, Holthofer H, Scharschmidt L, Epstein M, Schlondorff D (1989) Interactions of low density lipoprotein with rat mesangial cells. Kidney Int 35: 1168–1174
13. Wheeler DC, Persaud JW, Fernando R, Sweeny P, Varghese Z, Moorhead JF (1990) Effects of low density lipoproteins on mesangial cell growth and viability in vitro. Nephrol Dial Transplant 5:185–191
14. Keane WF, Phillips J, Kasiske BL, O'Donnell MP, Kim Y (1990) Injurious effects of low density lipoprotein on human mesangial cells. Kidney Int 37:509A.
15. Baud L, Hagege J, Sraer J, Rondeau E, Perez J, Ardaillou R (1983) Reactive oxygen production by cultured rat glomerular mesangial cells during phagocytosis is associated with stimulation of lipoxygenase activity. J Exp Med 158:1836–1852
16. Steinberg D, Parthasarthy S, Carew TE, Khoo JC, Witztum JL (1989) Modifications of low density lipoprotein that increase its atherogenicity. N Engl J Med 320:915–924
17. Kasiske BL, Cleary MP, O'Donnell MP, Keane WF (1985) Effects of genetic obesity on renal structure and function in the Zucker rat. J Lab Clin Med 106:598–604
18. O'Donnell MP, Kasiske BL, Cleary MP, Keane WF (1985) Effects of genetic obesity on renal structure and function in the Zucker rat II: Micropuncture studies. J Lab Clin Med 106:605–610
19. Schmitz PG, O'Donnell MP, Kasiske BL, Keane WF (1990) Glomerular capillary pressure is increased in old obese Zucker rats and is unchanged with enalapril. Kidney Int 37:520A.
20. Kasiske BL, O'Donnell MP, Cleary MP, Keane WF (1988)Treatment of hyperlipidemia reduces glomerular injury in obese Zucker rats. Kidney Int 33:667–672
21. Kasiske BL, O'Donnell MP, Garvis WJ, Keane WF (1988) Pharmacologic treatment of hyperlipidemia reduces glomerular injury in rat 5/6 nephrectomy model of chronic renal failure. Circ Res 62:367–374
22. Raij L, Azar S, Keane WF (1984) Mesangial immune injury, hypertension, and progressive glomerular damage in Dahl rats. Kidney Int 26:137–143
23. O'Donnell MP, Kasiske BL, Keane WF (1989) Risk factors for glomerular injury in rats with genetic hypertension. Am J Hypertens 2:9–13
24. O'Donnell MP, Kasiske BL, Schmitz PG, Katz SA, Keane WF (1990) Contrasting effects of lovastatin and enalapril and glomerular injury in Dahl salt-sensitive rats. Kidney Int 37:391A.
25. Hanchak NA, Karnovsky MJ, Diamond JR (1988) Cholestyramine resin lowers acute and recurrent proteinuria in chronic puromycin aminonucleoside necrosis. Kidney Int 33:376A.
26. Harris KPG, Purkerson ML, Yates J, Klahr S (1990) Lovastatin ameliorates the development of glomerulosclerosis and uremia in experimental nephrotic syndrome. Am J Kidney Dis 15:16–23
27. Schmitz PG, Kasiske BL, O'Donnell MP, Keane WF (1989) Lipids and progressive renal injury. Semin Nephrol 9:354–369
28. Kasiske BL, O'Donnell MP, Cleary MP, Keane WF (1989) Effects of reduced renal mass on tissue lipids and renal injury in hyperlipidemic rats. Kidney Int 35:40–48
29. Moorhead JF, Wheeler DC, Varghese Z (1989) Glomerular structures and lipids in progressive renal disease. Am J Med 87 (Suppl 5):12N–20N

Which Diet and When to Start It, in Patients with Chronic Renal Disease

Lamberto Oldrizzi, Carlo Rugiu, Vincenzo De Biase, and Giuseppe Maschio[1]

Summary. The effects of both early and late prescriptions of low-protein diets on the clinical course of chronic renal failure have been reviewed.

Many statistical tests showed that the clinical course of chronic renal failure was significantly worse in those patients to whom late conservative treatment was given.

This evaluation was carried out in an overall patient population of ($n = 450$) and in subjects with progressively declining renal function over time.

An analysis of the pros and cons of unsupplemented and supplemented low-protein diets is included in the second part of this review.

Introduction

Dietary treatment has been part of the conservative management of chronic renal failure (CRF) since the early 1960s. However, a renewed interest in the role of reduced protein intake has been shown in the last 10 years, mainly due to its regulating action on renal function when the nephron mass is reduced [1]. Nowadays, some important questions still remain to be answered regarding dietary treatment: when to use diets and how to use diets with CRF patients?

The presence in the early stages of CRF of well established functional and morphological damage [2] represents a valid motivation for early initiation of dietary protein restriction. Experimental evidence [3–7] exists that dietary treatment exerts the most positive effects when applied in the early stages of renal disease. Similarly, clinical studies [8] indicate a key role, at least as far as the progression of CRF is concerned, of early dietary treatment.

[1]Division of Nephrology, University of Verona, 37126 Verona, Italy

When to Diet

In line with these suggestions, we were looking for a value of renal function (we may call it "the point of no return") beyond which the positive effects of a low protein diet progressively decrease.

In general, we might discuss a zone, rather than a point, of no return; according to our 15-year clinical experience, we believe that such a zone should be identified within serum creatinine (SCreat) values ranging from 1.8 to 2.0 mg/dl.

This assumption is supported by a step-by-step statistical evaluation [9] performed on clinical data obtained from 450 patients with chronic renal failure, all kept on low protein diets.

Renal Survival Curves

Assuming a SCreat equal to or higher than 10 mg/dl to be "renal death," renal survival probability was computed by the Kaplan Meier method.

In the overall patient population, renal survival probability at 120 months was 62.4%. After stratifying the patients according to their initial SCreat values, two groups were identified regarding progression: patients with SCreat lower at the start than 1.8 mg/dl (EARLY group) and patients with SCreat higher at the start than 1.8 mg/dl (LATE group).

Renal survival probability at 120 months was found to be 79.1% in the EARLY group, whereas it was almost halved (48.4%) in LATE group patients. No overlapping in the relative survival trends was observed. The statistical comparison between the two curves was highly significant (Log Rank 33.96, Mantel 34.56, Wilcoxon 35.47, Prentice Peto 36.29 − P 0.0000).

General Characteristics

The follow-ups were, on average, nearly identical (57.9 vs 61.0 months) and there was no imbalance between the two groups regarding the underlying renal diseases.

Besides initial SCreat values (1.489 ± 0.198 vs 2.941 ± 1.135 mg/dl, t 18.81, P 0.000), the two groups differed in the duration of hypertension (22.8 ± 35.1 vs 32.1 ± 40.7 months − P 0.03), and duration of chronic renal failure (6.46 ± 15.01 vs 18.5 ± 25.6 months − P 0.000) before conservative treatment was started.

Clinical Course of CRF

The absolute increase in SCreat (1.623 ± 3.0 vs 3.176 ± 3.47 mg/dl, t 4.90, P 0.000), the monthly increase in SCreat (0.033 ± 0.07 vs 0.085 ± 0.114 mg/dl/month− t 5.77, P 0.000), and the percentage of patients requiring regular dialysis treatment (RDT) during follow-up (8.1% vs 30.6%, chi square 33.2, P 0.000) were significantly lower in the EARLY than in the LATE group.

The 95% confidence intervals of the mean monthly increase in SCreat in the two groups were 0.025–0.041 mg/dl per month (EARLY group) and 0.0725–0.0975 mg/dl per month (LATE group), respectively. As to the need for RDT, the outcome odds ratio between EARLY and LATE groups was 4.779; in other words, the risk of RDT within a 6-year follow-up was 5 times higher if conservative treatment had been delayed to a far advanced stage of CRF.

Multivariate Analysis

A statistical standardization (by dividing each single value for the SD of the mean) of all variables was required.

We plotted the monthly increase in SCreat (as an independent variable) against 35 variables, recorded at the start of follow-up on the low protein diet.

Multiple Regression Analysis

By means of a step-down procedure, we were able to identify two significantly independent variables: "entry" Screat (b 0.316, F 31.927) and duration of hypertension before conservative therapy (b 0.309, F 31.241) (r 0.482, P 0.000)

Cox Proportional Hazard Model

At variance with multiple regression, the Cox model pointed out one more prognostic factor: in addition to "entry" Screat (exp beta 1.81) and the duration of hypertension (exp 1.393), proteinuria (exp beta 1.66) was identified to negatively influence the course of CRF.

Selection of Patients with Proven Progressive CRF

It has been suggested that a definite percentage of patients with CRF may not experience any change in their renal function, regardless of conservative treatment [10]. In other words, there could be a population of patients affected with various renal diseases of a non progressive nature.

In order to eliminate this biasing factor, we decided to carry out the statistical analysis described above after removing from the sample those patients with no progression at all during follow-up (monthly increase in Screat lower than or equal to 0). This preliminary step cut out 116 of the 450 initial patients (60 from the EARLY and 56 from the LATE group).

Following the same procedural steps as those described above, we found that a preeminent influence on the history of CRF is the degree of functional deterioration present when dietary restriction is started.

Renal Survival Curves

Renal survival probability at 120 months was two times higher in the EARLY group, when compared with that observed in LATE group patients (69.2% vs 38.4% – Log

Rank 26.456, Mantel 27.00, Wilcoxon 28.273, Prentice Peto 28.94 – overall P 0.0000).

Clinical Course of CRF

Among the 334 selected patients, 72.6% of those in the EARLY group showed a very slow progression (monthly increase in Screat < 0.05 mg/dl per month), whereas only 36% of those in the LATE group had the same trend. The average monthly increase in Screat was significantly lower in EARLY (0.05±0.08 mg/dl per month) than in LATE patients (0.114±0.112 mg/dl per month) (*t* 5.76; P 0.000).

The 95% confidence intervals of the two means were 0.39–0.062 (EARLY) and 0.100–0.128 (LATE), respectively.

Seventeen patients in the early (12.8%) and 68 patients in the LATE group (39%) required RDT during follow-up. The outcome odds ratio was 4.377, a value quite close to that observed in the overall patient population and with the same prognostic implication as previously described.

Multivariate Analysis

Multiple regression analysis of standardized variables (step-down procedure) highlighted the influencing role of both "entry" Screat and duration of hypertension (F 31.3 and 22.49, respectively – *r* 0.476; P 0.000) on monthly increase in SCreat.

The Cox proportional hazard model confirmed the results obtained in the overall (*n*= 450) population (Scr exp beta: 1.774, U prot exp beta 1.554, hypertension exp beta 1.461).

The synopsis of this second statistical round may allow us to state that a positive role for an early dietary treatment is not overestimated by the presence of a hypothetical subgroup of non progressive patients.

Actually, a rough analysis of figures of survival rates, multivariate analysis, and odds ratios indicates the same risk of progression of CRF in the LATE group, either in the global or in the progressive patients' population.

Review

Clinical evidence exists to show that the natural history of patients with chronic renal failure is influenced by many factors, including conservative treatment of CRF.

Actually, this treatment means not only diet, but also administration of pharmacologic agents, more accurate and frequent clinical check-ups and, perhaps, significant changes in patients' life-style and mental habits [8,11]. But among the influencing factors, a critical one is the value of serum creatinine at which conservative treatment, namely a low protein diet, is prescribed. Thus, it appears useless or even dangerous for the patient to wait for a level of serum creatinine exceeding 1.8–2.0 mg/dl in order to make daily protein intake adequate to the reduced renal function. These conclusions, reached on a statistical basis, but also supported by daily empirical routine, put forward the second question. Which diet do we advise for patients with early CRF?

Which Diet?

In order to optimize the dietary treatment and thus the patients' compliance, two preliminary considerations have to be kept in mind: the characteristics of the diet and the patient's attitude toward the diet, this depending, in turn, on his/her psychosocial profile [11]. General guidelines for the dietary treatment of CRF must satisfy the following criteria: the diet must reduce the nitrogen intake, maintain nitrogen balance, cover essential aminoacid requirements, give a sufficient energy intake, and be palatable [11–13].

In line with these requirements, nephrologists face three possibilities: the unsupplemented low nitrogen diet with protein of high biologic value (HBV), the essential aminoacid supplemented diets and keto-acid supplemented diets.

Our experience with dietary treatment has been largely obtained with the use of the unsupplemented low-protein diet (LPD), mainly because we are convinced that this diet has some characteristics—namely palatability, simplicity, cheapness, long-term safety—which make it easy to follow, and therefore, well compliable. Thus its use appears suitable for early CRF patients [11].

However, we mustn't forget that the supplemented diets have been shown to be quite useful in renal patients, mostly in more advanced stages of CRF. Many positive effects have been obtained with these diets; however, a careful balance between the pros and cons suggests that their use in the very early stages of CRF is hardly suitable [14–18].

Pros	Cons
Slow progression rate	High Cost
No surface factor	Monotony
Improvement in metabolic state	Decreasing family support with time
Improvement of uremic neuropathy	Negative psychologic impact
Nitrogen sparing effect	Risk of malnutrition
Decrease in proteinuria	Careful and long lasting dietary education
Well-being of patients	Revolution in dietary habits
Decrease in S-PTH	Unknown effects on osteodystrophy

Turning to the LPD; this diet provides 35 KCal/kg body weight, 0.6 g/kg of proteins, 108 g/day of lipids, 320 g/day of carbohydrates, and 615 mg/day of phosphate. The requirements of trace elements and vitamins are satisfied [19].

With respect to proteins, 75% are HBV proteins. A quite peculiar characteristic of this diet is represented by the fact that 64% of the protein is of vegetable origin. The plant/animal protein ratio is 1.77, considerably higher than that recorded for current eating habits in European countries (< 1.0) [20]. Such a typical protein profile allows a low cholesterol and saturated fatty acid intake. While vegetable proteins have a slightly lower nutritive value than animal proteins, they might play a more effective protective role on the surviving nephrons, as already clinically and experimentally described [21,22].

The energy intake aims at well-established nutritional guidelines. As suggested by Kopple [23], patients with CRF who ingest 0.55–0.60 kg/kg of protein may have a neutral nitrogen balance and a reduced net urea generation only when the energy intake is above 30 KCal/kg per day.

The caloric support is given mainly by lipids (40%) and carbohydrates (53%). This division of energy supplies might arouse some controversy, since the fat and carbohydrate amounts are quite high. However, in the LPD, lipids are mostly of non-animal origin, the polyunsaturated to saturated fatty acid ratio is higher than 1, and the cholesterol intake is small. Moreover, there is no evidence that abnormalities of lipid metabolism in patients with CRF limit the usefulness of fat as an energy source.

Carbohydrates are provided as complex carbohydrates. The most likely metabolic effect of a high percentage of such substances in the diet is a direct effect on tryglyceride levels. Actually, the mean trygliceride level did not increase during follow-up in our patients, either in the EARLY or in the LATE groups.

At variance with some other more restricted low-protein diets [13], the essential aminoacid requirements are satisfied by this diet, which provides nearly 32 g/day of high biologic value proteins. A negative aspect might be, on the other hand, the quite high amount of sulfur-containing aminoacids, especially because of their acidotic effect [13].

Finally, we have to support our hypothesis that 0.6 g/kg (body weight i.b.w.), no more and no less, is the optimum protein intake for patients with early CRF.

Many previous studies have clearly demonstrated that the daily protein requirement in patients with CRF is close to 0.6 g/kg per day. In 1958 Herndorn demonstrated that to maintain a patient in nitrogen balance nearly 0.5 g/kg of protein was required, with the high/low quality protein ratio as high as 70%. These results were confirmed in the following years, by Giordano, Kerr, Ford, and Kopple [24].

On the other hand, in a self-controlled study [25] we have previously shown that patients with early CRF switched from 0.6 g/kg to a protein intake of 0.8–0.9 g/kg, under strict metabolic and dietary control, experienced a decrease in GFR and an increase in proteinuria over a 9-month period.

A diet providing less than 0.6 g/kg per day of protein and the same energy supply as the LPD, would probably have problems concerning negative nitrogen balance and would require, in order to be nutritionally adequate, some supplement with artificial foods. This latter fact might be linked with a progressively worsening compliance. Such a possibility seems, to some extent, supported by some data from the literature [26,27]: patients advised to have a protein intake of 0.4–0.5 g/kg showed, when urinary urea was checked, a daily protein intake averaging 0.6 g/kg. In our patients, compliance with the LPD is quite satisfactory and lasting over time. In this respect, we cannot sincerely deny that these results are improved by the similarity which exists between Italian dietary habits and the LPD scheme; the global figure, however, is impressive.

Moreover, nutritional data in a group of our patients [28] show that the supplies of the LPD are adequate for maintaining nutritional indices within normal ranges after a 5-year follow-up. On the other hand, the data also suggest that, if no care is paid to the caloric intake of patients, some nutritional parameters may worsen.

An unsupplemented low-protein diet is not like a panacea. Many problems are related to its use and the good results we showed you were not achieved as easily as it might appear. The following problems should be considered before starting a LPD program:

a) The scheme is fairly monotonous and implies a surface factor, due to the relatively small quantity of foods of animal origin.

b) Frequent clinical and dietary checks are required.
c) A careful survey of caloric intake is required, especially in younger patients.
d) As with supplemented diets, mental stress might arise over time due to some social limitations.
e) No information is available on the aminoacid muscle pattern in patients on long-term LPDs.
f) No protective effects have been shown in patients with nephrotic syndrome.

References

1. Mitch WE (1988) Nutritional therapy and the progression of renal insufficiency. In: Nutrition and the kidney, Mitch WE (ed) Little, Brown, Boston, pp 154–179
2. Diamond JR (1990) Effects of dietary interventions on glomerular pathophysiology. Am J Physiol 258:F1–F8
3. Ibels LS, Alfrey AC, Haut L (1978) Preservation of function in experimental renal disease by dietary restriction of phosphate. N Engl J Med 298:122–126
4. Friend PS, Fernandes G, Good RA, Michael AF, Yunis EJ (1978) Dietary restriction early and late. Effects on the nephropathy of the NZB × NZW mouse. Lab Invest 38: 629–632
5. Motomura K, Okuda S, Sanai T, Ando T, Onoyama K, Fujshima M (1988) Importance of early initiation of dietary protein restriction for the prevention of experimental progressive renal disease. Nephron 49:144–149
6. Nath KA, Hostetter M, Hostetter M, Hostetter TH (1986) Dietary protein restriction in established renal injury in the rat. J Clin Invest 78:1199–1205
7. Remuzzi G, Zoja A, Remuzzi A (1985) Low protein diet prevents glomerular damage in adryamicin treated rats. Proc Eur Dial Transplant Assoc 22:927–931
8. Maschio G, Oldrizzi L, Rugiu C (1989) Early dietary and nondietary intervention in chronic renal failure. Contrib Nephrol 70:163–171
9. Kramer MS (1988) Clinical epidemiology and biostatistics. Springer, Berlin, chapters 4–18
10. El Nahas AM, Coles GA (1986) Dietary treatment of chronic renal failure: ten unanswered questions. Lancet I:597–600
11. Oldrizzi L, Rugiu C, De Biase V, Maschio G (to be published) Factors influencing dietary compliance in patients with chronic renal failure on unsupplemented low-protein diet. Contrib Nephrol 81
12. Giovannetti S (1989) The purposes and rationale of nutritional treatment of chronic renal failure. In: Giovannetti S (ed) Nutritional treatment of chronic renal failure. Kluwer, Boston, pp 163–172
13. Gretz N, Lasserre JJ, Jerabek A, Strauch M (1989) Protein/aminoacid composition of low-protein diets. Contrib Nephrol 72:11–20
14. Lucas PA, Meadows JH, Roberts DE, Coles GA (1986) The risks and benefits of a low protein-essential amino acid -ketoacid diet. Kidney Int 29:995–1003
15. Druml W, Mitch WE (1988) Protein-restricted diets and progression of renal failure. Blood Purif 6:285–298
16. Persichetti S, Sagliaschi G, Clemenzia G, Bolletta A (1988) Considerazioni di psiconefrologia sulla dieta nella insufficienza renale cronica. Mienrva Med 79:1075–1078
17. Giovannetti S (1989) Supplemented diet for severe chronic renal failure: some controversial points. Contrib Nephrol 75:147–154
18. Strauch M, Gretz N (1988) Aminoacid and ketoacid supplements. In: Giovannetti S (ed) Nutritional treatment of chronic renal failure. Kluwer, Boston, pp 191–198

19. Maschio G, Oldrizzi L, Rugiu C (1986) The effects of protein restriction on the course of chronic renal failure. In: Mitch WE, Brenner BM, Stein JH (eds) The progressive nature of renal disease. Churchill and Livingstone, New York, pp 203–218
20. Strauch M, Lasserre JJ, Jerabek A, Gretz N (1989) The normal food intake. Contrib Nephrol 72:1–10
21. Wiseman MJ, Hunt R, Goodwin A, Gross JL, Keen H, Viberti GC (1987) Dietary composition and renal function in healthy subjects. Nephron 46:37–42
22. Williams AJ, Baker F, Walls J (1987) Effect of varying quantity and quality of dietary protein intake in experimental renal disease in rats. Nephron 46:83–90
23. Kopple JD, Monteon FJ, Shalb JK (1986) Effect of energy intake on nitrogen metabolism in nondialyzed patients with chronic renal failure. Kidney Int 29:734–742
24. Ford J, Phillips ME, Toye FE, Luck VA, de Wardener HE (1969) Nitrogen balance in patients with chronic renal failure on diets containing varying quantities of protein. Br Med J [Clin Res] 1:735–740
25. Oldrizzi L, Rugiu C, Maschio G (1989) Different protein diets in renal failure: a self-controlled study. Am J Nephrol 9:184–189
26. Rosman JB, Langer K, Brandl M, Piers-Becht TPM, van Derhem GK, ter Wee P, Donker AJM (1989) Protein restricted diets in chronic renal failure: a four years follow-up shows limited indications. Kidney Int 3(Suppl 27):S96–S102
27. Bergstrom J, Alvestrand A, Bucht H, Gutierrez A (1989) Stockholm clinical study on progression of chronic renal failure. An interim report. Kidney Int 36(Suppl 27):S110–S114
28. Guarnieri GF, Toigo G, Situlin R, Carrao M, Tamaro G, Lucchesli A, Oldrizzi L, Rugiu C, Maschio G (1989) Nutritional state in patients on long-term low-protein diet or with nephrotic syndrome. Kidney Int 36(Suppl 27):S195–S200

Low Protein Diet and Progression of Chronic Renal Failure: Results of Controlled Clinical Trials

N. GRETZ[1], S. GIOVANNETTI[2], and M. STRAUCH[1]

SUMMARY. As indicated by results from small scale trials, performed mostly in single centers, a low protein diet seems to delay the progression of chronic renal failure. Data from large scale controlled clinical trials, i.e., prospective randomized trials, are largely missing. Currently, quite a number of such trials are being conducted or are awaiting final evaluation. Preliminary data from the North Italian Trial seem to indicate that patients on a low protein diet display a much slower progression to end-stage renal failure than do patients on a free diet. This trial has a sufficient number of patients enrolled and thus exhibits considerable statistical value. The crucial point with all clinical trials is that due to the high number of patients needed they have to be multi-center trials. However, in such trials comparable degrees of compliance are difficult to achieve in the individual centers. Thus, with respect to this variable, a considerable center effect is a major confounding variable. Other problems in these trials are statistical in nature: a high rate of drop-outs has to be handled and the standard deviation of results has to be reduced by adequate stratification. A serious logistic problem arises in that it is difficult to recruit an adequate number of patients. In our opinion, however, it makes no sense to develop excellent statistical designs, to use refined methods of GFR determination, and to recruit an adequate number of patients, if sufficient dietary compliance cannot be achieved.

Introduction

Today, low protein diets (LPDs) are more and more frequently used in order to delay the progression of chronic renal failure (CRF). It is of note that earlier this century, Volhard [1] demonstrated that it was possible to postpone the increase of serum urea

[1]Clinic of Nephrology, Klinikum Mannheim, D-6800 Mannheim 1, Federal Republic of Germany
[2]1[a] Clinica Medica, Università di Pisa, I-56100 Pisa, Italy

concentrations for a prolonged period by restricting protein intake to 20 g, and allowing energy intake of at least 2000 kcal, per day. Thus, he was able to prevent uremic symptoms. When Kluthe, in 1974, pointed out for the first time that a LPD considerably delayed the progression of chronic renal failure, a new era in the use of these diets arose [2]. Subsequently, quite a number of studies have been performed. There has been, however, considerable criticism with respect to statistics, especially design problems and small sample size; there has also been criticism of the way GFR was determined and, recently, recognition of the fact that only poor compliance can be achieved. Despite that, most small single center trials have demonstrated that LPDs have a fair to excellent efficiency in delaying progression of CRF.

The aim of this paper is to survey observations on the impact of LPDs on the progression of CRF in controlled clinical trials. Before doing so, summarizing the results achieved so far from small scale trials seems to be warranted.

Results from Single Center Trials

In order to evaluate the results from single center trial, we introduced the so-called factor of delay (FD) [3]. The underlying idea was to have a comparable measure for all studies. Usually, different studies use quite different outcome measures, such as

Table 1. Summary of results obtained with different diets

Ref.	Diet		FD
	Protein	Phosphorus	
Early renal failure:			
[4]	C:free 95–125 g	1–1.8 g	1.5
	D:0.6 g/kg bw	12 mg/kg	
[4]	C:free 95–125 g	1–1.8 g	12.9
	D:0.6 g/kg bw	6 mg/kg	
[5]	C: 70 g	0.9 g	11.2
	D:0.6 g/kg bw	0.7 g	
Late renal failure: no supplement:			
[6]	C:free	?	2.3
	D:0.6 g/kg bw	0.6–0.7 g	
Late renal failure: eaa supplements			
[7]	C:40–60 g	?	10.5
	D:15–20 g	0.3–0.4 g	
[8]	C:0.5–0.7 g/kg bw	?	1.6
	D:0.5–0.7 g/kg bw	?	
Late renal failure: ka supplements:			
[9]	C:free	?	2.0
	D:0.4–0.5 g/kg bw	?	
[10]	C:0.6 g/kg bw	?	1.7
	D:0.4 g/kg bw	?	
[10]	C:0.4 g/kg bw	0.6–0.8 g	3.5
	D:0.4 g/kg bw	0.6–0.8 g	
[11]	C:0.3 g/kg bw	7–9 mg/kg bw	5.6
	D:0.3 g/kg bw	7–9 mg/kg bw	
[12]	C:1.2–1.4 g/kg bw	15–20 mg/kg bw	46.0
	D:0.2–0.6 g/kg bw	5–12 mg/kg bw	

Ref., reference number; Protein, protein intake; C, control; D, diet; FD, factor of delay

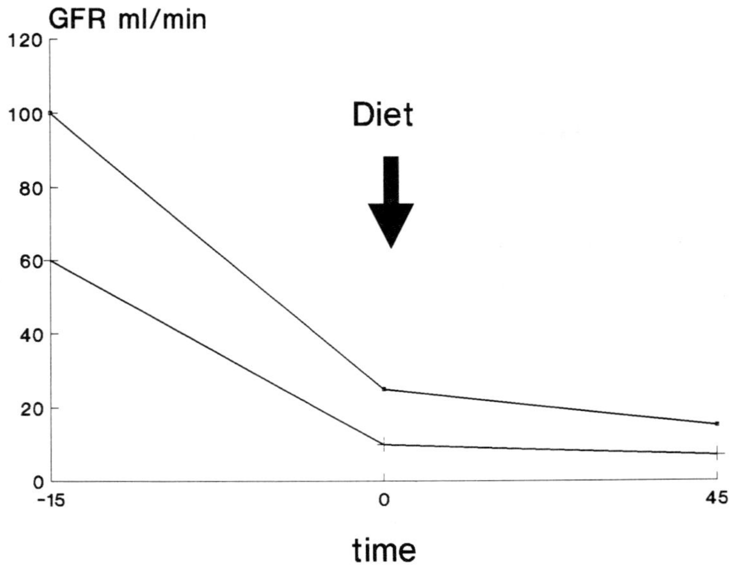

Fig. 1. Schematic drawing of the cross over of patients from free diet to LPD

1/SCR, creatinine clearance, or survival time, for the assessment of treatment efficiency. The FD is calculated as progression measure with diet, divided by progression measure without diet. Thus, the FD is the delay achieved with a LPD as a multiple of the progression in the control group. A list of studies providing data for control and treatment groups, thus allowing calculation of the FD, is shown in Table 1. From the table it is obvious that a wide scattering of FDs exists. It can, however, be concluded that at least an average FD of 2 can be achieved [4–12]. The trials presented, however, may be criticized for not being rigidly controlled clinical trials.

What is a "Controlled Clinical Trial?"

By definition the prerequisites for a controlled clinical trial are [13] that the study:

– is prospective,
– is randomized,
– contains a control group, and
– is double blind.

By definition, these trials are large scale, of necessity enrolling hundreds of patients. As it is impossible to recruit an adequate number of patients in a single center, controlled clinical trials are usually multicenter trials. Friedman et al. [13], however, noted that in some controlled clinical trials compromise was unavoidable. Thus, for example, a trial on dietary interventions can never be double-blind.

Cross Over Design in the Assessment of the Efficiency of LPDs

In some cases a cross-over design is used, thus the patient is his or her own control (Fig. 1). When applying such a design, the patient's decline in GFR is monitored before the start of a LPD and afterwards. Thereafter the rates of loss of GFR before and afterwards are calculated and compared. This cross over design, however, implies that all parameters influencing the progression of renal failure, e.g., blood pressure, hyperphosphatemia, hyperlipidemia, acidosis, etc., do not change while the disease progresses. This assumption, however, is highly improbable. On the other hand, such an analysis also implies that, as a linear regression analysis is used for the assessment of the slope of GFR, the decline in GFR is linear and an adequate and equal timing of blood sampling before and after start of LPD treatment is used. This, however, has only rarely been the case, as found when checking the literature. Despite these considerations, the cross-over approach is frequently used as the ensuing test statistics are reduced to a paired t-test and usually the sample size thought to be needed is fairly small. The significant P-values thus obtained, however, do not compensate for the inadequate design of studies. Thus, a cross over design is not suitable for assessment of the efficiency of a LPD in delaying the progression of CRF.

Stratification and Subgroups in Controlled Clinical Trials

From the statistical point of view, there is no way around the use of a prospective randomized trial, i.e., a controlled clinical trial, if the efficacy of a LPD in delaying the progression of CRF is to be analyzed. Thus, patients have to be randomly allocated to different types of treatment, e.g., no protein restriction, moderate protein restriction, or severe protein restriction. In order to reduce the often large standard deviation (SD) in these studies, adequate stratification before randomization is of utmost importance, as with larger SDs the size of sample needed increases (Fig. 2). As in patients with CRF different diets are used at different levels of renal function, it seems ethical to compare a LPD (e.g., 0.6 g/kg bw) in patients with good renal function versus patients with no protein restriction; while in the group with poor renal function, reducing protein intake in all subgroups seems to be warranted. Thus, the control group might be on a 0.6 g protein restricted diet while being compared with a group on a more restricted LPD with different amino acid or keto acid supplements. In addition to the stratification for renal function, in order to reduce SD, it seems appropriate to stratify for the underlying renal disease, as different renal diseases exhibit different progression rates [2,3,5]. Gender and age [14] are unsuitable as stratifying variables. This is underlined by the fact that in their final evaluation Rosman et al. [14] collapsed their initial strata into one group. It is, however, evident that the underlying renal disease, which to a certain extent is age and gender dependent, has a major impact on the average progression rate and differs from one renal

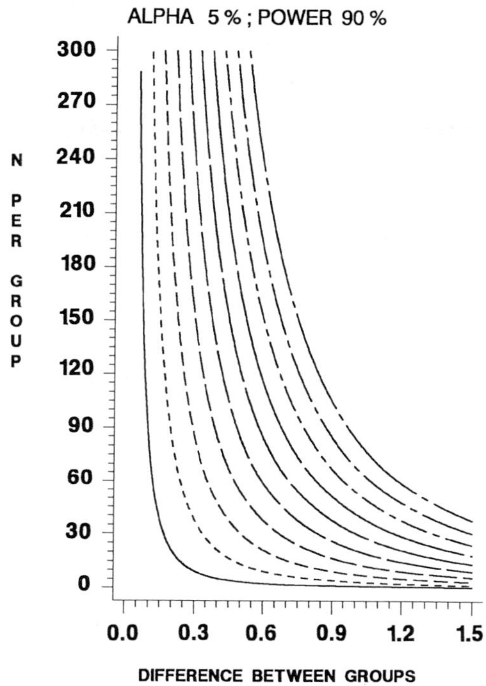

Fig. 2. Sample size calculation for given differences and standard deviations.

disease group to the other. Thus, ignoring this fact results in a considerable increase in the SD of the subgroups, or even results in missing an existing difference between groups.

Sample Size in Controlled Clinical Trials

The SD, however, is a major determinant for the sample size required in the study. Figure 2 shows the required sample size per subgroup on the y-axis, and the monthly difference in GFR (ml/min per month), between the groups on the x-axis. The individual curves represent the different SDs, starting from 0.1 (left curve) to 1 (right curve) in 0.1 steps. The diagram was calculated according to the formula given by Friedman et al. [13]. The assumptions used in this formula were also used for the calculation of the sample size in controlled clinical trials currently being conducted (see below).

Figure 2 may be used to recalculate whether, in a study, a difference between two groups of a given sample size really had the chance of being detected. The figure may also be used for the calculation of sample size in designing new trials. From the diagram it is obvious that in a trial where the impact of different LPDs on the progression of CRF is to be analyzed, sample sizes of at least 50–100 patients per subgroup are needed. Otherwise, the beta error, i.e., non detection of a difference between the groups, will be higher than ten percent.

Results from Multicenter Trials

Today, quite a number of controlled clinical trials are being conducted or are awaiting final evaluation. The 4 year follow up of the socalled Groningen Study [14] seems to provide a moderately optimistic view of the efficiency of the LPD in delaying the progression of CRF. It can be demonstrated, using survival analysis, that a significant difference between the control and the treatment group exists in the subgroup with poor renal function ($P=0.025$). Furthermore, the data seems to provide evidence that males benefit from LPDs, in contrast to females. As underlying renal disease influences progression rate, and the distribution of renal diseases is different in males and females, relating efficiency to gender seems inappropriate. The sex distribution in the different disease groups, however, is not given. Also the statement that only glomerular diseases benefit from a LPD is difficult to accept, as in this subgroup analysis, the sample size is sometimes extremely small. It is of note that in the analysis presented the problem of multiple testing might have confounded the results, as no adjustments for this problem were made, e.g., by using analysis of variance (ANOVA).

The preliminary results of the Northern Italian Trial, with a total enrollment of 456 patients, when evaluated using survival analyses, indicate that patients on 0.6 g protein restricted diets come to end-stage renal failure later than patients on a free protein intake [15]. This interpretation of the data presented seems to be valid, despite the fact that the calculated P-values sometimes reach only borderline significance. An analysis of the loss of renal function with respect to GFR slopes, however, it is still missing, as is the analysis of confounding factors.

None of the three ongoing trials: the French Cooperative Trial, the NIH-sponsored Modification of Diet in Renal Disease (MDRD) Trial, or the trial of the European Study Group for the Conservative Management of Chronic Renal Failure (ESG), can provide any data on progression. They will probably need some years to come to their projected end. In the meantime, the trial of the Medical Research Council of the United Kingdom has been cancelled, as the number of patients available for the study was too small.

Thus, there are only hints from one single center and from one multicenter trial that patients with chronic renal failure might benefit from low protein diets, insofar as progression to endstage renal failure is concerned. Final conclusions from large multicenter controlled clinical trials are still not available.

Major Problems in Ongoing Controlled Clinical Trials

The achievement of adequate compliance is probably the major difficulty found in ongoing controlled clinical trials. This is revealed by a survey of the literature (Table 2). In the ESG and MDRD trials an improvement of compliance, in the range of 0.2 g protein/kg body weight, has been noted over time. Rosman et al. [14] have also observed improved compliance over time. From the ESG and French Cooperative Study it became obvious that there was a considerable center effect with respect to compliance, indicating that the number of centers in a multicenter trial has to be as small as possible. This center effect also proves that it makes no sense to start dietary

Table 2. Compliance data from the literature

Ref.	Renal function	Protein intake (g/kg bw) Projected	Achieved[d]	Time of assessment
[16]	Good	Free	0.76 ± 0.47	Whole trial
		0.6	0.72 ± 0.66	
	Poor	0.6	0.68 ± 0.64	
		0.3[a]	0.63 ± 0.80	
[17]		Free	0.86[b] ± ?	18 months
		0.4	0.72[b] ± ?	
[18]	Good	1–1.4	1.04 ± 0.04	Whole trial
		0.58	0.91 ± 0.06	
		0.28[a]	0.69 ± 0.05	
	Poor	0.58	0.72 ± 0.03	
		0.28[a]	0.69 ± 0.03	
		0.28[a]	0.72 ± 0.03	
[14]	Good	Free	1.00[b] ± ?	18 months
		0.6	0.75[b] ± ?	
	Poor	Free	0.98[b] ± ?	
		0.4	0.86[b] ± ?	
[19]		Free	1.13 ± 0.26[c]	Whole trial
		0.55	0.67 ± 0.13[c]	

[a]Different amino/keto acid supplements
[b]Recalculated from figures in the paper, using Maroni's formula [19]
[c]Recalculated from SEM
[d]Means ± SD
Ref., reference number

management and a trial on the efficiency of a LPD at the same time in a center. This would result only in documentation of the process of learning dietary management.

Another problem is the recruitment of an adequate number of patients. The reader should be very concerned about results from small scale trials (see Fig. 2).

Acknowledgment. The authors appreciate the skillful help of Mrs. S. Redies in preparing the manuscript. Parts of this paper were made possible by grants from: Bundesministerium fuer Forschung und Technologie, FRG (Nr. 0704743).

References

1. Volhard F, Suter F (1931) Nieren und ableitende Harnwege. In: Mohr und Staehelin (eds) Handbuch der inneren Medizin, vol 5/1. Springer, Berlin, pp 804–811
2. Kluthe R, Oechslen D, Quirin H, Jesdinsky HJ (1972) Six years' experience with a special low-protein diet. In: Kluthe R, Berlyne G, Burton B (eds) Uremia. Thieme, Stuttgart, pp 250–256
3. Gretz N, Korb E, Strauch M (1983) Low-protein diet supplemented by keto acids in chronic renal failure: a prospective controlled study. Kidney Int 24(Suppl 16):S263–S267
4. Barsotti G, Giannoni A, Morelli E, Lazzeri M, Vlamis I, Baldi R (1984) The decline of renal function slowed by very low phosphorus intake in chronic renal patients following a low nitrogen diet. Clin Nephrol 21:54–59
5. Oldrizzi L, Rugiu C, Valvo E, Lupo A, Loschiavo C, Gammaro L, Tessitore N, Fabris A (1985) Progression of renal failure in patients with renal disease of diverse etiology on protein-restricted diet. Kidney Int 27:553–557

6. Bennet SE, Russel GI, Walls J (1983) Low protein diets in uraemia. Br Med J [Clin Res] 287:1344–1345
7. Alvestrand A, Ahlberg M, Bergstrøm J (1983) Retardation of the progression of renal insufficiency in patients treated with low-protein diets. Kidney Int 24(Suppl 16):268–272
8. Ando A, Orita Y, Nakata K, Fukuhara Y, Mikami H, Fujii M, Nakajima Y, Ueda N (1981) The effect of essential amino acid supplementation therapy on prognosis of patients with chronic renal failure estimated on the basis of the Markow process. Med J Osaka Univ 32:31–37
9. Gretz N, Meisinger E, Strauch M (1986) Influence of the underlying renal disease on the rate of progression. Contr Nephrol 53:92–101
10. Schmicker R, Frühling PT, Goetz KH, Kaschube I, Rakette I, Vetter K (1986) Influence of low protein diet supplemented with amino acids and keto acids on the progression of chronic renal failure. Contrib Nephrol 53:121–127
11. Walser M, LaFrance ND, Ward L, VanDuyn MA (1987) Progression of chronic renal failure in patients given ketoacids following amino acids. Kidney Int 32:123–128
12. Barsotti G, Ciardella F, Morelli E, Cupisti A, Mantovanelli A, Giovannetti S (1988) Nutritional treatment of renal failure in type 1 diabetes nephropathy. Clin Nephrol 29:280–287
13. Friedman LM, Furberg CD, DeMets DL (1982) Fundamentals of clinical trials. John Wright, PSG, Boston
14. Rosman JB, Langer K, Brandl M, Piers-Becht TPM, van der Hem G, ter Wee PM, Donker AJM (1989) Protein-restricted diets in chronic renal failure: A four year follow-up shows limited indications. Kidney Int 36(Suppl 27):S96–S102
15. Locatelli F (1989) Controlled study of protein-restricted diet in chronic renal failure. Contrib Nephrol 75:141–146
16. Giovannetti S, Gretz N, Attman PO, D'Amico G, Frühling PT (1990) Dietary compliance in the trial of the European Study Group: a preliminary analysis. Contrib Nephrol 81:61–70
17. Ihle BU, Becker GJ, Whitworth JA, Charlwood RA, Kincaid-Smith PS (1989) The effect of protein restriction on the progression of renal insufficiency. N Engl J Med 321:1773–1777
18. Kopple JD, Berg R, Houser H, Steinman TI, Teschan P (1989) Nutritional status of patients with different levels of chronic renal insufficiency. Kidney Int 36(Suppl 27):S184–S194
19. Walker JD, Bending JJ, Dodds RA, Mattock MB, Murrells TJ, Keen H, Viberti GC (1989) Restriction of dietary protein and progression of renal failure in diabetic nephropathy. Lancet II:1411–1415

Dietary Protein Restriction Retards Progressive Renal Failure in Type I Diabetes

KATHLEEN ZELLER[1], ELAINE WHITTAKER, LYNN SULLIVAN, PHILIP RASKIN, and HARRY R. JACOBSON[2]

Introduction

Diabetes mellitus is currently the leading cause of end-stage renal disease in the United States. Approximately 50% of patients with Type I (or insulin-dependent) diabetes mellitus develop progressive renal insufficiency, despite attempts to vigorously control blood sugar and treat co-existing hypertension [1–6]. Data accumulated from a number of studies in experimental animal models of diabetes, as well as data from models of other forms of progressive renal failure, have suggested that, despite different underlying disorders, the progression of renal disease may have a significant hemodynamic component and may be slowed by a reduction in dietary protein, and possibly phosphorus, intake [7–19]. Glomerular micropuncture studies performed in a number of models, but most commonly in rats subjected to subtotal nephrectomy or rats rendered diabetic with streptozotocin treatment, reveal that single nephron glomerular plasma flow is increased, as is glomerular capillary hydrostatic pressure. While some controversy exists, it is felt that these hemodynamic changes contribute to the progressive renal damage seen in these animal models. Dietary protein restriction has been shown to not only slow the progression of glomerular sclerosis and renal failure in these animal models, but also to normalize the elevated glomerular plasma flow and capillary hydrostatic pressure. Based on these observations, a number of clinical studies on humans have been performed [20–24].

Many reports have suggested that there is a beneficial effect of dietary protein and phosphorus restriction in humans with various forms of renal disease. The rates of progression of renal failure have been reduced from 2 to 10-fold in patients on a low protein diet [20–24]. Most of these studies, however, have been retrospective and uncontrolled and have dealt with patients exhibiting a variety of renal diseases. To

[1]Department of Internal Medicine, Center for Human Nutrition, University of Texas Southwestern Medical Center, Dallas, TX 75235, USA
[2]Division of Nephrology, Vanderbilt University Medical Center, Nashville, TN 37232, USA

address a potential beneficial role for dietary protein restriction in renal disease, we elected to study a single disease entity, namely Type I diabetes mellitus, which is known to cause progressive renal insufficiency in approximately 50% of patients with this disorder. We performed a prospective, randomized, controlled study, evaluating dietary protein restriction on the progression of renal failure in 35 subjects with Type I diabetes mellitus.

Methods

Patient Selection

Patients between the ages of 18 and 60 years, who had documented Type I diabetes mellitus with onset before the age of 30, were recruited for this study. Patients required evidence of diabetic nephropathy, manifested by significant proteinuria, concurrent retinopathy, and the absence of other potential causes for renal failure. All patients had initial glomerular filtration rates between 15% and 85% of predicted norms, as measured by ^{125}I iothalamate clearance. Patients who had a contraindication to a low protein diet, such as severe infection, malignancy, or pregnancy, and patients who had brittle, difficult to control diabetes, were excluded. All patients required a follow-up of at least 12 months for inclusion in the analysis.

We originally enrolled 47 patients with Type I diabetes mellitus in the study. Out of this initial group, 35 patients were able to comply with the study requirements and have been followed for a minimum of 12 months. A total of 6 patients were dismissed from the study for inability to comply; 2 of these were in the control group and 4 were in the low protein intake group. Two additional patients, one from each group, were dropped from the study subsequent to their move from the Dallas area. An additional control patient was excluded from the study after development of severe congestive heart failure, secondary to a myocardial infarction, and an additional patient on the low protein diet died suddenly and unexpectedly shortly after enrollment. Finally, 2 patients randomized to the low protein diet, on repeated occasions during which dietary protein intake was calculated from urine area nitrogen measurements, were shown to be non-compliant with the diet, i.e., they were consuming in excess of the 0.8 gm/kg per day cutoff. These patients were excluded from analysis with the remaining patients on the low protein diet. However, their results were analyzed separately. Baseline characteristics for the patients in both groups are summarized in Table 1. The groups did not differ with respect to mean age, initial glomerular filtration rate, or initial 24 hour urine protein excretion.

Table 1. Patient characteristics

	Control (15)	Low protein (20)	*P*
Age (years)	35 ± 2	33 ± 2	NS
Initial GFR (ml/min per 1.73m^2)	48.8 ± 7.1	46.3 ± 4.8	NS
Initial proteinuria (mg/24 h)	4266 ± 715	3144 ± 417	NS

Study Diet

Subjects were randomized to one of two diets. The low protein group consumed a diet containing 25–40 kcal/kg ideal body weight (IBW) per day with 0.6 gm/kg IBW per day protein, which was 70%–80% of high biologic value. The urinary losses of albumin were replaced gram for gram by increasing dietary protein intake. The diet also contained 2 grams of sodium, 500–1000 mg phosphorus and 1000 mg calcium. All subjects received a standard multi-vitamin preparation. Patients in the control group consumed their pre-study diet, with the stipulation that it contained 2 gms of sodium, 1000 mg of phosphorus, and $\geq$ 1 gm/kg IBW per day protein.

Measurements

Upon enrollment into the study, all patients underwent a complete history and physical examination, baseline renal function studies, dietary histories, determination of nutritional status, and measurement of glycemic control. Glomerular filtration rate was estimated by a number of parameters, including measurement of serum creatinine, collection of 24 hour urine for creatinine clearance, and measurement of radioisotopic tracer glomerular filtration rate, using ^{125}I iothalamate. Dietary protein intake was calculated by adding non-urea nitrogen losses (estimated at 31 mg/kg real body weight) to the measured urine urea nitrogen (UUN) and was adjusted for proteinuria [25]. A 24 hour urine collection was also made for measurement for sodium, potassium, calcium, and phosphorus. Nutritional status was evaluated by anthropometric measurements, determination of complete blood count, total protein and albumin. Diabetic control was assessed by measurements of glycosylated hemoglobin (HbA_{1c}), using high performance liquid chromatography [26] and lipid status was determined by measurements of serum cholesterol, triglycerides, and lipoproteins, via spectrophotometric analysis [27]. The laboratory measurements were performed monthly for three months and at three month intervals thereafter. Iothalamate determinations of glomerular filtration rate were performed at enrollment and at 3–6 month intervals. Iothalamate clearance determination was a standard procedure in our Renal Clinic and was performed as described previously [28]. Subjects were given an oral water load of 20 ml/kg and 10 drops of saturated solution of potassium iodine was administered to prevent thyroid uptake of radiolabelled iodine. Subsequently, ^{125}I labelled iothalamate was injected subcutaneously; clearance determinations were begun 60 minutes later. Three 30 min urine collections were obtained and were bracketed by collection of plasma samples for determinations of ^{125}I iothalamate. Urine and plasma were counted in an Abbott Autologic Gamma Counter and iothalamate clearances were calculated using the standard clearance formula. In some patients, significant scattering of clearance values between collection periods was observed, suggesting a problem with bladder emptying. In these patients, clearances were repeated after the insertion of a Foley catheter. The overall coefficient of variation for the iothalamate clearances was 8.4%.

At every visit, blood pressure was measured in the supine, sitting, and upright position, in the same arm. Every effort was made to maintain systemic blood pressure at a value of 140/85 mm/Hg or lower and patients were seen as often as weekly to obtain good blood pressure control. The use of angiotensin-converting enzyme (ACE) inhibitors was specifically avoided whenever possible, and only 2 patients received ACE inhibitors. As stated earlier, compliance with the prescribed dietary protein intake was assessed by repeated dietary history and measurement of UUN. Patients in the low protein group with protein intakes persistently > 0.8 gm/kg per day, or control patients with protein intakes persistently < 1 gm/kg per day were excluded from analysis.

Statistical Analysis

Data were analyzed, using ISP Software developed by the staff of the Academic Computering Services and by the General Clinical Research Center's statistician, using CLINFO and BMDP. The rate of decline of glomerular filtration rate was analyzed by three methods. First, regression lines for 1/serum creatinine were generated. Second, creatinine and iothalamate clearances over time were determined and mean slopes were calculated by regression analysis. Finally, initial renal function and final renal function, as assessed by creatinine clearance and iothalamate clearance, were determined and divided by the time interval between the measurements. When multiple values for a given parameter were obtained within a three month interval, the values were meaned to provide a single three month data point. The Student's two-tail *t* test was used to compare data between treatment groups if the variances were the same, and the Mann Whitney (MW) u test was used if they were not. Stepwise regression was performed, using data from the total study population, with the dependent variable being a change in glomerular filtration rate and the independent variables being protein intake, blood pressure, and hemoglobin A_{lc}.

Results

Progression of Renal Failure

The iothalamate clearances for the treatment and control groups are depicted in Fig. 1. The mean regression line for the groups is indicated by the "dashed" line. Those patients ingesting a low protein diet exhibited a rate of decline in renal function approximately four times slower than that exhibited by patients ingesting a normal protein diet. Numerical data are summarized in Table 2, where the reciprocal serum creatinine, the rate of decline of GFR with creatinine clearance, and the rate of decline of GFR with iothalamate clearance are depicted. The rate of decline of renal function was significantly slower in the low protein group, as assessed by iothalamate clearance (P = 0.02 by MW u test). Also, the rate of decline of renal function, as assessed by creatinine clearance, reached significance by *t*-test (P = 0.03). The rate of decline of renal function, as assessed by the reciprocal serum

Table 2. Decline in renal function assessed by linear regression analysis

	Control (15)	Low protein (20)	*P*
1/Cr ($1\mu Mol^{-1}mo^{-1} \times 10^6$)	-0.97 ± 0.27	-0.39 ± 0.15	NS
Creatinine clearance (ml/min per month)	-0.81 ± 0.20	-0.33 ± 0.12	<0.05
Iothalamate clearance (ml/min per month)	-1.01 ± 0.31	-0.26 ± 0.10	<0.05
Mean follow-up (months)	31.4 ± 2.5	37.1 ± 3.1	

Table 3. Changes in 24 h urinary protein excretion (mg/24 h)

	Control	Low protein
Initial	4266	3144
3 Months	5194	2384
Final	5290	2948

creatinine, was not statistically significant. When the data were expressed as a difference between initial and final clearances divided by time, the results were essentially the same. Of note, the two patients originally randomized to the low protein intake group, but whose mean protein intakes averaged 0.86 and 0.80 grams/kg per day were excluded from the overall data analysis, but had very stable renal function over a mean follow-up period of 44.5 months.

We subjected the data to analysis according to sub-groups of patients with initial glomerular filtration > or < 45 ml/min per 1.73 meters². In patients with GFR > 45 (n = 18, mean GFR 66.1 $\pm$ 4.1), the rate of decline of renal function, as assessed by the linear regression analysis of iothalamate clearances, was 0.003 $\pm$ 0.1 ml/min per month in patients ingesting the low protein diet. However, in patients ingesting the control diet, the rate of decline of GFR was 0.67 $\pm$ 0.22 ml/min per month (P = < 0.05). The data were not different when expressed as the difference between initial and final iothalamate clearances divided by time. In patients with an initial glomerular filtration rate < 45 ml/min per 1.73 meters² (n = 15, mean GFR 27.5 $\pm$ 2.0), the rate of decline of renal function was 0.51 $\pm$ 0.13 ml/min per month for patients in the low protein group and 1.41 $\pm$ 0.62 ml/min per month in patients ingesting the control diet. The difference between these two values, while large, did not quite make statistical significance.

Proteinuria

Approximately three months after initiation of the diet, urinary protein excretion in the protein restricted patients had fallen by a mean of 760 mg/24 h, whereas 24 h urine protein excretion in the control group had increased by 928 mg/24 h. At the conclusion of the study, the low protein intake patients had a mean 24 h urine protein excretion rate that was 196 mg/24 h less than their initial value, whereas the control group had a significantly elevated 24 h urine protein excretion rate that was 1024 mg/24 h above their initial value (Table 3).

Dietary Compliance

Protein intake over the entire study period was calculated for each patient from the UUN and was normalized for IBW. Control patients ingested a mean of 1.08 $\pm$ 0.10 gm/kg per day of protein, while protein restricted patients consumed a mean of 0.72 $\pm$ 0.06 gm/kg per day. Compliance, when expressed as the % intake in excess of that prescribed for each patient, came to 11% $\pm$ 2.3% over a mean follow-up of 37.1 months.

Sodium and potassium intake were estimated by 24 h urine collections and were not significantly different between the two dietary groups. However, in both groups the 24 h urine sodium excretion exceeded the prescribed 2000 mg/day.

Table 4. Effects of low protein diet on nutritional status

	Body weight (Kg)	Mid-arm muscle circumference (cm)	Albumin (g/l)
	+ 0.40 ± 0.77	+ 0.04 ± 0.30	+ 0.80 ± 0.90
P	NS	NS	NS

Diabetes Control

The hemoglobin A_{1c} in control patients throughout the study was 8.0% ± 0.4% and was not significantly different from the mean value on the low protein intake of 7.8% ± 0.2% (normal < 5.1%). There was no significant adjustment in the insulin requirements in either group.

Blood Pressure Control and Patient Visits

The average mean arterial pressure for control patients was 105.5 ± 0.9 mm/mercury, compared to 102.5 ± 1.2 mm/mercury in the protein restricted patients. This very small difference was significant at the P = 0.05 level. However, the contribution of this small blood pressure difference to the rate of progression of renal disease is likely to be minor.

Previous investigators have suggested that there is an inverse relationship between the number of patient visits with the physician and the rate of progression of chronic renal disease [30]. In the present study, the patients on the low protein diet were seen 10.6 ± 1.0 x/year, whereas control patients were seen 13.0 ± 1.8 x/year. This difference in patient visits was not significant.

Nutritional Parameters

Whether or not the prolonged intake of a low protein diet has adverse nutritional effects in subjects with Type I diabetes has not been evaluated. The results of those parameters followed in the present study—body weight, mean mid-arm circumference, and serum albumin—are listed in Table 4. The data are presented after one year follow-up because all patients were followed for a minimum of 12 months. It should be noted that in patients on low protein intake there were no significant changes in these parameters throughout the length of the study.

Listed in Table 5 are the lipid parameters, again after a follow-up period of 12 months. There were no significant changes in the serum cholesterol, triglycerides, or the LDL to HDL ratio.

Table 5. Effects of low protein diet on lipid status

	Initial	1 Year	*P*
Cholesterol (mMol/L)	5.1 ± 0.3	5.3 ± 0.3	NS
Triglycerides (g/l)	1.83 ± 0.33	2.05 ± 0.35	NS
LDL/HDL	2.91 ± 0.27	2.85 ± 0.25	NS

Discussion

A number of studies, in a number of experimental models of renal disease, have evaluated the efficacy of dietary protein restriction in preventing progressive renal failure and the associated hemodynamic changes thought to induce progression, (i.e., hyperfiltration) [7–16]. These experimental models include hypertension [10], renal mass ablation [8, 11–15], and diabetes [9]. A number of clinical trials in humans have suggested that there is a beneficial effect of protein and phosphorus restriction on the progression of renal failure, but the results of these trials have been challenged on several grounds [31,32]. Most studies have examined patient populations heterogeneous with respect to the cause of renal failure. In addition, in most studies, glomerular filtration rate has not been measured by what are currently the most acceptable and valid techniques, i.e., inulin clearance or radioisotopic tracer clearance, such as that of ^{125}I iothalamate. Indeed, many of these studies have relied on measurements of serum creatinine or on the determination of reciprocal serum creatinine, neither of which are accurate measures of glomerular filtration rate, especially when there is reduced intake of protein [33]. In addition, most of these studies have not reported anthropometric data to provide evidence for or against adequate maintenance of muscle mass and, presumably, nitrogen balance. While some studies have reported creatinine clearances, it is well known that this measurement may over-estimate GFR in patients with advanced renal insufficiency or decreasing muscle mass [34]. This is the first study which has assessed the impact of dietary protein intake on renal function, as determined by a well accepted technique for measuring GFR.

An additional advantage of the present study over previous reports is that compliance with the dietary protein intake was closely monitored by urine urea nitrogen measurements. In most previous studies, dietary compliance has been assessed predominantly by dietary history, which method is known to be inaccurate.

Finally, it is apparent that in the retrospective studies which have been reported previously, other uncontrolled variables may have played significant contributory roles in the progression of renal failure. This is especially true of blood pressure and, possibly, of sodium intake. The present study, because of its prospective design, paid attention to equally aggressive blood pressure control in both groups, as well as to equalization of dietary sodium intake.

The present study was specifically designed to address the effect of dietary protein intake on a single disease entity, namely, Type I diabetes mellitus. It was felt that choosing a single disease would increase the sensitivity of the study and, of course, the selection of diabetes is appropriate, since it is a major contributor to end-stage renal disease in the United States. The results of our study clearly demonstrate that a low protein diet can significantly influence the course of progressive diabetic nephropathy. The patients in the treatment group exhibited a four-fold decrease in the rate of progression of their chronic renal failure when compared to control patients. At the same time, nutrition has been well maintained and there has been no evidence of any dietary-related complications in nutritional status, diabetes control, or blood lipid control.

Previous studies [1,2] have shown that blood pressure control can reduce the progression of renal failure in Type I diabetic patients with clinical nephropathy. We observed a slight, but significant, difference in mean arterial pressure, of 3 mm/

mercury, between the treatment and control groups in the present study. While this may contribute somewhat to the difference in the rate of progression of renal failure, if one extrapolates from previous studies, where significant slowing of the decline of renal function was seen with reductions of mean arterial blood pressure of 12–14 mm/mercury, it is clear that the small differences in blood pressure cannot account for the major difference in the rate of renal function decline between the two groups.

While the present study clearly shows a beneficial effect of reduced dietary protein intake on progressive nephropathy of Type I diabetes, it cannot address the mechanism responsible for this beneficial effect. While the popular theory of hyperfiltration as the cause of progression, and the prevention of hyperfiltration by the low dietary protein intake, could explain our findings, we have no data to support this. Also, it is important to point out that while we are quite confident about our results, a tremendous amount of physician, nurse, and dietician effort is required to maintain a population of patients on such a dietary regimen. Thus, the practical and cost implications of such an approach should be considered. Also of importance is the fact that our subgroup analysis revealed that a beneficial effect of dietary protein restriction could be seen in patients with a mean initial glomerular filtration rate of 66 ml/min. Whether a beneficial effect can be seen in patients with even higher GFRs is unknown. Finally, we feel that a more complete understanding of the mechanisms responsible for the beneficial effect of dietary protein restriction will be important in helping to design possible alternative approaches, i.e., pharmacologic approaches, which can mimic the functional effects of low dietary protein intake.

References

1. Mogensen CE (1982) Long-term antihypertensive treatment inhibiting progression of diabetic nephropathy. Br Med J [Clin Res] 285:685–688
2. Parving HH, Anderson AR, Smidt UM, et al. (1983) Early aggressive antihypertensive treatment reduces rate of decline of kidney function in diabetic nephropathy. Lancet I:1175–1178
3. Knowles HC Jr (1974) Magnitude of the renal failure problem in diabetic patients. Kidney Int 6:1–7
4. Deckert T, Poulsen JE, Larsen M (1978) Prognosis of diabetics with diabetes onset before the age of thirty-one. Diabetologia 14:363–370
5. Dorman JS, LaPorte RE, Kuller LH, et al. (1984) The Pittsburgh insulin-dependent diabetes mellitus (IDDM) morbidity and mortality study. Diabetes 33:271–276
6. Anderson AR, Sandahl-Christiansen J, Anderson JK, Kreiner S, Deckert T: Diabetic nephropathy in type I (insulin-dependent) diabetes (1983) An epidemiological study. Diabetologia 25:496–501
7. Farr LE, Smadel JE (1939) The effect of dietary protein on the course of nephrotoxic nephritis in rats. J Exp Med 70:615–627
8. Hostetter TH, Olson JL, Rennke HG, Venkatachalam MA, Brenner BM: Hyperfiltration in remnant nephrons (1981) A potentially adverse response to renal ablation. Am J Physiol 241:F85–F93
9. Wen SF, Huang TP, Moorthy AV (1985) Effects of low-protein diet on experimental diabetic nephropathy in the rat. J Lab Clin Med 106:589–597
10. Dworkin LD, Feiner HD (1986) Glomerular injury in uninephrectomized spontaneously hypertensive rats. A consequence of glomerular capillary hypertension. J Clin Invest 77:797–809

11. Kenner CH, Evan AP, Blomgren P, Aronoff GR, Luft FC (1985) Effect of protein intake on renal function and structure in partially nephrectomized rats. Kidney Int 27:739–750
12. Kleinknecht C, Salusky I, Broyer M, Gubler MC (1979) Effect of various protein diets on growth, renal function and survival of uremic rats. Kidney Int 15:534–541
13. Laouari D, Kleinknecht C, Gubler MC, Broyer M (1983) Adverse effect of protein on remnant kidney. Dissociation from that of other nutrients. Kidney Int 24(Suppl 16):S248–S253
14. El-Nahas AM, Paraskevakou H, Zoob S, Rees AJ, Evans DJ (1983) Effect of dietary protein restriction on the development of renal failure after subtotal nephrectomy in rats. Clin Sci 65:399–406
15. Kikuchi H, Matsushita T, Hirata K (1983) Improved dietary treatment with low protein and phosphorus restriction in uremic rats. Kidney Int 24(Suppl 16):S254–S258
16. Neugarten J, Feiner HD, Schacht RG, Baldwin DS (1983) Amelioration of experimental glomerulonephritis by dietary protein restriction. Kidney Int 24:595–601
17. Ibels LS, Alfrey AC, Haut L, Huffer WE (1978) Preservation of function in experimental renal disease by dietary restriction of phosphate. N Engl J Med 298:122–126
18. Karlinsky ML, Haut L, Buddington B, Schrier NA, Alfrey AC (1980) Preservation of renal function in experimental glomerulonephritis. Kidney Int 17:293–302
19. Lumlertgul D, Burke TJ, Gillum DM, et al. (1986) Phosphate depletion arrests progression of chronic renal failure independent of protein intake. Kidney Int 29:658–666
20. Maschio G, Oldrizzi L, Tessitore N, et al. (1982) Effects of dietary protein and phosphorus restriction on the progression of early renal failure. Kidney Int 22:371–376
21. Barsotti G, Morelli E, Giannoni A, Guiducci A, Lupetti S, Giovanetti S (1983) Restricted phosphorus and nitrogen intake to slow the progression of chronic renal failure: A controlled trial. Kidney Int 24(Suppl 16):S278–S284
22. Mitch WE, Walser M, Steinman TI, Hill S, Zeger S, Tungsanga K (1984) The effect of a keto acid-amino acid supplement to a restricted diet on the progression of chronic renal failure. N Engl J Med 311:623–629
23. Rosman JB, ter Wee PM, Meijer S, Piers-Becht TP, Sluiter WJ, Donker AJ (1984) Prospective randomized trial of early dietary protein restriction in chronic renal failure. Lancet II:1291–1296
24. Evanoff GV, Thompson CS, Brown J, Weinman EJ (1987) The effect of dietary protein restriction on the progression of diabetic nephropathy. A 12-month follow-up. Arch Intern Med 147(3):492–495
25. Maroni BJ, Steinman TI, Mitch WE (1985) A method for estimating nitrogen intake of patients with chronic renal failure. Kidney Int 27:58–65
26. Nathan DM, Raskin P (1984) A convenient automated method for high performance liquid chromatography measurement of glycated (glycosylated) hemoglobin. Clin Chem 30:813–814
27. Petri A, Dunn FI, Raskin P (1980) The effect of improved diabetic control on plasma lipid and lipoprotein levels: A comparison of conventional therapy and continuous subcutaneous insulin infusion. Diabetes 29:1001–1005
28. Israelit AH, Long DL, White MG, Hull AR (1973) Measurement of glomerular filtration rate utilizing a single subcutaneous injection of ^{125}I-iothalamate. Kidney Int 4:346–349
29. Diabetic Retinopathy Study Research Group. Diabetic Retinopathy Study Report number 6. Design, methods, and baseline results. (1981) Invest Ophthalmol Vis Sci 21(1, pr2):149–209
30. Bergstrom J, Alvestrand A, Bucht H, Guttierrez A (1986) Progression of chronic renal failure in man is retarded with more frequent clinical follow-ups and better blood pressure control. Clin Nephrol 25:1–6
31. Zeller KR, Jacobson HR (1989) Reducing dietary protein intake to retard progression of diabetic nephropathy. Am J Kidney Dis 13(1):17–19

32. El Nahas AM, Coles GA (1986) Dietary treatment of chronic renal failure: Ten unanswered questions. Lancet I:597–600
33. Mitch WE (1984) Nutritional therapy in renal failure. Annu Rev Med 35:249–264
34. Schuster VL, Seldin DW (1985) Renal clearance. In: Seldin DW, Giebisch G (eds) The kidney: physiology and pathophysiology, vol 1. Raven, New York, pp 365–395
35. Walser M, Drew HH, LaFrance ND (1988) Creatinine measurements often yield false estimates of progression in chronic renal failure. Kidney Int 34:412–418

Proposed Mechanisms for Changes in Progression by Dietary Manipulation

WILLIAM E. MITCH[1]

SUMMARY. It has been known for at least 50 years that manipulation of the diet of rats with chronic renal disease slows progression of the disease. Understanding the mechanism for this effect could lead to modifications that would amplify any benefit proven effective in humans with renal disease. Proposed mechanisms can be divided into 1) nephrotoxicity of a constituent of the diet, including phosphate and lipids and 2) damage resulting from adaptive changes which occur in response to renal failure. The latter include hemodynamic, hypertrophic, and metabolic changes. Extensive investigation in rats has not yielded consistent results. In humans, even less is known, but tempting hypotheses include nephrotoxicity from excess dietary protein, plus a link to hypertension and hormonal responses.

Introduction

More than 50 years ago, it was shown that manipulation of the diet could affect the severity of progressive kidney damage, chronic renal failure (CRF), in rats subjected to subtotal nephrectomy or other types of experimental renal disease [1]. The mechanism for this effect remains obscure, but over the last several years growing evidence indicates that dietary manipulation can exert a similar beneficial effect in humans with progressive renal failure. Understanding the mechanism is important because the protective effect could be magnified by making more specific changes in the diet. Unfortunately, there is controversy surrounding the cause of progressive renal damage in even the most simple model: rats with renal failure after subtotal nephrectomy (the remnant kidney model). There is no uniform agreement about which nutrient(s) promotes progressive renal damage. It is not difficult to understand, therefore, why there is no uniform agreement about the cause of progressive damage in humans or about the way in which changing the diet could ameliorate the

[1]Renal Division, Emory University School of Medicine, Atlanta, GA 30322, USA

loss of renal function. I will assess the evidence that mechanisms proposed from studies in rats apply to humans with CRF.

Proposed mechanisms for the effect of dietary manipulation can be divided into groups: those related to a toxic effect of specific components of the diet; those related to adaptive responses to loss of kidney function; and those not obviously related to the diet.

Nephrotoxicity of the Dietary Constituents

In early studies of normal rats, it was noted that long-term feeding of a diet rich in liver, meat, or casein was associated with pathological damage to the kidney and loss of renal function. Moise and Smith documented that a high-casein diet (and hence, excess phosphorus) was associated with the development of glomerular and tubular lesions in uninephrectomized rats [1]. Chanutin and Ludewig showed that the severity of renal pathology, hypertension, and loss of renal function was related to the percentage of dried meat fed to remnant-kidney rats [2]. Subsequently, the opposite was noted, namely that restriction of dietary protein limited proteinuria and histological damage, preserved renal function, and prolonged survival even when renal damage was produced by immunologic methods [2,3]. Similar results have been obtained more recently. Since protein was restricted, one conclusion is that dietary protein led to accumulation of a nephrotoxin arising from metabolism of the protein. Another hypothesis was that the "work" required to excrete metabolites of excess protein led to kidney damage. To date, no nephrotoxin has been identified, nor is there persuasive evidence for the "renal work" hypothesis.

The only dietary nephrotoxin that has been manipulated experimentally is phosphate intake. The link with a high-protein diet is that such diets are almost invariably associated with a high phosphate intake. It has been suspected for many years that precipitation of calcium phosphate causes progressive deterioration of renal function and would account for interstitial rather than glomerular damage in experimental renal disease [4,5]. In 1937, Donohue and associates reported that excessive calcium deposition in residual renal tissue of remnant-kidney rats could be blocked by parathyroidectomy [6]. Ibels et al. reported that restriction of dietary phosphorus (plus aluminum hydroxide) in remnant-kidney rats preserved renal function and histology as well as survival [7]. One problem was that renal function was monitored by changes in serum creatinine, but low-phosphate diets induce weight loss so serum creatinine may not have accurately reflected renal function. To circumvent this problem, Lumlertgul et al. fed a normal diet plus a phosphate binder to remnant-kidney rats and found that rats receiving the phosphate binders exhibited less proteinuria and histologic damage and had improved renal function and survival [8]. In another manipulation, 3-phosphocitrate (an inhibitor of calcium phosphate precipitation and tissue calcification) dramatically limited calcium disposition and interstitial disease [9]. Collectively, the results suggest a prominent role for dietary phosphorus in progressive renal insufficiency in rats. However, the importance of dietary phosphate has been questioned. Critics argue that any benefit of low dietary phosphorus is due to reduced food and/or protein intake. Tapp and associates studied remnant-kidney rats, which were carefully pair-fed, in order to examine the influence of protein and food intake independently [5]. Note that pair-feeding has not been routine in many studies of progression in rats, hence interpretation of results is suspect. It was concluded that restriction of food intake prevented the development of end-stage renal pathology, regardless of whether dietary protein was restricted and it was concluded that mediators of growth might play an important role in this response.

In humans with CRF, it has been difficult to test the influence of dietary phosphate for two reasons: firstly, it is virtually impossible to restrict dietary phosphate without restricting protein, since foods rich in phosphate are generally rich in protein; and secondly, it is difficult to add phosphorus to the diet because of concern about inducing secondary hyperparathyroidism. Barsotti et al. fed the same low-protein diet to two groups of patients who also received either 6.5 or 12 mg phosphorus/kg per day [10]. Patients who had a low urinary phosphorus had no change or an improvement in creatinine clearance while those with values above 400 mg/day had a decrease in clearance. Although these results are impressive, they need to be confirmed.

Hyperlipidemia and Progression

Manipulation of the diet to avoid excess dietary protein (or phosphorus) could change the intake of other important nutrients such as lipids. Similarities between mesangial and smooth-muscle cells, which are so important in the pathogenesis of atherosclerosis, have led to the proposition that lipid accumulation in mesangial cells could stimulate proliferation and could ultimately induce focal glomerulosclerosis [11]. A central theme is that persistent proteinuria stimulates production of abnormal lipoproteins which perpetuate the proteinuria and promote glomerular damage.

Attempts to test the hypothesis by manipulating dietary lipids in rats have shown variable and sometimes conflicting results. A high-cholesterol diet has been associated with focal glomerulosclerosis in guinea pigs and in the obese Zucker rat; such a diet also seems to aggravate glomerular sclerosis in rats treated with puromycin. Other evidence for a nephrotoxic effect of dietary lipids includes decreased focal glomerulosclerosis in the remnant kidney model of rats treated with antihyperlipidemic drugs [11]. Exercise training of partially nephrectomized rats lowers serum lipids and decreases proteinuria and focal glomerulosclerosis.

Fatty acid metabolites could be mediators of progressive renal damage. Administration of a thromboxane synthesis inhibitor to remnant-kidney rats was associated with functional and histologic improvement [11]. However, a diet enriched with the arachidonic acid precursor, linoleic acid, had variable effects; in mice with immune complex nephritis [12] and in remnant-kidney rats, linoleic acid-enriched diets were reported to preserve renal function; other investigators report no beneficial effect of the regimen [13]. In mice genetically predisposed to develop immune-mediated nephropathy, a diet enriched with fish oils prevented proteinuria and increased survival, yet the same diet was associated with functional and histologic deterioration in remnant-kidney rats [14]. The mechanism for these conflicting effects induced by different types of polyunsaturated fatty acids is unknown.

For humans with renal disease, evidence that dietary lipids play an important pathogenetic role is lacking. Renal insufficiency is not a prominent feature of diseases associated with hypercholesterolemia. It is also disturbing to note that addition of specific lipids to the diet of rats has yielded such conflicting results.

Adaptive Responses and the Loss of Renal Function

The Hyperfiltration Hypothesis

In the 1980s it was proposed that the progressive loss of renal function in remnant-kidney rats was caused by the adaptive increase in glomerular perfusion which increased the function of less severely affected nephrons. Glomerular capillary hydrostatic pressure was associated with glomerulosclerosis. A link to the diet was provided when it was shown that protein restriction largely prevented glomerular capillary hypertension, proteinuria, and glomerular sclerosis [15]. Angiotensin II has been studied most intensively as a mediator of efferent arteriolar vasoconstriction. For example, remnant-kidney rats treated with an angiotensin converting enzyme inhibitor (CEI) had less systemic hypertension, nearly normal glomerular capillary hydrostatic pressure, and importantly, less proteinuria and glomerular damage than rats treated with a combination of reserpine, hydralazine, and hydrochlorothiazide [16]. A low-protein diet and CEI therapy has also been reported to benefit remnant-kidney rats given high doses of glucocorticoids and rats with diabetes mellitus.

In spite of the attractiveness of these experiments, other conditions have been studied in which glomerular sclerotic changes can be dissociated from glomerular hemodynamics. In rats given aminonucleoside drugs to induce proteinuria and sclerosis, administration of CEI reduced the degree of glomerular sclerosis without affecting intraglomerular pressure [17]. These studies employed a novel and technically demanding method of making serial measurements of glomerular hemodynamics in a single nephron, in order to analyze the relationship between glomerular hypertension and sclerosis; however the studies yielded no correlation between glomerular sclerosis and single nephron GFR (SNGFR) or glomerular pressure. These investigators also reported that enalapril and standard antihypertensive therapy (reserpine, hydralazine and hydrochlorothiazide) were equally effective at reducing glomerular sclerosis following subtotal nephrectomy, despite the more impressive reduction in glomerular pressure with enalapril [18]. In their view, glomerular hypertrophy appeared to be the primary determinant of sclerosis, hence growth stimuli cause progressive loss of renal function. Finally, a thromboxane synthesis inhibitor reduced systemic blood pressure, but markedly increased renal plasma flow and SNGFR in remnant-kidney rats [11]. Yet, in spite of hyperfiltration, treated rats had less proteinuria and glomerular damage than untreated rats, so stimuli other than glomerular capillary hypertension seemed to cause renal damage.

Besides these inconsistencies, there is the important question of how closely the subtotal nephrectomy model mimics the pathophysiology of CRF in humans. Many of the experiments have been performed in strains of rats with a high incidence of spontaneous glomerular sclerosis. Moreover, when dogs were subjected to 75% nephrectomy and followed for four years, renal pathology was minimal. Preliminary results from adult baboons fed high- vs low-protein diets and followed for one year after subtotal nephrectomy, showed no difference in progression despite a modest increase in proteinuria [19]. This raises the possibility that there may be important species differences with respect to the influence of dietary protein on renal function and morphology.

To assess the influence of adaptive changes in glomerular hemodynamics on progressive kidney damage in humans, normal subjects or CRF patients were fed a high-protein meal and changes in renal blood flow and GFR were measured. Bosch and associates concluded that CRF patients had little or no response because glomerular hemodynamics were maximally stimulated even in the resting state [20]. There have been a plethora of these studies, but few show such striking results. Hostetter evaluated the response to a meal consisting of 3.5 g protein/kg body weight and found that 4 of 10 patients had no increase in GFR above basal values [21]. Chan and associates performed an even more extensive analysis of the renal response to a high-protein meal and reached similar conclusions [22]. It should be emphasized that period to period measurements of GFR in humans have inherent variability (as expected with any biologic measurement). This fact raises questions about conclusions based on comparing baseline with the "peak" value following a high-protein meal.

The second method of assessing the influence of glomerular dynamics has been to evaluate renal function in patients with a unilateral nephrectomy. In kidney donors (who develop a compensatory increase in single kidney GFR and who are, presumably, eating a normal diet), there seems to be a slightly higher incidence of hypertension but little evidence for progressive renal failure [23].

Glomerular Hypertrophy

Following subtotal nephrectomy, there is a hypertrophic response and the development of glomerulosclerosis [11]. The diet could participate in the hypertrophic response because dietary protein modulates glomerular size in normal animals; high- or low-protein diets increase or decrease, respectively, the renal hypertrophy which occurs after nephrectomy or experimental diabetes. Although glomerular hypertrophy has been linked to abnormal glomerular hemodynamics, experimental support for this theory is lacking [18]. Administration of CEI to remnant-kidney rats markedly reduces glomerular hypertrophy which, according to some authors, is the primary determinant of sclerosis. In rats, Yoshida et al. performed a left nephrectomy, and either diverted the right ureter into the peritoneal cavity or performed a 2/3 right nephrectomy [24]. Despite a comparable degree of glomerular hypertension in both groups, glomerular hypertrophy and sclerosis was greater in remnant-kidney rats, suggesting that the loss of nephrons, and not simply the loss of excretory function, stimulates glomerular hypertrophy.

Nephron Hypermetabolism

Another hypothetical mechanism is based on the increase in cellular metabolism stimulated by loss of renal function. Remnant-kidney rats had increased oxygen consumption, which could not be accounted for by sodium reabsorption; the difference was eliminated in rats treated by verapamil or dietary phosphate restriction [4]. It was suggested that "nephron hypermetabolism" increases free radicals and membrane lipid damage, resulting in tubulointerstitial nephritis. The beneficial effect of verapamil suggested that changes in intracellular calcium, and hence abnormal signaling processes, are involved in the development of progressive renal damage. However, others find verapamil does not protect against progressive damage in the remnant-kidney model [25].

Intraglomerular Coagulation

A proposed mechanism that has little apparent relationship to the diet involves intraglomerular coagulation. Intraglomerular thrombosis is present in the remnant kidney and in glomeruli after immunologically-mediated nephritis is induced in rats. In similar models, anticoagulants or inhibitors of platelet aggregation can be shown to reduce glomerular injury and progression, suggesting that coagulation may contribute to loss of glomerular capillaries [11]. Fibrin deposits are found in glomerular capillaries of some patients with rapidly progressive glomerulonephritis and, apparently, the survival of platelets in subjects with membranoproliferative glomerulonephritis is shortened [26].

It is, therefore, interesting that heparin, independently of its anticoagulant properties, limits glomerulosclerosis in the remnant-kidney model. Since heparin also has antiproliferative properties [11], the beneficial effect may be due to suppression of mesangial growth and expansion.

Progression in Patients with Chronic Renal Failure

From the foregoing discussion, it should be obvious that the cause of progressive renal insufficiency in humans is not known. Two potential mechanisms have been suggested: damage from hypertension and damage from excess glucocorticoids. There is evidence that hypertension reduced GFR in experimental glomerulonephritis, even though glomerular morphology was unaffected [27]. In spite of these experimental results and results from patients with diabetic nephropathy, there is scarce evidence that hypertension exerts an important influence on the progression of renal disease in humans. Lindeman and associates found that hypertension was significantly correlated with the decline in creatinine clearance in elderly patients with evidence of renal dysfunction [28]. The association was weak, however, since only about 9% of the decline in clearance could be attributed to variation in mean blood pressure. Recently, Brazy et al., in a retrospective analysis of dialysis patients, reported that blood pressure was related to changes in renal function [29]. They found that patients with more rapid rates of progression had higher levels of systolic and diastolic blood pressure. Importantly, they also found that control of diastolic pressure below 90 mmHg was associated with slowing of the loss of renal function. The role of diet in these changes is unclear. Dietary restriction could limit intake of salt or some other factor causing hypertension. Alternatively, attention to the diet, with more frequent visits to the physician, could influence blood pressure control (and hence deterioration of renal function).

Finally, Walser and Ward reported that changes in GFR in CRF patients were related to the rate of excretion of glucocorticoid which in turn, was related to the type of diet; a ketoacid regimen was associated with the most benefit [30]. It seems unlikely that these results can be explained by the same factors shown to cause nephropathy in remnant-kidney rats, because the steroid dose used experimentally was quite high [31].

In summary, the exciting possibility that the diet can slow the loss of renal function in CRF patients has been widely studied in rat models, primarily in the remnant-kidney model. Several mechanisms have been proposed, but experiments in humans have lagged far behind. At present, there is no widely accepted explanation for the effect of dietary manipulation on preservation of renal function.

Acknowledgment. This work was supported by NIH grant DK 37175 and DK 40907.

References

1. Moise TS, Smith AH (1927) Effect of high protein diet on the kidneys. Arch Pathol Lab Med 4:530–560
2. Chanutin A, Ludewig S (1936) Experimental renal insufficiency produced by partial nephrectomy. V. Diets containing whole dried meat. Arch Intern Med 58:60–80
3. Farr LE, Smadel JE (1940) The effect of dietary protein on the course of nephrotoxic nephritis in rats. Am J Pathol 16:615–627
4. Schrier RW, Harris DCH, Chan L, Shapiro JI, Caramelo C (1988) Tubular hypermetabolism as a factor in the progression of chronic renal failure. Am J Kidney Dis 12:243–249
5. Tapp DC, Wortham WG, Addison JF, Hammonds DN, Barnes JL, Venkatachalam MA (1989) Food restriction retards body growth and prevents end-stage renal pathology in remnant kidneys of rats regardless of protein intake. Lab Invest 60:184–195
6. Donohue W, Springarn C, Pappenheimer AM (1937) The calcium content of the kidney as related to parathyroid function. J Exp Med 66:697–701
7. Ibels LS, Alfrey AC, Haut L, Huffer W (1978) Preservation of function in experimental renal disease by dietary restriction of phosphate. N Engl J Med 298:122–126
8. Lumlertgul G, Burke TJ, Gillum DM, Alfrey AC, Harris DC, Hammond WS, Schrier RW (1986) Phosphate depletion arrests progression of chronic renal failure independent of protein intake. Kidney Int 29:658–666
9. Gimenez L, Walker WG, Tew WP, Hermann JA (1982) Prevention of phosphate-induced progression of uremia in rats by 3-phosphocitric acid. Kidney Int 22:36–41
10. Barsotti G, Giannoni A, Morelli E (1984) The decline of renal function slowed by very low phosphorus intake in chronic renal patients following a low nitrogen diet. Clin Nephrol 21:54–59
11. Klahr S, Schreiner G, Ichikawa I (1988) The progression of renal disease. N Engl J Med 318:1657–1666
12. Kher V, Barcelli U, Weiss M, Pollak VE (1985) Effects of dietary linoleic acid enrichment on induction of immune complex nephritis in mice. Nephron 39:261–267
13. Keane WF, Kasiske BL, O'Donnell MP (1988) Hyperlipidemia and the progression of renal disease. Am J Clin Nutr 47:157–160
14. Scharschmidt LA, Gibbons NB, McGarry L, Berger P, Axelrod M, Janis R, Ko YH (1987) Effects of dietary fish oil on renal insufficiency in rats with subtotal nephrectomy. Kidney Int 32:700–709
15. Hostetter TH, Olston JL, Rennke HG, Venkatachalam MA, Brenner BM (1981) Hyperfiltration in remnant nephrons. Am J Physiol 241:F85–F93
16. Anderson S, Rennke HG, Brenner BM (1986) Therapeutic advantage of converting enzyme inhibitors in arresting progressive renal disease associated with systemic hypertension in the rat. J Clin Invest 77:1993–2000
17. Fogo A, Yoshida Y, Glick AD, Homma T, Ichikawa L (1988) Serial micropuncture analysis of glomerular function in two rat models of glomerular sclerosis. J Clin Invest 82: 322–330
18. Yoshida Y, Kawamura T, Ikoma M, Fogo A, Ichikawa L (1989) Effects of antihypertensive drugs on glomerular morphology. Kidney Int 36:626–635

19. Bourgoignie JJ, Gavellas G, Hwang KH, Disbrow MR, Sabnis SG, Antonovych TT (1989) Renal function of baboons (*papio hamadryas*) with a remnant kidney, and impact of different protein diets. Kidney Int. 36:S86–S90
20. Bosch JP, Lauer A, Glabman S (1984) Short-term protein loading in assessment of patients with renal disease. Am J Med 77:873–879
21. Hostetter TH (1986) Human renal response to a meat meal. Am J Physiol 19:F613–F618
22. Chan AYM, Cheng ML, Keil LC, Myers BD (1988) Functional response of healthy and diseased glomeruli to a large, protein-rich meal. J Clin Invest 81:245–254
23. Bay WH, Hebert LA (1987) The living donor in kidney transplantation. Ann Intern Med 106:719–727
24. Yoshida Y, Fogo A, Ichikawa I (1989) Glomerular hemodynamic changes vs hypertrophy in experimental glomerular sclerosis. Kidney Int 35:654–660
25. Brunner FP, Thiel G, Hermle M, Bock HA, Mihatasch MJ (1989) Long-term enalapril and verapamil in rats with reduced renal mass. Kidney Int 36:969–977
26. Donadio JV, Anderson CF, Mitchell JC, Holley KE, Ilstrup DM, Fuster V, Chesebro JH (1984) Membranoproliferative glomerulonephritis: A prospective clinical trial of platelet-inhibitor therapy. N Engl J Med 310:1421–1426
27. Blantz RC, Gabbai F, Gushwa LC, Wilson CB (1987) The influence of concomitant experimental hypertension and glomerulonephritis. Kidney Int 32:652–663
28. Lindeman RD, Tobin JD, Shock NW (1984) Association between blood pressure and the rate of decline in renal function with age. Kidney Int 26:861–868
29. Brazy PC, Stead WW, Fitzwilliam JF (1989) Progression of renal insufficiency: Role of blood pressure. Kidney Int 35:670–674
30. Walser M, Ward L (1988) Progression of chronic renal failure is related to glucocorticoid production. Kidney Int 34:859–866
31. Garcia DL, Rennke HG, Brenner BM, Anderson S (1987) Chronic glucocorticoid therapy amplifies glomerular injury in rats with renal ablation. J Clin Invest 80:867–874

Renal Diseases in Asia

Chair: Visith Sitprija (Thailand)
Wan-Yu Chen (Taipei, China)

Hepatitis B Virus Infection and Primary Glomerular Disease

LEISHI LI, JINHONG ZHANG, and ZHIHONG LIU[1]

SUMMARY. Since the first report of a possible pathogenetic association between persistent antigenemia and membranous Australian glomerulonephritis (GN) in 1951, the implications of hepatits B virus (HBV) on the pathogenesis of primary glomerular disease, particularly in the Asian region, have been extensively discussed.

Now the association of the HBV infection with membranous nephropathy (MN) in children is well established. There is a close relationship between the frequency of the HBsAg carrying state in MN and the underlying prevalence of HBsAg carriage in the general population. The HBV-MN in children is also unique in its clinical presentation, serology, and immunopathology, with HBeAg as the dominant type of HBV antigen deposited in glomeruli.

However, the investigation of HBV-GN relied mainly upon the demonstration of HBV specific antigens in the glomeruli which was subject to many technical errors and discrepancies. Opinions about the pathogenetic association between HBV and other types of primary GN (PGN) are still controversial.

Introduction

Since the first report of a possible pathogenetic association between persistent Australian antigenemia and membranous GN in 1951 [1], many studies have demonstrated the presence of HBsAg, HBeAg, and HBcAg in glomerular deposits of various morphological patterns [2,3]. The implications of HBV on the pathogenesis of PGN, particularly in the Asian region, have been extensively discussed.

In this review, we will briefly appraise the association of HBV infection with PGN, its incidence and salient features, and in particular, the experience obtained from China, in order to re-evaluate the significance of HBV infection on the immunopathogenesis of PGN [4–6].

[1]Department of Nephrology, Jinling Hospital, Nanjing University Medical School, Nanjing 210002, People's Republic of China

Evidence for the Etio-Pathogenetic Association of HBV Infection with PGN

Frequency of HBV Carriers among Patients with PGN

Statistics have shown that there is a greater than expected incidence of chronic HBsAg carriers among patients with MN, mesangio-capillary GN (MCGN) and, less frequently, mesangio-proliferative GN (MsPGN) (Fig. 1). Although the total positive rate of HBsAg antigenemia among PGN patients is not different from that in the general population, yet interestingly, HBV carriage in children with MN is in mutual relationship with the underlying prevalence of HBsAg carriage in the local region (Table 1). Also, the prevalence of MN among different types of PGN in children increases in relation to the rising frequency of HBV antigenemia in the local population. For instance, in Poland and China, where HBV antigenemia prevails, 86.7%–91.3% of children with MN are HBV carriers and MN accounts for 22%–28% in the whole group of PGN, values much higher than those in U.S.A. [3,5] (Table 2). This indicates a strong association between childhood MN and HBV infection. However, the frequency of HBsAg carriage in adults with MN is still significant but of a less magnitude (Table 3).

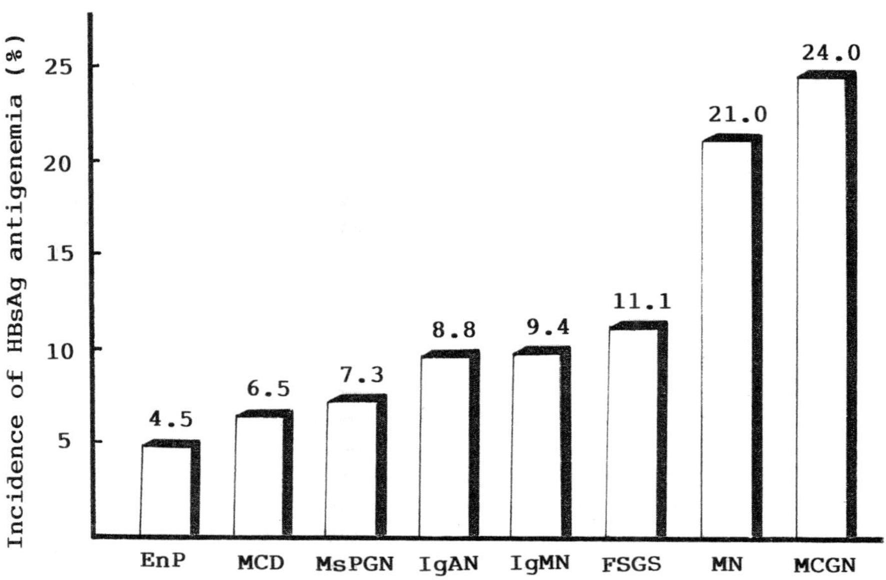

Fig. 1. Incidence of HBs antigenemia in 1375 Chinese patients with various types of PGN. EnP, endocapillary proliferative GN; MCD, minimal change disease; MsPGN, mesangio-proliferative GN; IgAN, IgA nephropathy; IgMN, IgM nephropathy; FSGS, focal segmental glomerular sclerosis; MN, membranes nephropathy; MCGN, mesangiocapillary glomerulonephritis

Table 1. Incidence of MN and HBV-MN in children

Country	Incidence of MN among PGN	Frequency of HBV-MN among children with MN
USA (Southwest Pediatric Nephrol Study Group, 1985)	5.5%	20%
China (Gou, 1989)	14.6%	86.7%
Poland (Slusarczyk, 1989)	23.5%	91.3%

MN, membranous nephropathy; HBV, hepatitis B virus; PGN, primary glomerular diseases

Regarding the types of serum HBV markers in PGN, there seem to be no significant differences between the positive rates of various HBV markers. Practically speaking, HBsAg is the type of serum marker most commonly recorded in the literature [7].

Demonstration of HBV Antigens in Glomerular Immune Deposits

Based on collective data in the literature, up to 1989 a total of 1578 patients with various GN with HBsAg antigenemia had been examined for HBV antigens in their glomerular immune deposits, among whom 497 patients (31.5%) showed positive results.

Three distinct antigens, HBsAg, HBcAg, and HBeAg were detected by immunofluorescence (IF) or immunoperoxidase (IP) techniques in renal biopsies from these patients. Different authors had conflicting reports on the nature and frequency of the glomerular HBV antigens which were identified in various glomerulopathic entities. Data are shown collectively in Figs. 2 and 3. More sophisticated assays, and the application of monoclonal antibodies have led to the strong suggestion that HBeAg is the dominant type of HBV antigen deposited in HBV-MN, and that HBsAg is common in MCGN [8,9,10].

Both HBeAg and HBsAg are large (10^6 daltons) in size and are anionic. They are of a size that is unlikely to penetrate the basement membrane into the subepithelial space. HBeAg, a part of viral nucleoprotein, was found in two forms, with molecular weights of 19000 and 300000. These two forms are also anionic, but induce anti-HBeAg, which are largely cationic (PI 5.8–10.2), that can shift the pI of HBeAg from 4.3–4.8 to the 6.4–8.4 range (bound to anti-HBe). HBeAg circulating immune

Table 2. Incidence of HBsAg antigenemia in children with MN

Country	General carrier rate (%)	HBsAg +ve (%)
USA	0.1–1.0	20
France	0.1–1.0	42
Italy	0.1–1.0	64
Poland	5–10	91–92
Japan	2–20	57–81
South Korea	10–15	80
China	10–15	86
South Africa	10–20	89–100
Hong Kong	10–20	94–100
Taiwan	10–20	100

MN, membranous nephropathy

Table 3. Incidence of HBsAg antigenemia in adults with MN

Country	Author	General carrier rate	n	+ve (%)
Great Britain	Rashid (1981)	1%	28	1(4.0)
Scotland	Mactier (1986)	1%	54	0(0)
France	Cahen (1989)	1%	69	0(0)
Hungary	Nagy (1979)	1–5%	17	3(18.0)
Hong Kong	Lai (1982)	5–10%	23	10(43.0)
Taiwan	Chen (1990)	20%	28	3(10.7)
South Korea	Lee (1988)	2–20%	49	10(20.4)
China	Li (1990)	10–15%	105	22(21.0)

MN, membranous nephropathy

complexes (CICs) are also small (2.5×10^5 daltons) and thus might be capable of localizing in the subepithelial space. HBeAg CICs have been identified in 44% of children with HBV-MN, and appear to correlate with disease activity. The potential importance of HBeAg in HBV-MN is further supported by observations that circulat-

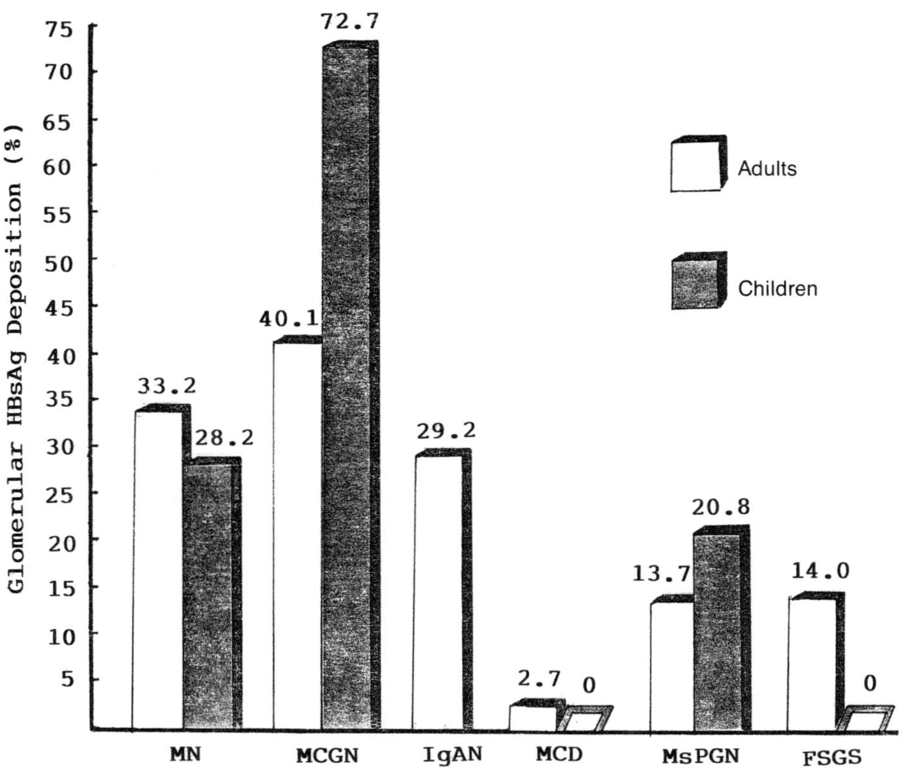

Fig. 2. Cumulative data on glomerular HBsAg deposition in various types of PGN. MN, membranous nephropathy; MCGN, mesangiocapillary glomerulonephritis; IgAn, IgA nephropathy; MsPGN, mesangio-proliferative GN; FSGS, focal segmental glomerular sclerosis

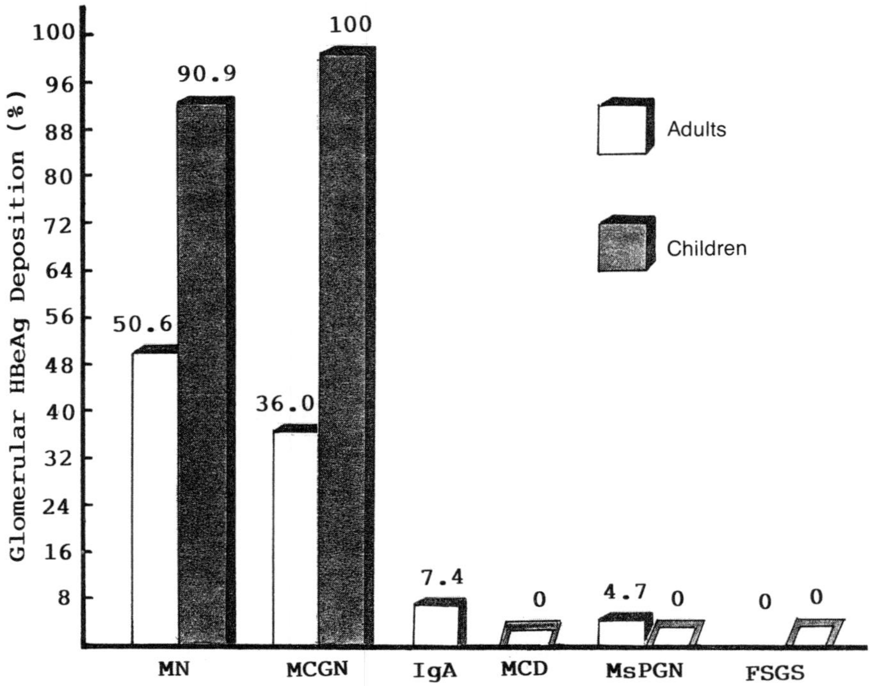

Fig. 3. Cumulative data on glomerular HBeAg deposition in various types of PGN. MN, membranous nephropathy; MCGN, mesangiocapillary glomerulonephritis; IgAN, IgA nephropathy; MCD, minimal change disease; MsPGN, mesangio-proliferative GN; FSGS, focal segmental glomerular sclerosis.

ing HBeAg frequently correlates with the activity of the disease and is the major antigen in the immune deposits [6,7,8,11].

Viral-like particles have been identified on electronic microscopy in the subepithelial and subendothelial areas of the glomerular basement membrane (GBM) as well as within endothelial cells, epithelial cells and mesangium [3]. Renal tissue elution studies have also shown that the glomerular bound Ig in HBV-MN contained antibody to HBV antigens, particularly to HBeAg [12].

The results of in situ hybridization study of HBV-DNA in glomeruli are conflicting. Lai et al. [6] confirmed its presence in 2 of the 6 cases studied, but Zhang [9] and Yu failed to prove its presence.

Controversies on HBV Associated GN

Some of the previous reports emphasized that in patients with glomerular diseases there is a significantly higher incidence of HBs antigenemia than that in the general population or in hospitalized patients, suggesting that HBsAg carriers were predisposed to glomerular disease. But survey statistics of large series collected from HBV endemic areas including China, Korea, and Taiwan did not confirm this phenomenon. In other words, the prevalence of GN in HBV carriers is not higher than that in the general population [10,13].

Although a number of authors reported that HBsAg or HBcAg could be identified by direct or indirect IF or IP techniques in the glomeruli of GN patients associated with HBV antigenemia, others could not confirm such observations [13]. Furthermore, the presence of HBsAg was demonstrated in the glomeruli of patients who had no detectable HBsAg in the serum [9]. Such conflicting results made many researchers doubt the specificity of fluorescent staining for HBsAg within the deposits [14].

In contrast to the accepted strong association of HBV with MN in children, opinions on the causal relationship between HBV infection and adult patients with MN are controversial; in particular, the reports from Taiwan and Korea did not favor such a concept. Chen et al. concluded that there was no significant association of HBV infection and PGN in adults except in MCGN [13]. Using a direct IF technique with monoclonal antibodies, they did not find any case showing immune deposits of HBV related antigens in renal biopsy specimens of PGN in adults.

Lai and others emphasized a significantly higher HBV carrier rate among patients with IgA nephropathy [8]. HBsAg and/or HBcAg were the chief type of HBV markers found in the glomeruli. Yet reports from China and Japan (Chen [13] and Iida [19]) respectively, failed to confirm this phenomenon [19].

Divergence of findings may be due, at least partly, to differences in staining techniques and quality of antisera, and may even be due to the methods of processing specimens [9,14,15].

Maggiore et al. found that the glomerular deposits contained immunoglobulin with antiglobulin activity which bound the Fc part of the anti-HBsAg antibody, thus the results described in the earlier studies may have been falsely positive [14].

Zhang et al. [9] compared results of HBV antigen deposition in adult GN patients with and without virus antigenemia. Not much difference was found between the groups, which included MN and lupus nephritis, while HBsAg could be more commonly detected in patients with virus antigenemia with MCGN and MsPGN. As far as technique factor is concerned, a series of studies using McAb to HBsAg, HBeAg, and HBcAg have shown that the 4-layer peroxidase antiperoxidase (PAP) method is too sensitive to identify HBV deposition in the kidney with some false positive findings. Indirect IP or IF and the avidin-biotin-complex (ABC) methods are fairly good techniques, although nonspecific staining is not entirely excluded.

Antibodies to HBV might have some false positive staining due to the contamination of antibodies to plasma proteins (Goodman et al. [15]). Besides, HBsAg may also bind horseradish peroxidase nonimmunologically and these entities may cause false positive staining. It is therefore essential to have well qualified antiserum and standard technique during the detection of HBV markers in glomeruli.

Theoretically, in order to ascertain whether a particular glomerular disease is etiologically associated with chronic HBV infection, it has to fulfill the following criteria:

1. Demonstration of HBV specific antigen(s) in the glomeruli.
2. Disappearance of the glomerular pathology with the eradication of the microorganism.
3. Experimental reproducibility of the morbidity in an animal model.

Unfortunately, at present the evidence for the presence of so-called "HBV associated GN" is founded basically on the demonstration of HBV specific antigen(s) in the glomeruli. Solid research work to confirm causal relationship between the therapeutic result and the effort to eradicate the HBV virus is still lacking although in anecdotal cases clearance of HBeAg was reported to be associated with resolution of the nephrotic syndrome [7].

For the purpose of staining glomerular HBeAg deposits more specifically, $F(ab')_2$ fragments of McAb raised against HBeAg were introduced into the study carried out by Hirose et al. [16]. In our laboratory, results obtained from a detailed comparison between the glomerular staining of McAb against HBsAg and its $F(ab')_2$ fragments in 12 cases with GN did show a marked difference between the two types of anti-sera being used. The positive rate of McAb against HBsAg was 75%; in contrast, the McAb-$F(ab')_2$ was only 33.3%.

Currently, the diagnosis of HBV-GN depends mainly on the demonstration of HBV specific antigens in the glomeruli. However, due to the different antibodies and various techniques used in histopathologic studies different authors reported wide variations in positive rates of glomerular deposition of HBV antigen. Investigators have pointed out that the glomerular staining of HBV antigens might be artifact, cross reactivity, or non-specific trapping [9,14,15]. Discrepancies between the HBV antigenemia and glomerular HBV deposits were also noticed in some reports.

Salient Features of HBV Associated MN in Children

Children with HBV-MN generally have no history or clinical evidence of ongoing liver disease. With rare exceptions, the liver pathology in children with HBV-MN usually shows chronic persistent hepatitis or minimal abnormality [4,7,17,18].

Despite a negative history for hepatitis, liver function tests and serum transaminases are usually mildly abnormal, in contrast to such values in idiopathic MN [4]. It is generally agreed that as many as 80%–100% of childhood HBV-MN patients are males [4,17]. Nephrotic syndrome or non-nephrotic proteinuria and microscopic hematuria are the common clinical presentations. Clinical remission, which mimics minimal change nephropathy, is quite common. HBV-MN in children usually follows a benign course. Only rarely do children with HBV-MN manifest renal insufficiency.

HBsAg and anti-HBc can almost always be demonstrated in the circulation [3,17]. Approximately 60%–80% of children will also have HBeAg, and the remainder will have anti-HBe antibody in their sera.

Serum C3 and C4 levels may be normal or depressed [17,18], CICs have been reported in up to 80% of cases of childhood HBV-MN. Staining of the glomerular capillary wall is usually positive for IgG (100%), C3 (75%), IgM (50%), and IgA (10%) [4,7]. In contrast to idiopathic MN, where deposits are seen in an exclusively subepithelial location, HBV-MN is characterized by the presence of subepithelial immune deposits in association with subendothelial and/or mesangial deposits. HBeAg has been identified to be the predominant type of HBV antigen deposited in the glomeruli of HBV-MN [7,17].

Clinical manifestations of adult HBV-MN tend to differ. Frequently there is a history of acute hepatitis, usually 6 months to several years prior to the onset of the kidney disease, and the typical liver pathology of chronic active hepatitis is common.

The nephrotic syndrome in adult HBV-MN patients usually does not respond to steroids and may progress to renal insufficiency.

Possible Immunopathogenesis of HBV-Associated GN

Several potential mechanisms for the development of HBV-MN have been suggested.

Immune Complex Formation

The observation that all 3 major HBV antigens, including HBsAg, HBeAg, and HBcAg have been identified in the glomeruli of patients with HBV-MN supports a mechanism involving HBV antigen-containing immune deposit formation either as a result of passive trapping of CICs or due to local IC formation.

CICs containing HBV antigens have been demonstrated in many patients with HBV-MN. However, CICs rarely result in subepithelial deposits, unless the CICs are very small and cationic. HBeAg CICs are small (2.5×10^5 daltons) and thus might be capable of localizing in the subepithelial space [6,7,20]. Immune complex-mediated GN requires a continuous supply of antigen and a maintained antibody response. Apparently, these requirements seem to be met in chronic HBV carriers. Thus, it is conceivable that MN, a GN with subepithelial deposits of HBeAg and antibody, could result from passive trapping of small cationic preformed CICs. The fact that HBeAg is the dominant type of HBV antigen deposited in HBV-MN also supports the above hypothesis [6,11].

Lai et al. [6] reported that HBeAg, rather than HBcAg, may play a pathogenetic role in the mesangial and subendothelial immune deposits commonly seen in MsPGN or MCGN associated with chronic HBV infection. However, there is currently little experimental evidence to support a preformed CIC trapping mechanism in the pathogenesis of HBV-MN.

A local mechanism of immune deposit formation in HBV-MN is also suggested. As anti-HBe antibodies are cationic, sequential localization of cationic antibody, followed by anionic HBeAg, could result in subepithelial IC formation in situ. The persistence of free antigen or antibody in the circulation may also favor this mechanism.

PGN and HBV Infection are Associated on the Basis of Genetic Predisposition

The association of PGN and HBV infection may not be caused by either HBV virus or by secondary liver disease, but rather may result from genetic predisposition or an underlying immunologic abnormality that increases the likelihood of these patients to develop both diseases independently of each other. Conditions associated with defective cell-mediated immunity do predispose HBV infected patients to become chronic HBsAg carriers, and defective cellular immunity has also been observed in cases with MN. Thus the possibility cannot be ruled out that MN and chronic HBV infection are not causally related, but rather are due to an inherent susceptibility of a subset of patients to develop both diseases. However, studies of human leucocyte antigen (HLA) patterns of patients with HBV-MN have not been reported [7].

Autoimmune Mechanism

Another possible pathogenetic mechanism for HBV-PGN involves the induction of autoantibodies to intrinsic glomerular antigens. Immunopathogenesis involving autoantibodies directed against glomerular antigens in MN has been established by both experimental and clinical studies. It was reported that many autoantibodies were demonstrated in patients with chronic HBV infection. Autoantibodies may contribute to some of the liver injuries in HBsAg positive chronic active hepatitis. Autoantibodies against glomerular antigens have also been identified. Thus, an autoimmune etiology for HBV-PGN should not be excluded.

Conclusions

The association of HBV infection with MN in children is now well established. There is a close relationship between the frequency of the HBsAg carrying state in MN and the underlying prevalence of HBsAg in the general population. The HBV-MN in children is also unique in its clinical presentation, serology, and immunopathology.

However, there is still controversy about the pathogenetic association in other types of PGN, even including HBV-associated MN in adults.

Currently, diagnosis and clinical research of HBV-associated PGN depends mainly on the demonstration of HBV specific antigens in the glomeruli, which demonstration is subject to many technical discrepancies. Improving the techniques and qualifying the immune reagents are mandatory to furthering the future understanding of these conflicting results.

References

1. Combes B, Stastny P, Shorey J, Eigenbrodt EH, Barrera A, Hull AR, Carter NW (1951) Glomerulonephritis with deposition of Australia antigen-antibody complexes in glomerular basement membrane. Lancet II:234
2. Brzosko WJ, Krawczynski K, Nazarewicz T, Morzycka M, Nowoslawski A (1974) Glomerulonephritis associated with hepatitis-B surface antigen immune complexes in children. Lancet II:477
3. Slusarczyk J, Michalak T, Mezer Teresa-Nazarewicz-de, Krawxzynski K, Nowostawski A (1980) Membranous glomerulopathy associated with hepatitis B core antigen immune complexes in children. Am J Pathol 98:29
4. Hsu HC, Lin GH, Chang MH, Chen CH (1983) Association of hepatitis B surface (HBs) antigenemia and membranous nephropathy in children in Taiwan. Clin Nephrol 20:121
5. Zhang YE (1986) An immunopathological study of hepatitis B immune complex glomerulonephritis in 33 cases. Chin J Nephrol 2:127
6. Lai KN, Lai FM, Chan KW, Chow CB, Tong KL, Vallance-Owen J (1987) The clinicopathologic features of hepatitis B virus-associated glomerulonephritis. Q J Med 18:411
7. Johnson RJ, Couser WG (1990) Hepatitis B infection and renal disease: immunopathogenetic and therapeutic considerations. Kidney Int 37:663
8. Lai KN, Lai FM, Tam JS, Vallance-Owen J (1988) Strong association between IgA nephropathy and hepatitis B surface antigenemia in endemic areas. Clin Nephrol 29:229

9. Zhang JH, Zhou H, Li LS (1990) Is there a hepatitis B virus (HBV)-associated GN? Identification of HBV in kidney with in situ hybridization and avidin biotin complex (ABC) methods (abstract). 4th Asian-Pacific Congress of Nephrology, 1990. Beijing, Peoples Republic of China p 165
10. Lee HS, Choi Y, Yu SH, Koh HI, Kim MJ, Ko KW (1988) A renal biopsy study of hepatitis B virus-associated nephropathy in Korea. Kidney Int 34:537
11. Anonymous (1987) HBV and glomerulonephritis. Lancet II:252 (editorial)
12. Hattori S, Furuse A, Matsuda I (1988) Presence of HBe antibody in glomerular deposits in membranous glomerulonephritis is associated with hepatitis B virus infection. Am J Nephrol 8:384
13. Chen WY, Chu TS, Chang CH, Chen YM, Tsal SL, Yen TS, Hsu HC, Lee SH (1989) Studies on adults primary glomerulonephritis and hepatitis B virus infection in Taiwan. The Eighth Asian Colloquium in Nephrology, 1989. Jakarta, Indonesia , p 263
14. Maggiore Q, Bartolomeo F, L'Abbate A, Misefari V (1981) HBsAg glomerular deposits in glomerulonephritis: Fact or artifact? Kidney Int 19:579
15. Goodman ZD, Langloss JM, Bratthauer GL, Ishak KG (1988) Immunohistochemical localization of hepatitis B surface antigen and hepatitis B core antigen in tissue sections. Am J Clin Pathol 89(4):533
16. Hirose H, Udo K, Kojima M, Takahashi Y, Miyakawa Y, Miyamoto K, Yoshizawa H, Mayumi M (1984) Deposition of hepatitis B e antigen in membranous glomerulonephritis: identification by F(ab')2 fragments of monoclonal antibody. Kidney Int 26:338
17. Southwest Pediatric Nephrology Study Group (1985) Hepatitis B surface antigenemia in North American children with membranous glomerulonephropathy. J Pediatr 106(4):571
18. Lin C-Y (1990) Hepatitis B virus associated membranous nephropathy: clinical features, immunological profiles and outcome. Nephron 55:37
19. Iida H, Izumino K, Asaka M, Fujita M, Takata M, Sasayama S (1990) IgA nephropathy and hepatitis B virus. IgA nephropathy unrelated to hepatitis B surface antigenemia. Nephron 54:18
20. Takekoshi Y, Tanaka M, Shida N, Sataka Y, Saheki Y, Matsumoto S (1978) Strong association between membranous nephropathy and hepatitis-B surface antigenaemia in Japanese children. Lancet II:1065

Snake Bite Induced Renal Disease

K.S. CHUGH and V. SAKHUJA[1]

SUMMARY. A variety of renal lesions have been documented following bites by viper, hydrophid, and colubrid snakes. Acute renal failure is the most frequent manifestation and complicates the course in 5–30% of victims of snake bite. The commonly encountered histological renal lesions are of acute tubular and acute cortical necrosis. Fibrin thrombi are often seen in the renal microvasculature in these cases. Less frequently, proliferative glomerulonephritis, interstitial nephritis and renal papillary necrosis are observed. The consistent presence of several hemostatic abnormalities in patients and animals, of which disseminated intravascular coagulation (DIC) is the most prominent, has focussed attention on the latter playing a significant role in the causation of renal failure. Other systemic effects including bleeding, hypotension, shock, and intravascular hemolysis could play a contributory role. Glomerular changes such as mesangiolysis, mesangial proliferation, and occasional crescent formation are most likely related to the toxic action of the "hemorrhagin" fraction of the venom on the glomerular capillaries. However, these lesions are inconsequential in most patients with renal failure. Severe glomerulonephritis has been documented in a few patients, but appears to be related to hypersensitivity to venomous or antivenomous proteins. Myoglobinuria is the major factor in the pathogenesis of renal failure in sea snake and Australian land snake envenoming. A consensus has not yet been reached on the precise role of the nephrotoxicity of venom in producing acute tubulo-interstitial lesions.

Introduction

Of the 2700 species of snake recognized the world over, fewer than 450 are venomous; the majority of these are distributed in the tropical and subtropical regions.

[1]Department of Nephrology, Postgraduate Institute of Medical Education and Research, Chandigarh-160012, India

The most frequent targets are farmers and fishermen, making snake bite a professional hazard. Less commonly, amateur collectors, cult followers, and others are affected. The world mortality from snake bites has been assessed to be around 40,000 per year.

Renal Lesions

Relatively recently, renal lesions following bites by venomous snakes have attracted attention; these lesions have been primarily associated with viperid, hydrophid, and colubrid snakes. Clinical reports on venom-induced renal disease have therefore appeared from geographical regions where snakes of these families are prevalent. The reported renal manifestations include acute renal failure, nephrotic syndrome, acute glomerulonephritis, necrotizing vasculitis, and papillary necrosis.

Acute Renal Failure (ARF)

The most frequently reported and devastating effect of envenomation on the kidney is the development of acute renal failure [1,2]. In Burma, where more than 1000 (3.3/100000) deaths occur annually from snake bite, Russell's viper envenomation constitutes 44%–70% of all cases of acute renal failure requiring dialysis and carries a mortality of 35% [3]. In Thailand, ARF has been recorded in 5% of patients bitten by Russell's viper and by sea snakes [4]. In Nigeria, ARF has been observed in 10% of puff adder bites [5] and in less than 1% of *Echis carinatus* envenoming [6]. In Israel, 6% of patients bitten by Palestinian viper [7] and in Sri Lanka, 26% of snake bite victims develop this complication [8]. In India, Russell's viper and *Echis carinatus* cause ARF in 13%–32% of those bitten by these two species [2,9,10]; patients bitten by these two species constitute nearly 3% of the total cases of ARF in our center. In some hospitals in Kerala [South India], snake poisoning accounts for 0.32%–1.4% of total hospital admissions and is responsible for 23% of cases of ARF amongst adults and children [11,12].

The histological entities encountered in envenomed patients with acute renal failure are:

Acute Tubular Necrosis

Cumulative data from several studies have shown that histological changes consistent with acute tubular necrosis [ATN] are seen in 60%–80% of envenomed patients [2,13]. On light microscopy, tubules appear dilated and lined by flattened epithelium. Severe cases exhibit cell necrosis and desquamation of necrotic cells from the basement membrane. Hyaline, granular, and pigment casts are seen in tubular lumina. Varying degrees of interstitial edema, hemorrhage, and inflammatory cell infiltration are seen. Later biopsies show regenerating tubular epithelium [1,2,9]. Fibrin deposits are seen in the glomerular capillaries in some cases [14].

Electron microscopy reveals dense intracytoplasmic bodies in the proximal tubules, which represent degenerating organelles or protein resorption droplets, distal tubular apoptosis, severe vascular lesions, and the presence of mast cells, eosinophils, and active fibroblasts in the interstitium, not observed in tubular necrosis due to other causes [14,15].

Acute Cortical Necrosis

Acute diffuse or patchy cortical necrosis has been reported in 20%–25% of patients bitten by *Echis carinatus* [1,2,10] and Russell's viper [1,2,16,17]. *Agkistrodon hypnale* [18] and *Bothrops* species [19,20] have also been associated with cortical necrosis. For reasons which are still not clear, cortical necrosis is observed more frequently among Indian patients than among Thais [2].

Under light microscopy, glomeruli and tubules appear necrotic and only their outlines can be discerned. Fibrin thrombi are present in the glomerular capillaries in 10%–25% of cases. The deeper cortical and medullary tissue shows changes of extensive tubular necrosis [1,2,13]. Calcification of necrotic areas may occur at a later stage [21]. In patchy cortical necrosis, varying numbers of glomeruli may be spared. With healing, fibroblastic proliferation and organization of the thrombi are seen [2,9].

Electron microscopy reveals collapsed capillary basement membrane denuded of foot processes. No viable mesangial or endothelial cells are seen, but capillary lumina may show swollen rounded cells, possibly of endothelial origin. Tubular basement membrane shows thickening and is lined by flattened epithelium. Fibroblastic proliferation is seen in the interstitium. Endothelial swelling of small arterioles and necrosis of peritubular capillaries is also seen [22].

Glomerular Lesions

Ballooning of the capillaries, mesangial proliferation, thickening and splitting of the basement membrane, swelling of endothelial cells, and crescent formation have been documented in some patients with renal failure. Seedat et al. [23] reported two patients with puff adder bite who developed oliguric renal failure soon after the bite; the renal histology showed changes consistent with crescentic glomerulonephritis. The authors suspected hypersensitivity to the venom as the basis for the renal lesions. Renal failure attributable to severe glomerulonephritis has also been reported in one case of Mamushi bite [24] and in four patients following Russell's viper or green pit viper bites [19]. IgM and C_3 deposits were seen in 63% of envenomed patients, C_3 alone was seen in 8% and no deposits were seen in 29% of patients.

Though other glomerular lesions are commonly seen in association with acute tubular necrosis, their precise contribution to the development of acute renal failure is not defined. Only an occasional patient has presented with evidence of overt glomerular disease.

Acute Interstitial Nephritis

In isolated renal failure patients, renal histology has shown a diffuse and intense mononuclear cell infiltration in the interstitium, suggesting the occurrence of acute interstitial nephritis. This has been observed in two patients bitten by Russell's viper [25,26] and in one bitten by *Echis carinatus* [9].

Acute Necrotizing Vasculitis

Necrotizing arteritis of the interlobular arteries has been observed in association with acute renal failure in two cases of Russell's viper bite. Other changes included thrombophlebitis of the arcuate veins and their tributaries. Immunofluorescence showed C_3 deposits in the afferent and efferent arterioles, but the significance of this finding is not clear [27].

Papillary Necrosis

A recent report has documented occurrence of papillary necrosis following snake bite, but the species was not identified [28].

Nephrotic Syndrome

A single case of nephrotic syndrome developing after an Australian snake bite has been reported by Steinbeck [29]. However, the renal histology was not studied in this case.

Pathogenesis of Renal Failure

One of the unresolved problems in snake venom research is the precise mechanism by which renal failure develops in envenomed patients. Several investigators have attempted to answer the question of whether or not the severe hemodynamic changes resulting from the vasculotoxic, hemotoxic, or myotoxic actions of the venom play a crucial role, or whether it is the nephrotoxic action of the venom on the glomeruli, interstitium, and the tubules which is vital to the development of acute renal failure. The available evidence is summarized.

Hemodynamic Changes

Significant hemodynamic changes result from the occurrence of several concurrent abnormalities in envenomed patients [1,2,6] and in animals [9]. These include bleeding, hypotension, shock, disseminated intravascular coagulation, hemoglobinuria, myoglobinuria, and hypersensitivity to venomous or anti-venomous proteins which are all known to cause acute renal failure individually or in combination.

Bleeding

Bleeding is a striking feature of most viperine bites and results from the direct vasculotoxic effect of the hemorrhagin component of the venom [30,31], which is caused by either a direct lytic action on the capillary endothelium [31,32], or by a widening of the intercellular junctions through which the erythrocytes and the plasma may escape [33]. The hemorrhagin component of *Echis carinatus* venom is ten times more potent than Russell's viper venom and has no effect on the coagulation cascade. Thrombocytopenia and consumptive coagulopathy, which are frequently present in viper-envenomed patients, enhance the tendency to bleeding initiated by hemorrhagin, and thus the tendency to produce ischemic tubular injury.

Hypotension and Shock

Hypotension and shock could be the consequences of bleeding or loss of plasma into the bitten extremity or could be due to hemodynamic effects directly attributable to the presence of certain enzymes such as bradykinin in Russell's viper or *Echis carinatus* venoms [34,35]. Puff adder (*Bitis arietans*) venom causes hypotension by causing myocardial depression, arteriolar dilatation, and increased vascular permeability [36].

Disseminated Intravascular Coagulation (DIC)

The consistent presence of several abnormalities in viper envenomed patients and animals [1–3,6,9,37–44], of which DIC is the most prominent, has focused attention on the latter playing a major pathogenetic role in the causation of renal lesions of acute tubular and cortical necrosis. The procoagulants in Russell's viper venom are known to cause a massive intravascular coagulation within minutes of the bite. Though the injected dose of the venom in human victims is generally insufficient to cause a rapid catastrophe, the deposition of microthrombi in the microvasculature may contribute significantly to the causation of acute renal failure. Carefully conducted histological studies have confirmed the presence of fibrin thrombi in the renal vasculature and occlusion of the glomerular capillaries in viper-envenomed patients and animals [1,3,14]. Intravascular coagulation and fibrin thrombi in the glomeruli are also a hallmark of the cortical necrosis associated with abruptio placentae, amniotic fluid embolism, and septic abortion [45,46]. Intra-glomerular fibrin deposition of lesser degree has been suspected to cause acute tubular necrosis by temporary interruption of the tubular blood supply [47]. In a recent study from our own center, acute disseminated intravascular coagulation was demonstrated in 56% of envenomed patients who developed acute renal failure [2].

Intravascular Hemolysis

Evidence of intravascular hemolysis was present in 50% of patients following bites by Russell's viper and *Echis carinatus* snakes [2,16]. The observation has been confirmed in Rhesus monkeys following administration of the venom of these two species of snakes [43,44]. In a study reported from Burma, hemolysis was absent in patients bitten by Russell's viper [3]. Hemolysis results from the action of phospholipase A2, which is present in almost all snake venoms. The occurrence of microangiopathic hemolytic anemia has also been documented in human victims of Russell's viper [1,2], puff adder [5], and gwardar snake [48], and also in animals given Malayan pit viper venom [49]. Intravascular hemolysis is known to be associated with acute renal failure [50].

Myoglobinuria

Sea snakes [51,52] and Australian land snakes [48,53,54] are myotoxic and renal failure may occur due to rhabdomyolysis and myoglobinuria.

Venom Nephrotoxicity

Glomerular Lesions

Current understanding of the pathogenesis of glomerular lesions is based on experimental studies which have been carried out with the venom of the Habu snake which is indigenous to Japan [55–59]. Habu venom contains a vasculotoxic factor "hemorrhagin" which has also been demonstrated in *Echis carinatus*, *Vipera palestinae*, *Agkistrodon halys*, and *Bothrops jararaca*. Within 6–24 h of administration of Habu venom, destruction of mesangium (mesangiolysis) occurs, resulting in segmental ballooning of capillaries. The capillaries become packed with red cells and fibrin, giving the appearance of "blood cysts." Within 3 days, proliferation of mesangial cells occurs which fills up the entire ballooned capillaries, giving an appearance resembling segmental proliferative glomerulonephritis. Rarely, crescents are also noted. Depending upon the period of envenomation, the histological lesions may resemble glomerular aneurysms or a focal proliferative glomerulonephritis.

In human victims of snake bite, mesangiolysis, which represents the earliest glomerular changes, has been documented in only one instance following *Agkistrodon halys* (Mamushi) bite [24]. This patient had presented with acute renal failure. Since renal histology is seldom studied in the first 24–48 hours, mesangiolysis is likely to be missed and this could account for the infrequent documentation of this lesion in snake-bite patients. These experimental studies have further suggested that the frequently observed proliferative changes in human biopsy and autopsy specimens of the kidney (which generally become available days or weeks after envenoming), are likely to represent a late stage in the evolution of glomerular changes. To what extent these changes contribute to acute renal failure is uncertain.

Tubulo-Interstitial Lesions

Despite several clinical and experimental studies, a consensus has still not been reached on the exact role of the nephrotoxicity of the venom in producing the tubular and interstitial lesions which are commonly seen in patients with renal failure. At least three experimental studies have supported a direct toxic action of the venom as an important factor in the causation of acute tubular necrosis. Schmidt et al. [60] observed proximal tubular damage in mice on electron microscopy after administration of rattlesnake venom, although the proximal tubular epithelium remained unaffected following administration of sea snake venom. Raab and Kaiser [61] attributed the increase in urinary alkaline phosphatase and aminopeptidase activity, following *Agkistrodon piscivorus* venom, to a direct effect of the venom on tubular epithelium. Ratcliffe et al. [62] documented characteristic changes, suggestive of acute tubular necrosis, in the urinary indices following exposure of isolated perfused kidney to Russell's viper venom.

Some studies have documented equivocal results, e.g., Hadler and Brazil [63] considered tubular damage following injection of crude *Crotalus terrificus* venom to be primarily due to shock and renal ischemia and partially due to the effect of lysolcithin formed by phospholipase A. Experimental studies with I^{125} labelled *Echis carinatus* venom and demonstration of venom antigen in envenomed patients using ELISA technique, have clearly shown that the venom may be excreted in urine without causing damage to the kidneys [64]. In two other studies carried out in rhesus monkeys, administration of lethal doses of *Echis carinatus* and Russell's viper venom was followed by acute tubular necrosis in only 20% of the animals, whereas following sublethal envenomation, more than 50% of animals showed significant renal lesions [2,9]. Fibrin thrombi were demonstrated in 50%–70% of glomeruli. The coagulation abnormalities and the histological changes were similar to those seen in human victims. The paucity of renal lesions in monkeys given lethal doses of viper venoms argues against a direct toxicity of the venom as a major factor contributing to the pathogenesis of acute renal failure.

Other Factors

At least three acute glomerulonephritis patients reported in the literature—two following puff adder bite [65] and one following Russell's viper bite [66]—appear to be examples of hypersensitivity to venomous or anti-venomous protein. Though significant complement abnormalities have been documented by us [66] and others [67], the role of these abnormalities in causing renal damage is far from clear.

Conclusions

Most of the studies have failed to provide convincing evidence in favor of a direct toxic action of the venom on the kidney as the predominant cause of the histological lesions of acute tubular and cortical necrosis which are frequently observed in human victims of snake bite. Instead, it has been found that hemodynamic changes, particularly DIC, resulting from systemic effects of envenoming, are likely to play a major role in the pathogenesis of acute renal failure. Mesangiolysis and proliferative changes in the glomeruli noted in some patients are likely to be due to the toxic action of the "haemorrhagin" fraction of the venom, but do not appear to play a significant role in the causation of acute renal failure. Efforts to solve the mysteries of this venomous disorder are continuing.

References

1. Chugh KS, Aikat BK, Sharma BK, Dash SC, Mathew T, Das KC (1975) Acute renal failure following snake bite. Am J Trop Med Hyg 24:692–697
2. Chugh KS (1989) Snake bite induced acute renal failure in India. Kidney Int 35:891–907
3. Myint-Lwin, Warrell DA, Phillips RE, Tin-Nu-Swe, Tun-Pe, Maung-Maung-Lay (1985) Bites by Russell's viper (*Vipera russelli siamensis*) in Burma: Hemostatic, vascular and renal disturbances and response to treatment. Lancet II:1259–1264
4. Sitprija V, Boonpucknavig V (1979) Snake venoms and nephrotoxicity. In: Lee CY ed, Snake Venoms. Springer, Berlin, pp 997–1018
5. Warrell DA, Ormerod D, Davidson N McD (1975) Bites by the puff adder (*Bitis arietans*) in Nigeria and value of anti venom. Br Med J [Clin Res] 4:697–700
6. Warrell DA, Davidson N McD, Greenwood BM, Omerod LD, Pope HM, Watkins BJ, Prentice CRM (1977) Poisoning by bites of the saw scaled or carpet viper in Nigeria. Q J Med 46:33–62

7. Efrati P, Reif L (1953) Clinical and pathological observations on 65 cases of viper bites in Israel. Am J Trop Med Hyg 2:1085–1108
8. Visuvaratram M, Vinayagamoorthy C, Balakrishnan S (1970) Venomous snake bites in North Ceylon – Study of fifteen cases. J Trop Med Hyg 73:9–14
9. Chugh KS, Pal Y, Chakravarty RN, Datta BN, Mehta R, Sakhuja V, Mandal AK, Sommers SC (1984) Acute renal failure following poisonous snake bite. Am J Kidney Dis 4:30–38
10. Mittal BV, Kinare SG, Acharya VN (1986) Renal lesions following viper bites. Indian J Med Res 83:642–651
11. Mathai TP, Date A (1981) Acute renal failure in children in snake bite. Ann Trop Pediatr 1:73–76
12. Jayarajan PM, Vijyakumar T, Leena Devi KR, Mathew MT (1979) Renal involvement in ophidism. J Assoc Physicians India 27:619–624
13. Chugh KS, Sakhuja V (to be published) Renal disease due to snake venom: In: AT Tu (ed) Handbook of natural toxins. Marcel Dekker, New York
14. Aung-Khin M (1977) Histological and ultrastructural changes of the kidney in renal failure after viper envenomation. Toxicon 16:71–75
15. Date A, Shastry JCM (1982) Renal ultrastructure in acute tubular necrosis following Russell's viper envenomation. J Pathol 137:225–241
16. Jeyarajah R (1984) Russell's viper bite in Sri Lanka – A study of 22 cases. Am J Trop Med Hyg 33:506–510
17. Sarangi A, Patnaik BC, Das GC, Tripathy N, Misra G, Swain AK, Das GK (1980) Renal involvement in viper snake bite. Indian J Med Res 71:918–923
18. Varagunam T, Panabokke RG (1970) Bilateral cortical necrosis of the kidneys following snake bite. Postgrad Med J 46:449–451
19. Sitprija V, Boonpucknavig V (1983) Glomerular changes in tropical viper bite in man. Toxicon 16:71–75
20. DaSilva OA, Lopez M, Godoy P (1979) Bilateral cortical necrosis and calcification of the kidney following snake bite: a case report. Clin Nephrol 11:136–139
21. Oram S, Ross SG, Pell L, Winteler J (1963) Renal cortical calcification after snake bite. Br Med J [Clin Res] 1:647–648
22. Date A, Shastry JCM (1981) Renal ultrastructure in cortical necrosis following Russell's viper envenomation. J Trop Med Hyg 84:3–8
23. Seedat YK, Reddy J, Edington DA (1974) Acute renal failure due to proliferative nephritis from snake bite poisoning. Nephron 13:455–463
24. Otsuji Y, Irie Y, Ueda H, Yotsueda K, Kitahara T, Yokoyama K, Higashi Y (1978) A case of acute renal failure caused by Mamushi (*Agkistrodon halys*) bite. Med J Kagoshima Univ (Jpn) 30:129–135
25. Sitprija V, Suvanpha R, Pochanugool C, Chusil S, Tung-sanga K (1982) Acute interstitial nephritis in snake bite. Am J Trop Med Hyg 31:408–410
26. Indraprasit S, Boonpucknavig V (1986) Acute interstitial nephritis after a Russell's viper snake bite. Clin Nephrol 25:111
27. Sitprija V, Benyajati C, Boonpucknavig PV (1974) Further observations of renal insufficiency in snake bite. Nephron 13:396–403
28. Mathew MT, Rajaratnam K (1987) Renal papillary necrosis in ophitoxemia (abstract). J Assoc Physicians India 35:20
29. Steinbeck AW (1960) Nephrotic syndrome developing after snake bite. Med J Aust 1:543–545
30. Taylor J, Mallick SMK (1935) Observations on poisoning with the venom of *Echis carinatus* and its treatment with a heterologous antivenom. Indian J Med Res 23:141–146
31. McKay DG, Moroz C, DeVries A, Csavossy J, Cruse V (1970) The action of hemorrhagin and phospholipase derived from *Vipera palestinae* venom on the micro-circulation. Lab Invest 22:387–399

32. Ownby CL, Bjarnason J, Tu AT (1978) Hemorrhagic toxins after rattle snake (*Crotalus atrox*) venom. Am J Pathol 93:201–218
33. Tsuchiya M, Ohshio C, Ohashi M, Ohsaka A, Suzuki K, Fujishiro Y (1974) Cinematographic and electron microscopic analyses of the hemorrhage induced by the main hemorrhagic principle HRI isolated from venom of *Trimeresurus flavoviridis*. Platelets, Thombosis, and inhibitors. In: Didisheim P, Shimamato T, Yamazaki H, Stuttgart FK (eds) F.K. Schattauer, pp 439–446
34. Chopra RN, Chowhan JS (1934) Action of the Indian daboia venom on the circulatory system. Indian J Med Res 23:493–506
35. Chopra RN, Chowhan JS, De NN (1935) An experimental investigation into the action of the venom of *Echis carinatus*. Indian J Med Res 23:391–405
36. Osman OH, Gumma KA (1974) Pharmacological studies of snake (*Bitis arietans*) venom. Toxicon 12:569–575
37. Than-Than, Hutton RA, Myint-Lwin, Khin-Ei-Han, Soe-Soe, Tin-Nu-Swe, Phillips RE, Warrell DA (1988) Hemostatic disturbances in patients bitten by Russell's viper in Burma. Br J Haematol 69:513–520
38. Shastry JCM, Date A, Carman RH, Johny KV (1977) Renal failure following snake bite. Am J Trop Med Hyg 26:1032–1038
39. Warrell DA, Pope HM, Prentice CRM (1976) Disseminated intravascular coagulation caused by the carpet viper: Trial of heparin. Br J Haematol 33:335–342
40. Lakier B, Fritz VU (1969) Consumptive coagulopathy caused by a boomslang bite. S Afr Med J 43:1052–1055
41. Nicolson IC, Ashby PA, Johnson ND, Versey J, Slater L (1974) Boomslang bite with hemorrhage and activation of complement by the alternate pathway. Clin Exp Immunol 16:295–300
42. Simon TL, Grace TG (1981) Envenomation coagulopathy in wounds from pit vipers. N Engl J Med 305:443–447
43. Chugh KS, Mohanthi D, Pal Y, Das KC (1979) Coagulation abnormalities induced by Russell's viper venom in the Rhesus monkey. Am J Trop Med Hyg 28:763–769
44. Chugh KS, Mohanthy D, Pal Y, Das KC, Ganguly NK, Chakravarty RN (1981) Hemostatic abnormalities following *Echis carinatus* (saw scaled viper) envenomation in the rhesus monkey. Am J Trop Med Hyg 30:1116–1120
45. Chugh KS, Singhal PC, Sharma BK, Pal Y, Mathew MT, Dhall K, Datta BN (1976) Acute renal failure of obstetric origin in Indian patients. Obstet Gynecol 48:642–646
46. Chugh KS, Singhal PC, Kher VK, Gupta VK, Malik GH, Narayan G, Datta BN (1983) Spectrum of acute cortical necrosis in Indian patients. Am J Med Sci 286:10–20
47. Clarkson AR, Macdonald MK, Fuster V, Cash JD, Robson JS (1970). Glomerular coagulation in acute ischemic renal failure. Q J Med 39:585–599
48. Harris ARC, Hurst PE, Saker BM (1976) Renal failure after snake bite. Med J Aust 2:409–411
49. Rubenberg ML, Bull BS, Regoeczi E, Dacie JV, Brain MC (1967) Experimental production of microangiopathic hemolytic anemia in vivo. Lancet II:1121–1123
50. Chugh KS, Singhal PC, Sharma BK, Mahakur AC, Pal Y, Datta BN, Das KC (1977) Acute renal failure due to intravascular hemolysis in North Indian patients. Am J Med Sci 274:139–146
51. Reid HA (1961) Myoglobinuria and sea-snake bite poisoning. Br Med J 1:1284–1289
52. Sitprija V, Sribhibhadh R, Benyajati C (1971) Hemodialysis in poisoning by sea snake venom. Br Med J 3:218–219
53. Rowlands JB, Mastaglia FL, Kakulas BA, Hainsworth D (1969) Clinical and pathological aspects of a fatal case of mulga [*Pseudechis australis*] snake bite. Med J Aust 1:226–230

54. Hood VL, Johnson JR (1979) Acute renal failure with myoglobinuria after tiger snake bite. Med J Aust 2:638–641
55. Suzuki Y, Churg J, Grishman E, Mautner W, Dachs S (1963) The mesangium of the renal glomerulus. Electron microscopic studies of pathologic alterations. Am J Pathol 43:555–578
56. Kitamura H, Hashiguchi T, Hamada R, Oyama M, Ikeda T, Inamori S, Mori T (1958) The pathological study of "Habu" (*Trimeresurus flavoridis*) venom II. The histopathological study of rabbit renal lesions caused by intravenous inoculation of "Habu" venom. Med J Kagoshima Univ (Jpn) 9:1586–1593
57. Sakaguchi H, Kawamura S (1963) Electron microscopic observations of the mesangiolysis. The toxic effects of "Habu snake" venom on the renal glomerulus. Keio J Med 12:99–106
58. Cattell V, Bradfield JWB (1977) Focal mesangial proliferative glomerulonephritis in the rat caused by Habu snake venom. A morphological study. Am J Pathol 87:511–524
59. Morita T, Kihara I, Oite T, Yamamoto T, Suzuki Y (1978) Mesangiolysis. Sequential ultrastructural study of Habu venom induced glomerular lesions. Lab Invest 38:94–102
60. Schmidt ME, Abdelbaki YZ, Tu AT (1976) Nephrotoxic action of rattle and sea snake venom: An electron microscopic study. J Pathol 118:75–81
61. Raab W, Kaiser E (1966) Nephrotoxic action of snake venoms. Mem Inst Butantan 33:1017–1020
62. Ratcliffe PJ, Purkittayakamee S, Ledingham JGG, Dunnill MS (1985) Acute renal failure in the isolated perfused kidney, induced by Russell's viper venom. Clin Sci 68(Suppl II):39–40
63. Hadler WA, Brazil OV (1966) Pharmacology of crystalline crotoxin nephrotoxicity. Mem Inst Butantan 33:1001–1008
64. Greenwood BM, Warrell DA, Davidson NMcD, Ormerod ED, Reid HA (1974) Immunodiagnosis of snake bite. Br Med J 4:743
65. Sitprija V, Boonpucknavig V (1980) Extracapillary proliferative glomerulonephritis in Russell's viper bite. Br Med J 2:1417
66. Chugh KS, Pal Y, Ganguly NK (1977) Complement depletion following envenomation by Russell's viper and *Echis carinatus* (saw scaled viper) in the Rhesus monkey. Am J Trop Med Hyg 26:1039–1043
67. Warrell DA, Greenwood BM, Davidson NMcD, Ormerod LD, Prentice CRM (1976) Necrosis, hemorrhage and complement depletion following bites by the spitting cobra. Q J Med 45:1–22

Acute Renal Failure in Asia

M. Rahman and M. Hossain[1]

Introduction

Acute renal failure (ARF) is an important nephrological disorder in most Asian countries, causing significant morbidity and mortality. Over the years the etiology of ARF has undergone considerable changes, particularly in Europe and developed Asian nations like Japan. In these developed countries ARF due to infection and septic abortion has practically disappeared, whereas, even today, infections of one kind or another, caused by bacteria, parasites, viruses, various toxins, and septic abortion remain as the major causes of ARF in most Asian countries. In addition, ARF following hypersensitivity reactions due to drugs, ARF due to immunological disorders such as primary glomerulonephritis and systemic lupus erythematosus (SLE) nephritis, and ARF due to hematological disorders such as myelomatosis etc. is as common in Asian countries as it is in Europe and in the United States. In this communication, we will briefly review different aspects of ARF in relation to Asia.

Definition and Prevalence

Acute renal failure is defined as deterioration of renal function, resulting in the rise of nitrogenous waste products, i.e., urea and creatinine, in blood [1]. Acute renal failure may occur in a previously healthy person; in such a person more than 50% deterioration in renal function is necessary to produce a rise in serum creatinine, whereas in a person with diseased kidneys (acute or chronic) a 10%–50% reduction of glomerular filtration will produce a rise in serum creatinine. Acute renal failure may progress slowly or rapidly (hypercatabolic) and may be associated with complete anuria, oliguria, or even with normal to high urine volume.

[1]Department of Nephrology and Paediatrics, Institute of Postgraduate Medicine and Research, Dhaka, Bangladesh

Prevalence of acute renal failure is variable, not only from one country to the other, but also in different parts of the same country and in different periods of the year [2]. In Bangladesh 4%–8% of admissions to nephrology units (dealing with adult patients) are due to acute renal failure [3,4]. In the years 1981–1989 children between the ages of 1–12 years were admitted to the Pediatric Nephrology unit of the Institute of Post-graduate Medicine and Research in Dhaka at the rate of 5–6 admissions a day. All these children presented with hypovolemic/ischemic acute renal failure with complete anuria of 1–13 days duration [5–8]. In most Asian countries the prevalence of acute renal failure due to gastroenteritis, septic abortions, malaria, leptospirosis, and snake bites, etc. is very common.

Specific Types of ARF in Asia

Acute renal failure is traditionally classified into (a) Pre-renal/Ischemic, (b) Renal due to intrinsic renal disease and various toxins, and (c) Post-renal/Obstructive groups. In the following chapters a brief description of specific types of ARF prevalent in Asia and due to various causes will be made.

Hypovolemic or Acute Ischemic Renal Failure (AIRF)

Fluid and electrolyte loss (producing hypovolemia), due to infective diarrhea, pyrexial illness, vomiting, and acute dysentery, remains the major causes of acute ischemic renal failure both in adults and children in countries like Bangladesh, India, Pakistan,

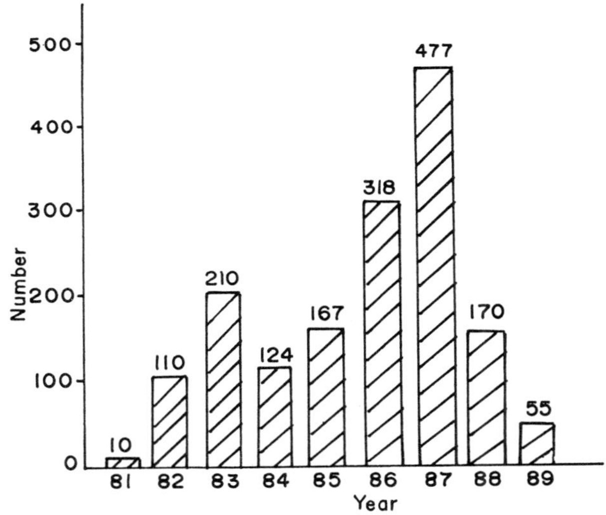

Fig. 1. Acute anuric non-obstructive renal failure in children of Bangladesh

Table 1. ARF in Bangladeshi children 1981–1989 (n = 1941)

Age range	Preceed illness	Duration of anuria	S. creat mean ±SD	Mortality
1–10 years	Pyrexia of unknown origin (PUO) 62% Diarrhea 28% Misc 10%	1–13 days	701±267.98 Micromol/l	87%

Indonesia, and Malaysia [9–13]. This form of acute renal failure is common in the densely populated developing countries of Asia which have mass poverty and illiteracy. Most of the patients are children and usually because of inadequate replacement of fluid and electrolytes, they develop oliguria, which usually goes unnoticed by illiterate parents; the children are generally brought to physicians after anuria has set in. During the period 1981–1989 in Bangladesh, there was almost an epidemic of ARF following pyrexial/diarrheal illness. In the year 1987 alone 477 children with ARF were admitted to the Paediatric Renal Unit of the Institute of Postgraduate Medicine and Research, Dhaka (Fig. 1). These children came with high serum creatinine and were treated with peritoneal dialysis; details are shown in Table 1. Overall mortality in this group of children suffering from AIRF was 87%–90%, compared to only 15% mortality in children suffering from ARF due to hemolytic uremic syndrome (HUS) [14,15].

Renal hypoperfusion is the mechanism responsible for producing acute renal failure in these cases. It seems likely that hypoperfusion which persists because of continued fluid and electrolyte loss may produce graded renal morphological changes, from none in pre-renal to acute or even cortical necrosis, depending on the severity of the insult and the delay in institution of corrective therapy. Therefore, it is reasonable to assume that this form of acute renal failure, which claims so many lives in Asian countries, is largely preventable. The pathogenic mechanisms, histological lesions, and methods of protection from this form of ARF have been the subject of extensive study in experimental animals [16–19].

Pregnancy Related Acute Renal Failure (PR-ARF)

In countries like Bangladesh, India, Thailand, Singapore, and Indonesia, ARF in pregnancy following severe hemorrhagic shock, with or without overwhelming infection, makes up about 15%–20% of all AIRF in adults [21–24], whereas in Western European countries the incidence of this form of AIRF has shown a ten-fold decrease, to about 3%, at the present time [25]. ARF during pregnancy occurs during the first trimester, due to toxemias of pregnancy (PE-E), abruptio placentae (AP), and post-partum hemorrhage (PPH). Disseminated intravascular coagulation (DIC) is a common association in this form of ARF. The histological lesion in PR-ARF is generally acute tubular necrosis; however, in severe cases there can be patchy or diffuse cortical necrosis. Patients with patchy cortical necrosis are usually left with renal insufficiency and those with diffuse cortical necrosis develop chronic renal failure, requiring dialysis for survival.

In most Asian countries PR-ARF patients are brought to hospital very late with severe manifestations, e.g., DIC with cerebral symptoms. The use of heparin is controversial, but recently, the use of fresh blood and fresh frozen plasma along with proteinine (antiprotiolytic agent) within 24–48 hours has been found to be beneficial. This group of ARF has a 30% mortality rate in Bangladesh. Legalization of abortion and institution of proper ante- and perinatal care would certainly reduce this form of ARF in Asian countries.

ARF Associated with Hemolysis

Acute renal failure due to severe hemolysis occurs following (1) *Plasmodium falciparum* malaria, (2) in G6 PD deficiency individuals when exposed to certain drugs, and in the (3) hemolytic uremic syndrome, etc.

Falciparum Malaria

Acute renal failure is a common complication of *Plasmodium falciparum* infection. In Thailand this infection is responsible for about 30% of ARF cases. Acute renal failure occurs in patients with partial loss of immunity and heavy parasitic infections. These patients are acutely ill with high pyrexia and jaundice; renal failure is generally hypercatabolic. Acute intravascular hemolysis may occur, which may be induced by antimalarial durgs, e.g., chloroquin, quinine, and pyrimethamine in patients with or without G6 PD deficiency. Black water fever is another possible cause of ARF due to severe hemolysis and can be diagnosed after drug-induced hemolysis has been excluded [26–28].

The pathogenic mechanism of ARF due to falciparum malaria has been extensively studied. The following factors: hypovolemia, hyponatremia, acute intravascular coagulation and hemolysis, hyperviscosity, activation of the renin-angiotensin system, and hyperbilirubinemia, have all been implicated [26,29]. These seriously ill patients need careful management with dialytic therapy. In places where hemodialysis facilities are not available, continuous equilibration peritoneal dialysis (CEPD) can be used [30,31]. With the return of malaria this form of ARF is becoming a potentially real threat in countries like Bangladesh and Burma.

G-6 PD Deficiency

Acute renal failure due to G-6 PD deficiency-associated hemolysis has been reported mostly from India. The incidence of G-6 PD deficiency has been variable among Asian nations: from the highest incidence, in Kurdish Jews (60%), to between 2%–15% in China and on the Indian subcontinent. In India this incidence constitutes about 20% of all patients with ARF needing dialytic therapy, who come to certain centers [32]. These patients usually have a history of febrile illness and have been exposed to analgesics and antimalarial drugs. The patients present with abrupt onset of hemolysis, anemia, reticulocytosis, jaundice, and hemoglobinuria. There are fragmented red cells in peripheral blood film. It is necessary to differentiate these patients from those with the hemolytic uremic syndrome.

Hemolytic Uremic Syndrome (HUS)

Hemolytic uremic syndrome is one of the common causes of ARF in children not only in developed countries, but also in certain Asian countries, including Bangladesh. It is characterized by sudden severe hemolysis with development of anemia and acute renal failure. This disease may precede diarrheal illness (Typical HUS) or may follow upper respiratory tract infection or vague non-specific symptoms (Atypical HUS). In Bangladesh, HUS has also been reported in children with shigellosis. The pathogenesis is not clear. However, it has been shown that intravascular platelet activation is associated with both typical and atypical forms of HUS [33,34].

This condition is also associated with fragmented and crenated red cells in the peripheral blood, anemia (at times very severe), thrombocytopenia, and reticulocytosis. This picture is consistent with that of micro-angiopathic hemolytic anemia and renal failure. Among Bangladeshi children, the recovery rate from HUS-caused ARF following fresh blood transfusion and peritoneal dialysis has been found to be 85%, in contrast to the recovery rate in acute ischemic renal failure, which was only 10%–13%. In certain cases, particularly in atypical HUS, relapse may occur and the patient may ultimately develop chronic renal failure.

Leptospirosis

Acute renal failure following leptospirosis is found in Bangladesh, Sri-Lanka, Philippines, Singapore, and Thailand [35,36]. The most prevalent serotype in The Philippines is L-autumnalis and in Thailand it is L-batavia. Acute renal failure occurs in 20%–66% of leptospirosis cases. The patients may have mild renal failure and may also develop severe renal failure requiring dialysis; this is found particularly in The Philippines and in Singapore [37,38]. Those patients with mild renal failure are anicteric; patients with severe renal failure are usually jaundiced, with thrombocytopenia, bleeding diathesis, and hepatic encephalopathy. In many cases there may be intravascular hemolysis with features of HUS.

In leptospirosis the predominant changes involve proximal tubules and interstitium. The glomerular and vascular changes are usually mild. The pathogenic mechanism is renal ischemia and direct nephrotoxicity. The overall mortality rate is around 10%.

Snake Bites

Acute renal failure is found in 5%–25% of patients following snake bite. The incidence of ARF among hospitalized snake bite patients has been highest in Sri Lanka, with 49% [39,40], about 28% in India, 5% in Thailand [41], and less than 1% in Bangladesh. In India, between 1965 and 1986, 3% of a total of 1962 ARF cases were due to snake bite. The snakes responsible for causing ARF were generally either Russell's viper or *Echis carinatus*. Following snake bite, ARF may be protracted, hypercatabolic, and often associated with jaundice and disseminated intravascular coagulation and bleeding manifestations. In this symposium a separate chapter has been devoted to this topic.

Rhabdomyolysis and ARF

Rhabdomyolysis and myoglobinuria (resulting from hyperpyrexia, heat stroke, multiple wasp stings, and crush syndrome) which cause ARF have been found in almost all countries of Asia. Extreme heat has been known to produce direct toxicity, causing dehydration, increased blood viscosity, disseminated intravascular coagulation, muscle damage, myoglobinuria, and in turn, acute renal failure [42,43]. Initially, hypokalemia is a predisposing factor for rhabdomyolysis; once muscle damage has been produced, intractable hyperkalemia is a feature. Tubular obstruction by myoglobin casts is regarded as the principal mechanism for producing ARF. Acute renal failure due to rhabdomyolysis can be diagnosed, apart from the history, by the elevation of creatinine phosphokinase and aldolase levels in the blood. In this condition hypocalcemia and calcium deposition in the damaged muscles during the oliguric/ anuric phase, and hypercalcemia during the diuretic phase, have been described as characteristic features [44].

Acute Renal Failure in Epidemic Hemorrhagic Fever

Epidemic hemorrhagic fever is characterized by sudden high temperature, hemorrhagic manifestations, and renal dysfunction, ranging from transient to established acute renal failure. This disease is due to a RNA virus (Hanta virus) and is found in Japan, Korea, and China [45]. The risk of Hanta virus infection is high among farmers in rural areas. Two to three weeks after contact with the infection the clinical syndrome, which can be divided into 5 phases as follows begins: febrile, hypotensive, oliguric, diuretic, and convalescent.

The acute febrile illness may be accompanied by abdominal pain and conjunctival hemorrhage. During this stage, leucocytosis, thrombocytopenia, raised serum GOT GPT, and LDH are found. Urinalysis may show proteinurea and hematuria. The stage of hypotension may be associated with shock; the majority of deaths occur in this phase

The renal lesion may be: (1) Mild glomerular alteration with mesangial cell proliferation, (2) Degeneration and necrosis of tubular epithelium, and (3) Lastly, congestion and hemorrhage into the renal tissue. Immunofluorescent studies show deposition of IgA, IgM, C3,C4 and C_{1q} along capillary basement membrane, indicating activation of both complement pathways [46,47].

The diagnosis is confirmed by demonstrating the rising titer of antibodies against Hanta viruses in two blood samples collected at intervals of one week. Recently, specific IgM antibodies have been more helpful in making the diagnosis possible quite early in the disease process in about 95% of cases. The introduction of peritoneal dialysis has reduced the mortality in this disease to about 10%.

Acute Renal Failure Due to Glomerular Nephritis (GN) and Toxic Agents

Acute renal failure due to intrinsic renal disease is the second most common cause of ARF in Asia. All forms of secondary glomerulonephritis, due to streptococcal infection [48,49], hepatitis β virus (HBV) infection [50], and primary glomerulonephritis, including even minimal change disease [57], have been reported to produce ARF in Asia. Rapidly progressive GN due to SLE [52] and Goodpasture's syndrome is also common. Acute renal failure due to malignant lymphoma [34] and myelomatosis [54] has also been reported. Acute renal failure due to various toxins, e.g., the raw bile of the grass carp [55], wasp stings [56,57], and toxins/infections of an undetermined nature has produced acute renal failure with, at times favorable outcome [58,59], and at other times the very unfavorable outcome of 100% mortality, which occurred in ARF presenting with anuria and intern developing neurological manifestations, involving the brain stem, causing death [60]. Acute renal failure due to copper sulphate has been reported, mostly from India [61]. Apart from this, drug-induced ARF, due to acute interstitial nephritis induced by drugs such as NSAIDs, aminoglycosides, and, currently, cyclosporin, is also not uncommon [62]. But the ARF of this group is relatively milder, having a comparatively better prognosis than AIRF.

Post-Renal ARF

Acute renal failure due mostly to bilateral ureteric obstruction, and, to a lesser extent, to lower urinary tract obstruction is quite common in countries like Bangladesh, India, and Pakistan [63]. This form of ARF makes up about 5%–9% of all cases of acute renal failure. The result of treatment, even in those patients with the most severe disease in this group are very rewarding.

Treatment Constraints

It is the experience of almost all Asian countries that patients come to hospital severely ill, in an advanced state of established ARF. In a few advanced countries like Japan, this pattern may be an exception. Most of these patients require dialytic forms of therapy immediately; with the introduction of peritoneal dialysis, the prognosis has greatly improved, even in hypercatabolic acute renal failure patients. But in remote areas of developing Asian countries the hospitals may not have the necessary biochemical facilities and even the facilities for peritoneal dialysis may be lacking; these factors coupled with poor referral systems and bad communication, may result in only conservative therapy, which leads to fatality in most of these cases. However, in most reported series, the mortality rate of ARF (18%–30%) has been comparable to that of the West.

Prevention and Mitigation

The acute renal failure which occurs in Asian countries due to infective causes, e.g., the ARF which is caused by diarrhea, malaria, leptospirosis, Hantaviruses, hepatitis viruses, and pregnancy-related septicemia, is no doubt mostly preventable. In addition, exposure to drugs and toxins can also be controlled to reduce this form of ARF.

This type of prevention can be called "Macroprevention" and is obviously dependent on the overall socioeconomic conditions in the country. Pretreatment with mannitol or furosemide of patients at high risk for development of ARF, e.g., those at risk for post-operative ARF, has been found to reduce its incidence, or at least lessen its severity [64–66]. Various agents, e.g., clonidine [67], Ca-antagonists [68], and ATP [69] used to prevent/mitigate ARF in experimental animals may be called "Microprevention" and as yet have no role in human disease.

Conclusion

The various types of acute renal failure prevalent in most Asian countries are largely preventable. Yet due to the developing nature of these countries and due to limited dialytic facilities a large proportion of these ARF cases prove to be fatal. It will be quite some time, probably even the twenty-first century before Asian nephrologists will be faced with the kind of ARF patients currently being faced by their Western counterparts. This difference in disease pattern has been clearly shown by Chugh et al. in their Chandigarh study [70].

References

1. Brezis M, Rosen S, Epstein FH (1986) Acute renal failure. In: The kidney, 3rd edn. W.B. Saunders, pp 735–779
2. Chugh KS, Singhal PC (1981) Acute renal failure in the Tropics. Asian Man Nephrol, SEAMIC, 181–194
3. Rahman M, Roy AC, Chowdhury D, Hossain M (1985) Clinicopathological spectrum of renal diseases in IPGMR. An analysis of 2000 cases in 11 years. J of BCPS III(No. 1)
4. Rashid HU, Azhar MA, Rahman A, et al. (1989) Pattern of acute renal failure in Bangladesh adults. Bang Ren J 6(1):16–20
5. Hoque M, Rashid HU (1982) Acute renal failure in children. Bang Ren J 1(2):12–15
6. Hoque M, Chowdhury D, Rahman M, Rashid HU, Talukder MQK, Khan MR (1985) Clinical course and outcome of acute anuric renal failure in children—A study of 275 cases. Bang J Child Health 9(1):5–9
7. Chugh KS, Narang A, Kumar L, Sakhuja V, Narayanan Unni V, Prizada R, Singh N, Pereira BJG, Singhal PC (1987) Acute renal failure amongst children in a tropical environment. Int J Artif Organs 10(2):97–101
8. Pereira BJG, Narang A, Pereira S, Gupta A, Sakhuja V, Chugh KS (1989) Acute renal failure in infants in the tropics. Nephrol Dial Transplant 4:535–538
9. Razzaque A, Ahmed S, Rahman M (1983) Profile of acute renal failure in adults. Bang Ren J 2(2):5–6
10. Malhotra UK (1989) Renal problems in India: Most prevalent kidney diseases and related problems. Proceedings of the eighth Asian colloquium of nephrology, Nov 17–21, 1989. pp 289–302
11. Sumanggar PS, Jose Roesma, Roemiati Oesman, Markum MS Gambaran gagal akut dibagian ilmu penyakit dalam FKUI/RSCM, Jakarta, (in Indonesian)
12. Herriyati S, Sukandar E Tinjauan Kasus Kegagalan ginjal mendadak disubagian ginjal-hipertensi bagianilmupe nyakit dalam RS hasan sadikin (in Indonesian) bandung SE lama 3 tahun (1977–79)

13. Azhar MA, Rahman MA, Rashid HU (1985) Acute renal failure following copper intoxication and its reversal after dialysis. 4(1):19–20
14. Rahman M, Chowdhury D, Hoque M, et al. (1982) Acute anuric renal failure in children. Bang Ren J 1(2):3–5
15. Rahman M, Chowdhury D, Islam KMN, Hoque M (1984) Acute anuric renal failure in children (abstract). IXth International Congress of Nephrology, Jun 11–16, 1984. p 120A
16. Schrier RW, Shapiro JI (1985) Current concepts in ischaemic acute renal failure. Proceedings of the sixth Asian colloquium of nephrology, Kuala Lumpur. pp 1–8
17. Raymond KH, Stein JH (1988) Acute renal failure: In vitro experimental models. Proceedings of the Xth international congress of nephrology, vol 2. pp 964–974
18. Fried TA, Stein JH (1984) Experimental acute renal failure: pathophysiology and methods of protection. Proceedings of the IXth international congress of nephrology, vol 1. pp 731–747
19. Himes HD, Hunt DA, Clark MJ, White MP, Weinberg JM (1984) Cellular mechanism of protection in nephrotic and ischemic acute renal failure. Proceedings of the IXth international congress of nephrology, vol 1. pp 770–783
20. Chugh KS, Singhal PC, Sharma BK, Yash P, Thomas MM, Kamla D, Datta Bn (1976) Acute renal failure of obstetric origin. 48(6)
21. Pravin C, Singhal VK, Kher, Gian I, Dhall, RL, Mehta, Kasi Visweswaran R, Narayanan Nampory MR, Kirpal S, Chugh (1982) Conservative vs surgical management of septic abortion with renal failure. Int J Gynaecol Obstet 20:189–194
22. Rakachanaran S, Jayatissa SK, Herath CA, Salgado M (1990) Aetiology and mortality of acute renal failure (ARF) in Sri Lanka (abstract). Conference, Beijing, China
23. Suleiman AB (1982) Clinical review of acute renal failure (1982) A 5 years experience at Kuala Lumpur. 11(1)
24. Suleiman AB, Morad S, Prasad S Prospective study of acute renal failure: In a general hospital Kuala Lumpur
25. Stratta P, Canavese C, Dogliani M, et al. (1989) Pregnancy related acute renal failure. Clin Nephrol 32:14–20
26. Boon PV, Sitprija V (1979) Renal disease in acute plasmodium falciparum infection in man. Kidney Int 16:44–52
27. Rahman H, Biswas GC, Rouf MA, Rashid HU (1988) Reversible acute renal failure following malaria—A case report. Bang Ren J 7(1):24–27
28. Sitprija V (1985) Acute renal failure in malaria and leptospirosis. Proceedings of the sixth Asian colloquium of nephrology, Kuala Lumpur. pp 15–40
29. Sitprija V (1989) Tropical diseases and acute renal failure: jaundice model. Proceedings of the eighth Asian colloquium of nephrology, Nov 17–21, 1989. pp 347–350
30. Hossain M, Chowdhury D, Rahman M (1986) Continuous equilibration peritoneal dialysis in hypercatabolic acute renal failure. Bang Ren J 5(2):63–65
31. Lanjona IA, Neidus OD, Daysog A Jr, et al. (1986) Continuous equilibration peritoneal dialysis (CEPD) in acute renal failure. Phil J Nephrol 1:90–96
32. Chugh KS, Singhal PC, Sharma BM, Mahakur AC, Pal Y, Datta BN, Das KC (1977) Acute renal failure due to intravascular hemolysis in North Indian patients. Am J Med Sci 274(2):139–146
33. Walters MDS, Levin M, Smith C, et al. (1988) Intravascular platelet activation in the hemolytic uremic syndrome. Kidney Int 33:107–115
34. O'Regan S, Blais N, Russo P, et al. (1989) Hemolytic uremic syndrome glomerular filtration rate, 6–10 years later measured by 99 MTC DTPA plasma slope clearance. Clin Nephrol 32:217–220
35. Sitprija V (1986) Acute renal failure due to tropical diseases. Phil J Nephrol 1:35–39
36. Ismael AE, Naidas OE, Daysog JA, et al. (1986) Acute renal failure in Leptospirosis. Phil J Nephrol 1:54–58

37. Estrada DR, Naidus OD, Daysog JA, et al. (1986) Nonoliguric acute renal failure. Its clinical features as observed at the Saint Thomas University Hospital. Phil J Nephrol 1:71–78
38. Ramachandran S, Rajapakse CNA, Perera MVF, Yoganathan M (1976) Patterns of acute renal failure in Leptospirosis. J Trop Med Hyg 158–160
39. Ramachandran S (1987) Renal failure: profiles and challenges. Ceylon Med J 32:59–74
40. Ramachandran S, Perera MVF (1974) Survival renal cortical necrosis due to snake bite. Postgrad Med J 50:314–316
41. Chugh KS (1989) Snake bite induced acute renal failure in India. Kidney Int 35:891–907
42. Honda N (1983) Acute renal failure and rhabdomyolysis. Kidney Int (Nephrology Forum) 23:888–898
43. Chugh KS, Singhal PC, Nath IVS, Pareek SK, Ubr HS, Sarker AK (1979) Acute renal failure due to non-traumatic rhabdomyolysis. Postgrad Med J 55:386–392
44. Han WH, Shieh S-D, Chen W (1983) A prospective study of soft tissue calcification in rhabdomyolysis induced acute renal failure. Taiwan I Hsueh Hui Tsa Chih 82:1139–1149
45. Lee HW (1988) Hantavirus infection in Asia. Proceedings of the Xth international congress of nephrology, vol 2. pp 816–830
46. Li LS (1986) Renal disease in China: An overview. Proceedings of the 3rd Asian Pacific congress of nephrology, Oct 5–10, 1986. pp 292–296
47. Kim MJ (1989) Hanta virus infection in Korea. Proceedings of the eighth Asian colloquium of nephrology, Nov 17–21, 1989. pp 303–313
48. Rahman M, Rahman H, Chowdhury D (1988) Post streptococcal acute glomerulonephritis in Bangladesh. A follow up study of 250 patients. Bang Ren J 7:46–51
49. Chugh KS, Malhotra HS, Sakheja V, et al. (1986) Prognosis of post-streptococcal GN-Chandigarth study. Proceedings of 3rd APCN, B 272–285
50. Rahman MA, Azhar MA, Rahman MH, Rashid HU (1985) Reversible acute renal failure associated with uncomplicated viral hepatitis – report of two cases. Bang Ren J 4(2):52–55
51. Haque A, Rahman M, Islam MN (1982) Reversible renal failure in minimal change neprhotic syndrome. Bang Ren J 1(1):1–3
52. Sultan M, Bari R, Rashid HU (1983) A case of acute renal failure following introgenic infection from a dextrose infusion. Bang Ren J 2(2):14
53. Roy AC, Rahman M (1983) Acute renal failure in malignant lymphoma. Report of a case. Bang Ren J 2(2):12–13
54. Dun-Lin Chen, Jong-Da Lian, Yun-Fu Yang, Kuo-Hsiung Shu, Chi-Hung Cheng, Lai-Ping Chen (1989) Acute renal failure in patients with multiple myeloma. J Nephrol ROC 3:221–226
55. Wan Yu Chen, Tsan Shin Yen, Jen Tse Cheng, Bor Shen Hsieh, Hey Chi Hsu (1976) Acute renal failure due to ingestion of raw bile of grass carp (*Clenopharyngodon Idellus*). Taiwan I Hsueh Hui Tsa Chih 75:149–157
56. Chiu-Ching Huang, Chi AU, Leung Chen, Swei Hsueh (1983) Acute renal failure and hepatic injury following multiple wasp stings – Report of 2 cases. Taiwan I Hsueh Hui Tsa Chih 82:623–628
57. Sakhuja V, Bhalla A, Pereira BJG, Kapoor MM, Bhusmurmath SR, Chugh KS (1988) Acute renal failure following multiple hornet stings (abstract). Nephrol 49:319–321
58. Chowdhury D, Kawser CA, Talukder MQK, Rashid HU, Rahman M (1982) Favourable outcome in four cases of anuric acute renal failure in children. Bang Paed J 6(1):31–33
59. Fatmi LE, Hoque M, Mannan MA (1985) Acute renal failure complicating Stevens-Johnson syndrome in a six year old child. Bang J Child Health 9(3):192–195
60. Rahman H, Chowdhury D, Rashid NU, Rahman M (1987) Acute renal failure in adults with central nervous system involvement – A new entity. Bang Ren J 6(2):53–58
61. Chugh KS, Sharma BK, Singhal PC, Das KC, Datta BN (1977) Acute renal failure following copper sulphate intoxication. Postgrad Med J 53:18–25

62. Schrier RW, Shapiro JI (1985) Drug-induced acute renal failure. Proceedings of the sixth Asian colloquium of nephrology, Kuala Lumpur, pp 9–14
63. Nagvi SAJ (1989) Regional problems in Pakistan – Most prevalent kidney diseases and related problems. Proceedings of the eighth Asian colloquium of nephrology, Nov 17–21, 1989. pp 283–288
64. Dawson JI (1965) Post-operatiave renal function in obstructive jaundice: Effect of mannitol diuresis. Br Med J [Clin Res] 1:82–86
65. Old CW, Lehrner LM (1980) Prevention of radio contrast induced acute renal failure with mannitol. Lancet I:885
66. Nuutimen LS, Kairabwoma M, Ruoonen S, et al. (1978) The effect of furosemide on renal function in open heart surgery. J Cardiovasc Surg (Torino) 19:471–479
67. Solez K, Racusen LC, Wheltoln A (1984) Clonidine, propranolol and the prevention of acute renal failure. Proceedings of the IXth international congress of nephrology, vol 1. pp 784–790
68. Burke TJ, Arnold PE, Schrier RW (1984) The role of calcium channel blockers. Proceedings of the IXth international congress of nephrology, vol 1. pp 791–799
69. Siegel NJ, Gandio KM, Mashgarian M (1984) Adenine nucleotides in the prevention of ischemic acute renal failure. Proceedings of the IXth international congress of nephrology, vol 1. pp 800–806
70. Chugh KS, Kjellstrand CM (to be published) The changing epidemiology of acute renal failure. Patterns in economically advanced and developing countries. In: International year book of Nephrology in press

Renal Stone Disease in the Middle East

WILLIAM G. ROBERTSON, VALERIE R. WALKER, HERBERT HUGHES[1], IMTIAZ HUSAIN, and SALAH AL-FAQIH[2]

SUMMARY. The pattern of urinary stone disease varies widely throughout the Middle East in terms of prevalence, site of formation, stone composition, diet, and urinary risk factors. In the developing countries, whose economies are still largely based on agriculture, ammonium urate-containing bladder stones in children are still a frequent finding, although this form of the disorder is decreasing with improving nutritional standards. In the more affluent Gulf states upper urinary tract stones in adults are extremely common—the life-time prevalence in men over the age of 60 being greater than 20%, the highest in the world. In these patients, the stones are composed mainly of calcium oxalate and/or uric acid. Calcium phosphate-containing calculi and infection stones are relatively uncommon. The high prevalence of calcium oxalate and uric acid stones can be attributed to the low urine volumes, more acid urines, hyperuricosuria, hypocitraturia, and extensive mild hyperoxaluria which are common in the region. These urinary abnormalities are due to the consumption of a diet over-rich in animal protein, purine, and oxalate but low in calcium. Addition of 1g/day calcium to the diet reduces urinary oxalate to normal without any major increase in urinary calcium.

Introduction

The pattern of stone disease in the Middle East is complex, but basically consists of two main themes which may be closely interwoven through different sections of society within the same country. Firstly, as a relic of the past history of the disease as it was known in the West in the last century, there is the formation of ammonium urate-containing stones in boys living in the developing countries of the region whose economies are still highly dependent on agriculture, e.g., Iraq, Jordan, and Egypt [1,2]

[1]Department of Biological and Medical Research, King Faisal Specialist Hospital and Research Centre, P.O. Box 3354, Riyadh 11211, Saudi Arabia
[2]King Khalid University Hospital, Riyadh, Saudi Arabia

and, secondly, there is the formation of calcium- and uric acid-containing upper urinary tract stones in adults (mainly men) in the more affluent, oil-rich states of the Arabian Peninsula, such as Kuwait, the United Arab Emirates (UAE), and the Kingdom of Saudi Arabia [3,4]. These forms of the disorder often occur together in the same country but, as nutritional standards improve, the incidence of bladder stones in children decreases [1,2] and that of upper urinary tract stones in adults increases [5,6].

Prevalence of Stones

There are few data on the actual prevalence of urolithiasis in the population and many studies have had to rely on hospital admission rates for stone disease as an indication of prevalence. Table 1 shows the data from various countries for adults and children. In general, these support the contention that stone-formation in adults is most common in affluent countries, but that its prevalence may be further aggravated by a number of environmental factors, such as living and/or working in a hot dry environment [5,6]. This factor, however, may only be of importance once the indigenous population concerned has reached a moderate level of affluence, as evidenced by data from various tropical countries in Africa and Asia where the climate is as hot as that in the more affluent countries of the Middle East but the prevalence of stones is considerably lower [6].

Table 1 shows that the Middle Eastern countries fall into three groups: (a) countries such as Iraq, Sudan, Turkey, Egypt, and Iran where bladder stones in children are still a frequent finding; (b) countries such as Jordan and Syria where bladder stones have largely disappeared and upper tract stone-formation in adults is now the predominant form of the disorder; and (c) countries such as Kuwait, the UAE, and Saudi Arabia where there are no bladder stones in children but where the occurrence of upper tract stones in adults and children is now of epidemic proportions.

In the few countries of the world where true prevalence studies have been carried out the pattern of the life-time risk of stones in men over the age of 60 (Table 2) is similar to that indicated in Table 1. Table 2 also contains data on the percentage of patients attending General Hospital Urology Clinics who have urolithiasis as their primary diagnosis. In general, they fit the pattern shown in Table 1, with the highest percentages occurring in the countries of the Arabian Peninsula.

The questions now arise—why do bladder stones in boys predominate at the lower end of the affluence scale, why do upper urinary tract stones in adults take over as the dominant form of the disorder as countries become industrialized, and why does the prevalence of upper tract stones continue to increase as these countries become more and more affluent?

Affluence and Stone-Formation

As a country develops and becomes more affluent, at least three factors are known to change which might influence the risk of stone-formation in the population. Firstly, both the standard of hygiene and supply of safe drinking water increase; secondly, the level of nutrition changes from one poor in energy to one richer in protein, refined carbohydrate, fat, and purine; and thirdly, the average level of physical

Table 1. Annual rate of hospitalization for urinary stone disease per 10000 population

Region	Annual hospital admissions in adults per 10000 adults in the population	Annual hospital admissions in children per 10000 children in the population
Thailand	1.0	8.0
India	1.0	7.0
Iraq	1.6	5.5
Sudan	2.1	5.4
Turkey	nd	5.0
Egypt	1.7	4.1
Iran	1.3	2.5
Indonesia	0.7	1.0
Pakistan	0.6	nd
South Africa (Bantu)	0.1	nd
Jordan	1.7	0.5
Sicily (1955)	2.5	0.5
Sicily (1970)	4.0	0.1
Syria	2.9	0.4
Czechoslovakia	1.6	nd
Nigeria	1.1	0.2
E. Mediterranean	2.0	nd
Japan	2.2	nd
Eire	3.0	nd
Austria	4.1	nd
Norway	4.3	nd
Italy	4.8	nd
UK	4.9	0.1
Finland	4.9	nd
Holland	5.0	nd
Australia	6.2	nd
W. Germany	6.3	nd
Denmark	7.0	nd
Sweden	7.5	nd
New Zealand	7.6	nd
Canada	10.1	nd
Kuwait	12.5	0.2
USA	15.0	0.1
United Arab Emirates	20.6	0.2
Saudi Arabia	22.1	0.2

nd, not determined

activity associated with the daily work routine decreases as people move from a rural to an urban lifestyle [1,2,5].

Hygiene and Drinking Water

One of the major changes in a country undergoing development is the increase in the overall standard of hygiene, including a safe supply of drinking water. The incidence of chronic diarrhea decreases and with it, probably, the risk of forming ammonium urate stones. Prior to the improvement in the level of hygiene the situation is analogous to that in cases of laxative abuse, as reported by Dick et al. [7], where ECF volume

Table 2. Occurrence of urolithiasis in various countries

Country	Urology patients with stones (%)	Life-time stone prevalence in men over 60 years (%)
China	–	1.5
Japan	–	5.4
UK	5–10	7.8
W Germany	–	8.0
Sweden	–	8.6
Canada	10–15	12.0
USA	10–20	13.0
United Arab Emirates	15–30	18.0
Saudi Arabia	20–50	20.1

depletion and intracellular acidosis produce a urine with a low volume and low sodium content and markedly reduced levels of potassium and citrate. Ammonia secretion into urine, in order to buffer hydrogen ions, is increased and the resulting high concentration of ammonium ions combines with urate to form ammonium urate crystals.

Nutrition

In children in many developing countries, where the level of hygiene is changing only slowly, this situation is aggravated by the consumption of a diet which is poor in meat protein, calcium, and phosphate and where rice is the staple constituent at an early age. The low intake of phosphate leads to a low urinary excretion of the ion which is normally required as a buffer. This promotes the production of ammonia and of a urine with a pH greater than 6. The combination of a high ammonium ion concentration in conjunction with a urinary pH between 6 and 7 is an unusual situation, which may be accentuated by the effects of chronic diarrhea, as described above. Furthermore, the total excretion of uric acid tends to be high in children, as result of rapid tissue turnover, and this will exist entirely in the form of urate in urine at pH values > 6. The resultant high ammonium and urate ion concentrations may lead to excessive supersaturation of urine with respect to ammonium urate.

In some countries, particularly in SE Asia, the addition of certain leaves which have a high content of oxalate to the diets of young children may lead to mild hyperoxaluria. This is often accentuated by the low intake of calcium. The resulting high concentrations of urinary oxalate may lead to calcium oxalate being deposited along with ammonium urate in the stones. As the level of hygiene and nutrition both improve, the risk of children forming ammonium urate-containing stones decreases and this form of the disorder may well disappear completely, as it has done previously in all developed countries, by the end of the century.

Why ammonium urate-containing stones should form mainly in the bladder and why only in boys is still a matter of conjecture. One possibility is that ammonium urate can exist as a colloid and only crystallizes relatively slowly, so that it is generally cleared from the kidney before crystalluria can develop. In the bladder, urine has a longer residence time in which to form abnormal crystals. These may occur in the urines of both boys and girls but, because of the wider urethra of the latter, the particles may be more readily expelled before they become large enough to be trapped and form the nucleus of a stone.

As countries develop and become more affluent, dietary composition changes quite markedly. Initially there is an increase in calcium intake as more dairy produce is consumed and this is accompanied by increases in the intakes of oxalate, refined carbohydrates, fats, purines, and animal protein. There is a concomitant decrease in dietary fiber. The strongest correlation at several demographic levels is between the consumption of animal protein (and purine) and affluence [6].

The effect of these dietary changes within a given population is to produce urine which is, on average, acidic and which is high in calcium, oxalate, and uric acid and low in citrate. Chemically this combination of urinary abnormalities increases the risk of calcium oxalate and uric acid crystalluria and stones. Most of these changes in urinary composition are attributable to the high consumption of animal protein and purine [8]. If, in addition, there are increases in the intakes of refined carbohydrates and oxalate, as mentioned above, then some of the effects on urine composition may be exaggerated, particularly in stone-formers, who appear to respond more sensitively to some of these dietary stimuli.

Conversely, it has been noted that if the consumption of animal protein and purine is reduced, the excretions of calcium, oxalate, and uric acid are also decreased and the biochemical risk of stones is low [8]. Vegetarians have a low predicted risk of stone-formation and a lower prevalence of the disorder than that in the general population [9].

Level of Physical Activity

One other factor which is influenced by increasing affluence in a given population is the average level of physical activity among the workforce. The movement away from the more active types of occupation associated with an agricultural economy and an increasing reliance on automation, office work, and more managerial types of activities, together lead to a reduction in the level of physical activity in the population. It has been considered for a number of years that stone disease is more prevalent among sedentary workers than among more physically active workers. Unfortunately, because individuals who have sedentary occupations are often more highly paid than those who perform more manual types of work, it is difficult to distinguish whether the higher prevalence of stones among the former is due to their more affluent lifestyle or to their less active occupations.

In this connection it has been suggested that the much lower prevalence of stones in women in developing countries (where the male/female ratio among stone-formers is about 5:1) than in their counterparts in the industrialized countries (where the male/female ratio is 2:1 or less) is due to the fact that the former lead much more physically active lives than the latter [2]. Again, however, the reasons are not clear-cut since the women from the industrialized countries are generally more affluent than those from the developing countries and this will affect the diets of the two groups.

Stone-Formation in the Arabian Peninsula

As indicated in Tables 1 and 2, the prevalence of stones in the populations of the oil-rich countries of the Arabian Peninsula is extremely high. The projected life-time

Table 3. Percentage occurrence of main constituents of stones

Stones containing	UK (1984)	USA (1964)	KSA (1989)
Uric acid	4.0	9.4	21.3
Calcium oxalate	77.7	72.1	73.1
Calcium phosphate	47.9	40.0	28.5
MAP	9.6	9.2	3.3
Cystine	1.6	0.9	2.1
Others	0.1	0.1	0.7

KSA, Kingdom of Saudi Arabia

risk of stone-formation in men over the age of 60 is at least 50% higher than the highest corresponding figures in the West.

In terms of stone composition, there is a considerable shift toward calculi containing calcium oxalate and/or uric acid, compared with data from the United Kingdom (Table 3). There are fewer calcium phosphate-containing stones and infection stones but more of the rare types of calculi which result from inborn errors of metabolism, such as cystinuria, xanthinuria and 2,8-dihydroxyadeninuria. Data from the United States lie between those of the United Kingdom and Saudi Arabia, but more recent figures suggest that the pattern in the United States over the past 25 years has shifted closer to that in Saudi Arabia (LH Smith, personal communication). Apparently there are now more uric acid-containing and fewer calcium phosphate-containing stones in the United States than in 1964.

The different patterns of stone composition between the Middle East and the West correlate well with the average composition of urine in the two regions (Table 4). Urine from men in the Arabian Peninsula has a lower volume, a lower pH, a lower calcium and citrate content, and a much higher oxalate and uric acid content than urine from men in the West. This leads to Middle Eastern men having generally higher levels of supersaturation of urine with respect to calcium oxalate and uric acid and lower levels of supersaturation with respect to calcium phosphate. This would explain the higher percentage of uric acid-containing stones and the lower proportion of calcium phosphate-containing stones in that part of the world.

In turn, the differences in urine composition can be accounted for by the differences in dietary intakes of the main nutrients influencing the excretion of stone-

Table 4. Comparison of 24-hour urine biochemistry in normal and stone-forming Middle Eastern and Western men

	Normals				Stone-formers			
Constituent	UK	USA	UAE	KSA	UK	USA	UAE	KSA
Volume (l)	1.60	1.55	1.44	1.25	1.76	1.70	1.68	1.56
pH	6.04	5.95	5.90	5.82	6.00	5.90	5.70	5.68
Calcium (mmol)	6.0	5.8	4.2	3.2	8.8	7.9	5.2	4.6
Oxalate (mmol)	0.33	0.41	0.46	0.53	0.43	0.49	0.63	0.69
Uric acid (mmol)	2.9	4.0	4.6	4.7	3.3	4.3	4.7	4.8
Citrate (mmol)	3.3	2.9	–	1.0	3.1	1.9	–	–

UAE, United Arab Emirates; KSA, Kingdom of Saudi Arabia

Table 5. Daily dietary intakes in male calcium stone-formers

Constituent	UK	USA	UAE	KSA
Animal protein (g)	61	85	"High"	87
Calcium (mmol)	24.5	25.0	23.0	13.0
Oxalate (mmol)	1.4	2.4	5.5	3.8
Purine (mg)	190	257	"High"	268
Oxalate/calcium (mmol/mmol)	0.06	0.10	0.24	0.29

UAE, United Arab Emirates; KSA, Kingdom of Saudi Arabia

forming minerals in urine. Table 5 shows that in the Arabian Peninsula male stone-formers consume more meat (i.e., a higher animal protein and purine intake), more oxalate, and less calcium than do their counterparts in the West.

Table 6 summarizes the data on normal men available from a number of countries. This shows that the life-time risk of stones rises in parallel with the ratio of oxalate/calcium in the diet and with the daily intake of animal protein. Diets high in oxalate and low in calcium have been shown to markedly increase the urinary excretion of oxalate, the most potent biochemical risk factor for stone disease next to a persistently low urine volume. Diets high in animal protein (and purine) have been shown to acidify urine, to increase the excretions of calcium, oxalate, and uric acid and to decrease the excretion of citrate. Where both dietary aberrations occur together, as in the affluent countries of the Arabian Peninsula, the risk of stone-formation explodes exponentially.

Table 6 also supports the observation that there is no relationship between the risk of calcium stone-formation and the urinary excretion of calcium [10]. Conversely, there is a high correlation between the prevalence of the disorder and the urinary excretion of oxalate [10].

Table 6. Relationship between life-time prevalence of urolithiasis in 60 to 70-year-old men and urinary and dietary composition in normal men in various countries

Country	Life-time stone prevalence in men > 60 years (%)	Urinary Ox (mmol/day)	Urinary Ca (mmol/day)	Diet Ox/Ca (mmol/mmol)	Diet AP (g/day)
China	1.5	–	3.5	–	21
Japan	5.4	0.31	4.1	–	39
UK	7.8	0.33	6.0	0.05	53
W Germany	8.0	0.36	5.8	0.06	59
Sweden	8.6	0.35	5.0	0.06	60
Canada	12.0	0.38	5.5	–	66
USA	13.0	0.41	5.8	0.10	76
United Arab Emirates	18.0	0.46	4.2	0.33	"Very high"
Saudi Arabia	20.1	0.53	3.2	0.29	82

Ox, oxalate; Ca, calcium; AP, animal protein

Treatment of Stone Disease in the Middle East

As indicated in Table 6, hypercalciuria is an uncommon finding in the Middle East. The reasons for this are two-fold – firstly, dietary calcium is lower than in the West (Table 5) and, secondly, hyperabsorption of calcium from a given oral load is rare [11]. The latter may be due to the paradoxically low vitamin D levels in Middle Eastern men. In terms of treatment, therefore, any measures designed to reduce urinary calcium excretion below the already low values are not likely to succeed.

Utilizing the above observations that calcium intake and absorption are low, a pilot study was carried out to determine the effects of adding 1 g/day, extra calcium (in the form of calcium citrate) to the diets of 12 recurrent idiopathic stone-formers. This regimen reduced the urinary oxalate excretions of all the patients. Only one value remained slightly above the normal range for urinary oxalate in the West. Since there was no major rise in urinary calcium, the biochemical risk of forming calcium oxalate stones was reduced. It is now the intention to extend this form of treatment by adding potassium citrate to the calcium citrate in order to alkalinize urine and increase the excretion of citrate. By this means it ought to be possible to further reduce the risk of calcium oxalate stones and, at the same time, to eliminate the risk of uric acid stones.

References

1. Andersen DA (1973) Environmental factors in the aetiology of urolithiasis. In: Cifuentes Delatte L, Rapado A, Hodgkinson A (eds) Urinary calculi. Karger, Basel, pp 130–144
2. Asper R (1984) Epidemiology and socioeconomic aspects of urolithiasis. Urol Res 12:1–5
3. Husain I, Badsha SA, Al-Ali IH, Walton M, Saheb A, Jafree S (1979) A survey of urinary stone disease in Abu Dhabi. Emirates Med J (Suppl) 1:17–33
4. Robertson WG, Nisa M, Husain I, Al-Faqi S, Chakrabarty A, Qunibi W, Taher S, Hughes H, Barkworth SA, Holbrow G, Louis S (1989) The importance of diet in the aetiology of primary calcium and uric acid stone-formation – the Arabian experience. In: Walker VR, Sutton RAL, Cameron ECB, Pak CYC, Robertson WG (eds) Urolithiasis. Plenum, New York, pp 735–739
5. Blacklock NJ (1979) Epidemiology of renal lithiasis. In: Wickham JEA (ed) Urinary calculous disease. Churchill Livingstone, Edinburgh, pp 21–39
6. Robertson WG (1982) Urolithiasis: epidemiology and pathogenesis. In: Husain I (ed) Tropical urology and renal disease. Churchill Livingstone, Edinburgh, pp 143–164
7. Dick WH, Lingeman JE, Preminger GM, Smith LH, Wilson DM, Shirrell WL (1989) Laxative abuse as a cause for ammonium urate renal calculi. In: Walker VR, Sutton RAL, Cameron ECB, Pak CYC, Robertson WG (eds) Urolithiasis. Plenum, New York, pp 303–305
8. Robertson WG, Peacock M, Heyburn PJ, Hanes F, Rutherford A, Clementson E, Swaminathan R, Clark PB (1979) Should recurrent, calcium-containing stone-formers become vegetarians? Br J Urol 51:427–431
9. Robertson WG, Peacock M, Marshall DH (1982) Prevalence of urinary stone disease in vegetarians. Eur Urol 9:334–339
10. Robertson WG, Peacock M (1980) The cause of idiopathic calcium stone disease: hypercalciuria or hyperoxaluria? Nephron 26:105–110
11. Walker VR, Bissada N, Qunibi W, Hughes H, Barkworth SA, Holbrow G, Phillips R, Robertson WG, Russell RGG (1989) Urinary calcium excretion in Saudi Arabia. In: Walker VR, Sutton RAL, Cameron ECB, Pak CYC, Robertson WG (eds) Urolithiasis. Plenum, New York, pp 717–719

Environmental Studies in Man in the Dead Sea Region

Ori S. Better[1]

Summary. The Dead Sea contains a hyperconcentrated solution and is an example of the salt lakes which abound along geological fault lines. It is important to study human exposure to such media because of intentional or accidental immersion in these lakes. The present communication reviews the effect of (1) experimental, neck out immersion (NI); and (2) accidental near drowning (ND) in the Dead Sea.

1) NI in Dead Sea water failed to produce the expected natriuresis, diuresis and hypotension that is seen during NI in fresh water. The reason is probably the tourniquet-like effect of the venous system in the lower limbs, due to the high head of pressure of Dead Sea water. Such an increased pressure head may prevent the rise in venous return from the lower body seen during immersion in fresh water.

2) ND in the Dead Sea causes much greater fatality and morbidity than ND in sea water. The reason for this increased danger is, at least partly, due to the augmented load of solutes on ND victims in the Dead Sea. Such an increased solute load may lead to extreme hypercalcemia and hypermagnesemia.

The Dead Sea is a lake that lies at the bottom (minus 400 m below sea level) of the hot, arid area of the Syrian-African Rift. Due to its geographic peculiarities and high rate of evaporation, its solute content is extremely high (specific gravity 1.2). Somewhat similar salt lakes abound along the entire length of the Syrian-African Rift and along other geological rifts, such as those found in the Western United States of America (including the Great Salt Lake of Utah). Many of these lakes are located in scenic environments and are used as recreation and resort areas as well as open mining regions for minerals. Man may be exposed to the water of these salt lakes either intentionally or accidentally. It is therefore important to learn the effects of immersion and of near drowning in hyperconcentrated solutions. The purpose of this communication is to review: (a) the effects of experimental immersion to the neck (NI)

[1]Department of Nephrology, Rambam Hospital, and Faculty of Medicine, Technion, Israel Institute of Technology, Haifa, 35254, Israel

on volume control; (b) plasma electrolyte disturbance during near drowning (ND) in the Dead Sea.

Immersion Studies

The extensive, pioneering studies of Gauer and Henry [1] and Epstein [2] have shown that NI in thermoneutral (34°C) fresh water is associated with natriuresis and diuresis, leading to negative salt and water balance. The mechanism of these changes was secondary to centripetal redistribution of body fluids with central (intrathoracic) hypervolemia. We decided to extend these experiments by comparing the effects of NI in Dead Sea water, (which is a hyperconcentrated medium) at 34°C, on volume regulation with those of NI in fresh water [3]. Our results, partially summarized in Fig. 1, show that NI in fresh water for 4 h did indeed produce the expected natriuresis, diuresis and weight loss (1.4 $\pm$ 0.4 kg). In marked contrast, and somewhat unexpectedly, NI in Dead Sea water failed to cause diuresis, natriuresis or change in body weight. Surprisingly, NI in Dead Sea water caused an increase in systolic and diastolic blood pressure, whereas NI in fresh water caused a decrease in systolic and diastolic blood pressure. The differences between the means of the blood pressure changes in the two immersion media were statistically significant.

We speculate that the absence of natriuresis and diuresis during NI in Dead Sea water is due to the following hydrostatic conditions: NI in the Dead Sea provides a 20% greater head of pressure on the body (specific gravity 1.2) than fresh water would. It may be calculated that the pressure on the body 1 m below the neck would be 91.2 mm Hg in Dead Sea water, compared with 76 mm Hg in fresh water. At 91.2 mm Hg external pressure, venous return from the lower limbs to the heart would be obliterated, and hemodynamic effects negated.

Information on the effect of immersion on arterial blood pressure is scant and conflicting. Epstein stated, in 1978, that "Immersion in fresh water was associated with significant, albeit slight, decrease in mean arterial blood pressure" [4]. A later study by the same author [5] also showed a decrease in mean arterial pressure during immersion in fresh water in, at least, certain individuals. Arborelius et al. [6], utilizing intraarterial manometry, found that immersion caused a mean increase in arterial pressure of 10 mm Hg. This was, however, less than the increase of pressure of 15 to 20 mm Hg in the ambient water surrounding the immersed arm in which the brachial artery was cannulated for the manometry. Moreover, their study was short and did not last for 100 min of immersion, which is when hypotension was seen in the present study.

Other independent studies have confirmed that NI in fresh water will lower blood pressure in the pregnant woman [7], in the normal man [8], and in patients with cirrhosis [9].

The cause of the hypotension of immersion appears to be the suppression, by NI, of at least three vasoconstrictor systems (AVP, catecholamine, and renin-angiotensin II), and the stimulation of the vasodilator system (atrial natriuretic factor). It is possible that minor changes in immersion medium temperature ($\pm$ 0.5° C) could affect blood pressure determination, thus explaining the controversy on this matter.

In summary, the specific gravity of the medium in which NI is performed has profound effects on the resulting hemodynamic influences. A high specific gravity

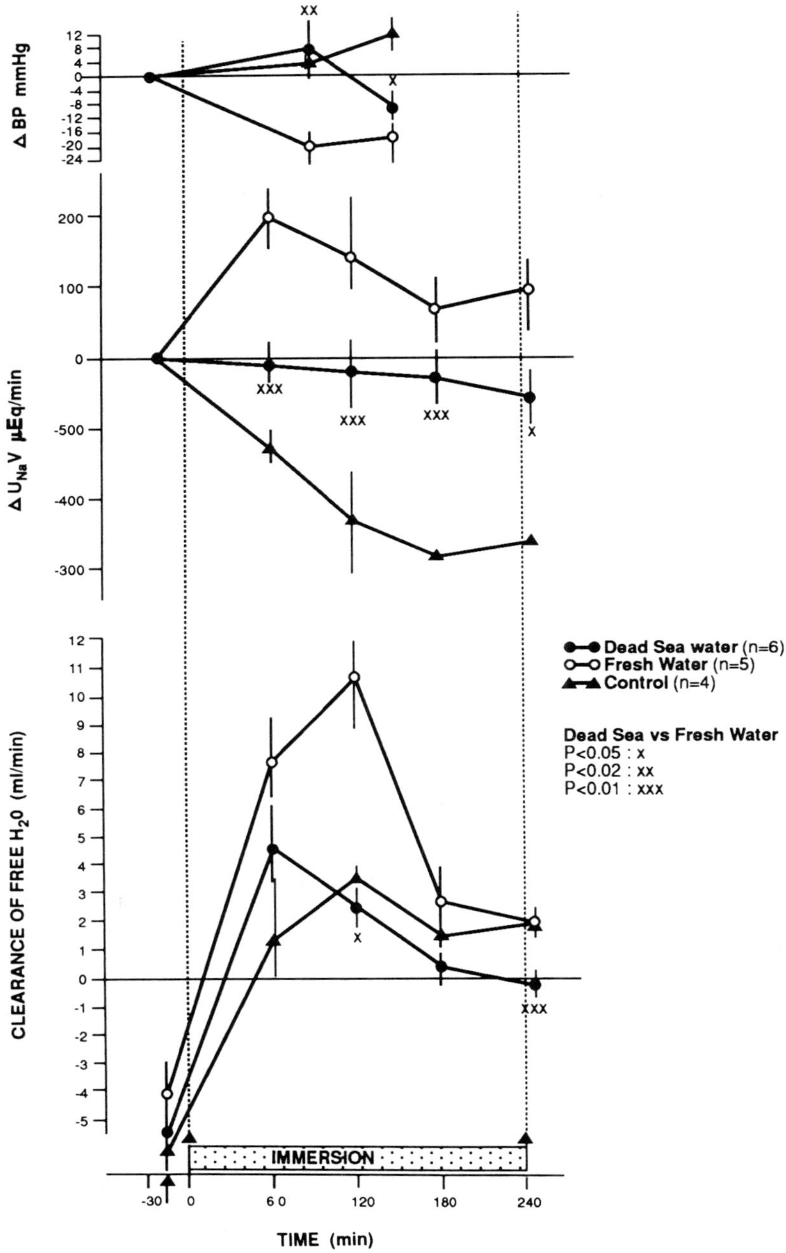

Fig. 1. Influence of neck-out immersion on systolic blood pressure (*BP*) (*top panel*), rate of urinary sodium excretion (*UNaV*) (*middle panel*), and clearance of free water (*bottom panel*). Note a fall in blood pressure and an increase in natriuresis and diuresis during immersion in fresh water. In contrast, immersion in Dead Sea water results in an increase in blood pressure not associated with increased natriuresis, and is associated only with moderately increased diuresis. Quiet sitting is not associated with changes in blood pressure or with increased natriuresis. Results are expressed as mean ± SD

medium may negate the hypotension, natriuresis and diuresis seen in NI in fresh water.

Near-Drowning (ND) in the Dead Sea

Drowning is defined as death due to submersion in water or other media. ND refers to at least temporary survival after asphyxia due to submersion [10]. Of patients with ND in fresh water or sea water, 91% survive; there are only minor changes in plasma electrolytes due to aspiration of fluids [9]. In marked contrast, ND in the Dead Sea (approximately 30% solutes, × 10 the concentration of the oceans), carries a mortality of at least 40% [11]. Such fatality is due, at least in part, to the load of solutes, which causes striking changes in the composition of the plasma, particularly in the concentration of divalent ions. The Dead Sea has extreme concentrations of calcium and magnesium. The hypercalcemia and hypermagnesemia after ND in the Dead Sea may reach 28.8 and 33.0 mg/dl (!) [12], respectively, values which separately, in other circumstances, are incompatible with life. Most patients, following ND in the Dead Sea, presented with disturbed sensorium, adult respiratory distress syndrome, tachyarrhythmia, and conduction disturbances. Surprisingly, the QTc interval in their ECG was normal in the face of extreme hypercalcemia and hypermagnesemia [12]. It is speculated that this co-intoxication with these divalent cations was mutually protective, since calcium and magnesium are physiological antagonists [13]. Moreover, intravenous calcium infusion was used as an emergency measure to protect against the otherwise refractory hypotension of extreme hypermagnesemia [14].

In general, the best single predictor of survival in ND in the Dead Sea was a serum calcium level below 15.5 mg%.

The recommended treatment of ND in the Dead Sea includes on-scene gastric suction for alert patients, respiratory support, and forced diuresis. The role of dialysis in ND is still being evaluated.

In summary, ND in the Dead Sea is dangerous, because it may cause extreme changes in plasma divalent ion concentration. Such changes in plasma composition are usually not seen in ND in the sea or in fresh water lakes.

References

1. Gauer OH, Henry JP (1976) Neurohumoral control of plasma volume. Int Rev Physiol 9:145–190
2. Epstein M (1978) Renal effects of head-out water immersion in man: implications for an understanding of volume homeostasis. Physiol Rev 58:529–581
3. Ish-Shalom N, Better OS (1984) Volume regulation in man during neck-out immersion in a medium with high specific gravity (Dead Sea water). Isr J Med Sci 20:109–112
4. Epstein M, Preston S, Weitzman RE (1981) Isoosmotic central blood volume expansion suppresses plasma arginine vasopressin in normal man. J Clin Endocrinol Metab 52:256–262
5. Epstein M (1978) Studies of volume homeostasis in man utilizing the model of head-out water immersion. Nephron 22:9–19

6. Arborelius M Jr, Balldin UI, Lilja B, Lundgren CEG (1972) Hemodynamic changes in man during immersion with the head above water. Aerospace Medicine 43:592–598
7. Kokot F, Ulman J, Cekauski A (1983) Influence of head out water immersion on plasma renin activity, aldosterone, vasopressin and blood pressure in late pregnancy and toxemia. Proc Eur Dial Transplant Assoc 20:557–561
8. Leung WM, Logan AG, Campbell PJ (1987) Role of ANP and urinary cGMP in the natriuretic and diuretic response to central hypervolemia in normal human subjects. Can J Physiol Pharmacol 65:2076–2080
9. Skorecki KL, Leung WM, Campbell P, Warner LC, Wong PY, Bull S, Logan AG, Blendis LM (1988) Role of atrial natriuretic peptide in the natriuretic response to central volume expansion induced by head-out water immersion in sodium retaining cirrhotic subjects. Am J Med 85:375–382
10. Modell JH, Graves SA, Ketover A (1976) Clinical course of 91 consecutive near drowning victims. Chest 70:231–238
11. Yagil Y, Stalinkowicz R, Michaeli J, Mogle P (1985) Near drowning in the Dead Sea. Electrolyte imbalances and therapeutic implication. Arch Intern Med 145:50–53
12. Porath A, Masseri M, Harman I, Ovsyshecher I, Keinan A (1989) Dead Sea poisoning. Ann Emerg Med 18:187–191
13. Levin BS, Coburn JW (1984) Magnesium, the mimic/antagonist of calcium (editorial). N Engl J Med 310:1523–1524
14. Mordes JP, Swartz R, Arky RA (1975) Extreme hypermagnesemia as a cause of refractory hypotension. Ann Intern Med 83:657–658

Progression and Chronicity of Acute Post-Streptococcal Glomerulonephritis (APSGN)

NOBUYUKI YOSHIZAWA[1] and INGE SAGEL[2]

SUMMARY. In a follow-up study of 33 patients who had had overt acute post-streptococcal glomerulonephritis (APSGN), 11 patients had intermittent or persistent hematuria and/or proteinuria with or without hypertension 2–15 years after onset.

In a prospective survey conducted in two separate areas of Japan, onset of asymptomatic APSGN after infection with β hemolytic streptococci was observed in 25% of the subjects studied. A follow-up of not less than two years was carried out on these patients. Progression of the disease into chronicity, as defined by persistent or intermittent hematuria, was observed in three of 10 patients. Repeat renal biopsies were performed in seven patients (three asymptomatic and four overt). Proliferative glomerulonephritis without deposition of IgA (non-IgA nephropathy) was diagnosed in all of these cases. Antibody titers were measured in 73 patients with non-IgA nephropathy detected as chance hematuria, using a streptococcal protein which we believe is the nephritogenic antigen. Titers against this antigen were, in our experience, uniformly elevated in patients with asymptomatic and overt APSGN. It was found that 14 of the patients (19%) had elevated levels as compared with normal subjects. These findings suggest that many of the non-IgAN patients may have progressed from asymptomatic APSGN.

Asymptomatic APSGN [1,2]

The author wishes to describe the results of a survey conducted in New York [3]. In the survey, 248 children with streptococcal infection were followed on a weekly basis with urinalysis and CH50 for at least 6 weeks. Of the 248 children, 194 developed no abnormal findings and were no longer followed. The remaining 54 children

[1]Department of Medicine, National Defense Medical College, 3-2 Namiki, Tokorozawa, 359 Japan
[2]Department of Pediatrics, New York Medical College, NY, USA

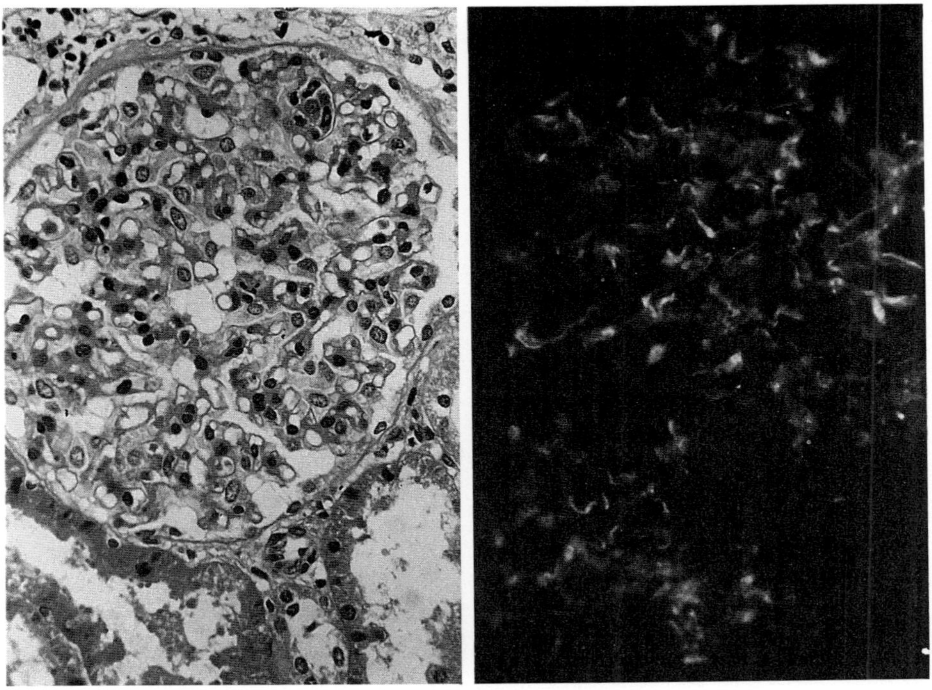

a b

Fig. 1. **a** Acute glomerulonephritis (AGN) (PAS), **b** AGN (C3)

showed one of the following abnormalities: 1] proteinuria and/or hematuria (15), 2] transient decrease in CH50 (19), 3] both of the above (20).

Renal histology in patients with both disorders showed that one was normal, seven had mild proliferative (+AGN), and nine had moderate proliferative change (++AGN). Three patients showed the classical pathology seen in APSGN (+++AGN). By immunofluorescence (IF) test five were negative, while the remainder showed positive segmental or diffuse granular deposition of IgG and C3 (Figs. 1,2). The infecting strains of group A, β hemolytic streptococci were mostly T type 4, 12, and Impetigo 19. All children were asymptomatic, except one who had mild periorbital edema.

These data indicate that the incidence of glomerular pathology among children infected by group A, β hemolytic streptococci is much higher than the reported incidence, and glomerulonephritis, even in the asymptomatic cases, is morphologically quite evident. In these asymptomatic APSGN cases, serum complement level decreased transiently at the early stage of the disease, together with the appearance of the urinary findings, suggesting development of nephritis subsequent to the streptococcal infection.

From 1978–1979 and from 1982–1984, a prospective survey was conducted, in the same manner as the survey in New York, in the Takanedai area of Funabashi City and

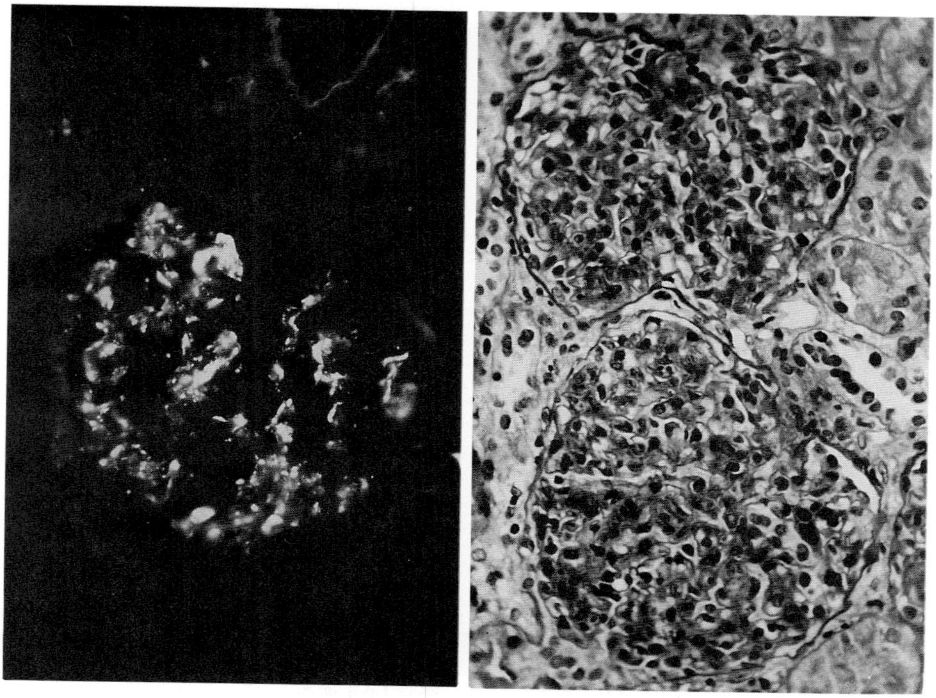

a b

Fig. 2. **a** AGN (PAS), **b** AGN (C3)

the Kanayamacho area of Tokorozawa City in Japan. Proteinuria and/or hematuria with or without decrease in CH50 were detected in 25% of the 44 patients with streptococcal upper respiratory infection (URI) in both groups [4] and all were asymptomatic. Table 1 shows the laboratory findings for our patients. In all cases, the presence of proliferative changes was confirmed by renal biopsy. The severity of these lesions varied, ranging from +AGN or mild, to classical +++AGN.

Incidence of Chronicity Following Asymptomatic and Overt APSGN

APSGN is considered to be a "curable nephritis" in most cases and is reported to progress into chronicity in only 5% of affected children and in about 20%–30% of affected adults. According to the diagnostic criteria published by the Ministry of Health and Welfare in Japan, chronic glomerulonephritis is defined as abnormal urinary findings or hypertension persisting over one year after onset of nephritis. As shown in Fig. 3, patients with overt APSGN may have normal urinary findings within one to two years after onset of the disease, therefore, we regard abnormal urinary findings of at least two years duration as progression into chronicity. Furthermore, as shown in Fig. 3, some patients, after an interval with normal urine, showed recur-

Table 1. Clinical and laboratory data of 13 patients with asymptomatic APGN

Patients		Latent period (W)	ASO	CH50	Urinalysis			Biopsy	Follow-up period	Outcome
					Protein	RBC	WBC			
1. S.M.	11F	3	500	24.5	+	0–1	0–1	+ AGN	2 Y	Recovered
2. U.H.	5F	7	1250	23.2	+	0–1	1–2	+ AGN	2 Y	Recovered
3. H.M.	26F	8	500	22.8	–	1–2	0–1	+ AGN	2 Y	Recovered
4. A.N.	11F	4	625	20.6	–	0–2	1–2	+ AGN	2 Y	Recovered
5. I.M.	34F	1	333	22.0	–	10–15	1–3	++ AGN	5 Y	Chronic
6. K.M.	11F	4	333	13.5	+	2–3	1–2	++ AGN	6 Y	Chronic
7. N.H.	11M	9	333	22.8	+	1–2	1–2	+ AGN	6.5 Y	Recovered
8. K.H.	16F	?	833	24.0	–	15–20	1–2	++ AGN	6.5 Y	Chronic
9. N.M.	13M	1	625	24.2	+	0–1	0–2	+ AGN	7 Y	Recovered
10. B.S.	8F	7	1250	<5	+	14–17	0–1	+ AGN	8 Y	Recovered
11. S.T.	13F	5	625	20.4	–	0–3	0–1	+ AGN	8 Y	Recovered
12. T.Y.	7M	2	625	17.5	+	0–1	1–2	+ AGN	8 Y	Recovered
13. S.M.	12F	2	625	<12	–	20–25	1–2	⧻ AGN	8 Y	Recovered

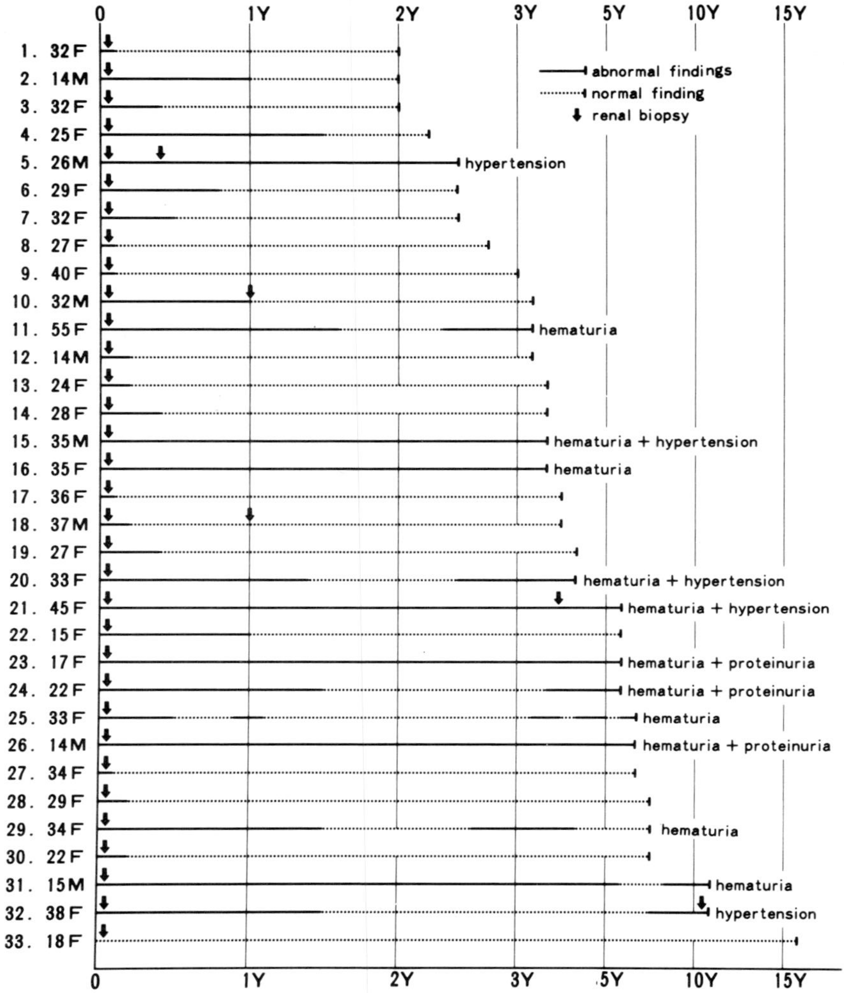

Fig. 3. Clinical course of 33 patients with overt APSGN

rence of abnormal urinary findings two–three years after the disease appeared to have healed, thus, the definition of chronicity is not easy.

The clinical course of thirteen Japanese patients with asymptomatic APSGN was followed up for 8 years. Three were lost to follow-up and three of the remaining 10 patients followed for at least 2 years had persistent or intermittent hematuria (Fig. 4). Of 33 patients with biopsy-proven overt APSGN, 11 (33.3%) progressed into "chronicity" by presenting with hematuria and/or proteinuria with or without hypertension (Fig. 3). Table 2 summarizes the results of renal biopsies in seven of these patients. Histology showed mild to moderate mesangial proliferative glomerulonephritis without IgA deposits, which is classified as Non-IgA nephropathy. The

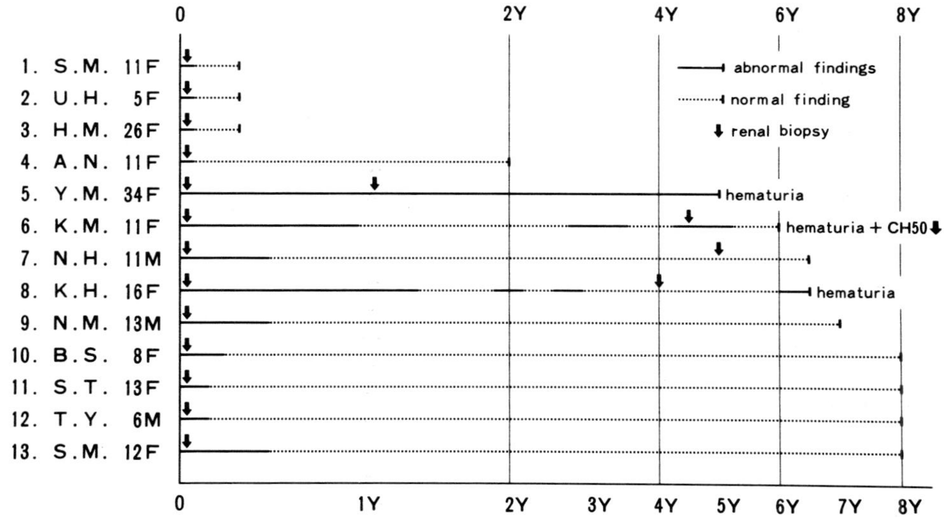

Fig. 4. Clinical course of 13 patients with asymptomatic APSGN

above-mentioned findings suggest that many patients with initially undetected streptococcal infections may present with chance hematuria and/or proteinuria in school or corporate physical examinations.

Non-IgA nephropathy is not an established entity; however, in Japan, 30%–40% of patients with chronic glomerulonephritis are of this type; this nephropathy along with IgA nephropathy, constitutes a principal type of nephritis, in the etiology of chance hematuria and/or proteinuria. Asymptomatic APSGN may develop insidi-

Table 2. Follow-up biopsies of 7 patients with chronic PSGN

Patient		Onset ↓ Biopsy	IF					LM
			C3c	G	A	M	Fib	
1. T.Y.	26M	20d	+++	++	−	++	−	+++ A G N
		110d	+	−	−	++	−	+ C G N
2. S.C.	38F	22d	++	+	(+)	−	−	++ A G N
		10y	−	−	−	−	−	+ C G N
3. W.K.	45F	31d	++	−	−	−	(+)	++ A G N
		4y	−	−	−	−	−	++ C G N
4. S.M.	39F	25d	++	−	−	−	−	++ A G N
		5y	−	−	−	−	−	+ C G N
*5. K.M.	11F	21d	+	+	−	+	(+)	++ A G N
		4.5y	+	+	−	±	(±)	+ C G N
*6. K.H.	16F	40d	+	±	(+)	±	(+)	+ A G N
		4y	+	±	(+)	±	(+)	+ C G N
*7. I.M.	34F	44d	++	+	(+)	+	(+)	++ A G N
		1.5y	+	−	(±)	±	(±)	+ C G N

*Asymptomatic
IF, immunofluorescence; LM, light microscopy
( ), focal

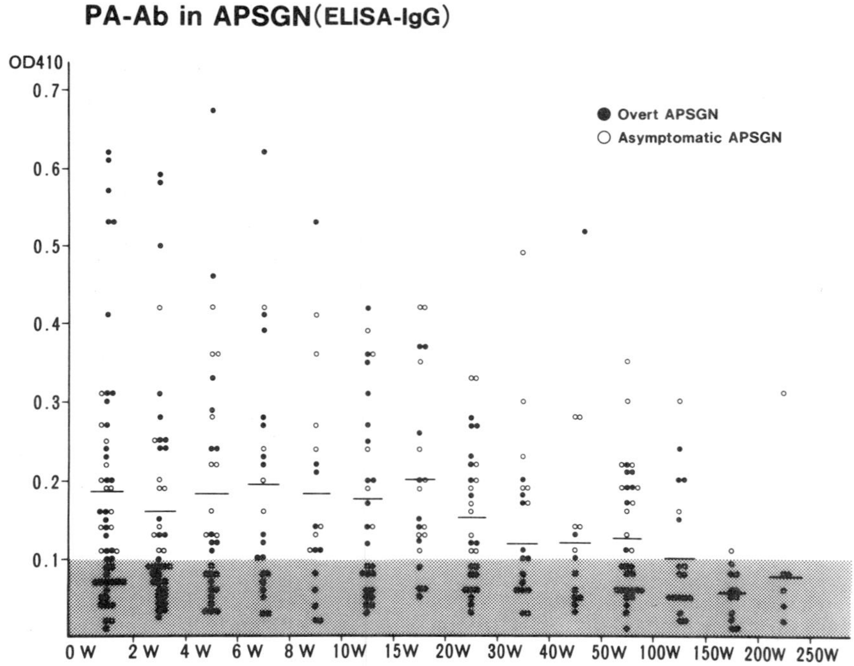

Fig. 5. Antibody to PA-Ag in APSGN (ELISA)

ously and may be detected accidentally as chance hematuria/proteinuria. For further clarification, we determined serum antibody titers against preabsorbing antigen (PA-Ag), using enzyme-linked immunoadsorbent assay (ELISA). In patients with asymptomatic and overt APSGN, mean titers of the antibody were significantly higher than those in normal adults and in patients with uncomplicated streptococcal infections. One third of the patients continued to have high titers for more than two years after onset (Fig. 5). Of 73 patients with Non-IgA nephropathy detected as chance hematuria, results were found to be positive in 14 (19%) patients (Fig. 6). This result suggests that streptococcal infection may have been the cause of the nephropathy detected as chance hematuria.

Preabsorbing antigen (PA-Ag) [5–7] is a protein fraction which we consider to have nephritogenic properties, isolated from nephritogenic streptococci. During the acute phase of APSGN this fraction was found to localize on the glomerular basement membrane and in the mesangium; the fraction is a purified form of endostreptosin [8,9] with a M.W. 43000 and pI 4.7.

Mechanism of Chronicity (Fig. 7)

Jennings and Earle [10] postulated that the severity of certain histologic lesions at disease onset was related to chronicity. According to these investigators, such lesions include (1) endothelial cell proliferation, (2) glomerular damage (lobular necrosis or

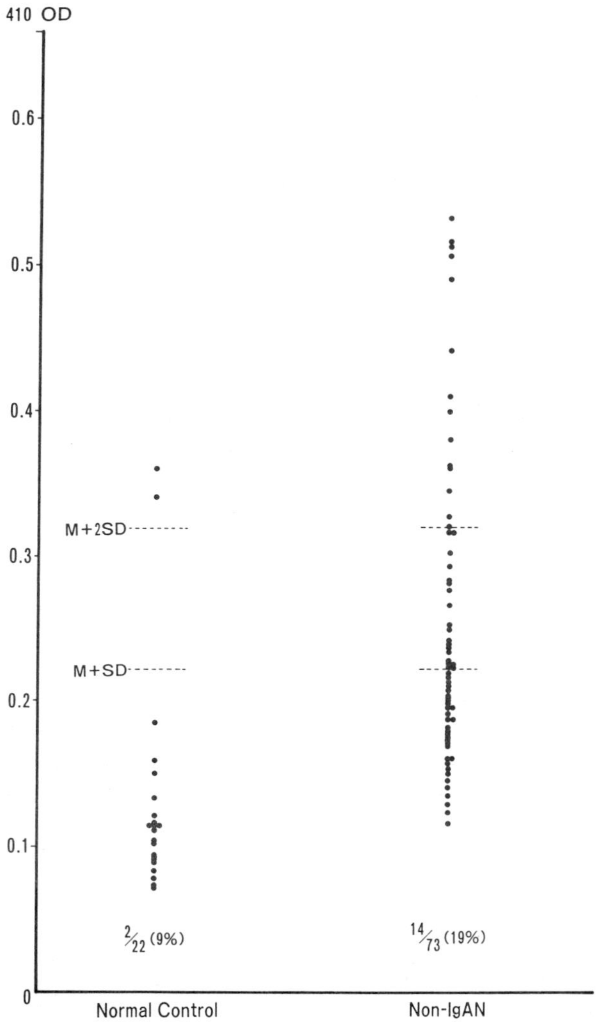

Fig. 6. Antibody titers to PA-Ag in patients with non-IgA nephritis detected by chance hematuria

scar, thrombosis, crescent, adhesion, or hyalinization), and (3) interstitial reaction. These authors postulated that the more severe and diffused these lesions, the more likely it would be that the disease would become chronic. Baldwin et al. [11] suggested that intrarenal vascular sclerosis can lead to glomerulosclerosis, and they proposed that ischemia might play an important pathogenetic role in the progression of APSGN to chronicity. In addition to the above, interstitial cellular infiltration [12,13] may also be an important factor in the development of chronic disease. We investigated interstitial cellular infiltration within the glomerulus and tubulointer-

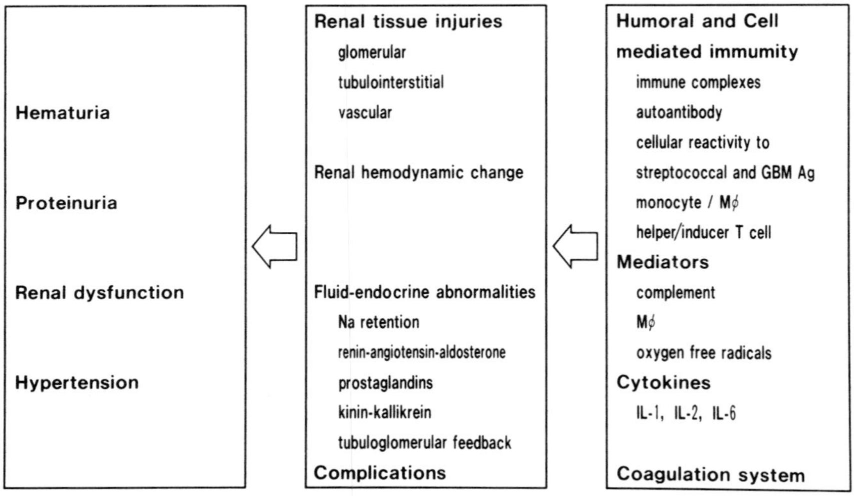

Fig. 7. Factors contributing to chronicity of APSGN

stitium (Fig. 8), using monoclonal antibody in various types of glomerulonephritis, and we found that there is little or no cellular infiltration in the glomerulus, except in APSGN. However, cellular infiltration, mostly of helper/inducer T cells and monocyte/Mϕ (Fig. 9), was increased in the interstitial tissue, with no apparent difference in the pattern of infiltration among various glomerulonephritides [14]. In ddition, there was a significant positive correlation between the extent of cell

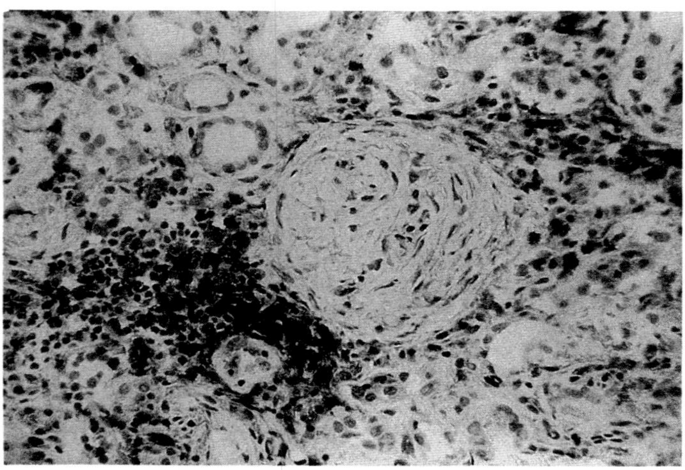

Fig. 9. Interstitial cellular infiltration (CD4 : helper/inducer T cell)

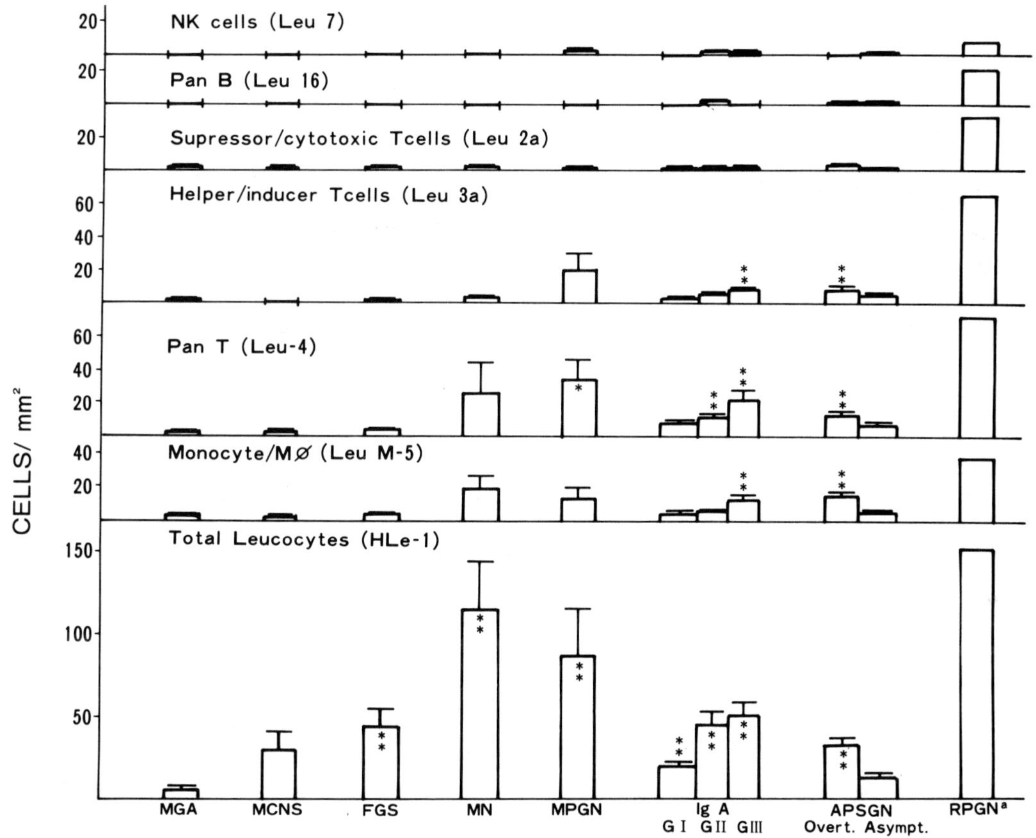

Fig. 8. Analysis of interstitial infiltrating leucocyte subpopulations in various glomerulonephritis. MGA, minor glomerular abnormalities; MCNS, minimal change nephrotic syndrome; FGS, focal glomerular sclerosis; MN, membranous nephropathy; MPGN, membranoproliferative glomerulonephritis; RPGN, rapidly progressive glomerulonephritis; * $P<0.05$ as compared with MGA; ** $P<0.01$

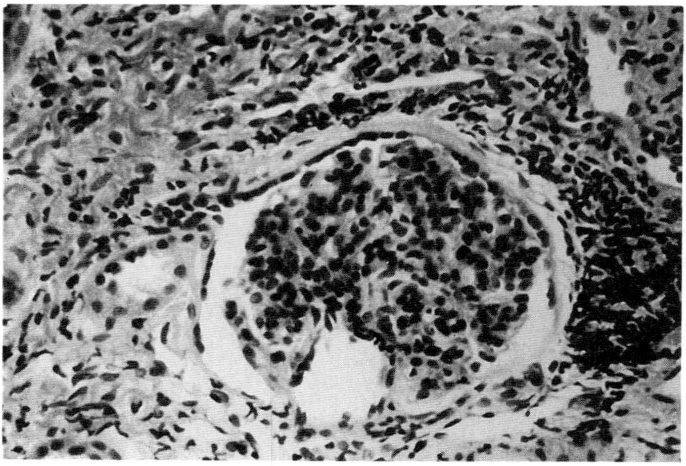

Fig. 10. Periglomerular cellular infiltration in APSGN (PAS)

infiltration and serum creatinine levels. That is, the more extensive the interstitial cellular infiltration, the more severe the renal dysfunction.

Tubular damage, caused by glomerular injury or other etiology, can unmask antigenic components of the tubules, thereby inducing antigenicity, which in turn induces delayed type hypersensitivity, resulting in the progression of tubulointerstitial damage. Interleukin-I (IL-1), released by Mϕ, is known to accelerate proliferation of fibroblasts, and it is possible that interstitial fibrosis can increase postglomerular capillary resistance and can cause deterioration in the glomerular circulation, thus reducing glomerular filtration rate (GFR) [15]. It is also possible that Na reabsorption disorders caused by dysfunction of the tubules can reduce GFR via tubulo-glomerular feedback mechanisms. These are mainly interstitial responses to aggravating factors, but generally, if the glomerular damage as described above is severe at the onset of the disease, periglomerular cellular infiltration may have occurred (Fig. 10). In this case the infiltrating cells are mostly T cells and monocyte/Mϕ, which can induce cell to cell interactions with infiltrating and mesangial cells.

Persistence and progression of such renal tissue injuries may be mediated by immunologic factors, namely humoral and cell-mediated immunity [16], as well as by complement, macrophages, cytokines, and the coagulation system.

References

1. Cohen JA, Levitt MF (1963) Acute glomerulonephritis with few urinary abnormalities. Report of two cases proved by renal biopsy. N Engl J Med 268:749–753
2. Freedman P, Meister HP, Co BS, Markowitz AS, Dubin A (1966) The subclinical renal response to streptococcal infection. New Engl J Med 275:795
3. Sagel I, Treser G, Yoshizawa N, Ty A, Kleinberger H, Yuceoglu M, Wasserman E, Lange K (1973) Occurrence and nature of glomerular lesions after group A streptococci infection in children. Ann Intern Med 79:492

4. Yoshizawa N, Oshima S, Takeuchi A, Sagel I, Treser G (1987) Occurrence of chronicity following asymptomatic and overt acute poststreptococcal glomerulonephritis (APGN). Proceedings of the Xth international congress of nephrology
5. Yoshizawa N, Treser G, Sagel I, Ty A, Ahmed U, Lange K (1973) Demonstration of antigenic sites in glomeruli of patients with acute poststreptococcal glomerulonephritis by immunofluorescein and immunoferritin techniques. Am J Pathol 70:131
6. Yoshizawa N, Oshima S, Takeuchi A, Takahashi K, Sagel I, Treser G (1985) Serological studies in poststreptococcal glomerulonephritis using streptococcal antigen (preabsorbing antigen, PA-Ag). In: Recent advances in streptococci and streptococcal diseases. Readbooks, Berkshire, p 251
7. Yoshizawa N, Oshima S, Takeuchi A, Takahashi K, Sagel I, Treser G (1985) A streptococcal antigen. (preabsorbing antigen, PA-Ag) causing in situ immune reaction in acute poststreptococcal glomerulonephritis (APGN). In: Recent advances in streptococci and streptococcal diseases. Readbooks, Berkshire, p 353
8. Lange K, Ahmed U, Kleinberger H, Treser G (1976) A hitherto unknown streptococcal antigen and its probable relation to acute poststreptococcal glomerulonephritis. Clin Nephrol 5:207
9. Lange K, Seligson G, Cronin W (1983) Evidence for the in situ of poststreptococcal glomerulonephritis: glomerular localization of endostreptotosin and the clinical significance of the subsequent antibody response. Clin Nephrol 19:3
10. Jennings RB, Earle DP (1961) Poststreptococcal glomerulonephritis: Histopathologic and clinical studies of the acute, subsiding acute and early chronic latent phases. J Clin Invest 40:1525
11. Baldwin DS, Melvin C, Gluck MC, et al. (1974) The long-term course of poststreptococcal glomerulonephritis. Ann Intern Med 80:342
12. Hooke DH, Gee DC, Atkins RC (1987) Leucocyte analysis using monoclonal antibodies in human glomerulonephritis. Kidney Int 31:964–972
13. Hotta O, Yoshizawa N, Oshima S, Takeuchi A, Kawamura O, Kondo S, Kubota T, Niwa H (1987) Significance of renal hyaline arteriolosclerosis and tubulointerstitial change in IgA glomerulonephritis and focal glomerular sclerosis. Nephron 47:262–265
14. Oda T, Yoshizawa N, Takeuchi A, Kubota T, Akashi Y, Oshikawa Y, Hotta O, Ohshima S, Niwa, H (1988) Significance of tubulo-interstitial (T-1) change in IgAGN (abstract). Kidney Int 35:372
15. Bohle A, Gise HV, Mackensen HS, Stark JB (1981) The obliteration of the post-glomerular capillaries and its influence upon the function of both glomeruli and tubuli. Klin Wochenschr 59:1043–1051
16. Zabriskie JB, Utermohlen V, Read SE, et al. (1973) Streptococcus related glomerulonephritis. Kidney Int 3:100

Pathobiology of Glomerular and Tubular Basement-Membranes

Chair: Yashpal S. Kanwar (USA)
Mitsumasa Nagase (Japan)

High Resolution Ultrastructure of the Basement Membrane

Zensuke Ota, Hirofumi Makino, and Kenichi Shikata[1]

Summary. The glomerular basement membrane (GBM) is thought to be a main filtration barrier in the glomerulus. However, its ultrastructure was unknown until recent years. In 1977, we were the first to demonstrate electron microscopically and by the negative staining method that the GBM is composed of a three-dimensional meshwork structure which has micropores approximately 3 nm in diameter. Since then, we have also found that alveolar basement membrane and other basement membranes exhibit a similar three dimensional meshwork structure, and we have advocated the molecular sieve theory of the basement membrane. In our subsequent studies, we established, by the ultrathin sectioning method, that type IV collagen forms the meshwork of the GBM. Since the diameter of micropores in the GBM is slightly smaller than the axis of albumin molecules, it is considered that GBM functions as a molecular sieve in the glomerulus. In the GBM of experimental nephrotic animals, it was observed that the meshwork was destroyed and the micropores were enlarged. Consequently, it is presumed that in nephrotic syndrome, the destruction of the molecular sieve is mainly responsible for the occurrence of proteinuria.

Introduction

Ultrafiltration takes place in the glomerulus, through which both water and low molecular weight solutes in blood are filtered nonselectively. On the other hand, however, substances of some magnitude, namely those larger than albumin molecules, are scarcely filtered through and remain in the blood. Human albumin has a molecular weight of 66248, which is the threshold value for the proteins; however, smaller proteins than this, such as β_2-microglobulin, are able to filter virtually completely through the glomerulus. If the glomerulus is observed under an electron

[1]The Third Department of Internal Medicine, Okayama University Medical School, Okayama, 700 Japan

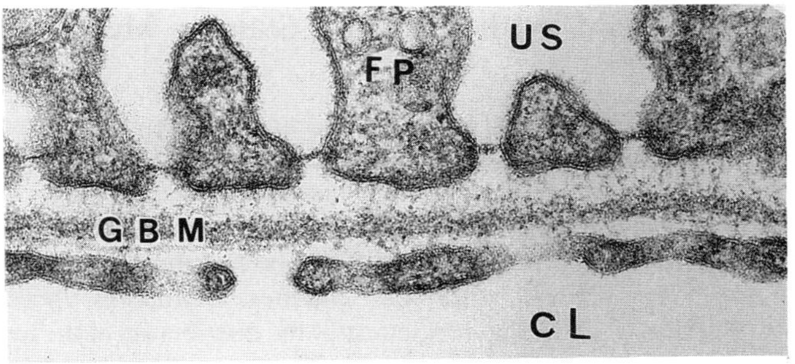

Fig. 1. Ultrathin section of the glomerular capillary wall from normal rat kidney GBM, glomerular basement membrane; FP, foot process; US, urinary space; CL, capillary lumen, ×80000

microscope by the standard ultrathin sectioning method, the ultrastructure of the glomerular basement membrane (GBM) can be observed as an amorphous substance [1] (Fig. 1), and, at the same time, if seen by the freeze etching replica method, its fine structure looks like microgranules approximately 4 nm in diameter [2]. For these reasons, the ultrastructure of the GBM remained controversial and was not understood until recent years, despite a large number of studies. In 1977, we demonstrated for the first time, under an electron microscope, that bovine GBM which had been treated by the negative staining method formed a three-dimensional structure and constituted a molecular sieve for blood components such as albumin [3]. In this paper we describe results obtained thereafter and the mechanism of the onset of proteinuria.

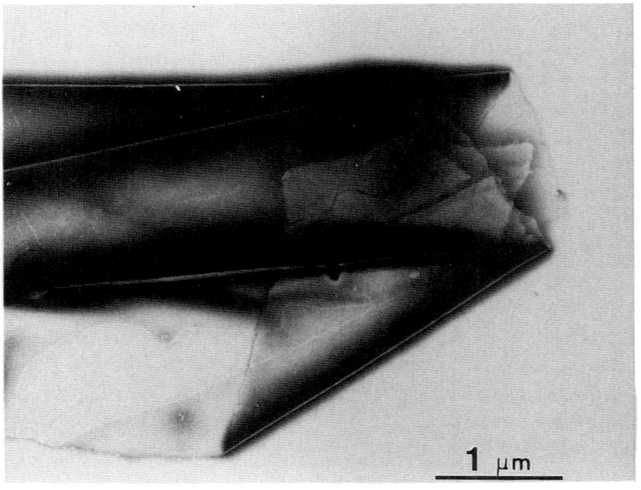

Fig. 2. Negative staining of unfixed rat glomerular basement membrane with 1% PTA. Note the broken folded paper-like appearance with felt-like surface, ×20000

Observation of GBM by the Negative Staining Method

We isolated GBM from bovine and rat kidney, according to Spiro's method [4]. The unfixed GBM thus isolated was observed, in 1% phosphotungstic acid (pH 7.3), electron microscopically by the negative staining method.

When observed at low magnification, the GBM appeared as felt-like paper pieces (Fig. 2). If seen at high magnification, the GBM showed a three-dimensional meshwork composed of fibrils in which there were countless micropores whose diameter was virtually identical (Fig. 3). Figure 4 indicates the distribution of the long dimensions and short dimensions of these micropores. Their mean long dimension was 3.1 $\pm$ 0.6 nm and their mean short dimension was 2.5 $\pm$ 0.3 nm [3,5–7]. We made further observations of GBM in the rat and human in the same fashion, and demonstrated that all the GBMs consisted of a three-dimensional meshwork composed of fibrils [5,8].

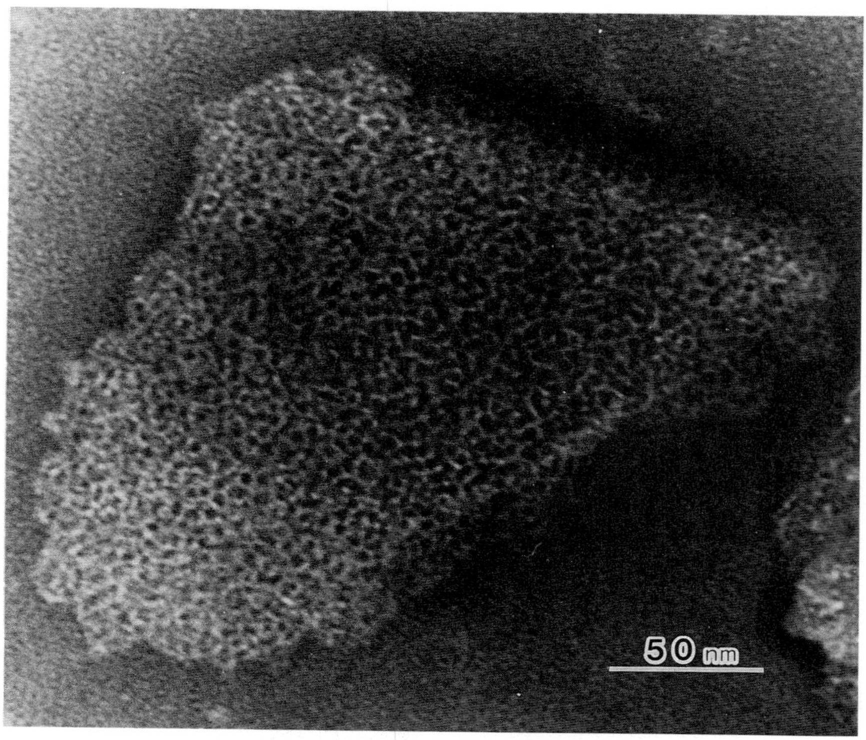

Fig. 3. Negative staining of unfixed bovine glomerular basement membrane at higher magnification. Note clearly discernible fibrils and micropores which form a meshwork structure, ×500000

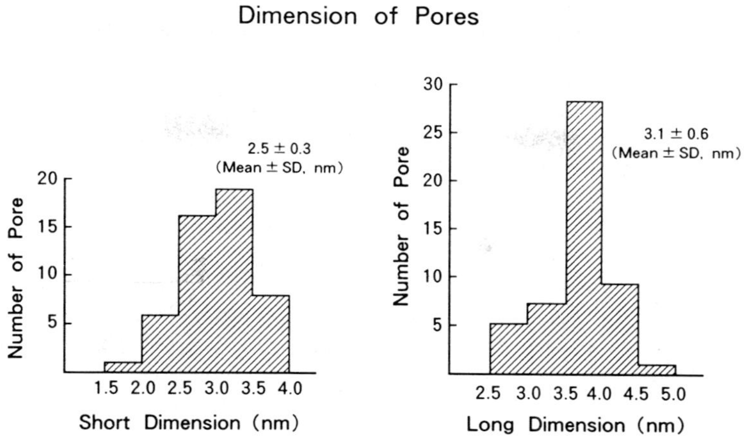

Fig. 4. Distribution of short and long dimensions in bovine glomerular basement membrane

Observation of Other Basement Membranes by the Negative Staining Method

When the unfixed tubular basement membrane (TBM) was isolated from the rat kidney and observed by the negative staining method, it was noted that in this membrane there was a meshwork structure composed of fibrils similar to that in the GBM [9,10] (Fig. 5). The micropores formed by the mesh had a larger diameter than did those in the GBM. This meshwork was also seen in the Descemet's membrane of bovine cornea and in alveolar basement membrane. Consequently, we proposed the molecular sieve theory of the basement membrane [11].

Observation of Chemically Treated GBM by the Ultrathin Sectioning Method

When an isolated GBM is untreated and observed by the ultrathin sectioning method, it is seen as amorphous and ribbon-like, and not as a meshwork structure. Because of this, in order to investigate the ultrastructure in more detail, we chemically treated GBM for observation and successfully demonstrated a meshwork structure even by the ultrathin sectioning method.

Observation by Treatment with Elastase

Rat GBM was isolated according to Spiro's method. The isolate was treated with 0.01% elastase (from porcine pancreas) at 37°C for 5 hours. The chemically treated GBM was fixed, embedded, and observed by the ultrathin sectioning method. In the specimen thus treated, there were fibrils that had disentangled from the GBM; they

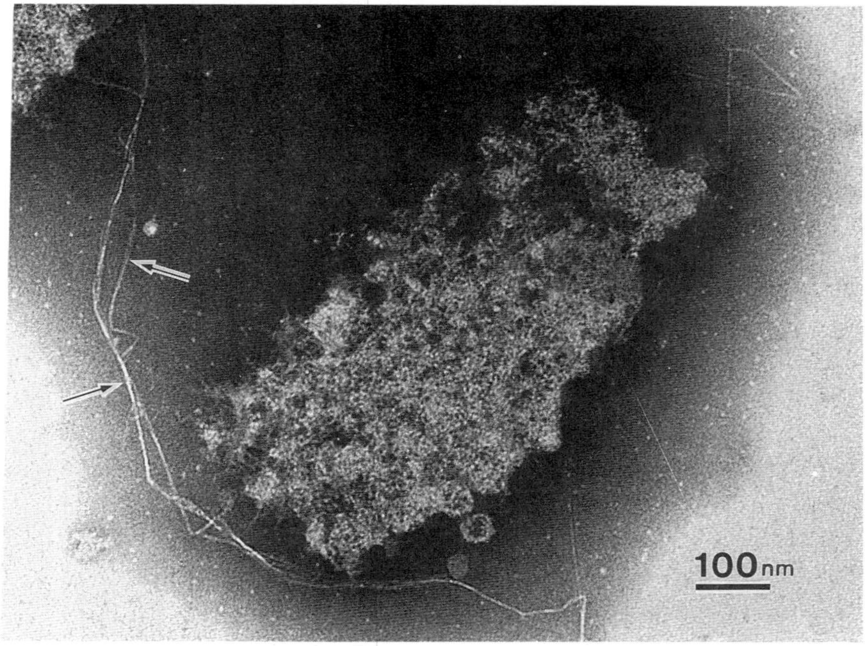

Fig. 5. An unfixed fragment of tubular basement membrane shows fine meshwork. Negative staining with 1% PTA. Note several long fine fibrils disentangling from around the fragment of basement membrane (*arrows*), ×120000

were approximately 3 nm in diameter. These fibrils were also seen in the interior of the GBM, forming a meshwork with micropores approximately 3 nm in diameter. Nodular structures, approximately 10 nm in diameter, were observed on the fibrils [12] (Fig. 6).

When the specimen was observed by immunoelectron microscopy, using anti-type IV collagen antibody obtained by the peroxidase labeled antibody method, the elastase-treated GBM was seen to be positively stained; thus indicating that the treated GBM consisted of type IV collagen [13].

Observation by Treatment with Elastase, Sodium Dodecyl Sulfate (SDS), and 2 Mercaptoethanol

Isolated GBM was treated with 0.01% elastase at 37°C for 24 hours, further treated with sodium dodecyl sulfate (SDS) and 2-mercaptoethanol at 37°C for 72 hours, and was observed by the ultrathin sectioning method. The treated specimen showed more clearly than did the previous method the structure of a meshwork, composed of fibrils over the GBM layer, along with nodular structures on the fibrils (Fig. 7). Stereographic observation revealed the three-dimensional form of this meshwork [14]. The micropores formed by the meshwork had a diameter of approximately 3–5 nm, which was very close to results obtained by the negative staining method.

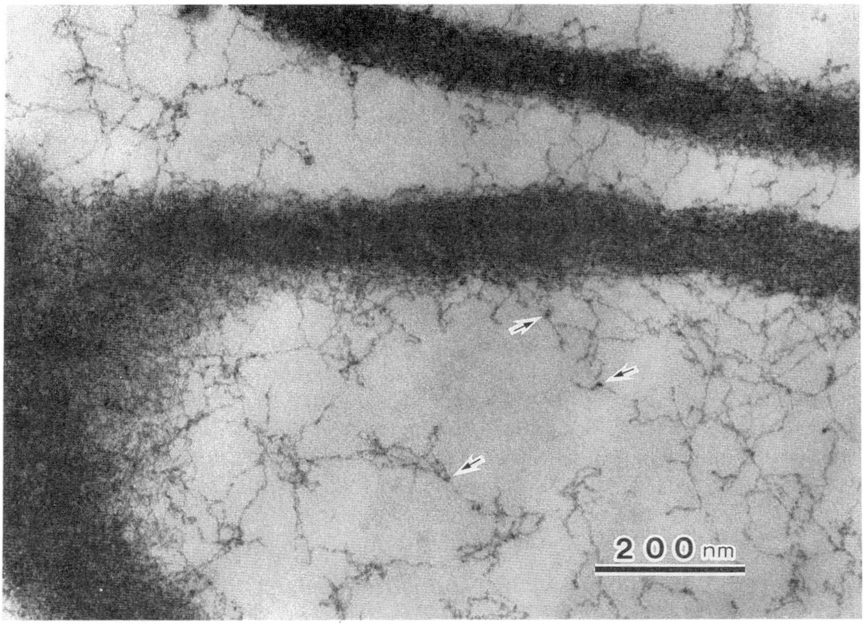

Fig. 6. An ultrathin section of isolated rat glomerular basement membrane (*GBM*) treated with elastase. Fibrils are drifting away from the surface of the GBM and nodular structures (*arrows*) are seen on the fibrils, ×120000

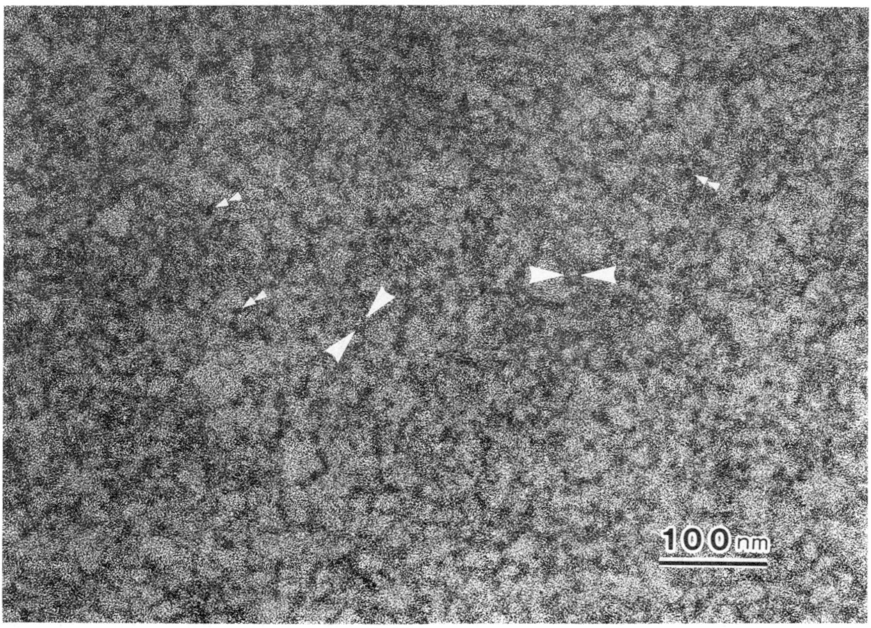

Fig. 7. An ultrathin section of bovine glomerular basement membrane treated with elastase, SDS, and 2-mercaptoethanol. Meshwork structure is composed of fibrils. Note the nodular structures (*double arrowheads*) and numerous micropores (*large arrowheads*), ×165000

These findings suggest that the GBM consists mostly of a three-dimensional meshwork structure, composed of type IV collagen, which contains micropores approximately 3 nm in diameter. The findings also support observations made according to the negative staining method.

In 1981, Timpl et al. confirmed that type IV collagen, the main constituent of the basement membrane, is a fibril similar to the fibrils we had found and that it forms a meshwork [15]. The meshwork that they showed was very large. They failed to demonstrate the micropores of approximately 3 nm in diameter which we had found in our experiments. Nevertheless, their findings serve as supporting evidence of the characteristics of GBM ultrastructure that we demonstrated. Since then, Lawrie et al. have shown the existence of fibrils called "cords" in an electron-microscopic observation of the GBM [16]. Kubosawa et al. have described the GBM by the deep-etch replica method [17]. In addition, Yurchenco et al. observed the tumor matrix of EHS sarcoma and established its meshwork [18]. Their results appear to support our molecular sieve theory.

Observation of the GBM in Nephrotic Rats

In accordance with the method of Arisz et al., nephrotic rats were prepared by inducing chronic serum sickness by means of bovine serum administration. When the isolated GBM was observed under an electron microscope by the negative staining method, the meshwork in the nephrotic rats was seen to be destroyed and the diameter of the micropores had enlarged significantly when compared with the GBM of control animals [19] (Fig. 8 and Table 1).

We have previously shown in the same manner that there is also an enlargement of the diameter of micropores in Masugi nephritis [20], in aminonucleoside nephritis [21], and in diabetic nephropathy. It is thought that the enlargement of micropore diameter is chiefly responsible for the occurrence of proteinuria.

GBM as a Size Barrier

The diameter of the micropores of the GBM is approximately 3 nm. However, the albumin molecule is a prolate ellipsoid, whose major and minor axes are 15.0 nm and 3.8 nm, respectively. In other words, the diameter of the micropores of the GBM is slightly smaller than the minor axis of the albumin molecule (Fig. 9). GBM, therefore, is thought to function as a molecular sieve in the production of filtrate in the glomerulus.

Another factor that affects filtration is static electric force. Since both the basement membrane and albumin are negatively charged, because of heparan sulfate proteoglycan, etc., and an isoelectric point, respectively, a repellent force is considered to occur between the GBM and albumin molecules on filtration [22]. On the basis of results of an experiment with dextran sulfate, etc., clearance increases as its electric charge shifts from negativity through neutrality to positivity. For this reason, it appears that the Coulomb force between electric charges cannot be ignored in the

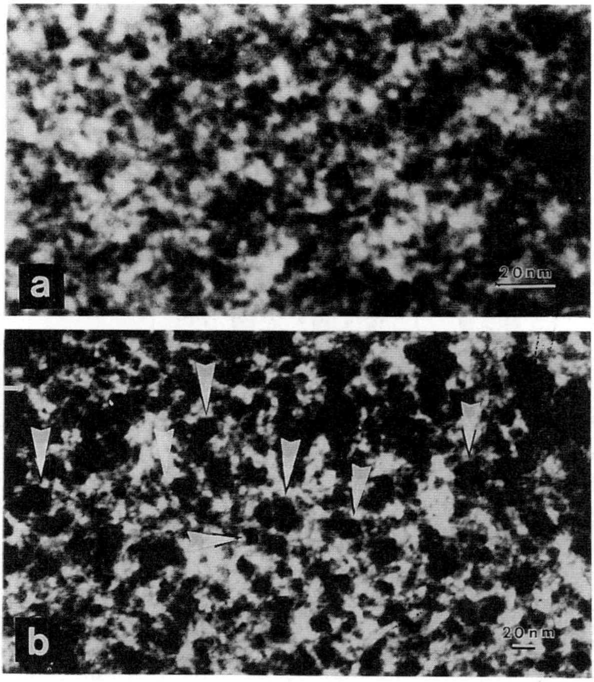

Fig. 8a,b. Negative staining of rat GBM with 1% PTA **a** control rat GBM, ×300000, **b** experimental rat GBM. Note enlarged micropores (*arrows*), ×125000

process of filtration [23]. Consequently, it follows that filtration involves two major barriers, namely the size barrier and the charge barrier.

When a massive amount of protein is filtered through in human nephrotic syndrome, which barrier would be involved more heavily? Based on the results of numerous studies of experimental nephritis, reduced charge of the GBM does not necessarily correlate with proteinuria. On the other hand, some results indicate an involvement of the size barrier [24]. Furthermore, our electron microscopic observations and results obtained from quantitative filtration experiments with ferritin

Table 1. Micropore and fibril diameters of glomerular basement membrane of rats with chronic serum sickness (CSS)

	Control	CSS
Long dimension, (nm)	4 ± 1	9 ± 5*
Short dimension, (nm)	3 ± 1	6 ± 3*
Diameter of fibrils, (nm)	3 ± 1	4 ± 1

a, Values are the means ± SD of 100 micropores or fibrils
*Statistically significant difference from controls ($P < 0.001$)

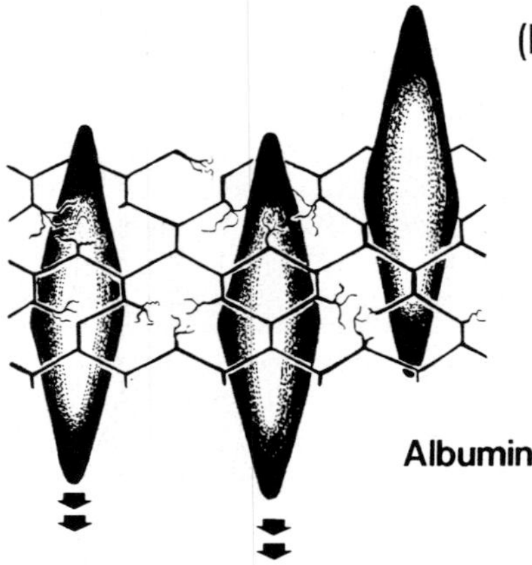

Fig. 9. Schematic representation of mechanism of proteinuria, from our studies (by Z. Ota)

monomers and polymers suggest that the size barrier is much more heavily involved in the filtration of proteins [25]. Therefore, it is presumed that the destruction of the molecular sieve of the basement membrane is chiefly responsible for such filtration.

Acknowledgment. This research was supported by a "Research Grant for Progressive Renal Disease" from diseases specially selected by the Ministry of Health and Welfare Research Project, the Ministry of Health and Welfare of Japan.

References

1. Farquhar MG, Palade GE (1961) Glomerular permeability. II Ferritin transfer across the glomerular capillary wall in nephrotic rats. J Exp Med 114:699–716
2. Ota Z (1975) Electron microscope studies on frozen kidney tissue (in Japanese). Cell 7:350–361
3. Ota Z, Makino H, Miyoshi A, Hiramatsu M, Takahashi K, Ofuji T (1977) Electron microscopic demonstration of meshwork structure in human and bovine glomerular basement membranes. Acta Med Okayama 31:339–342
4. Spiro RG (1967) Studies on the renal glomerular basement membrane. Preparation and chemical composition. J Biol Chem 242:1915–1922
5. Ota Z, Makino H, Miyoshi A, Hiramatsu M, Takahashi K, Ofuji T (1979) Molecular sieve in glomerular basement membrane as revealed by electron microscopy. J Electron Microsc (Tokyo) 28:20–28
6. Ota Z, Makino H, Takaya Y, Ofuji T (1980) Molecular sieve in renal glomerular and tubular basement membranes as revealed by electron microscopy. Renal Physiol 3:317–323
7. Ota Z, Makino H, Takaoka M, Soda K, Suzuki S (1985) Mechanism of proteinuria in rats with chronic serum sickness. In: Glomerular dysfunction and biopathology of vascular wall. Academic Press, Tokyo, pp 165–174

8. Makino H (1982) Molecular sieve in rat glomerular basement membrane as revealed by negative staining. Acta Med Okayama 36:371–382
9. Makino H, Ota Z, Takaya Y, Kida K, Miyoshi A, Hiramatsu M, Takahashi K, Ofuji T (1979) Ultrastructure of rat renal tubular basement membrane – meshwork structure demonstration by negative staining. Acta Med Okayama 33:133–136
10. Makino H, Ota Z, Takaya Y, Miyoshi A, Ofuji T (1981) Molecular sieve in rat tubular basement membrane as revealed by negative staining. Renal Physiol 4:180–190
11. Makino H, Toyofuku H, Mino Y, Takaoka M, Ota Z (1983) Molecular sieve in bovine Descemet's membrane as revealed by negative staining. Acta Med Okayama 37:155–157
12. Ichiyasu A, Takaoka M, Makino H, Takahashi K, Ota Z (1987) Fibrillar ultrastructure of the glomerular basement membrane of the rat kidney as revealed by digestive treatment. Acta Med Okayama 41:183–185
13. Ichiyasu M, Makino H (1988) Molecular sieve of the rat glomerular basement membrane: A transmission electron microscopic study of enzyme-treated specimens. Acta Med Okayama 42:317–325
14. Shikata K, Makino H, Ichiyasu A, Ota Z (1990) Three-dimensional meshwork structure of glomerular basement membrane revealed by chemical treatment. J Electron Microsc (Tokyo) 39:182–185
15. Timpl R, Wiedermann H, Van Delden V, Furthmayr H, Kuhn K (1981) A network model for the organization of type IV collagen molecules in basement membrane. Eur J Biochem 120:203–211
16. Laurie GW, Leblond CP, Inoue S, Martin GR, Chung A (1984) Fine structure of the glomerular basement membrane and immunolocalization of five basement membrane components to the lamina densa (basal lamina) and its extensions in both glomeruli and tubules of the rat kidney. Am J Anat 169:463–481
17. Kubosawa H, Kondo Y (1985) Ultrastructural organization of the glomerular basement membrane as revealed by a deep-etch replica method. Cell Tissue Res 242:33–39
18. Yurchenco PD, Ruden GC (1988) Type IV collagen lateral associations in the EHS tumor matrix – comparison with amniotic and in vitro networks. Am J Pathol 132:278–291
19. Makino H, Soda K, Komoda K, Ota Z (1988) Changes in the molecular sieve of the glomerular basement membrane of rats with chronic serum sickness. Acta Med Okayama 42:53–60
20. Makino H (1983) Changes in the molecular sieve of glomerular basement membrane in rats with Masugi nephritis. Renal Physiol 6:266–274
21. Takaya Y, Ota Z, Makino H, Kida K, Miyoshi A, Hiramatsu M, Takahashi K, Ofuji T (1980) Changes in the molecular sieve of glomerular basement membrane in rats with aminonucleoside nephrosis. Acta Med Okayama 34:67–70
22. Kanwar YS, Linker A, Farquhar MG (1980) Increased permeability of the glomerular basement membrane to ferritin after removal of glycosaminoglycans (heparan sulfate) by enzyme digestion. J Cell Biol 86:688–693
23. Bohrer MP, Deen WM, Robertson CR, Brenner BM (1977) Mechanism of angiotensin II-induced proteinuria in the rat. Am J Physiol 233:F13–F21
24. Kanwar YS (1984) Biology of disease. Biophysiology of glomerular filtration and proteinuria. Lab Invest 51:7–21
25. Ota Z, Kumagai I, Shikata K, Makino H (1989) Human liver ferritin as a new tracer for studying glomerular permeability. Act Med Okayama 43:363–365

Glomerular Basement Membrane: Molecular Structure of Type IV Collagen and Its Involvement in Diseases

Billy G. Hudson, Sripad Gunwar, Billie J. Wisdom, Jr., Mark D. Hudson, and Milton E. Noelken[1]

Summary. Glomerular basement membrane is a specialized extracellular matrix that functions as a molecular sieve in the nephron. Its function is altered in three notable human diseases that affect the kidneys, Goodpasture syndrome, Alport syndrome, and diabetes mellitus. Over the past decade, great advances have been made in understanding the supramolecular structure of this membrane and its role in the pathogenesis of these diseases. The membrane's major constituent is type IV collagen which provides tensile strength to the matrix and serves as a scaffold for the binding and alignment of several other macromolecular constituents. Recently, three new chains (α3, α4, and α5) of type IV collagen have been discovered, and they have been implicated in the pathogenesis of Goodpasture and Alport syndromes and potentially in that of diabetic nephropathy. This review will briefly describe the molecular structure of type IV collagen and its involvement in these diseases.

Introduction

Basement membranes are complex extracellular matrices that play key roles in diverse biological processes. The processes include: molecular sieving [1]; orchestration of embryonic development; and maintenance of tissue architecture during remodeling and repair [2,3]. Basement membrane function is altered in three notable human diseases that affect the kidneys, *Goodpasture syndrome*, *Alport syndrome* and *diabetes mellitus*, leading to serious and often fatal consequences. In these diseases, the molecular sieving function of the glomerular basement membrane (GBM) is altered (Fig. 1), which often leads to end-stage renal disease.

[1]Department of Biochemistry and Molecular Biology, University of Kansas Medical Center, Kansas City, KS 66103, USA

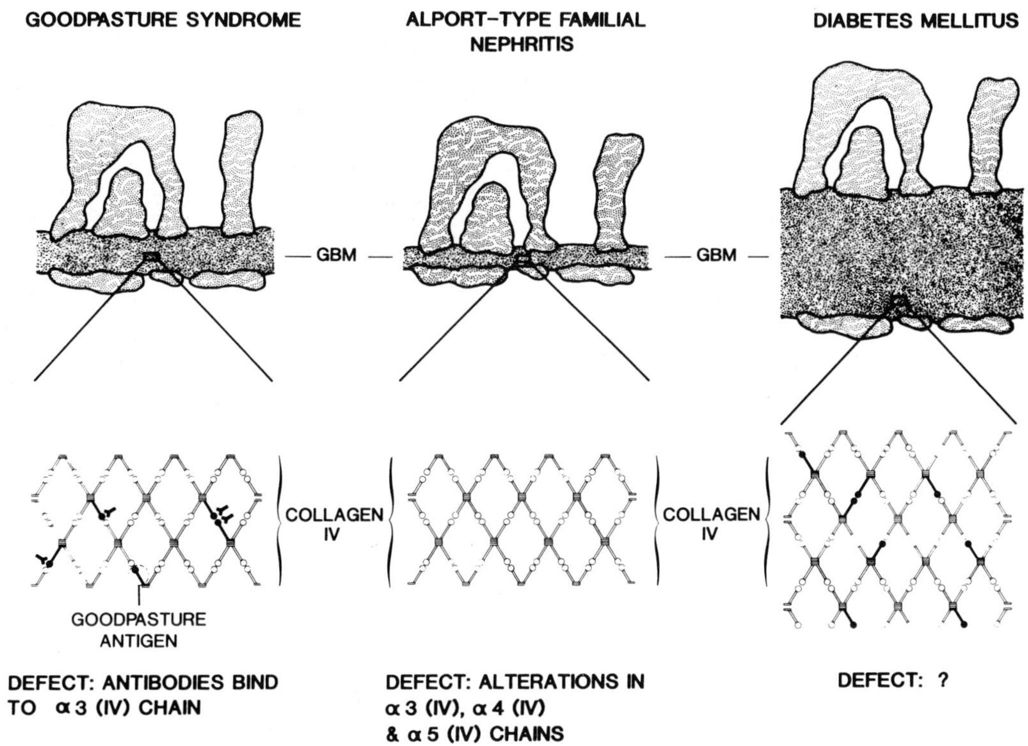

Fig. 1. Schematic illustration of the ultrastructural alteration and proposed molecular defect in GBM of 3 notable human diseases that affect the kidneys. In Goodpasture syndrome the autoantigen to which Goodpasture antibodies bind has been localized to the novel α3(IV) chain. In Alport-type familial nephritis (Alport syndrome) the GBM is characterized by thinning and sometimes multilamination. Evidence has been presented which shows that the α3(IV), α4(IV), and α5(IV) chains are either absent or are present in reduced amounts. In diabetes the GBM is unusually thickened, however the molecular defect which correlates to altered ultrafiltration has not been elucidated, but may involve type IV collagen. (Adapted from [5] with permission)

Over the last decade, great advances have been made by numerous investigators in advancing the understanding of basement membrane structure, function, and dysfunction. Recently, three new chains (α3, α4, and α5) of type IV collagen have been discovered and they have been implicated in the pathogenesis of Goodpasture and Alport syndromes [4–16]. Potentially, they may play a role in the development of diabetic nephropathy.

Molecular Structure of GBM

The molecular structure of GBM is very complex. The membrane is composed of several macromolecular constituents: type IV collagen, laminin, heparan sulfate proteoglycan, entactin, and fibronectin (Fig. 2). These interact to form a supramolecular complex. Type IV collagen, the major constituent, provides tensile strength to the matrix and its supramolecular structure serves as a scaffold for the binding and alignment of the other constituents [17,18]. A three-dimensional model of this suprastructure has been proposed [19]. The structure of GBM varies from that of other basement membranes, particularly with regard to the chemical nature of type IV collagen. This structural variation may be of fundamental importance in conferring a distinct function to GBM.

Supramolecular Structure of Type IV Collagen

The protomer, or building block unit, of type IV collagen is comprised of three α(IV) chains and is characterized by three distinct structural domains. These are: the NC1 domain at the carboxy-terminus; the triple-helical domain in the middle region; and the 7S domain at the amino-terminus (Fig. 3, lower panel) [4,17,18]. Protomers interact through covalent associations to form a supramolecular structure (Fig. 3, upper panel). Protomers associate in a head-to-head (NC1-to-NC1) fashion to form dimers, and in a tail-to-tail (7S-to-7S) fashion to form tetramers. Although these fundamental ways of connecting protomers are known, the three-dimensional structure of the collagen matrix remains largely unknown.

Several protomer subtypes, differing in the chemical nature of the α chains, exist in GBM (Fig. 4). The classical protomer, designated subtype A, is comprised of two α1 chains and one α2 chain, and is common to all basement membranes. The complete primary structure of these chains has been determined [20–25]. At least one other, and possibly several, protomer subtypes, exist in GBM because of the existence of the newly discovered α3, α4, and α5 chains. These are designated subtypes B, C, and D (Fig. 4), and correspond to protomers that contain these respective chains; however, the chain compositions are unknown.

The existence of several protomer subtypes introduces the possibility of several distinct arrangements in which protomers are interconnected and distributed in the supramolecular structure (Fig. 5). Different subtypes can be interconnected through their NC1 domains, forming homo- or hetero-dimers, and through their 7S domains, forming homo- and hetero-tetramers. The subtypes can be distributed in a regional or random fashion within the suprastructure [4]. In the extracellular matrix of the

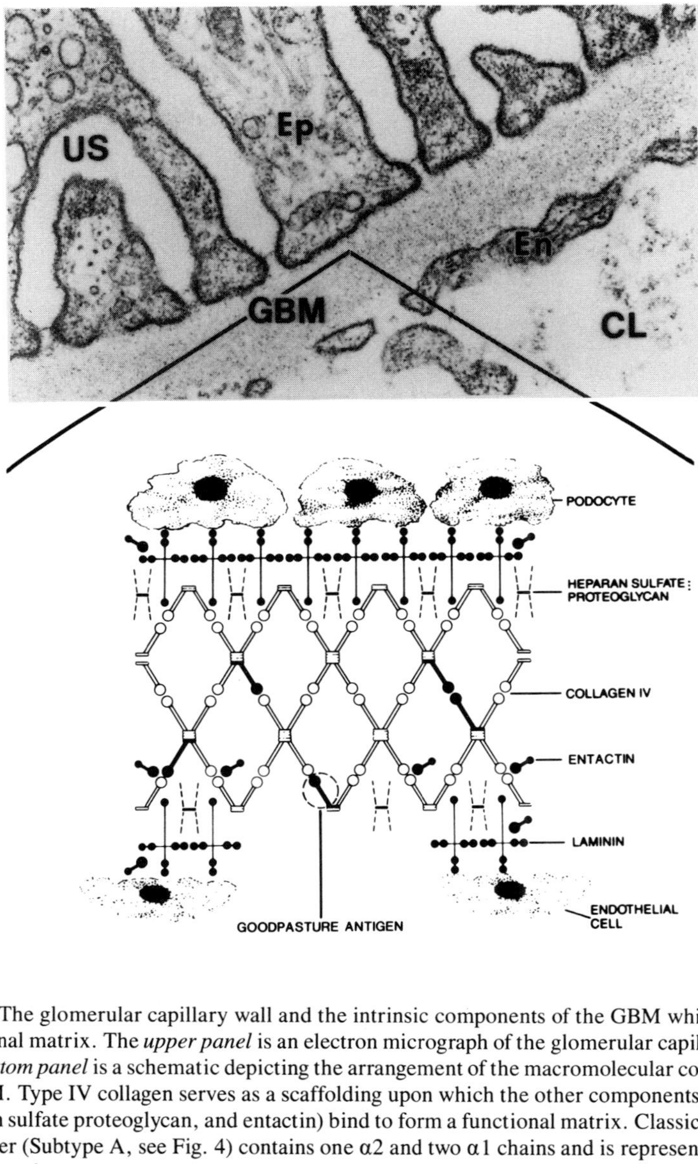

Fig. 2. The glomerular capillary wall and the intrinsic components of the GBM which form a functional matrix. The *upper panel* is an electron micrograph of the glomerular capillary wall. The *bottom panel* is a schematic depicting the arrangement of the macromolecular constituents of GBM. Type IV collagen serves as a scaffolding upon which the other components (laminin, heparan sulfate proteoglycan, and entactin) bind to form a functional matrix. Classical type IV protomer (Subtype A, see Fig. 4) contains one α2 and two α1 chains and is represented by the *undarkened protomers*. Protomers (Subtype B, see Fig. 4) containing the α3 chain (the Goodpasture antigen) are represented by the *darkened protomers*. Distribution of components represented within the matrix is preferential (but not exclusive). CL, capillary lumen; En, endothelium; Ep, epithelial podocytes; GBM, glomerular basement membrane; US, urinary space. (Adapted from [4] with permission)

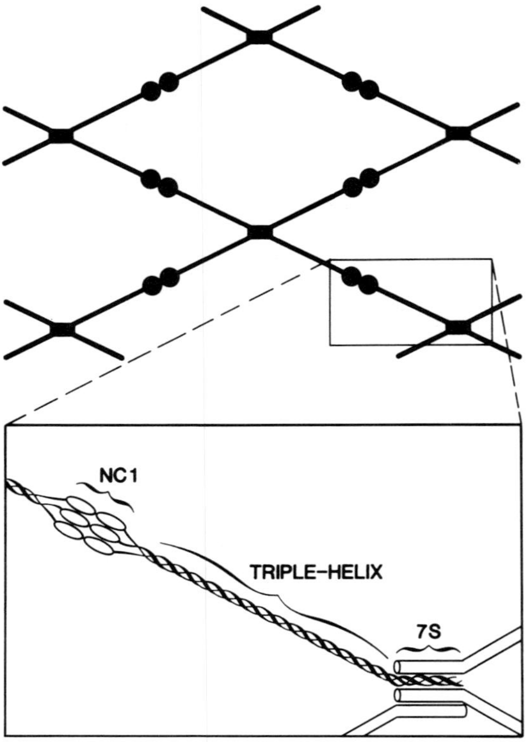

Fig. 3. Schematic drawing of the supramolecular structure of type IV collagen. The depicted model is based on studies of the basement membrane-like matrix produced by mouse Engelbreth-Holm-Swarm tumor. Several lines of evidence indicate that the model applies to GBM. The *upper panel* is a diagram of the type IV collagen supramolecular structure. The *boxed area* (*lower panel*) is an enlargement of a region of the structure to show the type IV collagen protomer and ways in which it is connected in the matrix. The protomer is a triple-helical molecule comprised of three polypeptide chains and has three distinct structural domains. These are the 7S domain at the amino-terminus, the triple-helical domain in the middle region, and the NC1 domain at the carboxy-terminus. Protomers are shown to associate in a head-to-head (*NC1*-to-*NC1*) fashion to form dimers and in a tail-to-tail (*7S-7S*) fashion to form tetramers. In addition to terminal interactions, helical or lateral interactions occur between type IV collagen protomers. (From [4] with permission)

glomerulus, subtype A appears to have a more endothelial/mesangial distribution, whereas subtype B is restricted to the GBM in the peripheral capillary loops [26]. The organization and function of these subtypes is unknown.

Evidence for the Existence of New Chains

Recently, we discovered the α3 and α4 chains of type IV collagen. The evidence is based on numerous chemical, physicochemical, and immunochemical studies of the NC1 domain (hexamer) of type IV collagen from GBM [4–9]. The chain identity was

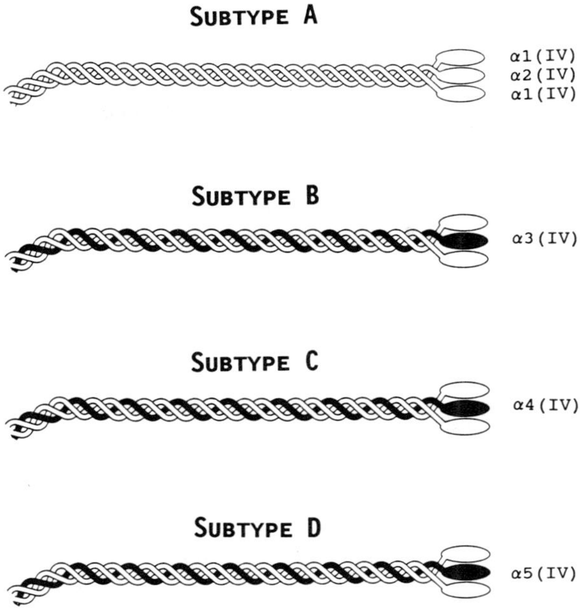

Fig. 4. Protomer subtypes of type IV collagen. The classical type IV collagen protomer (heterotrimer) is comprised of two α1 chains and one α2 chain (*undarkened chains*) and is designated as subtype A. Hypothetical type IV collagen protomers containing the α3, α4, or α5 chain (*darkened molecule*) are designated subtypes B, C, and D, respectively. (Adapted from [4] and [5] with permission)

deduced from amino-terminal sequences of NC1 monomers (Fig. 6) in which the sequences of α3 and α4 chains are highly related to, but distinct from, the collagenous-NC1 junctional regions of the classical α1 and α2 chains. Subsequently, we obtained chemical evidence for the collagenous domain of these chains [10]. The evidence is based on the molecular properties of a 60K collagenous component, extracted from GBM, that contains both a collagenous domain and the noncollagenous domain of the α3 chain (Fig. 7). The α5 chain was discovered by molecular cloning technologies and the primary structure of most of the chain has been elucidated [14–16].

Goodpasture Syndrome and Type IV Collagen

Goodpasture (GP) syndrome is an autoimmune disorder consisting of the triad of glomerulonephritis, lung hemorrhage, and anti-GBM antibody formation [27]. It includes a broad spectrum of clinical features, ranging from massive pulmonary hemorrhage with little overt evidence of renal disease to fulminant crescentic glomerulonephritis and little overt evidence of pulmonary hemorrhage. The nephritis is mediated by auto-antibodies that bind to the noncollagenous (NC1) domain of type IV collagen, and specifically to the NC1 domain of the α3 chain [4,6]. Many

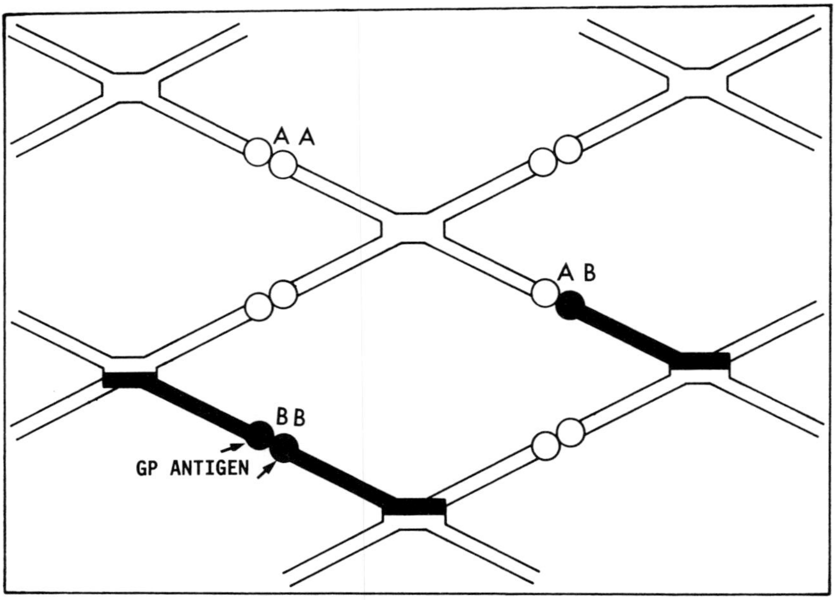

Fig. 5. End-to-end connections of protomer subtypes in type IV collagen supramolecular structure. Several different arrangements are possible, in which the subtypes are interconnected through their NC1 domains forming homo- or hetero-dimers and through their 7S domains forming homo- or hetero-tetramers in the type IV collagen matrix (see Fig. 3). *Undarkened protomer*, classical type IV collagen protomer; *Darkened protomer*, subtypes B containing the Goodpasture (*GP*) antigen. The darkened protomer also represents subtype C and D protomers (Fig. 4). (Adapted from [4] with permission)

important questions remain unanswered about the α3 chain, also termed the GP-antigen, with regard to its chemical nature, organization in the protomer, function, and role in the pathogenesis of Goodpasture syndrome.

Alport Syndrome and Type IV Collagen

Classical Alport syndrome in human beings is a heritable disorder that eventually causes kidney failure and deafness [28]. The nephritis is characterized by chronic hematuria with progression to end-stage renal disease, and by ultrastructural abnormalities (thinning, diffuse splitting, and multilaminations of the lamina densa) in the GBM (Fig. 1). The syndrome eventually leads to renal dialysis or transplantation because there is no known treatment that alters the clinical course or affects the underlying pathologic process. The ultrastructural abnormalities are widely accepted to reflect the primary molecular defect causing nephritis in all phenotypes.

There are several lines of circumstantial evidence for the absence or diminished quantity of one or more of the three new chains (α3, α4 and α5) of type IV collagen in Alport GBM. The binding of GP-antibodies to Alport GBM is frequently absent,

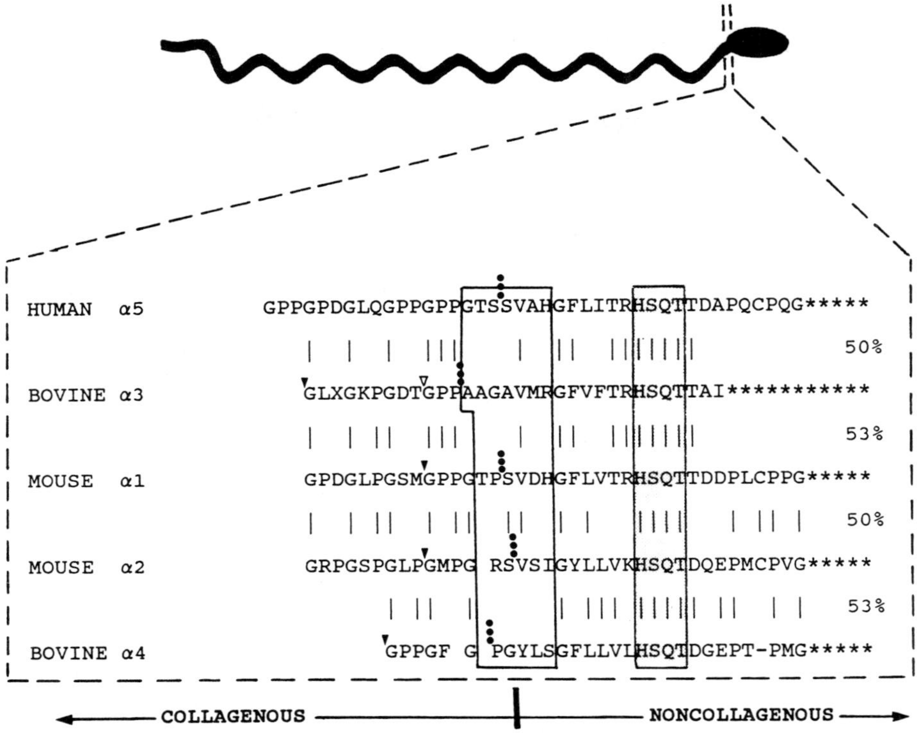

Fig. 6. Comparison of amino acid sequence of the collagenous-NC1 junction regions of the α1, α2, α3, α4, and α5 chains. The *darkened* α(IV) *chain* is drawn to show the region of sequence comparison. The five α(IV) chains have been aligned for maximal matching. The degree of homology between the upper and lower chains is given *at the right*. The *boxed areas* show positions of identity. The α1 and α2 sequences are taken from reference [22,25], the α3 and α4 are from reference [8,9], and the α5 is from reference [14]. *Lines* indicate identity of residues between sequences; *triangles* (*both undarkened and darkened*) represent collagenase cleavage sites; and *dots* indicate the junction region between the collagenous and NC1 domains. (Adapted from [5] with permission)

as determined by immunofluorescence of tissue sections [29–33]. The binding of a monoclonal antibody, directed to GP-antigen, to GBM is absent or diminished in 10 Alport patients [34]. Two components of the NC1 domain of collagen IV, M28+ and M28+++, which appear to correspond to the α3 and α4 chains [35], respectively, are absent from the GBM of three Alport patients [36]. Some Alport patients develop anti-GBM nephritis after renal transplantation, causing loss of allograft function. The alloantibodies show reactivity with unidentified dimer and monomer components of the NC1 domain of collagen IV [31,37–41]. A recent study reveals that genetic mutations in the α5 gene are present in kindred of Alport patients, which may relate to dysfunctional GBM [42]. Overall, these studies clearly implicate these new chains in the pathogenesis of the disease, particularly the α3 and α5 chains.

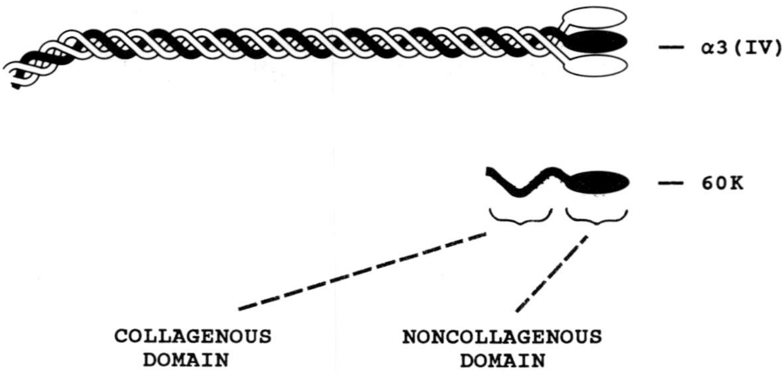

RESIDUES/1000	Collagenous domain	Noncollagenous domain
HoPro	111	2.5
HoLys	15	1.0
Gly	299	103.8

Fig. 7. Evidence for the collagenous domain of the α3 and α4 chains of type IV collagen. The 60K component was purified from a urea extract of GBM [10]. It contains a collagenous domain of 279 residues and a noncollagenous domain of 249 residues. Those amino acids indicative of a triple-helical collagen (HoPro, HoLys, Gly) are given for both the collagenous and noncollagenous regions

Conclusions and Perspectives

The structural knowledge of basement membrane constituents, particularly that of type IV collagen, has provided the necessary knowledge base from which we can begin to unravel the pathogenic mechanisms underlying the molecular sieving dysfunction of GBM in Goodpasture and Alport syndromes. Concurrent searches for the underlying mechanisms in these diseases have, in turn, provided deeper insights into the molecular complexity of this collagen, and into the molecular nature of GBM. A molecular commonality, which involves the new chains of type IV collagen, is emerging between the pathogenic mechanisms of Goodpasture and Alport syndromes. However, many questions about the molecular structure and assembly of this collagen, and its role in the pathogenic mechanism of these diseases, remain unanswered.

References

1. Farquhar MG, Courtoy PJ, Lemkin MC, Kanwar YS (1982) Current knowledge of the functional architecture of the glomerular basement membrane. In: Kuehn K, Schoene H, Timpl R (eds) New trends in basement membrane research. Raven, New York, pp 9–29
2. Hay ED (1984) Cell-matrix interaction in the embryo: cell shape, cell surface, cell skeletons, and their role in differentiation. In: Trelstad RL (ed) The role of extracellular matrix in development. Alan R Liss, New York, pp 1–32

3. Bernfield M, Banerjée SD, Koda JE, Rapraeger AC (1984) Remodeling of the basement membrane as a mechanism of morphogenic tissue interaction. In: Trelstad RL (ed) The role of extracellular matrix in development. Alan R Liss, New York, pp 545–572
4. Hudson BG, Wieslander J, Wisdom BJ, Noelken, ME (1989) Goodpasture syndrome: molecular architecture and function of basement membrane antigen. Lab Invest 61:256–269
5. Hudson BG, Wisdom BJ, Gunwar S, Noelken ME (to be published) Collagen IV: Role in Goodpasture syndrome, Alport-type familial nephritis, and diabetic nephropathy. In: Kang A (ed) Collagen, vol V: Pathobiochemistry. CRC, Boca Raton
6. Butkowski RJ, Langeveld JPM, Wieslander J, Hamilton J, Hudson BG (1987) Localization of the Goodpasture epitope to a novel chain of basement membrane collagen. J Biol Chem 262:7874–7877
7. Langeveld JPM, Wieslander J, Timoneda J, McKinney P, Butkowski RJ, Wisdom BJ, Hudson BG (1988) Structural heterogeneity of the noncollagenous domain of basement membrane collagen. J Biol Chem 263:10481–10488
8. Saus J, Wieslander J, Langeveld JPM, Quinones S, Hudson BG (1988) Identification of the Goodpasture antigen as the α3(IV) chain of collagen IV. J Biol Chem 263:13374–13380
9. Gunwar S, Saus J, Noelken ME, Hudson BG (1990) Glomerular Basement Membrane: Identification of a Fourth Chain, α4, of Type IV. Collagen. J Biol Chem 265:5466–5469
10. Fagg WR, Timoneda J, Schwartz CE, Langeveld JPM, Noelken M, Hudson BG (1990) Glomerular Basement Membrane: Evidence for Collagenous Domain of α3 and α4 Chains of Collagen IV. BBRC 170:322–327
11. Wieslander J, Langeveld J, Butkowski R, Jodlowski M, Noelken M, Hudson BG (1985) Physical and immunochemical studies of the globular domain of type IV collagen: Cryptic properties of the Goodpasture antigen. J Biol Chem 260:8564–8570
12. Butkowski RJ, Wieslander J, Wisdom BJ, Barr JF, Noelken ME, Hudson BG (1985) Properties of the globular domain of type IV collagen and its relationship to the Goodpasture antigen. J Biol Chem 260:3739–3747
13. Wieslander J, Barr JF, Butkowski RJ, Edwards SJ, Bygren P, Heinegard D, Hudson BG (1984) Goodpasture antigen of the glomerular basement membrane: Localization to noncollagenous regions of type IV collagen. Proc Natl Acad Sci USA 81:3838–3842
14. Hostikka SL, Eddy RL, Byers MG, Höyhtyä M, Shows TB, Tryggvason K (1990) Identification of a distinct type IV collagen α chain with restricted kidney distribution and assignment of its gene to the locus of X chromosome-linked Alport Syndrome. Proc Natl Acad Sci USA 87:1606–1610
15. Myers JC, Jones TA, Pohjolainen ER, Kadri AS, Goddard AD, Sheer D, Solomon E, Pihlajaniemi T (1990) Molecular cloning of α5(IV) collagen and assignment of the gene to the region of the X chromosome containing the Alport syndrome locus. Am J Hum Genet 46:1024–1033
16. Pihlajaneimi T, Pohjolanainen E-R, Myers JC (1990) Complete Primary Structure of the Triple-helical Region and the Carboxyl-terminal Domain of a New Type IV Collagen Chain, α5(IV). J Biol Chem 265:13758–17366
17. Martin GR, Timpl R, Kühn K (1988) Basement membrane proteins: molecular structure and function. Adv Protein Chem 39:1–50
18. Timpl R (1989) Structure and biological activity of basement membrane proteins. Eur J Biochem 180:487–502
19. Yurchenco PD, Schittny JC (1990) Molecular architecture of basement membranes. FASEB J 4:1577–1590
20. Brazel D, Oberbäumer I, Dieringer H, Babel W, Glanville RW, Deutzmann R, Kühn K (1987) Completion of the amino acid sequence of the α1 chain of human basement membrane collagen (type IV) reveals 21 non-triplet interruptions located within the collagenous domain. Eur J Biochem 168:529–536

21. Soininen R, Haka-Risku T, Prockop DJ, and Tryggvason K (1987) Complete primary structure of the α_1-chain of human basement membrane (type IV) collagen. FEBS Lett. 225: 188–194
22. Muthukumaran G, Blumberg B, Kurkinen M (1989) The complete primary structure for the α1-chain of mouse collagen IV: differential evolution of collagen IV domains. J Biol Chem 264:6310–6317
23. Brazel D, Pollner R, Oberbäumer I, Kühn K (1988) Human basement membrane collagen (type IV): The amino acid sequence of the α2(IV) chain and its comparison with the α1(IV) chain reveals deletions in the α1(IV) chain. Eur J Biochem 172:35–42
24. Hostikka SL, Tryggvason K (1988) The complete primary structure of the α2 chain of human type IV collagen and comparisons with the α1(IV) collagen. J Biol Chem 263: 19488–19493
25. Saus J, Quinones S, MacKrell A, Blumberg B, Muthukumaran G, Pihlajaniemi T, Kurkinen M (1989) The complete primary structure of mouse α2(IV) collagen: alignment with mouse α1(IV) collagen. J Biol Chem 264:6318–6324
26. Butkowski RJ, Wieslander J, Kleppel M, Michael AF, Fish AJ (1989) Basement membrane collagen in the kidney: regional localization of novel chains related to collagen IV. Kidney Int 35:1195–1202
27. Glassock RJ, Cohen AH, Adler SG, Ward HJ (1986) Secondary glomerular diseases. The Kidney 3:1014–1083
28. Atkin CL, Gregory MC, Border WA (1988) Alport syndrome. In: Schrier RW, Gottschalk CW (eds) Diseases of the Kidney, 4th edn. Little, Brown, Boston, pp 617–641
29. Jenis EH, Valeski JE, Calcagno PL (1981) Variability of anti-GBM binding in hereditary nephritis. Clin Nephrol 15:111–114
30. Jeraj K, Kim Y, Vernier RL, Fish AJ, Michael AF (1983) Absence of Goodpasture's antigen in male patients with familial nephritis. Am J Kidney Dis II:626–629
31. Kashtan C, Fish AJ, Kleppel M, Yoshioka K, Michael AF (1986) Nephritogenic antigen determinants in epidermal and renal basement membrane of kindreds with Alport-type familial nephritis. J Clin Invest 78:1035–1044
32. McCoy RC, Johnson HK, Stone WJ, Wilson CB (1982) Absence of nephritogenic GBM antigen(s) in some patients with hereditary nephritis. Kidney Int 21:642–652
33. Olson DL, Anand SK, Landing BH, Heuser E, Grushkin CM, Lieberman E (1980) Diagnosis of hereditary nephritis by failure of glomeruli to bind anti-glomerular basement membrane antibodies. J Pediatr 96:697–699
34. Savage COS, Pusey CD, Kershaw MJ, Cashman SJ, Harrison P, Hartley B, Turner DR, Cameron JS, Evans DJ, Lockwood CM (1986) The Goodpasture antigen in Alport's syndrome: studies with a monoclonal antibody. Kidney Int 30:107–112
35. Butkowski RJ, Shen G-Q, Wieslander J, Michael AF, Fish AJ (1990) Characterization of type IV collagen NC1 monomers and Goodpasture antigen in human renal basement membranes. J Lab Clin Med 115:365–373
36. Kleppel MM, Kashtan CE, Butkowski RJ, Fish AJ, Michael AF (1987) Absence of 28 kilodalton noncollagenous monomers of type IV collagen in glomerular basement membrane. J Clin Invest 80:263–266
37. Kashtan CE, Atkin CL, Gregory MC, Michael AF (1989) Identification of Variant Alport phenotypes using an Alport-specific antibody probe. Kidney Int 36:669–674
38. Shah B, First MR, Mendoza NC, Clyne DH, Alexander JW, Weiss MA (1988) Alport's syndrome: Risk of glomerulonephritis induced by anti-glomerular-basement-membrane antibody after renal transplantation. Nephron 50:34–38
39. Fleming SJ, Savage COS, McWilliam LJ, Pickering SJ, Ralston AJ, Johnson RWG, Ackrill P (1988) Anti-glomerular basement membrane antibody-mediated nephritis complicating transplantation in a patient with Alport's syndrome. Transplantation 46:857–859

40. Heuvel LPWJvd, Schröder CH, Savage COS, Menzel D, Assmann KJM, Monnens LAH, Veerkamp JH (1989) The development of anti-glomerular basement membrane nephritis in two children with Alport's syndrome after renal transplantation: characterization of the antibody target. Pediatr Nephrol 3:406–413
41. Savage COS, Noel LH, Crutcher E, Price SRG, Grunfeld JP, Lockwood CM (1989) Hereditary nephritis: immunoblotting studies of the glomerular basement membrane. Lab Invest 60:613–618
42. Barker DF, Hostikka SL, Zhou J, Chow LT, Oliphant AR, Gerken SC, Gregory MC, Skolnick MH, Atkin CL, Tryggvason K (1990) Identification of mutations in the COL4A5 collagen gene in Alport syndrome. Science 248:1224–1226

Relevance of Proteoglycans in Glomerular Matrix Pathology

Hirofumi Makino[1], Naoki Kashihara[1], Shuji Ikeda[1], Brigitte Lelongt[2], and Yashpal S. Kanwar[2]

Summary. Proteoglycans are one of the essential components of the extracellular matrices, i.e., glomerular basement membrane and mesangial matrix. Heparan sulfate-proteoglycan (HS-PG) appears to be the major proteoglycan present in the extracellular matrices, with small amounts of chondroitin sulfate-proteoglycans present in the mesangial matrix. The functions of the chondroitin sulfate-proteoglycans in the mesangium are unknown. The latter may play some role in glomerulosclerosis in various forms of nephritides, e.g., diabetes. The biologic relevance of HS-PG has been investigated extensively since its discovery a decade ago. Its biologic significance was first explored in glomerular permeability. Normally, anionic molecules such as plasma albumin are highly restricted during their passage across the glomerular capillary. With either the removal of or neutralization of the charge of HS-PG, the passage of albumin is greatly facilitated and the albumin appears in urine. Thus, the HS-PG imparts charge and size selectivity to the glomerulus. The loss of charge selectivity has been seen in several forms of glomerulonephritis, including diabetic nephropathy, where the synthesis of HS-PG has been found to be decreased. Moreover, intravenous administration of anti-HS-PG antibodies induces a proteinuric response and dramatically alters the extracellular matrices, thereby indicating that the HS-PG is nephritogenic. Another important role of HS-PG has been recently elucidated in renal morphogenesis. With the perturbation of proteoglycan metabolism, one finds failure in the development of the whole kidney in general, and also delayed maturation of the glomeruli as well as their extracellular matrices. Finally, several heparin binding domains on the laminin molecule have been described in in vitro systems, but their biologic significance is unknown.

[1]Third Department of Internal Medicine, Okayama University Medical School, 2-5-1 Shikata-cho, Okayama 700, Japan
[2]Department of Pathology, Northwestern University Medical, Chicago, IL, USA

Introduction

The glomerulus is comprised of three cell types: visceral epithelium, endothelium, and mesangium, and their two extracellular matrices: glomerular basement membrane (GBM) and mesangial matrix (MM). The visceral epithelium and endothelium cover the GBM from outside and inside, respectively; while the mesangial cell is embedded within its matrix. The GBM and MM, apparently synthesized by all the cell types of the glomerulus, are made up of various glycoproteins; these include: type IV collagen [1], laminin [2], entactin [3], heparan sulfate-proteoglycan (HS-PG) [4,5], chondroitin sulfate proteoglycan [6], nidogen [7], fibronectin [8], and amyloid P component [9]. The amyloid P component, fibronectin, and chondroitin sulfate-proteoglycan are exclusively located in the mesangium, while the remaining glycoproteins are present in both glomerular extracellular matrices. All these glycoproteins of the extracellular matrix play respective vital roles in various biologic and pathogenetic mechanisms involving the renal glomerulus. In this chapter certain mechanisms relevant to the pathobiology of the glomerular proteoglycans will be discussed.

What are Proteoglycans?

Proteoglycans are heterogeneous macromolecules distributed in most of the mammalian tissues, including extracellular matrices. A special type of proteoglycan, termed HS-PG, is found in the glomerular extracellular matrices. Its presence has been elucidated with the use of histochemical dyes (ruthenium red), selective binding with cationic proteins (cationized ferritin and lysozyme), and by labelling with isotopes, e.g., [^{35}S]-sulfate [5,6]. Evidence from several studies indicates that the molecular weight of proteoglycans varies greatly, depending upon the method of isolation and the source of the tissue. In general, they are made up of a core-protein to which glycosaminoglycan (GAG) chains are attached to the peptide via xylose-serine linkages. The GAG chains are made up of disaccharide units of glucuronic acid and glucosamine. The GAG chains are highly sulfated, which apparently imparts charge characteristics to the molecule. As ascertained by radiolabeling studies, the molecular weight of the intact HS-PG is 150–200,000 [10], while many other studies suggest that perhaps the de novo synthesized HS-PG is a smaller fragment of a relatively larger precursor macromolecule which has a molecular weight exceeding 1,000,000 [11,12]. Conceivably, the HS-PGs interact with one another by lateral or end to end associations; they also interact with other extracellular matrix macromolecules, thus forming the meshwork of the GBM. The mature GBM so assembled is endowed with charge and size-selective properties.

Role of Proteoglycans in Glomerular Ultrafiltration

The glomerular ultrafiltration unit is made of various strata. From the peripheral urinary space towards the inner capillary lumen they are: visceral epithelial foot processes with intervening diaphragms, GBM, and fenestrated endothelium. This

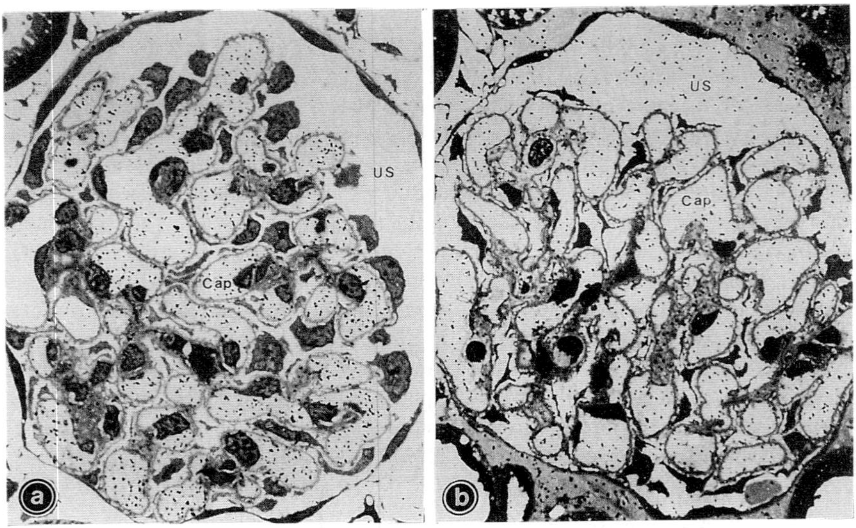

Fig. 1a-b. Light microscopic autoradiograms of glomeruli from control (**a**) and heparitinase-treated (**b**) kidneys that were subsequently perfused with ^{125}I-bovine serum albumin (*BSA*). Note that BSA molecules readily leaked into the urinary space (*US*) in glomeruli of the kidney treated with the heparitinase. Cap, capillary lumen

ultrafiltration unit is endowed with charge and size-selective properties which are partly due to the intrinsic presence of HS-PG in the GBM. Normally, the transcapillary passage of a given tracer with fixed molecular weight and varying degrees of charge would be as follows: cationic > neutral ≫ anionic. In in vivo situations, the anionic proteins such as plasma albumin have a highly restricted passage through the glomerular capillaries. With the removal of HS-PG from the GBM, the plasma albumin readily traverses into the urinary space [13] (Fig. 1). Similarly, the transcapillary passage of anionic ferritin is increased with the enzymatic digestion of HS-PG of the GBM. In the same manner, a proteinuric response is observed in rats with the constant intravenous infusion of hexadimethrine [14].

In addition to their critical role in ultrafiltration, the HS-PGs play an important role in protecting the GBM from assault by circulating plasma proteins [15]. They repulse the plasma proteins from the GBM by virtue of their electronegative charge. Also, they preserve the GBM matrix in a hydrated state by holding water molecules between the sulfate radicals. Thus, they prevent the non-specific adsorption of plasma proteins onto the GBM and do not allow it to become clogged by these proteins. In doing so, the HS-PGs allow a constant solute flow across the glomerular capillary, while keeping the GBM hydrophilic and keeping plasma proteins away from the GBM and in circulation. With the elimination of these anti-clogging functions of the GBM, one finds non-specific adsorption of anionic proteins, e.g., ferritin, albumin, and insulin, onto the GBM, resulting in an abrupt cessation of glomerular filtration (Fig. 2). Thus, it appears that under normal isoosmolar conditions, sulfated polyanionic macromolecules such as HS-PG act as anticlogging agents by preventing hydrogen bonding and adsorption of

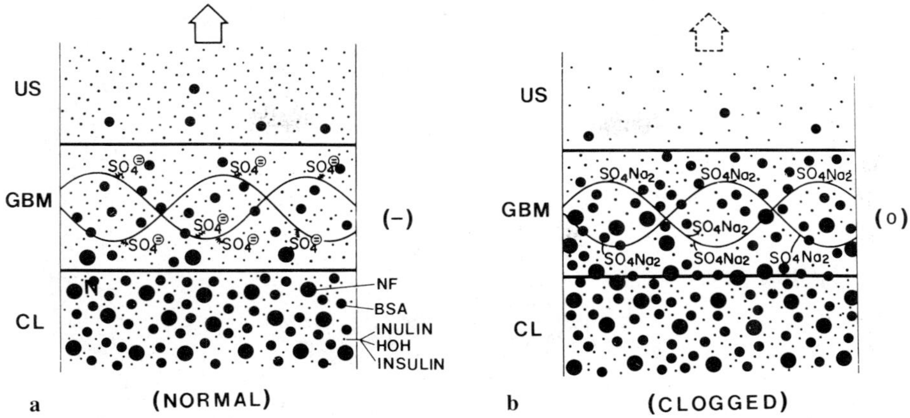

Fig. 2a,b. Schematic drawing of the phenomenon of clogging of glomerular basement membrane (*GBM*). Normally (**a**), anionic native ferritin (*NF*) and bovine serum albumin (*BSA*) do not adsorb onto the GBM, and small molecules like inulin or insulin or water pass through readily and reach the urinary space (*US*). With inactivation of sulfate radicals of proteoglycans (**b**), the NF and BSA adsorb onto the GBM and clog the filter; therefore, smaller molecules or plasma water do not pass through the glomerular capillaries readily. CL, Capillary lumen

plasma proteins onto the glycoproteins of the GBM; thereby a sustained transcapillary solute flow is maintained.

Proteoglycans in Diabetes Mellitus

Nonspecific adsorption of circulating plasma proteins, e.g., albumin and IgG, onto the GBM is seen in diabetic nephropathy. Such an adsorption has been attributed to the change in the biophysical/biochemical characteristics of the GBM. It has been shown that nonenzymatic glycation may interfere in the interaction of various glycoproteins of the GBM, but convincing data are not yet available in the literature. However, abnormalities in the metabolism of HS-PGs have been repeatedly demonstrated [16–20]. Usually, there is decreased incorporation of the precursor products (e.g., [^{35}S]-sulfate) of HS-PGs into the GBM in experimental diabetic states (Fig. 3) [16,19,20]. Similar biochemical abnormalities have been observed in human tissues as well. Also, it appears that the decrease is usually proportional to the degree of proteinuria and excretion of urinary proteins in diabetes (personal observations). Thus, it appears that there is a decrease in the synthesis of HS-PGs of the GBM, and this reduction probably relates to the increased spillage of proteins into the urine, at least in the nephrotic stage of diabetic nephropathy. However, the nature of the biochemical lesion in the early stages of diabetes, i.e., the microalbuminuric stage, is unclear. It is possible that insulin or insulin-like growth factors may possibly play some role in the hyperplasia/hypertrophy of the mesangial cells, which occurs in the pathogenesis of the early stages of diabetic nephropathy. Certainly, it seems that insulin-like and transforming growth factors upregulate the functions of glomerular

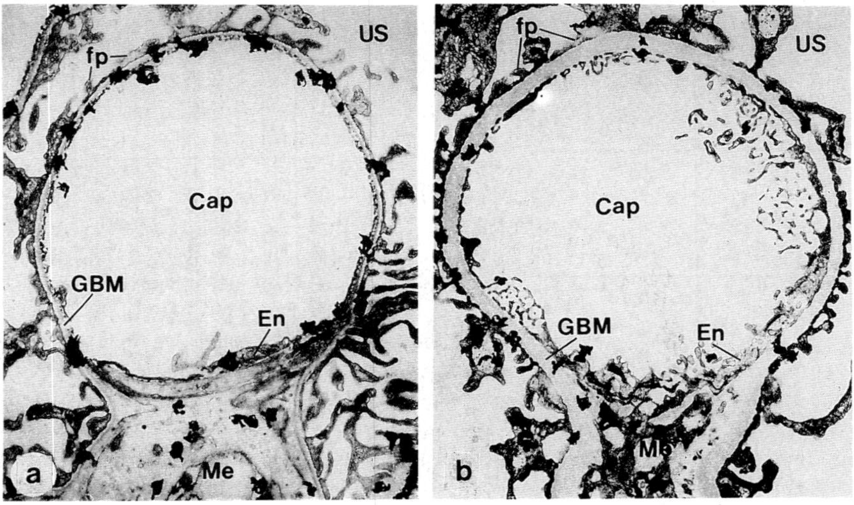

Fig. 3a,b. Electronmicroscopic autoradiograms of glomerular capillary loops of normal (**a**) and diabetic (**b**) rat kidneys radiolabelled with [^{35}S]-sulfate. Note the reduction in the autoradiographic grains overlying the glomerular basement membrane (*GBM*) of diabetic animal. US, urinary space; fp, foot processes; En, endothelium; Cap, capillary lumen; Me, mesangium

cells and increase the synthesis of proteoglycans specific to the mesangium [21,22]. At the moment, intensive investigatory efforts are being made in several laboratories to sort out various biochemical events which may shed some light on the pathogenesis of diabetic nephropathy.

Proteoglycans in Nephrotic Syndrome

Besides diabetes, the status of HS-PGs has been investigated in a wide variety of nephritides. Fractional clearance studies do provide the evidence of loss of charge-selectivity in various forms of glomerulonephritis. However, comparable histopathologic data are somewhat sparse. With the application of polyethylenemine, a dramatic decrease in the concentration of HS-PG was noted in patients with congenital nephrotic syndrome [23]. In regard to results obtained from experimental animals, there is much controversy. Aminonucleoside nephrosis in rats, a model of minimal change disease in man, has been exhaustively studied. The status of HS-PGs was investigated by the use of anti-HS-PG antibodies, and highly controversial results were obtained. The differences so observed can be reconciled if one takes into account the source of the antibody and the antigen. It is conceivable that in aminonucleoside nephrosis, certain antigenic epitopes, represented in a given antibody molecule, are lost while others remain preserved. This would likely be expected when the heterogeneous nature of the HS-PG macromolecule is taken into consideration during preparation of the antigens and antibodies.

Nephritogenicity of Anti-HS-PG Antibodies

The GBM as a whole is highly nephritogenic, i.e., anti-GBM antibodies, when administered intravenously, induce functional and structural alterations in the glomerulus which resemble those seen in Goodpasture's syndrome. Investigators have wondered about the glycoprotein or glycopeptide of the GBM which could be held responsible for the induction of the disease. Although the intact GBM is highly nephritogenic, the antibodies raised against its individual components, e.g., type IV collagen and laminin, evoke a weak proteinuric response. In view of these considerations, we investigated the nephritogenicity of proteoglycans in rats. Within a few hours of injection of anti-HS-PG antibodies, the animals showed a mild proteinuric response, minimal complement activation, and a transient influx of polymorphonuclear neutrophils (PMNs) into the glomerular capillaries. These changes regressed within a week. During the third week, tremendous ultrastructural alterations were observed, but without any proteinuric response. The changes included mesangial cell proliferation, irregular knob-like thickening of GBMs and occasional influx of monocytes and mesangial interposition (Fig. 4) [24]. The animals recovered completely 8 weeks after the administration of the antibodies. On the other hand, IgG-sensitized rats developed typical immune-complex nephritis within 7–10 days of injection of antibodies. After a week, subepithelial and subendothelial deposits were observed, along with complement activation. Subsequently, the subepithelial deposits enlarged in size and proteinuric response was accentuated (Fig. 4). The proteinuria was complement-dependent [25]. Finally, the deposits were reabsorbed by 3 months. Thus, it appears that the immune response and the formation of subepithelial immune-complex deposit is dependent upon the immune status of the animals. In this regard, we investigated the nephritogenicity of proteoglycans in various strains of mice and rats. The proteinuric response and ultrastructural alterations were dependent upon the genetically determined immune status of the animal. For example, Brown Norway rats and NZB/NZW (F1) mice exhibit maximal nephritogenic response as compared to other strains (unpublished work). Also, it appears that the degree of influx of monocytes into the glomerular capillaries is proportional to the severity of the disease; thereby indicating that inflammatory mediators somehow inflicted the damage to the glomerulus. In this regard, further investigatory efforts were made in order to delineate the nature of the mediator which could affect the HS-PGs of the GBM. The exposure of the glomerulus to interleukin-1 (IL-1) resulted in the degradation of the proteoglycan (unpublished work). In addition, a dramatic reduction in the incorporation of [^{35}S]-sulfate into the HS-PGs was observed, with the inclusion of reactive oxygen radicals in the medium (unpublished work). These experiments possibly suggest that a large number of inflammatory mediators can affect the integrity of the GBM HS-PG and that can result, conceivably, in a proteinuric response, which is observed in various forms of nephritides.

The other question which is relevant to the subject matter here pertains to the pathogenetic mechanisms involved in the formation of subepithelial immune-complex deposits. Recently, an attractive hypothesis has been advanced by Andres et al. [26]. According to this hypothesis, the antibodies bind to the antigenic epitopes present at the base of the visceral epithelial foot processes; this is followed by clustering of antigen-antibody complexes on the plasmalemma of the podocytes, with

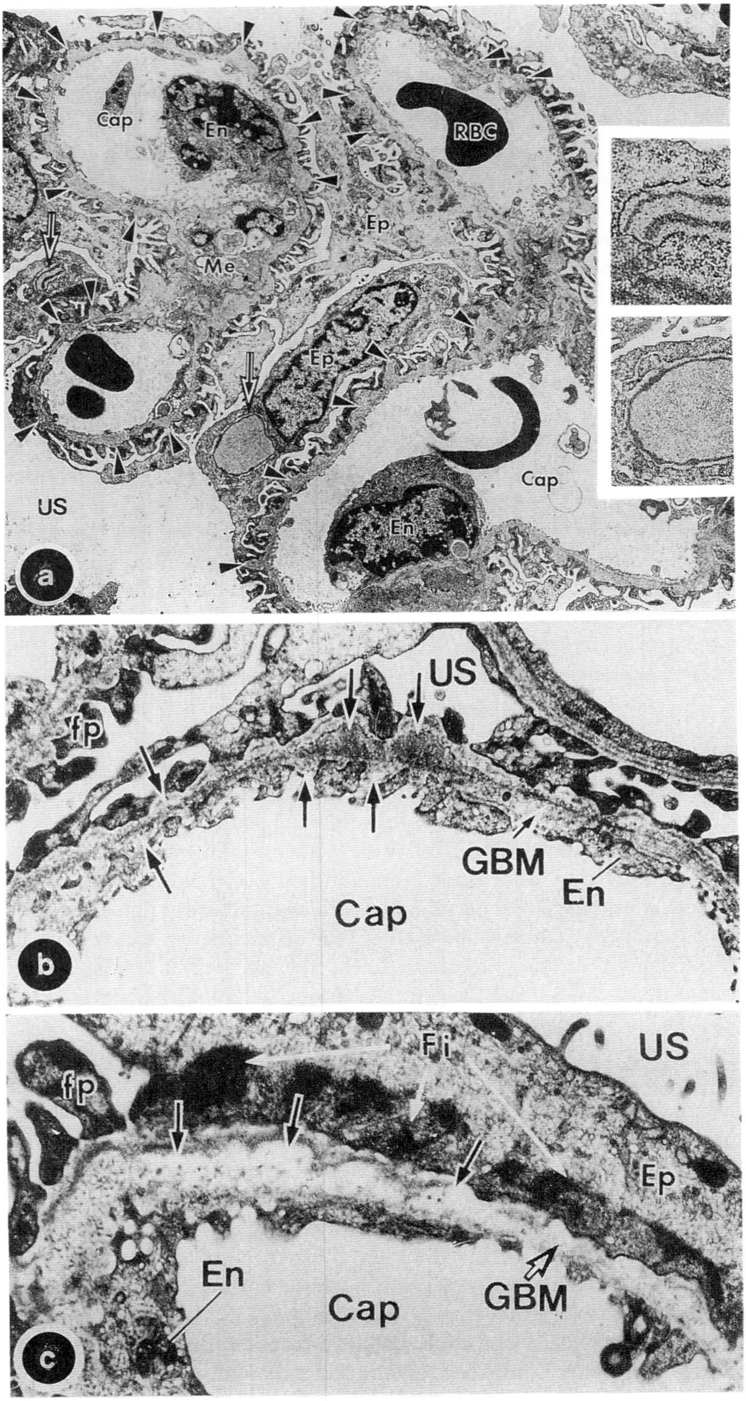
Cap
En
RBC
Ep
Me
Ep
Cap
US
En
a
US
fp
GBM
En
Cap
b
Fi
US
fp
Ep
En
Cap
GBM
c

consequential capping and shedding of the complexes into the subepithelial space with eventual immune-deposit formation. The second hypothesis takes into account the intrinsic hemodynamics of the glomerulus. According to this, shear forces of relatively greater magnitude are prevalent in the inner layers of the GBM and the velocity of these sweeping plasma fluid currents is weak in the outer layers of the GBM (Fig. 5) [25]. Therefore, the ligands bound in the subepithelial space would have a delayed clearance and a prolonged residence in the peripheral layers of the GBM, and thus could serve as a core nidus for the formation of immune-deposits. In support of this contention, the intravenously injected ligands first accumulate in the inner layers of the GBM; after 12–24 h they equilibrate on both sides of the GBM, and by 7th day they are exclusively seen in the outer layers of the GBM (Fig. 5). The ligands localized in the peripheral layers of the GBM would evoke an immune-response and would ultimately lead to the formation of subepithelial deposits.

Role of Proteoglycans in Renal Development

Presumably, all components of the extracellular matrices regulate organogenesis/morphogenesis. However, proteoglycans have attracted most of the attention in this field. As they regulate organogenesis in many other organs, the proteoglycans possibly regulate renal organogenesis. Evidence for this came from the studies by Lelongt et al. [27]. It was noted that with the interference in the metabolism of proteoglycans, the metanephric tissues did not mature normally. The ureteric bud branches were disorganized and the number of nephrons seen was relatively less than the number seen in the control metanephric kidney (Fig. 6). In addition, the glomerular extracellular matrices were poorly assembled, lacked ruthenium red staining granules, and had a dramatic reduction in the incorporation of [^{35}S]-sulfate. This meant that indeed the perturbed proteoglycan metabolism had some relationship with metanephric development. The other glycoproteins of the extracellular matrices, i.e., laminin and type-IV collagen, were minimally affected. Further investigation of the renal development was conducted using puromycin aminonucleoside (PAN). Here too, dysmorphogenesis of the metanephric tissues was observed, in association with a dramatic decrease in the synthesis of proteoglycans [28]. It is interesting to note here that the proteoglycans synthesized in metanephric tissue are much larger ($\gg 2.5 \times 10^6$) than those isolated from the adult rat kidney. Also, the embryonic renal proteoglycans contain substantial amounts of chondroitin sulfate. The reasons for such variations are unclear, but may be related to the fact that the

Fig. 4a-c. Electronmicrographs of glomerular capillary loops of kidneys from normal (**a**) and IgG-presensitized rats (**b,c**) injected with anti-HS-PG antibodies. Note the remarkable subepithelial thickening of the basement membrane (*arrow heads*) and basement membrane like material in the visceral epithelia (*arrows*) in glomeruli from normal rats. In the presensitized rats the immune-deposits are initially formed on both sides of the GBM (**b**); later on they are seen only in the subepithelial regions where they are being reabsorbed (**c**). US, urinary space; En, endothelium; Cap, capillary lumen; Me, mesangium; RBC, red blood cell; FP, foot processes; Ep, epithelium

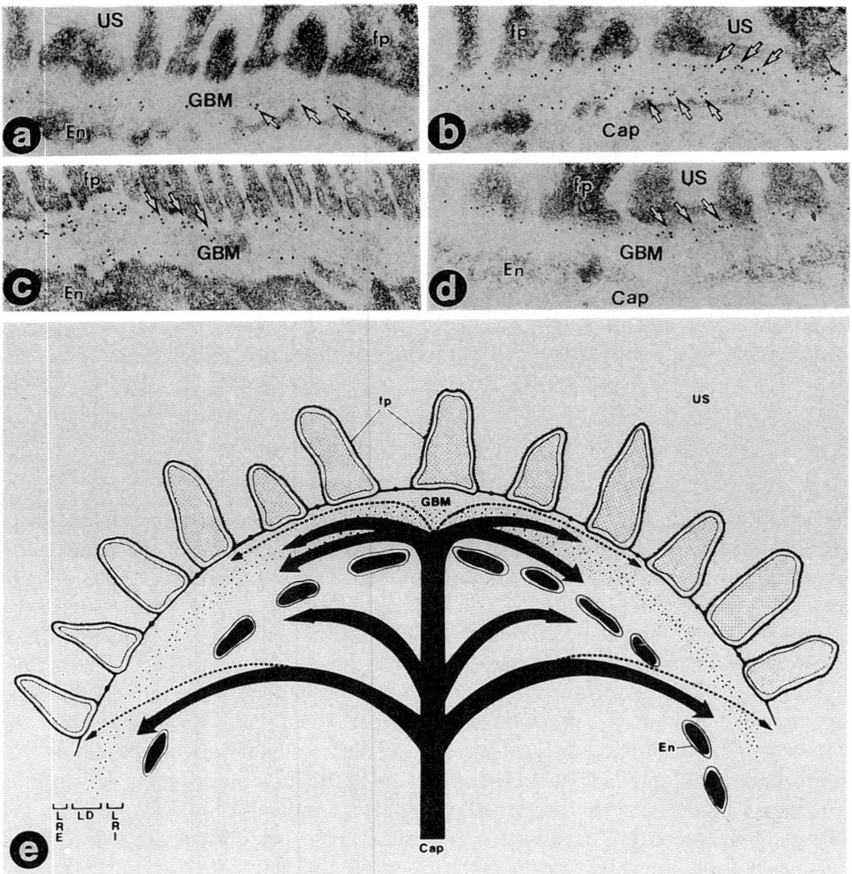

Fig. 5a-e. Electron micrographs of glomerular capillaries from kidneys of rats injected with anti-HS-PG antibody and sacrificed 1 h (**a**), 12 h (**b**), 3 days (**c**) and 7 days (**d**) later. The antibody was localized by immunogold method. Within one h the antibody localizes in the inner layers of the GBM (*arrows*); at 12 h it equilibrates on both sides of the GBM and remains there for three days; while on the 7th day the antibody molecules are exclusively localized in the outer layers of the GBM. **e** is a schematic drawing to indicate that the plasma fluid currents have relatively higher shear forces in the inner layers of the GBM than in the outer layers. This suggests that because of the higher shear forces the ligands present in the inner layers are easily cleared, while those in the outer layers remain localized and evoke a host immune-response and ultimately serve as a nidus for the formation of antigen-antibody immune complexes
US, urinary space; cap, capillary lumen; En, endothelium; FP, foot processes; LRE, lamina rara externa; LD, lamina densa; LRI, lamina rara interna

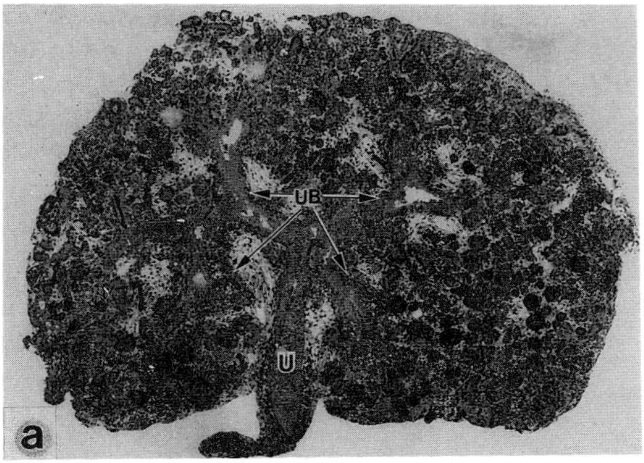

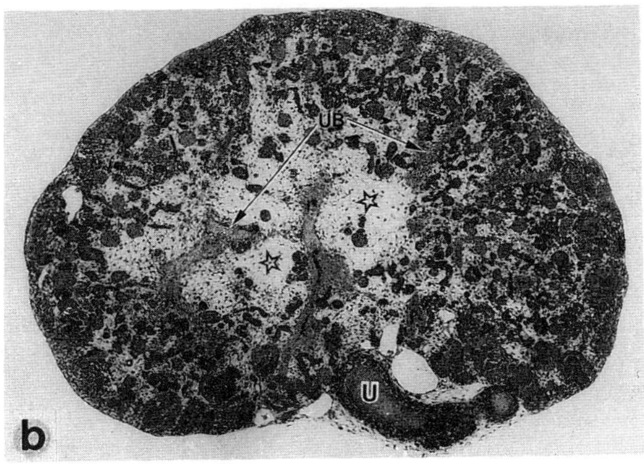

Fig. 6a,b. Light micrographs of normal (**a**) and beta-xyloside-treated (**b**) metanephric kidneys. Note in the xyloside-treated kidney the disorganization of the ureteric bud (*UB*) branches, looseness of the mesenchymal tissue (*) and reduction in the population of the nephrons as compared to the control metanephric kidney. U, ureter

embryonic tissues contain precursor proteoglycan macromolecules which later, in mature tissues, are modified to a smaller size via post-transcriptional or post-translational modifications.

Interactions of Proteoglycans with Other Glycoproteins

Several heparin binding domains have been localized on the various extracellular matrix proteins [29]. Presumably, these interactions may be relevant in the assemblage of the extracellular matrix. Proteoglycans, in general, accentuate the interactions among other matrix proteins. For instance, it has been shown that fibronectin bound to proteoglycans exhibits increased binding towards collagen. Similarly, the interactions of proteoglycans with other cell surface proteins have been investigated extensively. It appears that proteoglycans may serve as receptors which maintain communication between intracellular and extracellular matrix proteins [30]. Thus, it is possible that they may be responsible for some yet to be characterized transmembrane cellular signalling processes, and perhaps they also play a role in cell adhesion mechanisms. All these processes indicated above have been demonstrated in in vitro systems. Unfortunately, in vivo biologic proof, has so far yet to be elucidated.

In summary, we can say, with a certain degree of assurance, that proteoglycans play an essential role in regulating the morphogenesis and ultrafiltration of the renal glomerulus. Thus, derangements in the macromolecular structure of proteoglycans result in proteinuric responses which are seen in various forms of renal diseases.

Acknowledgments. Supported by grants from the Japanese Ministry of Education, Science and Culture (C-01570644) Japan, and NIH (DK28492) USA.

References

1. Keflides NA (1973) Int Rev Connect Tissue Res 6:63–104
2. Timpl R, Rohade H, Robey GP, Rennard SI, Foidart JM, Martin GR (1979) J Biol Chem 254:9933–9937
3. Carlin B, Jaffe R, Bender B, Chunh AE (1981) J Biol Chem 256:5209–5214
4. Kanwar YS, Farquhar MG (1979) Proc Natl Acad Sci USA 76:1303–1307
5. Kanwar YS, Veis A, Kimura JH, Jakubowski ML (1984) Proc Natl Acad Sci USA 81:762–766
6. Kanwar YS, Rosenzweig LJ, Jakubowski ML (1983) Lab Invest 49:216–225
7. Timpl R, Fujiwara S, Dziadek M, Aumailley M, Weber S, Engel J (1984) Ciba Foundation Symposium 108. London, Pitman, pp 25–43
8. Courtoy PJ, Kanwar YS, Hynes RD, Farquhar MG (1980) J Cell Biol 87:691–696
9. Houser MT, Scheinman JI, Basgen J, Steffes MW, Michael AF (1982) J Clin Invest 69:1169–1175
10. Kanwar YS, Hascall VC, Farquhar MG (1981) J Cell Biol 90:527–532
11. Hassell JR, Robey PG, Barrach HJ, Wilczek J, Rennard SI, Martin GR (1980) Proc Natl Acad Sci USA 77:4494–4498
12. Klein DJ, Brown DM, Oegema TR (1988) J Cell Biol 106:963–970
13. Kanwar YS (1984) Lab Invest 51:7–21
14. Hunsicker LG, Shearer TP, Shaffer SJ (1981) Kidney Int 20:7–17
15. Kanwar YS, Rosenzweig LJ (1982) J Cell Biol 93:489–494
16. Cohen MP, Surma ML (1981) J Lab Clin Med 98:715–720
17. Parthasarthy N, Spiro RG (1982) Diabetes 31:738–741
18. Rohrbach DH, Hassell JR, Kleinman HK, Martin GR (1982) Diabetes 31:185–188, 1982
19. Kanwar YS, Rosenzweig LJ, Linker A, Jakubowski ML (1983) Proc Natl Acad Sci USA 80:2272–2275
20. Klein DJ, Brown DM, Oegema TR (1986) Diabetes 35:1130–1142
21. Border WA, Okuda S, Languino LR, Ruoslahti E (1990) Kidney Int 37:689–695
22. Watanabe Y, Dalecki TM, Kanwar YS (to be published)
23. Vernier RL, Klein DJ, Sisson SP, Mahan JD, Oegema TR, Brown DM (1983) N Engl J Med 309-1001-1005

24. Makino H, Gibbons JT, Reddy MK, Kanwar YS (1986) J Clin Invest 77:142–156
25. Makino H, Lelongt B, Kanwar YS (1988) Kidney Int 34:195–219
26. Andres G, Brentjens JR, Caldwell PRB, Camussi G, Matsuo S (1986) Lab Invest 55:510–520
27. Lelongt B, Makino H, Dalecki T, Kanwar YS (1988) Dev Biol 128:256–276
28. Liu Z, Dalecki T, Kashihara N, Kanwar YS (to be published)
29. Ruoslahti E (1988) Annu Rev Cell Biol 4:229–255
30. Sanderson RD, Bernfield M (1988) Proc Natl Acad Sci USA 85:9562–9566

Pathobiology of Tubular Basement Membranes in Renal Cystic Disease

FRANK A. CARONE and YASHPAL S. KANWAR[1]

SUMMARY. The pathogenic role of the tubular basement membrane was studied in polycystic kidney disease (PKD) induced by diphenylthiazole (DPT) or its major urinary metabolite, phenol II, and in cyst-derived cells from human autosomal dominant PKD kidneys. DPT induced, in rats, progressive, but reversible cystic change of collecting tubules (CDs), characterized by thickening of the tubular basement membrane with marked reduction of the de novo synthesis of sulfated proteoglycans. The phenol II was administered for 4 days to determine the sequence of tubular cell and BM changes in the development of PKD. At day one, 12% of CDs were cystic and their BMs were altered. Over the 4 day interval, BMs remained structurally altered and cystic change increased progressively. Cell proliferation was not detected until day 2 and occurred both in cystic and in non-cystic renal zones; it did not increase as cystic change progressed. By immunofluorescence, there was a decrease in anti-heparin sulfate proteoglycan core protein reactivity and an increase in anti-fibronectin reactivity of the extracellular matrices of cystic tubules. In the in vitro studies, the growth rate, cell doubling time, and end cell number of cyst-derived autosomal dominant polycystic kidney disease (ADPKD) and normal human renal epithelial (NK) cells were the same; moreover, ADPKD cells did not exhibit any in vitro features of transformed cells. Post-confluent NK and ADPKD cells in vitro elaborated distinct BMs. By electron microscopy, BMs of NK cells were of uniform thickness with a regular pattern of ruthenium red (RR) binding sites indicative of proteoglycans. In contrast, BMs of ADPKD cells were less dense, thicker, and lacked RR sites; immunofluorescent reactivity to anti-HS-PG core protein was uneven and decreased while reactivity to anti fibronectin was increased. The findings suggest that BM components are in a dynamic metabolic state, capable of rapid modulation, and that PKD may be due to a defect in the synthesis/degradation of one or more basement membrane components, resulting in faulty tubular morphogenesis.

[1]Northwestern University Medical School, Chicago, IL, USA

Introduction

Polycystic kidney disease (PKD) presents as gigantic expansion of tubules and occasionally of glomeruli [1]. It is a localized, segmental event due to an aberration of one or more factors regulating tubular (or glomerular capsular) morphogenesis. PKD represents one of the most dramatic processes in biology, since some tubules increase in diameter from about 30 microns (not visible to the naked eye) to more than 5 centimeters. Furthermore, PKD is an excellent model to study the dynamics of transcellular fluid movement, cell growth, and the interactions and interdependence of tubular cells and their extracellular matrix. In some forms of PKD, cystic changes involve a specific segment of all nephrons, for example the collecting tubules in human autosomal recessive or infantile PKD. In other forms of PKD, cystic change involves random tubular sites of a small number of nephrons, for example in human autosomal dominant PKD, cystic change occurs only in a small percentage of nephrons where it can involve any segment of the nephron. Human PKD can pursue a rapid course with renal failure occurring early in life, or a benign course without renal failure developing during the natural life of the individual. Human acquired PKD develops in end stage kidneys that are atrophic and scarred. Clinical findings indicate that this form of PKD is reversible following renal transplantation with correction of the azotemic state [2]. Additionally, we have shown that PKD, induced experimentally by diphenylthiazole (DPT), reverses following withdrawal of the compound [3]. Whether other forms of human or experimental PKD are reversible remains to be determined. PKD occurs in the microenvironment of specific tubular segments. Baert microdissected two cases of ADPKD at an early stage of the disease [4]. Localized cystic dilatations were found in the proximal, distal, and collecting tubules and in Henle's loop. Many nephrons were normal. Cysts were localized distentions in otherwise normal tubules free of obstruction. Thus, expression of the gene defect in ADPKD is a localized event resulting in loss of tubular morphogenesis with extracellular matrix remodelling, tubular epithelial cell hyperplasia, and accumulation of tubular fluid.

Altered cell-BM interactions may be central to the pathogenesis of PKD. The epithelial cell is primarily responsible for synthesis/degradation of BM components, and the composition of the BM, in turn, plays a regulatory role in tissue morphogenesis and mobility, shape, differentiation, growth, and gene expression of the cell [5]. The tubular extracellular matrix is composed primarily of type IV collagen, laminin, sulfated proteoglycans (PGs), and fibronectin. These components have specific binding sites for each other and for structural components, both on the cell surface and in the underlying dense connective tissue [6]. Our studies on DPT or its hydroxylated metabolite phenol II and on autosomal dominant kidney disease (ADPKD) cells in vitro suggest that a faulty tubular extracellular matrix (basement membrane) plays a key role in the development of cystic change.

Materials and Methods

Two models of PKD were studies. 1. PKD was induced in rats by the oral administration of DPT [7] or its major urinary metabolite, 2-amino-4 hydroxyphenyl-5 phenyl thiazole, designated Phenol II [8]. Control animals were pair-fed. 2. In vitro methods

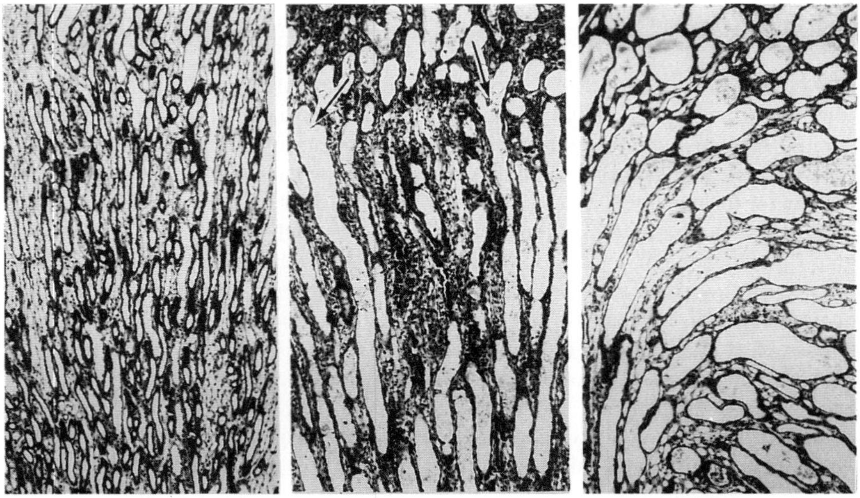

Fig. 1. Outer medulla of control and 4 day *DPT* and *phenol II* treated (*PKD*) kidneys, X 66 DPT, diphenylthiazole; PKD, polycystic kidney disease

were developed to isolate and propagate large numbers of cells from cysts of ADPKD kidneys and from normal human kidneys (NK) [9].

Rat kidneys were perfusion fixed and examined by light microscopy. For electron microscopy ruthenium red (RR) was added to the fixative [3]. To study the de novo synthesis of proteoglycans (PGs) in DPT-induced PKD, renal PGs were labeled with [^{35}S]-sulfate in a recirculating kidney-perfusion system [10]. The reactivity of tubules, tubular cells and extracellular matrices to anti-heparin sulfate-proteoglycan, -type IV collagen, -laminin and -fibronectin were ascertained by indirect immunofluorescence [11]. Standard tissue culture methods were employed to study the biological behavior of human ADPKD and NK cells in vitro [9].

Results and Discussion

We found that administration of DPT induced PKD, involving collecting ducts, in rats (Fig. 1); it occurred in the presence of normal glomerular and tubular function and normal intratubular pressure, and in the absence of tubular obstruction [7]. These findings suggest that cystic transformation is due to an inherent alteration in the wall of the tubule. By electron microscopy, BMs showed progressive thickening and loss of ruthenium red staining (indicative of loss of proteoglycans) with progressive development of cysts. Biochemical analysis of isolated, and purified tubular basement membrane (TBM), revealed an overall increase in the concentration of low molecular weight glycoproteins [12]. Immunochemical studies revealed a normal concentration of laminin, entactin and type IV collagen but an increased concentration of type 1 collagen and fibronectin; the latter components are probably not intrin-

Table 1.

	Control	Phenol II treated			
		Day			
		1	2	3	4
% Cystic tubules	0	12*	21*	25*	30*
Basement membrane					
Thickness	N	3+	3+	3+	3+
RR Staining	N	N	N	LOSS	LOSS
Cell proliferation					
% Thymidine labeling					
Cortex	.11	.43	2.5*	2.6*	1.4*
Medulla	.24	.57	5.9*	8.0*	6.4*

*, Significant, N, normal, RR, ruthenium red

sic to the TBM. These morphological and chemical alterations in DPT-induced PKD suggest that cystic transformation may be due to a change in TBM compliance. However, the deformability and viscoelastic creep of BM lining cysts induced by DPT were not significantly different from normal TBMs [13]. Immunofluorescence studies of BMs of cystic tubules in DPT-treated animals showed the following compared to controls: uneven staining for type IV collagen and laminin, weak or absent staining for heparin sulfate proteoglycans (HS-PG), and intense staining for fibronectin [11]. Further studies demonstrated a decreased de novo synthesis of PGs in DPT-induced PKD in rats [10]. The PGs of normal and cystic kidneys were labelled with [^{35}S]-sulfate in an organ perfusion system. Total radioactivity in cellular, basement membrane, and media fractions of cystic kidneys was reduced 9, 7, and 3-fold, respectively. PGs from cystic and normal kidneys had similar molecular weight profiles. In addition to heparin sulfate, 15–20% of glycosaminoglycans (GAGs) synthesized by cystic kidneys were chondroitin sulfate; PGs synthesized by cystic kidneys had a lower charge density, possibly related to decreased sulfation of the PGs. Quantitative autoradiography revealed a 2 and 2.5-fold decrease of grain-densities over the cellular and extracellular compartments, respectively, in cystic kidneys. Collectively, these data suggest that DPT alters the biosynthesis/degradation of one or more BM components, particularly HS-PG and fibronectin, resulting in a defective BM.

The major urinary metabolite of DTP, 4-hydroxyphenyl-5 phenyl thiazole, (phenol II) was administered for 4 days to determine the sequence of tubular cell and BM changes in the development of PKD [8]. Following *only* 4 days of treatment, phenol II induced a significantly greater degree of impairment of concentrating ability and cystic transformation than DPT (Fig. 1). BMs remained structurally altered and cystic change increased progressively up to day 4 (Table 1). Significant cell proliferation (thymidine labeling) was not detected until day 2; it occurred both in cystic (outer medullary) and non-cystic (cortical) zones, and it did not increase as cystic change progressed (Table 1). At days 3 and 4, by immunofluorescence, there was an apparent decrease in anti-heparin sulfate proteoglycan core protein reactivity, and an increase in anti-fibronectin reactivity of the extracellular matrices of cystic tubules. The findings suggest that BM components are in a dynamic state capable of rapid modulation. Highly significant is the observation that TBM changes occurred in tandem with cystic transformation of the tubules and preceded the onset of tubular cell proliferation.

We obtained comparable findings from in vitro studies with normal human renal epithelial cells (NK) and cyst-derived cells (ADPKD) from kidneys of patients with autosomal dominant PKD [9]. Post-confluent NK and ADPKD cells grown on collagen matrices synthesized basement membranes. BMs elaborated by NK cells were uniformly dense, exhibited regularly spaced ruthenium red positive granules (Fig. 2), and displayed uniform intense reactivity to fluorescein-tagged antibodies to fibronectin, laminin, type IV collagen and HS-PG core protein (Fig. 3). In contrast, BMs elaborated by ADPKD cells were thicker, less distinct, lacked ruthenium red positive granules, (Fig. 2) and had diminished reactivity to anti-HS-PG core protein and increased reactivity to anti-fibronectin (Fig. 3). Immunofluorescence studies in human ADPKD kidneys similarly revealed a loss of reactivity to anti-HS-PG and a greatly enhanced reactivity to anti-fibronectin in cystic tissue [11]. Thus, there is an apparent altered synthesis/degradation of PGs and fibronectin in both models of PKD, namely DPT-induced and ADPKD cyst derived cells in vitro. Collectively, these findings provide strong evidence that BM alterations are a key factor in the development of cystic disease.

Relevant to this concept are the data of Ebihara et al., who report abnormal regulation of BM gene expression in a murine model of congenital PKD [14]. Levels of mRNA for the alpha 1 (IV) chain of collagen IV were half normal one week after birth and then increased, while mRNA levels for laminin B1 and B2 chains were 80% of normal at one week but were maintained at that level. Identification of the alpha 1 chain mRNA by in situ hybridization with a radiolabeled cDNA probe revealed highest expression in cystic regions, with localization mainly to interstitial cells adjacent to cyst walls, suggesting that these cells are the source of elevated alpha 1 (IV) chain mRNA. These observations may be unique to PKD since interstitial cells are not usually associated with BM synthesis. As cysts developed rapidly between 1 and 2 weeks after birth, immunostaining for collagen IV, laminin and HS-PG around cysts appeared reduced and discontinuous. There was an apparent discrepancy between mRNA levels and protein content of cystic BMs, possible due either to defective translation or post-translation events, or to altered turnover of BM components. These data indicate an abnormal regulation of BM gene expression in congenital (autosomal recessive) PKD.

It has been proposed that PKD is due to hyperplasia and/or preneoplastic transformation of renal epithelial cells [12,15]. Cell proliferation is a feature of human and experimental PKD and increase in tubular cell number is a requirement for the growth of cysts. It has been shown that several proto-oncogenes are significantly over-expressed in cystic kidneys [16]. Moreover, a model of PKD was produced in transgenic mice by deregulation of the c-myc proto-oncogene [17]. However, in a recent in vitro study we found that cyst-derived cells from human kidneys with ADPKD did not exhibit accelerated growth or possess the phenotypic features of transformed cells, compared to renal epithelial cells from normal human kidneys [9]. Moreover, in a chronic study (30 weeks), DPT induced progressive cystic change in the absence of a detectable increased rate of tubular cell proliferation [18]. Similarly, in newborn 1–3 week-old cpk mice, when diffuse PKD involvement of collecting tubules was progressing at an alarming rate, no increase in the mitotic index was detected, even though epithelial cellularity of collecting ducts was obviously increased [19]. Thus, cell growth may be a secondary rather than a primary event in the pathogenesis of PKD.

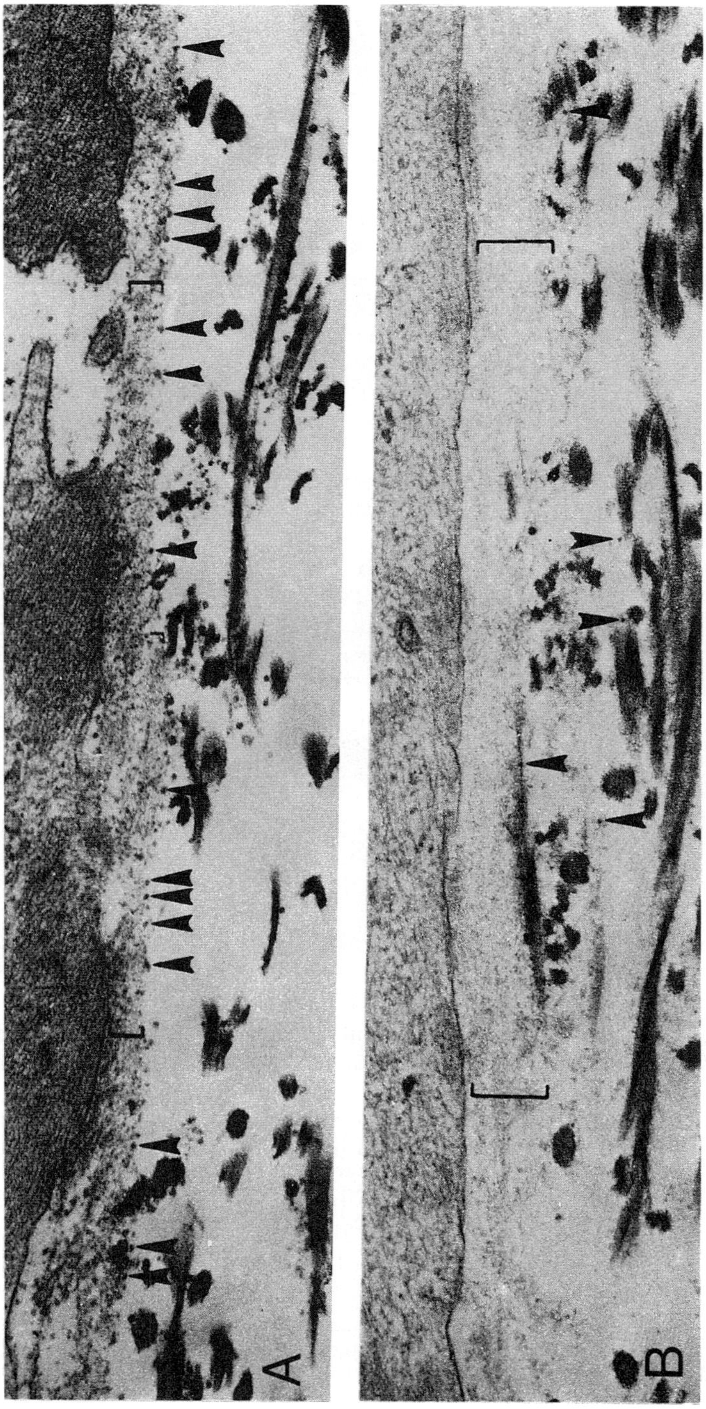

Fig. 2. Electron micrographs of basement membranes (*BM*) stained with ruthenium red (*RR*). *Panel A* shows *BM* of NK cells and *panel B* shows *BM* of ADPKD cells (*BM* delineated by brackets). *Arrow heads* indicate RR binding sites. X 45,000. NK, normal human renal epithelial cells; ADPKD, autosomal dominant polycystic kidney disease

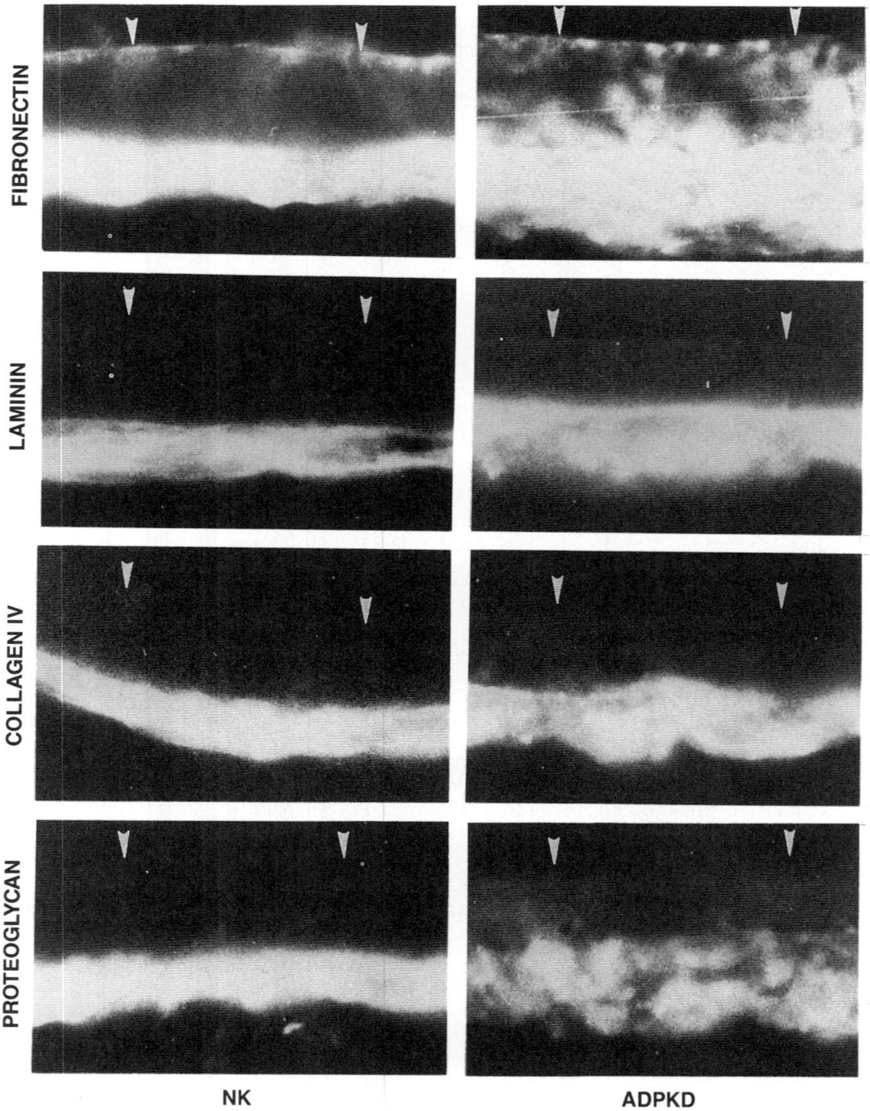

Fig. 3. Cell monolayers and basement membranes of *NK* and *ADPKD* cells stained with anti-fibronectin/laminin/collagen, type IV/HS-PG core protein (proteoglycan). (*Arrows* indicate the luminal membranes of the cell monolayers). X 500. NK, normal human renal epithelial cells; ADPKD, autosomal dominant polycystic kidney disease

Our findings support the concept that PKD may be due to a defect in the biosynthesis/secretion of one or more BM components, resulting in an altered composition and assembly of the BM and tubular dysmorphogenesis. The defect(s) could be transcriptional, translational or post-translational. Further attention should be directed to possible enzymatic defects in the biosynthesis/degradation of BM components and to tubular cell BM interactions in the pathogenesis of PKD.

Acknowledgments. Supported by NIH DK42304, DK28492, and Baxter Extramural Grants.

References

1. Grantham JJ (1983) A predominance of giant nephrons. Am J Physiol 224:F3–F10
2. Ishikawa I, Yuri T, Kitada H, Shinoda A (1983) Regression of acquired cystic disease of the kidney after successful renal transplantation. Am J Nephrol 3:310–314
3. Kanwar YS, Carone FA (1984) Reversible tubular cell and basement membrane changes in drug-induced renal cystic disease. Kidney Int 26:35–43
4. Baert L (1978) Hereditary polycystic kidney disease (adult form): A microdissection study of two cases at an early stage of the disease. Kidney Int 13:519–525
5. Hay ED (1984) Cell-matrix interaction in the embryo: Cell surface, cell skeletons and their role in differentiation. In: The role of extracellular matrix in development. A.R. Liss, New York, pp 1–31
6. Martinez-Hernandez A, Amenta PS (1983) The basement membrane in pathology. Lab Invest 48:656–677
7. Carone FA, Rowland RG, Perlman SG, Ganote CE (1974) The pathogenesis of drug-induced renal cystic disease. Kidney Int 5:411–421
8. Carone FA, Hollenberg PF, Nakamura S, Punyarit P, Glogowski W, Fluoret G (1989) Tubular basement membrane change occurs pari passu with the development of cyst formation. Kidney Int 35:1034–1040
9. Carone FA, Nakamura S, Schumacher BS, Punyarit P, Bauer K (1989) Cyst-derived cells do not exhibit accelerated growth or features of transformed cells in vitro. Kidney Int 35:1351–1357
10. Lelongt B, Carone FA, Kanwar YS (1988) Decreased de novo synthesis of proteoglycans in drug-induced renal cystic disease. Proc Natl Acad Sci USA 85:9047–9051
11. Carone FA, Makino H, Kanwar YS (1988) Basement membrane antigens in renal polycystic disease. Am J Pathol 130:466–471
12. Carone FA, Kanwar YS, Butkowski RJ (1987) Tubular cell and basement membrane changes in polycystic kidney. In: Hudson B, Price R (eds) Third International Symposium on Renal Basement Membrane. Academic, London, pp 413–423
13. Grantham JJ, Donoso VS, Evan AP, Carone FA, Gardner KD (1987) Viscoelastic properties of tubule basement membranes in experimental renal cystic disease. Kidney Int 32:187–197
14. Ebihara I, Killen PD, Laurie GW, Huang T, Yamada Y, Martin GR, Brown KS (1988) Altered mRNA expression of basement membrane components, in a murine model of polycystic kidney disease. Lab Invest 58:262
15. Bernstein J, Evan AP, Gardner KD (1987) Epithelia hyperplasia in human polycystic kidney diseases. Am J Pathol 129:92–101
16. Cowley BD, Smando FS Jr, Grantham JJ, Calvet JP (1987) Elevated c-myc proto-oncogene expression in autosomal recessive polycystic kidney disease. Proc Natl Acad Sci USA

17. Trundel M, D'Agati V, Costantini F (1989) The c-myc oncogene induces kidney cysts (KC) in transgenic mice. Kidney Int 35:364
18. Carone FA, Ozono S, Samma S, Kanwar YS, Oyasu R (1987) Renal functional changes in experimental cystic disease are tubular in origin. Kidney Int 33:1–6
19. Gattone VH II, Calvet JP, Cowley BD Jr (1988) Autosomal recessive polycystic kidney disease in a murine model. Lab Invest 59:231–238